Pediatric Surgery
Diagnosis and Management

System requirement:
- **Windows XP or above**
- **Power DVD player (Software)**
- **Windows Media Player version 10.0 or above**
- **Quick time player version 6.5 or above**

Accompanying DVD ROM is playable only in Computer and not in DVD player.

Kindly wait for few seconds for DVD to autorun. If it does not autorun then please follow the steps:
- Click on my computer
- Click the **drive labelled JAYPEE** and after opening the drive, kindly double click the file **Jaypee**

DVD CONTENTS

DVD – 1

- **Gastric Transposition** — *DK Gupta*
- **Colonic Interposition** — *A Hamza, DK Gupta*
- **Thal Fundoplication** — *KW Ashcraft*
- **Kasai's Portoenterostomy** — *R Ohi, M Nio*

DVD – 2

- **PSARP in a Male** — *A Pena*
- **PSARP in a Female** — *A Pena*
- **Common Cloaca** — *A Pena*

Pediatric Surgery
Diagnosis and Management
Volume 1

Editor

Devendra K Gupta MS, MCh, FAMS, FAAP, FRCSG (Hon.), DSc (Hon. Causa)
Professor and Head
Department of Pediatric Surgery
All India Institute of Medical Sciences
New Delhi, India

Associate Editor

Shilpa Sharma MS, MCh
Diplomate National Board
Assistant Professor of Pediatric Surgery
Postgraduate Institute of Medical Education and Research
(Dr RML Hospital, New Delhi)
PhD Scholar, Department of Pediatric Surgery
All India Institute of Medical Sciences
New Delhi, India

Guest Editor

Richard G Azizkhan MD, PhD (Hon.), FACS, FAAP
Surgeon-in-Chief
Lester W Martin MD Chair of Pediatric Surgery
Cincinnati Children's Hospital Medical Center
Professor of Surgery and Pediatrics
University of Cincinnati College of Medicine
Cincinnati, Ohio, USA

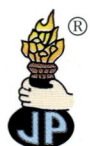

JAYPEE BROTHERS MEDICAL PUBLISHERS (P) LTD
New Delhi • Ahmedabad • Bengaluru • Chennai • Hyderabad • Kochi • Kolkata • Lucknow • Mumbai • Nagpur

Published by
Jitendar P Vij
Jaypee Brothers Medical Publishers (P) Ltd

Corporate Office
4838/24, Ansari Road, Daryaganj, **New Delhi** 110 002, India
Phone: +91-11-43574357

Registered Office
B-3, EMCA House, 23/23B Ansari Road, Daryaganj, **New Delhi** 110 002, India
Phones: +91-11-23272143, +91-11-23272703, +91-11-23282021, +91-11-23245672
Rel: +91-11-32558559   Fax: +91-11-23276490, +91-11-23245683
e-mail: jaypee@jaypeebrothers.com.   Website: www.jaypeebrothers.com

Branches

- 2/B, Akruti Society, Jodhpur Gam Road Satellite
  Ahmedabad 380 015   Phones: +91-79-26926233,   Rel: +91-79-32988717
  Fax: +91-79-26927094,   e-mail: ahmedabad@jaypeebrothers.com

- 202 Batavia Chambers, 8 Kumara Krupa Road, Kumara Park East
  Bengaluru 560 001   Phones: +91-80-22285971, +91-80-22382956, +91-80-22372664
  Rel: +91-80-32714073,   Fax: +91-80-22281761   e-mail: bangalore@jaypeebrothers.com

- 282 IIIrd Floor, Khaleel Shirazi Estate, Fountain Plaza, Pantheon Road
  Chennai 600 008   Phones: +91-44-28193265, +91-44-28194897,   Rel: +91-44-32972089
  Fax: +91-44-28193231,   e-mail: chennai@jaypeebrothers.com

- 4-2-1067/1-3, 1st Floor, Balaji Building, Ramkote Cross Road
  Hyderabad 500 095   Phones: +91-40-66610020, +91-40-24758498   Rel:+91-40-32940929
  Fax:+91-40-24758499,   e-mail: hyderabad@jaypeebrothers.com

- No. 41/3098, B & B1, Kuruvi Building, St. Vincent Road
  Kochi 682 018, Kerala   Phones: +91-484-4036109, +91-484-2395739, +91-484-2395740
  Fax: +91-844-2395740,   e-mail: kochi@jaypeebrothers.com

- 1-A Indian Mirror Street, Wellington Square
  Kolkata 700 013   Phones: +91-33-22651926, +91-33-22276404, +91-33-22276415
  Rel: +91-33-32901926   Fax: +91-33-22656075,   e-mail: kolkata@jaypeebrothers.com

- Lekhraj Market III, B-2, Sector-4, Faizabad Road, Indira Nagar
  Lucknow 226 016   Phones: +91-522-3040553, +91-522-3040554
  Fax: +91-522-3040553   e-mail: lucknow@jaypeebrothers.com

- 106 Amit Industrial Estate, 61 Dr SS Rao Road, Near MGM Hospital, Parel
  Mumbai 400012   Phones: +91-22-24124863, +91-22-24104532,   Rel: +91-22-32926896
  Fax: +91-22-24160828,   e-mail: mumbai@jaypeebrothers.com

- "KAMALPUSHPA" 38, Reshimbag, Opp. Mohota Science College, Umred Road
  Nagpur 440 009 (MS)   Phone: Rel: +91-712-3245220, Fax: +91-712-2704275
  e-mail: nagpur@jaypeebrothers.com

USA Office
1745, Pheasant Run Drive, Maryland Heights (Missouri), MO 63043, USA
Ph: 001-636-6279734   e-mail: jaypee@jaypeebrothers.com, anjulav@jaypeebrothers.com

Pediatric Surgery—Diagnosis and Management
© 2009, Editors

All rights reserved. No part of this publication and DVD ROM should be reproduced, stored in a retrieval system, or transmitted in any form or by any means: electronic, mechanical, photocopying, recording, or otherwise, without the prior written permission of the editor and the publisher.

> This book has been published in good faith that the material provided by contributors is original. Every effort is made to ensure accuracy of material, but the publisher, printer and editor will not be held responsible for any inadvertent error(s). In case of any dispute, all legal matters are to be settled under Delhi jurisdiction only.

First edition: **2009**

ISBN 978-81-8448-439-7

Typeset at JPBMP typesetting unit
Printed at: Ajanta Offset & Packagings Ltd., New Delhi.

Contributors

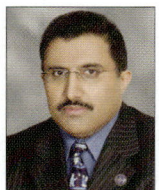

Aayed Al-Qahtani MD, FRCSC, FACS, FAAP
Associate Prof and consultant of
Pediatric surgery,
College of Medicine
King Saud University
PO Box-84147
Riyadh-11671, Saudi Arabia

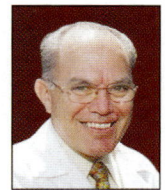

Alberto Pena MD
Director, Colorectal Division
Cincinnati Children's Hospital
Medical Center, University of
Cincinnati College of Medicine, 3333
Burnet Avenue, Cincinnati
Ohio/USA 45229-3039

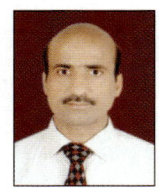

Abhinit Kumar MD
334, South Point Clinic
Vardman City Plus Mall
Dwarka
Sector 22
New Delhi-75

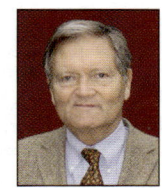

Alex Holshneider MD
Former Professor of Pediatric Surgery
Immenzaun, 6 A
51429 BERG
Gladbach, Koln
Germany

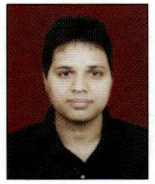

Ajay Kumar MD, PhD, DNB, MNAMS
Post-Doctoral Fellow, Pediatrics and
Neurology, Children Hospital of
Michigan School of Medicine,
Wayne State University, 3901 Beaubien
Street, Detroit MI, 48201, USA

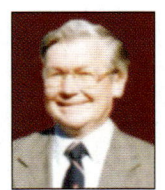

Alois F Scharli MD
Formerly, Professor and Head
Department of Pediatric Surgery
Pilatusstrasse 1 CH6003
Lucerne
Switzerland

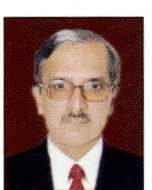

AK Mahapatra MS, MCh
Director
Professor and Head
Department of Neurosurgery
Sanjay Gandhi Postgraduate Institute
Lucknow, India

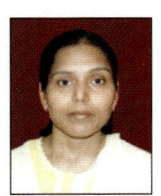

Alpana Prasad MS, MCh
Senior Consultant
Pediatric Surgeon
Fortis Hospital
Noida

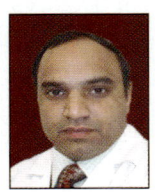

Akshay Chauhan MBBS, MCh
Fellow, Pediatric Urology
Surgical Services
Cincinnati Children Hospital and
Medical Center, Cincinnati
Ohio-45209

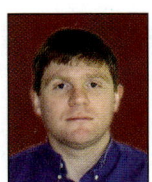

Alun R Williams FRCS
Consultant Pediatric Surgeon
Department of Pediatric Surgery
University Hospital
Queen's Medical Center Nottingham
NG7 2UH (UK)

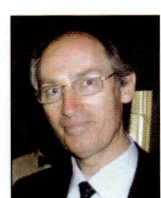

Alastair JW Millar MBBS
FRCS (Eng), (Ed) FRACS, DCH
Charles F M Saint Professor of
Pediatric Surgery, University of Cape
Town and Red Cross Children's
Hospital, University of Cape Town
Cape Town, South Africa

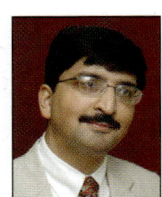

Amar Shah MS MCh, FRCS (Ped. Surgery)
Amardeep Multispeciality Children
Hospital, 65
Pritamnagar Society, Ellisbridge
Ahmedabad-06
India

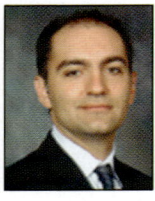
Amir Kaviani MD
Staff Surgeon
Vascular lab
Association of South Bay Surgeons
Torrance, CA

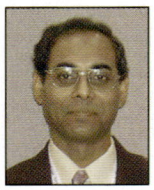
Amit K Dinda MD, PhD
Additional Professor
Department of Pathology and
Sub-Dean (examination)
All India Institute of Medical
Sciences, New Delhi-29

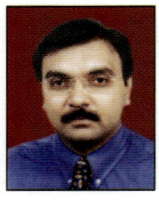
Amulya K Saxena MD, PhD
Associate Professor
Department of Pediatric and
Adolescent Surgery, Medical
University of Graz
Auenbruggerplatz-34
A-8036, Graz, Austria

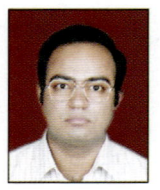
Anand Sharma MBBS, MD, FRCA
Specialist registrar, Anesthesia and
Intensive care, Addenbrookes
University Hospital, Hills Road
Cambridge, Cambridgeshire
CB22QQ, United Kingdom

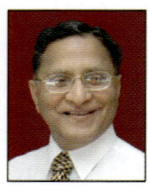
Anirudh Shah MS, FRCS(Eng), FRCS (Edin)
Director
Amardeep Multispeciality Children
Hospital, 65, Pritamnagar Society
Ellisbridge, Ahmedabad-380006
India

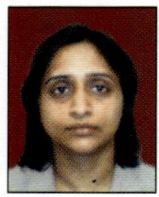
Anju Goyal MBBS, MS, MCh(Paed Surg), MRCS, FRCS(Paed)
Specialist Registrar in Pediatric
Surgery and Urology, Royal
Manchester Children's Hospital
Hospital Road
Manchester, M27 4HA, UK

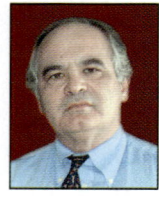
Antonio Dessanti MD, PhD
Professor of Pediatric Surgery
Head of Unit of Pediatric Surgery
University of Sassari, Azienda
Ospedaliero Universitaria. Viale S
Pietro, 43. 07100, Sassari, Italy

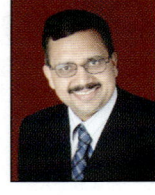
Anurag Bajpai MBBS, MD, FRACP
Consultant Pediatric Endocrinologist
Department of Endocrinology and
Diabetes, Royal Children's Hospital
Flemington Road, Parkville
Victoria, Melbourne-3052

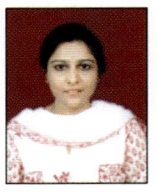
Archana Puri MS, MCh
Assistant Professor of Pediatric
Surgery, Lady Hardinge Medical
College and Associated Kalawati
Saran Children's Hospital
New Delhi-1

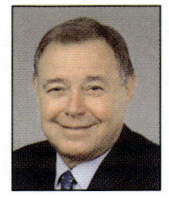
Arnold Coran AB, MD
Professor of Pediatric Surgery
University of Michigan Medical
School, C.S. Mott Children's Hospital,
F3970 Pediatric Surgery 1500 E
Medical Center Drive
Ann Arbor, MI, USA 48109-5245

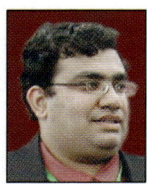
Arun Choudhary MD
Research Fellow in Medicine
(Gastroenterology), Center for
Swallowing and Motility Disorders
VA Boston Healthcare System
Harvard Medical School and Beth
Israel Deaconess Medical Center
Boston, USA.

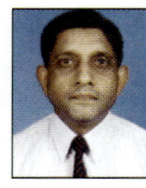
Arun Kumar Gupta MD
Professor and Head
Department of Radiology
All India Institute of Medical Sciences
New Delhi-29
India

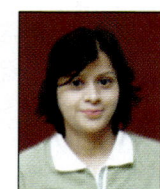
Arundhati Panigrahi MSc, PhD
Scientist, Department of
Transplantation and Immunogenetics
All India Institute of Medical Sciences
New Delhi-29
India

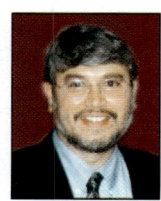
Ashley D'cruz MS, MCh
Former Professor and Head
Department of Pediatric Surgery
St John's Medical College Hospital
Bangalore-560034

Contributors vii

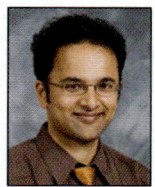

Ashok Srinivasan MD
Clinical Assistant Professor
Division of Neuroradiology
Department of Radiology
University of Michigan
USA

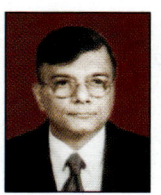

Ashoke K Basu MS, MCh
Consultant
Pediatric Surgeon
90, Ballygunge Place
Kolkata
West Bengal

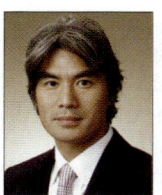

Atsuyuki Yamataka MD, PhD
Professor and Head
Pediatric General and Urogenital
Surgery, Juntendo University School
of Medicine, 2-1-1
Hongo, Bunkyo
Tokyo, 113-8421, Japan

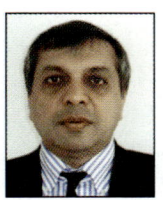

Azad B Mathur MS, MCh,
FRCS (Eng), FRCS (G)
Consultant Pediatric Surgeon
Jenny Lind Department of Pediatric
Surgery, Norfolk and Norwich
University, Hospital, Norwich Colney
Lane, NR4 7UY, United Kingdom

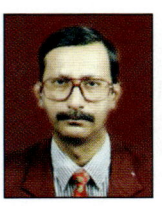

B Mukhopadhyay MS, MCh, FRCS
Professor and Head
NRS Medical College
Kolkata
West Bengal

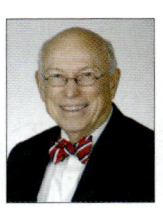

B Othersen Jr MD
Professor of Surgery and Pediatrics
Emeritus chief Pediatric Surgery
Medical University of South Carolina
Charleston, SC, USA

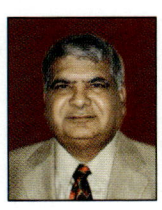

Bikramjit S Sangha MD
Attending Neonatologist
Kaiser Permanente–
Los Angeles Medical Center
USA

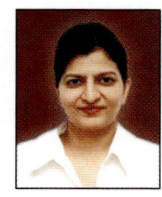

Bobby Batra MD
Director of Pediatrics
Detroit Medical Group
8125 Chatham Drive
Canton, MI
48187, USA

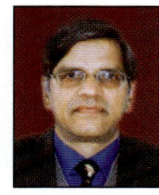

BS Sharma MS, MCh
Professor and Head
Department of Neurosurgery
All India Institute of Medical Science
Ansari Nagar
New Delhi

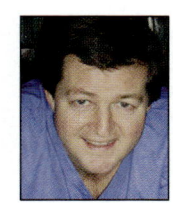

Carl F Davis MBMCh, FRCS(I)
FRCS (Glas), FRCS (Paed)
Consultant Pediatric Surgeon and
Neonatal Surgeon
Royal Hospital for Sick Children
Yorkhill, Glasgow G3 8 SJ
Scotland

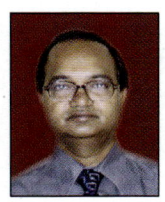

Chandersen K Sinha
MS, FRCS, MChMS, FRCS, MCh (Paed Surg)
Senior Specialist Registrar
Department of Pediatric Surgery
Denmark Hill
London SE5 9RS, UK

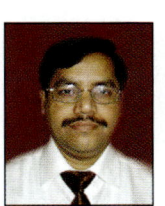

CS Bal MD
Professor
Department of Nuclear Medicine
All India Institute of Medical Sciences
New Delhi, India

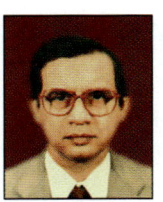

D Basak MS, MCh
Consultant Pediatric Surgeon
Pediatric Surgery
Peerless Hospital
223, C. R. Avenue
Kolkata

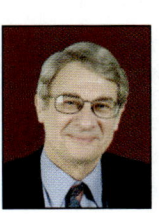

David A Lloyd MChir (Cantab)
FCS(SA), FRCS(Eng), FRCS(C), FACS
Professor of Pediatric Surgery
Department of Child Health
Alder Hey Children's Hospital
Eaton Road, Liverpool, L12 2AP

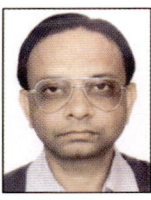
Deep N Srivastava MD
Professor, Department of Radiology
All India Institute of Medical Scinces
New Delhi-29, India

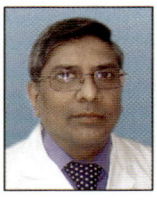
Devendra K Gupta MS, MCh
FAAP, FRCSG (Hon.), FAMS, DSc (Hon. Causa)
Professor and Head
Department of Pediatric Surgery
All India Institute of Medical Sciences
New Delhi-29, India

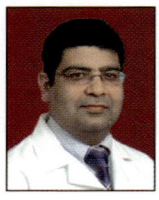
Dheeraj Gandhi MBBS, MD
Director
Interventional Neuroradiology
Assistant Professor of Radiology and
Neurosurgery, 1500 E Medical
Center Drive, Ann Arbor, MI 48109

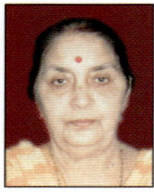
DK Agarwal MD
Ex-Prof and Head Pediatrics
Institute of Medical Sciences Varanasi
D-115, Sector 36
Noida- 201301

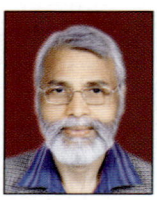
DK Pawar MD
Professor
Department of Anesthesiology
All India Institute of Medical Scinces
New Delhi-29, India

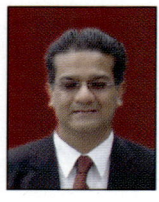
DN Jha MS
Consultant ENT Surgeon
Apollo Hospital
Colombo
Srilanka

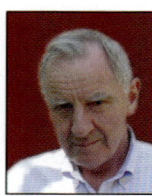
Edward Kiely FRCS
Consultant Pediatric Surgeon
The Hospital for Sick Children
Great Ormond Street
London
WC1N 3JH, UK

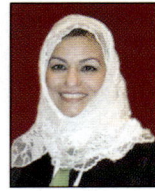
Enaam Raboei MD, PhD
Consultant Pediatric Surgeon
Chief of Pediatric Surgery
King Fahd Armed Forces Hospital
Jeddah 21159, PO Box-9862
Kingdom of Saudi Arabia

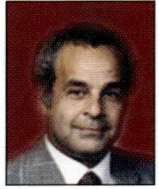
Essam El-Sahwi MD
5 Ahmed Abdel-Salam Street
El Sultan Hussein
El Attarin, Alexandria
Egypt

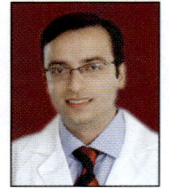
Faiz-ud-din Ahmad MBBS, MCh
Fellow, Pediatric Neurosurgery
Jackson Memorial Hospital
Miller school of Medicine, University
of Miami, Lious Pope Life Centre
1400 NW, 10th Avenue 2nd Floor
(Neurosurgery) Florida USA, 33136

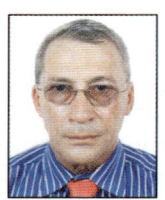
Gabriel O Ionescu MD, PhD
Professor, Iasi, Romania
Pretoria, RSA
Tawam Hospital
UAE

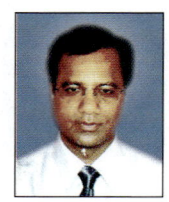
Ganga Prasad MD
Additional Professor
Department of Anesthesiology
All India Institute of Medical Sciences
New Delhi-29, India

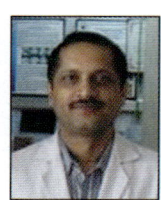
GD Satyarathee MS, MCh
Assistant Profeesor
Department of Neurosurgery
All India Institute of Medical Sciences
New Delhi-29, India

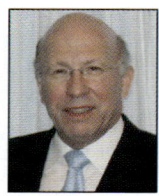
GH Willital MD, PhD
Chief of the International Institute for
Children's Surgery,
Münster Research Institute
Hansaring 94, Greven Münster 48268
Germany

Contributors ix

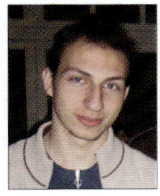
Giacomo Parigi BS
Department of Computer Sciences
Faculty of Engineering
University of Pavia
Italy

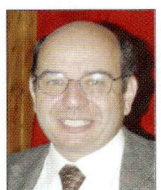
Gian Battista Parigi MD, FEBPS
Director, Specialization School in
Pediatric Surgery
Associate Professor of Pediatric
Surgery, University of Pavia
Pavia, Italy

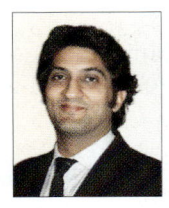
Gunninder Soin FRCS
Brownlow Group Practice
70 Pembroke Place
Liverpool
L69 3GF
UK

GVS Murthi
Department of Surgical Pediatrics
Royal Hospital For Sick Children
Yorkhill, Glasgow G3 8 55
Scotland

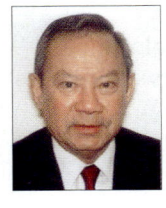
Htut Saing MD, PhD
Emeritus Professor
University of Hong Kong
2512 Aspen Valley Lane
Sacramento, CA 95835
USA

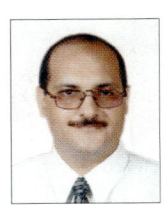
Hussam S Hassan MS, FRCS
Lecturer of Pediatric Surgery
Tanta University
Egypt

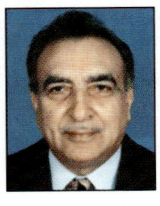
IC Pathak MS, FRCS
Professor Emeritus
Department of Pediatric Surgery
Post Graduate Institute of Medical
Education and Research
Chandigarh, India

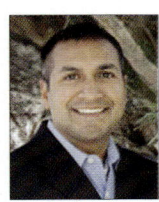
J Boix-Ochoa MD, PhD
Emeritus Professor
Can Tio
PO Box-308490
Tordera-BCN
SPAIN

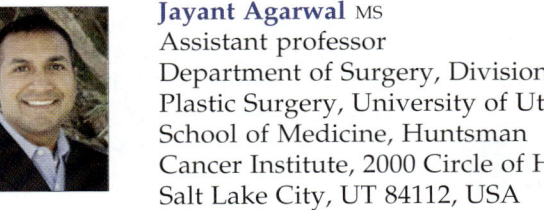
Jayant Agarwal MS
Assistant professor
Department of Surgery, Division of
Plastic Surgery, University of Utah
School of Medicine, Huntsman
Cancer Institute, 2000 Circle of Hope
Salt Lake City, UT 84112, USA

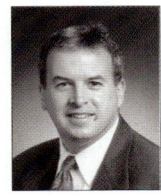
John J Aiken MD
Associate Professor
Division of Pediatric SurgeryMedical
College of Wisconsin Children's
Hospital of Wisconsin, 999 N
92nd Street, Ste. 320 Milwaukee
WI 53226

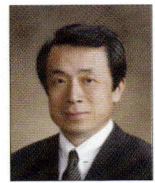
K Hashizume MD, PhD
Formerly, Professor and Head
Department of Pediatric Surgery
Graduate School of Medicine
The University of Tokyo
Tokyo, Japan

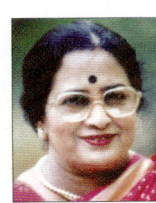
K Mathingi Ramakrishnan FRCS (Eng)
FRCS(Edin), MCh, DSc, DSc (Hon CAusa, BHU), FAMS
Director, CHILDS Trust Medical
Research Foundation, Chief of
Pediatric Burns Intensive Care Unit
and Department of Plastic Surgery
KK CHILDS Trust Hospital
Chennai-600034

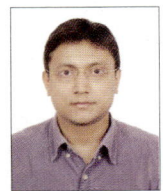
Kamalesh Pal MS, MCh
PO Box- 40129 Assistant Professor
Pediatric Surgery Division
King Fahad Hospital of the
University, Al Khobar 31952
Kingdom of Saudi Arabia

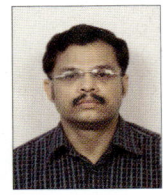
Kanishka Das MS, MCh
Professor and Head
Department of Pediatric Surgery
St John's Medical College Hospital
Bangalore-56003

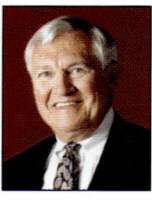
Keith Ashcraft MD
Emeritus Professor of Surgery
University of Missouri at Kansas City
School of Medicine, Former Surgeon-in-Chief, Children's Mercy Hospital
Kansas City, Missouri

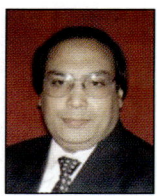
M Bajpai MS, MCh,
Diplomate National Board, PhD
Professor
Department of Pediatric Surgery
All India Institute of Medical Sciences
New Delhi-29, India

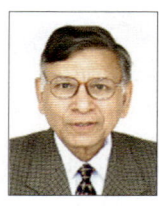
KN Agarwal MD
Hon. Scientist, Indian National
Science Academy and President
health Care and Res Ass for
Adolescents, D-115, Sector 36
Noida-201301

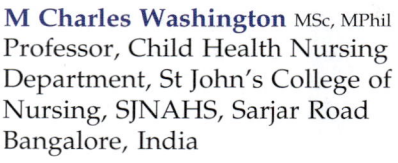
M Charles Washington MSc, MPhil
Professor, Child Health Nursing
Department, St John's College of
Nursing, SJNAHS, Sarjar Road
Bangalore, India

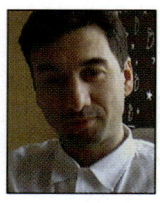
Kurush Paya MD
Associate Professor of Pediatric
Surgery, Dept of Surgery,
Div. of Pediatric Surgery
Medical University of Vienna
Waehringerguertel 18-20
Vienna, Austria

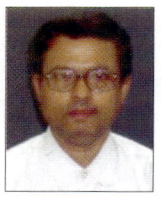
M K Bhattacharya MS, MCh
Asstt Professor
Department of Pediatric Surgery
Dr. B. C. Roy Memorial Hospital for
Children, Kolkata

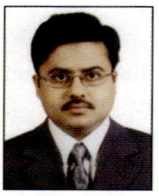
Lalit Parida MBBS, MCh
Pediatric Surgeon
King Fahad Specialist Hospital
PO Box-15215
Dammam 31444
Saudi Arabia

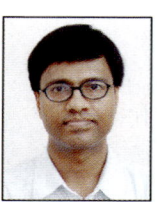
M Srinivas MS, MCh
Associate Professor
Department of Pediatric Surgery
All India Institute of Medical Sciences
New Delhi, India

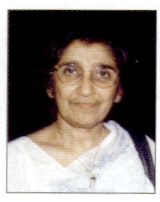
Leela Kapila FRCS, OBE
Formerly, Consultant Pediatric
Surgeon
University Hospital Queen's
Medical Centre, Nottingham
NG7 2 UH UK

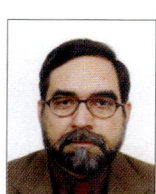
Mahesh K Arora MD
Professor
Department of Anesthesiology
All India Institute of Medical Sciences
New Delhi-29, India

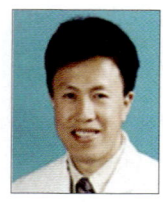
Li Long MD, PhD
Department of Pediatric Surgery
The Capital Institution of Pediatrics
Yabao Rd. 2, Beijing-100020
China

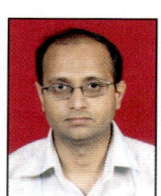
Manish Pathak MBBS, MCh
51, Shanti Niketan Colony
Barkat Nagar
Jaipur, Rajasthan-302015
India

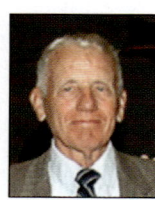
LW Martin MD
Chair of Pediatric Surgery, Cincinnati
Children's Hospital Medical Center
Professor of Surgery and Pediatrics
University of Cincinnati School of
Medicine, 3333 Burnet Avenue
Cincinnati, Ohio 45229

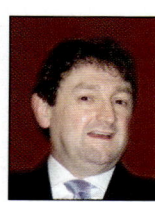
Mark Davenport ChM, FRCS (Paed Surg)
FRCS (Eng), FRCPS (Glas)
Consultant Pediatric Surgeon
Department of Pediatric Surgery
Kings College Hospital
Denmark Hill, London, SE5 9RS

Contributors xi

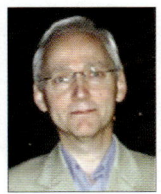
Mark Stringer BSc, MS, FRCS, FRCS (Paed.), FRCP, FRCPCH
Consultant Pediatric Surgeon Clinical Anatomist (Former Professor of Pediatric Surgery), Anatomy and Structural Biology, Otago School of Medical Sciences, University of Otago, Great King Street, Dunedin
New Zealand-9054

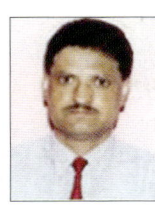
Nissar Ahmed Bhat MS, MCh
Assistant Professor
Department of Pediatric Surgery
Shere Kashmere Institute of Medical Sciences, Srinagar
Jammu and Kashmir, India

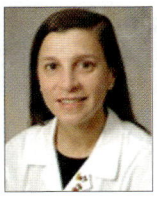
Mindy Statter FRCS
Associate Professor of Surgery and Pediatric Surgery
Section of Pediatric Surgery
University of Chicago
Chicago, IL, USA 60637

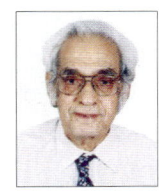
P Madhok MS, FRCS
Ashwani Nursing Home
15th Road
Khar
Mumbai-400052

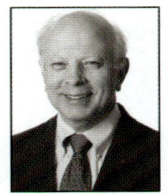
Moritz M Ziegler MD
Surgeon-in-Chief and the Ponzio Family Chair, The Children's Hospital, 13123 East 16th Avenue B323 Aurora, Colorado
USA 80045

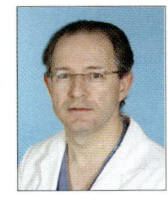
Paul D Losty MD, FRCSI, FRCS(Eng) FRCS(Ed), FRCS(Paed)
Professor, Department of Pediatric Surgery Institute of Child Health
Royal Liverpool Children's Hospital (Alder Hey) & The University of Liverpool, UK

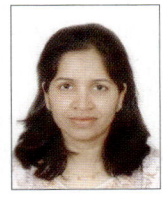
Mrunalini Chavarkar MD, MCh
Department Of Pediatrics
Louisiana State University
New Orleans
LA-70118, USA

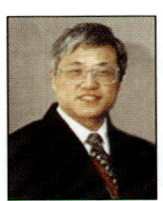
Paul KH Tam
Pro Vice Chancellor
Division of Pediatric Surgery
Department of Surgery
Queen Mary Hospital, K 15
Pokfulam, Hong Kong SAR
University of HongKong, China

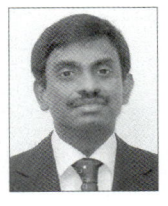
N Kumaran MS, MCh, FRCS
Formerly, Specialist Registrar in Pediatric Surgery, Mailpoint 44
Southampton General Hospital
Southampton SO16 6YD
United Kingdom

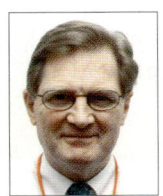
Peter AM Raine FRCS
Formerly, Professor
Royal Hospital for Sick Children
Yorkhill Glasgow
G3 8 SJ, Scotland

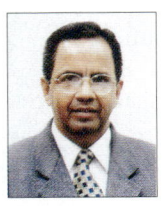
Narinder K Mehra MD, DSc
Professor and Head
Department of Transplantation and Immunogenetics
All India Institute of Medical Sciences
New Delhi-29, India

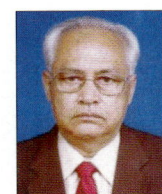
Pradip Mukherjee MS, MCh
Formerly, Professor and Head
Department of Pediatric Surgery
N. R. S. Medical College
Kolkata

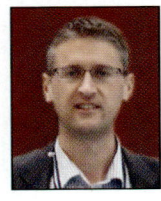
NC Featherstone FRCS
Specialist Registrar Pediatric Surgery
Norfolk and Norwich University
Foundation Trust Hospital
Colney lane, Norwich, UK

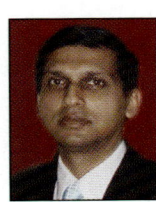
Prakash Agarwal MS, MCh
Associate Professor
Department of Pediatric Surgery
Sri Ramachandra University
Porur, Chennai-600116

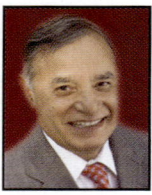
Prem Puri MS, FRCS
Consultant Pediatric Surgeon and
Director of Surgical Research
Children's Research Centre
Our Lady's Children's Hospital
Crumlin, Dublin 12, Ireland

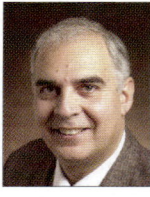
Richard Azizkhan MD, PhD, FACS, FAAP
Surgeon-in-Chief, Lester Martin Chair
in Pediatric Surgery, Cincinnati
Children's Hospital Medical Center
University of Cincinnati College of
Medicine, 3333 Burnet Avenue
Cincinnati, Ohio/USA 45229-3039

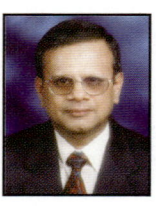
PSN Menon MD, MNAMS(Ped)
Consultant and Head
Department of Pediatrics
Jaber Al-Ahmed Armed Forces
Hospital, Kuwait

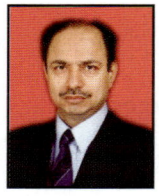
RK Batra MD
Professor
Department of Anesthesiology
All India Institute of Medical Sciences
New Delhi-29, India

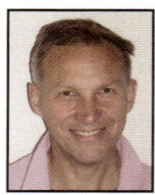
RA Wheeler MS, LLB, FRCS
Consultant Pediatric Surgeon
Lecturer in Medical Law Wessex
Regional Centre for Pediatric Surgery
Southampton General Hospital
Southampton
SO16 6YD, UK

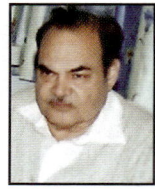
RK Tandon MS, MCh
Professor and Head
Department of pediatric Surgery
C.S.M. Medical University
Lucknow-226003

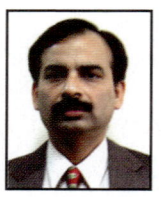
Rajesh Malhotra MS
Professor
Department of Orthopedics
All India Institute of Medical Sciences
New Delhi-29, India

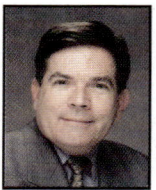
Robert Arensman MD, PhD
Emeritus Professor of Surgery and
Pediatrics, Northwestern University
and University of Chicago, Former
Surgeon-in-Chief, Children's
Memorial Hospital and the Wyler
Children's Hospital, Chicago, USA

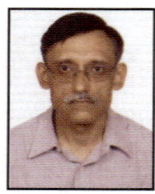
Rajiv Chadha DA, MS, MCh
Professor, Department of Pediatric
Surgery, Lady Hardinge Medical
College and Associated Kalawati
Saran Children's Hospital
New Delhi-01, India

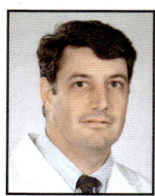
Robert Cywes MD, PhD, FRCS
Director Jacksonville Surgical
Associates, PA Wolfson
Children's Hospital
USA

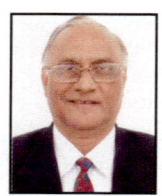
RC Deka MS, FAMS
Dean,
Professor and Head
Department of Otorhinolaryngology
All India Institute of Medical Sciences
New Delhi-29, India

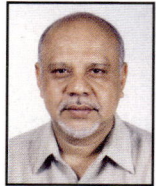
Supriyo Ghose MS
Professor and Head
Chief of Centre for Ophthalmic
Sciences
All India Institute of Medical Sciences
New Delhi-29, India

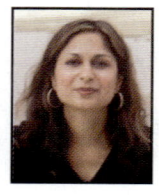
Reena Bhargava MD, FRCSC
Bariatric Health Centres
200 Fairview Road West
Toronto, Ontario
L5B 1K8, Canada

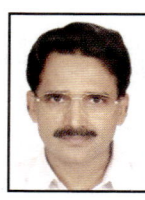
S N Kureel MS, MCh
Professor
Department of Pediatric Surgery
CS M Medical University
Lucknow-226003

Contributors **xiii**

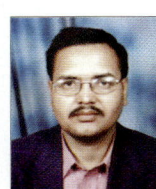
S Nainiwal MD, DNB, MNAMS
Asstt Professor, Ophthalmology
JLN Medical College
Ajmer, Rajasthan

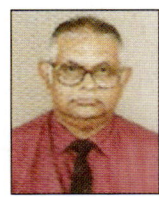
SK Mitra MS, MCh, FRCS
Formerly, Professor and Head
Department of Pediatric Surgery
Postgraduate Institute of Medical
Sciences, Chandigarh

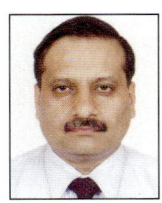
Sandeep Agarwala MBBS, MCh
Associate Professor
Department of Pediatric Surgery
All India Institute of Medical Sciences
New Delhi-29, India

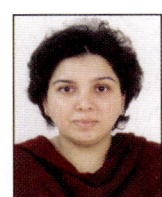
Sonika Aggarwal MD
Senior Resident
Department of Gynecology/
Obstetrics, All India Institute of
Medical Sciences, New Delhi-29
India

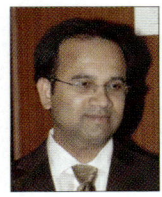
Sangamalai Manoharan FRCS
Specialist Registrar, Pediatric
Urology/Surgery, Nottingham
University Hospitals NHS Trust
Queens Medical Centre
Derby Road, Nottingham NG7 2UH
United Kingdom

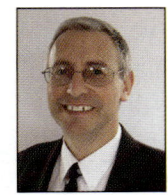
Spencer Beasley MBChB (Otago)
MS (Melb), FRACS
Consultant Pediatric Surgeon
Department of Pediatric Surgery
Christchurch Hospital
Christchurch, New Zealand

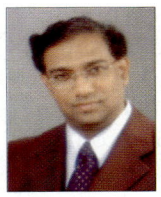
Sanjay Oak MS, MCh
Dean, Professor and Head
Dept of Pediatric Surgery
B Y L Nair Hospital
Mumbai

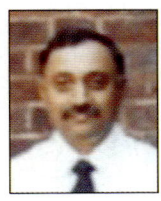
Sudipta Sen MS, MCh
Professor and Head
Department of Pediatric Surgery
Christian Medical College
Vellore

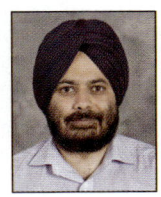
Shailinder Jit Singh MS, DNB, MCh, FRCSI
FRCS (Eng), FRCS (Paed. Surgery)
Consultant Pediatric Surgeon and
Programme Director, University
Hospital, Queen's Medical Centre
Nottingham (UK)
NG7 2UH

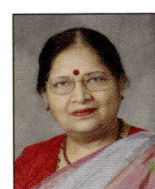
Suneeta Mittal MD, FAMA, FRCOG
FICOG, FICMCH, FIMSA
Professor and Head, Department of
Gynecology
All India Institute of Medical Sciences
New Delhi-29, India

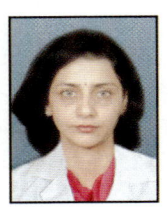
Shilpa Sharma MS, MCh, DNB
Assistant Professor
Postgraduate Institute of Medical
Education and Research
Dr RML Hospital, PhD Scholar
Department of Pediatric Surgery
All India Institute of Medical Sciences
New Delhi-29, India

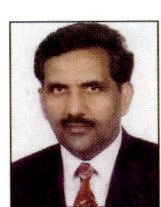
Suresh Chandra Sharma MS
Professor
Department of Otorhinolaryngology
All India Institute of Medical Sciences
New Delhi-29, India

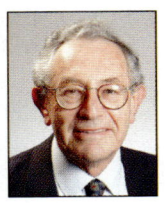
Sid Cywes MD, FACS (Ped), FRCS(Eng)
FRCS(Edin), FRCPS(Glas), FAAP (Hon.), FCS (SA)
(Hon), DSc (UCT) (Hon.)
Emeritus Professor, Department of
Pediatric Surgery, School of Child
and Adolescent Health, Red Cross
War Memorial Children's Hospital
University of Cape Town

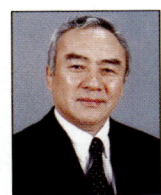
Takeshi Miyano MD, PhD
Emeritus Professor
Department of Pediatric Surgery
Juntendo University School of
Medicine, 2-1-1 Hongo, Bunkyo-ku
Tokyo-113-8421, Japan

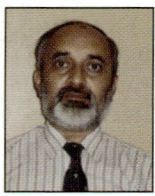
V Bhatnagar MS, MCh, FNASc, FIMSA, FAMS
Professor
Department of Paediatric Surgery
All India Institute of Medical Sciences
New Delhi 29, India

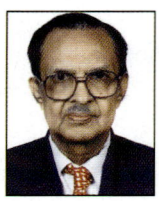
V Ravi Kumar MS, MCh
Consultant Peditatric Surgeon
GKNM hospital
Pappanayakkan palayam
Coimbatore-38

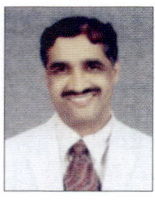
V Jayaraman MS, MCh
Consultant Plastic Surgeon, CHILDS Trust Hospital, Pediatric Burns Intensive Care Unit and Department of Plastic Surgery, K.K. CHILDS Trust Hospital, Chennai-600 034

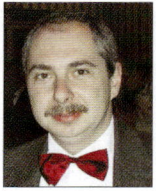
Vadim Kapuller MD, FRCS
Surgery Alef Department
Kaplan Medical Center
PO Box 1, Rehovot, Israel

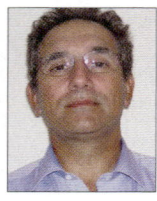
V Martinez Ibañez MD, PhD
Chairman, Department of Pediatric Surgery Hospital, Vall d'Hebron Autonomous University of Barcelona
Spain

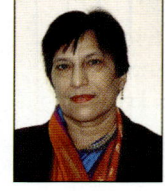
Veena Kalra MD, FAMS
Former Professor and Head
Department of Pediatrics
All India Institute of Medical Sciences
New Delhi-29, India

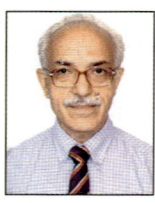
V P Choudhary
MD, FIAP, FIMSA, FIACM, FISHTM
Former Professor and Head
Department of Hematology
All India Institute of Medical Science
New Delhi-29, India

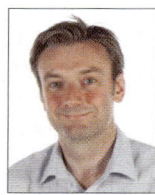
Walker Gregor M BSc(Hons), MBChB, MD FRCS(Ed), FRCS(Paed)
Consultant Pediatric Surgeon and Neonatal surgeon
Royal Hospital for Sick Children
Yorkhill, Glasgow, G3 8 SJ, Scotland

Foreword

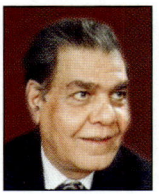

This book marks an important milestone in the growth of pediatric surgery in India. Its significance is indicated by the fact that it has been officially sponsored by IAPS, the Indian Association of Pediatric Surgeons.

The IAPS has grown, from a modest beginning in 1965, into a vibrant organization with more than 900 members. Thirty to thirty-five new members join each year after completing their training in 23 centers in the country. It is, therefore, time for it to have its own standard compendium of information relevant to the needs of its members. Trainees too need an authoritative textbook written by experts who are familiar with the needs of a developing country like India. Unfortunately, books written and published in the West are too exhaustive, often prohibitively expensive and largely unrealistic for our needs. I have no doubt that pediatric surgical trainees in neighboring countries of Asia will also appreciate the significance of this book.

There are more than 400 million children below the age of 12 years in India and the volume of surgical work is simply astounding. The kind of experience that a pediatric surgeon gets in India is the envy of many a surgeons in the developed world. Yet it is not very often that Indian authors find a place in the list of contributors to books published in the west and one gets the impression that children's surgery hardly exists in this vast subcontinent. Our authors need to be recognized for their rich and authentic experience. At the same time, our trainees need to be acquainted with the wide range of expertise from abroad. They need to have a broad vision, yet focused to the needs of a country like India. This is another valid reason for bringing out this book.

It is commendable that Professor Devendra K Gupta, Chief of pediatric surgery at the All India Institute of Medical Sciences has been chosen as the Editor. Professor Gupta is a highly regarded leader in pediatric surgery, recognized nationally and internationally for his writings. He has a wide base of valuable experience, which is admirably reflected in his editorship of this book. He has, very wisely, taken a younger colleague Dr Shilpa Sharma as Associate Editor to bring in, open-minded dynamism of the youth in the editing process. Significantly, he has also succeeded in getting the able guidance of Prof Richard Azizkhan, of Cincinnati, USA, as Guest Editor.

Professor Gupta has chosen contributors who are either working in India or who have been associated with Indian departments of pediatric surgery for some time. In fact, nearly one third of the contributors are working in countries abroad. It is noteworthy that authors have been selected not so much for their prominence in the profession as for proficiency in their fields of interest. In the fast changing world of medicine, dynamic young surgeons have acquired new expertise and amassed enormous experience that would be unimaginable in the West. I heartily welcome this move to include younger authors. They may not be well known today, but they certainly need to be taken note of, for they will be the leaders of tomorrow.

It usually takes several years to produce a multi-authored book – it is hard work collecting manuscripts and making the matter suitable for publication. Often, the information is outdated, if not obsolete, by the time the book is published. I would like to compliment the editors for bringing out this book as quickly as they have. The information provided is current, and presented with clarity of expression. Surgical techniques are described in a way that facilitates understanding. Wherever necessary, the subject has been discussed by more than one author so that varying points of view are accommodated.

I feel assured that this book will become an invaluable aid to pediatric surgeons not only in India but also in other parts of the world. With this book the editors have given an international identity to Indian pediatric surgery. This in itself is a commendable achievement.

Purushottam Upadhyaya MS, FRCS, FAMS
Emeritus Professor and Advisor
Himalayan Institute of Medical Sciences
Dehra Dun, India

Foreword

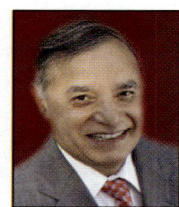

Professor Devendra Gupta deserves to be congratulated for his enormous effort in producing this valuable textbook in pediatric surgery. This book which comprises 130 chapters and 132 contributors from all five continents of the world provides an authoritative, comprehensive and complete account of various surgical conditions in children. This detailed reference text is suitable for both specialist pediatric surgeons as well as trainees in pediatric surgery as it covers both common and uncommon paediatric surgical conditions. The book has the added attraction because it covers recent developments in the care of children with congenital malformations and acquired surgical conditions. There are full chapters devoted to ethics in pediatric surgery, robotics, stem cell therapy, tissue engineering, laser applications in pediatric surgery, nanotechnology and computers.

Professor Gupta was successful in persuading well known pediatric surgeons to provide an authoritative and complete account of their respective topics. Pediatric surgical community should find this book a useful reference in the management of childhood surgical disorders.

We applaud the efforts of Professor Gupta and contributors for this comprehensive textbook in pediatric surgery.

Prem Puri MS, FRCS, FRCS (Ed), FACS
President, World Federation of Associations of Pediatric Surgeons

Preface

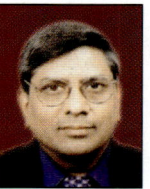

*" It is not enough to begin. Continuance is necessary.
The reason of failure in most cases is lack of perseverance."*

Though there are number of high quality books available in pediatric surgery, yet most of them are not accessible to the majority of pediatric surgeons in the world due to their high cost. The proposal from the Indian Association of Pediatric Surgeons (IAPS) to publish a multi-authored pediatric surgery book that was complete in all respects and still affordable, was quite a challenge. The Editor accepted this responsibility to bring out a book that would be of international quality, high in scientific value and still low in cost. To accomplish this task, the help and support received from Dr Shilpa Sharma as the Associate Editor and Prof Richard Azizkhan as the Guest Editor were simply outstanding and are greatly acknowledged.

The initial concept for the book was to include many pediatric surgical sub-specialties, e.g. General Pediatric Surgery, Neonatal Surgery, Pediatric Oncology, Pediatric Urology, Cardiothoracic Surgery and others, all in a single book. However, since the contents became too voluminous, this book was restricted to "Pediatric Surgery—Diagnosis and Management", primarily to cover general pediatric surgery; yet still these required two volumes to keep the book handy.

The scope of the book remains very broad and covers the spectrum of General Pediatric Surgery. It includes some relevant basic science, embryology and pathophysiology, diagnosis and management, as well as complications and includes long-term results. The descriptions and pictures of operative procedures have also been added wherever indicated. Many subjects have been covered by more than one expert still without duplicating the text.

The book with about 1200 figures (Clinical photographs, flow charts, X-rays and the ones drawn by the artist) makes it unique. The book also includes chapters on Nanotechnology, Minimal invasive procedures, Endoscopic procedures, Lasers, Robotic surgery, Stem cell regeneration, Tissue engineering, Computers and Molecular genetics to offer state-of-the-art information to the pediatric surgical community. The book also extends to adolescent surgery as it includes the chapters on Empyema, Intestinal obstruction, Bariatric surgery, Tuberculosis, Hydatid disease and Bezoars.

The authors in this book have been outstanding. Their contributions have been excellent. I was rather bestowed with faith to edit their work (Chapters, photographs, charts, tables, references, etc.), so as to maintain uniformity and regular flow of thoughts.

A foreword for this book has been written by Prof P Upadhyaya who had not only been my teacher and the Founder Professor and the Chief of the Department of Pediatric Surgery at the All India Institute of Medical Sciences, New Delhi, but also a perfectionist, and an academician with utmost human values. Prof Prem Puri, President of WOFAPS who is known internationally for his deep interest in research and surgical care has not only applauded our efforts but written a Foreword as well.

The support received from the colleagues and the staff from the department at All India Institute of Medical Sciences, New Delhi (AIIMS), especially from Mr Ved Grover, is greatly appreciated. I also thank my wife, Dr Rani and the daughters Dr Malvika and Deepika, for being the force behind to complete this book.

The book has been published by M/s Jaypee Brothers, the reputed exclusive Medical Publishers from New Delhi. Shri JP Vij, Chairman and Managing Director; Mr Tarun Duneja, the Director (Publishing), had shown special interest while publishing this book.

It is hoped that the book would serve its purpose if it reaches the pediatric surgical community in the developed and the developing world alike, for its scientific contents, quality of production, affordability and balanced approach.

When you light a lantern for another, it brightens up your path as well —Nichiren Daishonin.

Devendra K Gupta

Message

On behalf of the Indian Association of Pediatric Surgeons (IAPS), I take great honour and privilege to write a brief message for the long awaited book *"Pediatric Surgery—Diagnosis and Management"*, edited by Prof DK Gupta. The book published by Jaypee Brothers, New Delhi has been creditably supported by the rich experience of Prof Richard Azizkhan from Cincinnati Children Hospital, USA and Dr Shilpa Sharma from New Delhi.

It was the year 2000 that after the success of *"Textbook of Neonatal surgery"* published by Dr DK Gupta, the IAPS wanted more such books in the specialty and thus requested Dr Gupta to bring out the much needed book in Pediatric Surgery that would be complete, informative, affordable and at the same time matched with the best international standards in its presentation and scientific contents. It is commendable that the editors have accomplished this daunting task so well that would be beneficial for the pediatric surgical community.

This book, Pediatric Surgery—Diagnosis and Management, is first of its kind from the developing part of the world. It is well divided in sections, and covers the complete spectrum of diseases including recent advances. Despite being a multi-authored book, it has been dominated by the Indian contributors, reflecting the maturity of pediatric surgery specialty in India. Many chapters have been covered by more than one expert known for their professional standing in the field, so as to incorporate the differing views of various experts. Chapters have been supplemented generously with operative techniques, line diagrams, charts and clinical photographs to make the book educative and informative.

I am sure this book would be an asset and reach a large number of pediatric surgeons. It should serve as a reference book in general pediatric surgery not only to the postgraduates and the pediatric surgeons but also the institutional libraries across the world.

Anirudh Shah
President, Indian Association of Pediatric Surgeons
Ahmedabad

Acknowledgements

The Editors would like to thank the Indian Association of Pediatric Surgeons (IAPS), for giving us the singular honour and the major responsibility to write this book for the benefit of the pediatric surgical fraternity especially from the developing world.

The editors admire the support that has been received from the authors from around the world. The willingness, with which all of them gave us their valuable time, leaves us personally indebted.

The Editors acknowledge the blanket permission granted by MBD publishers to reproduce the published material free of charge (text, photographs, diagrams, charts, tables, etc.) from the Textbook of Neonatal Surgery, edited by DK Gupta, New Delhi 2000, in various chapters of this book. Though, every effort has been taken by the contributors to acknowledge the published text, color photographs, charts and diagrams reproduced/quoted from the books and the journals, an inadvertent error, if any, in any chapter of this book, would only be due to an oversight.

We also appreciate the support and the encouragement received from the World Federation of Association of Pediatric Surgeons (WOFAPS), Asian Association of Pediatric Surgeons (AAPS), the Federation of Association of Pediatric Surgeons from SAARC Nations (FAPSS) and the International Foundation for Pediatric Surgery and Research for producing the book aimed at improving the surgical care of children around the globe.

Finally, our appreciation to Shri JP Vij, Chairman and Managing Director of Jaypee Brothers, Mr Tarun Duneja, and members of the publishing team, including the artists, for their hard work and special interest taken to produce a book of this quality.

*To
The students of Pediatric Surgery,
"at all levels",
in their quest for knowledge*

Contents

VOLUME-I

SECTION 1: BASIC PEDIATRIC SURGERY

1. Pediatric Surgery—Overview of the Specialty 03
   DK Gupta
2. Evolution of Pediatric Surgery 10
   IC Pathak
3. Molecular Biology and the Pediatric Surgeon 21
   Arun Chaudhury, M Srinivas
4. Growth and Development in Pediatric Surgical Practice 34
   KN Agarwal, DK Agarwal
5. Fluid and Electrolytes in Pediatric Surgery 48
   V Ravikumar, M Srinivas
6. Shock in Children—Surgeon's Perspective 65
   DK Gupta, Archana Puri
7. Blood Component Therapy 82
   VP Choudhry
8. Ventilatory Support in Children 90
   DK Pawar
9. Pediatric Anesthesia—General Considerations 103
   Ravinder K Batra, Anand Sharma
10. Relief of Postoperative Pain in Children 123
    MK Arora, G Prasad
11. Common Radiological Procedures in Pediatric Surgery 131
    AK Gupta, Ashok Srinivasan
12. Nuclear Imaging in Pediatric Surgery 140
    CS Bal, Ajay Kumar
13. Pediatric Interventional Radiology 168
    Deep N Srivastava, Bobby Batra, Dheeraj Gandhi
14. Postoperative Care 180
    Bikramjit Singh Sangha
15. Antimicrobials and Antimicrobial Prophylaxis in Pediatric Surgery 199
    V Ravikumar, M Srinivas
16. Fungal Infections in Pediatric Surgical Patients 210
    Nissar A Bhat, DK Gupta
17. Ethics in Pediatric Surgery 215
    P Madhok
18. Esophagoscopy 222
    B Othersen Jr, HS Hassan
19. Pediatric Bronchoscopy 229
    DK Gupta, Shilpa Sharma
20. Management of Terminal Illnesses 238
    Kanishka Das, M Charles, Ashley L J D'Cruz

SECTION 2: TRAUMA

21. Pediatric Trauma 253
    Azad B Mathur, NC Featherstone
22. Head Injuries in Children 264
    BS Sharma, Feiz Uddin Ahmad
23. Pediatric Abdominal Trauma 272
    David A Lloyd, Gunninder Soin
24. Soft Tissue Trauma 286
    DK Gupta, Lalit Parida
25. Vascular Injuries in Children 298
    Nagarajan Kumaran, Rob A Wheeler
26. Pediatric Burns 307
    K Mathingi Ramakrishnan, V Jayaraman
27. Traumatic Hemobilia in Children 321
    Shilpa Sharma, DK Gupta

SECTION 3: THORACIC SURGERY

28. Gastroesophageal Reflux in Children 329
    J Boix-Ochoa
29. Thal Fundoplication 357
    Keith W Ashcraft
30. Achalasia Cardia 363
    Shilpa Sharma, DK Gupta
31. Esophageal Strictures 369
    Shailinder J Singh, Leela Kapila
32. Esophageal Replacement with Colon 382
    D K Gupta, Shilpa Sharma
33. Gastric Tube Esophageal Replacement 391
    Gabriel O Ionescu
34. Gastric Transposition 409
    D K Gupta, Shilpa Sharma
35. Jejunal Interposition as a Substitute of Esophagus 422
    Kohei Hashizume, Antonio Dessanti
36. Colon Patch Esophagoplasty 426
    Enaam Raboei
37. Esophageal Perforation 432
    HS Hassan, B Othersen
38. Principles of Lung Resection 437
    DK Gupta, Shilpa Sharma
39. Lung Anomalies 448
    John Aiken
40. Bronchiectasis and Lung Abscess 471
    Shilpa Sharma, DK Gupta
41. Pulmonary Tuberculosis in Children 478
    Shilpa Sharma, DK Gupta
42. Chylothorax 491
    Spencer W Beasley

43. **Empyema Thoracis** 495
    Shilpa Sharma, DK Gupta
44. **Chest Wall Deformities** 510
    Amulya K Saxena, Günter H Willital

SECTION 4: GASTROINTESTINAL SURGERY

45. **Disorders of the Umbilicus** 523
    Sudipta Sen
46. **Inguinal Hernia and Hydrocele** 527
    AR Williams, SJ Singh, L Kapila
47. **Rare Pediatric Hernias** 534
    DK Gupta, Shilpa Sharma, Kamlesh Pal
48. **Peritonitis in Childhood** 544
    Rajiv Chadha
49. **Infantile Hypertrophic Pyloric Stenosis** 564
    Sengamalai Manoharan, Azad B Mathur
50. **Gastric Volvulus** 570
    Shilpa Sharma, DK Gupta
51. **Gastrointestinal Bleeding** 575
    AK Basu, D Basak
52. **Idiopathic Primary Intussusception** 581
    Essam El-Sahwi
53. **Meckel's Diverticulum** 587
    M Gregor Walker, F Carl Davis
54. **Appendicitis** 596
    Kurosh Paya
55. **Short Bowel Syndrome** 618
    DK Gupta, Shilpa Sharma
56. **Intestinal Obstruction** 633
    Alpana Prasad, Rajiv Chadha
57. **Abdominal Tuberculosis** 646
    Shilpa Sharma, DK Gupta
58. **Alimentary Tract Duplications** 659
    Richard G Azizkhan
59. **Bezoars in Children** 671
    Shilpa Sharma, DK Gupta
60. **Ascariasis Lumbricoides** 678
    Essam-El-Sawhi
61. **Hirschsprung's Disease** 681
    Edward Kiely
62. **Total Colonic Aganglionosis** 696
    Lester W Martin
63. **Variant Hirschsprung's Disease** 701
    Prem Puri
64. **Swenson's Pull-through** 709
    DK Gupta, Shilpa Sharma

65. Duhamel's Pull-through 717
    Sandeep Agarwala
66. Soave's (Boley Scot) Endorectal Pull-through 723
    DK Gupta, Manish Pathak, Shilpa Sharma
67. Transanal Endorectal Pull-through 733
    DK Gupta, Shilpa Sharma
68. Crohn's Disease 741
    Robert Cywes, Arnold G Coran
69. Ulcerative Colitis 758
    Robert Cywes, Arnold G Coran
70. Polyposis Syndromes 771
    AF Scharli
71. Anorectal Malformations: Anatomy and Physiology 776
    Pradip Mukherjee, MK Bhattacharyya
72. Anorectal Malformations: Diagnosis and Management 787
    SN Kureel, RK Tandon
73. Anorectal Malformations: Pena's Perspectives 816
    Shilpa Sharma, Alberto Pena
74. Anomalies Associated with Anorectal Malformations 825
    DK Gupta, Shilpa Sharma
75. Complications Following PSARP 833
    Alex Holschneider, DK Gupta
76. Congenital Pouch Colon 846
    Shilpa Sharma, DK Gupta
77. Persistent Cloaca 857
    DK Gupta, Shilpa Sharma, Alex Holschneider
78. Anorectal Malformations: Current Perspectives 874
    DK Gupta, Shilpa Sharma
79. Rectal Ectasia 884
    Shilpa Sharma, DK Gupta
80. Fecal Incontinence and Constipation 889
    Anju Goyal, Paul D Losty
81. Bowel Management 899
    Shilpa Sharma, DK Gupta, Alberto Pena

VOLUME-II

SECTION 5: HEPATOBILIARY SYSTEM

82. Diseases of the Gallbladder in Children 909
    Mark Devenport
83. Hepatic Hemangiomas 918
    Mark Devenport
84. Liver Abscess in Children 925
    Mark D Stringer
85. Hydatid Disease 936
    SN Oak, Prakash Agarwal, M Chavarkar
86. Liver Resections and Allograft Preparation 949
    Mark D Stringer

87. Transplant Immunogenetics 969
Narinder K Mehra, Arundhati Panigrahi

88. Liver Transplantation 988
AJW Millar, S Cywes

89. Biliary Atresia 1002
CK Sinha, DK Gupta, Mark Davenport

90. Choledochal Cyst 1013
Takeshi Miyano, Long Li, Atsuyuki Yamataka

91. Pancreatic Pseudocyst 1026
Shilpa Sharma, DK Gupta

92. Pancreatitis 1033
GVS Murthi, PAM Raine

93. Management of Portal Hypertension 1044
M Bajpai

94. Persistent Hyperinsulinemic Hypoglycemia of Infancy 1051
Shilpa Sharma, DK Gupta

95. Pancreas and Intestinal Transplantation 1058
V Martinez Ibanez

96. Spleen 1066
Amir Kaviani, Moritz M Ziegler

SECTION 6: VASCULAR DISORDERS

97. Hemangiomas 1079
Richard G Azizkhan

98. Vascular and Lymphatic Anomalies 1099
Robert Arensman, Jayant Agarwal, M Statter

99. Picibanil (OK-432) in Lymphangiomas 1108
DK Gupta, Shilpa Sharma

SECTION 7: PEDIATRIC NEUROSURGERY

100. Hydrocephalus 1117
DK Gupta, Shilpa Sharma

101. Encephaloceles 1148
AK Mahapatra, GD Satyarthee

102. Microcephaly 1163
Shilpa Sharma, Veena Kalra

103. Spina Bifida 1168
DK Gupta, Shilpa Sharma

SECTION 8: HEAD AND NECK SURGERY

104. Craniosynostosis 1193
M Bajpai

105. Cleft Lip and Palate 1201
Peter AM Raine

106. Neck Anomalies 1222
B Mukhopadhyay, SK Mitra

107. Torticollis 1230
DK Gupta, Manish Pathak, Shilpa Sharma

SECTION 9: PEDIATRIC SURGICAL SPECIALITIES

108. **Common Eye Problems in Children** 1239
     Supriyo Ghose, Sanjeev Nainiwal
109. **Pediatric Otolaryngology** 1257
     RC Deka, DN Jha
110. **Pediatric Larynx and Trachea** 1265
     Abhinit Kumar, Suresh C Sharma
111. **Orthopedic Problems in Children** 1299
     Rajesh Malhotra
112. **Conjoined Twins** 1349
     Htut Saing, DK Gupta
113. **Heteropagus Twinning** 1364
     DK Gupta, Shilpa Sharma
114. **Gynecological Problems in Children** 1370
     Suneeta Mittal, Sonika Agarwal
115. **Ovarian Cysts** 1381
     Shilpa Sharma, DK Gupta
116. **Vaginal Anomalies and Reconstruction** 1387
     Akshay Chauhan, Shilpa Sharma, DK Gupta
117. **Adrenal Disorders** 1404
     Anurag Bajpai, PSN Menon
118. **Childhood Obesity** 1415
     Anurag Bajpai, PSN Menon
119. **Surgery for Pediatric Morbid Obesity** 1421
     Reena Bhargava, Shilpa Sharma, Azad B Mathur

SECTION 10: RECENT ADVANCES

120. **Molecular Genetics of Hirschsprung's Disease** 1433
     Paul KH Tam, Mercè Garcia-Barcelo
121. **Duhamel's Pull-through Using Staplers** 1450
     SN Oak, Prakash Agarwal
122. **Pediatric Laparoscopy** 1455
     Anirudh Shah, Amar Shah
123. **One Port Laparoscopically Assisted Appendectomy** 1463
     Vadim Kapuller
124. **Robotic Pediatric Surgery** 1468
     Aayed R Al-Qahtani
125. **Tissue Engineering: Present Concepts and Strategies** 1482
     Amulya K Saxena
126. **Stem Cell Therapy** 1491
     DK Gupta, Shilpa Sharma
127. **Nanotechnology: Technology to Revolutionize the Future of Medicine** 1503
     Amit K Dinda
128. **Laser Applications in Pediatric Surgery** 1512
     V Bhatnagar
129. **Pediatric Surgeon and the Computer** 1518
     Gian Battista Parigi, Giacomo Parigi
130. **Pediatric Surgery in Europe: Problems and Perspectives** 1552
     Gian Battista Parigi

     Index 1565

SECTION 1

Basic Pediatric Surgery

Pediatric Surgery—Overview of the Specialty

DK Gupta

The mere formulation of a problem is far more essential than its solution, which may be merely a matter of mathematical or experimental skills. To raise new questions, new possibilities, to regard old problems from a new angle requires creative imagination and marks real advances in science.
—Albert Einstein

Recently, when pediatrics was separated from the general medicine, a strong need was also felt, though much later, that children need the services of a specialized surgeon to deal with their surgical problems. The reasons being the different anatomical and physiological parameters, smaller size of the organs needing intricate surgical skills, special dosage schedules, difficult venous access, and especially the spectrum of surgical diseases much different from those seen in adults.

The World Federation of Associations of Pediatric Surgeons had signed a document during the council meeting of the World Federation of Association of Pediatric Surgeons (WOFAPS) held in Kyoto, 2002, to protect the rights of the surgical child. It is popularly known as "Kyoto Declaration", reproduced as below:

- Children are not just small adults and have medical and surgical problems and needs that are often quite different from those encountered by adult physicians. Infants and children deserve the very best medical care available. Every infant and child who suffers from an illness or disease has the right to be treated in an environment devoted to their care by a pediatric medical or surgical specialist.
- Pediatric Surgeons are specially trained physicians with extensive experience and expertise in treating infants and children of all ages (from birth to adolescence) with surgical disorders. Because of their unique training, pediatric surgical specialists provide a wide range treatment options and the highest quality care to children.
- Pediatric Surgeons diagnose, treat, and manage children's surgical needs including: surgical repair of birth defects, serious injuries in children, childhood solid tumors, conditions requiring endoscopy and minimally invasive procedures, and all other surgical procedures in children.
- In order to provide the best surgical care for infants and children, complex pediatric surgical procedures should be carried out in specialized pediatric centers with appropriately equipped intensive care facilities staffed 24 hours per day seven days per week. In addition to the trained pediatric surgeons, these facilities should be staffed with other pediatric specialists including radiologists, anesthesiologists and pathologists. These specialized centers should provide post-graduate education and research.

There are many children's hospitals and pediatric centres in the developed world that are celebrating their 200 years of establishments. However, developing world is yet to have adequate facilities to treat large volume of work related to congenital malformations, trauma, tumors, transplants, infections and many other pediatric surgical problems.[1-5]

WHO SHOULD DO PEDIATRIC SURGERY?

Only the Pediatric Surgeons who are qualified by virtue of their training in the field, should tackle the surgical cases in newborns, infants and children up to adolescents. There are however, many variations depending on local circumstances, practices and compulsions. Many institutions with a heavy workload, would accept children only up to 12-year of age. However, all newborns with emergencies (Acute Intestinal obstructions, respiratory distress) would normally be referred to the qualified pediatric surgeons who are all trained in the sub-specialty of newborn surgery.[6] In absence of availability of the trained pediatric surgeons in all the centers, at all times, in all sub-specialties, the common pediatric surgical problems have been treated by general surgeons. This is true even in developed world. In the best interest of the patient, the treating general surgeon dealing with such routine cases should not only be familiar with the latest approach but also should have enough experience dealing with their special requirements.

WHAT IS THE SCOPE OF PEDIATRIC SURGERY?

Parents are becoming now more aware about the scope and the postsurgical results. Pediatric surgery is a wide field and deals with most body parts and organs in newborns, infants and children. These include various sub-branches like; neurosurgery (spina bifida, hydrocephalus, cranisynostosis), head and neck lesions, thoracic surgery (various congenital lung anomalies, empyemas, hydatid cysts, eventration of diaphragm, congenital diaphragmatic hernia, tracheo-esophageal fistula, esophageal replacements using gastric tube, colon transposition, stomach pullup, and rarely the tumors), abdominal surgery related to the disease of the liver, biliary tract, spleen, large and small bowel, anorectal malformations, Hirschsprung's disease, abdominal wall defects, undescended testis, hernia, torsion of testis, and others), plastic surgery (dealing with defects like cleft lip and palate, hypospadias, syndactyly, reconstruction of various flaps), urologic surgery (pyeloplasty, ureteric reimplantation, reconstruction of epispadias and exstrophy complex, vesico-intestinal fissure, partial and complete nephrectomies, urinary bladder augmentation, colon conduits and many more). Even in centers with well developed sub-specialties, a general Pediatric Surgeon is allowed to operate on patients with neonatal emergencies, trauma and routine surgical procedures to remain in stream.

Thus, the spectrum of the pediatric surgery is very wide and covers whole body except the open heart surgery, brain tumors, orthopedic anomalies, ophthalmology and ear, nose and throat. Presently, there are only few centers, mostly in developed nations, where the pediatric surgical specialists devote most of their time to a particular sub-specialty and they are satisfied with the volume as well the returns. Others would like to continue as general pediatric surgeons to cater to large spectrum of diseases. In the interest of patient care it is important now to define and develop the sub-specialties as the distinct disciplines, e.g. urology, neurosurgery, hepatobiliary, oncology, thoracic surgery, and may be in the neonatal surgery also.[7] This may be feasible only in fully funded centers and the teaching institutes of national importance.

WHERE SHOULD PEDIATRIC SURGEONS FUNCTION?

Congenital anomalies differ from region to region and so the spectrum of anomalies seen in a developed country differ from those in a developing countries. Ideally each newborn should have the facility of being seen by a pediatric surgeon without having to travel long distances. In many countries, it is not the distance but the mode of transport what is most important. To travel even small distances (from hills, remote areas which are not well connected with roads, air and rail network), parents might take many hours or even days to bring the baby to the nearest center for medical care.

Generally, a group of 3 Pediatric Surgeons is required for a center catering to the general population of one million. Similarly, there should be a neonatal surgical ICU for the same sized population. Though, the future need would be to have Pediatric Surgeons even at the district level to manage general pediatric surgical problems, presently, all medical colleges, referral centers and institutes of national importance should have a teaching department of pediatric surgery with at least 3-5 teachers and supporting staff (resident, nursing and technical staff).

In urban areas, with the good antenatal ultrasonography, a large percentage of anomalies, can be diagnosed well in time and thus can be referred to a tertiary center as the case may be. The types of patients managed in a rural center are different from those seen in an urban center. The facilities in a government center would also differ from those in a private set up and similarly the type of surgeries would also be quite different in different places.

TRAINING IN PEDIATRIC SURGERY

The pediatric surgical specialty is different from others, requiring involvement, commitment and dedication. Presently, it is neither paying nor glamorous. Only those with a zeal and interest to serve the delicate babies should opt for it. The pattern of training differs in different parts of the world.[8] The learning becomes meaningful with the depth of involvement, large volume of workload faced and the surgical experience gained in managing various types of anomalies during the limited period of surgical training.

In most setups the surgeons first trains himself/herself in general surgery to acquire the basic principles and the skill of general surgery. One should then get training in pediatric surgery to acquire experience and finer skills. The period of training also varies from place to place. In India, it is minimal period of 12 years including the medical graduation, to become a qualified pediatric surgeon. However, this does not include the period required for the fellowships (urology, neonatal surgery, oncology, laparoscopy, etc.). As there may be more than one technique for diseases like Hirschsprung's disease, hypospadias, pyeloplasty, esophageal replacement and bladder augmentation. It is ideal that a pediatric surgeon is posted to work under the supervision of at least 3-4 pediatric surgeons to get exposed and experience the different techniques. Then he can adopt the one he feels most comfortable. Training courses should also be imparted to teachers to keep them updated on the subject.

AGE GROUP FOR A PEDIATRIC SURGICAL PATIENT

This varies from 12-18 in different parts of the world. Most developed countries however limit the upper age to 18 while developing countries keep it as 12. This depends on the doctor to patient ratio. Countries with limited workload, allow children up to 18 years to be included in the pediatric surgical group, while others with major workload, would like to restrict the admissions only up to 12 or 14 years of age. Despite all this, many a times, patients present very late with pediatric surgical index diseases like Hirschsprung's disease, anorectal anomalies, hepatobiliary disorders, lung pathologies, genitourinary requiring reconstructions and others. These have either been missed or mismanaged in the past. Due to their expertise, it is desirable that the pediatric surgeons should either accept the responsibility to treat index cases, irrespective of age, and operate upon them. Else, they should help their counterparts to achieve the best surgical results.

RECENT ADVANCES

Since 1980, the Stem cell research has taken a lead and is currently recognized as one of the main areas of interest to explore its potential in congenital anomalies, renal dysplasias, tumors, cirrhosis, testicular dysgenesis and many more.[9] The very fact that the infant's bone marrow is quite rich with mononuclear cells (mostly hemopoetic and less of mesenchymal cells), which if modulated by appropriate regulators (unfortunately not well known till yet) may have the potential to repair or regenerate the damaged tissues in the body.

Minimal invasive surgery and endoscopy with much finer instruments have become popular to suite the pediatric surgical patients.[10] However, their indications in newborns and infants still remain limited in general practice. Robotic surgery, though really useful and a preferred tool for deep pelvic surgery (e.g. radical prostectomy in adults and anorectal anomalies in children) has been used even for other procedures like pyeloplasty. Parents are aware of the global developments and demand for laparoscopy and even robotic surgery. These are becoming popular for use in pediatric surgical practice. Telesurgery has also become feasible with surgeons operating from distant places even across continents.

Laser technology has been applied to bronchial, esophageal and urethral valves, renal, ureteric and bladder stones and surface anomalies like hemangiomas. The harmonic scalpel has enabled liver resection, tumor surgery without much blood loss.

Most infants with biliary atresia would ultimately require Liver transplant (Ltp) in almost 80-90% children by 2-year of age, even after an initial successful porto-enterostomy. Currently, biliary atresia is the most common indication for Ltp, followed by other indications like, tumors, trauma, and hepatic failure. However, the facility remains limited to developed nations, supported by the governmental or other program for an otherwise very expensive life long proposition for surgery and maintenance of immunosuppression. Though, renal transplant can now be performed even in smaller babies, the problem remains to find a suitable donor to fit in the recipient's small abdomen. With the ongoing research and interest in tissue engineering, it might just take another 5-10 years when the most of the organs in the body of the appropriate sizes and shapes would be made available on shelf for children also.

Indications of fetal surgery have now become well defined with the lessons learnt from the experiences during the past two decades.[11] There are few conditions where fetal intervention can improve the morbidity and even the mortality. Small instruments assisted by minimal access surgery have been utilized for thoracic procedures, urinary tract decompression in babies with obstructive uropathy, ligation of the main vessel supplying the large tumors (e.g. Sacrococcygeal tumors), tracheal occlusion in babies with diaphragmatic hernia associated with lung hypoplasia and so on with the development of newer anesthetic agents and proper tocolysis, fetal surgery has been considered safe without much risks to both the fetus and the mother.

The management of pediatric tumors has been revolutionized both in investigations and in treatment. Positron Emission Tomography has been recognized as an important new modality of treatment.[12] It is now possible to cure at least some of these if not all. Renal tumors, lymphomas, are a good example with almost 80-95% survival. Newer chemotherapeutic drugs and regimes are not only more effective but with less side effects also. Sarcomas need not have amputations any more. Radiotherapy is also considered only in selected cases if the chemotherapy is not sufficient. Intra-operative implants or brachytherapy can be considered in children with residual tumors, e.g. neuroblastoma, so as to have less of side effects usually associated with postoperative wider field of radiation. Detection of new microarrays may help in newer ways to classify tumors and detect their recurrences.

The electronic world of computers has not only improved the communication faster, easier and economical but also the skills amongst the experts. Many offices have already gone paperless. Telemedicine and teleconferencing has brought the whole world close to each other, enabling bilateral exchange of ideas from different centers and different parts of the world at an affordable cost.

PEDIATRIC SURGICAL SPECIALTY IN INDIA

The exact past of the specialty of Pediatric surgery is not known. However, in India, it may date back to ancient times. Sushruta, the father of Indian surgery and Plastic surgery had written large volumes of literature and recently retrieved from Turkey, may be as old as 3000 BC (Fig. 1.1). Others feel it is only 600 year BC and may well coincide with the Hippocratic era. Sushruta is known to have the knowledge about pediatric surgical conditions like anorectal malformations, intussusception, a condition resembling Hirschsprung's disease, bladder outlet obstruction in children, vesicoureteric reflux, vesical calculus, phimosis, congenital hydrocele, inguinal hernia and pelvic tumors. He had also reasoned the etiology of intersex due to non-dominance of either the sperm or the egg.

Sushruta also wrote, "Only the union of medicine and surgery constitutes the complete doctor. The

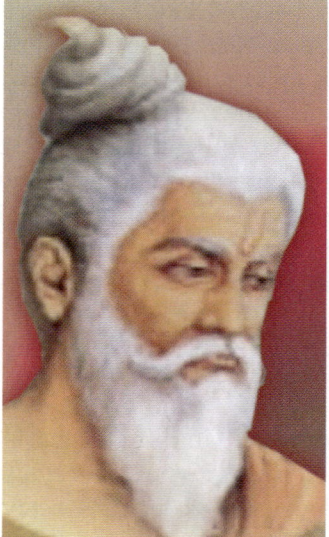

Fig. 1.1: Sushruta who lived in Kasi was an ancient Indian medical practitioner who was one of the first to study the human anatomy

doctor who lacks knowledge of one of these branches is like a bird with only one wing." Thus the need for collaboration between a pediatrician and pediatric surgeon is evident. He understood the high mortality in pediatric surgery in absence of anesthesia and antibiotics and warned that any surgeon should operate upon children only after obtaining due permission from king, lest it will amount to the offense of infanticide.

The pediatric surgical specialty in India, first established in 1965, as a section of Association of Surgeons of India (ASI), has a present strength of more than 800 members and collectively 30-40 pediatric surgeons are added each year from 23 teaching departments. After the improvement seen in the care of patients with trauma, malignancy and serious infections, the infrastructure for providing care to the surgical. Newborns is also improving with the survival of the newborns even with major malformations. Our specialty is very demanding and the facilities, including the trained faculty, nursing and technical staff is limited. The services are also restricted mostly to the urban areas. Most patients have to travel long hours even for short distances.

National Scenario

Our National Health Policy draft plan of 1983 was recently revised in the year 2002. The nation spends only 2.6% of its annual budget on health care. It increases to 5.2% if the expenditure incurred on providing preventive public health and hygiene is also included. The Government still has to focus on controlling the communicable diseases through various national health programs and treat malnutrition, diarrhea and infectious diseases on priority. Small pox has been eradicated. Polio is on the verge of eradication. There has been substantial drop in the total fertility rate and the infant mortality rate. Present population in India has already crossed 1 billion and we add 17-18 million newborns each year, almost equal to the existing population of Australia. The life expectancy has also increased from 36.7% in 1951 to 64.6% in year 2000.

Pediatric surgery is new and yet to be recognized for the role the specialty plays in providing quality care and reducing the national Infant Mortality Rate (IMR). Pediatric surgical services are presently limited only to the urban cities with very little or no pediatric facilities available in the rural sector. Also, almost 70-80% of pediatric surgical procedures are being performed by the general surgeons as the pediatric surgical specialists are not available in most centers or the medical colleges. It is aimed at developing pediatric surgery, in each and every Medical college in the country in the near future, and the facility needs to be extended later at the district level.

The main strength of pediatric surgery in India is the massive clinical work load dealing with more than 400 million children less than 14 years of age, constituting about 39% of population. This offers vast training opportunities to the residents in almost all aspects of surgical disciplines except open heart surgery and advanced neurosurgery.

Teaching and Training

The teaching program in pediatric surgery in India was started way back in 1969. It was only in 1972 that the American Board of Surgery was approved for the certification in Pediatric Surgery. This was followed by Canada and Great Britain in 1976. The Inter Collegiate Board of Royal Colleges in UK started its examination only in 1990s. India is proud of the postgraduate training program in pediatric surgery, following the British system, is now considered one of the best in the world. India, have not only the intense postdoctoral teaching program, dedicated curriculum and the syllabus but also have the expertise to offer in many sub-specialties.

Challenges

The clinical workload in the specialty is immense and is mostly directed to institutions, for seeking free, fair and seasoned service. The private sector is expensive especially for the newborn surgery and malignancy, remaining beyond the reach of the common man. The insurance cover is for less than 2% population. Antenatal care is limited and only 10-15% anomalies can be detected pre-natally. Folic acid prevention therapy is yet to take off. Challenging anomalies like spina bifida, exstrophy bladder, gross hydrocephalus, large abdominal wall defects, multiple anomalies incompatible with life, require ethical considerations. Finally, the job opportunities even for the most qualified and the talented staff are also rare. This has contributed to the professional dissatisfaction and sometimes even frustration amongst the younger generation opting for the specialty.

In a vast country like India, with lots of diversity in clinical workload, teaching and the research priorities, we have the following objectives:
1. To provide specialized pediatric surgical services to over 400 million pediatric population at an affordable cost and safety, ethically and professionally.
2. To provide rigorous and uniform training including sub-sections, at least in apex and centers of excellence.
3. To utilize the available limited financial resources to conduct only need based research to understand the common diseases in the region.

India being a vast country, all facilities are not likely to be available in each and every center. The quality of teaching and training also differs from place to place. Most our residents become quite trained and adequately competent after receiving the rigorous 3 year training. To meet any shortcoming, inter-departmental and the interstate exchanges have been established to widen their horizons and also keep the specialty vibrant and attractive. The talented faculty can excel in any field of medicine with proper planning and utilization of services.

In the recent past, the trend has been reversed. Not only the residents but also the faculty from developing and developed countries have been visiting key departments like that at AIIMS, New Delhi for higher training and patient care. This is only going to grow in future, with many teaching departments improving their teaching and training programs.

It is important that all postgraduate students in pediatric surgery are exposed to the research methodology to make them better teachers of tomorrow.[13,14] Unfortunately, Animal experiments are conducted only in a few institutions in India. Recently, various Govt. and the non-Government organizations are objecting to the experiments on animals. This has seriously affected the ongoing animal experimental research programs in major institutions. However, animal research is essential, and these should be performed following the strict guidelines as laid down by various ethical committees. Alternately, experiments in the field of molecular biology, stem cell research and Tissue Engineering are quite exciting.

Antenatal diagnosis is still not very common and only 10-20% anomalies are being diagnosed, that to mostly after 20 weeks of gestation, offering limited scope for termination even for major defects.[15] Organ transplantation remains a major challenge due to lack of facilities, shortage of donors and the high maintenance cost involved. India also has infrastructure and the well developed expertise in the field of endoscopy, urology, oncology and neonatal surgery but again only in the limited centers.

There is acute need to develop pediatric surgery in all Medical Colleges for teaching and patient care. Also, there should be at least one major tertiary care level center, one in each state. There should be apex centers at the national level to train the teachers and offer advanced surgery like transplant programs, conduct clinical and experimental research in the field of molecular biology, tissue engineering, stem cell therapy and others. These centers should be independent with complete autonomy for efficient delivery of advanced patient care, quality teaching and need based research.

Thus, Pediatric Surgery has come a long way in last few decades.[16] It has taken a better shape, yet we have to go a long way to establish ourselves and the specialty, solve many hurdles, develop infrastructure and refine treatment methodologies suiting to each nation.

It is not enough to begin. Continuance is necessary. The reason of failure in most cases is—lack of perseverance.

REFERENCES

1. Chatterjee SK. Is Pediatric Surgery a sinking specialty? J Indian Assoc Pediatr Surg 2002;7:103-4.
2. Dorairajan T. Future of Pediatric Surgery. J Indian Assoc Pediatr Surg 2002;7:115-16.
3. Gupta DK. Pediatric Surgery. Is it a sinking or growing specialty? J Indian Assoc Pediatr Surg 2002;7:105-8.
4. Rao KLN, Chowdhary SK. Shortcomings of Pediatric Surgery. J Indian Assoc Pediatr Surg 2002;7:109-14.
5. Gupta DK, Editorial. The much awaited Baby is born with a smile. Journal of Pediatric Surgical Specialties March 2007;1(1):3.
6. Upadhyaya P Foreword, in Textbook of Neonatal Surgery, Modern Publishers, DK Gupta (Ed), New Delhi 2000.
7. Gupta DK, Editorial. Sub-specialization in Pediatric Surgery—Who, When, Where ? Journal of Indian Association of Pediatric Surgeons 2006;11(2):70-72.

8. Gupta DK. Official document of the Indian Association of Pediatric Surgeons (IAPS)— Recommendations of the Curriculum Committee, for M Ch training Program in Pediatric surgery in India, submitted to Medical Council of India, 1998.
9. Gupta DK, Sharma Shilpa. Stem Cell Therapy — Hope and scope in pediatric Surgery. Journal of Indian Association of Pediatric Surgeons. July - September 2005:10(3);138-41.
10. Gupta DK, Editorial. Make Pediatric Laparoscopy a surgeon's armamentarium. Journal of Indian Association of Pediatric Surgeons. October - December 2006:11(4);198-200.
11. Gupta DK, Sharma Shilpa. Fetal surgery, in Recent Advances in Surgery, Ed. Roshal Lal Gupta, 2006;chapter 6;10:116-29.
12. Gupta DK, Pathak M, Kumar R, Sharma S, Agarwala S, Bajpai M, Bhatnagar VB. PET-CT in staging and determining treatment response in Neuroblastoma and Rhabdomyosarcoma, Abstracted in the proceedings of the 8th Congress of European Pediatric Surgeons Association. Turin Italy 2007;54.
13. Gupta DK, Editorial. Research in Pediatric Surgery — Who should light the flame. Journal of Indian Association of Pediatric Surgeons. July-September 2006;11(3):127.
14. Gupta DK Editorial. Research in Pediatric Surgery in the developing countries. African Jour Pediatr Surg, 2008 (in press).
15. Sharma Shilpa, DK Gupta. Discrepancies between the Antenatal and Postnatal Diagnosis of Pediatric Surgical Conditions. Journal of Indian Association of pediatric surgeons 2006;11:183.
16. Pathak IC. Editorial. Is'nt it time to get started? Journal of Indian Association of Pediatric Surgeons. July-September 2005;10(3):135-36.

Evolution of Pediatric Surgery

IC Pathak

Surgery of children has been known to be practiced since times immemorial. It is, however, only during the twentieth century after the 2nd World War that it was recognized as a distinct and independent entity and practiced exclusively by surgeons who felt attracted to treat conditions neglected or treated ineffectively by adult general surgeons. Before World War II there were very few surgeons who devoted their energies exclusively to the care of children. Breathtaking advances in science and technology during the last century almost over shadowed the development of the new specialty. The development of pediatric surgery after 1945 is therefore astonishing. It has been likened to the evolution of an Oak tree from an acorn, growing from humble beginnings to a well-recognized surgical specialty. Robert E Gross (Fig. 2.1) one of the founding fathers of pediatric surgery in North America had written in 1953 that "the care of the children requires a certain indefinable something which might well be called the 'art' of pediatric surgery; it cannot be quantitated or characterized any more than one can describe adequately the tints of Titian or the bold strokes of Michel Angelo. This extra something is a priceless attribute which is most sought for in members of the visiting or house staff".[1] Willis Potts (Fig. 2.2), another pioneer of the newly emerging specialty in North America had in his inimitable style said in 1959 that pediatric surgery born of the lawfully wedded parents need and demand is now joining the family of specialties. After slow progress during infancy the specialty has grown into a lusty child howling for recognition and demanding a place at the table.[2]

Pediatric surgery is surprisingly popular as a career because as compared to many other newer surgical specialties that have come up during the last 50 years the professional rewards are not as great nor the specialty as glamorous as Cardiac or Neurosurgery. Inspite of the fact that pediatric surgery is still struggling to gain recognition as a distinct entity in many developing countries as India, the number of candidates seeking admission to MCh training programs in our country is astounding. It is I believe,

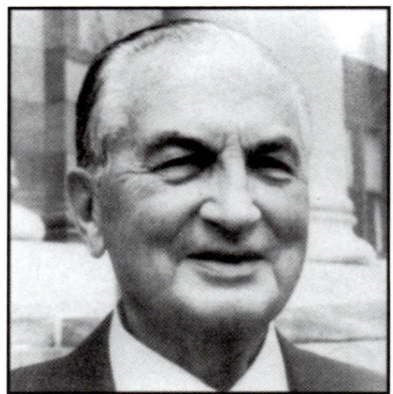

Fig. 2.1: Robert E Gross

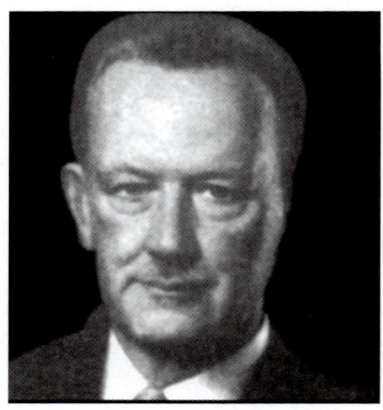

Fig. 2.2: Willis Potts

the fascination of dealing with children, that grip those who care for them.

WHAT IS PEDIATRIC SURGERY?

Herbert E Coe (Fig. 2.3) possibly the first American to practice pure pediatric surgery at the Children's Orthopedic Hospital in Seattle, addressing the 9th International Congress of Pediatrics at Montreal in July, 1959 had said, that Pediatric Surgery may be defined "as the application of sound surgical principles in the treatment of an organism which is in the most rapidly changing state of its entire lifespan. Pediatric Surgery is the surgery of evolution as contrasted with involution. It is the surgery of the transition period between the protected intrauterine existence and a world of an infinite number of more or less violent external stimuli, the period of adjustment of neuro-muscular mechanism, of heat regulation, of nutrition, of fluid and electrolyte balance, where arithmetical computation of requirement based on those of 150 pound adults is completely fallacious. The patient frequently does not understand our language, cannot or will not cooperate and has emotional or mental reaction which are often unpredictable."[3]

Isidor Ravdin, the highest ranking Medical Officer in the US Army in India during the 2nd World War once used a mathematical equation when he claimed that "a Surgeon is a Physician and something more".

$$\text{A Surgeon} = (\text{A Physician})^{SM}$$
RAVDIN

Dr Henry Bahnson, in his presidential address before the American Association for Thoracic Surgeons, enlarged upon this metaphor and said "a Thoracic Surgeon is a Physician and something more" and raising the equation by another exponential power and something more.[4]

$$\text{A Thoracic Surgeon} = (\text{A Physician})^{SM\ SM}$$
BAHNSON

Judson Randolph while addressing the 16th annual meeting of the American Pediatric Surgical Association at Hawii in 1985 said that "when one considers the exacting technical requirements for surgery in 1000 G infant, it is not illogical to take Dr Bahnson's analogy one step further: "a pediatric surgeon is a physician and something more and something more and something yet again."[5]

$$\text{A Pediatric Surgeon} = (\text{A Physician})^{SM\ SM\ SM}$$
JUDSON RANDOLPH

RECORDED EARLY HISTORY OF PEDIATRIC SURGERY

Medical care of children has existed since time began. Old writings make it clear that it has included surgical procedures, Pediatrics as a medical specialty, however, did not come into existence before the middle of 19th century. Pediatric surgery distinct from surgery of the adult came much later. The Egyptian petroglyphs dating as far back as 2500 B C depict circumcision and surgery of the head and extremities. An Egyptian Papyrus dating back to 1450 BC is perhaps the oldest known treatise on pediatrics consisting of prescriptions and incantations for the protection of mothers and babies. But "The first consistent body of pediatric doctrine, particularly on hygiene and nutrition is in the Indian Sushruta, compiled in the 5th century BC; it describes about 120 surgical instruments".[6] Indian historians believe that there were two Sushrutas, a senior and a junior, and it would seem that the author of the original Sushruta samhita, flourished as early as 1000 BC and the later, the younger Sushruta, the author of most of the chapters in the present Sushruta samhita taught surgery in Kashi (Varanasi) during the 6th century BC. Sushruta samhita is the first ancient treatise, which advocated dissection of the human cadavers much against the prejudices, which must have flourished in his times. He is to be credited to be the first who described the removal of bladder stone by the perineal route. He described operations for anal fistula but his description

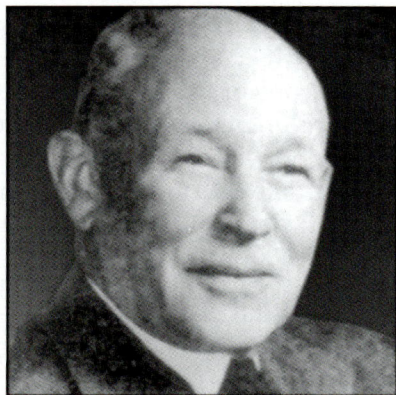

Fig. 2.3: Herbert E Coe

of repair of a cut nose by rotating a flap of skin from the cheek was the most original concept. Other aspects of plastic surgery dealt by Sushruta were repair of ear lobules and lips and are described in meticulous details.

Hippocrates (460-370 BC) considered to be the Father of Medicine and Pediatrics described special problems inherent in head injuries of children and gave advice for the treatment of hematomas and fractures.[7]

Aulus Cornelius Celsus who wrote "De re Medica" around 30 AD believed by Western historians as the first classical medical work was in fact a compilation from the Greek, included were a few passages mentioning diseases in children stating that the "children are required to be treated entirely differently from adult".[8] He described tonsillectomy, uvulotomy, frenotomy and the repair of the hare lip and nasal defects.

One of the largest and most complete medical encyclopedia written in the middle ages, Kitab at-Tasrif was authored by Abu I - Quasim Khafaf, known to historians by the distorted Latin name of Albucasis. He was an Arab by descent. Cardoba in Spain where he was born in 912, was famous all over Europe in those days by its teachings of Islamic religion, humanities, literature, pharmacology and medicine. The encyclopedia comprised 30 volumes, the last one dealing with surgery. Albucasis book on surgery was considered by the developing European World to be a basic work of reference for many centuries throughout the renaissance. There were numerous translations and editions of this famous work. Pediatric surgery was known to Albucasis and the subjects covered were cauterization of hare lip, care of hydrocephalus, removal of ranula, treatment of imperforate urinary meatus and treatment of hypospadias. A detailed description is given on circumcision of boys and correction of their erroneous treatment.[9]

In 1465, Serafeddin Subuncuoglu published the earliest known Pediatric surgical Atlas "Cerrahiye-I ilhaniye" in Turkish describing surgical technique and instruments. Serafeddin was born in Amasya in Northern Turkey. This book contained many miniature drawings concerning the operative procedures. It is believed by many historians that Serafeddin made only a faithful translation of Albucasis' book of surgery, the only addition being the miniatures depicting the surgical technique. This has been contested and it has been claimed that the book "contain not only the pictures or miniatures of surgical and pediatric surgical procedures but also many important and major new contributions to the surgical literature originally described by Subuncuoglu himself.[10]

The first textbook in Pediatric Surgery is, however, credited to the Swiss Surgeon Felix Wurtz published in 1563. In 1612, a new edition of the book 'An experimental Treatise of surgery' appeared with a pediatric appendix including references to orthopedic problems.[11]

PEDIATRIC SURGERY IN THE NINETEENTH CENTURY

Nineteenth century saw an increasing interest in the surgery of the children. This was due to many reasons. Opening of hospitals exclusively for children, publication of books and periodicals on the surgical diseases of children, increasing interest in saving new born babies suffering from medical and surgical conditions and exciting individuals contributions of surgeons and physicians in treating children. An awareness was thus gradually generated amongst the medical profession on surgery of children heralding the beginning of Pediatric Surgery.

Europe is considered to be the cradle of Pediatric Surgery. Many children's hospitals came up all over Europe mostly during the 1st half of the nineteenth century. The first being the hospital des infant malades in Paris in 1802. The World famous Hospital for Sick Children Great Ormond Street was established in 1852. In North America Hospitals for children came up much later mostly during the latter part of the nineteenth century. The famous Boston Children Hospital modeled after the Hospital for Sick Children, London, opened in 1882.

Pediatric Surgeons of the nineteenth century to a large extent were engaged in orthopedic surgery. Tuberculosis of bones, osteomyelitis, congenital anomalies of bones like club foot, fractures and dislocation of bones, and deformities of extremities due to poliomyelitis were rampant in those days. "This tradition persisted in certain countries like France, where all Professors of Pediatric Surgery in Paris from Kirmisson in 1901 to the great Ombradanne in 1923 were largely, although not entirely orthopedically oriented."[12]

Inspite of the fact that children's hospitals existed in most European countries during the 19th century, very few surgeons devoted their work only in children. The reasons were mostly economical. Many once appointed to the staff of children's hospitals were lured by the lucrative practice in adult surgery and tried their level best to leave. This phenomenon is seen even today in many parts of our country.

Many books exclusively on diseases of children were published during the nineteenth century in Europe and England. JN Coley published his 'A practical treatise of children' in 1846 in London. And between 1856 and 1877, there were atleast fifteen publications in English, French and Italian on the subject.[13] One of the first textbooks of Pediatric Surgery in the English language "The Surgical Diseases of Children" was published by John Cooper Forester in 1860. Forester a Fellow of Royal College of Surgeons was an Assistant surgeon to Guys Hospital and Surgeon to the Royal Infirmary in London. In 1870, after fifteen years as Assistant Surgeon he became the Surgeon to the Guys Hospital in London. He favored the use of chloroform and felt that as it was safe there was no justification for inflicting pain in children needing surgery. By 1874 he had changed his views and preferred ether for babies. He was one of the few surgeons of his time who did tracheostomies in children and was the first to perform a gastrostomy for stricture of the esophagus in children. For stone bladder he made lateral perineal incision as advocated by Sushruta in India in the hoary past. He classified imperforate anus and described fistulous communication to vagina and urinary bladder . He was aware of the good results in low lesions and described a simple incision into the perineum. He had also advocated bringing the rectum down and suturing it to the skin. Forester's book is largely descriptive but contains excellent lithographs reproducing in great detail many anomalies including hemangiomas of arm, lip, vulva and face.[14]

A more detailed book on children's surgery was compiled from a series of lectures given between 1840 and 1860 by MP Guersant, Honorary Surgeon of the Hospital des Enfants Malades, Paris. Richard Dunglison of Philadelphia translated the text from the French in 1873. Guersant described many congenital lesions like harelip, hypospadias and spina bifida. His description of congenital absence of the anus with fistula to an "abnormal position" indicated an increasing recognition of the various types of the malformation. He advocated making a puncture in the perineum, directing it to the side of the sacrum to avoid wounding the vagina or the bladder in cases of simple anal imperforate anus which we now refer to as "low anomaly". He described various trocars and stents used to maintain the opening made in the perineum.[15]

Prior to 1870 the management of sick babies did not constitute a problem at all. Since antiquity they were left to die. The Franco Prussion War took place in 1870-71 and this changed the attitudes of medical profession toward these babies. The reason was the enormous loss of human life on the French side and consequently the great reduction in the birth rate. The already weakened French nation could not persist in the future against a victorious Germany more populous and much more fertile. Every life saved thus became an asset. It is not surprising therefore that the first improvements in the neonatal care came almost entirely from France. There were 3 main dangers to the neonates particularly the premature ones; hypothermia, infection and faulty feeding habits. All of these were systematically tackled. In 1878 Odite Martin, the Director of the Paris Zoo constructed a warming chamber for hatching of eggs. Tarnier, the Paris obstetrician was fascinated by the device. In close collaboration the two men built the first incubator heated by warm air which was installed in 1880 in the Paris Maternity Hospital. Isolating babies in special units controlled infection and careful sterilization of feeding bottles was successful in saving many a baby.[16]

The first half of the nineteenth century witnessed the contribution of two eminent French Surgeons, a contribution which is considered a landmark in the evolution of surgical treatment of imperforate anus. In 1834, JN Roux operated on a case of imperforate anus through a midline longitudinal incision in the perineum.[17] In 1835, JZ. Amussat operated on a girl using a T shaped incision. The rectum was pulled down to the perineum and stitched to the skin. This innovative procedure was heralded as the "great break through in the management of imperforate anus.[18]

The latter half of the nineteenth century was an exciting time in the development of modern surgery. Ether anesthesia was introduced in 1846, the origin of surgical sepsis from bacteria discovered by Pasteur and its prevention by scrubbing the operative skin site and scrupulous hand washing described by Lister. Billroth wrote about his success in gastric resection, esophageal surgery and bowel resection. Despite these advances, the general principles of surgical care established during the latter-half of the nineteenth century, almost uniformly benefited adult patient, and rarely if ever did a newborn with a major congenital anomaly or child with an acute surgical abdomen, large tumor and serious injury survive.[15]

Toward the close of nineteenth century the contribution of a pediatrician interested in surgical matters who often attended surgical operative procedures, exemplified the keen interest and knowledge of a pediatric surgeon. Harald Hirschsprung whose name is familiar to pediatricians and surgeons today was born in Copenhagen in 1830. He qualified MD in 1855 and was appointed the Chief Physician to the First Children's Hospital in 1870. As a pediatrician Hirschsprung was interested in a wide range of neonatal problems. In 1886, he reported before the Society of Pediatricians in Berlin on "constipation in newborn due to dilatation and hypertrophy of the colon". Although he failed to recognize the cause of congenital megacolon, a condition that bears his name even today, the contribution does not detract from his keen observation and far ranging interest in surgical matters. Earlier in 1861, he had described four cases of esophageal atresia with tracheoesophageal fistula occurring over a 7-month period in a town with a population of only 100,000. His report on cases of hypertrophic pyloric stenosis in 1887, established this condition as a distinct clinical entity. But perhaps his most imposing contribution was the use of hydrostatic reduction of ileocolic intussusception published in 1876. His results were so superior to previously published reports of surgical intervention that many doubted his conclusion. His final report in 1905 of 107 cases, substantiated a 35% mortality rate for a condition that up to that time was fatal in over 80% of cases. Hirschsprung's observations regarding a number of potentially correctable surgical conditions gives him the distinction of being recognized as a modern day pediatric surgeon. His interest in surgical matters makes one suspect his unspoken desire to have been a Surgeon.

MODERN PEDIATRIC SURGERY

Modern pediatric surgery is largely the work of three generations of surgeons. The founders, notably

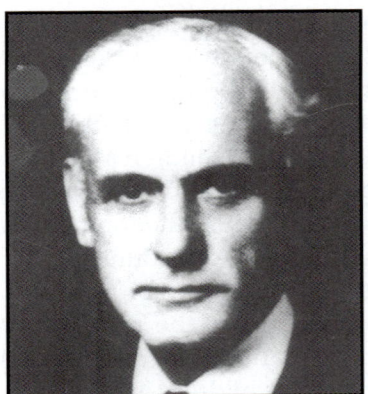

Fig. 2.4: William Ladd

William Ladd (Fig. 2.4) and Robert Gross in Boston and Sir Dennis Browne in London, a middle generation of 50-60 surgeons who were responsible for founding the surgical section of the American Academy of Pediatrics and the British Association of Pediatric Surgeons; and the third generation of very large number of surgeons all over the world.

Surgery of infants and children in the USA began with William Ladd. He is regarded as the Father of the Pediatric Surgery in North America. Born in 1880, he graduated from Harvard College in 1902 and Harvard Medical School in 1906 and joined the staff of the Boston Children's Hospital in 1910.

"On December 6, 1917, during World War I, a munition ship exploded in the harbor at Halifax, Nova Scotia, causing many casualities among whom were many children. A plea was made to physicians from Boston. William Ladd was among those who responded. It is said that this heart wrenching event helped influence Ladd to concentrate his efforts in the field of child surgery.[19] In 1941 after nearly 15 years as Head of the Surgical Services at Children's Hospital, he was honoured by the Medical School, the hospital and his colleagues and friends by the creation of the Ladd's professorship of child surgery. He held this chair until his retirement in 1945. Not only he was recognized as the authority in pediatric surgery at Harvard but also he became the acknowledged leader throughout North America.

Ladd had an almost unique group of qualities in that he developed new and sound methods of surgical treatment; he was a superb teacher at all levels, from medical students to residents as well as to practicing medical and surgical community. The result of all these attributes was to attract an enthusiastic group of

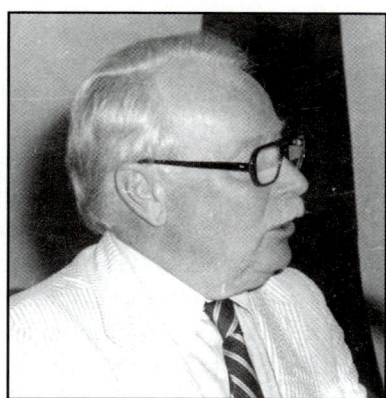

Fig. 2.5: Orvar Swenson

trainees. Of his trainees by far the greatest is his former resident and immediate successor Robert E Gross. Gross followed directly in Ladd's footsteps although more as a great innovator of surgery and as a teacher. His other trainees included Orvar Swenson (Fig. 2.5), H William Clatworthy and Everett Koop.

Robert Gross became surgeon in Chief at the Children's Hospital, Boston in 1947, during his career he made great contributions in the field of pediatric surgery. In 1938, when he was Chief Surgical Resident, he successfully divided a patent ductus arteriosus. Unfortunately, the operation was done when Dr Ladd was on vacation. Ladd never forgave him for doing the operation when he was out of town. Thus began an estrangement that probably slowed the development of pediatric surgery more than we will acknowledge. Nevertheless Ladd and Gross published in 1941, the first American Textbook on Child Surgery "Abdominal surgery of infancy and childhood". Because of the antagonism between the two, Ladd made it difficult as he possibly could for Gross to ascend to the chair that bore his name. It was only after two years of Ladd's retirement in 1947 that Gross was finally appointed the Chief since his accomplishments were overwhelming and he was acclaimed internationally. In 1953, Gross published his matchless textbook, "The surgery of infancy and Childhood".

The founder of Modern British Pediatric surgery Sir Dennis Browne was born in Australia where he studied medicine at the University of Sydney, New South Wales. He qualified in medicine in 1914 and having volunteered for the Australian expeditionary Force spent the whole of 1914-18 world war in France as an Army Medical Officer. He came to England after the war and continued his surgical training at the London and Middlesex Hospital and trained in orthopedic surgery under Sir Robert Jones in Liverpool. Surgery of childhood always fascinated him and he therefore joined the staff of the Hospital for Sick Children, Great Ormond Street, London, as a registrar and a resident surgical officer. He was elected as a consultant surgeon to that hospital in 1928 and retired in 1957.

Dennis Browne was the first surgeon in England to confine his practice to children. After second world war the fame of his work spread all over the globe and young Pediatric Surgeons from all over the world came to him to learn. He was one of the founders and the first President of the British Association of Pediatric Surgeons.

Dennis Browne had a truly original mind and left his mark on virtually every branch of pediatric surgery. Among them one can recall his operations for harelip and cleft palate in plastic surgery, the operation for hypospadias and undescended testis in urology, his work on talipes equinovarus and congenital dislocation of hip in orthopedic surgery and his investigations and operations for anorectal malformation in Proctology. In 1957, the surgical section of the American Academy of Pediatrics awarded him the Ladd Medal for his services to Pediatric Surgery. In 1961, he was knighted.

CURRENT STATUS

It is amazing that inspite of the great struggle initially the specialty has grown up during the last 50 years all over the world and has shown signs of maturity and independence denied to them in the forties and fifties of the last century. Though independent pediatric surgical departments have come up and are well established in many medical institutions and universities all over the world there are disturbing trends which are likely to change the practice of peditric surgery in future. The founding fathers and pediatric surgeons of yester years, were interested in orthopedic, in many a plastic procedures, treatment of congenital cardiac anomalies, and congenital malformations of central nervous system. Many of the pioneers in the treatment of cardiac anomalies started their professional career in pediatric surgery like Robert Gross and Willis Potts in North America,

Christian Barnard in South Africa and Waterston in England.

The present day pediatric surgeons have gradually shied away from the management of facial anomalies like harelip and cleft palate and malformations of central nervous system. The plastic and Maxillofacial surgeons have taken over the management of the former and neurosurgeons are now managing the latter. Many pediatric surgeons have duly recognized the increasing complexity of operative procedures for cardiac malformation and their management now is entirely in the hands of cardiac surgeons.

Another disturbing trend is the lack of interest of the present generation in the newly emerging sub-specialties of transplant surgery and intrauterine fetal surgery.

There has also been a very rapid development of organ specialties in recent years. Specialties like urology, microvascular and transplant surgery have successfully made inroads into the specialty of pediatric surgery. The dangers of such a development have probably not been appreciated. Admission of children to highly specialized departments of urology, microvascular and transplant surgery, under the care of surgeons, and the supporting staff unaware of the special needs of sick children can often be disastrous. Pediatric surgeons of the future would have to either receive training in these sub-specialties which obviously is likely to lengthen the course of their training or practice in a field which is already shrunk by the fragmentation of the specialty. Both these alternatives are difficult to choose. Newer knowledge and complexity of the surgical procedures of the newly coming up sub-specialties will make it difficulty for many to master the complicated procedures.

In recent years, the popularity of laparoscopic surgery in adults has stimulated the pediatric surgeons to adopt this newly emerging specialty in their own field. It is inevitable that in the foreseeable future, laparoscopic surgery will also become a major and important component of our specialty.

THE INDIAN SCENARIO

Pediatric surgery as a specialty is only about 40 years old in India. Essentially it is no different than the development of this specialty in other countries. In the fifties of the last century very few general surgeons were interested in the surgical diseases of children particularly the severe congenital anomalies. The result was that nearly all such babies either died in the hospitals they were admitted to or were sent home to die.

In those days there were only a few surgeons who were exclusively practicing pediatric surgery in India. Prof UC Chakraborty of Calcutta Medical College, Dr Raman Nair (Fig. 2.6) at Trivandrum Medical College and Prof O Anjaneyulu at Niloufer Hospital at Hyderabad were perhaps the only ones in the whole country. Two other distinguished general surgeons of that era namely Dr Arthur E Desa at Bombay and Col RD Ayyar at Delhi who were interested in children surgery did more for the development of Pediatric Surgery in the fifties and sixties of the last century than any other surgeon of the day by their encouragement and moral support to the young talented surgeons. Both of them were influential in the Health Services of the country and helped behind the scenes to promote and establish independent pediatric surgical centers in the country. Encouraged by the guiding spirit of surgeons like Arthur Desa and Col Ayyar a number of young surgeons therefore, decided to practice surgery exclusively in children. Many of them went abroad for training in the specialty since there were hardly any facilities in the country. They had heard and read about the great masters like Dennis Browne in London, William E Ladd, Robert E Gross and Orvar Swenson in Boston, Wills Potts in Chicago, C Everett Koop in Philadelphia and some others in Canada and Australia and to these masters or their successors our young surgeons went. After varying periods of training they returned home with great hopes of settling down to practice the new specialty.

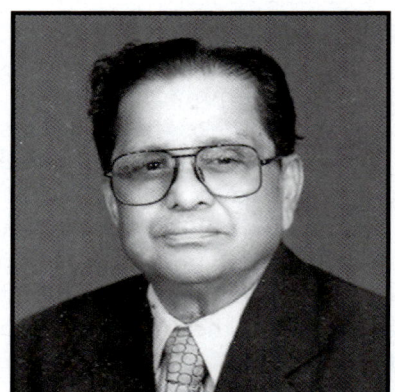

Fig. 2.6: Raman Nair, Calicut

Many of them were soon disillusioned, as they were not received with open arms as they expected. In fact there was a stiff resistance not only from the Health administrators but also from the general surgeons. The general surgeons felt threatened that their specialty already fragmented by the newer specialties of cardiac, neuro and plastic surgery could not accept further fragmentation.

Two very significant developments took place at this point of time in initiating the process of development of the new specialty. One was the formation of an independent pediatric surgery section within the frame work of Association of Surgeons of India in 1964 and the other was the institution of Postgraduate degree in Pediatric surgery at the University of Madras in 1966.

It was during the Silver Jubilee Conference of Association of Surgeons of India (ASI) at Mumbai in December 1964, that Dr RK Gandhi (Fig. 2.7) of Mumbai thought of putting up a proposal for establishing an independent pediatric surgery section within the ASI, Dr Gandhi hurriedly cornered like minded youngsters who had returned from abroad after training in Pediatric surgery to seek their opinion. About 30 young surgeons enthusiastically received the suggestion and it was decided to put up a proposal before the General Body Meeting. Dr KK Gandhi, Dr T Dorairajan from Madurai, drafted the proposal with the help of late Dr MS Ramakrishnan (Fig. 2.8) of Madras. The resolution was presented before the General Body Meeting of the ASI. The proposal, as expected, encountered stiff opposition from the surgeons but was finally adopted after a strong plea made by one of the past Presidents of the ASI late Prof. BN Sinha.[20]

The institution of a postgraduate course at the University level leading to a degree in the specialty was the other noteworthy event, which had a vast impact in the development of the specialty. The late Prof MS Ramakrishnan was able to plead for such a course at the Madras University and because of his efforts, this University was the first in the country to institute such a course in 1966. The first MCh degree in the country was awarded in 1968. Gradually other Universities and Postgraduate Institutions followed suit and by the end of the 1972, as many as seven Institutions were awarding MCh degrees in Pediatric surgery. Starting of such courses gave an academic recognition and professional status to the specialty and helped train pediatric surgeons within the country. As a consequence the flow of surgeons going out of the country for higher training in pediatric surgery virtually dried up and till 1998 as many as 500 Pediatric Surgeons had been trained at various centers in the country.

Besides these two significant and fortuitous events, I believe there was an additional element, which made Pediatric surgery a popular, and a dynamic specialty. It was the pioneering spirit of a handful of young surgeons of those days. The contributions made by Prof RK Gandhi and Prof SS Deshmukh from Mumbai, Prof MS Rama Krishnan and Prof T Dorairajan from Tamil Nadu, Prof Raman Nair from Trivandrum, Prof Subir K Chatterjee (Fig. 2.9) from Kolkata, Prof Purushottam Upadhyaya (Fig. 2.10) from New Delhi, Prof IC Pathak from Chandigarh (Fig. 2.11), Prof KC Sogani from Jaipur (Fig. 2.12) and Prof Meera Bai from Hyderabad are legendary.

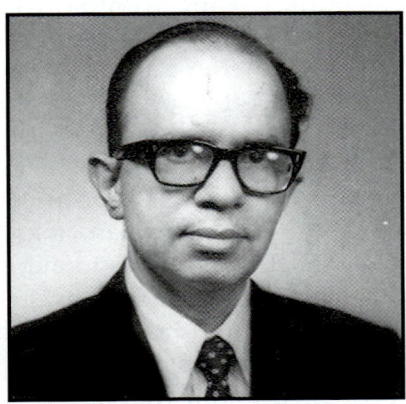

Fig. 2.7: RK Gandhi, Mumbai

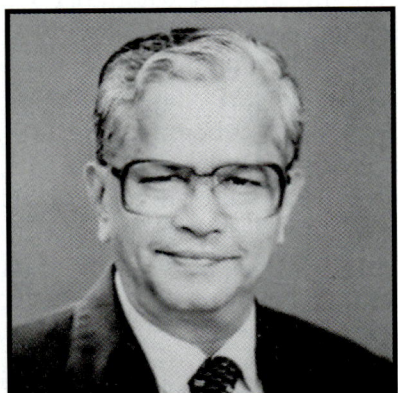

Fig. 2.8: MS Ramakrishnan, Chennai

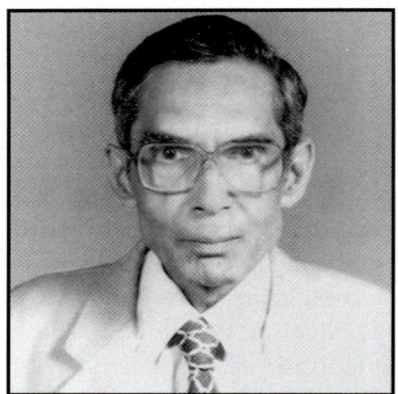

Fig. 2.9: Subir K Chatterjee, Kolkata

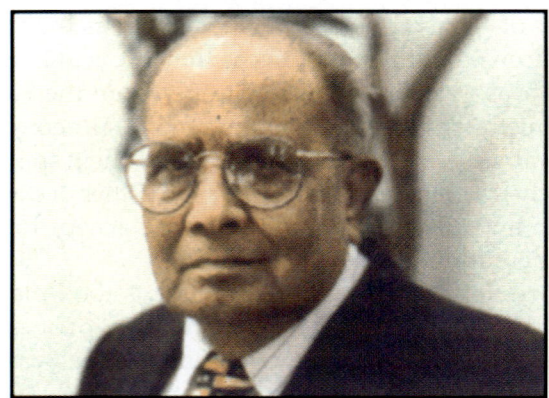

Fig. 2.12: KC Sogani, Jaipur

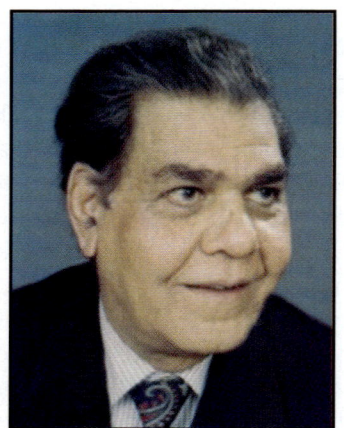

Fig. 2.10: P Upadhyaya, New Delhi

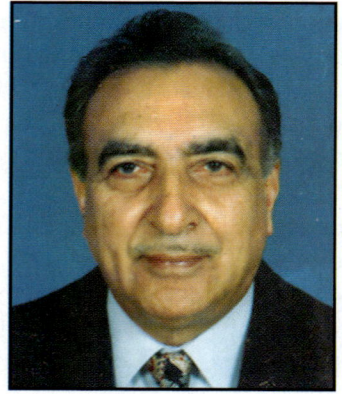

Fig. 2.11: IC Pathak, Chandigarh

Besides establishing independent Pediatric surgical centers for Postgraduate training all over the country these pioneers involved themselves actively in the organizational activities of the Association of Surgeons of India (ASI), Asian Association of Pediatric Surgeons and World Federation of Association of Pediatric Surgeons which gave them an opportunity of having a voice in several policy decisions. It is a remarkable historical fact that three of these pioneer pediatric surgeons of the country namely Prof MS Rama Krishnan from Chennai, RK Gandhi from Mumbai and T Dorairajan from Madurai were elected Presidents of the ASI in 1979-80 and 1981 respectively. Prof SS Deshmukh from Mumbai joined their illustrious company a few years later.

At the meeting of the Pacific Association of Pediatric Surgeons in Tokyo in 1972, the first meeting of the Asian Pediatric Surgeons was also held and elected adhoc office bearers to formalize the Association. Two of the three crucial offices were secured by Prof MS Ramakrishnan as founder Vice President and Prof RK Gandhi as founder Secretary General. India managed to maintain its pre-eminence by continued representations and occupying key positions in the Asian Association of Pediatric Surgeons. Prof RK Gandhi was its President from 1980-82, Prof P Upadhyaya was the President for the years 1984-86 and Prof SK Chatterjee was the Vice President for the years 1986-88.

The individual contributions of some of these pioneers during the early days of pediatric surgery in the country have been no less significant. Prof Upadhyaya's work on splenic trauma, inventing the first low priced indigenous shunt valve for the management of hydrocephalus and innovative new surgical techniques for the treatment of rectal atresia and anterior perineal anus has been internationally recognized. He was the first surgeon to successfully separate conjoint twins in the country in 1969 and established a neonatal ICU, the first of its kind in the country in 1971 at the AIIMS, New Delhi. Prof Subir

Chatterji was the first one in the country to save a baby with esophageal atresia in 1964 and also separated successfully two sets of conjoint twins in the mid-eighties.[21] He is the author of a popular book "Anorectal malformation" published in 1993 and is the founding Chief Editor of the "Journal of the Indian Association of Pediatric Surgeons" since 1995. Prof Pathak and his associates from Chandigarh drew the attention of Pediatric surgeons to a peculiar variant of anorectal Malformation, now popularly known as "Pouch Colon" for the first time in 1972.[22] This anomaly since then has been found to be common in the northern belt of the country and large series have been reported from this geographical area during the last 35 years.

The present day leaders of the specialty in various Medical Institutions in the country are the students of these first generation Pediatric Surgeons. They have not only maintained the high standards of competence laid down by their teachers but have by their diligence and hard work improved and expanded the specialty in all aspects of patient care, training and research. The future of Pediatric Surgery I believe is in their hands and in turn in the hands of their students.

The progress made by the specialty during the last three decades has been tremendous both by individual surgeons as well as the Pediatric Surgical Centers in some parts of the country. These centres have raised the standards of surgical care of children and many of them compare favorably with the best centers in the world. It must, however, be emphasized that these are isolated islands of excellence. India is a big country and we are still woefully short of well established centers in most parts of the country. Presently, there are 21 teaching departments of Pediatric surgery in the country producing about 30 pediatric surgeons each year.

What is the lot of pediatric surgeon in the country that we have trained during the last 30 years? I understand it is not very happy situation. In a recent survey conducted by Dr KL Narasimhan and his colleagues from the Postgraduate Institute of Medical Education and Research, Chandigarh, it was found that the trained and qualified pediatric surgeons in the country were a dissatisfied lot.[23] Only 50 percent of them were economically satisfied. Nearly 1/4th had to resort to general adult surgery work to augment their income. Nearly two thirds felt the need for a change in the training program. It was the opinion of many of the Pediatric Surgeons that uniform curriculum, better hands-on experience and a rotation through 2-3 centers of training in the country was desirable. It was found that the cities were overcrowded with pediatric surgeons and there were very few and insufficient numbers in the rural areas. It was also the opinion of many that majority of general surgeons had inadequate training to operate on children and there was a need for better cooperation with pediatricians.

I hope the present day leaders of the profession in our specialty would take note of this dissatisfaction amongst the practitioners of this specialty and make efforts to rectify the deficiencies in our training programs. It does not brook any delay and sooner we address these inadequacies better it will be for our specialty.

REFERENCES

1. Gross RE. The surgery of infancy and childhood. Philadelphia, Saunders 1953.
2. Potts WJ. The Surgeon and the child. WB Saunders Company, Philadelphia and London 1959.
3. Coe HE. Cited by Simpson JS. History of Medicine. The Canadian Journal of Surgery 1976;19:551-58.
4. Bahnson HT. Our obligation to developing nations. J Thor and Cardiothoracic Surg 1977;74:168.
5. Randolph J. The first of the best. J Pediatr Surg 1985; 20:580-91.
6. Garrison FH. Introduction to history of Medicine, 4th ed. Philadelphia Saunders 1929.
7. Mettler LC, Mettler FA. History of Medicine, Correlative text, arranged according to subjects, Philadelphia, Blakiston 1947.
8. Still FG. History of Paediatrics. Progress of study of diseases of children up to the end of XVIIIth Century, New York, Oxford 1931.
9. Montagnani CA. Pediatric surgery in Islamic Medicine from the Middle ages to the renaissance Prog in Paed Surg 1986;20:39-51.
10. Unver AS. Quoted by Buyukunal SNC and SARI N, Serafeddin subuncuoglu, the author of the earliest pediatric surgical Atlas:CERRAHIYE-1 Ilhaniye. J Pediatr Surg 1991;26:1148-51.
11. Wurtz F. Quoted by Simpson GS. History of Medicine. The Canadian Journal of Surgery 1976;19:551-58.
12. Rickham PP. An analysis of Pediatric Surgery in North America and North Western Europe 1972, J Pediat Surg 7:475-81.
13. Simpson JS. History of Medicine. Pediatric Surgery: Old Art and New Science. The Canadian J of Surg 1976;19: 551-58.
14. Raffensperger JG. A review of the first Textbook of Pediatric Surgery in the English language, Jr Pediat Surg 1969;4:403-05.

15. Touloukian RJ. Pediatric Surgery between 1860 and 1900, 1995. J Pediatr Surg 30:911-16.
16. Rickham PP. Thoughts about the past and future of Neonatal Surgery, J Pediatr Surg 1992;27:1-6.
17. Roux JN (1834). Cited by DeVries PA and Pena A. Posterior sagittal anorectoplasty, J Pediatr Surg 1982;17:638-43.
18. Amussat JZ. Cited by DeVries PA and Pena A. Posterior Sagittal Anorectoplasty, 1982, J Pediatr Surg 1835;17:638-43.
19. Hendren WH. From an acorn to an Oak, J Pediat Surg. 34 Supplement; 1999;1:46-58.
20. Gandhi RK. Birth and Growth of Pediatric Surgery in India. Society for promotion of Pediatric Surgery, Mumbai.
21. Chatterjee SK, Sarangi BK, Ghosal SP. Congenital oesophageal atresia with oesophageo-tracheal fistula. Jr Indian Med Assoc 1966;47(2);75-76.
22. Pathak IC. Pouch colon syndrome: A changing scenario. Ann Natl Acad Sci (India) 1999;35(2):69-81.
23. Narasimhan KL, et al. A survey of the training, professional status and career opportunities of pediatric surgeons in the Indian context, J Indian Assoc Pediatric Surgeons 2000;5:3-9.

CHAPTER 3

Molecular Biology and the Pediatric Surgeon

Arun Chaudhury, M Srinivas

We are presently in the era of Molecular Medicine and for a busy Pediatric Surgeon it is difficult to be updated on molecular biology concepts and applications. For better understanding of the following text, it is imperative to understand the commonly used terms in Molecular Medicine. Therefore, the glossary given at the end of this chapter has commonly referred terms.

There are several pediatric surgical conditions where we encounter defects at the genetic and the molecular level. For example, duodenal atresia may be seen in Down's syndrome, which is one of the commonest chromosomal abnormality. There are numerous other situations, where study of molecular biology may enhance our basic understanding of the disease, structure diagnostic tests, and identify appropriate molecular therapeutic targets. The DNA for molecular diagnosis may be obtained from a variety of living tissues including peripheral and umbilical blood lymphocytes, epithelial cells lining the buccal mucosa, chorionic villus and amniotic fluid. The principal limitation in using these molecular techniques for diagnosis is the heterogeneity of genetic changes that underlie the inherited disorder.

The *gene* is the basic unit of heredity and contains the information for a particular *protein* and/or *RNA* (ribonucleic acid) molecule. This gene consists of a *continuous stretch of DNA* (deoxyribonucleic acid), which in turn forms part of a larger microscopically visible genetic unit associated with acidic and basic proteins, the *chromosome*. Even bacteria and virus require thousands of different genes and their products to carry out its biological function.

The term gene was first used by Danish geneticist Wilhelm Johannsen in 1911. Thomas Hunt Morgan predicted that these genes were carried on chromosomes. The three-dimensional structure of DNA was elucidated in 1953 in an exciting way by James Dewey Watson and Francis Harry Compton Crick in collaboration with Maurice Hugh Frederick Wilkins and Rosalind Franklin. They demonstrated (using X-ray diffraction studies) that DNA existed as a *double helix* consisting of 2 *polynucleotide* chains held together by hydrogen bonds. The key components of the DNA molecule with respect to its role as the carrier of transmissible information were the four *nitrogenous bases* which were the alphabets of heredity and reproduction - A, T, G, C - and it was the sequence of the bases along one of the two polynucleotide chains (the coding strand) that carried the information in the form of a *genetic code*, and was the essential blueprint of life.

The two complementary strands of the double helix are held together by specific number of hydrogen bonds (with low bond energy) between A-T and G-C (Table 3.1). The complementary nature of the two strands ensures that the information stored within a gene can be transmitted to the next generation by the process of DNA replication with complete fidelity.

Genes are the blueprints for all RNA and protein molecules within a cell. Some genes encode RNA as the final product (genes for r RNA, t RNA, sn RNA) whereas others encode polypeptide chains, which are synthesized by way of the intermediate m RNA. These blueprints may be modified by *mutation,* which alters the genetic information encoded by the gene through alteration of the base sequence of the DNA.

The genetic information stored within a gene is downloaded in a couple of sequential processes: *transcription,* whereby a linear portion of the gene is copied into a single-stranded RNA molecule, and

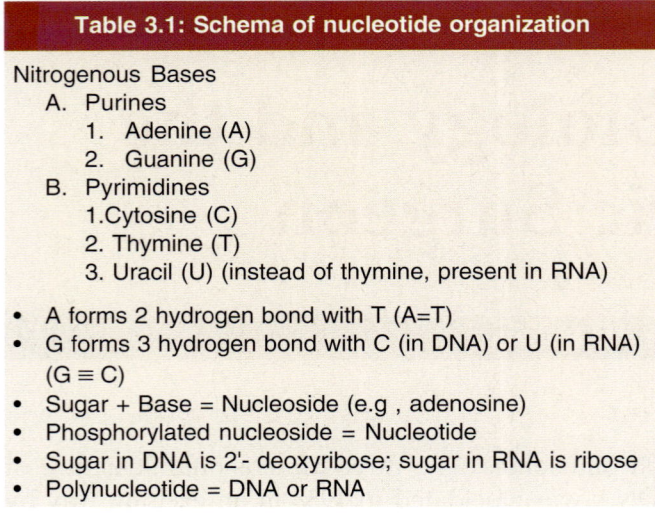

Table 3.1: Schema of nucleotide organization

Nitrogenous Bases
- A. Purines
  1. Adenine (A)
  2. Guanine (G)
- B. Pyrimidines
  1. Cytosine (C)
  2. Thymine (T)
  3. Uracil (U) (instead of thymine, present in RNA)

- A forms 2 hydrogen bond with T (A=T)
- G forms 3 hydrogen bond with C (in DNA) or U (in RNA) (G ≡ C)
- Sugar + Base = Nucleoside (e.g , adenosine)
- Phosphorylated nucleoside = Nucleotide
- Sugar in DNA is 2'- deoxyribose; sugar in RNA is ribose
- Polynucleotide = DNA or RNA

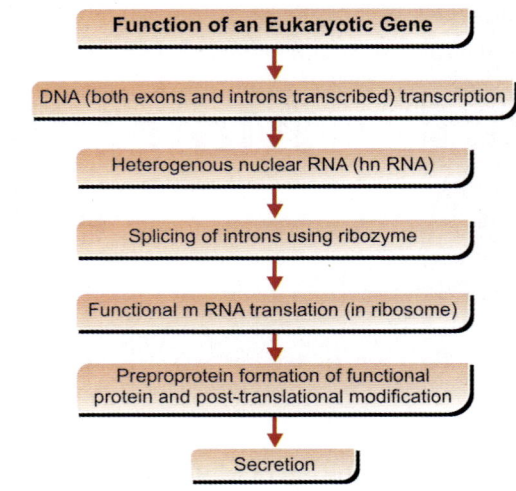

Fig. 3.2: Function of an eukaryotic gene

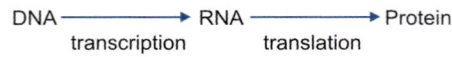

Fig. 3.1: Central dogma of molecular biology

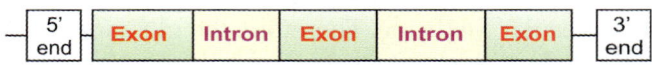

Fig. 3.3: Split gene in an eukaryote

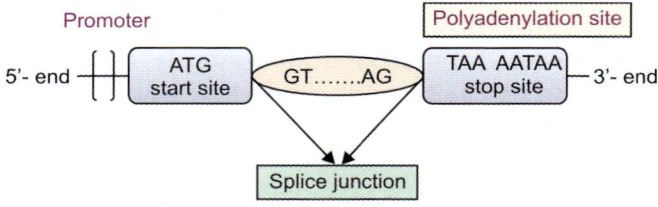

Fig. 3.4: Eukaryotic gene construct

translation of the information into a functional protein molecule (Fig. 3.1). At the ribosome the coded genetic message in m RNA is translated into an equivalent string of covalently linked amino acid, a polypeptide chain.

The flow of genetic information from DNA to RNA to protein is highly regulated in all cell types. The process of gene expression is highly regulated, thus ensuring that the cell does not spend excessive energy in synthesizing a gene product until that product is required by the cell.

With the advent of the DNA cloning technology, and DNA sequencing methodologies, scientists were ultimately able to unfold the organization of the gene to the level of the single base pair.

A typical eukaryotic gene (Fig. 3.2) consists of the coding region *(exon)* and the non-coding region *(intron or the selfish DNA)*. The coding region contains the genetic code that is read by the translational setup in the cytoplasm and is defined by the initiation codon (normally, AUG, codes for methionine, and GUG, codes for valine) and one or other of the three *termination codons (UAA, UGA and UAG)*. The nitrogenous sequences in introns appear to have no role in gene expression *per se* (Figs 3.3 and 3.4) and are discarded during the process of primary RNA transcript *(RNA splicing)*. In the 3 billion base pairs of the human genome, there are about 30,000 - 40,000 genes and the coding region is less than 5%. The number of genes may be just over twice the number in *Drosophila or Cenorhabditis*. The promoter region is required to promote the enzyme RNA polymerase to bind to the gene at the correct position with respect to the region that needs to be transcribed, i.e. the transcription unit.

Genes that encode polypeptides are generally present in one or two copies per haploid genome, that is they are single-copy genes, whereas genes encoding tRNA, rRNA and histones are often present in multiple copies to ensure that sufficient gene product is available to the cell.

As mentioned earlier, DNA is a linear polymer of 4 different building blocks (nucleotides) of which the variable parts are adenine(A), guanine(G), cytosine(C), thymine(T). Proteins are linear polymers of 20 different amino acids. The amino acid sequence of a protein must be encoded by the sequences of bases in the corresponding DNA. The four-letter alphabet of DNA is correlated with the 20 letter alphabet of amino acid by a 3-letter nonoverlapping code. Each consecutive triplet of bases in RNA is called a *codon*. The codon is unpunctuated and correct translation of a sequence depends on the starting at the right place so that the sequence is read in the correct reading frame. *tRNA* is the adaptor molecule - within its nucleotide sequence is a 3 nucleotide *anticodon* which binds to a particular codon and at its 3' end it carries the appropriate amino acid. The *aminoacyl t RNA synthetase* are responsible for attaching the correct amino acid to the corresponding t RNA. 61 of the 64 (4 to the power 3) codons correspond to an amino acid. AUG/GUG are chain initiating signals (start codon). Most amino acids (excepting methionine and tryptophan) are encoded by more than one triplet. This is called *degeneracy of the codon*. Synonymous codons defining the same amino acid differ only by the last base (wobble hypothesis). With few exceptions, the genetic code is universal and eukaryotic genes can be accurately transcribed in *Escherichia coli*. This forms the basis of recombinant DNA technology, resulting in a directed and predetermined alteration in the genotype of an organism.

An organism's characteristics are specified by its genetic information represented as a precise nucleic acid sequence, the sum total of this information being its *genome*. Genome organization is related to the functional demands placed upon it by the organism's biological characteristics. Definition of the complete nucleic acid sequence of an organism's genome is expected to identify its every gene product, their relative arrangements and organization, and the sequences required for controlled gene expression and replication, thus leading to a much greater understanding of the organism's biology.

The goal of genetics and molecular biology is to study the structure and function of genes and genomes. Although it is relatively easy to isolate DNA from living tissue, DNA in a test tube looks like a mass of mucus. How could it be possible to isolate a single gene from this tangled mass of DNA threads? Recombinant DNA technology provided us the technique for just doing that.

Gene isolation is important because it enables us to determine the nucleotide sequence and reflect on the internal landmarks (introns, etc), and also enable us to predict the function of the gene. For example, it was know from pedigree analysis that cystic fibrosis is inherited as an autosomal recessive disorder. However, the function of the gene product (CFTR) was known only after the gene was isolated and sequenced.

MAKING RECOMBINANT DNA

The basic procedure comprises of extracting and cutting DNA from a donor genome into fragments containing from one to several genes and allow these fragments to insert themselves individually into opened - up small autonomously replicating DNA molecules such as *plasmids*. These small circular DNA molecules act as carriers, or *vectors*, for the DNA fragments (Fig. 3.4). The vector molecules with their inserts are called *recombinant DNA* because they consist of unique combination of DNA from the donor genome (which can be from any organism) with vector DNA from a completely different source (bacterial plasmid or viruses). The recombinant DNA is then used to transform bacterial cells, and it is common for single vector molecule to find their way into individual bacterial cells. Bacterial cells are plated and allowed to grow into colonies. An individual transformed cell with a single recombinant vector will divide into a colony with millions of cells, all carrying the same recombinant vector. This colony containing a very large population of identical DNA inserts is called a DNA *clone*. Thus, cloning allows the amplification and recovery of a specific DNA segment from a large, complex DNA sample such as a genome. The clone with the specific gene of interest is isolated in bulk and subjected to analyses.

For cloning, the plasmid DNA can be isolated by the differential binding of ethidium bromide to the circular plasmid DNA, making it denser than the chromosomal DNA, and the plasmids form a distinct band on centrifugation in cesium chloride gradient and separated out, to be used as cloning vectors. Phage lambda can also be used as a vector for cloning.

All DNA molecules, from viral to human, have *restriction-enzyme target sites* purely by chance and may

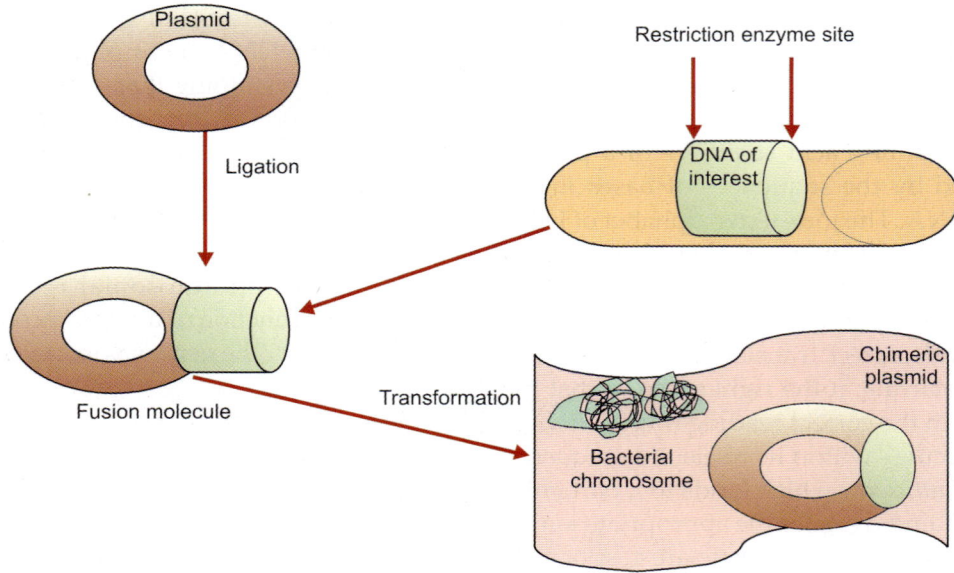

Fig. 3.5: Formation of a chimeric molecule of DNA

be cut into defined fragments of a size suitable for cloning. For example, the restriction enzyme Eco RI (obtained from *E coli*) can cut the following 6-nucleotide pair sequences in DNA of any organism:
5' - GAATTC - 3'
3' - CTTAAG - 5'

The segment is a DNA *palindrome* with similar sequences in antiparallel orientation (for, e.g. the statement - Madam , in Eden, I'm Adam - reads the same when read from either direction). This enzyme cleaves between G and A, leaving single stranded sticky ends with enhanced cohesiveness, which can from recombinant DNA.

The donor DNA and vector DNA after cleavage by restriction enzymes (and leaving sticky ends) are mixed in a test tube to form fusion DNA molecules. Once introduced into a bacterial cell, the *chimeric molecule* (Fig. 3.5) undergoes enormous proliferation (the plasmid has a replication origin) and the donor DNA is automatically replicated along with the vector.

Salient Characteristics of Vector

1. Small manipulable molecule
2. Prolific replication capacity
3. Possess restriction site.

For example - plasmid, phage lambda, cosmid, yeast artificial chromosome(YAC), bacterial artificial chromosome (BAC) (can carry 45 kb DNA insert). Special vectors called *expression vectors*, may detect a specific cloned gene, by detecting their protein products expressed in the bacterial cell.

The next step is collection of clones in a genomic library or a *c DNA (complementary DNA)* library. The advantage of c DNA is that it is made from m RNA using *reverse transcriptase* and is devoid of upstream and downstream regulatory sequences and introns. A genomic library is useful during cloning an entire genome.

Pulsed field gel electrophoresis (PFGE) may be used to construct a *chromosome specific library*. The library may further be probed using a DNA probe, which, when denatured, will complementarily bind to the single strand of the denatured library transferred onto a nitrocellulose membrane. The sequence of probe DNA can be made from several sources. The probe is usually labeled by radioactive agent or fluorescent dye and the signal subsequently detected.

Information about a gene's position in the genome may be used to bypass the tenacious work of assaying an entire library to find the clone of interest. *Positional cloning* is a term hat can be applied to any method that makes use of such an information. A common starting point is the availability of another cloned gene or other markers known to be closely linked to the gene being sought. The linked markers acts as the departure point in a process called *chromosome walking*, that will terminate at the target gene. Cloned DNA has several uses. They may be used as a probe, or can be used to find a specific nucleic acid in a mixture.

There are several ways of *fractionating* DNA (Figs 3.6 and 3.7, Table 3.2). The most extensively used method is gel electrophoresis. If a mixture of linear DNA molecules is placed in a well cut into an agarose gel and the well is placed near the cathode (negative electrode) of an electric field, the molecules will move through the gel to the anode (positive electrode) at speeds dependent on their size. If there are distinct size classes in the mixture, these classes will form distinct bands on the gel. The bands can be visualized by staining the DNA with ethidium bromide which causes the DNA to fluoresce in ultraviolet light. If bands are well separated, then purified bands can be cut from the gel and the purified DNA sample can be recovered from the gel matrix. Thus, DNA electrophoresis can be either diagnostic or preparative.

Polyacrylamide gels are most effective for separating small fragments of DNA (5-500 bp), and they can resolve DNA fragments that differ in size by 1 bp. Agarose gels have a lower resolving power but a greater range of separation (200 bp - 50 kbp).

Detecting specific nucleic acid sequence uses a technique called *hybridization*. After electrophoresis, the gel is placed in buffer and covered by a nitrocellulose filter and a stack of paper towels. The fragments are denatured to single strands so that they can stick to filter. They are carried to the filter by the buffer. The filter is then removed and incubated with

Table 3.2: Analytical blot transfer techniques

Blot technique	Molecule analyzed	Fractionation	Detection
Southern	DNA	electrophoresis	Nucleic acid hybridization
Northern	RNA	electrophoresis	Nucleic acid hybridization
Western	Protein	electrophoresis	Immunoblot method using antibody

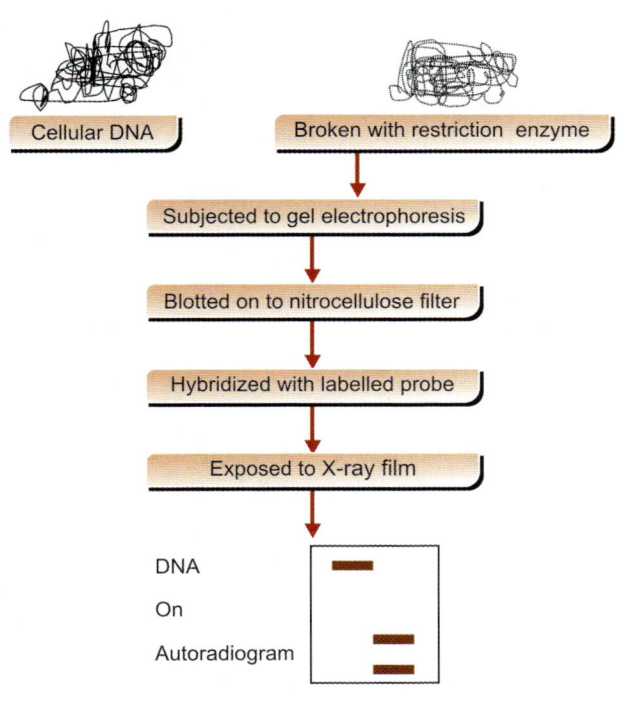

Fig. 3.6: Southern Blotting

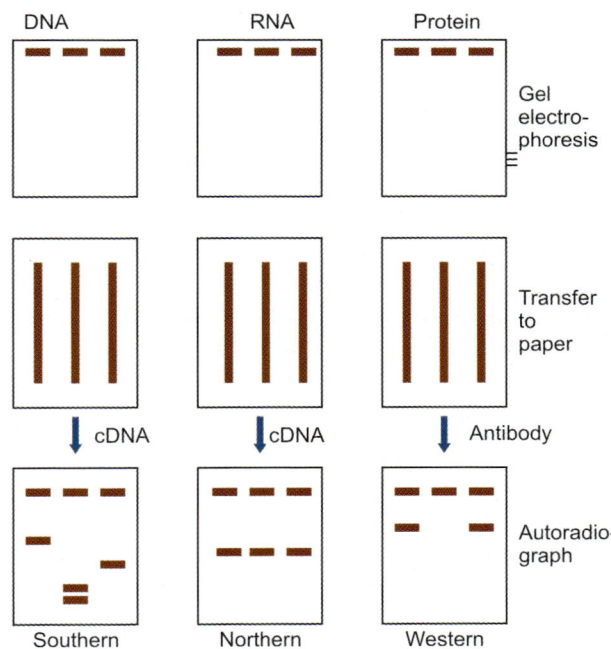

Fig. 3.7: Blot transfer techniques

a radioactively labelled single stranded probe that is complementary to the targeted sequence. Unbound probe is washed away, and X-ray film is exposed to the filter. Because the radioactive probe has hybridized only with its complementary restriction fragments, the film will be exposed only in bands corresponding to those fragments. Comparison of these bands with labelled markers revels the number and size of the fragments in which the targeted sequences are found. This procedure is called *Southern blotting* (Fig. 3.6) named after E M Southern, when DNA is transferred to the nitrocellulose paper and *Northern blotting* when RNA is transferred (Fig. 3.7).

A parallel technique called *Western blotting* has been developed to transfer electrophoretically fractionated protein from a gel and then to visualize with antibodies (polyclonal, prepared from animals, or monoclonal, prepared by *hybridoma technology*). Proteins can be separated based on molecular weight by technique of SDS - PAGE (*polyacrylamide gel electrophoresis*). SDS (sodium dodecyl sulfate) coats the protein, gives them a negative charge, and facilitates migration in an electric field. The proteins are denatured in the presence of SDS and the migration is made smooth. After electrophoresis, the specimen is detected by staining with silver, Sypro Ruby or Coomassie blue, or by performing Western blotting (Western blot increases the preciseness of detection).

Further analysis after cloning is to characterize the structure and function of that gene. The *DNA sequencing* now most commonly used was developed by Fred Sanger (Fig. 3.8). His method is based on DNA synthesis in the presence of dideoxynucleotides, which differs from normal deoxynucleotides in that they lack a 3' - OH group. The dideoxynucleotide triphosphates (ddNTPs) can be incorporated into a growing chain, but when incorporated, they terminate synthesis because they lack the 3'-OH group necessary to bind to the next nucleotide triphosphate. Each of the four reaction tube is prepared with single stranded DNA template for the sequence of intent, DNA polymerase and primers. Each tube receives different ddNTP, and 4 normal d NTP. In any given tube, various truncated chain lengths will be produced, each corresponding to the point of insertion of dd NTP. These lengths are in turn clear indications of where the bases complementary to the dd NTPs are in the template strand. The fragments can be visualized by electrophoresis of the 4 samples in 4 lanes on an acrylamide gel, where the fragments form bands. The base sequence can be determined by scanning up the gel, encompassing all four lanes, and recording which ever base occupies the terminus in the next band. Instead of radioactive labels, fluorescent dyes can be tagged to the oligonucleotide probes and automated sequencing performed. The data is fed into computers, and based on the *open reading frames (ORFs)*, the prospective candidate genes are predicted.

Newer advances like reverse genetics (gene knockout) and organism containing introduced foreign DNA (transgenics) will provide wonderful tools for research at baseline levels. The latest excitement is genomics: Structural Genomics, characterizing the physical nature of the whole Genome and Functional Genomics, characterizing the transcriptosome (the entire range of transcripts produced by an organism) and the proteome (the entire array of encoded proteins).

Now, how do we analyze small amounts of DNA sample? Polymerase chain reaction provides for the amplification of this sample and facilitates its analysis by techniques elucidated in this chapter. The *polymerase chain reaction (PCR)*, the repetitive bi-directional DNA synthesis via primer extension of a

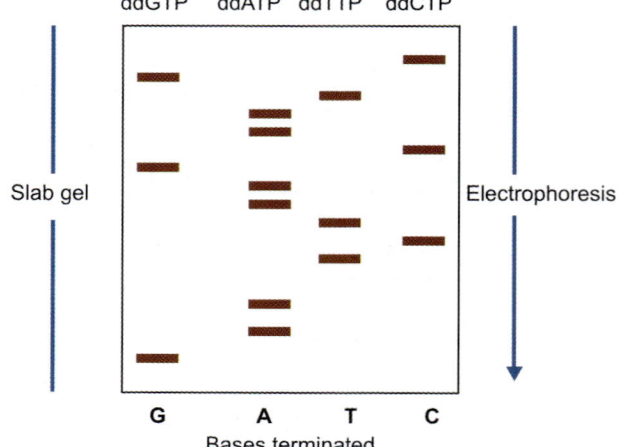

Fig. 3.8: Sequencing of DNA by Sanger's method

Read the sequence of original strand as follows:

* - GAATCTTAAGCAATGC –3'

The sequence of the other strand will follow from the base pairing rules (A-T, G-C) of Watson and Crick:
CTTAGAATTCGTTACG

region of nucleic acid, is simple in design and has revolutionized molecular biology. After 25 cycles, there is a 10 (5) fold increase in DNA. PCR amplification of a template requires two oligo-nucleotide primers, the four dNTPs, Mg^{++} ion in molar excess of dNTPs, and a thermostable DNA polymerase to perform DNA synthesis. The reaction samples are usually between 20 and 100 microliters.

There are 3 distinct steps of PCR cycle (Fig. 3.9):

a. *Denaturation of template:* Reaction is heated to 92 - 96 degree Celsius. The time required usually depends on complexity, thermal cycler, geometry of tube and the volume of reaction.

b. *Primer annealing:* After denaturation, the oligonucleotide primers hybridize to their complementary single stranded sequences. The temperature of this step varies between 37-65 degree celsius, depending on the homology of the primers for the target sequence as well as the base composition of the oligonucleotide. Primers are present at a significantly higher concentration than the target DNA, and are shorter in length; as a result, they hybridize to their complementary sequences at an annealing rate much faster than the target DNA duplex can reanneal. Optimizatioin of annealing temperature begins with the calculation of Tm value of the primer-template pairs

$$Tm = 4(G+C) + 2(A+T)$$

c. *DNA synthesis by a thermostable DNA polymerase*: This is carried out at 72 degrees Celsius. Thermostable Taq polymerase is often used for this step. The time required to copy the template fully depends on the length of the PCR product.

Because of the nature of the PCR it is critical that the only DNA that enters the reaction is the template added by the investigator. Thus, PCR must be performed in a DNA free, clean environment. DNA generated by previous amplification of the same target sequence can cause carryover contamination and adequate precaution should be taken about this to avoid false positive results. An ideal PCR would have high specificity, fidelity and yield.

Virtually all forms of DNA and RNA are suitable substrates for PCR. They include genomic, plasmid, and phage DNA, previously amplified DNA, c DNA, and m RNA. Typically, 0.1-1 microgram of mammalian genomic DNA is utilized per PCR. Samples prepared

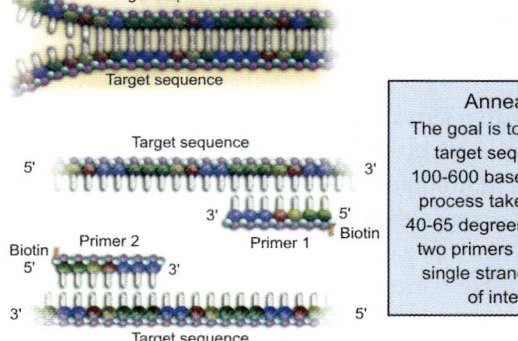

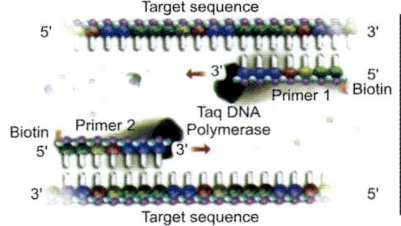

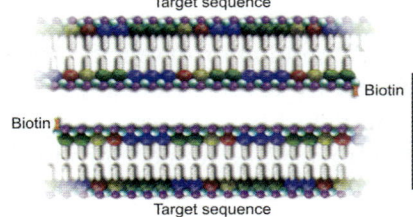

No. of cycles of PCR	Copies of target
1	2
2	4
3	8
4	16
5	32
6	64
20	1048576
30	1073741824

Fig. 3.9: Steps of PCR

by standard molecular methodologies are sufficiently pure for PCR. Now, *rapid isolation of DNA* may be done from whole blood spot, whole blood, and whole tissue with the aid of *Genereleaser*. The suspension is composed of 20% suspension of an activated hydrophilic proprietary polymer in aqueous 0.01 M Tris-HCl, 0.05 M KCl, 10% DMSO, pH 7.4-7.6. The hydrophilic polymer aids in cell disruption and serves as a nucleation site for precipitation and absorption of proteins.

PCR can also simultaneously amplify multiple loci in the human dystrophin gene. *Multiplex PCR* has been widely used in linkage analysis, template quantitation, and genetic disease diagnosis.

After performing PCR, the PCR product may be detected using agarose gel electrophoresis. The appearance of a discrete band of the correct size suggests a successful reaction. Following PCR, a portion of the reaction is subjected to digestion with the appropriate restriction enzyme and electrophoresed to detect the DNA fragments of the predicted size. An oligonucleotide probe that hybridizes to the template and is located between the two primers employed in PCR may be used to detect the PCR product. This probe can be used to detect the PCR product after transfer to a solid support (Southern Blotting). Other approaches to the detection of PCR product include systems using a nonradioactive ELISA - based format.

The amplification and quantitation of specific RNA species can be performed by reverse transcriptase - PCR *(RT-PCR)*. This can detect or measure a defined RNA species, ranging from m RNAs for gene products to levels of viral RNA in plasma (e.g. hepatitis C virus, HIV, etc). Quality RNA template is converted to complementary DNA using RT, which is then subjected to PCR. This method can also be used for studying gene expression.

Single nucleotide polymorphism (SNP) is the commonest type of polymorphism in the genome where variation is at only one nucleotide. It is detected by PCR using a common primer at one end and a variable primer at the other end, 3' end of which anneals to the polymorphic base. Depending on the base at that position, only one of the variable primers will successfully amplify the locus and determine the base at that position. Using fluorescent probes and *Real Time PCR,* SNPs can be detected during PCR without running a gel. Once the linkage between a particular polymorphism with a disease or phenotype is established, it can be used as an inexpensive way of determining susceptibility to the disease and predict the probability of the disease in the offspring arising from a given match. The DNA obtained from polar body, blastomere or blastocyst biopsy during preimplantation diagnosis may be studied by PCR, gene sequencing or *in situ* hybridization, or the protein and enzymes identified and assayed.

PCR (polymerase chain reaction) has gained much importance in diagnostics. This highly sensitive molecular technique permits amplification of DNA without cloning that can be analyzed for gene alteration by techniques such as single stranded conformation polymorphism, denaturing gradient gel electrophoresis, etc. For example, *single stranded conformation polymorphism (SSCP)* have been used to detect genetic defects in sodium channels and resultant prolonged QT interval in sudden infant death syndrome (SIDS).

PCR and *fluorescence in situ hybridization (FISH)* have surpassed other non-isotopic *in situ* hybridization techniques *(NISH)* and have proved to be very powerful in the detection of genetic alterations. Oligonucleotide-primed *in situ* DNA synthesis (PRINS), an alternative procedure to conventional *in situ* hybridization, and direct incorporation of labelled nucleotides by PCR greatly improve the detection of small DNA probes, thus rendering a high sensitivity to these procedures.

FISH have been particularly useful in identifying microdeletions. For example, FISH has been used to diagnose Prader-Willi syndrome/Angelman syndrome, Miller-Deiker syndrome, etc. It is a precise technique for localization of single sequences within metaphase chromosome. The contrast enhancement of diaminophenylindole (DAPI) banded chromosome images permit the direct visualization of fluorescent signal on G-like bands. A variety of cDNA or genomic probe is used for the purpose. Some tissues, like amniotic fluid cells, chorionic villus and fetal blood are particularly refractile to hypotonic treatment, colcemid arrest, and yield chromosomes of unsatisfactory morphology. So, *interphase FISH* can be used to study these cells, especially for facilitating prenatal diagnosis. Interphase FISH has also been used to study minimal residual disease in cancer patients, diagnosis and prognostication of cancer, and assessment of radiation induced damage. FISH can also detect the microdeletions in chromosome 22 in velocardiofacial syndrome.

Multiplex FISH uses digital images acquired separately for each fluorochrome using a charged couple device camera and analysed using an image analysis software. FISH can also be used to detect nuclear RNA. *Spectral karyotyping (SKY)* can be used for precise identification of chromosomes involved in complex arrangements. Digital fluorescence ratio (FR) may be used to quantify and discriminate fluorescent probes. *Comparative genomic hybridization (CGH)* is an analytical technique based on FISH and FR measurements that allow us to compare cytogenetically the entire genome of malignant and normal cells, as well as to assess gain and loss of DNA in tumor cells.

There are several other upcoming techniques in molecular biology which have broadened our horizon. *Denaturing high performance liquid chromatography (DHPLC)* can detect single nucleotide substitutions, small deletions, insertions, genotyping, LOH determination and gene expression analysis. *Serial analysis of gene expression (SAGE)* is a computer based technique for analysis of gene expression, and may be useful in studying the gene products of many tumors, including pancreatic cancer. There are several other techniques for detecting known and unknown mutations, which are helpful in academic and diagnostic purpose.

DNA chips have revolutionized genetics in the same way that semiconductor chips have revolutionized the information industry a few years back. DNA chips are samples of DNA laid out in regimented arrays bound to a glass chip the size of a microscope cover slip. Robotic machines with multiple printing tips resembling miniature fountain pen nibs deliver microscopic droplets of DNA solution to specific positions (addresses) on the chip. The DNA is dried and treated so that it will bind to the glass. Thousands of samples can be applied to one chip. The arrays of DNA are known cDNAs from different genes. For probing, fluorescent label is used, and the binding of probe molecules to the glass chip is optically monitored automatically by laser beams.

DNA chips can also be used to detect mutation. With the complete DNA sequence of human genome in hand, it will be possible to survey the expression links of all gene products during the formation and progression of a particular type of tumor. This systemic information will be a source of much greater insight into the panorama of gene expression disturbances that characterize the malignant state. Further, these microarrays can be utilized to study the expression of various genes during development, and may provide useful insights into the aberrations of development.

Conventional cytogenetics and karyotyping have helped us in understanding the genotypic makeup in several situations including ambiguous genitalia. For example, 46 XY pattern is seen in male pseudohermaphrodite and 46 XX is seen in congenital adrenal hyperplasia in more than 80% of cases. 46 XY pattern with mosaicism, 45 XO/XXO is seen in mixed gonadal dysgenesis and dysgenetic male pseudohermaphroditism. Molecular biology has taken us one step ahead - it has given us insight into the chaos in function at the cellular level. The molecular techniques will be powerful as diagnostic tool, and provide insights into possible therapeutic targets for a wide range of diseases. A protocol for identifications of mutations is given in Table 3.3 and an algorithm for analysis of genetic diseases is given in Figure 3.10. Most common Pediatric surgical conditions having genetic abnormality have been enumerated in Table 3.4.

Table 3.3: Identification of mutations

I. Direct Methods

A. Detecting known mutations
1. Base sequence specificity of restriction endonucleases
2. Oligonucleotide hybridization
3. Amplification refractory mutation system (ARMS) (useful for detecting point mutation as in thalassemia and sickle cell anemia)
4. Detection of deletion using multiplex PCR
5. Southern blot and PCR based methods for detecting triplet expansion as in fragile X syndrome, myotonic dystrophy.

B. Detecting unknown mutation
1. Single stranded conformation polymorphism (SSCP)
2. Heteroduplex analysis
3. Denaturing gradient gel electrophoresis (DGGE)
4. Chemical and Enzymatic Mismatch Cleavage (CCM)
5. Protein Truncation Test (PTT)
6. Denaturing high performance liquid chromatography (DHPLC)

II. Indirect Methods

Linkage analysis
1. RFLP (Restriction fragment length polymorphism)
2. VNTR (Variable number tandem repeat)

Table 3.4: Most common pediatric surgical conditions along with the genetic abnormality

Disease / Syndrome	Abnormality	Remarks
Wilms' tumor	WT1 WT2 WT3	WT1 : 11p13, WT2 : 11p15, WT3 : 16q
	Familial Wilms' tumor loci FWT1 and FWT2[2]	Loss or inactivation of tumor suppressor gene at 11p13[1]
	Mutations of p53 implicated for anaplastic variant, drug resistance[5]	WT2 gene maps to 11p15 in the region of Beckwith - Wiedemann locus.
		WT1 is also expressed in fetal gonad and it can lead to genitourinary malformations[3]
		Loss of chromosome 22 identifies high risk for Wilms' tumor[4]
WAGR [Wilms' tumor, aniridia, genitourinary malformations, mental retardation]	AN gene on chromosome 11p13[6]	
Neuroblastoma	Amplification of MYCN oncogene ? 1p36.1-2, 1p32-34, 1p36.3[7]	
Hepatoblastoma	Trisomy 2 , Trisomy 20[8] P27/KIP 1 gene expression[9]	
Rhabdomyosarcoma	Embryonal type: Allelic loss at chromosome 11p 15.5 Alveolar type: Chromosomal translocations: 2;13, 1;13[10]	
Congenital anomalies of urinary tract	? Angiotensin type 2 receptor gene on X chromosome[11]	
Vesicoureteric reflux	Genetic heterogeneity at chromosome 1[12]	
Cryptorchidism	? Insulin 3 gene (INSL3) in mice[13]	No evidence in human beings
Extrahepatic biliary atresia	Jagged 1 gene (JAG1)[14]	
Orofacial cleft	? Clefting gene 2q11.1-q13.2[15]	
Craniosynostosis syndromes	Fibroblast growth factor receptor 2 gene (FGFR2)[16] 7p21 deletions[17]	
Pyloric stenosis	Partial trisomy: 9q22.1-q31.1[18]	
Duodenal atresia	Down's syndrome	25% association
Congenital diaphragmatic hernia	Deletion 15q24-26[19]	
Anorectal malformations	Mutations of sonic hedgehog (Shh) in mice[20]	
Currarino syndrome (ARM, presacral mass, urogenital malformations)	HLXB9 geneautosomal dominant sacral agenesis[21]	
Omphalocele	? Autosomal dominant transmission[22]	
Hirschsprung's disease	Deletion in chromosome 13q Homozygous mutations in Endothelin B receptor gene (EDNRB) on 13q22.[23] RET proto oncogene mutations[24]	

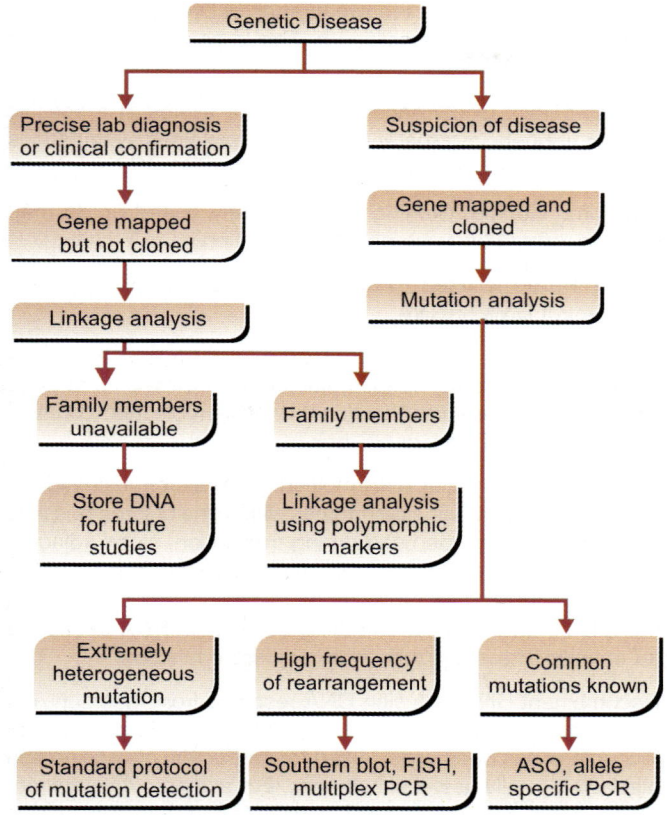

Fig. 3.10: Algorithm for approach to a genetic disease

The need for dedication at bedside, appropriate observation, analysis and holistic approach to patient care has no alternative in practice of medicine. There are several diseases including cancer, autoimmune diseases and congenital malformation, whose pathogenesis and evolution are still in the grey zone. Basic medical research has enormous prospects in finding the molecular aspects and the cellular susceptibility to such conditions. However, in a country like India, the tools of biotechnology may be directed at present for improving food supplies, development of basic vaccines and diagnostic agents for infectious diseases. Also, the heterogeneous population of India is a big genetic laboratory in itself. Thus, the need for integration of the concepts of molecular biology in surgical sciences is justified.

GLOSSARY

Allele: One of the two alternative forms of a DNA sequence, each one inherited from father and mother.

Autosome: Chromosomes not involved with sex differentiation. In human beings, chromosomes numbering from 1 - 22.

Anticodon: A trinucleotide sequence on a transfer RNA which is complementary to codon that is present on messenger RNA.

Base pairing: The bond between adenine and thymine or guanine and cytosine of a double stranded DNA.

Bacteriophage : Virus that infects a bacteria.

Clone: Colony of cells descended from a single ancestral cell. In a noun sense it means — a population of recombinant DNA molecules all of them carrying the same inserted genetic code. To clone (as a verb) means to use *in vitro* recombination techniques to insert a particular gene or other DNA sequence into a vector molecule.

Cloning vector: It is used to carry foreign DNA molecule.

Coding sequence: Portion of a DNA that specifies a particular amino acid sequence, many of such would result in a particular protein.

Codon: A triplet of nucleotides in messenger RNA that specifies a particular amino acid. Each protein would have a specific ladder of amino acids.

Complementary: Each strand of the human DNA is said to be complementary to the another strand of DNA as it is base paired with hydrogen bonds.

Complementary DNA: DNA complement of an RNA sequence. This is synthesized by the enzyme RNA-primed DNA polymerase of reverse transcriptase. The single stranded DNA product of this enzyme may be converted into the double stranded form by DNA-primed DNA polymerase and inserted into a suitable vector to make a complementary DNA clone.

DNA finger printing: This is a method to generate a pattern of DNA restriction fragments that are unique to an individual. DNA from blood, semen etc is isolated and fragmented with enzyme - restriction endonuclease. That is further separated and documented by gel electrophoresis. Fragments of a specific nucleotide sequence are detected by hybridization with an appropriate DNA probe to produce the unique pattern.

DNA polymerase: This enzyme synthesizes DNA by copying a template strand.

DNA topoisomerase: This enzyme alters DNA by change in the supercoiling of double stranded DNA. In single stranded DNA it is capable of converting it to rings or knots.

Electrophoresis: A technique that separates DNA/RNA/protein based on ionic solute's differential migration after application of electric field.

Endonuclease: Enzymes that cleave nucleic acids at specific positions within the chain.

Euchromatin: Lightly staining regions of chromosomes that contain less condensed chromatin.

Exon: Expressed region of a gene. This encodes a protein as opposed to intron.

Fluorescence *in situ* hybridization (FISH): A method to label DNA probes for *in situ* hybridization utilizing non-isotropic fluorochrome.

Gene: A segment of DNA invlolved in a specific RNA molecule or a specific protein.

Heterochromatin: Condensed chromatin in certain chromosome regions that do not contain actively tanscribed genes.

Heterozygote: Individual with two different alleles (genes) at a single locus.

Histones: Proteins found in the nuclei of all eukaryotic cells where they are complexed to DNA. These may act as a non-specific repressors of gene transcription.

Homologus chromosome: Chromosomes that pair with each other. They contain most of the same genes from a common ancestor.

Homozygote: An individual with two identical alleles (genes) at a single locus.

Hybridization: Annealing of a labelled nucleic acid probe to DNA or RNA for detecting the particular nucleic acid sequence.

Intron: Part of the gene that is not represented in the protein product. This means intron sequences are transcribed into RNA and then excised - intron splicing - before translation of RNA to protein.

Karyotype: Chromosomal number, size and morphology etc detected by light microscopy by stains.

Linkage: Tendency to inherit together two or more nonallelic genes or DNA markers than is to be expected by independent assortment. Genes/DNA markers are linked because they are sufficiently close to each other on the same chromosome.

Microarray: Chip technology for profiling of function of many genes or for screening for multiple genetic abnormalities.

Mutation: Change in the nucleotide sequence or arrangement of DNA

Northern blot: A method for studying RNA; RNA is transferred from an agarose gel to a nitrocellulose filter, on which the RNA can be detected using a specific probe.

Operon: Set of coordinately controlled genes adjacent to one another in the genome.

Palindrome: The sequence of double stranded DNA that is the same when read in opposite direction; e.g, "NURSES RUN"

Plasmid: Small circular DNA present outside the chromosome and replicates independent of the host DNA; responsible for conferring antibiotic resistance in bacteria; is used extensively as a vector in recombinant DNA technology.

Polymerase chain reaction: This discovery by Kary Mullis has opened several new vistas. This utilizes thermostable enzymes for repeated copying of the two strands of DNA (of a particular gene) and ultimately amplifies it. The large amount makes it easy for analysis of the DNA.

Polymorphism: Occurrence of 2 or more alleles at a specific locus in frequencies greater than can be explained by mutations alone; polymorphisms are common in introns.

Positional cloning: Cloning a gene purely based on its map position without knowing about the function

Probe: Probe is used to detect the presence of a specific fragment of DNA or RNA.

Promoter: Site located upstream of gene where RNA polymerase II and transcription factors assemble so that gene can be transcribed into functional m RNA molecule; contains TATA box, CAAT box, or GC box.

Reading frame: In a m RNA molecule, the exact nucleotide at which translation begins determines which one of three possible reading frames will be used during translation, since adjacent groups of three nucleotides are passed by the translation of machinery. Insertions or deletions of nucleotides that are not multiples of three shift the reading frame of m RNA to encode an entirely different protein with a different function.

Recombinant DNA: A fusion DNA resulting from insertion of a sequence of nucleotides into a separate molecule of DNA; the technology has been widely used for production of vaccine and other biologically useful substances. For example recombinant collagen is now being used as Vasostat to seal bleeding vessels and thus perform sutureless surgery.

Restriction enzyme: A bacterial endonuclease which cleaves both strands of DNA at very specific sites of the base sequence (4-10 base pairs).

sn RNA: Small nuclear RNA.

Southern blot: Used for detection of DNA.

Splicing: The removal of introns from RNA followed by the ligation of the exons; splicing involves some RNA molecules which act as enzymes(ribozymes).

StIcky ended DNA: Complementary single strands with high affinity for each other.

Transcription: DNA -directed synthesis of RNA using RNA polymerase enzyme.

Transgenic: Introduction of new DNA into germ cells by direct injection into the nucleus of ovum.

Translation: Synthesis of protein on a m RNA template.

Transposon: Mobile DNA sequences that jump from one place in the genome to another, e.g. Alu and LINE - 1 sequences. Transposable elements affect the genetic variability.

Vector: A plasmid or bacteriophage in which foreign DNA can be introduced for cloning.

Western blot: An immunoblot transfer technique for detecting protein.

REFERENCES

1. Tay JS. Molecular genetics of Wilms' tumour. J Paediatr Child Health 1995;31(5):379-83.
2. Dome JS, Coppes MJ. Recent advances in Wilms tumor genetics. Curr Opin Pediatr 2002;14(1):5-11.
3. Nordenskjold A, Friedman E, Tapper-Persson M, Soderhall C, Leviav A.
4. Svensson J, Anvret M. Screening for mutations in candidate genes for hypospadias. Urol Res 1999;27(1):49-55.
5. Bown N, Cotterill SJ, Roberts P, Griffiths M, Larkins S, Hibbert S, Middleton H, Kelsey A, Tritton D, Mitchell C. Cytogenetic abnormalities and clinical outcome in Wilms tumor: A study by the UK cancer cytogenetics group and the UK. Children's Cancer Study Group. Med Pediatr Oncol 2002 Jan;38(1):11-21.
6. Brownlee NA, Hazen-Martin DJ, Garvin AJ, Re GG. Functional and gene expression analysis of the p53 signaling pathway in clear cell sarcoma of the kidney and congenital mesoblastic nephroma. Pediatr Dev Pathol 2002;5(3):257-68.
7. Drechsler M, Meijers-Heijboer EJ, Schneider S, Schurich B, Grond-Ginsbach C, Tariverdian G, Kantner G, Blankenagel A, Kaps D, Schroeder-Kurth T, et al. Molecular analysis of aniridia patients for deletions involving the Wilms' tumor gene. Hum Genet 1994;94(4):331-38.
8. Hiyama E, Hiyama K, Ohtsu K, Yamaoka H, Fukuba I, Matsuura Y, Yokoyama T. Biological characteristics of neuroblastoma with partial deletion in the short arm of chromosome 1. Med Pediatr Oncol 2001;36(1):67-74.
9. Hu J, Wills M, Baker BA, Perlman EJ. Comparative genomic hybridization analysis of hepatoblastomas. Genes Chromosomes Cancer 2000;27(2):196-201.
10. Brotto M, Finegold MJ. Distinct patterns of p27/KIP 1 gene expression in hepatoblastoma and prognostic implications with correlation before and after chemotherapy. Hum Pathol 2002;33(2):198-205.
11. Xia SJ, Pressey JG, Barr FG. Molecular pathogenesis of rhabdomyosarcoma. Cancer Biol Ther 2002;1(2):97-104.
12. Hiraoka M, Taniguchi T, Nakai H, Kino M, Okada Y, Tanizawa A, Tsukahara H, Ohshima Y, Muramatsu I, Mayumi M. No evidence for AT2R gene derangement in human urinary tract anomalies. Kidney Int 2001;59(4):1244-49.
13. Baker LA, Nef S, Nguyen MT, Stapleton R, Pohl H, Parada LF. The insulin-3 gene: lack of a genetic basis for human cryptorchidism. J Urol 2002;167(6):2534-37.
14. Kohsaka T, Yuan ZR, Guo SX, Tagawa M, Nakamura A, Nakano M, Kawasasaki H, Inomata Y, Tanaka K, Miyauchi J. The significance of human jagged 1 mutations detected in severe cases of extrahepatic biliary atresia. Hepatology 2002;36(4):904-12.
15. Riegel M, Schinzel A. Duplication of (2)(q11.1-q13.2) in a boy with mental retardation and cleft lip and palate: Another clefting gene locus on proximal 2q? Am J Med Genet 2002;111(1):76-80.
16. Wong LJ, Chen TJ, Dai P, Bird L, Muenke M. Novel SNP at the common primer site of exon IIIa of FGFR2 gene causes error in molecular diagnosis of craniosynostosis syndrome. Am J Med Genet 2001;102(3):282-85.
17. Gripp KW, Kasparcova V, McDonald-McGinn DM, Bhatt S, Bartlett SP, Storm AL, Drumheller TC, Emanuel BS, Zackai EH, Stolle CA. A diagnostic approach to identifying submicroscopic 7p21 deletions in Saethre-Chotzen syndrome: fluorescence *in situ* hybridization and dosage-sensitive Southern blot analysis. Genet Med 2001;3(2):102-08.
18. Heller A, Seidel J, Hubler A, Starke H, Beensen V, Senger G, Rocchi M, Wirth J, Chudoba I, Claussen U, Liehr T. Molecular cytogenetic characterisation of partial trisomy 9q in a case with pyloric stenosis and a review. J Med Genet. 2000;37(7):529-32.
19. Schlembach D, Zenker M, Trautmann U, Ulmer R, Beinder E. Deletion 15q24-26 in prenatally detected diaphragmatic hernia: increasing evidence of a candidate region for diaphragmatic development. Prenat Diagn 2001;21(4):289-92.
20. Mo R, Kim JH, Zhang J, Chiang C, Hui CC, Kim PC. Anorectal malformations caused by defects in sonic hedgehog signaling. Am J Pathol 2001;159(2):765-74.
21. Lynch SA, Wang Y, Strachan T, Burn J, Lindsay S. Autosomal dominant sacral agenesis: Currarino syndrome. J Med Genet 2000;37(8):561-66.
22. Kanagawa SL, Begleiter ML, Ostlie DJ, Holcomb G, Drake W, Butler MG. Omphalocele in three generations with autosomal dominant transmission. J Med Genet 2002;39(3):184-85.
23. Shanske A, Ferreira JC, Leonard JC, Fuller P, Marion RW. Hirschsprung's disease in an infant with a contiguous gene syndrome of chromosome 13. Am J Med Genet 2001;102(3):231-36.
24. Pasini B, Rossi R, Ambrosio MR, Zatelli MC, Gullo M, Gobbo M, Collini P, Aiello A, Pansini G, Trasforini G, degli Uberti EC. RET mutation profile and variable clinical manifestations in a family with multiple endocrine neoplasia type 2A and Hirschsprung's disease. Surgery 2002;131(4):373-81.

Growth and Development in Pediatric Surgical Practice

KN Agarwal, DK Agarwal

Growth is observed in measurable units postnatally as increase in length/height, skull circumference and weight. It stretches from:

a. Conception— intrauterine growth period to infancy (Most rapid growth period— >70% of total human brain growth is completed),
b. Followed by a long phase of slow juvenile growth, and
c. Finally by 10-12 years in girls and 12-15 years in boys there is initiation of puberty – adolescent growth spurt lasting for 2.5-3.0 years (in this phase girls gain 25-26 cm and boys 28-30 cm in height).

TOOLS FOR ASSESSMENT OF GROWTH AND NUTRITIONAL STATUS

Intrauterine Assessment

Ninth week of gestation onward growth is measured as crown-rump and crown-heel length, later as biparietal and occipitoparietal measurements of skull using ultrasonography.

Infancy–Childhood—Adolescence

Anthropometric tools can be used not only for *growth monitoring* but also for nutritional status assessment. It is the repeated measurement only that can give the clue on assessment of growth. For minimizing errors measurements should be taken preferably by the trained workers; using accurate techniques and standardized instruments. The knowledge of *exact age* is very essential to evaluate growth in a child. The measurements used for growth monitoring are, skull circumference, height and weight.

For assessment of *nutritional status* midarm circumference is another good measurement. Skin fold thickness is useful in assessment of thinness and obesity in later years of childhood, particularly adolescence. In this age group to diagnose overweight/obesity and thinness the internationally used index is BMI weight kg/height meter.

Head Circumference

A very important growth measure, it *enlarges* rapidly in hydrocephalus/raised intracranial tension. *Small head* size with little gain in circumference with palpable ridge on suture(s) could be diagnostic of craniostenosis.

In infants and small children it can be measured in the lap of the mother/caretaker. On older children it can be measured with head in Frankfort plane (see measurement of height) with arms relaxed and legs apart. A *fiber glass tape (nonstrechable)* is passed over the occipital protuberance of the head at the back and most anterior protuberance at the front, tightly so as to compress the hair. Some recommend that tape be passed over glabella in front and occiput at the back. The objective is to record maximum of the head circumference. Measure twice to ensure the correct reading.

Stature (Length/height)

In children below 2 years of age recumbent length on an *infantometer* be accurately measured by two persons. Infantometer has an horizontal board with scale markings; two side perpendicular boards of which one is sliding allows child in lying position (Supine), with child's knees extended firmly and feet are flexed at right angles to the lower legs for proper measurement (accuracy 0.1 cm). The upright sliding feet sideboard is moved to closely touch the heels (without shoe and shock) and length is recorded. Height is measured (For children above 2 years of age), on a vertical-measuring rod called *anthropometric rod*, it has a flat small horizontal arm to be fixed on head for exact measurement.

Weight

The child should be weighed in minimal (Standard weight) clothing. The weighing scale should be checked for zero error each time the subject is weighed. Placing known weight everyday can check it. The weighing scales used commonly are (i) beam balance, (ii) spring balance and (iii) electronic scale. The beam balances are more sturdy, but heavy to carry. The lighter spring balances are easy to carry but likely to give fallacious reading, due to elasticity of spring, if proper care is not taken in its maintenance. Electronic weighing scale gives reading upto 10 gm, but it should also be tested before use against a known weight.

There are beam-weighing scales with fitted anthropometric rod. Child with standard minimum clothing without shoe and shocks stands with feet parallel on the even flat platform, stretching upward to the fullest, arms hanging on the sides; buttocks and heels touching against the rod. The head should be held comfortable, erect, with lower border of the orbit of the eye in the same horizontal plane as the external canal of the ear (Frankfort plane). The headpiece (flat small horizontal arm) of the measuring device should be gently lowered to make contact with the top of the head. The measure should be calibrated unto 175 cm with markings of 0.1 cm.

Arm Circumference

Midarm circumference is recorded midway between tip of acromian process and olecranon. The tape is passed around the arm at the marked level, but no pressure is applied.

Measurement in the age group 1-6 years changes < 1.0 cm. The following cut off are accepted by the WHO to diagnose under/malnutrition
- >13.5 cm — Normal
- 12.5 - 13.4 cm — Mild to moderate
- < 12.4 cm — Severe.

Skin Fold Thickness (SFT)

Half of body fat is located directly under the skin. Measurement of skinfold gives the estimate of the body fat. Triceps and biceps SFT measure peripheral fat and subscapular and suprailiac SFT measure central fat.

Growth in Head Circumference (Cm)

In normal full-term child.

At birth	3 mo	6 mo	9 mo	12 mo	2 yr	5 yr	12 yr
34-35,	40	42-43	44-45	46-47	48	50.3	52 cm

The increment is 2 cm/month in first 3 month; 1 cm/month between 3 - 6 month; 0.5 cm/month between 9-12 month. Thereafter gain in head circumference is very slow, only 5 cm after first birth day to 12 years of age (Tables 4.1 and 4.2 give percentiles for head circumference for boys and girls – Birth until 6 years of age). Figure 4.1 shows percentile curves for boys. These can be used for girls also as data (Tables 4.1 and 4.2) do not show much difference.

Tables 4.1 and 4.2 are based on data published by the author in 1992 and 1994 that were the results of a large multicenter survey of growth and development of Indian Children.[1,2] Though various studies have tried to formulate reference data in the past, but in all

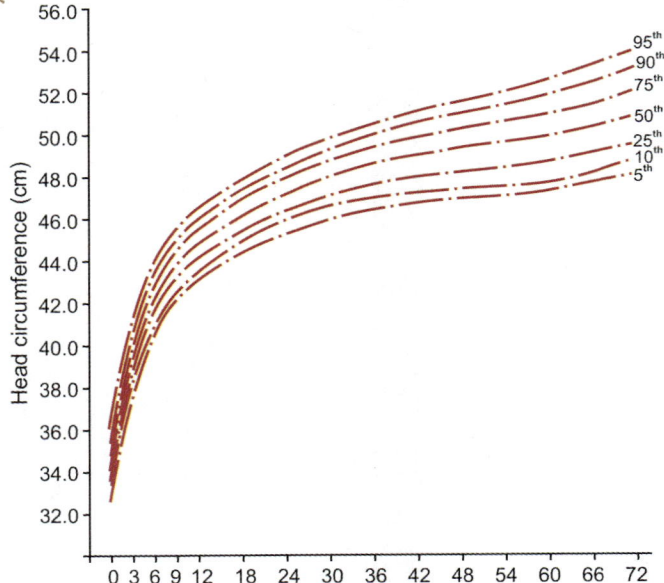

Fig. 4.1: Smoothen percentile curves of head circumference by age for boys (cubic spline least square method)

Table 4.1: Head circumference (cm) percentiles, with ± 3SD values for girls (Birth - 6 years of age)

Age (months)	N	3rd	5th	10th	20th	25th	30th	40th	50th	60th	70th	75th	80th	90th	95th	97th	−3SD	−2SD	−1SD	Median	+1SD	+2SD	+3SD
0	269	33.1	33.2	33.6	33.9	34.1	34.2	34.4	34.6	34.8	35.0	35.2	35.2	35.5	36.0	36.4	32.1	32.9	33.3	34.6	35.5	36.3	37.2
3	299	37.4	37.9	38.2	38.8	39.0	39.1	39.4	39.6	39.9	40.1	40.3	40.5	41.8	41.3	41.4	36.4	37.5	38.6	39.6	40.7	41.8	42.8
6	308	39.7	40.1	40.3	41.6	41.3	42.0	42.2	42.4	42.6	42.8	42.9	43.0	43.4	43.8	44.0	39.3	40.3	41.4	42.4	45.5	44.5	45.6
9	302	42.2	42.5	42.3	43.2	43.4	43.5	43.7	43.9	44.1	44.3	44.5	44.6	44.9	45.3	45.5	41.4	42.2	43.1	43.9	44.7	46.6	46.4
12	290	43.1	43.5	44.1	44.4	44.6	44.7	44.9	45.1	45.3	45.5	45.7	45.8	46.1	46.4	46.5	42.4	43.3	44.2	45.1	46.0	47.0	47.9
18	135	43.9	44.4	44.9	45.5	45.7	45.9	46.0	46.4	46.7	46.9	47.0	47.2	47.8	48.0	48.0	42.7	44.6	45.2	46.4	47.6	48.9	50.1
24	179	44.7	45.0	45.5	46.0	46.2	46.5	46.9	47.0	47.3	47.5	47.7	47.9	48.3	48.7	48.9	43.5	44.6	45.8	47.0	47.1	49.3	50.5
30	206	44.9	45.4	45.8	46.5	46.7	47.0	47.5	47.3	48.0	48.2	48.4	48.5	49.1	49.7	50.0	43.3	42.1	46.5	47.8	49.1	50.5	51.8
36	266	45.3	45.7	46.0	46.8	47.0	47.3	47.6	48.0	48.5	48.9	49.0	49.1	49.9	50.4	50.9	43.7	45.1	46.6	47.9	49.9	50.8	52.3
42	370	45.9	46.0	46.5	17.2	47.5	47.7	48.0	48.4	48.9	49.4	49.7	49.9	50.5	51.0	51.5	43.3	45.4	46.9	48.4	50.0	51.5	53.0
48	432	45.9	46.4	46.9	47.5	47.7	47.9	48.4	48.9	49.3	49.9	50.2	50.4	51.0	51.8	52.0	43.5	45.3	47.1	48.9	50.7	52.5	54.3
54	459	46.2	46.9	47.2	47.9	48.1	48.3	48.8	49.2	49.5	50.0	50.4	50.8	51.5	52.0	52.5	44.2	45.9	47.5	49.2	50.9	52.6	54.2
60	381	46.6	47.2	47.5	48.4	48.7	48.9	49.1	49.5	49.9	50.4	50.7	51.0	51.9	52.6	53.0	44.5	46.2	47.9	49.2	51.2	52.9	54.5
66	245	47.4	47.5	48.0	48.7	48.9	49.1	49.5	50.0	50.5	51.0	51.3	51.5	52.1	53.0	53.3	45.0	46.6	48.3	50.0	51.5	53.3	55.0
72	98	47.5	47.7	48.1	48.9	49.2	49.6	50.4	51.3	51.8	52.0	52.2	52.4	53.1	54.2	54.9	45.3	47.3	49.3	51.3	53.3	55.3	57.3

Indian Pediatrics1994;31:377 (Agarwal and Agarwal)[2]

Growth and Development in Pediatric Surgical Practice

Table 4.2: Head circumference (cm) percentiles, with ± 3SD values for boys (Birth - 6 years of age)

Age (months)	N	3rd	5th	10th	20th	25th	30th	40th	50th	60th	70th	75th	80th	90th	95th	97th	−3SD	−2SD	−1SD	Median	+1SD	+2SD	+3SD
0	329	33.2	33.5	33.9	34.1	34.2	34.3	34.4	34.7	34.9	35.1	35.3	35.4	35.9	36.3	36.5	32.1	33.0	33.3	34.7	35.5	36.3	37.1
3	386	38.1	38.2	38.6	39.1	39.3	39.5	39.7	40.0	40.2	40.5	40.7	40.9	41.4	42.0	42.5	36.5	37.6	38.8	40.0	41.1	42.3	43.5
6	398	40.3	40.7	41.3	47.9	42.2	42.2	42.5	42.7	42.9	43.1	43.3	43.4	43.3	44.2	44.7	39.6	40.6	41.7	42.7	43.7	44.8	45.8
9	386	42.5	42.9	43.2	43.6	43.7	43.8	44.0	44.2	44.4	44.6	44.8	44.9	45.3	45.8	42.2	41.6	42.4	43.3	44.2	45.1	46.0	46.9
12	378	43.7	44.0	44.4	44.8	44.9	45.0	45.2	45.4	45.5	45.8	45.9	46.0	46.5	46.9	47.3	42.2	43.7	44.5	45.4	46.2	47.1	48.0
18	136	44.8	44.9	45.4	46.0	46.1	46.2	46.7	47.0	47.5	47.9	48.0	48.0	48.4	48.7	48.9	43.4	44.6	45.8	47.0	48.2	49.4	50.6
24	202	45.5	45.8	46.3	46.8	46.9	47.0	47.3	47.7	48.0	48.4	48.5	48.5	49.0	49.5	49.9	44.3	45.4	46.6	47.7	48.8	50.6	51.2
30	266	46.2	46.4	46.8	47.3	47.4	47.5	47.9	48.2	48.5	48.8	48.9	48.9	49.6	49.9	50.4	44.8	46.0	47.0	48.2	49.3	50.4	51.3
36	363	46.1	46.7	47.0	47.8	47.9	48.0	48.4	48.7	49.0	49.4	49.5	49.7	50.0	50.9	51.0	44.8	46.1	47.4	48.7	50.6	51.3	52.6
42	470	46.9	47.1	47.5	48.0	48.2	48.4	48.9	49.3	49.6	49.9	50.1	50.3	50.9	51.0	51.4	45.5	46.8	48.20	49.3	50.6	51.8	53.2
48	523	46.9	47.1	47.9	48.5	48.7	48.9	49.4	49.9	50.0	50.5	50.7	50.9	51.2	52.0	52.1	45.6	47.0	48.5	49.9	51.3	52.7	54.1
54	523	47.4	47.7	48.0	48.8	48.9	49.2	49.6	50.0	50.4	50.9	51.0	51.2	52.0	52.5	52.9	55.5	51.0	58.5	60.0	61.4	62.9	64.4
60	450	47.5	47.9	48.4	48.9	49.2	49.5	50.0	50.3	50.6	51.0	51.2	51.5	52.3	52.8	53.0	45.6	47.1	48.7	50.3	51.8	53.4	55.5
66	277	47.7	48.3	48.8	49.4	49.6	49.9	50.4	50.9	51.3	51.6	51.9	52.1	53.0	53.5	53.9	46.1	47.6	49.3	50.9	52.5	54.1	55.7
72	124	47.9	48.3	48.8	49.5	49.8	50.1	50.8	51.1	51.6	52.0	52.2	52.4	53.3	54.2	54.5	45.9	47.6	49.4	51.1	52.8	54.6	56.3

Indian Pediatrics1994;31:377 (Agarwal and Agarwal)[2]

these studies, the sample size was very small and they were more regional rather than representative of the whole country.[3,6]

Skull circumference is important in pediatric surgical practice: The causes of variations are:

Large Head

Big infant, familial feature, hydrancephaly, hydrocephalus (progressive or arrested), subdural effusion, cerebral tumor, storage diseases megacephaly (abnormal storages of substances within the brain parenchyma- lysosomal diseases, e.g. Tay-Sachs, gangliosidosis, mucopolysacchridosis chondrodystrophies, metachromatic leucodystrophies, etc.

Small Head

Small infant, familial, microcephaly- skull size below 2 SD (primary brain growth failure), craniostenosis (ridge is palpable on the suture line).

Head Circumference in Pre-term Babies

Gestation age (wk)	Mean head circumference (cm)
26	24.0
27	25.6
30	27.6
32	29.6
34	31.6
36	33.0

Length/Height Growth

At birth length is 50 cm it becomes 73-75 cm by first birth day; 86-87 cm by 2nd year and 100 cm at 4 years of age. Until puberty sets in gain in length (height velocity) is 5-7 cm every year. If gain is less than 4 cm/year possibility of growth hormone deficiency be kept in mind. Percentile growth curves for height given in Figure 4.2 are for children up to 36 months of age (same curve can be used for girls) and in Figures 4.3A and B for children up to 12 years of age. By the age of 12 years 'Puberty' sets in majority of girls and in some boys. Therefore, percentiles in relation to sexual maturity rating are given in Tables 4.3 and 4.4 . These figures and tables will assist us in plotting the child's measured valve and if the value is closer to the 50th

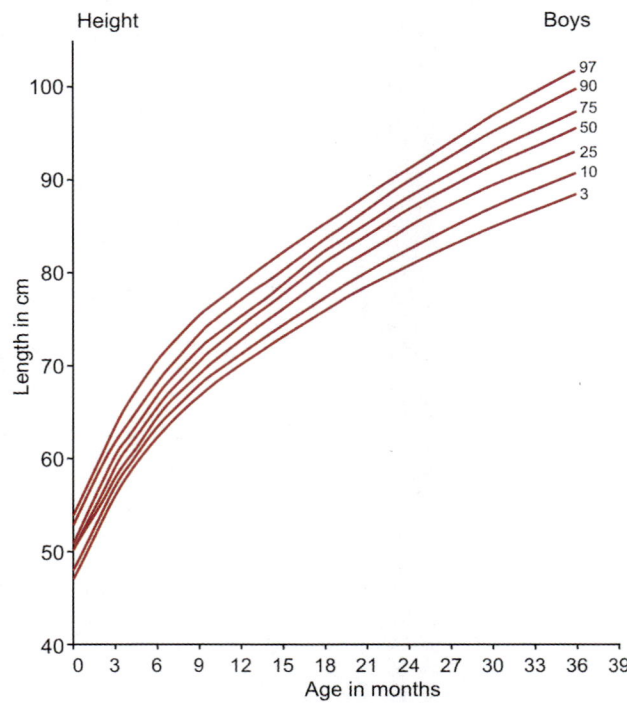

Fig. 4.2: Shows percentiles for length/height of children < 90% value of the 50th percentile value are "stunted" (chronic undernutrition)

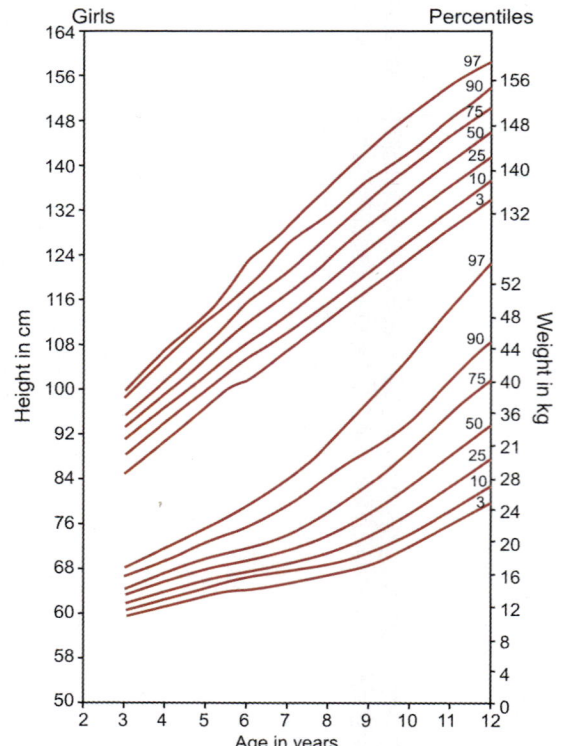

Fig. 4.3A: Agarwal's growth curves (Percentile curves for height and weight on affluent in Indian children)

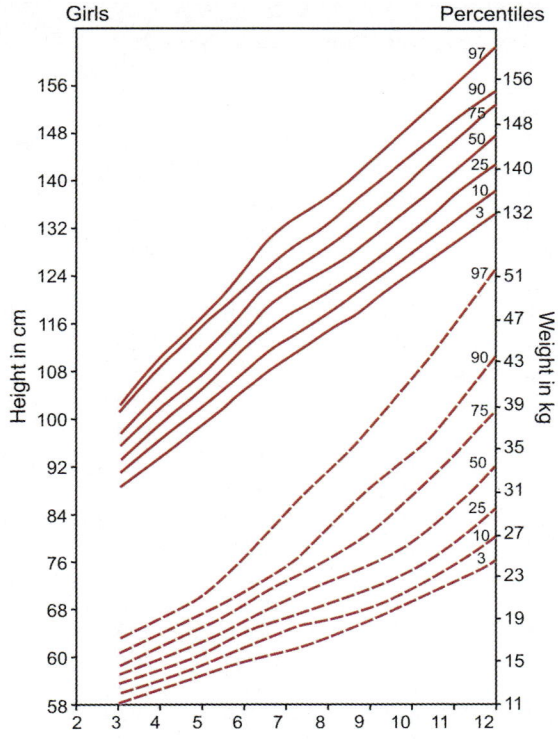

Fig. 4.3B: Agarwal's growth curves (Percentiles for height and weight in Indian affluent children)

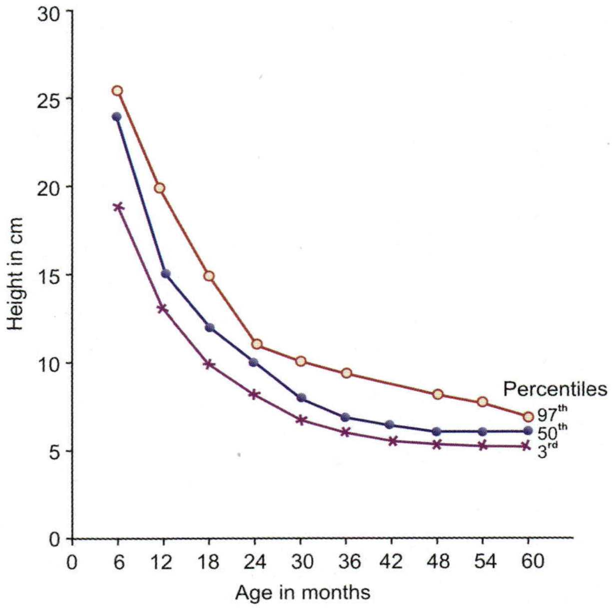

Fig. 4.4: Height-velocity Chart for boys and girls (Indian Pediatr 1994;31:377)

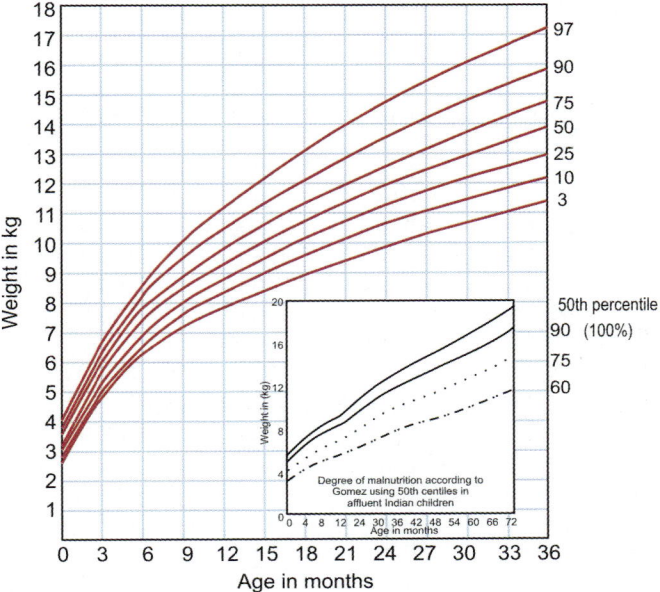

Fig. 4.5: Growth and nutrition assessment: The inset graph has 50th centile weight as 100% of weight and lines for 90%, 75% and 60% are to identify normal in weight for age (> 90%), grade I (< 90–75%), grade II (< 75–60%) and < 60% are in grade III, Gomez's classification for malnutrition (Birth-3 years) Indian pediatr 31:377-412, 1994. Weight, height, skull and mid-arm centiles for boys and girls are very close, thus the graphs can be used for girls, also

Table 4.3: Showing weight and height percentiles in relation to breast development and age in girls									
Age (years)		3	10	25	50	75	90	97	Number
Breast development stage– (SMR-2)									
10	Wt.	23.8	26.4	29.3	32.3	36.5	42.3	46.9	383
	Ht.	127.7	131.5	135.4	139.4	143.9	147.3	151.0	
11	Wt.	24.5	26.7	29.0	32.2	36.8	42.1	50.6	353
	Ht.	131.1	134.3	137.7	142.5	146.2	149.7	154.7	
12	Wt.	25.8	27.2	29.9	33.2	37.4	43.0	48.7	195
	Ht.	134.9	137.6	140.0	144.5	149.1	152.6	157.7	
13	Wt	27.0	29.1	30.7	36.1	41.0	46.8	50.9	53
	Ht.	139.9	141.3	144.9	149.5	153.7	161.0	165.2	
Breast development stage– (SMR-3)									
10	Wt.	29.0	31.2	33.1	37.6	43.0	48.9	53.0	131
	Ht.	134.9	138.5	141.0	144.3	147.5	150.5	153.7	
11	Wt.	30.1	32.4	34.8	38.8	43.5	47.3	56.2	316
	Ht.	138.0	140.0	143.2	147.0	150.5	154.5	157.1	
12	Wt.	30.9	33.6	35.9	39.4	44.5	51.2	57.2	330
	Ht.	140.00	143.5	146.0	150.2	153.5	157.3	162.0	
13	Wt.	32.0	33.5	36.3	40.0	45.0	50.6	60.6	242
	Ht.	141.5	154.0	148.0	151.9	156.7	160.1	163.3	
14	Wt.	32.4	34.2	38.8	42.9	47.0	52.1	58.3	143
	Ht.	144.0	145.8	150.0	154.2	157.0	161.7	164.5	
15	Wt.	34.8	37.8	39.1	43.0	46.5	48.2	53.2	71
	Ht.	146.5	149.0	150.6	155.0	157.3	162.7	164.9	
16	Wt.	36.2	37.2	38.2	43.0	46.8	52.6	55.2	34
	Ht.	147.1	148.9	152.0	155.2	158.4	163.5	168.3	
Breast development stage– (SMR-4)									
11	Wt.	29.9	35.5	39.3	43.6	49.6	58.7		115
	Ht.	138.2	142.7	147.0	150.3	154.5	156.3	161.7	
12.	Wt.	34.4	37.8	40.2	44.5	49.3	53.9	59.1	244
	Ht.	142.7	145.3	148.5	152.0	156.0	159.3	161.9	
13	Wt.	33.4	37.6	40.5	44.3	49.6	55.3	64.3	304
	Ht.	144.0	146.2	150.1	153.3	157.1	160.6	164.2	
14	Wt.	35.7	38.0	40.9	44.4	50.3	55.3	63.6	264
	Ht.	145.1	146.5	150.5	154.5	157.7	161.6	167.0	
15	Wt.	35.7	38.7	42.3	45.8	50.4	56.0	64.5	142
	Ht.	146.2	148.2	152.0	155.0	159.0	161.7	167.7	
16	Wt.	38.2	39.5	43.5	48.0	53.3	57.3	66.4	89
	Ht.	147.1	148.7	152.7	156.0	159.9	163.0	167.1	
17	Wt.	37.4	39.7	43.0	47.7	51.5	54.2	59.3	44
	Ht.	148.0	149.3	152.0	155.5	159.0	165.0	166.8	
Breast development stage– (SMR-5)									
12	Wt.	39.0	42.7	47.3	52.8	58.6	63.3	66.1	88
	Ht.	142.8	147.5	149.8	152.6	156.8	161.1	163.2	
13	Wt.	39.4	42.0	45.7	51.8	59.3	66.2	71.5	178
	Ht.	143.0	147.5	150.5	155.1	160.5	163.8	167.8	
14	Wt.	37.1	41.5	45.4	51.4	57.3	65.0	73.2	189
	Ht.	145.6	147.8	151.4	155.0	159.5	162.2	165.6	
15	Wt.	36.5	41.5	44.9	49.9	58.5	66.2	72.4	187
	Ht.	146.2	148.1	151.5	156.0	160.8	164.5	168.0	
16	Wt.	38.4	41.8	46.4	50.8	58.0	64.8	75.2	148
	Ht.	147.1	148.2	152.8	156.6	159.9	163.0	166.9	
17	Wt.	41.2	43.4	48.0	53.2	57.7	62.8	77.0	60

Indian Pediatr 2001; 38:1217[7]   Ht.= Height   Wt. = Weight

Table 4.4: Showing weight and height percentiles in relation to genital development and age in boys

Age (Year)	3	10	25	50	75	90	97	
\multicolumn{9}{c}{Genital development stage– (SMR-2)}
10 Wt	23.0	25.3	27.5	31.1	35.3	40.8	48.2	259
Ht	128.2	130.8	135.5	139.7	144.6	148.5	151.3	
11 Wt	24.5	27.0	29.4	32.6	37.0	42.9	51.0	480
Ht	130.7	134.7	138.5	142.4	146.8	151.0	155.3	
12 Wt	26.1	28.1	31.0	34.9	39.9	46.3	55.8	518
Ht	133.8	137.3	141.7	145.5	150.0	154.5	159.3	
13 Wt	28.2	30.2	32.5	36.5	41.5	52.2	61.2	287
Ht	136.5	141.0	145.0	149.0	152.2	156.0	160.6	
14 Wt	31.4	32.2	35.0	38.9	42.5	49.0	62.1	91
Ht	142.4	145.7	148.6	153.4	156.6	159.9	166.6	
\multicolumn{9}{c}{Genital development stage– (SMR-3)}
10 Wt	23.8	26.2	28.9	34.7	40.2	45.4	49.1	64
Ht	127.8	134.6	137.8	145.6	151.8	155.1	159.1	
11 Wt	28.4	29.7	32.8	36.4	41.8	46.7	50.9	165
Ht	134.2	139.6	143.6	148.0	153.1	158.5	163.0	
12 Wt	28.7	32.4	35.4	39.0	44.2	50.6	59.4	366
Ht	139.6	143.4	148.2	152.2	156.4	160.5	163.0	
13 Wt	30.4	23.7	35.8	39.9	45.6	51.7	61.9	467
Ht	141.5	142.2	149.5	154.1	158.5	162.1	166.9	
14 Wt	32.8	34.7	38.2	42.8	48.6	54.4	64.8	311
Ht	145.7	149.3	153.5	157.8	161.8	165.6	169.1	
15 Wt	37.2	38.0	42.0	46.1	51.3	61.6	77.0	116
Ht	152.5	152.5	156.1	161.1	166.0	169.3	172.7	
16 Wt	39.6	41.8	44.1	50.2	55.3	63.7	71.9	45
Ht	154.6	157.0	157.4	162.0	165.6	172.8	179.6	
\multicolumn{9}{c}{Genital development stage– (SMR- 4)}
11 Wt	27.9	35.8	39.7	43.2	49.0	54.3	58.6	28
Ht	138.8	147.4	150.9	156.4	161.3	163.0	166.0	
12 Wt	32.1	35.1	38.4	43.0	47.7	54.1	61.0	156
Ht	143.0	148.4	153.1	157.9	162.5	167.0	168.9	
13 Wt	33.8	36.8	41.1	45.6	51.1	59.4	71.1	430
Ht	147.0	151.5	156.0	160.2	165.0	168.5	172.6	
14 Wt	34.8	38.5	42.5	47.7	52.7	58.9	65.6	555
Ht	148.5	154.0	158.0	162.6	167.58	171.2	174.8	
15 Wt	39.2	41.7	45.2	50.8	56.5	65.7	75.2	407
Ht	154.0	157.0	161.0	165.5	169.3	172.8	176.3	
16 Wt	41.8	43.5	47.8	52.6	60.2	69.5	76.6	210
Ht	156.7	159.0	162.5	166.5	171.5	175.0	178.9	
17 Wt	43.9	45.7	47.4	55.1	62.9	68.6	76.2	68
Ht	160.3	161.0	164.1	167.8	173.7	177.5	184.3	
\multicolumn{9}{c}{Genital development stage– (SMR-5)}
13 Wt	39.3	41.3	45.8	50.5	57.2	65.7	71.3	80
Ht	152.9	157.6	160.5	164.9	169.1	173.0	177.4	
14 Wt	40.5	42.9	46.8	52.0	57.7	65.8	77.3	316
Ht	153.7	158.0	162.0	166.0	170.7	174.1	178.2	
15 Wt	41.6	44.0	47.3	52.3	59.6	69.2	77.9	461
Ht	156.5	159.2	163.5	167.0	171.5	174.5	179.4	
16 Wt	42.5	45.4	50.0	55.0	62.5	70.5	82.3	420
Ht	157.9	160.2	164.7	168.9	173.5	177.2	181.5	
17 Wt	44.8	47.1	52.3	57.1	63.1	70.9	80.6	259
Ht	160.3	162.0	165.4	169.3	173.3	176.5	181.0	
18 Wt	43.9	46.5	51.7	58.3	64.5	74.7	84.9	75
Ht	147.5	163.8	166.5	170.0	173.0	177.9	183.2	

Indian Pediatr 2001;38:1217[7]

Table 4.5: Showing degree of malnutrition

Weight for age (KG)			Weight range for malnutrition		
Age	50th percentile	Normal >90%	Grade I 90-75 %	II 75-60%	III <60%
3 m	5.7	5.1	5.1-4.3	4.3-3.4	3.4
6 m	7.4	6.7	6.7-5.6	5.6-4.4	4.4
9 m	8.5	7.7	7.7-6.4	6.4-5.1	5.1
12 m	9.3	8.4	8.4-7.0	7.0-5.6	5.6
18 m	10.7	9.6	9.6-8.0	8.0-6.4	6.4
24 m	11.9	10.7	10.7-8.9	8.9-7.1	7.1
30 m	12.9	11.6	11.6-9.7	9.7-7.7	7.7
36 m	13.8	12.4	12.4-10.4	10.4-8.3	8.3
42 m	14.6	13.1	13.1-11.0	11.0-8.8	8.8
48 m	15.4	13.0	13.0-11.6	11.6-9.2	9.2
54 m	16.2	14.5	14.5-12.2	12.2-9.7	9.7
60 m	17.1	15.4	15.4-12.8	12.8-10.3	10.3
66 m	18.1	16.3	16.3-13.8	13.8-10.9	10.9
72 m	19.2	17.3	17.3-14.4	14.4-11.5	11.5

Gomez et al 1956, J Trop Pediatr Env Ch Hlth. 2:77
(Used by the National Nutrition Monitoring Bureau in India)[8]

centile, no problem. But in case of values away from the median valve it is advisable to record measurements every three monthly, three such readings will allow to calculate the height velocity (Fig. 4.4). There may be rapid increase in velocity to catch up after the surgical cause is treated, e.g. adrenal tumor, vesicourethral reflux, etc.

What are Percentile Growth Curves?

To follow a child regularly percentile growth curves are used. The percentile refers to the position of an individual on a given reference distribution. The percentiles are calculated foe 3rd, 10th, 25th, 50th, 75th, 90th and 97th etc; the data between 3rd and 97th include 94% children (this covers children within + 2 SD from the mean). The 50th centile value for any age indicates that 50% vaues lie above and remaining 50% below this value. In case there is gaussian distribution mean and median values will be the same.

Weight Gain

Birth weight is around 3.0 kg, it doubles by 5 months of age (wt = 6.0 kg) and trebles (wt = 9.0 kg) on first birthday. At 2 yr of age it is 4 times (wt = 12 kg) of the birth wt. It becomes five times at 3 yr (wt = 15 kg) and 6 times (wt = 18 kg) at 5 year of age. The percentile growth curves for children upto 36 months and 12 year of age are in Figure 4.5. In the Figure , the nutritional status curve is inset to grade the malnutrition according to Gomez et al (Table 4.5).

The National Child Health Survey (NCHS) percentiles available for American children are also given in Tables 4.6 A and B. Our children have similar height as those of Japanese, Thai, Hongkong—thus closer to Asian children. But are shorter than Caucasian children from Europe and USA.

Sexual Maturity

This can be assessed by using Tanner's criteria given in Tables 4.7 and 4.8.

DEVELOPMENTAL MILESTONES

Control of body movements is thru the coordinated activities of nerves, nerve centers and the muscles. These motor movements develop in a definite sequence the direction being *cephalocaudal*. The first step in gross motor development is head control, involving the neck muscles. It is development of spinal muscle coordination that makes child sit with straight back instead of a round one. Child develops coordinated movements of hands, allowing him to crawl, followed by the leg movement, e.g. standing and walking. The development is proximodistal also, e. g. movement coordination develops first in trunk muscle followed by shoulder, arm, hand and fingers. The aimless movements of arms and legs of the first six months are replaced by the specific movements of locomotion and manipulation. In surgical practice – 'Neck holding, sitting, standing, walking' are easy to observe. The gross motor, fine motor (Manipulation), vision and hearing(personal social) and language development are summarized in Table 4.9.

ESSENTIAL MILESTONES

4–6 weeks:	Smiles, vocalises 1-2 weeks later.
12–16 weeks :	Head control/holds objects placed in hands converses with mother
12–20 weeks:	Hand regard
20 weeks:	Goes for objects and gets them
26 weeks:	Transfers objects from one hand to another
28–30 weeks:	Sits unaided
9–10 months:	Index finger approach (Points index finger to the object).

Table 4.6A: Length (mm), weight (kg) and head circumference (cm) by age for boys and girls: Birth to 36 months (NCHS-Data)

Percentiles	Boys							Measurement	Girls						
Age	5th	10th	25th	50th	75th	90th	95th		5th	10th	25th	50th	75th	90th	95th
Birth	46.4	47.5	49.0	50.5	51.8	53.5	54.4	Length, mm	45.4	46.5	48.2	49.9	51.0	52.0	52.9
	2.54	2.78	3.00	3.27	3.64	3.82	4.15	Weight, kg	2.36	2.58	2.93	3.23	3.52	3.64	3.81
	32.6	33.0	33.9	34.8	35.6	36.6	37.2	Head C cm	32.1	32.9	33.5	34.3	34.8	35.5	35.9
1 months	50.4	51.3	53.0	54.6	56.2	57.7	58.6	Length, mm	49.2	50.2	51.9	53.5	54.9	56.1	56.9
	3.16	3.43	3.82	4.29	4.75	5.14	5.38	Weight, kg	2.97	3.22	3.59	3.98	4.36	4.65	4.92
	34.9	35.4	36.2	37.2	38.1	39.0	39.6	Head C cm	34.2	34.8	35.6	36.4	37.1	37.8	38.2
3 months	56.7	57.7	59.4	61.1	63.0	64.5	65.4	Length, mm	55.4	56.2	57.8	59.5	61.2	62.7	63.4
	4.43	4.78	5.32	5.98	6.65	7.14	7.37	Weight, kg	4.18	4.47	4.88	5.40	5.90	6.39	6.74
	38.4	38.9	39.7	40.6	41.7	42.5	43.1	Head C cm	37.3	37.8	38.7	39.5	40.4	41.2	41.7
6 months	69.4	64.4	66.1	67.8	69.7	71.3	72.3	Length, mm	61.8	62.6	64.2	65.9	67.8	69.4	70.2
	6.20	6.61	7.20	7.85	8.49	9.10	9.46	Weight, kg	5.79	6.12	6.60	7.21	7.83	8.38	8.73
	41.5	42.0	42.8	43.8	44.7	45.6	46.2	Head C cm	40.3	40.9	41.6	42.4	43.3	44.1	44.6
9 months	68.0	69.1	70.6	72.3	74.0	75.9	77.1	Length, mm	66.1	67.0	68.7	70.4	72.4	74.0	75.0
	7.52	7.95	8.56	9.18	9.88	10.49	10.93	Weight, kg	7.00	7.34	7.89	8.56	9.24	9.83	10.17
	43.5	44.0	44.8	45.8	46.6	47.5	48.1	Head C cm	42.3	42.8	43.5	44.3	45.1	46.0	46.4
12 months	71.7	72.8	74.3	76.1	77.7	79.8	81.2	Length, mm	69.8	70.8	72.4	74.3	76.3	78.0	79.1
	8.43	8.84	4.49	10.15	10.91	11.54	11.99	Weight, kg	7.84	8.19	8.81	9.53	10.23	10.87	11.24
	44.8	45.3	46.1	47.0	47.9	48.8	49.3	Head C cm	43.5	44.1	44.8	45.6	46.4	47.2	47.6
18 months	77.5	78.7	80.5	82.4	84.3	86.6	88.1	Length, mm	76.0	77.2	78.8	80.9	83.0	85.0	86.1
	9.59	9.92	10.67	11.47	12.31	13.05	13.44	Weight, kg	8.92	9.30	10.04	10.82	11.55	12.30	12.76
	46.3	46.7	47.4	48.4	49.3	50.1	50.6	Head C cm	45.0	45.6	46.3	47.1	47.9	48.6	49.1
24 months	82.3	83.5	85.6	87.6	89.9	92.2	93.8	Length, mm	81.3	82.5	84.2	86.5	88.712	90.8	92.0
	10.54	10.85	11.65	12.59	13.44	14.29	14.70	Weight, kg	9.87	10.26	11.10	11.90	74	13.57	14.08
	47.3	47.7	48.3	49.2	50.2	51.0	51.4	Head C cm	46.1	46.5	47.3	48.1	48.8	49.6	50.1
30 months	87.0	88.2	90.1	92.3	946	97.0	98.7	Length, mm	86.0	87.0	88.9	91.3	93.7	95.6	96.9
	11.44	11.80	12.63	13.67	14.51	15.47	15.97	Weight, kg	10.78	11.21	12.11	12.93	13.93	14.81	15.35
	48.0	48.4	49.1	49.9	51.0	51.7	52.2	Head C cm	47.0	47.3	48.0	48.8	49.4	50.3	50.8
36 months	91.2	92.4	94.2	96.5	98.9	101.4	103.1	Length, mm	90.0	91.0	93.1	95.6	98.1	100.0	101.5
	12.26	12.69	13.58	14.69	15.59	16.66	17.28	Weight, kg	11.60	12.07	12.99	13.93	15.03	15.97	16.54
	48.6	49.0	49.7	50.5	51.5	52.3	52.8	Head C cm	47.6	47.9	48.5	49.3	50.0	50.8	51.4

Table 4.6B: Percentiles of stature (cm) and weight (kg) by age [NCHS-data] for boys and girls

Age (Yr)	5th	10th	25th	50th	75th	90th	95th
2.0+	82.50 / 10.49	83.50 / 10.96	85.30 / 11.55	86.80 / 12.37	89.20 / 13.36	92.00 / 14.38	94.40 / 15.50
							93.60 / 14.15
2.5+	85.40 / 11.24	86.50 / 11.77	88.50 / 12.55	90.40 / 13.52	92.90 / 14.61	95.60 / 15.71	97.80 / 16.61
							96.60 / 15.76
3.0	89.00 / 12.05	90.30 / 12.58	92.60 / 13.12	94.90 / 14.62	97.50 / 15.78	100.10 / 16.95	102.00 / 17.77
							100.60 / 17.22
3.5	92.50 / 12.84	93.90 / 13.41	96.40 / 14.46	99.10 / 15.68	101.70 / 16.90	104.30 / 18.15	106.10 / 18.98
							104.50 / 18.59
4.0	95.80 / 13.64	97.30 / 14.24	100.00 / 15.39	102.90 / 16.69	105.70 / 17.99	108.20 / 19.32	109.20 / 20.27
							108.30 / 19.91
4.5	98.90 / 14.45	100.60 / 15.10	103.40 / 16.30	106.60 / 17.69	109.40 / 19.06	111.90 / 20.50	113.50 / 21.63
							112.00 / 21.24
5.0	102.00 / 15.27	103.70 / 15.96	106.50 / 17.22	109.90 / 18.67	112.80 / 20.14	115.40 / 21.70	117.00 / 23.09
							115.60 / 22.62
5.5	104.90 / 16.09	106.70 / 16.83	109.60 / 18.14	113.10 / 19.67	116.10 / 21.25	118.70 / 22.96	120.30 / 24.66
							119.20 / 24.11
6.0	107.70 / 16.93	109.60 / 17.72	112.50 / 19.07	116.10 / 20.69	119.20 / 22.40	121.90 / 24.31	123.50 / 26.37
							122.70 / 25.75
6.5	110.40 / 17.78	112.30 / 18.62	115.30 / 20.02	119.20 / 21.74	122.20 / 23.62	124.90 / 25.76	126.60 / 28.16
							126.10 / 27.59
7.0	113.00 / 18.64	115.00 / 19.53	118.00 / 21.00	121.70 / 22.85	125.00 / 24.94	127.90 / 27.36	129.70 / 30.12
							129.50 / 29.68
7.5	115.60 / 19.52	117.60 / 20.45	120.60 / 22.02	124.40 / 24.03	127.80 / 26.36	130.80 / 29.11	132.70 / 32.73
							132.90 / 32.07
8.0	118.10 / 20.40	120.20 / 21.39	123.20 / 23.09	127.00 / 25.30	130.50 / 27.91	133.60 / 31.06	135.70 / 34.51
							136.20 / 34.71
8.5	120.50 / 21.31	122.70 / 22.34	125.70 / 24.24	129.60 / 26.66	133.20 / 29.61	136.50 / 33.22	138.80 / 36.96
							139.60 / 37.58
9.0	122.90 / 22.25	125.20 / 23.33	128.20 / 25.40	132.20 / 28.1	136.00 / 31.46	139.40 / 35.57	141.80 / 39.58
							142.90 / 40.64
9.5	125.30 / 23.25	127.60 / 24.38	130.80 / 26.88	134.80 / 29.73	138.80 / 33.46	142.40 / 38.11	144.90 / 42.35
							146.20 / 43.85
10.0	127.70 / 24.33	130.10 / 25.52	133.40 / 28.07	137.50 / 31.44	141.60 / 35.61	145.50 / 40.80	148.10 / 45.27
							149.50 / 47.17

Contd...

Contd...

Age (Yr)	5th		10th		25th		50th		75th		90th		95th	
10.5	130.10	130.40	132.60	132.50	136.00	136.70	140.30	141.50	144.60	146.10	148.70	150.40	151.50	152.80
	25.15	25.75	26.78	27.32	29.59	30.57	33.30	34.72	37.92	40.17	43.63	46.84	48.31	50.57
11.0	132.60	133.50	135.10	135.60	138.70	140.00	143.33	144.80	147.80	149.30	152.10	153.70	154.90	156.20
	26.80	27.24	28.17	28.97	31.25	32.49	35.30	36.95	40.38	42.84	46.57	49.96	51.47	54.00
11.5	135.00	136.60	137.70	139.00	141.50	143.50	146.40	148.20	151.10	152.60	155.60	156.90	158.50	159.50
	28.24	28.83	29.72	30.71	33.08	34.48	37.46	39.23	43.00	45.48	49.61	53.03	54.73	57.42
12.0	137.60	139.80	140.30	142.30	144.40	147.00	149.70	151.50	154.60	155.80	159.40	1600.00	162.30	162.70
	29.85	30.52	31.46	32.53	35.09	36.52	39.78	41.53	45.77	48.07	52.73	55.99	58.09	60.81
12.5	140.20	142.70	143.00	145.40	147.40	150.10	153.00	154.60	158.20	158.80	163.20	162.90	166.10	165.60
	31.64	32.30	33.41	34.42	37.31	38.59	42.27	43.84	48.70	50.56	55.91	58.81	61.52	64.12
13.0	142.90	145.20	145.80	148.00	150.50	152.80	156.50	157.10	161.80	161.30	167.00	165.30	169.80	168.10
	33.64	34.14	35.60	36.35	37.74	40.55	44.95	46.10	51.79	52.91	59.12	61.45	65.02	67.30
13.5	145.70	147.20	148.70	150.00	153.60	154.70	159.90	159.00	165.30	163.20	170.50	167.30	173.40	170.00
	35.85	35.98	38.03	38.26	42.40	42.65	47.81	48.26	55.02	55.11	62.35	63.87	65.51	70.30
14.0	148.80	148.70	151.80	151.50	156.90	155.90	63.10	160.40	168.50	164.60	173.80	168.70	176.70	171.30
	38.22	37.76	40.64	40.11	45.21	44.54	50.77	50.28	58.31	57.09	65.57	66.04	72.13	73.08
14.5	152.00	149.70	155.00	152.50	160.10	158.80	166.20	161.20	171.50	165.60	176.60	169.80	179.50	172.20
	40.66	39.45	43.34	41.83	48.08	46.28	53.76	52.10	61.58	58.84	68.76	67.95	75.66	75.59
15.0	155.20	150.50	158.20	153.20	163.30	157.20	169.00	161.80	174.10	166.30	178.90	170.50	181.90	172.80
	43.11	40.99	46.06	43.38	50.92	47.82	56.71	53.68	64.72	60.32	71.91	69.54	79.12	77.78
15.5	158.30	151.10	161.20	153.60	166.20	157.50	171.50	162.10	176.30	166.70	180.80	170.90	183.90	173.10
	45.50	42.32	48.69	44.72	53.64	49.10	59.51	54.96	67.64	61.48	74.98	70.79	82.45	79.59
16.0	161.10	151.60	163.90	154.10	168.70	157.80	173.50	162.40	178.10	166.90	182.40	171.10	185.40	173.30
	47.74	43.41	51.16	45.78	56.16	50.09	62.10	55.89	70.26	62.29	77.97	71.68	85.62	80.99
16.5	163.40	152.20	166.10	154.60	170.60	158.20	175.20	162.70	179.50	167.10	183.60	171.20	186.60	173.40
	49.76	44.20	53.39	46.54	58.38	50.75	64.39	56.44	72.46	62.75	80.84	72.18	88.59	81.93
17.0	164.90	152.70	167.70	155.10	171.90	158.70	176.20	163.10	180.50	167.30	184.40	171.20	187.30	173.50
	51.50	44.74	55.28	47.04	60.22	51.14	66.31	56.69	74.17	62.94	83.58	72.38	91.31	82.46
17.5	165.60	153.20	168.50	155.60	172.40	159.10	176.70	163.40	181.00	167.50	185.00	171.10	187.60	173.50
	52.89	45.08	56.78	47.33	61.61	51.33	67.78	56.71	78.32	62.89	86.14	72.37	93.73	82.62
18.0	165.70	153.60	168.70	156.00	172.30	159.60	176.80	163.70	181.20	167.60	185.30	171.00	187.60	173.60
	53.97	45.26	57.89	47.47	62.61	51.39	68.88	56.62	76.00	62.78	88.41	72.25	95.76	82.47

Table 4.7: Breast development and pubic hair changes in various sexual maturity stages (SMR) in girls

SMR Stages	Breast (Mean ages)	Pubic hair (13.6 years)
1.	Preadolescent	Preadolescent
2.	Bud stage and papilla elevated as small mound, areolar diameter increased (10.2 yrs)	Sparse lightly pigmented straight, medial border of labia
3.	Areola enlarged (11.6 yrs) no contour separation	Darker, beginning to curl, increases in amount
4.	Areola and papilla form secondary mound (13.5 yrs)	Coarse, curly abundant but amount less than in adult
5.	Mature nipple projects, areola part of general breast contour (15.6 yrs)	Adult feminine triangle spread to medial surface of thigh

Table 4.8: Development of sexual organs and pubic hair in boys

SMR stages	Penis	Testes	Pubic hair (14.2 years)
1.	Preadolescent	4 ml = 0.9	None
2.	Slight or no enlargement (113 yrs)	Enlargement of scrotum, pink texture altered = 2.5	Scanty long slightly pigmented
3.	Longer (12.8 yrs)	Testes 6-8 ml = 3.4	Daker start to curl, small amount
4.	Larger, glans and breadth increase in size (14.1 yrs)	Testes 10-12 ml, scrotum dark = 5.2	Resembles adult type but less in quantity, coarse curly
5.	Adult size (16.4 yrs) (Mean ages) Testosterone level ng/ml	Adult size 5.7 Minimum= 12 ml Average = 18.6 ± 4 ml	Adult distribution spread to medial surface of thigh Axillary (14.9 yrs); Facial (14.8 yrs)

Table 4.9: Developmental pattern (modified Gesell's development schedule)

Gross motor	Manipulation (Fine motor)	Vision and hearing (Personal social)	Language
Head control 6 wk-at level 8 wk- above the body complete 3 ½-4 m **Sitting** – 6-7 m 11m– with pivoting **Standing** 12 wk bears much wt 24 wk bears most wt 28 wk-full wt 36 wk-stand holding furniture 52 wk–**Walks** with one hand held 13 m–Walks with support 2 yr- **Climbs** steps with 2 feets on each step 2½ yr– **Runs** 3 yr – Climbs one foot one each step 4-5 yr– **Skips**	Hand closed -4 weeks Primitive grasp disappear 8-12 wks) 12 wk looks object, wants to grasp/holds toy placed in hand (hand open). 16 wk–hands come together in mid-line but overshoots the objects, plays with rattle 20 wk- grasps an object, takes to mouth plays with toes **Grasp** first 6 months (Immature gras-ulnar) 24-32 wk–Radial index, ring+little fingers (Intermediate grasps) 6 m– **Transfers objects** from one hand to another/feeds on a biscuit 40 wk–**Index approach** Points the objects as he picks 10 m – **Index + thumb apposition**	6 wk-3 m **Social smile** (Sight/shound) Fixation/convergence+ focussion improves progressively 3-16 m (12-24 wk) **Hand regard** 20 wk- smiles mirror reflexion 28 wk-Pats mirror image 6m– 2 yr– recognises familiar ones 2-3 yr– stubborn 3-5 yr– Plays with other children	12-16 wk converses with mother 28 wk-monosyllables ba, da, ka 32 wk-dada 40 wk-obeys 'No' and simple command 1 yr– 2-3 words with meaning

REFERENCES

1. Agarwal DK, Agarwal KN, Upadhyay SK, Mittal R, Prakash R, Rai S. Physical and sexual growth pattern of affluent Indian children from 5 to 18 years of age. Indian Pediatr 1992;29:1203-68.
2. Agarwal DK, Agarwal KN. Physical growth of Indian affluent children (Birth - 6 years). Indian Pediatr 1994;31: 377-413.
3. Katiyar GP, Sehgal D, Khare BB, Agarwal DK, Tripathi AM, Agarwal KN. Physical growth characteristics of upper socioeconomic adolescent boys of Varanasi. Indian Pediatr 1985;22:915-22.
4. Datta Banik ND. Semilongitudinal growth evaluation of children from birth to 14 years in different socioeconomic groups. Indian Pediatr 1982;19:353-59.
5. Kaul. KK, Taskar AD, Madhavan S, Mukerji B, Parekh P, Sawhney K, et al. Growth in height and weight of urban Madhya Pradesh adolescents. Indian Pediatr 1976;13: 31-39.
6. Rath B, Ghosh S, Man Mohan, Ramanujacharyulu TKTS. Anthropometric indices of children (5-15 years) of a privileged community. Indian Pediatr 1978;15:653-59.
7. Agarwal KN, Saxena A, Bansal AK and Agarwal DK. Physical Growth Assessment in Adolescence Indian Pediatrics 2001;38:1217-35.
8. Gómez F, Galvan RR, Frenk S, et al. Mortality in second and third degree malnutrition. J Trop Pediatr 1956;2:77-83.

Fluid and Electrolytes in Pediatric Surgery

CHAPTER 5

V Ravikumar, M Srinivas

Billions of years ago the life started in the sea as unicellular organism and the cell was surrounded by the sea water. The sea water protected the cells as a shell. In human beings the extracellular fluid (ECF) compartment has the composition of fluids similar to that of sea water and it protects the cells. Primary disturbances in fluid and electrolytes affect mainly the extracellular compartment. Though minor disturbances in the extracellular environment are compensated by renal and other mechanisms, gross changes in ECF lead ultimately lead to alterations in the intracellular fluid (ICF). This may affect the cell function and cell survival depending upon the severity of the deleterious changes.

Fluid and electrolyte imbalances occur much more quickly in children than in adults. Newborn babies, infants and children present unique problems in managing fluids and electrolytes.[1-5] Differences in the rate of metabolism and body surface area are two unique aspects of them that contribute to special circumstances. Children and adults obviously are different in size, but children are not miniature adults. A child's body composition and homeostatic controls differ from those of an adult very much. The younger the child, the greater the differences and it posed the greater challenge to manage. Fluid and electrolyte requirements vary, not only with the size of a patient, but also with the child's age and clinical condition. The pediatric surgeon needs to be alert to the potential problems of these children and this would have a tremendous effect on patient outcome.[4] It is necessary to be alert to fluid and electrolyte imbalance so they necessary intervention could be instituted before the situation turns out to be too critical.[5]

FLUID BALANCE

Fluid is well balanced in all living organisms by nature. "Fluid balance" refers to total body water, which stays constant with consistent distribution among the main fluid compartments - that is ECF, ICF and interstitial fluid. Water and electrolytes are balanced together and each one of them in each compartment is important and all of them together determine the fluid equilibrium. The ICF and ECF composition is shown in Table 5.1.

In summary, the body is comprised two fluid compartments – ECF and ICF. The ECF has extracellular fluid compartment, which is intravascular fluid (plasma) and extravascular or interstitial fluid (lymph and cerebral spinal fluid). For these the major electrolyte is sodium (Na^+). The ICF is within cell walls, and here the major electrolyte is potassium (K^+). Water balance is maintained in the body in an almost constant amount, and under normal circumstances, water taken in is close to the amount of urine excreted in a 24-hour period. The water in food and from oxidation balances the water lost in feces and evaporation. These auto-regulated events keep the body's fluids in balance.

Table 5.1: Intracellular and extracellular fluid composition		
	Intracellular (mEq/L)	Extracellular (mEq/L)
Na^+	20	133 - 145
K^+	150	3 - 5
Cl^-	-	98 - 110
HCO_3^-	10	20 - 25
PO_4^{3-}	110-115	5
Protein	75	10

The premature infant's body is approximately 90% water, the newborn infant's body is 70-80% water; and the adult's body is approximately 60% water.[6] By the time a child is almost 3 years old, the total body water is approximately 60%. However, although an infant has more total body water than an adult, the infant is not protected from excessive fluid loss. In fact, the opposite is true. An infant may exchange half his extracellular fluid daily, whereas an adult may exchange only one sixth in the same day. This means the infant has a greater fluid requirement and is able to keep only a small amount of fluids in reserve. Any increase in fluid loss can quickly cause an infant to become dehydrated. Insensible water losses (fluids lost through the skin and lungs) are higher for infants and children than for adults. Because an infant has relatively greater body surface area than does an adult, an infant will lose more insensible fluids. For example, compared to an older child, a premature infant has almost five times as much body surface area in relation to its weight; the newborn has three times the body surface area. Consequently, any situation that causes an increase in loss of water and electrolytes through the skin threatens the body fluid balance of the infant and small child to a greater degree than it would an older child or adult. Insensible water losses may increase as much as 50-70 ml for each degree Celsius above normal body temperature in an infant. Fever increases insensible water losses by about 0.42 ml/kg/degree Celsius for each degree above 37°C. It also is important to consider any additional sources of fluid loss that can increase evaporation losses through the skin, such as the use of radiant heat warmers or phototherapy lights.[7-9]

BASAL METABOLIC RATE

The basal metabolic rate (BMR) for infants and children is higher than for adults because of larger body surface area in relation to the mass of active tissue. Another reason BMR is higher in infants is to support growth. Infants expend 100 calories per kilogram of body weight. An adult expends 40 calories per kilogram. Any condition that increases metabolism causes greater heat production, greater insensible fluid loss, and an increased need for water for excretion of wastes. An infant's high BMR means the fluid intake per kilogram body weight per day actually must exceed the per kilogram fluid requirements of an adult.

In addition, infant kidneys are not mature enough to concentrate urine efficiently.

MAINTENANCE FLUID THERAPY

Maintenance fluids provide water and electrolytes equal to those lost during normal activities, such as breathing, urination, stool formation, and regulating body temperature. Holliday and Segar devised a formula in 1957 that is still used to estimate maintenance water requirements. It is important to keep in mind that the amounts calculated from the formula does not take into consideration the increase or decrease in water excretion secondary to illnesses. Also, it is important to keep in mind those maintenance fluid needs to be supplemented with deficits. For this it is imperative to assess whether the baby already has deficits. Assessment skills are important for the pediatric surgeon to recognize subtle clues before an infant or child gets into serious fluid and electrolyte imbalance. Assessing physical data, the results of laboratory tests, body weight, and intake and output charts are some of the important aspects in this regard.

PHYSICAL ASSESSMENT

When if child is dehydrated, extracellular fluid volume decreases, which leads to a decrease in peripheral circulation. As circulation becomes compromised, skin color changes from normal to pale. Capillary filling time also increases. Skin turgor will be dry, and tenting of the skin may be noticed. A decrease in the production of secretions may also be noted. As fluid volume decreases small arterioles vasoconstrict to keep blood flow to vital organs resulting in cool extremities. The mouth is a good place to assess fluid deficit. Watch for a decrease in saliva, dry lips and nares, and cracked mucous membranes. The tongue may become red, rough, dry, and wrinkled. Pulse rate is another sensitive indicator of fluid status. If a pulse rate is greater than 160 beats per minute (bpm) for infants and 120 bpm for children, hypovolemia should be strongly suspected. Fontanels of infants will be depressed with a moderate fluid deficit. Fluid volume deficit causes a mild metabolic acidosis. Children often will hyperventilate to compensate for the acidosis. An increased respiratory rate will increase insensible water loss, worsening the fluid volume deficit. Blood pressure is the last vital sign to show changes and should not be relied on as an assessment indicator of dehydration.

LABORATORY DATA

Laboratory values and physical assessment data are a necessary for diagnosing and treating fluid and electrolyte imbalances. Normal serum laboratory value ranges may differ from one laboratory to another, so it is imperative to keep in mind the values of the local laboratory. Common normal values for this purpose are given in Table 5.2.

BODY WEIGHT

Body weight is an important variable in guiding diagnosis and treatment. An accurate baseline weight is essential. Frequent follow-up weight measurements are critical to the treatment of an infant or child with a fluid and electrolyte imbalance.

INTAKE AND OUTPUT CHARTS

Calculating and documenting accurate intake and output are critically important. Though these charts are maintained by the nurses, pediatric surgeon should cross check and utilize them for calculating the fluid and electrolyte requirements of the baby. The number, consistency, and character of stools must be documented. Urine, emesis, gastric suctioning, and wound drainage also should be included in output amounts.

OVERVIEW OF ELECTROLYTES

The most crucial electrolytes for all cell life are potassium (K^+), sodium (Na^+), and chloride (Cl^-). Another electrolyte to be closely monitored in children is calcium. Although not an electrolyte, serum glucose plays an important role in the hemodynamic monitoring of the pediatric patient. Electrolytes are lost in different amounts with normal body fluids, except insensible losses. For example, more potassium is lost in stool than are sodium and chloride. To effectively monitor infants and children, we need a basic knowledge of important electrolytes and signs and symptoms of imbalances. The normal values along with important biochemical parameters are listed in Table 5.2.

Table 5.2: Normal range of important parameters related to the fluid and electrolyte imbalance

Biochemical parameter	Normal value (Range)
Sodium (Na^+)	135 - 145 mEq/L
Potassium (K^+)	3.5 - 5.0 mEq/L
Chloride (Cl^-)	98 - 108 mEq/L
Calcium (Ca^{++})	9.0 - 11.5 mg/dl
Phosphate	4.5 - 5.5 mg/dl
Magnesium	1.3 - 2.0 mEq/L
Blood urea nitrogen (BUN)	5 - 20 mg/dl
Creatinine	0.5 - 1.5 mg/dl
Serum osmolality	270 - 285 mOsm/kg
Urine specific gravity	1.002 - 1.030
Urine pH	5 - 8
Blood sugar	60 - 100 mg/dl

Sodium

Sodium is the most abundant electrolyte in extracellular fluid. When a decrease in serum sodium concentration (hyponatremia) produces an acute decrease in intravascular osmolality, free water moves from the intravascular to the interstitial space until the osmolality of the compartments are the same. Thus, an acute decrease in serum sodium will result in an acute shift, which may lead to significant cerebral edema.

Sodium concentration of extracellular fluid profoundly influences the kidneys' regulation of body water and electrolyte status. For example, when sodium concentration falls, the kidneys promote water excretion under the influence of aldosterone. When sodium concentration increases, the release of antidiuretic hormone causes the kidneys to retain more water and dilute the sodium to normal levels.[10] Hyponatremia is associated with acute respiratory distress in infants with bronchopulmonary dysplasia. Other causes of hyponatremia include gastrointestinal fluid losses coupled with increase water replacement, adrenal insufficiency, water enemas, potent diuretic therapy, and factors predisposing to syndrome of inappropriate anti-diuretic hormone secretion from drugs, tumors, or central nervous system disorders. Signs and symptoms of hyponatremia are apprehension, headache, abdominal cramps, convulsions, oliguria or anuria, diarrhea, muscle twitching or weakness, increased deep tendon reflexes, lethargy or confusion, tachycardia, and cold clammy skin. Hypernatremia may be caused by an excessive intake of sodium or an increased water loss related to sodium loss. Signs and symptoms are dry, sticky mucous membranes; flushed skin; intense thirst; rough and dry tongue; irritability when stimulated; firm tissue turgor; and coma. When treating hypernatremia, eliminate the cause of excess intake, if possible; give infusates to dilute the serum level; and monitor closely.

Hyponatremia

The causes and laboratory data of hyponatremia is summarized in the Table 5.3.

Treatment

It is important to look for the losses and replace the losses appropriately. The original cause for the hyponatremia needs to be treated. If there is an increase in the body weight along with the hyponatremia, fluid restriction is recommended.

Syndrome of Inappropriate Antidiuretic Hormone (SIADH) Secretion

Conditions associated CNS disease or injury (head injury, meningitis, subarachnoid hemorrhage, meningoencephalitis, brain tumors, neurosurgery may result in SIADH.

The treatment includes normovolemia with fluid restriction, to maintain normovolemia and an addition of diuretic (e.g., furosemide). It needs administration of insensible fluid losses plus isotonic fluid to replace hourly urine output.

Hypernatremia

The causes and laboratory data of hypernatremia is summarized in Table 5.4.

Clinical Management

Predominantly neurological symptoms: Lethargy, weakness, altered mental status, irritability, and seizures. Additional symptoms may include muscle cramps, depressed deep tendon reflexes, and respiratory failure. Treatment includes, replacement of free water losses based on calculations in present text and treat the cause. Natriuretic agent may be considered if there is an increased weight.

Potassium

Potassium is the predominant intracellular electrolyte. Potassium activates several enzymatic reactions, helps regulate acid-base balance, influences kidney function and structure, and maintains neuromuscular

Table 5.3: Causes and laboratory data in hyponatremia

Decreased weight		Increased or Normal weight
Renal losses	Extra-renal losses	
Causes		
Na⁺ losing nephropathy	GI losses	Nephrotic syndrome
Diuretics	Skin losses	Congestive heart failure
Adrenal insufficiency	Third space loss cystic fibrosis	SIADH
		Acute/chronic renal failure
		Water intoxication
		Cirrhosis
		Excess salt-free infusions
Lab data		
↑ Urine volume	↓ Urine volume	↓ Urine volume
↓ Specific gravity	↑ Specific gravity	↑ Specific gravity
↓ Urine osmolality	↑ Urine osmolality	↑ Urine osmolality

Table 5.4: Causes and laboratory data in hypernatremia

Decreased weight		Increased or Normal weight
Renal Losses	Extra-renal losses	
Nephropathy	GI losses	Exogenous Na
Diuretics use	Skin losses	Mineralcorticoid excess
Diabetes Insipidous	Respiratory	Hyperaldosteronism
Postobstructive diuresis		
Diuretic phase of ATN		
Lab data		
↑ Urine Na⁺	↓ Urine Na⁺	Relative ↓ Urine Na⁺
↑ Urine volume	↓ Urine volume	Relative ↓ Urine volume
↓ Specific gravity	↑ Specific gravity	Relative ↑ Specific gravity

excitability. Potassium exists normally in the serum in a narrow range (3.5 mEq/l - 5.5 mEq/l), thus small deviations in either direction can have disastrous consequences. Even for children who are only mildly ill, a potassium imbalance can quickly become surprisingly severe. Fortunately, potassium levels usually stay within normal limits, despite a great fluctuation in fluid and electrolyte intake. There may be a reciprocal relation between sodium and potassium: A large intake of sodium increases the loss of potassium and *vice versa*. The kidneys are the main compensatory and regulatory mechanism responsible for this hemodynamic state. Potassium is the electrolyte most affected by intestinal illness such as diarrhea.[11] Children have a reservoir of potassium in their extracellular fluid that the body uses when needed. Thus, when a drop in the serum potassium (intracellular) level is observed, the pediatric surgeon can assume the extracellular supply is gone, and the child could be headed for serious trouble. Adults are at risk for cardiac arrhythmias when their potassium levels drop below 3.5 mEq/l. However, children do not usually show cardiac symptoms until their level is below 3.0 mEq/l.

Hyperkalemia

Hyperkalemia is a dangerous electrolyte disturbance because of the potential for cardiac arrest. Hyperkalemia may result from excessive intake (particularly intravenously), changes in acid-base balance, cell destruction (releases intracellular potassium), or reduced renal excretion (such as renal failure).[12] This is summarized in Table 5.5. Hyperkalemia is a common, but poorly understood, problem in premature infants, with an incidence reported as high as 60% of all infants of very low birth weight. Signs may appear within the first 6 hours of life. Hyperkalemia may also represent an intravascular shift of potassium ions that occurs in acidosis or it may be associated with renal failure. If the serum potassium level does not decrease during rehydration, renal failure should be suspected. Signs and symptoms of hyperkalemia include tall T-waves and prolonged P-R intervals. Ventricular arrhythmias or ventricular fibrillation can occur anytime. These following measures are recommended to manage hyperkalemia:

1. Administer calcium gluconate to alter cardiac effects.
2. Decrease serum K^+ by increasing extracellular volume.
3. Decrease serum K^+ by sending it into the cells (sodium bicarbonate, insulin, glucose) and
4. Remove excessive serum K^+ (with the administration of sodium polystyrene sulfonate).

The following is the algorithm for management of hyperkalemia (Fig. 5.1).

Table 5.5: Causes of hyperkalemia		
Increased stores		Normal stores
Increased urinary K^+	Decreased urine K^+	
Blood transfusion	Congenital adrenal hyperplasia	Improper blood sampling (thin needle)
Exogenous K^+	Renal failure	Rhabdomyolysis/crush injury
	Hypoaldosteronism	Thrombocytosis
	Aldosterone insensitivity	Metabolic acidosis

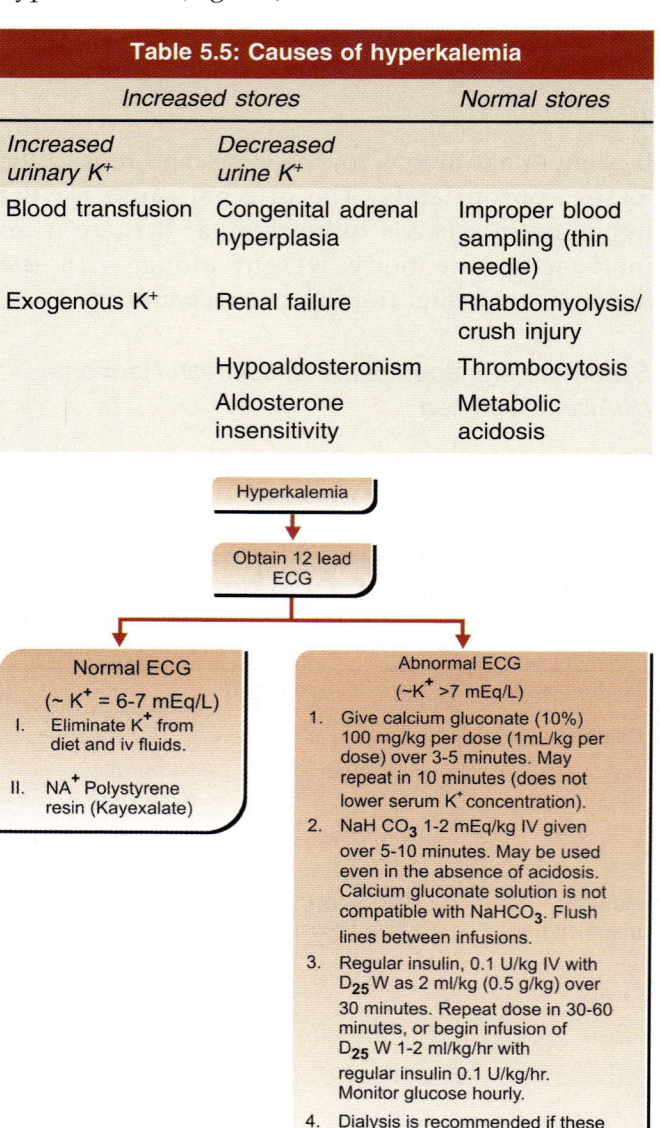

Fig. 5.1: Management of hyperkalemia in children

Hypokalemia

Hypokalemia also is a dangerous situation. Pediatric patients in danger of becoming hypokalemic are those with large gastrointestinal losses, such as from protracted vomiting, prolonged gastric suctioning, or diarrhea. Patients receiving chronic loop or thiazide diuretics also are at risk because of potassium loss. Other common causes of hypokalemia include shifts into the cell that may occur with TPN, alkalosis, or excessive secretion or administration of insulin (Table 5.6.). Signs and symptoms include thirst, malaise, muscle weakness, tremors, diminished reflexes, tachycardia, hypotension, and myocardial irritability. Treatment is the administration of potassium, either parenterally or orally. The clinical manifestations are summarized in Table 5.7.

Calcium

Infants and children are more prone to hypocalcemia than adult patients. When an infant is stressed, more growth hormone is secreted, which results in increased deposits of calcium in the bone. Because of low stores, the infant often is unable to keep up with the demand to deposit calcium in bones. The result is systemic hypocalcemia. Hypocalcemia also may be caused by acute pancreatitis, excessive infusion of citrated blood, malabsorption syndrome. Cow's milk given to newborns, alkalosis, hyperphosphatemia, hypomagnesemia, and vitamin D deficiency are also in the list. Signs and symptoms are tingling of fingers and toes, tetany, abdominal cramps, muscle cramps, and seizures. Infusions of calcium gluconate are administered to correct this electrolyte imbalance. Hypercalcemia usually is the result of immobilization, excessive use of diuretics, or malignant neoplastic disease. Signs and symptoms include constipation, dehydration, and dry mouth, polyuria, and muscle hypotonicity. Cardiac arrest is possible in severe hypercalcemia. Treatment includes decreasing the serum calcium level by administering IV fluids and promoting renal excretion. Calcium disequilibrium is summarized below.

Hypocalcemia

Hypocalcemia can be caused by pancreatitis, malabsorption states (malnutrition), hypoparathyroidism (decreased parathyroid hormone (PTH) levels or ineffective PTH response), vitamin D deficiency, hyperphosphatemia (i.e. secondary to excessive use of sodium phosphate enemas), drug therapy (anticonvulsants, cimetidine, aminoglycosides, Ca^+ - channel blockers), hypomagnesemia/hypermagnesemia, maternal hyperparathyroidism if patient is a neonate, Calcitriol (activated vitamin D) insufficiency, tumor lysis syndrome. Clinical features include — Tetany, neuromuscular irritability with weakness, paresthesias, fatigue, cramping, altered mental status, seizures, laryngospasm and cardiac dysrhythmias, ECG changes (prolonged QT interval), Trousseau's sign—carpopedal spasm after arterial occlusion of an extremity for 3 minutes and Chvostek's sign—muscle twitching with percussion of facial

Table 5.6: Causes of hypokalemia

Hypertension	Normal Blood Pressure		Normal stores
	Renal	Extrarenal	
Renovascular disease	Renal tubular acidosis	GIT losses	Metabolic alkalosis
Excess rennin	Fanconi's syndrome	Skin losses	Increased insulin
Excess Mineralocorticoid	Diabetic ketoacidosis	High carbohydrate diet	Leukemia
Cushing's syndrome	Antibiotics Diuretics	Enema abuse Malnutrition	Hypokalemic Periodic paralysis
Lab data			
↑ Urine K^+	↑ Urine K^+	↓ Urine K^+	↑ Urine K^+

Table 5.7: Clinical manifestation of potassium disturbances

Serum K^+ (mEq/L)	ECG changes	Other symptoms
~2.5	AV conduction defect, prominent U wave, ventricular dysrhythmia, ST- segment depression	Apathy, weakness, paresthesias
~7.5	Peaked T waves	Weakness, paresthesias
~8.0	Loss of P wave, widening of QRS	—
~9.0	ST-segment depression, further widening of QRS	Tetany
~10	Bradycardia, sine wave QRS, first degree AV block, ventricular dysrhythmias, cardiac arrest	—

nerve. Treatment in acute setting includes the administration of, calcium gluconate, or calcium chloride intravenously but slowly in a diluted form.

Hypercalcemia

Hypercalcemia is caused by hyperparathyroidism, vitamin D intoxication, excessive exogenous calcium administration, some malignancy cases, prolonged immobilization, with the use of some diuretics (thiazides), granulomatous disease (i.e., sarcoidosis) and hyperthyroidism. Clinical features include weakness, irritability, lethargy, seizures, coma, abdominal cramping, anorexia, nausea, vomiting, polyuria, polydipsia, renal calculi, pancreatitis and ECG changes (shortened QT interval). Management includes the following:

1. Treat the underlying disease.
2. Hydrate to increase urine output and Ca^{2+} excretion.
3. Diuresis with furosemide.
4. Consider hemodialysis for severe or refractory cases.
5. Steroids may be indicated in malignancy, granulomatous disease, and vitamin D toxicity to decease vitamin D and Ca^{2+} absorption.
6. For severe or persistently elevated Ca^{2+} give calcitonin or bisphosphonate.

Chloride

Chloride imbalances are seen as acid-base disturbances. For homeostasis, blood pH, the patient's arterial carbon dioxide tension ($PaCO_2$), and serum bicarbonate concentrations must be in balance. Any disturbance in that balance tells the body to immediately compensate. For example, a child loses a great deal of bicarbonate in diarrhea, which lowers the serum bicarbonate level. The body responds by increasing alveolar ventilation, which lowers $PaCO_2$. If the diarrhea is not severe, the blood pH will remain normal because the homeostasis-compensatory mechanism has worked.

Acid-base imbalances are classified as metabolic, respiratory, or mixed, depending on which concentration ($PaCO_2$ or bicarbonate) has been disturbed. Metabolic acidosis usually occurs in pediatric patients because they lose too much bicarbonate in diarrheal stools. High fevers or ketosis of starvation (such as failure to thrive or neoplastic disease) also cause increased metabolic rates that change the acid-base balance. Metabolic alkalosis in pediatric patients usually is related to loss of acid from vomiting or excessive gastric suction. Alkalosis is a common occurrence in children on diuretic therapy attributable to losses of Na^+, Cl^-, and water without a proportional loss of bicarbonate.

DEHYDRATION

Being alert for developing dehydration is an important aspect of caring for infants and children. Dehydration often is characterized as mild, moderate, or severe. In children, dehydration usually is attributable to vomiting or diarrhea.

The clinical signs and symptoms of classic dehydration are the result of extracellular fluid volume depletion: Hypovolemia and decreased tissue perfusion. The child usually is lethargic. Hands and feet are cold and may be cyanotic because of constriction of peripheral arterioles caused by hypovolemia. Tachycardia and other responses to hypovolemia are the body's efforts to keep cardiac output supported. Dehydrated patients occasionally are mildly febrile, although young infants may be hypothermic. Oliguria may be present, and the urine osmolality usually is high unless renal failure is present.

Types of Dehydration

Isotonic Dehydration (Isonatremic)

Electrolyte and water deficits are approximately equal. This is the most common dehydration in children and may be life threatening. The child with isotonic dehydration has signs and symptoms characteristic of hypovolemic shock.

Hypotonic Dehydration (Hyponatremia)

Electrolyte losses are greater than water losses. Hypotonic dehydration also presents with signs and symptoms of hypovolemia.

Hypertonic Dehydration (Hypernatremic)

Hypernatremic dehydration is caused by water losses that are greater than electrolyte losses or large electrolyte intake. Gastroenteritis, vomiting, and diarrhea in children usually leads to hypernatremic dehydration. Burns, high fever, diabetes insipidous, aggressive diuresis, and diabetic ketoacidosis also may produce fluid loss that is more than sodium loss. Hypernatremic dehydration also occurs in infants with diarrhea who are given fluids by mouth that contain large amounts of solute and in children receiving high protein nasogastric tube feedings that place an excessive solute load on the kidneys.

Degree of Dehydration

Treatment of dehydration is determined by the degree of the dehydration. This has be elaborated in the following section (fluid deficits).

Rehydration

Intravenous fluids remain the treatment of choice for fluid volume deficit in children as well as adults. The ability to select from different types of fluids and customize the infusion prescription to the patient's needs is a large part of ensuring positive patient outcomes. However, there is an alternative therapy for some patients after their conditions have been stabilized with IV treatments.

Oral Rehydration Solutions

Intravenous rehydration is commonly used to replace lost fluids and electrolytes. After initial stabilization, oral rehydration solutions may be used in the hospital or home setting.

Oral solutions are successful in treating many children with isotonic, hypotonic, or hypertonic dehydration. Vomiting is not a contraindication. A child who is vomiting should be given frequent, small doses of oral rehydration solutions. After successful IV rehydration, oral rehydration solutions may be used during the maintenance fluid therapy phase. Alternating an IV solution with a low-sodium fluid, such as water, breast milk, lactose-free formula or half-strength lactose containing formula, is an effective treatment plan.

Diarrhea

Generally, diarrhea is present when there is an increase in stool frequency accompanied by increased water content. The impact of diarrhea changes with its severity, duration, associated symptoms, the age of the child, and the child's nutritional status.

Chronic diarrhea usually is secondary to chronic conditions, such as malabsorption syndromes, inflammatory towel disease, immune deficiency, food allergy, lactose intolerance, and chronic, nonspecific diarrhea. Chronic diarrhea also may be the result of inadequate management of acute infectious diarrhea.

Water Intoxication (Acute Symptomatic Hyponatremia)

Water intoxication, or water overload, is observed less often than dehydration. However, it is important to be aware that water intoxication can occur and be alert of the possibility in certain situations. Infants are especially vulnerable to fluid overload. Because their thirst mechanism is not well developed, they are unable to turn off fluid intake appropriately. Decreased glomerular filtration rate prevents their immature kidneys from excreting more fluid when faced with an increased water load. Consequently, infants are unable to excrete a water overload effectively. The immediate danger of water intoxication is from brain swelling. Infants with water intoxication have a serum sodium level of less than 130 mEq/l. Hyponatremia not associated with dehydration results from an infant having too much water in proportion to sodium. The infant with water intoxication has received too much water parenterally, orally, or by enema. Another factor is a history of diarrhea. It is not unusual to discover that the infant has been given inappropriate fluids {such as dilute low-solute formulas, water, juices, tea, or soft drinks} to keep the infant from become dehydrated. Water intoxication also can occur during acute IV fluid overloading, too rapid dialysis, or with too rapid reduction of glucose levels in diabetic ketoacidosis. Administration of improperly prepared formula is another common cause of water intoxication. Families who cannot afford to buy formula may dilute the formula to increase the volume or may substitute water for the formula. In addition, water sometimes is used for pacification. Water intoxication may occur in infants who receive overly vigorous hydration during a febrile illness.

When we order for fluids for a patient, we have to make sure that we answer the following three questions:
1. How much fluid to give?
2. What fluid to give?
3. How to give?

HOW MUCH FLUID TO GIVE?

This depends on the maintenance requirements and the deficits.

Maintenance Requirements

Maintenance requirements stem from basal metabolism. Metabolism produces two by-products: Heat and Solute. Most by-products are taken out of the body. Heat dissipation through insensible losses and solute excretion in urine each can be considered as representing 50% of maintenance needs. In the management of children who have anuric renal failure, maintenance fluid needs decrease by 50% because the only fluids that need to be replaced are insensible losses. This can be calculated by the following methods.

Holiday and Segar Method

The Holliday and Segar method (Table 5.8) estimated caloric expenditure in fixed weight categories; it assumes that for each 100 calories metabolized, 100 mL of H_2O will be required. For each 100 kcal expended, about 50 mL of fluid is required to provide for skin, respiratory tract, and basal stool losses, and 55-65 ml of fluid is required for the kidneys to excrete an ultra-filtrate of plasma at 300 mOsmL without having to concentrate the urine. This method is not suitable for neonates. It generally overestimates fluid needs in neonates compared with the caloric expenditure method.

Caloric Expenditure Method

The caloric expenditure method is based on the understanding that water and electrolyte requirements more accurately parallel caloric expenditure. For this standard basal calorie (SBC) expenditure as approximated by resting energy expenditure is calculated, and then adjustments by various factors (e.g. fever, activity) is done. For each 100 calories metabolized in 24 hours, the average patient will need 100-120 mL H_2O, 2-4 mEq Na^+, and 2-3 mEq K^+.

Body Surface Area (BSA) Method

The BSA method is based on the assumption that caloric expenditure is related to body surface area. It is not recommended for infants. In this method, water requirements are 1500 $mL/m^2/24$ hr, Na^+ requirements are 30-50 $mEq/m^2/24$ hr and K^+ requirements are 20-40 $mEq/m^2/24hr$. The surface are can be calculated by the following formula:

Surface area = [4w + 7] divided by [w + 90]

Approximately the following chart depicts the surface area for the various weight measurements:

Surface Area Simplified

0.3 kg	=	0.2 sq m
10 kg	=	0.5 sq m
30 kg	=	1.0 sq m
50 kg	=	1.5 sq m
60 kg	=	1.65 sq m
70 kg	=	1.75 sq m
80 kg	=	1.85 sq m
90 kg	=	1.95 sq m
100 kg	=	2.05 sq m

Since the calculation of surface area in the ward on the weight basis is difficult, a method has been evolved to administer fluid based only on weight. Hence Holliday and Segar method is the most popular method to calculate the fluid requirements.

Table 5.8: Holliday and Segar method of fluid requirement estimation

Body weight	ml/kg/day	ml/kg/hr
First 10 kg	100	4
Second 10 kg	50	2
Each additional kg	20	1

For example, the correct fluid requirement of a child of 10 years old with a body weight of 25 kg would be :
For the first 10 kg = 10 × 4 ml/h = 40 ml/h
Plus
For the second 10 kg = 10×2 ml/h = 20 ml/h
Plus
For the last 5 kg = 5×1 ml/h = 5 ml/h
So, the total would be 40 +20+5 = 65 ml/h

Deficits

Assessment of the deficits may be done my calculated assessment and clinical assessment. To this the ongoing losses need to be added up.

Calculated Assessment

The most precise method of assessing fluid deficit is based on preillness weight:

Fluid deficit (L) = Preillness weight (kg) - Present weight (kg)

Percentage of dehydration = [(preillness weight illness weight)/pre illness weight] × 100%

If the accurate weight is not known, the clinical observation as described below is used.

Clinical Assessment

This requires a good clinical examination. Table 5.9 elaborates this.

Table 5.9: Correlation of degree of dehydration with clinical assessment

Examination	Older child		
	3% (30 ml/kg)	6% (60 ml/kg)	9% (90 ml/kg)
	Infant		
	5% (50 ml/kg)	10% (100 ml/kg)	15% (150 ml/kg)
Dehydration	Mild	Moderate	Severe
Skin turgor	Normal	Tenting	None
Skin (touch)	Normal	Dry	Clammy
Buccal mucosa/lips	Moist	Dry	Parched/Cracked
Eyes	Normal	Deep Set	Sunken
Tears	Present	Reduced	None
Fontanelle	Flat	Soft	Sunken
CNS	Consolable	Irritable	Lethargic/Obtunded
Pulse rate	Normal	Slightly/Increased	Increased
Pulse quality	Normal	Weak	Feeble/Impalpable
Capillary refill	Normal	2 sec	More than 3 sec
Urine output	Normal	Decreased	Anuria

Ongoing Losses

In pediatric surgical practice, this constitutes an important component of the fluid calculations. The following table (Table 5.10) would give an idea about the losses and this needs to kept in mind during the calculation.

Role of ECF and ICF

Na^+ deficit is the amount of Na^+ that was lost from the Na^+ containing ECF compartment during the dehydration period. Na^+ deficit (mEq) = fluid deficit (L) × proportion from ECF × Na^+ concentration (mEq/L) in ECF. (Intracellular Na^+ is negligible as a proportion of total; therefore, it can be disregarded).

K^+ deficit is the amount of K^+ that was lost from the K^+ containing ICF compartment during the dehydration period. K^+ deficit (mEq) = fluid deficit (L) × proportion from ICF × K^+ concentration (mEq/L) in ICF. (Extracellular K^+ is negligible as a proportion of total; therefore it can be disregarded).

Role of Distribution Factor

Electrolyte deficits (in excess of ECF/ICF electrolyte losses).

$$mEq\ required = (CD - CP) \times fd \times wt$$

where, CD = concentration desired (mEq/L), CP = concentration present (mEq/L), Fd = distribution factor as fraction of body weight (L/kg).

The FD of HCO_3 is 0.4 - 0.5, Cl^- is 0.2 - 0.3 and Na^+ × 0.6 - 0.7.

WHAT FLUID TO GIVE ?

Fluids are classified into:
1. Electrolytes such as NaCl, KCl, $NaHCO_3$, $CaCl_2$.

Table 5.10: Electrolyte composition of various body fluids

Fluid	Na^+ (mEq/l)	K^+ (mEq/l)	Cl^- (mEq/l)
Gastric	20-80	5-20	100-150
Pancreatic	120-140	5-15	90-120
Small bowel	100-140	5-15	90-130
Bile	120-140	5-15	80-120
Ileostomy	45-135	3-15	20-115
Diarrhea	10-90	10-80	10-110
Burns	140	5	110

2. Non-electrolytes like glucose, fructose, and mannitol.

Electrolytes are solutions which contain electrically charged particles and they are always in electroneutrality. The positively charged ions (Ca^+ ions) are equivalent to the negatively charged ions (anions). For example, 0.9% NaCl has Na: 154 mEq/L and Cl:154 mEq/L. Blood is an electrolyte and its major biochemical parameters pertinent to this chapter are tabulated in Table 5.2.

Chemical substances can also be expressed as milli moles. A mole is atomic weight in grams. A milli mole is one thousandth of a mole. In a monovalent ion like sodium one millimole is equivalent to one milli equivalent. In a bivalent ion like calcium one milli mole is equivalent to 2 milli equivalents.

In the SI system of units the concentration of substances of known and exact composition will be expressed as moles/liter where as substances of ill defined composition such as protein will continue to be expressed by weight in milligrams/liter (Table 5.11).

Tonicity of Solutions

A solution is described as isotonic or iso-osmotic if it has the same tonicity or osmolality of the blood. For example, 0.9% NaCl is isotonic with blood. However, it is not physiological since it contains more chloride than the blood.

	Na	Cl
Blood	142 mEq	102 mEq/L
0.9% NaCl	154 mEq	154 mEq/L

Table 5.11: Conversion to SI units

Plasma concentration	Old	New
Calcium	10 mg/dl	2.5 mmol/L
Magnesium	1 mEq/L	0.5 mmol/L
Sodium	140 mEq/L	140 mmol/L
Chloride	100 mEq/L	100 mmol/L
Bilirubin	1 mg/dl	18 mmol/L
Urea	10 mg/dl	3.6 mmol
Creatinine	1 mg/dl	88 mmol/L
Glucose	100 mg/dl	5.5 mmol/L

There is a balance of chlorides and bicarbonates in the blood. If the chloride level goes up as in Hyperchloremic acidosis, the bicarbonate level comes down. Hence administration of large amounts of 0.9 NaCl to patients who lose more chlorides than sodium in diarrhea develop hyperchloremic acidosis. Ringer's lactate solution on the other hand is physiological. The chloride content is only 102 mEq/L and bicarbonates are formed from metabolization of lactate ions.

The composition of various well known fluids is shown in Table 5.12.

It is preferable to use acetate salt than lactate as acetate ions are metabolized at the peripheral tissues and muscles. They require less oxygen for metabolism into CO_2 and bicarbonate ions. This is important especially if shock is present. In Ringer's lactate a part of the lactate is converted into glycogen by the liver hence the available bicarbonate is less. Ringer's Lactate is superior to isotonic saline and acetated ringer is preferable to lactated ringers solution. In shock 0.9% normal saline mixed with sodabicarbonate can also be used. Multiple electrolyte solutions are now available in the market like Isolyte P. (Pediatric maintenance) Isolyte M, Isolyte G and Isolyte R. It is necessary to make sure what they contain. Salient features of these are noted below.[13-16]

Isolyte M (half isotonic): Contains Na 40 mEq/l, K 35 mEq/l. It is a potassium rich solution. Isolyte P is one-third isotonic and sodium poor solution. It contains 26 mEq of Na per liter of solution. Normal saline, 0.9% NaCl, has more chlorides than chlorides-in the blood.

Ringer's Lactate (Isotonic)

Lactate has to be metabolized to bicarbonate, it has low potassium. Unless specified it does not contain any sugar-glucose.

Isolyte G

Gastric replacement solution has an acidifying solution containing ammonium chloride as the acidifying salt. NH_4Cl is contraindicated in patients with cirrhosis liver or any liver dysfunction, azotemia, congestive cardiac failure. It can precipitate metabolic acidosis if given in large amounts. Most often Isolyte G is given for metabolic alkalosis which can be treated better by sodium chloride and potassium chloride solutions.

Fluid and Electrolytes in Pediatric Surgery

Table 5.12: Composition of frequently used parenteral fluids

Liquid	CHO (gm/100 mL)	Protein (gm/100 mL)	Cal/L	Na^+ (mEq/L)	K^+ (mEq/L)	Cl^- (mEq/L)	HCO_3^- (mEq/L)	Ca^{2+} (mEq/L)	MOsm/L (mEq/L)
D5 W	5	–	170	–	–	–	–	–	252
D10 W	10	–	340	–	–	–	–	–	505
NS (0.9% NaCl)	–	–	–	154	–	154	–	–	308
½ NS (0.45% NaCl)	–	–	–	77	–	77	–	–	154
D5 ¼ NS (0.225% NaCl)	5	–	170	34	–	34	–	–	329
3% NaCl	–	–	–	513	–	513	–	–	1027
8.4% sodium bicarbonate	–	–	–	1000	–	–	1000	–	2000
Ringer solution	0-10	–	0-340	147	4	155.5	–	4	
Lactated Ringer	0-10	–	0-340	130	4	109	28	3	273
Amino acid 8.5%	–	8.5	340	3	–	34	52	–	880
Albumin 25% (salt poor)	–	25	1000	100-160	–	<120	–	–	300
Intralipid	2.25	–	1100	2.5	0.5	4.0	–	–	258-284

In actual practice Isolyte G is used as the gastric replacement fluid when the gastric aspirate is bile stained. Bile is an alkaline solution and isolyte G which is an acid solution should not be used as the replacement solution.

Potassium Containing Solutions

The commercially available ampoules are 15% KCl. It is highly concentrated solution and unless it is adequately diluted it can kill the patient. Each ml provides 2 mEq of K and 2 mEq of chloride. 2 ml of the above solution diluted with 100 ml of dextrose or normal saline will give a concentration of 40 mEq/liter and is the safe limit. At no time the concentration of the K in the solution should exceed 80 mEq/liter (40 ml of 15% KCl in 1000 ml) but even this concentration has to be given under strict monitoring of the vital functions. The safe limit is 40 mEq/liter (20 ml of 15% KCl in 1000 ml of fluid). The isolyte M gives 40 mEq/liter of K and is one of the potassium rich solutions available in the market within the safe limits of administration. The basic rule is even in severe hypokalemia, not more than 20 mEq of K should be given in an hour.

Alkaline Solutions

Sodium bicarbonate is available in the market as a hypertonic solution. It is available as 7.5% solution and should be used adequately diluted. One-sixth molar (isotonic) sodium lactate can be used instead of bicarbonate if there is no fluid restriction in the administration of fluids. However, the lactate has to be metabolized into bicarbonate in the liver and hence cannot be used in liver dysfunction or in shock, since the metabolism of the lactic acid is impaired. THAM (Tromethamine) has been used in metabolic acidosis. It is an amino alcohol and has side effects if large amounts are used. It can produce severe hypoglycemia, hyperkalemia and is not available in India.

Amongst the volume expenders that are available pooled plasma is a good physiological expander. However, it carries the risk of hepatitis unless it is stored at 34°C for six months. Plasmonate contains human plasma protein fraction and heat treated to destroy the hepatitis virus. Patients with low serum albumin level can be treated with albumin containing solutions which are salt free. Dextrose 5% in water if used as volume expander, it will be distributed evenly in all ICF and ECF. Three liters of 5% dextrose will be needed to expand the ECF by one liter. One liter of isotonic saline will expand the ECF by one liter. But because of their relative size one liter of isotonic saline will expand the plasma volume by one quarter of liter. Plasma, whole blood or plasma expanders—all these will expand the plasma volume by one liter. Albumin is also a plasma expander but diffuses into interstitial fluid in clinical practice.

PREOPERATIVE FLUID NEEDS

During surgery, isotonic fluids are the most preferred and recommended fluids. For minor procedures 6 ml/kg/h, for moderate procedures, 8 ml/kg/h and for major procedures 10-15 ml/kg/h is the fluid recommended.[17]

HOW TO GIVE FLUIDS?

This is very important in fluid administration of neonates or when the fluid used is diluents to give certain drugs like dopamine. One conventional drop is equivalent to 4 micro drops. Algorithm for dehydration correction is shown below (Fig. 5.2).

ACID-BASE DISTURBANCES

Introduction

An acid is a hydrogen ion donor where as a base is hydrogen ion acceptor. The strength of an acid depends on the concentration of hydrogen ions and the degree with which is dissociates. The hydrogen ion power is expressed as pH (Puissance hydrogen).

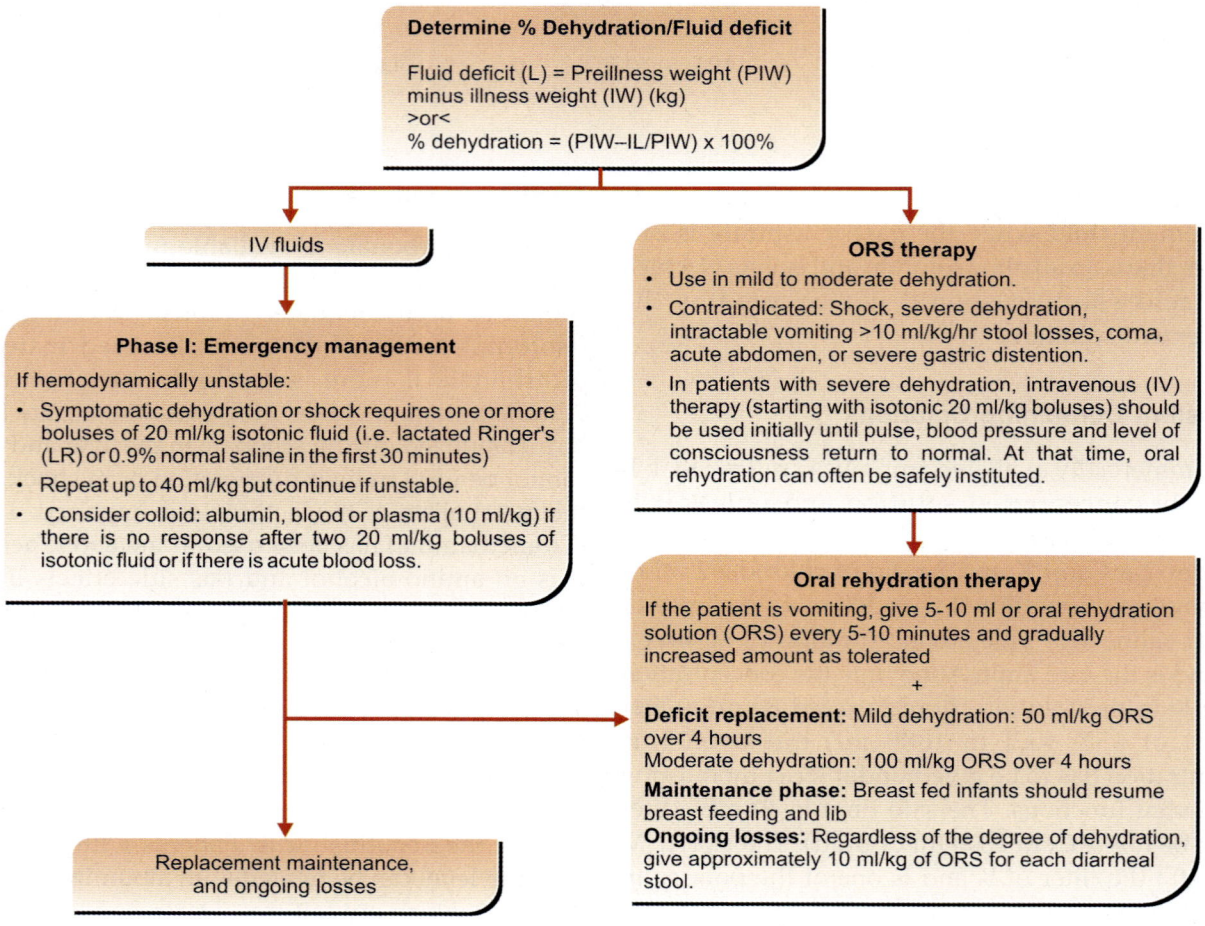

Fig. 5.2: Algorithm for dehydration correction

Table 5.13: Relationship between pH and hydrogen ion concentration	
pH	Hydrogen ion concentration
7.0	100
7.1	80
7.4	40
7.7	20

Blood pH

Normal range of plasma pH is 7.36 - 7.44. The extreme range of pH compatible with life is 6.7 - 7.9. It is acidosis if the pH is below 7.36 and it is alkalosis if the pH is above 7.44.

pH Calculation

pH = [6.1 + log (HCO_3)] divided by [H_2CO_3 + CO_2)]

This can be rewritten by stating that the pH is equivalent to the bicarbonate–carbonic acid ratio. Relationship of pH and hydrogen ion concentration expressed as nanomole. Since hydrogen ion concentration in the plasma is very small it is measured in terms of nano equivalents (or nanomole). The following table gives the values of Hydrogen ion concentrations at different pH (Table 5.13). It will be observed from the Table that the hydrogen ion concentration is 40 nanomole at 7.4 pH of the blood. But it increases two fold when the pH is 7.1 (80 nanomole). But similar increase in pH-7.7 does not reduce the hydrogen ion. It is obvious that the changes in hydrogen ion concentration are profound in acidosis.[18,19]

Chemical and Physiological Regulation of the pH of Body

The following mechanisms regulate the acid base balance:
1. Chemical buffers (immediate).
2. Respiratory buffers (slow).
3. Renal buffers (slowest).

Chemical buffers react with strong acids and bases formed within the body or which enter the body. The three buffers are :
1. Bicarbonate carbonic acid system.
2. The phosphate buffer system.
3. Protein and hemoglobin buffer system.

The respiratory buffer system deals primarily with the carbon dioxide elimination and regulation which in turn determines the blood carbonic acid. The partial pressure of the CO_2 is one of important parameters in acid base status of the individual. The kidneys are the most important buffering mechanism and not only compensate the buffering deficiencies in the chemical and respiratory system but it also eliminates certain acids that cannot be buffered by other systems like sulphuric and phosphoric acids produced by the protein catabolism.

Base Excess

This represents the amount of strong base or acid per liter of blood which has been added as a result of metabolic disturbances. This describes the presence of an excess base or a deficit of base. Positive values indicate an excess of base negative values indicate a deficit of base. The normal value for base excess is 0 (+2.5 to –2.5) mEq /L.

Standard Bicarbonate

Standard bicarbonate represents the concentration in plasma of blood which has been equilibrated at PCO_2 of 40 mm of Hg with oxygen to saturate the hemoglobin. The normal value s of standard bicarbonate is 24 mEq/l. If actual bicarbonate is higher than standard bicarbonate it will indicates respiratory acidosis. If f actual bicarbonate is lower than standard bicarbonate it will indicate respiratory alkalosis.

Disturbances in Acid-Base Balance

1. Respiratory acidosis (that is, ventilatory failure). The drop in pH is explained by the change in $PaCO_2$.
2. Respiratory alkalosis (that is, alveolar hyperventilation)-the decreased $PaCO_2$ explains the increased pH.
3. Metabolic acidosis: Reduced pH not explained by increased $PaCO_2$. It is usually associated with an increased anion gap due to the accumulation of renal acids, lactic acids, and ketoacids (from diabetes or starvation).
4. Metabolic alkalosis: Raised pH out of proportion to changes in $PaCO_2$. It is associated with hypokalemia, volume contraction, or exogenous alkali administration.

Relation between pH and PaCO$_2$

Acute changes in PaCO$_2$ result in predictable changes in pH (the negative log of hydrogen ion concentration) and plasma carbonic acid. This represents the respiratory acid base change. Although the relation is not completely linear, within clinically relevant ranges it is sufficiently linear to allow the following guideline to estimate the degrees of abnormality resulting from acute changes in PaCO$_2$:

For every increase in PaCO$_2$ of 20 mm Hg (2.6 kPa) above normal the pH falls by 0.1.

For every decrease of PaCO$_2$ of 10 mm Hg (1.3 kPa) below normal the pH rises by 0.1. Any change in pH outside these parameters is therefore, metabolic in origin.

Anion Gap Concept

Cells exist in a state of electroneutrality with major and minor cations balanced by similar anions. The anion gap is an artificial disparity between the concentrations of the major plasma cations and anions routinely measured–normally sodium, chloride, and bicarbonate. The anion gap is calculated as Na$^+$(Cl$^-$ +HCO$_3^-$).

The anion gap is normally 8-16 mmol/l, of which 11 mmol/l is typically due to albumin. A decreased anion gap is usually caused by hypoalbuminemia or severe hemodilution. Less commonly, it occurs as a result of an increase in minor cation concentrations such as in hypercalcemia or hypermagnesemia. Increased anion gap acidosis is caused by dehydration and by any process that increases the concentrations of the minor anions, lactate, ketones, and renal acids, along with treatment with drugs given as organic salts such as penicillin, salicylates, and with methanol and ethylene glycol. Rarely an increased anion gap may result from decreased minor cation concentrations such as calcium and magnesium. Metabolic acidosis without an increased anion gap is typically associated with an increase in plasma chloride concentrations; chloride ions replace plasma bicarbonate. Hyperchloremic acidosis is usually caused by gastrointestinal loss or renal wasting of bicarbonate.

Definitions

Serum Osmolality

Number of particles per liter. Can be calculated as follows:

2 [Na$^+$] + glucose (mg/dL)/18 + BUN (mg/dL)/2.8

Normal range: 275-295 mOsm/L.

Serum Osmolar Gap

Calculated serum osmolality - laboratory measured osmolality.

May be elevated in some anion gap acidosis, but a markedly elevated osmolar gap in the setting of an anion gap acidosis is highly suggestive of acute methanol or ethylene glycol intoxication.

Anion gap (AG)

Represents anions other than bicarbonate and chloride required to balance the positive charge of Na$^+$, K$^+$ is considered negligible in AG calculations. Clinically, it is calculated as follows:

AG = Na$^+$ - (Cl$^-$ + HCO$_3^-$)
(Normal: 12 mEq/L ± 2 mEq/L)

Rules for Determining Primary Acid-Base Disorders

1. *Determine the pH:* The body does not fully compensate for primary acid-base disorders; therefore, the primary disturbance will shift the pH away from 7.40. Examine the pCO$_2$ and HCO$_3$ to determine whether the primary disturbance is a metabolic acidosis/alkalosis or respiratory acidosis/alkalosis.
2. Calculate the anion gap: if the anion gap is > 20 mmol/L, there is a primary metabolic acidosis regardless of pH or serum bicarbonate concentration (The body does not generate a large anion gap to compensate for a primary disorder).
3. Calculate the excess anion Gap (i.e. "ΔGap" or "Gap-Gap"):

ΔGap = [calculated anion gap - normal anion gap (i.e., 12) mmol/L] + measured HCO$_3^-$.

If the ΔGap is greater than a normal serum bicarbonate concentration (>30 mmol/L), there is an underlying metabolic alkalosis.

If the ΔGap is less than a normal bicarbonate concentration (< 23 mmol/L), there is an underlying nonunion gap metabolic acidosis (1 mmol of unmeasured acid titrates 1 mmol of bicarbonate) (+Δ anion gap = –Δ [HCO$_3^-$])

All this is summarized in the Flow chart (Fig. 5.3.)

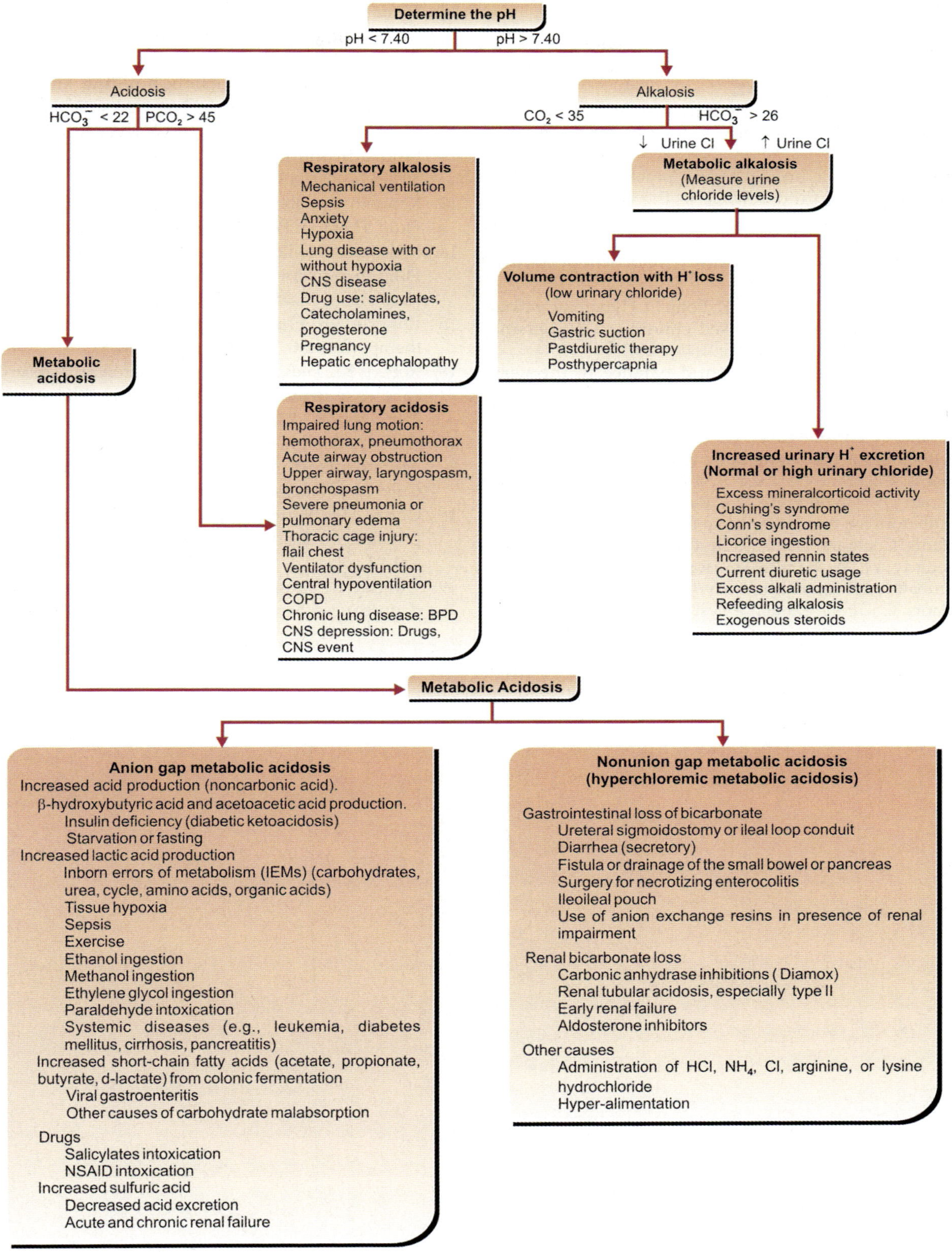

Fluid and Electrolytes in Pediatric Surgery

```
                        Determine the pH
                    pH < 7.40      pH > 7.40
                    ┌──────────────────────┐
                    ▼                      ▼
                Acidosis                Alkalosis
            HCO₃⁻ < 22 | PCO₂ > 45      CO₂ < 35 | HCO₃⁻ > 26
                                          ↓ Urine Cl    ↑ Urine Cl
```

Respiratory alkalosis
- Mechanical ventilation
- Sepsis
- Anxiety
- Hypoxia
- Lung disease with or without hypoxia
- CNS disease
- Drug use: salicylates, Catecholamines, progesterone
- Pregnancy
- Hepatic encephalopathy

Metabolic alkalosis
(Measure urine chloride levels)

Volume contraction with H⁺ loss
(low urinary chloride)
- Vomiting
- Gastric suction
- Pastdiuretic therapy
- Posthypercapnia

Metabolic acidosis

Respiratory acidosis
- Impaired lung motion: hemothorax, pneumothorax
- Acute airway obstruction
- Upper airway, laryngospasm, bronchospasm
- Severe pneumonia or pulmonary edema
- Thoracic cage injury: flail chest
- Ventilator dysfunction
- Central hypoventilation
- COPD
- Chronic lung disease: BPD
- CNS depression: Drugs, CNS event

Increased urinary H⁺ excretion
(Normal or high urinary chloride)
- Excess mineralcorticoid activity
- Cushing's syndrome
- Conn's syndrome
- Licorice ingestion
- Increased rennin states
- Current diuretic usage
- Excess alkali administration
- Refeeding alkalosis
- Exogenous steroids

Metabolic Acidosis

Anion gap metabolic acidosis
Increased acid production (noncarbonic acid).
  β-hydroxybutyric acid and acetoacetic acid production.
    Insulin deficiency (diabetic ketoacidosis)
    Starvation or fasting
Increased lactic acid production
    Inborn errors of metabolism (IEMs) (carbohydrates, urea, cycle, amino acids, organic acids)
    Tissue hypoxia
    Sepsis
    Exercise
    Ethanol ingestion
    Methanol ingestion
    Ethylene glycol ingestion
    Paraldehyde intoxication
    Systemic diseases (e.g., leukemia, diabetes mellitus, cirrhosis, pancreatitis)
Increased short-chain fatty acids (acetate, propionate, butyrate, d-lactate) from colonic fermentation
    Viral gastroenteritis
    Other causes of carbohydrate malabsorption
Drugs
    Salicylates intoxication
    NSAID intoxication
Increased sulfuric acid
    Decreased acid excretion
    Acute and chronic renal failure

Nonunion gap metabolic acidosis
(hyperchloremic metabolic acidosis)

Gastrointestinal loss of bicarbonate
    Ureteral sigmoidostomy or ileal loop conduit
    Diarrhea (secretory)
    Fistula or drainage of the small bowel or pancreas
    Surgery for necrotizing enterocolitis
    Ileoileal pouch
    Use of anion exchange resins in presence of renal impairment
Renal bicarbonate loss
    Carbonic anhydrase inhibitions (Diamox)
    Renal tubular acidosis, especially type II
    Early renal failure
    Aldosterone inhibitors
Other causes
    Administration of HCl, NH₄, Cl, arginine, or lysine hydrochloride
    Hyper-alimentation

Fig. 5.3: Flow chart for determination of primary acid-base disorders

REFERENCES

1. Aggarwal R, Deorari AK, Paul VK. Fluid and electrolyte management in term and preterm neonates. Indian J Pediatr 2001;68(12):1139-42.
2. Friedman AL. Pediatric hydration therapy: historical review and a new approach. Kidney Int 2005;67(1):380-88.
3. Hartnoll G. Basic principles and practical steps in the management of fluid balance in the newborn. Semin Neonatol 2003;8(4):307-13.
4. Barcelona SL, Coté CJ. Pediatric resuscitation in the operating room. Anesthesiol Clin North America. 2001;19(2):339-65.
5. Choong K, Kho ME, Menon K, Bohn D. Hypotonic versus isotonic saline in hospitalised children: A systematic review. Arch Dis Child 2006;91(10):828-35.
6. Modi N. Management of fluid balance in the very immature neonate. Arch Dis Child Fetal Neonatal Ed 2004;89(2):F108-11.
7. Flenady VJ, Woodgate PG. Radiant warmers versus incubators for regulating body temperature in newborn infants. Cochrane Database Syst Rev 2000;(2):CD000435.
8. Flenady VJ, Woodgate PG. Radiant warmers versus incubators for regulating body temperature in newborn infants. Cochrane Database Syst Rev 2003;(4):CD000435.
9. Flenady VJ, Woodgate PG. Radiant warmers versus incubators for regulating body temperature in newborn infants. Cochrane Database Syst Rev 2002;(2):CD000435.
10. Trimarchi T. Endocrine problems in critically ill children: An overview. AACN Clin Issues 2006;17(1):66-78.
11. de Silva NT, Young JA, Wales PW. Understanding neonatal bowel obstruction: building knowledge to advance practice. Neonatal Netw 2006;25(5):303-18.
12. Moghal NE, Embleton ND. Management of acute renal failure in the newborn. Semin Fetal Neonatal Med 2006;11(3):207-13.
13. Kenneth B, Roberts. Fluid and Electrolytes: Parenteral Fluid Therapy. Pediatrics in Review 2001;22:380-87.
14. Malcolm A Holliday1, Patricio E Ray, Aaron L Friedman. Fluid therapy for children: Facts, fashions and questions. Archives of Disease in Childhood 2007;92:546-50.
15. Roberts KB. Fluid and electrolytes: parenteral fluid therapy. Pediatr Rev 2001;22(11):380-87.
16. Roberts KE. Pediatric fluid and electrolyte balance: Critical care case studies. Crit Care Nurs Clin North Am 2005;17(4):361-73.
17. Paut O, Lacroix F. Recent developments in the perioperative fluid management for the paediatric patient. Curr Opin Anaesthesiol 2006;19(3):268-77.
18. Corey HE. Bench-to-bedside review: Fundamental principles of acid-base physiology. Crit Care 2005;9(2):184-92.
19. Quigley R, Baum M. Neonatal acid base balance and disturbances. Semin Perinatol 2004;28(2):97-102.

CHAPTER 6

Shock in Children— Surgeon's Perspective

DK Gupta, Archana Puri

The clinical syndrome of shock is one of the most life threatening problems faced by the treating doctor in the critical care unit. Shock is an acute complex state of circulatory dysfunction that results due to the discrepancy in oxygen need and supply. The metabolic demands of body are not met leading to multiple organ failure and death. Although untreated shock carries a very high mortality, yet with early diagnosis and prompt management, the mortality is considerably reduced.

PATHOPHYSIOLOGY

Normal circulatory function is maintained by the complex interplay between cardiac output and systemic vascular resistance. Cardiac output is the most important determinant of tissue perfusion. Delivery of oxygen to tissue (DO_2) is a direct function of cardiac output and arterial oxygen content CaO_2.[1]

$$DO_2 = CO \times CaO_2$$

Where CO = HR × SV (HR-heart rate, SV-stroke volume)

$$CaO_2 = (Hgb \times 1.39 \times SaO_2) + (0.003 \times PaO_2)$$

Thus inadequate oxygen delivery can result from either limitation or misdistribution of blood flow or due to increased oxygen demand (fever, sepsis etc). When oxygen delivery fails to meet cellular oxygen demands, patient goes in a state of shock and various compensatory mechanisms are activated. There are three phases of shock, namely:
a. Compensated
b. Uncompensated
c. Irreversible.

Compensated Shock

In compensated shock, vital organ function is maintained by various intrinsic hemostatic mechanisms. Hence, blood pressure, cardiac function and urine output may appear to be normal. Thus, early stages of all types of shock may be difficult to identify and requires a high index of clinical suspicion.

The compensatory mechanisms aim to increase the intravascular volume and blood pressure. Various compensatory mechanisms are triggered by the baroreceptors, chemoreceptors and by renin angiotensin system (RAS).

Baroreceptors

Stretch receptors are located in the atria and in the carotids. The carotid sinuses, aortic arch receptors, receptors in the walls of right and left atria (at the entrance of the superior and inferior venae cava) and in the pulmonary circulation, monitor the arterial circulation. They are stimulated by distension of these structures in which they are located and so they discharge at increased rate when the pressure in these structures rises. Their afferent fibers pass via the glossopharyngeal and vagus nerves to the medulla. Most of them end in the nucleus of the tractus solitarius (NTS), and the excitatory transmitter they secrete is probably glutamate.[2] Impulses generated by stimulation of baroreceptors excite the vagal innervation of the heart, producing vasodilatation, bradycardia and decrease in cardiac output. Hypotension causes decreased in stretching of these receptors leading to diminished firing of impulses which results in increased sympathetic activity and decreased vagal discharge of heart.

Increased sympathetic discharge causes increased cardiac contractility and vasoconstriction starting from small venules, veins and progressing to arterioles of skin, subcutaneous fat, muscle, splanchnic vessels and kidney. The vessels last to be affected are those of heart and brain.

Chemoreceptors

Chemoreceptors are located in the carotid and aortic bodies. Afferents from the chemoreceptors exert their main effect on respiration, but they also have affect on vasomotor area. Shock leads to tissue anoxia due to inadequate local perfusion, thereby stimulating the chemoreceptors. The cardiovascular response to chemoreceptor stimulation consists of peripheral vasoconstriction.

Renin Angiotensin Aldosterone System (RAAS)

Renal hypoperfusion, in shock leads to stimulation of renin angiotensin aldosterone system (RAAS), as shown in Figure 6.1.

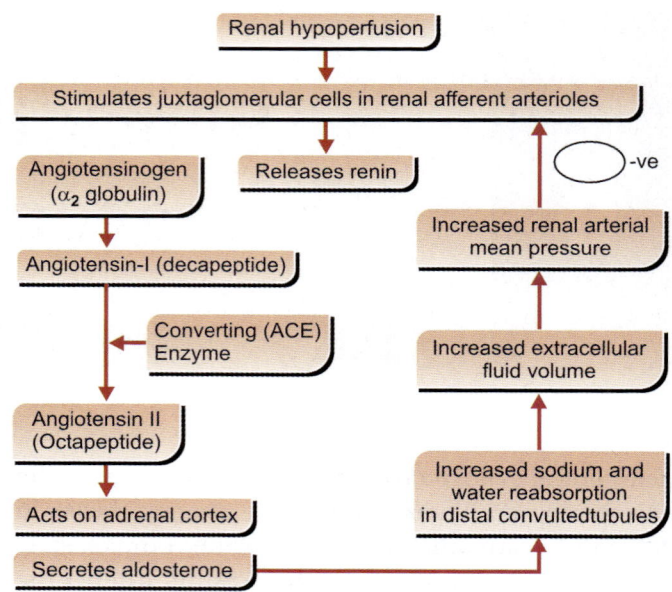

Fig. 6.1: Stimulation of RAAS

Decompensated Shock

If these early compensatory mechanisms are not enough, shock progresses on to a decompensated state. In uncompensated shock the effects of cellular ischemia with associated release of vasoactive and inflammatory mediators begins to affect the microcirculation and the child shows sign of brain, kidney and cardiovascular compromise.

Irreversible Shock

Terminal or irreversible shock implies damage to the vital organs of such magnitude has occurred, that death occurs even if therapy returns cardiovascular measurement to normal levels.

PATHOGENESIS AND MULTISYSTEM EFFECT OF SHOCK

Shock is a multisystem disease. Initially the body tries to compensate it by various mechanisms as mentioned earlier. If, however, intravascular volume loss, surpasses the body's compensatory mechanisms, then decompensation appears with profound ischemia and anaerobic metabolism.

Due to anaerobic metabolism and hypoxia the capillary endothelium gets damaged with exudation of proteins and fluids from circulation. This not only worsens the state of hypovolemia but also stimulate microcirculatory dysfunction, release of biochemical and vasoactive mediators, leading to multiple organ failure and death.[3] Mortality in shock has been related to multiple organ system involvement. Lung, kidney, GIT and heart are the most common organs to be involved initially. If one system is involved mortality is 30-50%, with 2 system involvement it increases to 50-60%, with 3 systems involvement it rises further to 60-80% and with 4 or > systems more than four involvement, mortality is 100%.[4]

Microcirculatory dysfunction is common to all type of shock. It is characterized by maldistribution of capillary blood flow, altered capillary permeability and mechanical obstruction of capillary beds with cellular debris (aggregation of platelets and granulocytes). Anaerobic metabolism in shock leads to accumulation of lactic acid. The resultant metabolic acidosis causes efflux of intracellular potassium into ECF (leading to hyperkalemia) and an influx of sodium and calcium with an obligate influx of water into the cells. This cellular swelling further potentiates the cellular dysfunction.

Biochemical Mediators in Shock

Biochemical mediators play an important role in the development and continuation of all types of shock. These vasoactive mediators are usually endogenous (host derived), primarily from cells of nervous and hemopoetic system. In septic shock these mediators are released in response to exposure to microbial products (e.g. endotoxin) and play a primary role in initiating shock. In hypovolemic and cardiogenic shock, they are released secondarily in response to ischemic cellular injury.

These biochemical mediators are vasoactive and exert their effect by induction of severe vasoconstriction and vasospasm, induction of platelet aggregation, increased capillary permeability and thrombus formation, as shown in Table 6.1.

Inflammatory Mediators in Shock

Endogenous inflammatory mediators are the major culprits in the pathogenesis of septic shock. The most potent stimulus for the activation of the inflammatory cascade is the outer cell membrane of gram-negative bacteria, *lipopolysaccharide antigen* also called endotoxin. Once in blood stream the LPS, attaches to a plasma protein called LPS binding protein (LBP). This complex LPS-LPB binds to CD14 receptors on the surface of monocytes/macrophages which leads to stimulation of tumor necrosis factor (TNF) and interleukin 1 (IL-1). TNF is capable of inducing a broad range of vasoactive and inflammatory mediators. Treatment of shock with anti-TNF antibodies has been attempted with mixed results. The various inflammatory mediators in shock are as described in Table 6.2.[3]

Nitric Oxide

Literature reports increased level of nitric oxide in circulatory shock. After exposure to TNF and IL1 variety of cells like macrophages, vascular endothelium, vascular smooth muscle, hepatocyte and cardiac myocytes are induced to produce increased nitric oxide. Nitric oxide causes vasodilatation, vascular hyporesponsiveness and hypotension. Trials are ongoing to determine whether drugs that inhibit nitric oxide production may be helpful in controlling shock.

Complement Activation

Tumor necrosis factor (TNF) and bacterial antigens activate the complement system. Vasoactive affects are seen with C3 and C5 fragments which promote the release of histamine and other vasoactive mediators, producing vasodilatation, increased capillary permeability and platelet aggregation leading to blockage of capillaries.

Table 6.1: Endogenous vasoactive mediators in shock[3]

	Mediator	Stimulus	Source	Major action
1.	Norepinephrine	Hypovolemia	Sympathetic nervous system	Vasoconstriction
2.	Epinephrine	Hypovolemia	Adrenal medulla	β stimulation vasoconstriction
3.	Angiotensin	Hypovolemia	Kidney	Vasoconstriction
4.	Arachidonic acid metabolites, e.g.			
	Leukotriene	Tumor necrosis factor [TNF]	Macrophages Platelet	Increased capillary permeability Vasoconstriction Release of lysosomal enzymes
	Thromboxane A_2	Hypoxia	Platelet	Vasoconstriction platelet aggregation
	Prostaglandin F_2	Hypoxia	Platelet	Vasoconstriction
5.	Myocardial depressant factor	Ischemia	Pancreas	Negative inotropic effect
6.	Opiates (β endorphin)	Hypoxia	Pituitary	Decreased myocardial contractility

Table 6.2: Endogenous inflammatory mediators in shock[3]

Mediator	Stimulus	Major source	Major action
TNF	Bacterial antigen	Macrophage	– Induce other mediators – Adhesion to endothelium
Interleukin-1 (IL-1)	TNF bacterial Ag	Mononuclear cells	– Leukocytosis – Acute phase reactant
Interleukin 6	TNF IL-1	Monocytes Endothelial cells	– Leukocytosis – Fever – Thrombosis
Interleukin 8	TNF Endotoxin	Monocytes Endothelial cells	– Neutrophil activation
Complement fragments	TNF Endotoxin	Alternate pathway	– Chemotactic
Platelet activating factor	TNF Bacterial Ag	Platelet, WBC	– Thrombosis Increased permeability

Myocardial Depressant Factor

All types of shock are accompanied with myocardial dysfunction of varying severities. Investigations have revealed that a small peptide called myocardial depressant factor (MDF) is released by the pancreas when they are ischemic and hypoperfused. MDF acts directly on myocardial tissue causing a negative inotropic effect.

SYSTEMIC EFFECT OF SHOCK

Shock, if uncorrected can affect almost all the systems of body like respiratory, renal, hepatic, gastrointestinal, cardiac, CNS and endocrinal.

Respiratory: Respiratory failure is a frequent complication of shock. It may be due to dysfunction of alveolar endothelial interface (ARDS) or due to respiratory muscle fatigue. Management options include increasing the inspired oxygen and positive pressure ventilation in selected cases.

Renal: Shock syndromes may be associated with renal failure. The shock related renal failure syndromes are usually due to pre-renal causes. Acute tubular necrosis can however, result if the ischemic results are continued for too long. Renal failures associated with shock are mostly oliguric, but, one should remember that high output renal failure can also occur in these patients.

Renal support for these patients consists of volume augmentation, diuretics (e.g. frusemide, mannitol) and low dose dopamine (3-5 µg/kg/min).

Hepatic and gastrointestinal tract: Prolonged hypoperfusion and stress in shock can lead to hepatic dysfunction, GIT bleeding, ileus and bacterial translocation. It is usually recommended that patients with shock should receive prophylactic H_2-receptors blockers in order to prevent stress ulcers.

Another devastating condition which can occur in shock syndrome is acute nonocclusive mesenteric ischemia. This is characterized by prolonged splanchnic vasoconstriction, intestinal mucosal hypoxia, acidosis, mesenteric ischemia, transmural necrosis of bowel, bacterial translocation, sepsis and eventually multisystem organ dysfunction. Prevention of gut ischemia is advocated to prevent bacterial translocation.

Cardiac: Myocardial dysfunction, both due to hypoxia, hypovolemia and myocardial depressant factor is known to occur in all shock syndromes.

Coagulation abnormalities: Disseminated intravascular coagulation (DIC) can occur to various extents in all forms of shock. DIC is usually secondary to intravascular thrombosis which is induced in response to activation of TNF and platelet aggregation factor. Replacement therapy specifically for various absent clotting factors, vitamin K, fresh frozen plasma, and cryoprecipitate and platelet transfusion are some of the advisable management options for these patients.

Endocrine: Multiple endocrine problems may arise and complicate the management of shock in children like problems with fluid electrolyte, mineral balance and calcium homeostasis.

CNS: Shock if prolonged for too long can lead to cerebral anoxia, altered sensorium and mental obtundation.

CLASSIFICATION OF SHOCK

For purpose of description, shock can be classified into following four major categories.

a. Hypovolemic Shock

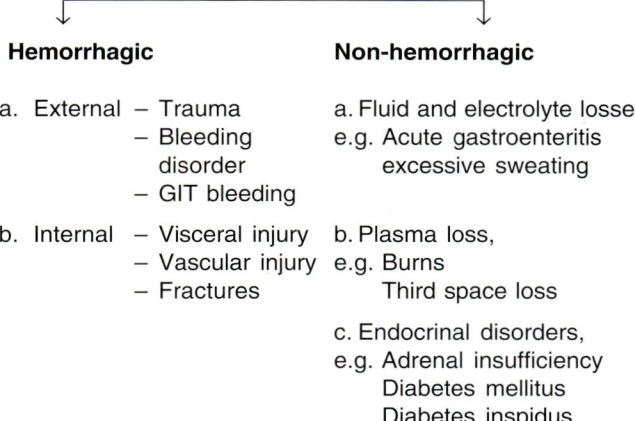

b. Septic shock

c. Distributive shock
 e.g. Anaphylaxis
    Neurogenic shock
    Drug toxicity

d. Cardiogenic shock

Cardiac insufficiency	Obstructive lesions
e.g. Myocarditis	e.g Pericardial temponade
Cardiomyopathy, dysrhythmias	Tension pneumothorax
Metabolic: hypoxia, hypoglycemia	Pulmonary embolism,
Congenital heart disease	Aortic stenosis
Drug intoxication, e.g. anthracycline	Pneumopericardium
β-blocker, tricyclic antidepressant	Critical pulmonary stenosis
Cardiac surgery	

Various Types of Shock can be Remembered by the Mnemonic as follows:[4]

S - Sepsis
H - Hypovolemia (intrinsic/extrinsic, hemorrhagic/nonhemorrhagic)
O - Obstructive (e.g. cardiac temponade, tension pneumothorax, massive pulmonary embolism)
C - Cardiogenic (primary pump failure)
K - Kinetic/distributive.

Diagnosis and Monitoring of Shock

Early diagnosis of shock requires a high index of suspicion. Identification of a full blown case of shock with hypotension, cold extremities and poor peripheral perfusion are usually suggestive of a decompensated shock.

Clinical assessment usually begins with a proper history taking. History of excessive fluid loss because of trauma, diarrhea, vomiting, burns etc is suggestive of hypovolemic shock. It is important to elicit details of environmental exposure, previous medical problems, allergies and potential drug ingestion. Septic shock is suspected in a child with history of fever, features suggestive of infection and circulatory collapse. Previous history of disorders such as congenital heart disease offers clue to the etiology.

On clinical examination features of decreased perfusion are assessed. Decreased perfusion affects the temperature, capillary filling time and vital organ function. Cold extremities with peripheral core temperature of > 2 °C indicates decreased perfusion to skin.

Impaired capillary filling time is a more sensitive indicator of poor peripheral tissue perfusion. The refill is determined by blanching an area over face, sternum, and forehead by firm compression with finger tip for > 5 seconds, and then noting the time for the blanching to disappear. Normally it should be < 3 sec, if it is > 5 seconds, it is a nonspecific indicator of tissue hypoperfusion.

Hypoperfusion of vital organs may manifest as oliguria (renal hypoperfusion) or altered sensorium (CNS hypoperfusion). Urine output measurement is one of the most important indicator for shock. In children urine output of < 1 ml/kg/hr is considered as oliguria.

Most significant physical findings in shock result from autonomic response to stress. It must be emphasized that "hypotension is not the sine qua non of shock". BP may be recorded as normal in early phases of shock. A rough estimate of minimal acceptable systolic BP in children is: systolic BP (mm Hg) = 70 + [age (yrs) × 2]. Hypotension, if present, strongly supports the diagnosis of shock. Initially the pulse pressure is decreased, later both systolic and diastolic pressure fall.

In children, tachycardia occurs early and is the sole determinant of cardiac output. Respiratory rate may also be increased in shock due to metabolic acidosis (Kussamaul's respiration). However, one should remember that respiratory rates and heart rate vary considerably with age as shown in Table 6.3.

It has to be emphasized that acute volume deficiency of us little as 10% may cause tachycardia while a gradual loss of 10-15% of volume produces minimal changes. However, hypotension may not occur until there is volume loss of 30% or more. Hemodynamic variables in different shock status are as shown in Table 6.4.

MONITORING THE PATIENT OF SHOCK

All children with shock are best managed in a pediatric intensive care unit (PICU). The aim of monitoring is to detect the alternation, in the physiological status and to assess the response of intervention.

It is noteworthy, that clinical monitoring is most crucial in the management of shock. It is probably, the most sensitive and effective monitoring technique. Clinical monitoring must include repeated and careful examination of the following parameters:
1. Color-pink/dusky/blue
2. Temperature – skin, core
3. Pulse rate
4. Respiratory rate
5. Capillary filling time
6. Blood pressure
7. Level of consciousness
8. Urine output (intake-output changes) (one should aim for urine output of >1-2 ml/kg/hr.

Based on these clinical parameters, shock can be categorized in compensated, decompensated and irreversible shock as shown in Table 6.5.

INVASIVE MONITORING

This is also sometimes required in management of shock. It includes the following:
a. CVP measurement (central venous pressure monitoring).
b. PCWP measurement (pulmonary capillary wedge pressure monitoring).
c. Arterial blood gas analysis.

CVP Measurement

The role of CVP monitoring in management of shock in basically in patients with myocardial compromise or renal failure, in order to avoid volume overload. In

Table 6.3: Age related upper normal limit for respiratory rate

Age	RR (per minute)	HR (per min)
Infant	50	160
Toddler	30	140
School age	25	120
Adolescent	20	110

Table 6.4: Hemodynamic variables in different shock status

	Shock type	Skin	UO	JVP	CO	SVR	PCWP
1.	Hypovolemia	Cool (pale)	↓	↓	↓	↑	↓
2.	Cardiogenic	Cool (pale)	↓	↑	↓	↑↑	↓
3.	Obstructive	Cool (pale)	↓	↑	↑	↑	↑
4.	Distribution (neurogenic)	Warm pink	↓	↓	↑	↓↓	N/↓
5.	Septic						
	- Early	Warm (pink)	↓↑	↓↑	↑	↓	N
	- Late	Cool (pale)	↓	↓	↓	↑	↑
6.	Anaphylactic	Cool (pale)	↓	↓	↓	↑	↓

UO-urine output, JVP-jugular venous pressure, CO-cardiac output, SVR-systemic vascular resistance, PCWP-pulmonary capillary wedge pressure

Table 6.5: Staging of shock

Parameters	Stage I Compensated	Stage II Decompensated	Stage III Irreversible
HR	↑	↑↑	↑↑↑
RR	N	↑	↑↑
BP	N	↓	↓↓
Pulse pressure	N	↓	↓↓
Urine output	N	↓	0
Skin	Cool	Mottled	Cold, cyanotic
Mental status	Anxious, thirsty	Obtunded	Coma

pure hypovolemic shock it is unlikely that CVP measurement may add anything significant to careful evaluation of peripheral perfusion, BP, HR and urine output. CVP monitoring also helps the surgeon to differentiate between hypovolemic and septic shock.

CVP catheter can be placed via the external or internal jugular, femoral, basilic or subclavian vein. Before using CVP measurement, it is essential to confirm the position of the tip of catheter in the right atrium. Normal CVP is described as > 10 mm Hg (5-8 mm Hg) and it reflects intravascular volume, right ventricular contractibility and right ventricular pressure CVP should not be taken as a guide of left ventricular function. Poor correlation has been reported between CVP and pulmonary artery occlusion pressure. Reported complication of internal jugular or subclavian vein catheterization include bleeding, pneumothorax, hemothorax, chylothorax, pericardial temponade, in advent arterial puncture, dysrhythmias, sepsis and thrombosis. Complications of indwelling catheter occur in approximately in 5% of children mostly < 5 year of age.[5] Line sepsis is reported as 1.4 septic episodes per 100 catheterization.[5] Line patency can be prolonged with continuous infusion of a solution containing 0.25-1U/ml of heparin.

Pulmonary Artery Swan-Ganz Catheter

Pulmonary artery catheters are required in the management of cardiogenic shock and in cases of refractory shock resistant to usual forms of treatment. Swan-Ganz catheters are currently used for pulmonary artery catheterization. They have a proximal side hole to monitor right atrial pressure, a thermostar to estimate cardiac output by thermodilution, as well as an end hole to measure pulmonary artery pressure. When the balloon is inflated the pulmonary artery wedge pressure (PAWP) which is as reflection of left atrial pressure can also be recorded.

Insertion of such catheter is usually done either from the left subclavian or right internal jugular vein, using the Seldinger's technique. Normal PAWL is 2-8 mm Hg. Reported complications with these catheters are minimal in children.[5,6]

Arterial Blood Gas Analysis

Arterial blood gases should be frequently monitored in patients with shock. It helps in determining the adequacy of ventilation and also about tissue perfusion. In shock patients usually have metabolic acidosis (lactate acidosis) with increased anion gap. The best treatment for such patient is restoration of intravascular volume.

Therapeutic Approach

Management of shock irrespective of the causes is aimed at optimizing the vital organ perfusion and in correcting the metabolic abnormalities due to tissue hypoperfusion. However, for proper treatment of shock, determining the etiology and management of the underlying cause is mandatory. Certain therapies are however common to all the forms of shock. They are as follows:

a. *Correction of hypoxemia:* All patients with shock should receive supplemental oxygen. Endotracheal intubation and mechanical ventilation is, however, not needed in all cases of shock. This is only indicated under following circumstances:
  i. Patients with non-cardiac pulmonary edema (ARDS).
  ii. Respiratory fatigue (decreased respiratory muscle function).
  iii. Children with cardiogenic shock and pulmonary edema.

Intubation and intermittent positive pressure ventilation aids myocardial function by improving pulmonary compliance, decreasing intrapulmonary shunting and by decreasing after load.[7]

b. *Fluid therapy:* In all patients of shock intravenous access should be established at the earliest. Initially percutaneous peripheral IV cannulation should be tried. In case of failure, central veins like femoral, saphenous or internal jugular should be tried. If such attempts are unsuccessful the intraosseous route should be resorted to without wasting time for performing cut down. If unfortunately the child sustains a cardiopulmonary arrest before establishment of IV assess then resuscitative drugs like epinephrine and atropine can be given via endotracheal tube. In children less than 5 years old, needle placement into the marrow space of the medial portion of proximal tibia, angulated away from the growth plate and 1-2 inches below the tibial tuberosity, is indicated. In older children, needle placement 1-2 inches above the medial marrow is indicated. Veiasoo et al found that intraosseous route is helpful in resuscitation of hypovolemic shock.[8] Intravenous fluids, blood products, bicarbonates are among the other drugs that can be given using this technique. He also showed that efficacy of intraosseous route is comparable to central and peripheral intravenous routes.

Initial fluid for all types of shock is crystalloid, i.e. Ringer's lactate or normal saline. Subsequently, depending on the cause of shock fluid can be changed as described later, e.g. in dehydration crystalloid is continued, in sepsis or trauma blood products or colloids are given judiciously. Initial bolus of crystalloid in shock is 20 ml/kg over 6-10 min. On reassessment if peripheral perfusion and BP improves and the patient passes urine, maintenance fluids should be continued. If, however, patients fails to pass urine or hypotension persist then a repeat bolus of 20 ml/kg of crystalloid is given. If anuria still persists, another bolus of 20 ml/kg is advisable before further interventions.[4] Thus, it is apparent that upto 60 ml/kg of fluid can be administered while managing patients with shock, hypotension and anuria. Beyond this, CVP monitoring should be instituted and cardiac status should be evaluated before giving further fluid therapy as mentioned later. Further treatment of shock is specific to the type of shock and is mentioned with them.

HYPOVOLEMIC SHOCK

Hypovolemic shock is the most common cause of shock in infants and children.[1] There is decrease in intravascular blood volume, leading to a decrease in preload, thereby causing fall in stroke volume and cardiac output. Various etiological factors leading to hypovolemic shock are mentioned earlier in the classification of shock.

Acute loss of 10-15% of the circulatory blood volume may be well tolerated in healthy children. Based on the amount of blood volume loss hypovolemic shock can be classified into three classes as shown in Table 6.6. Class I shock or early hypovolemic shock are characterized by normal BP and normal heart rate. With continued loss of blood volume as in class II and III shock, fluid loss surpasses body's compensatory abilities and signs of circulatory and organ dysfunctions appears.

Therapy of Hypovolemic Shock

Initial treatment of hypovolemic shock is similar regardless to etiology and includes establishment of adequate oxygenation, ventilation and restoration of circulatory blood volume as mentioned earlier. Initial volume resuscitation is with crystalloids (Ringer's lactate or 0.9% sodium chloride) as shown in Figure 6.2.

Use of Colloids in Hypovolemic Shock

Administration of colloids in hypovolemic shock is a controversial issue. Colloids may be used after the

Table 6.6: Classification of hypovolemic shock				
	Class I	Class II	Class III	Class IV
Blood loss %	<15	15-30	30-40	>40%
HR/min	<100	100-120	120-140	>140
BP (mm Hg)	N	N	↓	↓
Pulse pressure	N	↓	↓↓	↓↓
CFT	N	Delayed	Delayed	Delayed
RR/min	N (14-20)	20-30	30-40	>40
UO ml/hr	>30	20-30	5-15	Negligible
Mental status	N, thirsty	Slightly anxiety	Confusion	Lethargy

HR-heart rate, BP-blood pressure, CFT-capillary filling time, RR-respiratory rate, UO-urine output

Shock in Children—Surgeon's Perspective

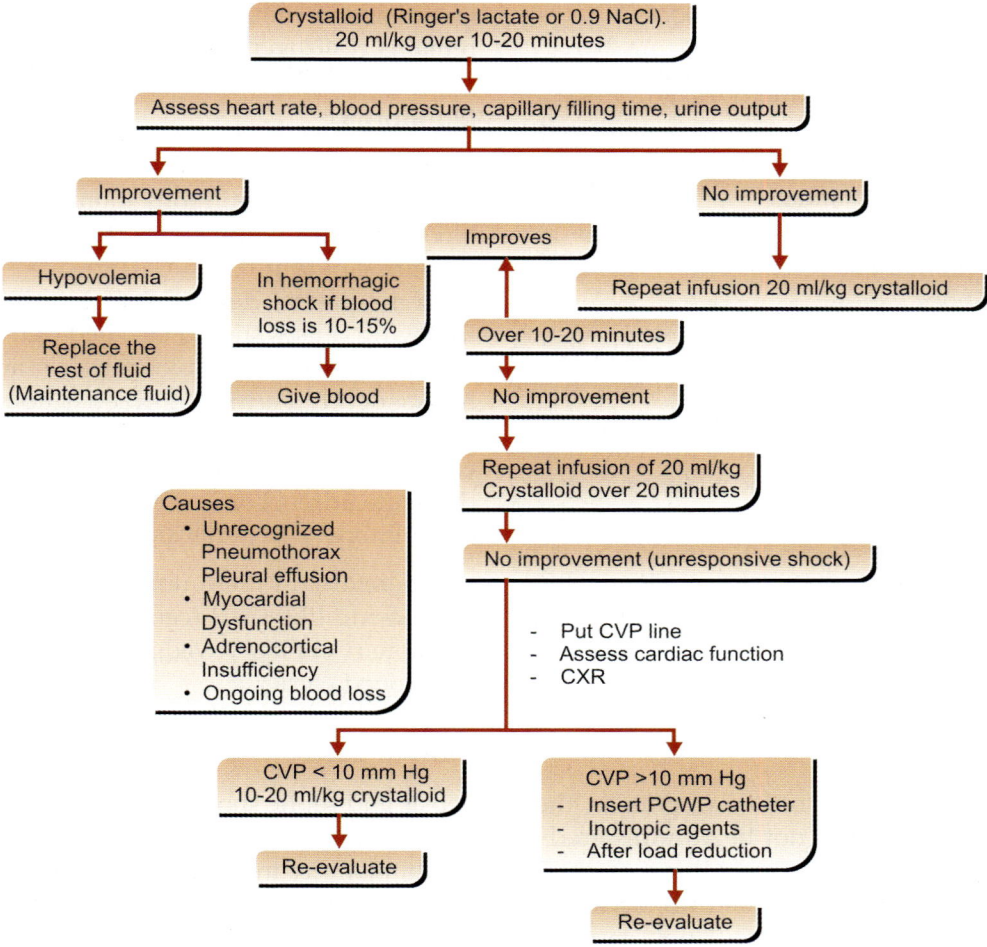

Fig. 6.2: Fluid management in hypovolemic shock

child has received 60 ml/kg of crystalloid and continues to have ongoing fluid loss. Colloids like 5% albumin or hydroxyethyl starch may allow for more rapid volume expansion and may decrease the amount of interstitial edema. However, a meta-analysis of several clinical studies concluded that hypovolemic shock should be managed with crystalloid resuscitation as colloid administration leads to increased intravascular volume at the expense of interstitial fluid.[9]

Use of Blood and Blood Substitutes

Hemorrhagic variety of hypovolemic shock warrants blood transfusion, especially if blood volume lost is > 15%. Type specific cross matched blood should be arranged for these patients. Failing which they can receive type specific uncross matched blood, and if even this is not available then in emergency setting, as a life saving measure, they can be transfused 0 negative blood.

Recently artificial blood substitutes like perfluorocarbons (PFC), perfluorodecalin and highly purified stoma free hemoglobin (SFH) have also been tried in the management of patients with acute blood loss.

Role of Vasopressors in Hypovolemic Shock

Vasopressors are not indicated in the treatment of uncomplicated hypovolemic shock. Vasopressors raise blood pressure by increasing peripheral vascular resistance which is already elevated in hypovolemic shock. Thus, these agents aggravate the deleterious effect of hypovolemic shock and as such are unwarranted in these patients.

Role of Positioning in Hypovolemic Shock

Most first aid courses teach that patients in shock should be placed in the head down position (Trendelenburg). Although, this position is efficacious in neurogenic shock yet its role in hypovolemic shock has not been of much advantage.

Role of MAST Garment In Hypovolemic Shock

Military antishock trousers (MAST) are mentioned in the management of hypovolemic shock to be condemned. MAST[10] causes compression of inferior vena cava, impairs ventricular function, decreases blood supply to gastrointestinal and abdominal viscera and is known to cause compartment syndrome in limbs. Because of these disadvantages, MAST is no longer used in the management of hypovolemic shock. It may, however, have some role in the management of bleeding pelvic fracture.

Use of Analgesics and Antibiotics in Hypovolemic Shock

Analgesics are needed for reducing pain in these patients. Analgesics should not be administered by intramuscular or subcutaneous routes as due to reduced blood supply to these structures, these drugs would not reach the systemic circulation. However, once the circulation gets improved the doses previously administered are suddenly reabsorbed and may result in profound sedations which may be life threatening.

Antibiotics were used in the treatment of hypovolemic shock for many years and were thought to exert a protective mechanism against the ravages of hypovolemia. Subsequent data, however, fails to support this hypothesis. Presently there is no role for the use of prophylactic antibiotics in these patients. Antibiotics are advocated only in presence of contaminated and infected wounds.

Role of Steroids in Management of Hypovolemic Shock

Routine use of steroids in management of hypovolemic shock is not indicated. Only in patients with Addison's disorders and post-adrenalectomy states who present with hypovolemic shock, steroids can be used. The use of steroids in complicated unresponsive shock states remains controversial.[11]

Monitoring

Response to treatment in hypovolemic shock is determined by continuous monitoring of heart rate, blood pressure, peripheral perfusion, saturation (SaO_2) and urine output.

If the patient develops unresponsive shock then following causes should be ruled out:
a. Unsuspected loss of blood in chest and or abdomen.
b. Associated unrecognized pneumothorax, or pericardial effusion
c. Myocardial dysfunction
d. Acute adrenocortical insufficiency
e. Pulmonary hypertension

Therefore, in these unresponsive patients special monitoring like CVP (central venous pressure) and pulmonary capillary wedge pressures are required as mentioned earlier.

SEPTIC SHOCK

Sepsis and septic shock are among the leading causes of mortality in children. Septic shock is often a combination of multiple problems like hypovolemia, maldistribution of blood flow, myocardial depression and cellular derangements that makes cells and tissues unable to utilize the substrates delivered to them.

The definitions used for the description of sepsis are highly variable. In order to resolve this ambiguity the American College of Chest Physicians and Society for Critical Care Medicine (1991) have stated following definitions of sepsis and its related syndromes and they are universally accepted.[12] They are as follows:
a. *Sepsis (systemic inflammatory response syndrome):* It is the systemic response to infection. Two or more of the following conditions manifests this systemic response-
   - Temperature > 38 °C or < 36 °C
   - Heart rate > 2 SD than normal
   - Respiratory rate > 2 SD above normal
   - WBC count >12,000 cells/ml^3, < 4000 cells/ml^3 or band count >10%
b. *Severe sepsis:* Sepsis associated with organ dysfunction, hypoperfusion or hypotension.

c. *Septic shock:* Sepsis with hypotension despite adequate fluid resuscitation along with the presence of perfusion abnormalities, which includes lactic acidosis, oliguria and or an acute alteration in mental status.

Septic shock is usually highly fatal with a reported mortality in neonates of around 20% and in older children it ranges from 10 - 50%.[13,14] Although bacteria, virus, fungi and parasite may result in septic shock, yet the most common organisms causing septic shock are gram-negative organisms, e.g. *E. Coli, Klebsiella pneumoniae, Enterobacter* and *Pseudomonas aeruginosa*. The most common source of gram-negative bacteria is the genitourinary system, followed by respiratory tract and alimentary tract (especially biliary tract). Gram-positive bacteria responsible for septic shock include *Staphylococci, Pneumococcus* and *Neisseria meningitidis. Staphylococci* are common isolates in nosocomial sepsis and in sepsis secondary to indwelling vascular catheters. Besides these organisms sometimes anaerobic organisms are also implicated in sepsis especially after abdominal surgeries.

Pathophysiology

The pathophysiology of septic shock is as described earlier in the chapter. Lipopolysaccharide (LPS) antigen of endotoxin binds to lipopolysaccharide binding protein (LBP). This LPS-LBP complex than attach to CD14 receptors on macrophages and leads to stimulation of fibrinolytic system, coagulation system, complement system, vasoactive and biochemical mediators resulting in vasodilatation, increased capillary permeability and myocardial dysfunction. Endotoxin, tumor necrosis factor and interleukins stimulate nitric oxide synthatase in macrophages and vascular smooth muscle cells leading to profound peripheral vasodilatation. Various causes have been attributed to myocardial dysfunction that is seen in septic shock. Some of those mechanisms are as follows:
  i. Myocardial ischemia due to shock
  ii. Defective myocardial calcium metabolism
  iii. Presence of cardioinhibitory substances in circulation like myocardial depressant factor (MDF), histamine, endorphins, complement, interleukins and prostaglandins.
  iv. Endocardial endothelial injury
  v. Nitric oxide production by endocardium/myocardium.

Thus, it is important to note that myocardial dysfunction appears to occur not only in preterminally sick patients but also in the early stages of septic shock.[15]

Endotoxin also activates the intrinsic coagulation cascade along with fibrinolytic system. Platelets are activated, natural anticoagulant like antithrombin 3; protein C and protein S are depleted leading to disseminated intravascular coagulation (DIC). Adrenal insufficiency is common in children with septic shock. In a study by Hatherill et al adrenal insufficiency is documented in 52% of children with septic shock.[16]

Clinical Features of Septic Shock

Early stages of septic shock (early septic shock) are characterized by an elevated or a normal cardiac output decreased systemic vascular resistance, widened pulse pressure with warm extremities and a normal BP. This phase is also called pink shock or warm shock. If, sepsis is uncorrected then these patients progress on to a classical pale shock characterized by hypotension, decreased cardiac output and metabolic acidosis. The features of early and late septic shock are elaborated in Table 6.3.

Investigations

Laboratory work up for patients of septic shock includes the following:
1. Hb, TLC, DLC: Total leukocyte count (TLC) >12,000 or < 4000 cells/ml^3, blood count of > 10%, vacualotion of neutrophils, toxic granules and presence of dohle bodies are suggestive of sepsis.
2. Acute phase reactants, ESR, C-reactive protein, platelet count.
3. Coagulation profile - With the occurrence of DIC in sepsis platelet count decreases and PT, APTT prolong. (PT - prothrombin time, APTT - activated partial thromboplastin time).
4. Arterial blood gas analysis — reveals hypoxia and acidosis.
5. Blood, urine and cultures from all the catheters and IV line is also required. CSF analysis may be required in selected patients to rule out associated meningitis.

6. Procalcitonin is a new diagnostic tool in the management of septic shock. It is a polypeptide, which is present in plasma at concentration of 0.5 mg/ml. It is markedly increased in invasive bacterial infections. It is not elevated in viral and in non-invasive bacterial colorization. Harbath S et al revealed the mean concentration of procalcitonin in SIRS (0.6 ng/ml), sepsis (3.5 ng/ml), severe sepsis (6.2 ng/ml) and in septic shock as (21.3 ng/ml).[17] The sensitivity of procalcitonin is 97% and specificity is 78%.[17] Serial estimation of serum procalcitonin can be used to monitor the response of infection to antimicrobials.
7. Polymerase chain reaction (PCR): PCR has been found to be more sensitive than blood cultures in detecting bactremia.[18]

Therapy

Initial treatment of septic shock includes establishment of adequate oxygenation, ventilation and fluid management as mentioned earlier.

Fluid Therapy

Crystalloids (Ringer's lactate or isotonic saline) are the preferred fluid of choice in septic shock. However, in these patients signs of volume overload should be closely monitored with the help of central venous pressure (CVP). Judicious use of colloids and blood products to maintain hemoglobin, clotting factors and colloid oncotic pressure is also advocated for these patients. Colloids may be used after the child has received 60 ml/kg of crystalloids. 5% albumin in saline is used in dose of 5 ml/kg in septic shock. So far no additional benefit has been documented with its use.[19] Hemodynamic monitoring is required to prevent pulmonary edema, which is known to occur with its excessive use.

Antibiotics

Before putting the patient of septic shock on broad-spectrum antibiotics, cultures of blood, urine and any other potentially infected site should be sent. Broad-spectrum antibiotics covering gram-positive, gram-negative and anaerobic bacteria can be started empirically in these patients; depending on the bacterial flora of the hospital or nursery.

Cardiovascular Support – Role of Vasopressors

Vasopressor agents are indicated if cardiac output remains low despite adequate fluid infusion, as predicted by CVP of >10 mm Hg or if the child develops pulmonary edema. Some of the commonly used vasopressors in management of septic shock are dopamine, dobutamine, epinephrine and isoproterenol.

Dopamine: Dopamine is the most commonly used vasopressor agent in shock. It stimulates α, β and dopaminergic receptors at varying dose. At low dose (3-5 µg/kg/min) it improves renal perfusion by selectively stimulating the dopaminergic receptors of renal and mesenteric vessels. At dose of 5-10 µg/kg/min it stimulates β-receptors along with dopaminergic receptors, thereby having direct inotropic affect on heart. At higher doses (>10 µg/kg/min) it acts mainly on α receptors and causes systemic vasoconstriction. In management of septic shock it is usually used in dose of 3-5 µg/kg/min or uptil 10 µg/kg/min.

Dobutamine: Dobutamine acts on β-receptors and causes an inotropic effect on heart. Besides improving myocardial contractility, it causes peripheral and pulmonary vasodilatation. Therefore, dobutamine should be used in the patients only after they have been infused with adequate amount of fluid, otherwise significant vasodilatation and intrapulmonary shunting, caused by dobutamine can lead to fall in cardiac output. It is usually used in doses of 1-20 µg/kg/min.

Epinephrine: Epinephrine is the reserve inotrope to be preferred as last choice in cases where there is no response to other inotropes.[19] It acts on α and β 1, 2 receptors resulting in increased cardiac output, heart rate and blood pressure. The potential complications of epinephrine are ventricular tachyarrhythmias and renal ischemia.

Norepinephrine and Isoproterenol: In patients with low peripheral vascular resistance as in anaphylaxis and septic shock, enhancing peripheral vascular tone with nor epinephrine may be beneficial. However, the potential vasoconstrictor effect of norepinehprine requires careful hemodynamic monitoring. Isoproterenol is best reserved for patients requiring potent inotropic stimulation especially in conjunction with pulmonary vasodilatation.

Renal Support in Septic Shock

Renal support is essential to avoid renal failure in hypoperfusion states. Fluid therapy and use of low dose dopamine (3-5 µg/kg/min) improves renal blood flow. If there is oliguria/anuria even after fluid management and CVP is >10 mm Hg then loop diuretics (frusemide) can be given in dose of 1-2 mg/kg. If, however patient goes in a state of renal failure then peritoneal or hemodialysis is required.

Nutritional Support in Septic Shock

Parenteral or enteral nutrition should begin as soon as cardiovascular stability is achieved. Many surgeons advocate the early use of minimal enteral nutrition (MEN) to prevent gut mucosal atrophy and bacterial translocation.[20]

Role of Steroids in Management of Septic Shock

Several large trials have failed to show the beneficial effect of steroids in treatment of septic shock.[21] Current studies suggest that replacement therapy with hydrocortisone may alleviate the symptoms of SIRS.

Newer Management Strategies in Septic Shock

With better understanding of the pathophysiology of sepsis and septic shock, new management strategies have been proposed and are presently under trial. They are as follows:

Antiendotoxin Antibody

Monoclonal antibody against bacterial endotoxin may be helpful in preventing the stimulation of various immunological pathways in sepsis. Trials with murine monoclonal antibody E5 have not shown encouraging results.[22]

Anti-TNF Antibody

Monoclonal antibodies against tumor necrosis factor (TNF) have been tried in the management of septic shock. Afelimomab, the murine monoclonal antibody against TNFα has been tried and phase I results have revealed a sustained rise of blood pressure.[23]

Lenercept

Lenercept is the human recombinant p55 tumor necrosis factor receptor immunoglobulin G1 fusion protein. It decreases the effect of TNF by blocking its receptor protein. Abraham E et al tried it in 1342 patients with severe sepsis and found that mortality in Lenercept group is 27% as against 28% in placebo group.[24]

Activated Protein C

Recombinant human activated protein C (rh APC) has antithrombotic, anti-inflammatory and profibrinolytic properties. Trials have been conducted with rh APC in patients with severe sepsis, and they have shown an absolute reduction in risk of death by 6.1% but its use is associated with increased risk of bleeding.[25]

Antithrombin III

Antithrombin III inhibits thrombin, intrinsic and extrinsic clotting cascade, besides having anti-inflammatory properties. Warren BL et al administered antithrombin III in patients with severe sepsis and septic shock and found that overall mortality was not much different in the treated and placebo group.[26]

Tissue Factor Inhibitor

Tissue factor inhibitor (TFI) inhibits the action of tissue factor, factor 10A and factor 7A, thus affecting both the intrinsic and extrinsic pathways. Kemme MJ et al showed a dose dependent reduction of thrombin with TFI.[27]

Intravenous Immunoglobulin

Intravenous immunoglobulins (monoclonal or polyclonal) are used as an adjunctive therapy in septic shock. The Cochrane database reviewed 27 studies of use of IV immunoglobulins in septic shock and found that beneficial effect were apparent in children who received polyclonal immunoglobulins.[28] Mortality did not decrease in children who received monoclonal antibodies.

Nitric Oxide Synthase Inhibitor

Nitric oxide synthase inhibitor, N (G)-methyl-L-arginine hydrochloride (546 C88) has been tried in patients with septic shock (1-20 mg/kg/hr) along with norepinephrine and dobutamine.[29] Usage of 546C88 is associated with 60-80% reduction of requirement of NE to control hypotension.

Angiotensin II

Yunge et al used angiotensin II in two children with septic shock who remained hypotensive despite fluid management and high dose of conventional inotropes and vasopressors.[30] In both cases angiotensin II could stabilize the blood pressure and both the patients survived the septic shock. Thereby, proving the beneficial effect of angiotensin II in septic shock.

Recombinant Granulocyte Colony Stimulating Factor (rh G-CSF)

Rh G-CSF has been used as a prophylactic agent in some trials with encouraging results.[31] However, larger studies are needed to document the benefit of rh G-CSF (Filgrastim) in severe sepsis.

Vasopressin

Some workers have advocated the use of vasopressin infusion in dose of 0.01-0.04 U/min in patients with septic shock refractory to other agents.

Pentoxyfylline

Pentoxyfylline inhibits cytokine-mediated inflammation. Lauterbach R et al infused pentoxyfylline in dose of 5 mg/kg/hr for 6 hrs for 6 days in 100 premature babies with sepsis, and found that 1 out of 40 patients died in pentoxyfylline group as compared to 6 out of 38 in placebo group.[32] Also in pentoxyfylline group complication of DIC, anuria and metabolic acidosis were less common.

High Volume Hemofiltration (HVH)

HVH can be used in septic shock for supporting hemodynamics and also for removing complements, cytokines, interleukins and other activated inflammatory reactants. In study conducted by Cole et al use of HVH has shown to decrease the requirement of vasopressors in septic shock.[33]

Management of Complications Related to Septic Shock

The following complications are known to occur in the course of septic shock:

Adult Respiratory Distress Syndrome (ARDS) or Shock Lung

The inflammatory mediators increase the pulmonary capillary permeability resulting in pulmonary edema, and capillary thrombi, leading to ventilation perfusion mismatch. It manifests clinically with hypoxemia, hypocarbia, and metabolic acidosis. Early mechanical ventilation with PEEP is recommended for supporting respiratory function.

Disseminated Intravascular Coagulation (DIC)

Septic child may present either with thrombocytopenia in the initial stage of sepsis or with DIC in the late stage with bleeding from multiple sites. In such patients platelet counts, BT, CT, PT, APTT should be assessed. In these patients blood transfusion, fresh frozen plasma (FFP) and platelet transfusions may be required along with vitamin K supplementation.

Gastrointestinal, Renal and Cardiac Related Complications

Shock can lead to stress ulceration in the fundus and body of stomach. They can be prevented and treated with H_2 blockers. Renal and cardiac support also needs to be given in these patients as mentioned earlier.

Conclusion

Inspite of advance in the management of septic shock, mortality continues to be high (10-50%) and the main cornerstone of treatment continues to be antibiotics and cardiovascular support.

DISTRIBUTIVE SHOCK

It results from maldistribution of blood flow to the tissue. The important causes are anaphylaxis, neurogenic shock and drug over dosage (spine/epidural anesthesia).

Anaphylactic shock: Results in previously sensitized host when an antigen reacts with fixed IgE antibody, thereby, triggering mast cells, eosinophil, complement and vasoactive mediators, leading to widespread vasodilatation decreased venous return, increased capillary permeability and shock. Treatment consists of IV fluid administration, along with steroid (+) vasopressor.

Management of neurogenic shock consist of positioning the patient in head low position, IV fluid and vasopressors.

CARDIOGENIC SHOCK

Cardiac shock is the pathophysiological state in which abnormality of cardiac function is responsible for the failure of the cardiovascular system to meet the metabolic demand of body. This disease mainly comes in the jurisdiction of physicians. Therefore, a detailed description of this entity is beyond the scope of this book. We shall briefly mention an outline of management in these patients.

Cardiogenic shock can be caused by multiple etiologies as mentioned earlier in the classification of shock. Early recognition of congestive heart failure or cardiac shock in infancy requires a high index of suspicion. The initial workup of these patients is as shown below:

History

1. Excessive respiratory effort
2. Prolonged feeding time
3. Poor weight gain
4. Excessive sweating
5. Frequent respiratory tract infections

Physical Examination

1. Tachycardia/Tachypnea
2. Gallop rhythm
3. Cold extremities, weak peripheral pules
4. Wheezing, rales
5. Cyanosis
6. Diaphoresis
7. Hepatomegaly
8. Neck vein distension
9. Peripheral edema
10. Hypotension

Investigation

1. Chest X-ray
    - Cardiomegaly
    - Pulmonary venous congestion
    - Hyperinflation
2. Echo
    - Size thickness and performance of the heart
3. CVP, PCWP --Raised

In contrast to hypovolemic shock, compensatory mechanisms can have a deleterious effect in patients with cardiogenic shock as shown below:
a. Increased systemic vascular resistance causes increased myocardial after load. This along with increased heart rate and contractility raises the myocardial oxygen demand and ischemia.
b. The diastolic filling is impaired because of tachycardia leading to decrease in myocardial perfusion.
c. Fluid retention causes increase in preload, pulmonary congestion and hypoxemia.
d. Increased myocardial demand of oxygen and other subtracts in setting of decreased perfusion leads to worsening of ischemia.

Therapy

General principles in the management of cardiogenic shock are as shown below:
1. Minimize myocardial oxygen demands
    - Intubation, mechanical ventilation
    - Maintain normal temperature
    - Provide sedation
    - Correct anemia
2. Maximize myocardial performance
    - Correct dysrythmias
    - Optimize preload
    - Salt + water restriction
    - Diuretics, vasodilatation
3. Improve myocardial contractility
    - Provide oxygen
    - Ventilation
    - Correct acidosis and other metabolic abnormalities
    - Inotropic drugs (Digitalis, amrinone, milirone)
4. Reduce after load
    - Sedation
    - Vasodilator

Inotropic Agents used in Cardiogenic Shock

The catecholamines like norepinehprine, epinephrine, dopamine, dobutamine and isoproterenol are some of the most potent positive inotropic agents. Digitalis glycosides augment myocardial contractility but because of narrow therapeutic to toxic ratio, their use in patients with cardiogenic shock should be avoided. Newer drugs Amrinone and Milirone decease myocardial intracellular cAMP degradation by inhibiting phosphodiesterase type III, thus augmenting myocardial contractility. Amrinone is administered intravenously (a bolus of 1-3 mg/kg our 1-3 min followed by continuous infusion of 1-20 mg/kg/min).

After Load Reduction

Nitroprusside is more potent than nitroglycerin as afterload reducing agents. Nitroglycerin is a more potent arterial vasodilator effect.

Cardiac Obstructive Shock

Obstructive shock is caused by the inability to produce adequate cardiac output despite normal intravascular volume and myocardial function. The various causative factors have been enumerated earlier in the chapter. Out of the various causes cardiac temponade and tension pneumothorax are of relevance in a surgical setting.

Cardiac Temponade

Cardiac compression caused by accumulation of fluid, blood or gas in pericardium

Clinical features are characterized by Becks triad
- Hypotension
- Increased jugular venous pressure
- Silent heart (barely audible hearts sound).

Besides these signs patient also has pulsus paradoxus and pericardial rub. Echocardiography is confirmatory. Emergency management consists of pericardiocentesis in an unstable patient. Pericardiocentesis is usually done by a subxiphoid approach on left side in 6th intercostals space monitored by echocardiography.

Definitive treatment of cardiac temponade is removal of pericardial fluid by surgical drainage.

PROGNOSIS IN SHOCK

Aggressive management of shock especially hypovolemia can be quite rewarding. However, septic shock still continue to have a high mortality rate of around 50%. Adverse outcome is anticipated in following situations:
1. Multiple organ failure
2. Major myocardial damage
3. DIC
4. Renal failure
5. Respiratory failure
6. Uncontrolled sepsis.

Thus, to conclude early detection, immediate intervention, close monitoring and systemic approach to reverse the pathophysiological abnormalities are the key points in the successful management of shock.

REFERENCES

1. McConnell MS, Perkin MR. Shock states. In: Pediatric Critical Care. Fuhrman BP, Zimmerman JJ (Eds). 2nd ed. Mosby 1998;293-305.
2. Ganong WF. Cardiovascular regulatory mechanisms. In: Review of Medical Physiology. Lange JD (Ed). 15th ed., Lange 1991;550-61.
3. Bell LM, Shock. In: Textbook of Pediatric Emergency Medicine. Gary R Fleishner, Eudwig S (Ed). 4th ed. Lippincott Williams and Wilkins, Philadelphia 2000; 47-57.
4. Singh D. Shock in children. Pediatric Today 2000;5: 354-60.
5. Ejchelberger M, Rous P, Hoelzer D, et al. Percutaneous subclavian venous catheters in neonates and children. J Pediatr Surg 1981;16:547-53.
6. Smith WD, Green T, Lock J. Complication of vascular catheterization in critically ill children. Crit Care Medicine 1984;12:1015-17.
7. Lodha R, Menon PSN. Shock. In: Medical emergencies in children. Mehraban S (Ed) 176-91.
8. Velasco AL, Delgado PC, Templeton J. Intraosseous infusion of fluids in the initial management of hypovolemic shock in young subjects. J Pediatr Surg 1991;26:4-8.
9. Velonovich V. Crystalloid versus colloid fluid resuscitation: A Meta-analysis of mortality. Surgery 1989;105:65.
10. Mattox KL, Bickwell W, et al. Prospective MAST study in 911 patients. J Trauma 1989;29 (8):1104.
11. Claussen MS, Landercasper J, et al. Acute adrenal insufficiency presenting as shock after trauma and surgery. J Trauma 1992;32(1):94.
12. Bone RC. Definition for sepsis and organ failure and guideline for the use of innovative therapies in sepsis. The ACCP/ SCCM consensus conference committee. Chest 1992;101:1647.
13. Ferrieri P. Neonatal susceptibility and immunity to major bacterial pathogens. Rev Infectious Disease 1990;12(4):48.

14. von Rosenstiel N, et al. Management of sepsis and septic shock in infants and children. Pediatric Drugs 2001;3(1):9-27.
15. Parker JL, Adam R. Development of myocardial dysfunction in endotoxin shock. Am J Physiol 1985;248:818.
16. Hatherill M, Tibby S, et al. Adrenal insufficiency in septic shock. Arch Dis Child 1999;80(1):51-55.
17. Harbath S, et al. Diagnostic value of Procalcitonin, interleukin 6, interleukin 8 in critically ill patients admitted with suspected sepsis. Am J Resp Critical Care Medicine 2001;1:164.
18. Curson, et al. The use of polymerase chain reaction to detect septicemia in critically ill patients. Critical Care Medicine 1999;27(5):937-40.
19. Rao MMU. Sepsis and septic shock in children: current concepts. Pediatrics Today 2002;(1):6-18.
20. Moore FA, Feliciano DV, Andressy R. Early enteral feeding compared with Parenteral reduces postoperative septic complications. The result of a meta-analysis. Ann Surg 1992;216:172.
21. Bone RC, Fischer CJ, Clemmer JP, et al. Methyl prednisolone severe sepsis study group. A controlled clinical trail of high dose methyl prednisolone in the treatment of severe sepsis and septic shock. N Engl J Med 1987;317:653.
22. Angus DC, Birmingham MC, et al. ES Murine monoclonal Antiendotoxin antibody in gram-negative sepsis: A randomized controlled trial JAMA 2000;283:1723-30.
23. Natanson C. Selected treatment strategies for septic shock based on proposed mechanisms of pathogenesis. Ann Intern Med 1994;120:771.
24. Abraham E, Laterre PF, Garbino J, et al. Lenercept (p 55 tumor necrosis factor receptor fusion protein) in severe sepsis and septic shock: A randomized double blind placebo-controlled multicenter phase III trial with 1342 patients. Crit Care Med 2001;29(3):503-10.
25. Bernard GR, Vincet JL, Laterre PF, La Rossa SP, et al. Efficacy and safety of recombinant human activated protein C for severe sepsis. N Engl J Med 2001;344:699-709.
26. Warren BL, Eid A, Pillay SS, et al. Caring for critically ill patients. High dose antithrombin 2 in severe sepsis: a randomized controlled trial. JAMA 2001;286(15):1869-78.
27. Kemme MJ, Burggraf J, Shoemaker RC, et al. The influence of reduced liver blood flow on the pharmacokinetics and pharmacodynamics of recombinant tissue factor inhibitor pathway. Clin Pharma Therapy 2000;67:504-11.
28. Alejandria MM, et al. Intravenous immunoglobulin for treating sepsis and septic shock. Cochrane Database Syst Rev 2001;2:3-5.
29. Grover R, Zaccardelli D, Colice G, Guntupalli K, et al. An open label dose circulation study of nitric oxide synthase inhibitor, 546C88 in patients with septic shock. Glaxo Wellcome International Septic Shock Study Group. Critical Care Medicine 1999;27(5):913-22.
30. Yunge, et al. Angiotensin for neither septic shock unresponsive to nor adrenaline. Archive Dis Child 2000;82(5):388-99.
31. Wunderink R, Leeper K, Schein R. Filgrastim in patients with pneumonia and severe sepsis or septic shock. Chest 2001;119(2):523-29.
32. Lauterbach R, Pawlik D, et al. Effect of immuno-modulating agent Pentoxyfylline in the treatment of sepsis in prematurely delivered infant: a placebo controlled double blind trial. Critical Care Medicine 1999;27(4):807-14.
33. Cole L. High volume hemofiltration in human septic shock. Int Care Med 2001;27:978-86.

Blood Component Therapy

VP Choudhry

Transfusion of blood and its components requires careful consideration in children as a result of continuous anatomical and physiological developments. A correct diagnosis is essential for proper choice and use of various components. The weight and age of the patient determines the transfusion requirements and risks of complications. Potential problems often arises because of the small intravascular volume and difficulty in administration of larger amounts blood products if the concentrates are not available. Premature infants and neonates under the age of four months present unique problems in pediatric transfusion therapy. Premature infants are often over transfused.[1] With the better understanding of the pathophsiological changes and advances in the management of critically ill newborns have necessitated changes in the blood banks policies and preparation of smaller units. The administration of blood components have been altered to suit their special needs. Appropriate pediatric transfusion practice requires the understanding of neonatal physiology.

A full-term neonate has an average blood volume of 85 ml/kg and a premature infant has about 100-110 ml/kg of the body weight. The blood volume reduces after birth as a result of transudation of the plasma. A newborn cannot compensate for volume depletion or over transfusion as well as an adult can because of limited cardiovascular adaptive capabilities. Normal hemoglobin (Hb) level in the neonates varies between 16-18 g/dL and normal levels varies significantly. Neonatal hemoglobin is not able to deliver oxygen to tissues as effectively as an adult hemoglobin. The bone marrow shows poor response to anemia, primarily due to low erythropoietin level and poor reticulocyte response to anemia.

Metabolic problems may arise as a result of immature kidneys which has poor capability of excreting potassium and acid and/or calcium loads. Similarly, acidosis or hypocalcemia may occur because of immature liver which cannot metabolize citrate efficiently.

BLOOD COMPONENTS

The various blood components used for pediatric transfusion are shown in Table 7.1. All these components can be leucodepleted, irradiated or saline washed as per requirements.

Red Blood Cells (RBCs)

There are marked differences in transfusion practices in children and adults:
1. Children require relatively small quantities of blood and blood products, usually 10-15 ml/kg body weight of and thus require only fraction of unit.

Table 7.1: Blood components
Unmodified components

1. Cellular components
   a. Red cells
   b. Platelets
   c. Granulocytes

2. Plasma components
   a. Fresh frozen plasma
   b. Cryoprecipitate
   c. Factor concentrates

2. Repeated blood sampling, even of small quantities, can lead to volume depletion in a neonate. Some times red cell transfusions are needed following iatrogenic blood loss for laboratory tests and blood gas analysis.[1] The sicker infant more often requires blood sampling and thus may require red cells, plasma and platelet products.[1] It is generally recommended that micromethods should be used for various investigations such as biochemical parameters, blood gas analysis blood cultures etc. specially for neonates and infants.
3. Since neonates have maternal antibodies, in addition to their own, until the age of 3-6 months, therefore, it is preferable that red cells intended for transfusion should be crossmatched with the mother's serum, as well.

Currently the knowledge of hematopoiesis during neonatal, perinatal period and that of response to RBC (i.e. packed red cells) transfusion is limited. The tissue need for oxygen cannot be measured directly and presence of high fetal hemoglobin cannot release the oxygen to tissues as freely as adults. Therefore, the indications for red cell transfusions are not well defined.[1,2] However, packed red cell transfusions in presence of cardiorespiratory failure secondly to anemia is unquestioned. Role of packed red cell transfusion in situations such as poor weight gain, respiratory difficulties, apnea, patent ductus arteriosus or maintenance of a predetermined blood hemoglobin concentration etc. remains controversial.

The concept of 'fresh' red cells needs to be clarified. Freshness is a vague form as its definition is variable. Platelets and factor VIII are lost within 48 hours of storage at 4°C. There is an increase in potassium and ammonia along with a reduction in pH after 5-7 days of storage. Blood less than 5 days old is often used for large volume transfusions, e.g. exchange transfusion in neonates. Blood less than 5 days old ensures that the plasma electrolyte concentration is within tolerable limits for infants and is now considered as fresh blood.

Indications for Red Cell Transfusions

The indications of red cell transfusion are given in Table 7.2. Pediatricians can modify them according to the general condition of the patient and their hospital transfusion practices.

Table 7.2: Guidelines for red blood cell transfusions

Neonates

a. Physiologic anemia of infancy/anemia of prematurity
b. Hemoglobin (Hb) < 10 g/dL, if neonate is symptomatic
c. Hb < 13.0 g/dL, in cardiopulmonary disease
d. Hb < 10.0 g/dL, in cases of failure to thrive
e. Replacement of iatrogenic blood loss
f. Situations requiring large volume transfusions, e.g. exchange transfusion

Infants and older children

a. Hb < 7 g/dL, or in presence of symptomatic anemia
b. Blood loss due to hemorrhage

Neonates

Physiologic Anemia of Infancy

The anemia, resulting from the decrease in red cell mass due to physiological factors during the first eight weeks of life is termed as "physiologic anemia of infancy." Hemoglobin values in term infant fall to about 11 ± 2 g/dL by 8 weeks of age.[1] The erythropoietin (EPO) response to anemia is relatively diminished and the drop in hemoglobin is variable, with the lowest values (9 ± 2 g/dL).[1] Clinical trials with recombinant human erythropoietin (rhEPO) for the physiological anemia of infancy have been encouraging.[3]

Hb < 10 g/dL, if Symptomatic

In neonates, particularly with respiratory distress, red cell transfusions should correct systemic hypoxia, improve peripheral oxygen delivery and assure adequate oxygen perfusion. The adequacy of transfusion is assessed by hemoglobin level or hematocrit.

Hb <13.0 g/dL, in Cardiopulmonary Disease

Neonates requiring oxygen and ventilator support for longer period should be transfused red cells containing adult hemoglobin. It will provide satisfactory oxygen delivery during the period of illness associated with diminished pulmonary function. It has been recommended that hemoglobin should be maintained above 13.0 g/dl. This level of hemoglobin ensures optimal oxygen delivery in severe cardiac disease with cyanosis or congestive heart failure while in patients with patients ductus arteriousus the rise in hemoglobin levels following red cell transfusion has been found to be useful as it increases pulmonary vascular resistance which enhances the ductal closure and alleviates high output failure. Red cell transfusion should be given slowly and should be monitored closely as transfusion may transiently increase blood volume leading to cardiac failure.

Hb < 10 g/dL in Infants with Failure to Thrive

Anemia is one of the several possible causes for growth failure, especially in presence of other signs of distress (e.g. tachycardia, respiratory difficulty, less vigorous cry and activity and poor sucking). RBC transfusion is recommended in infants having anemia with growth failure, if Hb level is less than 10 g/dL in the absence of other causes for poor weight gain.

Replacement of Iatrogenic Blood Loss

Red blood cells transfusion for iatrogenic blood loss account for about 90% of transfusions during the neonatal period.[4] Repeated blood sampling may be necessary for laboratory monitoring in the intensive care unit. Therefore, it is recommended that only minimal necessary investigations should be undertaken. Secondly these investigation should be done by micromethods to prevent anemia. It is generally advised that red cells should be replaced on volume to volume basis.

Infants and Older Children

Symptomatic Children with Hb < 7 g/dL

Causes of severe anemia could be secondary to diminished erythropoiesis in conditions such as leukemia, aplastic anemia, following chemotherapy, infiltration by tumor cells, myelofibrosis or due to ineffective erythropoiesis secondary to various hemolytic anemia, congenital dyserythropoietic anemia, hemoglobinopathies etc. The usual practice is to raise Hb above 10 gm/dL. Red cells transfusions may be required in asymptomatic infants with anemias, e.g. radiotherapy, which requires adequate Hb for optimal effectiveness and for children undergoing major surgery.

Blood Loss due to Hemorrhage

Blood loss usually occurs during surgical procedures and more in presence of thrombocytopenia or following accidents. The aim of transfusion is to replace the red cell mass and to maintain the oxygen carrying capacity with adequate tissue perfusion. In massive transfusion (> 1 blood volume replacement in 24 hours) whole blood may be given as it also provides plasma for maintaining oncotic pressure.

Transfusion of the RBC Product

Packed red cells (hematocrit 70-80%) in a dose of 10-15 ml/kg body weight is the product of choice for neonates. Clinical and laboratory evidence suggest that RBCs preserved in extended storage media (AS-1 or AS-3) are safe for neonatal transfusions until the units have been preserved for over 42 days.[5,6]

Donor exposure should be limited by collecting RBCs in a multiple bags (e.g. triple bag or pentapack) and splitting the bag into individual small volume units, which retain the expiry date of the original red cell unit. Alternatively the required amount of red cells can be transferred to a transfer bag using a sterile connecting device under all aseptic measures to ensure sterility.

The age of blood does not matter for small volume top-up transfusions. Hyperkalemia is not a common complication because of higher amounts of plasma potassium in stored RBCs except when large volume transfusions are given.[7] Storage of blood often results in depletion of 2, 3-DPG (2,3-diphosphoglycerate) and the resultant high oxygen affinity is a theoretical disadvantage of aged blood, but does not constitute any significant problem in clinical practice. The 2,3-DPG rapidly regenerates following transfusion. 2,3-DPG is greater than 70% during the first 5 days of storage, therefore it is preferable that blood collected within 5 days should be used for exchange and other massive transfusions.

For other infants and older children the dose for transfusion is 15 ml/kg body weight, irrespective of the age. It results in rise of Hb by 2 to 2.5 g/dL. Smaller repeat doses (5 ml/kg) spread over 24 hours may be given in children with severe anemia. Children may be given 15 ml/kg of body weight. Very slow transfusion with constant monitoring and use of frusemide may be undertaken in infants with severe anemia. Otherwise a partial exchange should be done to avoid volume overload.

Platelet Transfusion

Platelet concentrates may be either random donor platelet (RDP) units or single donor platelet (SDP) units. RDP units are prepared from one unit of whole blood and contain 5.5×10^{10} platelets in 40-60 ml of plasma. SDP units are harvested from a donor connected to the cell separator (apheresis) and contain 3×10^{11} platelets. Both are stored at +22°C on a platelet agitator and have a short shelf-life for 3-5 days depending on the type of the bag.

The normal platelet count in infants and children is similar to adults with a range of $150\text{-}450 \times 10^9/L$. General guide lines for platelet therapy are given in Table 7.3. The primary indication for platelet transfusion is thrombocytopenia with active bleeding. Thrombocytopenia may result from decreased platelet production, increased platelet destruction or following massive blood transfusion. There is no absolute threshold or critical value below which bleeding always occurs. However, the risk of bleeding is high when platelet count is below $10 \times 10^9/L$ and very high when platelet count is below $5 \times 10^9/L$. In actively bleeding patients or those undergoing major surgical procedures the platelets should be transfused if the platelet counts is below $50 \times 10^9/L$. Platelet counts should be maintained above $20 \times 10^9/L$ in those who have thrombocytopenia following bone marrow failure or undergoing minor surgical procedures. Consensus Conference Statement (1998) recommended that platelet count should be maintained above $10 \times 10^9/L$ for stable thrombocytopenic patients and $20 \times 10^9/L$ for those with fever infection and related conditions with prophylactic platelet support.[8] In neonates, the Consensus suggests a higher threshold should be maintained as there is considerable danger of hemorrhage. However, in developing countries, it is more practical to treat clinical bleeding rather than platelet count in view of poor availability of platelet concentrates, high cost and limited facilities.

Platelet transfusions may also be required in the neonatal immune thrombocytopenia (secondary to maternal idiopathic thrombocytopenic purpura (TIP) or neonatal alloimmune thrombocytopenia).

In thrombocytopenia secondary to maternal ITP the platelet antibodies have broad reactivity against all platelets. Transfusion of platelets from all donors including the mother and family members have uniformly short survival. It should be given only in life threatening situations. Intravenous immunoglobulin is effective therapy for both the categories of immune thrombocytopenia. In neonatal alloimmune thrombocytopenia, maternal platelets can be used as they are the most readily available source of compatible platelets. Platelet can be washed to remove incompatible plasma and irradiated to avoid graft-versus-host disease (GVHD). If PLA–1 negative platelets are necessary SDP should be preferred.

Platelets should be rapidly infused over 30-40 minutes. One unit of RDP unit/5 kg body weight is sufficient to stop hemorrhage. Platelets have a lifespan of 7 days but are probably hemostatically effective for only the first 4 or 5 days. About two-third remain in the circulation while the rest comprise a freely exchangeable splenic pool. Determination of a 1 hour post-transfusion corrected count increment (CCI) has been suggested to assess the response to platelet therapy. However, the cessation of hemorrhage is the way to determine the effectiveness of platelet therapy. If the adequate platelet therapy does not arrest the bleeding in the absence of infection and other causes such as disseminated intravascular coagulopathy, platelet refractoryness should considered. In these cases one should investigate for platelet antibodies. Special platelet products like HLA-matched platelets, should be considered to control the bleeding episodes in presence of platelet alloantibodies.

Table 7.3: Guidelines for platelet transfusion

1. Platelet count < 50 x 10^9/L in premature infants
2. Platelet count < 10 x 10^9/L
   a. active bleeding or
   b. major invasive or surgical procedure
3. Platelet count < 20 x 10^9/L
   a. marrow failure or
   b. minor surgical procedure
4. Cardiovascular bypass surgery
5. Excessive hemorrhage, regardless of the platelet count
6. Immune thrombocytopenia
7. Neonatal thrombocytopenia
   a. Neonatal alloimmune thrombocytopenia
   b. Secondary to maternal ITP

Random donor platelet (RDP units) are usually given irrespective of ABO and Rh blood group if the RDP is not visibly contaminated with red cells. It has been observed that platelet survival is better when ABO compatible platelets are transfused. Heal et al found a higher median CCI with ABO identical transfusions and the lowest with platelet incompatible transfusion, i.e. when recipient has antibodies to donor ABO antigens.[9,10]

Transfusion of ABO incompatible plasma is more dangerous in the pediatric recipients, especially in the neonates, than in adults due to their smaller blood volume. If necessary the plasma volume of platelets (RDP) can be reduced. Volume reduction is also necessary to prevent volume overload.

There is a possibility of recipient sensitization to Rh-(D) antigen in Rh-(D) negative patients as small numbers of donor erythrocytes are always present in platelet products. Although the ability of the host to respond to immunogenic stimuli may be compromised by disease or by therapy, but it is essential to administer the anti D immunization to Rh negative individuals.

Granulocyte Transfusions

The quantitative and qualitative abnormalities in myelopoiesis and circulating neutrophils present in the newborn have suggested a possible role for granulocyte transfusions in addition to microbial therapy for treatment of overwhelming sepsis. Neonates are more susceptible to severe bacterial infections than older individuals.

Optimal use of granulocyte transfusion for neonatal recipients is under investigation and is yet to be established beyond doubt. The only granulocyte preparations whose efficiency is documented in the clinical trials are those harvested by leukopheresis. The average cells per leuukopheresis unit is 2×10^{10}, nearly two times of daily production in neonates and about 10% of the daily granulocyte production in adults. It should be borne in mind that septic neonates need granulocyte transfusion urgently.

Stauss has analyzed the data from seven reports of granulocyte transfusions.[11] He has concluded that the precise role of granulocyte transfusion for neonatal sepsis is unclear. Some patients of neonatal sepsis respond to antibiotics alone but have high mortality.

The dose of granulocytes transfused should be at least $1-2 \times 10^9$/kg body weight given once in 24 hours or more frequently as required. The volume of infusion is usually 10-15 ml/kg. The granulocyte product should be red cell compatible and preferably irradiated if the infant is premature or immunodeficient. Since granulocyte function deteriorates with storage, they should be transfused within a few hours of collection.

Fresh Frozen Plasma (FFP)

FFP is the fluid portion of the blood which is separated and frozen at lower than –30°C within 6-8 hours of collection. In general FFP is used to replace coagulation factors in infants with acquired or congenital deficiencies (Table 7.4).

Since maternal clotting factors do not cross the placenta, hereditary deficiencies of clotting factors may be apparent at birth. Hemorrhagic disease of the newborn, caused by deficiency of vitamin K dependent coagulation factors (factor II, VII, and IX and X) may result in significant cutaneous, gastrointestinal or CNS hemorrhage at 2-4 days of age. Now this disease is rare as intramuscular vitamin K is routinely given at birth. Vitamin K deficiency may also occur in pediatric patients in the setting of malnutrition and/or alteration of the gut microflora following broad spectrum antibiotics therapy or interference of vitamin K metabolism by certain newer cephalosporins.

Coagulopathy is also a feature of disseminated intravascular coagulation (DIC) or impaired hepatocellular function. Management of DIC includes of treatment of the underlying cause and transfusion of FFP and platelets till the process of DIC is

Table 7.4: Recommendation for transfusion of FFP
1. Vitamin K dependent coagulopathy in hemorrhagic disease of newborn (HDN) with significant hemorrhage
2. Replacement of isolated factor deficiencies, when specific component therapy is not available (Factor VIII, Factor IX, fibrinogen deficiency, Factor X, V, II deficiency etc)
3. Replacement therapy in antithrombin III, protein C or S deficiency
4. DIC
5. Reversal of hemostatic disorders following massive transfusion
6. Therapeutic plasma exchange in thrombotic thrombocytopenic purpura (TTP)
7. Coagulopathy secondary to L-asparaginase therapy

controlled.[12] Hemorrhage prior to invasive procedures in patients with impaired hepatocellular function (e.g. hepatitis or hepatotoxicity due to chemotherapy) is also managed with FFP. In thrombotic thrombocytopenic purpura (TTP), the first line therapy is plasma exchange with large volume FFP infusion, or cryo-poor plasma. FFP is more effective as it is able to provide a labile platelet aggregation inhibitor.[13] FFP also reduces the incidence of coagulopathy associated with L-asparaginase therapy in acute lymphoblastic leukemia (ALL).

Each unit of FFP contains 1 unit of activity/ml of therapeutically useful clotting factors, FFP is administered usually in the dose of 10 ml/kg body weight over 1-2 hours and repeated every 30 minutes as necessary to control the hemorrhage. The dose can be repeated every 12 or 24 hours depending on the clinical situation.

FFP should not be used for the sole purpose of treating hypovolemia as the FFP carries the risk of transfusion transmitted infections. FFP would definitely be preferred for infants who require both plasma volume expansion and clotting factor replacement, as occurs in septic shock or nercotizing enterocolitis.

Cryoprecipitate

It is prepared by thawing FFP at 4°C. The cryoprecipitate provides a concentrated form of fibronogen, F VIII, vWF and F VIII as compared to FFP (approximately a five fold increase in factor VIII concentration). A commonly used dose is 20 ml/kg.

Cryoprecipitate is a useful for acquired hypofibrinogenic states besides for management of bleeding episodes in factor VIII deficiency, von Willebrand's disease (Table 7.5).[14]

Modified Components

Gamma-irradiated Blood Products

Transfusion associated graft-versus-host disease (TA-GVHD) is due to the immune response mounted by the donor T-lymphocytes against host tissues. Gamma-irradiation in doses of 25-30 Gy prevents the GVHD by inactivating these T cells.[15] Irradiated blood products are also indicated in severely immuno-deficient patient fetus requiring intrauterine transfusions and children getting transfusion from first degree relatives. Though occasional instances of TA-GVHD have been reported in the neonates. There is no definitive data to suggest the need for irradiated blood to be given to healthy term infants.[16] Deleterious effects of irradiation have been noted on recovery of red cells and on extracellular potassium which increases with the storage. Therefore, it is preferable to irradiate blood products prior to dispensing.

Table 7.5: Recommendations for use of cryoprecipitate
1. Hemophilia A
2. von Willebrand's disease
3. Hypofibrinogenemia or dysfibrinogenemia
4. DIC
5. Preparation of fibrin glue (fibrin sealant)

Besides whole blood, the blood components can cause TA-GVHD. It is usual practice is to irradiate (with a minimum of 25 Gy) these blood components used for intrauterine transfusions or for neonatal patients with birth weight < 1200 grams or whenever the donor and recipient are first-degree relatives.[9] Components that have been frozen (deglycerolized RBCs, fresh frozen plasma, and cryoprecipitae) or blood products such as albumin, plasma protein fraction, and gammaglobulin need not be irradiated.

Use of Special Filters and Leucocyte Depleted Blood

Currently available third generation leucodepletion filters achieve a 3 log depletion, i.e. they remove 99.9% of the leucocytes. Leucocyte depletion diminishes the chance of alloimmunization to WBC antigens, decreases the risk of CMV transmission, and possibly also reduces the effects of immuno-modulation. Several studies have failed to confirm the postulated high risk of transfusion-transmitted CMV in the neonates as the recipients of CMV seropositive blood and blood products do not have an increased mortality or morbidity.[17]

The genuine benefits of WBC reduction are limited. In view of the technical difficulties and high costs of filters the routine use of leucocyte depletion for all transfusions is not justified.

Saline-washed Red Blood Cells and Platelets

Washing of RBCs removes about 90% of the leucocytes and 99% of plasma proteins and electrolytes. Saline-washed red cells are recommended in patients who are hypersensitive to plasma to prevent urticarial reactions in IgA deficient patients to avoid anaphylaxis, in multitransfused patients, e.g. thalassemia, to prevent nonhemolytic febrile transfusion reactions and in babies with paroxysmal nocturnal hemoglobinuria to remove the compliment.

Saline-washed platelets reduces the plasma content by 95% without any significant platelet loss. Saline washed platelets are of great benefit in patients with severe allergic reactions. Similarly, washed platelets of the mother are recommended in neonates with alloimmune thrombocytopenia.

TRANSFUSION IN DISEASE STATES REQUIRING MULTIPLE TRANSFUSIONS

Thalassemia

The aim of management in thalassemia is to maintain the Hb level above 10 gm/dL. Packed red cell transfusions may be required initially at short intervals to achieve the required hemoglobin levels. Subsequently packed red cell transfusions are given at 2-3 weekly intervals.[18,19]

Generally, RBC units that have been stored for fewer than 7-10 days are advocated for two reasons: (a) Higher 2, 3 DPG levels and (b) better transfusion survival in these units compared to units stored for 35-42 days. However, both these reasons are not valid as red cell stored for relatively short periods do not increase TLC post-transfusion survival or decrease the transfusion requirements.

Thalassemics may develop allergic and/or febrile non-hemolytic trasnfusion reactions following multiple transfusions. Leucocyte filters are used are recommended with the first RBC transfusion to prevent the development of these side effects. Since the cost of filters is high and the fact that all patients do not develop these reactions. Therefore, practical strategy for a developing country is to use the filters when children develop these reactions. Alternatively saline washed red cells, which have negligible plasma proteins and less than 10% of the leukocytes has been recommended.

Sickle Cell Disease (SCD)

Red cell transfusions are given to patients with SCD with the objectives to (a) to correct anemia which increases the oxygen carrying capacity in the anemic patients and (b) To replace the abnormal HbS by normal HbA to reduce the viscosity of blood which in turn reduces the incidence of blood sequestration. Reduction of sickle cells to 40% in the blood alleviates the pain, prevents local hypoxia and prevents pooling of blood in the spleen and at other sites.

The red cells can be given as a simple transfusion or exchange transfusion depending upon the severity of disease. In a simple transfusion, red cells (10 ml/kg) are given at 12 hourly intervals till hemoglobin level attains normal range. Subsequently blood may be given at 3-4 weekly interval to ensure that the proportion of sickle cells in the blood are kept below 40%. Exchange transfusion may be undertaken in infants during acute crisis.

Hemolytic Disease of the Newborn (HDN)

In HDN, the red cells of the fetus are coated with IgG alloantibodies of maternal origin resulting in accelerated destruction fetal red cell at birth. Exchange transfusion is performed in severe hemolytic disease of the newborn (HDN) with the objectives of:

1. Reducing the load of accumulated bilirubin and of antibody molecules by removal of the plasma from the newborn.
2. Reducing the antibody/coated cells prevents the hemolysis of red cells. There by reduces the bilirubin production;
3. Provides additional albumin to bind residual bilirubin; and
4. Restoring the hemoglobin level.

In severe HDN, inspite of a successful exchange, bilirubin may reaccumulate in the intravascular space due to continued hemolysis or redistribution of bilirubin from other compartments. Exchange transfusion can be repeated if required.

Hemophilia

The availability of factor concentrates has drastically reduced the use of cryoprecipitae as the source of coagulation factors.[14] The factor concentrate are much safer as they are virally inactivated. Recombinant factor concentrates are now available. However, in developing countries, due to limited availability of factor concentrates and its high cost, fresh frozen plasma (FFP) is being used in majority of cases.

The dose of Factor VIII for hemophilia A is calculated as follows: 0.5 units of factor VIII/kg body weight raises the plasma levels by 1%. Factor VIII has a short half-life of 8-12 hours. Therefore, factor VIII is administered at 12 hourly. The indication of factor replacements for various situations has been reviewed recently.[20] Currently few centers are using factor replacement prophylactically to ensure near normal life and to prevent development of arthropathy.

In hemophilia B, the dose of Factor IX is 1 unit/kg body weight to raise the Factor IX level by 1%.

Oncology Patients

Patients especially with leukemia and other malignancies present with anemia. Chemotherapy may also lead to anemia and thrombocytopenia. These children need repeated red cell and platelet transfusions for several weeks or months during and after chemotherapy. These cases need to be monitored periodically. Leucodepleted blood products are advisable if the bone marrow transplant is being considered for treatment of cancer to reduce the risk of alloimmunization and CMV disease. Irradiated blood products are recommended to prevent TA-GVHD.

REFERENCES

1. Strauss RG. Transfusion therapy in neonates. Am J Dis Child 1991;45:904-11.
2. Strauss RG, Sacher RA, Blazina JF, et al. Commentary on the small volume red cell transfusion for neonatal patients. Transfusion 1990;30:565-70.
3. Messer J, Haddad J, Donate I, et al. Early treatment of premature infants with recombinant human erythropoietin. Pedaitrics 1993;92;519-23.
4. Choudhry VP, Krishnamurti L. Hemato-oncologic emergencies in Principles of Pediatric and Neonatal emergencies Ed. Sachdev HPS, Puri RK, Bagga A, Choudhry P. Publication of Ind. Pediatrics. Jaypee Publishers 1994;201-20.
5. Strauss RG, Burmeister L, James T, Miller J, et al. A randomized trial of fresh versus stored RBCs for neonatal transfusion (abstract): Transfusion 1994;34(suppl):66S.
6. Strauss RG, Burmeister LF, Johnson K, et al. AS-1 red cells for neonatal transfusions: A randomized trial assessing donor exposure and safety. Transfusion 1998;38:873-78.
7. Voak D, Cann R, Finney RD, et al. Guidelines for administration of blodo products: Transfusion of infants and neonates. British Committee for Standards in Haematology Blood Transfusion Task Force. Transfusion Medicine 1994;4:63-69.
8. Consensus Conference on Platelet Transfusion. Br J Cancer 1998;78:290-91.
9. Heal J, Rowe J, McMican A, et al. The role of ABO matching in platelet transfusion. Eur J Haematol 1993;50:110-17.
10. Heal JM, Blurnberg N, Masel D. An evaluation of crossmatching. HLA and ABO matching for platelet transfusions to refractory patients. Blood 1987;70:23-30.
11. Strauss RG. Current issues in neonatal transfusions. Vax Sang 1986;51:1-9.
12. Choudhry VP, Sharma LM, Kashyap R. Disseminated intravascular coagulation in Recent Advances in Pediatrics. Ed Gupte S. Jaypee Publications 2001;11:75-86.
13. Rock GA, Shumak KH, Buskard NA, et al. Comparison of plasma exchange and plasma infusion in the treatment of thrombotic thrombocytopenic purpura. N Engl J Med 1991;325-393.97.
14. Kashyap R and Choudhry VP. Management of hemophilia in developing countries. Ind Pediatr 2001;68;151-57.
15. Rosen NR, Weidner JG, Bolot HD, Rosen DS. Prevention of transfusion associated graft-versus-host disease: Selection of an adequate dose of gamma irradiation. Transfuson 1993;33:125-27.
16. Strauss RG. Practical issues in neonatal transfusion practices. AM J Clin Pathol 1997;107(suppl 1):557-83.
17. Preiksaitis JK. Indications for use of cytomegalovirus seronegative blood products. Trans Med Rev 1991;5:1-17.
18. Marous RE, Wonke B, Bantock HM, et al. A prospective trial of young red cells in 48 patiens with transfusion dependent thalassemia. Br J Hematol 1985;60:153-59.
19. Choudhry VP, Ahlawat S and Pati HP. Current management protocol in thalassemia in current management protocols in pediatric practice. Ed Kukreja S Publishers CBS 1995;178-86.
20. Kashyap R and Choudhry VP. Inhibitors in hemophilia in Recent Advances in Pediatrics Ed. Gupte S. Jaypee Publications 2001;11:314-23.

Ventilatory Support in Children

DK Pawar

Ventilatory support may be defined as supporting the ventilation of the patient partially or completely to maintain blood gas tension homeostasis within acceptable physiological limits. It may be achieved by moving the air and oxygen into and out of the lungs, by an external device such as a resuscitation bag or a mechanical ventilator through ET tube, tracheostomy or a facemask.

Ventilatory support is not curative. It is a supportive technique. It's purpose is to provide adequate alveolar ventilation, optimal systemic oxygenation and decreased work of breathing till such time the primary cause of respiratory failure such as, atelectasis, pulmonary edema, respiratory muscle paralysis, etc. resolves.

Vasaline in 1955 was one of the first to suggest that artificial respiration in humans was possible by blowing air through a tube of Reed or cane positioned in the trachea. Though Crafoord, a Swedish surgeon first used positive pressure ventilation during thoracic surgery in 1930s, the polio epidemic of 1950s established the role of intermittent positive pressure ventilation (IPPV) to support ventilation and save life. Subsequently a variety of mechanical devices for ventilating the lungs by IPPV were designed.[1] In recent years, tremendous technological advances have been made in design and sophistication of mechanical ventilators.[2]

By and large the practice of mechanical ventilation in children is an extrapolation of adult techniques. There are no well-designed prospective, randomized studies in pediatric patients, which validate any mode of conventional ventilation as safe and efficacious.

In this article, relevant applied respiratory physiology will be reviewed the basic principles of ventilators will be explained, and patients who might benefit from the support device identified and care of the children on ventilator and the ventilator will be described.

APPLIED RESPIRATORY PHYSIOLOGY

During spontaneous respiration, a pressure gradient is created between the proximal airway and the pleural space due to diaphragmatic and inspiratory muscle contraction, resulting in gas flow in to the lungs. The volume of gas that is moved in and out of the lungs per breath is called a tidal volume (6-8 ml/kg). The airways act to conduct gas, which passes in aliquots to the alveolar space and back. The volume of gas that remains in the lungs at the end of quiet expiration is called the functional residual capacity (FRC). The normal FRC is about 30 ml/kg. This volume of gas primarily takes part in gaseous exchange. The smaller conducting airways have a tendency to collapse at lower volumes on expiration. The volume of gas present in the lungs when airways begin to collapse is called the closing capacity (CC). In children over the age of 6 years FRC exceeds CC, which allows the small airways and alveoli to remain open throughout the respiratory cycle. In children less than 6 years CC generally exceeds FRC, which leads to an increased incidence of atelectasis in infants and young children. That's why these children benefit from CPAP. Gas exchange from the alveoli to pulmonary circulation occurs entirely by diffusion of gases across the alveolar capillary barrier.

FRC is decreased in respiratory failure from alveolar or interstitial disease. A major goal of ventilatory support is to return the FRC to normal value and thereby improve systemic arterial oxygenation.

Pulmonary Compliance

Compliance of the lungs is defined as the change in volume per unit change in distending airway pressure and is determined by elastic forces within the lungs.[3] Lung compliance is therefore a measure of 'stiffness' of lungs. Chest compliance is the change in thoracic cage volume produced by a unit change in transthoracic pressure. Respiratory system compliance is defined as total of lung and chest wall compliance.

Airway Resistance

Airway resistance is the pressure difference between mouth and alveoli or the driving pressure needed to move respiratory gases through the airways at a constant flow rate.[3] The most important determinant of airway resistance is the airway radius. The resistance is inversely related to the 4th power of the radius as defined by Poiseuelle's Law, which means a 50% decrease in the radius would increase the resistance by 16 times. Even minor decrease in airway lumen size due to edema, mucous plug or bronchospasm can lead to significant increase in airway resistance.

Time Constants

The time constant of the respiratory system is a measure of how quickly the lungs fill or how long it takes for the alveolar and proximal airway pressure to equilibrate. The product of airway resistance and pulmonary compliance defines the time constant. Knowledge of time constants aids greatly in choosing the safest, most effective ventilator respiratory time and inspiratory time for a particular patient.[4] In a healthy lung 3-5 time constants are necessary to allow complete filling or emptying of alveoli. In a healthy infant one-time constant equals 0.15 sec. Three time constants (0.45 sec) allow approximately 80% filling of all alveolar units. Increasing the inspiratory time beyond 5 time constants does not yield more than 95% alveolar filling.

A patient with increased airway resistance is at risk of gas trapping the end of expiration. Appropriate ventilator setting must be selected to prolong the expiratory phase as much as possible for the child's tidal volume to be expelled completely.

Work of Breathing

The work of breathing is entirely performed by muscles of inspiration during normal tidal breathing. Normally <5% of total oxygen delivery is consumed to meet the work of breathing by the respiratory muscles. In lung disease the work of breathing is markedly increased. The oxygen demand to meet the increased work of breathing may increase to 25-50% of total oxygen delivery. The increase in oxygen demand causes a redistribution of oxygen delivery. In such circumstances mechanical ventilation may decrease the work of breathing, reroute the oxygen delivery to other vital organs and reverse the respiratory muscle fatigue.[5]

UNDERSTANDING THE VENTILATOR

The ventilator is a device to provide artificial respiration that is to move gases in and out of the lungs. Understanding the ventilator is important in order to choose the right one for a hospital set up or to use it correctly in a particular patient.

Anatomy

The ventilator has basically three parts: (a) face, (b) brain and (c) limbs.

Face

This is the control panel, which is what is seen on the front of the ventilator with the control knobs and keys, manometers and dials. The respiratory parameters are set by using these knobs. In new generation ventilators, the control panel is divided in to three areas, which are separately color coded and displayed. One area shows the set parameters for a patient, the second area shows the actually delivered parameters, e.g. pressures and gas flow, rates which are measured by a pressure transducer at the patient end and a flow transducer. The third area shows the alarm system. It provides audiovisual alarms when set parameters are not achieved. Some of the ventilators have the facility for numeric as well as graphic display.

Brain

Brain of the ventilator is not seen from outside. It's within the box. It consists of the mechanical component of the early ventilators or the electronic logic of the new ventilators, which control all the functions. With the advent of microprocessor technology, the control of all the respiratory parameters can be performed more precisely. For example, the opening of valves used to take seconds in mechanical ventilators where it now can be done in microseconds with the help of microprocessors. The sensing of pressure generated by the older mechanical ventilators was crude thereby a patient triggering an inspiratory breath use to increased work of breathing.

Limbs

This is the external components, which protrude out of the ventilator box, are called limbs. They have four basic components:

i. *Filters:* These are incorporated into the pneumatic component of the ventilator for prevention of contamination of the patient from ventilated gas (inspiratory limb filter) and atmosphere air from the patient (expiratory limb filters). The expiratory limb filter needs to be changed after every patient use where as inspiratory one can be used for many patients.

ii. *Valves:* These are present at either end of the breathing system. When the inspiratory valve opens and expiratory one closes inspiratory takes place. During expiration, the inspiration valve closes and expiratory one opens.

iii. *Humidifiers:* These are provided for humidification of inspired gases. The nose that normally humidifies inspired gases is bypassed with endotracheal intubation or a tracheosotomy. It is important to maintain humidification for optimal mucociliary activity and softening and elimination of the normal secretions of the tracheobronchial tree. The servocontrolled heated humidifier is the common one used in most ventilators. Heating vaporizes water and it delivers 40-80% humidified gas. The size of the water vapor has to be smaller than 1 micron to reach the respiratory bronchioles.

iv. *The corrugated tubing:* These are small bore (15 mm) non-kinkable low compliant tubings to conduct gases from the ventilator to the patient and from the patient to the atmosphere. In babies and small children where the tidal volume is low, there might be considerable volume loss if the tubing is too compliant.

Physiology

As the ventilator provides artificial inspiration, it has to mimic normal phases of respiration in it's optimal functioning. Like in normal respiration the ventilator should have the following features:

i. Energy to breathe (driving energy)
ii. Inspiration has to be initiated (inspiration phase)
iii. After desired volume is delivered, inspiration has to stop (cycling inspiratory phase to expiratory phase)
iv. Expiration phase
v. Means of cycling expiratory phase to inspiratory phase.

  i. *Drive:* The ventilator derives its energy or power either from a gas source ("pneumatically" driven, e.g. Bird) or electricity (as in most of the new ventilators).

  ii. *Inspiration:* Inspiration is initiated by ventilators by basically two mechanisms:

    a. *Pressure generators (Fig. 8.1):* Ventilators using this mode have a small driving pressure. The pressure difference between the alveolar pressure and driving pressure determines flow and volume of ventilation. With change in lung characteristics such as low compliance or high airway resistance the pressure difference is low and consequently the flow is reduced and the volume delivered would be less.

    b. *Flow generators (Fig. 8.2):* In this mechanisms of inspiration, the driving pressure is much greater and the pressure difference between the alveolar pressure and driving pressure is so large that change in lung and airway characteristics have negligible effect on the flow pattern and therefore by the volume delivered is unaltered.

Most of the new generation ventilators utilize this mechanism for initiation of inspiration.

Ventilatory Support in Children

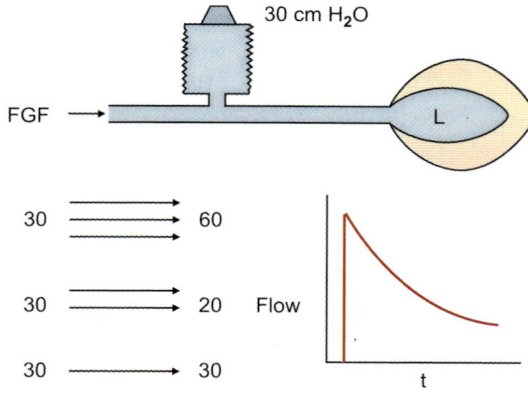

Fig. 8.1: Constant pressure generator

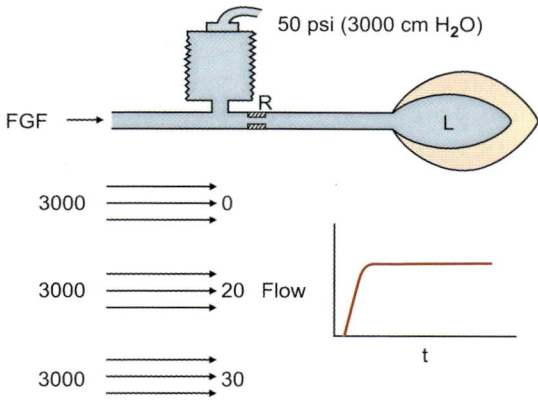

Fig. 8.2: Constant flow generator

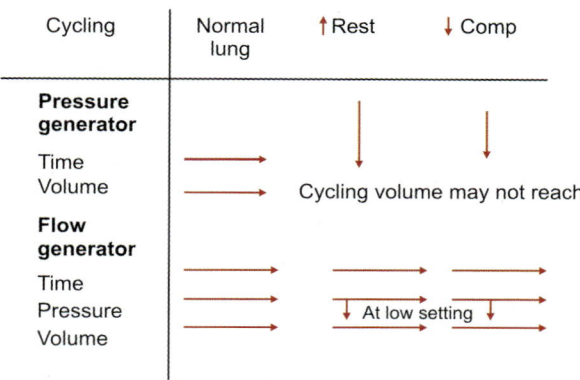

Fig. 8.3: Effect on tidal volume of flow and pressure generator ventilators

The effect of the flow and pressure generator ventilators with the various mechanism of cycling on the delivery of tidal volume is shown in Figure 8.3.

iii. *Cycling inspiration to expiration:* During inspiration, a flow is delivered over a time to a preset volume. As a result a pressure is generated in the airway and lungs. All these parameters, i.e. time, volume, pressure and flow have been utilized to terminate inspiration and cycle to expiration.
   a. *Pressure cycled:* Inspiration ends when the preset pressure is reached in the lungs and the breathing system. This mechanism does not take into account the inspiratory time, flow and volume delivered.
   b. *Volume cycled:* Inspiration ends when a particular preset volume are delivered. The duration of inspiration and airway pressure depends on the airway and lung characteristics.
   c. *Time cycled:* Inspiration ends after a particular preset time elapses. The volume delivered and pressure generated again depends on the characteristics of the lung of airways.
   d. *Flow cycled:* The inspiration ends whenever a particular flow rate is achieved. Normally this is 25% of the peak inspiratory or initial inspiration flow.
   e. *Time cycled volume preset:* Certain ventilators though essentially time cycled can deliver a preset volume during a particular inspiratory period because of the power of the machine. They are called time cycled volume preset ventilators. Most of the new generation ventilators offer this mechanism. Flow generator and time cycled volume preset ventilators best achieve maintenance of a steady level of alveolar ventilation in the face of changes in lung compliance or airway resistance.

iv. *Expiration:* Expiration usually takes place passively to atmosphere. Sometimes the passage of expired gas is modified to provide CPAP, PEEP or NEEP (negative end-expiratory pressure).

v. *Cycling expiration to inspiration:* In most of the ventilators, this is achieved by a time cycling mechanism.

These simple explanations of the basic principle of functioning of ventilator are for the sake of understanding. The new generation ventilators adopt a variety of complex mechanisms.

MODES OF VENTILATION

The versatility of a ventilator in patient care depends on the availability of different modes of ventilation.

The initial development of ventilation was in the field of negative pressure ventilators like Tank, Jacket and Cuirass ventilators. They generated negative pressure around the chest. The function is normal physiologically but it impedes access to the patient. If a tight seal is not achieved especially in infants and children, it cannot deliver an adequate tidal volume. These types of ventilators are not common. Most of the present day ventilators use intermittent positive pressure ventilation (IPPV) to provide alveolar ventilation. In 1950s and 60s it was believed that IPPV is a God sent blessing to save patients lives. With more use in a variety of patient conditions, it was realised that it was not enough; other ventilatory strategies have to be adopted to manage oxygenation and prevent complications. A plethora of ventilatory modes have been designed from very simple to complex.[6] Not many of them have been subjected to critical analysis by controlled trials. So claims of protagonists for a particular mode have to be seen from that point of view. Few representative modes will be discussed here.

They can be classified as:
a. Basic modes: IPPV controlled, Assist, spontaneous
b. Modes to increase FRC and improve oxygenation: CPAP, PEEP, APRV.
c. Modes that allow interaction with patient: IMV, SIMV, auto, proportional assist.
d. Modes, which help in weaning by decreasing the work of breathing: Pressure support, BIPAP.
e. Modes especially useful in children: Pressure limiting, PRVC, HFV, volume support.

Basic Modes

Intermittent Positive Pressure Ventilation (IPPV)

In this mode, positive pressure generated in the ventilator is utilized to deliver a flow and volume over a period of time. In a healthy lung the pressure needed to deliver an adequate volume is around 20 cm H_2O. This mode alters the normal respiratory physiology from negative to positive (Figs 8.4A and B). It leads to impedance in venous return.[7] As the primary goal of ventilation is to maintain oxygenation, ventilatory parameters are often aggressively adjusted to high setting (if necessary) to achieve normal PaO_2 (tidal volume, inspiratory pressures, inspired oxygen concentration).

Assist Controlled

Mechanical breaths are activated by patients' spontaneous inspiratory efforts. In this mode the haemodynamic effect is less marked. However, if the patient effort is insufficient or there is apnoea for more than 12 seconds, the preset mechanical rate is maintained automatically.

Modes to Increase FRC

CPAP/PEEP

When oxygenation is not maintained despite the use of high concentration of oxygen supplementation,

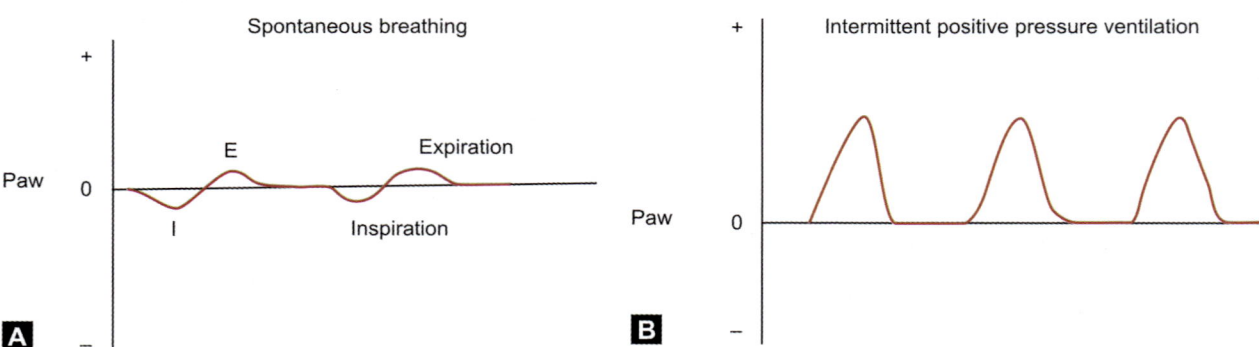

Figs 8.4A and B: Intrathoracic pressure changes in **A.** spontaneous and **B.** IPPV

these modes are applied to increase the FRC. CPAP and PEEP are usually defined as airway pressure above atmosphere maintained throughout the respiratory cycle during spontaneous (CPAP) and controlled respiration (PEEP) respectively, so the airway pressure is always positive. (Figs 8.5A and B) These modes are chieved by application of a continuous gas flow source or a valve, a reservoir or a restriction to the out flow of gases at expiration to produce above atmospheric expiratory pressures. CPAP is most commonly applied through an ET tube, however it can be applied through a mask or nasal prongs. Excessive CPAP/PEEP has been shown to reduce venous return and decrease cardiac output, increase right ventricular after load and shift the interventricular septum into the left ventricular.[8] The use of CPAP/PEEP may result in increase in intracranial hypertension or cerebral ischaemia. The increased intrathoracic pressure obstructs venous return to the thorax and mean venous pressure in the central veins increase. These changes are directly correlated with the level of end expiratory pressure applied.[9,10]

CPAP/PEEP may produce injury to the lungs by over distending the more compliant alveoli.

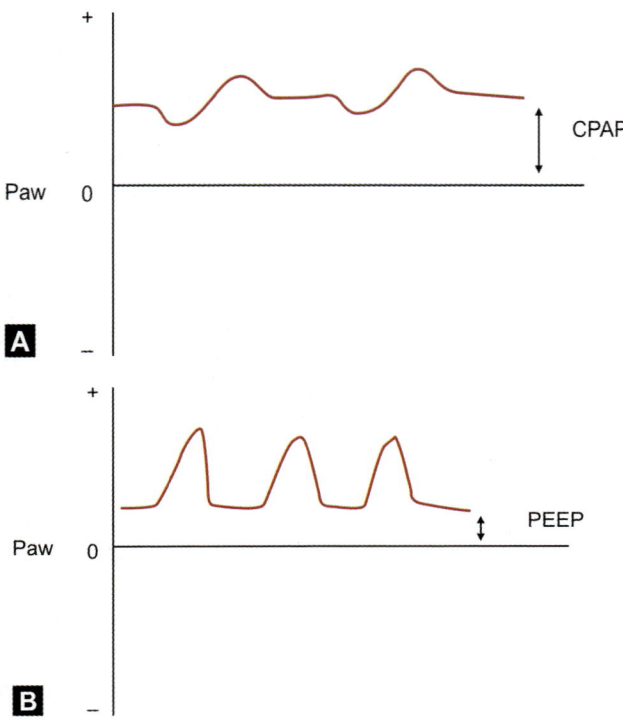

Figs 8.5A and B: Intrathoracic pressure changes with application of **A.** CPAP, **B.** PEEP

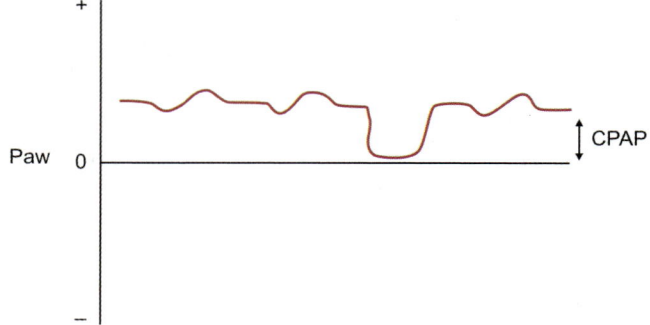

Fig. 8.6: Pressure changes in APRV mode

Airway Pressure Release Ventilation (APRV)

This mode utilizes two levels of pressure during spontaneous breathing.[11] CPAP is maintained at a pre determined level and periodically decreased to a lower pressure. The periodic decrease in intrathoracic pressure theoretically minimizes the haemodynamic compromise (Fig. 8.6).[12]

Modes that allows Patient — Mechine Interaction

Intermittent Mandatory Ventilation (IMV)

This mode delivers a preset mechanically generated breath regardless of patients' inspiratory efforts. This mode was designed to support inadequate ventilation of spontaneously breathing patients.[13] As this mode does not recognize the patient's effort or the breathing pattern, it leads to asynchronous breathing between the patient and ventilator. In order to avoid this complication SIMV mode was designed (Fig. 8.7).

Synchronized Intermittent Mandatory Ventilation (SIMV)

In this mode the ventilator presets the mechanical breaths but patients' own inspiratory efforts are used to synchronise the intermittent mandatory breath (Fig. 8.8).

Proportional Assisted Ventilation

In this method, the ventilator output is modified to meet the patient's respiratory demands.[14] It functions only in spontaneously breathing patients. The ventilator senses and monitors patients' respiratory efforts and provides the pressure support needed. If a

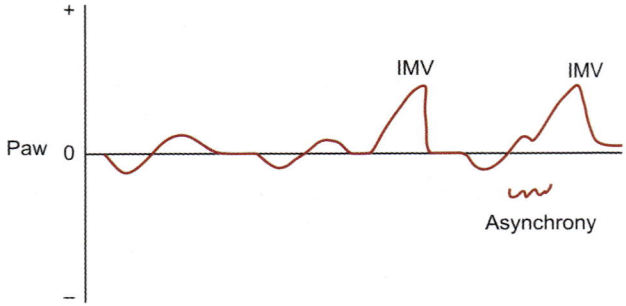

Fig. 8.7: Pressure changes in IMV mode

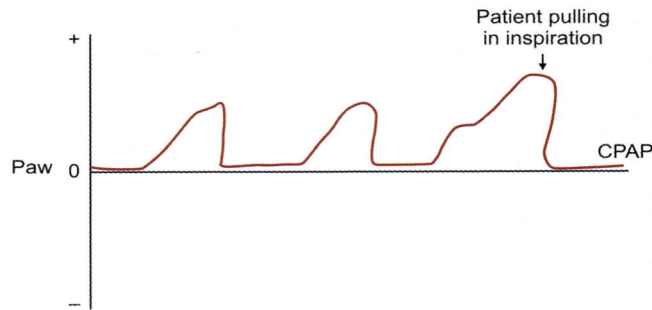

Fig. 8.9: Proportional assist ventilation

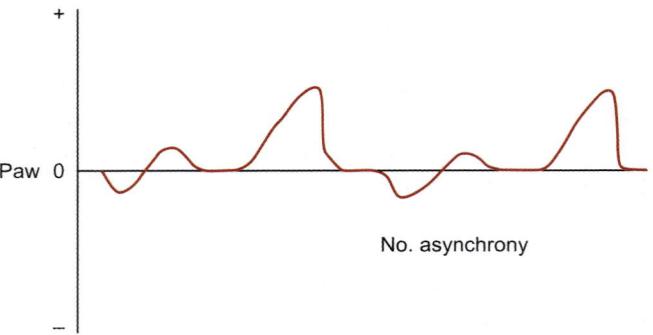

Fig. 8.8: Pressure changes SIMV mode

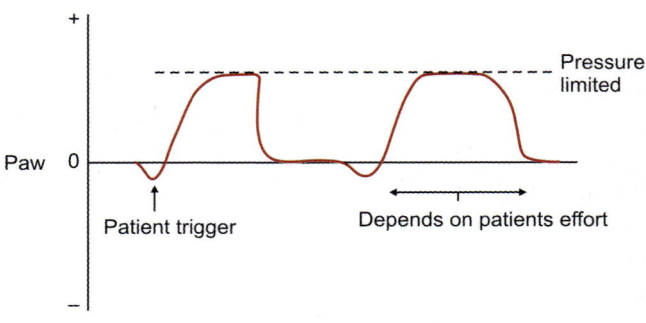

Fig. 8.10: Pressure support

patient generates more negative pressure on inspiration, at respiration, the ventilator provides higher-pressure support compared to SIMV. This mode decreases the Peak Inspiratory Pressure. Though this mode is very promising it is still in experimental stage (Fig. 8.9).

Automode

This mode serves the patients respiratory pattern and changes from support ventilation (controlled SIMV) to non-support ventilation (spontaneous). This mode has recently been introduced by Siemens (300 A) and has undergone a few favorable trials.

Modes Useful in Weaning

Pressure Support (PS, ASV)

This mode provides a predetermined pressure assist from the ventilator once the patient triggers an inspiration. The patient determines the respiratory rate, I: E ratio and part of the resultant tidal volume.

When upper pressure is reached, the pressure assist is maintained at the preset level until the inspiratory flow rate decreases to 25% of maximum inspiratory flow, when the inspiration ceases and passive exhalation takes place (Fig. 8.10).[15,16]

This mode is useful at the weaning phase after prolonged ventilation. In patients with respiratory muscle weakness or fatigue, this mode is used along with SIMV. As the weakness decreases, the SIMV rate needs to be reduced and patients can be successfully weaned.[17]

BIPAP

This mode delivers bilevel positive pressure and ventilatory assistance to a spontaneously breathing patient. When the patient initiates a breath, the device delivers a small assistance to the ventilation along a positive pressure gradient. Unlike CPAP system it can deliver different pressure at inspiration and expiration. This mode has not been studied in children.

Modes Useful for Children

Pressure Limiting

In this mode, the peak inspiration pressure is limited to a preset level.[18,19] Once the pressure is reached, inspiration is terminated irrespective of the volume of gases delivered. It leads to hypoventilation unless the pressure limit is raised. In children there is a variable leak around the endotracheal tube and with increased airway resistance or decreased compliance when the PIP increases, this leak around the tube increases with resultant reduced tidal volume.

Pressure Control Ventilation

In this mode in case of the pressure reaching the preset level, the flow would be diverted from inspiration to produce an inspiratory plateau at that level of pressure.[20] This mode was designed to deliver adequate tidal volume without producing excessive peak inspiratory pressures (PIP), which are considered to be responsible for producing barotrauma (Fig. 8.11).

Pressure Regulated Volume Controlled (PRVC) Ventilation

This is a relatively new mode of controlled ventilation (Siemens 300) in which the ventilator analyses tidal volume on a breath-to-breath basis and resets the peak inspiration pressure (PIP) level needed to assure the target tidal volume (Fig. 8.12). The ventilator accomplishes this by regulating inspiratory pressure to a value based on the volume pressure relationship derived from the previous breath and compared with the target tidal volume.

The advantage of this mode is that the tidal volume is guaranteed at the lowest PIP necessary to achieve it.[21] It thereby minimizes the possibility of barotrauma and variation in tidal volume delivery due to change in compliance and airway resistance. This mode has a special advantage in children as there is a leak around the tube and there is loss of volume due to compression of gases and compliance of the tubing. This mode guarantees the delivery of a preset tidal volume.

High Frequency Ventilation (HFV)

There are three types of high frequency ventilation (HFV) (frequency 60-400/mt): High frequency oscillation (HFO); high frequency positive pressure ventilation (HFPPV) and high frequency jet ventilation (HFJV). HFO has been extensively studied by physiologists but it remains and experimental method of mechanical ventilation. Till recently only HFPPV and HFJV have defined clinical applications. Compared to conventional techniques, the advantage is that they enable adequate gas exchange to occur using small tidal volumes, approximating dead-space volume.[22,23] In ICU patients they reduces peak inspiratory pressure (PIP). So long as adequate humidification and warming of the gas mixture is delivered it offers attractive alternatives to conventional ventilation in a limited number of indications such as:

1. Bronchopleura fistula with large air leak
2. Tracheal lesions secondary to trauma
3. Respiratory failure with elevated peak airway pressure (> 50 cm H_2O) and reduced respiratory compliance.

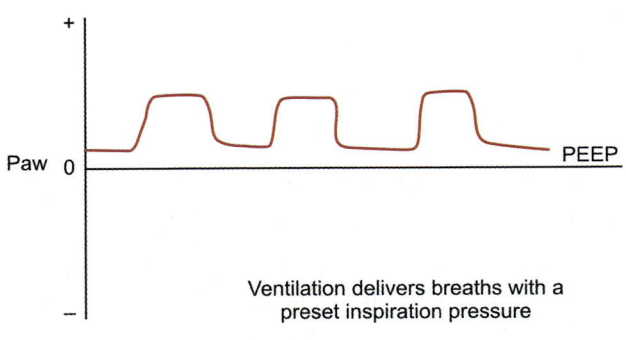

Fig. 8.11: Pressure control ventilation

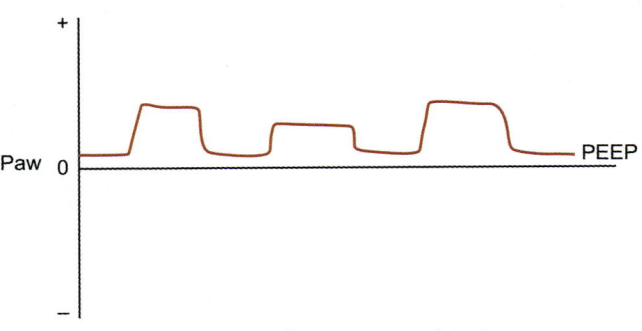

Fig. 8.12: Pressure regulated volume controlled ventilation

HFV is contraindicated in obstructive diseases like Bronchial asthma or in the presence of bronchospasm.[24]

Volume Support Ventilation

In this mode the patient spontaneously triggers the ventilator to provide a pressure limited, flow cycled breath with a condition to provide a tidal volume (as in Bird) or minute ventilation (as in Siemens). These modes have the theoretical benefits of pressure support along with guaranteed minute ventilation. The clinical experience with this attractive mode has not however been published.

INDICATIONS

The vast majority of surgical patients do not require pre or post operative ventilation. The indication is primarily the inability to maintain oxygenation.

Preoperative

i. Children with respiratory failure either due to previous lung pathology, chest infection or trauma. Ventilation is needed to stabilize the patient prior to surgery and CDH, HMD.
ii. Following cardiopulmonary resuscitation specially in trauma victims.

Postoperative

It should be understood that a large number of patients might unexpectedly need postoperative ventilation. Postoperative ventilation improves left ventricular function and decreases the work of breathing thereby allows redistribution of oxygen to vital organs.

A. *Elective preplanned ventilation is carried out in*
  i. Patients already on ventilator preoperatively. (e.g. TOF with chest infection or trauma patients).
  ii. Neonates following major surgery (e.g. diaphragmatic hernia, omphalocele or gastroschisis
  iii. Following surgery after head injury with the possibility of raised intracranial pressure.
  iv. Following major cranial surgery, e.g. craniosynosteosis.

B. *Residual effect of anesthetics*
  i. Inadequate reversal of muscle relaxants. This is seen in patients with electrolyte disturbances, metabolic acidosis and hypothermia.
  ii. Narcotics.

C. *Preoperative conditions may require ventilation:*
  i. Sleep apnea-often come for removal of adenoid and tonsillectomy.
  ii. Neurological disease like myasthenia and muscle dystrophy after major surgery.

D. *Intraoperative complication*
  i. *Aspiration of gastric contents*: These patients are electively ventilated even if the lesion is minor in the intraoperative or immediate postoperative period, as the area of damage is only radiologically evident after some hours.
  ii. *Massive blood loss*: When blood volume loss is more than two blood volumes and in any situation where adequate replacement has not been provided.
  iii. *Cardiovascular instability:* It occurs primarily in children with preoperative cardiac lesions. The commonest cause in previously healthy children is untreated hypovolemia.
  iv. *Hypothermia:* It is a common everyday occurrence in surgery lasting for more than two hours, because of dry gases, cold fluids and cold environments and non-availability of warming devices. If the temperature goes below 34 °C there is possibility of severe metabolic acidosis and inadequate reversal of muscle relaxants.
  v. *Phrenic nerve injury:* It is a complication following cardiac surgery often only recognized in the postoperative period due to failure to wean the child off the ventilator.
  vi. *Postcardiac arrest:* Until such time that the child is stabilized and raised intracranial pressure reduced.

ICU Indication

i. Neonates lung resuscitation.
ii. Preterm HMD.
iii. CDH.

VENTILATORY STRATEGY

Choosing the Right Ventilator and the Mode of Ventilation

For most postoperative patients any type of ventilator and mode used are good enough because of healthy lung conditions. The only consideration should be prevention of the complication of ventilation namely barotrauma.

However, in children with lung disease with altered compliance and airway resistance the ventilator and mode, which guarantees adequate ventilation with minimal PIP should be selected. A time-cycled volume preset ventilator with a pressure-limiting device is the one most desirable. The new supportive modes like PRVC, volume support, and proportional assist ventilation theoretically hold promise. However, more clinical experience is needed to assess their efficacy.

ENDOTRACHEAL TUBE OR TRACHEOSTOMY

If the patient is likely to require long term ventilation for over two weeks and the airway is maintained by ET tube, injury to the larynx and cords might occur.

A nasal ET tube provides more comfort to the patient and is more acceptable. It can also be better secured to the face. It is the preferred route in neonates. However, the tube obstructs the opening of the sinuses in the nose and produces sinusitis in older children. An oral tube is preferred in these age groups.

The tube size (below size 6 mm ID) should be such that, there is an audible leak around the tube. This recommendation was made following the observation that fitting tubes can lead to postoperative stridor due to oedema of the larynx and trachea. Use of cuffed tubes in children in recent reports has not shown such injury. Cuffed tubes might avoid loss of volume, which usually accompanies a leak.

However, child specific ET tube have only recently being designed (kimberly) and not freely available.

ROLE OF MUSCLE RELAXANT ANALGESIA AND SEDATION

Children need to be sedated or paralysed to accept a tube and ventilation. Recent reports implicate the use of muscle relaxants with development of post-operative myopathy.[25] It has not been reported with use for less than 48 hours. So use of muscle relaxant should be avoided and if it cannot be avoided it should be limited to 48 hours. As all the surgical patients have some degree of pain, morphine infusion at the rate of 10-20 ug/kg/hr provides good analgesia, sedation and ventilator acceptance. In some patients a midazolam infusion might be used to supplement. Sedative and analgesics have to be used when children are paralyzed with muscle relaxants.

PERMISSIVE HYPERCAPNIA

The goal of ventilation is to provide adequate oxygenation and reverse respiratory acidosis.

For many years conventional strategy was to achieve these goals by using a volume oriented approach to normalize blood gases. Now we understand that in patients with reduced compliance, (because of atelectasis or collapse of lungs), adequate lung volume is not available for ventilation. The tidal volume is delivered to a small amount of aerated lung. This may lead to over-distension of alveoli and progressive lung injury. There is enough evidence in animal studies to show that mechanical ventilation can result in acute paranchymal lung injury, which is histologically similar to ARDS (in addition to conventional barotrauma).[26] This ventilator induced lung injury occurs by a number of mechanisms: (i) inspiratory over distension due to high volume (volutrauma) (ii) high pressure may result in very high shear forces at the interface between collapsed and aerated lung areas during reinflation. To prevent lungs injury for both these reasons, it is necessary to use low tidal volume (often 6 ml/kg) with optimal PEEP. This may lead to hypercarbia. Hypercarbia does not produce any gross physiological changes and can be tolerated up to a level of 80-90 mm Hg. This ventilatory strategy is called permissive hypercapnia.[27] This may not be applicable in children with head injury and raised intracranial pressure.

COMPLICATIONS OF VENTILATION

i. *Repeated extubation:* It usually occurs inadvertently due to inadequate sedation or improper fixation. It may lead to episodes of hypoxia with resultant morbidity and mortality. Repeated intubation may lead to trauma of larynx and cords.
ii. *Barotrauma (rupture of lung parenchyma):* It is believed to be due to excessive positive pressure. The strategy adopted to prevent barotrauma is to maintain a low PIP, with a Pressure Limiting mode.[28] However, barotrauma is seen more commonly at the interface of a healthy and an adjacent collapsed lung. This leads to asymmetric ventilation and higher shear force at the interface.
iii. *Volutrauma:* is because of over distension of the alveoli at end of inspiration, which leads to injury of the lung.[26] Probably most of the lung injury is due to volutrauma though higher pressures were earlier blamed for it.

iv. *Infection:* The retention of secretions often leads to infection if proper airway toilet in an aseptic manner is not performed. Immuno-compromised patients are more prone to develop infection.

CARE OF THE VENTILATOR

Certain components of the ventilator need to be taken care of on a regular basis by the nursing personnel, respiratory therapists or technical staff. These activities are often supervised or even performed by doctors.

Breathing System

i. The filters need to be changed as per the recommendations of the manufacturer. It could be every 24-48 hours or more depending on the presence of infection.
ii. The humidifier water level has to be maintained by regular refilling with distilled water. The temperature setting has to be adjusted. After every patient it should be cleaned and autoclaved.
iii. Corrugated tubing needs to be changed every 48 hours. In some tubing there are moisture traps, which need to be emptied at regular intervals.

The ventilator tubing should be positioned in such a way that there is no drag and no pressure on the patient's body. Whenever some procedures are carried out, (like physiotherapy or X-ray of the patient), there is the possibility of drag on the tubings and ET tube dislodgment.
iv. Cleaning and sterilization of the reusable components.

CARE OF THE PATIENT ON VENTILATOR

The patients who are put on ventilator are usually sick and cannot breathe. They are either unconscious or paralysed and/or sedated. So they cannot look after themselves and need to be taken care of. Patient care is basically two types:

i. **Care of the unconscious patient:** This involves care of skin, eye, bladder and bowels. Prevention of contracture (by providing regular physiotherapy) and bed sores (by regular turning of patients) is important
ii. **Care of the "ventilator" aspects of the patient:**
   a. *Care of the ET tube:* When an endotracheal tube or tracheostomy is used, the nose is bypassed. The nose normally provides humidification to the tracheobroncheal tree and is essential to maintain the normal defense mechanism of the lungs. So provision of adequate humidification is essential. A conscious person coughs out secretions, which unconscious patients cannot. Repeated endotracheal suctions need to be performed preferably associated with chest physiotherapy. It should be performed aseptically with sterile gloves and sterile catheters. The catheter size should be less than 1/2 the internal diameter of endotracheal tube with a non-traumatic tip and multiple holes, preferably transparent. A tightly fitting suction catheter might generate excessive negative pressure and cause atelectasis. The catheter should be inserted without connecting to suction. After insertion, suction is applied for not more than 10 seconds at a time. Along with the secretions, it sucks out oxygen, which might cause hypoxia. The negative pressure generated may collapse the alveoli causing further hypoxia. Patients should be ventilated with 100% oxygen prior to ET suction, Humidifier, a servo controlled heated humidifier should be incorporated is the inspiratory limb.

   Inadequate humidification leads to reduced or thick secretions. Both doctors and nurses should be able to provide chest physiotherapy such as percussion and vibration.
   b. *Care of the lines (IA, CVP, IV):* Each of these is a potential route of infection. The intravenous, intra arterial, central venous lines should be properly sealed and non-communicating to atmosphere. (All ports should be closed by sterile blockers) and only handled if necessary. The urinary catheters, chest and tube drains should be sealed completely. All the tubing should be changed 24-48 hrs. to prevent any ascending infection.

   The care of the nasogastric tube is very important especially when enteral feeding is provided.
   c. *Nutrition:* To prevent muscle weakness, better wound healing and control of infection a good nutritional status needs to be maintained.

   In the last decade parenteral nutrition in the form of intravenous fat emulsions, proteins and aminoacids and carbohydrates was widely used. This may lead to many complications such as infection, acidosis, electrolyte disturbances, embolisation etc. It is also very expensive. Now most of the patients receive enteral feeding either prepacked one or prepared. These feeds need to be given through nasogastric tube continuously or feeding at regular intervals.

d. *Monitoring:* Patients on ventilator are extensively monitored and it's the responsibility of the ICU personal to observe continuously and maintain a record of it. Common monitoring is:
  i. CVS: Heart rate, blood pressure, central venous pressure, (Cardiac output).
  ii. Respiratory system: Respiratory rate, tidal volume and minute volume, oxygen saturation.
  iii. Temperature and urinary output.
  iv. Ventilator monitors tell us about airway pressure, minute volume, inspired oxygen concentration, compliance and resistance of the lungs and airways. Pressure, flow and volume are important parameters monitored usually at the expiratory limb of the breathing system at the patient end.
  v. Laboratory: Blood gas analysis and electrolytes, kidney function test, culture and sensitivity.

e. *Fluid balance and transfusion:* Maintaining the fluid infusion or blood transfusion record is the nursing responsibility. Besides the record keeping the nurse should assess the adequacy of the fluid therapy and provide proper feed back to the treating surgeons.

f. *Prevention of infection:* Besides providing aseptic care in all the techniques and procedures performed in these patients, some simple but important measures are important in preventing the infection.
  – Barrier nursing, only one nurse should be touching and handling one patient at a time.
  – Before and after touching the patient every one should wash their hands with soap and water followed by use of 70% ethyl alcohol or any similar disinfectant solution.

WEANING

An attempt to wean a child from the ventilator should be made after the cause of ventilation shows improvement, the patient is in minimal oxygen (< 40%) and inotropic support is < 5 ug/kg of dopamine or dobutamine and a PEEP. There should not be any sternal recession, intercostal indrawing or diaphragmatic breathing. Surgical patients after short-term ventilation normally do not need a prolonged process of weaning process unlike long-term ventilated patients.

i. 'T' piece weaning is the conventional method of weaning.[29] Once the patient meets all the criteria for weaning the ventilator is disconnected and the patient connected to a 'T' piece with oxygen. If patient respiratory status does not deteriorate for a period of 2-4 hours ventilation delivery is no more needed.

ii. Gradual weaning is necessary in patients who have been on a ventilator for a long-time, or who-have muscle weakness or fatigue.[30,31] In this technique, once spontaneous effort comes back the ventilator is set to SIMV mode with pressure support from IPPV mode. The support from the SIMV breaths is gradually decreased as the patient's respiratory effort improves. Once it is decreased to a rate of 4/mt no support is needed and only pressure support upto 20 cm H_2O is provided. Pressure support gradually decreased and when it reaches 10 cm H_2O the patient can manage on his own.

The weaning process basically consists of three steps:
  i. Weaning from the ventilator (described above).
  ii. Weaning from the ET tube. Once the ventilator is disconnected the ET tube should be left in situ for at least 2-4 hours and proper humidification maintained. The ventilator should be kept ready should there be a need. If the respiratory parameters, (clinical and oxygen saturation) are maintained, the patient is extubated.
  iii. Weaning from the oxygen: Normally weaning attempts start when the patient maintains oxygenation at a FiO_2 of 0.4. Hence after extubation, all children should be administered humidified oxygen (40%) either through hood, mask or nasal prongs. Gradually the oxygen percentage is decreased.

The criteria of weaning in children are more clinical oriented than adults.

CONCLUSION

The basic principles in mechanical ventilator are:
1. To protect the ventilated lung (healthy or diseased) using adequate ventilatory support as soon as

possible and for as short a lime as necessary.
2. To prevent oxygen toxicity using the lowest FiO_2, applying complimentary means of support, which can lead to an improvement PaO_2. For example, PEEP/CPAP.
3. To recruit the infiltrated, atelectatic and consolidated lung using adequate PEEP level.
4. To maintain gas exchange, accepting a PaO_2 level between 50-70 mm Hg and moderate hypercapnoea ($PaCO_2$ 45-55 mm Hg).

REFERENCES

1. Spearman CB, Sanders HG. The new generation of mechanical ventilators, Rspr Cone 1987;32:403-18.
2. Cane RD, Choppies BA. Mechanical ventilatory support, JAMA 1985;254:87-92.
3. Demling RH, Knov JB. Basic concepts of lung function and dysfunction' Oxygenation, ventilation and mechanics. New horizons 1993;1:362-70.
4. Pawar D. Choice of ventilator. In Recent advances in Intensive Care. Editor Kaul H L, et al.1990;118-22.
5. Bersten AD, Rertten AJ, Vedig AF, et al. Additional work of breathing imposed by endotracheal tubes, breathing circuits and intensive care ventilators. Crit Care Med 1989;17:671-77.
6. Marraro GA, New modes of ventilation in pediatrics. In: Anesthesia and Intensive Care in Neonates and children. Salvo I, Vidyasagar D Editors Springer 83-97.
7. Perkin RM, Levin DL. Adverse affect of positive pressure ventilation in children. In Gregory G Ed. Respiratory Failure in the child. Clinics of critical care medicine. New York; Churchill Livinstone 1981;3.
8. Gregory GA, Edmunds LH, Ketterman JA, et al. Continuous positive airway pressure and pulmonary and circulatory function after cardiac surgery in infants less than three months of age, Anesthesiology 1975;43: 426-31.
9. Gattinoni L, Pesenti A, Bombino N, et al. Relationship between lung computed tomographic densities, gas exchange and PEEP in acute respiratory failure. Anesthesiology 1988;69:824-32.
10. Apostolakos MJ, Papadakos PJ. High inflation pressure and positive end-expiratory pressure injurious to the lung? Yes – Crit Care Clin 1996; 12: 627-34.
11. Stock MC, Dowm JB, Frolichn DA. Airway pressure release ventilation, Crit Care Med 1987;15:462-66.
12. Smith RA, Smith DB. Does airway pressure release ventilation alter lung function after acute lung injury? Chest 1995; 107:805-08.
13. Downs JB, Klein EF, Desautels DA, et al. Intermittent mechanical ventilation, a new approach to weaning from mechanical ventilation, Chest 1973;64:331.
14. Younes M, Puddy A, Roberts D, et al. Proportional assist ventilation; Results of an initial clinical trial, Am Res Respr Dis 1992;145:121-29.
15. Mac Intyre NR. Respiratory function during pressure support ventilation. Chest 1986;89:677-83.
16. Brochard L. Pressure support ventilation, Intensive Care World 1989;59:257-61.
17. Bronchard L, Rera F, Lori no H, et al. Inspiratory pressure-support compensates for the additional work of breathings caused by the endotracheal tube. Anesthesiology 1991;5:739-45.
18. Tsuno K, Prato P, Kolobow T. Acute lung injury from mechanical ventilation at moderately high airway pressures. J Appl Physiol 1990;69:956-61.
19. Kolobow T, Moretti MP, Fumagalli R, et al. Severe impairment in lung function induced by high peak airway pressure during mechanical ventilation. Am Rev Respir Dis 1987;135:312-15.
20. Papadakos PJ, Lachmann B, Bohm S. Pressure control ventilation review and new horizons. Clin Pulm Med 1998;5:120-23.
21. Passor Amato MD, Valente Barbas CS, Bonassa J, et al. Volume assured pressure support ventilation: A new approach for reducing muscle workload during acute respiratory failure. Chest 1992;102:1125-34.
22. Rouby JJ, Viars P. Clinical use of high frequency ventilation. Anaesthesiol Scand (suppl. 90) 1989;33: 134-39.
23. Bancalori E, Goldberg RN. High frequency ventilation in the neonate. Clin Perinal 1987;14:581-95.
24. Lunkenheimer PP, Whimster WF, Sykes MK (Editors). High frequency ventilation 20 years of endeavor reviewed: final stress or departure to achievement. Acta Anaesth Scand 1989;90:33.
25. Hansen Flaschen J, Cowen T, Raps EL. Neuromuscular blockade in the intensive care unit. Am Rev Respir Dis 1993;147:234-36.
26. Amato MBP, Barbas CSV, Modeiros DM, et al. Effect of a protective ventilation strategy on mortality in the acute respiratory distress syndrome. N Eng J Med 1998;338: 347-54.
27. Tunem DV. Permissive hypercapnoea ventilation. Am J Respr Crit Med 1994;150:870-74.
28. Haake R, Schlichtig R, Vlstad DR, Henschen RR. Barotrauma: Pathophysiology, risk factor and prevention. Chest 1987;91:608-13.
29. Esteban A, Alia I, Ibanez J, et al. Modes of mechanical ventilation and weaning: A national survey of Spanish hospitals. Chest 1994;106:1188-93.
30. Bronchard L, Rauss L, Benito S, et al. Comparison of three methods of gradual withdrawal from ventilatory support during weaning from mechanical ventilation. Am J Respr Cut Med 1994;150:896-903.
31. Esteban A, Frutos F, Tobin M, et al. A comparison of four methods of weaning patients from mechanical ventilation. N Engl J Med 1995;332:545-50.

CHAPTER 9

Pediatric Anesthesia—General Considerations

Ravinder K Batra, Anand Sharma

Pediatric anesthesia has progressed rapidly throughout the years. The first recorded case of pediatric anesthesia occurred in 1842 when Crawford W Long, MD, of Jefferson, Georgia, administered ether to an 8-year-old boy for the amputation of a toe.[1] With this introduction, surgical procedures that would previously have been impossible for children could now be performed. Ether seemed to be the anesthetic of choice for use on infants and children. The success of ether can largely be attributed to its wide margin of safety between ventilatory and cardiovascular depression and its lack of dangerous toxic effects.

Beginning in the 1930s and through the 1950s, several new anesthetic agents and new methods for their administration were introduced. Also introduced in the 1930s was thiopental, which caused a rapid induction of anesthesia by intravenous injection. After halothane debuted in the 1950s, there was rapid change in pediatric anesthesia.[2]

Pediatric Anesthesia has progressed rapidly throughout the years. This has allowed us to do the difficult and complicated surgery. Today, pediatric anesthesia has grown to include new anesthetic agents, more advanced technology and sophisticated equipment, and special training that provides education in all aspects of pediatric anesthesia. Teaching and communication came to forefront augmenting the growing base of clinical research.

Ways to control children's (and parent's) fears were explored, and more predictable medications were developed. Safety was enhanced, initially by use of the pre-cordial stethoscope, BP cuff (or arterial lines), ECG, continuous temperature monitoring and better fluid management. Greater control of blood volume and pain management allowed for even more complex and life saving surgery. Though introduced in the 1970s, pulse oximetry became the national standard of care, enhancing patient monitoring, and greatly reducing the morbidity and mortality in children. Out patient surgery and patient/child controlled analgesia are now common place. Organ transplantation and surgery of the neonates (and more recently the fetus) are the cutting edge.

Anesthesia for children requires consideration of how development affects patients psychology, anatomy, physiology and response to drugs. Infants always prove a challenge to the anesthetist because of their special needs, size or congenital abnormalities.

ANESTHETIC CONSIDERATIONS

Unlike popular belief, children are not mini-adults. They have a different anatomical and physiological make up. This means a great difference in anesthetic options and a lesser margin of error.

The respiratory system is capable of supporting life from 26 weeks. However, alveolar growth continues till 8 years of age.[3] Smaller airway diameter means high airflow resistance. Oxygen consumption is as high as 7 ml/kg/m in neonates. Due to the highly compliant chest wall, functional residual capacity is low, and airway closure can occur at end expiration.[4] Immature respiratory centers are prone to fatigue. This means the rapid development of hypoxia. Also, the smaller functional residual capacity and high respiratory rate speeds up induction with inhalational agents. The large tongue, "higher" glottis, angulated vocal cords and long U shaped epiglottis can make tracheal intubation difficult in infants.[4]

Higher resting cardiac outputs in children speed up anesthetic induction. Predominance of parasympathetic control at birth explains the onset of bradycardia with noxious responses.

Maturation of renal function takes 2 years. The ability to handle solute loads and excretion of anesthetic agents is impaired till such time hepatic metabolism, notably conjugation, takes 3 months to develop, while oxidation reduction appears earlier. Following 3-4 months, hepatic metabolism is increased and is comparable to adults at 3 years of age.

PREOPERATIVE ASSESSMENT

Most centers offer opportunities for preanesthetic assessment of children through preanesthesia clinics prior to surgery. The time constraints of these clinics may preclude confidence building measures, but wherever possible, the first interview between the anesthetist and the child and his parents can help to build a rapport with the former and allay anxiety of the latter. The anxiety is specially marked in parents of infants going in for their first surgery. Arrangement of organized trips to the hospital with film or puppet shows for patients and their attendants may help inform them about the procedure planned, though in children with past anesthetic exposure, anxiety is not decreased by such efforts.

A detailed history, with examination of past medical records is essential. Physical examination in children is successful in degrees depending on the co-operation and age of the child. Standard examination of the airway may be difficult in small children except when they are crying with a wide open mouth. History of loose deciduous teeth, needless to say, must not be omitted.

Most children appearing for surgery fall into ASA I-II groups. Earlier routine requirements of a hemoglobin and urine analysis are being questioned, because the return of medical information is significantly less compared to the costs, and the trauma of needles adds another anxiety to a frightened child.[5,6] However, exceptions to the rule occur where a baseline hemoglobin would serve for postoperative comparison. Examples include surgery with anticipated blood losses (vascular lesions), or clinical anemia. Included are also infants of less than 6 months of age with physiological anemia, specially preterm babies.[6] Laboratory testing would depend on the preoperative disease process, and surgery contemplated, with an emphasis being laid on avoidance of blanket testing.

Children with upper respiratory tract infections (URTI) form a controversial subgroup. Airway hyper-reactivity present for 2 weeks after an episode of URTI, may manifest as intraoperative desaturation, laryngospasm and bronchospasm are other adverse events.[7] Complications are higher among younger children.[7,8] The irritability of the respiratory mucosa takes 6-8 weeks to diminish. Interestingly, most complications, were associated with endotracheal intubation.[7] However, mortality from the intra operative complications is low, as most are readily treatable.[9,10] Since children develop URTI at the rate of 5-10 episodes per year, postponing for 4-6 weeks till the end of airway reactivity may not be totally feasible. Also, allergic rhinitis may mimic viral rhinitis.

Faced with such a situation, it is prudent to consider a risk benefit ratio for the child. A child with frank purulent secretions, running fever should probably be postponed, as also children with bronchospasm at the time of surgery. Children with improving symptoms could probably undergo surgery without a major event. Also, discharge times in daycare surgery for children with URTI can be increased to allow for a greater period of postoperative monitoring.

FASTING

In recent years the whole approach to preoperative fasting has undergone extensive evaluation (Table 9.1) (Table 9.1). As infants have a higher BMR and a larger body surface area/weight ratio than adults, they tend to dehydrate more easily. A number of studies have found no difference in gastric residual volume/pH when children are allowed to ingest clear fluids up to 2-3 hours prior to induction.

Table 9.1: Fasting guidelines[11]		
	Fasting time (hours)	
Age	Milk and solids	Clear fluids
< 6 months	4	2
6-36 months	6	3
> 36 months	8	3

The finding that clear liquids are rapidly emptied from the stomach have questioned earlier fasting guidelines. Fear of hypoglycemia, specially in infants also led to a revision of previous guidelines advocating prolonged fasting preoperatively. This has increased patient and parental comfort. The guidelines apply to healthy patients of all ages, undergoing elective procedures. Clear liquids include water, fruit juices without pulp, carbonated beverages, black coffee and clear tea. Light meals consist of toast and clear liquid. The amount of light meal or nonhuman milk ingested is important prior to recommending fasting periods.

PREMEDICATION

Children in the age group of 6 months to 6 years are in need of effective premedication as they are traumatized by parental separation and are difficult to reassure by strangers. An entire gamut of drugs are available though the oral, intranasal, rectal routes, have gained popularity (oral ketamine, midazolam, diazepam, phenergan, chloral hydrate, fentanyl lollypops, midazolam and diazepam suppository). Injectable narcotics and sedatives can be administered in older children.

Pharmacological alleviation of preoperative distress and anxiety is challenging in a pediatric patient, who are non-co-operative due to anxiety and fear of needles driving children away from the health care provider deeper into the arms of the accompanying parent.

Traditional intramuscular premedication combines an opioid with an antisialogogue. Intramuscular ketamine 3-4 mg/kg with anticholinergic and benzodiazepine produces a dissociative state within 5 minutes of injection lasting 15-20 min.[12] Intramuscular midazolam (0.05 - 0.15 mg/kg) achieves an onset of action in 1-2 min. However, intra-muscular injections are painful and best reserved for uncontrollable children.[6]

Oral premedication is popular with both physician and patients alike. It is non-invasive, usually cheaper, easy to administer and causes less anxiety. Diazepam, at 0.13 mg/kg as either tablets or syrup achieves the desired effect after 60 minutes. Oral midazolam 0.3 – 0.7 mg/kg is rapidly gaining popularity as a premedicant, acting in 30-45 min.[13] However, commercial preparations are few, and disguising the bitter taste of the drug is a challenge. Honey, fruit juice and 25% dextrose have all been tried to suppress the taste. Ketamine though not specifically marketed in an oral form, has nevertheless been used in doses from 4-6 mk/kg, either alone or with midazolam, with better results in the combination.[14] Ketamine orally has a rapid onset within 10-15 min, and should be combined with an antisialagogue (atropine 0.02 mg/kg) to reduce secretions.[14]

Rectal short acting barbiturates achieve a sedated patient with a risk of airway obstruction. Diazepam, midazolam and ketamine, alone or in combination have also been attempted. However, the route may be uncomfortable for older children and the erratic absorption due to fecal contents may blunt the effect.[15]

For children with a functional intravenous access, midazolam 0.05-0.07 mg/kg, morphine 0.1 mg/kg, fentanyl 0.25-0.5 ug/kg or ketamine 0.5-2 mg/kg produce rapid onset within 5-10 min. Nasal sufentanyl, midazolam and ketamine have been attempted, though the route is uncomfortable and may be associated with increased injury.[16]

INHALATIONAL AGENTS

Halothane

Revolutionizing volatile agent usage, halothane was the first in a series of fluorinated hydrocarbons providing a rapid onset of action and clear headed recovery.[17] Metabolism of halothane lead to the formation of Trifluro Acetyl radicals, implicated in the development of halothane hepatitis. This condition, postulated to be immune mediated, is a diagnosis of exclusion.[18] Avoiding re exposure to individuals with prior histories of adverse reactions like pyrexia and jaundice or those with a positive family history limits this complication.

Isoflurane

Isoflurane has a lower blood gas solubility than halothane accounting for a faster onset and recovery.[19] This makes it a useful agent in the outpatient setting, but not good for induction of anesthesia.

Dose dependent ventilatory depression exists, and bronchoconstriction is attenuated.[20] Increased sympathetic activity leads to a lesser depression of myocardial contractility, tachycardia and vasodilatation.[22] Cerebral autoregulation is maintained at higher concentrations than halothane.

It does not sensitise the myocardial to catecholamines, so the arrhythmogenic potential is low.[22] Hepatic perfusion is better maintained than halothane.

Sevoflurane

Sevoflurane is a potent, non-pungent liquid. No trifluoroacetic radicals are formed with its metabolism. Low blood gas solubility leads to a fast induction and recovery. Alone, it produces conditions for intubation at lower inhaled concentrations than halothane and has been suggested as an alternative to muscle relaxants in cases where rapid recovery is needed.[23,24]

Lesser tachycardia than isoflurane and lesser cardiac depression than halothane, without coronary steal is an attractive feature.[25-27] Arrhythmias are uncommon. Dose dependent respiratory depression is as common as with other fluorocarbons.

Desflurane

A minimally metabolized, cardiostable agent, Desflurane has the lowest blood gas partition coefficient among volatile agents, accounting for a speedy onset and recovery.[28] However, it is irritant to the airways, causing laryngospasm, breath holding and coughing, hence not recommended for inhalational induction.[29] It exists as a gas at room temperature in most tropical countries and has to be dispensed through specialized delivery systems.

Dose dependent respiratory depression is observed so is a lesser negative inotropic effect than other fluorocarbons. There is no arrhythmogenic potential. The awakening is rapid and smooth, unassociated with apneic spells in infants.[30]

Nitrous Oxide

The only inorganic compound in wide usage used for general anesthesia, Nitrous oxide is a gas (boiling point –88.5°C) with low solubility. Since, nitrous oxide alone is insufficient to produce unconsciousness, it is combined with more, potent volatile agents as an adjunct, and helps reduce their dosage. Nitrous oxide is a potent analgesic. It produces cardiovascular and respiratory depression that is clinically unimportant in healthy subjects.

Diffusion of nitrous oxide into closed spaces during administration may increase the volume of pneumothorax, in bowel and endotracheal cuffs. Similar effects in the middle ear cavity may be the reason for postoperative nausea and vomiting seen with the agent. Also, prolonged exposure can lead to bone marrow suppression and vitamin B_{12} deficiency.

INTRAVENOUS AGENTS

Thiopentone

This derivative of barbituric acid, since its introduction by Ralph Waters and John Lundy, has revolutionized anesthetic technique. It replaced the slow, unsteady induction of ether with a smooth rapid onset. It is commonly used in a concentration of 2.5% as higher concentrations are progressively irritating to veins.[31]

However, hypovolemic subjects may experience a severe drop in blood pressure that may not be compensated. Common with most anesthetics, thiopentone causes a dose dependant depression of respiration and myocardial contractility. Accidental intra-arterial injection causes vasospasm and severe pain, leading to gangrene in the absence of timely therapy, which includes dilution of the drug, pharmacological vasodilation or surgery.

Thiopentone induces a reduction in cerebral metabolism, reducing oxygen requirements. It has been mooted as a brain preservative following hypoxic insults, but studies are inconclusive.[32]

Propofol

Propofol a substituted isopropylphenol, is marketed as 1% emulsion in lipid with long chain triglycerides. It has a fast redistribution from blood to tissues and a faster elimination than thiopentone, accounting for a clear headed, rapid recovery.

Pain on injection is a distressing feature of an otherwise rapid and smooth induction. Propofol causes myocardial and respiratory depression to a greater degree than thiopentone.[32] Bradycardia, associated with the drug is probably due to a resetting of the baroreceptor reflex arc. It suppresses pharyngeal and laryngeal reflexes effectively, so it is the preferred agent for LMA insertion.

The high systemic clearence of propofol enables it to be used in infusions, promoting faster recovery at the end of surgery. Nausea and vomiting are reduced.[33]

Ketamine

First used in 1965, ketamine holds a unique place among the plethora of induction agents. It is a powerful analgesic and induces a phenomenon of dissociation characterized by apparent wakefulness while withdrawal from surroundings. This is brought about by a dissociation of the thalamocortical and limbic systems.[31]

Used in a variety of routes (intravenous, intramuscular, oral, nasal), ketamine has a rapid onset of action with a rapid clearance. Oropharyngeal reflexes are preserved though silent aspiration has been reported. Central sympathetic stimulation causes tachycardia and hypertension. Respiration is depressed though to a lesser degree than other anesthetics. Bronchodilation and increased secretions are seen.[34] An increase in intracranial pressure with the drug makes it an unlikely selection for patients with intracranial disease.

Emergence delirium during discontinuation has been reported in adults, though not in children.[35] However, absence in the latter has been postulated to be due to their failure to communicate.

Neuromuscular Blocking Agents

Neuromuscular blocking agents allow muscle relaxation in surgery, allowing for greater ease of operation. They facilitate tracheal intubation and are used in intensive care units to effectively control a patient's respiration when on a ventilator.

Neuromuscular transmission is carried out by acetylcholine released by prejunctional neurons in the synaptic cleft, where it binds to acetylcholine receptors in the motor end plate, triggering a chain of events leading to muscle contraction. Acetylcholinesterase present in the synaptic cleft rapidly clears acetylcholine, terminating its actions. Acetylcholine receptors differ in morphology between newborns and adults, and mature to adult levels in 2 years. Also, prejunctional acetylcholine reserves are small in neonates, making them highly sensitive to neuromuscular blockade. However, a high volume of distribution leads to a lower plasma concentration so the net dose of the relaxant, according to body weight is unchanged.

Depolarizing agents, commonest of which is succinylcholine, causes an initial weak stimulation, manifests as fasciculation, followed by paralysis. Succinylcholine has a rapid onset (45–60s) and fast, spontaneous recovery, making it the drug of choice in situations where rapid intubation is required as well as it is essential for the treatment of laryngospasm. However, it increases serum potassium, a greater rise encountered in paraplegia, burns, muscle dystrophies. It can lead to bradycardia due to enhanced vagal tone, specially with a second dose in the same patient and is known to trigger malignant hyperthermia. These factors dampened enthusiasm for its use.

Non-depolarizing agents are free of such side effects. The relaxant molecule directly occupies the acetylcholine receptor and inhibits acetylcholine binding, producing muscle relaxation not preceeded by fasciculations. However, compared to succinylcholine, most non-depolarizing agents have a longer onset and duration of action. Depending on their clearence, they have variously been divided into the longer acting (e.g. pancuroneum), intermediate acting (e.g. vecuroneum) or short acting (mivacurium).

While depolarizing blockade wears off by itself, non depolarizing blockade has to be reversed with anticholinesterases. These drugs inhibit the acetylcholinesterase enabling high concentration of acetylcholine to accumulate at the neuromuscular junction and over come blockade. Danger of stimulation of muscarinic along with nicotinic receptors means that muscarinic receptor inhibitors like atropine or glycopyrrolate are given concomittantly.

Opioids

Synthetic or natural derivatives, opioids act on receptors throughout the body to produce a variety of effects. Their chief role in anesthetic practice involves their analgesic properties, and their ability to attenuate stress responses to noxious surgical stimuli. The latter attribute is only partly achieved, though to a greater degree than other anesthetic agents.

Morphine, isolated commonly from the opium poppy is used through intramuscular, intravenous, subarachnoid, epidural and oral routes. The effect of opioids on different receptors is shown in Table 9.2. Both intermittent boluses and continuous infusions are described.[36] Pethidine with an inherent Atropine – like

Table 9.2: Effect of opioid on different receptors

Receptor	Effect	Agonist
μ	μ1 supraspinal analgesia μ2 respiratory depression muscle rigidity physical dependence	Morphine and endorphin
k	Sedation Spinal analgesia	Morphine, nalbuphine butorphanol, dynorphin
δ	Analgesia, euphoria convulsions	β-endorphin
Σ	Dysphoria, hallucinations, Respiratory stimulation	Pentazoine, nalorphine ketamine

structure is associated with tachycardia. However, later developments like fentanyl, alfentanyl, and Sufentanil and remifentanil are highly lipid soluble. Hence, they have a rapid onset and shorter duration of action, making them attractive choices in neonates, who have an increased depression of respiration with opioids.[37]

Beyond 1 month to 2 years, the increase in the volume of distribution and rapid elimination of opioids calls for an increase in drug doses by almost 1.5 times if based on weight (but the same if on body surface area).[38]

Most opioids are cardiovascular stable in the well hydrated, normal patient. Fentanyl and it's congeners can provoke bradycardia, specially when used with propofol and vecuronium. However, in shock, opioids can cause an additional myocardial depression. Respiratory depression is usually gradual with a rise in apneic threshold and accumulation of CO_2. Constipation and histamine release leading to bronchospasm and anaphylaxis may be seen in those susceptible with morphine. Antagonism is best achieved with naloxone at 2-4 μg/kg. Since duration of action is short, an infusion of 1–10 μg/kg/hr is recommended.[36]

LOCAL ANESTHETICS

These group of drugs achieve an inhibition of nerve conduction. Commonly classified as ester or amide, based on structural features, local anesthetics can achieve sensory, motor and autonomic blockade, depending in the area chosen.

Lignocaine, bupivacaine and the recently introduced ropivacaine are the prime agents in current usage. Maximum doses for lignocaine with or without adrenaline are 7 and 4 mg/kg while the same for Bupivacaine are 3 and 2 mg/kg. The addition of adrenaline causes localized vasoconstriction and delays the clearance, prolonging action. The more rapid onset of block attributed to adrenaline is unsubstantiated.

Inadvertent intravascular injections, or over doses can lead to convulsions, coma and death. Bupivacaine is singularly cardiotoxic and can cause resistant ventricular arrhythmias. Ropivacaine, a congener of bupivacaine apparently lacks the cardiotoxicity while retaining the increased duration of action. Hence, all local anesthetic administrations should occur in the presence of equipment for cardiopulmonary resuscitation.

MONITORING

With the advent of extensive monitoring equipment, the safety standards during the perioperative period have reached a new high. But, one should not forget the value of the precordial stethoscope, tactile palpation of fontanelle and skin for fluid status and most importantly constant observation of the pattern of respiration and skin color.

The measurement of O_2 saturation is an invaluable perioperative tool. The probe is available in different sizes for neonates and older children (wrap around or clip on). Measurement of end tidal CO_2, continuous temperature monitoring, invasive pressures (CVP and arterial) should be done where indicated. Continuous temperature monitoring especially in neonates, very sick children or in those undergoing major surgical procedures is must. Operating Room temperature should be maintained appropriate to age of the children as their capacity for thermoregulation is poor.

MANAGEMENT OF ANESTHESIA

Given the variation in children, anesthetic management differs from adult practice in certain areas, though the basic techniques remain the same.

Compared with adults, intravenous induction in children is reserved for those cooperative enough to allow a needle, or with pre-existing intravenous access prior to their entry into the theatre. The use of EMLA (eutectic mixture of local anesthetic) with Lignocaine and Prilocaine or Amethocaine cream applied on the intended puncture site reduces the pain of needle entry. However, some children may be frightened by the very sight of the needle.

For this subgroup of patients an inhalation induction appears to be non-invasive and pain free. The concentration of anesthetic agent is either gradually stepped up or is increased to a maximum and a co-operative child asked to inhale to vital capacity and hold his breath (the single breath technique). Intubation if required is performed under deep inhalational anesthetic agent or after a muscle relaxant is administered, after confirmed ease of mask ventilation. Muscle relaxants are usually avoided in children with obvious or potential difficult intubation in whom intubation can be attempted while spontaneously breathing using deeper planes of anesthesia. Newer inhalation agents like sevoflurane are rapidly acting and less irritant.

Recently, parental participation at the time of induction has made anesthesia more smooth and less traumatic for the children. In Europe this practice is preferred than in US.

Large occiput, small head size and large tongue make pediatric mask ventilations challenges for the uninitiated. Part of the solution lie in pillows or rolls under the neck to provide appropriate extension. Laryngoscopy can be hampered by the large tongue size and the overhanging, omega shaped epiglottis, making visualization of the larynx difficult.

Appropriate size of face mask, airway, laryngoscope blade, tube is now available for neonates and children. However, the 15-22 mm connections on masks, tracheal tubes and anesthesia circuit remain standardized to avoid confusions. Laryngeal mask airway is being used in all age groups starting from the neonates to older children for all types of surgery wherever possible. Fiberoptic bronchoscopes is useful in difficult airways situations as well as in assessing the correct placement of double lumen tubes which are now available in pediatric sizes for thoracic surgery.

The cricoid cartilage is the narrowest point of the airway in children below the age of 5 years. Cuffed tracheal tubes are avoided in this age group to prevent post intubation croup. The correct internal diameter of a tracheal tube for a child older than 2 years is approximately given by the formula.

$$\frac{\text{Age (years)}}{4} + 4 = \text{Tube internal diameter (mm)}$$

While the depth of insertion (tube length) till mid trachea from the mouth (more than 2 years) as

$$\frac{\text{Age (years)}}{2} + 12 \text{ Tube length (cm)}$$

Circuits for delivery of anesthetic gases to children should be light weight, safe and with a reduced dead space. The Mapleson F, or the Ayre's T piece is the most popular circuit in use among pediatric anesthetists, fulfilling all the above criteria. Mapleson D and A systems have also been used in children. Circle absorber systems with reduced diameter of tubings are fast emerging in pediatric anesthesia as a reliable method for conservation of heat, humidity and anesthetic agents.

The development of the laryngeal mask airway (LMA) in 1988 has revolutionized anesthetic practice. The LMA when inserted is sited above the larynx and forms a seal around the laryngeal inlet with the tip resting against the upper esophageal sphincter. It requires a lesser depth of anesthesia compared to a tracheal tube for both insertion and toleration during maintenance of anesthesia. Insertion of the LMA is easily learnt and usually does not require a laryngoscope. This, coupled with the non-invasiveness of the device leads to less pharyngeal and laryngeal stimulation, a boon in patients with reactive airways and cardiac disease.[39] With the availability of pediatric sized laryngeal masks (size 1, 11/2, 2, 21/2). For routine surgery and patient's with difficult airways, pediatric sized laryngeal masks have become very popular.

Maintenance of anesthesia usually involves ventilating the child with an anesthetic gas mixture with muscle relaxation, if required. Newer intravenous agents like propofol have a faster recovery and infusions of these can be used instead of halogenated anesthetics for maintenance of anesthesia. The respiration in majority of children is controlled or assisted, as the immaturity of respiratory centers and lung dynamics makes a spontaneously breathing child more prone to respiratory depression.

Emergence from anesthesia involves reversal of muscle relaxation and ventilation with anesthetic free oxygen to reverse the concentration gradient and promote clearance. Preterm neonates with high incidences of apnea in the postoperative period require intensive monitoring after surgery.

Intravenous Fluids

Perioperative fluid therapy has following purposes:
1. To supply water and thereby to create enough urine volume to excrete solutes.
2. To replace insensible fluid losses.
3. To replace electrolytes lost from the urine, skin and gut.
4. To supply calories to reduce tissue catabolism.

Infants have a total body water of 75% as compared to 60% in adults. Also their extracellular fluid volume is 44% as compared to 15-20% in adults. Therefore, combined with their high metabolic rate they are prone to dehydration. Neonates have poor energy reserves and immature enzyme system and do not withstand starvation well. It is hence imperative to supplement glucose in the perioperative period. Intraoperatively dextrose and balanced salt solutions are used for this purpose. Ringer's lactate is considered a good replacement fluid in older children.

Various calculations involving body weight surface area, or caloric expenditure have been used to determine fluid therapy in children undergoing surgery. Assessment of fluid and electrolyte imbalance is performed during preoperative evaluation and it should consider the cardiopulmonary status, renal function, and any existing systemic abnormalities that may have an impact on fluid and electrolyte management.

The estimated fluid deficit (EFD)
= Hours fasting × Maintenance fluid requirement (MFR) (ml/kg/hr)

First hour fluid = MFR + ½ EFD
Second hour fluid = MFR + ¼ EFD
Third hour fluid = MFR + ¼ EFD

Fasting fluid is taken as 3 ml/kg/hr

Maintenance fluid requirement
For superficial surgery   1-2 ml/kg/hr
For abdominal procedure   6-10 ml/kg/hr
For thoracic surgery   4-5 ml/kg/hr

Infants less than 4 years of age who are kept fasting for more than 6 hours may become hypoglycemic and irritable.[40] Whereas Nilsson et al have failed to demonstrate hypoglycemia in infants less than 2 years of age including those who fasted for 6-8 hours.[41] So it is advisable to do blood glucose in these infants who are fasting for longer periods and if blood glucose < 40 mg/dl, glucose solution should be infused. However, preterm infants who are receiving glucose containing solution should be observed for hyperglycemia. The metabolic need for glucose in the infant is 5 g/kg/day.

Blood transfusion is recommended in neonates with HCT < 30 and in infants or children when HCT < 25.

POSTOPERATIVE PAIN MANAGEMENT

Since, prehistoric times, the emotional component of pain and meaning of the sensory experience of the pain has been interpreted in the greater context of the time. This has been true for infant children who are unable to articulate their pain. Pain in the mid - 19 century was considered very real in infant. Today, the concept of neonatal and pediatric pain is well established. The development of rectal analgesia has also helped in reducing the pain in the postoperative period.

Pain is an "unpleasant sensory and emotional experience associated with actual or potential tissue damage or described in terms of such a damage".[42] The development of pain pathways have been elucidated in neonates and older children and infants challenging earlier erroneous beliefs that pain transmission was under developed in children. A multimodal approach using opioid and non-opioid based analgesics, with regional anesthesia works best in the pediatric age group.[43] Included within these are steps to involve both the child and parents in the management along with sympathetic support and child friendly surroundings to cope with the negative emotional falling out commonly associated with pain.

Clinical assessment of pain in children is challenging. Depending on the age, children may not communicate their discomfort due to a various reasons, ranging from a stranger anxiety to fear of needles. Bear in mind that assessments of the degree of pain are incomplete till they are associated with therapeutic measures.

Since pain is a subjective phenomenon, self-reporting by patients remain the gold standard of assessment.[44] By 18 months children develop words for pain, while by 3-4 yr, cognitive development is sufficient to allow the child to quantify the pain.[45] Other modes include observational assessment for behavioral changes, agitation, reported by either healthcare worker or parents themselves. The limitation here being the inability to differentiate, in certain scenarios, between signs due to pain and these due to anxiety. Another measure is a quantification of physiological responses to monitor the degree of pain. These methods may be expensive and nonspecific, though are effective in those with cognitive disability or immaturity.[44] Instead of a single parameter, most pain scales incorporate a multi-dimensional assessment, based on the age of the child, sensitivity of illness and the surgical procedure carried out.

Clinical Assessment of Pain in Children— Infants and Adolescent in Table 9.3.

PHARMACOLOGICAL INTERVENTIONS

Non-steroidal anti-inflammatory agents (NSAIDs) include inhibitors of prostaglandin synthesis and weaker opioids. Prostaglandin are mediators of inflammation derived from arachidonic acid by cyclo-oxyenase. These act on free nerve endings to stimulate pain receptors and are patent vasodilators within action, compiled with increased capillary permeability, leads to edema and erythema. They are also responsible for platelet aggregation, pyrexia and increased renal blood flow.

PROSTAGLANDIN SYNTHETASE INHIBITORS (PSI)

PSI form the most commonly used analgesic medication worldwide, with most available over the counter. The agents, inhibit cyclo-oxygenase pathways, reduce the production of prostaglandins and thromboxanes and attenuate the effects of the inflammatory mediators. Compared to opioids, they lead to no depression of consciousness, respiration or hemodynamics, and are free of addictive potential making them attractive choices for outpatient therapy.

Acetaminophen, due to its convenience, effectiveness for mild to moderate pain and safety, is the most commonly used analgesic agent in children.

Table 9.3: Clinical assessment of pain in children

	Scale	Age	Indicator	Pain Stimulus
Infants				
1.	Behavioral pain score[46]	Preterm and full-term	Facial expression, body movements, response to handling / consol ability rigidity of limbs	Procedural pain in ventilated neonates
2.	Pain assessment tool (PAT)[47]	Full-term neonates	Posture, tone, sleep pattern, expression, color, cry, respiration, heart rate, oxygen saturation, blood pressure, nurses perception of infant pain	Postoperative pain
3.	CRIES[48]	Full-term neonates	Crying, oxygen saturation heart rate, blood pressure, expression, sleeplessness	Postoperative pain
4.	NAPI[49] postoperative neonatal assessment of pain inventory	Infants 1-36m	Smiling, sleeping, response to touch, crying, respiration	Postoperative pain 1-36 months
Children and Adolescents				
5.	Children's Hospital[50] East Ontario Pain Scale (CHEOPS)	1-7 yrs	Crying, facial expressions mobilisation, activity whether and how child touches wound, by position	Postoperative pain
6.	Visual Analogue[51] Scale (VAS)	> 4.5 yrs	A single line marked with descriptions of pain at each end. Subject marks on the line to indicate pain intensity	Postoperative pain
7.	Comfort Scone[52]	All ages	Alertness / calm / agitation, respiratory response, physical movement, heart rate, blood pressure muscle tone, facial tension	Used in critical care
8.	Colored Analog[53] Scale (CAS)	5-16 yrs	Visual analogue scale with graded coloring :pale pink (less pain) to dark red (more pain)	Postoperative

Acting on the central cyclo-oxygenase, rather than peripheral, its anti-inflammatory activities are limited, so too its adverse effects on renal, platelets and gastrointestinal function.[54] It is available as oral, rectal, intramuscular preparations, though the later would not be the mode of choice in children. An intravenous prodrugs proparacetamol has also been developed but is not yet licensed for use.[55]

The analgesic concentrations of acetaminophen in children have not yet been accurately evaluated.[56]

Paracetamol Dosing in Children[44,56]

Oral

Load 20 mg/kg, then 15 mg/kg 4-8 hrly max 90 mg/kg/d (neonates 60 mg/kg/d).

Rectal

- Load 30-45 mg/kg (20 mg/kg in neonates). Then 20 mg/kg 6-8 hrly to a maximum 90 mg/kg/day (60 mg/kg/day neonates)
- Taper after 48-72 hrs
- Watch for evidence of hepatotoxicity, specially in dehydrated, malnourished subjects.

Ibuprofen and diclofenac are available in oral suspension and offer effective pain relief for mild to moderate pain. However, administration round the clock and not as and when required maintains a steady state concentration.

The important NSAID doses are summarized in Table 9.4.

Contraindications to PSI[44]

- True allergy
- Peptic ulcer disease

Table 9.4: NSAID doses in children (Oral)[44,57]

NSAID	DOSE (mg/kg)	Maximum daily dose
Diclofenac	1	3
Ibuprofen	10	40
Indomethacin	1	3
Ketorolac	0-5	2
Naproxen	7-5	15
Piroxicam	0-4	0-4

- Renal failure
- Uncorrected hypovolemia
- Bleeding dyscrasia
- Qualitative/Quantitative platelet dysfunction
- Asthma
- Ongoing or risk for surgical bleeding
- Proven influenza or variable infection.

Weak Opioids

Combined with PSIs, weak opioids receptor agonists provide superior analgesia compared with either drug alone.

Codeine in doses of 0.5 mg/kg orally 4-6 hourly combined with PSIs is suitable for pediatric outpatients. A high oral bioavailability and partial demethylation to morphine increase analgesic efficacy. Parenteral preparations are associated with allergic reactions, and are not preferred.[44] Oxycodine and hydrocodone, semi-synthetic variants at 0.1 mg/kg 3-4 hourly are acceptable alternatives.

Tramadol a μ receptor agonist is another option to control mild to moderate pain. Additional mode of action is inhibition of serotonin uptake. Dose ranges include 1-1.5 mg/kg parenterally. Oral preparations, for pediatric use are not marketed by the manufacturer, who limit the drug for pediatric use. Table 9.5 shown Adverse effects of opioids.

REGIONAL ANESTHESIA IN CHILDREN

Rapid strides in safer anesthetics, development of better techniques and recognition of pain pathways in children have lent focus on regional anesthesia among children. Usually supplemented with General

Table 9.5: Adverse effects of opioids

Side Effects	Therapy
Sedation, respiratory depression	Oxygenate, maintain airway and ventilate
Constipation	Hydration, stool softness, cathartics
Nausea, vomiting	Phenothiazine, metoclopramide (0.15 mg/kg)
	Ondansetron (0.15 mg/kg)
	Change opioid
Pruritis	Diphenhydramine (0.5 mg/kg) Change opioid, e.g tramadol with low histamine release

anesthesia, it helps provide a smooth emergence and comfortable recovery.

Anatomic variations in the central nervous systems in children compared to adults make regional techniques in children an independent entity, not just a scaling down of adult procedures. Incomplete myelinization of nerves, completing only at the second year of life, reduced diameter of nerves and decreased distances between the nodes of Ranvier alter pharmacodynamics of local anesthetics.[59] The spinal cord occupies the entire spinal canal in the embryo, but is gradually drawn upwards with the rapid growth of the axial skeletons. At birth, the lower end of the spinal cord is situated at L3, reaching L1 in the first year of life. Correspondingly the dural sac is shifted from S3-4 in a newborn to S1-2 by 1 year of age.[59] The distinct vertebral pieces of the sacrum are not fused till 25-30 years. Loose attachments of nerve trunks of fascial planes promotes wider spread of drug.[60]

Regional anesthesia is well tolerated in children, with no major hemodynamic side effects till 8 years of age. However, patient co-operation for seeking paresthesias is often not possible, due to non comprehension by frightened children. Hence, Dalens recommends nerve stimulation or loss of resistance techniques coupled with sedation or general anesthesia.[60]

Contraindications include infections at puncture site, bleeding allergy to the drugs being used and hypovolemia in case of central neuraxial blockade.

Complications commonly arise as a result of inadvertent intravascular injection. Respiratory compromise can occur with overdosage with opioids or excessive spread in central neuraxial blockade. Local trauma, pneumothorax, accidental subarachnoid injections and nerve injuries depend on the particular block used.

COMPLICATIONS FOLLOWING REGIONAL ANESTHESIA

Prevent

Aspirate prior to injection
Slow injection (10 ml/min)
Do not inject against resistance
Monitoring during injection.

Treat

Common

Oxygenate: Face mask or endotracheal intubation if needed.

Hemodynamic support, external cardiac compression, fluid bolus, and inotropes.

Convulsions

Thiopentone 4-5 mg/kg IV, Diazepam 3-5 mg, Midazolam 1-2 mg IV and
Muscle relaxant and intubate if convulsions persist.

Arrhythmias

Treat according to nature of arrhythmia
Defibrillate first, for ventricular fibrillation/tachycardia at 3J/Kg.

CAUDAL ANESTHESIA

Caudal epidural analgesia with Bupivacaine 0.25 - 0.125% as per requirement with volumes ranging from 0.5-1.25 ml/kg depending on surgical site administered at the time of induction provides good intraoperative and post operative analgesia. A variety of adjuncts can be used like morphine, fentanyl or ketamine. Caudal catheters can be used for thoracotomy and extensive laparotomy for pain relief where High Dependency Unit Care is available. Caudal epidural is relatively an easy procedure in children because the landmarks are better defined.

Non-union of the vertebral arches of S_{4-5} creates a hiatus flanked on either side by two easily identifiable bony crests, the sacral cornu. The sacral hiatus provides an easily palpable access to the caudal epidural space in children. Caudal anesthesia is commonly used for surgery on the urogenital tract, perineum and lower extremities.

The block can be performed with patient prone or commonly lateral. The needle is advanced through the cornu, piercing the sacrococcygeal membrane at right angles, then directed rostrally to a depth of 3 mm in the sacral canal. Proximity of the anus has limited catheter insertions for prolonged anesthesia among practitioners, though proponents of catheter techniques are present.[61,62]

Like most epidural blockade, caudal anesthesia is volume dependent. A variety of schemes for drug volumes have been devised, among which the most popular is that of Armitage.[63] 0.5 ml/kg of local anesthetic blocks of sacral, 1 ml/kg high lumbar, and 1.25 ml/kg provides a midthoracic spread. However, if higher volumes are to be used morethan 20 ml then the caudal route is best avoided due to the risk of high cephalad spread of anesthetic.[64]

Misplacement of needle tip can cause intravascular or subarachnoid injections, "failed" blocks and rectal perforations.

Both local anesthetic blocks and infusions, as well as opioids, have been successfully used to provide anesthesia through this route.[62,65]

LUMBAR EPIDURAL BLOCKADE

Special equipment has been designed for children up to 4 years of age (5 cm 19G Touhy needle). For older children the routine 8-9 cm 18G Touhy needle can be used. It should be remembered that the distance from skin to epidural space is short and the ligaments are soft. Loss of resistance using air is more sensitive in children. The epidural fat in young children is very loose. It is therefore, advisable to thread catheters to appropriate thoracic levels from lumbar or caudal space to avoid potential dural punctures or cord damage.

The degree of difficulty experienced in performing an epidural blockade increases proportionately with increasing height progressively from the sacral hiatus up the vertebral column.[66] Vertebral spinous processes horizontally afford greater working interspace for the negotiating needle in the lumbar region. Introduction of a catheter allows indefinite prolongation of anesthesia. The technique can be used as a safe anesthetic in older, cooperative children and adolescents or as a supplementation with general anesthesia, reducing opioid and volatile agent dosages. The high quality of analgesia provided in the post-operative period promotes faster recovery specially since it enables patient movement and cooperation for procedures like chest physiotherapy.

The patient can be positioned lateral, sitting or prone, with rolls under the iliac crests. Adequate flexion in the sitting and lateral positions is brought about by on assistant if the patient is anesthetized or sedated. The puncture site can be L3,4 or L2, 3 in older children, but Dalens recommends a puncture at the L4, 5 or L5, S1 in children below 10 years to avoid direct trauma to the cord.[67] The line joining the Iliac crests crosses the L5 in neonates and in older children, and corresponding vertebrae are thus located.

The Tuohy needle with a curved hubbard tip is popular among epidural enthusiasts. The curve at the tip prevents dural puncture, while the laterally facing outlet allows easy threading of the catheter. Various sizes are available, 16G or 17G needles threading 18G catheters are commonly used in adults and adolescents. 19G needles with 22G catheters are appropriate in children upto 25 kgs. 22 and 20 G needles and smaller catheters are available. Spinal infusion catheters have been used in the epidural space with smaller needles. However, increased resistance to injection, difficulty in visualizing cerebrospinal fluid or blood in cases of misplacement, and difficulties in placement have dampened enthusiasm for their use.[66,67]

Localization of the epidural space is done through documentation of loss of resistance through saline, or air, or the detection of negative pressure by indrawing of a hanging drop at the needle hub. Epidural lignocaine, bupivacaine, with or without opiates like morphine and fentanyl have been used either as boluses or infusion.[62] However, intravenous opioid usage concomitant with neuraxial opioids is not advisable due to synergistic respiratory depression.[66]

SPINAL ANESTHESIA

Spinal anesthesia is commonly used for lower abdominal or lower limb procedures like inguinal hernia repair and orthopedic limb surgery. The advantages it enjoys in children include better hemodynamic stability then adults and decreased incidence of postdural puncture headache. Nevertheless, the duration of the block is significantly reduced. (Bupivacaine 45 min compared from 3 hrs in adults) Spinal anesthesia used without sedation in preterm infants leads to a lesser incidence of postoperative apnea and bradycardia compared to general anesthesia.[68]

Most technical features remain the same as epidural anesthesia. The important difference lying in the use of a thin bore needle to deliberately puncture the dura with the smallest hole possible .Onset is usually faster, within 4-5 minutes, with reversal of block and recovery of sensations after around three hours.[60] Intrathecal opioids are associated with a significant risk of respiratory depression postoperative and warrant careful monitoring for 24 hours after surgery.

Older children have been shown to suffer postdural puncture headache, specially after large bore needle usuage, but the headache is short lasting.[64] Epidural blood patches have been used to produce good results in dural puncture headaches in adolescents.[69]

Subarachnoid block is useful in lower abdominal or perineal surgery in ex-premature babies to avoid risk of post operative apnea. Care should be taken to puncture dura below L3 to avoid damage to the cord. The distance from skin to dura is approximate 0.5 - 1 cm in premature and term neonates respectively. Special 2.5 cm; 25 G, short bevelled needles are to be used for spinal anesthesia.

Bupivacaine alone or with fentanyl or morphine can be used in doses as given in Table 9.6.

NERVE BLOCKS

Ilioinguinal, iliohypogastric, infraorbital, dorsal nerve of penis block, and intercostal nerve block are administered at the beginning of surgery which provide good intraoperative and postoperative analgesia.

Penile Block

Circumcision, urethroplasty, hypospadias repairs can be undertaken with this technique, though the limited range of blockade means that it is totally adequate only for the first of the above mentioned surgery. The penile block anesthetizes the terminal branch of the nerve as it courses under the symphysis pubis. The anesthetic is injected in the subpubic space, between the pubic and perineal membrane on one side and the fibrous envelope covering the crura or corpora cavernosa on the other. The injection is made with the penis stretched downwards to keep scarpa's fascia intact. The two puncture sites are located below each pubic rami, on either side of the pubic symphysis, and the needle is introduced perpendicular to the skin and then medially and caudally till the "give way" of scarpa's fascia is located.[60,66]

DAY CARE SURGERY

Day care surgery is gaining popularity in pediatric practice surgery today as it cuts costs, avoids nosocomial infection and causes least disruption to family life. Improving standards of postanesthesia care units, better monitoring facilities and newer short acting agents like propofol, midazolam, fentanyl and remifentanil have made day care surgery possible. It is recommended that the surgery should be of short duration, with minimal blood loss. Day care surgery is however, contraindicated in premature infants less than 44 weeks post-conceptual age, extensive/painful surgery and children with poorly controlled and associated comorbid conditions (asthma, diabetes, seizure). Newer, rapid acting anesthetic agents like desflurane, propofol and sevoflurane as well as improved monitoring have made hospital stay times shorter than before.

SPECIFIC CONSIDERATIONS

Congenital Hypertrophic Pyloric Stenosis

The regular "projectile" vomiting in infants within the first week of life heralds the beginning of dehydration and dyselectrolytemia, if not adequately corrected. hypovolemic children experience episodes of hypotension intraoperatively, and are poorly compensated for intraoperative fluid shifts. Dyselectrolytemia may predisposes to unpredictable, delayed responses to anesthetic agents, prolongs recovery and increases risks of intraoperative cardiac rhythm disturbances.

The large gastric volume preoperatively make these patients ideal candidates for pulmonary aspiration during induction of anesthesia when protective airway reflexes are absent and the endotracheal tube is not in place yet. Decompressions, reduce the risk but do not obliterate it entirely. Nasogastric tubes for gastric lavages and decompressions can be left open to atmosphere at the time of induction. Since the presence

Table 9.6: Dosage schedule of bupivacaine (0.5%) for spinal anesthesia			
Wt of Patient kg	Dose (mg/kg)	Volume (ml/kg)	Duration (min)
0-5	0.5	0.1	75
5.15	0.4	0.08	80
7>15	0.3	0.06	85

of the tube hampers lower esophageal integrity, some practioners remove it preinduction.

Safest among pediatric induction routines is the rapid sequence approach. After adequate preoxygenation an induction agent with short acting muscle relaxant are injected to provide rapid loss of consciousness with relaxation. A backward pressure on the cricoid, the Sellick's maneuver prevents regurgitation while the patient is anesthetized. It is generally applied by an assistant till the airway is secured.

Uncooperative children, absence of intravenous accesss, anticipated difficulties in intubation, operator inexperience, deem alternative methods of induction, based on operator preference and patient status. Thus, induction techniques may range from inhalation induction with Sellick's maneuver applied by an assistant, to awake intubation in a moribund infant with a difficulty airway.

Maintenance is with a combination of O_2, N_2O and volatile agent. Muscle relaxation is usually provided with a non-depolarizing agent. Intraoperative opioid usage mandates vigilant postoperative monitoring of respiratory function. Analgesia for intra and post-operative periods can effectively be provided with local infiltrations of anesthetic agents or caudal epidural blocks.

Bowel Artesia

Patients in this group are managed similarly to pyloric stenosis, bearing in mind that optimization of pre-operative dyselectrolytemia and fluid deficit is essential to avoid intraoperative hemodynamic instability and postoperative morbidity. Rapid sequence, or similar induction techniques are safe approaches to avoid pulmonary aspiration. Maintenance can be with oxygen air and volatile agent plus opioid supplementation. The propensity for nitrous oxide to enter and expand closed cavities is the basis for the wisdom behind it's avoidance.

Regional anesthesia, either as wound infiltrate or lumber and caudal epidural blocks provides satisfactory analgesia. Catheter techniques allow the analgesia to be continued in the postoperative period as well.

Gastroschisis and Exomphalos

The hypothermic and dehydrated state that these babies commonly present will necessities rapid securing of intravenous access and fluid resuscitation with crystalloids like Hartman's solution and colloids. Preoperative investigation are necessary to reveal current physiological status which has to be optimized.

Anesthetic induction techniques remain the same as previously described. The use of nitrous oxide during maintenance of anesthesia is strongly discouraged to avoid distention of the gut. To avoid oxygen toxicity the addition of air in the inspiratory mixture is utilized.

Parenteral opioids, as well as epidural catheters have been described for intra and post operative analgesia. Abdominal wall closure under tension may be associated with increased airway pressures, and in extreme cases, reduced blood pressures. In such condition a delayed secondary closure of the abdominal wall may be decided upon. Tense closures of the abdomen may necessitate elective postoperative ventilation.

Inguinal Hernia

Most institutions undertake this procedure as a day care surgery. Premedication is thus avoided. Pain from venipuncture is provided with EMLA cream used carefully.

Induction of anesthesia by intravenous or inhalation routes is dependent on the cooperation of the child and the preference of the anesthetist. Short acting agents like propofol, sevoflurane and desflurane contribute to a clear headed, faster recovery. Intubation can be avoided and a laryngeal mask airway or a face mask used to keep the airway patent. Pain relief is commonly provided by caudal epidural, lumbar spinal or local anesthetic infiltration into the wound.

Esophageal Atresia and Tracheosophageal Fistula

Tracheoesophageal fistula repair form a daunting challenge to the anesthetist both during induction and maintenance. The problems of securing an airway in a neonate is compounded by the uncertain ventilatory path once the endotracheal tube is presumably in place. Endotracheal tube openings facing the fistula can direct ventilation into the stomach, or the blind pouch, if present.

Either inhalational or intravenous induction is practiced on these children, based on operator ease. The tip of the endotracheal tube is carefully positioned beyond the fistula to allow adequate ventilation. Any alterations in this arrangement as caused by jerky positional changes from supine to central or unmonitored head flexion or extension is to be guarded against vigilantly.

General anesthesia with a volatile agent and opioid is most commonly used in our institution. Nitrous oxide is avoided by some to prevent added gastric distention. Ventilation with low tidal volumes and high frequencies till the fistula is ligated prevents excessive gastric insufflation.

Epidural catheters threaded into the thoracic region via lumbar or caudal route provide good quality analgesia, their continuation in the postoperative period speeds recovery and reduces the incidence of pulmonary complication.

The surgery necessitate a close cooperation at all time between the surgeon and the anesthetist. The extrapleural surgical approach requires a constant communication to prevent tearing the pleura. The upper esophageal pouch is identified with a large catheter which has to be securely fixed for appropriate anastomosis. Intermittent release and ventilation of retracted lung is important whenever deoxygenation commences. Tracheal compression during surgery is immediately recognized by the high inflation pressure required to ventilate, it is important to readjust the retractor or check the clamps, prior to proceeding. Tense, distended stomach impeding ventilation may need to be decompressed prior to closure of the fistula.

Congenital Diaphragmatic Hernia

Notwithstanding current advances in ventilation like the extracorporeal membrane oxygenation, mortality from this condition can be between 30-50%.

Current outlooks prefer to stabilize the child's oxygenation and hemodynamics prior to surgery. The best time for which is arrived at on discussion between the surgeon and anesthetist. Sick babies on ECMO, Nitric oxide or high frequency oscillatory ventilation may be operated in the ICU, if the logistical problems of transporting the patient in the OT is insurmountable.

Most neonates taken up for surgery are already intubated, sedated and have intravenous access for surgery. Anesthetic induction for children not intubated yet must avoid the dangers of nitrous oxide and the risks of mask ventilation. Both of these can increase pressures in the herniated gut contents and cause hemodynamic compromise.

Maintenance of anesthesia is with both opioids and muscle relaxants. Children hand ventilated during surgery mandate the availability of an airway pressure gauge to avoid barotrauma.

Epidural anesthesia with catheters have been described but is avoided in children with ECMO who are anticogulated.

Neurosurgery

Children with repair of neural tube defects, or cranially (encephalocele) or along the spine (meningomyelocele) may pose challenges in intubation. Large lesions impair supine positioning. Intubation in such cases is either in the lateral position or supine after positioning the child with pillows and towels. Latex precautions are essential.

Anesthesia can be induced either intravenously or by inhalational route if airway difficulty is anticipated. However, inhalational induction may increase intracranial pressures. Nitrous oxide, volatile agent and opioids with a muscle relaxant provide balanced anesthesia for all cases. Extubation is preferred only in an awake patient with satisfactory recovery of airway reflexes.

Increasing depth of anesthesia at times of noxious stimuli (Laryngoscopy, surgical stimulation) prevents sharp rises in intracranial pressures. Most induction agents, barring ketamine when used alone, lower ICP. Among volatile agents, Isoflurane has the most favorable profile in cerebral hemodynamics.

Bronchoscopy

Children with recently aspirated foreign bodies namely food, pose the dual risk of aspiration pneumonitis due to full stomach, and the danger of intrapulmonary swelling of the vegetable body. Older bodies are associated with pulmonary consolidations. If an acute respiratory compromise is not present, regular chest physiotherapy preoperatively reduces intra and postoperative morbidity.

Spontaneously breathing children during bronchoscopy may prevent distal dislodgement of foreign bodies. On the other hand, control of ventilation with muscle relaxants allows a lighter plane of anesthesia to be developed, leading to a faster recovery. The ventilatory side ports of bronchoscopes enable connection to anesthetic circuits, but the large amount of leak often created necessitates high gas flow and pollution. Interrupting ventilation during surgical manipulation can cause sharp falls in oxygenation which has to be constantly monitored and communicated to the surgeon to allow transient cessation of surgery and resumption of ventilation.

Upper airway edema postoperatively is reduced by steam inhalation, nebulized epinephrine and steroids. Chest physiotherapy needs to be continued postoperative in patients with pulmonary complications.

Trauma

Basic principles of trauma management in a child remain the same as an adult. A rapid assessment followed by securing the airway and ventilation remains the first essential step. Younger children, with larger occiputs have a greater neck flexion than desired. With polytrauma, usage of shoulder rolls and pillows for optimal head positioning may not always be possible. Nasal intubation, airways and nasogastric tubes are avoided with evidences of basilar skull fractures like otorrhea, CSF rhinorrhea or perorbital ecchymosis.

As in adults all pediatric trauma cases are considered as full stomach, and appropriate anti aspiration precautions are taken. Rapid sequence "crash" induction are essential for commencement of anesthesia. Agents used for anesthesia are chosen carefully and titrated to avoid hemodynamics compromise while maintaining hypnosis and analgesia. Ketamine has been an attractive choice in hypovolemic patients, and carries a low risk of emergence delirium in children.

Biliary Atresia

It is characterized by a lack of patency of the extrahepatic bile duct with an incidence is 1:15,000 live births. In 10-15% of patients, it is associated with other abnormalities like absent inferior vena cava, intestinal malrotation, polysplenia and preduodenal portal vein.

Biliary atresia presents in infants from 1-6 weeks of age – these patients comes for Kasai Operation (Hepatic portoenterostomy). Preoperatively, these infants should be assessed for liver function tests. Liver function is fairly well preserved in the first few months of life. Ductal fibrosis begins as the infant grows and liver function deteriorates. The degree of liver dysfunction and the drugs ability to bind to plasma proteins are important variables in determining drug kinetics in patients with liver disease. Prothrombin time should be within normal limits. Fresh Frozen Plasma should be infused if there is any deviation from normal values.

Intravenous induction with thiopentone (4-5 mg/kg as 1%) can be achieved if venous access is present. Otherwise sevoflurane is the inhalational agent of choice for the induction. Before the introduction of sevoflurane, majority of our patients were induced with halothane when venous access was not present.

Anesthesia can be maintained with oxygen-nitrous oxide, isoflurane or sevoflurane and fentanyl. Air can be replaced with nitrous oxide as the bowel distension caused by nitrous oxide may caused technical problems to the surgeon. Atracurium is the muscle relaxant of choice as it is metabolized by Hoffman's elimination.

Standard monitoring and care provided to the infants undergoing surgery should be provided. CVP and arterial cannulation are not necessary for uncomplicated cases. Intraoperatively care should be taken at the time of retraction of liver. Hypotension due to decrease venous return and bradycardia (vagal stimulation) should be noted and corrected immediately.

Intraoperative fluid should be replaced by Ringer's lactate 6-10 ml/kg/hr. Repeated Blood Sugar estimations are done and 5% dextrose is added to Ringer's lactate when the blood sugar is low.

It has been seen that liver blood flow and oxygen supply are better maintained during isoflurane than during halothane anaesthesia.[70]

At the end of surgical procedure, if major fluid shifts have not occurred, blood loss has been minimal and the patient is warm, muscle relaxation is reversed with neostigmine (0.05 mg/kg) and atropine

(0.02 mg/kg) and the trachea is extubated. Postoperative ventilation may be required in infants with other organ system failures (sepsis, cholangitis, or pneumonia) hypothermia and blood loss of more than one blood volume. These should be recovered in a high dependency unit.

Liver Tumors

Children with hepatic tumors usually present with abdominal mass. Infrequently they will have anemia, jaundice, and ascites. Liver function tests are frequently within normal limits. Hepatoblastoma has also been associated with sexual precocity due to liver's exotrophic gonadotropic production and the Beckwith-Wiede-Mann syndrome.

Other associated disease with hepatocellular carcinoma are Von-Gierke's disease, type I glycogenesis, cystinosis, extrahepatic biliary atresia, α–1-antitrypsin deficiency, hypoplasia of intrahepatic bile ducts, Wilson's disease, Giant cell hepatitis, and Soto's syndrome.

The principles about the anesthetic management of these patient is similar as those with biliary atresia. Cardiovascular evaluation and ECHO should be done to rule out any cardiomyopathy in patients who receive adriamycin before coming for surgery.

Hepatic resection is usually associated with massive blood loss, so invasive monitoring should done to measure arterial and central venous pressure. The blood loss is reduced with the use of ultrasonic aspirator. Two large bore peripheral intravenous cannulae and 2-3 lumen internal jugular vein cannulation should be achieved. Frequently ABG, chemistry and coagulation profile may be required. Urine output should also be monitored. Massive blood loss may require replacement of Fresh frozen plasma, and platelet concentrate in addition to blood transfusion. These patients may require ventilatory support postoperatively.

Thoracic Surgery

Alterations in lung ventilation perfusion ratios occur with changes in body posture. In the lateral position as in surgery, perfusion and ventilation is superior in the dependent and non-dependent lung respectively, in spontaneously breathing individuals. Altered chest wall compliance can account for these changes. Airway closure during tidal volumes can occur due to low functional residual capacity. A high metabolic rate and oxygen consumption, with low lung volumes vital capacities and residual capacities make lung separation a difficult proposition.

Preoperative assessment to deduce baseline physiological status is essential. A history and examination with baseline blood biochemistry and hematology is the same as for an adult. However, pulmonary function tests, though having been devised for children, may be hampered by poor cooperation. Pulse oximetry is a reliable non-invasive substitute for arterial blood gas analysis. Optimization and chest physiotherapy needs to continue to reduce postoperative morbidity.

One lung ventilation techniques, while widespread in adults are limited in children due to non-availability of equipment methods. These include:[71]

- Simple surgical retraction – most commonly practiced, but can lead to anatomic damage.
- Double lumen tubes : size 28 or 32 french sizes are available for older children. Muraro tubes, consisting of two separate tubes attached to each other are available in sizes for smaller children.
- Bronchial blockers, either specialized univent tubes, or Fogarty catheters or single lumen tubes guided by fiberoptic bronchoscopic techniques provide alternatives.

Caution is recommended with usage of nitrous oxide, specially in relation to gas filled cysts in lobar emphysema. Positive pressure ventilation may expand an emphysematous lobe causing mediastinal shift.

Good postoperative analgesia is mandatory else the reduced chest wall movement consequent to pain promotes atelectasis. Older children can be motivated for chest physiotherapy once good relief is achieved. Epidural catheters, threaded through the lumbar and caudal route up the thoracic interspaces provide effective postoperative pain control with opioid or local anesthetic combinations. Opioids intravenously by boluses or infusions can depress respiration and consciousness. Intercostal and interpleural local anesthetic can provide temporary relief, but carry the risk of systemic absorption of the drug.

Craniosynostosis

It is the premature fusion of one or more cranial sutures and cause an abnormal skull shape. Most often it involves only the sagittal suture and results in a deformity that is primarily cosmetic. These patients have normal ICP and intelligence. Without treatment, this may result in intracranial hypertension as the brain grows. Multiple suture craniosynostosis is most commonly seen in association with craniofacial anomalies, particularly Apert's and Crouson's syndromes which are also associated with hypoplasia of the orbits and midportion of the face.

The anesthetic problems in patients coming for craniectomy and frontal advancements are difficult intubation, fixation of endotracheal tube, blood loss, increased ICP (for this furosemide and mannitol may be required).

Repairs range from multiple craniectomies to removal of a single strip. Blood losses from scalp incisions can be significant necessitating transfusions Venous air embolism may occur and vigilance is essential.[72]

SUMMARY

With the progress in different aspects of anesthesia, complicated pediatric surgical procedures are possible today. Better understanding of the physiology and pharmacology of the newer drugs has led to the advancement in anesthetic techniques. Rapid acting inhalational agent like sevoflurane has made induction and recovery quick and smooth. Parental participation in the induction procedure has made induction less traumatic. Intravenous induction has been facilitated by EMLA cream. Laryngeal mask airway has revolutionized the airway management in children, whereby tracheal intubation is avoided in majority of patients. It is also listed as a tool in difficult pediatric airway management. The concept of fluid therapy has recently being changed to infusion of balanced salt solution as primary maintenance and replacement fluid.

Postoperative pain relief is provided more by regional blocks and the child/parent/nurse can also control the analgesia demand to suit patient comfort.

REFERENCES

1. Long CW. An account of the first use of sulphuric ether by inhalation as an anesthetic in surgical operations. South Med J 1849;5:710.
2. Steward DJ. History of Pediatric Anesthesia. In: Gregory GA. Ed. Pediatric Anesthesia. Second Edition. New York, NY: Churchill Livingstone Inc 1983:1-14.
3. Davies G, Reidl. Growth of alveoli and pulmonary arteries in childhood. Thorax 1970;25:669.
4. Mansell A. Bryan C, Levinson H. Airway closure in children. Journal of Applied Physiology 1972;33:711-14.
5. American Society of Anesthesia Guidelines.
6. CJ Cote. Pre-operative preparation and premedication. British Journal of Anaesthesia 1999;83(1):16-28.
7. Tait AR, Ketcham TR, Klun MS, Knight PR. Preoperative respiratory complications in patients with upper respiratory tract infection: Anaesthesiology 1983;24 A (433):3.
8. Cohen M, Camerone B. Should you cancel the operation when a child has upper respiratory tract infection? Anaesthesia Analgesia 1991;72:282-88.
9. Empey DW. Effect of Airway infections on bronchial reactivity. European Journal of Respiratory Disease (supplement) 1983:128:366-68.
10. Hunt JN, MacDonald M. The influence of volume on gastric emptying. Journal of Physiology 1954;126:459-74.
11. Practice guidelines for sedation and Analgesia by non Anesthesiologists, Anesthesiology 2002;96:1004-17.
12. Green S. Dissociative Agents Kraus BK, Brostowicz RM. Pediatric Procedural Sedation and Analgesia, Lippin Cott Williams and Wilkins 1999;49.
13. Funk W, Jakob W, Riedl T, Taeger K. Oral preanaesthetic medication for children : double blind and randomized study of a combination of midazolam and ketamine Vs. midazolam or ketamine alone. British Journal of Anaesthesia 2000;84:335-40.
14. Gingrich BK. Difficulties encountered in a comparative study of orally administered midazolam and ketamine anesthesiology 1994;80:1414-15.
15. Lejus C, Renaudin M, Testa S, Malinousky JM, Vigier – T, Souron R. Midazolam for premedication in children: nasal Vs. rectal administration. European Journal of Anesthesiology 1997;14:244-49.
16. Karl HW, Keifer AT, Rosenberyer JL, Larach MG, Ruffle JM. Comparison of the safety and efficacy of intranasal midazolam or sufentanil for preinduction of anesthesia in pediatric patients. Anesthesiology 1992;76:209-15.
17. Eger EI, Smith NT, Stoelting RK. Cardiovascular effects of Halothane in man. Anesthesiology 1970;32:396-409.
18. Brown BR. Hepatotoxicity of inhaled Anesthetics Current Opinions in Anesthesiology 1989;2:414-17.
19. Eger EI. Isoflurane a review. Anesthesiology 1981;55: 559-76.
20. Eger EI. The Pharmacology of Isoflurane. British Journal of Anaesthesia 1984;56:715-995.
21. Jones RM. Clinical comparison of inhalation anaesthetic agents. British Journal of anaesthesia 1984;56:575.
22. Priebe HJ. Isoflurane and coronary hemodynamics, Anesthesiology 1989;71:960-76.
23. O Brien K, Kumar R, Morton NS. Sevoflurane compared with Halothane for tracheal intubation in children. British Journal of Anaesthesia 1998;80452-55.
24. Jackson D, Sidhu VS, Lomax DM. Sevoflurane–an alternative to routine use of suxamethonium in children. Anaesthesia 1997;52:189.

25. Frink EJ, Malan TP, Atlas m, Dominguez LM, Navdo JX, Brown BR. Clinical comparison of sevoflurane and isoflurane in healthy patients. Anaesthesia and Analgesia 1992;74:241-45.
26. Holzman RS, Vander Velde ME, Klans SJ. Sevoflurane depresses myocardial contractility less than Halothane during induction of Anaesthesia in children. Anesthesiology 1996;85:1260-67.
27. Kester JR, Brayer AP, Pagel PS, Tessmer JP, Warltier DC. Perfusion of ischemic myocardium during anaesthesia with sevoflurane. Anesthesiology 1994;81:995-1004.
28. Smiley RM, Orn Stein E, Matteo RS, Pantuck EJ, Pantuck CB. Desflurane and Isoflurane in surgical patients : A comparison of emergence time. Anesthesiology 1991;74:425-28.
29. Taylor RH, Lerman J. Induction, maintenence and recovery characteristics of Desflurane in infants and children. Canadian Journal of Anaesthesia 1992;39:6-13.
30. Wolf AR, Lawson RP, Dryden CM, Davies FW. Recovery after Desflurane anaesthesia in the infant: comparison with Isoflurane. British Journal of Anaesthesia 1996;76:362-64.
31. Stoelting RK. Nonbarbiturate induction drugs. Pharmacology and physiology in Anaesthetic practise. Philadelphia JB Lippencott and company 1991.
32. Aun CST, Sung RYT, O'meara ME, Short TG, Oh TE. Cardiovascular effects of iv induction in children: A comparison between propofol and Thiopentone British Journal of Anaesthesia 1993;70:647-53.
33. Crawford MW, Lerman J, Sloan MH, Sikich N, Halpernl, Bissonnette B. Recovery characteristics of propofol anaesthesia with and without nitrous oxide: a comparison with Halothane/nitrous oxide anesthesia in children. Pediatric Anaesthesia 1998;8:49-54.
34. Hamza J, Ecottey C, Gross JB. Ventilatory response to CO_2 following Intravenous Ketamine in children. Anesthesiology 1989;70:422-25.
35. Gardner AE, Olson BL, Lichtiger M. Cerebrospinal fluid pressure during dissociation anaesthesia with ketamine. Anesthesiology 1971;35:226-28.
36. Morton NS. Prevention and central of Pain – British Journal of Anaesthesia 1999;83:118-29.
37. Scott JC, Ponganis KV, Stanski DR. EEG quantitation of narcotic effect. The comparative pharmacodynamics of Fentanyl and alfentanyl. Anaesthesiology 1985:62:234-41.
38. Gvay J, Gavdneault P, Tang A, Goolet B, Varin F. Pharmacokinetics of sufentanil in normal children. Candian Journal of Anaesthesia 1992;39:14-20.
39. Pennat J, White P. The laryngeal mask airway. It's uses in anaesthesiology. Anesthesiology 1993;79:144-63.
40. Thomas DKM. Hypoglycemia in children before operations: its incidence and prevention. Br J Anaesth 1974;46:66.
41. Nilsson K, Lavsson EL and other. Blood glucose concentration during anaesthesia in children. Br J Anaesth 1984;56:375.
42. Merskey H, Aibc – Fessard DG, Bonica JJ, et al. Pain tenns respiration: A list with definition and notes M usage: Recommended by ASP subcommittee on Taxonomy Pain 1979;6:249.
43. Morton NS. Prevention and control of pain in children. British Journal of Anaesthesia 1999;83(1):118-29.
44. Frank L-S, Greenlary CS, Stenens B. Pain assessment in infants and children. Pediatric clinics of north America Acute Pain in Children 2000;347(3):487.
45. Harbeck C, Peterson L. Elephants dancing in my head : A developmental approach to children's concept of specific pairs. Child development approach to children's concept of specific pairs. Child Development 1992;63:138-49.
46. Pokela M. Pain relief can reduce hypoxemia in distressed neonates during routine treatment procedures. Pediatrics 1994;93:379.
47. Hodogkenson K, Bear M, Thorn J. Measuring pain in neonates Evaluating an instrument and developing a common language. Austration Journal of Advanced Nursing 1994;12:17.
48. Krechel Sir, Bidner J. CRIES. A new neonatal postoperative pain management score: Initial testing of validity and inability. Pediatric Anaesthesia 1995;5:53.
49. Schade JG, Joyee BA, Gerkensmeyer J. Comparison of three preverbal scales for postoperative pain assessment in a diverse pediatric sample. Journal of pain symptom management 1996;12:348.
50. Mebrath PJ, Johson G, Goodman JT, et al. CHEOPS: A behavioural scale for rating postoperative pain in children. Advances in pain research and therapy 1985;9:395.
51. Tyler DC, Ti A, Douthit J, et al. Towards validation of pain measurement to old for children: a pilot study. Pain 1993;52:301-09.
52. Ambuel B, Hamlett KW, Marx AN. Assessing distress in pediatric intensive care environment: The comfort scale. Journal of Pediatric Psychology 1992;17:95.
53. Mc Grath PA, Scifert CE, Speechley KN, et al. A new analogue scale for assessing children's pain: An initial validation study. Pain 1996;64:435.
54. Rumack BH. Aspirin versus acetaminoptic: A comparative view pediatrics 1978:62;943-46.
55. Delbos A. Boccard and the morphine sparing effect of propara cetamol in orthopedic postoperative pain. Journal of pain symptom management 1995;10:279.
56. Birmingham D, Tobin M, Henthorm T, Fisher D, Derkelhamer M, Smithi, Fanto K, Cote CJ. Twenty four hour pharmacokineties of rectal sctammophen in children: An old dry with new recommendatory. Anesthesiology 1997:87:244-52.
57. Tay CLM, Tan S. Diclofenac or Paracetamol for Analgesia in pediatric nysingotomy operations: Anaesthesia Intensive Care 2002;30:55-59.
58. Kokki H, Karrinen M, Jekunen A. Pharmacokmetics of a 24 hour intravenous ketoprofen infusion in children. Acta Anaesthesiological Scandinavica 2002;46:194-98.
59. Dalens B. Anatomy in Regional Anaesthesia in infants, children and adolescents. Bernard Dalens (Editor).

60. Dalens B. Regional Anaesthesia in children. Anaesthesia Ronald D. milter (Editor) Churchill livingstone
61. Mc Nelly JK, Trentadue NC, Rusy LM, Farbar NE. Culture of bacteria from lumbar and caudal epidural catheters used for postoperative analgesia in children. Regional Anaesthesia 1997;22:428-31.
62. Jylli L, Lunderberg S, Olsson GL. Retrospective evaluation of continuous epidural infusion for postoperative pain in children. Acta Anesthesiologica Scandinavica 2002;46:654-59.
63. Armitage EN. Regional Anesthesia in paediatrics. Clinical Anesthesiology 1985;3:553.
64. Dalens B, Harnaonti A. Caudal anaesthesia in paediatric surgery: Success rate and adverse effects in 750 patients. Anesthesia and Analgesia 1989;68:83.
65. Haberkern CM. Epidural and intravenous bolus morphine for postoperative analgesia in infants. Canadian Journal of Anesthesia 1996;43:1203-10.
66. Brown TCK, Eyres RL, McDovgall RJ. Local and Regional anaesthesia in children. British Journal of Anaesthesia 1999;83:65-77.
67. Dalens B. Lumbar Epidural Anaesthesia. Regional Anaesthesia in infants, children and adolescents. Bernard Dalens (Editor), Williams, wilkins and wanerly Europe.
68. Welborn LG, Rice LJ, Hannallah RS, Broadman LM, Rottimann UE, Fink R. Postoperative Apnea in Former preterm Infants : Prospective comparison of Spinal and General Anaesthesia. Anesthesiology 1990;72:838-42.
69. Ylonen P, Kokki H. Epidural blood patch for management of postdural puncture headache in adolescents. Acta Anaesthesiologica Scandinavica 2002;46:794-98.
70. Gelman S, Fowler KC, Smith LR. Liver circulation and function during Isoflurane and halothane anesthesia. Anesthesiology 1984;61:726.
71. Nicoll SJB, Bingham R. Pediatric Thoracic anaesthesia: in Thoracic Anesthesia: principles and practise. S Ghosh, R D Latimer (Editors). Butterwan theinmann, Oxford 1999.
72. Fabevouski LW, Black S, Mickle JP. Incidence of venous air embolism during craniectomy for craniosynostosis repair. Anesthesiology 2000;92:20-23.

CHAPTER 10
Relief of Postoperative Pain in Children

MK Arora, G Prasad

For years acute pediatric pain management has been practiced without a clear rationale of analgesic therapy. Improved understanding of opioid and local anesthetic pharmacology in infants and children has led to the development of formal analgesic regimens for the management of pain particularly postoperative pain.[1,2]

Despite the advances in analgesic therapy, numerous studies show that postoperative pain is still inadequately treated in children, adolescents and almost ignored in infants due to following reasons (Table 10.1).

Every child, irrespective of age, must get adequate pain relief after as his/her right. A multimodal approach in pain relief has better pain relief with lesser side effect. This can be achieved by using combination of local or regional anesthesia unless contraindicated, opioids, and nonsteroidal antiinflammatory drugs (NSAID) or paracetamol. The parents' emotional involvement and child friendly environment also play an important role in pain management.

DEVELOPMENT OF PAIN IN THE FETUS AND THE NEONATE

Very little is known about the perception of pain by the fetus and the newborn. Early studies of neurological development concluded that the fetus and the newborn were not capable of having organized response to painful stimuli and could not perceive or localize pain.[3] They had no memory of pain and therefore did not require analgesia even for very painful procedures. Recent studies however have shown that a fetus reacts to stimuli in utero and that newborn demonstrates hormonal changes in response to surgery that can be decreased by intraoperative use of narcotics and deep anaesthesia.[4,5]

New evidence suggests that inhuman fetus pain pathways as well as cortical and subcortical center necessary for pain perception are well developed late in gestation and the neurochemical systems now known to be associated with pain transmission and modulation are intact and functional.[6]

PAIN ASSESSMENT

Pain assessment is necessary before prescribing analgesics. This gives information about efficacy of drugs, individual requirement, time to intervene for analgesia, deciding the route of administration and helps in the studies of analgesics drugs.

The assessment of pain is difficult in neonates and nonverbal age as they can not self-report about pain. The most accurate methods of rating pain are when child can himself report the site and intensity. Emphasis was placed on behavioral indicators (facial expression, cry and body movement), physiological parameters (heart rate, respiratory rate, oxygen saturation and intracranial pressure) and biochemical parameters (ACTH, beta endorphins, cortisol).

The following physiological and behavioral distress measures have been investigated in children as potential pain measures (Tables 10.2 and 10.3).[7]

Table 10.1: Factors responsible for under treatment of pain in children

- Opioid induced respiratory depression
- Potential for addiction
- Difficulty in assessing pain by physicians
- Inability to communicate pain by older children
- Fear of shot in some children

Table 10.2: Potential Pain Measures

Physiological methods
- Heart rate
- Palmer sweat response
- Blood pressure
- Endorphin level

Behavioural methods
- Overt distress scale
- Procedural behavioral rating scale – revised
- Observation scale of behavioral distress
- Children's hospital of Eastern Ontario pain scale (CHEOPS)

Projective methods
- Color
- Shapes
- Drawing
- Cartoons

Table 10.3: Objective pain score (OPS)[9]

Parameter	Findings	Points
Systolic blood pressure	Increase < 20% of preoperative blood pressure	0
	Increase > 20% of preoperative blood pressure	1
	Increase >30% of preoperative blood pressure	2
Crying	Not crying	0
	Responds to tender loving care	1
	Does not responds to tender loving care	2
Movements	Not moving	0
	Restless moving in bed	1
	Thrashing	2
Agitation	Asleep/calm	0
	Can be comforted to lessen the agitation (mild)	1
	Can not be comforted to the agitation (hysterical)	2
Complain of pain	Asleep/no pain	0
	Can not localize	1
	Can localize	2

Table 10.4: Direct report methods

- Pocker chip tool
- Faces scale
- Oucher scale
- Pain thermometer
- Visual analogue scale (VAS)

In neonates, a number of tools have been developed using facial expression, body posture, crying, heart rate, oxygen saturation and state of sleep. Neonatal infant pain scale (NIPS), and CRIES postoperative pain assessment scale is being used for validating neonatal pain. CRIES scale is valid for 32 - 60 weeks of gestation and uses parameters of C-Crying; R-Requires oxygen to maintain saturation greater than 95%; I-Increased vital signs; E-Expression; and S-Sleeplessness. 0-2 points given for each parameter with total score of 10 and score of 4 and above require analgesic supplementation.[8]

Pain in younger children (< 4 yrs) can be assessed by objective pain score (OPS). In this 0-2 points allotted for each physiological parameters, i.e. systolic blood pressure, crying, movement, agitation (confused excited), complains of pain and 4 or above to be treated for pain (Table 10.3).

The following methods are also used for pain assessments in children above 3 years (Table 10.4).

VAS (visual analogue scale) is used for pain assessment in children above 4 or 5 years depending upon education and understanding of the child. This has 0-100 mm marking on the horizontal scale, 0 is no pain and 100 is worst imagine pain. Child reports their pain on the scale.

DESIGN ISSUES

In designing a comprehensive plan for postoperative analgesia the objectives need have to be clearly defined for each patient. These are dependent on various considerations as given below.

1. Type and site of surgery
2. Severity of pain expected
3. Predicted recovery course
4. Abilities of the patient
5. Patient and family needs and desires
6. Associated medical and psychological issue
7. Technical aspects of interventions
8. Environment.

Decision regarding postoperative pain needs to be made with a complete understanding of the surgical procedures and expected convalescence.

Type and Site of Surgery Planned

For example, superficial surgical procedure such as excision of small nevi produces significantly less discomfort and pain compared to more invasive procedure such as excision of abdominal or thoracic masses. Additionally patient undergoing superficial procedures may be discharged hours after the surgery while the patient following more invasive procedure may have prolonged recovery including a period of time in the intensive care unit.

Severity of Pain

Mild analgesics are appropriate for the patient following superficial operations but are inappropriate for patients undergoing major operations like laminectomy or rhizotomy. As a result analgesic plan needs to be tailored specifically to the procedure. The benefit of epidural analgesia may far outweigh the potential disadvantage of urinary retention.

Abilities of Patients

In contrast to most adult patients, the age maturity and development level of pediatric patients vary with each child. Blanket assessments based on the surgical procedure and expected convalescent period ignore the needs of various pediatric patient populations that results from vide spectrum of development and cognitive abilities.

Needs and Desires of the Family

Past experiences of family members resulting from inadequate pain management of their child may require a more efficient management in future. Similarly, beliefs held by the family regarding the utility of analgesic and need for pain control also merit consideration, e.g. some families view opioid analgesics as routinely dangerous and addicting.

Associated Medical and Psychological Issue

For medical conditions such as severe liver or renal disease alter the metabolism and excretion of analgesics and have necessitated modification in standard pain management protocols. In the face of altered pharmacokinetics, doses and dosing intervals of analgesics may need to be varied.

Hospital environment can lead to significant behavioral and psychological changes leading to depression, anxiety and fear. This may be mistaken for pain in the postoperative period. Similarly, the behavioral issues surrounding children with known drug abuse problems further complicate postoperative pain management.

Technical Aspect

The technical issue revolves around procedures and equipments required for various pain control therapies. Regional analgesia continuous infusion using syringe pumps and more recently patient controlled analgesia (PCA) requires special equipment as well as technical skills.

THERAPEUTIC MODALITIES FOR PAIN MANAGEMENT

An effective systemic analgesic as well as route of administration already exists for pediatric pain management. Unfortunately the adequate analgesics and delivery systems are underutilized because of prevalent and persistent misconceptions regarding the propensity for respiratory depression and addiction in children and the actual presence of pain in certain age group. Similarly, potent and safe regional anesthesic/analgesic techniques so often used in adults are sparingly used in children due to lack of adequate skill and nursing facilities.

Nonopioid Analgesics

These agents provide relief of mild to moderate pain when used alone and provide additive analgesic when combined with opioids. Ketorolac, a recently released parenterally administered NSAID has shown analgesic potency similar to opioids. Ketorolac 2 mg is considered equipment to 1 mg of morphine by the IM route.[10] Unlike opioids, ketorolac does not produce respiratory depression, reduction of gastrointestinal motility or addiction (Table 10.5).

Opioids

Opioids analgesics are the mainstay of pain management in the postoperative pediatric patient. No matter what opioid or administration technique is selected, careful titration and adjustment is usually needed.

Oral Route

Presence of nausea, vomiting and delayed gastric emptying due to the effect of surgery and anesthesia

Table 10.5: Recommended starting doses for analgesic medication drugs

Non-opioids	Dose, Routes and Frequency
Acetaminophen	10 - 15 mg/kg po q 4 hr
	15 - 20 mg/kg sos PO q 4 hr
	20 - 30 mg/kg rectal 4 hr
Diclofenac	1 mg/kg (>1yr of age) PO q 8 hr
	1 - 2 mg/kg rectal
Ibuprofen	4 - 10 mg/kg PO q 6-8 hr
Ketorolac	0.5 mg/kg, IM/IV q 6-8 hr
Opioids oral	
Codeine	0.5 - 1 mg/kg po q 4 hr
Morphine	0.05 - 0.2 mg/kg po q 4 hr
	Pethidine 1 mg/kg po a 4 hr
Methadone	0.1 mg/kg po q 6-8 hr
Intramuscular	
Pethidine	0.8 to 1.3 mg/kg IM/SC q 3-4 hr
Morphine	0.1 -0.15 mg/kg IM q 3-4 hr
Intravenous Intermittent	
Pethidine	0.5 - 1 mg /kg IV q 2 hr
Morphine	0.05 - 0.1 mg /kg IV 2 hr Prn
Fentanyl	0.5 - 2 mcg /kg IV q 1-2 hr
Methadone	0.1 mg /kg IV q 4 hr initially then Q 6 - 12 hr

Continuous IV Infusion Morphine

Less than
3 months old   Initially 50 mcg/kg IV Q 15 - 20 SOS
                         Maintenance 10 - 15 mcg/kg/hr

Older than 3 months of age
- Initially 100 mcg /kg IV q 15 - 20 min sos
- Maintenance 10 - 50 mcg/kg/hr

Morphine NCA
- 1 mg/kg in 50 ml saline (20 mcg/kg/ml)
- Rate: 1ml/hr. bolus: 1ml. lockout time: 20 min

Morphine PCA
- 1 mg/kg in 50 ml saline (20 mcg/kg/ml)
- Rate: 0.2 ml/hr. bolus: 1ml. lockout time: 5 min

precludes the use of oral analgesic in the immediate postoperative period. Codeine is the most commonly used oral opioid for relief of mild to moderate pain.[11] Morphine can also be used for relief of moderate to severe pain.[12]

Parenteral Medication

Intravenous is the best route for analgesic administration wherever available and there is little of any indication for IM route in such children. Drugs can be administered as boluses or as continuous infusions. It is much easier to administer boluses and provide rapid relief of pain. The disadvantage includes short periods of analgesia followed by periods of inadequate analgesia before the next dose is administered. Besides side effects associated with higher blood level are common. Continuous infusion on the other hand provides continuous analgesia with low plasma level even in newborn and infants.[13] Probably the best way to administer drug is to give a loading dose to provide patients comfort followed by an infusion.[14] Morphine and pethidine are the most commonly used narcotics in India.

Use of Opioids in Analgesia

Paediatric anesthesiologists have noted more frequent ventilatory problems in neonates when opioids are used. Possibly this may be due to the fact that the clearance of opioids is decreased in neonates, leading to unexpected high blood levels and a greater risk of respiratory depression.[15] Additionally infants may be more sensitive to opioids as a result of a more rapid transfer of a opioids across the blood brain barrier. Yet neonate after major surgery suffers pain and requires opioid administration. As a result of these altered pharmacokinetics and pharmacodynamics slow titration of small incremental doses and careful observation is required to safely provide adequate opioid analgesia to the postoperative neonate.

Patient Controlled Analgesia (PCA)

Intravenous PCA is a novel method where a microprocessor operated infusion pump is programmed to deliver predetermined safe amount of intravenous opioid at specified interval on patient demand.

The introduction of PCA in the pediatric population seems promising because it is self limiting when pain free patients go off to sleep, they can no longer medicate themselves. Unfortunately PCA is not applicable to children less than 7 years of age or those with minimal Cognitive skills. Another drawback is that it is an expensive device. PCA has been used in children 11 years and older with varying results but most adolescent use PCA responsible and with satisfaction.[16] Morphine is the drug of choice. Instead of patient controlled, the same technique can be used as nurse controlled analgesia (NCA) is smaller children. The regimes are given Table 10.4.

Side Effects

Respiratory depression is the most feared and potentially serious side effect of opioids. The incidence of respiratory depression with μ-agonists is directly related to the dose of drug used. Minor side effect such as nausea, vomiting, urinary retention, drowsiness, hallucination, nightmare, light headedness and ileus occur no more frequency in children than in adults.

Tolerance is an uncommon clinical problem in children when opioids are used in appropriate doses for short period of time.

Regional Anesthesia/Analgesia

Although, opioids are simple to administer, convenient and inexpensive means of managing postoperative pain the judicious use of specific regional anesthetic techniques offer better pain relief for some specific surgical procedures. Nerve block produces reliable and effective analgesia without the risk of sedation and respiratory depression. Such features make most neural blockade techniques suitable for outpatient surgery.

Peridural Administration

Peridural administration of local anesthetics significantly diminishes or abolishes nociceptive impulses from entering the Central Nerve System. Placing local anesthetics at the level of the spinal cord produces profound analgesia without producing the systemic sedation seen with opioid therapy. Caudal and epidural administration of local anesthesia are the chief route of peridural administration.

Local anesthetics can be given either as a single bolus or as a continuous infusion through a catheter. Single caudal injection of bupivcaine with epinephrine provides prolonged analgesia in children undergoing superficial inguinal and penile procedures lasting up to 23 hrs in children under 5 years and 6-10 hrs in older children.

Continuous infusion of local anesthetics through epidural or caudal catheters provides the opportunity to produce pain relief during the period of infusion. Infusion of bupivacaine in concentration from 0.1 - 0.25% at low rate of infusion provides excellent analgesia with bupivacaine level well under the toxic range.[17]

Peridural Narcotics

Peridural delivery of opioids analgesics produces prolonged and profound analgesia as they occupy opioids receptors in substantia gelatinosa of the spinal cord.[18,19] Either administered as a single dose or as a constant infusion peridural opioid administration (Epidural, caudal or intrathecal) delivers concentrated amounts of opioids to the receptors of the cord.

Single dose of opioid administration at the beginning or end of a surgical procedure either in epidural or intrathecal space provides prolonged analgesia for up to 24 hours for in excess of IV opioids or epidural bupivacaine. Through catheters, continuous infusion and repeated intermittent loses can be administered. Catheters can be placed epidurally in thoracic, lumbar intrathecally. Combination of local anesthetic and morphine may potentiate the analgesic effect of spinal morphine. Combination of low dose of morphine 30 μg/kg along with bupivacaine 0.25% given caudally has been reported to give prolonged analgesia lasting about 16–30 hours with minimal or no side effects. Respiratory depression has not been reported with this low dose.[20]

REGIONAL ADMINISTRATION

Local Infiltration

Wound infiltration with local anesthetic provides pain relief following surgery especially in superficial procedures. The effect may last as long as 4-6 hours with bupivacaine and lignocaine.

Peripheral Nerve Blocks

Peripheral nerve blockade by local anesthetic allows interruption of sensory transmission along specific nerves or nerve groups. Systemic effects often seem with epidural techniques can be avoided since the specific region affected by surgery is targeted and the dose of local anesthetic used is likely to be smaller. Various types of nerve blockade use are given in the below (Table 10.6).

Penile Block

Penile block is being commonly used for circumcision and distal urethral surgeries. A short bevelled needle

Table 10.6: Peripheral Nerve Blockade in Postoperative Pain Management

Body region	Peripheral or regional nerve to be blocked
Head and Neck	Cranial nerves
Upper extremity	Brachial plexus, specific nerves of arm
Chest / upper abdomen	Intercostals Interpleural catheter
Lower abdomen / Pelvis	Ilioinguinal Iliohypogastric Penile
Lower Extremity	Femoral, sciatic lumbar plexus Specific nerve of leg

is inserted in the midline at the penile pubic junction and advanced slightly laterally till fascia is penetrated. At this point, 1-3 ml of 0.25% bupivacaine with out adrenaline is injected and same is done on other side.

Caudal Block

Caudal anesthesia/analgesia is the most widely used neural blockade in children for the management of postoperative pain following surgical procedures on the lower abdomen, perineum and lower extremity. The clinical experience suggests that caudal anaesthesia/analgesia is simple to perform, reliable and safe.[21,22]

Positioning and Landmarks

It is quite easy to perform in children. To aid positioning and performance of the techniques it is customary to give a light general anesthetic. The patient can be positioned in the lateral (sims) position, prone or the knee chest. In the lateral position the lower leg is only slightly flexed at the hip. The upper leg is flexed to a greater extent so that it lies over and above the lower leg. The advantages of lateral sims position include comforts for the patient, comfortable and familiar workstations for anesthesiologist and easy access to the airway.

Procedure

Confirmation of the bony landmark is the key to successful performance of the technique. In most children, the protrusion of sacral cornua can be seen without palpation. The shallow depression of the sacral hiatus can be seen between the cornua. In land marks are not easily visible, the coccyx may be palpated and the finger moved cephalad until the fingertip overlies the sacral hiatus with cornua on each side. The chosen needle (22 or 23 G, 2-3 cm long) is inserted at an angle of 45°–60° to sacrococcygeal ligament. The penetration of sacrococcygeal ligament has a characteristic feel or pop. The anterior wall of sacral canal is contacted and the needle is redirected so that it is line with long axis of the spinal canal. The needle is then advances 2-5 mm further.

Choice and Dosing of Local Anesthetic

Bupivacaine is the most commonly used agent for postoperative pain management, though there are various formulae to calculate the dose. Armitage has reported 98 percent success rate with a simple and easily remembered method of calculating effective analgesic volume of 0.5 ml/kg is used for sacral analgesia 1 ml/kg for lower thoracic analgesia and 1.25 ml/kg of 0.25% bupivacaine for midthoracic analgesia. Caudal morphine in dose of 30–50 mcg/kg has been found to be safe. The duration of analgesia lasts nearly 24 hours but close monitoring for respiratory depression is recommended for a minimum of 24 hours, particularly in infants.

The duration of caudal block analgesia can be extended use of additives like clonidine, preservative free ketamine, and preservative free morphine with bupivacaine. Caudal morphine is not used for day care procedures due to fear of delayed respiratory depression and urinary retention.

POSTOPERATIVE ANALGESIA

The plan of postoperative analgesia is decided before starting of procedures. Minor procedures are managed with infiltaration of local anesthetic or regional blocks. Analgesia supplemented with rectal or injectable analgesics. Oral analgesics to be given at regular interval when orally allowed to the child. Major procedures require multimodal treatment for pain relief. Infusion or boluses of mixture of local anesthetic and narcotic through epidural or caudal catheter is the main stay of severe pain management. Intravenous infusion of morphine or fentanyl via patient controlled or nurse controlled analgesia is an alternative if epidural catheter is not *in situ*. Morphine, pethidine or fentanyl was also given as rescue analgesic. It has

Table 10.7: Practical guidelines for postoperative analgesia

Day care surgery/minor procedure
- Regional/Local anesthetic block
- Oral/rectal paracetamol
- Oral Ibuprofen q 6 hrly
- Oral codeine/Inj ketorolac

Major surgical procedure (multimodal approach)
- Regional (caudal, epidural catheter)
- Epidural infusion of bupivaciane + morphine/fentanyl
- Morphine injusion IV, SC
- Patient/Nurse controlled analgesia
- IV morphine/pethidine/fentanyl for rescue analgesia

NSAIDs
- oral
- rectal

been observed that addition of NSAIDs rectal/oral by injection will improve quality of analgesia (Table 10.7).

INHIBITION OF CENTRAL HYPERSENSITIZATION

The Concept of Pre-emptive Analgesia

The surgical trauma creates a barrage of nociceptive afferent transmission which may alter the excitability of both peripheral and central neurons.[23] Under general anesthesia the spinal cord is lightly anesthetized and receives massive afferent nociceptive input from the site of the surgery. Under regional anesthesia the spinal cord receives no nociceptive transmission. Prevention of the afferent "barrage" associated with the surgical stimulus may be accomplished by application of regional anesthetic techniques prior to incision. It has been hypothesized that pre-emptive analgesia can prevent neuroplastic changes within the spinal cord and the attendant physiologic sequelae.

It has also been hypothesized that the pre-emptive analgesia may produce prolong effects that long outlast the initial neural blockade. In laboratory models very high doses of opioids are necessary to suppress central hypersensitization once established. However, small doses of opioid administration prior to the barrage of nociceptive transmission can prevent the center hyperexcitability of dorsal horn neuron. This taken to its extreme conclusion, a single preoperative dose of analgesic could conceivably completely prevent postoperative pain.

The results of the several clinical studies have supported the concept of pre-emptive analgesia.

Mc Quay et al studied the effects of preoperative opioids premedication and regional anesthesia on the time to first request for postoperative analgesia often elective orthopedic surgery. If opioid premedication and regional anesthesia were not used, the median time to request the postoperative analgesia was less than 2 hours. Use of opioid premedication and regional anesthesia extended the median time to more than 9 hours.[24] Pretreatment therefore decreased the need for postoperative analgesia.

To involve the management of pediatric pain, the attitude of doctors, nurses and parents must change. Children should not be denied pain relief as it will be unreasonable to expect a child to cope up with pain of a procedure that are treated with analgesics, local or general anaesthesia in adults. This subject needs further evaluation particularly in view ethnic and socio economic groups. Regional analgesia techniques in children are an important part of anesthesiologist armamentarium today. One thing is very clear that children also need adequate postoperative pain relief "to relieve pain in divine".[25,26]

REFERENCES

1. Anand KJS, Hickey PR. Pain and its effects in the human neonate and fetus. New Engl. J Med 1987;317:1321-29.
2. Schechter NL, Allen D. Physicians' attitude towards pain in children. Develop Behav Pediatr 1986;7:350-54.
3. Levy, DM. The infant earliest memory of inoculation. A contribution to public health procedures. J Genet Pay Chol 1960;96:37-46.
4. Anand KJS, Hickey PR. Randomized trial of high dose sufentanil anaesthesia in neonates undergoing cardiac surgery hormonal and hemodynamic stress response (abstract). Anaesthesiology 1987;67:A501.
5. Holve RL, Brom berger PJ, Grovession HD, et al. Regional anaesthesia during new born circumcision. Effection infant pain response. Clin Pediatr 1983;22:813.
6. Valman HB, Pearson JF. What the fetus feel? Br Med J. 1980;280:233-34.
7. MC Grath PJ, Unruh AM. The measurement and assessment of pain. In pain in children and adolescents. Elsevier Amsterdam 1987;72.
8. Krechel SW, Bildner J. CRIES: A new postoperative pain measurement score. Initial testing of validity and reliability. Pediatr Anesth 1995;5:53-65.
9. Yee JP, Koshiver JE, Albon C, Brown CR. Comparison of intramuscular ketorolac trimethamine and morphine sulphate for analgesia for pain after major surgery. Pharmacotherapy 1986;6:253.

10. Hanallah RS, Broadman LM, Belman AB. Comparison of caudal and ilioinguinal/iliohypogastric nerve blocks for control of postorchidopexy pain in pediatric ambulatory surgery. Anesthesiology 1987;66:832-34.
11. Koren G, Maurice L. Pediatric use of opioids. Pediatric Clin North Am 1989;36:1141.
12. O'hara M, McGrath PJ, D Astous J, Vaor CA. Oral morphine verses injected meperidine for pain relief in children after orthopedic surgery J. Pediatric Orth. 1987;7:78.
13. Koren G. Butt W, Crinyanga H. et al. Postoperative morphine infusion in new born infants: assessment of disposition characteristics and safety. J Pediatric 1985;107:963-67.
14. Bray J. Postoperative analgesia provided by morphine infusion in children. Anaesthesia 1983;38:1075.
15. Lynn AM, slattery JT. Morphine Pharmacokinetics in early infancy. Anaesthesiology 1987;66:131-39.
16. Brown RE, Broadman LM. Patient controlled (PCA) for postoperative pain in adolescents, (abstract). Anaesth. Analg 1987;66:S22.
17. Warner MA, Kunkel SE, Offered KO, Atchism SR, Dawson B. The effects of age, epinephrine and operative site on duration of caudal analgesia in pediatric patients. Anaesth Analg 1987;66:995-98.
18. Shapiro LA, Jedeikin RJ, Shalev D, Hoffman S. Epidural morphine analgesia children. Anaesthesiology 1989;71:48-52.
19. Krane EJ, Tylar DC, Jacobson LE. The dose response of caudal morphine in children. Anaesthesiology 1989;71:48-52.
20. Arora MK, Rajeshwari S, Kaul HL. Comparison of Caudal Morphine and Bupivacaine for postoperative analgesia in children (abstract). J Pain Symp Manag 1991;6:165.
21. Yaster M, Maxwell LG. Pediatric regional anaesthesia. Anaesthesiology 1989;70:324.
22. Broadman LM, Hannallah RS, Norden JM, McGill WA. "Kiddie Caudal" experience with 1154 consecutive cases without complicating (abstract). Anaesth. Analg, 1987;66:518.
23. Coderre TJ, Melzack R.Cutaneous hyperanalgesia-Contributions to peripheral and central nervous systems to the increase in pain sensitivity after injury. Brain Res 1987;404:95.
24. Mcquay HJ, Carroll D, Moore RA. Postoperative orthopedic pain: the effect of opiate premedication and local anesthetic blocks pain 1988;33:291.
25. Arora MK. Pediatric Pain (Editorial). Journal of Anaesthesiology Clinical Pharmacology 1992;8:1-4.
26. Arora MK. Regional Anaesthesia in Paediatrics (Editorial). Journal of Anaesthesiology Clinical Pharmacology. 1997;13:95-98.

CHAPTER 11

Common Radiological Procedures in Pediatric Surgery

AK Gupta, Ashok Srinivasan

Imaging plays a crucial role in the evaluation of pediatric surgical conditions. In this chapter, we will discuss some of the common imaging procedures, their indications, contraindications and techniques, without going into the specific diseases and their imaging patterns. The procedures covered are: Micturating cystourethrography (MCU), retrograde urethrography (RGU), intravenous urography (IVU), investigation of anorectal malformations (ARM), genitography, ultrasound (US), computed tomography (CT), magnetic resonance imaging (MRI), magnetic resonance cholangiopancreaticography (MRCP), conventional X-rays and barium studies. Before proceeding further it is important to know about two aspects: Intravenous contrast agents and Radiation protection.

WATER SOLUBLE INTRAVENOUS CONTRAST MEDIA[1]

Of the radiopaque atoms examined, only three have so far been proven useful as a basis for the development of contrast media: Barium, bromine and, in particular, iodine because of the favorable position of the K-edge in the absorption spectrum. Of these iodine is the key atom whose properties have been exploited in the manufacturing and clinical application of contrast media. Iodine is the only element that has proved satisfactory for general use as an intravascular contrast agent.

The present day iodinated contrast media can be divided into four categories:

Ionic Contrast

a. Ionic monomer, e.g. diatrizoate, iothalamate
b. Ionic dimer, e.g. ioxaglate

Nonionic Contrast

a. Nonionic monomer, e.g. iohexol, iopamidol
b. Nonionic dimer, e.g. iotrolan, iodixanol

The classification above is based on whether the molecule ionizes in solution (i.e. body water) and whether it is a monomer or dimer. These two properties—ionization and dimerization confer upon the molecule certain advantages and disadvantages and cause a significant impact in clinical application as well. As a rule, nonionic contrast agents are preferred over ionic agents for intravenous injections because of significantly low rate of side effects.

Adverse reactions to these agents can be divided on the basis of the mechanism into: (1) Idiosyncratic anaphylactoid reactions, (2) Non-idiosyncratic reactions and (3) Combined reactions. They can be classified into minor, intermediate, severe life threatening reactions and deaths. These include flushing, nausea, vomiting, headache, urticaria, hypotension and bronchospasm. Although the nonionic compounds cause lesser incidence of adverse reactions, they are much more costly than the ionic compounds.

RADIATION PROTECTION[2]

Ionizing radiation has harmful effects–which may be non-stochastic (acute) and stochastic (chronic). Some of these include cataract, cancer, genetic mutations and even deaths. Therefore, there is a need to keep radiation exposure down to a minimum both for the patient as well as the radiation worker. Some of the measures that should be taken are:

1. One should take care to order investigations involving ionizing radiation only if other non-

radiating modalities like US or MRI cannot provide the requisite information.
2. During performance of X-ray examinations or CT scans, the minimum level of radiation exposure should be used. To reduce radiation, collimation of the X-rays should be done to include only the field of interest.
3. During fluoroscopic examinations, the exposure time should be kept down to a minimum and spot films taken only when required.
4. Use of digital radiography, if available, helps in reducing radiation exposure.
5. Lead aprons should be worn by the persons in the radiation environment (operator, child's parents, others) for personal protection.

MICTURATING CYSTOURETHROGRAPHY (MCU)[3]

Indications

- Recurrent urinary tract infections
- Posterior urethral valve
- Vesicoureteral reflux disease
- Neurogenic bladder
- Developmental anomalies like ectopic ureter.

Contraindications

- Acute urinary tract infection.

Procedure

Sedation is rarely required: The procedure is performed on an outpatient basis. Usually antibiotic cover is provided prior to the procedure and continued thereafter as and when required. Appropriate aseptic precautions are followed when performing the procedure. An initial radiograph of the Kidneys, Ureters, Bladder (KUB) area is essential for the following reasons.
- It provides an idea of the exposure factors in the individual patient.
- Any abnormal radiodensities like calculi can be detected
- Bone anomalies like spina bifida, hemi vertebrae can be identified which may be responsible for urinary problems.

MCU can be performed in two ways:
a. *Catheter technique:* After obtaining the preliminary radiograph, the perineum and periurethral area is cleansed using an antiseptic solution. Then the urethra is anesthetized using 1-2% lignocaine jelly and the child is catheterized using a 5 F or 6 F infant feeding tube. Sometimes, there might be resistance in advancing the catheter at the level of the external sphincter, wherein gradual injection of normal saline while advancing the catheter usually helps in solving this problem. After the urinary bladder has been entered 1:1 diluted water soluble contrast medium is injected gradually until full bladder sensation is achieved. Then the catheter is removed and the patient asked to void the contrast. In infants, there is usually spontaneous voiding when the bladder capacity has been achieved and hence it is essential to be ready to monitor the voiding by fluoroscopy and to take spot films.
b. *Suprapubic puncture technique:* An 18G Venflon needle can be placed into the urinary bladder via the suprapubic approach with or without US guidance. The suprapubic area is cleaned with an antiseptic solution and the needle is passed into the urinary bladder. If necessary, US can be used for guidance of the needle. The advantages of this technique are that trauma to the urethra can be avoided and this is especially suitable for very young children. During MCU the following spot films are generally obtained:
    - The full bladder film: anteroposterior projection
    - The voiding film: Bladder and urethra
      – bilateral anteroposterior obliques (males) (Fig. 11.1)
      – anterior and occasionally lateral (females)
    - Spot films of the kidney area to look for vesicoureteric reflux
    - Postvoid film to assess for residue.

RETROGRADE URETHROGRAPHY (RGU)[3]

RGU is performed in boys to assess anterior urethral strictures, postoperative status of urethral reconstructions, infrasphincteric rectourethral fistulas in patients with anorectal malformations and anterior urethral injuries. Water soluble contrast media are used in the same concentration as for MCU. The tip of

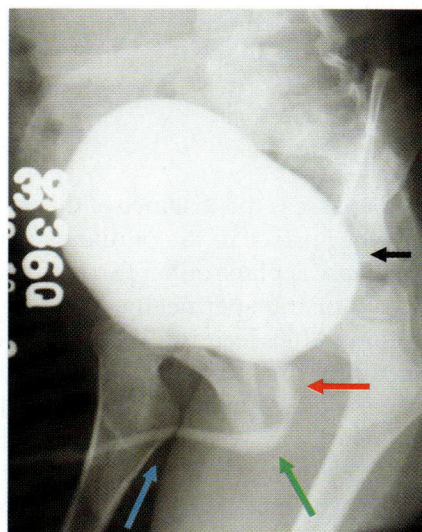

Fig. 11.1: Normal MCU in a 8-year-old male: black arrow – urinary bladder, red arrow – posterior urethra green arrow – bulbar urethra, blue arrow – penile urethra

a Foley's catheter is placed in the distal urethra and the balloon is gently inflated in the fossa navicularis. Alternately, an infant feeding tube can be placed at the same location and the tip of the penis pinched gently to prevent leakage of contrast. Contrast medium is then injected from a syringe. The patient is positioned in a steep oblique or lateral projection. Good coning of the area is important for a superior image. It is performed only in boys and accurately evaluates only the anterior urethra. Because of inadequate filling, the urethra proximal to the external sphincter cannot be evaluated satisfactorily.

INTRAVENOUS UROGRAPHY (IVU)[1,3]

The IVU should not be the first examination of the renal tract; it should be performed only when less invasive methods suggest it may be helpful and then is tailored to the problem at hand. This results in the need for fewer radiographs and a lower radiation dose, and yields specific answers for the clinician.

The IVU is Indicated in the Following Special Cases

- Complicated duplex kidney
- To visualize the nondilated ureter in exstrophy bladder
- Intermittent pelvi-ureteric junction (PUJ) obstruction (If US is normal)
- Medullary necrosis (following acute renal failure)
- Calyceal abnormalities.

Contraindications

- Acute renal failure
- Neonates in the first 24-48 hours.

Technique

Fluid and food are withheld for a few hours prior to the IVU. Only in older children bowel preparation with a laxative like pegelac or dulcolax is performed for 1-2 days before the IVU in order to get a good visualization of the renal areas. Blood urea and creatinine measurements should be obtained before IVU to assess renal function since contrast is contraindicated in patients with high blood urea and creatinine values. A preliminary (plain) radiograph is obtained before intravenous injection in order to

- Assess radiographic exposure factors
- Detect renal calculi
- Detect nephrocalcinosis
- Identify vertebral anomalies
- Detect bone density alterations as in renal osteodystophy.

Nonionic contrast medium is preferred to ionic medium: Intravenous contrast (IV) injection is made at a maximum dose of 3 ml/kg body weight. The exact timing of the films varies with the indication for the examination since every IVU now carried out is undertaken only to answer a specific question after a full US examination and an isotope study has been carried out (Fig. 11.2). It is important to remember that the visualization of the kidney on the IVU may be delayed in the neonate and radiographs taken at 2, 6 and 18 hours after the IV injection may be useful.

ANORECTAL MALFORMATIONS[4-6]

Imaging plays an important role and is directed to define four things:
- Exact level of anomaly
- Anatomy of the anomaly
- Integrity of the perineal nerve supply
- Muscle mass available for reconstruction.

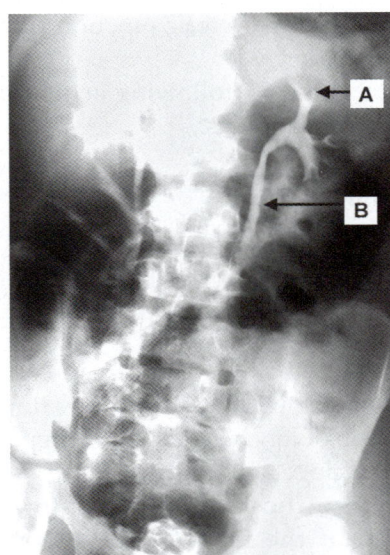

Fig. 11.2: Normal IVU in a 10-year-old male: A— left upper polar calyx, B— left ureter

Plain Radiography

Conventional invertogram

It was first described by Wangensteen and Rice.

Technique

A radiopaque marker is placed at the anal pit. Then the infant is held upside down for atleast 6 minutes with hips flexed. X-rays are performed in the lateral and anteroposterior projections with the centering at the level of the greater trochanter. Three lines, namely *the PC line, I line, and anal pit line,* are considered for interpretation.

An invertogram has a number of potential pitfalls which may give a false impression of the level of anomaly, e.g. due to contraction of the puborectalis at the time of X-ray, escape of air through a fistula from the blind rectal pouch, etc.

The Prone Cross Table Lateral View

The infant is put face down in a prone position with their hips flexed in the genupectoal position for at least 3 minutes. A cross table lateral film is obtained with centering over the greater trochanter. Relation of the level of blind rectal pouch with the PC and I line are assessed, as in conventional invertogram. The advantages of this technique over the invertogram include less time consumption, and more patient comfort.

ULTRASOUND (US)

It can be used to assess the distance of the rectal pouch in relation to the surface of the perineum. The scan is performed in sagittal plane either through the anterior abdominal wall or transperineally, with the infant in supine position. After locating the rectal pouch, the relationship of the distal portion of the pouch to the bladder base is determined. Pouch-perineal distance of < 1.5 cm is indicative of low anomalies. However, the distinction between high and intermediate anomalies cannot be made with this technique. Besides being operator dependent, the technique has a number of possible pitfalls and hence is not in much use.

Computed Tomography (CT)

CT may be used for:
  i. CT invertography
  ii. CT pelvis, for muscle attachment

  i. *CT invertography:* The baby is placed in prone position for a few minutes. A midline, direct sagittal section is taken after AP topogram.
  ii. *CT pelvis:* The patient is placed in the supine position and a lateral scout film is taken. Contiguus 4 mm axial sections are obtained parallel to the pubococygeal line, from the superior margin of the pubic bone to the perineum. Intravenous, oral or rectal contrast are not required. CT is useful in assessing the muscular anatomy of the anorectal region both prior to and after surgery.

Magnetic Resonance Imaging (MRI)

It is superior to CT in providing images in multiple images without the risk of ionizing radiation. There is also excellent soft tissue contrast resolution and the anorectal muscle complex can be exquisitely demonstrated. It is important to remember that the use of body coil is associated with poor results due to poor resolution and so it is essential to use special coils like endorectal or wrapped around coils for this purpose.

Prudent set of investigations are required for the diagnosis and follow-up of patients with anorectal malformations. The following provides a guideline for the same:

Day 1

Conventional invertogram, prone cross table lateral view, US, CT invertogram.

Postcolostomy

- Distal cologram and MCU/RGU— to assess presence, level and type of fistula
- CT or MRI pelvis—for assessment of pelvic musculature.

Postpull-through in Patients with Fecal Incontinence

CT pelvis with rectal contrast or MRI pelvis – to assess muscle thickness, muscle damage, retracted fat, eccentrically located neorectum or neorectum lying outside the sling.

GENITOGRAPHY[7,8]

Indications

- Ambiguous external genitalia (Intersex disorder).

Contraindications

- Local perineal infections.

Technique

Perineum is first outlined by placing and taping an opaque catheter in the midline. A radiopaque marker is placed at the external genital opening. Water soluble contrast medium is injected by retrograde route via the external genital opening so as to opacify the internal genital and urethral anatomy, i.e. vagina, uterus, tubes, urethral length, site and junction between the urethra and vagina and the length of the urogenital sinus. It can be performed by two techniques.

Flush Technique

This was first described by Schopner. A 10 ml syringe filled with a water-soluble contrast medium is placed

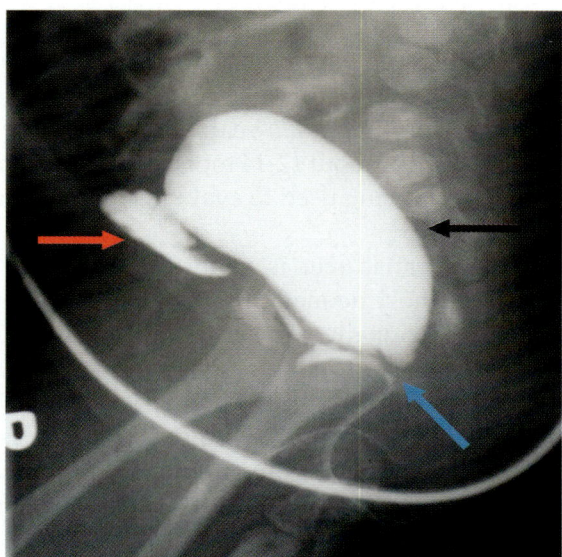

Fig. 11.3: Genitogram in intersex disorder: red arrow – compressed urinary bladder, blue arrow – common channel, black arrow – mullerian remnant

at the external opening. With gentle pressure, an injection of 3-4 ml is made under fluoroscopy and spot films are obtained in lateral projection. AP view is only occasionally required. The process may be repeated several times if necessary.

Catheter Technique (Fig. 11.3)

A single hole catheter is used, whose tip should be placed in the common urogenital sinus. Water soluble contrast is injected via a syringe attached to the catheter and spot films are obtained. Catheter tip must be well compressed by hand to prevent leakage.

ULTRASOUND

Ultrasound is a very useful modality in the evaluation of pediatric diseases, both as a screening modality and for characterization of the disease. Ultrasound can be used to detect disease in the head, neck, chest, abdomen as well as to assess vascular system of the limbs. The basic technique and indications in various areas are described below.

Cranial Sonography: Equipment and Technique

Standard brain scanning includes sagittal and coronal planes. Non-standard planes can, and should, be used if they are helpful to outline pathologic states.

Currently most brain sonographic examinations are performed through the anterior fontanelle in both coronal and sagittal planes. Anterior fontanelle remains open until about 2 years, but is suitable for scanning only until about 12-14 months. More recently, color Doppler is being used to evaluate neonatal brain and vasculature.

A 5 MHz transducer is generally adequate for evaluation of most neonatal brains through anterior fontanelle. Occasionally, a lower frequency transducer is needed to ensure adequate penetration, especially in larger infants or older infants with closing fontanelles. Higher frequency transducers such as 7.5 or 10 MHz are helpful to evaluate superficial structures in the near field such as extracerebral spaces or cortex or in preterm babies.

Transducers with very small foot plates are well suited for premature infants because of smaller fontanelles. These transducers are also useful when scanning from posterior mastoid area or foramen magnum. Small linear array or convex transducers can provide quality images for scanning in axial plane through the squamous portion of temporal bone. This thin bone window usually requires a 3.5 MHz transducer.

Although cranial sonography can be used in any intracranial pathology, its main use is in the following diseases:
- Hypoxic ischemic encephalopathy
- Hydrocepalus
- Congenital brain malformations

US can also be used to study diseases in the abdomen and pelvis for detection of disease and for characterization of masses as cystic, solid or complex, assess vessels, detect metastases and for guidance of FNAC (Fine Needle Aspiration Cytology) or biopsy procedures. It can be used to detect pleural effusions and for guidance of FNAC or biopsy procedures wherein a chest lesion contacts the chest wall.

Special Applications of US

US including color flow imaging and Doppler have been studied in the diagnosis of vesicoureteric reflux, differentiating obstructive and nonobstructive dilatation of the renal collecting system, and in diagnosing high pressure hydrocephalus.

TRACHEOESOPHAGEAL FISTULA (TEF)

Plain film of the chest taken soon after birth reveals distended proximal esophageal pouch. In equivocal cases, a thin soft rubber catheter is passed into the proximal pouch and about 5 cc of air is injected. A lateral radiograph, centering on cervico-thoracic area is taken. Dilated proximal pouch with round distal margin is diagnostic. Presence of air in the stomach and the small intestine indicates esophageal atresia with a distal TEF. Use of radiopaque positive contrast in the proximal pouch should be avoided owing to the possibility of aspiration. Swallowed air or nasogastric tube with negative contrast (air) is usually adequate for the diagnosis and to demonstrate the extent of the proximal pouch. If positive contrast examination needs to be done then nonionic isotonic contrast medium or dilute barium is preferred with continuous fluoroscopic monitoring. The best way to demonstrate a H-type fistula is to inject radiopaque contrast (dilute barium or nonionic media) through a catheter with its tip just above the GE junction. Under fluoroscopic guidance, the catheter is gradually pulled out with continuous contrast injection at each level in succession. The patient should be evaluated in the lateral or steep prone position.

BARIUM STUDIES[1,4,6]

Barium studies are performed in suspected intestinal tract disorders especially abnormalities like hypertrophic pyloric stenosis, colonic aganglionois (Hirschsprung's disease) and emergencies like midgut volvulus.

Hypertrophic Pyloric Stenosis

Nowadays US is usually the screening modality of choice. Although sonography is usually done without a NG tube, it would be preferable to do the examination with an empty stomach by aspiration through a nasogastric tube. During the study, the child is given a clear feed or preferably, normal saline can be injected through the NG tube. This distends the stomach providing a good window, improves visualization of the pylorus and stimulates peristalsis thereby maximizing pyloric muscle thickening.

In order to obtain a technically satisfactory barium study, a nasogastric tube should be passed and the

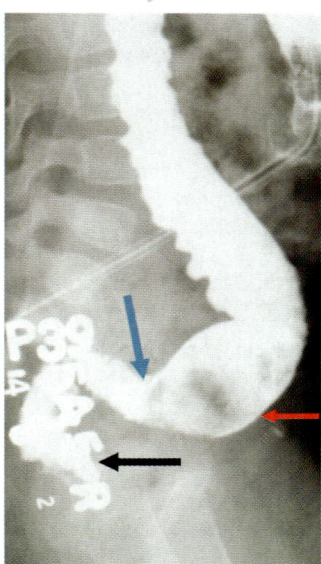

Fig. 11.4: Barium enema in Hirschsprung's megacolon: black arrow – rectum, red arrow – sigmoid colon, blue arrow - transitional zone

stomach emptied. With the patient in the prone oblique position the tube is placed in the antrum so that large amounts of contrast material are not required. Barium is injected via the tube under fluoroscopic control and spot films are taken. Raising the head end of the table would help to distend the pyloric region.

Hirschsprung's Disease (Fig. 11.4)

Plain films may demonstrate a distal large bowel obstruction. Gasless rectum or at times a small gas filled rectum may be seen, especially on prone films and may help with diagnosis except where digital examination has introduced rectal air. The dilated colon proximal to the aganglionic segment can be recognized by its lumen.

Barium enema is used for confirmation of the clinical diagnosis. It is performed on the unprepared patient by inserting a straight tipped catheter to a point just beyond the anal sphincter. With the patient in the lateral position, barium suspension is introduced slowly, preferably by gravity drip infusion, under fluoroscopic monitoring. The infusion is stopped as soon as the transitional zone is demonstrated. Rapid infusion of barium can distend and mask the transitional zone. An immediate post-evacuation film as well as a 24 hours late film should be done to assess the degree of contrast clearance.

Intussusception

An intussusception is a prolapse of one portion of the bowel into another. The segment of the intestine that prolapses is called the intussusceptum and the receiving segment is the intussuscipiens. In children, the intussusception is usually ileocolic (90%); ileoileocolic intussusceptions make up most of the rest.

If the clinical diagnosis of intussusception is fairly certain, an enema is the most useful initial investigation since it is both diagnostic and therapeutic in all those who show no evidence of peritonism. Sonography can diagnose intussusception as a mass with a dense central echogenic area surrounded by the concentric sonolucent rim. Barium, water-soluble contrast, gas, or carbon dioxide have all been used for reduction, which can be performed either fluoroscopically or under US guidance.

Rarely children with chronic abdominal pain may have recurring jejuno-jejunal or ileo-ileal intussusception. These require barium follow through for diagnosis.

COMPUTED TOMOGRAPHY (CT)

The basic advantage of CT is that it demonstrates tissue anatomy with precision and clarity. The spatial resolution and anatomical detail of CT are superior to that of US. However, it has a lesser contrast resolution than MRI. It is not operator dependent and permits accurate measurement of tissue attenuation.

Patient preparation: Food and liquids should be withheld from all infants and children who will be sedated and/or receive intravenous contrast. This achieves two goals: 1. The child is thirsty enough to drink oral contrast and 2. It diminishes nausea during IV bolus contrast injection. Usually solids are withheld 4 hours and liquids 3 Hours before the procedure. Sedation is almost always required under age 5 and might be required in older, uncooperative or anxious children.

Table 11.1 summarizes the important indications for CT examination in the pediatric age group.

MAGNETIC RESONANCE IMAGING (MRI)

MRI is a sectional imaging technique that depends on proton density, T1 and T2 relaxation, flow phenomena, magnetic susceptibility and diffusion. Image quality

Table 11.1: Indications and abnormalities detected by CT in children

CNS and craniofacial structures
- Hydrocephalus
- Intracranial hemorrhage
- Infarction/infection
- Gross congenital malformations
- Craniosynostosis
- Head/facial/orbital trauma
- Sinusitis
- Choanal atresia
- Temporal bone lesions
- Spinal column abnormality.

Chest
- Mediastinal tumor involvement
- Mediastinal adenopathy
- Metastases
- Opaque hemithorax
- Diffuse lung disease
- Primary pulmonary 'masses'.

Abdomen
- Blunt trauma
- Neoplasms of viscerae
- Adenopathy
- Abscesses, infections, complex fluid collections
- Portal hypertension
- Extent and complications of inflammatory bowel disease.

Musculoskeletal system
- Osteoid osteoma
- Developmental hip dysplasia
- Soft tissue tumors
- Tarsal coalition.

Table 11.2: Indications for MR in children

Brain
- Developmental anomalies
- Myelination disorders
- Neoplasms
- Infections, inflammations
- Vascular malformations
- Seizures
- Unexplained hydrocephalus, seizures.

Spine
- Developmental malformations
- Neoplasms
- Infections, trauma
- Atypical scoliosis.

Chest
- Vascular rings
- Congenital heart diseases
- Mediastinal masses
- Diaphragmatic hernia
- Foregut malformations
- Chest wall pathology.

Abdomen and pelvis
- Anorectal malformations
- Congenital anomalies of the genitourinary tract
- Neoplasms, infections
- Liver transplant evaluation
- Budd-Chiari syndrome
- Hemosiderosis.

Musculoskeletal system
- Trauma to joints
- Infections
- Neoplasms
- Osteonecrosis.

is determined by homogeneity of the magnetic field and gradient strength, magnetic field strength and utilization of surface or specifically designed coils to increase signal to noise ratio. The standard imaging planes include the axial, coronal and sagittal planes though there are infinite planes possible and appropriate planes can be chosen according to the body part imaged. The advantages of MRI include good spatial resolution, excellent contrast resolution, multiplanar imaging and the lack of ionizing radiation.

Patient sedation is required in very young patients in order to obtain sufficient immobility during the scan. Table 11.2 lists the indications for MR in children.

Table 11.3 compares CT and MRI for their advantages (√) and disadvantages (×):

Table 11.3: Comparison of CT and MRI

	CT	MRI
Cost	√	×
Ionizing radiation	×	√
Shorter examination time	√	×
Multiplanar imaging	×	√
Detection of calcification	√	×
Spatial resolution	√	×
Contrast resolution	×	√
Contrast requirement	×	√

Special Applications of MRI

In recent times, MRI has been used for demonstration of bile duct anatomy in a fashion that is similar to what is seen on ERCP. The technique is called MRCP (Magnetic Resonance Cholangiopancreatography). It uses heavily T2 weighted images to render the bile ducts hyperintense. 3D reconstruction of these ducts can then be performed and displayed for analysis. It plays an important role in differentiating the various causes of neonatal jaundice, e.g. neonatal hepatitis versus biliary atresia.

REFERENCES

1. Grainger RG, Allison DJ. Grainger and Allison's Diagnostic Radiology. A textbook of medical imaging. 3rd edn. Volumes 1,2. Churchill Livingstone.1997
2. Seith A, Gupta AK. Technical considerations in pediatric imaging. In Berry M et al (Eds) Diagnostic radiology. Pediatric imaging. Jaypee brothers, New Delhi 1997;chap 1:1-15.
3. Chapman S, Nakielny R. A guide to radiological procedures. 3rd edn. Prism India 1997.
4. FN Silverman, JP Kuhn. Caffey's Pediatric X-ray diagnosis. An integrated imaging approach. 9th edn. Mosby publishers 1993; vol. 1 and 2.
5. Donald R Kirks. Practical pediatric imaging. Diagnostic radiology of infants and children. Lippincott-Raven, 3rd Edn, 1998.
6. Saxena AK, Katarayia S. Anorectal malformations. In Berry M et al (Eds) Diagnostic radiology. Pediatric imaging. Jaypee brothers, New Delhi 1997;chap 6:86-97.
7. Schopner CF. Genitography in intersex problems. Radiology 1964;82:664-74.
8. Gupta AK, Sharma S. Radiology of intersex disorders. In Berry M, et al (Eds). Diagnostic radiology. Pediatric imaging. Jaypee brothers, New Delhi 1997; chap 12: 223-37.

Nuclear Imaging in Pediatric Surgery

CS Bal, Ajay Kumar

Nuclear Medicine is a medical specialty that uses safe, painless, and cost-effective techniques to both image the body and treat diseases with the help of radioisotopes/radiopharmaceuticals. Pediatric nuclear medicine encompasses diagnostic, investigational and therapeutic applications of nuclear medicine technology in children. An isotope is a variant of an element, having the same atomic number but different atomic weight. The chemical behavior of an element is dictated by its atomic number and therefore all isotopes of the same element have identical behavior. Biological systems fail to recognize the differences between atomic weights and treat all isotopes in the same fashion. Radioactive isotopes are those isotopes, which emit radioactivity. The radioisotope or radiotracers can be detected *in vitro* or *in vivo* with ease, because it is possible to detect radioactivity with a great deal of sensitivity and precision by means of modern electronic equipment such as gamma or PET cameras. These cameras work in conjunction with computers used to form images and provide data and information about the area of body being imaged. Nuclear medicine imaging is unique in that it documents mostly organ function and to a lesser extent structure, in contrast to diagnostic radiology, which is based upon anatomy.[1,2]

Nuclear medicine imaging is among the safest diagnostic imaging modalities available. A patient only receives an extremely small amount of a radiopharmaceutical, just enough to provide sufficient diagnostic information. Radiopharmaceuticals are physiologically innocuous and do not produce toxic or pharmacological effects or allergic reactions; nor do they result in hemodynamic or osmotic overload. In addition, the amount of radiation from a nuclear medicine procedure is comparable to, or often several magnitude less than, that of a diagnostic X-ray.[3,4] The complex physiology and biochemistry of growth and development, the types of diseases in children, differences in body and organ sizes, radiation dose considerations, and even the behavior of the patients during the examinations all require special expertise, interest, training, dedication, equipment, and facilities for providing care for children, who may range in age from premature infants to adolescents. Sedation is not needed for most nuclear medicine procedures in children, but it is helpful if a child is unable to cooperate, especially when the procedures, such as SPECT or whole body imaging, require the patient to be still for 30-60 minutes. Sedated patients, both inpatients and outpatients, must be closely monitored by a physician or a nurse until they are fully awake.

Administered radiotracer doses in pediatric nuclear medicine have been developed by experience, taking into account the absorbed radiation dose, type of examination, available photon flux, instrumentation, and examination time. There is not a single formula to calculate administered doses in children. Dose estimation for pediatric patients based on adult dose corrected for body weight or body surface area is generally a good guide for most children over 1 year of age.[1] The administered dose should be the lowest that will make it possible to obtain the needed information from the examination. For example, a skeletal scintigram to detect metastatic cancer in an infant can be performed with 18.5 MBq (0.5 mCi) of technetium-99m methylene diphosphonate (^{99m}Tc-MDP); however, if the problem is the diagnosis of osteomyelitis, a radionuclide angiogram of the involved region is needed as part of the examination, and a dose of 74-111 MBq (2 - 3 mCi) should be used. Premature infants and newborns require special consideration and the concept of minimal total dose should be applied. Minimal total dose is the minimal dose of radiopharmaceutical below which the study will be inadequate regardless of the patient's body weight or surface area.[1,3,5] For example, the usual pediatric dose of technetium 99m pertechnetate ($^{99m}TcO_4$) for radionuclide angiography is 0.2 mCi/kg of body weight. However, a radionuclide angiogram obtained on a premature baby who weighs 900 gm requires a minimal total dose of 2 mCi. Attention to technical performance of the examinations ensures that the doses are as low as possible. This chapter deals with non-nephrourological uses of radiopharmaceuticals in pediatric conditions.

NUCLEAR IMAGING IN PEDIATRIC ONCOLOGY

Nuclear medicine plays an important role in the management of childhood malignancy. This is particularly true in the solid tumors of childhood. Scintigraphy is a complementary investigation to other radiological techniques. Scintigraphy is used in the initial diagnosis, staging, assessment of tumor response to treatment, detection of recurrence and the diagnosis of complications.

The major tumor imaging agents and radionuclides used in pediatric oncology are ^{99m}Tc-phosphates, Gallium-67 Citrate (67-Ga), Thallium-201 (201-Tl), ^{99m}Tc-sestamibi (MIBI), and Iodine-131 Metaiodo benzyl guanidine (131-I-MIBG). The somatostain analogue octreotide has been labelled with Indium-111 (111-In) or Iodine-123 (123-I) and has been investigated for use in neuroendocrine tumors namely the pituitary adenomas, carcinoids, pheochromo-cytoma, medullary thyroid carcinoma, para-gangliomas, neuroblastomas, and islet cell carcinomas.

Chemotherapy is very effective for the cure and palliation of cancer; however drug resistance of malignant cells through various mechanisms is a major problem despite the use of multidrug therapy. One mechanism involves the "multidrug resistance" or MDR gene. This gene encodes for a membrane glycoprotein complex (PGP), which causes the active extrusion of certain chemotherapeutic agents from the cell, preventing their effects. Expression of this gene is a poor prognostic factor for children with soft tissue sarcomas and primary bone tumors. Radionuclide imaging can be used for the assessment of chemotherapy resistance. MIBI has been recognized to act as a substrate for the glycoprotein complex coded for by the MDR gene and is actively extruded from the cells expressing the gene. The potential advantage of MIBI tagged with ^{99m}Tc lies in the noninvasive detection of the presence of PGP and therefore, predict response to therapy before initiation of therapy.[6,7]

Lymphoma

Lymphoma in pediatric oncology accounts for approximately 10% of pediatric solid tumors; and usually presents with enlarged unexplained painless lymph nodes. The prognosis in lymphoma depends on accurate staging of the disease, adequate primary therapy, early detection of recurrent or nonresponding disease and the early commencement of secondary treatment.[8,9]

Gallium (67-Ga) is well established in the management of lymphoma in children. 67-Ga has a sensitivity of 90%, specificity of 85% and accuracy of 84% in the detection of childhood lymphoma. 67-Ga has been reported to have 100% sensitivity in Burkitts lymphoma of childhood.[10] Bone involvement occurs in 10-15% of lymphoma patients at some time during the disease and can be efficiently demonstrated by 67-Ga scan (Fig. 12.1). Few feel that bone scintigraphy has the same sensitivity as 67-Ga in detecting bone involvement and recommend that 67-Ga only be used in follow-up. Lymphoma may be seen on both bone scan and 67-Ga scintigraphy as focal or diffuse symmetrical metaphyseal abnormalities. 67-Ga has been found to be an accurate monitor of treatment response in lymphoma patients, However, others advocate the use of 201-Tl in lymphoma patients with bone involvement as the 201-Tl reflected response to treatment more accurately than 67-Ga. Accuracy of 88% for mediastinal disease, 82% for cervical and 88% for axillary disease and 81% for supraclavicular disease have been reported for 201-Tl. Use of ^{99m}Tc-MIBI can predict the response to chemotherapy. While MIBI positive cases respond well, MIBI negative cases respond poorly. The somatostatin analogue 111-In

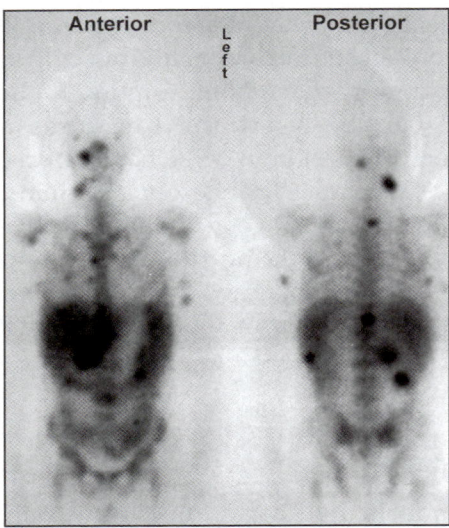

Fig. 12.1: Ga-67 whole body scan showing multiple sites of involvement (area of increased radiotracer uptake) in a case of lymphoma

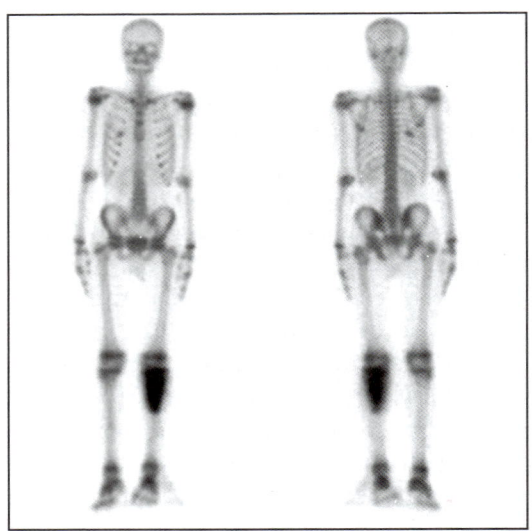

Fig. 12.2: ^{99m}Tc-MDP bone scan showing intense radiotracer uptake in Left tibia in a case of osteogenic sarcoma

pentatreotide (octreotide) has been used in non-Hodgkins lymphoma and Hodgkins disease and has a sensitivity of 87 and 98%, respectively. In follow-up both CT and MRI may have difficulties determining whether a mass is residual active tumor, recurrent disease or fibrotic/scar tissue. Positive uptake of 67-Ga scintigraphy is often the first indicator of recurrent disease.

Osteogenic Sarcoma and Ewing's Sarcoma

Osteogenic sarcomas commonly occur in the metaphyseal region of the long bones (Figs 12.2 and 12.3). Pain in the region of the primary tumor is the usual presentation. A palpable or visible mass may be present. Ewing's sarcoma may occur anywhere in the skeleton. It is usually in the bones of the lower extremities and pelvis but may affect flat bones, i.e. ribs, scapula, vertebra and pelvis. There is usually a soft tissue mass associated with the tumor and the initial presentation is usually due to pain, which may be accompanied by fever and tenderness. The bone scan is often requested to exclude osteomyelitis.

Osteogenic sarcoma and Ewing's sarcoma of bone show intense osteoblastic reaction on bone scintigraphy.[6,8] The radionuclide bone scan is the primary method to detect skeletal metastases. Photopenic malignant bone tumors have been reported but are very rare. The diagnosis of primary

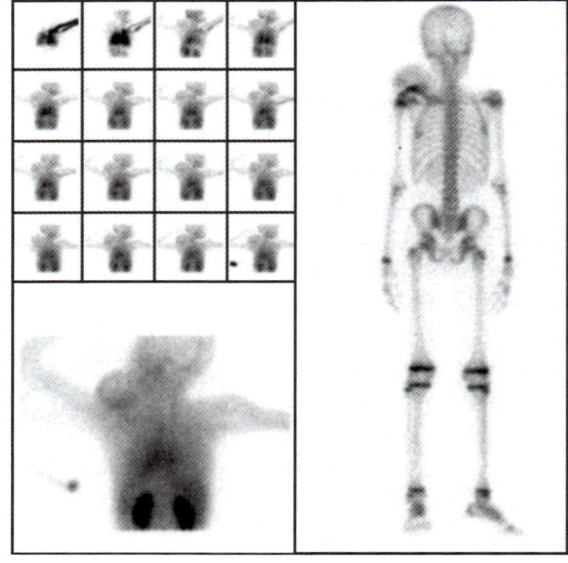

Fig. 12.3: A case of Ewing's sarcoma of the clavicle: three phase ^{99m}Tc-MDP bone scan showing intense radiotracer uptake

bone tumors is usually made on the plain radiograph. However, CT and MRI are important modalities to define the local extent of tumor. MRI defines the local soft tissue extension and invasion of the bone marrow; however, will often overestimate bone marrow involvement due to edema. CT assesses the bony aspect of the tumor and shows periosteal reaction, cortical destruction and mineralization of the matrix.

Bone scintigraphy is used primarily to detect skeletal metastases and the extent of the primary bone tumor. The bone scan however, does overestimate the size of active tumor due to the increased blood flow. radionuclide bone scintigraphy will show a vascular primary tumor and variable uptake from patchy irregular bone reaction to a markedly intense focal uptake. Osteogenic sarcoma and Ewing's sarcoma may present with metastatic disease usually to the lungs and bone. Bone metastases in osteogenic sarcoma are uncommon at diagnosis (2%), but due to longer survival with current therapy, bone metastases are more common after treatment. Patients with Ewing's sarcoma more commonly have skeletal metastases at diagnosis.

67-Ga has been used but is not accurate in defining the extent of the bone tumor as 67-Ga will accumulate in repairing bone also. However, normal 67-Ga study is highly specific for no active tumor tissue. 201-Tl is a better agent as there is no uptake in reactive bone. 201-Tl is helpful in differentiating benign from malignant bone lesions. In the majority of patients with osteogenic sarcoma, major surgery has been performed often with amputation of a lower limb followed by a prosthesis or allograft limb reconstruction. There may be reactive bone for many months on plain X-ray and bone scan at the operative junction of bone or prosthesis. Increased uptake may be seen at the stump site, in the ipsilateral hip joint and sacroiliac joint on bone scans. There may be increased uptake in soft tissues adjacent to the prosthesis and in the contralateral limb due to altered weight bearing. 201-Tl is particularly useful in these situations as there is no uptake of 201-Tl in reactive bone unless there is recurrence of tumor. Persistent intense uptake at an amputation site usually indicates recurrent disease. Occasionally a destructive bone lesion, e.g. osteomyelitis in the sacroiliac joint may appear similar to a primary bone tumor on X-ray. These are negative on 201-Tl scans indicating a benign lesion.

Assessment of response to treatment is important. Radiological studies are of limited use in predicting response to therapy because they do not accurately reflect the amount of viable tumor cells in residual tissue because of edema, hemorrhage and necrosis in the tumor. 201-Tl more accurately reflects viable tumor burden than CT, MRI, ^{99m}Tc bone scans and 67-Ga. Poor tumor response shows persistence of 201-Tl uptake. The early identification of poor responders may lead to a change in therapy or alternate treatment, e.g. radiotherapy or surgery. It has been reported that 201-Tl has sensitivity of 100%, specificity of 87.5 and 96.5% accuracy for detection of recurrent disease after therapy and differentiation from post-therapy changes on other imaging modalities. CT and MRI are found to have a sensitivity of 95%, specificity of 50% and accuracy of 82.7%.

Soft Tissue Sarcomas

Rhabdomyosarcoma (RMS) is the commonest soft tissue sarcoma in childhood and is a highly malignant tumor arising from embryonal mesenchyme. The tumor usually presents with a solid mass. The tumor may metastasize to lymph nodes or hematogenously to the lungs and bone.

Bone and gallium-67 scintigraphy in RMS has a sensitivity of 100% and specificity of 95% for bone metastases. 67-Ga uptake is found in 86% of primary tumors. If the primary tumor is 67-Ga avid then in the detection of metastatic disease, 67-Ga shows a sensitivity of 94% and a specificity of 95%. 67-Ga is found to be useful in detection of local recurrence before other modalities and often prior to clinical detection. Bone scans are reported to be more sensitive than 67-Ga for skeletal metastases but 67-Ga is better for soft tissue metastases. 201-Tl can also be used for this purpose. There is no difference in tracer uptake relating to histologic cell type. Other agent that has been used in Soft tissue tumors have been pentavalent ^{99m}Tc DMSA (dimethyl succinic acid).[6,8]

Neuroblastoma

Neuroblastoma is a malignant disease of the sympathetic nervous system and is the most common solid tumor in the first decade of life. Neuroblastoma can occur anywhere along the sympathetic nervous system from head and neck to pelvis, however occurs most commonly in the abdomen. Fifty percent of infants and 70% of older children have metastases at presentation. The tumor metastasises readily to local lymph nodes, bone, bone marrow and liver. Patients present due to the structural effect of the tumor mass and the consequences of metastases, including bone pain, proptosis or periorbital bruising and anemia or

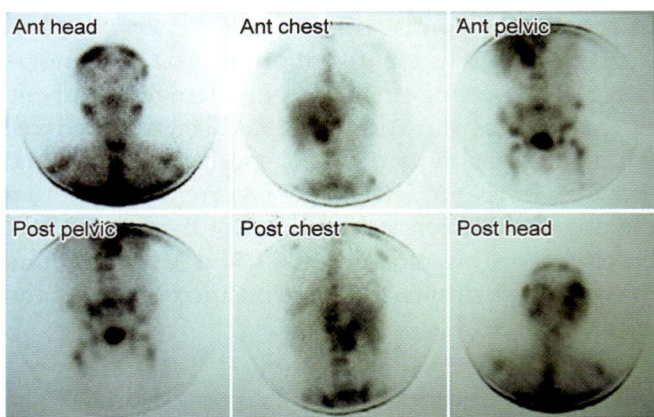

Fig. 12.4: 131-I MIBG whole body scan in a child with neuroblastoma showing extensive skeletal involvement

pancytopenia due to marrow invasion. Humoral affects are rare but may result in diarrhea due to VIP secretion or paraneoplastic syndromes such as opsoclonus-myoclonus syndrome.

Nuclear scintigraphy using 123/131-I-MIBG scintigraphy plays an invaluable role for the detection of metastatic disease anywhere in the body in a single procedure (Fig. 12.4). It is used in conjunction with bone scans, which clearly delineate skeletal involvement and the anatomical imaging modalities (ultrasound, CT and MRI), which provide superior detail regarding attachment and relationship of tumor to vital structures (e.g. vessels, spinal cord and orbits) and the presence of hepatic metastases. MIBG is concentrated by normal sympathetic adrenergic tissue within neurosecretory granules as well as in tumors derived from the neural crest, proportional to the number of neurosecretory granules. Sensitivity is over 90% in patients with neuroblastoma at presentation, with near absolute specificity (99%) due to its tumor specific uptake.[6-8] MIBG imaging is therefore essential for the initial staging of disease and has been recommended by the International Neuroblastoma Staging System. Tumor uptake non-invasively establishes the diagnosis and rules out other tumors such as Wilms' tumor, lymphoma and rhabdomyosarcoma. This is particularly helpful when tumors are inaccessible to biopsy or when histology is non-diagnostic, as may be the case with small round cell tumors of childhood. Although an MIBG positive tumor in childhood is most likely to be neuroblastoma, other tumors of the neural crest, such as ganglioneuroblastoma and, in approximately 50% of cases ganglioneuroma, pheochromocytoma, medullary thyroid carcinoma and retinoblastoma may also accumulate MIBG.

MIBG studies are also used to assess response to treatment and to distinguish post-therapeutic changes on CT/ultrasound from residual or recurrent viable disease. Recurrent disease is detected in the majority of cases on the MIBG scan; however, recurrent disease may be MIBG negative, particularly when recurrence occurs in the primary site. CT surveillance of the primary site is therefore recommended in addition to MIBG scans during follow-up.

Langerhans' Cell Histiocytosis

Langerhans' cell histiocytsosis (LCH) is pathologically characterised by abnormal idiopathic proliferation of histiocytes and granuloma formation. LCH commonly occurs in childhood and has a broad spectrum of clinical and radiological features. LCH may involve any organ however, affects the skeleton in 60-80% of cases.

The initial workup in LCH should be done by a total body radiological skeletal survey and whole body bone scan. Bone scan should be preferred as the follow-up method. However, lesions not seen on bone scan, particularly in the skull should be followed by X-ray. 67-Ga and 201-Tl have also been used in LCH. More aggressive forms of LCH are more 67-Ga avid. This is particularly in the patients with soft tissue involvement, i.e. lungs, lymph nodes and multiple organ. The use of 201-Tl in LCH may play a role in assessing therapeutic response similar to its application in primary bone tumors.

Wilms' Tumor

Wilms' tumor shows avid uptake of 67-Ga and 201-Tl in 75% of cases. Bone metastases in classical Wilms' tumor are rare and mainly occur in patients with clear cell sarcoma, which accounts for 4-5% of Wilms' tumor patients. However, bone scan are usually performed in patients with Wilms' tumor at initial diagnosis to exclude metastatic disease.

Hepatoblastoma

The main imaging modalities for liver tumors are CT and MRI. 67-Ga or 201-Tl has been used to assess hepatoblastomas and these tumors classically show

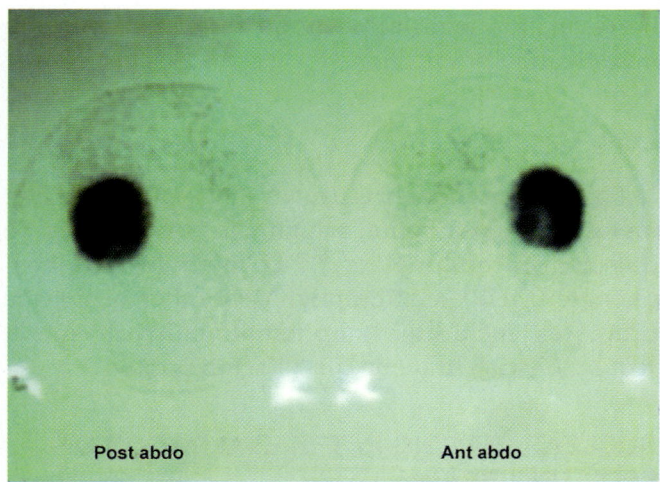

Fig. 12.5: 123-I MIBG scan showing pheochromocytoma (Lt)

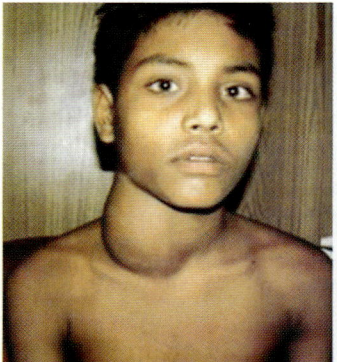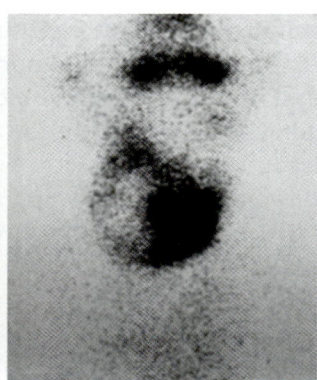

Fig. 12.6: $^{99m}TcO_4$ thyroid scan showing cold nodule in the right lobe of thyroid

avid uptake on scintigraphy. 67-Ga is an important adjunct in the follow-up and detection of recurrence of disease particularly using SPECT. Most patients with liver tumors will have a total body bone scan at presentation to exclude skeletal metastases.

Endocrine Tumors

Carcinoids and Pheochromocytoma

They are imaged by 123 or 131-I-MIBG (Fig. 12.5). Octreotide can also be used. MIBG has the sensitivity and specificity similar to CT scans for the detection of pheochromocytoma in children. Faint uptake of 131-I MIBG is seen normally in the adrenal glands and must be differentiated from the moderate to intense uptake seen in pheochromocytoma.

Thyroid Cancer

^{99m}Tc pertechnetate thyroid scan is used in the investigation of thyroid carcinoma and tumor is seen as a cold nodule on scan (Fig. 12.6). ^{99m}Tc pertechnetate uptake in the neck lymph node, although very rare in the presence of intact thyroid gland, is highly suggestive of metastatic thyroid cancer. Approximately 60% of children with thyroid carcinoma are found to have regional lymphadenopathy and around 25% will have pulmonary metastases at the time of initial presentation. After thyroidectomy whole body scanning with 131-I is done to detect any local and/or distant metastases. Prior to 131-I imaging, exogenous thyroid medications must be discontinued for at least 4 - 6 weeks to allow the endogenous TSH blood levels to rise and to ensure an adequate accumulation of radioiodine by the lesions.

Adrenal Carcinoma

67-Ga is found to be very useful in a child with adrenal carcinoma and accurately detects recurrence before other modalities do.

Brain Tumors

In childhood, brain tumors account for 15-20% of all malignancies and comprise the most common solid tumors. The spectrum of brain tumors in the pediatric population is diverse and quite different from that seen in adults. In contrast to adult brain tumors, the majority of pediatric brain tumors arise within the confines of the posterior fossa. Anatomical imaging modalities (CT, MRI) provide invaluable information regarding tumor location and relationship to vital structures and the presence of leptomeningeal metastases. However, the appearance of the tumor does not reflect its grade nor can postsurgical changes or postradiotherapy necrosis be accurately distinguished from viable tumor.

201-Tl has been investigated as a marker of tumor behavior and viability posttherapy.[6,8] 201-Tl tumor uptake relates to its affinity for the Na/K ATPase pump, increased blood flow and disruption of the blood brain barrier. The intensity of 201-Tl accumulation reflects tumor histological grade, proliferative activity, biological behavior and viable tumor burden. An index based on the ratio of uptake in tumor compared to normal brain can be calculated and it has been found that an index greater than 1.5 is compatible with high-grade malignancy with 89% accuracy. In evaluating post-therapy changes, 201-Tl has high sensitivity for residual/recurrent tumor, however suffers from low specificity. Supratentorial gliomas occur in children but many are of low-grade and may not demonstrate 201-Tl accumulation. Pilocytic astrocytomas show intense 201-Tl accumulation, which would imply high-grade malignancy in the adult glioma group; however, they are of very low malignant grade. This highlights the importance of carefully correlating the result of the 201-Tl scan with the histopathology before implying a relationship between 201-Tl accumulation and tumor behavior. The relationship between the intensity of 201-Tl accumulation and tumor aggressiveness is not simply related in the childhood brain tumors as a whole as it is with a majority of adult brain tumors.

^{99m}Tc-MIBI has also been found to accumulate in a variety of pediatric brain tumors. A major limitation of MIBI is the accumulation of tracer within the choroid plexus, which may prevent diagnosis of adjacent tumor activity. Also, MIBI has lower sensitivity in detecting recurrence in comparison with 201-Tl, especially in low-grade tumors.

Leukemia

Leukemia commonly involves the skeleton. Patients may present with bone pain and are referred due to skeletal symptoms or recurrent fevers. A bone scan may be requested to exclude osteomyelitis or arthritis. As bony involvement does not affect prognosis or outcome, radiographic or scintigraphic evaluation of the skeleton is not routinely performed. In patients who have leukemia with focal clinical signs and symptoms, a bone scan will help to determine the cause of pain and exclude other pathologies, e.g. infection, fracture and avascular necrosis. Leukemic changes on bone scan are seen as a diffuse metaphyseal uptake of the radiotracer with blurring of the growth plates and is often symmetrical; however focal abnormalities may also be seen. Photopenic areas (reduced radiotracer uptake) in the bone have been described in acute ALL and AML and during treatment particularly with high dose steroids causing avascular necrosis. 67-Ga has been used in leukemia; however, the main application for 67-Ga is in the investigation of infection.

Lung Cancer

Lung cancer in children is usually metastatic, including metastic osteosarcoma, which can occasionally be detected in the lungs by ^{99m}Tc methylene diphosphonate (MDP) scintigraphy. Most other neoplastic processes, including lymphomatous involvement, require 67, Ga citrate or 201-T1 scintigraphy.

NUCLEAR IMAGING IN THE EVALUATION OF PEDIATRIC BRAIN

Radiotracers used for brain imaging can be divided into several distinct classes either by the type of instrumentation used [for example, single-photon emission computed tomography (SPECT) or positron emission tomography (PET)] or by the function being measured (cerebral blood flow, blood-brain barrier studies, metabolism studies, receptor studies, and so forth).

Blood-brain Barrier Defects Imaging

In healthy brain tissue, most hydrophilic radiotracers that are not transported into the brain via active or facilitated transport are excluded by the BBB. However, under a variety of pathological conditions, including cerebral tumors, abscesses, and intracranial injury such as subdural hematoma or intracerebral hemorrhage, the integrity of the BBB is disrupted, and these water soluble tracers can diffuse from the circulation into the damaged tissue.

Presently, ^{99m}Tc pertechnetate, ^{99m}Tc diethylenetriaminepentaacetic acid (DTPA) and ^{99m}Tc glucoheptonate (GHA) are used for imaging studies of the BBB. ^{99m}Tc DTPA has advantages over 99mTc pertechnetate in that it is rapidly cleared from the circulation by glomerular filtration, allowing images to be obtained earlier with better target-to-background ratios. ^{99m}Tc GHA offers advantages over both ^{99m}Tc DTPA and pertechnetate since it is removed from the circulation even faster than DTPA by both glomerular filtration and tubular secretion, providing even higher lesion-to-background ratios.

Usual administered doses: 0.2 mCi/kg (7.4 MBq/kg); minimum dose 10 mCi (370 M13q), maximum dose 20 mCi (740 MBq).[6,8,9]

Abscess Imaging

X-ray CT and MRI are useful in the diagnosis of cerebral abscesses but cannot always differentiate abscesses from other types of lesions such as tumors, infarcts, or hematoma. Indium-111 labeled granulocytes have been reported to provide a sensitive method for the detection of cerebral abscesses. However, localization of 111-In granulocytes in cerebral abscesses can be inhibited in patients receiving corticosteroid treatment. Also, weak or moderate uptake of 111-In granulocytes is seen in some patients with brain tumors.[7,9,10]

Tumor imaging

201-Tl

Thallium-201 (monovalent cation) is widely and commonly used for the evaluation of myocardial perfusion. Besides, it also appears to be the method of choice for grading gliomas, assessing residual viable tumors following radiation therapy, and detecting malignant degeneration of low grade gliomas.

Usual administered doses: 0.03-0.05 mCi/kg body weight; minimum dose 0.5 mCi (18.5 MBq), maximum dose 2.0 mCi (74 MBq).[7]

^{99m}Tc MIBI/TF

These are myocardial perfusion agents, which also accumulate in brain tumors. Like 201-Tl, tumor uptake before treatment may indicate the potential to use this tracer as a marker of residual tumor after treatment. The spectrum of tumor avidity is similar to that of 201-Tl, while clearer identification of boundaries with MIBI/TF may be an advantage in some applications such as radiotherapy port planning.[7]

^{99m}Tc GHA

We at AIIMS are using this radiopharmaceutical very successfully, particularly in cases of residual/recurrent tumor post Sx/CT/RT (Fig. 12.7).

Usual administered doses: 0.3 mCi (11.1 MBq)/kg body weight, minimum dose 1 mCi (37 MBq), maximum dose 20 mCi (740 MBq).[7]

Cerebral Perfusion

A positron emission tomography measurement of CBF is done by infusion or a bolus injection of oxygen-15 (O-15). However, theoretically, this tracer is not ideal, and other positron emitting radiotracers for CBF imaging had been developed, including krypton-77 and C-11 Butanol.

SPECT Measurement of Brain Perfusion

Tracers used for this purpose must have the following characteristics:

1. Radiotracers must be lipophilic, allowing them to cross the BBB via passive diffusion with nearly complete firstpass extraction in the brain.
2. Their extraction must approximate unity and be independent of flow so that their initial distribution will be proportional to regional cerebral blood flow.
3. They must be retained within the brain in their initial distribution long enough for statistically valid tomographic images to be obtained. After diffusion into the brain, they must be retained by some mechanism such as binding to nonspecific receptors or metabolism to a significantly less lipophilic species that cannot readily wash out of the brain.
4. For high extraction efficiencies to be achieved, log P (a measure of lipophilicty) must be at least 0.5 and the molecular weight of the tracer must be < 650 and preferably < 400 KD.
5. It is also important that the tracer have low plasma protein binding.

Technetium-99m-hexamethylene propylamine oxime (Tc-99m-HMPAO)

^{99m}Tc HMPAO, a lipophilic complex, is rapidly cleared from the blood after intravenous injection. Brain uptake is 3.5-7.0% of the injected dose within 1 minute after administration.[1,7] Maximum uptake is at 10 minutes. After diffusion of HMPAO into the brain, it is converted to a second, more hydrophilic complex that cannot diffuse back out of the brain. The formation

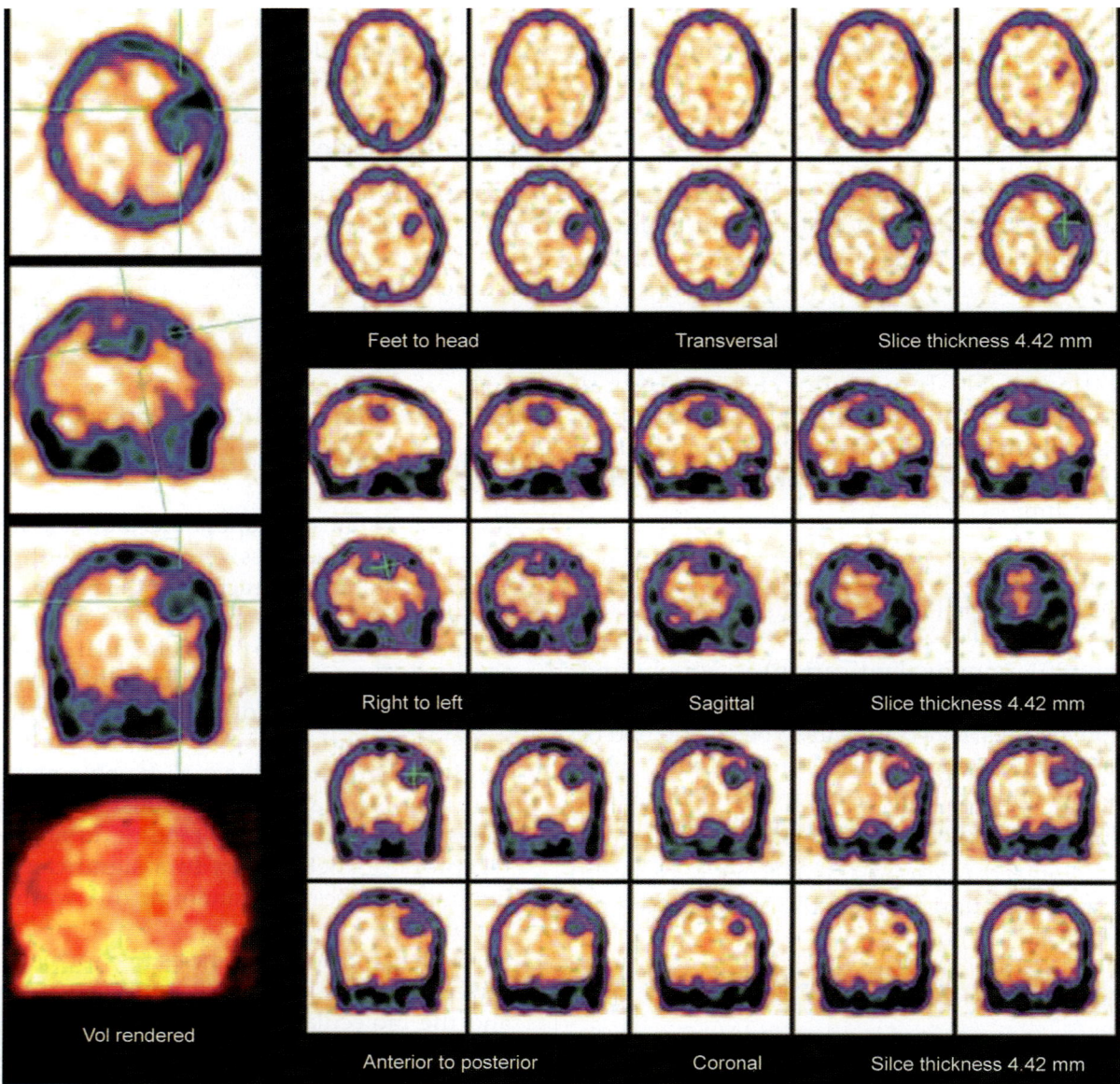

Fig. 12.7: ^{99m}Tc-GHA brain SPECT showing recurrent GBM in the parietal lobe

of the hydrophilic complex that is trapped in the brain is thought to be the result of a simple chemical reaction with glutathione, which is present in millimolar concentration in brain cells, although other mechanisms have been proposed. Approximately 15% of the initial cerebral uptake is cleared in 2 minutes, the other 85% remains in the brain for 24 hours. Redistribution of HMPAO within the brain does not occur for at least 8 hours and wash out is insignificant-only 0.4%/hr. Extracerebral uptake is distributed throughout the body, particularly in the muscles and soft tissues. Approximately 30% of the administered tracer activity is found in the gastrointestinal tract a few minutes after injection, and approximately 50% is eliminated by this route in 24 hours. Approximately 40% of the tracer activity is eliminated in the urine within 48 hours.

Technetium-99m Ethylcysteine Dimer (^{99m}Tc-ECD)

ECD is a lipophilic agent that rapidly concentrates in the brain following intravenous injection at approximately 6% of the administered dose. Peak uptake is at 5 minutes. After entering the brain, selective enzyme catalyzed hydrolysis of one of the ester groups to a carboxylic acid results in the formation of a negatively charged complex, which can't diffuse out. The primary route of excretion of this agent is the urinary tract, and approximately 50% is cleared by the kidneys within the first 2 hours after administration. Approximately 11% of the tracer is eliminated via the gastrointestinal tract over 48 hours.[1,7]

This agent has following advantages over ^{99m}Tc HMPAO:
  i. A 6 hours shelf life,
 ii. More rapid blood clearance (shorter biological half-life,
iii. Lower background activity and
 iv. Less radiation to the patient.

Because of the 6 hour shelf life, this radiopharmaceutical can be administered at any desired time required by the clinical problem being investigated. For example, it can be given during an ictal episode to map the regional cerebral perfusion during the ictus. A similar advantage may hold for performing SPECT during the time of abnormal brain activity in other paroxysmal disorders, such as migraine or transient cerebral ischemic episodes.

Cerebral Metabolism

Several metabolic substrates have been labeled with positron emitting radionuclides and used for PET studies of brain metabolism, including tracers for glucose metabolism, oxygen utilization, dopamine metabolism, protein synthesis, and amino acid transport.

Receptor Specific Radiopharmaceuticals

Mapping of brain receptor distribution has been done with PET and can also be achieved with SPECT. Several conditions of childhood may have an important component of receptor dependency. In the common problem of attention deficit disorder, dysfunction of the dopaminergic system may play a major pathogenic role. 123-I iodobenzamide, a dopaminc D_2 receptor antagonist detectable by SPECT, may prove useful for investigating these hypotheses in this common disorder of the school going child.

CLINICAL APPLICATIONS

Normal Brain Development

Metabolism is initially more intense in the sensorimotor cortex, thalamus, brainstem, and cerebellar vermis; later it involves the parietal, temporal, and occipital cortex, basal ganglia, and cerebellar cortex, and finally the frontal cortex. By 1 year the pattern resembles that of adult and cerebral cortical areas approximately display a parallel evolution.[11,12] These developments can be assessed and followed by Fluorine-18 Fluorodeoxyglucose (F-18-FDG) PET. The cerebellum/mean cerebral cortex index has shown to be higher in the neonatal period, slightly lower between 2 months and 15 years and thereafter is more or less identical to the adults.

Childhood Epilepsy

Epilepsy in children is treated with considerable success by medical means (anticonvulsants administered with appropriate clinical and pharmacologic monitoring). Some patients, however, do not respond to medical therapy. Surgical removal or disconnection of a portion of brain believed to contain the epileptogenic focus may control seizures. Interictal PET studies with temporal lobe epilepsy reveal a characteristic zone of decreased metabolism in the region of the epileptogenic focus. However, ictal studies demonstrate a more focal region of increased metabolism. These ictal and interictal changes in brain metabolism are found to be matched by corresponding changes in perfusion, revealed by SPECT. These functional abnormalities are frequently accompanied by normal or almost normal CT or MRI scans. In other instances the perfusion abnormalities are seen to extend far beyond the limits of structural lesions. Perfusion brain SPECT studies with temporal epilepsy have revealed characteristic time dependent changes in regional cerebral perfusion following a partial seizure (Fig. 12.8). During the earliest postictal period, there is increased perfusion involving the medial temporal lobe, succeeded by hypoperfusion of the lateral temporal cortex, and later of the entire temporal lobe. Ictal perfusion SPECT provides an opportunity to localize an epileptogenic focus. Ictal SPECT must be performed with tracer injection at the onset of ictus. Delayed injections of the tracer may demonstrate activation of secondary epileptogenic tissue and may lead to erroneous conclusion.

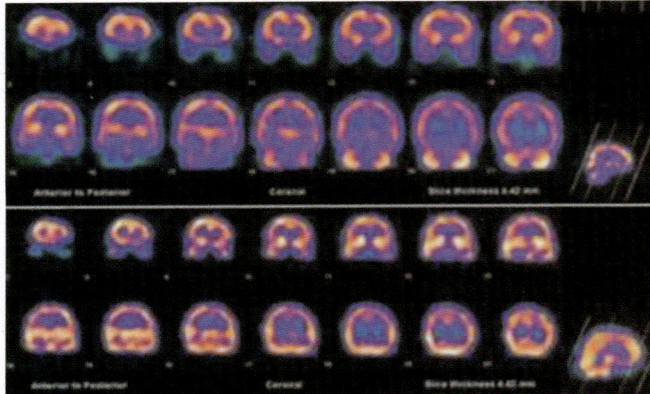

Fig. 12.8: ^{99m}Tc-ECD interictal (upper rows) and ictal (lower rows) brain SPECT showing lesion in right temporal lobe

Traumatic Brain Injury

rCBF studies have a role in those children with brain trauma, who have any neurological consequences in the follow-up, but structural imagings are normal. In these children, usually abnormalities are seen throughout the brain but more frequently in the frontal, parietal and temporal lobes (Fig. 12.9).

Moya Moya Disease

Moya moya is a form of cerebrovascular disease occurring predominantly in children and characterized by an angiographic pattern of supraclinoid internal carotid artery stenosis, followed ultimately by a luxuriant pattern of collateral vascularization. This angiographic appearance has been likened to a puff of cigarette smoke. Serial cerebral perfusion studies can document the changes in cerebral blood flow that occur during the course of the disorder. The SPECT abnormalities are partly congruent with MRI and CT findings but show larger perfusion defects than those revealed by the other modalities. Hence brain SPECT offers an effective way of following the natural history of moya moya disease, and its noninvasive nature may offer an attractive alternative to serial arteriography. SPECT may play an important role in evaluating the success of proposed treatments for the disorder, such as superficial temporal artery middle cerebral artery bypass.

Complications of Extracorporeal Membrane Oxygenation

In newborns undergoing extracorporeal membrane oxygenation (ECMO) for refractory respiratory failure,

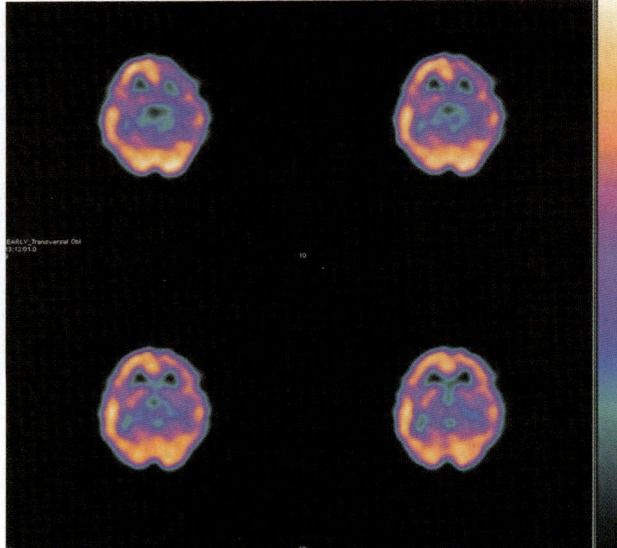

Fig. 12.9: ^{99m}Tc-ECD brain SPECT showing hypoperfusion in the frontoparietal lobe (L) in a case of head injury

^{99m}Tc HMPAO/ECD SPECT can be used to investigate the status of cerebral perfusion. Significant perfusion defects in either the ipsilateral or contralateral hemisphere are documented, whereas only few patients show abnormalities on ultrasonography, CT or MRI.

Effect of Hypothermia and Hypoxia

Surgical repair of complex congenital heart disease in very small children is possible today because of advances in anesthesia and techniques of hypothermia with hypoxia. This method, however, carries a risk of brain damage. A known complication of hypothermia with hypoxia is the choreoathetosis syndrome (CAS). In these patients, SPECT may show striking focal rCBF abnormalities at both the cortical (frontal, parietal, and temporal cortex) and subcortical (anterior basal ganglia) levels. The distribution of the perfusion abnormalities is not predictable from clinical examination and CT and MRI are usually normal or show only generalized nonspecific abnormalities. These cerebral perfusion abnormalities may have important implications for developmental outcome in these children.

BRAIN TUMORS

Cancer continues to be the second leading cause of death in children under age 15 years, with central nervous system tumors constituting the most fatal group of solid tumors in children. Some may be cured with combined surgery and external beam irradiation, hyperfractionated therapy, or stereotaxic radiosurgery. The promise of these new approaches to treatment of childhood brain tumor increases the importance of developing accurate methods for the assessment of residual disease after primary therapy.

Both CT and MRI have high sensitivity and specificity in the diagnosis of brain tumors in children, but these structural imaging methods have limitations in their ability to detect tumor viability. CT is often unable to distinguish between tumor presence and nonspecific brain injury. MRI, likewise, frequently cannot differentiate radiation effect from residual or recurrent brain tumor. Functional imaging (SPECT and PET), on the other hand, may detect the presence of active tumor. In combination with CT and MRI, this ability is useful for diagnosing residual brain tumor following therapy and differentiating between recurrent tumor and radiation necrosis.

Cerebrospinal Fluid Studies

Radionuclide evaluation of the cerebrospinal fluid (CSF) kinetics includes radionuclide cisternography (Fig. 12.10) and the evaluation of diversionary shunts. It can be helpful in the detection and localizalion of CSF leaks such as rhinorrhea or otorrhea. Indium-111-diethylenetriaminepentaacetic acid (DTPA) is the agent most commonly used in cysternography. The pediatric dose is 1 mCi for ^{99m}Tc-DTPA and 50-100 µCi for 111-In-DTPA. The technetium-99m radiopharmaceutical has a lower radiation dose and better imaging characteristics, but the observation period is limited to 24 hours after administration of the tracer. This is rarely a problem in the evaluation of children's CSF dynamics. Both agents are administered into the subarachnoid space via lumbar puncture. Other sites of injection include the cisterna magna or a lateral ventricle.[7] Immediately following injection of the tracer, a static image of the area of administration is obtained to ensure proper injection technique. Serial imaging at 1, 2, 4-6, and 24 hours is carried out, including anterior, posterior, and lateral views. In the assessment of CSF leaks, more frequent imaging is required, with attention to patient positioning in order to maximize the chances of identifying "leaking" tracer with CSF.

In CSF diversionary shunts, 70-500 µCi of ^{99m}Tc as pertechnetate in 0.1-0.2 ml is injected in the appropriate site of the shunt tubing, depending on the question being asked. When a CSF shunt is patent, tracer is absorbed rapidly within the body. Rapid absorption of the tracer takes place in the peritoneum with ventriculoperitoneal shunts. Similarly, rapid absorption of pertechnetate occurs in patent ventriculoatrial shunts. Careful technique to avoid extravasation of the tracer is critical. If the shunt is occluded, pertechnetate remains within the shunt tube and is not absorbed. CSF shunt flow can be evaluated visually by observation of the serial images. A region of interest over the injection site permits the measurement of the half time of tracer disappearance. Normal values for T 1/2 are 0.5-6.0 minutes. CSF flow rates can be calculated if the volume of initial distribution of the shunt reservoir is known. CSF shunt flow rates are normally in the range from 0.2 - 0.3 ml/minute. If the shunt does not seem to flow after a few minutes of observation, the patient may be moved or the shunt reservoir can be pumped and additional images obtained to ascertain whether there is any flow under these conditions.

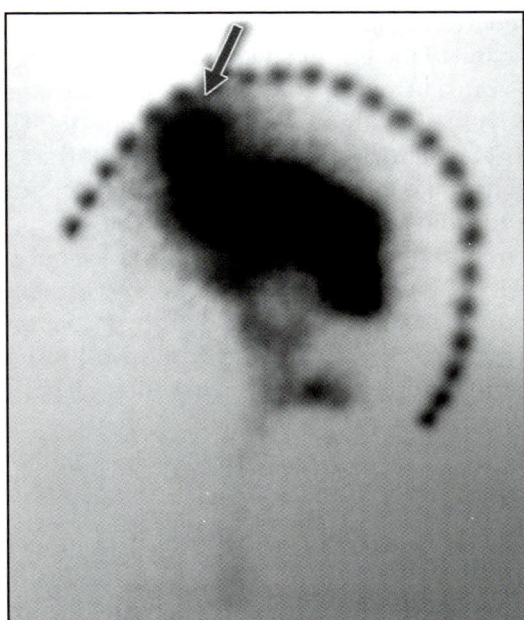

Fig. 12.10: Cisternography (ventriculography) showing abnormal tracer accumulation in the ventricles (arrow) in a case of communicating hydrocephalus

IMAGING OF THE THYROID

Thyroid scintigraphy in children is indicated in the evaluation of thyroid and neck masses in order to determine their level of function and in the detection of ectopic thyroid tissue. Radionuclide assessment of thyroid function is used in the 131-I treatment planning for hyperthyroidism in pediatric patients in whom medical therapy has failed or when the patient (or parents) refuses surgery. 131-I whole body scan is very useful in the detection of local recurrence and metastatic disease as well as in 131-I treatment planning and follow up in children with thyroid cancer.

In India, thyroid scintigraphy and uptake for the assessment of children with benign conditions are carried out using 131-I, as 123-I, which is the agent of choice for this population, is very costly and not available. Imaging is done 24-48 hours after the oral administration of 25-50 µCi of 131-I. However, for the assessment of metastatic disease and iodine turnover measurement in patients with thyroid cancer prior to treatment, 131-I is more suitable. The biochemical behavior of 131-I is identical to that of stable iodide. Organification defects can also be diagnosed with this tracer using the perchlorate discharge test.[7,13]

^{99m}Tc pertechnetate is trapped by the thyroid in the same fashion as iodide but is not organified. It is released from the gland after trapping and can be washed out of the thyroid by perchlorate. Scintigraphic images must be obtained while ^{99m}Tc-pertechnetate is in relatively high concentration in the plasma. Thyroid imaging is complicated by the fact that ^{99m}Tc pertechnetate is taken up by the salivary glands as well as the thyroid and is eliminated in the saliva. ^{99m}Tc pertechnetate activity in the saliva may be intense enough to overshadow uptake by an ectopic, hypofunctioning gland. Imaging of the thyroid following ^{99m}Tc-pertechnetate administration begins 5-10 minutes after intravenous injection of 2-5 mCi of the radiotracer.

Normal Thyroid Gland

The normal thyroid gland reveals a homogeneous distribution of tracer activity (Fig. 12.11). Slight asymmetry in lobe size is common, with the right lobe usually being larger. In most patients, tracer activity in the region of the isthmus is not seen. Rarely, a pyramidal lobe is seen extending up from the isthmus.

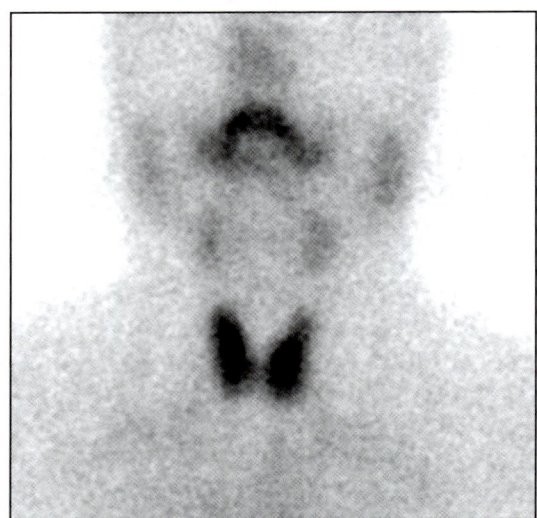

Fig. 12.11: Normal ^{99m}TcO$_4$ thyroid scan

Radioiodine thyroid uptake is calculated at 2 and 24 hours after administration of 5-10 µli of 131-I. Normal values for radiotracer uptake ranges at AIIMS are from 5-15% at 2 hours and from 15-35% at 24 hours.

Hyperthyroidism

Hyperthyroidism in children with a diffuse goiter is usually because of Graves' disease. In Graves' disease radiotracer uptake is high; however, when iodine turnover is very rapid, the radiotracer leaves the thyroid and 24-hour uptake values may be normal. Scintigraphy although not needed in children with obvious Graves' disease, reveals diffusely increased radiotracer uptake with markedly reduced radiotracer concentration in salivary glands (Fig. 12.12). Toxic nodular goiter, either uninodular or multinodular, is another cause of hyperthyroidism. In patients with a nodular thyroid, thyroid scintigraphy can reveal toxic adenomas, which appears as increased focus of radiotracer with decreased/no radiotracer uptake in rest of the gland.[13]

Thyroid Nodule

Thyroid nodules are classified as "functioning" or "nonfunctioning," depending on the amount of radiotracer accumulation. In children with thyroid nodules, scintigraphy differentiates solitary from multinodular goiters and can identify lesions not palpable in patients originally thought to have a

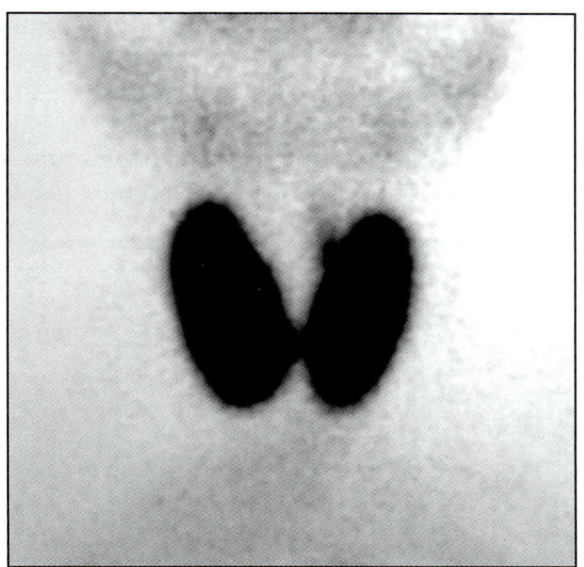

Fig. 12.12: $^{99m}TcO_4$ thyroid scan showing increased radiotracer uptake in a case of Graves' disease (almost no uptake in salivary glands)

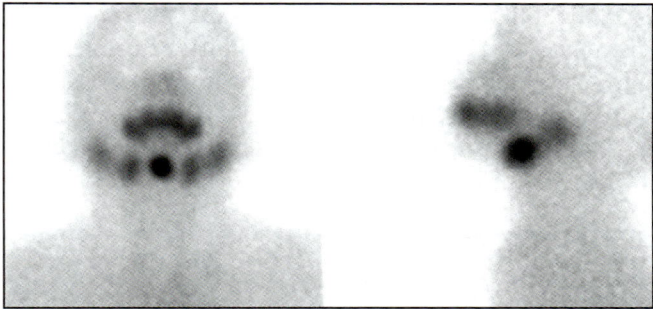

Fig. 12.13: Sublingual thyroid: $^{99m}TcO_4$ scan

solitary nodule. A neck mass that does not accumulate radioiodine may coexist with a normally located, bilobed thyroid gland. The problem for the physician is to determine whether the mass is a lymph node, cyst, hemorrhage, abscess, metastatic deposit, or benign or malignant neoplasm. Ectopic thyroid tissue can be identified if it accumulates the radiotracer (Fig. 12.13). In nongoitrous hypothyroidism, the incidence of ectopic thyroid tissue in children ranges from 22-75%. Therefore, an important use of thyroid scintigraphy in patients with a midline neck mass is to identify and locate functioning thyroid tissue prior to surgery in order to avoid inadvertent excision of an ectopic thyroid gland.[13]

Chronic Lymphocytic Thyroiditis (Hashimoto's disease)

Chronic lymphocytic thyroiditis (Hashimoto's disease) is a cause of hypothyroidism in children. The 2 hour and 24 hour radioiodine uptake may be low, normal, or elevated. Patients are usually found to have diffuse thyroid enlargement. The scintigraphic appearance varies, depending on the stage of the disease. In the acute phase, the thyroid silhouette may appear enlarged and radiotracer uptake may be greater than normal. With time, images begin to have patchy or diffuse radiotracer distribution. Discrete areas of increased uptake can result from islands of hypertrophic thyroid tissue, with decreased or absent uptake elsewhere in the gland.

Subacute (de Quervain's) Thyroiditis

In subacute (de Quervain's) thyroiditis scintigraphy helps to distinguish the hyperthyroidism of subacute thyroiditis from that due to Graves' disease and may reveal patchy radiotracer uptake. The 2 and 24 hour radioiodine uptake is also very low. With clinical recovery, the scintigraphic abnormalities disappear.[13]

IMAGING OF THE LUNG

Nuclear medicine offers imaging methods to assess regional pulmonary blood flow and ventilation, gas and fluid transport across the alveolocapillary membrane, mucociliary clearance, pulmonary aspiration, and parenchymal disease. Indications for pulmonary scintigraphy in children are pulmonary artery agenesis, hypoplasia, stenosis; pulmonary aplasia, hypoplasia; pulmonic valve stenosis, pulmonary sequestration, pulmonary embolism, alpha-antitrypsin deficiency, congenital diaphragmatic hernia, arteriovenous malformation, bronchopulmonary fistula, pectus excavaturn, lobar emphysema, human immunodeficiency virus (HIV) related pathology, cyanosis, asthma, tumor, sarcoidosis, pneumonia, burns, irradiation, cystic fibrosis, bronchial occlusion, infection or inflammation, scimitar syndrome, swyer james syndrome and prior to and/or following lung surgery.[7]

Pulmonary perfusion scintigraphy is performed with ^{99m}Tc labeled macroaggregated albumin (MAA) (Fig. 12.14). Radiolabeled macroaggregates define the pattern of pulmonary perfusion by the principle of capillary blockade. Radiolabeled particles ranging in size from 10-90 μ occlude precapillary arterioles and some capillaries. Untoward effects are not observed, since only a small percentage (0.1%) of the arterioles is embolized. The biological half-life of the particles in the lungs is approximately 7 hours. Peripheral venous injection of ^{99m}Tc MAA is performed during normal breathing. The administered dose of radioactivity and number of particles are adjusted according to the patient's age, weight, and clinical status. The patient receives 1.85 MBq/kg (50 μCi/kg), with minimum and maximum doses of 7.4 MBq (200 μCi) and 111 MBq

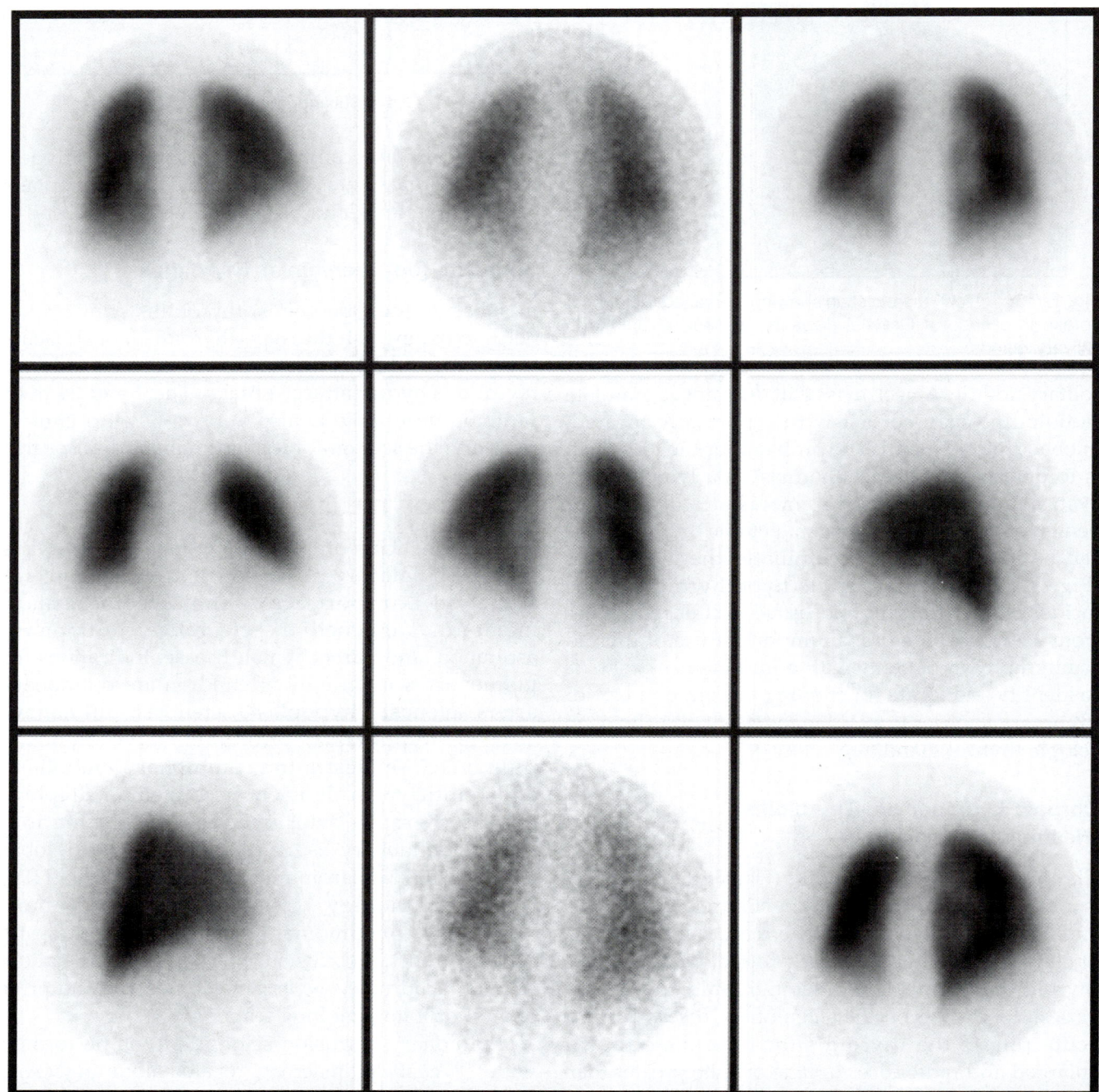

Fig. 12.14: Normal pulmonary perfusion scan

(3 mCi), respectively. Newborns should be injected with no more than 50,000 particles, 150,000 at 1 year of age, and 500,000 thereafter to adulthood. Patients with severe pulmonary disease and those with suspected right to left shunts should be injected with smaller numbers of particles (<10,000). Following injection, SPECT or eight view planar images are obtained in the anterior, posterior, right and left lateral, and anterior and posterior oblique projections. Fewer views are adequate when the only purpose of the study is to determine left to right differential perfusion ratios. Multiple views are evaluated by subjective criteria and regional lung perfusion between the two lungs and in various lung regions can be quantified by computer analysis.

To measure alveolocapillary permeability, low molecular weight compounds that can cross the alveolocapillary membrane, such as ^{99m}Tc DTPA, can be used to detect membrane abnormalities. Such studies may be helpful in children with immunodeficiency virus. For ^{99m}Tc DTPA aerosol studies, the patient breathes the nebulizer output through a facemask. Usually no more than 10% of the 1.11 GBq (30 mCi) of radiopharmaceutical placed in the aerosol device is delivered to the patient. Posterior planar images are obtained, and regional washout rates are measured and used to detect increased permeability of the alveolar epithelium. Normal values are not available for children.

In patients with pulmonary hemorrhage, arteriovenous malformation, or lung sequestration, ^{99m}Tc pertechnetate or other ^{99m}Tc agents, including red blood cells, DTPA, or sulfur colloid, are used.

Inflammation and Infection

In patients with recurrent localized pneumonia, a ^{99m}Tc-MAA perfusion scan can help reveal a possible structural abnormality. Gallium-67 citrate or 111-In or ^{99m}Tc granulocyte imaging can document and quantify infections in children. With 111-In oxime, the patient's leukocytes are labeled and readministered. Imaging is performed after 24 hours. A disadvantage of 111-In white blood cell (WBC) scintigraphy, particularly in children, is the radiation dose to the spleen, liver, and bone marrow. ^{99m}Tc HMPAO labeled WBCs or ^{99m}Tc antigranulocyte antibodies result in much less radiation exposure than do 111-In WBCs (Fig. 12.15).

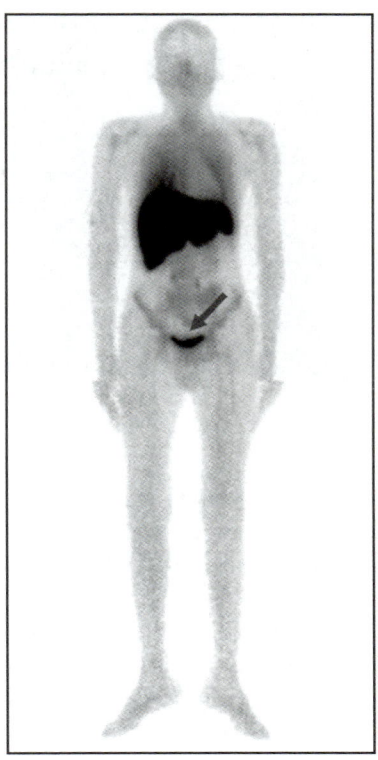

Fig. 12.15: ^{99m}Tc-HMPAO labeled WBC scan revealing source of infection in the terminal ileum (arrow)

The administered dose in the case of 67-Ga is 3.7 MBq/kg (100 µCi/kg). The usual total administered dose of ^{99m}Tc HMPAO WBCs is 37-296 MBq (1-8 mCi), depending on patient size and labeling efficiency.[7]

IMAGING OF THE CARDIOVASCULAR SYSTEM

In children with congenital heart disease, planning appropriate therapy often requires the detection and quantification of left to right shunts, determination of regurgitation in valvular insufficiency, and assessment of right and left ventricular ejection fraction.

First pass radionuclide angiocardiography is used in the detection and quantitation of left to right shunts and in the assessment of right and left ventricular ejection fraction (Fig. 12.16). Gated blood pool angiography is useful for the determination of regurgitation in valvular insufficiency and is the most accurate way to make this measurement.[14] Radionuclide angiocardiography can be performed in children of any age, including premature infants. Detection and quantitation of left to right shunting

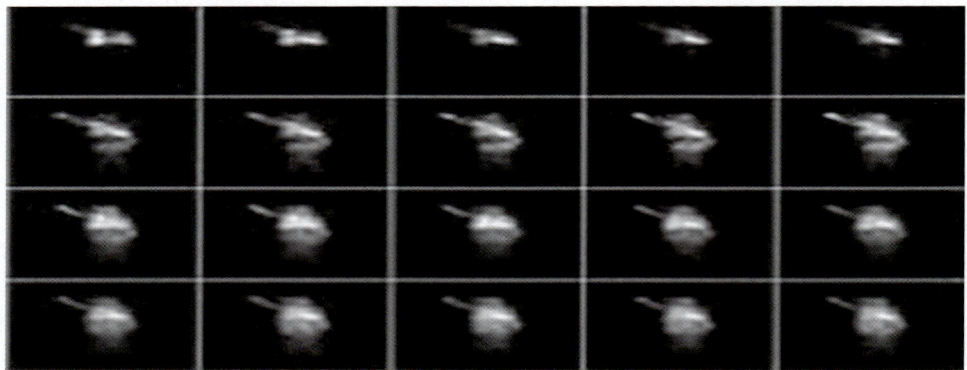

Fig. 12.16: First pass radionuclide angiocardiography

require experience, understanding of cardiovascular anatomy and physiology, and meticulous attention to technical details. The method consists of the rapid (< 2 seconds) intravenous injection of pertechnetate. Poor bolus injections result in poor studies. Deconvolution methods permit evaluation of shunt studies resulting from bolus inadequacies to a certain degree, but it is better to inject a sharp bolus. Technetium-99m sodium pertechnetate in a minimum total dose of 148-185 MBq (4 to 5 mCi), 7.4 MBq/kg (200 µCi/kg) is often used, but other ^{99m}Tc radiotracers can be used as long as the volume injected is small. Ultrashort lived radionuclides such as iridium-191m result in a low radiation dose and permit multiple serial evaluations.

Monitoring the passage of the bolus through the cardiovascular system for 20 seconds is adequate for detection of shunts and measurement of ejection fraction in children. Visual assessment is supplemented by quantification in the diagnosis of shunts, measuring ejection fraction, and detecting major structural abnormalities. Appropriate regions of interest are selected. Left to right shunts can be expressed as pulmonary to systemic flow ratios (Qp:Qs) by analysis of a pulmonary time activity curve.

Ejection fraction of the right and the left ventricles can be estimated rapidly and accurately (Figs 12.17 and 12.18). One must identify the chambers of the right and left heart as the tracer passes through them. Summed end diastolic and end systolic images are utilized to increase the statistical reliability of the results. Ventricular ejection fraction is calculated as the difference of end diastolic counts and end systolic counts divided by end diastolic counts. Parametric images, such as the stroke volume image, can be used to display regional ventricular contraction.

Left ventricular ejection fraction can be obtained in children by gated blood pool angiography. Indications in children are measurement of regurgitant fraction, cardiomyopathies, cystic fibrosis, thalassemia, prelung transplantation assessment, assessment of doxorubicin (Adriamycin) toxicity, postoperative assessment in congenital heart disease. Gated blood pool angiocardiography does not require special attention to the speed or the volume of radiopharmaceutical injected and provides better image resolution because longer observation times are possible. In children, the longer duration of the study, 20-30 minutes, presents problems not encountered by the shorter radionuclide angiocardiography for simple determination of left ventricular ejection fraction. Because of anatomical overlap of the cardiac chambers, there is greater variation of estimated ejection fractions. Right ventricular ejection is difficult to estimate with this method.

Indications for myocardial perfusion scintigraphy are postoperative evaluation of arterial switch operation for TGA (transposition of the great arteries), Tetralogy of Fallot repair, Mustard-Senning operation, Mucocutaneous lymph node syndrome (Kawasaki disease), Anomalous left coronary artery, cardiomyopathies, and thalassemia. SPECT can effectively detect myocardial perfusion abnormalities in patients with anomalous origin of the left coronary artery from the pulmonary artery, which is often accompanied by myocardial ischemia or infarction. Mucocutaneous lymph node syndrome (Kawasaki disease) also impairs myocardial blood flow. In

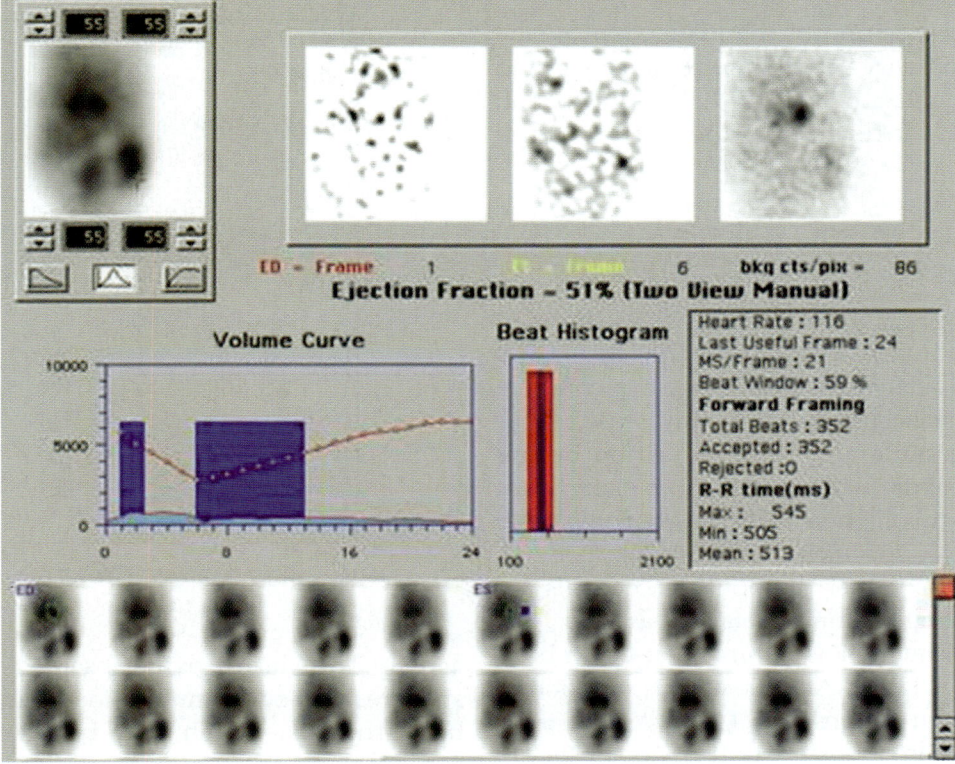

Fig. 12.17: MUGA scan to calculate left ventricular ejection fraction

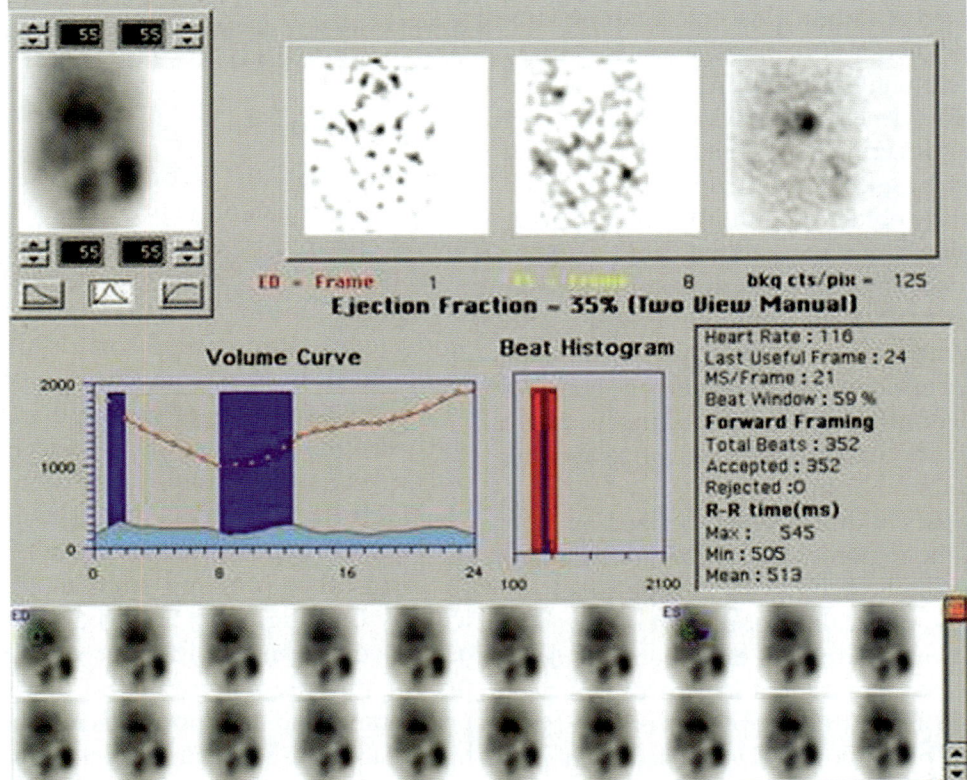

Fig. 12.18: MUGA scan to calculate right ventricular ejection fraction

surgery for transposition of the great arteries, the origins of the coronary arteries are reimplanted and scintigraphy done with Tl-201/^{99m}Tc. Tetrofosmin provides unique information about myocardial perfusion.

IMAGING OF THE MUSCULOSKELETAL SYSTEM

Skeletal scintigraphy with the ^{99m}Tc labeled phosphates is a valuable technique for diagnosing and determining the extent of skeletal disease in children. These radiopharmaceuticals are highly sensitive for demonstrating skeletal pathology, often before radiographs are abnormal. In the absence of pertinent clinical history, this high sensitivity is accompanied by a relatively low specificity for most disorders. To improve specificity, other radiopharmaceuticals are useful in evaluating certain skeletal diseases.

Technetium-99m MDP is commonly used for bone scintigraphy (Fig. 12.19). An intravenous injection of ^{99m}Tc-MDP is given in a dose of 7.4 MBq/kg (200 µCi/kg), with a minimum total dose of 18.5 MBq (500 µCi). Blood levels of ^{99m}Tc-MDP fall to 4 - 10% of the injected dose by 2 hours and to 3-5% by 3 hours. Optimal imaging is obtained at 4 hours post-tracer administration. By this time, about 60% of the injected activity will have been eliminated in the urine with normal renal function. In selected cases when findings at 4 hours are unclear, imaging at 24 hours may be helpful to elucidate findings. Delayed imaging may be performed either by obtaining multiple "spot" planar images or by using a moving gamma camera. Other useful techniques include pinhole magnification scintigraphy with a 2-3 mm pinhole aperture and SPECT. The importance of using the pinhole collimator to improve spatial resolution in pediatric bone imaging cannot be overemphasized. An example of its usefulness is in the early diagnosis of avascular necrosis of the femoral head.[7,15]

Bone imaging in children is characterized by high tracer uptake in the region of the physes, reflecting a high level of metabolic activity. Although this may obscure pathology, physeal tracer uptake is normally symmetrical. Patient positioning must be meticulous if one is to use asymmetry as a sign of disease. Abnormally high focal tracer uptake reflects both increased regional blood flow and increased metabolic

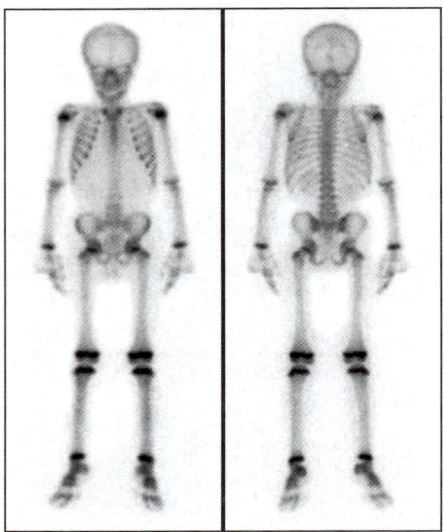

Fig. 12.19: Normal ^{99m}Tc MDP bone scan

activity. Focal increases are observed in osteomyelitis, stress reaction or fracture, eosinophilic granuloma, and bone tumors, which may be primary (Ewing's sarcoma, osteosarcoma) or metastatic. Foci of decreased tracer uptake are observed in early avascular necrosis, early osteomyelitis, acute infarct, simple benign cysts, and radiotherapy fields (very early or late stages).

Osteomyelitis

Bone imaging with ^{99m}Tc MDP is a sensitive indicator of childhood osteomyelitis (Figs 12.20 and 12.21). Intense tracer uptake occurs within 24-48 hours of the onset of symptoms. In the long bones, the abnormality is usually found in the metaphysis. The three-phase study helps differentiate soft tissue inflammatory involvement from osteomyelitis, with a specificity of 94% and a sensitivity of greater than 90%. When the study is normal or there is little tracer uptake in acute osteomyelitis, the possible cause is a reduction in focal blood flow as a result of edema. In such rare cases, it is helpful to repeat the bone scan after 48 hours or perform other imaging such as 67-Ga or labeled leukocyte scintigraphy. Some believe that in neonatal osteomyelitis there is little tracer accumulation. With proper pinhole magnification, meticulous patient positioning, and attention to technique, the method is highly accurate for neonatal osteomyelitis.

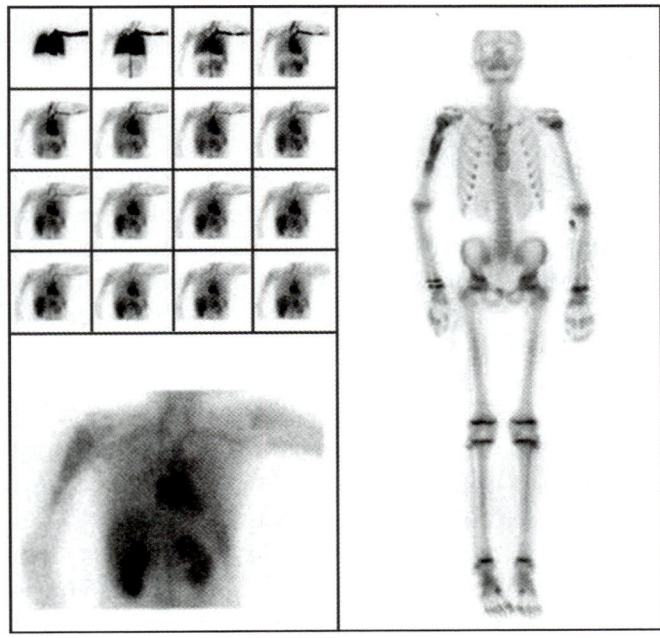

Fig. 12.20: Triple phase ⁹⁹ᵐTc-MDP bone scan in a case of acute osteomyelitis right humerus

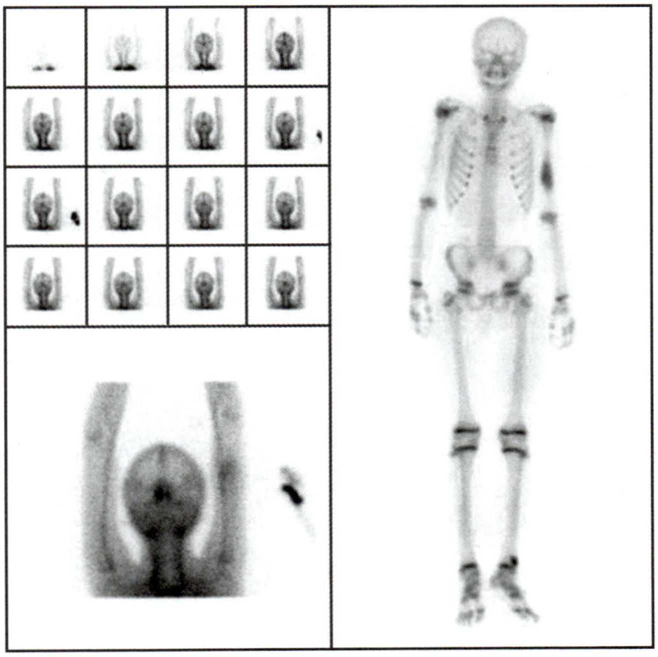

Fig. 12.21: ⁹⁹ᵐTc-MDP bone scan in a case of chronic osteomyelitis

Septic Arthritis

In the absence of concomitant osteomyelitis, septic arthritis is characterized by increased tracer uptake in periarticular areas, a pattern that can be readily differentiated from osteomyelitis. In osteomyelitis, the abnormal tracer uptake is more focal, while septic arthritis results in activity on both sides of the joint together with signs of inflammation in the early images of the radionuclide angiogram. The usual benefit of the study is to exclude concomitant osteomyelitis rather than to make a definitive diagnosis of septic arthritis, which is usually based on joint aspiration.

Avascular Necrosis of Femoral Head

Avascular necrosis involving the proximal femoral capital epiphysis may be seen in Legg-Calve-Perthes disease and other conditions producing increased intracapsular pressure, such as synovitis, high dose steroid therapy, and Gaucher's disease. An interruption of the blood supply from the medial femoral circumflex artery to the femoral head is believed to be responsible for the changes seen radiographically and scintigraphically. Early detection of femoral head avascular necrosis is important so that treatment can be promptly started and disability minimized. Initially, radiographs are normal. It is only during healing and revascularization that the density of bone increases and modeling and sclerosis become prominent. Absence of ⁹⁹ᵐTC MDP uptake may be demonstrated prior to any plain film changes and may be noted at the time of initial symptomatology. This may involve the entire femoral head or just its anterolateral aspects (Fig. 12.22). Pinhole imaging is useful in establishing a diagnosis. SPECT, particularly coronal images, is essential for detailed delineation of articular structure. In osteochondritis dissecans there is epiphyseal ischemic necrosis affecting the appendicular skeleton, most commonly the medial femoral condyles, and begins between 15-25 years of age. Focal increased uptake of tracer usually occurs at the involved site in bone scan.

Trauma

After trauma to bone, the reparative response begins immediately and a bone scan can reveal the increased uptake within 24-48 hours of injury, even though a radiograph may rarely be normal for several days after the accident. Usually, the scintigraphic findings are nonspecific, but in some cases a characteristic

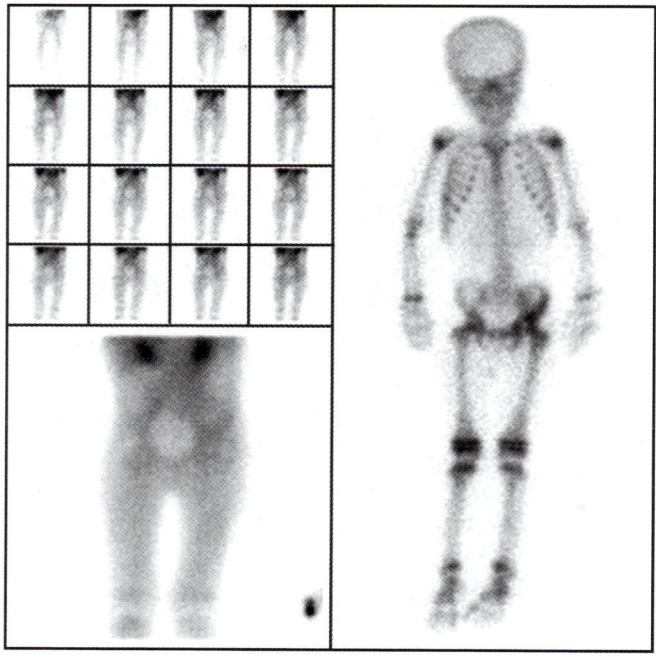

Fig. 12.22: Avascular necrosis head of femur (Left): Triple phase ^{99m}Tc-MDP bone scan showing photopenic area in the region of head

appearance of the lesions in the proper clinical setting makes possible a specific diagnosis (e.g., in tibial torsion fractures in toddlers). Another characteristic finding occurs later in some fractures. In reflex sympathetic dystrophy, which is the result of denervation of the limb, one observes diffusely increased or decreased tracer activity throughout the extremity. Bones are often subject to stress in athletes, ballet dancers, or other active persons. When osteoclastic activity exceeds osteoblastic repair, the result can be cortical disruption. In stress fractures, the scintigraphic abnormality can appear as much as 3 weeks before any radiographic abnormalities.

Bone Cysts and Fibrous Dysplasia

Bone scans are usually normal in small cysts or are characterized by a zone of decreased tracer activity compared to their surroundings. Increased uptake may occur in the bone surrounding a cyst with associated stress or trauma. Fibrous dysplasia, characterized by the absence of mature bone, affects multiple skeletal regions, chiefly the femora, tibiae, and pelvis. Fractures and deformities are common complications. Typically, skeletal scintigraphy reveals multiple areas of markedly increased focal tracer uptake.

Osteoid Osteoma

Osteoid osteoma is the most common benign tumor of bone in children and is characterized by a core of osteoid (the nidus) with a surrounding zone of reactive bone. Osteoid osteomas are most commonly cortically located but can also be cancellous or subperiosteal in location. While plain films are often diagnostic, the radiographic appearance of osteoid osteomas is variable, reflecting differences in reactive bone formation related to lesion location. The typical radiographic appearance of a cortical osteoid osteoma is a small central lucency with surrounding sclerosis and cortical thickening. Skeletal scintigraphy is often requested in patients with suspected osteoid osteomas when the classic radiographic findings are not present or when referred pain results in the initial radiographic examination missing the lesion completely. The typical scintigraphic appearance of an osteoid osteoma is intense tracer localization in the nidus surrounded by less prominently increased tracer uptake in surrounding reactive bone (Fig. 12.23). Intraoperative bone scanning has greatly reduced the recurrence of the disease after surgical resection. After performance of a preoperative baseline study, the same regions are imaged in the operating room during the progress of the surgery. Serial views obtained with a mobile gamma camera with pinhole collimation ensure the completeness of the resection.

IMAGING OF THE GASTROINTESTINAL TRACT

Gastroesophageal Reflux

Gastroesophageal reflux is a common occurrence in children. The child may present with vomiting, loss of appetite, weight loss, and failure to thrive. There may be irritation, erosion, or ulceration of the mucosal lining of the esophagus, which may cause bleeding. One fifth of patients suffering from gastroesophageal reflux have respiratory symptoms, including allergic bronchitis, asthma, or bronchitis. These symptoms are due to aspiration of refluxed gastric contents. Direct irritation of the esophageal mucosa with acid can cause respiratory symptoms, even in the absence of aspiration. Aspiration of gastric contents causes

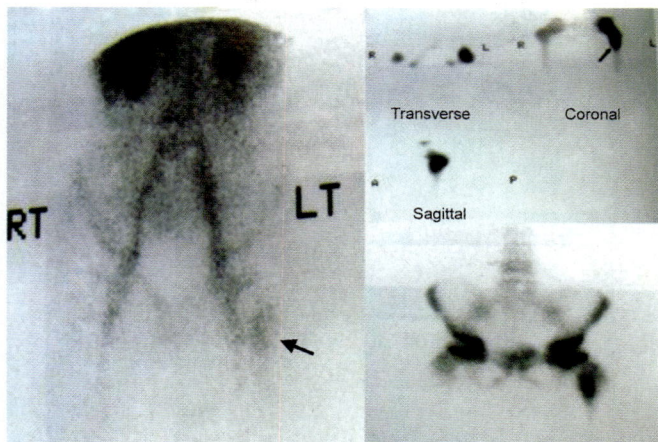

Fig. 12.23: ^{99m}Tc-MDP bone scan in a case of osteoid osteoma in femur (arrow)

coughing, vomiting, dyspnea, apnea, and cyanosis. About two thirds of patients are asymptomatic up to the age of 18 months. The rest exhibit symptoms by the age of 4 years. Less than 5% eventually have esophageal damage.

Gastroesophageal reflux and gastric emptying can be documented by adding ^{99m}Tc sulfur colloid to food. The minimum dose is 7.4 MBq (200µCi), and the maximum dose is 37 MBq (1 µCi); or 0.185 MBq (5µCi) ^{99m}Tc per ml of liquid food. The radiotracer is mixed with the child's formula or in milk.[7,8] The gamma camera is placed under the table on which the infant lies supine. The stomach, chest, and oropharynx are included in the field of view. Serial images are obtained using a 64×64 or a 128×128 matrix at one frame per 30 seconds for 1 hour (Fig. 12.24). The study is best portrayed using a computer generated cinematic display. Levels of activity 5% above background should be portrayed in order to visualize small volumes of reflux. If there is no patient motion, regions of interest are drawn over the gastric and esophageal regions in order to generate time activity curves. Gastroesophageal reflux detected scintigraphically correlates closely with esophageal probe pH monitoring.

Gastric emptying can be evaluated by observing the gastric time activity curve (Fig. 12.25). Normal gastric emptying times are highly variable and depend on the type of meal, patient position, and anxiety. There is no correlation between gastric emptying times and the presence of gastroesophageal reflux. Only significantly delayed or significantly rapid gastric

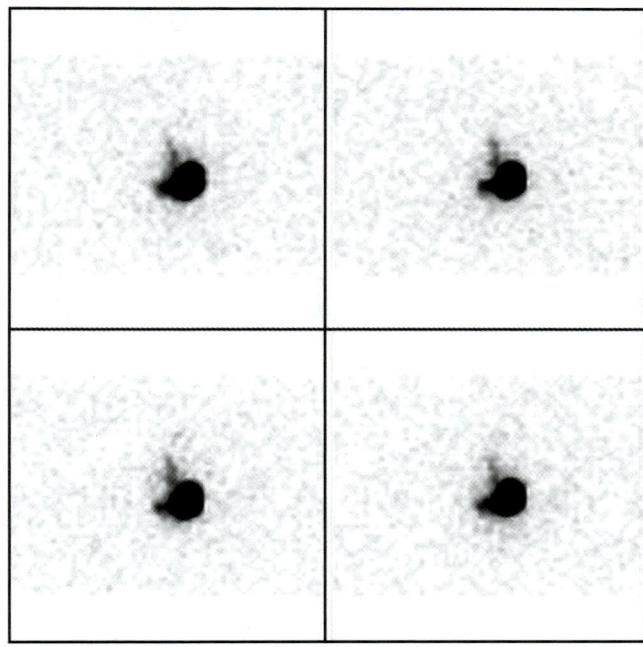

Fig. 12.24: ^{99m}Tc-sulfur-colloid scan showing GER

emptying times can be interpreted as abnormal and reported with confidence. The patterns of gastric emptying curves are also variable. The sensitivity of detecting pulmonary aspirations in patients suspected of this condition is low.

Meckel's Diverticulum

Meckel's diverticulum is a frequent cause of gastrointestinal bleeding in children. Following intravenous administration, ^{99m}Tc-pertechnetate is rapidly and actively taken up by gastric mucosa, accumulating approximately 20% of the injected dose.[6,7] ^{99m}Tc-pertechnetate also concentrates in functioning ectopic gastric mucosa within a Meckel's diverticulum. Scintigraphy with pertechnetate is quite effective in the detection of such ectopic tissue. The patient should fast for at least 4 hours prior to the examination in order to reduce the tracer activity in the stomach. No sodium or potassium perchlorate should be administered to the patient because it reduces gastric uptake of tracer. Potassium perchlorate can be administered orally after the imaging procedure to decrease thyroidal accumulation of the tracer. Barium contrast studies of the abdomen should not be performed before scintigraphy because the contrast agent will absorb gamma radiation and can interfere

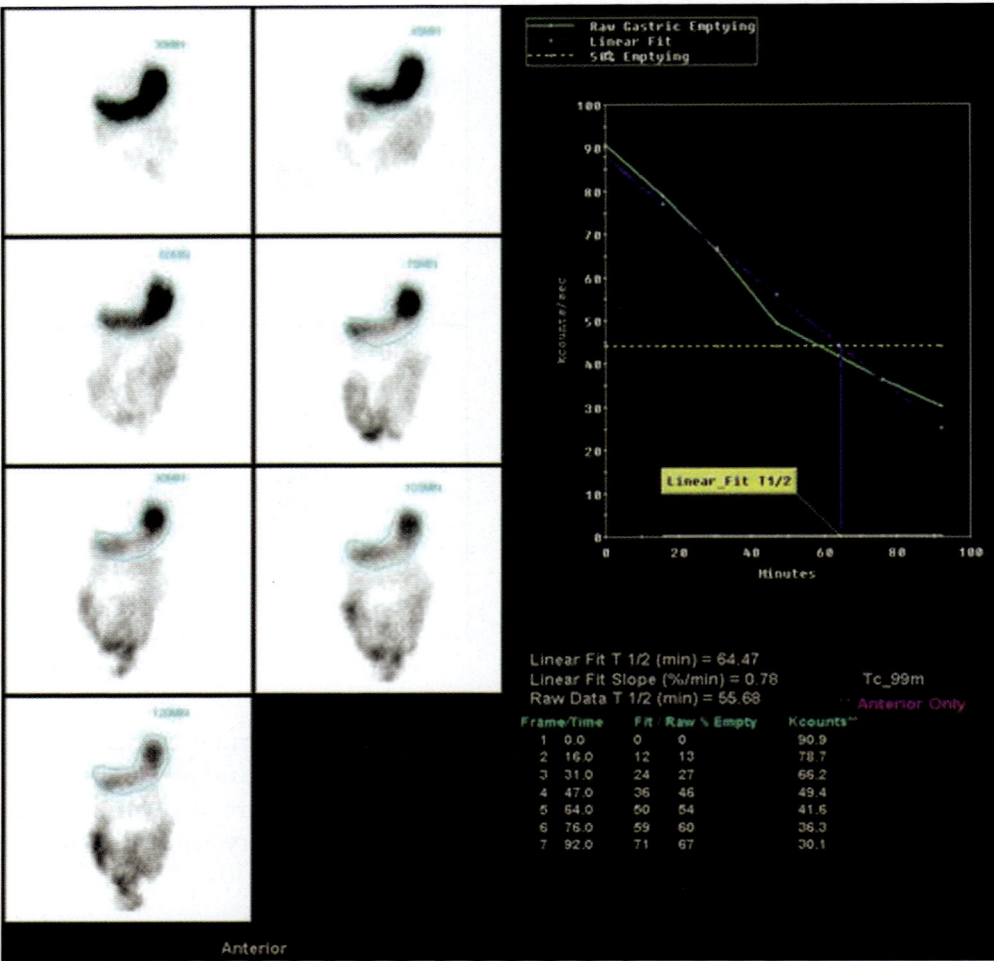

Fig. 12.25: Gastric emptying time calculation by generating gastric time activity curve

with detection of the ectopic gastric mucosa. Pentagastrin (6 µg/kg) is administered subcutaneously approximately 15 minutes before administration of the tracer to increase gastric mucosal uptake of the tracer and to reduce background activity. The patient lies supine, with the gamma camera viewing the entire abdomen. The tracer is administered intravenously, and recording begins immediately thereafter. A radionuclide angiogram is obtained with one image per second for 60 seconds, followed by serial imaging at one frame per 30 seconds for 30 minutes. The radionuclide angiogram helps detect highly vascular lesions such as hemangiomas; the serial imaging with 30 second frames is used to detect the ectopic gastric mucosa. If abnormal, intense extragastric accumulaton of tracer occurs, multiple projections (right lateral, posterior, obliques) should be obtained in order to better localize the abnormal uptake.

Tracer within functioning gastric mucosa in Meckel's diverticulum is easily identified by its location. Paralleling gastric uptake of the tracer is the progressive increase in focal activity in the right lower quadrant of the abdomen (Fig. 12.26). Other locations within the abdomen can occur. One must be aware that pertechnetate secreted into the stomach moves into the intestinal tract and also is excreted by the kidneys. These sites can be confused with uptake in ectopic tissue. Abnormal accumulation of radiopertechnetate in the abdomen can also be seen in intestinal obstruction, intussusception, inflammation, vascular malformations, ulcers, some tumors, and various urinary tract abnormalities. The appearance is different from the typical appearance of ^{99m}Tc uptake in ectopic gastric mucosa in a Meckel's diverticulum. Failure to see ectopic activity does not completely eliminate the possibility of a Meckel's diverticulum.

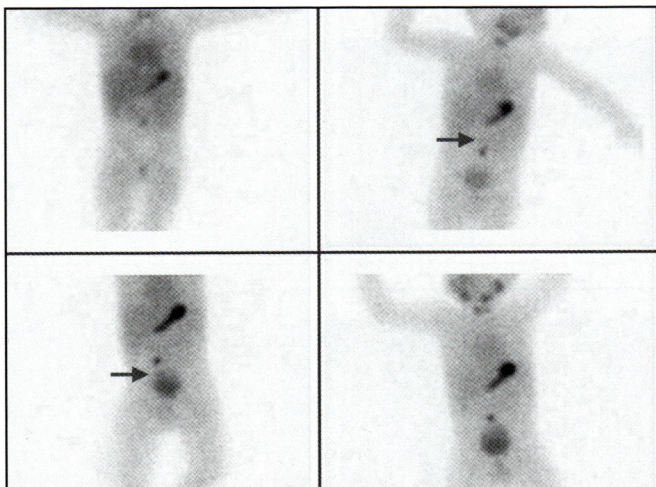

Fig. 12.26: $^{99m}TcO_4$ scan showing Meckel's diverticulum (arrow)

Rarely, necrosis, fibrosis, ischemia, atrophy, dysfunction of ectopic gastric mucosa, or severe anemia may prevent its detection by pertechnetate imaging.

GI Bleed

Abdominal bleeding can be detected by serial blood pool imaging using ^{99m}Tc labeled red blood cells (Fig. 12.27). In case of GI bleed, compared with angiography and endoscopy, scintigraphy is well tolerated, easy to perform, requires no patient preparation, is low risk, highly sensitive at low bleeding rate (scintigraphy can detect bleeding as low as 0.1-0.2 ml/min, whereas angiography can locate GI bleeding at a rate greater than 1 ml/min) and can detect intermittent bleeding.[7] The administered dose of radiolabeled red blood cells is the same as that for gated blood pool scintigraphy. The patient is examined in the supine position, with the camera field viewing the entire abdomen. Following intravenous administration of the blood pool tracer, serial imaging at one frame per 15-30 seconds is carried out for 60 minutes. Additional images at hourly intervals are obtained if the site of bleeding has not been localized during the first hour of imaging. Cinematic viewing of the serial images is often helpful. ^{99m}Tc-sulfur colloid can also be used in the detection and localization of lower abdominal bleeding. Because of the rapid blood disappearance of the radiocolloid, bleeding can be detected with the advantage of high target to nontarget ratios, but the method is limited to patients with severe, acute bleeding.

HEPATOBILIARY SCINTIGRAPHY IN PEDIATRIC PATIENT

The relatively non-invasive methods for the evaluation of the biliary system, like ultrasonography, computed tomography, oral cholangiography, cholecistography, provide excellent anatomic information. Hepatobiliary scintigraphy however, is the only technique providing real-time assessment of hepatocytes function and bile progression from the liver to the intestine.[16] Iminodiacetic acid analogs (IDA) are rapidly taken up by hepatocytes from circulating blood and are excreted into the biliary tree without conjugation. ^{99m}Tc-labeled IDA analogs provide liver and biliary tract images showing a progression from uptake to elimination. It can assess vascularity, parenchymal function, biliary drainage, possible presence of a bile leak, obstruction and many other disorders of the liver and the biliary tract in children and specifically in infancy. It has very good sensitivity and specificity for the detection and evaluation of neonatal jaundice (neonatal hepatitis vs biliary atresia (BA)), acute cholecystitis, bile leak, gallbladder dysfunction, trauma, choledocal cyst and liver transplantation. The most widely used IDA is mebrofenin. The recommended administered activity is a fraction of the adult dose (150 MBq) calculated in function of body surface area, with a minimum of 20 MBq in neonates. Patient should fast for at least 3-4 hours before the examination, so that gallbladder is not contracted. When study is done in neonates with hyper-bilirubinemia, it is necessary to administer the oral Phenobarbital (5 mg/kg per day in two divided doses) and/or beta methasone (oral drops) for 3-5 consecutive days prior to the study. Phenobarbital increases the the hepatic parenchymal uptake and the biliary excretion of the tracer. The combination greatly reduces the false positive diagnosis of BA.

Normal Findings

The scintigraphic appearance of the liver uptake in the abdominal field of view occurs rather rapidly, following that of kidneys and spleen, since the predominant part of liver perfusion comes from the

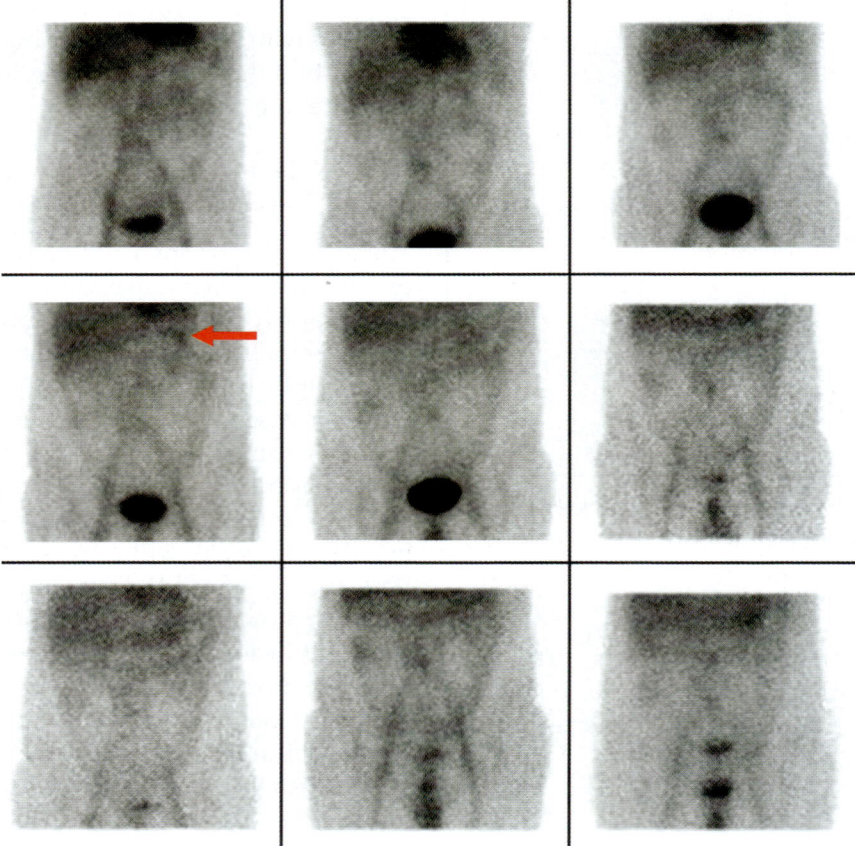

Fig. 12.27: Blood pool imaging with ^{99m}Tc labeled RBC for GI bleed in the splenic flexture (arrow)

portal venous system. In any case, in normal subjects, the area normalized ratio of liver to heart uptake at 5 minutes is higher than 1.0. The biliary tree visualization occurs 15 minutes postinjection, while its elimination into the duodenum is generally present at 30-45 minutes and the gallbladder is seen within one hour (Fig. 12.28).

The liver of neonates and infants is round-shaped as compared to that of adults; the gallbladder is easily identified, but not always the right and left main hepatic ducts. Care must be taken to distinguish the signal coming from overlapping structures of the urinary tract; this may be of some difficulty in liver insufficiency, because of the compensatory increase of urinary tracer excretion.

Persistent Hyperbilirubinemia

Hyperbilirubinemia can be divided into two main groups, based on the presence of predominant conjugated or unconjugated serum bilirubin levels.

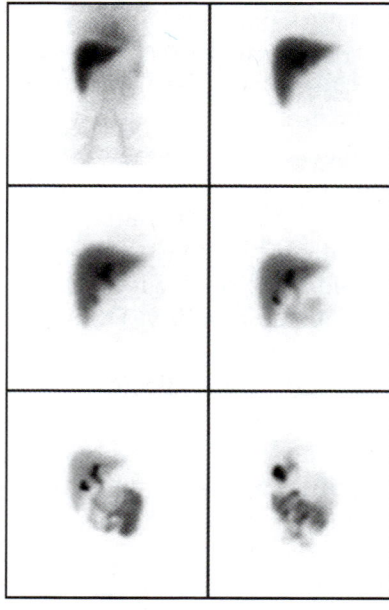

Fig. 12.28: Normal ^{99m}Tc-mebrofenin hepatobiliary scintigraphy

Physiologic neonatal jaundice, breast milk jaundice and erythroblastosis fetalis are relatively common causes of unconjugated hyperbilirubinemia. The hepatobiliary scan is not indicated generally in these circumstances. Conjugated and persisting hyperbilirubinemia most often occurs in the presence of biliary tract obstruction, the so-called "cholestatic" or "obstructive" jaundice. This, in neonates, may be due to biliary malformations; however, other causes may be involved, like hepatocellular disorders or bilirubin transport defects. Laboratory investigations easily establish the diagnosis in cases of infection, toxic or metabolic diseases. Ultrasound may well support the diagnosis of biliary anomalies, like choledocal cyst, gallbladder absence or hypoplasia, bile plugs. The evaluation of neonatal jaundice has to differentiate between those diseases, which can improve with Surgery, such as BA, from others in which medical treatment is preferable, such as neonatal hepatitis. The differential diagnosis between BA and neonatal hepatitis cannot be done with confidence without hepatobiliary scintigraphy. The sensitivity of hepatobiliary scintigraphy for BA is reported to be from 91-100% (Fig. 12.29); Percutaneous liver biopsy instead is known to reach 60-90% sensitivity. Moreover, histological similarities often exist between BA and neonatal hepatitis, making the diagnosis difficult. In these instances, surgical exploration of the portal region is indicated. Its correct diagnosis indicates prompt surgical correction, being this of paramount importance for the prognosis of the patient. The tracer appearance in the small intestine by 24 hours imaging, certainly rules out the diagnosis of BA; if no radiopharmaceutical is noted in the bowel, a distinction between inspissated bile syndrome and BA is more difficult to make. However, good point is that both need surgical exploration.[7]

Common bile duct cyst or choledoclal cyst is known to be an uncommon cause of neonatal cholestatic jaundice. Indeed, it is associated with distal biliary tract obstruction and presents a clinical picture that is indistinguishable from BA. Choledochal cysts usually manifest during infancy and childhood, the clinical findings including jaundice, right upper quadrant pain and masses. They are considered congenital because do occur in fetuses and neonates. Their origin may be related to an abnormal connection between the pancreatic duct and common bile duct and chronic

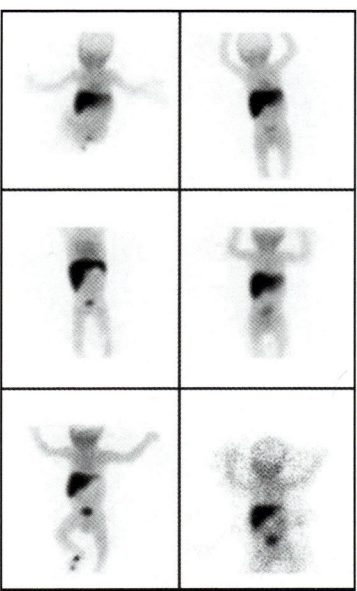

Fig. 12.29: ^{99m}Tc-mebrofenin hepatobiliary scintigraphy

reflux of pancreatic juice into the bile duct, resulting in irritation of the duct and subsequent dilatation.

Choledochal cysts appear as cystic or fusiform dilatation of the common bile duct at radiography. Ultrasonography is the best initial method of evaluating the intra- and extrahepatic bile ducts dilatation. Computed tomography is considered to be more accurate in delineating the intrahepatic biliary tree. Early detection and treatment of choledochal cyst in neonates are important for preventing serious complications due to biliary obstruction. Hepatobiliary scintigraphy provides physiologic information on hepatic uptake and accumulation of radionuclide in the dilated biliary tree.[6-9] The scintigraphic demonstration of tracer accumulation within the choledocal cyst (delayed 24 hours imaging) serves to exclude other cystic right upper quadrant masses from the differential diagnosis (Fig. 12.30).

Congenital biliary ectasia or Caroli's disease consists of segmental saccular intrahepatic bile ducts dilatation and may present with hyperbilirubinemia; the complicated form of Caroli's disease, bile ducts dilatation plus congenital hepatic fibrosis, is more common. Hepatobiliary scintigraphy confirms the diagnosis in most cases, showing multiple photopenic areas in initial images, and then gradual accumulation of tracer in the same areas as radiopharmaceutical is excreted into the biliary system (Fig. 12.31).

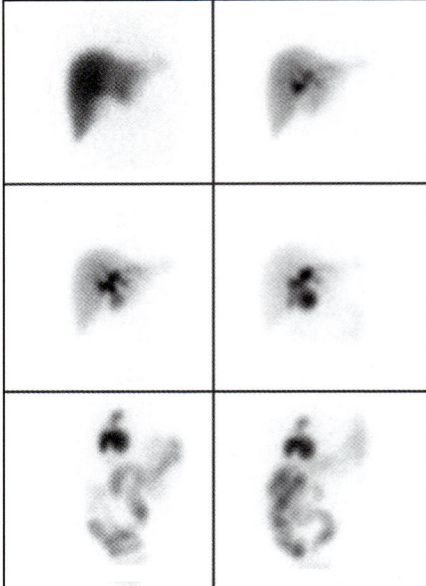

Fig. 12.30: ^{99m}Tc-mebrofenin hepatobiliary scintigraphy showing choledochal cyst

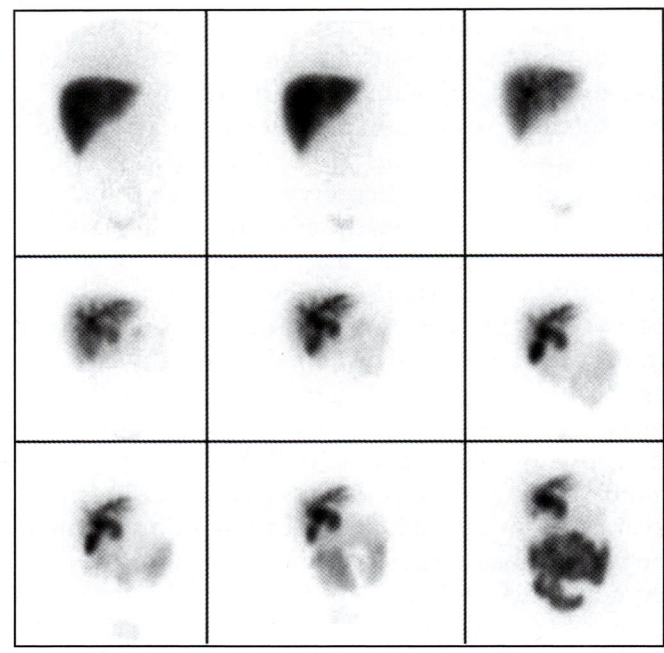

Fig. 12.31: ^{99m}Tc-mebrofenin hepatobiliary scintigraphy in a case of caroli's disease intrahepatic photopenic area (dilatation) filling up with time

Liver Transplantation

Liver transplantation (LT) is an accepted and successful mode of treatment for pediatric end-stage liver disease. Hepatobiliary imaging in children who have undergone LT is of major importance. As already described, it can assess vascularity, parenchymal function, biliary drainage, possible presence of a bile leak, and obstruction. In suspected bile leak, hepatobiliary imaging provides information generally not available by other techniques, except for direct cholangiography.[8,9] If the amount of intraperitoneal accumulation of the tracer is greater than that entering the gastrointestinal tract, surgery is usually indicated. Hepatobiliary scintigraphy has good sensitivity and specificity for the detection of biliary leak and biliary stricture after transplantation: no patient with normal scintigraphy requires biliary intervention; some patients with biliary leaks and few with strictures suggested by scintigraphy require intervention.

Imaging of the Spleen

Indications for splenic scintigraphy in children include evaluation of abdominal trauma, detection of accessory spleens, polysplenia, asplenia, heterotaxia, functional asplenia, splenosis, infarction, left upper quadrant mass, splenomegaly, splenic abscess, and diaphragmatic eventration.[6,7]

Specific splenic imaging with ^{99m}Tc labeled denatured red blood cells is preferable in most instances. The usual dose of ^{99m}Tc denatured red blood cells is 3.7-18.5 MBq (100-500 µCi) given intravenously 0.5 - 1.0 hour before imaging. Anterior, posterior, right anterior, left anterior, and left lateral projections should be obtained. Delineation of small defects, such as splenic fracture, or small accessory spleens can be made more effectively using a 3 mm pinhole collimator or SPECT imaging.

In abdominal trauma, splenic scintigraphy is effective in diagnosing splenic fracture or rupture. Although, accessory spleens and splenosis can be detected with ^{99m}Tc-sulfur colloid, 99mTc heat denatured red blood cells are the agent of choice in these conditions (Fig. 12.32).

Non-visualization of the spleen means that the spleen is not functioning, not the absence of the spleen. In these patients, splenic scintigraphy plays a role in the identification of functional splenic: Tissue and assists in the decision whether to place the patient on a long-term prophylactic antibiotic regimen. Patients suffering from sickle cell disease may have functional asplenia. Functional asplenia is diagnosed by non-visualization of the spleen with ^{99m}Tc sulfur colloid or, better, with ^{99m}Tc denatured red blood cell imaging.

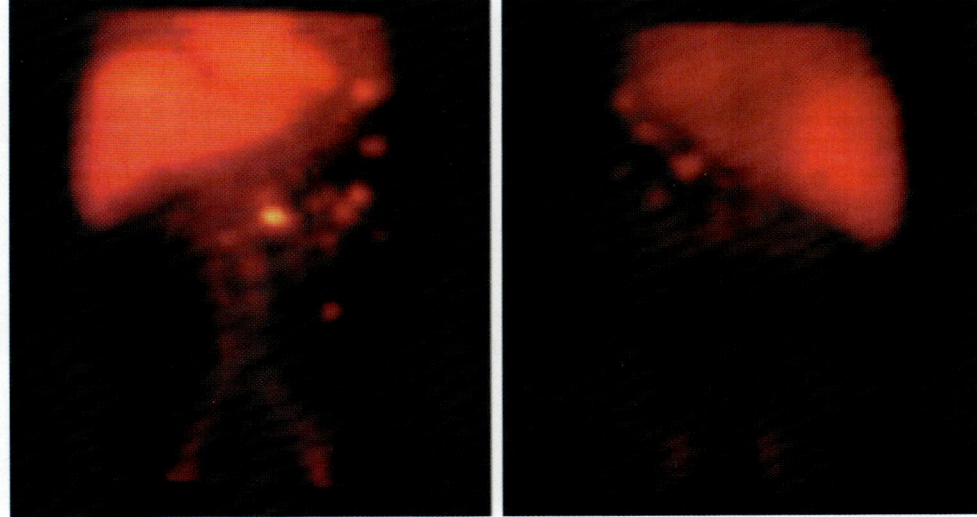

Fig. 12.32: ^{99m}Tc-heat denatured RBC scan showing multiple accessory spleen

PET IMAGING IN PEDIATRICS

Positron Emission Tomography (PET) is a medical imaging technology, which has an unparalleled capability to generate images of body function and metabolism. In PET, positron-emitting radionuclides are used. Many PET tracers are physiologically identical to natural biological substrates. As a result, a PET tracer in the body follows the same physiological pathways as the non-radioactive natural substrate that it mimics. Quite often, internal chemical or physiological changes related to metabolism predate or exceed changes in the structural appearance of tissue or organ. PET uses internal tracers to measure the rate of internal processes and can often distinguish between normal and abnormal physiology in cases where no anatomical change has occurred. PET applications in children have provided useful insights into the physiology and pathophysiology of various diseases and conditions. As are most nuclear medicine and radiological procedures in children, PET scans are challenging to perform in the pediatric age groups and particular attention to preparation and detail are necessary to optimize image quality.[11]

REFERENCES

1. Sorensen JA, Phelps MF, Eds. Physics in Nuclear Medicine. Grune and Stratton, New York, 1996.
2. Ramesh Chandra, Ed. Nuclear Medicine Physics, Williams and Wilkins, Philadelphia. 1998.
3. Living with Radiation, National Radiological Protection Board 1981.
4. Treves S T, Ed. Pediatric Nuclear Medicine, Springer-Verlag, New York 1995.
5. Early P J, Sodee D B, Eds. Principles and Practice of Nuclear Medicine, Mosby, Philadelphia 1995.
6. Henry N Wagner Jr, Ed. Principles of Nuclear Medicine, WB Saunders Co, Philadelphia 1995.
7. Murray I P C, Ell P J, Eds. Nuclear Medicine in clinical diagnosis and treatment, Churchill Livingstone, Edinburgh 1998.
8. Henkin R E, Eds. Nuclear Medicine, Mosby, St Louis 1996.
9. Harbert J C, Eckelman W C and Neuman R D, Eds. Nuclear Medicine: diagnosis and therapy, Thieme Medical Publishers, Inc., New York 1996.
10. Wilson M A, Ed. Textbook of Nuclear Medicine, Lippincott-Raven Publishers, Philadelphia 1998.
11. Wieler H J, Coleman R E, Eds. PET in clinical oncology, Springer, Berlin 2000.
12. Duncan R, Ed. SPECT imaging of the brain, Kluwer Academic Publishers, London 1997.
13. Braverman L E, Utiger R D, Eds. Werner and Ingbar's. The Thyroid- A fundamental and Clinical text, Lippincott Williams and Wilkins, Philadelphia 2000.
14. Gerson M C, Ed. Cardiac Nuclear Medicine, McGraw-Hill, New York-New Delhi 1997.
15. Collier B D, Fogelman I, Rosenthall L, Eds. Skeletal Nuclear Medicine, Mosby, St. Louis 1996.
16. Krishnamurthy G T, Krishnamurthy S, Eds. Nuclear Hepatology, Springer, Berlin 1996.

Pediatric Interventional Radiology

Deep N Srivastava, Bobby Batra, Dheeraj Gandhi

Over the past two to three decades, there has been rapid growth of a new and intrusive subspecialty of Radiology called *'Interventional Radiology'*. Interventional radiology has become an umbrella description of all types of radiological procedures that are invasive in nature. While many of these procedures are therapeutic or curative, others are of purely diagnostic in nature.

It is difficult to classify the various interventional techniques in radiology in a logical and comprehensive fashion. We intend to provide a general overview of common interventional procedures in pediatric practice.

PRE-PROCEDURE PLANNING

The most important part of pediatric interventional procedure is adequate planning and good sedation. The sedation protocols and regimes in pediatric patients vary widely. Most pediatric interventional studies require some form of sedation or anesthesia. A physician who is trained to handle the subsequent complications (if any) and intubation should administer the drugs. The patients' vitals must be monitored continuously during the examination and we usually monitor with a pulse oximeter during entire study. An oxygen saturation of 45% or above is adequate oxygen saturation, however a value below 80% is suggestive of significant desaturation. Premedication using phenobarbitol and meperidure is beneficial in children over 18 month's.[1] In our institution, we frequently use a cocktail regimen of chlorpromazine, pethidine and phenergan. If there are no contraindications, ketamine also provides a good combination of sedation and immobility. General anesthesia may be necessary if intravenous sedation has failed or in procedures requiring longer time.

CLASSIFICATION OF PEDIATRIC INTERVENTIONAL STUDIES

As has been pointed out earlier, it is difficult to classify the vast array of interventional techniques in a rational and comprehensive manner. However, broadly the interventional techniques may be classified) into vascular and non-vascular procedures (Table 13.1). Some of these techniques have been described below.

PEDIATRIC ANGIOGRAPHY

Pediatric vascular procedures require a number of technical modifications of standard adult angiography.[1-4] With the advent of Doppler Ultrasound, CT, CT angiography, MRI and Magnetic Resonance Angiography the need for angiography has decreased markedly. Many pediatric angiograms are now performed with an aim of endovascular intervention. Table 13.2 sums up most of the current indications of diagnostic angiography in pediatric patients.

Arterial access, especially in small children, is often the most difficult part of the procedure. Percutaneous cannulation of the femoral artery, using the modified Seldinger technique is the most commonly utilized route.[5] In the newborn, the umbilical artery may be used for arterial access.[2]

It is advisable to use the smallest and least traumatic needles and catheters wherever feasible. The femoral arteries of young children are small, easily

Table 13.1: Pediatric interventional procedures

Vascular

Diagnostic
- Angiography
- Venography

Therapeutic
- Angioplasty
- Embolization
- Sclerotherapy
- Central venous line insertion
- Foreign body retrieval
- Transjugular route interventions

Non-vascular
- Aspiration: Abscess, pleural effusion, ascites, fluid collections
- Drainage: Abscess, pleural effusion, fluid collections
- Biopsy
- Procedures related to gastrointestinal tract:
  - Percutaneous gastrostomy/Gastrojejunostomy
  - Balloon Dilatation of esophagus, bile duct
  - Foreign body removal
  - PTC and PTBD procedures
- Procedures related to genitourinary tract:
  - Percutaneous nephrostomy
  - Balloon dilatation of ureter
  - Stone removal

Table 13.2: Common indications of diagnostic angiography in children	
Cerebral angiography	Subarachnoid hemorrhage, unexplained cerebral ischemia, vascular complication of trauma, vascular anomaly
Thoracic angiography	Congenital heart disease, hemoptysis, AV fistula, pulmonary thromboembolism
Visceral angiography	Hypertension, GI bleeding, vascular ischemia after organ transplanation
Extremity angiography	Penetrating injury, vascular malformation, correction of complex congenital anomalies

traumatized and prone to thrombosis and spasm.[6] The puncture is usually made 1 cm below the inguinal crease with needle directed nearly horizontally to enter the common femoral artery just below the inguinal ligament. Small gauge needles (19-22G) are used, depending upon patient's size and weights. They can accept small guidewires. When repeated catheter exchanges are anticipated, use of 4-5 Fr sheaths are recommended. Most of the pediatric interventional procedures can be accomplished with 3 and 4 - For catheters. A bolus of 100 U of heparin per kilogram of body weight is given as soon as the catheter has been inserted.

At the end of the procedure, the catheter is removed. If the catheter cannot be easily withdrawn, it may indicate spasm of the artery. Infiltration of lidocaine around the artery or intra-arterial injection of dilute nitroglycerine will usually relieve the spasm.[2] After removal of the catheter, pressure is applied to puncture site for 10-15 mins. to stop the bleeding. Peripheral pulses of the lower limbs must be monitored for 24 hours after the study.

In experienced hands, major complications of pediatric angiography are rare.[5] Major complications are usually observed at the site of puncture. Thrombosis of femoral artery is a grave complication, which may necessitate immediate surgery.[5] Spasm of the artery and excessive bleeding from the puncture site are also seen occasionally. The other potential complications are false aneurysm formation, AV fistula, infection and systemic embolization. Infants and small children are particularly susceptible to dehydration, fluid overload and hypothermia.

PEDIATRIC VENOGRAPHY

The venography in pediatric patients is sometimes done to look for venous element in venous malformations or in cases of varicosities to look for Klippel-Trenaunay syndrome or deep vein thrombosis (Figs 13.1A to C).[7]

PEDIATRIC VASCULAR INTERVENTIONS

Angioembolization

Angioembolization has been described extensively in the radiological and surgical literature. Various embolising materials both temporary and permanent are used for this purpose. Most common indications of embolization in children are listed in Table 13.3.

The technique of embolization in children is similar in general to those used in adults. It requires superselective catheterization of supplying arteries.[8] Small arterial sheaths and catheters, especially microcatheters of variable stiffness are used.[9] For

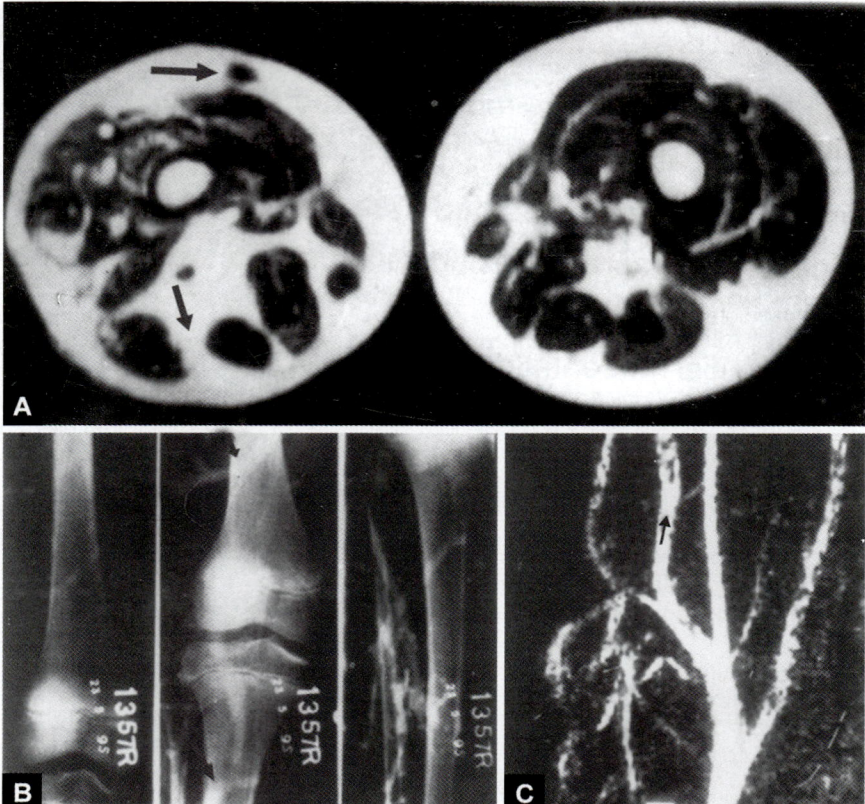

Figs 13.1A to C: Klippel–Trenaunay syndrome right leg **A.** Axial T1 MR shows atrophy with patchy increase in signal intensity affecting all muscle groups. There is increase in the fat in intermuscular planes (small arrow). One Klippel-Trenaunay vein (large arrow) is also seen **B.** MR angiogram shows Klippel-Trenaunay veins as well as their communications with the popliteal and superficial femoral vein **C.** Ascending phlebogram shows two Klippel-Trenaunay veins, one communicating with the popliteal vein (arrow) and the other with the superficial femoral vein (arrow). (hypoplastic deep veins in the leg are also seen)

Table 13.3: Indications of angioembolization in children

- Congenital vascular malformations[10] (Figs 13.2A to 13.3C)
- Presurgical or primary treatment of hypervascular
  Tumors: Hepatoma, hepatoblastoma, hemangiosarcomas, hemangioendothelioma non-responsive to non-invasive therapy, angiolipomas, angiomyolipoma, etc.[11]
- Acute or chronic bleeding:
  - Gastrointestinal bleeding[12] (Fig. 13.4)
  - Hematurea (Figs 13.5 to 13.6B)
  - Post-traumatic (Figs 13.7A to 13.8B)
- Ablation of splenic tissue (in hypersplenism)
- Portosystemic surgical shunts[13] (Figs 13.9A and B)
- Ablation of renal tissue (hypertension)
- Anomalous or hypertrophied arteries to lungs
- Systemic-pulmonary shunts.

short-term embolization, autologous clot is often used. The most commonly used agents are Gelfoam and Ivalon (polyvenyl alcohol particles). For long-term occlusion, isobutyl cyanoacrylate, steel coils and detachable balloons are used. The soft tissue venous malformations can also be treated by percutaneous injection of sclerosing agent like alcohol, sodium tetradecyl sulphate, etc. (Figs 13.10A to D).[14]

Transcatheter embolization provides a quick and relatively simple means of therapy and avoids potentially difficult surgery. The hazard of embolizing tissues other than the target organ is a constant concern in the interventional radiology and account for most of its significant complications.[15]

Angioplasty

The percuatenous transluminal angioplasty (PTA) is used infrequently in children due to the absence of atherosclerotic disease.[16] PTA, however, has been successfully employed in treatment of renal artery stenosis.[16,17] Postrenal transplant anastomoses and surgically created access fistulae have also been treated. Venous obstructions, such as catheter related stenosis, IVC stenosis and hepatic venous stenosis (Budd-Chiari syndrome) also constitute the indications of PTA.

This procedure involves passing of a balloon catheter through the area of vascular stenosis. With constant monitoring of the pressure within the balloon, successive dilatation of stenosis is performed under fluoroscopic guidance.

The hazards of PTA include arterial spasm, occlusion and perforation, embolization to the target organs and intimal dissection.[16]

PTA has many advantages over surgery. It is usually performed under local anesthesia. The length of hospital stay is short and repeat procedure can easily be performed if the stenosis recurs.

Thrombolysis

Majority of pediatric vascular occlusion is the result of catheterization.[6] Thrombolytic therapy is effective

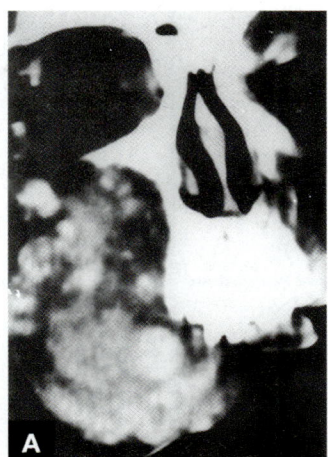
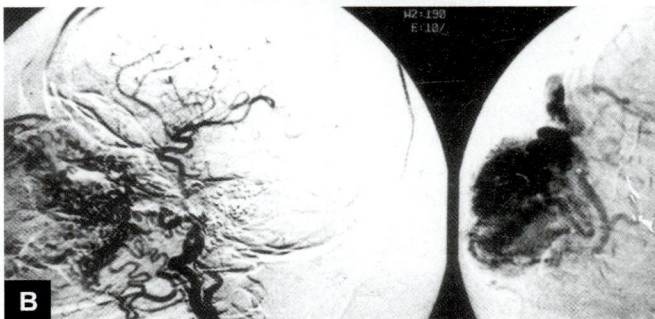

Figs 13.2A and B: Arteriovenous malformations (AVMs) of cheek. **A.** CT shows soft tissue vascular mass overlying maxilla, mandible, and inferior orbital margin **B.** On DSA the mass is supplied by branches of left external carotid artery with early venous filling

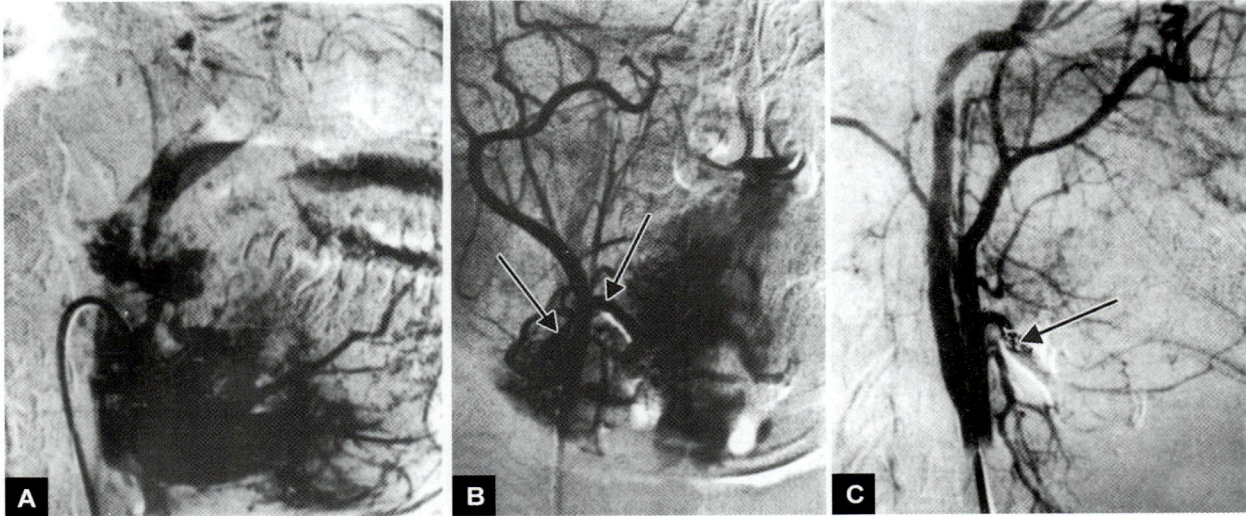

Figs 13.3A to C: A. Hemangioma submandibular region **B.** supplied by right facial and lingual arteries (arrows), **C.** the common origin of which was embolized by steel coils (arrow)

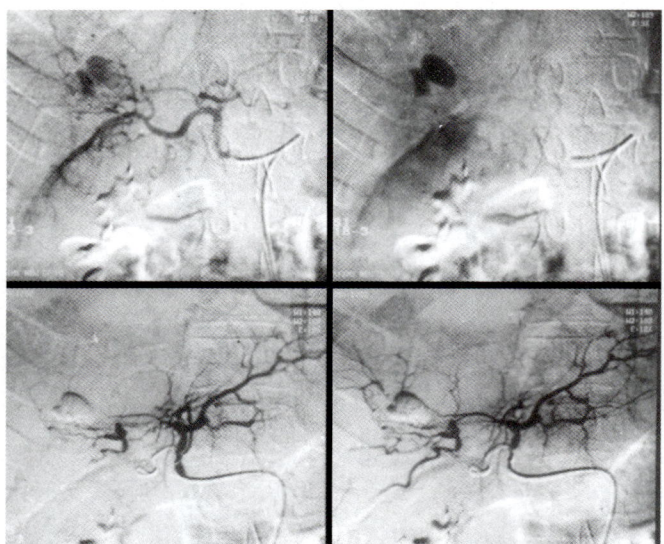

Fig. 13.4: Common hepatic angiogram in a case of hemobilia following a road traffic accident showing a bleeding vessel in right lobe of liver (upper images). Post embolization angiogram is not showing leakage of contrast (lower images)

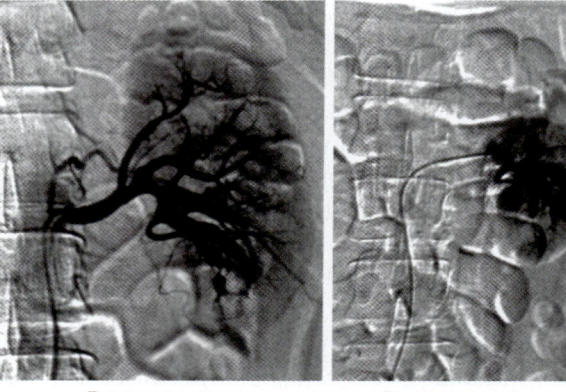

Fig.13.5: Left renal angiogram in a case of postrenal biopsy with massive hematuria is showing a small aneurysm near lower pole. Postembolization angiogram is not showing the aneurysm. The hematuria was stopped after embolization

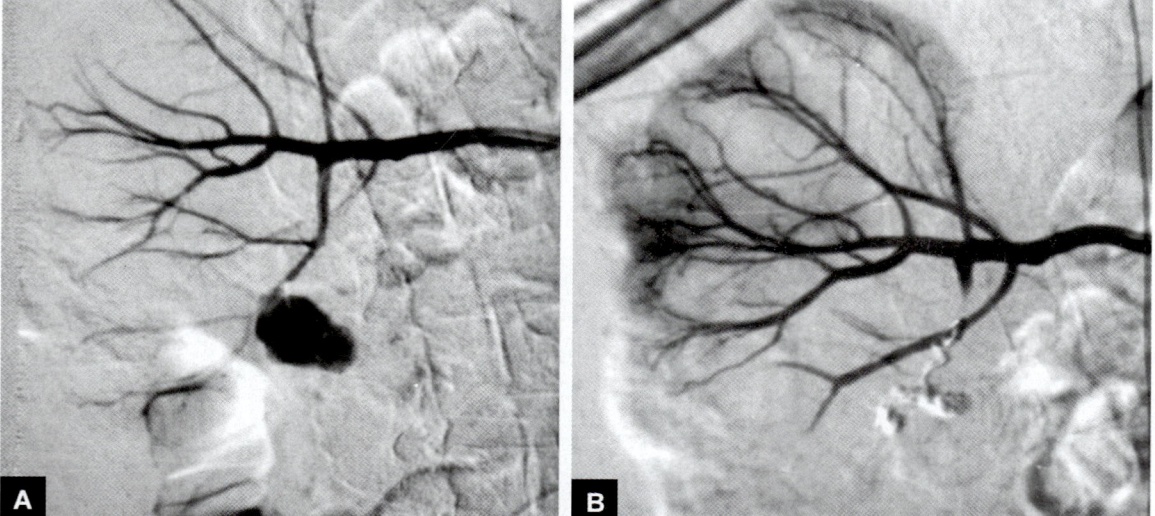

Figs 13.6A and B: A. Right renal angiogram in a case of post-pyelolithotomy with hematuria is showing a large aneurysm **B.** This aneurysm was embolised with steel coils. Postembolization angiogram is not showing the aneurysm (the hematuria was stopped after embolization)

in restoring lower extremity circulation in 70-84% of patients with femoral artery thrombosis after cardiac catheterization.[18] Other indications include central venous thrombosis, neonatal aortic thrombosis,[19] renal vein and dural sinus thrombosis, pulmonary artery thrombosis and other vascular anastomosis.[2]

The techniques of administration include systemic high-dose infusion of streptokinase, urokinase and selective direct infusion into the clot. Low-dose direct clot infusion is used in the presence of contraindications to high dose IV thrombolytic therapy and after failure of IV treatment. The bleeding from the

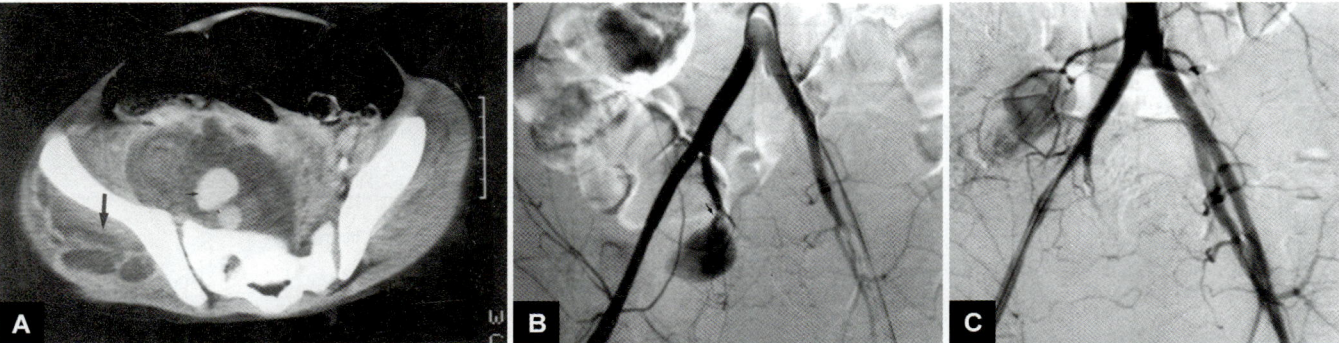

Figs 13.7A to C: A. CT of a eight year-child a road traffic accident victim is showing a large hematoma on right side of the pelvic cavity with extravasation of contrast (small arrow) with associated soft tissue injury (large arrow) **B.** The right common iliac angiogram is showing bleeding from right internal iliac artery trunk (arrow) **C.** Post-embolization aortogram shows complete stoppage of bleeding

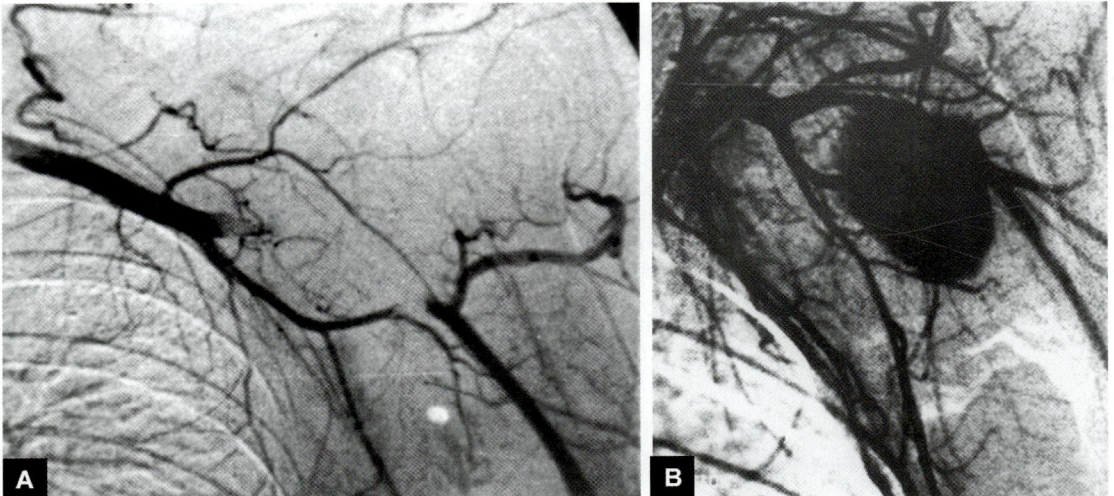

Figs 13.8A and B: A. Road traffic accident victims showing thrombozed left axillary artery with filling of brachial artery from collaterals, **B.** large pseudoaneurysm from axillary artery

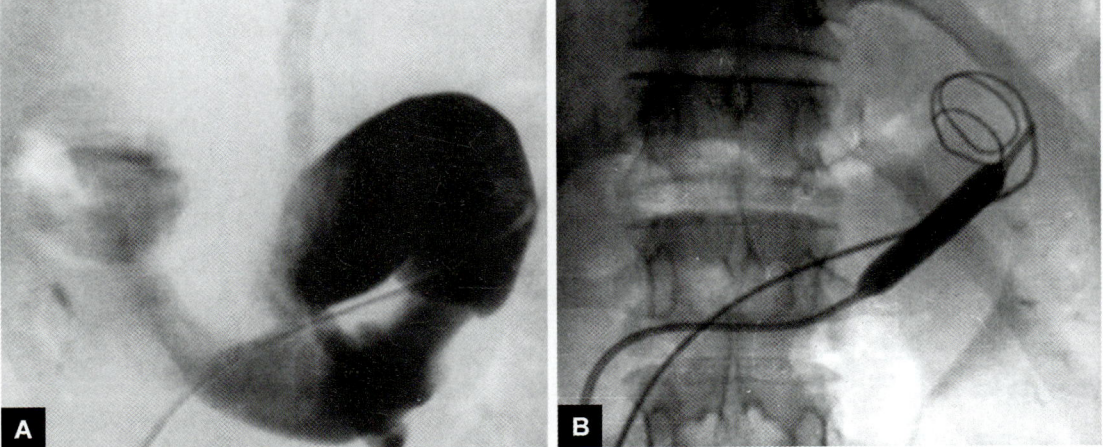

Figs 13.9A and B: A. Angiogram of a patient of hepatic failure and encephalopathy after creation of portosystemic shunt few years' back shows distal splenorenal shunt with patient anastomosis **B.** This shunt was embolized by releasing steel coil after inflating 10 mm balloon at anastomotic site (there was complete occlusion of surgical shunt after embolization procedure)

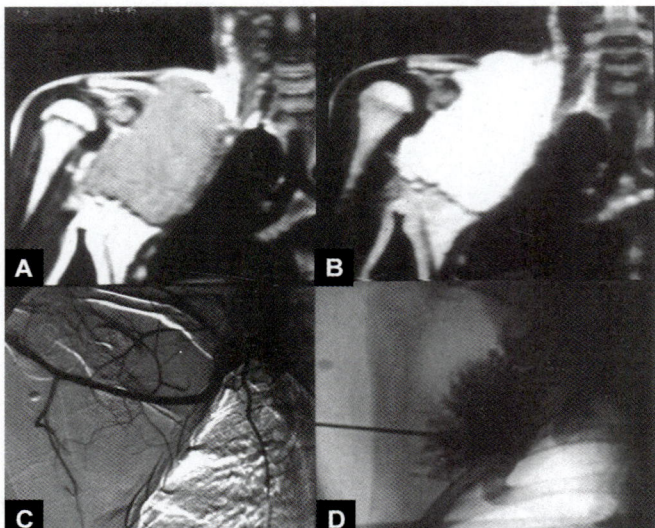

Figs 13.10A to D: Venous hemangioma of axilla with supraclavicular extension. **A.** The mass is mildly hyperintense to muscles on T1, **B.** and hyperintense on T2, **C.** On DSA the mass is not vascular with mass effect over axillary artery with splaying of its lateral thoracic and subscapular branches. There is no venous filling, **D.** Percutaneous aspiration and injection of contrast shows multiple dilated vascular spaces. (The pain disappeared and the size was reduced after injection of sclerosing agent through the same needle)

arteriotomy site is rare in children undergoing thrombolytic infusion.[2]

Intravascular Foreign Body Retrieval

The need to remove foreign bodies is well documented. Sepsis, thrombosis, myocardial perforation and systemic embolization have all been reported[16] as complications of retained foreign bodies. Most frequent device encountered is a broken CVP catheter. Subclavian IV lines, ventriculo-atrial shunts and bullets have been removed angiographically, obviating a major surgery. Loop snare technique[20] is probably the most widely used method. It involves positioning the introducing catheter near the foreign body and snaring with the closed loop. Two other popular approaches are modified bronchoscopic forceps and an adaptation of Dormia basket.[16]

New Applications

Transjugular liver biopsy is indicated in the presence of undiagnosed severe liver disease complicated by coagulopathy.[16] Transjugular intrahepatic porto-systemic shunting (TIPS) may be performed in patients with GI bleeding from esophageal varices, not controlled by endoscopic sclerotherapy[21] (Figs 13.11 to 13.14C).

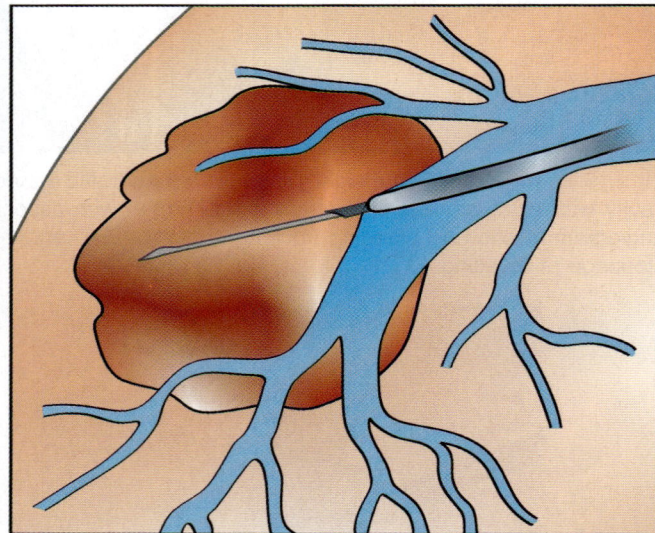

Fig. 13.11: Diagrammatic representation of technique of transjugular biopsy shows that the biopsy is obtained by passing the needle through the wall of the hepatic vein. The shaded area is the hepatic mass and the needle shown is quick core biopsy needle

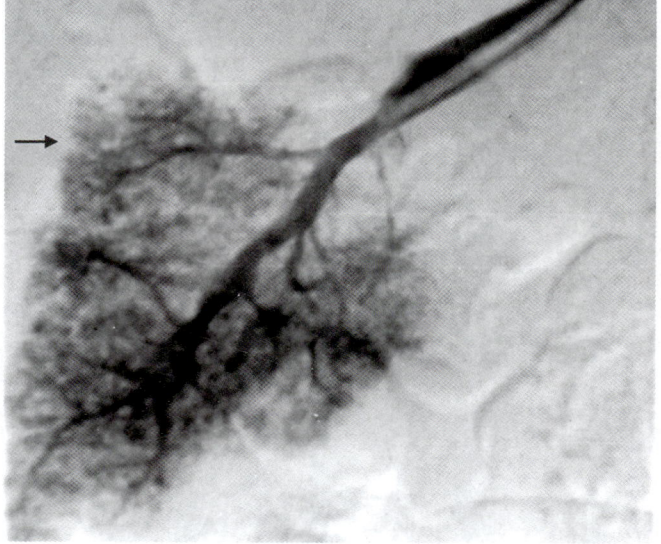

Fig. 13.12: Fulminant hepatic failure secondary to hepatitis B. The hepatogram obtained prior to liver biopsy shows a small shrunken liver. There is increased space (arrow) between liver and the abdominal wall due to ascites

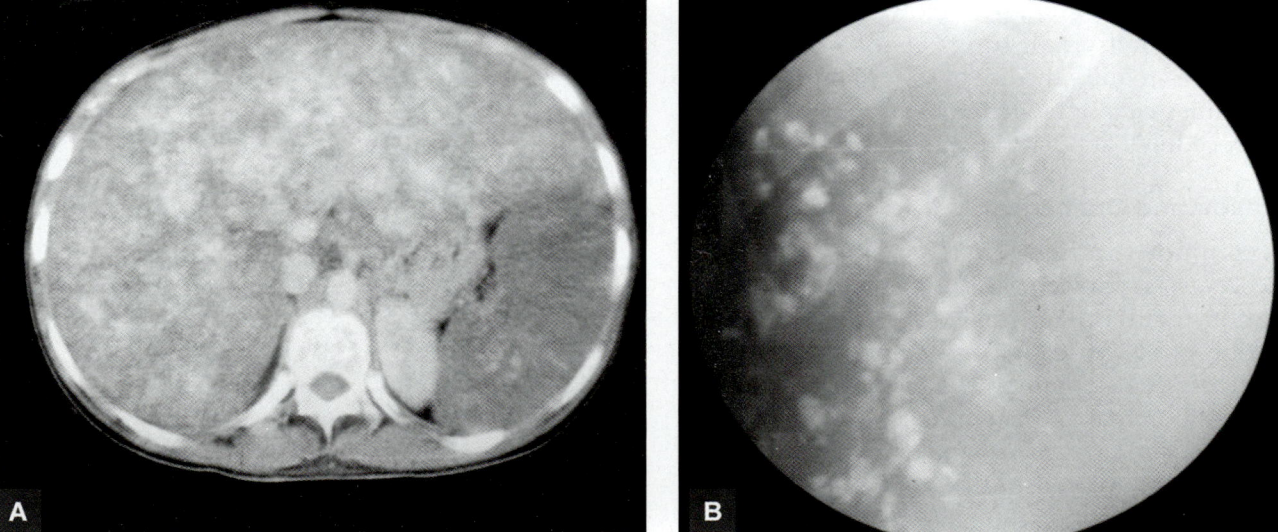

Figs 13.13A and B: Non-Hodgkin's lymphoma liver. Contrast enhanced CT liver **A.** showing diffuse and nodular hepatic involvement. Liver biopsy was taken through transjugular route **B.** because of increased prothrombin time

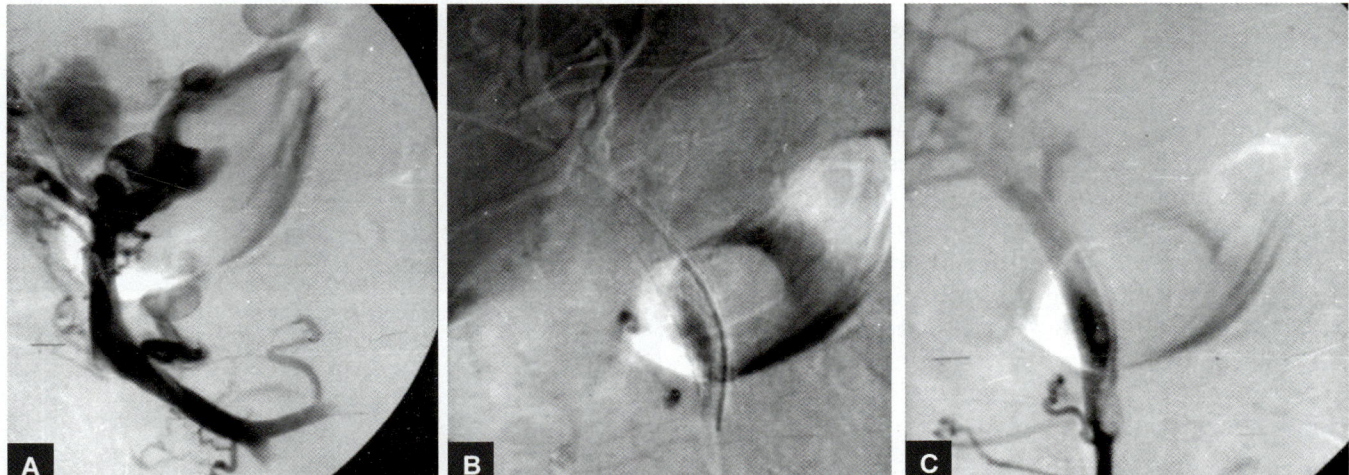

Figs 13.14A to C: The angioplasty and wall stent placement in a periportal collateral in a patient of portal hypertension with recurrent variceal bleeding not responding to medical or endoscopic treatment, **A.** Transjugular portal hepaticovenogram showing that the main portal vein is replaced by multiple periportal collaterals with marked hepatofugal flow in left gastric vein, which is dilated, **B** and **C.** A wall stent has been placed after dilating one of the periportal collateral

Radiologic insertion of central venous catheters is becoming more common. The procedures involve the use of sonographic or venographic guidance of venous cannulation and subsequent fluroscopic catheter placement.

PEDIATRIC NONVASCULAR PROCEDURES

In many clinical situations non-vascular interventional procedures can provide an effective alternative to surgery without being as invasive and usually with less morbidity and rapid recovery. It is important to review all preprocedure imaging studies before starting the interventional procedure. Review of previous images is helpful in planning the correct and safest approach to the abnormality. It is important to distinguish viable from necrotic tissue, for biopsy. A vast number of procedures can be easily performed using ultrasonography (USG) and fluoroscopy. At our center, we prefer to use USG wherever possible as it provides real time guidance. However, very small lesions, parenchymal lung lesions and bony abnormalities require the use of CT guidance as these abnormalities cannot be imaged using USG. Some of these procedures are described below.

Aspiration and Drainage

The common indications of aspiration are thoracocentesis, paracentesis, ultrasound guided hip aspiration for the diagnosis of septic arthritis and aspiration of abscesses (e.g. amoebic and pyogenic liver abscess). The common indications for drainage are intra-abdominal and pelvic abscesses, obstructive hydronephrosis, lung abscess and empyema.[2,22,23] Less frequently encountered indications are drainage of lymphocoeles, infected biliomas and urinomas.

These procedures are done under real time guidance using USG or under the guidance of CT. The aspiration needle is inserted into the abnormality for aspiration and drainage procedures, taking care to avoid neurovascular structures and bowel loops. Spinal needles (18-22G) or Chiba needles are frequently used for aspirations depending on the viscosity of the fluid. In drainage procedures, the initial puncture is done by Chiba needle. With a modified Seldinger's technique, over a 0.018" wire, a 4-Fr coaxial dilating system (Micropuncture introducer set, COOK) that accepts a 0.038" guide wire is placed. After sequential dilatations, 8 to 14-Fr catheter is placed in the collections.

Biopsy Procedures

The accurate positioning of biopsy needles and instruments in the areas of interest has been greatly facilitated by improvements in imaging equipments in recent years. The accurate guidance of biopsies by biplane angiography, ultrasound, CT and, more recently MRI[24] has made it possible to obtain samples from sites previously thought inaccessible. Most of these biopsies in pediatric patients can be accomplished under sedation and local anesthesia.

The indications of percutaneous biopsy in children may be to determine and establish the cause of general organ dysfunction (hepatitis, glomerulonephritis etc.), to determine the pathology of a tumor or infections process (Figs 13.15A to C).

In adult patients, cytology from a fine needle aspiration (FNAB) is often adequate to diagnose

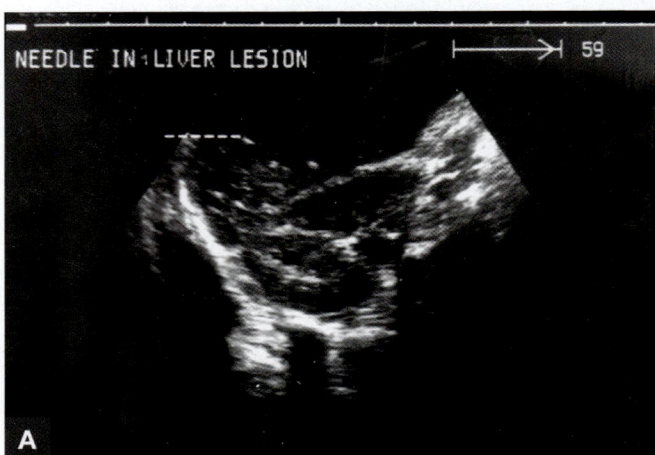
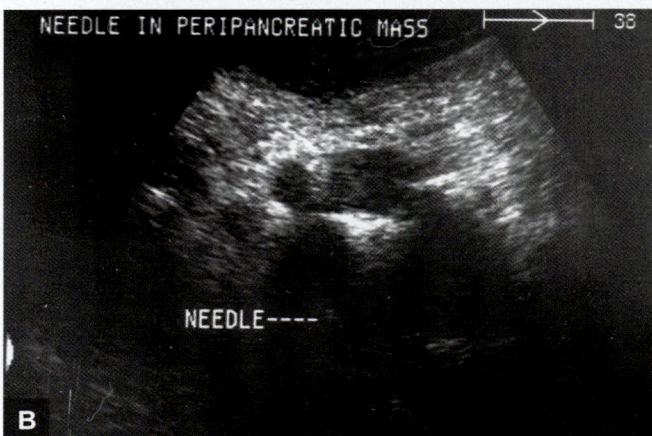
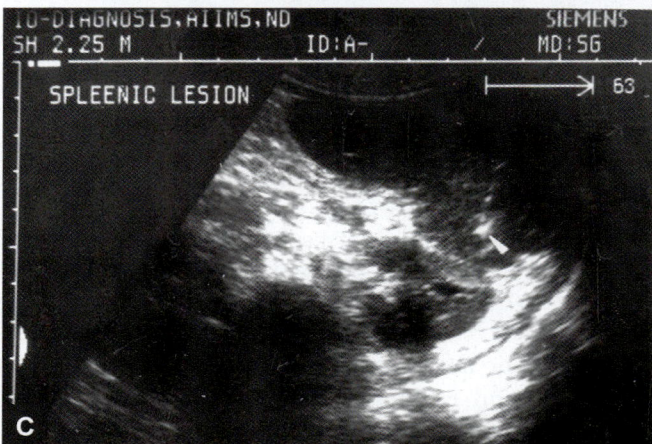

Figs 13.15A to C: Ultrasound guided biopsy taken from **A.** liver mass **B.** peripancreatic mass **C.** splenic mass

carcinomas. In children, however, frequently there is a need to obtain a core biopsy[2] because neoplasms are often sarcomas and round cell tumors. In addition, there may be a need to establish cytogenetic findings, which aid in diagnosis and prognosis of tumor for example neuroblastoma.[2]

We always try to utilize real time ultrasound image guidance to biopsy the lesions. Lesions of solid abdominal viscera (liver, kidney) or of retroperitoneum are easily amenable to US guided biopsies. Biopsy of thoracic lesions, bony lesions and lesions which are not well visualised on USG are best performed using CT guidance.

Solid core biopsies at our center are usually performed with 20-16G needles with either trucut action or spring loaded automated needles. Bone biopsies (e.g. vertebral biopsy) is performed with a 14G trephine needle. FNAB can be performed using Chiba or small gauge spinal needles.

Biopsy techniques should be used with the great caution inpatients with a bleeding diathesis or who are on anti-coagulant therapy. Inpatients in whom hemorrhage is a likely complication, the biopsy track can be embolized at the end of the procedure.[25]

The potential complications of biopsy procedures include infection, hemorrhage, tumor dissemination along needle tracks and in adverting puncture of adjacent organs. In clinical practice, the incidence of serious complications following biopsy procedures by experienced operators is low.

PROCEDURES RELATED TO GASTROINTESTINAL TRACT

Percutaneous Gastrostomy (PG)

Towbin RB et al. has developed an effective technique for percutaneous placement of (Sacks-Vine) gastrostomy tubes in infants and young children.[26] The indications of percutaneous gastrostomy include patients with major swallowing difficulties or debilitating diseases where maintaining adequate nutrition can be a major problem. Majority of the techniques described in the literature involve inflating the stomach with gas or fluid-filled balloon, followed by puncture of the inflated organ through the anterior abdominal wall. The complications of PG include looping of guidewires and catheters in the peritoneum, dislodgement of catheters, acute gastric dilation and leakage of the gastric contents.

Dilatation Procedures

Balloon catheter dilatation of tracheobronchial stenosis in infants and children has been successfully performed for both congenital and postsurgical strictures of the airways.[1] Balloon dilatation of esophageal strictures in children is a very successful form of treatment of congenital stenosis or postoperative stricture following repair of tracheoesophageal fistula.[26]

Removal of Foreign Bodies

Removal of foreign bodies (e.g. coins) from the esophagus with the help of balloon catheters have also been reported.

PERCUTANEOUS TRANSHEPATIC CHOLANGIOGRAPHY (PTC) AND PERCUTANEOUS TRANSHEPATIC BILIARY DRAINAGES (PTBD)

In patients with jaundice, the two most important imaging techniques relevant to potential drainage procedures are ultrasound and direct-contrast cholangiography. A percutaneous cholangiogram is carried out prior to biliary drainage. If the bile ducts are known to be dilated, it is best to apply suction while gradually withdrawing the needle through the liver until bile is aspirated; this is preferable to intermittent injections of contrast medium, which might obscure the image. Puncture of right-sided ducts can easily be done under fluoroscopic guidance; however, left-sided ducts are better punctured with US guidance. Initial puncture is usually done with a 21 or 22 G needle followed with sequential changes of increasingly larger guidewires and catheters.[27] If an external drainage is desired, a catheter with multiple side holes is placed deep in the biliary tree. It is best to use an entirely closed biliary drainage system,[28] as this is associated with significant reduction in the incidence of bacteriemia following the procedure. In many cases, the stage of external drainage is superseded by the establishment of external-internal drainage at the first session: A catheter is advanced through the stricture, and side holes above and below the obstruction bypass the obstruction and drain internally into the duodenum. The indications of PTBD are same as in adults, both preoperative as well as palliative (Figs 13.16A to 13.17).

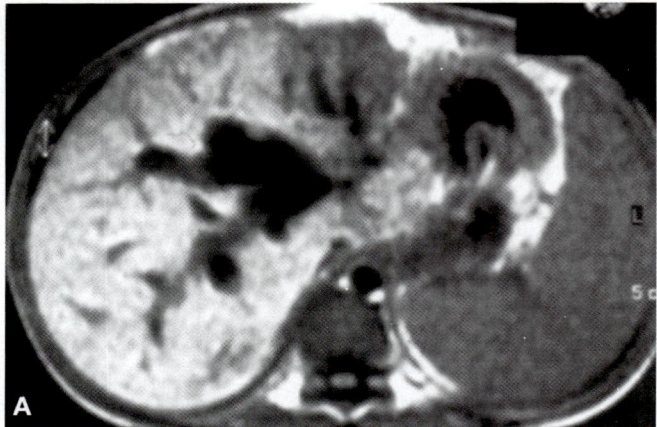

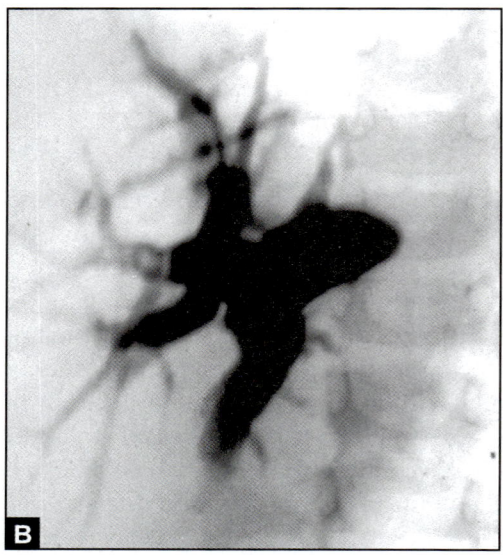

Figs 13.16A and B: Eight-year-old child with progressive jaundice due to right hepatic duct inflammatory stricture. **A.** MR is showing dilated right hepatic ducts, **B.** Preoperative right sided external biliary drainage was done

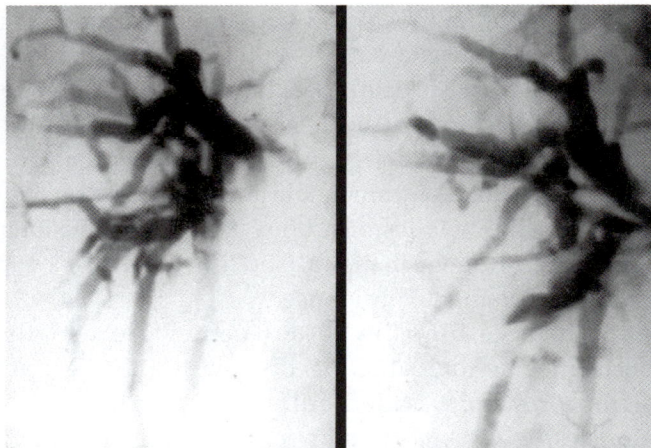

Fig. 13.17: Progressive jaundice due to a malignant mass at porta. Preoperative right-sided external biliary drainage was done using two catheters

REFERENCES

1. Hubbard AM, Fellows KE. Paediatric interventional radiology: Current practice and innovations. Cardiovasc Intervent Radiology 1993;16:267-74.
2. Chung T, Kirks DR. Techniques. In: Practical Pediatric Imaging. Kirks DR (Ed), Lippincott Raven Publishers, Philadelphia 1998;50-63.
3. Burrows PC, Robertson RL, Bames PD. Angiography and the evaluation of cerebrovascular disease in childhood. Neuroimaging Clin N Am 1996;6:561-88.
4. Tonkin IL, Stapleton FB, Roy SL. Digital substraction angiography in the evaluation of renal vascular hypertension in children. Paediatrics 1988;81:150-58.
5. Stanley P. Angiographic procedure. In Stanley P, ed. Paediatric Angiography, Baltimore: Williams and Wilkins 1982;1-34.
6. Burrows PE, Benson LN, Williams WG, et al. Iliofemoral arterial complications of balloon angiography for systemic obstruction in infants and children. Circulation 1990;82:1697-704.
7. Srivastava DN, Gulati M, Thulkar S, Berry M. Klippel - Trenaunay Syndrome: Unusual MR features. Australasian Radiology 1998;42(1):88-89.
8. Lasjaunias P, Berenstein A. Endovascular treatment of craniofacial lesions. Surgical neuroangiography. Berlin: Springer Verlag 1987;2.
9. Burrows PE, Lasjaunias PL, Ter Brugge KG, Flodmark O. Urgent and emergent embolization of lesions of head and neck in children: indications and results. Paediatrics 1987;80:386-94.
10. Srivastava DN. Angiography in musculoskeletal lesions. In: Berry M, Chowdhury V and Suri S, (Eds). Diagnostic Radiology: Musculoskeletal and Breast Imaging, Ist edn. New Delhi: Jaypee Brothers Medical Publishers (P) Ltd. 1998;22-37.
11. Srivastava DN. Advances in imaging and therapeutic interventions in liver tumours. In: Berry M, Chowdhury V and Suri S (Eds). Diagnostic Radiology: Advances in imaging technology, Ist edn. New Delhi: Jaypee Brothers Medical Publishers (P) Ltd. 2000;169-85.
12. Srivastava DN. Gastrointestinal Haemorrhage- protocols for evaluation. In: Berry M, Chowdhury V and Suri S (Eds). Diagnostic Radiology: Hepatobiliary and Gastrointestinal Imaging, Ist edn. New Delhi: Jaypee Brothers Medical Publishers (P) Ltd. 1997;302-19.
13. Srivastava DN, Yadav S, Sahni P, Pande G. Emergency percutaneous occlusion of surgical porosystemic shunt using steel coils and balloon catheter. Am J Roentgenol 1999;172(5):1453-54.

14. Allison DJ, Adam A. Percutaneous liver biopsy and track embolisation with steel coils. Radiology 1988;169:261-63.
15. Levin DC, Beckman C, Hillman B. Experimental determination in of flow patterns of gelfoam emboli: Safety implications. Am J Roentgenol 1980;134:525-28.
16. Pentecost M. Interventional Radiology and recent advances. In Pediatric Angiography. Stanley P (Ed). Baltimore, Williams and Wilkins 1982:401-28.
17. Saddekni S, Sniderman KW, Hiltons S, Sos TA. Percutaneous transluminal angioplasty of non-athersclerotic lesions. A JU 1980;135:975-82.
18. Wessel DL, Keane JF, Fellows KE, et al. Fibrinolytic therapy for femoral arterial thrombosis after cardiac catheterization in infants and children. Am J Cardiol 1986;58:347-51.
19. Corrigan JJ Jr, Jeter M, Allen D, Malons JM. Aortic thrombosis in a neonate: failure of urokinase thrombolytic therapy. Am J Paediatr Hematol Oncol 1982;4:243-47.
20. Rossi P. "Hook catheter" technique for transfemoral removal of foreign body from right side of the heart. Am J Roentgenol 1970;169:101-06.
21. Srivastava DN. Hepatic interventions through transjugular route. In: Berry M, Chowdhury V and Suri S, Eds. Diagnostic Radiology: Advances in imaging technology, Ist Edn. New Delhi: Jaypee Brothers Medical Publishers (P) Ltd, 2000;186-93.
22. van Sonnenberg E, D' A gostin H B, Casola G, et al. Lung abscess. CT-guided drainage. Radiology 1991;178:347-51.
23. Lee KS, Im JG, Kim YH, et al. Treatment of thoracic multi-loculated empyemas with intracantary urokinase: a prospective study, Radiology 1991;179:771-75.
24. Mueller PR, Stark DD, Simeone JF, et al. MR guided aspiration biopsy: needle design and clinical trials. Radiology 1986;161:605-09.
25. Towbin RB, Ball WS Jr, Bissett GS III. Percutaneous gastrostomy and percutaneous gastrojejunastomy in children. Antegrade approach. Radiology 1988;168:473-76.
26. Hoffer FA, Winter HS, Fellows KE, Folkman J. The treatment of post-operative and peptic oesophageal strictures after oesophageal atresia repair: a program including dilatation with balloon catheters. Paediatr Radiol 1987;17:454-58.
27. Cope C. Conversion from small (0.018") to large (0.038 inch) guide wires in percutaneous drainage procedures. Am J Roentgenol 1982;138:170-71.
28. Strosberg SM, Soper NJ. Laparoscopic Cholecystectomy. Current Op Gastroenterol 1993;9:823-34.

Postoperative Care

Bikramjit Singh Sangha

The postoperative period is very critical and carries specific problems. Early in this transitional period, the patient recovers from anesthesia and regains homeostasis. Later the patient repairs the operative and disease injury. Very often, early rehabilitation starts before discharge and continues until the patient is ready to resume normal duties. The postoperative care varies depending upon the severity of disease, nature of the operation, and the patient's health, age, and special needs. Many patients need prolonged postoperative care in the hospital. Sometimes, the patient can be discharged early if close follow-up and extra help at home is assured. Patients with same day surgeries are discharged after brief observation and verification of normal spontaneous respiration, consciousness, and intact gag reflex. Patients, operated with regional anesthesia are usually discharged faster than those operated under general anesthesia. Adequate postoperative pain management and follow up are integral parts of the postoperative care. The patient and guardians should be educated about possible complications, their initial treatment, and telephone numbers or places of contacts, where they can come in case of deterioration.

TRANSPORT TO INTENSIVE CARE UNIT (ICU)

The patient can be observed postoperatively in different locations (PICU, SICU, NICU) depending upon the needs and facilities of an individual institution. A case could be made to transport critical patients to the ICU under mild anesthesia where they can be awakened and deparalyzed in a more controlled environment. This decreases the problems of transition during transport. The transport to ICU should be in a well-controlled manner. Equipment for emergency resuscitation should always be carried, even for transports over short distances. The transport kit should contain a working laryngoscope, a pair of extra endotracheal tubes (current size and a size smaller), bag and appropriately sized mask, stylet, oxygen source, and important emergency drugs. Similarly, it is important that a team, well versed in resuscitation, should accompany the patient during the transport, preferably with ICU nurse and respiratory therapist. Prior to transport, the endotracheal tube (ET) should be secured in good position. Similarly, no patient should be transported until temporary pulmonary and cardiovascular stability is established. Adequate monitoring of the patient during transport is of utmost importance. Heart rate (HR) and oxygen saturation must be monitored; if available and indicated, carbon dioxide (CO_2) (transcutaneous or endtidal) and blood pressure (BP), indirect or invasive, should also be monitored. If ventilating with a bag and mask, it is important to use a manometer to avoid excessive pressures. Extracaution should be taken with exchanging monitors and medication drips on admission to ICU. Only one monitor or vital drip should be changed at a time. For closer control of ventilatory pressures, equipment like the Neopuff® or portable ventilator is preferred over manual bag and mask ventilation.

The importance and need of communication between the caretakers in the operating room (OR) and the ICU cannot be overemphasized. The patient's intravenous fluids, anesthesia, sedation, drugs, vasomotor stability, urine output, laboratory examinations, temperature, and ventilation problems during the operation should be discussed in detail. The patient's need for equipment, intravenous fluids, medication drips, ventilation settings, chest tubes, and any other special items should be related to the ICU staff before the transport is initiated. This enables the ICU staff to plan a smooth admission. The ICU staff should set up equipment well before the patient's arrival. It is important to continue the same level of support after transport as during it, unless the clinical condition demands otherwise. Then changes should be made slowly to adjust to the patient's changing needs. To maintain stability, small but frequent changes are preferred over large and sudden ones. Making one change at a time, instead of several, allows assessment of its net effect. The intensivist's detailed communication with the surgeon and the anesthesiologist greatly aids initial assessment. Some variability in vital signs during transport and admission to the ICU is universal. Usually these changes are transient and do not require specific treatment.

INITIAL ASSESSMENT

Ventilatory assessment should begin by observing the chest movement. Lungs are auscultated to assess the condition of the lungs and the position of the ET. Although pressures used during manual positive pressure ventilation are good guides, one should not try to duplicate those exact pressures on the ventilator. Breathing patterns with mechanical ventilation differ from those with manual bag ventilation. Oxygen (O_2) and CO_2 monitors can help the intensivist optimize ventilator settings. If facilities are available, bedside lung function testing (tidal volume, percent leak, compliance, resistance, and pressure volume curves) can greatly help to reduce ventilator complications. Otherwise, adequate but not excessive chest movements assure optimal tidal volumes. A chest X-ray on admission is mandatory to assess position of the ET, diaphragm, chest tubes, drains, and vascular catheters. In addition, it enables evaluation of heart size, evidence of air leak, plural fluid, atelectasis, pulmonary vascular markings, edema, and other pulmonary conditions.

Simultaneously, the cardiovascular assessment includes heart rate (HR), its rhythm, murmurs, BP, pulses, central venous pressure (CVP), and capillary filling. The abdomen should be assessed for distension, erythema, discoloration, bowel sounds, tenderness, or masses. Measuring the abdominal girth at regular intervals gives a good objective measure of abdominal distension. The neurological exam is important even with the use of narcotics, anesthesia, and muscle relaxants, because markedly abnormal or asymmetrical tone, movement, or pupillary reactions may still indicate a catastrophic complication needing, further evaluation.

It is better to wait for 20-60 minutes before initiating laboratory studies to assess baseline ventilation and metabolic status. They should include arterial blood gas (ABG), serum glucose, electrolytes, blood urea nitrogen (BUN), creatinine, complete blood count (CBC), differential, and platelets. The hematocrit may be spun in the unit to get an immediate result. If bleeding excessively, investigate disseminated intravascular coagulation (DIC) by a DIC-panel including prothrombin time (PT), partial thromboplastin time (PTT), fibrinogen, and fibrin split products (FSP) or D-Dimer. Suspect multiorgan failure in case of prolonged hypoxic or ischemic insult during or before surgery and baseline investigations of liver, kidney, heart, and brain may be indicated.

Precise urinary output measurement is an important monitoring tool in evaluating renal and, indirectly, cardiac function. It also helps to assess electrolyte and fluid needs. Unfortunately, iatrogenic neuromuscular blockade, anesthesia and sedation hamper voluntary micturition. It is advisable to insert a urinary catheter before surgery to measure urinary flow, during and after surgery, in critical patients and the patients with prolonged or complex surgery. A closed drainage system is mandatory to ensure the system's sterility. Once the patient regains the ability to micturate voluntarily, the catheter should be removed promptly.

MONITORING

The level of monitoring varies greatly depending upon the level of observation needed and available equipment. Basic monitoring addresses ECG (heart rate and rhythm disturbances). Particular bed assignment to the patient may also depend on the needs of the patient. Monitor the blood pressure (BP) by continuous direct (Intra-arterial line) or intermittent indirect methods. The frequency of BP monitoring depends upon the condition of the patient. Most patients need to be assessed every fifteen to twenty minutes until stable. Adequate cuff size is very important in order to accurately measure BP. It is also important to change the site of the cuff periodically. The indwelling intra-arterial catheter is the most accurate method for measuring continuous BP. Most commonly, the radial artery is used. Alternatively, the posterior tibial or dorsal pedis artery may be used. Axillary or ulnar arteries are also used occasionally. Avoid using the brachial and temporal arteries. The frequent calibration of arterial lines is necessary to maintain accurate measurements. When confronted with abnormal BP, a dampened arterial line should be suspected; measurements should be verified with other methods while the arterial line is recalibrated. BP is slightly higher in peripheral arteries due to increased resistance.

The central venous pressure (CVP) is used to assess intravascular volume and right ventricular function. Trending rather than any absolute number is important.[1] The tip of the catheter should be in the Superior Vena Cava (SVC) close to right atrium (RA). The catheter is usually inserted percutanously via subclavian, jugular, or femoral veins. Rarely other veins are also used; the catheter may be inserted by cut down as well. Continuous O_2 saturation, partial pressure of oxygen and carbon dioxide in blood (PO_2, PCO_2), pH monitoring by indwelling catheter is possible by keeping the tip in the RA, PA, aorta or peripheral artery. Its cost is prohibitive except in the extremely critical patient who needs frequent blood gases, when it saves money, blood, and infection chances.

The pulmonary artery (PA) is used to measure pulmonary capillary wedge pressure and cardiac output. Mixed venous oxygen (PVO_2) measures the oxygen saturation in the pulmonary artery. Decreased PVO_2 is secondary to either increased metabolic demand or decreased cardiac output (decreased oxygen delivery). Sometimes, the RA blood sample is used, as a substitute of sample from PA line, although it is not a true mixed venous sample. Cardiac output can be measured using Fick's M method.[2]

Approximate Arterial (Art) O_2 Content/100 ml = 1.34 × Hgb × Art O_2 sat (ml of O_2)

Because one gram of oxyhemoglobin carries 1.34 ml O_2

Approximate venous (Ven) O_2 content/100 ml = 1.34 × Hgb × Ven O_2 sat (ml of O_2)

Oxygen consumption = Arterial oxygen content–venous oxygen content

Thus, oxygen consumption = Cardiac output × 1.34 × Hgb (Art O_2 sat–Ven O_2 sat)/100

Or, Cardiac output = K × (Art O_2 sat – Ven O_2 sat)

Where K= constant assuming oxygen consumption stays constant

Thus, cardiac output is inversely proportional to the difference between arterial and mixed venous saturation. Increased mixed venous O_2 saturation indicates improved cardiac output.

The cardiac echocardiogram is also a useful tool to assess cardiac output, cardiac contractility, and blood volume in a hypotensive patient. End diastolic volumes are good indirect measure of intravascular volume and venous return. Visualizing closely touching ventricular walls (the "Kissing's sign") is indicative of low ventricular filling. Tricuspid regurgitation, increased right-sided volumes and pressures, and atrial or ventricular septal bulging toward the left, indicates pulmonary hypertension.

Initially monitor respiration rate at least. It is also important to assess retractions, which are usually secondary to metabolic acidosis, upper airway obstructions, secretions, worsening respiratory status, and atelectasis. The respiratory rate may decrease falsely due to drugs (e.g. narcotics) rather than improving in respiratory status. Fever, anxiety, pain, agitation, drugs, hypoxia, obstruction, or worsening lung disease can increase the respiratory rate.

Intermittent ABG remains the gold standard for evaluating the patient's ventilation and oxygenation. Because this information reflects the patient's status at the moment of sample draw and can change fast, continuous trending monitors are used in addition to isolated ABG sampling. Capillary or even the venous samples can be used to assess pH and ventilation status but they cannot assess oxygenation. The transcutaneous (TCM) monitoring to measure CO_2 and O_2 or alternatively endtidal carbon dioxide ($ETCO_2$) and pulse oximetry can be used as a very important means for continuous evaluations of the ventilation and oxygenation. Verify these measurements periodically with blood gas evaluations. Pulse oximetry is a simple and noninvasive means of pulmonary monitoring but it is not useful in extreme PO_2 ranges. For example, O_2 saturation may not change much when the PO_2 exceeds 100 torr, although it indicates a significant change in clinical condition. Pulse oximetry may not work if perfusion is very low. TCM measurement is perfusion dependent. Decreased perfusion will artificially increase CO_2 and decrease PO_2 readings. TCM can also be used to trend change in perfusion by observing the electricity (miliamperes) needed to keep the probe temperature constant. Increased miliamperes used indicates improved perfusion due to increased cooling of the probe by blood. The trend, rather than any absolute number is more useful. Evaluating the differences of CO_2 and PO_2 in TCM and arterial blood gas can also be used to assess perfusion. Increasing differences in TCM and ABG indicate worsening perfusion, unless it is due to TCM malfunction. Similarly, false high O_2 and low CO_2 may be due to an air leak at the TCM site.

Many devices are currently available to measure continuous or intermittent lung functions. Peak Inspiratory Pressure (PIP), Peak End Expiratory Pressure (PEEP), Mean Airway Pressure (MAP), fraction of the inspiratory oxygen (FIO_2), tidal volume (TV), minute ventilation and intermittent mandatory ventilation (IMV) are used to monitor progress in pulmonary disease. Similarly, compliance, resistance, pressure volume curves can be used to find optimal pressures and inspiratory time (IT). Ideally, IT should be five times the time constant (TC). TC is the product of compliance and resistance. At higher IMV, a shorter IT may be preferred to give enough time to expire. Increased tidal volume leak (inspiratory volume minus expiratory volume) measurement, continuous or intermittent, can give clues to the worsening compliance or obstruction in the ET tube. Increased PIP requirements may indicate atelectasis, pneumonia, edema, pneumothorax, secretions, and obstructed ET tube or ventilator circuit. Noninvasive $ETCO_2$ is also helpful to measure CO_2 continuously. There are some technical difficulties in measuring $ECTO_2$ in the very small patients. Normally, there is a 5-10 torr gradient in between the arterial carbon dioxide pressure (PCO_2) and $ECTO_2$ due to mixing of anatomical dead space. Increased gradient indicates increased dead space, e.g. atelectasis, pulmonary embolism and excessive PEEP. Failure to reach plateau or an extremely low $ETCO_2$ may indicate bronchospasm, as there is minimal expiratory volume or ET slipping into esophagus. Similarly, extremely low cardiac output conditions can also show artificially low $ETCO_2$ despite very high PCO_2 as not much CO_2 is excreted into alveoli. Ventilator leak may cause artificial decrease in $ETCO_2$ also.

Pulmonary artery catheterization is used to measure cardiac output (COP), intracardiac and pulmonary artery pressures. It is also used to continuously monitor mixed venous oxygen saturation and for ventricular pacing. Multiple lumen catheters are available in different sizes (5-7 Fr). Because of desired minimal distance required between different ports to use thermodilution method for COP measurement, it can be used only in preteens or teens. However, a single lumen, thin catheter inserted in the PA, RA, or RV during cardiac surgery is often used in small children including neonates to measure pressure and blood sampling. Small children need special order custom-made catheters with small distance between proximal and distant ports. It has different lumens for right atrium, pulmonary artery occlusion pressure, pulmonary artery blood pressure, floatation and occlusion of balloon and distal thermodilution sensor (for COP). Some also have fifth port for mixed venous oxygen saturation, right ventricular pressure or pacing. Pulmonary artery occlusion is an indirect reflection of left ventricular end-diastolic pressure (LVEDP). The safety or efficacy of these applications to reduce mortality and morbidity in pediatric population is not yet well documented. Similarly, small catheters in the left atrium (LA) put during cardiac surgery have been used to measure LA pressures in critical small children briefly. One should use them with special care as it could generate emboli.

Level of consciousness, pupillary reactions, and responses to verbal commands constitute the basic neurological monitoring. Various methods of monitoring intracranial pressure (ICP) are used to calculate cerebral perfusion pressure (CPP) in head injury and neurosurgical patients. CPP can be calculated by subtracting the ICP from the mean arterial blood pressure (MABP). ICP can be measured noninvasively using external appliance attached directly to the open fontanel of the newborn. Direct ICP measurement is invasive and its use requires the benefits to exceed the risks. Usually it is limited to patients who are nonverbal and the computerized tomogram (CT) determines increased ICP. Nuclear brain scan and transcranial Doppler flow studies can also evaluate cerebral blood flow. Intermittent or continuous EEG monitoring helps diagnose and modify therapy for seizures in comatosed patients.

COMMON PROBLEMS OF POSTOPERATIVE CARE

Metabolic Problems

Patients receive minimal potassium (K) during surgery. Excessive fluids if administered could also dilute serum K. Furthermore, increased urination secondary to excessive fluids or diuretic, could lower the serum K. Alkalosis, as a result of inappropriately excessive ventilation or HCO_3 administration, also decreases serum K. Conversely, metabolic and respiratory acidosis, tissue damage, hemolysis, and decreased renal function (direct or related to cardiovascular insufficiency) can cause hyperkalemia. It is important to have a baseline potassium level postoperatively and reassess it depending upon metabolic, cardiovascular, and renal stability. It is important to establish a reasonable urine output before adding potassium in intravenous fluids. Depending upon the emergency hyperkalemia is treated by holding K, using sodium exchange resins (sodium polystyrene sulfonate), and insulin along with glucose. In critical patients, it is temporarily dealt with by raising pH and Ca infusion. Sustained effects are achieved by dialysis only. In few cases, salbutamol has also been used successfully to reduce serum K for few hours. Because hypokalemia is much easier to treat than hyperkalemia, it is also advisable to keep the serum K at a low normal level until cardiovascular and renal stability is assured. If impending renal insufficiency cannot be ruled out but there is hypokalemia, warranting treatment, infuse 0.5 mEq/kg potassium chloride (KCl) over 1-2 hours. Potassium can never be given by intravenous push, as it can cause death by asystole. Potassium should be kept in a remote secure place such as the pharmacy, separate from routine medications, to avoid accidental intravenous administration.

Hypokalemia can cause ileus and cardiac arrhythmias, more so if the patient is also taking digoxin. One must consider the patient's metabolic status at the time of blood sampling for potassium and ionized calcium (Ca). The serum K or ionized Ca can change significantly with the pH of the sample without much change in whole-body K or total Ca. Alkalosis decreases and acidosis increases both K and ionized Ca. In general, 2-4 mEq/kg/day of K is needed.

Depending upon the amount and type of fluids received during surgery and renal function, the patient may become hypo- or hypernatremic postoperatively. Review of the anesthesia record and discussion with the anesthesiologist can help anticipate the sodium (Na) status and future Na needs of the patient. The sodium status should also be confirmed on admission. Avoid allowing the serum sodium to rise above 155 mEq/L, but if it is present, it should be corrected slowly over 12-24 hours to prevent cerebral edema and subsequent seizures.[3] A sudden decrease in the serum sodium decreases the serum osmolality faster than the osmolality of brain cells, therefore causing cerebral edema by shifts of water. Loop diuretics decrease the serum sodium by increasing Na losses. Suspect inappropriate antidiuretic hormone (ADH) secretion in unexpected hyponatremia. The diagnosis is supported if the serum osmolality falls below 280 mOsm/L while the urine osmolality greater than 400 mOsm/L and is treated by restricting fluids. Increased urine output, diuretics, third spacing, or low intake also causes hyponatremia. The usual Na intake is 3-5 mEq/kg/day.

Magnesium, phosphorus, and calcium should be assessed postoperatively in critical patients, and these may be low due to low intake. Patients with hypoxic insult are at increased risk for hypocalcemia due to endogenous phosphate release. Total calcium may be spuriously low in the case of low serum albumin. Although ionized calcium is a better measure of calcium activity, it is affected by the pH of the sample. Alkalosis will lower the ionized calcium and vice versa. In case of persistent and treatment resistant hypocalcemia, the serum magnesium should be measured, as hypocalcemia is difficult to treat in a patient with hypomagnesemia due to altered parathyroid function. In newborns with persistent hypocalcemia, especially with congenital conotruncal heart disease, one should also consider DiGeorge's syndrome. Generally, it is diagnosed with chromosomal analysis and patient phenotype. Not all cases of DiGeorge's syndrome are complicated by hypocalcemia, or have abnormal chromosomes. Calcium is a potent cardiotonic drug, and hypocalcemia may adversely affect myocardial contractility. Treatment consists of either calcium gluconate or calcium chloride. When calcium is needed urgently, calcium chloride is preferred because all of the calcium is available in the ionized form immediately. Conversely, with calcium gluconate, the calcium ion is released slowly as the gluconate is metabolized. Because of their different molecular weights, the calcium chloride requirement by weight (mg) is only one-third that of calcium gluconate, to deliver the same number of milliequivalents. Calcium chloride is also more irritating than calcium gluconate, so it must be given slowly after diluting, then infused preferably in a central line. When calcium is infused into a peripheral IV, patency of the IV must be confirmed to avoid severe chemical burns in the case of infiltration. There is some concern about long-term aluminum toxicity from calcium gluconate formulations in parenteral nutrition (excessive aluminum is leached from the glass container of calcium gluconate as an impurity). Alternatively, calcium chloride contains very little aluminum.

Hypotension, decreased perfusion, decreased cardiac output; increased metabolic demand, and cold stress can cause metabolic acidosis. Mostly this is self-limited and is treated by treating the primary cause. Renal dysfunction and renal tubular acidosis may also contribute to metabolic acidosis. Use of sodium bicarbonate or sodium acetate should be reserved for extreme cases, using small aliquots and frequent blood gases to avoid overcorrecting. The maximum amount of bicarbonate needed to buffer acidosis is calculated by the following equation:

mEq of HCO_3 = weight (kg) × (0.3) × (base deficit)

Sodium acetate has a slow onset but prolonged effect. Acetate is metabolized, outside liver, in isomolar ratio into HCO_3. It also increases the patient's buffer capacity. Excessive use of bases (HCO_3/acetate) or diuretics may cause metabolic alkalosis due to excessive excretion of chloride. If NaCl or KCl is contraindicated, hypochloremia is treated with ammonium chloride (NH_4Cl), lysine chloride, or arginine chloride. Similarly, tromethamine (THAM) may be used to buffer acidosis instead of the sodium or potassium salts, but renal toxicity often limits its use.

Hyperglycemia

Hyperglycemia from surgical stress, even with adequate pain management, is extremely common in the immediate postoperative period. Such hyperglycemia is usually self-limited to 4-8 hours. Because they can cause hyperglycemia, intravenous lipids should be avoided until the glucose is more stable. Steroid use can complicate hyperglycemia further. Most postoperative patients should receive 5% glucose initially to keep the blood glucose below 250 mg/dL. The nondiabetics patients rarely need insulin. Tight control of diabetic patients improves their outcome significantly.[4] Head trauma patients require even tighter glycemic control (less than 150 mg/dL).[5] When needed, insulin should be given intravenously rather subcutaneously because of uncertain perfusion in the postoperative patient. If resistant to intermittent insulin, a continuous insulin drip with a sliding scale may be considered. When infusing insulin, the blood glucose should be monitored frequently enough to avoid hypoglycemia. Spontaneous hypoglycemia in nondiabetics outside NICU is rare and often treated easily with increased glucose intake. Critical or symptomatic hypoglycemia should be treated by 2 ml/kg of 10% glucose in infants and 1ml/kg of 25% glucose in older children. The serum glucose should be closely monitored until stable. Hardly ever, endocrinal investigation of the persistent hypoglycemia, with serum insulin, peptide C and growth hormones, is needed.

Clotting

Immediate postoperative focal bleeding is usually surgical in nature, especially if closure is done in markedly hypotensive patients, because bleeding recurs at untreated bleeding points when the hypotension resolves. On the other hand, generalized oozing from mucosal surfaces or wounds, or excessive bleeding during needle sticks, suggests DIC. In a patient with excessive bleeding, PT and PTT are measured. Suspect surgical etiology if the bleeding continues despite normal PT, PTT and platelets. Most patients do not bleed despite slight increases in PT and PTT and decrease in platelets. Platelet counts as low as 50,000/mm^3 in the immediate postoperative period and 20,000/mm^3 in the delayed postoperative period are rarely a cause of bleeding. In actively bleeding patient, platelets are maintained above 100,000/mm^3. Newborns have slightly prolonged PT and PTT compared to adult norms, and premature infants have even more prolonged values. These studies should be repeated after treatment or for clinical deterioration. D-dimer and FSP persist 24-48 hours after successful treatment of DIC. A "corrected PTT" excludes the effect of endogenous or exogenous inhibitors like heparin, which sometimes contaminates the blood specimen. The PTT is corrected by repeating the test on the same sample after mixing with an equal volume of normal serum. A normal corrected PTT indicates true prolongation due to deficient clotting factors, because the PTT becomes normal with factors of normal serum. On the other hand, persistence of prolongation suggests an inhibitor like heparin. Use fresh frozen plasma (FFP) only to treat lab documented (PT or PTT at least 1½ times normal) and clinically suspected DIC. Because of its risks and cost, never use FFP as a blood volume expander or protein source.[6] The usual dose is 10-20 ml/kg. If kept in the refrigerator, one can use thawed FFP for up to 24 hours. Cryoprecipitate may be considered in a patient with restricted fluids or DIC associated with marked fibrinogenemia. One or two units of platelet concentrate per 10 kg body weight are given for thrombocytopenia (< 50,000/mm^3) in a bleeding patient. The newborns receive 10-20 ml of platelets per kg. Failure to significantly increase the platelet count within one hour after transfusion indicates a refractory state from antiplatelet antibodies or hypersplenism. In such cases, HLA-matched platelets may be used. However, fast destruction in few hours indicates sepsis or DIC. Risks of transfusion, including producing antiplatelet antibodies, should be weighed against the temptation to transfuse platelets in a non-bleeding thrombocytopenic patient. The amount of blood replacement in an actively bleeding patient depends upon rate of bleeding. The actively bleeding patient requires both volume and hemoglobin, supplied by whole blood or a combination of FFP and packed red blood cells (PRBC). Usually 7-8 ml/kg of whole blood or 3-4 ml/kg of PRBC increases the hemoglobin (Hgb) by 1gm/dL and the hematocrit by 3-4%. The potassium load of old PRBC presents a problem in patients needing massive transfusion or having renal insufficiency. Such patients should receive washed PRBC. Washed cells may also be indicated in severe allergic reactions. Massive blood transfusion can produce granulocytopenia, thrombocytopenia, and labile clotting factor deficiency. There is no evidence of any beneficial effect of prophylactic platelet transfusion while massive blood transfusion.

Renal

Blood urea nitrogen (BUN) and serum creatinine measurements are good measures of fluid status and renal function. Absorption of blood from the gut can artificially elevate the BUN. Significant renal dysfunction can occur before the serum creatinine rises. Decreased BUN and creatinine may reflect decreased muscle mass. The frequency of follow up depends upon the initial laboratory values, cardiovascular stability, renal function, and the use of nephrotoxic drugs such as gentamicin.

Oliguria and anuria are the most common renal problems in the postoperative period. Their diagnosis is confirmed by palpating the absence of a full bladder because of failure to empty. It is mostly prerenal in nature due to decreased renal perfusion, secondary to hypotension. Increased vasoconstriction, iatrogenic or otherwise, makes oliguria worse. Rarely it may be secondary to thromboembolic phenomenonae in the renal vessels, especially in patients with deep catheters. Renal ultrasound or renal scan can be used to visualize them. Acute tubular necrosis may develop after prolonged ischemia or hypotension. Ureteral obstruction or intra-abdominal leakage is rare. Blockage of the urinary catheter or inaccurate measurement or recordings of urinary volumes are other causes of oliguria.

Principally oliguria treatment addresses the primary causes, like hypovolemia and hypotension. Inotropes are used to treat poor cardiac contractility, but it is prudent to also avoid excessive vasoconstriction from high dosages dopamine, epinephrine, or norepinephrine. Renal dose dopamine (2-5 mcg/kg/min), along with a loop diuretic, is a useful addition to treating the primary cause. A bolus of 10-20 ml/kg normal saline, with or without small dose of loop diuretic, may be tried, even if hypovolemia is not that evident. If the anuria continues despite maximal treatment, fluid intake is decreased to insensible water loss and urine output.

Polyuria is extremely rare. Mostly it is caused by the polyuric phase of acute tubular necrosis. Rarely diabetes insipidus, following head injury or surgery, can produce polyuria. Adequate fluid and electrolyte replacement is necessary to avoid dehydration and electrolyte imbalance. Usually one-half to three-quarters of the urine out put is replaced. Mild polyuria may also develop due to excessive fluid intake, diuretics, and during the recovery phase following the third spacing (capillary leak syndrome). Serum electrolytes should be followed closely in these patients.

Urine specific gravity, blood urea nitrogen (BUN) and serum creatinine measurements are a good measure of blood volume (fluid status) and renal function. Absorption of blood from the gut could artificially elevate the BUN. Significant renal dysfunction can occur before the serum creatinine rises. Decreased BUN and creatinine reflects decreased muscle mass. The frequency of follow up depends upon the initial laboratory values, renal function, and the use of nephrotoxic drugs such as gentamicin.

Hypothermia

Hypothermia is a relatively common problem during and immediately after an operation. Usually it is due to cold operation rooms or excessive exposure of the patients or their bowels. Relatively cold intravenous fluids, especially if given in large amounts can also contribute to hypothermia. It is also caused by cardiovascular instability. Infants, especially premature or malnutrition children are more prone to hypothermia. Core temperature is routinely assessed by rectal, sublingual or tympanic membrane temperature.[6] In critical patients, it is best assessed by temperature probes in pulmonary artery or urinary bladder. Hypothermia can complicate postoperative care significantly. It is associated with metabolic acidosis due to decreased perfusion. It compromises the patient's coagulation system. Both the PT and PTT may be elevated despite normal coagulation factors.[7] Further, the patient may bleed excessively during hypothermia despite normal PT and PTT also.[8] Low temperature also decreases platelet functions.[9,10] It also decreases cardiac function and may contribute to bradycardia or arrhythmias. Intense vasoconstriction may even cause hypertension and significant tissue hypoperfusion leading to metabolic acidosis. This metabolic acidosis is usually further exaggerated during warming as reperfusion collects the lactic acidosis of vasoconstricted tissue; but this decrease in pH may not be a sign of deterioration. Therefore, sufficient fluids should be given during rewarming to compensate for the vasodilatation and increase in vascular volume. A decrease in temperature increases the hemoglobin's affinity for oxygen because of the leftward shift of the hemoglobin dissociation curve. Although it increases the oxygen saturation at the pulmonary level, delivery of oxygen to tissues decreases due to decrease of oxygen release. Shivering should be avoided to prevent its associated sudden increase in oxygen demand.[11] Cerebral profusion also decreases significantly during hypothermia. It also affects immune systems adversely at many levels, thus increasing the risk for infections and sepsis. It depresses liver functions including drug metabolism. It also impairs insulin release thus causing hyperglycemia. As always, prevention is much better than treatment. Even mild decrease in temperature can have significant effect on clotting.[11] Increasing ambient room temperature, keeping most of the body including the head dry and covered and warming infused fluids and gases to room temperature will prevent hypothermia in many cases. Warming devices like The Bear Hug®, warm water bags or mattress, etc can prevent hypothermia as well. Postoperatively, aggressively treat it using warming blankets and heating lamps. On the other side, mild hypothermia may have some protective effects against decreased availability of oxygen by decreasing oxygen demands. The role of cooling the head in an asphyxiated patient is not well defined yet.

Endocrine

Exact mechanisms of the effects of different hormones due to stress and its effects on the healing and immune systems of the patients are very complex and not well understood yet. Rarely mild adrenal insufficiency may cause hypotension, hyponatremia, hyperkalemia, hypothermia, and eosinophilia postoperatively. Hyperpigmentation in a patient may indicate primary adrenal insufficiency. The patients who have received glucocorticoids in last 12-18 months are at high risk for secondary adrenal insufficiency and will need replacement therapy for stress. Dosage and duration of steroids will define the chances of adrenal suppression.

Corticotrophin (ACTH) stimulation test can help diagnose it. It is performed by measuring plasma cortisol concentration immediately before and 30 minutes after small dose of alpha 1-24 corticotrophin. If in doubt or while waiting for results, give hydrocortisone or hydrocortisone 60 mg/M^2/dose initially, IV then give 30 mg/M^2 every 4-8 hours depending upon the patient sickness. It is weaned over 4-7 days. The patients receiving high chronic dose glucocorticoids, for asthma or autoimmune disease, need double or triple the daily usual dose for several days until stable. Wean to presurgical dose in 5-7 days. Perioperative coverage depends upon dosage, duration of glucocorticoids therapy, and nature and length of surgery. One should weigh negative effects of glucocorticoids on immune systems, growth, and healing against benefits. Role of growth hormones for improved wound healing, weight gain and positive nitrogen balance in selected cases is still controversial. Prolonged catecholamine used may cause decreased response in adenergic receptors, and then non-adenergic inotropic agent should be used. Hypocalcemia could be multifactorial, including illness-associated hypoparathyroidism, change in vitamin D metabolism, hypomagnesemia, and change in acid base status. Certain stress responses including fever actually enhances immune functions so should not always be truncated.

Cardiovascular

Neuromuscular blockade and the sedative effect of anesthesia decreases the metabolic demand thus protects the heart during anesthesia. The postoperative patient's metabolic demand increases due to the decreasing anesthesia and increasing catecholamines due to pain, anxiety, and agitation despite reasonable pain management.

Tachycardia is a cause and effect of increased metabolic demand. It may be due to decreased perfusion, blood volume loss, hypotension, hypoxemia, airway obstruction, and the stress of pain, anxiety, and agitation. Certain drugs used during anesthesia like pancuronium and atropine can cause tachycardia. Rarely it may be due to direct irritation of SA node, if a tip of central line is in right atrium. It may also be due to tachyarrhythemia and can be diagnosed by EKG.

The absolute number defining bradycardia is age dependent. It is much less common but have much more serious consequences. It may also be due to excessive sedation. Bradycardia, if due to hypoxemia, is always critical and needs immediate relief. Heart block especially in postcardiac surgery can cause bradycardia that can be diagnosed by EKG. Sudden increases in blood pressure due to any reason also cause bradycardia, though transient, due to negative feedback by carotid bodies. It is also important to consider the preoperative baseline as many athletic patients may have low baseline heart rate. During deep sleep and pain relief, heart rate may fall significantly. Many drugs can also decrease heart rate. Neostigmine without atropine, when used to reverse muscle relaxants, causes bradycardia and will be relieved by atropine only.

Hypertension is rather rare and usually due to pain, anxiety and agitation. Hypertension due to excessive volume infusion, especially colloid, is rare, mild, and transient. Excessive use of pressors or its sudden accidental bolus during drip change is a common cause of transient hypertension in ICU. Patients on steroids can also become hypertension. Steroids increase sensitivity of dopanergic receptors for endogenous and exogenous catecholamines. Renal vaso-occlusive disease, especially when patient have central catheters, should be ruled out by ultrasound and serum rennin levels. Severe hypertension if not treated can cause cardiac failure and worsen respiratory status. The hypertensive crisis is initially best treated by sodium nitroprusside. It could be titrated easily for the desired effect, because of its quick onset and short duration of action. Once the BP is controlled, an angiotension converting enzyme (ACE) inhibitor is commonly used for the subacute hypertension management.

Hypotension is an emergency and always need immediate intervention. Decreased cardiac output or decreased vascular tone is the most common cause of hypotension. Decreased venous return or decreased myocardial contractility causes decreased cardiac output. Decreased venous return may be secondary to increased intrathoracic pressure (ventilation), decreased blood volume, or decreased vascular tone. Inadequate fluid intake or excessive losses including third spacing due to leaky capillaries can cause decreased blood volume. Routine chest X-ray may give many clues for causes of hypotension. Small heart on routine chest X-ray, provided it is not due to excessive intrathoracic pressure, indicates decreased blood volume. Similarly, large heart may point toward dilated, poorly contractile heart. Hyperexpanded and hypolucent lungs may indicate increased intrathoracic pressure. Chest X-ray may also ruleout any air leak, which can be the cause of hypotension and needs urgent treatment. In case of sudden severe hypotension, along with deteriorating ventilation and oxygenation, a tension pneumothorax or cardiac temponade should be suspected. Signs of mediastinal shift and unilateral decreased breath sounds help make the diagnosis of tension pneumothorax. Similarly, fast thready pulses, engorged neck veins, distant muffled heart sounds, and initial tachycardia followed by terminal bradycardia may indicate cardiac temponade. In small infants with thin chest wall, transillumination may help make the diagnosis of air leak. However, negative transillumination does not rule out air leak. If suspicion is very high and patient is extremely critical, trial of needle aspiration may be indicated and may be life saving. Patients with central line tips in heart are at higher risk for cardiac temponade. Most often, a chest tube is needed after needle aspiration, but if a patient appear stable, it may reasonable to wait, especially when the patient is on high frequency oscillator. Blood volume expansion may partially compensate for decreased venous return during early phases of air leaks.

Preferably hypovolemia should be treated by crystalloid and if indicated blood products. Use of 5% albumin should be avoided as in sick child with leaky capillaries it immediately leaks into third spaces and takes water to extravascular spaces and this edema is difficult to manage later.[12,13] Pressors are used for poor myocardial contractility. Dobutamine increases cardiac output and tissue perfusion yet it may not always improve hypotension. On the contrary, dopamine in moderate and high doses increases BP. Due to vasoconstriction it may not necessarily increases or sometimes even decreases the cardiac output and the tissue perfusion. Epinephrine and norepinephrine though potent drugs and always increase the blood pressure. These should be avoided until last effort, as BP elevation benefits may not be enough to justify their use, due to negative effects of vasoconstriction and increased metabolic demand associated with tachycardia. Mild hypotension in congestive heart failure patient can be treated by milrinone (Primacor), as it increases cardiac contractility but decreases the peripheral resistance, so giving dual benefits. Load it with 50-100 mcg/kg over 15-30 minutes then use continuous drip at 0.5 - 0.75 mcg/kg/minute.[14] Dopamine in low doses (2-5 mcg/kg/min) has renal effect, while in higher doses (10-20 mcg/kg/min) has more vasoconstrictive effect that may have negative effect on cardiac output and glomerular filtration rate (GFR). Often, a combination of these drugs is needed to get the optimum effect. Sometimes, both pressors and after load reducers, like nitroprusside, are used to increase cardiac output. There is sudden peripheral venous pooling after neuromuscular blockade. It causes the hypotension, tachycardia, hypoperfusion, and occasionally desaturation and hypercapnia. Fluid bolus can compensate decreasing venous return, because of venous pooling. Third spacing due to leaky capillaries in sepsis or ischemia can decrease blood volume significantly and needs extra fluids to maintain normal blood volume. CVP and pulmonary artery pressure monitoring help assess blood volume in critical patients. Trends rather than any absolute numbers in CVP measurement are used. In extremely compromised patient, an intra-aortic balloon pump is placed in aorta via femoral artery, in between left subclavian and renal artery. It is inflated in diastole to support perfusion of vital organs proximal to balloon.

Pulmonary

Desaturations or hypoxemia and hypercapnia are the commonest pulmonary problems of the postoperative time. Both can be due to accidental extubation, slipping ET into the main stem bronchus, aspiration, secretions, ET blockade, hypoventilation. It may also be due to lack of changes in the ventilator settings in response to changing conditions of the lung, or changing metabolic needs of the patient after wearing off of neuromuscular blockade and anesthesia. Furthermore, agitation, fighting against ventilator, inadequate relief of pain, pneumothorax, pneumopericardium, and hydrothorax can also cause hypoxemia and hypercapnia. It can also be due to premature extubation, atelectasis, laryngeal edema, excessive narcotics or resurgence of reversed narcotic or neuromuscular blockade. Pulmonary edema due to excessive water intake, heart failure, renal failure and increased negative intrathoracic pressure in retracting patient can cause initially hypoxemia and ultimately hypercapnia also.[15] Similarly, pulmonary hemorrhage and infections can also cause these problems. Lot of evidence has accumulated recently regarding the negative effects of hyperventilation, especially in newborns. It is always iatrogenic, thus evaluate ventilation plan every time PCO_2 is less than 30-35 torr. Similarly, keeping PO_2 high increases morbidity and can be catastrophic in premature newborns.

VENTILATOR MANAGEMENT

Detailed management of individual ventilator is out of the scope of this chapter. Still concise general principles of ventilation will be discussed here. Mechanical ventilation is usually indicated for inability to oxygenate, ventilate, or keep airway open. Spontaneous breath, with negative intrathoracic pressure in inspiration is very different from ventilator breath. As a principle, use ventilator as an adjuvant rather than replacement of spontaneous breathing and aim for gentler and minimal ventilator therapy. Prefer ventilator, nasal continued positive airway pressure (CPAP), and nasal cannula or oxyhood in reverse order. Avoid unnecessary use of sedation and muscle relaxants considering genuine pain relief.

In general, mean airway pressure (MAP) increase by any means improves oxygenation unless there is an excessive intrathoracic pressure causing V/Q mismatch. MAP is the average pressure of the airway during respiratory cycle. Alternatively, increasing FIO_2 improves oxygenation. Usually positive end expiratory pressure (PEEP) of five is enough and then positive inspiratory pressure (PIP) is chosen to achieve enough visual chest movement or desired measured tidal volumes. Tidal volumes are the volume of gas moved in and out during a single breath. Normally 8-10 ml/kg in children and 5-7 ml/kg in newborns are adequate tidal volume.

Initially, start at rate of 20-25 breaths per minute, and then change it to attain desired CO_2. Increasing breathing rate or intermittent mandatory ventilation (IMV) is the commonest means to lower PCO_2. Lung expansion, seen in chest X-ray, may also help monitor pressure settings on ventilator. Usually high diaphragm, especially with high FIO_2, may indicate need to increase pressures and vice versa. Often, FIO_2 can be decreased by increasing MAP or vice versa. In general, somewhat balance is maintained between FIO_2 and MAP, although occasionally two definite strategies favoring either high FIO_2 or high MAP are used.

High lung volume or alveolar recruitment strategy is used in patients with high FIO_2, who often have diffuse alveolar collapse causing V/Q mismatch. Initially, it was proposed for high frequency oscillation ventilator (HFOV), its principles can be used in conventional ventilation also. In this strategy, PEEP and MAP are slowly increased, which allow FIO_2 lowering. During this, lung expansion through 10th posterior rib is achieved, which opens collapsed alveoli. Usually FIO_2 is decreased to 0.4 (40%) during this, and then MAP is decreased slightly without need to increase FIO_2. If significant or sudden increase (5-10%) in FIO_2 requirement occurs with further decrease in MAP, probably too much MAP was decreased. MAP should be increased again to open the recent atelectasis until FIO_2 is decreased. After one-two hours lower the MAP slowly.

On the other hand, air leak strategy is used in a patient with air leaks. In this, higher FIO_2 is tolerated so MAP can be kept lowers. High MAP and tidal volumes are the major factors in production and continuance of air leaks. Lungs are kept at no more than eighth posterior rib expansion.

Usually a PEEP of five is enough but a PEEP up to eight can be safely used in selective case in noncompliant lung requiring high FIO_2. Normally increasing PEEP increases oxygenation and decreases ventilation by reducing Tidal volumes. However, in an atelectic lung raising PEEP may open new alveoli thus increasing the lung's tidal volume and decreasing PCO_2.

PRESSURE SUPPORT VENTILATION (PSV)

Certain predetermined pressure is delivered above PEEP, to support each spontaneous breath, triggered by the initiation of breath. It is a useful tool to wean the patient from ventilator. It also helps patients who are fighting ventilator or are on very low IMV rates. Pressure support depends upon the needs of the patient and slowly weaned as the patient contributes more. Once PSV is around 10 cm of water, it could be stopped just before extubation. Depending upon the spontaneous breathing rate even a small pressure support may contribute significantly to MAP and ventilator support. It is also used to reduce WOB by compensating for the resistance of ET and respiratory system in low IMV. Similarly, each spontaneous breath can also be supported by predetermined tidal volumes.

High Frequency Oscillation Ventilator (HFOV)

HFOV uses tidal volumes much smaller than dead space at extremely high rates (360-900 breaths/seconds). It is mainly used to treat resistant hypercapnia, prevention and treatment of air leak syndromes. Its role in decreasing chronic lung disease is not established yet. In this mode also, increase in MAP and FIO_2 are the main means to improves oxygenation. Increase in amplitude (ΔP) improves ventilation. Frequency of breath has minimal and paradoxical role. Increased frequency increases PCO_2, because it decreases the IT that reduces the tidal volumes significantly. In small infants, the ET size change can make a big difference in ventilation.

Use of Nonendotracheal PEEP (CPAP)

Atelectasis reduces functional residual capacity (FRC) that significantly Function residual capacity (FRC) is a volume of gas left after normal breath, increases work of breathing. Patient adapts to it by decreasing TV and compensates reduced TV by increasing respiratory rate. Increasing PEEP will reverse it by clearing, atelectasis and recovering FRC. Change in pressure (ΔP) needed for a particular TV (ΔV) will decrease thus decreasing WOB, retractions, and increasing compliance ($\Delta V/\Delta P$). PEEP also distends airway that can reduce airway resistance, which decreases respiratory work. Low-level PEEP can help expiration even in chronic obstructive lung disease patients by distending the airway. However, higher PEEP may hurt these patients by overdistending lung and increases V/Q. Optimum PEEP for a patient has to be individualized and changes with changing conditions of lung. Need for close titration and frequent evaluation cannot be over emphasized.

PEEP also helps patients with diffusion problems due to pulmonary interstitial disease like pulmonary edema or pneumonia. Nasal prongs or facemask could apply PEEP. Complete seal is very important in facemask. PEEP may cause significant gastric distension especially at higher level. Stomach could be decompressed by gastric tube in these cases. Although most patients needs PEEP of 5-8 cm of water but rarely PEEP up to 15 cm of water have been successfully utilized. Excessive PEEP causes hyperinflation and increases V/Q ratio reducing arterial PO_2. It also decreases the venous return to heart and decreases cardiac output, which increases the oxygen extraction, seen by decreasing mixed venous oxygen saturation. Difficulty in expiration secondary to excessive peep increases work of breathing and metabolic needs of patient. It may significantly increases the dead space lowering ventilation, but this increase may not appropriately show on endtidal CO_2 due to dilution by increased dead space. Appropriate PEEP in a sick lung may become excessive as the lung compliance improves. Although in general, PEEP helps inspiration but it makes expiration difficult. Nevertheless, it can help expiration in reactive or malaciac airway patients by keeping airway open. Decreased venous return by PEEP due to its transmitted pressure on veins could be partially compensated by increasing preload with fluids. However, consider the deleterious effects of increasing fluids. Barotrauma of PEEP is minimal on a spontaneously breathing patient specially when compared to alternatives like intubation.

Work of Breathing (WOB)

Although the ET size depends upon the size of the patient still at times one of the two ET sizes could be chosen for a particular patient. Smaller size ET could increase work of the breathing significantly. As discussed earlier optimal PEEP can decrease WOB significantly. Pressure support ventilation can also lower the work of breathing. Ventilators with demand flow, which have different flows for inspiration and expiration, decrease work of breathing. Keeping the patient slight upright (brings diaphragms down), decreasing edema (diuretics) or correcting atelectasis by increasing PIP or PEEP can also decrease the work of breathing. Similarly, sometimes bronchodilators can significantly decrease WOB.

Atelectasis

Atelectasis may be focal or diffuse. Reduced lung volume helps its differentiation from edema or consolidation, on chest X-ray, but still it is not always that easy. FRC decreases significantly in spine position, which increases likelihood of atelectasis postoperatively. It also increases the risk of infection. Early ambulation, mobilization, deep breathing exercises and incentive spirometry can help to maintain the FRC. Nasal or facemask CPAP may be used alternatively in patients who cannot cooperate. Effective pain control also helps maintain FRC as pain may inhibit cough mobilization and discourages deep breathing. General anesthesia, obesity, diaphragm dysfunction, abdominal and thoracic surgery also decrease FRC. Closing capacity is the lung volumes at which small airway begin to close during expiration. Residual anesthetics and narcotics inhibit respiratory drive and decreases ventilatory response to hypercapnia and hypoxia. Defense mechanism of cough, mucociliary transport are also impaired postoperatively, increasing risk of pulmonary infection. Lack of humidity, intubation and high FIO_2 further hampers mucociliary transport. Atelectasis decreases force of cough that in return increases atelectasis. It can be treated by chest physiotherapy (CPT), hydration, bronchodilators, and postural drainage. Occasionally a brief treatment with mucolytics may be used in selected patients. Rarely bronchoscopy is needed in persistent atelectasis. Atelectasis, infection, and pulmonary edema worsen the existing chronic lung disease and prolong ventilatory support. Obesity, smoking, existing chronic lung disease, pre-existing URI, and prolonged anesthesia increase the risk of pulmonary complications.

Nitric Oxide (NO)

Nitric oxide has good dilatation effect on pulmonary circulation with effect on systemic circulation.[16] Its prompt and short duration of action, along with it ability to be delivered directly into alveoli makes it an excellent choice for treatment for pulmonary hypertension. It is mixed with the inspired oxygen in very low concentration. Usually, NO in 5-20 parts per million (ppm) dose affectively reduces the pulmonary artery pressure. NO up to 80 ppm has been used for brief time but higher doses rarely have higher effect but significantly increase the chance of toxicity due to methemoglobinemia. These patients should be monitored for methemoglobinemia and nitric dioxide (NO_2). Methemoglobinemia when present is treated by methyline blue. Use NO in minimal affective dose. Some times, NO although initially ineffective with conventional ventilation may response positively with high frequency ventilation due to recruitment of alveoli so NO can act on more surface.

Extubation

Decision to extubate should be deliberate and not a hurried one. Assessment of preoperative lung condition, nature of secretions, gag reflex, conscious level, sedation needs, residual neuromuscular blockade and level of needed ventilator support should help make decision to extubate. When patient is extubated in ICU, it is advisable to wait until initial chest X-ray and initial blood gas is done. The chest X-ray helps to rule out atelectasis and assess overall lung condition. Clear the atelectasis completely before extubation.

If the neuromuscular blockade is reversed recently, wait for at least an hour to avoid return of neuromuscular blockade. Mixture of neostigmine (0.025-0.1 mg/kg) and atropine (0.02 mg/kg) is usually used to reverse neuromuscular blockade. However, we have usually been be able to reverse it using neostigmine alone by diluting dose in 2-5 ml solution and administer slowly over 5-10 minutes. This way we could avoid tachycardia and drying of secretion caused by atropine. Neostigmine increases bronchial secretion so suction the ET after using it.

When surgery is done around or on trachea and larynx, surgeon should be consulted regarding time of extubation. Similarly, prospective of abdominal distension should be considered before extubation also. Avoid aspiration by emptying stomach and stopping feed during this transient period. Similarly, when extensive surgery is done on chest and abdomen, pain management and altered breathing pattern may delay extubation considerably.

When there is history of difficult intubation, laryngeal and vocal cord edema and potential difficulty for reintubation should be considered before extubation. Benefits of steroids (dexamethasone 0.5-1 mg/kg/day in four divided doses) use should be weighed against negative effect on healing and metabolism. Usually two doses each are given before and after extubation.

Patient may be placed on humidified air or O_2 after extubation. If there is any inspiratory stridor, retractions indicating laryngeal edema, nebulized racemic epinephrine can be used. These treatments if beneficial and tolerated without excessive tachycardia or hypertension can be used as often as every hour for short period. Rarely a mixture of helium and oxygen is used as inspired gas, for lower gas density of helium as compared to nitrogen makes this admixture easy to breath through edematous airway.

Obstructed Endotracheal Tube

While partial obstruction of the ET may pose only a subtle difficulty in ventilation, complete obstruction can cause major emergency needing prompt relief. Thick secretion and mucus are the most common culprits. Kinked ET or other ventilator tube may also cause obstruction. Small size ET, if used in children and infants' can complicate it further. Sudden deterioration in ventilation and hypercapnia are earlier indications of obstructed tube. Partially obstruction may initially increase oxygenation by increasing FRC but ultimately oxygenation also deteriorates. Lack of observed chest expansion, marked retractions and decreased breath sounds, on auscultation suggest near complete obstruction. Decreased tidal volumes especially expiratory also indicate obstruction. If obstruction is below ET in airway, large leaks will be observed and similarly obstruction in one of main bronchus will indicate decreased breath sounds on that side. Mediastinal shift may differentiate bronchus obstruction that can lead pneumothorax. Total bronchus obstruction will lead to collapse but partial obstruction may cause hyperinflation due to the ball-valve action.

When ET obstruction is suspected, it should be immediately suctioned with a big catheter. Failure to pass suction catheter confirms major obstruction. On the other hand, if suction catheter continued to be advance much more than usual, one may suspect accidental extubation. Bronchoscopy may be of great help if immediate bronchoscopic examination to diagnose and treat, obstruction is possible. Otherwise, ET should be replaced immediately. Sometimes, suction with a bigger catheter on direct laryngoscopy is indicated to remove the big mucus plug that could not be suctioned through ET.

Reintubation

All equipment needed for intubation with different size ET's and laryngoscope blades should be kept, in a single mobile case, in the ICU that can be immediately pulled to the patient's bedside for intubation. The patient can be effectively ventilated with bag and mask, using manometer, until equipment and personnel are available for intubation. Deep oral suction also helps airway patency. Intubation should be attempted only after directly visualizing vocal cords in full view. Blindly pushing ET can do serious harm. While miller (straight) blade is put under epiglottis to extend its tip to glottis, Macintosh (curved) blade is placed in valecula. Choosing a relatively bigger ET reduces airway resistance and work of breathing.

ET position is usually certain when an experienced personnel intubates under direct visualization. Still bilateral auscultation is mandatory to confirm equal bilateral breaths for normal ET position. If advanced too far ET commonly moves to right main bronchus. It causes significantly reduced breaths on left side. ET tube in position should always be confirmed by chest X-ray. If available, a capnograph or disposable CO_2 detector can be used, in doubtful cases, to rule out esophagus intubation. Intermittent CO_2 detected in expired air over many breaths confirms endotracheal intubation.

INFECTION

Infection plays a major role in the postoperative period. Strict hand washing before and after touching the patient remains the hallmark of prevention of infection. Universal precautions should be strictly followed. Sterility, including cap, gown, mask, gloves and drapes, is very important during invasive procedures including inserting deep lines. Fever always brings attention toward infection. Decreased temperature may be the presenting symptom of sepsis in neonates and debilitated patients. Changes in the cardiovascular, respiratory or mental status also indicate sepsis. Leukocytosis, leukopenia, thrombocytopenia, and left shift on differential count are reasonable causes to look for infection. Detailed physical examination is the most important means in quest of infection causes. Change in color (purulent) and amount of endotracheal secretions raises suspicions of pneumonia, leading to Gram stain and culture of tracheal secretions. Chills and rigor often indicate bacteriemia. When present, central lines are always suspected as the cause of sepsis and should be removed or replaced if symptoms persist. Wound and suture lines should be carefully evaluated. Sometimes, rather moderate abscesses are not evident until surgical wound or suture line is explored. Abnormal abdominal examination with ileus, tenderness, or redness may indicate abdominal pathology. If redness or pus is present around the insertion site, remove the line. In case of thrombophlebitis, the vein should be pressed toward insertion site. In severe case, surgical excision of the vein should be considered. Urine culture, Gram stain will help diagnose UTI. Suspect meningitis or cerebral abscess if there is mental alteration or seizures. CBC, chest X-ray, tracheal aspirate, and one or two sets of aerobic and anaerobic peripheral blood culture should be done in sepsis suspect patients. The central line blood cultures should be done only at the time of insertion or in addition to peripheral blood culture. Complete blood count usually shows leukocytosis but leukocytes count may be depressed in overwhelming infection and patients on chemotherapy or steroids. Thrombocytopenia is usually a late sign in sepsis and more often indicate Gram negative or fungal sepsis. We have seen isolated thrombocytopenia in the otherwise asymptomatic surgical newborns due to very small abscesses, which were found only on detailed examination of the suture line. The platelets dramatically improved after opening these abscesses. Chest X-ray may help diagnose pneumonia, fluid effusion and lung abscess. An X-ray may be negative early in the disease. Abdominal investigation starts with plain KUB film, which may show free air, ileus, bowel displacement showing mass effect, or collection of peritoneal fluid pushing bowel in the center. Persistent sentinel bowel loop in same place may be the only indication of abscess. Elevated right diaphragm may indicate subphrenic abscess. Ultrasound and CT scan are indicated in the difficult cases. In difficult patients with suspect abscess, interventional radiologist can aspirate it percutanously under ultrasound guide. Nuclear scan can also be used to investigate abdominal abscess. Gram stain and cultures of ascitic fluid can help tailor the therapy. Severe cardiovascular collapse usually accompanies alternation in mental status and if it is out of proportion to cardiovascular instability or accompanied by signs of focal neurological deficit then lumbar puncture (LP) is indicated. CT scan or MRI may be useful, if brain abscess is suspected. Consider blind laparotomy if abdominal pathology is highly suspected despite negative investigation as it can be lifesaving.

Initial increase in indirect bilirubin, in the first week of postoperative period, is usually not related to infection. On the other hand, direct bilirubin accompanied by clinical picture of sepsis indicates infection. The bilirubinemia associated with infection usually appears and resolves fast. Direct bilirubinemia secondary to total parenteral nutrition (TPN) related to cholestasis is seen at least after 2-3 weeks of TPN and is slow and progressive. Worsening of lung disease during sepsis is due to pneumonitis or the increased capillary leak by the toxic or ischemic effects of sepsis. Clinically both act by decreased compliance and increased diffusion block, needing high pressure and FIO_2. The tracheal aspiration examination shows large amount of neutrophils and organisms in the pneumonia. If only one organism predominates it helps establish diagnosis and treatment of pneumonia. Chest X-ray showing focal changes also gravitates toward pneumonia; but generalized opaqueness does not rule out pneumonia. In case of valvular disease patients with sepsis, echocardiogram investigation of the heart should be done to rule out vegetation. New or changing nature of murmur may be due to vegetation.

Routine blood or tracheal aspirate cultures are not that helpful. However, index of suspicion should be very low in a patient with the central lines or ET. Never the less, colonization if known by previous cultures may help you to cover the right organisms in case of deterioration. Yeast and staphylococcal infections are usually undulating.

Although a broad coverage is started initially, treatment should be narrowed down depending upon the culture results and clinical response. Monitor drug levels of antibiotics like vancomycin, and gentamicin in patients treated for more than 48 hours. High trough level indicates need for increased duration between doses and low peak indicate need of increasing dose. The patients with third spacing have higher volume of distribution and needs less frequent doses but higher dosage for the drug levels to be in the therapeutic range. Evidence is accumulating in favor of higher but less frequent dosage for higher efficiency and lower toxicity.[17]

PAIN MANAGEMENT

Although, the pain relief has been the main stay of medicine since early times, but lately there is increased awareness to the pain. Most of the times still, the pain is not adequately treated. The pain management, in a nonverbal postoperative patient is an amalgam of science and art. It becomes even more complicated in a critical patient with vasomotor instability, because of decreased margin of safety. Furthermore, confusion, hesitation, anxiety, individual variability to tolerate pain, and new environment make it even harder to assess the exact status of the pain. Inadequate relief of the pain and anxiety can increase metabolism, prolong hospitalization, delay extubation and healing. Increased oxygen consumption, because of pain, can worsen the ischemic condition of heart and body. It may cause hypercoaguabilty and adversely effects immune system. It can cause water retention due to increased ADH and rennin secretion. It may also delay return of bowel function. Severe pain decreases ambulation, cough and ventilation, which increase the chances of atelectasis, pneumonia, and thromboembolic complications. It can also alter responses to acute and chronic pain, later in the life. The important signs as tachycardia, hypertension, and tachypnea can be wrongly assessed during clinical assessment of the patient.

Preoperatively, discuss the pain management with the patient and family to relieve anxiety and make plans for the postoperative pain. The importance of pain prevention and need for continuous relief of discomfort cannot be over emphasized. Once the pain is well established, it takes much larger dose to control. Sometimes increased catabolism, because of decreased insulin with the pain, causes hyperglycemia. Periodic pain reassessment after treatment can confirm its adequate effect. Nonpharmacological methods of pain relief are as important as medications. Simple processes like, parents holding patient's hand during blood draw have shown to soothe even newborns. Multidisciplinary team approach, including physician, nurse, parents, pharmacist, and many other allied health professionals, is the best approach. Pain assessment is considered as fifth vital sign and should be assessed and recorded whenever vital signs are taken. There are many approaches to assess the pain; commonly used, one to ten pain-scale is most practical. The pain level of ten is the most severe pain and zero score being no pain at all. Usually a pain level of four and more warrants intervention. Most commonly, opioids as morphine and fentanyl are used for the pain. Sudden respiratory deterioration along with reduced chest movement just after fentanyl suggests chest wall and laryngeal rigidity, which can be promptly reversed with naloxone.[18] For early onset and predicted levels, secondary to independence from absorptive process, prefer intravenous route in acute pain. Chronic pain is treated by long acting preparations including transdermal opioids. Occasionally, an intramuscular route can be used according to the choice and needs of the patient. In acute pain, continued infusion avoids yo-yo phenomenon but it needs close observation to prevent its toxicity. On the other hand, the too infrequent doses can cause breakthrough pain.

The patient controlled analgesia (PCA) is ideal for pain control in the older postoperative patient. In this, the patient controls pain by self-administering medication by small boluses in addition to a baseline drip. Usually, two-third the anticipated daily dose is given as a continuous infusion and remained one-third dose is given as many boluses by pushing a button. PCA has been used successfully in young children as young as seven years old. It is important in these cases that only the patient administer the bolus. The parents should abstain pushing button to administer medication by assessing pain on the child's behalf. Either these cases have no baseline infusion or very low dose baseline infusion is used to avoid accidental overdose.

Opioids with local anesthetics infusion, through the epidural catheter, can decrease the individual doses and side effects in selected high-risk patients. Similarly, nerve blocks by local anesthetics are also used effectively to reduce postoperative pain. Nonsteroidal anti-inflammatory drugs (NSAID) can help wean opioids in mild-to-moderate pain conditions. It acts mainly inhibiting prostaglandins and decreasing inflammatory reactions at tissue injury site. Although, benzodiazapines do not have any analgesic effects, still they help release anxiety and it's secondary pain. When using benzodiazapines in addition to opioids, especially in the newborns and unstable patients, be aware of its additive effect on respiratory and cardiovascular depression.

Nonpharmacological methods of massage, soothing music, quite environment, acupuncture, and hypnosis are used more often nowadays. Pain management teams and consultative services are becoming common sites in the most US hospitals. The pain transmission through efferent peripheral nerve can be blocked by regional and local anesthesia. Intrathecal and epidural anesthesia blocks pain at spinal cord level. Nonnociceptive input from larger mylenated nerve fibers can prevent entry of nociceptive stimulus. The pain can be assessed indirectly by physiological response of heart rate, blood pressure, respiration, diaphoresis, face grimace, and tearing, or crying. The patient can also verbally communicate by direct description of pain or using visual analog scales. It is important to use standardized approach to have consistency in pain assessment and pain management.

Proper recording of periodic pain assessment, treatment rendered and pain reassessment to evaluate its therapeutic response has become an important part of the postoperative charting. Physician may consider writing orders; to give pain medications at regular intervals rather than as needed doses in the immediate postoperative patient. Patient with as needed orders may not receive adequate pain relief as some nurses may feel uncomfortable giving narcotics. Different opioids agonists activate separate opioid receptors. Individual pain tolerance and pharmacological variability can make ideal drug administration, with minimal breakthrough pain and toxicity, very difficult. The tolerance to opioids (except constipation) develops rather soon. Thus, increased doses may be needed for the same therapeutic response only after few days.

NEUROMUSCULAR BLOCKADE

Many times neuromuscular blockade, from the operation room, is continued in the ICU in critical patients for stability. Sometimes, it is also used in a patient fighting ventilator or when patient movement causes clinical instability. It can be administered intermittent or by continuous drip. Never use it without adequately addressing pain, anxiety, and breathing issues. The neuromuscular blockade causes decrease in peripheral vascular tone and peripheral venous pooling, which may cause decreased blood return, lower cardiac output, hypotension, and tachycardia. Infusing fluid bolus to increase blood volume can compensate it effectively. Intermittent doses make above mentioned changes every time the patient receive the dose and could initiate a cardiovascular instability in a critical patient. It can also make sudden changes in oxygenation and ventilation. Conversely, the continuous drip has the potentials of using excessive dose. Similarly, during continuous drips, drugs may accumulate in secondary compartment (e.g. fat), which may increase the prolonged duration of action even after drip is stopped.

Neuromuscular blockade also decreases the lymphatic drainage, causing progressive edema by third spacing. It can be avoided by closely monitoring the status of blockade by nerve stimulation test or decreasing the dose periodically to evaluate the continued need of the blockade. The aim of the treatment is using the minimum level of neuromuscular blockade required. Reverse neuromuscular blockade with neostigmine and atropine.

TOTAL PARENTERAL NUTRITION (TPN)

TPN provide nutritional requirements in supplement to enteral feeding to maintain basal metabolism, avoid negative nitrogen balance, promote optimal repair of injured tissue, and growth. Continue maximum tolerated enteral feeding, how small it may be.

Enteral feeding is held postoperatively in all critical patients for variable periods. In these patients, TPN becomes essential to avoid catabolism and promote healing and positive nitrogen balance unless adequate enteral feeding is expected soon. It is even more important in malnourished and growing children. The patient has negative nitrogen balance in the immediate postoperative period. There is not enough good evidence that starting TPN very early can prevent or reverse this catabolism. Still, a case could be made to start TPN after few hours, once the hyperglycemia resolves indicating against catabolism. It can be given as peripheral intravenous solution if enteral feeding is expected within 7-10 days. Peripheral route limits the glucose concentration (12.5%) and calories administered, especially in patients with restricted fluids. On the other hand, give hypertonic solutions (1000-1500 mOsm/L) via central line only. More than 20% glucose or 4% amino acids are used rarely.

Amino acids are essential to compensate the catabolism of stress and injury. Fasting newborns lose 1.2 gm/kg/day of proteins (1% of body protein mass) for every day without TPN. This deficit soon becomes difficult to catch despites maximal TPN. It can be avoided by early TPN use. Usually, non-protein calories are increased slowly along with increasing protein intake. Ideal ratio between non-protein calories and grams of nitrogen is 150-200:1. In sick patients, it may decrease up to 100:1. One gram of nitrogen is found in 6.25 gm of protein, which can constitute nearly 30 g of wet muscles. Newborns and infants require 3-3.5 g/kg/day of protein. Older children need slightly less proteins (2.5-3 g/kg/day). Adults need only1-2 g/kg of proteins daily. Protein requirement is higher than average in premature newborns, surgical cases and patients with malnutrition, excessive protein loss, stress, and sepsis. One gram of protein produces four calories. Start with 1.5-2 g/kg of amino acids and quickly advance to full requirement in 1-2 days. The premature newborns have transient higher BUN and creatinine when they are on full protein intake but it does not have any long-term deleterious effect. Replacing some chloride with acetate easily treats premature newborns, which may have some metabolic acidosis on higher dose of amino acids.

Fat is provided by intravenous, isomolar and dense caloric lipid emulsions. The lipids can prevent essential fatty acid deficiency. It decreases the irritative nature of protein solution. Thus, relatively hyperosmolar solutions can be used peripherally if given with lipid emulsions. Lipid metabolism produces less CO_2 than carbohydrate for similar amount of calories. Thus, lipids may be preferred in a patient with difficulty in excreting CO_2. In addition, fewer calories are wasted when fat is synthesized from triglycerides rather than carbohydrate. 20% lipid solution is better tolerated than 10% solutions. 20% lipid emulsions contain one Kcal/ml. Initially start 1-1.5 g/kg of lipids daily and increase daily depending upon serum glucose. Lipid infusion increases serum glucose. Lipids more than 3-3.5 gm/kg/day are rarely used. Although, lipids are relatively contraindicated during sepsis, thrombocytopenia, and hyperglycemia and in a newborn with indirect hyperbilirubinemia, still one gram/kg of lipids can be used in most patients.

Glucose solution is used as the preferred source of energy. Commonly 4-6 mg/kg/min, depending upon age and activity, of glucose is needed to maintain basic metabolic rate. The patients who do not tolerate even this much glucose infusion are considered catabolic. Protein and lipids are held in these patients. Initially start 6-9 mg/kg/min of glucose infusion and then increase glucose intake depending upon serum glucose levels on previous days up to 24 mg/kg/min. Monohydrate glucose used in intravenous solutions provides 3.4 Kcal/g.

When TPN is infused through a central line, 0.5 units/ml heparin is added to increase the patency of the catheter. Most commercially available vitamins and trace-element preparations adequately provide the daily requirements. Copper and manganese intakes are reduced in the cholestatic patients because of decreased excretion. The patients with increased gastrointestinal losses may need increased zinc intake.

The patients who are discharged home with TPN, total daily TPN is infused over 10-14 hours daily during night. The TPN is consolidated slowly over many days monitoring serum glucose. Infusion is terminally tapered over 1-2 hours to avoid hypoglycemia caused by abrupt stopping of glucose solution. Utilize drug incompatibility charts to administer drugs in TPN. Alternatively, infuse the compatible drugs very close to the patient.

Monitor frequently serum electrolytes, BUN, creatinine, glucose until stable TPN with stable electrolytes is achieved. Then monitor once weekly. Serum triglycerides are measured to verify tolerance of lipids initially when lipids are given in a high dose. Similarly, CBC is monitored routinely once weekly for scouting anemia and infection. Liver functions could be screened by weekly direct bilirubin measurement. If cholestatic jaundice is suspected, detailed investigation of the liver by enzyme assay, ultrasound and nuclear scan of gallbladder and liver is indicated, to rule out other causes. Infection plays the major role in cholestasis secondary to TPN. Enteral feeding, lowering glucose load and infection prevention are the most important methods in its prevention. It has been also treated with cholecystokinin, ursodeoxycholic acid, cyclic TPN, and gut decontamination.[19-21]

In conclusion, postoperative care is a complex mixture of managing medical, surgical, social, and psychological problems of a patient after surgery. It's planning starts before surgery in assessing and discussing the potential postoperative problems and may continue at home as prolonged rehabilitation. Close monitoring, complication prevention and their treatment, and adequate pain management are its important parts. Social support of family including arrangements of teaching in the convalescent patient should be incorporated in the postoperative care.

REFERENCES

1. Matthay MA. Invasive homodynamic monitoring in critically ill patients. Clin Chest Med 1983;4:233-49.
2. Mahette CK, Jaffe MB, Sasse SA, et al. Relationship of thermodiluation cardiac output to metabolic measurements and mixed venous oxygen saturation. Chest 1993;104:1236-42.
3. Kaieda R, Toded MM, Cook ALN, et al. Acute effects of changing plasma osmolality colloid oncotic pressure on the formation of brain edema after cryogenic injury. Neurolsurgery 1989;24:671-78.
4. The Diabetes Control and Complications Trial Research Group: The effect of intensive treatment of diabetes on the development and progression of long-term complications in insulin-dependent diabetes mellitus. N Engl J Med 1993;329:977-86.
5. Andrews BT. The intensive care management of patients with head injury in neurosurgery intensive care. Andrews BT, eardrum, New York McGraw-Hill 1993;227-32.
6. Shinozaki T, Deane R, Perkins FM. Infrared tympanic thermometer: evaluation of a new clinical thermometer. Crit Care Med 1988;16:148-50.
7. Rohrer MJ, Natale AM. Effect of hypothermia on the coagulation cascade. Crit Care Med 1992;20:1402-05.
8. Krause KR, Howells GA, Buhs CL, Hernandez DA, Bair H, Schuster M, Bendick PJ. Hypothermia-induced coagulopathy during hemorrhagic shock. Am Surg 2000; 66(4):348-54.
9. Bogdonoff DL, Williams ME, Stone DJ. Thrombocytopenia in the critically ill patient. J Crit Care 1990;5:1186-205.
10. Watts DD, Trask A, Soeken K, et al. Hypothermic coagulopathy in trauma: effect of varying levels of hypothermia on enzyme speed, platelet function, and fibrinolytic activity. Jour of Trauma 1998;44(5):846.
11. Pflug AE, Aashiem JM, Foster C, et al. Prevention of post-anesthesia shivering, Can Anaesth Soc J 1978;25:43-49.
12. Cochrane Injuries Group Albumin Reviewers. Human albumin administration in critically ill patient: systematic review of randomised controlled trials. BMJ 1998;317: 235-40.
13. Velanocich V. Crystalloid versus colloid fluid resuscitation: a meta-analysis of mortality. Surgery 1989;105: 65-71.
14. Allen. Moss and Adam's Heart Disease in infants, children and Adolescents 2001;1460-68.
15. Lang SA, Duncan PG, Shephard DAE, et al. Pulmonary edema associated with airway obstruction. Can J Anaesth 1990;37:210-18.
16. Rossaint R, Falke K, Lopez F, et al. Inhaled nitric oxide for the adult respiratory distress syndrome. N Engl J Med 1993;328:399-405.
17. Kapusink JE, Sand MV. Challenging conventional aminoglycoside dose regimens, Am J Med 1986;80:908.
18. Fahnenstich. Fentanyl-induced chest wall rigidity and laryngospasm in preterm and term infants. Crit Care Med 2000;28:836-39.
19. Martinez-Pellux AE, Merino P, Bru M, et al. Can selected digestive decontamination avoid the endotoxemia in cytokine activation promoted by cardiopulmonary bypass? Crit Care Medi 1993;21:1684-91.
20. Teitelbaum. Treatment of Parenteral Nutrition-Associated Cholestatsis with Cholecystokinin-Octapeptide. J Pediatr Surg 1995;30:1082-85.
21. Bhatt DR, Bruggman DS, Thomas JC, et al. Neonatal drug formulary. (5th edn), Kaiser Permanente; Fontana, California 2002.

CHAPTER 15
Antimicrobials and Antimicrobial Prophylaxis in Pediatric Surgery

V Ravikumar, M Srinivas

The pattern of surgical infections in children is changing and this requires the need to define the problems in surgical infections and to find out efficient means to prevent varieties of bacterial, fungal and viral infections. Despite the use of modern antibiotics, there is significant persistence of postoperative and nosocomial infections due to increase in the definitive surgical procedures in neonates, surgical procedures in grossly premature and very low birth weight babies whose immune mechanisms are not well developed, development of new and complex surgical techniques, complex invasive, therapeutic techniques and preoperative resuscitative measures like extracorporeal membrane oxygenation (ECMO) and surgery in immunocompromised children. The aim of the treatment in a child with infection is to destroy the microorganism without significantly harming the child.

Antisepsis surgery in the Listerian era involved chemicals like carbolic acid, iodine, etc. This was followed by various heavy metals and dyes like– mercury, trypan, prontosil, etc. Epoch making research by *Sir Alexander Fleming* gave way to the first antibiotic – Penicillin. Strictly speaking, the term antibiotic is applied only to the naturally occurring substance produced by one microbial species that is capable of inhibiting the growth of another microbe. Whilst the term *antimicrobial* agent is used to the synthetic substance that inhibits the growth of the microorganisms. Such a distinction is rather academic and hence many authors use them interchangeably. Antibiotic is a substance that is capable of inhibiting the growth of bacteria (a *prokaryotic* cell). Fungi are *eukaryotic* cells and the agents which inhibit their growth are called as *antifungals*. Agents inhibiting viral replication are called as *antivirals*.

ANTIBIOTICS

Antibiotics either stop multiplication or destroy the bacteria acting at various levels of bacterial cell structure, metabolism and/or nucleic acids. Broadly mode of action is:
1. By destroying the bacterial cell wall – *Bactericidal*.
2. By preventing multiplication of the cells – *Bacteriostatic*. Here, the bacteria are prevented to replicate and this eventually permits the host immune mechanism to over come the infection.

Exact Mode of Action

Interference with Cell Wall Synthesis

Inhibition of cell wall synthesis affects osmotic gradient across the cell membrane and the microbe swells up and bursts. *Penicillins* bind to the cell membrane enzymes involved in synthesizing peptidoglycan, and *Vancomycin* prevents cell membrane cross linkage process. Gram-negative bacteria have less peptidoglycan in their cell membrane and therefore are not amenable for treatment by penicillin.

Disruption of the Cell Membrane

Fungal cell membrane is rich in cholesterol and the agents like *Nystatin* disrupt the cell membrane. Human cells also have cholesterol and hence most of the potent antifungals are restricted as topical agents.

Interference with Nucleic Acid Synthesis

Nucleic acids are the building blocks of the nucleotides and any interference with their synthesis would stop the growth of the bacteria. Trimethoprim prevents the synthesis of folic acid in the bacteria, *Rifampicin* inhibits the transcription of DNA into RNA. *Gyrase* is an enzyme, which is involved in the coiling and uncoiling of the DNA strands, and it is affected by the quinolones.

Interference with Protein Synthesis

Few antibiotics selectively bind to the bacterial ribosomes there by affecting the protein synthesis. Most aminoglycosides affect protein synthesis.

Pharmacokinetics of Antibiotics

When an antimicrobial is introduced in the body it gets distributed into two compartments, the vascular (central) and the tissues (the peripheral) compartments. What ever be the route of administration the vascular compartment is filled either by vascular, oral or intramuscularly route.

The amount of drug available in the vascular compartment as percentage of the total dose given is termed *Bioavailability*. The drug diffuses from the vascular to the peripheral regions and then undergoes metabolic changes or excreted. Part of the drug reaches the vascular compartment by redistribution. When the drug is administered the drug reaches the peak in serum concentration in phase one called *alpha phase* from where the drug gets distributed into the tissues. The rise in the tissue concentration, which is initially lower than the vascular compartment but subsequently goes above, is called the *beta phase* where the drug gets eliminated by metabolism or excretion.

MAIN GROUPS OF ANTIBIOTICS

Penicillin

Penicillin was discovered and initially manufactured by fermentation process and the need to make the drug by chemical means resulted in the manufacture of synthetic penicillins where side chain to the Beta lactam was altered with broader spectrum of activity. Penicillin is active only against gram-positive cocci where as the synthetic penicillins are active against gram-negative organisms also. The cell wall of gram negative bacteria is more complex and resistant to conventional penicillin. Synthetic penicillin can more readily penetrate outer lipid membrane of gram-negative bacteria and hence are effective against gram-negative bacteria. Salient features of this group are summarized in Table 15.1.

Cephalosporin

The cephalosporins have chemical structure similar to the penicillins and the most important agents are summarized in Table 15.2.

Other Beta Lactams

Monobactems (e.g. Imipenem) are effective against a wide range of gram-positive and gram-negative organisms and do not cause hypersensitive reactions in patients who are sensitive to penicillins.

Table 15. 1: Important penicillins and their spectrum and uses

Subgroup	Name	Main spectrum of activity	Remarks
Natural penicillin	Benzylpenicillin	Gram +ve bacteria	Intravenously for meningitis
	Penicillin V	Gram +ve bacteria	Oral administration Prophylaxis-postsplenectomy
Broad spectrum penicillin	Ampicillin	In addition, enterococci	Oral for mild infections IV for moderate infections
	Amoxycillin Co-amoxiclav	In addition, good for penicillinase producing organisms	Clavulanic acid binds with penicillinases
Penicillinase resistant penicillins	Flucloxacillin	Gram +ve bacteria, especially for *Staphylococcus aureus*	Better absorbed from gut
	Oxacillin		
Antipseudomonal penicillins	Mezlocillin Piperacillin Azlocillin	Especially for *Pseudomonas aeruginosa* Usually used in combination with	For serious gram-negative and anaerobic infections aminoglycosides

Table 15.2: Important cephalosporins and their spectrum and uses

Generation	Name	Main spectrum	Remarks
First	Cephradine Cephalexin Cefaclor	Gram –ve and gram +ve organisms	Staphylococcal cephalosporin Useful for mild to moderate infections Oral preparations
Second	Cefuroxime Cefamandole	Gram –ve and gram + ve organisms	Useful for moderate to severe infections, prophylaxis against infections
Third	Cefotaxime Ceftazidime Ceftizoxime Ceftriaxone	Better activity against Gram –ve organisms. Less effective against Gram +ve organisms	Colifrom cephalosporin. Useful for serious infections. Very good for *pseudomonas* and *acinetobacter*. Ceftazidime - Pseudomonal cephalosporin Ceftriaxone has long half-life
Third oral	Cefixime	Better activity against Gram –ve organisms. Less effective against Gram +ve organisms	Oral administration Not useful for *Staphylococcus* and *Pseudomonas* Primarily for switch over therapy from parenteral third generation preparations
Fourth	Cefepime Cefpirome	Both Gram +ve and Gram –ve organisms	Useful for serious infections

Carbapenems, in addition to the above spectrum, are also effective against anaerobes. These agents have a broad spectrum of action except *Pseudomonas* and *Proteus mirabilis.* Important disadvantage is that the therapeutic-toxic ratio is low and myoclonic seizures can develop.

Meropenem is closely related to imipenem and has been approved for use in children. It has greater activity against gram-negative bacteria and lack of association with seizures which is a distinct advantage.

Aminoglycosides

Aminoglycosides are active against all gram-negative organisms. Anaerobes are resistant to aminoglycosides. These drugs are generally used in combination with another antibiotic to provide activity against broad spectrum. Aminoglycosides are not absorbed orally and hence need to be given parenterally. However, given orally they are useful in gut "Sterilization". The drugs available are –

Gentamicin, Amikacin, Tobramycin and Netilmycin, etc. Many of this group are active against *Pseudomonas.* Nephrotoxicity and ototoxicity are main drawbacks and hence should be used with caution. Drugs with lesser toxicity and same spectrum if available should be chosen and aminoglycosides should be used as a second line therapy based on culture and sensitivity reports.

Macrolides

These drugs inhibit bacterial protein synthesis by biding to the ribosomes reversibly and hence these are bacteriostatic. These agents are effective against most gram-positive organisms and a range of anaerobes. They are also effective against intracellular pathogens such as chlamydia and rickettsia. Erythromycin is commonly advised for children who are sensitive to penicillins.

Quinolones

Quinolones have wide spectrum of activity including gram-negative aerobic coliforms and those organisms that tend to get localized in the intracellular regions like *Salmonella, Mycoplasma, and Cshlamydia.* Though initial fears have been expressed on the role of these drugs on joint cartilage damage in children, the drug has been used in critical situations including meningitis in newborn and infants. *Ciprofloxacin, Ofloxacin, Pefloxacin, Enoxacin* are good even when administered orally. *Trovofloxacin* is a fluroquinolone with an exceptionally broad spectrum of activity.

Glycopeptides

Vancomycin is active only against gram-positive organisms. They are poorly absorbed from the gut and Vancomycin given intramuscularly is very painful and hence needs to be given intravenously. Rapid infusion results in flushing of upper body called *red man syndrome*. Ototoxicity has been reported. It can be used in penicillin hypersensitive patients for treatment or prophylaxis of *Staphylococcal endocarditis*. Anti staphylococcal drugs like *Vancomycin* and *Teicoplanin* are very effective against most methicillin resistant strains of *Staphylococci*.

Sulphonamides

These are synthetic chemicals that interfere with para amino benzoic acid (PABA), an enzyme involved in the production of folic acid, which is essential ingredient for the production of nucleic acids. They are very popular as topical preparations especially in burns. *Trimethoprim* does also affect folic acid synthesis and because it enhances the activity of the sulphonamides, it is generally used in combination as *Co-trimoxazole*. This is excreted in urine and is useful in urinary tract infections especially as a chemoprophylactic agent.

Imidazoles

Metronidazole is the original drug of this group and it is the drug of choice for anaerobes. Most of the anaerobes are sensitive and is the drug of choice in such situations since resistance to metronidazole is rare. It is well absorbed from gastrointestinal tract with the bioavailability of 90%. It could penetrate abscesses and interferes with nucleic acid synthesis of the bacterial cells. It can be used for oral bowel preparation for GI surgery. *Tinidazole* is another similar drug with longer half-life.

Antifungal Therapy

Fungi have a potential to cause various infections ranging from superficial skin and mucous membrane to serious systemic infections. These are generally seen in immunocompromised children. *Amphotericin B* is a broad-spectrum antifungal agent most commonly used for serious systemic infection. Nephrotoxicity of this drug is the most limiting factor. *Flucytosine* disrupts protein synthesis of eukaryotic cells there by prevents the growth of the fungi and is used for systemic infections from yeasts. *Fluconazole* is the antifungal of choice for prophylactic treatment in immunocompromised children.

Antiviral Therapy

Viruses are intracellular organisms and utilize the host cell to replicate themselves. Important antiviral agents are summarized in the Table 15.3.

PROPHYLAXIS

Antibiotics are used to protect children at risk during surgery. Prophylaxis aims to protect the child from local infection as well as distant infection. This has a particular role in children who are vulnerable for infective endocarditis. The objective for quality standard for antimicrobial prophylaxis in pediatric surgical patients is to provide an implementation mechanism that will facilitate reliable administration of prophylactic antimicrobial agents to children undergoing operative procedures in which such a practice is judged to be beneficial and to provide a guideline that will help local hospital committees to formulate policies and set up mechanisms for their implementation. A prophylactic antibiotic does not reduce the chances of infections if proper surgical principles are not adhered to. A good antibiotic will not cover a bad surgery. In choosing the antibiotic the endogenous and exogenous flora likely to cause infection should be considered and appropriate antibiotic chosen. It is preferable to choose a single antibiotic rather than multiple combinations unless the type of surgery needs it. Proven antibiotics should be chosen and additional new antibiotics should not be introduced unless there is proof of its efficiency in a

Table 15.3: Important antiviral agents used in children

Antiviral agent	Remarks
Amantadine	Used prophylactically to prevent influenza infection
Idoxuridione	Topical usage – For skin and corneal Herpes infection
Acyclovir	Useful for herpes simplex and varicella zoster
Ganciclovir	Drug of choice for cytomegalovirus infection in immunocompromised children. Induces neutropenia
Vidarabine	Comparatively less toxic
Zidovudine	Inhibits DNA polymerases. Commonly used for HIV infection and prophylaxis
Sequinavir / Ritonavir / Indinavir	Protease inhibitors. Effective for retroviruses. Used in combination with others for HIV

specific situation. A single shot prophylaxis is as effective as multiple doses, as unnecessarily prolonged administration increases the likelihood of resistant strains and serious nosocomial infections.

Timing of Antibiotic Prophylaxis in Pediatric Surgery

Intrapartum prophylactic measures are necessary to prevent infections to the newborn baby as it prevents infections from the amniotic fluid and genitalia of the mother. After birth, the chosen antibiotic should be administered at the time of induction of anesthesia so that maximum tissue concentration of drug is present at the site of surgery. If the surgery is prolonged a repeat administration of antibiotic should be given depending on the half-life of the drug initially used. Full dose of chosen antibiotic should be used so that its concentration is more than *minimal inhibitory concentration* (MIC) and *minimal bactericidal concentration* (MBC). Prophylactic antibiotics need not be continued in the postoperative period, unless the host defenses are compromised or a drain is kept or a prosthesis is implanted. Antibiotics, however, may be continued if a focus of infection is found at the time of surgery or there is a high risk of infection. If the same drug is used for prolonged period for prophylaxis, it is pertinent to aware of the resistant strains that might develop. The decision to change the antibiotics is purely based on the clinical course, evidence of overt or covert infection. Ideally it should be based on the emerging resistant strains. A good antibiotic should have wide spectrum of activity both against aerobic and anaerobic organisms, should be least toxic, should have high degree of diffusion in the tissues with bactericidal action, and should be at an affordable cost to the patient. The agent is selected depending upon the site of surgery. For example, children undergoing resection and end-to-end anastomosis of bowel would require protection against aerobic coliforms and anaerobes. So the agents used would be — A penicillin/cephalosporin to kill gram-positive aerobes, an aminoglycoside to kill gram-negative organisms and metronidazole to protect against anaerobes. It should be given close to the time of incision to ensure that the levels of the agents are adequate during the bacteriemia. Prophylactic therapy is generally not continued beyond 24 hours after surgery.

Antibiotic Resistance

Bacteria are described as *sensitive* to a particular antibiotic if their growth is inhibited or they are killed by a concentration of the drug in the body that could be achieved by the usual dose regimen. *Resistant* bacteria are not inhibited by this concentration of the agent. The bacteria can acquire resistance to antibiotics by means of one or more of the following mechanisms:

1. By altering the permeability to the agent at cell membrane level.
2. By producing enzymes that inactivate the agent (e.g. *Beta lactamases* destroy penicillins and cephalosporins).
3. The drug may be actively expelled from the cell.
4. *By plasmids:* Plasmids are small molecules of DNA independent of the chromosome, which can be replicated between cells by conjugation, transformation, or transduction. *Plasmids* provide a highly effective means of spreading resistance genes, both within a species and to other species.
5. *By transposons:* Transposons are specific sequences of DNA that can insert into both plasmids and chromosomes, and can transfer or jump between them. They have a potential to carry genes encoding for resistance to a wide variety of antibiotics and play a key role in the dissemination of antibiotic resistance, especially where species develop resistance to more than one drug. *Multiple drug resistance* (MDR) is a term used to describe bacteria that have developed resistance to several antibiotics.

Agricultural use of antibiotics, wide spread use of antibiotics, unnecessary prescription of antibiotics and prolonged usage of antibiotics have contributed to the drug resistance and this has become a significant health problem today.

Intrapartum Prophylaxis

Prophylactic intravenous ampicillin-sulbactam has been shown to reduce intra-amniotic fluid infection and this is likely to decrease the potential consequences of it to the newborn baby. HIV infection is becoming one of the major serious neonatal infectious diseases in many parts of the world and 40-80% of perinatal HIV transmission occurs during or close to intrapartum period.[1,2] Antiviral agent – *Zidovudine* is reported to reduce transmission risk by 70%. In this regard, WHO/UNICEF expert group recommends the following:[3]

Zidovudine, 200 mg thrice a day, is recommended from 14 weeks of pregnancy. A loading dose of 2 mg/k over first hour is followed by maintenance dose of 1 mg/k/h over intrapartum period. The newborn baby, once delivered, is administered syrup Zidovudine (2 mg/k every 6 h for 6 weeks).

Mothers with symptomatic *genital herpes* infection have a significant risk of infecting the newborn baby. *Acyclovir*, 400 mg thrice a day, is started from 36 weeks of pregnancy and it is given until delivery to reduce this risk.[4]

SPECIFIC PROPHYLAXIS IN PEDIATRIC SURGERY

An ideal prophylactic agent should target the entire spectrum, easily administerable, well tolerated and should have minimal side effects. Children would like to have a single oral dose of the drug rather than multiple doses/parenteral preparations.

The factors that influence efficacy of the prophylaxis regimen are related to the potential pathogen, the prophylactic agent and the host and these are summarized in the Table 15.4.

Table 15.4: Factors related to the efficacy of the prophylaxis regimen

Pathogen factors
- Nature of the potential pathogen
- Number of potential pathogens
- Sources of potential pathogens
- Load of the potential pathogen

Antimicrobial agent factors
- Type of agent
- Activity spectrum of the agent
- Pharmacokinetics and pharmacodynamics of the agent
- Dosage of the agent
- Timing of the drug administration
- Duration of the prophylaxis
- Drug resistance

Host factors
- Immune status of the individual
- Congenital / acquired immune deficiency disorders
- Severity of the surgical intervention
- Target organs that need to be protected

It is imperative to keep all these factors in mind while deciding the antimicrobial agent.

Intravascular Catheters

Staphylococcus epidermidis is a normal commensal and the infection with this pathogen is likely to occur in newborn babies. Premature babies, very low birth weight babies and babies receiving parenteral nutrition are more vulnerable. Studies have shown that low dose vancomycin significantly reduces such infection.[5-7] Mupirocin is a topical antibiotic with high anti-staphylococcal activity. Mupirocin applied to the insertion site significantly reduces the risk of *Staphylococcus aureus* skin and catheter colonization, exit site infection, *Staphylococcus bacteriemia* in with intravenous catheters.[8] A randomized, multicenter, double blind trial has shown to decrease complications associated with central venous catheters by Vancomycin and Ciprofloxacin in addition to heparin used as a flush solution.[9]

Bacterial Endocarditis

All children, who are at risk of endocarditis, undergoing any intervention that is likely to produce bacteriemia are given prophylaxis.[10] Poor oral hygiene and oral infections need to be tackled before any elective surgical procedures. Perioperative prophylaxis (from shortly before surgery to about 10 hours) is recommended. Alpha hemolytic *Streptococci* are the most common organisms responsible for endocarditis after upper respiratory, oral and upper GI procedures. The drugs recommended are: Amoxcillin (50 mg/kg) given orally 1 hour before the surgery *or Ampicillin* (50 mg/kg) IV/IM 30 minutes before the surgery. For children hypersensitive to penicillin *Azithromycin* (15 mg/kg) orally 1 hour before the procedure is recommended. Prophylaxis for genitourinary (including endoscopic interventions/ voiding cystourethrography) or GIT surgery should cover enterococci. *Ampicillin* (50 mg/kg) PLUS *Gentamicin* (2 mg/kg) intravenously 30 minutes before the procedure is recommended. For children hypersensitive to penicillins, *Vancomycin* (20 mg/kg) by infusion (starting 1 ½ hour before surgery and lasting for 1 hour) *and Gentamicin* (2 mg/kg) intravenously 30 minutes before the procedure is recommended.

In addition to the above, children who undergo surgical procedures where in prosthetic material is likely to be placed inside the body, should receive

Vancomycin perioperatively and not more than 48 hours after the procedure.

Antimicrobial Prophylaxis for Urinary Tract Infections

Many of pediatric urology patients require prophylactic antibiotics to prevent recurrent urinary tract infections. Though treatment of acute UTI is based upon the urine culture reports, the chemoprophylaxis is straight forward and generally involves choosing from a short list of antibiotics. There are good published guidelines and in December 2000, an expert group meeting of the Indian Pediatric Nephrology recommended the following guidelines.[11-14] The recommended drugs are summarized in Table 15.5.

The expert group meeting also reached the following consensus regarding the indication and duration of the chemoprophylaxis that depends upon number of episodes of infection, reflux status and renal scarring. The committee also felt that there is no role for cyclic therapy. The recommendations are summarized in Table 15.6.

Circumcision in boys, particularly in infants with VUR, has been shown to reduce the risk of urinary tract infections.[15] A review of 18-year experience from Royal Free Hospital School of Medicine has shown that long-term nitrofurantoin is effective, safe and tolerable in urinary infections.[16]

Asplenia/Splenectomy

Functions of the spleen may be deficient in congenital asplenia syndromes, surgical removal for hypersplenism/trauma or auto splenectomy in sickle cell disease. Absence of spleen predisposes to overwhelming post splenectomy infections (OPSI). Approximately 80% of fatal infections occur within 2 years of splenectomy and 80% of the infections are due to bacteria with capsular polysaccharides – *Strepto pneumonia, Hemophilus influenza* and *Nissieria meningitidis*.[17-18]

Penicillin V, given twice daily, significantly decreases the frequency of invasive pneumococcal infections. Penicillin prophylaxis would definitely decrease the chances of pneumococcal sepsis but does not completely eliminate the risk of fulminant sepsis as the resistant strains are well known. Erythromycin/ Trimethoprim Sulfamethoxazole combination are alternatives for children hypersensitive to penicillins. Chemoprophylaxis is recommended for all children, especially for those under 5 years of age, for at least 1 year following splenectomy. However, prophylaxis

Table 15.5: Chemoprophylaxis for urinary tract infections in children

Agent	Dose	Remarks
Cephalexin	10 mg/kg/d	Drug of choice in infants below 6 months of age
Co-trimoxazole	1-2 mg/kg/d of trimethoprim	Not recommended for infants below 3 months of age. Avoid in G-6 PD deficiency
Nitrofurantoin	1-2 mg/kg/d	Avoid in G-6 PD deficiency Avoid in renal insufficiency

Table 15.6: Indications and duration for chemoprophylaxis for UTI

Main finding	Additional finding(s)	Age of child	Duration/Remarks
First episode of UTI			
	No reflux, No renal scar	< 2 years	6 months ‡
	No reflux, No renal scar	> 2 years	No prophylaxis
	Grade I and II reflux	< 5 years	Until 5 years of age
	Grade III and U/L grade IV	< 5 years	Until 5 years of age
	Grade III and U/L grade IV	> 5 years	Surgery
	B/L grade IV, grade V	< 1 year	Until 1 year of age
	B/L grade IV, grade V	> 1 year	Surgery
	No reflux, renal scar +	All ages	6 months. ‡
Recurrent UTI			
	No reflux and no scar	All ages	6 months
Legend:			
‡ [After 6 months of treatment, if no reflux and no scar are found – stop chemoprophylaxis].			

is continued indefinitely in immunocompromised children.

Prophylaxis Related to the Specific Surgical Interventions

Epidemiologists have stratified surgical procedures based on the risk of infection as—
1. *Clean cases:* There are primarily elective cases in which wound is primarily closed without any drain and respiratory, alimentary, or genitourinary tracts are not breached. The expected infection rate in this category is less than 2%.
2. *Clean contaminated cases:* Respiratory, alimentary, or genitourinary tracts are breached and/or the wound is drained. The expected infection rate in this category is around 5%.
3. *Contaminated cases:* Gross spillage from gastrointestinal tract, gross infection, or open traumatic wounds are present. The expected infection rate in this category is around 15%.
4. *Dirty cases:* Perforated viscera at the site of operation, delayed treatment of traumatic wounds, or gas gangrene is present. The expected infection rate in this category is around 40%.

Generally, clean operations such as herniotomy, orchidopexy does not require antibiotics. However, even in clean operations if prosthesis is being contemplated, then antibiotic cover is necessary. Antibiotics should also be used in all immune compromised children and children who are at risk for infective endocarditis.

Pediatric Neurosurgical Procedures

Insertion of ventriculo-peritoneal shunt is one of the most common pediatric neurosurgical procedures and most infections manifest within 15 days to 2 months of surgery.[19]

Coagulase – negative *Staphylococci* are the most common organisms and account for 70% of shunt infections. A meta-analysis of 12 randomized controlled clinical trials has indicated that short-term perioperative antibiotic prophylaxis at the time of shunt insertion significantly decreases the postoperative infections.[19]

Duration of this perioperative prophylaxis should not exceed 48 hours. A single dose of second generation cephalosporin has been shown to be enough in shunting procedures.[20]

Pediatric Oral Surgery

Preoperative local decontamination by Povidone Iodine solution has been found to be beneficial in a randomized clinical trial.[21] Perioperative prophylactic coverage with Ampicillin/Amoxcillin/Azithromycin (in Penicillin sensitive children) is sufficient for cleft lip and palate surgery and recently cefuroxime has been shown to be better than the conventional antibiotics.[22]

Pediatric Thoracic Surgical Procedures

Monotherapy prophylaxis utilizing a third generation Cephalosporin is acceptable which is started 30 minutes before surgery and is given for not more than 48 hours. However, prophylactic antibiotics are continued if thoracostomy tubes, vascular catheters or endotracheal tubes are placed until their removal. In 1995, a survey of North American academic centers with pediatric cardiovascular surgery programs revealed that most popular regimen was monotherapy with a first or second generation cephalosporin used for less than 2 days or until transthoracic medical devices were removed.[23]

Pediatric GI Surgery

Bacteria are involved in the pathogenesis of necrotizing enterocolitis (NEC). Presently, oral administration of non-absorbable aminoglycosides like Kanamycin is not recommended to prevent NEC. Though oral Vancomycin given for 48 hours before introduction of oral feeds in neonates at risk has been shown to of benefit until multicentric trials prove it conclusively, it is better not to recommend this drug routinely for prevention of NEC.[24]

A single dose of cefuroxime (30 mg/k) at induction of anesthesia has been reported to reduce infection in infantile pyloromyotomy.[25]

A single dose of intravenous vancomycin prophylaxis in permanent peritoneal dialysis catheter placement is reported to be superior to single dose of cefazolin in reducing the risk of postoperative peritonitis.

Appendectomy

In a suspected or overt inflammation confined to appendix alone, a single dose of antibiotic at the time of induction of anesthesia is enough. Cefazolin and Metronidazole will cover the usual pathogens of the appendix. If it is perforated or evidence of localized or generalized peritonitis is present a third generation cephalosporin along with an aminoglycoside and metronidazole is started. Generally Metronidazole is stopped after 5 days and others after 7-10 days depending on the clinical course and evidence of persistence of infection. Study from Karolinska Institute had concluded that a single preoperative dose of Metronidazole alone significantly decreases the rate of postoperative infectious complications in children with appendicitis. No further improvement was noted if cefuroxime was added in that study.[26]

Pediatric Colorectal Surgeries

Antibiotic prophylaxis is necessary not only to prevent wound infection but also to minimize the complications such as leaks at the site of anastomosis and wound dehiscence. It is imperative to decrease the bacterial load by promoting purgation. Wash outs with Polyethylene glycol (PEGLEC) — 25 ml/kg/h for 4 hours or with normal saline — 10 ml/kg is very important. Perioperative prophylaxis with a third generation cephalosporin along with an aminoglycoside and metronidazole provides a good cover.

Antibiotics may be used empirically in situations without waiting for the culture reports in clinical situations like lacerations, liver abscesses, peritonitis, etc based on the earlier knowledge of the type of organism and the antibiotic sensitivity. Anaerobic cover is also required in situations like liver abscess where the cavity will harbor amoebae and anaerobic bacteria.

Many children develop febrile neutropenia during chemotherapy for cancer. In lower risk neutropenic children receiving anticancer therapy, oral Cefixime given for 4 days after 72 hours of intravenous Ceftriaxone plus Amikacin has been shown to be safe and cost effective compared to the conventional protocols.[27]

Pediatric Transplantation Surgery

Perioperative prophylaxis is very important in children undergoing transplantation as they are predisposed to infections arising out of immunosuppressive therapy. Nystatin is started few days before the transplantation to prevent oropharyngeal candidiasis.[28] Standard antibiotics – a third generation cephalosporin and an aminoglycoside along with Metronidazole are followed by long-term Trimethoprim – Sulfamethoxazole combination to prevent pneumocystis carinii pneumonia. Few transplant centers are adding antiviral prophylaxis by administering ribavirin as well.[29]

TOPICAL AGENTS

Mupirocin is a topical antibiotic with high anti-staphylococcal activity. Mupirocin applied to the insertion site significantly reduces the risk of *Staphylococcus aureus* skin and catheter colonization, exit site infection, *Staphylococcus* bacteriemia in hemodialysis patients.[8] Nasal mupirocin has been reported to be an effective method of controlling Methicillin resistant *Staphylococcus aureus* outbreak in neonatal intensive care unit.[30]

Povidone Iodine gel alcohol (PGA) is reported to be an effective skin–preparation formulation for use.[31]

A topical antimicrobial gel containing cetrimide, bacitracin and polymyxin B sulfate has been shown to reduce the incidence of clinical infections in minor accidental wound.[32] It needs to be seen whether this has any applicability in the routine surgical wound.

Although, short duration prophylaxis is scientifically proven to be cost effective and provides maximum benefits in most of the elective surgeries, many centers in this country do prolong the antibiotic usage. We hope that this review article would convince us to adhere to the recommended prophylactic regimens. In addition to the antibiotics, we should remember Sir William Osler's aphorism – Soap, water and commonsense are the best disinfectants. Antibiotics are not the panacea. For example, it has been shown that systemic antibiotics do not consistently eradicate gram-negative bacillary air way colonization in mechanically ventilated newborns.[33] This shows the importance of preventive measures like proper hand washing, etc. In future, computerized pediatric anti-infective decision support programs are likely to benefit clinicians dealing with infections in children.[34]

REFERENCES

1. Adair CD, Sanchez-Ramos L, McDyer DL, Gaudier FL, Del Valle GO, Delke I. Predicting fetal lung maturity by visual assessment of amniotic fluid turbidity: comparison with fluorescence polarization assay. South Med J 1995;88:1031-33.
2. Lyall EG, Blott M, de Ruiter A, Hawkins D, Mercy D, Mitchla Z, Newell ML, O'Shea S, Smith JR, Sunderland J, Webb R, Taylor GP. Guidelines for the management of HIV infection in pregnant women and the prevention of mother-to-child transmission. HIV Med 2001;2:314-34.
3. WHO/UNICEF statement on breast feeding and HIV. WHO / UNICEF consultative meeting. Weekly epidemiol Rec 1992;67:177-84.
4. Scott LL, Sanchez PJ, Jackson GL, Zeray F, Wendel GD Jr. Acyclovir suppression to prevent cesarean delivery after first-episode genital herpes. Obstet Gynecol 1996;87:69-73.
5. Kacica MA, Horgan MJ, Ochoa L, Sandler R, Lepow ML, Venezia RA. Prevention of gram-positive sepsis in neonates weighing less than 1500 grams. J Pediatr 1994;125:253-58.
6. Spafford PS, Sinkin RA, Cox C, Reubens L, Powell KR. Prevention of central venous catheter-related coagulase-negative staphylococcal sepsis in neonates. J Pediatr 1994;125:259-63.
7. Cooke RW, Nycyk JA, Okuonghuae H, Shah V, Damjanovic V, Hart CA. Low-dose vancomycin prophylaxis reduces coagulase-negative staphylococcal bacteremia in very low birthweight infants. J Hosp Infect 1997;37:297-303.
8. Sesso R, Barbosa D, Leme IL, Sader H, Canziani ME, Manfredi S, Draibe S, Pignatari AC. Staphylococcus aureus prophylaxis in hemodialysis patients using central venous catheter: effect of mupirocin ointment. J Am Soc Nephrol 1998;9:1085-92.
9. Henrickson KJ, Axtell RA, Hoover SM, Kuhn SM, Pritchett J, Kehl SC, Klein JP. Prevention of central venous catheter-related infections and thrombotic events in immuno-compromised children by the use of vancomycin/ciprofloxacin/heparin flush solution: A randomized, multicenter, double-blind trial. J Clin Oncol 2000;18:1269-78.
10. Brook MM. Pediatric bacterial endocarditis. Treatment and prophylaxis. Pediatr Clin North Am 1999;46:275-87.
11. Bollgren I. Antibacterial prophylaxis in children with urinary tract infection. Acta Paediatr Suppl 1999;88:48-52.
12. Jodal U, Lindberg U. Guidelines for management of children with urinary tract infection and vesico-ureteric reflux. Recommendations from a Swedish state-of-the-art conference. Swedish Medical Research Council. Acta Paediatr Suppl 1999;88:87-89.
13. Elder JS, Peters CA, Arant BS Jr, Ewalt DH, Hawtrey CE, Hurwitz RS, Parrott TS, Snyder HM 3rd, Weiss RA, Woolf SH, Hasselblad V. Pediatric Vesicoureteral Reflux Guidelines Panel summary report on the management of primary vesicoureteral reflux in children. J Urol 1997;157:1846-51.
14. Bagga A, Babu K, Kanitkar M, Srivastava RN. Consensus statement on management of urinary tract infections. Indian Pediatr 2001;38:1106-15.
15. Cascio S, Colhoun E, Puri P. Bacterial colonization of the prepuce in boys with vesicoureteral reflux who receive antibiotic prophylaxis. J Pediatr 2001;139:160-62.
16. Brumfitt W, Hamilton-Miller JM. Efficacy and safety profile of long-term nitrofurantoin in urinary infections: 18 years' experience. J Antimicrob Chemother 1998;42:363-71.
17. Lynch AM, Kapila R. Overwhelming postsplenectomy infection. Infect Dis Clin North Am 1996;10:693-707.
18. Siddins M, Downie J, Wise K, O'Reilly M. Prophylaxis against postsplenectomy pneumococcal infection. Aust N Z J Surg 1990;60:183-87.
19. Langley JM, LeBlanc JC, Drake J, Milner R. Efficacy of antimicrobial prophylaxis in placement of cerebrospinal fluid shunts: meta-analysis. Clin Infect Dis 1993;17:98-103.
20. Zentner J, Gilsbach J, Felder T. Antibiotic prophylaxis in cerebrospinal fluid shunting: a prospective randomized trial in 129 patients. Neurosurg Rev 1995;18(3):169-72.
21. Summers AN, Larson DL, Edmiston CE, Gosain AK, Denny AD, Radke L. Efficacy of preoperative decontamination of the oral cavity. Plast Reconstr Surg 2000;106:895-900.
22. Alfter G, Schwenzer N, Friess D, Mohrle E. Perioperative antibiotic prophylaxis with cefuroxime in oral-maxillofacial surgical procedures. J Craniomaxillofac Surg 1995;23:38-41.
23. Lee KR, Ring JC, Leggiadro RJ. Prophylactic antibiotic use in pediatric cardiovascular surgery: a survey of current practice. Pediatr Infect Dis J 1995;14:267-69.
24. Ng PC, Dear PR, Thomas DF. Oral vancomycin in prevention of necrotising enterocolitis. Arch Dis Child 1988;63:1390-93.
25. Nour S, MacKinnon AE, Dickson JA, Walker J. Antibiotic prophylaxis for infantile pyloromyotomy. J R Coll Surg Edinb 1996;41:178-80.
26. Soderquist-Elinder C, Hirsch K, Bergdahl S, Rutqvist J, Frenckner B. Prophylactic antibiotics in uncomplicated appendicitis during childhood—a prospective randomised study. Eur J Pediatr Surg 1995;5:282-85.
27. Paganini HR, Sarkis CM, De Martino MG, Zubizarreta PA, Casimir L, Fernandez C, Armada AA, Rodriguez-Brieshcke MT, Debbag R. Oral administration of cefixime to lower risk febrile neutropenic children with cancer. Cancer 2000;88:2848-52.
28. Garcia S, Roque J, Ruza F, Gonzalez M, Madero R, Alvarado F, Herruzo R. Infection and associated risk factors in the immediate postoperative period of pediatric liver transplantation: a study of 176 transplants. Clin Transplant 1998;12:190-97.
29. Kapelushnik J, Or R, Delukina M, Nagler A, Livni N, Engelhard D. Intravenous ribavirin therapy for

adenovirus gastroenteritis after bone marrow transplantation. J Pediatr Gastroenterol Nutr 1995;21(1): 110-12.
30. Hitomi S, Kubota M, Mori N, Baba S, Yano H, Okuzumi K, Kimura S. Control of a methicillin-resistant *Staphylococcus aureus* outbreak in a neonatal intensive care unit by unselective use of nasal mupirocin ointment. J Hosp Infect 2000;46(2):123-29.
31. Jeng DK, Severin JE. Povidone iodine gel alcohol: a 30-second, onetime application preoperative skin preparation. Am J Infect Control 1998;26:488-94.
32. Langford JH, Artemi P, Benrimoj SI. Topical antimicrobial prophylaxis in minor wounds. Ann Pharmacother 1997;31(5):559-63.
33. Cordero L, Sananes M, Ayers LW. Failure of systemic antibiotics to eradicate gram-negative bacilli from the airway of mechanically ventilated very low-birth-weight infants. Am J Infect Control 2000;28:286-90.
34. Mullett CJ, Evans RS, Christenson JC, Dean JM. Development and impact of a computerized pediatric antiinfective decision support program. Pediatrics 2001;108:E75.

CHAPTER 16

Fungal Infections in Pediatric Surgical Patients

Nissar A Bhat, DK Gupta

The incidence of major fungal infection in recent years has paralleled the increasing use of immunosuppressive drugs, broad-spectrum antibiotics, indwelling catheters and prostheses. Severe burns, hyperalimentation, renal failure and other debilitating conditions also predispose to invasive mycosis.[1-2] The immature immune system of neonates is partially responsible for same specific disease and pose unique management problems. These infants are increasingly stressed to degrees not previously seen in intensive care nurseries. The frequent uses of longterm indwelling catheters contribute to the potential for fungal infection in pediatric population.[3] An aggressive diagnostic approach is particularly important and tissue specimen is often necessary to establish diagnosis. Meticulous surgical techniques and minimization of the predisposing factors are crucial in the prevention of these infections and prophylactic antimycotic agents may be of value in selected high risk patients. Some mycotic wound infections can be managed effectively without systemic therapy but when systemic agents are needed, Fluconazole is used for most patients because of its efficacy. However, for the most critically ill patient Amphotericin remains the treatment of choice.[4]

BACKGROUND

Prior to the 1960, invasive opportunistic fungal infection was a rare diagnosis. The recovery of *Candida* from human tissue or body fluids was viewed as contamination and was of little importance. Fungemia was seen in patients with severe burns and in patients with malignancy, usually at the time of terminal events. Despite this timing, the fungal infection was not thought to increase the risk of mortality. The invasive potential of *Candida* was documented in 1968 when Krause et al[4] recovered *Candida* in both urine and blood following the ingestion of the organism into normally functioning intestines. Subsequently autopsy studies in the 1970 proved that *Candida* could infiltrate solid organs without causing clinical organ dysfunction.[5] In 1980, clinical studies demonstrated *Candida* as an important pathogen that could affect the outcome in critically ill patients.[6] Currently, the management of fungal infection is equally important as that of bacterial infection in the intensive care unit.

EPIDEMIOLOGY

Candida is the most commonly found fungus in isolates. The National nosocomial infection surveillance system of the centers for disease control (CDC) reported that the incidence of *Candida* as a nosocomial pathogen is increasing steadily.[7] During the past decade, *Candida* has increased in rank from the eighth to the fourth most common nosocomial pathogen isolated from blood, and accounts for 8-15% of all hospital acquired bloodstream infections.[8] This 480% rise is second only to coagulase negative *Staphlococcus*.[9] The morbidity and mortality associated with these infections is striking, with a median intensive care unit/hospital stay increasing by 30 days and death rates rising from 30-80%.[10]

Fungi

The medically important fungi are divided into two categories, *pathogenic fungi* and *opportunistic fungi*. The pathogenic fungi or virulent fungi, which include Histoplasma, Blastomyces and Coccidomyces, are usually located in endemic areas and cause infection in hosts with a normal immune function. Opportunistic fungi like Candida, Torulopsis, Aspergillus, Mucormycetes, Eryptococcus and Phycomycetes are often commensial with humans and are less virulent. The genus *Candida* and *Torulopsis* are the major pathogens causing nosocomial fungal infection in surgically ill patients.[10] The various subtypes of *Candida* are:

i. *C. albicans*, colonizes the mucosal tissue of gastrointestinal and genitourinary tracts. It is the primary fungal pathogen isolated from blood, tissue and other body fluids.
ii. *C. tropicalis*, is the second most common species responsible for fungal infection and is commonly seen in patients with hematopoietic malignancies and diabetes. It is often associated with the presence of a characteristic embolic lesion. Biopsies of these lesions can prove dissemination of the infection.[11]
iii. *C. parapsilosis*, the third most common isolate and is best known for its association with hyperalimentation and indwelling catheters. It is commonly seen in patients with solid tumors. This organism appears less virulent and its infection has a better prognosis.[10]
iv. *C. krusei* is being reported in 1-3% of isolates. It is an important pathogen among patients with neutropenia in hematological malignancies. This organism is resistant to flucanazole.[12]

Torulopsis: It can be found colonizing mucosal surfaces of the gastrointestinal and genitourinary tracts in human. *T. glabrate* is thought to be less virulent and its infection is associated with a high mortality rate of 50-70% and has a predilection for causing renal infection in diabetes patients.[13]

RISK FACTORS AND PATHOGENESIS

The most common risk factors to acquire a fungal infection are, severity of illness (APACHE II SCORE > 10, ventilator use > 48 hours), use of broad-spectrum antibiotics, indwelling central venous catheters, malnutrition, immunosuppression and burns.

Broad-spectrum Antibiotics and Fungal Translocations

Broad-spectrum antibiotics are being used with increasing frequency in the intensive care unit setting. Presumably antibacterial antibiotics suppress the growth of the normal intestinal flora and therapy promotes the overgrowth of *Candida*. When bacteria counts decrease secondary to suppression by antibiotics, the *Candida* in then able to bind and take the first important step toward translocation.[14] Decreased intestinal mucosal integrity caused by surgery, low perfusion of the bowel and endotoxin release caused by sepsis, increases the risk for translocation of fungi across the mucosal membranes. Other sites of the digestive system (pancreas, liver, gallbladder) have been implicated as sources of fungal invasion.

Central Venous Access

The overgrowth of *Candida* in the gastrointestinal tract coincides with skin colonization, any break in the epithelial barrier are important risk factors in the development of fungal invasion.

Nutritional Support

TPN has been shown to reduce complement-mediated fixation of immunoglobulins and suppress macrophage function. It also produces intestinal mucosal atrophy, possibly secondarily to deficient glutamine content in TPN fluid.[15] These factors along with presence of central venous catheter increase the risk for the development of fungal infection.

Immunosuppression

Immunosuppression can result from major surgery, trauma, burns, cancer, bacterial sepsis, hypoperfusion, corticosteroids, chemotherapy, diabetes and post-transplant immunosuppressive therapy.[6] The immunocompromised state leads to increased risk of invasion by opportunistic pathogens. Defence against fungal invasion at both superficial and deeper lesion layer is provided primarily by cellular immune function.

Burns

These patients have increased susceptibility to the fungal infection and dissemination because of following factors:
- Loss of mechanical barrier
- Gastrointestinal mucosal atrophy
- Prolonged ileus

- Decreased number of complement system, CD3, CD 4 and CD 8 T cells
- Decreased phagocytic function
- Decreased interleukin 2 production and receptor affinity
- Increased complement degradation products and burn specific polypeptides
- Use of antibiotics and indwelling central venous and urinary catheters

Overall risk factors for disseminated fungal infection and acute renal failure are:
- Age > 40 years
- Second and third degree burns
- Antibiotics for > 7 days
- Treatment with three or more antibiotics
- Gram-negative sepsis
- Acute peritonitis
- Intra-abdominal abscess
- Diabetes mellitus
- Malignancy
- Multiple organ trauma
- Parenteral nutrition
- Serum glucose > 200 mg/dl
- Severe head injury
- Steroids

High-risk > 3 risk factors
Low-risk < 3 risk factors

DIAGNOSIS

Once the diagnosis of fungal infection is entertained, the most difficult task is to differentiate colonization from invasion/disseminated disease. A firm laboratory diagnosis is difficult. Histological examination demonstrating both forms of Candida, yeast and pseudohyphae is considered diagnostic. Except for skin and burn wounds, the acquisition of tissue for histological diagnosis may require an invasive procedure. Therefore, the diagnosis of invasive/dissemination relies more on inferential rather rather than direct tissue evidence of disease.

The initial workup for the patients suspected of having fungal invasion/dissemination starts with sampling of many sites (e.g. urine, sputum, open wound, drain site, stool, stomach contents) for evidence of colonization. Although blood culture is routinely done, its interpretation can be misleading for several reasons. First, *Candida* is difficult to grow and concomitant bacterial infection may decrease its recovery from blood cultures. Second, only 50% of patients with invasive candidiasis have positive blood cultures and positive cultures do not necessarily indicate dissemination.[16] Methods of increasing sensitivity of blood cultures include lysis centrifugation and sampling of arterial instead of venous blood.[17] Lysis centrifugation increases the yield of positive cultures by 30 - 40%. Positive cultures of urine, drain sites, burns, open wounds or peritoneal fluid at the time of surgery are difficult to interpret. Each may be indicative of colonization only but may be indicative of invasive disease in the appropriate setting. Candiduria can occur in absence of candidiasis, but candidiasis without candiduria is highly unlikely.[18]

DIAGNOSTIC CRITERIA FOR DISSEMINATED FUNGAL INFECTION

Definitive Criteria

- Culture of fungus from tissue (e.g. kidney or lungs)
- Endophthalmitis
- Burns wound invasion
- Culture from peritoneal fluid.

Likely Criteria

- Two positive cultures at least 24 hours apart, without a central venous catheter
- Two positive blood cultures with a second obtained more than 24 after removal of central venous catheter.
- Three or more colonized sites.

FUNGAL INFECTION OF URINARY TRACT

Is relatively uncommon in infants and children. However, their incidence has shown an increase in recent years; probably because of better survival of LBW and premature babies.[19] The major risk factors include prematurity, LBW, contamination of urethral catheters, long-term antibiotic therapy, and obstructive uropathy.[20]

Three groups of fungi may lead to urinary tract infection.[21]

i. Opportunistic fungi like candida, aspergillus and cryptococcus

ii. Environmental fungi including coccidiodes, blastomyces and histoplasma and
iii. Rare fungi like mucormycae

Candida is the most common causative agent in UTI. The urinary tract may be involved primarily but is usually implicated secondary to systemic fungal infection. The kidneys are affected in more than 85% of cases.[22]

Patients may present with urosepsis and its common manifestation is oliguria or anuria secondary to a fungus ball obstructing the urinary tract. Diagnosis is based on clinical features, urine examination and serum precipitin titers. The presence of a fungal bezoar may be confirmed by demonstrating an echogenic mass on ultrasonography or a filling defect in the collecting system on an intravenous urogram. Observation of the mycelial or yeast form of a fungus on microscopic examination or a colony count of more than 15000/ml on culture of a properly collected urine specimen is diagnositic.[21]

Treatment of fungal UTI has been highly difficult principally due to lack of a effective and safe antifungal medication that can achieve adequate concentration in the urine. This choice is further limited by a state of compromised renal function. The initial step in management includes removal of any indwelling catheter and discontinuation of antibiotic therapy. As fungi thrive at a low pH, alkalinisation of urine with sodium bicarbonate may be helpful.[21] Upper urinary tract obstruction by a fungal bezoar often necessitates nephrostomy drainage in addition to antifungal therapy.

TREATMENT AND PROPHYLAXIS

The successful treatment of fungal infection requires a combination of the surgical principles of drainage and debridement and systemic therapy with antifungal agents. In addition the removal of infected vascular access catheters and sometimes prosthesis is necessary to cure infection. Currently, there are three indications for the use of antifungal therapy:
  i. *Prophylaxis:* Use of antifungals prior to colonization in high-risk patients.
 ii. *Early presumptive treatment:* Initiation of treatment after colonization is documented in order to prevent invasion and dissemination.
iii. *System therapy:* Treatment of documented invasive or disseminated fungal disease.

The action of most antifungal agents is targeted at the cell membrane, which is vital to cell function and viability. The major cell membrane inhibitors are:
- Polyenes: Amphotericin-B and Nystatin
- Azoles:
  - Imidazoles-Ketoconazole, Miconazole and Fluconazole
  - Triazoles – Itraconazole
- Antimetabolites: 5 Fluorocytosine

Amphotericin-B

Is a lipophilic fungicide produced by *Streptomyes nodosus*. Selective permeability to ions especially potassium and vital metabolites account for its lethality. Currently it is the drug of choice for invasive and disseminated fungal infection in critically ill patients. It is active against *Candida* and *Torulopsis*, and resistance is rare. Its route of administration is intravenous, intrathecal or intravesical as a colloid suspension with deoxycholate. To avoid hypersensitivity related reactions, which occur in 20% of patients, it is mandatory to give a test dose of 1 mg and observe for allergic reactions for at least 20 minutes before administration of therapeutic doses. Blood levels are not influenced by renal or hepatic failure. However, the dosage should be decreased or treatment stopped if renal function deteriorates.

Side effects include fever, rigors (incidence decrease with pre-treatment), renal toxicity, hypokalemia, hypomagnesemia and occasionally mild anemia. .

Nystatin

Its primary use is as a topical agent in the treatment of cutaneous fungal infection and infected burns and as a rinse in the treatment of thrush. It should not be administered parentally because of its toxicity. It is not absorbed from the gastrointestinal tract and hence its main efficacy is in reducing overgrowth at that site.

Ketoconazole

It is administered orally and requires gastric acidity for its absorption. It is highly bound to plasma proteins and metabolized in the liver. Its use as a systemic therapy in the surgical patients is debated. For prophylaxis, 200 mg once a day significantly reduces colonization. Side effects include gastrointestinal intolerance, decreased steroidogenesis leading to gynecomastia and occasionally adrenal insufficiency. It is a hepatotoxic drug therefore, weekly transaminase monitoring is recommended.

Miconazole

It is mainly used as a topical agent but it is sometimes used intravenously.

Fluconazole

It is well absorbed from the gastrointestinal tract regardless of the pH and its bioavailability is excellent (> 90%) by oral and intravenous route. Because it is excreted in urine, its dosage requires adjustment for creatinine clearance in presence of renal failure. Heptotoxicity has also been reported.

Itraconazole

It has greater than 70% bioavailibity following oral ingestion. Absorption is increased by foods, decreased by antacids and not influenced by H_2 blockers.

Drug interaction includes decreased levels of rifampicin, theophylline, digoxin, cyclosporin phenytoin and oral hypoglycemics. Clinically, it is the drug of choice for the treatment of endemic fungi (Histoplasmosis and Blastomyces).

5-Fluorocytosine

Usual dosage is 5-150 mg/kg/day in four divided doses. Toxicity are related to alteration in hematological parameters.

REFERENCES

1. Nagar H. Mycotic Infections and the Pediatric Surgeon. Mycopathologia 1990;112(3):147-55.
2. Codish SD, Sheridan ID, Monaco AP. Mycotic wound infections. A new challenge of the surgeons. Arch surgery 1979;114(9):831-35.
3. Hilfiker ML, Aziz Khan RG. Mycotic infection in Pediatric surgical pts. Seminars Pediatr Surg 1995;4(4):239-44.
4. David AD, Kenneth WB. Fungal infection in surgical patients. Am J Surg 1996;171:374-82.
5. Hickey WF, Sommerville LH, Schoen FJ. Disseminated candida glabrata, a report of a unique severe infection and a literature review. Am J Clin Pathol 1983;80:724-27.
6. Burchard KW, Minor LB, Slotman GJ, Gann DS. Fungal Sepsis in surgical patients. Arch Surg 1983;118:217-21.
7. Horan T, Culver D, Jarvis W. Pathogens causing nosocomial infections; surveillance system antimicrob. Newslet 1988;5.
8. Beck-Sagne CM, Jarvis WR. Secular trends in the epidemiology of nosocomial fungal infections in the United States, 1980-1990. J Infect Dis 1993;167:1247-51.
9. Banerjee SN, Emori TG, Culver DH, et al. secular trends in nosocomial primary blood stream Infections in the United States, 1980-1989. Am J Med 1989;91(Suppl 3B): 86S-89S.
10. Fraser VJ, Joves M, Dunkel J, et al. Candidiasis in a tertiary care hospital: Epidemiology of risk factors and predictors of mortality. Clin Infect Dis 1992;15:414-21.
11. Bodey GP, Lano M. Skin Lesions associated with disseminated candidiasis. JAMA 1974;222:1466-68.
12. Wingard JR, Merz WG. Rinaldi MG, et al. Increase in candida Krusei infections among patients with bone marrow transplantation and neutropenia treated prophylactically with Fluconazole: NEJM 1992;325: 1274-77.
13. Kauffman CA, Tan JS. Torulopsis glabrata renal infection. J Clin Microbiol 1984;20:813-14.
14. Samonis G, Gikas A, Toludis P, et al. Prospective study of the impact of broad-spectrum antibiotics on yeast flora of the human gut. Eur J Clin Microbiol infect. Dis 1994;13: 665-67.
15. Alvedy J, Aoys E, Weiss- Carrington P, Burk DA. The effect of glutamine enriched TPN on gut immune cellularity. J Surg Res 1992;52:34-39.
16. Gaines JD, Remington JS. Disseminated candidiasis in surgical patients. Surgery 1972;72:730.
17. Geha DJ, Roberts GT. Laboratory detection of fungemia. Clin Lab. Med 1994;14:83-97.
18. Rutledge R, Mandel SR, wild RE. Candida Sepsis. Insignificant contaminant or Pathologic species. Am Surg 1986;52:299.
19. Rehan VK, Dandisan DC. Neonatal renal candidal bezoar. Arch Dis child 1992;67:63-64.
20. Robinsen PJ, Knirsch AK, Joseph JA. Fluconazole for life threatening fungal infection in patients who cannot be treated with conventional antifungal agents. Rev Infect Dis 1990;12(Suppl 3):349-63.
21. Wise GJ. Amphotericin in urological practice. J Urol 1990;144:215-23.
22. Irby PB, Stoller MZ, MC Aninch JW. Fungal bezoars of the urinary tract. J Urol 1990;143:447-51.

CHAPTER 17

Ethics in Pediatric Surgery

P Madhok

Ethics and medicine were born together. In the olden days when medicine was learnt by apprenticeship, the founding fathers formulated a set of rules on the basis of which pupils were selected. This was necessary in view of the closeness and intimacy that the physician enjoyed with his patient. The incumbent had to be of a good moral character, respect his teachers, be fair to his peers and kind to his patients. He had to act in the best interest of the patient and avoid doing any harm.

Infact the Hippocratic Oath (500 BC) remains even today the mother of all oaths and prayer of physicians. Its three cardinal principles:

a. Benefecience
b. Nonmalfecience and
c. Autonomy remain enshrined in all later modifications, which became necessary due to change of circumstances and advances of science.

A modern version of the Oath is detailed as follows:

THE WORLD MEDICAL ASSOCIATION DECLARATION OF GENEVA (1985)

Physicians' Oath

- At the time of being admitted as a member of the medical profession.
- I solemnly pledge myself to consecrate my life to the service of humanity.
- I will give to my teachers the respect and gratitude which is their due.
- I will practice my profession with conscience and dignity; the health of my patient will be my first consideration.
- I will maintain by all the means in my power, the honour and the noble traditions of the medical profession; my colleagues will be my brothers.
- I will not permit considerations of religion, nationality, race, party politics or social standing to intervene between my duty and my patient.
- I will maintain the utmost respect of human life from the time of conception, even under threat, I will not use my medical knowledge contrary to the laws of humanity.
- I make these promise solemnly, freely and upon my honor.

With science advancing at a rapid pace it is likely that the oath will be changed from time to time.

Hippocratic forbiddance to abortion is likely to be transgressed by people struggling to keep population levels down and by women who feel that it infringes upon their fundamental right. Be that as it may the principles enunciated by Hippocrates remain supreme. Another piquant situation can arise with a patient coming for an HIV test: If postitive, do we tell only the patient and or/his spouse?

The Pediatric Surgeon faces a more complex situation. His patient is too small to take autonomous decision. So in his place the parents act as proxy. Also, benefecience may be limited to treatment of a single defect. The child may still remain with other defects (duodenal atresia and trisomy), similarly beneficence to one twin may mean maleficence to another, when you have to treat conjoint twins and only one is salvagable. Chemotherapy is the greatest thing that has happened to cancer treatment in the last fifty years. It is especially effective in pediatric malignancy. Yes, it has side effects (beneficence is tainted by maleficent). In situations like neural tube defects, pre and perinatal surgery, intersex and advance malignancy ethical issues are apt to arise. These are discussed briefly in the ensuing pages.

RIGHTS OF PATIENTS

'Treat me right' is the title of a book written by Ian Kennedy, a medico legal authority, in which he discusses fundamental rights of patients. He further elaborates that the patient is entitled to good treatment delivered in a competent manner. Even in India, the constitution grants right to life as a fundamental right (Article 21).[1] The Supreme Court has elaborated that right to life includes proper diagnosis, proper medicine, proper attendance. It also precludes any unfair or wrong treatment. In dealing with emergencies, it has instructed primary centers to be well equipped, district hospitals to be upgraded, a competent ambulance service to be provided and health personnel to be well trained. Non-availability of a bed is not to be used as an excuse to deny admission.

Treatment may be denied by individual doctors on grounds of non-competence or lack of equipment but certainly not on financial grounds. Every person is entitled to emergency first aid, and payment cannot be insisted upon. The "Baby Doe" case, when the parents refused surgery on a Mongol Child with esophageal atresia, raised a storm in the USA.[2] The Department of Health and Human Resources ruled that no child can be refused treatment, because of a handicap. In our country where children are considered family wealth, level of education is poor, and most people have strong belief in religion and miracles, telling the truth may not be easy. The Consumer Protection Act of 1986, advises the medical practitioner to take "informed" consent from both parents before any surgical procedure. It should be done preferably in the presence of a witness. The total implications of surgery must be explained as well as risks of operation. All records must be maintained and patient must have access to them. Medical negligence will be punished.

Of late, the US Congress has taken a pragmatic view of some of the situations a pediatric specialist can face. In 1985 it amended the Child Abuse and Neglect Preventive Act and excluded from its purview, medical negligence in the following situations:[3]
a. Child is chronically and irreversibly comatosed.
b. When the condition is such that prolonging life might mean prolonging death.
c. Treatment is worse than disease. The "right to die with dignity". Society of India is also seized of this matter. Hopefully there will be similar legislation in our country soon.

PRENATAL DIAGNOSIS

Advances in renal time ultrasonography have made it possible to diagnose several congenital defects prenatally. Although several interventional techniques are available like aminocentesis, cord blood sampling, chorionic villus biopsy and fetoscopy, most structural defects show up in the early middle trimester on a good sonography machine. Those of interest to the Surgeons are: Neural tube defectsm PU valves, PUJ obstruction, diaphragmatic hernia, sacrococcygeal teratoma, lung defects and intestinal atresia.

The Indian society for prenatal diagnosis (ISPAT) has done commendable work to improve the standard of prenatal diagnosis and laid down guidelines regarding treatment. They advise formation of a core group consisting of sonologist, a perinatalogist, pediatric surgeon, geneticist, ethicist, psychologist and social worker. Because, fetal intervention carries some risk to both baby and mother, it is desirable that all matters concerning fetal intervention be referred to them. Let the core group consider the pros and cons and take a decision in their collective wisdom.

Four Options are Available

1. Fetal abortion, e.g. Spina bifida, multiple defects, trisomy.
2. Fetal intervention because of increasing organic damage for, e.g. PU valves, diaphragmatic hernia
3. Early cesarian section, e.g. PUJ obstruction with E/o increasing renal cortical thinning.
4. Await delivery: Early operation on the newborn, e.g. Intestinal atresia.

Option two carries a risk of death of fetus, maternal infection, evisceration and injury.

Guidelines on ethical problems involved in fetal therapy have been clearly laid down in the International Conference on Fetal Medicine (1987) and are as follows:
1. Most defects are best treated at birth.
2. Select the fetus most likely to benefit.
3. Adhere to selection criteria.
4. Minimal intervention.

In cases of doubt whether fetal intervention will help or not, the benefit should be given to fetus and the pregnancy continued. No cesarian section must be done unless 34 weeks or unless the baby is 2 kgs.

After informed consent, if the mother refuses any intervention it is her prerogative. The courts can intervene, in case the mother is biased, e.g. divorced couple in which case fetal rights become paramount, so long as there is no risk to the mother.

It must be admitted that most fetal surgery in India at present is experimental. In cases where the fetus clearly stands to benefit for, e.g. PU valves and intervention is minor; it should be carried out after fully explaining the risks to the mother.

One looks forward to the day when endoscopic and minimal invasive surgery will come, carrying lesser risk to mother and fetus.

NEONATES

The availability of surfactants ventilators and other technology, made it possible for physicians to save very small babies, asphyxiated babies and newborn with multiple congenital defects. Many of them would not have survived a few years back. After survival some of them may end up with cerebral palsy, blindness and deafness.

An informed consent from the parents may be difficult because of the short time lag between birth and decision making. Most of the time, therefore, one is apt to over treat these babies. In 1993, Jobe put forth a disturbing finding that although surfactant treatment increased the survival of small infants, the morbidity between treated and untreated infants was the same.[4] Strong suggests a multidisciplinary approach in such cases to include the physician, parents and relative; ethicist, and/or a religious person.[5]

To resuscitate or not in the delivery room can be another problem. CPR (cardiopulmonary resuscitation) must be available to all babies if clear guide lines are not available. Jones has suggested DNR (Do not resuscitate) to children with easily recognisable diseases, incompatible with life or poor quality survival, e.g. hydrocephalus, holoprosencephaly, anancephaly, trisomy 13, 18. Renal agenesis, short limb dwarfism, Meckel-Gruber syndrome, triploidy and sirenomelia.

All these cases are obvious or diagnosis can be confirmed soon after birth. Additionally the severely asphyxiated neonate or the very low birth weight child also may be not resuscitated if parental consent is available.

MULTIPLE DEFORMITIES

A child with multiple defects is not an unusual problem for the Pediatric Surgeon. Request for treatment throws up four options: Full cure, life with acceptable handicap, life with unacceptable handicap and death. Acceptable handicap will depend on the cerebral function of the survivor and the socio-economic status and mental attitude of the parents.

Infants with multiple malformations can be divided into six groups:
1. Malformations are curable. Only one is life threatening (e.g. imperforate anus with hypospadias). Obviously threat to life must be removed and other problem sorted out later.
2. Both malformations are life-threatening and curable. (e.g. Esophageal atresia and imperforate anus). Treatment must be staged and cost factor discussed with the parents.
3. Both malformation are life-threatening. Only one is curable (e.g. imperforate anus and neural tube defects). Threat to life must be removed. Long-term implication of the other defect must be discussed.
4. One life threatening and one non-life threatening but not curable (e.g. Duodenal atresia + trisomy). Removal of life threatening defect, results in a permanent handicap. Options must be given to parents.
5. Neither malformation is life-threatening. One can be cured (e.g. Cleft palate; Down's syndrome). Treat the treatable.
6. Both malformation are life-threatening and incurable (e.g. Neural defect and gross cardiac malformation).

This is basically a situation for euthanasia. Parents must be helped to take a decision. In this situation the words of Willis Potts, in his book "The Surgeon and the Child" are worth recalling.[6]

"An infallible answer to the question of performing or with holding life saving operations for extensively deformed infants is not always available. Each case is different. Religious belief, philosophy of life and economic consideration alter decisions. Life is the most precious thing in the world. Is it so to the individual born without a brain capable that make social seclusion necessary, and marital live impossible? Our duty as doctor is crystal clear to preserve life. And yet when looking at a hopeless little mass of deformed humanity, compassion wrestles with duty".

Should such infants be encouraged to live or die with dignity? Euthanasia may be practised passively by withholding treatment or actively (rarely) by administering lethal doses of drugs. The second will need state sanction and legislation. Also whether such drugs should be given surreptitiously or openly is a matter of debate. Abandonment of defected babies by parents is not uncommon. Sometimes even orphanages refuse to take them because they are unfit for adoption.

NEURAL TUBE DEFECTS

Neural tube defects, myelomeningocele is one of the most common and tragic congenital abnormality. Not only is the child paralysed below the waist, he is also incontinent of urine and faeces. Because of Arnold-Chiari malformation, there is also hydrocephalus. Associated defects like club foot and heart disease are not uncommon. Treatment is life-long beginning with repairing the meningocele and putting in a shunt. Later an orthopedic operations to enable the patient to walk. Lastly urinary diversion may be required to control incontinence. It is perfectly possible that some of these operations may have to be repeated. Mental status is unpredictable. Under these circumstances we have to fit in this disease with parental thinking, Hippocratic principles, child rights and quality of life. The Baby Doe case in America brought in legislation of rights of the handicapped. So even the courts may be involved in decision making.

Because of widespread public awareness, two groups have emerged, right to life versus death with dignity. 'Baby Doe' regulations versus quality of life judgement. Individual approach versus socialistic approach. Some even question whether doctor, parents and nurse should decide the future of the child or social worker, courts and ethics board should decide. Dr John Lorber was the first who advocated diagnostic indicators and selection of cases. Today prenatal diagnosis is available and if the sonography is convincing about the presence of myelomeningocele with hydrocephalus, these cases are best aborted. Recent work has shown that folic acid given in adequate doses to married women before and in the first trimester pregnancy can prevent neural tube defects. After birth if the patient has no associated anomalies and good power in the hip joints, the chances of walking with support are high. These children must be given the benefit of operation after speaking clearly with the parents regarding the nature and duration of disease. Expensive investigations should be kept at a minimum and parental education must continue parapassu with treatment so that parents can take on increasing responsibility of nursing care. Gross deformities associated with myelomeningocele, minimum earning capacity of parents and social ostracization is a tragedy that many will face unless clear guidelines come regarding euthanasia.

INTERSEX

Ethical issues in intersex are complicated by medical, social and even emotional factors.
1. Diagnosis can be difficult even for an experienced clinician, e.g. congenital adrenal hyperplasia with labial fusion.
2. Some patients may present at prepuberty for, e.g. Androgen insensitivity, 5-Alpha reductase deficiency.
3. Some children may present late, and the parents may already have assigned gender to them. Conversion to another gender may be non-acceptable.
4. Registration of birth.
5. The fixation of Indian families to have a male child.
6. Even after treatment many of these patients will end up being reared as females.
7. Fertility, mensturations and procreation may not be achievable.
8. Lastly, counseling parents and the patients.

Types of Intersex are as Follows

- Female pseudohermaphrodite
- Male pseudohermaphrodite
- True hermaphrodite.

Female Pseudohermaphrodite

This is the commonest type of intersex and they are all genetic females (46 XX) born with hypertrophic clitoris, virilization due to 21- hydroxylase deficiency.

Additionally there may be labial fusion and poorly developed vagina. Diagnosis is easy and is possible at birth by estimating 17-alpha ketosteroids and karyotyping. Properly treated with corticosteroids they have a good fertility potential and can function as normal females. Reduction clitoroplasty with or without vaginoplasty can be done in early infancy. Should the parents have already assigned sex, they should be persuaded to reverse it because to convert them to a functional male is very difficult.

Male Pseudohermaphrodite

These are genetic males (46×y) and raise serious ethical as well as surgical problems. They are basically of two types: Complete androgen insensitivity and incomplete androgen insensitivity and 5-alpha reductase deficiency.

a. *Complete androgen insensitivity:* As the external genitalia are completely feminine, babies are not bought to the doctor at birth. They may present later for inguinal hernia with a palpable gonad or for primary amenorrhea. Family history of sterility and scanty hair in the patient and mother may be suspicious. Karyotyping would confirm the diagnosis. These patients have male gonad that produces estrogens. These children require gonadectomy after the breast has developed. Also vaginoplasty. These children look like females but do not have the internal organs of females. Vaginoplasty will give them ability for coitus but they are unable to reproduce or mensturate. It is difficult for parents to understand and accept this situation so a multidisciplinary approach with a gynecologist and psychologist will be required.

b. *Incomplete androgen insensitivity and 5-alpha reductase deficiency:* These children are incompletely Masculinized and have small genitals. It is necessary to distinguish between the two conditions. Androgen insensitivity will produce female sexual characters where as alpha reductase deficiency may get virilized after puberty. Decision to rear them as male and female will depend on the size of phallus and response to testosterone therapy. In case of a good phallus and good response to testosterone, the hypospadias should be corrected and the boy brought up as a male. In incomplete androgen insensitivity, it is better to rear up the child as a female. Corrective surgery can be done in infancy. Parents find it very difficult to accept that although the patient is a genetic male how and why should it be reared up as female. This is the hard core of the intersex problem.

True Hermaphrodites

These children have ambiguous genitals; complicated genetic picture and are often brought late. Assigning gender takes time and a full coterie of tests with or without laparatomy. If they have prominent male external genitals, (which is rare) they must be reared as males. Otherwise females. Fertility potential either way is poor. These are tragic situations and will tax the patience of both, parents and surgeon. Transsexuality is being slowly accepted in this country.

Two other questions need to be addressed. Registration of birth, normally required within 40 days of birth can always be extended by giving a suitable medical certificate. Secondly the possibility of malignancy must be explained in case of androgen insensitivity and gonadel dysgenesis.

Telling the child patient is the most difficult of all. Help of a child conseller is in order.

PEDIATRIC MALIGNANCY

Most liquid and embryonic tumors in the pediatric age group are curable with multimodal therapy. Ethical problems that may arise in the treatment of malignancy are:

1. Should costly investigations be ordered?
CT/MRI have become the gold standard of diagnosis and staging of the disease. In view of the radiation and the cost involved only minimal cuts must be ordered. Repeat investigations in the course of treatment must be kept to a minimum.

2. Financial involvement:
Cancer being a chronic ailment, treatment is apt to be prolonged. As it is a disease of the under five, parents are usually young. Financial resources may be limited. As and when need to they should have access to the poor fund and the social service department. There is a tendency in some parents to become martyrs and sell property and other assets in the hope of a cure for the child. They must be clearly advised as to what to expect from treatment.

Chemotherapy

Because of advances in chemotherapy patients are living longer. Most chemotherapy has side effects which cannot be avoided. So beneficence and malfecience may coexist. Similarly, no advance is possible without drug trials which may involve animals or human volunteers. Elements of risk and malfecience are always there in newer drugs, needless to say the child cannot take his own decision and the parents have to be led into believing that chemotherapy will help. So even autonomy is questionable. In advanced cancer, recurrent cancer and terminal cases the choice of euthanasia must lie with the parents.

Euthanasia

For patients with advanced malignancy, multiple organ failure, bed sores and incontinence, euthanasia is a clear option. It is mostly of a passive nature and involves with holding treatment. Only symptomatic and pain relieving treatment need be given. Because of emotional bonding and religious taboo permission for active euthanasia practically never comes from the parents. In fact their belief in supernatural miracles, saints and seers is so high that the message of terminal disease is often lost of them. In such cases the doctor can only be a passive observer of the event.

EUTHANASIA FOR OTHER CASES

Deliberately causing death in an easy manner is called Euthanasia. It is usually meant for terminal patients who have incurable diseases involving a lot of suffering.[7] It may be voluntary, if requested by the patient or involuntary when decided by others, usually the dear and near ones. It can be active, e.g. Injection of lethal drug or passive, by withdrawing of life saving systems.

Euthanasia has always been debated by ethicists, but has received a fresh impetus after the Supreme Court of India ruled, that attempted suicide is not punishable by law.

Advances in technology have made it possible to prolong life although it may have lost its meaning. Sometimes by prolonging life we are prolonging death. Life must be meaningful and pain free and the patient must be capable of responding to the demands of living. Once cerebral function is lost (brain death) the other organs follow suit. In such cases drugs, drips dialysis and artificial ventilation should not be used to prolong life. In this debate on euthanasia two groups have emerged: One which believes in terminating life if its purposeless, handicapped and painful. The other believes in leaving it to God.

In the pediatric context when autonomy is not the principle involved but decision has to be taken by others, there is room for euthanasia in special situations, e.g.

1. Prenatal: Multiple defects, poor brain function and likelihood of a dependant life.
2. Child having some correctable and some uncorrectable defects leading to handicapped life. Parents unable to cope.
3. Advanced malignancy.

In such cases it is difficult to decide whether saving the life is beneficence or malfecience!!

ETHICS IN RESEARCH

Nowhere are the principles of Hippocratic Oath so stretched as in conducting research. This include development of new techniques, not all of them may be successful. Research is the bass of progress in science. It involves:

1. *Animal experiment:* Here the rights of animals must be kept in mind. Animal to be used as last resort and suffering kept to a minimum.
2. *Embryo research:* The unresolved question is what makes an embryo? Is embryo a person ? As most of these questions are unresolved only removing cells from the embryo for research purpose is justified. Transfer of animal embryos into human or vice versa is not justified. Cloning is not justified.

Development of newer techniques like tissue cultures and computer developed models will reduce the need for experimental animal. One looks forward to a future which will be animal free and pain free. At present only research on aborted embryos is justified.

HOSPITAL ETHICS COMMITTEE

Now that high technology has made inroads into the practice of medicine, doctors are getting more and more technical and less and less humane. The art of bed side manner is a thing of the past and communicating with the patients is left to the junior most echelons of the medical pyramid. This often results in frustration, bitterness and sometimes litigation.

Most hospitals in the West have an ethics committee which goes into quality patient care, medical research, publication and even ethical dilemmas that may arise in dying patients. This committee should include physicians, surgeons, departmental heads, matron, social worker and ideally should be presided by a person with a religious background.

Our own ethical norms in this country are confused. We have codified or tried to codify, principles of ethical behavior based, on Judaeo Christian thought that was imbided by Indians educated by Western minds and exposed to Western literature. The time has come for our Medical Councils to face this issue head on and formulate ethical norm as that will encourage practice in keeping with our traditional and modern Indian values.

The committee should concern itself with improved patient care. How to cut down out patient procedures, the location and design of various departments by easily understood symbols. Improve the paging system of doctors. Over see medical audit and reduce beaurocratic obstacles in issuing certificates specially death certificates.

Publish or perish should not be the motto. Publication must be quality controlled and be relevant to the local problems. Meager resources that we have should not be dissipated in duplicating work done abroad. Even if the committee meets once a month it will have a lot to do specially as time goes on.

REFERENCES

1. Constitution of India. Govt of India Publication 1972; Article 21.
2. In Re Doe: 418 SE 2nd (Ga 1992) cited by Camiano DA + Clayton EW Paed. Surg by Oniel, Rowe etal Vol 1, VII ed, Mosby and Co, Missouri PP. 229–33.
3. Ramsey P. Benign Neglect of Defective Infant : Ethics in the edges of life. New Haven, Conn, Yale Univ Press. 1978
4. Jobe A. Pulmonary Surfactant Therapy. New Eng Jour Medicine 1993;328:861-68.
5. Strong A. The Neonatologist duty to parents and patients: Hastings Cent Rep (August) 1984;10-16.
6. Willis Potts. The Surgeon and the Child Philadelphia. WB Saunders 1959.
7. Madhok PD and Karmarkar SJ. Ethics in Paed Surgery; IAPS: Hoescht M Russell Hoescht House, Mumbai.

CHAPTER 18

Esophagoscopy

B Othersen Jr, HS Hassan

The ability to visualize the lumen of the gastrointestinal tract added an extra dimension to the diagnosis and management of various pathological conditions affecting it. Rarely in the history of medicine has a new technology so influenced a major specialty, as has gastrointestinal endoscopy influenced gastroenterlogy. Within less than 50 years, endoscopy has reoriented diagnostic approaches to numerous clinical problems, facilitated ingenious therapeutic development, permitted new physiological studies and modified long held concepts of gastrointestinal disease events.[1] The refinement of the endoscope and ancillary diagnostic techniques has led to an increased ability to diagnose and treat patients with diseases of the esophagus. The addition of biopsy and brush cytology techniques further augments its abilities. The use of absorptive stains that are sprayed on the mucosa during endoscopy has been described by several groups and can assist in the detection and definition of abnormalities. Endoscopic ultrasonography has expanded the diagnostic capabilities of endoscopists by imaging the wall layers of the esophagus as well as the surrounding structures. Additional techniques that appear to have endoscopic applications include molecular biologic investigation of specimens obtained at endoscopy, tissue autofluorescence, and magnetic resonance imaging during endoscopy.[2]

INDICATIONS OF ESOPHAGOSCOPY

Diagnostic

Esophagitis

Endoscopic findings of esophagitis include erythema, loss of the superficial vascular pattern that can be seen just below the mucosal surface, erosions, ulceration or nodularity, mucosal bleeding on contact, white plaques of various configurations surrounded by an erythematous border and cobblestone appearance of the mucosa.[3] However, histologic changes of esophagitis may be found in a grossly normal mucosa, and conversely, subjective gross endoscopic findings including erythema, edema, increased vascularity and friability do not predict abnormal histology.[4,5] Diagnosis of esophagitis is based on histologic criteria in biopsies obtained during endoscopy in infants and children. The sine qua non of histologic esophagitis is intraepithelial neutrophils.[6] The finding of only one neutrophil per high power field in a section of a punch biopsy is reported to be pathologic and sufficient to make a diagnosis of histologic esophagitis Intraepithelia neutrophils are regarded as less specific than eosinophils.[7,8] Boyle JT suggested a grading of esophagitis that incorporates both gross and histological findings:[9]

Grade	Gross Finding	Histologic Finding
0	Normal	Normal
1	Normal or subjective mucosal changes erythema, edema, friability increased vascularity	1-19 eosinophils and/or neutrophils/ hpf or basal hyperplasia or papillary elongation
2	Same as grade 1	> 20 eosinophils and / or neutrophils/ hpf
3	Definite esophageal erosions or exudate	
4	Definite esophageal ulcer	
5	Stricture	Barrett's esophagus

Gupta et al found that vertical linear indentations in distal esophageal mucosa might be a highly specific endoscopic feature of esophagitis in children.[10] Isaac et al found that endoscopy also help in treatment of esophagitis by specifying a specific etiology.[11]

Corrosive Ingestion

Endoscopic examination is necessary to determine whether or not there has been an esophageal burn. Studies have shown that signs and symptoms are unreliable guides to the presence or severity of an esophageal injury.[12,13] It should be performed the next day (12-24 hours after ingestion) not immediately because the extent of injury may be difficult to determine, and because if the patient has a full stomach, regurgitation of caustic may produce further injury.[14,15] As many as 75 % of patient will be found to have no esophageal injury. The most likely sites of injury are at points of natural narrowing of the lumen: the cricopharyngeus, the aortic arch, the left main stem bronchus, and the diaphragm. It is not possible to accurately evaluate the depth of the burn at esophagoscopy. Although ulceration is usually associated with full thickness damage, apparently mild mucosal changes may conceal a transmural injury. The risk of perforation is minimal if the examination is stopped when evidence of mucosal burn is seen.[14-16]

Endoscopic grading of corrosive esophageal and gastric burns:

Grade 1 = Mucosal hyperemia and edema
Grade 2 = Limited hemorrhage, exudate, ulceration and pseudomembrane formation
Grade 3 = Sloughing of mucosa, deep ulcers, massive hemorrhage, complete obstruction of lumen by edema, charring, and perforation

There are several limitations to esophagoscopy.[17] At times it may be difficult to evaluate the depth of any burn with absolute certainty by observing superficial epithelial necrosis.[13] When a severe burn is encountered in the upper-third of the esophagus, the esophagoscope is not passed beyond this area and the involvement of the middle and lower thirds cannot be ascertained.[14] The area of burn may not be visualized, thus delaying the diagnosis. The areas of ulceration may be more easily visualized if a dilute solution of methylene blue is instilled into the esophagus at the time of esophagoscopy. The normal epithelium will be stained blue, whereas the areas of ulceration will not.[18]

Diagnosis of Tracheoesophageal Fistula (TEF) and Other Anomalies

The symptoms of choking and coughing with feedings, excessive tracheal secretions, and recurrent atelectasis or pneumonitis should direct attention to the possibility of an H- or N-type tracheoesophageal fistula, or a recurrent fistula in a patient with a previous repair.[19,20] TEF is one of the rare congenital anomalies of the trachea and esophagus. It constitutes 4-5% of these anomalies. Seventy percent of H-type TEF occurs at or above the level of the second thoracic vertebra and extends in an oblique course like the letter N, from the posterior membranous wall of the trachea to the anterior wall of the esophagus.[21] Although congenital, the condition may present late; this may be explained by various theories; an occlusive valve like mucosal flap, which may close during swallowing because of the oblique direction of the tract, or spasm of the muscular layer occluding the lumen during swallowing.[21] The key to repair of isolated (H-type) and recurrent TEF is identification of the level of the fistula. This is important both before operating, so that the correct exposure can be planned, and intra-operatively, so that the fistula can be localized and repaired.[22]

TEF can be diagnosed by endoscopy either directly or by using some techniques.[22-28] Although better seen by a bronchoscope, an esophagoscope can also be used to visualize the esophageal opening of the fistula.[19,20]

Other anomalies as congenital stenosis, leiomyomas, cystic duplication, esophageal diaphragm and epiphrenic diverticulae can also be confirmed by esophagoscopy.[29,30]

Upper GIT Bleeding

A variety of etiologic factors may be responsible for an upper GIT bleeding. Commonly esophageal varices, severe peptic esophagitis, peptic ulcer or Mallory-Weiss syndrom. Esophagoscopy can determine the etiology and, in certain instances as esophageal varices, may be used in management.

Esophageal Perforation

Esophageal perforation may be intraluminal, as occurs druing instrumentation: Endoscopy, dilatation, intubation (nasogastric or Sengstaken tubes, or sclerotherapy, or due to foreign body impaction, or caustic ingestion; or may be extraluminal as in cases of penetrating wounds, blunt trauma, operative injuries, and fracture spine. Spontaneous perforation (Boerhaave's syndrome) may also occurs in newborn and older children.

Although diagnosed by plain X-ray, contrast study or even CT scaning, esophagoscopy can identify major tears or complete disruption.[31-34]

Dysphagia

Esophageal causes of dysphagia include esophageal strictures (Figs 18.1A and B) and webs; vascular anomalies as aberrant right subclavian artery, double aortic arch and right aortic arch with left ligamentum; trauma: either external or trauma during intubation and endoscopy; neurologic defects: as occurs in head trauma and hypoxic brain damage or peripheral nervous system congenital or traumatic diseases; neuromuscular diseases as myasthenia gravis or miscellaneous causes as achalasia and esophageal spasm.

Esophagoscopy is an aid to diagnosis of many of these causes. Some lesions of the esophagus are sometimes amenable to endoscopic treatment. Endoscopy may be a useful adjunct in the diagnosis of vascular anomalies, because pressure with the tip of the scope on the vessel indenting the esophagus may abolish one or more distal pulses, thereby helping to identify the offending vessel.[35]

Miscellaneous

Esophagoscopy is an aid to diagnosis of many other conditions as hiatus hernia, achalasia, stenosis, and Barrett's esophagus (Fig. 18.2).[30]

Therapeutic

Esophageal Dilatation

For patients with narrow esophageal lumen for whatever etiology, esophageal dilatation is an important therapeutic modality.[36] There is no perfect

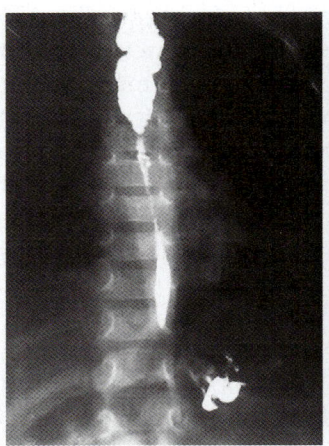
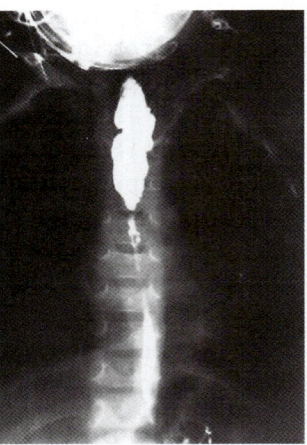

Fig. 18.1A: Barium swallow showing corrosive stricture esophagus

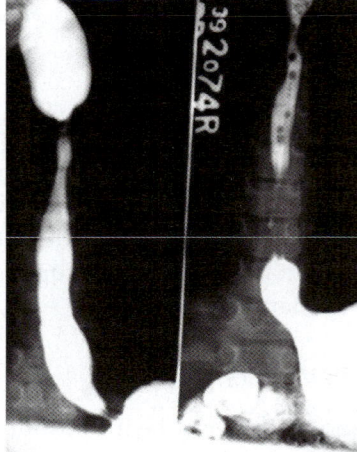

Fig. 18.1B: Barium swallow showing severe corrosive stricture esophagus

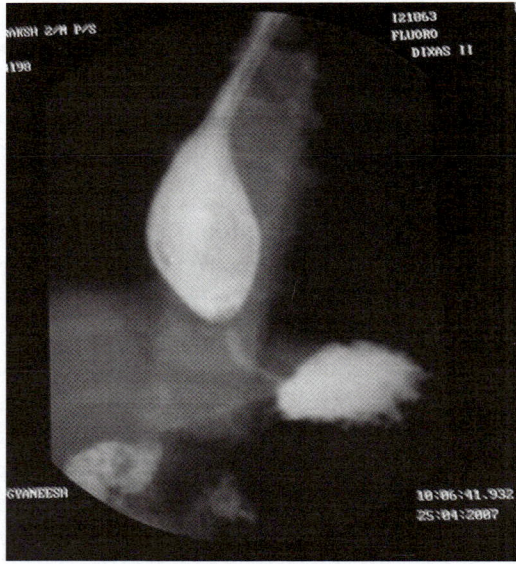

Fig. 18.2: Barium swallow of 2-year-old child showing narrowed lower esophagus with dilated proximal part suggesting congenital esophageal stenosis

dilator or dilating procedure for the management of peptic esophageal strictures. Successful dilatation requires versatility in technique and instrumentation. Until recently, a common means of dilatation was the passage of dilators via the rigid esophagoscope under general anesthesia, modern equipment has made the routine use of this technique obsolete, and it is reserved for special situations such as uncooperative patients, high cervical esophageal strictures, or dilatations that have been unsuccessful under local anesthesia and sedation.[37]

Several types of dilators are available: Gum elastic dilators (Jackson), mercury filled dilators (Maloney), Eder-Puestow dilators, Savary-Gilliard dilators or balloon dilators. All these dilators require esophagoscopy for pre-evaluation, insertion of the dilator and examination after the dilatation setting.

Esophageal Foreign Body Removal

Ingestion of foreign bodies is a common problem in pediatric patients, and the majority of these objects are coins (Fig. 18.3). Because the esophagus is the narrowest portion of the pediatric alimentary tract, a significant number of ingested coins will lodge here. Esophageal perforation and aspiration are well-documented complications of retained esophageal foreign bodies, and this risk, although of low incidence (9.1 %) mandates immediate extraction.[38,39]

Foreign body ingestion is a relatively common problem in the United States, with an estimated incidence of 120 per 1 million population, resulting in approximately 1500 deaths each year.[40] Swallowed objects may be true foreign bodies) such as coins, plastic toys, bones, pins, or disc batteries.[41-43]

Prior to the 1960s, esophagoscopy was the accepted method of managing esophageal foreign bodies. In 1966, however, Bigler reported a method of extracting smooth esophageal foreign bodies using a Foley balloon catheter.[44] Subsequently, several authors have reported the technique of esophageal bougienage to dislodge coins into the stomach.[45,46] Each of these methods has its proponents, and all of them are effective.

Those advocating balloon catheter or bougienage techniques cite the following advantages over esophagoscopy: (1) avoidance of the use of an operating suite, (2) avoidance of hospitalization, (3) avoidance of the risks of general anesthesia and endotracheal intubation, and (4) avoidance of the risks of esophagoscopy. At a glance, these may seem to be worthwhile arguments, but on closer examination their foundation is not strong. For instance, the alternative methods are recommended only for blunt foreign bodies, usually coins, of short duration without pre-existing esophageal disease or other factors that make complications more likely. These are precisely the foreign bodies that are the easiest and safest to remove by esophagoscopy. Any foreign body that can be removed by a Foley catheter or a bougie can be removed just as easily and perhaps more safely under direct vision with esophagoscopy. Foreign bodies with any suggestion of complications are not considered candidates for the alternative blind methods of extraction. It seems logical that the safest technique for removal of complicated foreign bodies should also be the safest technique for removal of uncomplicated foreign bodies.[47]

Kelly et al, however, noticed a striking difference in cost between esophagoscopy and the use of Foley catheter or bougienage.[38] He developed a protocol for management for esophageal coins utilizing either Foley catheter (for proximal 1/3 of the esophagus) or bougienage (for distal 2/3), and reverting to esophagoscopy only on failure of those techniques. He applied the protocol selectively, adopting the criteria developed by Jona et al; thus excluding from this protocol all cases seen after 24 hours form impaction, those patients with respiratory distress or history of esophageal pathology, and in the presence of more than one coin.[48,49]

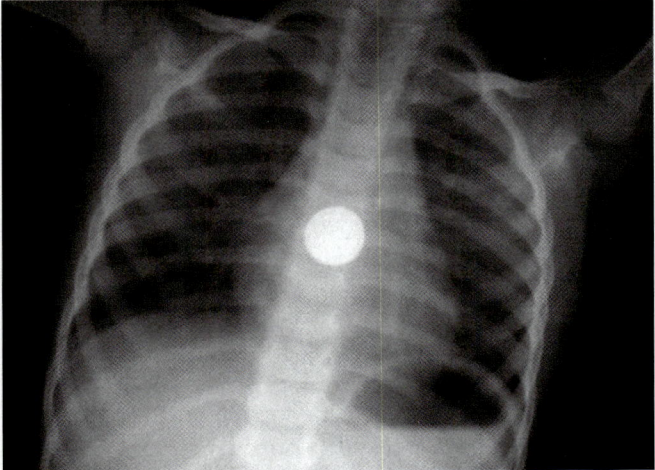

Fig. 18.3: Chest X-ray showing radio opaque battery in esophagus

Finally, pharmacological methods to manipulate the muscular tone of the esophagus, allowing passage of an impacted foreign body, have been attempted.[50-53] Glucagon and nifedipine have been used with varying degrees of success.[52] Gas-forming agents have been tried; the idea being that increased pressure from the gas would force the object into the stomach. Magnets were used to pull metals as pins, rings and batteries.[53] Enzymatic digestion of a meat bolus with papain has largely been abandoned because of an unacceptable complication rate.[50-53]

Sclerotherapy for Bleeding Esophageal Varices

Bleeding from esophageal varices is the most common cause of serious gastrointestinal bleeding in children. It is associated with a considerable morbidity and a reported mortality of 12-21% even in the absence of liver disease.[54-58]

The first report of the injection of sclerosant into esophageal varices for the control of bleeding came in 1939 from the two Swedish surgeons Crafoord and Frenckner, who used this technique in a 19 years old female to control bleeding esophageal varies, utilizing a rigid esophagoscope and a specially deviced needle.[59]

Techniques of injection sclerotherapy presently in use can be divided into those aiming to inject sclerosant into the varix to obliterate the lumen, and those injecting into the submucosa alongside the varix (paravariceal) to produce a layer of fibrosis to cover the vessel. With both methods the flexible fiberoptic endoscope and injection needle has largely replaced the rigid esophagoscope, although the latter instrument is still favored by some, especially in the presence of active bleeding when the field of vision and the control of the bleeding point by the tip of the esophagoscope are superior. More elaborate methods of injection sclerotherapy have included a means of balloon tamponade in order to maintain a blood-free field during the procedure. This has been achieved in two ways. Firstly, by applying traction to the large gastric balloon of the Linton's tube and then injecting the varices immediately above the gastroesophageal junction by means of the fiberoptic endoscope and, secondly, by incorporating a balloon onto the distal end of a fiberoptic endoscope which is inflated against the injection site to prevent any post-injection bleeding.[60]

A verity of sclerosants might be used, including: 5% sodium morrhuate, 5% ethanolamine, 1.5% sodium tetradecyl, and 50% dextrose.[61] Complications include retrosternal pain and burning at the time of injection, fever, esophagodynia, superficial ulcers and pleural effusion.[62]

Recently, endoscopic variceal ligation has been shown to be just as efficacious and is associated with fewer complications.[63,64] Endoscopic variceal clipping is also a promising; Ohnuma et al successfully used a clipping apparatus to stop bleeding in 99.3% of cases of his series.[65]

Miscellaneous

Other miscellaneous authors report successful endoscopic management of some diseases. Hoelzer and Luft reported successful occlusion of a recurrent tracheoesophageal fistula using fibrin glue, applied endoscopically in a 6 years old child.[66] Kim et al successfully used chemocauterization to occlude the opening of a pyriform sinus fistula by endoscopically applied trichloroacetic acid, and suggests this technique as a reasonable alternative in the management of pyriform sinus fistula.[67]

INSTRUMENTATION

Flexible Esophagogastroscope

The use of the flexible esophagogastroscope is indicated in most instances. The apparatus have a working channel through which graspers, biopsy cups, scissors, etc. can be passed through. It is also prepared with air insufflation, suction and irrigation capabilities. The tip of the scope can be moved in four directions controlled from the handle. Operator may use the eyepiece or a video camera may be mounted on the eyepiece to deliver the picture to a monitor. Illumination is provided by an external light source with a xenon arc or halogen -filled tungsten filament lamps. A pediatric size is now available by many manufacturers.

Rigid Esophagogastroscope

Since the first flexible fiberoptic endoscope was constructed by Basil Hirschowitzl in 1957, the technique of flexible endoscopy has been the primary method employed by gastroenterologists for investigating patients with complaints involving the upper digestive tract. With the technical advances that followed the original design gastroenterologists abandoned the rigid endoscope for the flexible version. It has proven easier to use, with fewer complications.[68] However, rigid esophagoscope still have a place in clinical practice, particularly for foreign body removal.

Complications

Complications include esophageal perforation, impaction in the esophagus, aspiration pneumonia and infection.[17,69-71]

Contraindications

Strict contraindications include agitated patient, shock, inexperienced endoscopist, defective instruments and absent CPR equipment. The relative contraindications include neck deformities, large pharyngeal pouch, aortic arch aneurysm, recent surgery and perforated esophagus.

REFERENCES

1. Blackstone MO. Endoscopic interpretation. Normal and pathologic appearance of the gastrointestinal tract. Raven press. New York, 1984.
2. Edmundowicz SA. Endoscopy in Castell DO, Richter JE. The Esophagus, third edition. Lippincott Williams and Wilkins, Philadelphia 1999;89.
3. Johnson DG. Esophagoscopy and other diagnostic techniques in O'neill JA, Rowe MI.
4. Goldman H, Antonioli DA. Mucosal biopsy of the esophagus, stomach, and proximal duodenum. Hum pathol 1982;13:423.
5. Biller A Winter HS, Grand RJ, et al. are endoscopic changes predictive of histologic eophagitis in children? J pediatr surg 1980;15:74.
6. Grosfeld JL, et al, Eds. pediatric surgery, fifth edition. Mosby St. Louis 1998;927.
7. Winter HS, Madara JL, Stafford TL, et al. Intraepithelial eosenophils: a new diagnostic criterion for reflux esophagitis. Gastroenterology 1982;83:818.
8. Shub MO, Ulshen MH, Hargrove CB, et al. Esophagitis: a frequent consequence of gastroesophageal reflux in infancy. J Pediatr 1985;107:881.
9. Boyle J. gastroesophageal reflux in the pediatric patient. Gastroent clin north America 1989;18(2)315.
10. Gupta SK, Fitzgerald JF, Chong SKF, et al. vertical lines in distal esophageal mucosa VLEM): a true endoscopic manifistation of esophagitis in children? Gastrointest endos 1997;45(6):485.
11. Isaac DW, Parham DM, Patrick CC. The role of esophagoscopy in diagnosis and management of esophagitis in children with cancer. Med Ped oncol 1997;28:299.
12. Mansson I. Diagnosis of acute corrosive lesions of the oesophagus. J Laryngol Otol 1978;92:499.
13. Gaudreault P, Parent M, McGuigan MA, et al. Predictability of esophageal injury from signs and symptoms: A study of caustic ingestion in 378 children. Pediatrics 1983;71:767.
14. Leape L. Chemical Injury of the Esophagus in Ashcraft KW and Holder TM (Eds): Pediatri.c esophageal. surgery. Grune and Stratton, Inc Orlando 1986;73-88.
15. Anderson KD. Corrosive Injury-early management. In: Pearson GF, Deslaauries J, Ginsberg RJ, et al. Esophageal Surgery. Churchill Livingstone NewYork 1995;465-86.
16. Postlethwait RW. Chemical Burns of the esophagus in Postlethwait RW: Surgery of the Esophagus 2nd (Eds). edition. Appleton-Century-Crofts/Norwalk, Connecticut.
17. Beauchamp G, Duranceau A. Diagnostic and therapeutic esophagoscopy. Indications, contraindications and complications. Surg Clin North America 1983;63(4):801.
18. Kirsh MM, Peterson A, Brown JW, et al. Treatment of caustic injuries of the esophagus: A ten year experience. Ann Surg 1978;188:675-78.
19. Gans SL, Berci G. Inside tracheoesophageal fistula: new endoscopic approach. J Ped Surg 1973;8(2):205.
20. Gans SL, Johnson RO. Diagnosis and surgical management of " H-type" tracheoesophageal fistula in infants and children. J Ped Surg 1977;12(2):233.
21. Karnak I, Senocak ME, Hicsonmez A, et al. The diagnosis and treatment of H?type tracheoesophageal fistula. J Ped Surg 1997;32(12):1670.
22. Garcia NM, Thompson JW, Shaul DB. Difinitive localization of isolated tracheoesophageal fistula using bronchoscopy and esophagoscopy for guide wire placement. J Ped Surg 1998;33(11):1645.
23. Williams J. Diagnosing tracheoesophageal fistula without esophageal atresia. Clin Pediatr 1996;35:103-04.
24. Andrassy RJ, Ko P, Hanson BA, et al. Congenital tracheoesophageal fistula without esophageal atresia. Am J Surg 1980;140:731-33.
25. Karnak 1, Senocak ME, Hicsonmez A, et al. The diagnosis and treatment of H-type tracheoesophageal fistula. J Pediatr Surg 1997;32:1670-74.
26. Benjamin B, Pham T. Diagnosis of H-Type tracheoesophageal fistula. J Pediatr Surg 1991;26:667-71.
27. Gans SL, Johnson RO. Diagnosis and surgical management of "H-Type" tracheoesophageal fistula in infants and children. J Pediatr Surg 1977;12:233-36.
28. Killen DA. Endoscopic catheterization of H-type tracheoesophageal fistula. Surg 1964;55:317-20.
29. Gilat T, Rozen P. Fiberoptic endoscopic diagnosis and treatment of a congenital esophageal diaphragm. Am J Dig Dis 1975;20(8):781.
30. McBroom GL. Experience with conventional upper gastrointestinal endoscopy. Gastroint endos 1970;16(4)213.

31. Panzini L, Burrell MI, Traube M. Instrmental esophageal perforation: chest film findings. Am J Gastroent 1994;89(3):367.
32. Goh GJ. Pilbrow WJ. Youngs GR. The use of gastrografin for esophageal perforation [letter; comment] Gastroenterology 1995;108(2):618.
33. Phillips LG, Cunningham J. Esophageal perforation. Radiol Clin North America 1984;22(3):607.
34. Ben-Ami T, Rozenman J, Yahav J. Computed Tomography in children with esophageal and airway trauma. J ped Surg 1988;23(10):919.
35. Weiss MH. Dysphagia in infants and children. Otol Clin North America 1988;21(4)727.
36. Dumon JF, Meric B, Sivak MV, et al. A new method of esophageal dilatation using Savary-Gilliard bougies. Gastroint endos 1985;31(6):379.
37. Rice TW. Dilatation of peptic stricture in Pearson FG, Deslauriers J, Ginsberg RJ, et al (Eds): Esophageal Surgery. Churchill Livingstone Inc. NewYork 1995;293.
38. Chaikhouni A, Kratz JM, Crawford FA. Foreign bodies of the esophagus. Am Surg 1985;51:173.
39. Kelley JE, Leech MH, Carr MG. A safe and cost effective protocol for management of esophageal coins in children. J Ped Surg 1993;28(7):898.
40. Ratcliff KM. Esophageal foreign bodies. Am Fam Physician 1991;44:824-31.
41. Crysdale WS, Sendi KS, Yoo J. Esophageal foreign bodies in children: 15 year review of 484 cases. Ann Otol Rhinol Laryngol 1991;100:320-24.
42. Hawkins DB. Removal of blunt foreign bodies from the esophagus. Ann Otol Rhinol Laryngol 1990;99:935-40.
43. Thompson N, Lowe-Ponsford F, Mant TGK, Volans GN. Button battery ingestion: a review. Adv Drug React Acute Poison 1990;9:157-80.
44. Bigler FC. The use of a Foley catheter for removal of blunt foreign bodies from the esophagus. J Thorac Cardiovasc Surg 1966;51:759-60.
45. Banadio WA, Jona JZ, Glicklich M, et al. Esophageal bougienage technique for coin ingestion in children. J Pediatr Surg 1988;23:917-18.
46. Jona JZ, Glicklich M, Cohen RD. The contraindications for blind esophageal bougienage for coin ingestion in children. J Pediatr Surg 1988;23:328-30.
47. Hawkins DB. Removal of blunt foreign bodies from the esophagus. Ann Oto Rhinol Laryngol 1990;99:935.
48. Banadio WA, Jona JZ, Glicklich M, et al. Esophageal bougienage technique for coin ingestion in children. J Pediatr Surg 1988;23:917-18.
49. Jona JZ, Glicklich M, Cohen RD. The contraindications for blind esophageal bougienage for coin ingestion in children. J Pediatr Surg 1988;23:328-30.
50. Berggreen PJ, Harrison ME, Sanowski RA, et al. Techniques and complications of esophageal foreign body extraction in children and adults. Gastroint endos 1993;39(5):626.
51. Richardson JR. A new treatment for esophageal obstruction due to meat impaction. Ann Otol Rhinol Laryngol 1945;54:328.
52. Ferrucci JT, Long JA. Radiologic treatment of esophageal food impaction using intravenous glucagon. Radiology 1977;125:25.
53. Equen M. A new magnet for removal of foreign bodies from the food and air passages. Ann Otol Rhinol Laryngol 1944;53:775.
54. Howard ER, Stamatakis JD, Mowat AP. Management of esophageal varices in children by injection seclrotherapy. J Ped Surg 1984;19(2):2.
55. Howard ER. Paediatric liver disease: Surgical aspects, in Wright R, Alberti KGMM, Karren S, et at (Eds): Liver and Biliary Disease (2nd ed) (Chap 43). London, WB Saunders (in press).
56. Arcari FA, Lynn HB. Bleeding esophageal varices in children. Surg Gynecol Obstet 1961;112:101-05.
57. Foster JH, Holcomb GW, Kirtley JA. Results of surgical treatment of portal hypertension in children. Ann Surg 1963;157:868-80.
58. Clatworthy HW. Extrahepatic portal hypertension, in Child CG (Ed): Portal Hypertension: Major Problems in Child CC (Ed): Portal hypertension: major problems in clinical surgery. WB Saunders, London 1974;243.
59. Crafoord C, Frenckner P. New surgical treatment of varicose veins of the esophagus. Acta Otolaryngol 1939;27:422.
60. Westaby D, Williams R. Endoscopic sclerotherapy for esophageal varices. Gastrointest endosc 1983;29(4):303.
61. Jensen DM. Evaluation of sclerosing agents in animal models. Proceedings of the Third International Endoscopy Symposium 1983:46-49.
62. Lewis J, Chung RS, Allison J. Sclerotherapy of esophageal varices. Arch Surg 1980;115:476.
63. Price MR, Sartorelli KH, Karrer FM, et al. Management of esophageal varices in children by endoscopic variceal ligation. J Ped Surg 1996;31(8):1056.
64. Hall RJ, Lilly JR, Stiegmann GV. Endoscopic esophageal varix ligation: technique and preliminary results in children. J Ped Surg 1988;23(12):1222.
65. Ohnuma N, Takahashi H, Tanabe M, et al. Endoscopic variceal ligation using a clipping apparatus in children with portal hypertension. Endos 1997;29(2):86.
66. Hoelzer DJ, Luft JD. Successful long term endoscopic closure of a recurrent tracheoesophageal fistula with fibrin glue in a child. Int J Ped Otorhinolaryngol 1999;48(3):259.
67. Kim KH, Sung MW, Koh TY, et al. Pyriform sinus fistula: management with chemocauterization of the internal opening. Ann Otol Rhinol Laryngol 2000;109(5):452.
68. Glaws WR, Etzkorn KP, Wenig BI. Comparison of rigid and flexible esophagoscopy in the diagnosis of esophageal disease: diagnostic accuracy, complications and cost. Ann Otol Rhinol Laryngol 1996;105:262.
69. Berry BE, Ochsner JL. Perforation of the esophagus. A 30 years review. J Thorac Cardiovasc Surg 1973;65:1.
70. Parker LS. impacted fibroscope in the esophagus. J laryngol 1969;83:1123.
71. Meyers MA, Ghahremani GG. Complications of fiberoptic endoscopy. I. Esophagoscopy and gastroscopy. Radiol 1975;115:293.

CHAPTER 19

Pediatric Bronchoscopy

DK Gupta, Shilpa Sharma

The development of the Hopkins rod lens has revolutionized the field of bronchoscopy. The reduction in the size of the fiberoptic bronchoscopes has expanded its utility from the diagnostic to its use in operation theatres, casualty, neonatal/pediatric intensive care units, assisting endotracheal intubations and diagnostic procedures such as bronchoalveolar lavage and transbronchial biopsy. Pediatric bronchoscopy is now being performed even while on high-frequency oscillatory ventilation the development of narrow-caliber flexible fibreoptic bronchoscope has enabled diagnostic bronchoscopy in premature and newborns in the neonatal Intensive Care Unit.[1,2] The rigid bronchoscope however can not be replaced and is of immense use for removal of foreign bodies. While rigid bronchoscopy is performed by only Pediatric Surgeons, a flexible bronchoscopy is performed by Pediatric Surgeons, Otorhinolaryngologists, Pneumologists, Anesthetists and Pediatricians.[3]

PEDIATRIC AIRWAY ANATOMY

The infant larynx is placed more anteriorly in the neck compared to the adult. The epiglottis has a U shaped curvature and the arytenoid cartilages may be very prominent in the infant. The subglottic space is the narrow portion of the airway in infants and young children as compared to the glottis in the adults. This should be taken into consideration during selection of bronchoscope.[4]

In children the trachea is nearly round, with the cartilages extending visibly through an arc of approximately 320 degrees. Some inward protrusion of the membranous portion of the trachea and main bronchi may be seen. The main carina is keel shaped and oriented in an anteroposterior plain. In the adult the main carina is sharp and a widened carina in adults may indicate subcarinal lymphadenopathy. In the child the main carina is often quite blunted. The right mainstem bronchus is immediately visible on passing the scope down the trachea (Fig. 19.1).

The right upper lobe division takes off just beyond the carina at an angle of approximately 100 degrees. The right upper lobe bronchus itself may have a small length before dividing into the anterior, posterior and apical segmental bronchi. Beyond the origin of the right upper lobe bronchus, the right main stem bronchus continues as the bronchus intermedius, after which it gives rise to the middle lobe bronchus anteriorly, the superior segment of the right lower lobe posteriorly and right lower lobe bronchus that divides into basilar segments. It is however not possible to negotiate the bronchoscope into the terminal bronchioles in children.

The left main bronchus can be visualized in its entirety from the carina, after turning toward the left, and even then it takes a curving course so that its bifurcation may not be seen from the carina.

The left mainstem bronchus terminates into the upper lobe and lower lobe bronchi. As the left upper lobe bronchus ascends superiorly, the lingular bronchus arises and extends slightly downward in an inferior-lateral direction. The upper division bronchus of the upper lobe passes beyond the orifice of the lingula and gives rise to the apicoposterior and the anterior segments. Immediately on entering the left lower lobe bronchus arises the superior segment of the left lower lobe that descends posteriorly and then the basal bronchi.

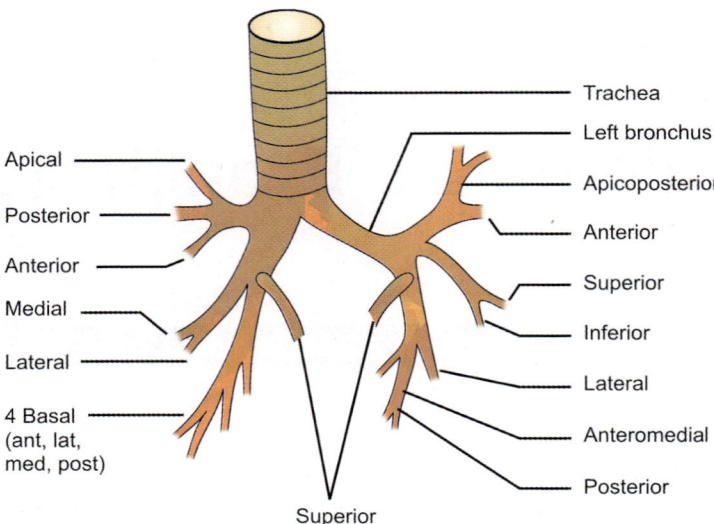

Fig. 19.1: Anatomy of bronchial tree

INDICATIONS FOR BRONCHOSCOPY

Although pediatric bronchoscopy has become a well-accepted routine procedure with a high diagnostic yield, it is important that the most appropriate means of access to the airways is chosen according to the indications and the age of the child.[5]

Diagnostic

1. Tracheobronchial foreign body.
2. Stridor, wheezing and persistent cough.
3. Persistent pneumonia, persistent atelectasis.
4. Persistent opacity on the chest radiograph.
5. Use in the intensive care unit.
6. Suspected mucus plug blocking the bronchus.
7. Hemoptysis.
8. Diagnose H-type tracheoesophageal fistula.
9. Bronchoalveolar lavage—pneumonitis.
10. Respiratory symptoms in immunocompromised child.

Confirm Suspected Diagnosis

1. Recurrent laryngeal nerve injury—Vocal cord palsy.
2. Laryngomalacia.
3. Tracheomalacia.
4. Subglottic stenosis.
5. Tracheoesophageal fistula.

Therapeutic

1. Removal of foreign body.
2. Removal of mucous plugs.
3. Bronchoalveolar lavage for persistent pneumonitis.
4. Guide to surgical interventions - H-type tracheo-esophageal fistula.
5. Treat H-type tracheoesophageal fistula—fibrin glue/laser/coagulation, deflux.
6. Interventional —Balloon dilatation.
7. Tracheobronchial prosthesis—stents.
8. Tracheostomy care.
9. Aid in intubation.

Stridor forms one of the most common indications for bronchoscopy in children.[6] Bronchoscopy is indicated when stridor is severe, persistent or worrisome. The common causes of stridor are laryngomalacia, tracheomalacia, vocal cord paresis, subglottic cysts or stenosis and extrinsic compression of the trachea (vascular ring or innominate artery compression.[7] The common causes of acute stridor in children are croup, epiglottitis or a laryngeal foreign body. In a series of 90 infants, the causes of stridor diagnosed with fiberoptic bronchoscopy were subglottic stenosis in 21, tracheobronchomalacia in 20, laryngomalacia in 20, tracheal stenosis in 17, cervical hemolymphangiomas in 5, vocal cord palsies in 4, and glottic edema in 3.[8] More than half of these patients

(51%) required surgery.[8] The severity of stridor does not always correlate with the severity of the lesion.[8]

In presence of persistent cough, bronchoscopy may reveal unsuspected foreign bodies, tracheomalacia, bronchomalacia, extrinsic compression in the tracheobronchial tree or gastroesophageal reflux . Unilateral or a localized wheeze is a definite indication for bronchoscopy. In case of bilateral wheezing, bronchoscopy is indicated if it were persistent or poorly responsive to optimal bronchodilator therapy.[9] The common findings in these situations are unsuspected foreign bodies, tracheomalacia, bronchomalacia or airway stenosis.

In cases of tracheostomy, the trachea may be examined for the presence of granulation tissue or stenosis at the site of tracheostomy. Retrograde laryngoscopy may be performed through the tracheostomy stoma to evaluate the subglottic area and larynx. Flexible bronchoscopy may be used for endotracheal intubations for patients with a difficult airway.

Bronchoscopy may also be used in confirming the diagnosis and identifying a tracheoesophageal fistula.

BRONCHOALVEOLAR LAVAGE

Bronchoalveolar lavage (BAL) is a safe and sensitive technique for investigating infectious causes of respiratory disease. Bronchoalveolar lavage allows the recovery of both cellular and noncellular components from the epithelial surface of the lower respiratory tract and differs from bronchial washings, which refer to aspiration of either secretions or small amounts of instilled saline from the large airway.[10] When the pulmonary pathology is diffuse, BAL is performed from the lingula and right middle lobe due to their favorable anatomical location, ease of obtaining a good wedge, and a higher volume of returning fluid as compared to other lobes.[11] When the pathology is localized, BAL is obtained from the affected segment.

In children over 3 kg of weight, 1-3 aliquotes of 5-10 ml each are used upto a maximum of 3 ml/kg.[6] Some authors restrict the amount of lavage fluid to no more than 5-15% of the functional residual capacity (FRC). The FRC may be measured by spirometry or estimated from the patients height using the following equation: FRC = 1.3 to 1.5 ml × height or length in centimeters.

In the immunocompromized child BAL is used to obtain samples for microbiology and cytology studies. The most common indications for BAL in immunocompromised children are fever, hypoxia, and abnormality on chest auscultation. The safety and diagnostic yield of BAL in this set of patients has been reported to be relatively high with a rate of > 60% positivity.[12] In immunosuppressed patients with diffuse lung infiltrates, *P. carinii* can be identified in BAL with a sensitivity of up to 85%.[13]

DISINFECTION OF BRONCHOSCOPE

High level of disinfection, defined as a procedure that inactivates all fungi, viruses, and vegetative microorganisms, bacteria but not necessarily all bacterial spores, can be achieved with 2% glutaraldehyde. Immersion in glutaraldehyde for 10 minutes will destroy bacteria, viruses, and 99.8% of mycobacterial organisms. Immersion in glutaraldehyde for 45 minutes at 25 °C will destroy all mycobacterial organisms.

CARE OF HOPKINS ROD LENS TELESCOPE

Prior to use, the Hopkins rod lens telescope must be carefully and meticulously cleaned and sterilized or disinfected. For machine cleaning, only special procedures may be used which have been tested and approved (maximum temperature 93 °C). Use a cleanser with a neutral pH (e.g. enzymatic cleanser). After a program is completed, remove the telescopes form the machine immediately if possible. All Hopkins rod lens telescopes should be routinely gas sterilized or chemically disinfected (soaked). Following routine gas sterilization, no aeration is required. The telescopes must be positioned securely. Any careless and slight bending of the rigid telescope may damage the rod lens system making it foggy or even unusable. The telescope should not remain for more than 60 minutes in any solution, including sterile water. Otherwise there is a risk of making it foggy. Similarly, the body and the tip of the telescope should not be touched with a heat source like laser fiber, diathermy coagulation, etc.

Due to foreign matter in the steam, stubborn films of deposit may in time develop on the cover glasses of the optical end faces after autoclaving. These deposits can be removed with the special cleaning paste enclosed with scopes. Polishing may be done to remove even stubborn films of deposits. Cleaning with special cleaning paste should only be performed if the image as viewed is clouded and not as a matter routine after every cleaning.

Hopkins telescopes that are marked "Autoclave" can be steam autoclaved at 134 °C (272 °F) for 5-8 min at three atmospheric pressure. When the autoclave cycle is complete, remove the container from autoclave and allow telescopes to cool to room temperature before removing top container.

During the steam autoclaving, the telescopes should not come into direct contact with metal instruments, trays, etc. Sudden changes in temperature may fracture the glass components of telescopes. The telescope should not be immediately exposed to air after removal from the autoclave. Never attempt to cool telescopes by pouring cool, sterile liquid over them. Forced cooling will cause severe damage to the telescope.

FLEXIBLE FIBEROPTIC BRONCHOSCOPY

The flexible fiberoptic bronchoscope is relatively atraumatic as compared to rigid bronchoscope. It is of immense utility for diagnostic purposes especially in the intubated child in the intensive care unit. It allows visualization of the natural dynamics of the palate and larynx. The upper lobes can be easily visualized. The limitations include partial occlusion of the airways and limited instrumentation.

The various sizes of flexible bronchoscopes available for pediatric flexible bronchoscope range from 2.2 mm - 4.9 mm (outer diameter). Bronchoscopes that are 3.2 mm or more in diameter usually have a working channel, which facilitates suction and also allows passage of biopsy forceps. Bronchoscopes that are 2.2 mm or less in diameter, do not have a working channel and are particularly useful in the intensive care units, for neonates, in assessing nasal space and laryngeal/vocal cord pathology.[7]

The different parts of the flexible broncho-scope are: (i) the eye piece; (ii) angulation control lever; (iii) angulation lock; (iv) working channel; (v) suction connector; (vi) insertion tube: at the distal end has objective lens, light guides and instrument channel (which is also the suction channel) and has a bending section at the tip of the endoscope; and (vii) universal cord which connects to the light guide connector section.

A laryngeal mask airway has been used as an alternative to endotracheal intubation for flexible fiberoptic bronchoscopy in children.[14] The major complications reported with its use have include airway obstruction and failure to place the laryngeal mask airway in the appropriate position, laryngospasm, bronchospasm, and oxygen desaturations have been reported.[15,16]

The advantages to the use of a laryngeal mask airway include secured airway, accommodation of a larger bronchoscope with a suction channel and less resistance to gas flow compared to a conventional endotracheal tube and greater visibility of the glottis and supraglottic structures.[17] Also, with a larger bronchoscope, transbronchial biopsies can be performed in younger children.

The disadvantages of the laryngeal mask airway include increased work of breathing when compared to endotracheal intubation.[18] However, these effects may be lessened once the bronchoscope is inserted into the artificial airway. The laryngeal mask airway is relatively contraindicated in presence of severe respiratory.[17]

RIGID BRONCHOSCOPY

The rigid bronchoscope will remain the gold standard treatment for removal of foreign bodies. The system offers a large lumen, removable telescope, adjustments for various types and sizes of the foreign body forceps and enough space for ventilation. The posterior commissure of the larynx is better visualized with the rigid bronchoscope as it approaches the larynx from an anterior angle. There is an excellent control of the airway. Figures 19.2 and 19.3 show the parts of a rigid bronchoscope.

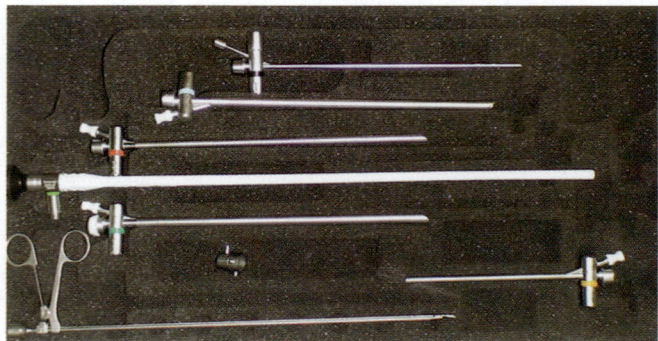

Fig. 19.2: Rigid bronchoscope set — different sized sheaths, telescope and an optical foreign body removal forceps fitting well with the scope

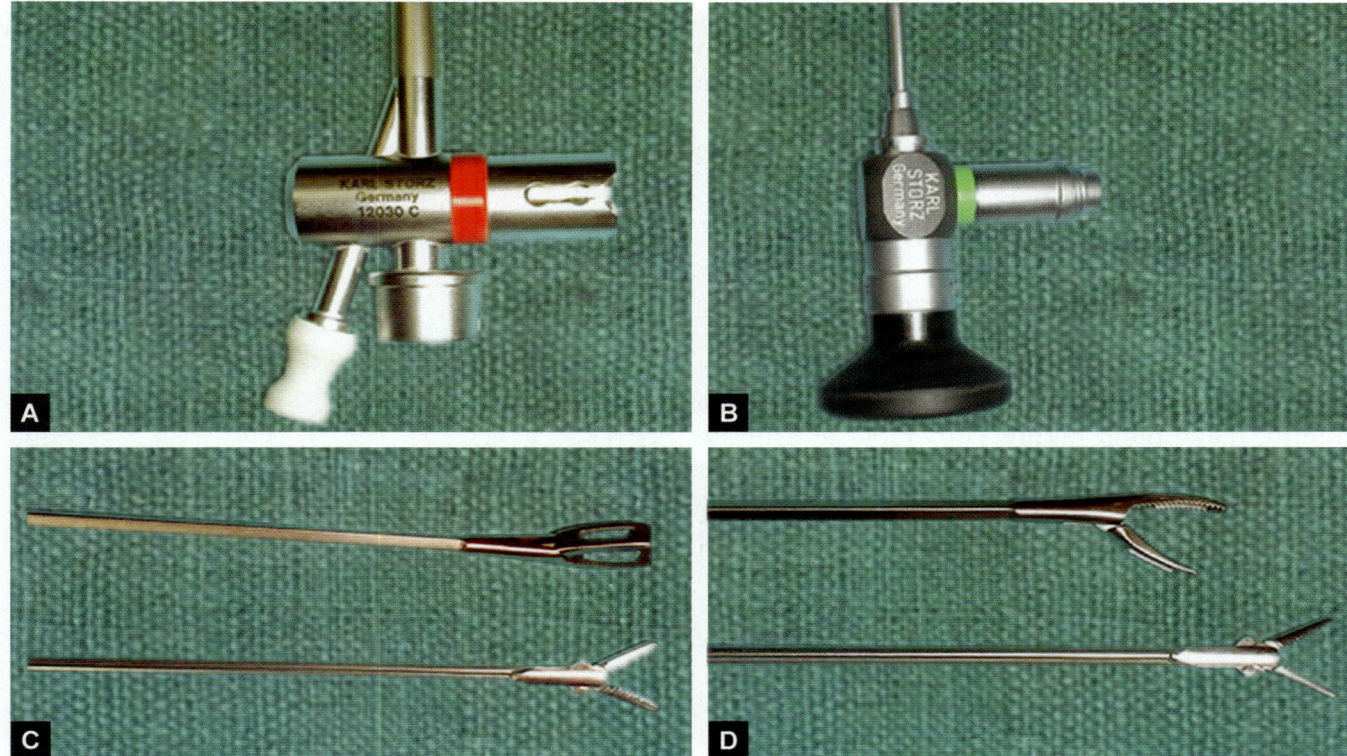

Figs 19.3A to D: Parts of a rigid bronchoscope: **A.** Bronchoscope sheath with large lumen, a side working channel for guiding catheters and side channels for attaching the prism and connecting the airway, **B.** Matching Telescope with side attachment for light source, **C** and **D.** Foreign body removing forceps (peanut and alligator) matching the sheath and telescope lengths

All therapeutic interventions can be done with ease as there is facility to pass instruments through the brochoscope sheaths. There is however a risk of trauma to the airway and inability to pass the scope into the distal airways. It is also difficult to visualize the right upper lobe bronchus with the rigid system as it opens at a right angle in the trachea.

THERAPEUTIC BRONCHOSCOPY

Bronchoscopy has been the time tested modality to confirm the diagnosis of tracheoesophageal fistula.[19] Bronchoscopy is a useful adjunct to guide the surgical treatment of H-type tracheoesophageal fistula by identification and passing a catheter for easy identification of the fistula peroperatively. Recently, various therapeutic attempts have been made at the time of bronchoscopy to treat the tracheoesophageal fistula. These have included fibrin glue, Laser and diathermy coagulation.[20,21] The authors have recently used deflux injections in 4 cases, tracheoesophageal fistulas, (three of them complicated with prematurity, serious ongoing chest infections making him unfit for major surgery, and a recurrent TEF). The outcome had been satisfactory and none required surgery during the followup ranging from 8 months to 2 years.

Tracheoscopy and bronchoscopy has also been used to guide the extent of surgical manipulations intraoperatively for aortopexy/tracheopexy procedures.

Peroperative fiberoptic tracheoscopy assisted repair of tracheoesophageal fistula has been reported to be useful for the surgeon with regards to identification of the fistula and proper fistula ligation.[22] Fiberoptic bronchoscopes with an outer diameter of 2.0, 2.4 and 2.8 mm were passed through the lumen of the endotracheal tube into the fistula that helped the surgeon to rapidly identify and dissect the fistula. Bronchoscopy assisted neonatal tracheostomy as been described as a new technique that restricts dissection strictly to the midline and ensures accurate placement of the tracheostomy below the first tracheal ring, preventing potential for damage to adjacent neurovascular structures.[23] Preliminary experience with the use of balloon dilatation and expandable metallic airway stents for tracheobronchial stenosis in the pediatric population has been reported to be encouraging.[24-26]

Foreign Body

Children are more prone to aspirate foreign bodies due to the decreased ability to chew the food sufficiently. Also the propensity to talk, laugh, and play around while chewing and the habit of putting objects in the mouth, make them highly vulnerable to aspirate despite of the defense mechanisms operating against the lodgment of a foreign body (motility of the epiglottis and arytenoid cartilages in closing the airway, intense spasm of the vocal cords and cough reflex) in the respiratory tract. However, none of these mechanisms is full proof and foreign bodies do lodge frequently in the pediatric airways.

The peak ages for aspiration of foreign bodies are 2-4 years, though accidental aspiration may occur at all ages. Even relatively younger immobile infants have been victims of foreign body aspiration while playing with small objects or due to the acts of their siblings, who may put the wrong objects/foods in the baby's mouth in an attempt to help feed them. The authors have even seen infants aspirate jewellery items of the mother like pendants and earrings and even the nails, beads, nuts and safety pins while playing with them (Fig. 19.4). The uncommon foreign bodies removed by the authors include screws, torch bulbs and pieces of whistles (Fig. 19.5).

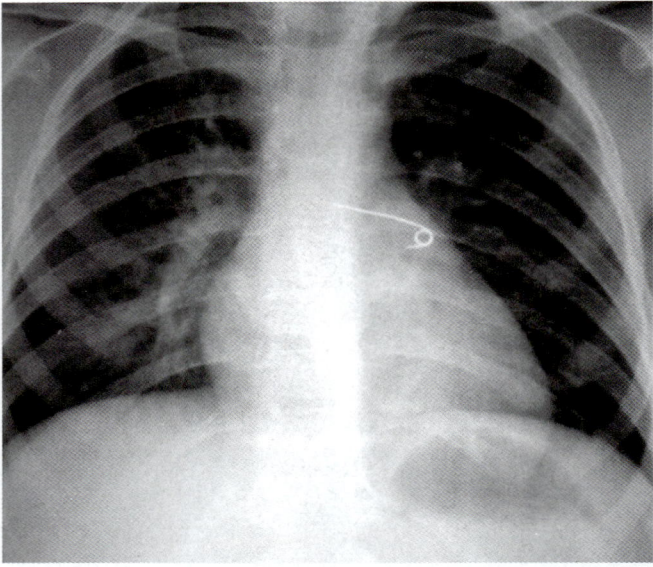

Fig. 19.4: Skiagram chest showing a radiopaque broken safety pin in the left main bronchus lying for more than 6 months. Foreign body could be removed after clearing the bronchus from granulation tissue

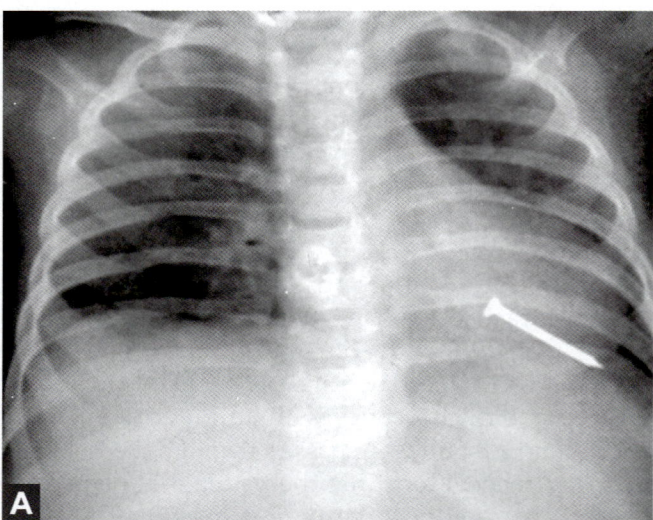
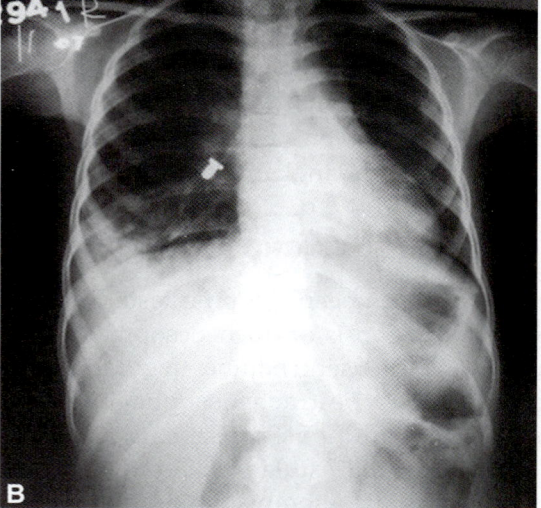

Figs 19.5A and B: A. Skiagram chest showing a radiopaque nail in the left bronchus left for many months inviting local reaction and partial blockage of the lumen and recurrent chest infection. The "head" of the nail projecting proximally was in a unfavorable position and could not be grasped bronchoscopically. A thoracotomy and bronchotomy incision was made "over the head" of the nail and the rusted nail was removed successfully. Distal bronchus was suction cleaned, **B.** Skiagram showing a metallic nut in the right main bronchus, with the head facing proximally and making the grasping impossible with the foreign body forceps. A thoracotomy and the bronchotomy incision over the head of the nut successfully delivered the foreign body

The most common aspirated materials are small food items such as groundnuts and seeds. Food items that are small, round, smooth, or both, such as grapes and balloons, are more likely to cause tracheal obstruction. Dried foods may cause progressive obstruction as they absorb water. Free floating foreign bodies in the trachea are more dangerous than the ones lodged in one of the bronchi. Old foreign bodies, vegetable or metallic, invite local reaction, inflammation and granuloma formation with the blockade of the lumen resulting in collapse consolidation, abscess formation or even the bronchiectetic changes in the corresponding lobe or the lung.

In a child in the upright and supine position, the right main bronchus is wider and has a more direct entry from the trachea, thus is a more common site for housing the foreign bodies and aspiration.

There may be a definite history of observation of accidental aspiration or sudden episode of coughing or choking while eating with subsequent wheezing, coughing, or stridor. However, in most cases, the episode is not witnessed or recalled and the diagnosis depends on a high index of suspicion. In delayed cases the child may present with persistent wheezing, persistent or recurrent pneumonia, lung abscess, focal bronchiectasis, or hemoptysis. A foreign body in the subglottic space may present with stridor, recurrent or persistent croup, and voice changes.

On auscultation, adventitial sounds like wheezes may be heard. There may be stridor or decreased breath sounds. The coarse wheeze is often unilateral, but not as a rule. The sounds are inspiratory if the foreign body is in the extrathoracic trachea. If the lesion is in the intrathoracic trachea, noises are symmetric expiratory stridor, more prominent in the central airways. Once the foreign body passes the carina, the breath sounds are usually asymmetric. It should however be remembered that a lack of findings on physical or radiological examination does not preclude the possibility of an airway foreign body.

If the child has respiratory distress and is unable to speak or cry, complete airway obstruction is likely present, and the likelihood of morbidity or mortality is high. In those cases, a Heimlich maneuver may be tried. If the child is able to speak, the Heimlich maneuver would be contraindicated, as it might dislodge the material to an area where it could cause complete airway obstruction.

Most aspirated foreign bodies are radiolucent. Thus, indirect signs of the foreign body aspiration have to be looked for. These include an area of focal overinflation or an area of atelectasis, depending on the degree of obstruction. If the airway is completely occluded, the radiograph should show opacification of the distal lung because the residual air is absorbed and there is no air entry. If the obstruction is partial with progressive ball valve obstruction, there is focal overinflation in the area of the lung directly connected to the affected airway.

An anteroposterior expiratory radiograph, lateral decubitus or fluoroscopy of the chest may be helpful in showing focal air trapping.

A chest CT scan may demonstrate the material in the airway, focal airway edema, or focal overinflation not detected in the plain radiographs. However, if the degree of suspicion is high one may straight away proceed with bronchoscopy, without wasting time. No routine investigations are required for this life saving procedure.

The differential diagnosis includes gastro-esophageal reflux, asthma, bronchitis and pneumonia.

Rigid bronchoscopy is the therapy of choice for diagnosis and removal of foreign bodies. Flexible bronchoscopy should not be encouraged for dealing with the foreign bodies. However, the flexible bronchoscopy may have a theoretical advantage that it can be used to detect the foreign bodies in moribund patients in the emergency room without the need for general anesthesia. Once, the foreign body has been confirmed at flexible bronchoscopy, the rigid bronchoscopy is warranted to remove the firm, large and solid foreign bodies. The fact that the rigid system has a wider lumen, the instruments of appropriate size and length can be adapted to suit the removal of the foreign body. On the contrary, the flexible bronchoscopes have a narrow side channel and at the best can accommodate only a thin sized instrument (foreign body removal and biopsy forceps) suitable, if at all, only to remove the thin peels or the covers of whistle or the ground nut.

Predictive signs of a bronchial foreign body have been reported as a radiopaque foreign body, and associated unilaterally decreased breath sounds and obstructive emphysema (positive predictive value = 0.94).[27] Some authors prefer to perform a rigid bronchoscopy first, in all cases presenting with asphyxia, localized wheezing or atelectasis.[27,28] This algorithm has been thought to decrease the negative first rigid bronchoscopy rate to 4%.[27] However, flexible bronchoscopy can also be performed first for diagnostic purposes.[27,28] Fiberoptic bronchoscopy has a diagnostic accuracy rate of 100% but played a poor therapeutic role with 10.7% complete resolution of cases.[29]

Rigid bronchoscopy has been successful in the removal of the tracheobronchial foreign body in 97.2% of patients.[29] The authors' preference has been to use the rigid system for the removal of all types of foreign bodies. It requires combination of skill and innovations to grasp the foreign body and take it out without slipping or harming the child. A Fogarty catheter may be employed to remove a rounded bead with a central hole large enough to permit the deflated catheter to negotiate through it. Vegetable nuts impacted in the respiratory tract swell up and become large enough to be retrieved in one piece. These may be first broken or divided in pieces before removal. Also a larger section of the same may be retrieved en block with the bronchoscope system holding the foreign body firmly all through. Authors resorted to open bronchotomy in many cases presenting late with sharp and dangerously impacted foreign bodies with presence of lot of granulation tissue in the bronchi, which bled to touch with the scope. A decision for thoracotomy and open bronchotomy exactly over the head of the impacted nail (directed upwards) is much better and safer procedure to the repeated attempts on rigid bronchoscopy. It may be extremely difficult to grasp the head of the nail as its sharp edges would get lodged in the wall of the bronchus. Similarly, a ragged long wire or a broken safety pin impacted in the bronchus may have to be divided first with a wire cutter before the same could be retrieved safely, holding the same on either side with artery forceps to avoid its dislodgement.

VIRTUAL BRONCHOSCOPY

This is a new noninvasive diagnostic modality that has enabled to view tracheobronchial anomalies in fair detail and accuracy. This has been found useful in cases of tracheal atresia and tracheoesophageal atresia to see the exact opening of the fistula in the trachea.

Three-dimensional computed tomography bronchoscopy has been reported to demonstrate accurate anatomical structures in 2 cases of prenatally diagnosed congenital lobar emphysema caused by bronchial atresia at the left upper lobar bronchus.[30]

REFERENCES

1. Babbitt CJ, Khay C, Maggi JC. Pediatric bronchoscopy performed on high-frequency oscillatory ventilation. Intensive Care Med. 2007 Aug 1; [Epub].
2. Nakano T, Shikada M, Nomura M, et al. Feasibility of fiberoptic bronchoscopy for small infants including newborns. Tokai J Exp Clin Med. 2004;29(1):1-5.
3. Pollina JE, Ibarz JA, MartÃnez-Pardo NG, et al. Pediatric endoscopy: state of the art Cir Pediatr 2007;20:29-32.
4. Rovner MS, Stillwell PC. Pediatric flexible bronchosopy for the adult bronchoscopist. In: Flexible Bronchoscopy. Eds. Wang KP, Mehta AC. New York, Blackwell Science 1995;339-62.
5. Niggemann B, Haack M, Machotta A. How to enter the pediatric airway for bronchoscopy. Pediatr Int. 2004;46(2):117-21.
6. Wood RE. Spelunking in the pediatric airways: Exploration with the flexible bronchoscope. Pediatr Clin North Am 1984;31:785-99.
7. Chhajed P N. Cooper P Pediatric Flexible Bronchoscopy Indian Pediatrics 2001;38:1382-92.
8. Parente Hernajndez A, Garcaa-Casillas MA, Matute JA, et al Is stridor a banal symptom in infants? An Pediatr (Barc). 2007 Jun;66(6):559-65.
9. Wood RE, Postma D. Endoscopy of the airway in infants and children. J Pediatr 1988;112:1-6.
10. American Thoracic Society. Clinical role of bronchoalveolar lavage in adults with pulmonary disease. Am Rev Respir Dis 1990;142:481-86.
11. Reynolds HY. State of the art: Bronchoalveolar lavage. Am Rev Respir Dis 1987;135:250-63.
12. Kasow KA, King E, Rochester R, et al. Diagnostic yield of bronchoalveolar lavage is low in allogeneic hematopoietic stem cell recipients receiving immunosuppressive therapy or with acute graft-versus-host disease: the St. Jude experience, 1990-2002. Biol Blood Marrow Transplant 2007;13:831-7.
13. Frankel LR, Smith DW, Lewiston NJ. Bronchoalveolar lavage for the diagnosis of penumonia in the immunocompromized child. Pediatrics 1988;81:785-88.
14. Slonim AD, Ognibene FP. Enchancing Patient Safety for Pediatric Bronchoscopy Alternatives to Conscious Sedation Chest 2001;120:341-42.
15. Tunkel, DE, Fisher, QA. Pediatric flexible fiberoptic bronchoscopy through the laryngeal mask airway. Arch Otolaryngol Head Neck Surg 1996;122:1364-67.

16. Bandla, H, Smith, D, Kiernan, M (1997) Laryngeal mask airway facilitated fiberoptic bronchoscopy with bronchoalveolar lavage in young children [abstract]. Chest 112(suppl),59S
17. Smyth, AR, Bowhay, AR, Heaf, LJ, et al. The laryngeal mask airway in fiberoptic bronchoscopy. Arch Dis Child 1996;75:344-45.
18. Keidan, I, Fine, GF, Kagawa, T, et al. Work of breathing during spontaneous ventilation in anesthetized children: a comparative study among the face mask, laryngeal mask airway and endotracheal tube. Anesth Analg 2000;91:1381-88.
19. Brookes JT, Smith MC, Smith RJ, et al. H-type congenital tracheoesophageal fistula: University Of Iowa experience 1985 to 2005 Ann Otol Rhinol Laryngol 2007;116(5): 363-8.
20. Gutierrez San Roman C, Barrios JE, Lluna J, et al. Long-term assessment of the treatment of recurrent tracheoesophageal fistula with fibrin glue associated with diathermy. J Pediatr Surg 2006;41:1870-3.
21. Bhatnagar V. Laser application in Pediatric Surgery In Neonatal Surgery. Ed. D K Gupta. Modern publishers. New Delhi 2000;83:554-6.
22. Deanovic D, Gerber AC, Dodge-Khatami A, et al. Tracheoscopy assisted repair of tracheoesophageal fistula (TARTEF): a 10-year experience. Paediatr Anaesth 2007;17(6):557-62.
23. Pereira KD, Weinstock YE. Bronchoscopy assisted neonatal tracheostomy (BANT): a new technique Int J Pediatr Otorhinolaryngol 2007;71(2):211-5. Epub 2006 Nov 13.
24. Wood RE, Prakash UBS. Pediatric flexible bronchoscopoy. In: Bronchoscopy, 1st edn. Ed. Prakash UBS. New York, Raven Press, 1994;345-46.
25. Filler RM, Forte V, Frage JC, Matute J. The use of expandable metallic airway stents for tracheobronchial obstruction in children. J Pediatr Surg 1995;30:1050-55.
26. Depasquale KS, Tucker JA, Wolfson B, Varlotta L. Tracheobronchial stenting in an infant with an anomalous right main bronchus. Ear Nose Throat J. 2007;86(4):240-3.
27. Martinot A, Closset M, Marquette CH, et al. Indications for flexible versus rigid bronchoscopy in children with suspected foreign-body aspiration Am. J. Respir. Crit. Care Med., 1997;155(5):1676-79.
28. Righini CA, Morel N, Karkas A, et al. What is the diagnostic value of flexible bronchoscopy in the initial investigation of children with suspected foreign body aspiration? Int J Pediatr Otorhinolaryngol 2007;71: 1383-90.
29. Divisi D, Di Tommaso S, Garramone M, et al. Foreign bodies aspirated in children: role of bronchoscopy. Thorac Cardiovasc Surg 2007;55:249-52.
30. Seo T, Ando H, Kaneko K, et al Two cases of prenatally diagnosed congenital lobar emphysema caused by lobar bronchial atresia J Pediatr Surg 2006;41:17-20.

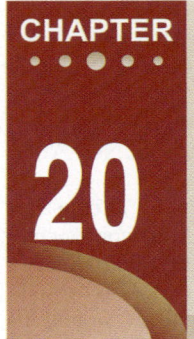

Management of Terminal Illnesses

Kanishka Das, M Charles, Ashley L J D'Cruz

A child is a gift from God - a promise for the future.

Irrespective of the geographic or socioeconomic milieu, the child remains the focus of a family. A sick child is even more vulnerable and deserves the full support of the family and society to make a recovery. If recovery is not possible, death in dignity is his right. It is an erroneous and callous thought that children are neglected in the poorer societies; the apparent neglect is the result of poverty and not the lack of concern. Society associates children with growth, activity and hope and in the natural order of things children are not supposed to die. Hence, it is difficult to accept terminal illness and death in childhood. Further, the hospital setting for preterminal and terminal care reduces the inbuilt support from family and society.

Despite the advances in neonatal and pediatric care, a sizeable number of children with complex anomalies, chronic disease cancer and HIV infection eventually succumb to their illness. With life sustaining critical care, a number of such children remain on pre-terminal support for varying periods, particularly in the developed world. Many undergo various operative procedures on routine or emergency basis for effective palliation.

Since the causes (trauma, lethal congenital anomalies, extreme prematurity, heritable disorders and acquired disease) and patterns of death are different from the adult, adult palliative care guidelines are not suitable for the child and specific approaches are still being developed. Given its socioeconomic, linguistic and cultural diversity, the complex emotions of the grieving process is very different in the Indian context. Grief counseling guidelines adopted in the western world are not entirely appropriate for the child in a developing country.

Empathy, pain relief and optimal palliation of the terminally sick child have a dramatic effect on the psychosocial recovery of the family.

NEED FOR FORMAL TRAINING

Parents of terminally ill children have a right to know about the diagnosis, treatment and prognosis of their child's illness.

Studies of medical school curricula, textbooks and residency programs showed absence of an integrated approach to systematically address the complexities of terminal care and death. A study on practices of pediatric oncologists regarding terminal care revealed a lack of confidence in dealing with various core issues. In the absence of formal training, they relied on a trial and error learning method with inputs from senior role models. The acknowledgement of impending death was considered a daunting task and many were unsure of the meaning of euthanasia. Hence they chose to maintain a distance so as to be able to discharge their duties in a detached manner. An equal proportions of health personnel report terminal cares as the 'best' or 'worst' parts of the job.

Similarly, well-designed studies reflect the dissatisfaction of parents with the overall management of such cases. A striking difference was noted between the physician's perception of the child's pain and that of the child/parent. Physicians often communicated in vague and confusing language, particularly during the transition from curative to palliative care.

Identified obstacles in terminal care are communication difficulties, unrealistic expectations of parents/family regarding outcome, extreme emotional burden on family for decision making, symptom management, difficulties in pain assessment and control and impact on care providers. This is further impacted by the prevalent financial and sociocultural influences. There is evidence that many bedside manners (communication and psychological skills) for terminal care can be taught. It is recommended that palliative care be integrated into curative care as early as the prognosis becomes clear. It is not advisable to set it aside till all curative options are exhausted since by such time an opportunity to enhance the quality of life (QoL) is lost.

CHARACTERISTICS OF TERMINAL ILLNESS

Terminal illnesses in Pediatric surgical practice may be due to congenital conditions complicated benign illnesses and malignant diseases. The following is a brief characterization of its peculiarities.

Classification

Terminal illness in children has been classified into the following broad categories depending on the nature of medicosurgical care required.

Palliative Care from Time of Diagnosis

Congenital anomalies and advanced metastatic malignancies that carry a very poor prognosis and a predictably short life expectancy (months/years) are included here. They involve major systemic afflictions that need support for survival like nutrition. For example, in Trisomy 18 (Edward's syndrome), neonates have considerable feeding and respiratory difficulties and a gastrostomy tube may be placed for feeding.

Treatment Available, Uncertain Prognosis

This comprises pediatric malignancies where treatment has reached the stage of trial therapeutic protocols and HIV infections. The life expectancy is not predictable and depends on various factors. Vascular access for chemotherapy/parenteral nutrition and minor procedures for complications of the disease warrant surgical intervention, e.g. abscess drainage in HIV infection.

Chronic Course with Short Life Expectancy

Neuromuscular degenerative disorders and congenital metabolic disorders typify the prototype of this group. They exhibit a variable progression of disease to a terminal crippling event resulting in premature death, e.g. meconium ileus with cystic fibrosis. Even if these children survive the neonatal intestinal obstruction and are maintained with pancreatic enzyme supplementation and respiratory care, they succumb to pulmonary compromise by the third decade of life. In their lifetime, they may require surgical attention for intussusception, bronchiectasis, cholecystitis, etc.

CAMPBELL AND DUFF'S SCHEMA—COST BENEFIT ANALYSIS

The dilemma to continue or forgo life-sustaining measures in managing critically ill children has ethical, psychosocial and financial implications. Campbell and Duff have proposed a schema, which defines three groups according to prognosis of the illness (Fig. 20.1). With prognosis changing from good to poor, the benefits of treatment decline while the costs increase.

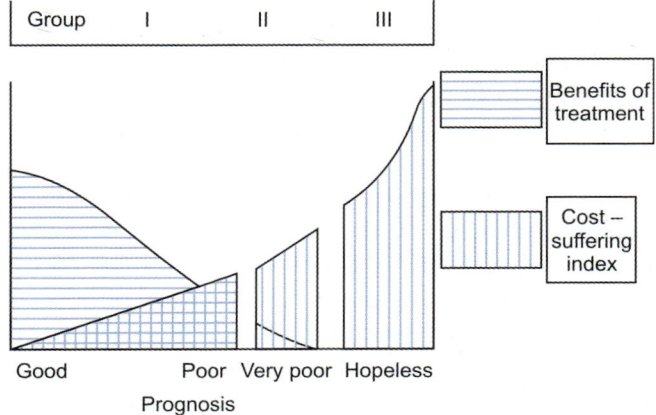

Fig. 20.1: Scheme defining three groups on the basis of prognosis (abscissa), benefits (horizontal bars) and costs of treatment (vertical bars). (Adapted from Duff RS, Campbell AGM.
Moral communities and tragic choices. In: McMillan RC, Englehart HT, Spicker SF (Eds). Euthanasia and the newborn. Dordrecht. The Netherlands: D Reidel Publishing 1987:273- 89.

In Group II and III circumstances where the prognosis is poor, benefits of treatment are uncertain, and life sustaining measures personally and economically burdensome, active family involvement is desirable in deciding to provide/limit/forgo further treatment. Decisions are most difficult to make in Group II. Though originally described for neonatal critical care, this scheme exemplifies the problem of costbenefit in critical care of the terminally ill child.

ETHICAL ISSUES

Numerous moral and ethical dilemmas confront the caretaker and the physician caring for the terminally ill child. Advances in medical technology, increasing cost of health care and free access to medical literature has moved the conventional patient-physician toward a consumerist focus. Despite this development, the following ethical principles are to be adhered to in resolving issues concerning disclosure, informed consent, shift of treatment to palliative care, etc.

- Autonomy – right to self-determination
- Beneficence – duty to do good and avoid harm
- Nonmaleficence – duty not to harm
- Fidelity – making and keeping promises
- Justice – fairness
- Veracity – truth telling and integrity.

The child rights need to be remembered at every stage. These include the right not to endure ineffective therapy, not to have a poor quality of life extended artificially, to have access to palliative interventions and to have the terminal goals met.

Another practical concern is the rationing of resources. Rationing is of two types. The first involves a greater efficiency in the delivery of care. The care that is less expensive, yet as effective as the more costly care is chosen. The second involves refusal of needed and wanted care because of unaffordable expense. All rationing decisions including those involving costly extraordinary measures to preserve life in the face of significant risk of death or severe debility are governed by the ethical principles outlined earlier.

Despite the primary obligation to sustain life, situations arise where medical interventions no longer prove to be in the patient's best interests. In such cases, the decision to shift the goal of management from curative to palliative intent is reached after repeated consultations with the family and inputs from ancillary-quarters, e.g. ethical committee, religious personnel, etc. This does not mean withdrawal of care or decrease in concern and is distinct from euthanasia or intentional termination of life.

The fine balance between physician responsibility to inflict no harm (non-maleficence), do good (beneficience) and respect for the patient's wishes (autonomy) may occasionally be impossible, e.g. the decision to withdraw life support systems. When the physician is not satisfied with the decision, he may withdraw from the case/handover the case to an alternative physician or seek medicolegal assistance.

The birth of a child is the beginning of life and modern society expects children to outlive their parents. The death of a child is met with resistance and the impact ripples across generations. It is important that events surrounding death are dealt with diligently, lovingly and humanely with utmost consideration for the overall well being of the dying child, the parents, siblings, extended family, community and care providers. The terminal phase is remembered and choices made are reviewed many a times in the minds of bereaved parents.

HASTENING DEATH

Euthanasia is the intentional termination of life and is commonly referred to as 'physician assisted suicide'. Much of the available literature refers to the adult population; the dynamics in pediatric practice could be more complex. When a child/adolescent requests euthanasia, the health care team should respond with a renewed focus on holistic palliative care. With the provision of adequate analgesia and sedation for the treatment of rapidly progressive symptoms, requests to hasten death are generally abandoned. Although the topic lends itself to personal interpretation, national regulatory bodies such as the AAP do not support the practice of Physician assisted suicide or euthanasia in children.

Sometimes, medications provided for the relief of suffering may through a foreseeable, unintended consequence hasten death. This 'rule of double effect' has been generally accepted. This rule justifies the liberal use of opioids and sedatives to alleviate symptoms and suffering in terminal illness and is distinct from euthanasia.

PATTERNS OF DEATH

The pattern of death in terminally sick child may be broadly characterized as –
a. Brain death – where clinical and investigative tests confirm brain death and the patient is 'alive' on life support systems such as ventilation/ ionotropes.
b. Failed cardiopulmonary resuscitation – where death occurs after failure of the normal resuscitative attempts in the face of a cardiopulmonary arrest consequent to the primary disease.
c. Death following a Do Not resuscitate order – as in 'b', but no resuscitation is attempted in the presence of the order.
d. Death following a withholding/withdrawal of therapy – death follows partial/complete restriction of life sustaining measures.

The proportion of cases in each category depends on various factors.

PALLIATIVE CARE

'Palliative care' is defined as comprehensive, interdisciplinary care of patients and families facing a terminal illness, focussing primarily on comfort and support. It affirms life and seeks to enhance the quality of life (QoL) in the face of an ultimately terminal condition. Palliative care begins with the diagnosis of a life-threatening disease and continues regardless of whether the child is receiving curative treatment for the primary disease.

It implies active total care of the child's body, mind and spirit as well as support for the child's family. The family get time and space to begin the process of anticipatory grieving. The goal is to add life to the child's years and not simply years to the child's life.

The key principles of palliative care are –
1. Respect for the wishes, preferences and dignity of the patient and family.
2. Compassionate, coordinated competent health care at the hospital/home/extended care facilities/ daycare centers, etc.
3. Personalized care aiming at maximizing patient determined quality of life.
4. Family centered care that extends through bereavement time to ensure that the family unit remains functionally intact.
5. Meticulous symptom control.
6. Improved professional and social support-regulatory, educational, insurance, etc.
7. Psychosocial and spiritual care.
8. Caregiver support.
9. Continuing research and education of involved personnel.

Hospice Care

This embodies a philosophy and attitude that aims at maximizing the quality of life of the child, family and caregivers. It is a holistic approach incorporating inputs from psychological, social and spiritual angles. The personnel involved include the primary physician/surgeon, child psychiatrist, child psychologist, social worker, nutritionist, religious personnel and volunteers. Palliative care is not reserved for hospices, but can be provided in hospitals, community health centers and in the child' home.

Home Care

The home is the most appropriate place for the child and least disrupts the family life. Considerations include the child's desire to be at home, parental commitment to have the child at home, sibling perspectives and the health care team's willingness to participate in home care. Besides lower costs and individualized parental attention, it is a source of pride and accomplishment for the family.

The medical team (nurse, doctor, psychologist, etc) act as facilitators and assure the family of advice and support at all times. Even trial drugs and experimental therapies may continue in the home setting. The facilitators help in the procurement of drugs not available over the counter, particularly narcotics. They provide instructions on the procedures to be followed in the event of death. Families are encouraged to care at home till the time of death though the option to return to hospital always exists.

However, home care cannot be adopted in all families. Some parents and children feel safer in the hospital or the family circumstances may not be conducive to optimal home care. Many misconceptions (belief that hospitalization for terminal illness is the best, confusion about the appropriate time for home/hospice care) and logistic difficulties (lack of physician support/resource personnel for this care, family conditions such as single parent, poverty, unstable family structure) restrict the adoption of home/hospice care.

Respite Care

This is the provision of care to an ill child by qualified caregivers other than the family members to allow the family time to rest and renew. It may be offered at anytime in the course of the illness for varying time periods.

COMPONENTS OF PALLIATIVE CARE

Procedural Aspects

These attain enhanced significance in the light of delicate ethical and psychosocial issues involved. Some of these routine *formalities* which pose practical problems in care of the terminally ill are discussed.

Disclosure

A suitable time and place is chosen to make an honest attempt at disclosure about the child's condition to the family and, if appropriate, the child. Compassionate communication, sensitive discussion and thorough attempts to support the family facilitates acceptance. Miscommunication and misinterpretation can foster anger, isolation and abandonment in the family. Delicate issues such as termination of treatment, resuscitation, Do Not resuscitate orders and autopsy should not be designated to junior personnel. Active participation of the family is sought on pain and comfort management.

Talking to a Child about Death

Adults, physician and parents alike, have preconceptions that children are incapable of understanding death. Although they may not overtly express it, awareness of death develops over time. Since there exists a general pervasiveness of death themes in children games, media exposures and daily experiences, the idea is certainly not alien to children. By the age of 3 years, a child is aware of death. At 5 years, they are increasingly curious and by 6-10 years they view death as irreversible, final and a personal experience. By 10-12 years their concept and comprehension of death is similar to adults, though variations occur. The adult concept of death is universal (happening to everyone), irreversible (impossible to change) and permanent (for all time). Children attain this concept through a process more dependent on developmental level rather than chronological age.

An assessment of the child's developmental level and the family's communication pattern is necessary before attempts at broaching the subject. Overprotection, lying, covering up or evading the issue does not make his life easier. It is useful to take clues from the child and respond accordingly. Guidelines in discussing death with children include physician conviction about the need to do so, involvement of the family member, and use of non-verbal/symbolic communication such as play, drama, art, stories and schoolwork. There has to be a willingness to respond to that occasional question 'Am I dying?' with such questions, children are only seeking emotional support and companionship; they are forgiving of faltering adults if they care to communicate.

Decision Making

This is crucial at every stage of management and must involve the entire treating team, the family and in select circumstances the sick child. The child should participate to the fullest extent possible depending on his illness experience, developmental status and level of consciousness.

The factors that are evaluated prior to any form of therapy include nature of the indication, cost-benefit analysis, surgical and anesthetic risks, overall prognosis and informed consent. Individually, each is a difficult assessment and all decisions are made after thorough discussions with the parents. A multidisciplinary approach with a significant time commitment by team members is needed. Such counseling time and place must be consciously scheduled amidst busy mainstream pediatric practice. Impromptu, fleeting conversations cannot address these issues comprehensively.

Consent

Conventionally, a child is not legally competent to decide on his/her medical care. The law of the land determines such competence. In a child who is legally not competent, the parent/legal guardian acts in the best interest of the child. This proxy decision maker is termed "surrogate". However, the medical fraternity respects the involvement of the child in the decision making process (autonomy) depending on the child's comprehension and maturity. Adolescents, who have decision-making capacity, are considered separately.

Informed consent implies respect for patient autonomy and right to decide where possible. There are two situations where a child can give informed consent. Firstly, when he/she is an *emancipated minor* (self-supporting, married, pregnant or a parent, member of military, declared by court) or secondly when the child is a *mature minor*, capable of making decisions for self or seeking treatment for specific health care concerns such as venereal diseases or drug abuse.

DNR (Do Not Resuscitate) Order

A DNR order is written by the primary physician in children with terminal conditions after extensive discussions with the surrogate decision-maker. This prevents resuscitation of the child in the event of a cardiopulmonary arrest. It is formulated in the best interests of the child on the assumption that a cardiopulmonary arrest will be a spontaneous event in the dying process and not of iatrogenic origin.

DNR orders are not empirically reversed as such a step disregards patient autonomy/surrogate decision making. In certain special situations such as anesthesia, DNR orders may need specific modifications or temporary suspension. These are based on cure and comfort care policies and are individualized. Such 'required reconsideration' of DNR orders are instituted after the family discuss the options preoperatively with the surgical team .Two such modified orders are 'goal directed DNR orders' and 'procedure specific DNR orders'. A goal directed DNR order is based on the physician's intimate knowledge of the patient and allows for resuscitative measures to achieve the child's /family's goal. It honors the child's/family's wishes but also provides the medical staff with management flexibility. The major limitation of this order is the reliance on physician's intimate knowledge of the patient and interference of his personal feelings. In contrast, procedure specific DNR orders provide clear and strict guidelines for the performance of specific resuscitative measures (e.g. ionotropic support) as per the child's/family's wishes. It limits the scope of resuscitative measures irrespective of the cause of arrest or potential for reversal.

PAIN RELIEF

Pain (Greek-'poine') means punishment and the immature mind may wrongly blame himself for the pain. Mc Caffney writes-'Pain is whatever the experiencing person says it is and exist wherever he says it does'. Children do experience and remember pain.

The pain may be from the disease or from diagnostic/monitoring procedures or therapy. Psychological variables should not be blamed where physical causes have not been exhaustively addressed. Individual perceptual variation, lower verbal fluency and changing development add to the complexities of pain assessment. Insufficient knowledge of pharmacology of analgesics, irrational fear of overmedication, difficulties in pain assessment and evaluation has resulted in undermedication.

"The quality of mercy is essential to the practice of medicine"— Angell. The vulnerability, powerlessness and dehumanization that accompany pain must be controlled. The goal of pain management is to keep the patient pain free and as alert as possible to enjoy precious time. There is no one way of pain management and frequent evaluation of drug choice, dosage and frequency is warranted till the child is pain free.

Effective pain relief facilitates earlier mobilization, shortened hospitalized stay and reduced costs.

Pain Assessment

Three primary components of pain assessment are cognitive (self- report), behavioral manifestations and psychological responses.

Cognition and evaluation of pain is influenced by multiple factors such as the meaning of pain to the individual, prior experience with pain, expectation of the painful experience and cultural attitudes .The expression of pain may take on several forms- vocalization, verbal statements, facial expressions and body posture and the manner in which the child interacts with the environment. All children do not overtly express their pain and unlike adults, self-report can vary greatly in children. Depending on the age and developmental level, various formal assessment tools are used to quantify the cognitive component of pain.[1,2] Self-report for the 4-7 years group and Wong and Becker's Faces Pain Rating Scale (WBPRS) for > 7 years children are illustrative examples. The POPMP (postoperative pain measure for parents) is a simple pain assessment tool for parents in home care.

Behavioral responses like 'projecting' the pain onto dolls/drawings, restlessness, sleeping, irritability and poor quality/destructive activity/play in the young child signify unrelieved pain and pain coping mechanisms. FLACC scale the Toddler-Preschooler Postoperative Pain Scale (TPPPS) for the preverbal/nonverbal children are behavioral assessment tools.[3] However, one must be cautioned to interpret behaviors cautiously. Behaviors such as playing, sleeping or even watching television may be strategies that the child uses for coping with pain.[4-6] Pain behaviors are also obscured in the child with continued severe pain or in situations such as depression, fatigue, extreme illness, and the use of sedatives or hypnotics.

Physiological signs such as sweating palms, tachypnea and tachycardia can be used as adjuncts to self-reports and behavioral observation measure but they are neither sensitive nor specific as indicators of pain. Despite all these measures when one is unsure and there is reason to suspect pain, a diagnostic trial of analgesics is strongly recommended.

Treatment Modalities

Cognitive behavioral techniques: These are taught during the pain free interval and guide the child to a better sense of control. For example, passive relaxation with mental imagery, cognitive distraction/focussing, music therapy, hypnosis, deep breathing, progressive muscle relaxation. Cognitive behavioral techniques are used in conjunction with pharmacotherapy for optimal pain relief.

Physical methods: Like holding, rocking, massaging, position change and TENS (transcutaneous electrical nerve stimulation) all increase the child's comfort. Activities like playing/watching TV may distract from pain. Parents are a source of help in the event of pain. They are termed as extremely powerful analgesic agents.

Table 20.1: Opioid and non-opioid analgesics

Non-opioid analgesics

DRUG	DOSAGE, ROUTE
Paracetamol	10-15 mg/kg, orally, every 4-6 hours
Ibuprofen	5-10 mg/kg, orally, every 6-8 hours
Naproxen	5 mg/kg, orally, every 8-12 hours

Opioid analgesics

DRUG	DOSAGE, ROUTE
Codeine	0.5-1 mg/kg, orally, every 3-4 hours
Pethidine	0.75 mg/kg, sc/iv, every 2-4 hours
Morphine	0.15-0.3 mg/kg, orally, every 4 hours
	0.05-0.1 mg/kg, sc/iv, every 2-4 hours
	0.03 mg/kg/hr continuous IV infusion
Fentanyl	0.5-2 µg/kg/hr continuous IV infusion
Controlled Release morphine	0.6 mg/kg, orally, every 8 hours/ 0.9 mg/kg, orally, every 12 hours

- Pethidine is not recommended for chronic use because of its long half-life and cumulative toxicity of metabolite.
- For > 50 kg children, normal adult doses are advised.

Adapted from- Cancer pain relief and palliative care in children, WHO, Geneva 1998.

Pharmacologic methods: The World Health Organization's three-step ladder of analgesia is applicable to children. Non-opioid analgesic for mild pain (e.g. Paracetamol), weak opioids for moderate pain (e.g. Codeine) and strong opioids for severe pain (e.g. Morphine sulfate) forms the standard steps. NSAIDs and opioids are commonly employed. They are administered around the clock (ATC) based on the duration of action and are supplemented by additional breakthrough/rescue dose in between. An "as needed basis" is often suboptimal and associated with under medication. Analgesics are administered prophylactically before chest physiotherapy, suctioning and other potentially painful procedures. Additional local anesthesia decreases the dose of analgesics during invasive procedures. It is useful to consult the pain clinic personnel when needed. Table 20.1 summarizes dosages and routes of administration of analgesics in common use.

Paracetamol has been conventionally used in subtherapeutic doses (10 mg/kg). An initial loading dose of 30 mg/kg and a ceiling dose of 90 mg/kg/

day is currently accepted. Doses above 150 mg/kg/day cause liver toxicity. Paracetamol-codeine combination is superior to paracetamol alone. Bleeding is of particular concern in the cancer patient on NSAIDs. Non-opioid analgesics have a 'ceiling effect' whereby increasing the dose beyond the recommended therapeutic level has little additional analgesia but a significant increase in side effects and toxicity.

Opioids are used in severe pain. Dosages are calculated using 0.1 mg/kg/dose of morphine sulfate as standard. These are dosages to begin with and except codeine, increasing doses of opioids provide increased analgesia. There is no ceiling effect with opioid analgesics. Therefore, unless adverse drug reactions are observed, the opioid dose may be increased till adequate pain relief is obtained.

Drug administration should be by the simplest, most effective and the least painful route. If oral intake is not preferred, intermittent parenteral route is used. An indwelling central venous line is useful and precludes patient discomfort and fear of needles. A continuous infusion gives consistent therapeutic blood levels. Bolus or as needed infusions may be used. Multimodal analgesic regimens, long acting oral formulations, transdermal delivery systems and patient controlled analgesia are newer patient and physician friendly management options. Such medication can be instituted in home care too.

The physician and family must note the difference between dependence/tolerance and addiction. Physical dependence is the physiological need for a substance in order to function; characterized by signs and symptoms of withdrawal if the body is suddenly deprived of the narcotic. Tolerance is habituation to a substance such that larger doses of the narcotic are required to attain the original level of effectiveness. Addiction is a psychological and/or physiological dependence on a narcotic, characterized by an intense craving for the drug and an overwhelming involvement in obtaining it and using it for purposes other than pain relief. Addiction never occurs unless drug abuse was present prior to the onset of disease. Paradoxical fears of addiction (opiophobia) lead to under medication. It must be clarified to parents that increasing dosages of narcotics to achieve pain control does not necessarily mean worsening disease.

Side effects of opioids need careful control. Constipation is managed with dietary changes, laxatives and enemas. Vomiting and itching are occasionally seen and rarely need specific therapy. Respiratory depression with standard opioid doses is a problem in the infant. In mild depression, doses are to be withheld/reduced and the child stimulated to breathe. In severe depression, airway support, oxygen and reversal with carefully titrated opioid antagonist (Naloxone) are required.

The analgesics may be combined with adjuvants in pain management. These include.
- Tricyclic antidepressants (e.g. imipramine), anticonvulsants (e.g. carbamazepine, gabapentin) and systemically administered local anesthetics (oral mexiletine, parenteral lignocaine) in refractory neuropathic pain.
- Psychostimulants to counteract the sedative effects of opioids (e.g. dexamphetamine, methylphenidate)
- Biphosphonates and radioisotopes (e.g. strontium-89) in pain associated with bony metastases.
- Medications to relieve muscle spasm (e.g. benzodiazepines and baclofen) in neuro-degenerative disorders.
- Local anesthetics-topical local anesthetic, e.g. Emla cream (lignocaine and prilocaine) to reduce pain from peripheral venous cannulation, etc.
- Other pain relieving procedures such as nerve blocks and spinal (epidural, intrathecal) analgesia
- Corticosteroids are useful initially but the long-term side effects outweigh it's benefits.

SYMPTOM CONTROL

Assessing symptoms involves discussion with the child, review of parental reports and formal assessment tools. This is relatively difficult for preverbal and developmentally challenged children.

Dealing with symptoms is challenging, more so if home care is instituted. A delicate balance is struck between preparing a family to recognize problems and arousing unfounded fears. Keeping calm, initiating specific first aid measures and contacting the hospital staff for advice is stressed. In certain instances, the patient may need to be shifted to hospital for therapy.

Children find it difficult to take large number/amounts of drugs and complicated regimens are not feasible to implement. A careful choice between the various routes (oral/rectal/transdermal/subcutaneous/intramuscular/intravenos) and formulations (tablet/capsules/crushed tablets/liquid mixtures/

long acting formulations) is made to suit patient and physician acceptability.

Constipation/diarrhea, fatigue, pain, dyspnea and poor appetite are commonly reported problems. Symptoms of treatment related complications cause more suffering and are less alleviated than those did attributable to progressive disease.

Anxiety and Delirium

This is commonly seen and gets exacerbated with events such as external bleeding, seizures and dyspnea. It reflects the child's needs to express his/her fears and distress. Benzodiazepines and haloperidol provide relief in the final stages of life. Neuroleptics such as haloperidol and chlorpromazine improve the thinking in both agitated/delirious and confused/tranquil patients.

Depression

Common in terminal illness, it is under recognized and under treated. Physicians must assess patients for depressive signs (e.g. late night sleeplessness that is not due to pain) that cannot be attributed to the primary illness. It has a biological basis and is treated with psychostimulants such as dexamphetamine or methylphenidate which have a rapid onset of action.

Fatigue

A common symptom in cancer patients, physicians often pay little attention to this. Causes include progression of disease, anemia, poor nutritional status and depression.

Feeding

Sucking and eating are part of the normal development of a child and provide comfort, pleasure and stimulation. Children with brain tumors or neurodegenerative disorders will require assisted feeding with a nasogastric tube or gastrostomy.

Anorexia

Since appetite is equated with good health, anorexia is disturbing. The anxiety during eating is eased by helping the family accept the child's natural loss of appetite. Small frequent feeding of the child's favorite food with modifications to increase their nutritional and caloric value yields better results. Progestational agents, such as megestrol acetate, and glucocorticoids improve anorexia.

Nausea and Vomiting

They are often exhausting. Anti-emetics (prokinetics, serotonin antagonists) are selected according to their site of action and probable cause of nausea (Table 20.2). Oral/parenteral/rectal routes are used as appropriate. Careful hydration is essential with frequent emesis.

Constipation

Inactivity and high doses of narcotics lead to constipation. Increasing fiber and bulk in the diet and use of stool softeners are useful. An oral, poorly absorbed opioid antagonist, such as naloxone, is useful in opioid associated constipation when the above measures fail.

Fever

In neutropenic patients, fever heralds potentially life threatening complications. Besides sponging with tepid water and antipyretics, sensitivity based antibiotics are indicated. The desire to treat vigorously is dictated by the family's wishes.

Dyspnea

Nebulization/steam inhalation, provision of humidification/O_2 can reduce the distress.

Benzodiazepines are used in extreme anxiety. Oropharyngeal suctioning must be 'gentle' especially inpatients with thrombocytopenia.

Table 20.2: Antiemetic drugs	
Cause of vomiting	Antiemetic drug
Gastrointestinal stimuli	Metoclopramide Domperidone Ondansetron
Drugs and biochemical upset	Phenothiazines Metoclopramide Domperidone Ondansetron
Raised intracranial pressure and cortical stimuli (anxiety)	Cyclizine Ondansetron Dexamethasone (resistant cases)

Bleeding

Visible external bleeding is most frightening to the family. External bleeds are managed with packs, topical agents (thrombin, gelatin sponge) and blood product transfusion as indicated.

Convulsions

Protection of the child's body and head during a convulsion is essential. Rectal diazepam and subcutaneous midazolam are useful at home in emergencies. Readjustment of anti-convulsant dosage as the disease progresses and relief of increased intracranial pressure (brain tumors) with medication/shunts may be required.

SURGICAL CARE

A number of surgical procedures, minor and major, are likely to be performed on terminally ill children. The procedure may be palliative/elective or both.[7] Palliative procedures aim at patient comfort and improved quality of life, e.g. gastrostomy and tracheostomy in a neurologically impaired child. Elective procedures aim at limiting/curing an unrelated associated condition (not considered to be a usual terminal event) with the aim of prolonging life, e.g. surgery for an obstructed inguinal hernia in a child with Stage 4 neuroblastoma. The distinction is often blurred and different members of the treating team may disagree on the scope of each. This is more so when the prognosis is unknown or questionable.

ANESTHETIC CARE

Anesthetic care is as demanding as surgical care for the terminally ill. A compromise between hemodynamic stability and optimal anesthesia is often elusive. Generally low risk strategies such as regional anesthesia or monitored anesthesia care (MAC) is preferred where possible. However, general anesthesia may be required in certain circumstances. Anesthetic care may be individualized according to the underlying disease, pathophysiologic state and risk-benefit analysis. A compromised pulmonary status and consequent risk of pulmonary failure is the prime concern.

Existing DNR orders will need reconsideration. During anesthesia, hemodynamic instability may lead to cardiopulmonary arrest and measures to reverse the same should not be withheld in the presence of a DNR order. In fact a blanket DNR order encourages the use of anesthetic options with inferior patient comfort.

PSYCHOSOCIAL SUPPORT

The commonly heard statement 'There's nothing more we can do for the child' is out of place and much can be done even for a dying child. Hope needs to be fostered in the child and the family. The hope for happy times with the family— an important conversation, a good meal, a game while the family could see the child comfortable and free of pain is the essence of palliative care.[8]

The process of preparing a child/parents for survivorship/death begins when they learn the diagnosis. A degree of emotional distancing is needed to facilitate anticipatory grieving. Early introduction of intervention programs positively affects later adjustment. Liaisons with schools and community resources and certain flexibility in professional approach ease the work. Knowledge of the child and the family's beliefs about life and death and sources of emotional support helps in providing psychological support. Such an approach is central to the concept of palliative care.

Bereavement is a state of loss of a significant other through death or as a process that individuals must work through or recover from. Grieving is the emotional response to bereavement. Grief is a dynamic process; a continuum that begins at the point of diagnosis of the terminal illness. The situation elicits stressful behavior from all quarters— the patient, the siblings, parents and physicians. The responsibility of the bereaved families should not be overlooked after the death of the child. The family will often feel the need to discuss/clarify thoughts and notions during the process of bereavement. Providing compassionate knowledgeable information during this period is crucial. An introduction to bereavement intervention programs involving self-help groups, religious establishments, etc. is useful.

Patient

The responses are primarily dependent on the developmental level with the adolescent reacting quite differently from the toddler. The infant and preschooler are entirely dependent on the parents and the immediate family and have not established a relationship beyond this insular environment. The majority have little/no fun, are sad, afraid and not calm or restful. One needs to decipher symbolic communication in many instances. At every step, an effort is made to involve personal artifacts of the child/family and personalize the care.

Adolescence is a transition from child hood to adulthood and the dying adolescent is acutely aware of the reality of losing everything suddenly. Marked physical deterioration imparts a wasted child like appearance; however, intellectual maturity and adult like insight leads to significant depression in the terminally ill. Signs of depression (e.g. sadness, irritability, multiple aches, deranged sleep patterns) may overlap with symptoms of the illness and are easily missed. Frequent hospitalization, school absenteeism, social isolation from peers, parental overprotection and parental dependence throttles the emerging independence of adolescence. Most adolescents are aware of the impending death and raise issues that are realistic and not existential. Their queries are directed to members of the healing team they perceive as 'competent' to answer. Inappropriate efforts to hide the knowledge from them are counterproductive. The young have less tolerance to pain and identify deficiencies in pain control.

These issues can be managed by encouraging normal adolescent activities (school participation, education, peer interaction), frank communication (expression of fear/anxiety, essential information about care and prognosis, encouraging questions), 'permission giving atmosphere', ensure patient confidentiality and adequate pain control (patient controlled analgesia), desires and wishes. Sick children need the opportunity to pursue their interests and have short-term goals for as long as possible.

Parental Grief

When a child is diagnosed to have a terminal condition, the family undergoes a myriad of changes. Parents initially react with disbelief, anguish, and despair and feel loss of control not only over their lives but also of their child's life. Anxiety, fright and a sense of uncertainty loom large. Parental grief is severe, long lasting and manifests itself with a multitude of psychological (e.g. shock, numbness, apathy, anger, etc) and physical reactions (e.g. lethargy, weight loss or gain, crying spells, etc.). The degree of parental grief varies with the age of the child at the time of death and the attachment bonds between the deceased and the bereaved. A change in parental relationships is inevitable with the death of an offspring. Interparental relationship, change in family structure and concerns about surviving children influence parental grief.

Intervention for bereaved parents include helping them to accept the reality of their loss, facilitate the expression and interpretation of feelings and assistance in finding resources for continuing support. Providing parents with complete and honest information about the child's condition is essential to anticipatory grieving. Clarity and accuracy should substitute for euphemisms. Dysfunctional and persistent denial states may be challenged. Silent presence, empathy and personal use of the self are the need. Parents should be assisted in dealing with sibling concerns. The families of children with an inherited condition have additional problems of guilt and blame; they need genetic counseling and information regarding prenatal diagnosis in the future.

Sibling Grief

The sibling may feel confused, ignored, betrayed or isolated. Other behaviors observed include acting like the deceased, psychosomatic illness, regression and depression. An adolescent sibling is developmentally more unstable and vulnerable. Factors influencing sibling grief are sudden death, developmental age, pre-existing psychological difficulties, family-community support systems and disruption of routine.

Facilitating anticipatory grieving with parental support, sibling participation in care of the sick child and receiving consistent information all along can alleviate sibling grief. Home care is more suited to these tasks.

Caregiver Grief

Attending physicians tend to perceive the terminal illness and death of their patient as a personal failure and an affront to one's abilities to preserve life. It reminds us of our limitations and vulnerability.

Physicians and nurses may blame themselves overtly or covertly for the death. Each caregiver has to introspect and come to term with his/her personal pain and sentiments. They may experience a grief similar to that with the death of a loved one; the extent of such a reaction is proportional to the degree of their involvement in the care of the patient.

This is often ignored and needs to be tackled. Taking personal care is an obligation to oneself and the patients. The physician should know his limitations and reach for help when needed. This is influenced by an individuals's stage of personal and professional development. Overinvolvement/underinvolvement are defined with years of experience and introspection and a continuing review of one's personal philosophy.

INTERVENTIONS AROUND A CHILD'S DEATH

This is a sensitive phase and is of critical importance. It must be ensured that the child dies with the parents /loved ones in attendance. At this moment it is necessary to guard against protecting the parent and allow them to 'parent their child'. If the child dies alone, the staff should take the family aside and relate the events surrounding the death.

Focus on Religious Beliefs of the Family

Health care professionals are faced with varied cultural and religious beliefs of families during the terminal phase of their child's life. It is necessary to enquire about these beliefs and restrictions and prepare to offer whatever possible in the event of death. Illustrative examples are presented below.

Hinduism[9]

- A devout Hindu receives solace from hymns/ readings from the Bhagavad Gita
- A desire for performance of a holy rite such as sprinkling of sacred water from the Ganges over the person.

Islam[10]

- The dying patient may wish to sit or face Mecca
- The body is considered a belonging of God; so post-mortems/ organ transplants are prohibited unless legally binding.

Sikhism[11]

- Special regards should be given to the special K's (Kesh- unshorn hair; Kara- iron wrist band; Kirpan- a short sword; Kanga- wooden comb). The hair is covered, the body is straightened and covered with a white shroud with a religious emblem.
- Newborns and still births are buried while others are cremated, preferably within 24 hours.

Catholicism[12]

- Baptism of great significance before and even at death
- The sacraments are given great importance – sacraments of the sick is a symbol of Christ's healing.

Free churches and other significant Protestant churches:
- Visit from leaders of community is an essentiality.

Zoroastrianism (Parsees)[13]

- Last rites include thourough cleansing of the body, covering it with a cloth (sadra) and a sacred kusti, covering the head with a cap/scarf
- Burial/cremation/disposal of body by water is considered inappropriate, instead they have bodies placed in the tower of silence.

Jehovah's Witness[14]

- Postmortem, body/organ donation is based on individual's desire. They are strictly against blood transfusions.

Time should be provided for the family to grieve over the child's body in private and as they wish. Allow the family to talk about their feelings and to cry. There is no right way to react— extreme shock; anger, withdrawal and denial are all ways of expressing grief. Denial is a form of emotional protection, which disappears once the individual is ready to accept.

It is necessary to acknowledge parental grief and say 'I'm sorry'. It only exhibits the concern health professionals have for such families. Avoid unthinking comments or inadvertently blaming anything/anyone for the death. Recount the positive aspects of the child's life and discuss sibling needs, participation and bereavement. The parents could be offered limited bereavement time with the health personnel who were intimately involved with the child during the follow-up.

POSTDEATH INTERVENTIONS

These are aimed at facilitating grieving and preventing dysfunctional consequences of bereavement. Areas of continuing misunderstandings are clarified, questions answered and preventive bereavement counseling provided. They include:
- Self-help programs
- Person to person contact with another bereaved individual/group
- Referral to a mental health professional

Most families do not need specialist counseling but general support and reassurance from those who know the family and the illness.

REFERENCES

1. Wong DL, Baker CM. Pain in children: Comparison of assessment scales. Pediatric Nursing 1988;14 (1):9-16.
2. Eland JL. Pain in children. Nursing Clinics of North America 1990;25(4):871-83.
3. Merkel SI, Shayevitz JR, Voepel-Lewis T, Malviya S. The FLACC: A behavioral scale for scoring postoperative pain in young children. Pediatric Nursing 1997;23(3):293-97.
4. Heiney SP. Helping children through painful procedures. AJN 1991;20-24.
5. Nancy OH, Jacox A, Miaskowski C, Ferrel B. The management of pain in infants, children and adolescents undergoing operative and medical procedures. MCN 1992;17:146-52.
6. Tarbell SE, Cohen T, Marsh JL .The toddler- preschooler postoperative pain scale: an observational scale for measuring postoperative pain in children aged 1-5 years. Preliminary report. Pain 1992;50:273-80.
7. Berlandi JLH. Ethical issues in pediatric perioperative nursing. Nursing Clinics of North America 1997;32(1): 153-67.
8. Whittam EH. Terminal care of the dying child. Psychosocial implications of care. CANCER Supplement 1993, 71(10): 3450-62.
9. Green J. Death with dignity-Hinduism. Nursing Times 1989 Feb 8-15;51.
10. Green J. Death with dignity- Islam. Nursing Times 1989 Feb 1-7;56.
11. Green J. Death with dignity- Sikhism. Nursing Times 1989 Feb 16-23;56.
12. Green J. Death with dignity-Catholicism. Nursing Times 1992;28-29.
13. Green J. Death with dignity-Zoroastrianism. Nursing Times 1992;12-18;44.
14. Green J.Death with dignity-Jehovah's witness. Nursing Times 1992;36.

SECTION 2

Trauma

CHAPTER 21

Pediatric Trauma

Azad B Mathur, NC Featherstone

Trauma is the principle cause of death in children aged 1-14 years in the developed world.[1] Its management has improved considerably over the past 30 years; whilst there will always be some injuries incompatible with life, effective early institution of care can significantly reduce morbidity and mortality.[2]

In 1979, Cowley defined the 'Golden Hour', the first hour following traumatic injury, as being critical for treatment to ensure optimal care for patients.[3] Subsequently, common systematic approaches to injury assessment and management have been developed (Advanced Trauma Life Support/Advanced Pediatric Life Support) which begin treatment of life threatening injuries or problems as soon as they are detected.[4,5] Knowledge, experience, rehearsal, and practical experience of the procedures involved makes for a smooth effective delivery of care in an otherwise stressful time for doctor, nurse and the patient.

Motor vehicle accidents, pedestrian accidents, falls, bicycle accidents and child abuse are the most common causes of injury in children. Non-accidental injury (NAI) is particularly important in children under 1 year of age.[1] Transmitted energy during injury delivers more force per unit volume resulting in multisystem injuries in children.

We aim to give an informative background explanation of areas specific to pediatric trauma, followed by a revision of the treatment protocols.

Many aspects of the initial resuscitation of children depend on the child's weight.[6,7] This is not always easy to estimate or practical to measure in the emergency situation, hence the development of the Broselow Pediatric Resuscitation Measuring Tape (Fig. 21.1) which relates height to weight, and gives fluid and drug doses appropriate for the size of the child.[8,9] In addition, if the age of the child is known, the following formula can be used to derive an estimate of weight:[5]

$$\text{Weight (kg)} = 2 \times (\text{Age} + 4)$$

ANATOMICAL AND PHYSIOLOGICAL DIFFERENCES IN CHILDREN

The anatomy and physiology of children differs significantly from that of adults. It is vital to have a sound appreciation of these differences because they alter the types of injury sustained and permits prediction of outcome. Body proportions, structures and normal physiological parameters change with age.

Head

Children have a large head to body size ratio, which needs to be considered, in relation to heat loss, and surface area of burns patients. The head is 19% of surface area at birth, reducing to 9% at the age of 16 years.

The size of the head also affects safe positioning of the unconscious child. If a child lies on a flat surface the large size of the occiput relative to the chest causes a flexion of the neck potentially compromising the airway.[10] The airway is best protected with the midface moved anteriorly and superiorly (the 'sniffing position'). A child's trunk can also be supported on a raised pad to avoid this happening. However, the neck must not be over extended as the trachea is short and soft, and over-extension of the neck may result in tracheal compression. The relatively large size of the head also puts children at greater risk of head and high cervical spine injuries.

254 Pediatric Surgery—Diagnosis and Management

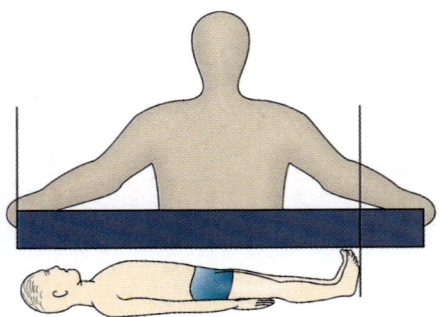

Fig. 21.1: Broselow pediatric emergency tape

Upper Airway

Infants less than 6 months are obligate nasal breathers. The face and mandible are small leading to a small oral cavity, whilst the tongue is large tending to obstruct the airway in the unconscious child.[10] The tongue may also obscure the glottis during intubation. The floor of the mouth is easily compressed by extrinsic pressure, so a mask being used on the face needs to be held carefully.

Narrow airways are often obstructed by mucus, loose teeth are at risk of being lost into the bronchial tree, and adenotonsillar hypertrophy is frequently present between 3-8 years, adding to the difficulties of securing the airway.

The epiglottis is more U-shaped in the child, projecting posteriorly at 45 degrees. The larynx is cephalad and anterior at the level C2-3 in the infant, as compared with C5-6 in the adult. It is therefore easier to intubate children younger than 12 months with a straight bladed laryngoscope. The narrowest point of the upper airway is the cricoid ring, which is lined with pseudostratified ciliated epithelium, which is prone to edema if cuffed tubes are used for intubation. Uncuffed tubes are used for all children who have yet to reach puberty, and the sizing of the tube should allow a small leak of gas past the tube during inflation of the lungs.[10]

The trachea is short, in neonates 4-5 cm and in infants 7-8 cm; therefore tubes can easily become displaced accidentally or during transport, entering the relatively straight right main bronchus.

Neck

In children, the interspinous ligaments and joint capsules are more flexible; the vertebral bodies are wedged anteriorly, so tend to slide forward with flexion and the vertebral facet joints are flat. Cervical spine radiographs in children can cause some concern due to normal physiological appearances mimicking fracture or dislocation. It is important to correlate clinical examination and radiological findings. It is unusual to find a fracture without physical signs.

Pseudosubluxation (anterior displacement C2 on C3 or sometimes C3 on C4) is a common finding in approximately 40% of children less than 7 years old and up to 20% of children up to 16 years.[11] There is normally more than 3 mm of movement when the joint is studied in flexion/extension. To differentiate pseudosubluxation from cervical spine injury, the flexion of the spine needs to be removed by positioning the head in a neutral position, bringing the head forward to a 'sniffing position'.

Skeletal growth centers can also be confused with fractures.[11] The basal odontoid synchondrosis has a radiolucent area at the base of the dens in children less than 5 years, whilst the tip of the odontoid epiphyses appears separate in children age 5-11 years. The growth center of the spinous process can itself be mistaken for a fracture.

Spinal injuries in children are rare but can occur; most affect the cervical spine.[12] Spinal cord injury without radiological abnormality (SCIWORA) occurs almost exclusively in children < 8 years old.[13] SCIWORA mainly affects the cervical spine and to a lesser extent the thoracic spine (the upper cervical spine is more susceptible due to its increased mobility). *Seriously injured children should be immobilised until full neurological assessment is possible.* Magnetic resonance imaging (MRI) may have to be used.

Cardiovascular

The young cardiovascular system has an increased physiological reserve compared to adults and able to tolerate significant blood loss without obvious outward distress. As a consequence, there may only be subtle signs of severe shock. Early assessment and recognition of shock is essential to the appropriate management of the injured child. Tachycardia and reduced capillary refill are frequently the only signs available. It is important to note that the normal physiological parameters vary with age (Table 21.1). Anxiety and pain in the injured child can confound tachycardia as a sign of shock.

The child's heart has a limited capacity to increase stroke volume, so cardiac output is mostly dependant on heart rate. With a typical blood volume of 80 ml/kg, an amount of blood, which would otherwise be considered a minor blood loss in an adult could severely compromise a child.[14]

The child initially responds to reductions in intravascular volume by increased heart rate and vasoconstriction, thereby maintaining cardiac output. Thus, shock in a child is difficult to recognise below 25% volume loss, but may be suggested by a weak thready pulse, increased heart rate, lethargy and irritability, and cool clammy skin. There would be a slight reduction in urine output if measured.

As volume loss approaches 25-45% the heart rate remains raised, but there is a definite reduction in consciousness and a dulled response to pain. The skin becomes cyanotic, with reduced capillary refill time (CRT) and the extremities become cold. If measured there would be minimal urine output.

Finally above 45% volume loss the child can no longer compensate and there is a point at which the child becomes hypotensive and bradycardiac, and the child is comatose. These are late signs and signify a grave situation.

An idea of a child's normal parameters is required. As an approximate guide:

Systolic Blood Pressure (mm Hg) = 80 + (Age in years × 2)
Blood volume (ml) = 80 × Weight (kg)

Thermoregulation

With a large surface area to body mass ratio and a relative lack of adipose tissue children cool down rapidly in a cold environment. This may affect their conscious level, hemostasis through deranged clotting and reduce their response to treatment.

Every effort should be made to reduce exposure and keep the child warm and comfortable, without compromising safe resuscitation, primary and secondary surveys. The patient should be kept warm

Table 21.1: Normal physiological parameters					
Age	Weight (kg)	Heart Rate/min	Blood pressure (mm Hg)	Respiratory rate/min	Urinary output ml/kg/hr
0 – 6 months	3 – 6 kg	180 – 160	60 – 80	60	2
Infant	12	160	80	40	1.5
Preschool	16	120	90	30	1
Adolescent	35	100 – 50	100	20	0.5

with heaters, thermal blankets as appropriate, and all intravenous fluids, and preferably, inhaled gases used in treatment should be warmed.

Compliant Skeleton

The child's skeleton is more elastic and compliant compared to that of the adult. As a result, injuries to internal organs may be encountered without external signs of trauma or fracture (e.g. pulmonary contusions without rib fractures).

Structured Approach to the Seriously Injured Child

The accepted structured approach has been developed and refined by surgeons in recent decades and is one which all doctors ought to be familiar. Greater detail can be found in the manual of the Advanced Pediatric Life Support group.[5]

It consists of the following basic sequence:
1. Primary survey
2. Resuscitation
3. Secondary survey
4. Emergency treatment
5. Definitive care.

HISTORY

A brief description of the suggested mechanism of injury or the circumstances in which the child was found gives the trauma doctor an idea of what injuries to expect. Children are frequently too distressed to give a coherent story, and relatives are often extremely distressed. The ambulance crew who have been at the site of the accident can usually give a good account.

PRIMARY SURVEY

The aim of which is a rapid assessment to identify immediate life threatening problems and prevent secondary injury.
A Airway and cervical spine control
B Breathing
C Circulation and hemorrhage control
D Disability
E Exposure.

Airway and Cervical Spine Control

The airway should be assessed to ensure its patency. This is done by *looking* for chest and/or abdominal movement, *listening* for breath sounds and *feeling* for breath.

Cervical spine injury should be assumed present until excluded; the C-spine protected by immobilisation. The airway is optimised by correct positioning of the head relative to the neck using either a head tilt/chin lift or jaw thrust maneuver. The mouth and oropharynx are cleared and oxygen is supplied. If the child is unconscious then an oral airway is inserted under direct vision curving it over the tongue, to prevent trauma to the palate.

If the child is unable to maintain their own airway or has a Glasgow Coma Score (GCS) of 8 or less, or requires assisted ventilation, then the child needs to be intubated with rapid sequence induction. The child should be preoxygenated beforehand as children rapidly desaturate. Prolonged bag and mask ventilation may result in gastric distension which could splint the diaphragm and make abdominal examination difficult. Passage of an **orogastric** tube may be useful in this situation.

The endotracheal tube (ETT) should be close to the diameter of the little finger or the size of the nares. The following formula can also be utilised to calculate the approximate ETT size:

Endotracheal tube size (mm) = (Age / 4) + 4

An *uncuffed* tube is used which sits in position at the cricoid ring. In children less than 8 - 12 years the glottis is cone shaped and the use of an uncuffed tube prevents later subglottic stenosis secondary to intubation.[10] Auscultation over the chest and stomach helps avoid selective endobronchial intubation or tube misplacement.

Cricothyroidotomy is unlikely to be required in a child, and if necessary, needle cricothyroidotomy is the preferred first step, using oxygen jet insufflation.[10]

Breathing

Once the airway is secured and the cervical spine controlled, breathing should be assessed. Its adequacy is established by looking at the *effort, efficacy* and *effects* of inadequate breathing on other systems.

Normal ventilatory rate varies and reduces with age. Tidal volume is of the order 7-10 ml/kg. Care should be taken when assisting ventilation to match these parameters without using excessive force, which may result in barotrauma or volutrauma. In an effort to avoid this, many bag-valve-mask devices have pressure-limiting valves to limit insufflation pressures. Hypoventilation is the most common cause of cardiac arrest in children, resulting from the ensuing respiratory acidosis.[5,15]

The chest needs to be assessed for the presence of pneumothorax/hemothorax and definite treatment planned.

Circulation and Hemorrhage Control

Circulatory assessment consists of a rapid assessment of the following parameters:
- Heart rate
- Systolic blood pressure
- Capillary refill time
- Skin color
- Temperature
- Respiratory rate
- Mental status.

Capillary refill time (CRT) is measured by squeezing and elevating an extremity, great toe or thumb, above heart level, for 5 seconds, then releasing it. A CRT > 2 seconds, skin mottling, and low peripheral temperature are signs of shock.

When shock is suspected, a 20 ml/kg bolus of warmed crystalloid solution is given. Failure to improve suggests either ongoing hemorrhage or gross fluid depletion. A 20 ml/kg bolus represents 25% of blood volume, but as this volume becomes distributed into other body fluid compartments up to three boluses of 20 ml/kg may be necessary to achieve 25% blood volume replacement. Blood replacement (whole blood or packed cells) should be considered if a third bolus is required.[5]

Venous access in a young child is often difficult at the best of times. In the emergency situation, two attempts at peripheral cannulation, lasting 90 seconds, should be made. If these are unsuccessful, then either placement of an intraosseous needle (Fig. 21.2) into the proximal tibia in children less than 6 years, or a venous cutdown should be used. Placement of an intraosseous needle is relatively safe, quick and effective, and allows marrow to be taken for blood grouping. Once alternative vascular access has been established it should be removed. The preferred site for cut down is the saphenous vein at the ankle. An experienced anesthetist may place a percutaneous central line or femoral line using the Seldinger technique.

Disability

A brief assessment of the child's conscious level is undertaken and also to determine the pupil size and reactivity. The AVPU scale can be used to assess disability with ease:
- **A** Alert
- **V** Responds to voice
- **P** Response to pain
- **U** Unresponsive.

Exposure

All surfaces of the child need to be inspected during the course of the primary survey, but this can be done region by region to avoid distress and heat loss.

Resuscitation

Treatment of life-threatening injuries should be undertaken as they are identified during the primary survey.

Standard Investigations

Standard trauma bloods are taken during placement of intravenous access and the primary survey. Seriously injured children should undergo a series of radiological investigations (trauma series).

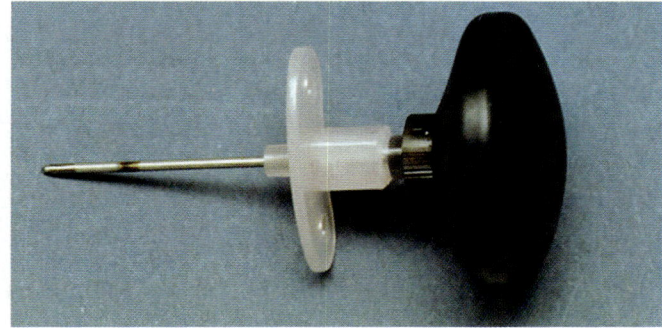

Fig. 21.2: Intraosseous infusion needle

Blood:
- Full blood count (FBC), electrolytes (U and E), glucose (Glu), amylase (Amy)
- Blood for group and save (G and S) or urgent cross match (XM)
- Arterial blood gases (ABGs)

X-ray:
- Trauma series (Chest, lateral C-spine, pelvis)
Additional investigations are taken once the patient is stabilized.

SECONDARY SURVEY

The secondary survey is a head to toe assessment, including reassessment of vital signs. A complete neurological exam including the Glasgow Coma Scale (GCS) should be carried out. A brief medical history needs to be recorded. A useful mnemonic being used is AMPLE:

A Allergies
M Medications
P Past illnesses/pregnancy
L Last meal/drink
E Events related to the injury.

EMERGENCY TREATMENT

Emergency treatment is that required to stabilise the child prior to transfer to an appropriate referral centre, theatre for operative treatment or the ward for conservative expectant observation. These interventions are not as urgent as those provided during the resuscitation phase, but important nevertheless.

DEFINITIVE CARE

Definitive care is the final phase in the structured approach to trauma; others than the admitting trauma team may provide it. The patient may require transfer to receive definitive treatment in a tertiary center; consequently, it is essential that good written records are maintained throughout the admission process.

HEAD TRAUMA

Head injury is the most common reason for hospital admission in children, and the most common cause of death in children after the age of 1 year.[16] Vomiting is frequently used as a justification for admission for observation in young children because of the association with raised intracranial pressure, but even very minor injuries may cause children to vomit. Children may sleep fairly heavily and not wake as promptly as adults, especially when subjected to hourly neurological observations, leading the less experienced to assume a reduced conscious level.

In infancy, the possibility of non-accidental injury (NAI) should be considered. Older children are more likely to suffer from falls either around the house or at play. Road traffic accidents are the commonest cause of fatal head injury. The use of cycle helmets has led to a significant reduction in the severity of head injuries.[17,18]

Unfortunately significant head injuries do occur. The standard trauma and resuscitation approach is used in the assessment and early treatment of these patients and the aims of emergency treatment are directed at preventing secondary brain injury, and referring early to a neurosurgical unit for definitive treatment.

PRIMARY AND SECONDARY BRAIN INJURY

Neurosurgical referral is indicated if there is a deteriorating conscious level, Glasgow Coma Score (GCS) < 12, focal neurological signs, depressed skull fracture, basal skull fracture or penetrating injury. Definitive treatment is directed at the cause of the raised intracranial pressure or injury. This may involve the evacuation of hematoma or elevation of depressed fracture in addition to other intensive care measures.

Any child with a GCS of 8 or less should be intubated and ventilated with rapid sequence anesthesia. If the conscious level deteriorates rapidly despite all other supportive measures then urgent referral is indicated and measures intended to increase cerebral perfusion in the short-term are used. These include the use of:

1. IV mannitol 0.5-1 g/kg.
2. Hyperventilation to a $PaCO_2$ of 3.5 - 4.0 KPa.
3. 20 degree head up position to promote venous drainage.
4. Plasma expanders to avoid cerebral hypotension.

A focal seizure is considered as a focal neurological sign. Generalised fits are of less concern but should be controlled if they have not stopped within 5 mins. IV diazepam is preferred.

In many cases, head injuries are restricted to minor scalp hematomas. Injuries are often associated with self-limiting vomiting and normal neurology. If the head injury appears stable, a period of close observation for 24 hours is appropriate.

The assessment of head injuries in children depends on the age of the child, their ability to describe the mechanism of injury, and the history obtained from reliable witnesses. Potentially serious injuries are suggested by significant energy transfer, e.g. RTA or fall from height > 2 m, loss of consciousness (LOC), an altered state of consciousness, obvious neurology, or penetrating injury. The conscious level should be documented using the appropriate scale for the age of the child.

THORACIC TRAUMA

Children have compliant, elastic ribs and the thorax can absorb significant amounts of energy without obvious external signs of injury.[19] An apparently normal chest radiograph cannot exclude significant thoracic injury. Rib fractures suggest a significant transfer of energy and other associated organ injuries should be suspected.[20-22]

The provision of high flow oxygen via a reservoir mask allows a FiO_2 of greater than 60% to be achieved and should be used routinely in chest trauma. Chest injuries can be immediately life threatening or only become apparent at a later stage.

Clinical examination and assessment should be swift. Early identification of injuries and their treatment can maximise outcomes.[23,24] We discuss the management of immediately life threatening injuries in this section.

Tension Pneumothorax

Air is drawn into the pleural space compressing the mediastinum and compromising venous return to the heart. Cardiac output reduces, such that the child becomes hypoxic and shocked, and the jugular veins become distended.

There will be hyper-resonance and reduced air entry on the side of the pneumothorax. As the mediastinum is pushed to the opposite side the trachea is said to deviate away from the side of the pneumothorax.

Treatment should be immediate needle thoracocentesis in the 2nd intercostals space mid clavicular line, relieving the tension and converting the injury into a simple pneumothorax. Definitive treatment is insertion of a chest drain.

Major Hemothorax

Bleeding into the pleural space from damage to the lung vessels or chest wall can be a source of a large volume of blood loss. In addition to the reduction in lung volume, shock and hypoxia may be evident if significant blood volume has been lost. There will be reduced chest movement, reduced air entry and reduced resonance to percussion on the side of a hemothorax. Treatment requires volume replacement and the insertion of a large bore chest drain.

Open Pneumothorax

The presence of penetrating wounds to the upper body, between the umbilicus and root of the neck should alert the clinician to the possibility of an open pneumothorax.

There will be reduced chest movement, reduced breath sounds and hyper-resonance on the side of the pneumothorax. Air may be heard to suck and blow through the wound. Treatment requires the creation of a flap valve using a air tight dressing secured on three of four sides, to allow air out but not in, thereby preventing a tension pneumothorax from developing. A chest drain is required, followed by surgical exploration, debridement and repair.

Flail Segment

In the child, a flail chest is a very significant injury due to the amount of energy required to create it and the degree of underlying lung injury. Abnormal chest movement may be seen over the flail segment and crepitus may be felt. Early involvement of an anesthetist is advised. Treatment should consist of endotracheal intubation and ventilation.

Cardiac Tamponade

Injury that results in bleeding into the pericardial sac reduces the volume available for cardiac filing. As the pericardial sac fills with blood, the cardiac output is reduced. Shock develops, the heart sounds become muffled and the neck veins may become distended. Treatment is emergency needle pericardiocentesis.

Even aspiration of a small volume of blood from within the pericardium can increase cardiac output.

ABDOMINAL TRAUMA

The abdomen is more exposed in children than in adults. The soft elastic rib cage offers less protection to the liver, kidneys and spleen. The pelvis is shallow and the bladder is intra-abdominal in the younger child. The most common organs to be damaged following blunt trauma are in order, spleen, liver, kidney, gastrointestinal tract, genitourinary tract and pancreas. Penetrating trauma most commonly affects the gastrointestinal tract, liver, kidneys and bloods vessels. The significant morbidity and mortality following splenectomy has lead to a more conservative approach with regard splenic trauma.[25] Experience has shown that the majority of abdominal injuries can be treated conservatively, provided they receive close observation, repeated assessment and monitoring. Attention should be paid to vital signs, fluid balance and blood factors. A pediatric surgeon should be available during this period if required.

Operative intervention is required if the child exhibits:
1. Hemodynamic instability after replacement of 40 ml/kg of fluid.
2. A penetrating abdominal injury
3. A non-functioning kidney on contrast study (warm ischemic time for a kidney is 60 mins)
4. Signs of bowel perforation

The abdomen is only considered in the primary survey under circulation if shock does not respond to volume replacement and no other obvious site of hemorrhage can be found. In children a nasogastric tube or orogastric tube should be passed, as air swallowing occurs during crying and can cause significant gastric distension. This may result in splinting of the diaphragm making breathing and/or ventilation difficult.

During the secondary survey the abdomen is inspected for bruising, laceration and penetrating injury. The external genitalia must also be examined and the external urethral meatus inspected for blood. If blood is seen, this is an indication for retrograde urography and passage of urethral catheter must not be attempted by anyone other than a Consultant Urologist. Rectal examination on children is carried out only if it is considered appropriate by the pediatric surgeon who would be operating.

FRACTURES

Skeletal injuries in young children are common; up to 42% of boys and 27% of girls will sustain a fracture during childhood.[26] In the early stages of resuscitation, fractures should be thought of as a potential source of volume loss. Grossly displaced fracture/dislocations should be reduced. The blood loss from a long bone or pelvic fractures is proportionately greater in a child than adult and should be considered.

The majority of children's fractures heal rapidly and well. Whilst the bones are still growing there is a good capacity for bone remodeling, so some angulation of a reduced fracture can be accepted. Fractures of the soft springy immature bones in children are often the classic greenstick fracture. In very young children small buckle fractures also known as torus fractures are seen as small defects in the cortical surface.

Some injuries such as crush injuries to the epiphysis are very difficult to diagnose radiologically, yet they can have serious consequences on the future growth and therefore symmetry of the limbs.[27] Other fractures have well-established association with vascular and neurological injury, which should be sought once such a fracture is seen.

PSYCHOLOGICAL ASPECTS OF TRAUMA

Our aims are to try to establish useful communication to assess the mechanism of injury, extent of injury, and response to treatment, whilst calming and reassuring the child. Communication with an injured child in pain and distress, in an unfamiliar environment is a challenge to the most empathetic experienced doctor. A younger child has a limited ability to describe and localise pain, and is less able to give a clear history. They will become distressed at interventions required during the course of the resuscitation, investigation and treatment of injuries. The medical team should be sympathetic to the needs of the child, and co-operation may be better gained if one nurse is focused on communication and comforting the child.

Accompanying relatives are frequently distressed and need careful consideration. In appropriate circumstances, providing they are calm enough to be of comfort to the child they should be encouraged to stay in attendance and given as much explanation as is required so that they understand what is happening and why.

NON-ACCIDENTAL INJURY (NAI)

The abuse of children by their carers is a regrettable fact of life. It can take many forms, physical, sexual, emotional or neglect. It is important to have a high index of suspicion of the possibility of abuse and be aware of the patterns of presentation, explanations and injury seen.[28]

Factors which should alert the doctor to the possibility of NAI include, odd times of presentation for treatment, delayed presentation, presenting without the prime carer, inconsistent accounts and imprecise times for the mechanism of injury. The injury may not be compatible with the mechanism of injury, or the carer's attitude or focus of concern does not seem right. Perhaps the child's interaction with the adult is abnormal, or their behavior seems inhibited or withdrawn.

Injuries seen in NAI include head injuries, including occipital fractures and intracranial injury. Fractures of long bones and particularly multiple fractures at different stages of healing may be seen. Bruising and finger marks in a hand print distribution, burns, scalds, cigarette burns, belt and bite marks should all be carefully examined.

Sexual abuse may present as frank injury, genital infection, or may present with odd inappropriate behavioral or other emotional problems.

Assessment of any child with suspected child abuse needs great care and sympathy, and the involvement of seniors at the earliest point of concern.

TRAUMA SCORES

Trauma scores are used as a predictor of survival and for comparative purposes.[29] They include the following:

Pediatric Trauma Score

	Coded value		
Patient factors	+2	+1	-1
Weight (kg)	> 20	10 - 20	< 10
Airway	Normal	Maintained	Not Maintained
Systolic BP	> 90	50 - 90	< 50
CNS	Awake	Obtunded	Coma
Open wound	None	Minor	Major
Skeletal trauma	None	Closed	Open/multiple

Revised Trauma Score

This is a physiological scoring system consisting of a weighted combination of Glasgow Coma Scale, Systolic blood pressure and Respiratory Rate.

Glasgow coma scale score	Systolic blood pressure	Respiratory rate	Coded value
13 – 15	> 89	10 – 29	4
9 – 12	76 – 89	> 29	3
6 – 8	50 – 75	6 – 9	2
4 – 5	1 - 49	1 – 5	1
3	0	0	0

RTS = 0.94 GCS + 0.73 Systolic BP + 0.29 Respiratory Rate

The RTS can be in the range 0 - 7.84. When RTS is plotted against survival a sigmoid shaped curve is produced.

Trauma Score – Injury Severity Score (TRISS)

TRISS is used to estimate probability of survival of a patient obtained from multiple regression analysis of a large trauma outcome database. It uses weighted values of revised trauma score, injury severity score and age.

IMMUNE DYSFUNCTION FOLLOWING TRAUMA

Severe trauma can cause life-threatening complications after immediate survival and resuscitation due to the dysfunction of the immune system.[30] The normal response to trauma is to restore homeostasis. This is achieved initially by hemostasis, followed by increased regional blood flow to allow removal of waste material and the repair of tissue ('the classical ebb and flow phases of stress response').

Following major trauma, the excessive immune activation in response to tissue damage, necrosis, hemorrhagic shock, and infection can have an adverse effect on otherwise healthy tissue and organs. This may result in Systemic Inflammatory Response Syndrome (SIRS), which may progress leading to Multiple Organ Failure (MOF). This may also be complicated by sepsis. Multiple organ failure typically occurs in a progressive sequence affecting the lungs (Adult Respiratory Distress Syndrome ARDS), gastrointestinal tract, kidneys, heart and liver.

The immune system is a complex inter-related defence system that is influenced by a multitude of molecular messengers, released in response to a variety of stimuli. Multiple feedback loops are involved in the system. SIRS following massive trauma is thought to develop due to the excessive release of pro-inflammatory mediators in response to tissue damage, disrupting the existing balance between pro- and anti-inflammatory mediators.[30]

The initial response observed is macrophage activation leading to the release of cytokines and complement response to tissue damage.[31] Endothelial cells are stimulated by complement breakdown products to release additional factors, which are chemotatic for leucocytes. Monocytes arrive and mature into tissue macrophages.

Cytokines are low molecular weight proteins effective at very low concentrations, which act by binding with cell surface receptors. Their effects may be multiple and overlapping - growth factors, modulators of leukocyte chemotaxis, modulators of lymphocyte function and modulators of inflammatory response (either pro or anti-inflammatory).

Cytokines such as TNF-α, IL-1, IL-6, and INF-γ are released in response to tissue damage and other, second messenger compounds, platelet activating factor (PAF), intercellular adhesion molecules (ICAMs) etc, are produced in response.[30] This can lead to a massive uncontrolled activation of the complement and cellular based immune system. Cytokines cause rapid activation of non-specific monocytes and macrophages, alter production of cell surface adhesion molecules, induce enzyme production at distant sites (including nitric oxide) and depress cell-mediated specific immune systems. For example, TNF-α increases the phagocytic and respiratory burst activity of macrophages and increases neutrophil adhesion.[32]

Activation cascades result in the production of acute phase reaction proteins, which have systemic effects on thermoregulation, metabolism, catabolism, and liver protein synthesis. There is reduced production of albumin and coagulant proteins.

Nitric oxide synthase activity is increased due to proinflammatory activation; levels of nitric oxide increase as a result. Nitric oxide (NO) is a transmitter molecule of multiple cell types including vascular endothelium, smooth muscle cells, fibroblasts, and macrophages. It is also involved in regulating platelet aggregation, platelet adhesion, and neutrophil adhesion to endothelial cells, and can produce highly reactive molecules when combined with superoxide radicals.

An understanding of the basis of SIRS and the need for prompt treatment to avoid hemorrhage, hypoxic tissue damage, and the stimulus of necrotic tissue may reduce its occurrence. Ultimately the development of drugs and antibody therapy to control or limit the immune activation may be possible in the form of immunomodulation, but is still under evaluation.[33]

The treatment of SIRS remains supportive; this may include nutritional support in the form total parental nutrition (TPN), mechanical ventilation, renal support, hemo-correction of coagulopathy, and antibiotic treatment of infection.

REFERENCES

1. Browne GJ, Cocks AJ, McCaskill ME. Current trends in the management of major pediatric trauma. Emergency Medicine 2001;13:418-25.
2. Stafford PW, Blinman TA, Nance ML. Practical points in evaluation and resuscitation of the injured child. Surg Clin North Am 2002;82:273-301.
3. Cowley RA. Emergency Medical Services in the State of Maryland. Echelons of trauma care. Am Surg 1979;45:77-78.
4. American College of Surgeons. Advanced Trauma life Support of the American College of Surgeons: Advanced Trauma Life Support for Doctors (ed 6). Chicago, IL, American College of Surgeons 1997.
5. Mackway-Jones K, Molyneux E, Phillips B, Wieteska S, (Eds). Advanced Pediatric Life Support – The Practical Approach. 3rd edition. London: BMJ Publishing Group 2001.
6. Greig A, Ryan J, Glucksman E. How good are doctors at estimating children's weight? J Accid Emerg Med 1997;14:101-04.
7. Harris M, Patterson J, Morse J. Doctors, nurses and parents are equally as poor at estimating pediatric weights. Pediatr Emerg Care 1999;15:17-18.
8. Hofer CK, Ganter M, Tucci M, et al. How reliable is length-based determination of body-weight and tracheal tube size in pediatric age group? The Broselow tape reconsidered. Br J Anaesth 2002;88:283-85.
9. Luten RC, Wears RL, Broselow J, et al. Length-based endo-tracheal tube and emergency equipment in pediatrics. Ann Emerg Med 1992;21:900-04.
10. Stone DJ, Gal TJ. Airway management. In Miller RD (Ed): Anesthesia Philadelphia, PA, Churchill Livingstone, 2000;1414-51.
11. Lustrin ES, Karakas SP, Ortiz AO, et al. Pediatric cervical spine: normal anatomy, variants and trauma. Radiographics 2003;23:539-60.

12. Hall DE, Boydston W. Pediatric neck injuries. Pediatr Rev 1999;20:13-19.
13. Martin BW, Dykes E, Lecky FE. Patterns and risks in spinal trauma. Arch Dis Child 2004;89:860-65.
14. Kincaid EH, Chang MC, Letton RW, et al. Admission base deficit in pediatric trauma: A study using the national trauma data bank. J Trauma 2001;51:332-35.
15. Reis AG, Nadkarni V, Perondi MB, et al. A prospective investigation into the epidemiology of in-hospital pediatric cardiopulmonary resuscitation using the international Utstein reporting style. Pediatrics 2002;109:200-209.
16. Lee LK. Controversies in the sequelae of pediatric mild traumatic brain injury. Pediatr Emerg Care 2007;23:580-83.
17. Attewell RG, Glase K, McFadden M. Bicycle helmet efficacy: a meta-analysis. Accid Anal Prev 2000;33:345-52.
18. Berg P, Westerling R. A decrease in both mild and severe bicycle-related head injuries in helmet wearing ages – trend analyses in Sweden 2007;22:191-97.
19. Allen GS, Cox CS Jr. Pulmonary contusion in children: diagnosis and management. Soc Med J 1998;91:1099-1106.
20. Black TL, Snyder CL, Miller JP, et al. Significance of chest trauma in children. South Med J 1996;89:494-96.
21. Nakayama DK, Ramenofsky FL, Rowe MI. Chest injuries in childhood. Ann Surg 1999;210:770-75.
22. Peclet MH, Newman KD, Eichelberger MR, et al. Thoracic trauma in children: an indicator of increased mortality. J Pediatr Surg 1990;25:961-66.
23. Bliss D, Sileen M. Pediatric thoracic trauma. Crit Care Med 2002;30:S409-S15.
24. Haller JA Jr., Shermeta DW. Major thoracic injury in children. Pediatr Clin North Am 1975;22:341-47.
25. Keller MS. Blunt injury to solid abdominal organs. Seminars in Pediatric Surgery 2004;13:106-11.
26. Lindin LA. Fracture patterns in children. Acta Orthop Scand 1983;54:1.
27. Gladden PB, Wilson CH, Suk M. Pediatric Orthopedic Trauma: Priciples of management. Seminars in Pediatric Surgery 2004;13:119-25.
28. Speight N. Non-accidental injury. BMJ 1989;298:879-88.
29. Furnival RA, Schunk JE. ABCs of scoring systems for pediatric trauma. Pediatr Emerg Care 1999;15:215-23.
30. Hietbrink F, Koenderman L, Rijkers GT, et al. Trauma: the role of the innate immune system. World Journal of Emergency Surgery 2006;1:15.
31. Hernandez LA, Grisham MB, Twohig B, et al. Role of neutrophils in ischemia-reperfusion-induced microvascular injury. Am J Physiol 1987;253: H699-H703.
32. Martin TR. Lung cytokines and ARDS: Roger S. Mitchell Lecture. Chest 1999;116:2S-8S.
33. Bastian L, Weimann A. Immunonutrition in patients after multiple trauma. Br J Nutr 2002;87:S133-34.

CHAPTER 22

Head Injuries in Children

BS Sharma, Feiz Uddin Ahmad

Head injures in children differ from adults on account of age related differences in its etiological mechanisms, clinicopathological responses, type, management, prognosis and sequelae.[1]

ETIOLOGY

Head injuries in children can occur due to accident, fall or abuse. Most common cause of head injury in children is a fall from height. The commonest cause of severe head injury in children is motor vehicle related trauma. The peak incidence under the age of 1 year largely due to non-accidental trauma – birth trauma and "battered child" being the major causes. At 1-4 years of age, falls from lap, cot, windows and stairways and injury by siblings are common. Recreational, automobile and other vehicular injuries are commoner after the age of 4 years.[1]

MECHANISMS

Motor vehicle accidents with acceleration/deceleration forces results in a diffuse injury, whereas trauma produced by low velocity focal contact injuries produce local injury. The pliability of skull and compressibility of brain in infants allows focal absorption of energy rather than causing acceleration of fluid wave across the intracranial cavity producing a contrecoup injury, which is relatively uncommon in young children. Most injuries in the perinatal period result from low momentum deforming forces that lead to tears of structures such as falx, tentorium, venous sinuses or the bridging veins. This static loading allows surface injuries and makes contracoup lesions rare.[2]

PATHOPHYSIOLOGY

Structural differences in a thin, flexible and elastic skull capable of undergoing much deformation, open fontanelles and sutures, a large subarachnoid and extracellular space immature developing brain, more water content of brain, incomplete myelination, low ratio of brain to CSF, low cerebral blood flow and cerebral metabolic rate for oxygen in young children result in special physiological response to trauma. Children tolerate a rapidly expanding intracranial mass lesion better and the onset of features heralding impending disaster are delayed. The elastic skull can withstand a considerable amount of distortion without fracture and the degree of deformation is sufficient to produce local brain damage. Cerebral trauma in the linear growth period from 1-4 years after birth may disrupt brain development and functional maturation, resulting in defects of behavior, intellect and seizures. The child's brain is more susceptible to edema formation and physiological reactions are more rapid and intense but of a shorter duration.[1-3]

Great majority (86%) of head injuries are mild. Severe head injuries in children are less likely to involve surgical mass lesions compared to adults.[4]

TYPES OF INJURIES

Birth Injuries

These are of two types :
i. Injuries produced by normal forces of labor and delivery, e.g. ping-pong fracture, subarachnoid hemorrhage, subdural hemorrhage and caput succedaneum.

ii. Injuries produced by obstetrical instrumentation, i.e. misapplication of forceps, e.g. linear and depressed fractures with or without dural laceration and hemorrhage.

Common birth injuries are:[1]
 a. *Caput succedaneum* is localized swelling of scalp due to edema rather than a hematoma. It is typically seen in midline posterior parietal area. No therapy is required.
 b. *Cephalohematoma* is collection of blood between perisoteum and skull and is limited by sutures. It usually resolves spontaneously. If it doesn't resolve by 6 weeks and plain X-ray skull shows calcification, surgical removal may be indicated.
 c. *Subgaleal hematoma* is bleeding into loose connecting tissue layer between galea aponeurotica and pericranium. It shouldn't be aspirated unless there is impending compromise of scalp circulation.
 d. *Ping-pong fracture* is produced by steady pressure of ischial tuberosity against skull. Lesions larger than 3 cm. require corrective surgery. After 2-3 cm. scalp incision, periosteum elevator is inserted between dura and bone beyond deepest part of depression to get adequate leverage to pop the fracture out.

Skull Fractures

 i. *Linear:* These fractures may be single, multiple, branched, circumferential (blow-out type) or stellate.
 ii. *Growing skull fracture:* Also called the craniocerebral erosion or traumatic leptomeningeal cyst, is progressive diastatic enlargement of fracture line (Fig. 22.1).[5-8] Dural laceration conciding with diastatic skull fracture of 4 mm or more, under the age of 3 years are essential factors for its production. Growth of fracture line is due to resorption of adjacent bone as a result of continuous pulsatile wedge pressure from tissues herniating through the fracture line. Arachnoid prolapses out through dural tear and is trapped. A ball valve mechanism with easy ingress than egress of CSF and arachnoid adhesions form a cyst. When arachnoid is also torn, brain herniates. Repair of growing fracture requires removal of bony edge circumferentially until normal dura is

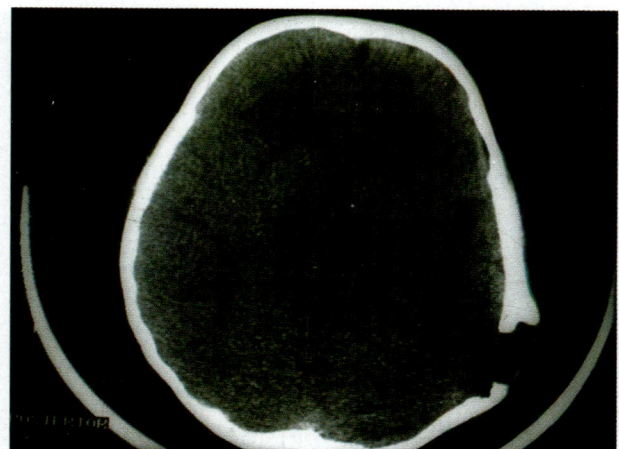

Fig. 22.1: CT scan head showing growing skull fracture with sclerosed margins

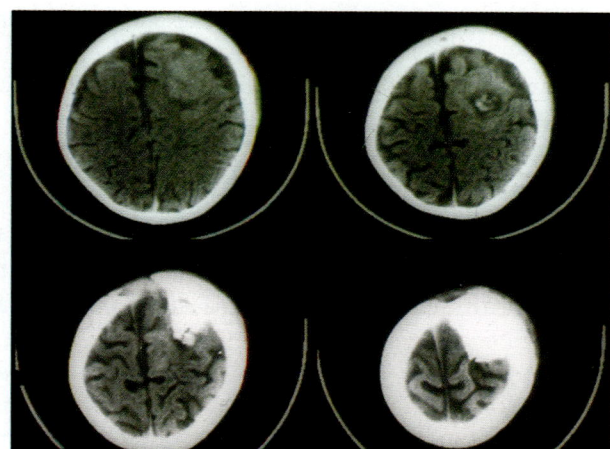

Fig. 22.2: CT scan head showing depressed fracture frontal bone

defined all around. Cyst is drained and gliosed brain scar is excised. Dura is separated from brain and duraplasty is done with pericranium or facialata followed by cranioplasty with split clavarial or rib graft.
 iii. *Basal fracture and CSF liquorrhea:* CSF otorrhea and early onset CSF rhinorrhea generally subside spontaneously within 2-3 weeks. Episode of pyogenic meningitis, persistent or recurrence of liquorrhea and late onset rhinorrhea would require surgical repair.[2]
 iv. *Depressed fracture (Fig. 22.2):* Closed depressed skull fractures require surgery when the depression is more than 5 mm located over motor or sensory cortex, compound or there is an associated foreign body. Depressed fracture is

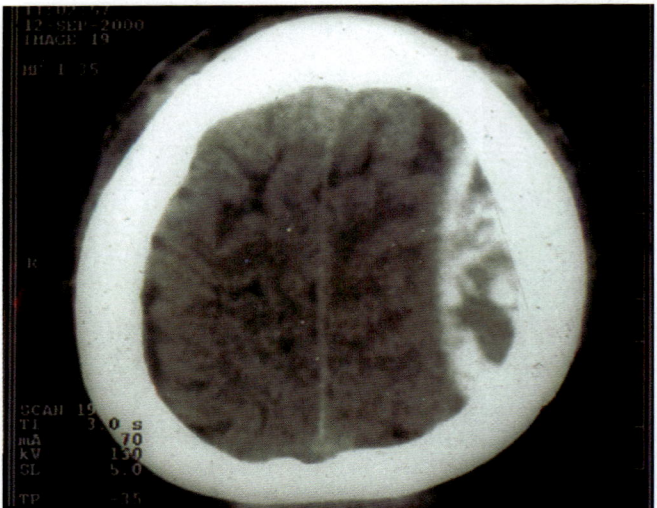

Fig. 22.3: CT scan head showing acute epidural hematoma

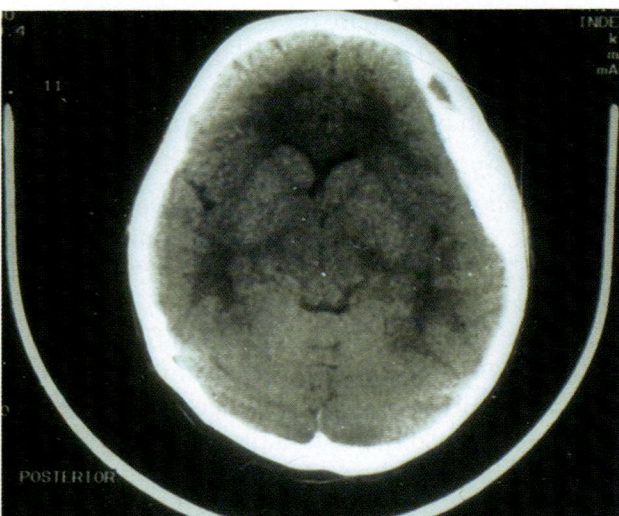

Fig. 22.4: CT scan head showing acute subdural hematoma

elevated and bone fragments are replaced back after duraplasty and thorough wound toilet.

Hematomas

Intraventricular and subarachnoid hemorrhage is more common in younger children, as compared to intracerebral, acute epidural and subdural hematomas.[4]

i. *Acute epidural hematoma (Fig. 22.3):* It is less common in children because harp edged fractures are unusual, dura is tightly adherent to the suture lines and middle meningeal vessel grooves in the inner table of skull are not yet formed. The location of such a hematoma in a child is higher in the parietal region than in adults and a typical low temporal burr hole may miss it. Fall from < 3 feet is most common mechanism in children below 2 years. It occurs following multiple blows to the head, such as a fall down the stairs. Tachycardia may occur as clot expands because of acute anemia associated with blood loss in epidural space.[1-2]

ii. *Acute subdural hematoma (Fig. 22.4):* These are usually seen with traumatic breech delivery. The hallmark is a rapid clinical deterioration. A neonate with acute subdural hematoma in an acute neurological distress should have diagnostic bilateral subdural aspirations.

iii. *Shaken baby syndrome or "Child Abuse:"* These children have bulging fontanelles and retinal hemorrhages.[9-12] They may develop apnea, decrebration or fixed dilated pupils requiring immediate fontanelle tap. CT scan shows acute subarachnoid hemorrhage and convexity or posterior interhemispheric triangular shaped subdural hematoma produced by tearing of parasagital bridging veins by violent shaking of the child. Diffuse or focal hypoattenuation of brain suggest poor outcome and survivors later develop infarcts.

iv. *Chronic subdural hematoma:* It is common in infants of 3-6 months of age. Lethargy, vomiting, failure to thrive, delayed milestones, chronic anemia, increasing cephalofacial disproportion, large square shaped head, tense fontanelle with distended scalp veins and setting sun eyes, or subhyaloid hemorrhages are suggestive of chronic subdural hematoma. Respiratory embarrassment is an early sign of posterior fossa subdural hematoma.

v. *Intracranial hematoma:* An intracerebral hematoma in children may cause mass effect, seizures or progressive deterioration in alertness/neurological deficits.

Diffuse Axonal Injury[2]

Under the age of 5 months, stress to the head sufficient to cause damage to cerebral tissue results in tears of the white matter rather than contusions or hemorrhages, which are most often found beyond this

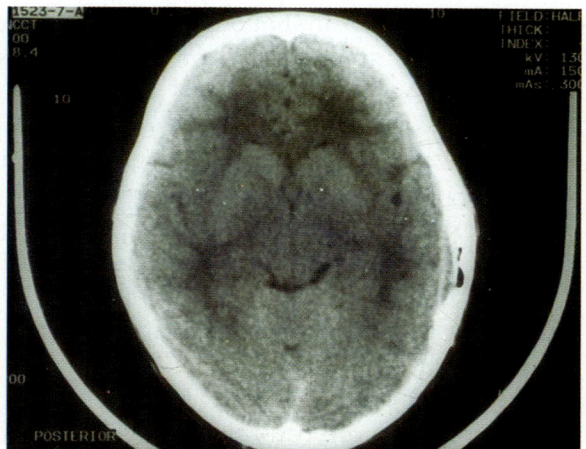

Fig. 22.5: CT scan head showing diffuse brain swelling

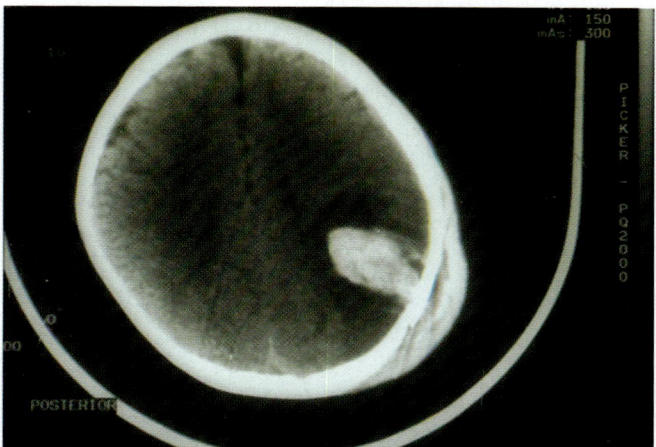

Fig. 22.6: CT scan head showing brain contusion

age. This response is probably due to different elastic properties of the immature brain, compliance of skull and smoothness of the intracranial fossae. This is most common post-traumatic entity in children with severe head injury. Motor vehicle accident is the exclusive cause. Immediate unresponsiveness and minute to minute fluctuation in neurological examination are common. Emergence from coma waxes and wanes. CT scan may reveal small hemorrhages in the head of caudate nucleus, corpus callosum, superior cerebellar preduncle or around the aqueduct.

Diffuse Brain Swelling (Fig. 22.5)

This syndrome of malignant brain edema may occur after trivial trauma or delayed deterioration may occur due to seizures, SIADH, hypoxia or fluid overload. History of apnea or shock is often present and neurological examination has been impaired from the outset. It is exacerbated by hypoxia or ischemia from hypovolemic shock due to scalp laceration or subgaleal hematoma. Ischemia and hypoxia in infants with non-accidental injuries show hypodensity in CT scan, so called "big black brain". Children with diffuse axonal injury develop severe brain swelling as a result of vascular engorgement due to paralysis of resistance vessels or increased cerebral blood flow and vasodilatation. Within hours of head injury 20-40% children who are comatose show cerebral swelling cisterns, and non-visualization of Sylvian fissures, gyri and perimesencephalic cistern. It is associated with primary subarachnoid hemorrhage or acute subdural hematoma. Brain swelling appears within 2-4 hours and subsides in 3-5 days, while brain edema appears about 24 hours following injury reaching its peak in 3-10 days. Brain swelling, on CT appears as low or isodense and diffusely spread, whereas brain edema appears as low density spread from contusions into surrounding white matter as finger-like projections. Brain swelling with low density brain suggests injury and poor prognosis. Normal or increased density of brain carries good prognosis.[2,13-16]

Brain Contusion or Laceration (Fig. 22.6)

Due to smooth intracranial fossae and rarity of centracoup injury. Contusion or laceration of brain is less common in children. They are usually treated conservatively. When the contusion is large in size producing, altered sensorium, mass effect and midline shift, surgery is indicated.

Pediatric Concussion Syndrome

It occurs following injury sufficient to produce loss of consciousness or amnesia. Child appears well shortly after trauma but sow clinical worsening during subsequent hours, child may appear in sleep, waking briefly and reluctantly to noxious stimuli then falling promptly back to sleep. This may be punctuated by vomiting, intermittent agitation and confusion. Impact seizures may occur in 12% cases which are not predictive of early or late post-traumatic epilepsy. No treatment is required unless recurs. Transient post-concussion blindness may occur from impact to back of head, vision usually returns within minutes or hours with no long-term sequelae. Asymmetry of basal-cisterns in CT scan is predictive of subsequent swelling and deterioration.[2]

MANAGEMENT

Objectives

1. Reduction of risk of exacerbation of existing brain damage by prevention or control of hypoxia or ischemia.
2. Recognition of intracranial hematoma/contusion as early as possible.
3. Control of intracranial hypertension.
4. Reduction of complications like epilepsy, infection, etc.

A. *General:* The 'ABC' system : A – airway; B – breathing; C – circulation, is aimed at rapidly assessing and initiating the life supports urgently needed followed by detailed diagnosis and adjustment of treatment. Respiratory evaluation, support and maintenance of free airway and paO$_2$ above 100 torr is the aim.

B. Control of scalp bleeding and correction of hypovolemic shock. Anemia if present is corrected by blood transfusion. Intubation is indicated in presence or hypoventilation maxillofacial injuries severe head injury with raised intracranial pressure. During intubation neck movement is minimized even if lateral cervical spine. X-ray is normal because of high incidence of ligamentious injury in children.[17]

C. Circulator support with intravenous fluid should never involve the use of 5% dextrose in water, because inappropriate antidiuretic hormone secretion is common in children with severe head injury, and dextrose adds to osmotic load, causes dehydration and hyperglycemic nonketotic coma which may confuse neurological signs and also cause massive cereberal edema.

Fluid overload should be avoided. The preferred intravenous solution is 5% dextrose in one-half normal saline or ringer lactate maintained at half the normal daily amount of 1500 ml per square meter per day. ICP monitoring is required to detect large swings in ICP when both shock and coma are present.

D. Quick and careful examination for associated chest, abdominal and spinal injury or fracture of long bones.

E. *Neurological Examination:*
   1. History and progress of neurological condition
   2. Level of consciousness.
   3. Seizures, hyperpyrexia, bleeding from orifices.
   4. Vital sings-pulse respiration, blood pressure temperature.
   5. Pupils, size, shape and reaction subhyaloid hemorrhages.
   6. Palpation of fontanelles and suture.
   7. Examination of postural changes in tone and primitive reflexes.
   8. Any evidence of weakness of any limb, cranial nerve palsy and meningeal signs.
   9. Local scalp examination – subgaleal hematoma, depressed fracture, palpation of scalp laceration with gloved finger, echymosis over mastoid region (Battle's sign) or periorbital discoloration (raccoon sign).
   10. Glasgow coma scale (GCS) is applicable in older children. It is of limited value in infants and young children as it relies on fully developed language skills and patient's cooperation. However, modified pediatric Glasgow coma scale grade more limited responses with maximum score of less than 15. Pediatric GCS or Adelaide pediatric coma scale are useful for assessment of initial depth of coma and its progress.

Modified Glasgow Coma Scale[2,18,19]

Eye Opening

- 4 – Spontaneous
- 3 – Speech
- 3 – To pain
- 1 – None.

Motor Response

- 6 – Obeys commands (reaches)
- 5 – Localizes
- 4 – Withdraws
- 3 – Abnormal flexion
- 2 – Abnormal extension
- 1 – Flaccid.

Verbal Response

- 5 – Babble/gestures
- 4 – Cries for needs
- 3 – Cries – nonspecific
- 2 – Sounds
- 1 – None.

There is no reliable method to discover the occasional child who will develop intracranial hematoma, other than careful repeated observations of evolution of specific neurological signs. The mother's opinion that the child is not well should never be dismissed. One major clinical indication of an intracranial mass lesion is the occurrence of seizures in the first 24 hours after a traumatic delivery. Any trauma to the head involving moderate momentum, i.e. automobile accidents or falls from several feet has the potential to produce rapid deterioration in a child who is initially alert and ambulatory. Acute deterioration in consciousness may occur due to seizure, acute brain swelling or expanding clot. Progressive agitation appearance or strange behavior, persistent vomiting and intermittent lethargy must be considered as a harboring of intracranial hematoma. The classical signs suggestive of coning and raised ICP seen in adults are rarely seen in children. The Cushing reflex or hypertension and bradycardia seen in adults may be not clear cut in children, in whom tachycardia and increasingly shallow respirations may be the first sign of cerebral compression. A child who deteriorates or fails to show steady improvement in neurological condition should be suspected to have intracranial hematoma unless proved otherwise.

Indications of Hospitalization for Children with Head Injury

1. More than momentary unconsciousness
2. Trauma of moderate momentum
3. Change in level of sensorium
4. Abnormal vital signs
5. Skull fracture – particularly traversing the middle meningeal vessel groove or sinus
6. Suspicion of child abuse
7. Neurological deficit–drowsy, irritable, hemiparesis
8. Persistent vomiting, increasing headache, fever
9. Seizures
10. A pale or anemic looking child
11. CSF liquorrhea
12. Unreliable parents to monitor child at home
13. Depressed fracture skull
14. Associated injury.

Spontaneous bicycling movements of lower limbs may be seen in association with major head injury and should not be interpreted as normal. Hyperpyrexia is common in children with cerebral concussion and temperature above 40°C need vigorous therapy. Pallor, vomiting and tachycardia are extremely common following concussion injury in the child.

Indications of CT Scan

1. All unconscious children
2. All children with deteriorating level of consciousness/fail to show expected recovery/ deterioration of consciousness after initial movement
3. All children with depressed fracture – to know about underlying parenchymal injury
4. Persistent or increasing headache or vomiting
5. Seizure within 24 hours of traumatic deliver or head injury
6. Letharginess
7. Full anterior fontenelle
8. Split fracture on plain X-ray
9. Low hematocrit
10. Focal neurological deficit.

Standard lines with Glasgow Comma Score of 8 or less are intravenous line, arterial line, endotracheal tube and Foley's urinary catheter. If GCS is 5 or less, ICP monitor should be inserted. Repeat CT scan is indicated in presence of new focal findings or change in alertness.

Treatment of Raised ICP[1,20]

Conservative or Non-surgical

The aim is to keep the ICP below 20 torr in children with diffuse swelling.
1. Elevation of head to 30 degree
2. Controlled ventilation –$PaCO_2$ around 30-35 torr.

If still there is no change in ICP and CT scan shows diffuse brain swelling:
1. Furosemide 1 mg/kg
2. Pentobarbital
3. Mannitol 1 gm/kg

4. In children with diffuse swelling mannitol is avoided except in presence of midline shift. Hyperventilation and dehydration are avoided because they exacerbate ischemia.

If CT shows brain edema, then elevation of head, megadose steroids, mannitol, furosemide, hyperventilation and barbiturates are used stepwise, if the ICP is not responding.

All unconscious children require proper nursing care. The position should be changed frequently and pressure at bony points should be avoided to prevent bed sores. Anticonvulsant therapy should be given in patients who have history or high risk of seizures. Unconscious children on prolonged ventilation or intubation may require tracheostomy for tracheal toilet, chest infection and reduction of dead space. Nasogastric tube may be required for feeding. Glycerol by mouth or nasogastric tube is given to children with chronic or persisting cerebral edema.

Surgical Treatment

1. Evacuation of acute EDH, SDH large ICH or contusion.
2. Decompressive craniotomy or lobectomy in cases refractory to medical treatment.

PROGNOSIS[21-25]

The initial low Glasgow come score may be due to reversible causes and in children with scores above 5 with no associated injury or shock the mortality rate should be very low. Outcome after severe head injury is more favorable in children as compared to adults. Children do better than adults for the same type and severity of head injury. Reported mortality rate in children varies from 10-40%. Common cause of death is secondary brain edema. Primary are flexia denotes poor outcome. Brain contusion and subdural hematoma increase mortality rate by producing secondary brain edema. Mortality is highest in infants, decline until 12 years, then rises again in teenager and probably reflects mechanism of injury. Other factors associated with poor outcome include – low GCS at 72 hours, appearance of big black brain in CT, associated extracranial trauma, hypoxia, shock or iscemia, raised ICP and long duration of coma. Intellectual memory, attention behavioral and emotional defects may occur but are less permanent than in adults. Children below 2 years of age have a better potential for functional recovery.

SEQUELAE

1. *Epilepsy:* Children below 2 years of age with severe head injury and low GCS who are unconscious for more than 12 hours have higher risks of developing post-traumatic seizure. Incidence of post-traumatic epilepsy is < 5%. Psychogenic seizures can also occur.[26,27]

2. *Attention deficit hyperactivity disorder:* It may develop in children with moderate or severe closed head injury particularly, with thalamic and basal ganglion injury.[28]

3. *Persisting headache, dizziness and fatigue:* These are more common in children with pre-existing learning difficulties, previous head injury, psychiatric or family problem.[29]

4. *Intellectual, cognitive and behavioural disturbances:* It may occur.[30-32]

Rehabilitation – Post-injury motor, cognitive, memory, deficit, learning difficulties behavioral problems and poor scholastic performance require neuropsychological assessment and integrated rehabilitation services.

Prevention – Community programs of school children education like national *SAFE KIDS* campaign and *THINK FIRST* are efforts toward prevention of accidents. Improvement in suboptimal social or environmental factors, use of proper passenger restrains – seat belt, window lock, proper fit bicycle helmet may help in prevention.[33,34]

REFERENCES

1. McLaurin RL, Towbin R. Diagnosis and treatment of head injury in infants and children. Chapter 68, Youman's Neurological Surgery. WB Saunders Company Philadelphia 1990;3:2149-93.
2. Duhaime AC, Sutton LN. Head injury in the pediatric patient. In the practice of Neurosurgery. Tindall GT, Cooper PR, Barrow DL. Williams and Wilkins, Baltimore, Chapter 103. 1996;2:1553-77.
3. Bruce DA : Pediatric head injury in Neurosurgery second edition. Vol. II, Eds. Wilkins RH, Rengachary SS. McGraw-Hill. Health professions division. New York, Chapter 266. 1996;2709-15.

4. Teasdale GM, Murray G, Anderson E, et al. Risk of acute traumatic intracranial hematoma in children and adults: implications for managing head injuries. BMJ 1990;300: 363-67.
5. Tandon PN, Banerji AK, Bhatia R, et al. Cranio-cerebral Erosion (Growing fracture of the skull in children). Acta Neurochir (Wien) 1987;88:1-9.
6. Miwa T. Growing skull fractures. In: Youman's Neurological Surgery, Vol.4, 3rd edn, Ed. Youman JR, WB Saunder Company Philadelphia Chapter 73. 1990;2662-8.
7. Tomita T. Growing skull fractures of childhood. In: Neurosurgery, Wilkins RH, Rengachari SS eds. Vol. II, Second edition, McGraw-Hill Health professions division, New York, Chapter 272. 1996;2757-61.
8. Gupta SK, Reddy NM, Khosla VK, et al. Growing skull fractures : A clinical study of 41 patients. Acta Neurochir (Wien) 1997;139:928-32.
9. Duhaime AC, Gennarelli TA, Thibault LE, et al. The shaken baby syndrome: A clinical, pathological and biochemical study. J Neurosurg 1987;66:409-15.
10. Duhaime AC, Alario AJ, Leander WJ, et al. Head injury in very young children : mechanism, injury types and ophtalmological findings in 100 patients younger than 2 years of age. Pediatrics 1992;90:179-85.
11. Gilles EE, Nelson MD Jr. Cerebral complications of non-accidental head injury in childhood. Paediatric Neurology 1998;19:119-28.
12. Reece RM, Sege R. Childhood head injuries: accidental or inflicted ? Archives of Pediatrics and Adolescent Medicine 2000;154:11-15.
13. Bruce DA, Alavi A, Bilaniuk LT, et al. Diffuse cerebral swelling following head injury in children. The syndrome of "malignant brain edema". J Neurosurg 1981;54:170-78.
14. Yoshino E, Yamaki T, Higuchi T, et al. Acute brain edema in fatal head injury : analysis by dynamic CT scanning. J Neurosurg 1985;63:830-39.
15. Aldrich EF, Eisenberg HM, Saydjari C, et al. Diffuse brain swelling in severely head injured children. A report from the NIH traumatic coma data bank. J Neurosurg 1992;76:450-54.
16. Levin HS, Aldrich EF, Saydjari C, et al. Severe head injury in children : experience of the traumatic coma data bank. Neurosurgery 1992;31:435-44.
17. Pang D, Wilberger JE Jr. Spinal cord injury without radiographic abnormalities in children. J Neurosurg 1982;57:114-29.
18. Raimondi AJ, Hirschauer J. Head injury in infants and toddlers coma scoring and outcome scale. Child's Brain 1984;11:12-35.
19. Simpson DA, Cockington RA, Hanieh A, et al. Head injuries in infants and young children : the value of the pediatric coma scale. Child Nerv Syst 1991;7:183-90.
20. Raphaely RC, Sivedlow DB, Downes JJ, et al. Management of severe pediatric head trauma. Pediatr Clin North Am 1980;27:715-27.
21. Walker ML, Meyer TA, Storrs BB, et al. Pediatric head injury : factors which influence outcome. Concepts Pediatr Neurosurg 1985;6:84-97.
22. Alberico AM, Ward JD, Choi SC, et al. Outcome after severe head injury. Relationship to mass lesions, diffuse injury and ICP course in pediatric and adult patients. J Neurosurg 1987;67:648-56.
23. Michand LJ, Rivara FP, Grady MS, et al. Predictors of survival and severity of disability after severe brain injury in children. Neurosurgery 1992;31:254-64.
24. Levi L, Guilburd JN, Bar-Yosef G, et al. Severe head injury in children – analyzing the better outcome over a decade and the role of major improvement in intensive care. Child Nerv Sys 1998;14:195-202.
25. Feickert HJ, Drommer S, Heyter R. Severe head injury in children : impact of risk factors on outcome. Journal of Traum-Injury Infection and Critical Care 1999;47:33-38.
26. Pakalins A, Paolicchi J. Psychogenic seizures after head injury in children. J Child Neurol 2000;15:78-80.
27. Dulac O, Nabbout R, Plouin P, Chiron C, Scheffer IE. Early seizures: causal events or predisposition to adult epilepsy? Lancet Neurol 2007;6(7):643-51.
28. Gerring J, Brady K, Chen A, et al. Neuroimagng variables related to development of secondary attention deficit hyperactivity disorder after closed head injury in children and adolescents. Brain Injury 2000;14:205-18.
29. E wing – Cobbs l, Minner ME, Fletches JM, et al. Intellectual, motor and language sequelae following closed head injury in infants and preschoolers. J Pediatr Psychol 1989;14:531-47.
30. Ong LC, Chandran V, Zasmani S, et al. Outcome of closed head injury in Malaysian children: neurocongnitive and behavioral sequelae. J Pediatr and Child Health 1998;34:363-68.
31. Ponsford J, Willmott C, Rothwell A, et al. Cognitive and behavioral outcome following mild traumatic head injury in children. J Head Trauma Rehab 1999;14:360-72.
32. Luis CA, Mittenberg W. Mood and anxiety disorders following pediatric traumatic brain injury: a prospective study. J Clin Exp Neuropsychol 2002;24(3):270-79.
33. Rivara FP, Astley SJ, Claren SK, et al. Fit of bicycle safety helmets and risk of head injury in children. Injury Prevention 1999;5:194-97.
34. Mitra B, Cameron P, Butt W. Population-based study of pediatric head injury. J Pediatr Child Health 2007;43: 154-59.

23 Pediatric Abdominal Trauma

David A Lloyd, Gunninder Soin

MECHANISMS OF INJURY

The axiom "a child is not a small adult" is nowhere more pertinent than in relation to abdominal injuries, which account for approximately 10% of deaths from injury in childhood. In a child the kinetic energy from an external force is absorbed by a body mass that is considerably smaller than that of an adult, and there is a higher risk of multiple organ injury. Knowledge of the mechanism of injury as well as the anatomical site of impact is important for predicting the pattern of injury in an individual patient. Thus, when a car hits a child, it is very likely that the abdomen will be injured as well as other body regions (Fig. 23.1). In a child the relatively large, superficial liver, the spleen and the kidneys are not well protected from blunt trauma by the pliable ribs and thin abdominal wall muscles, and organ injury may occur without fracture of the overlying ribs. The kidney, being surrounded by less fat and connective tissue, is more mobile and therefore, susceptible to deceleration injury with traction on the renal pedicle, while the bladder lies in the lower abdomen and is vulnerable to direct trauma. In addition, an understanding of how children differ from adults physiologically and psychologically is essential for anticipating the effects of the injuries and their potential complications.

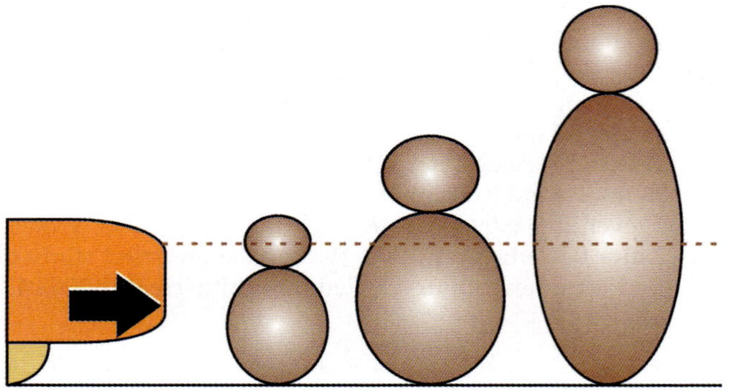

It is not surprising, therefore, that road traffic accidents (RTA) account for most of the deaths from injury. More than 50% of fatal RTA victims are pedestrians or cyclists struck by a vehicle and sustaining multiple injuries, most commonly of the head, neck, and limbs, but also of the abdomen.[1] Within the vehicle, abdominal injuries may be caused by seatbelts that often are not correctly used and are not suitable for a small child. Cyclists may sustain abdominal injuries from direct contact with the bicycle handlebars. It is important to bear in mind that as many as 10% of abdominal injuries in children result from non-accidental (intentional) injury.

ASSESSING THE CHILD WITH ABDOMINAL INJURY

Clinical Assessment

This begins with the Advanced Trauma Life Support (ATLS) and Advanced Pediatric Life Support (APLS) Primary Survey ABCD sequence and concurrent resuscitation.[2,3] When the Primary Survey reveals evidence of bleeding without an obvious injury to account for this, an intra-abdominal or pelvic injury must be suspected. In children, who are able to compensate for blood loss better than adults and maintain a normal blood pressure, early signs of

Fig. 23.1: The distribution of a motor vehicle impact on children of different sizes, illustration why a small child is at greater risk of multiple injuries

bleeding are tachycardia and peripheral vasoconstriction (indicated by cold peripheries, and prolonged capillary refill time > 2 seconds).

In the Secondary Survey the child is methodically examined for injuries. The abdominal examination begins by looking for any external evidence of injury, including the marks of tyres or seatbelts, the circular bruising of a cycle handlebar, or a penetrating wound. In an infant, bruises and abrasions of the abdominal wall or perineum may be an evidence of non-accidental injury and must be recorded. Abdominal distension may be due to acute gastric distension (which is common in the injured child), pneumoperitoneum or fluid (such as blood or bowel content); these may be distinguished by abdominal percussion for evidence of free air or fluid and by passage of a nasogastric tube to decompress the stomach. Tenderness and guarding are an evidence of intra-abdominal pathology, including hemoperitoneum or intestinal contusion or perforation. The presence or absence of bowel sounds is of no practical significance in the acute situation. Worsening abdominal signs suggest progressive peritonitis from bleeding or intestinal or bladder injury. Blood in the perineum may be due to a superficial straddle injury but could also be from the urethra, vagina or anus, indicating injury of the relevant organ system. We do not advise routine rectal or vaginal examination during the Secondary Survey in a conscious child, because this is traumatic for the child and often is inadequate; if indicated this examination should be done under general anesthesia. Finally, the child is logrolled to examine the spine.

Intentional/Non-accidental Injury (NAI)

The possibility of NAI must always be borne in mind, in particular for infants less than one year of age. All abdominal organs are at risk of injury.[4] Common mechanisms of abdominal organ injury include tightly squeezing the abdomen while shaking or sexually abusing the infant (the marks of fingers may be visible), or punching, kicking or dropping the child. Suspicion must be aroused when the child is brought to hospital after an unreasonable delay, when inconsistent explanations are given for the cause of the injury or delay in presentation, when there are suspicious associated injuries and when there is evidence of previous injuries. If there is suspicion of NAI the child must be admitted to hospital regardless of the severity of the injuries, so that a full investigation can be undertaken by social workers and pediatricians trained in managing NAI. Referral to these experts must be made urgently so that appropriate investigations can be done before possible evidence is lost. This applies particularly to sexual abuse, when examination under anesthesia may be required to detect injuries, to take swabs for evidence of spermatic fluid, and to obtain photographs of the injuries.

LABORATORY INVESTIGATIONS

Laboratory investigations provide useful supportive information, but in a previously healthy child may be relatively normal on admission and serial measurements are necessary to detect evolving pathology. A falling haemoglobin level and hematocrit may be an evidence of continuing hemorrhage, but it must be interpreted in the clinical context, for example a large volume of intravenous crystalloids may lead to hemodilution. Serum amylase levels that rise progressively suggest pancreatic duct injury, while persistent metabolic acidosis may indicate hypovolemia or tissue ischemia as with intestinal injury.[5]

IMAGING

With the reduced use of exploratory laparotomy, which provides an opportunity to rapidly examine the organs within the abdominal cavity and pelvis, there is increasing reliance on imaging to identify intra-abdominal injuries. While modern imaging techniques have become increasingly sensitive, their limitations must be appreciated, and there is no substitute for careful and repeated clinical evaluation for recognising intra-abdominal injury and the need for operation. The initial clinical examination may not reveal the true extent of visceral injury, particularly of the intestine, and repeated abdominal examination on several occasions is essential to detect evolving signs of peritonitis.

According to ATLS guidelines, the initial *emergency X-rays* must include an AP view of the pelvis for evidence of a fracture, which may be the source of hidden bleeding.[2] In children the abdomen can be included on the same film and this is useful for identifying pneumoperitoneum or acute gastric dilatation, a common occurrence in the injured child.

Computed tomography (CT) with intravenous contrast enhancement is the preferred method for identifying abdominal and retroperitoneal injuries. This single non-invasive investigation shows the distribution and degree of solid organ injuries, presence of intraperitoneal fluid, and the status of retroperitoneal structures. CT is indicated in a stable patient with suspicion of abdominal trauma based on clinical signs or on the mechanism of injury. This includes patients who are hypotensive on admission and respond to fluid replacement or who have signs of slow continuing bleeding but are hemodynamically stable. CT is also indicated in patients in whom there is a risk of abdominal injury who either cannot be assessed clinically because of their depressed level of consciousness, or who require urgent operation for extra-abdominal injuries. CT is contraindicated when there is respiratory or hemodynamic instability or if there is an extra-abdominal injury (usually a head injury) requiring immediate intervention. Intravenous contrast enhancement highlights the major blood vessels and the blood supply to specific organs (Fig. 23.2). CT is superior to other methods for identifying intra-abdominal injuries provided it is of high quality and is interpreted by an experienced radiologist.[6-8] However, it is noteworthy that if the CT is done in immediate post-injury period, it may not identify pancreatic injuries, even with contrast enhancement.[5]

The routine use of oral contrast has been recommended in emergency CT to identify duodenal injuries.[9] In our experience oral contrast has not been useful, largely because of delayed gastric emptying.[10] The presence of free intraperitoneal fluid in the absence of an injury to the solid organs must raise suspicion of a hollow organ injury.

Ultrasound scanning (USS) has the advantage of speed and ease of execution and in adults is used to screen patients for abdominal organ injury.[11] USS demonstrates intraperitoneal free fluid, an indicator of intra-abdominal injury, and may show injuries of the kidney, liver, spleen and pancreas. But in children the specificity and sensitivity of USS are inferior to CT.[8,12] USS is useful for the follow up of solid organ injuries.[13]

Intravenous pyelography and *angiography* are useful in selected situations.

Tc^{99} *radioisotope scanning* is rarely used but may have a value Tc^{99} if CT is not available.

DIAGNOSTIC PERITONEAL LAVAGE (DPL)

DPL will demonstrate the presence of blood or bowel contents, but is not recommended in children for the following reasons: firstly, hemoperitoneum in pediatric trauma is not in itself an indication for operation; secondly, DPL is painful and makes further clinical assessment of the child's abdomen impossible, and thirdly, the presence of residual lavage fluid in the peritoneal cavity may cause confusion in the interpretation of subsequent CT or USS.[6] DPL may be useful for evaluating the abdomen of a child who is unconscious and is not sufficiently stable for CT to be done, or in situations where imaging is not available.[14]

MANAGEMENT (FIG. 23.3)

Resuscitation

The general principles of emergency management of the injured child should follow ATLS[2] and APLS[3] guidelines. Vital signs are monitored, bearing in mind age-related normal values, especially blood pressure.[3] In seriously injured children with evidence of abdominal injury, two large bore intravenous lines are inserted so that fluids can be infused rapidly; one of these must be above the level of heart in case of inferior vena cava injury. A nasogastric tube is introduced to empty the stomach and a urethral catheter is inserted to measure the urine output accurately. If there is blood at the urethral meatus, a suprapubic catheter

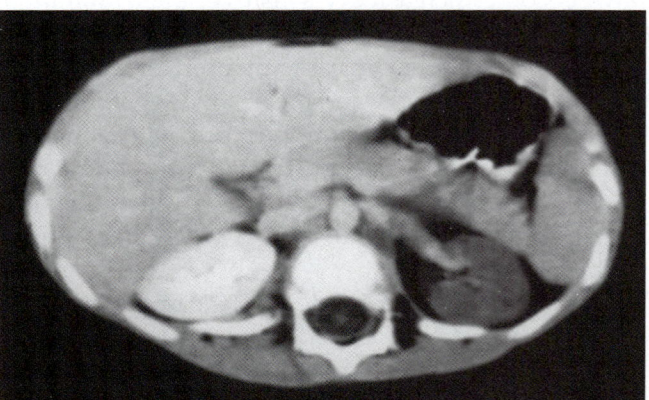

Fig. 23.2: CT scan with intravenous contrast showing absence of arterial perfusion of the left kidney due to an intimal tear, seen as a filling defect in the left renal artery

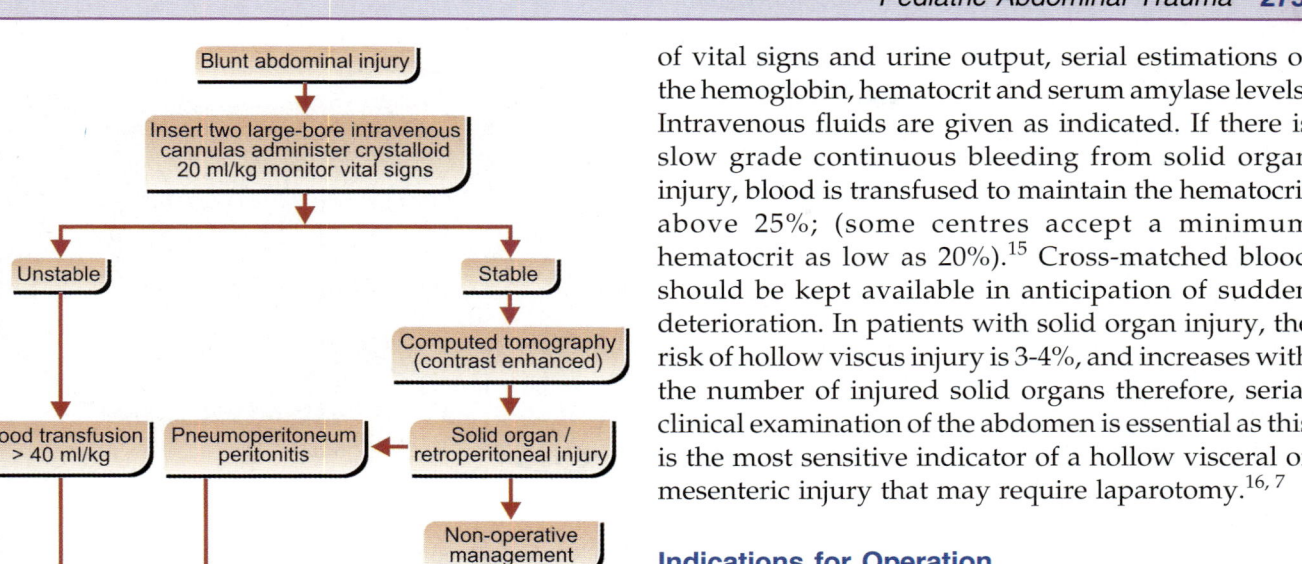

Fig. 23.3: Algorithm for the management of blunt abdominal injury

of vital signs and urine output, serial estimations of the hemoglobin, hematocrit and serum amylase levels. Intravenous fluids are given as indicated. If there is slow grade continuous bleeding from solid organ injury, blood is transfused to maintain the hematocrit above 25%; (some centres accept a minimum hematocrit as low as 20%).[15] Cross-matched blood should be kept available in anticipation of sudden deterioration. In patients with solid organ injury, the risk of hollow viscus injury is 3-4%, and increases with the number of injured solid organs therefore, serial clinical examination of the abdomen is essential as this is the most sensitive indicator of a hollow visceral or mesenteric injury that may require laparotomy.[16,7]

Indications for Operation

Following initial stabilisation, operation is indicated for continuing hemorrhage requiring blood transfusion exceeding 40 ml/kg or when there is evidence of intestinal, mesenteric or a major pancreatic injury. Immediate laparotomy is indicated in major intra-abdominal bleeding or penetrating injuries.

Emergency Laparotomy

The skin preparation extends from the clavicles to the groins to allow thoracic extension without delay if needed. A vertical midline incision is used; this provides rapid access to the whole abdominal cavity, and can be extended easily into the mediastinum or pleural cavity. In the newborn infant, a wide transverse supraumbilical incision is advised because the distance from umbilicus to pubis is relatively short and the bladder extends to the umbilicus. The abdomen of an infant is square and a transverse incision will allow access to the whole peritoneal cavity. On opening the abdomen the tamponade effect is released and the rate of bleeding may increase; it is essential to ensure that intravenous infusions are on flow before making the incision.

The first objective is to identify and control the source of bleeding. Since the liver and spleen are common sources of bleeding, the upper abdomen should be examined first, by retracting the costal margins and removing free blood using suction and large swabs. If a source of bleeding is discovered it is initially controlled by direct pressure. The intestine must be retracted or exteriorised to enable inspection

may be required (*see* 'urethral injuries', p.26). The normal urine output for infants is 2 ml/kg/hr, for children 1.5 ml/kg/hr and for adolescents 1 ml/kg/hr. Early surgical consultation is important.

For hypovolemic shock, an initial bolus of 20 ml/kg of crystalloid is given, using normal saline or Ringer lactate; the latter is preferred in infants because of its lower sodium load. If the response is not satisfactory, a second bolus of either crystalloid or blood (whole blood or packed cells) is infused depending on the rate of hemorrhage and the degree of shock; this equates to replacement of 50% of the circulating blood volume (approximately 80 ml/kg). If hypovolemia still persists, a further bolus of 20 ml/kg whole blood or packed cells is given and urgent laparotomy must be considered. A severely shocked child would require intubation and mechanical ventilation.

Nonoperative Management

Most children with blunt abdominal injury do not require an operation. The child must be admitted for repeated clinical assessments, continuous monitoring of the retroperitoneum and pelvis, and both the intestine and the mesentery are examined. As a general rule a retroperitoneal hematoma should not be disturbed unless it is rapidly expanding. If there is suspicion of duodenal injury, the duodenum is kocherised and carefully inspected. The pancreas is exposed by entering the lesser sac through the gastrocolic ligament. The management of specific organ injuries is discussed below.

Finally the abdomen is closed with a strong continuous suture to the midline fascia. A tight closure carries the risk of abdominal compartment syndrome, in which case temporary closure of the skin only or with a synthetic patch to the fascial layer may be advisable.

Damage Control Surgery (Abbreviated Laparotomy)

Most patients undergoing operation for blunt abdominal trauma are relatively stable and the procedure is straightforward. On the other hand, the outcome following a prolonged, difficult operation associated with massive blood loss and hemodynamic instability is generally poor, mainly due to progressive intraoperative hypothermia, acidosis and coagulopathy, which in turn exacerbate bleeding. This has lead to the concept of damage control surgery or abbreviated laparotomy.[18-20]

Damage control surgery is a staged protocol in which the first operation is limited to life saving procedures, followed by transfer to the ICU for resuscitation and stabilisation for 24-48 hours, and then a second definitive operation. At the initial operation, bleeding is controlled by ligation and tamponade. For example, with hemorrhage from major liver lacerations, tamponade is achieved using perihepatic packing to "close the book" and compress the laceration (Fig. 23.4).[21] Contamination from intestinal injury is controlled by ligation and stapling. It may not be possible to close the abdomen primarily. Experience in children with liver trauma shows an increase in survival from less than 40% to over 80% using this approach.[20]

Laparoscopy

The role of laparoscopy in evaluation of an injured child is yet to be defined. Chen and Schopp[22] used

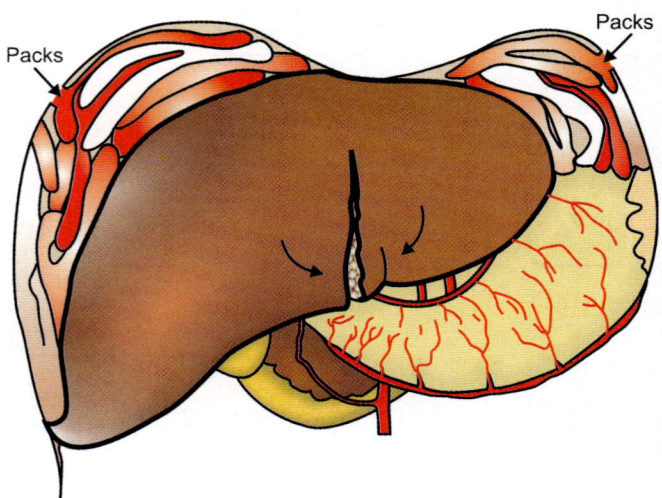

Fig. 23.4: Perihepatic packing: The triangular ligaments are divided and packs are placed above the right and left lobes to compress the liver laceration

laparoscopy to identify and treat children with hollow viscus injuries and to assess stable children with penetrating wounds of the abdominal wall.[22] Others have recommended laparoscopy as an alternative to laparotomy in children and adults.[23,24]

MANAGEMENT OF SPECIFIC ORGAN INJURIES

Liver

The child's relatively large and unprotected liver is vulnerable to blunt or penetrating injury to the right lower chest or upper abdomen. Adjacent organs may also be injured, notably the lung, kidney and spleen. Injury to the porta hepatis may be associated with damage to the duodenum and pancreas. The extent and pattern of liver injury may be graded according to CT or operative findings (Table 23.1) but management depends on the hemodynamic stability of the patient and not on anatomical grade of the injury.[25-27]

Nonoperative Management

In children, most injuries to the liver parenchyma (linear fractures as well as stellate fractures and hematomas) will stop bleeding spontaneously. In about 90% of children with liver injury a policy of selective nonoperative management is effective and safe, provided the child remains hemodynamically

Table 23.1: Grading of liver injuries[25,26]

Surgical grade		Injury description
I	Hematoma	Subcapsular, <10% surface area
	Laceration	Capsular tear, <1 cm deep Parenchymal depth
II	Hematoma	Subcapsular, 10-50% surface area; intraparenchymal, < 10 cm in length
	Laceration	1-3 cm parenchymal depth, < 10 cm length
III	Hematoma	Subcapsular, > 50% surface area or expanding; ruptured subcapsular or parenchymal hematoma Intraparenchymal hematoma > 10 cm or expanding
	Laceration	> 3 cm parenchymal depth
IV	Laceration	Parenchymal disruption involving 25-75% of hepatic lobe or 1-3 Couinaud's segments within a single lobe
V	Laceration	Parenchymal disruption involving > 75% of hepatic lobe or > 3 Couinaud's segments within a single lobe
	Vascular	Juxtahepatic venous injuries; i.e. retrohepatic vena cava/major hepatic veins
VI	Vascular	Hepatic avulsion

Computed Tomography Grade

I Subcapsular hematoma
II Simple laceration 1-3 cm small, 1-3 cm hepatic confusion
III Simple or complex lacerations > 3 cm deep. Peripheral in location. Large intrahepatic hematoma.
IV Hepatic transection. Extensive laceration, stellate dome, or posterior segment right lobe.
V Not applicable

stable after resuscitation. Patients are monitored as described above; admission to an Intensive Care Unit is not necessary for stable patients.[15] In a review of children with isolated liver or splenic trauma more than 97% of patients with Grade I to III injuries recovered without operation; of these between 2% and 10% required a blood transfusion.[28]

Following nonoperative management the risk of complications is approximately 10% which includes delayed hemorrhage, abscess formation and bilioma.[27,29-31] Follow-up imaging with CT or USS has been recommended to identify residual hematoma or other fluid collections in symptomatic patients but is not necessary in all patients.[13,27] A minor bile leak from a parenchymal laceration usually will resolve with or without percutaneous drainage. A rare but significant delayed complication is late hemorrhage from the parenchymal injury. Shilyansky et al and Berman et al described three patients with severe hemorrhage 3 and 10 days after liver injuries initially treated non-operatively, of whom two died.[31-32] Risk factors for this complication included a high Injury severity score, on-going requirement for blood transfusion, and persistence of right abdominal and shoulder tip pain. Hemobilia is diagnosed by selective angiography and controlled by embolization.

Operative Management

Intra-abdominal bleeding is the major cause of death from liver injury, and surgical efforts to control the bleeding may be associated with significant blood loss. Massive blood transfusion results in coagulopathy, which further aggravates bleeding. Gross et al reported that a transfusion requirement in excess of 25 ml/kg in the first 2 hours was a strong indicator of major hepatic vascular injury requiring operation; these patients had a mortality of up to 70%.[33]

At operation, hemostasis is the immediate priority. A thorough understanding of the anatomy of the liver is important. Major bleeding from liver injury usually is venous in origin from deep parenchymal lacerations of major intra-hepatic vessels, disruption of retro-hepatic hepatic veins and the inferior vena cava, or from the porta hepatis. Adequate exposure and mobilisation of both liver lobes by dividing the triangular ligaments are necessary. Direct ligation or coagulation of bleeding points is more effective and causes less tissue damage than mass sutures or hepatic artery ligation. Formal anatomical resection has a high mortality and non-anatomic resection is preferred with resection of non-viable tissue. Cross-clamping the portal triad by Pringle's maneuver provides temporary hepatic inflow occlusion while bleeding points are controlled. Temporary occlusion of the vena cava may be necessary using vascular clamps or intraluminal balloon tamponade using a Foley catheter.[34] a procedure that requires a degree of expertise. Median sternotomy may be required for access to the proximal inferior vena cava. In general, when bleeding cannot be controlled with straightforward methods, temporary perihepatic packing is advised (see Damage Control Surgery, p 11). This allows time for the patient to be stabilized, and is followed by delayed secondary laparotomy for definitive treatment. This procedure also enables the patient to be transferred to a tertiary care unit if appropriate.[18,21]

Extra-hepatic Biliary Tract

Injuries to the extra-hepatic bile ducts are rare. Those, which are associated with blunt pancreatico-duodenal injury, may be identified during initial investigations or at operation, or may present later with a biloma or biliary fistula. Biliary tract injuries may also be caused by penetrating trauma or iatrogenic trauma during open or laparoscopic operative procedures or endoscopy. If not recognized early, this may lead to the formation of a biliary stricture causing obstructive jaundice. The diagnostic methods include USS, CT, Tc^{99} iminodiacetic acid (IDA scan), endoscopic retrograde cholangio pancreatography (ERCP) or magnetic resonance cholangio-pancreatography (MRCP). Injuries to the gallbladder may require cholecystectomy. For injuries to the bile ducts, primary repair with t-tube drainage or stenting, or Roux-en-Y choledocho-enterostomy may be required; these are easier and safer to perform if postponed until the patient is stable. Endoscopic insertion of a nasobiliary drain has been reported.[35]

Spleen

In children the spleen is not well protected by the overlying ribs and is frequently injured as a result of blunt trauma (Table 23.2). More than 50% of children with splenic trauma have multiple solid organ injuries, mainly to the liver and left kidney, and up to 85% have extra-abdominal injuries.[30]

The clinical features of splenic injury include left upper quadrant pain and tenderness, and pain referred to the left shoulder. With hemoperitoneum, the tenderness becomes generalised. Chest X-ray may show contusion in the lower lobe of left lung, often without overlying rib fracture. CT confirms the diagnosis of splenic injury. USS or radio-isotope scan may also identify a splenic fracture but are less sensitive than CT.

The immediate consequence of splenic trauma is hemorrhage. Routine splenectomy is not recommended because of the risk of postsplenectomy sepsis and it is now established that in about 90% of childhood splenic injuries the bleeding will stop spontaneously within hours of injury.[36,37] Management of splenic trauma is nonoperative in patients who remain stable following initial resuscitation.

Table 23.2: Grading of Splenic Injuries[25,26]

Grade		Injury description
I	Hematoma	Subcapsular, < 10% surface area
	Laceration	Capsular tear, < 1 cm Parenchymal depth
II	Hematoma	Subcapsular, 10 – 50% surface area; intraparenchymal, < 5 cm in diameter
	Laceration	1 – 3 cm parenchymal depth which does not involve a trabecular vessel
III	Hematoma	Subcapsular, > 50% surface area or expanding; ruptured subcapsular or parenchymal hematoma intraparenchymal hematoma > 5 cm or expanding
	Laceration	> 3 cm parenchymal depth or involving trabecular vessels
IV	Laceration	Laceration involving segmental or hilar vessels producing major devascularization (> 25% of spleen)
V	Laceration	Completely, shattered spleen
	Vascular	Hilar vascular injury which devascularises spleen

Nonoperative Management

Patients are admitted for bed rest and monitoring, until the abdominal signs have resolved and normal gastrointestinal function has returned. Most patients can be discharged within a week after injury. Gandhi et al. formulated a clinical pathway for nonoperative management of splenic injury.[38] Use of this pathway showed that in hemodynamically stable children, isolated blunt splenic injuries could be treated safely with a 4 day hospital stay, followed by 3 weeks of quiet activities at home and then 3 months of light activity (including avoidance of contact sport) before returning to a full, normal lifestyle. Similar guidelines stratified according to grade of injury on a CT have been proposed by the American Pediatric Surgical Association.[28]

Concerns that nonoperative management would increase the need for blood transfusion have not been confirmed and the studies suggest nonoperative management is associated with a reduced need for blood transfusion compared to patients who undergo splenectomy.[39,40] Fewer than 10% of patients with isolated splenic injury require a blood transfusion.[38]

Delayed complications of nonoperative management of splenic injuries are rare. Acute hemorrhage due to secondary bleeding or rupture of a subcapsular hematoma may necessitate blood transfusion and splenectomy; fatal delayed hemorrhage is a very rare but a devastating complication. Splenic abscesses can be drained percutaneously.[41] Routine follow-up CT or USS may not be necessary for stable uncomplicated injuries,[28] but may be required in selected patients based on clinical assessment, in particular to exclude residual hematoma, which if present, needs a close follow-up.[28] Shafi et al reviewed the use of follow-up CT scanning in 72 children with splenic injuries.[42] In five, the CT showed a worsening radiological picture; however, only one of these children required operation, and the decision to operate was made on clinical grounds and not the imaging appearances. The authors concluded that routine CT follow-up of all patients was not beneficial.

Operative Management

Operation is indicated for continuing hemorrhage requiring blood transfusion exceeding 35-40 ml/kg (50% of the circulating blood volume). Patients with pre-existing disease predisposing to continuing hemorrhage, for example coagulation disorders or infective mononucleosis, are at particular risk but Cosentino et al reported successful nonoperative management of splenic injury in a child with Factor VIII deficiency and another with Factor XII deficiency.[43] The goal at operation is to control the bleeding while conserving as much splenic tissue as possible; attempts to preserve the spleen are justified providing the patient is stable. The impact of the splenic injury on associated injuries must be taken into consideration, but in spite of the theoretical risk that a head injury might be aggravated by hypotension if bleeding is not rapidly controlled, nonoperative management of splenic and liver injuries is not contraindicated in this situation.[44] The techniques for splenic preservation include topical hemostatic agents such as fibrin glue, splenic wrapping using synthetic mesh to tamponade the splenic fragments, partial splenectomy, splenorraphy, splenic artery ligation and selective splenic artery embolization.[45-46] Partial splenectomy is done along anatomical planes, and an understanding of the anatomy of the spleen and its segmental blood supply is necessary. Operative salvage rates of 20% and higher have been reported, and in Toronto the overall rate of splenic preservation was 96%.[30,36] Splenic remnants transplanted into the omentum will survive with reduced but demonstrable reticuloendothelial function.[47]

Post-splenectomy Prophylaxis

The spleen provides defence against infection, by production of antibodies and opsonising peptides, and clearance of circulating bacteria by the reticuloendothelial cells. The latter is particularly important in young children, who have a limited ability to mount a humoral response to infection. Overwhelming post-splenectomy sepsis (OPSI), an important complication of splenectomy occurs in only 0.05 - 3% of patients but has a mortality of approximately 50%.[48,49] In a 25-year retrospective review the incidence of OPSI following splenectomy for trauma in 883 patients less than 16 years of age was 2% and the mortality 1%.[50] OPSI did not occur in 395 older patients. While young children are at greater risk than adults, the risk is lowest when a previously normal spleen is removed, as in trauma, compared to splenectomy for hematological or malignant disease.

Strep. pneumoniae accounts for more than 50% of post-splenectomy infections, but various other bacteria have been associated with OPSI, including *H. influenzae* and *N. meningitidis*. Holdsworth et al.[50] suggest that the pattern and possibly the incidence of post-splenectomy *Strep. pneumoniae* infection reflects the natural history of these infections in the general population. Following splenectomy, prophylactic antimicrobial therapy is recommended using an antibiotic effective against capsulated bacteria, for example amoxycillin, in a single daily dose until the age of at least 5 years. Compliance is variable and it is important to ensure that the parents fully understand the risks to their child. In particular, acute pyrexial episodes should be treated promptly with therapeutic doses of the antibiotic, which should be readily available.

Polyvalent pneumococcal vaccine is recommended, but all serotypes are not covered.[51] *H. influenzae* type 6 vaccine and meningococcal vaccine are also available.

Pancreas

Pancreatic injuries occur in 2-10% of children with blunt abdominal trauma. The pancreas is well protected in the retroperitoneum but may be crushed against the vertebral column by an external force, typically a fall onto the handlebar of a bicycle or a deliberate blow or kick.[52] The injuries range from minor contusion to severe crush injury with complete transection of the pancreatic duct (Table 23.3). Injuries to the head of the pancreas may be associated with duodenal and bile duct injury, while injury to the tail of the pancreas may be associated with splenic injury.

There may be bruising of the skin in the epigastrium and the mark of a bicycle handlebar may be visible. Initially there may be little if any clinical evidence of injury to the pancreas and it is not unusual for a patient to be sent home, only to return a few hours later with vomiting and abdominal pain. Deep epigastric tenderness due to retroperitoneal injury must be distinguished from abdominal wall tenderness and guarding. Trauma to the tail of the pancreas is associated with tenderness in the left costovertebral angle. Serum amylase levels measured within 3 hours of injury may not be elevated, a progressive rise in serum amylase levels during the first 24-48 hours strongly suggests major pancreatic duct injury; however the correlation is not consistent, and a moderate elevation of the serum amylase does not exclude a major duct disruption.[5,54] Injury to the parotid gland may also cause elevation of the serum amylase level; when head and abdominal injuries coexist. In such cases serum or urinary lipase level, which is specific for pancreatic injury, should be measured.

As with other abdominal solid organs, CT with contrast is the preferred method for identifying pancreatic injury. CT and USS may give false negative findings in the early post-injury period, even with complete transection of the pancreas, possibly because the pancreatic capsule maintains the alignment of the pancreatic fragments, which cannot be distinguished until inflammatory changes have occurred.[5] Associated duodenal injury may be detected by the presence of retroperitoneal free air or fluid on abdominal imaging. The key to managing pancreatic injuries is maintenance of integrity of the main pancreatic duct. This is best visualised by ERCP or MRCP. With ERCP there is a risk of pancreatitis or perforation.[55,56] MRCP has the advantages of being non-invasive, sensitive, and safer.[57]

Most contusions and lacerations of the pancreas with an intact main pancreatic duct will heal without complications, and hyperamylasemia will resolve. The majority of patients therefore can be treated non-operatively, with bowel rest and intravenous feeding. Urgent operation is our treatment of choice when the main pancreatic duct has been transected, with or without associated duodenal injury. At operation, retroperitoneal edema may be the only evidence of pancreatic injury and pancreatic transection may be overlooked unless the pancreas is carefully palpated for the transverse groove at the site of the fracture. If pancreatic transection is confirmed, we perform distal pancreatectomy with preservation of the spleen.[5,58] The proximal pancreatic stump is oversewn; with a previously healthy pancreas, it is not necessary to ligate the pancreatic duct or anastomose it to the small bowel.[58] If a less severe pancreatic injury is found at operation the pancreas should not be disturbed. A suction catheter is placed in the lesser sac to reduce the risk of pseudocyst formation. ERCP with stenting of the main pancreatic duct is an alternative.[56] An associated duodenal injury must be treated on it's own merits. Non-operative management of pancreatic duct transection is recommended by some.[59-61] Pseudocyst may be drained percutaneously or by open operation (see below). The disadvantages of percutaneous

Table 23.3: Grading of Pancreatic Injuries[53]

Surgical grade	Injury description
Grade I	Contusion or hematoma (minimal parenchymal damage)
Grade II	Capsular or parenchymal disruption without major ductal injury
Grade III a	Capsular or parenchymal disruption with ductal involvement distal to the superior mesenteric vessels. The duodenum is intact.
Grade III b	Capsular or parenchymal disruption with ductal involvement to the right of the superior mesenteric vessels. The duodenum is intact.
Grade IV	Combined extensive pancreatic and duodenal crush injuries

drainage are the need for prolonged intravenous feeding and considerably longer hospital stay of 44-161 days as compared to 10-17 days after distal pancreatectomy.[52,58-60]

Other complications of pancreatic injury include pancreatic abscess, fistula, duct stricture and chronic pancreatitis. Patients are followed with serial serum amylase estimations and USS or CT scanning to monitor resolution of the pancreatic injury and to detect pseudocyst formation. A pseudocyst may present after a previously unrecognised pancreatic injury with loss of appetite, vomiting, epigastric pain and an epigastric mass. The serum amylase is elevated and imaging studies show the typical lesser sac mass (Fig. 23.5). More than 50% of pseudocysts will resolve with nonoperative management.[62] Those that persist beyond 3-4 weeks or become symptomatic may be drained by ultrasound guided percutaneous drainage.[63] Operative management includes cystogastrostomy or distal pancreatectomy.[64] Endoscopic cystogastrostomy is a less invasive mode of treatment.[65] A persistent pancreatic fistula may require excision. Duct stricture is treated by endoscopic dilatation and stenting, or by operation.

Gastrointestinal Tract

Blunt injuries to the gastrointestinal tract in children are commonly due to a localised blunt force such as a seat belt, cycle handlebar or deliberate blow or kick). GIT injuries occur in 1-5% of injured children often in association with injuries to other intra-and extra-abdominal injuries.[17,66,67] In a report by Canty et al, 19% of GIT injuries were non-accidental.[66] With the trend toward the non-operative management of injuries to the solid organs in retroperitoneum there is a risk that injuries to the intestine may not be recognised early. In patients with multiple solid organ injuries, the chance of missing intestinal injuries is high[17] because signs and symptoms of gastrointestinal injury may be masked by abdominal wall tenderness or by the effects of other injuries. Also, there is no specific imaging modality, which could reliably identify intestinal or mesenteric injuries. CT and USS may show thickening of the bowel or mesentery or fluid filled loops of bowel, but their sensitivity is low.[68,69] CT with oral contrast may show extravasation from a perforation of the stomach or duodenum, but this is not a reliable test and we no longer use oral contrast.[10] The presence of free fluid in the abdominal cavity on a CT without evidence of injury to the solid organs must raise suspicion of intestinal or mesenteric injury and may be an indication for laparoscopy or laparotomy.[22,23,66,67,70] The most important and sensitive method for diagnosing intestinal or mesenteric injury is by serial abdominal examination.

Intestinal contusion or intramural hematoma may cause temporary intestinal obstruction but usually heal without complication. Immediate operation is required for intestinal perforation. Severe bowel contusion or avulsion of the mesentery may lead to ischemia and delayed perforation, in which case signs of peritonitis may appear after admission. This emphasi the importance of repeated clinical assessment. Fortunately, delayed diagnosis of intestinal injury does not appear to increase the risk of complications.[66] Complex pancreatic-duodenal injuries are particularly difficult to recognise clinically and a high index of suspicion is needed. CT and MR scans may be useful in these cases, but exploratory laparotomy is the only certain way to clarify the situation.[71]

Operation usually involves repair of perforations with or without intestinal resection, depending on the degree of contusion. Defunctioning stomas are seldom required except for distal colonic and rectal injuries, when proximal colostomy is recommended. For duodenal injuries simple repair may be adequate, but

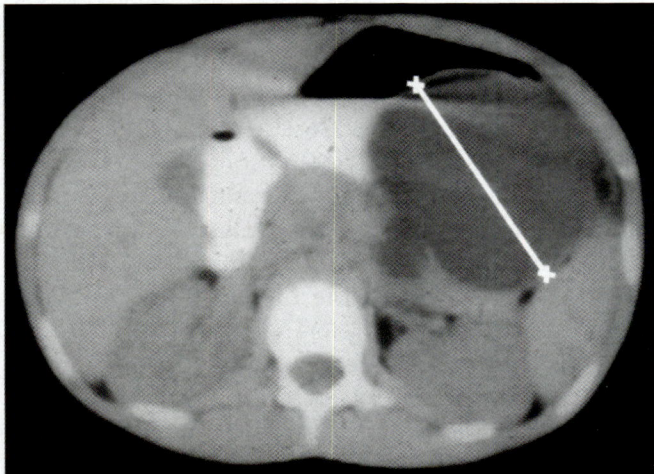

Fig. 23.5: Abdominal CT scan with contrast demonstrating a large pancreatic pseudocyst three weeks after transection of the body of the pancreas from a bicycle handle bar injury. The defect in the pancreas is clearly visible

more complex injuries will require more complex treatment, including duodenal diversion.[71]

Kidney

Although apparently well protected by its retroperitoneal position, the kidney is susceptible to injury in children because of the compliance of the overlying ribs and the paucity of perinephric fat to absorb the energy of an impact. As a result, renal injuries are more common in children than in adults.[72] Injuries range from contusion to parenchymal lacerations with fragmentation (Table 23.4). Disruption of the collecting system will lead to extravasation of urine. Further, the kidney is mobile in an anteroposterior plane and apparently trivial acceleration or deceleration forces may stretch the renal pedicle causing an intimal tear and sometimes completely avulsing the renal artery. A pre-existing anomaly such as a congenital obstruction, malformation or tumor may be present in the injured kidney.

Hematuria strongly suggests renal injury and should lead to further investigation of the urinary tract, but the degree of the hematuria does not correlate with the severity of the renal injury.[73,74] Clinical examination may reveal loin tenderness, and a palpable renal lump consistig of hematoma or extravasated urine. USS will identify the anatomical injury and the presence of perinephric fluid. It is useful for screening patients with suspected renal injury but does not assess function. CT with intravenous contrast will demonstrate parenchymal lesions, a perinephric hematoma, urinoma, as well as renal perfusion defects and any separated fragments. (Fig. 23.2). Importantly, the presence of a normal, perfused contralateral kidney will be confirmed at the same time. Intravenous pyelography or radionuclide scan will also demonstrate lack of function, but ultrasound examination is then needed to confirm the presence of the kidney.

Most contusions or lacerations of the renal parenchyma, with or without extravasation, will heal with nonoperative management, Margenthaler et al[74] reported successful non-operative management in 48 of 55 (87%) children with grade I–V blunt renal injury. Patients should be admitted to hospital for assessment and monitoring until the gross hematuria resolves. Perinephric hematoma or urinoma should be monitored by USS. In patients with major hemorrhage, ongoing heavy hematuria or an expanding flank mass, angiography with selective embolisation is the treatment of choice. Surgical exploration for hemorrhage after results in nephrectomy and should be avoided if possible. A retroperitoneal perinephric hematoma identified at operation should not be explored unless there is a strong indication for this such as major bleeding. Injury to the renal vascular pedicle requires immediate repair if the kidney is to be salvaged. However, in our experience renal salvage is rarely achieved and even if the kidney does survive, renal function is significantly impaired and there is a risk of hypertension. Nonoperative management may therefore be justified in most cases. There is controversy over the management of a major parenchymal injury extending into the collecting system with urinary extravasation. Some recommend immediate exploration but there is the risk of intra-operative bleeding necessitating nephrectomy.[75] Others prefer monitoring by USS, with delayed exploration after few days if the urinoma persists.[73] By this time the patient would have stabilised, the bleeding ceased and devitalised tissue become clearly apparent and can be removed along with repair of the collecting system. An exception is pelvi-ureteric disconnection, for which urgent repair is advised. Hypotension is a possible late complication after renal trauma and long-term follow up is

Table 23.4: Grading of renal injuries[25]

Surgical grade		Injury description
I	Contusion	Microscopic or gross hematuria; urologic studies normal
	Hematoma	Subcapsular, nonexpanding without parenchymal laceration
II	Hematoma	Nonexpanding perirenal hematoma confined to renal retroperitoneum
	Laceration	< 1.0 cm parenchymal depth of renal cortex without urinary extravasation
III	Laceration	>1.0 cm parenchymal depth of renal cortex without collecting system rupture or urinary extravasation
IV	Laceration	Parenchymal laceration extending through the renal cortex, medulla and collecting system
	Vascular	Main renal artery or vein injury with contained hemorrhage
V	Laceration	Complete shattered kidney
	Vascular	Avulsion of renal hilum which devascularises kidney

advised.[76] Other complications that may develop following nonoperative management include abscess formation, urethral obstruction, renal cyst and dystrophic calcification.

Ureter, Bladder and Urethra

The diagnosis and management of these injuries in children is similar to that in adults. In infants the bladder is an intra-abdominal organ and may be injured by a blunt or penetrating abdominal trauma, leading to intra- or extraperitoneal rupture. A cystogram may confirm the diagnosis, but the perforation may be very small and not easily visible on contrast X-ray.

Injury to the anterior urethra commonly occurs as a result of a straddle injury to the perineum that crushes the urethra against the symphysis pubis. The typical presentation is with a perineal or scrotal hematoma, which may need aspiration. In girls following a straddle injury there often is an associated bruise or laceration to the vaginal introitus and perineum; the possibility of non-accidental intentional injury must be borne in mind and examination under anesthesia for evidence of sexual abuse is advised. Injury to the posterior urethra associated with a pelvic fracture presents with blood at the urethral meatus and inability to void. In this situation a suprapubic catheter should be inserted and urethral catheterization must not be attempted till the investigations to assess the integrity of the urinary tract, like ascending urography, have been performed.

REFERENCES

1. Injury Prevention. British Medical Association, London 2001.
2. Advanced Trauma Life Support. American College of Surgeons Committee on Trauma. Chicago 1997.
3. Advanced Paediatric Life Support. British Medical Journal Publishing Group, London 1993.
4. Ng CS, Hall Cm, Shaw DG. The range of visceral manifestations of non-accidental injury. Arch Dis Child 1997;77:167-74.
5. Smith SD Nakayama, DK Gantt, N, et al. Pancreatic Injuries in Childhood Due to Blunt Trauma. Journal of Pediatric Surgery 1988;23:610-14.
6. Federle MP, Crass RA, Jeffrey RB, Trunkey DD. Computed Tomography in Blunt Abdominal Trauma. Archives of Surgery 1982;117:645-50.
7. Taylor GA, Eichelberger MR, O'Donnell R, Bowman L. Indications for Computed Tomography in Children with Blunt Abdominal Trauma. Annals of Surgery 1991;213: 212-18.
8. Richardson MC, Hollman AS, Davis CF. Comparison of computed tomography and ultrasonographic imaging in the assessment of blunt abdominal trauma in children. Br J Surg 1997;84:1144-46.
9. Cox TD, Kuhn JP. CT scan of bowel trauma in the pediatric patient. Radiol Clin North Am 1996;34:807-18.
10. Shankar KR, Lloyd DA, Kitteringham L, Carty HML. Oral contrast with computed tomography in the evaluation of blunt abdominal trauma in children. Br J Surg 1999;86: 1073-77.
11. Stengel D, Bauwens K, Sehouli J, et al. Systematic review and meta-analysis of emergency ultrasonography for blunt abdominal trauma. Br J Surg 2001;88:901-12.
12. Coley BD, Mutabagani KH, Martin LC, et al. Focused abdominal sonography for trauma (FAST) in children with blunt abdominal trauma. The Journal of Trauma: Injury, Infection and Critical Care 2000;48:902-906.
13. Navarro O, Babyn PS, Pearl RH. The value of routine follow-up imaging in pediatric blunt liver trauma. Pediatr Radiol 2000;30:546-50.
14. Porras-Ramirez G, Ramirez-Reyes F, Hernandez-Herrera MH, Porras-Hernandez JD. Clinical Recognition and Management of Pediatric Blunt Abdominal Trauma without Ultrasound or Computed Tomography Scan in Community Hospital in Mexico. J Pediatr Surg 1999;34: 1700-1702.
15. Siplovich L, Kawar B. Changes in the Management of Pediatric Blunt Splenic and Hepatic Injuries. Journal of Paediatric Surgery 1997;32:1464-65.
16. Morse MA, Garcia VF. Selective non-operative management of pediatric blunt splenic trauma: Risk for missed associated injuries. J Pediatr Surg 1994;29:23-27.
17. Nance M, Keller MS, Stafford PW, Predicting Hollow Visceral Injury in the Pediatric Blunt Trauma Patient With Solid Visceral Injury. Journal of Pediatric Surgery 2000;35:1300-1303.
18. Krige JEJ, Bornman PC, Terblanche J. Therapeutic perihepatic packing in complex liver trauma. British Journal of Surgery 1992;79:43-46.
19. Moore EE, Burch JM, Franciose RJ, et al. Staged physiologic restoration and damage control surgery. World J Surg 1998;22:1184-91.
20. Stylianos S. Abdominal packing for severe hemorrhage. J Pediatr Surg 1998;33:339-42.
21. Losty PD, Okoye BO, Walter DP, et al. Management of blunt liver trauma in children. Br J Surg 1997;84:1006-1008.
22. Chen MK, Schropp KP, Lobe TE. The Use of Minimal Access Surgery in Pediatric Trauma: A Preliminary Report: Journal of Laparoendoscopic Surgery 1995;5: 295-301.
23. McKinley AJ, Mahomed AA. Laparoscopy in a case of pediatric blunt abdominal trauma:Surg Endosc 2002;16(2):358.

24. Simon RJ, Rabin J, Kuhls D. Impact of increased use of laparoscopy on negative laparotomy rates after penetrating trauma. J Trauma 2002;53(2):297-302.
25. Moore EE, Shackford SR, Pachter HL, McAninch JW, Browner BD, Champion HR, Flint, LM, Gennarelli TA, Malangoni MA, Ramenofsky ML, Trafton PG. Organ Injury Scaling: Spleen, Liver and Kidney: Journal of Trauma 1989;29:1664-66.
26. Moore EE, Cogbill TH, Jurkovich GJ, Shackford SR, Malangoni MA, Champion HR. Organ Injury Scaling: Spleen and Liver: Journal of Trauma: Injury, Infection and Critical Care (Revision) 1994;38(3):323-24.
27. Pryor JP, Stafford PW, Nance ML. Severe Blunt Hepatic Trauma in Children. J Pediatr Surg 2001;36:974-79.
28. Stylianos S. The APSA Trauma Committee: Evidence-Based Guidelines for resource utilization in children with isolated spleen or liver injury. J Pediatr Surg 2000;35:164-69.
29. Oldham KT, Guice KS, Ryckman F, Kaufman RA, et al. Blunt liver injury in childhood: Evolution of therapy and current perspective. Surgery 1986;100:542-49.
30. Oldham KT, Caty MG. Liver and Spleen Trauma in Children in: Oldham, KT Coran, AG and Harris BH. Eds Pediatric Trauma: Proceedings of the Third National Conference. JB Lippincott Company 1990.
31. Shilyansky J, Navarro O, Superina RA, et al. Delayed haemorrhage after 'non-operative management of blunt hepatic trauma in children: A rare but significant event. J Pediatr Surg 1999;34:60-64.
32. Berman S, Mooney E, Weireter Jr L. Late Fatal Hemorrhage in Pediatric Liver trauma. Journal of Pediatric Surgery 1992;27:1546-48.
33. Gross M, Lynch F, Canty Sr T, et al. Management of Liver Injury - A 13 year Experience at a Pediatric Trauma Center. Journal of Pediatric Surgery 1999;34:811-17.
34. Chandrasekar R, Wu A. Control of Haemorrhage during Liver Resection - A Simple but Effective Technique. British Journal of Surgery 1994;81:97.
35. Poli ML, Lefebvre F, Ludot H, et al. Non-operative management of biliary tract fistulas after blunt abdominal trauma in a child. J Pediatr Surg 1995;30:1719-21.
36. Pearl RH. Wesson DE. Spence LJ, et al. Splenic Injury: A 5-Year Update with Improved Results and Changing Criteria for Conservative Management. Journal of Pediatric Surgery 1989;24:121-25.
37. Wisner DH, Blaisdell FW. When to save the ruptured spleen. Surgery 1992;111:121-22.
38. Gandhi RR, Keller MS, Schwab CW. Stafford PW. Pediatric Splenic Injury – Pathway to Play? Journal of Pediatric Surgery 1999;34:55-59.
39. Avanoglu A, Ulman I, Ergun O, et al. Blood Transfusion Requirements in Children with Blunt Spleen and Liver Injuries. European Journal of Pediatric Surgery 1998;8:322-25.
40. Patrick DA, Bernard DD, Moore EE, Karrer FM. Non-operative management of Solid Organ Injuries in Children Results in Decreased Blood Utilization. Journal of Pediatric Surgery 1999;34:1695-99.
41. Frumiento C, Sartorelli K, Vane D. Complications of Splenic Injuries – Expansion of the Non-operative theorem. Journal of Pediatric Surgery 2000;35:788-91.
42. Shafi S, Gilbert J, Irish M, Glick P, Canty M. Follow-up Imaging Studies in Children with Splenic Injuries. Clinical Pediatrics 1999;273-76.
43. Cosentino CM, Luck SR, Barthel MJ, et al. Transfusion Requirements in Conservative Non-operative Management of Blunt Splenic and Hepatic Injuries During Childhood. Journal of Pediatric Surgery 1990;25:950-54.
44. Keller M, Sartorelli K, Vane D. Associated Head injury should not prevent non-operative management of spleen or liver injury in children. Journal of Trauma 1996;41:471-75.
45. Fingerhut A, Oberlin P, Cotte JL, et al. Splenic salvage using an absorbable mesh: feasibility, reliability and safety. British Journal of Surgery 1992;79:325-27.
46. Tristan J, Poenou D, Lagares F, et al. Selective Splenic Artery Embolization or use of Polyglycolic Acid Mesh in Children with Severe Splenic Trauma. European Journal of Pediatric Surgery 1995;5:310-12.
47. Traub A, Giebink GS, Smith C, et al. Splenic Reticuloendothelial Function after Splenectomy, Spleen Repair, and Spleen Autotransplantation. The New England Journal of Medicine 1987;317:1559-64.
48. Luna GK, Dellinger EP. Non-operative Observation Therapy for Splenic Injuries: A Safe Therapeutic Option? The American Journal of Surgery 1987;153:462-68.
49. Meckes I, van der Staak F, van Oostrum C. Results of Splenectomy performed on a group of 91 children. European Journal of Pediatric Surgery 1995;5:19-22.
50. Holdsworth RJ, Irving AD, Cuschieri A. Postsplenectomy sepsis and its mortality rate: actual versus perceived risks. British Journal of Surgery 1991;78:1031-38.
51. Lawton J, Baddeley PG, Finn AHR, Barnes R, Hann IM, Burnett A, Davies JM. The Prevention and Treatment of Infection in Patients With An Absent or Dysfunctional Spleen: British Committee for Standards in Haematology Guideline update.
52. Arkovitz MS, Johnson N, Garcia VF. Pancreatic trauma in children. Mechanisms of injury. Journal of Trauma, Injury, Infection and Critical Care 1997;42:49-53.
53. Classification of Pancreatic Injuries. In: Management of Pediatric Trauma Ed Buntain WL. WB Saunders Company, Philadelphia 1994.
54. Takishima T, Sugimoto K, Hirata M, et al. Serum amylase level on admission in the diagnosis of blunt injury to the pancreas. Annals of Surgery 1997;226:70-76.
55. Rescorla FJ, Plumley Da, Sherman S. The efficacy of early ERCP in pediatric pancreatic trauma. J Pediatr Surg 1995;30:336-40.
56. Canty TG, Weinman D. Management of major pancreatic duct injuries in children. Journal of Trauma, Injury, Infection and Critical Care 2001;50:1001-1007.

57. Fulcher AS, Turner MA, Yelon JA, et al. Magnetic Resonance cholangiopancreatography (MRCP) in the assessment of pancreatic duct trauma and its sequelae: preliminary findings. Journal of Trauma 2000;48:1001-17.
58. McGahren Ed, Magnuson D, Schaller RT, Tapper D. Management of transacted pancreas in children. Aust NZ J Surg 1995;65:242-46.
59. Ohno Y, Ohgami H, Nagasaki A, Hirose R. Complete disruption of the main pancreatic duct: A case successfully managed by percutaneous drainage. J Pediatr Surg 1995;30:1741-42.
60. Lucaya J, Vazquez E, Caballero F, et al. Non-operative management of traumatic pancreatic pseudocysts associated with pancreatic duct laceration in children. Pediatr Radiol 1998;28:5-8.
61. Kouchi K, Tanabe M, Yoshida H, et al. Non-operative management of blunt pancreatic injury in childhood. J Pediatr Surg 1999;34:1736-39.
62. Vitas GJ, Sarr MG. Selected management of pancreatic pseudocysts: Operative versus expectant management. Surgery 1992;111:123-30.
63. Rescorla FJ, Cory D, Vane DW, et al. Failure of Percutaneous Drainage in Children with Traumatic Pancreatic Pseudocysts. Journal of Pediatric Surgery 1990;25:1038-42.
64. Wilson RH, Moorehead RJ. Current management of trauma to the pancreas. British Journal of Surgery 1991;78:1196-02.
65. Kimble RM, Cohen R, Williams S. Successful endoscopic drainage of a post-traumatic pancreatic pseudocyst in a child. J Pediatr Surg 1999;34:1518-20.
66. Canty TG Sr, Canty TG Jr, Brown C. Injuries of the gastrointestinal tract from blunt trauma in children. A 12 year experience at a designated paediatric trauma center. Journal of Trauma, Injury, Infection and Critical Care 1999;46:234-40.
67. Allen GS, Moore FA, Cox CS, et al. Hollow visceral injury and blunt trauma. Journal of Trauma, Injury, Infection and Critical Care 1998;45:69-78.
68. Albenese CT, Meza MP, Gardner MJ, et al. Is computed tomography a useful adjunct to the clinical examination for the diagnosis of pediatric gastrointestinal perforation from blunt abdominal trauma in children? Journal of Trauma, Injury, Infection and Critical Care 1996;40:417-21.
69. Kurhchubasche AG, Fendya DG, Tracy TF. Blunt intestinal injury in children. Arch Surg 1997;132:652-58.
70. Ng AKT, Simons RK, Torreggiani WC, et al. Intra-abdominal free fluid without solid organ injury in blunt abdominal trauma: An indication for laparotomy. Journal of Trauma, Injury, Infection and Critical Care 2002;52:134-40.
71. Degiannis E, Boffard K. Duodenal injuries. Br J Surg 2000;87:1473-79.
72. Brown SL, Elder JS, Spirnak JP. Are pediatric patients more susceptible to major renal injury from blunt trauma? A comparative study. Journal of Urology 1998;160:138-40.
73. Thompson-Fawcett M, Kolbe A. Paediatric renal trauma: caution with conservative management of major injuries. Aust N Z J Surg 1996;66:435-40.
74. Margenthaler JA, Weber TR, Keller MS. Blunt renal trauma in children: Experience with conservative management at a pediatric trauma center. Journal of Trauma, Injury, Infection and Critical Care 2002;52:928-32.
75. Cass AS. Blunt Renal Trauma in Children. The Journal of Trauma 1983;23:123-27.
76. Elshihabi I, Elshihabi S, Arrar M. An overview of renal trauma. Current Opinions in Paediatrics 1998;10:162-66.

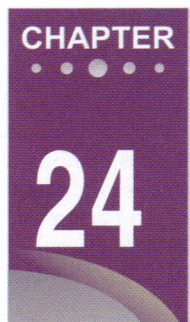

Soft Tissue Trauma

DK Gupta, Lalit Parida

While assessing children with soft tissue trauma we must exclude relatively serious and sometimes occult injuries that will take precedence in management. Factors to be taken into consideration include history of the injury, child's tetanus immunization status, whether the child has any medical problems or allergies, any medications that the child takes, what wound care was received prior to arrival in the hospital and any indication of child abuse—the **"Ample"** history

A: Allergies
M: Medications
P: Past medical history
L: Last meal
E: Environments and events.

MECHANISM OF TRAUMA

A. **Blunt trauma,** shearing forces are the most common mechanisms of injury.

However, compressive forces, such as contusions and crush injuries are more threatening for wound complications. The stellate wound resulting from compression should prompt more aggressive debridement and antibiotic prophylaxis because much of the tissue injury may be clinically occult.

B. **Penetrating trauma** may result from low-velocity or high-velocity wounds.
1. Low-velocity penetrating wounds are caused by stab wounds. Damage to the underlying structures, rather than the missile itself, is responsible for wound morbidity.
2. High-velocity gunshot wounds (> 2500 feet/sec) have the propensity to create enormous tissue damage, and only rarely should high-velocity wounds be closed primarily.
3. Distance is a key determinant of energy transfer in shotgun wounds. At < 2 inches, a single shotgun fire represents a high-velocity missile. Most shotgun missiles at < 20 feet distance will produce a single wound, whereas those at > 20 feet will produce multiple discrete wounds. In addition to the multiple or single projectiles delivered by a shotgun, hot gases and wadding can play a major role in the morbidity of the shotgun wound.

Soft tissue trauma can be considered in the following categories:
- Skin and subcutaneous tissue injury
- Vascular injury
- Nerve injury
- Muscle injury
- Tendon injury
- Ligament injury
- Synovial injury.

SKIN AND SUBCUTANEOUS TISSUE INJURY

Clinical Type

- Abrasions
- Contusions and hematomas
- Lacerations
- Penetrating injuries
- Crush injuries
- Foreign bodies
- Bites.

Mechanism of Wound

- Sharp versus blunt
- High energy versus low energy.

Condition of Wound

- Tidy versus untidy: Tidy wounds are created by sharp objects and do not contain devitalized tissue or debris. An untidy wound usually results from more forceful impact, crush, tearing or avulsion. As a result there is usually devitalized tissue, loss of tissue, and more frequently injury to deeper structures.
- Clean versus contaminated: Represents a general assessment of the number of bacteria in the wound and therefore the likelihood of a subsequent infection.

The child will usually present clinically as pain in the injured area, bleeding and limited mobility of extremity in case of extensive soft tissue injuries. The child should be assessed systemically and locally. A history of injury (mechanism of injury, when it occurred, where it occurred, past medical history) and an initial examination (pre-anesthesia) should be carried out. The final evaluation of the injury should be done following anesthesia. The type of wound and extent of injury is noted. Injury to bone, joint, ligaments tendons, nerves and muscles should be looked for and assessed.

Wound Assessment[1]

A. Assesmnent of wound viability may be difficult in early stages of resuscitation. Repeat examination is essential. Physical examination of the wound must include assessment of the length and depth of the injury, circulatory status, motor and sensory function, the presence of foreign bodies and contaminants, and the involvement of underlying structures (nerves, tendons, muscles, ligaments, vessels, bones, joints and ducts).

B. Skin can be assessed by color, capillary refill, quality of bleeding, sensory and bleeding response to pin prick, and intravenous fluorescein injection using a Wood's light.

C. Muscle is the most difficult tissue to assess for viability. Color, capillary bleeding, and contractile response to stimulation are not totally reliable. Muscle conservation is prudent during initial debridelnent. Tendons, muscles, and ligaments are tested distal to an injury, with special attention to hand and forearm injuries

D. Fat is difficult to assess for viability, but it can be readily removed at the first debridement as long as care is taken not to devascularize skin.

E. Nerve viability can be ascertained by inspection and electrical stimulation.

If primary nerve repair is not indicated (e.g. in high-velocity wounds), nerve ends should be identified and tagged for later suture repair. Although the sensorimotor examination must precede the administration of anesthesia, the remainder of the examination should rarely be performed without adequate anesthesia. Sensation is tested by measurement of two-point discrimination distal to an injury. For children younger than 3 years of age, the use of a noxious stimulus, such as a pinprick, may be necessary to provide a sensory and partial motor assessment. Since normal autonomic tone produces a degree of normal sweating. Denervated fingers do not sweat, which provides a clue to injury. The ophthalmoscope can assist in spotting sweat beads on the fingers.

F. Parotid or lacrimal duct continuity should be ascertained.

G. Circulation is evaluated by palpation of peripheral pulses and skin temperature, observation of skin color, and rapidity of capillary refill. Any clinical sign of vascular injury (minimal ooze or large hematoma, distal vascular skin insufficiency, absent distal pulse) should be followed up by diagnostic testing (Doppler flowmeter, arteriograms, CT scan, stabograms-contrast study through injury tract).

H. Adequate tetanus immunization must be assured for all wounds.

I. Extremities: All extremities are examined for deformity, contusions, abrasions, sensation, penetrating injuries, pulses, and perfusion. The presence of a pulse does not exclude a proximal vascular injury or a compartment syndrome. The long bones are palpated circumferentially, assessing for tenderness, crepitation, or abnormal movement. Open fractures and wounds should be covered with sterile dressings. Soft tissue injuries are inspected for foreign bodies and irrigated to minimize contamination, and devitalized tissues are debrided. Tendons, muscles, and ligaments are tested distal to an injury, with special attention to hand and forearm injuries. With cooperative older children, it is possible to test these structures' functions individually; however, with younger, less cooperative children, one must rely on observation of posture, symmetry, and function and on exploration of the wound. A toy or penlight that requires manipulation by the child can be used to help in evaluating motor function.

J. Skin: The skin is examined for evidence of contusions, penetration sites, burns, petechiae, and signs of abuse. A traumatized child may have concomitant burn or inhalation injuries. The depth, location, and types of burns and the extent of body surface area involved need to be documented. The burns should be covered with sterile dressings and intravenous fluid resuscitation initiated appropriate for the extent of the burns.

K. Compartment syndrome: Increased pressure within enclosed soft-tissue compartments of the extremities can cause irreversible muscle and nerve injury. The incidence of compartment syndrome is related to the severity of the trauma. The lower leg and forearm are the commonest sites. Compartment syndrome can occur with open fractures, with pain that is either out of proportion to the injury and requires frequent strong analgesia, or is exaggerated by passive stretching of the distal joints, being the earliest indicator. Other important findings are swelling and tenseness of the compartment. Pallor, paralysis, paraesthesia and pulselessness are late findings, and the diagnosis should not be excluded if these are absent. Once the diagnosis is suspected, measurement of compartment pressures and/or fasciotomy should be performed.[2-5]

L. Photograph significant wounds, then apply a sterile dressing.

The priorities of managing a child with a soft tissue injury in sequence are:
1. Stabilization of the patient against life threatening conditions.
2. General history and physical examination.
3. Assessment of the tissue injury.
4. Treatment plan.
5. Institution of wound care.
6. Follow-up and reassessment.

MANAGEMENT OF TRAUMATICALLY AMPUTATED PARTS

Management of the amputated part is focused on reducing warm ischemia time.

Urgent transfer of the patient and the part must be organized unless the patient is already in a specialist center. The temperature of the part should be lowered as much as possible, without allowing it to freeze. This is best achieved by taking the following steps:
- Gross contamination is gently removed, but damage caused by rubbing is avoided
- The part is covered in a single layer of damp (not dripping-wet) gauze
- The covered part is placed in a plastic bag and the bag is sealed
- The sealed bag is placed in a container of water/ice mix

The amputated part should never be allowed to come into direct contact with ice, as this will cause frostbite.

The tissue priorities include
- Skin cover
- Skeletal stabilization
- Musculotendinous repairs
- Nerve and vessel repair.

TREATMENT PLAN

1. General measures
2. Wound closure.

General Measures

I. RICEM procedure for management of soft tissue injury for first 48-72 hours.
   R: Rest—the child should stop moving the injured part.
   I: Ice—cryotherapy (ice-packs, crushed-ice, ice-towels, ice-massage, gel-packs, refrigerant-gases and inflatable splints) for 10-20 minutes, 2-4 times a day for the first 2-3 days.

C: Compression of the injured area may squeeze some fluid and debris out of the injury site.

E: Elevation of the injured area in combination with ice and compression limits circulation to that area and therefore helps limit internal bleeding and minimizes the swelling.

M: Mobilization.

II. The use of NSAIDs for its analgesic and anti-inflammatory effects should be restricted to the first 3 days.

III. Prophylactic antibiotics

Indications
- Traumatic wounds with heavy contamination.
- Untidy wounds in which adequate debridement cannot be completed or must be delayed.
- Wounds entering joint spaces or compound fractures.
- Wounds in which treatment has been delayed (beyond 6-12 hrs).
- Most animal and all human bite wounds.
- The immunocompromised host.

General Rule for Selecting a Prophylactic Antibiotic[6-8]
- Use a bactericidal drug if possible
- Give in therapeutic doses for 3-5 days
- Use drugs based on wound culture reports. Gram-positive cocci are the most common organisms found in tissue wounds.

IV. Tetanus immunisation status must be checked.

V. Gas gangrene management.

VI. In case of animal bites vaccination for rabies must be considered.

VII. The detection and removal of foreign bodies like wood splinters, glass, metal and plastic can be done with the help of plain X-rays, image intensified fluoroscopy and ultrasound.

VIII. Physiotherapy/Rehabilitation.

Early mobilization, guided by the pain response, promotes a more rapid return to full functional recovery. Progressive resistance exercises (isotonic, isokinetic and isometric) are essential to restore full muscle and joint function.

Analgesia/Anesthesia in Wound Management

Open wounds are irrigated with large amounts of normal saline, RL or sterile water. The wound is covered with sterile dressing, moistened with saline or RLS. The extremity is splinted. Blood loss is reduced by application of manual pressure and pressure bandages. The hair around a wound should be trimmed closely with a pair of scissors, not shaved.

A. For the uncooperative child an effective combination of local analgesia is :
- Pethidine 2 mg/kg IM
- Promethazine 1 mg/kg IM
- Chlorpromazine 1 mg/kg IM.

It is important to wait for at least 30 minutes following IM injection before proceeding with care. Very young children or uncooperative children might require general anesthesia for wound closure.

Provision of local anesthesia is both a science and an art form. Lidocaine with epinephrine at 0.5-1.0% concentrations can be provided at a maximal dose of 7 mg/kg of body weight. Epinephrine is added to provoke vasoconstriction, thereby prolonging the effect of lidocaine.

1. Epinephrine should be avoided in the digits or in patients with severe arteriosclerotic vascular disease. The maximal dose of lidocaine without epinephrine is 4 mg/kg of body weight.
2. Warming the solution or adding bicarbonate and injecting slowly can significantly reduce the pain of injection.
3. Infiltrating the proximal portion of the wound can reduce discomfort of infiltrating the distal portion.
4. Allowing adequate time for local anesthetic to be effective can reduce discomfort and enhance vasoconstriction.

B. Regional nerve blocks are underutilized, but they can be helpful, especially on the distal extremities and face.

C. Judicious intravenous sedation or analgesia is useful.

Wound Management

Debridement

Sharp debridement is essential, removing obvious dead skin, muscle and fat. In wounds free of specialized tissue, early sharp resection of the wound edges and underlying tissues can be accomplished at the first debridement.

Wound Cleansing

Wounds containing specialized tissues such as nerves, tendons, and vessels may not lend themselves to extensive sharp debridement. In these circumstances, high-pressure irrigation followed by open treatment with wet saline soaks and frequent Operating Room inspection is preferred.

Irrigation

High-pressure irrigation at a minimum of 8 pounds per square inch is useful. A variety of devices, including a large syringe with a small needle or catheter, pressurized fluid bag attached to an 18-gauge catheter, or commercially available pulse irrigators, have proved effective in wound management.

Packing

Aggressive, precise packing of external traumatic wounds can be effective in securing hemostasis in a traumatized patient with coagulopathy. Packing is primarily for hemostasis control and not for debridement. Subsequent wound care after packing removal is best done with either delayed closure or saline soaks. Most skin wounds do not need to be packed for hemostasis because they can be temporarily sutured or stapled closed.

Wound Closure

Traumatic wounds and surgical wounds in trauma patients are closed according to time from injury, amount of tissue available and degree of contamination.
1. Primary closure (primary intention) is appropriate for most superficial wounds. This implies that the wound is closed within the first 6-8 hours of incision or laceration.
2. Secondary closure (sometimes called secondary intention) implies that a wound is left open and allowed to close by subsequent granulation and contraction.
3. Tertiary closure (delayed primary closure) is used for class III (contaminated) or class IV (dirty or infected) wounds. Wound edges are left open for 4 - 5 days with application of wet saline dressings. The wound is then reapproximated with suture, tape, or staples.
4. Suture closure
   a. Wounds in cosmetic areas of the body usually undergo layered closure comnonly incorporating subcuticular absorbable suture material with Steri-strips or fine skin sutures.
   b. In non-cosmetic areas of the body, simple closure of the skin is satisfactory, assuming underlying fascial layers have been reapproximated when appropriate.

Tissue Transfer

a. Split-thickness skin grafts are commonly used for traumatic wound closure. In general, full-thickness skin grafts are used for the face. Local flaps are most useful for the extremities and face, and myocutaneous flaps are designed primarily for the central part of the body.
b. Free-tissue transfer is most useful for defects in the distal extremities, although it can be used in many parts of the body.

Suture Removal

Varies with location of wound, size of wound, and pre-existing disease.
a. Face: 3-5 days
b. Abdominal wall: 5 - 7 days
c. Scalp: 10 days
d. Vertical torso wounds or wounds over movable joints: 2 weeks
e. Delay suture removal in patients with multiple organ dysfunction syndrome and immuno-compromised patients.

Non-surgical modalities to enhance healing and care of soft tissue wounds.[9-13]
- Exogenous application of growth factors
- Cultured keratinocyte grafts
- Electrical stimulation
- Hyperbaric oxygen
- Vacuum Assisted Closure System (VAC).

VASCULAR INJURY

The incidence of pediatric vascular trauma is increasing as a result of more invasive diagnostic and therapeutic procedures on children and because children are more frequently the victims of domestic violence. Attempts at diagnosis should initially be made non-invasively, because anteriography has the potential of further injury. Arterial repair of major arteries should be undertaken to avoid growth retardation.

Mechanism of Injury Producing Vascular Injury[14]

I. Trauma
   A. Penetrating trauma
      - Gunshot wounds
      - Stab wounds; including lacerations from sharp objects like broken glass windows.
   B. Blunt trauma
II. Iatrogenic
      - Cardiac catheterization and indwelling umbilical arterial catheters (and is most often seen in children under 2 years of age).
III. Long bone fractures involving the humerus and femur.

In the urban civilian experience, extremity vascular injuries comprise less than 50% of arterial trauma. Extremity arterial injuries predominate in the rural environment reflective of the higher incidence of blunt mechanisms and farming/industrial type injuries.

In the urban set-up, both upper and lower extremities have equal incidence of involvement. But in the rural set-up, the upper extremity is more commonly involved. The brachial artery is more commonly involved than the axillary artery in the upper extremity. The femoral artery is more commonly involved than the popliteal artery.

Trauma to blood vessels results in systemic, regional and local pathophysiologic imbalance. The systemic effects are produced by blood loss, which if not controlled will result in hypovolemic shock. The local and regional effects will be determined by the type of vessel injury, which is usually determined by the mechanism. A laceration is the most frequent type of injury to both arteries and veins.

Diagnosis

History

The work up should be expeditious with the goal being reperfusion of the ischemic limb within six hours or less. A history of pulsatile, bright red bleeding from the wound that ceased after a period of minutes suggests arterial injury; while the history of a steady flow of dark blood from the wound suggests a venous injury. Because peripheral pulses may be palpable in upto 33% of the patients with arterial injuries, a history suggesting vascular injury may be the most important diagnostic indicator at the time of initial evaluation. The most important differential diagnosis in pediatric vascular trauma is between thrombosis and spasm of the injured vessel. Spasm may be associated with adjacent injury to soft tissue, blunt trauma to the vessel wall, and hemorrhage into surrounding tissue. Nevertheless, spasm as the only cause of absent distal pulses is uncommon and will usually disappear within three hours. If the pulses remain absent beyond three hours, vascular occlusion is likely. When the pulses remain absent longer than six hours, thrombosis or transaction of the vessel is certain.

Physical Examination

The physical findings are extremely variable. The signs indicative of ischemia or ongoing hemorrhage, and which if present indicate the need for operative exploration are as follows:
- Pulsatile bleeding
- Expanding hematoma
- Palpable thrill
- Audible bruit
- Evidence of regional ischemia
  - Pallor
  - Paresthesia
  - Paralysis
  - Pain
  - Pulselessness
  - Poikilothermia

The signs suggestive of vascular injury, but without definitive evidence of ischemia or hemorrhage and which, if present, indicates the need for further evaluation are as follows:
- History of moderate hemorrhage
- Injury (fracture, dislocation, or penetrating wound) in proximity to a major artery
- Diminished but palpable pulse
- Peripheral nerve deficit

Ultrasonic Flow Detection

The easily performed segmental pressure Doppler, combined with the flow velocity wave forms, is a useful instrument in determining peripheral vascular problems.

Absence of palpable distal pulses and measurement of the ankle systolic pressure with a Doppler ultrasonic flowmeter alone provide reliable and non-invasive, objective evidence of arterial insufficiency.

Other Diagnostic Modalities

- Duplex scanning
- Arteriography: In most series, the most common indication has been proximity of an injury to a major artery.
- Intra-arterial digital subtraction arteriography
- Digital venous angiography
- Magnetic resonance angiography
- Venography.

Vessel Repair[15-17]

Figure 24.1 shows the incision of choice for exposure and gaining proximal and distal vascular control.

Before proceeding with a definitive arterial repair any thrombus that may have accumulated in either the proximal or distal artery during the period of ischemia is removed. Thrombectomy should be performed passing the smallest Fogarty catheter (2F or 3F) first proximally and then distally through the previous arteriotomy or puncture site. Systemic heparinization should be given unless it is absolutely contraindicated.

Vascular repair is indicated for pseudo-aneurysms and arteriovenous fistulae. Rupture of the pseudo-aneurysm is the most likely complication with resulting hemorrhage and compartment syndrome. Failure to repair an arteriovenous fistula in a growing child may result in marked hemihypertrophy of the affected leg from the increased growth of bones and soft tissue.

Arterial repair is accomplished by:
- Resection with end—end anastomosis
- Primary autogenous repair with interrupted 6-0 prolene sutures after debridement to native intima.
- Autogenous reconstruction with vein patch or vein graft.

Special considerations during vascular repair:
- Use of generous spatulations of anastomosis
- Fine vascular suture (polypropylene, 6-0 to 8-0)
- Placement of vein bypass grafts when necessary
- Interrupted sutures for vascular anastomosis are used when substantial remaining skeletal growth is anticipated
- Systemic heparinization is used for vascular repairs when not contraindicated by associated injuries
- Local infusion of papaverine is used effectively to alleviate vasospasm when this was found to contribute to ischemia
- Liberal use of fasciotomy.

NERVE INJURY

Acute traumatic damage to a peripheral nerve may occur as a result of traction, contusion, compression, or laceration. A nerve trunk can be stretched by as much as 15% of its length without injury. As the nerve is stretched beyond this limit, the axons (efferent) and dendrites (afferent), which have little tensile strength, fail before the surrounding connective tissues (epineurium and perineurium), which are stronger. Traction injuries may be associated with fractures, at the time of injury or during reduction or fixation; with dislocations and stretch injuries; and with gunshot wounds. Although spontaneous recovery is typical of most of these injuries, complete nerve loss can also occur.

Contusion injuries from a blunt blow to the nerve carry a similar prognosis to traction injuries, with spontaneous functional recovery being the normal

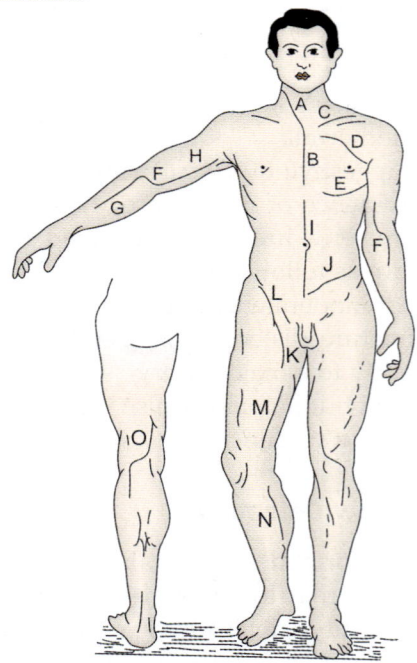

Fig. 24.1: Incisions of choice for exposure and gaining proximal and distal vascular control

Table 24.1: Tests of peripheral nerve gunction

Test	Effect of Neurotmesis	Comment
Sudomotor activity	Loss of sweating in affected distribution	Test by starch-iodine, ninhydrin, or palpation; correlates loosely with sensory loss
Wrinke test	Deinnervated skin immersed in warm water for 30 min will not wrinkle	
Volitional muscle action	Lost distal to lesion	Palpate the muscle belly rather than simply looking at distal motion. Test all muscles (distal to proximal) to localize lesion. Nerve block of parallel nerves may be useful
Electromyography	Fibrillation action potentials in deinnervated muscle	Seen several weeks after neurotmesis
Nerve conduction velocity	Stimulus distal to lesion is not seen proximally, or velocity is reduced in partial lesion	A true sensory test independent of cortical integration
Static and moving two-point discrimination	Lost; recovery shows increasing acuity	May be confused by overlapping receptive fields; difficult to administer consistently
Semmes-Weinstein monofilaments	Lost; recovery shows increasing acuity	This and the tuning fork test are threshold tests, best suited to follow nerve status after compression injury when nerve is intact
Tuning fork or vibrometer	Lost; recovery shows increasing acuity	
Tinel's sign	In recovery, percussion over regenerating front produces tingling in area of distribution	Failure to progress distally is indication for surgery
Pick-up test	Lost; with recovery, speed and accuracy improve	Reflects functionality of the repair (combined sensory, motor, and cortical function)

prognosis. Recovery from compression injuries depends on how long the nerve has been compressed and the degree of compression.

A lacerated nerve has no chance of spontaneous recovery, and the discontinuity must be surgically repaired. Results of nerve repair in children are always better than those in adults. More distal injuries have a better prognosis for recovery than proximal ones, and a pure motor or sensory nerve has a better prognosis than a mixed nerve.

Classification of Nerve Injuries

In the Sunderland classification, the following terminology and definitions are used:[18]

1. *Neuropraxia:* A localized conduction block without axonal disruption. Tinel's sign is present, and complete recovery should occur.
2. *Isolated axonotmesis:* The axon is disrupted, but the Schwann's cell tubes are intact. Wallerian degeneration occurs distal to the site of injury. Recovery is usually complete if the lesion is not too proximal for successful reinnervation.
3. *Axonal injury with endoneurial scarring:* The nerve is in continuity, but there is enough disruption of the axons that incorrect reinnervation occurs. This leads to a partial recovery, but one that is better than with excision and end-to-end repair.
4. *Neuroma in continuity:* The nerve sheath is intact, but the axons have been disrupted, and there is scarring across the nerve. The treatment is excision and repair by end-to-end anastomosis or interposition nerve grafting.
5. *Neurotmesis:* The nerve is completely divided, and repair is required.
6. Combination of the above injuries exist within a single nerve.

Tests of Peripheral Nerve Function

These are outlined in Table 24.1. A combination of tests may be done to elicit the function.

Nerve Repair[19-21]

An acute primary repair may be undertaken if the wound is clean, the mechanism of injury is a sharp laceration, the patient's condition is stable, and the surgical team and its facilities are available. If this constellation of circumstances is not encountered, perform a delayed primary repair within 8-15 days. Early repair is preferable in a clean wound because extensive nerve retraction has not yet occurred and less mobilization is required.

Secondary repair (> 2 weeks after injury) is indicated in heavily contaminated wounds if soft-tissue coverage is poor and requires flaps, if the amount of nerve damage cannot be assessed early (e.g. in patients with gunshot sounds, head injuries), or if the diagnosis is initially missed. Some motor recovery may be expected after repairs as late as 1 year after injury; partial sensory recovery may result from repairs as late as 2 years after injury. Success diminishes with delay, however, because muscle atrophies and endoneurial tubules undergo fibrosis. The anatomic goal of neurorrhaphy is, simply, to exactly realign the axons so that regenerating axon sprouts will reconnect to their preinjury end points.

Figure 24.2 depicts the cross-sectional anatomy of a peripheral nerve.

Three surgical techniques of neurorrhaphy are in current use epineurial repair, fascicular repair, and group fascicular repair (Figs 24.3 to 24.4B).

Epineurial repair is the standard method of nerve repair carried out by placing several sutures peripherally in the epineurium after aligning the nerve ends according to fascicular pattern and epineurial landmarks (Fig. 24.3). This technique has the advantage of being less technically demanding, being less traumatic to the nerve ends, and placing less suture material in the repair site. Epineurial repair is indicated for small nerves, for nerves with only one or two fascicles, and for primary repair of a clean laceration in a larger nerve.

In fascicular (also called funicular) repair, individual fascicles are dissected free of enveloping epineurium and sutured fascicle to fascicle through the perineurium (Figs 24.4A and B). This repair is not widely used because of the increased amount of suture material required at the site of repair and the difficulty in confirming the actual alignment of each of the fascicles.

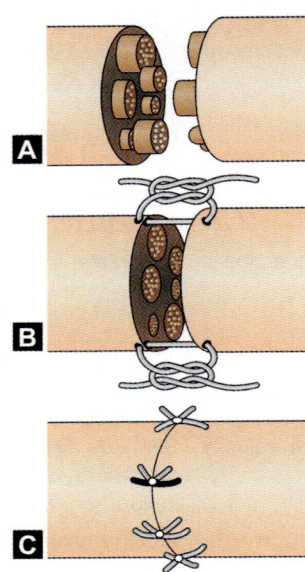

Figs 24.3A to C: Steps involved operative epineurial repair

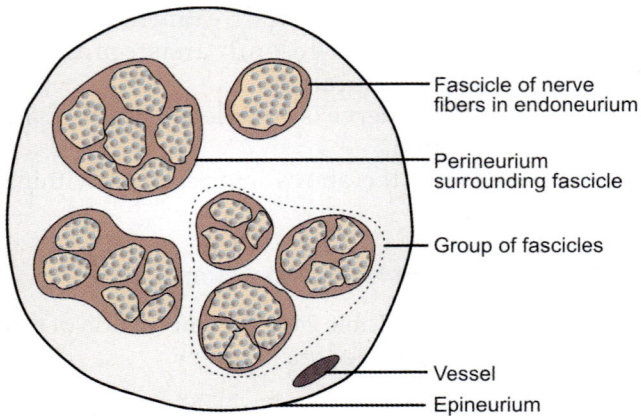

Fig. 24.2: Cross-section of a peripheral nerve, showing principal structures

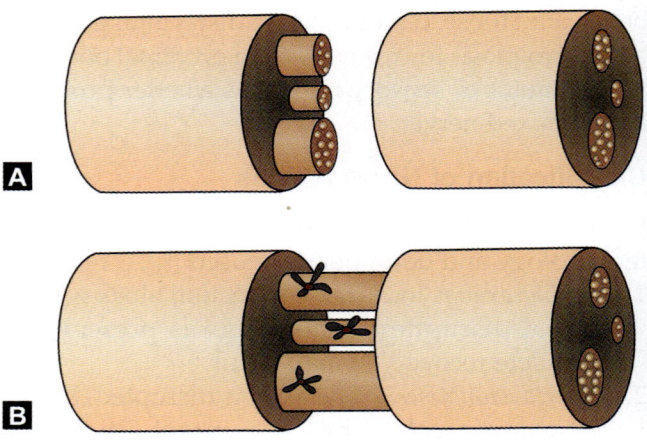

Figs 24.4A and B: Operative steps involved in fascicular repair

Group fascicular repair is similar in principle to fascicular repair except that recognizable groups of fascicles are joined instead of individual fascicles. The repair of more than five fascicles or groups is impractical, because it excessively injures the nerve end and leaves too much suture material within the wound. Group fascicular repair is the technique employed in nerve grafting. Group fascicular repairs work best when there has been a crushing component of the nerve injury or a delayed repair requiring the trimming of a portion of the nerve ends.

Nerve grafting:[22] If segmental loss prohibits end-to-end repair without excessive tension, interfascicular nerve grafting is indicated. The sural nerve is typically used as the graft. The lateral antebrachial cutaneous nerve can also be used.

MUSCLE INJURY

A strain is an injury to the musculotendinous unit. Muscle injuries are classified as either (a) acute muscular strains and avulsions, (b) contusions, or (c) exercise-induced muscle injury or delayed-onset muscle soreness (DOMS).

Muscle injuries can be caused by strain or by a direct blow. Muscle strain may be generated by passive overstretching or by sudden voluntary eccentric or concentric concentration.

The severity of muscle strains is categorized similar to ligament injuries: first-degree (mild) strains are defined by minimal structural damage, minimal hemorrhage, and early resolution; a second-degree (moderate) strain is defined as a partial tear, most often at the myotendinous junction, accompanied by pain, significant hemorrhage, inflammatory pain, and functional loss; and third-degree (severe) strains are accompanied by ovious hemorrhage, swelling, and, often, complete and palpable muscle tissue disruption.

A muscle contusion results from an external force that is sufficient to cause muscle damage. Contusions may be graded in severity according to the restriction of motion (ROM) of the subtended joints. A mild contusion causes a loss of less than one-third of the normal ROM of the adjacent joint, whereas severe contusions limit motion to less than one-third of normal excursion. Contusions result in vascular disruption, producing two types of injury intermuscular hematoma (a hemorrhage occurring along large intermuscular septa or fascial sheaths) and intramuscular hematoma (a hemorrhage occurring within muscle substance). Intermuscular hematomas are more likely to disperse and be reflected by distal ecchymosis and difusion of degradating blood components. Intramuscular hematomas are more difficult to resolve and are associated with scar contraction or myositis ossificans.

Treatment of muscle strains should be administered with an understanding of the anatomy of the particular muscle injured, the severity of injury, and the sequence of healing following partial muscle tears. The RICEM measures are applicable.

The most common injury seen in children in contact sports, particularly football and soccer, is the muscle contusion. This injury normally causes considerable pain and temporary disability in some cases, it also requires prolonged rehabilitation. Contusions typically occur in the lower extremities and are most common in the quadriceps (charley horse) and anterior tibial muscles. Massage is definitely contraindicated in the management of contusions and the RICEM measures are applicable in contusions also.

TENDON INJURY

Because of their prevalence in sports, injuries to tendons and tendon insertions have received considerable attention. Normal tendon has a tensile strength that measures 45-98 N per millimeter, but tendon begins to fail at 8-10% strain. Available evidence from surgical biopsy suggests that inflammation occurs after a tendon tear. Table 24.2 outlines the terminology used to describe tendon injury.

Management

The first principle is to diagnose the tendon injury by careful clinical examination. A second principle involves adequate exposure of the wound site. The third basic principle in the treatment of tendon injuries is to identify any associated injuries to the adjacent bones, nerves, or blood vessels. If possible, repair all the injured structures during the initial surgery. The sequence of repair is usually bone, ligament, tendon, nerve, and important blood vessels.

Table 24.2: Terminology of tendon injury

New	Old	Definition	Clinical Signs and symptoms
Paratenonitis	Tenosynovitis Tenovaginitis Paratenonitis	An inflammation of only the paratenon, either lined by synovium or not	Cardinal inflammatory signs: swelling, pain, crepitation, local tenderness, warmth, dysfunction
Peritendinitis with tendinosis	Tendinitis	Paratenon inflammation associated with intratendinosis degeneration	Same as above, with often palpable tendon swelling, and inflammatory signs
Tendinosis	Tendinitis	Intratendinous degeneratin due to atrophy (aging, microtrauma, vascular compromise, and so on)	Often palpable tendon nodule that can be asymptomatic, but may also be point tender, swelling of tendon sheath is absent
Tendinitis	Tendon strain or tear	Symptomatic degeneration of the tendon with vascular disruption and inflammatory repair response	Symptoms are inflammatory and proportional to vascular disruption, hematoma, or atrophy-related cell necrosis. Symptom duration defines each subgroup: acute (< 2 wk), subacute (4-6 wk), and chronic (> 6 wk)

Table 24.3: Schemes for assessing ligament injury

Grade	Severity	Degree	Structural Involvement	Examination	Performance Deficit
1	Mild	1°	Negligible only joint stable	No visible injury; locally tender	Minimal to a few days
2	Moderate	2°	Partial tenderness stability	Visible swelling, marked	Up to 6 wk (may be modified by protective bracing)
3	Severe	3°	Complete	Gross swelling, marked tenderness, antalgic posture; unstable	Indefinite, minimum of 6-8 wk

Tendon Repair[23,24]

The basic objective of tendon surgery is to appose the lacerated tendon ends to allow the healing process to reestablish the continuity of the disrupted collagen bundles and the smooth gliding surface of the tendon. Restore the tubular form to the tendon, avoiding both gapping and bulging of tendon tissue at the repair site.

Numerous suture techniques have been described for tendon repair (Fig. 24.5). Most of them include a "core" suture, which passes through the endotendon substance of the tendon ends across the laceration site to provide strength and stability to the repair until healing takes place. Additionally, a peripheral suture is placed circumferentially around the laceration site.

LIGAMENT INJURY

A sprain is an injury to a ligament. Disruption of ligament is followed by hematoma and soft tissue inflammatory repair. Full recovery may take more than 1 year, and the ultimate tensile strength may be reduced by 30 - 50%. An increased amount of ligament scar helps to counteract mechanical weakness, but other biomechanical properties (e.g. bending stiffness) are not improved. Therefore, once a ligament is damaged, "normal" ligament tissue is not restored. Collagen fibers straighten completely at about 4% elongation.

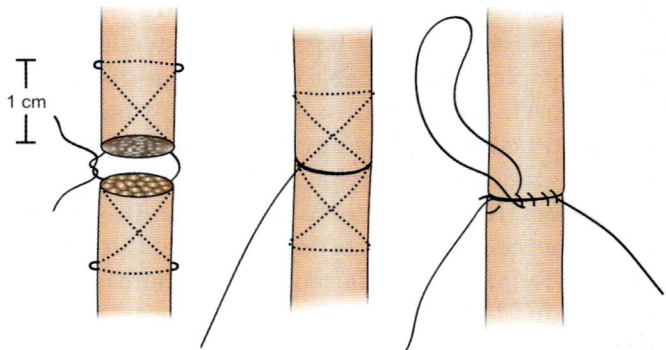

Fig. 24.5: Modified Bunnell core suture and circumferential running suture

Schemes for Assessing Ligament Injury

These have been described in Table 24.3.

SYNOVIAL INJURY

The synovial membrane is a thin layer of cells loosely classified as a specialized form of connective tissue. Synovitis is a frequently associated complaint of tendon and ligament sports-induced injury. Medications such as corticosteroid injections or NSAIDs reduce synovial inflammation through direct suppression of the arachnoid acid cascade.

REFERENCES

1. Landry GL, Gomez JE. Management of Soft Tissue Injuries. Adolesc Med 1991;2(1):125-40.
2. Vitale GC, Richardson JD, George SM Jr, Miller FB. Fasciotomy for severe, blunt and penetrating trauma of the extremity. Surg Gynecol Obstet 1988;166(5):397-401.
3. Naidu SH, Heppenstall RB. Compartment syndrome of the forearm and hand. Hand Clin 1994;22:427-32.
4. Tiwari A, Haq AI, Myint F. Acute compartmental syndromes. Br J Surg 2002;89(4):97.
5. Gulli B, Templeman D. Compartment syndrome of the lower extremity. Orthop Clin North Am 1994;25:677-84.
6. Patzakis MJ, Wilkins J. Factors influencing infection rate in open fracture wounds. Clinical Orthopedics 1989;243:36-40.
7. Eron LJ. Targeting lurking pathogens in acute traumatic and chronic wounds. J Emerg Med 1999;17(1):189-95.
8. Feng LJ, Eaton C. Soft-tissue infection in lower-extremity trauma. Clin Podiatr Med Surg 1990;7(3):449-65.
9. Morykwas MJ, Argenta LC. Nonsurgical modalities to enhance healing and care of soft tissue wounds. J South Orthop Assoc 1997 Winter;6(4):279-88.
10. Herscovici D Jr, Sanders RW, Scaduto JM, Infante A, DiPasquale T. Vacuum-assisted wound closure (VAC therapy) for the management of patients with high-energy soft tissue injuries. J Orthop Trauma 2003;17(10):683-88.
11. Mooney JF 3rd, Argenta LC, Marks MW, Morykwas MJ, DeFranzo AJ. Treatment of soft tissue defects in pediatric patients using the VAC system. Clin Orthop Relat Res 2000;(376):26-31.
12. DeFranzo AJ, Argenta LC, Marks MW, Molnar JA, David LR, Webb LX, Ward WG, Teasdall RG. The use of vacuum-assisted closure therapy for the treatment of lower-extremity wounds with exposed bone. Plast Reconstr Surg 2001;108(5):1184-91.
13. Hopf HW, Humphrey LM, Puzziferri N, West JM, Attinger CE, Hunt TK. Adjuncts to preparing wounds for closure: hyperbaric oxygen, growth factors, skin substitutes, negative pressure wound therapy (vacuum-assisted closure). Foot Ankle Clin 2001;6(4):661-82.
14. Qiang J, Liu Y, Qing-Sheng Z, Ming-Quan L, Li Z, Guang-Yue Z, Yun-Yu H. Orthopedic trauma of limbs associated with vascular injuries. Chin J Traumatol 2007;10(6):371-75.
15. Eren N, Ozgen G, Ener BK, et al. Peripheral vascular injuries in children. J Pediatr Surg 1991;26:1164-68.
16. Reichard KW, Reyes HM. Vascular trauma and reconstructive approaches. Sem Pediatr Surg 1994;3:124-32.
17. LaQuaglia MP, Upton J, May JW. Microvascular reconstruction of major arteries in neonates and small children. J Pediatr Surg 1991;26:1136-40.
18. Sunderland S. A classification of peripheral nerve injuries producing oss of function. Brain 1951;74(4):491-516.
19. McAllister RM, Gilbert SE, Calder JS, Smith PJ. The epidemiology and management of upper limb peripheral nerve injuries in modern practice. J Hand Surg [Br] 1996;21(1):4-13.
20. Berger A, Mailänder P. Advances in peripheral nerve repair in emergency surgery of the hand. World J Surg 1991;15(4):493-500.
21. Portincasa A, Gozzo G, Parisi D, Annacontini L, Campanale A, Basso G, Maiorella A. Microsurgical treatment of injury to peripheral nerves in upper and lower limbs: a critical review of the last 8 years. Microsurgery 2007;27(5):455-62.
22. Park HD, Kwak HH, Hu KS, Han SH, Fontaine C, Kim HJ. Topographic and Histologic Characteristics of the Sural Nerve for Use in Nerve Grafting. J Craniofac Surg 2007;18(6):1434-38.
23. Strickland JW. Flexor tendon repair. Hand Clin 1985;1(1):55-68.
24. Bernstein MA, Taras JS. Flexor Tendon Suture: A Description of Two Core Suture Techniques and the Silfverskiöld Epitendinous Suture. Tech Hand Up Extrem Surg 2003;7(3):119-29.

CHAPTER 25
Vascular Injuries in Children

Nagarajan Kumaran, Rob A Wheeler

Vascular injuries in children are relatively uncommon. When they do occur they pose difficulties in recognition and the results could be catastrophic if appropriate measures are not instituted early.

Ligation of the major bleeding vessel was the only treatment available until early half of 20th century and the amputation rate in World War II was 49%. In the Korean War, reconstructive techniques were implemented and the amputation rate fell to 13.6%. With ever increasing civilian trauma, attention has been given to primary repair of nerves and skeletal fixation during the primary injury thus improving functional limb salvage. Presently trauma is the leading cause of pediatric mortality in USA. It is to be noted that gunshot injuries are one among the leading causes of such trauma.

The true incidence of vascular trauma in India is difficult to estimate. A study by Tandon JN et al from Agra suggests that falls and traffic accidents are the most common causes of childhood accidents and mortality due to trauma.[1] This is consistent with the experience from Ohio.[2] With the very high number of bicycle and motorcycle usage in India, the potential for handlebar injuries causing blunt arterial trauma should be borne in mind. Another major source of injuries could be child labor where sharp objects (e.g. in carpet weaving) or mechanical accidents lead to occupational trauma.

CHARACTERISTICS OF PEDIATRIC INJURIES

Prolonged arterial spasm is characteristic of vascular trauma in the pediatric age group. This is a common phenomenon and lasts at the most up to three hours. It should reverse after this time-period. Nevertheless, the commonness of this situation could induce a false sense of security in the attending physician and precious time may be lost before beneficial treatment could be instituted. Children cannot communicate subtle complaints of weakness and paresthesia. Absence of atherosclerotic process as seen in adult vascular system and *rich collaterals* mean that children could partially compensate for arterial occlusion. Hence, they could maintain a viable limb and could even have normal distal pulses in the presence of significant arterial injury. However, this collateral circulation may be inadequate for a normal growth and these children may develop claudication or limb length discrepancies later on in life if normal circulation is not restored. Ironically, formation of A-V fistulas could result in local hypertrophy of limb. These factors together mean that the attending physician should maintain *'high level of suspicion'* to avoid long-term disabilities. In addition, the small caliber of the blood vessels pose challenges for surgical repair.

MECHANISMS OF TRAUMA (TABLE 25.1)

Vascular injuries can occur in two different settings in children. Under the age of 2 years, they are usually *iatrogenic* and occur in children who are ill owing to the coexisting conditions that necessitated the potentially harmful interventions [e.g. cardiac catheterization or arterial access] in the first place. Rarely vascular injuries could occur as a complication of major operative procedure.

Children who are more than 2 years of age are prone to different types of injuries since their increased

Table 25.1: Mechanism of trauma

Iatrogenic
- Access, e.g. umbilical artery catheters, arterial catheters
- Cardiac catheterization
- Arteriography
- Angioplasty

Blunt Trauma
- Joint displacement
- Bony fracture
- Contusion

Penetrating wounds
- Gunshot, shotgun
- Stab
- Glass (vehicular accident)

} Adjacent to a major artery

mobility is not accompanied by improved judgement. They could have multiple system injuries or coexisting musculoskeletal injuries. Children could be victims of direct abuse or could sustain violence being innocent bystanders.

Blunt Injuries: It could cause intimal disruption, dissection, contusion and thrombosis. Surrounding hematomas and tissue swelling can cause a tamponade effect on the vessel as well as impede formation of effective collaterals.

Bony Fractures: It could cause secondary damage to anatomically vulnerable vascular structures and nerves. This may be in the form of vascular traction, penetration by bony spikes or entrapment of vessel wall. The edema accompanying the injury could impede venous return in the closed muscle compartments of extremities. The vicious cycle progresses to impede arterial flow and leads to muscle ischemia, necrosis and fibrosis (Volkmann's ischemic contracture).

Penetrating Injuries: Are commonly caused by glass, knives and other sharp objects. Vehicular accidents can create flying sharp objects which act as low velocity missiles causing vascular injury. Vessels could be completely transected causing hematoma which allows vascular contraction and temporary cessation of bleeding. If a tangential injury is sustained, such an outcome is precluded and incessant bleeding results. Associated venous injury facilitates formation of an arteriovenous fistula, which limits distal run-off leading to limb ischemia by causing an 'arterial steal' and could potentially result in high output cardiac failure. High-velocity missiles as in gunshot wounds cause temporary cavitation and arterial and venous thrombosis due to the absorption of kinetic energy. In shotgun injuries, pellets can enter vascular system and could embolise to extremities.

ASSESSMENT

The interests of child with injuries is best served by a team approach. Children with vascular trauma could have associated airway (e.g. penetrating neck injuries), breathing (e.g. hemothorax) or circulation problems which could be life-threatening and need prompt recognition and treatment. Fluid resuscitation takes precedence when the child is in shock. In cases where IVC injuries are considered possible, it is prudent to obtain vascular access through the upper limb veins and vice versa. Often associated injuries like skeletal fracture may distract the examiner's attention and vascular injuries may not be recognized unless specifically looked for. Palpation of pulses and assessment of skin temperature could provide early clues. Lack of spontaneous movement of the limb and tenderness elicited during passive movement of major joints could provide corroborative evidence that a vascular injury exists. Physical examination is very sensitive especially when repeated and combined with noninvasive Doppler assessment.

IMAGING MODALITIES

Doppler Studies

Doppler signals can be used to examine clinically feeble pulses especially in an edematous extremity. Ankle-Brachial pressure Indices (ABI) can be determined by recording accurate blood pressures. A comparison of resting and post-exercise ABIs can give an idea of critical stenoses. A Duplex scan (ultrasound combined with Doppler) can be used to measure the diameters at critical sites such as vascular and graft anastomosis. Also they may be useful in identifying pseudoaneurysms. Color flow is an additional facility to measure turbulence of flow. Combined with clinical symptoms and examination these can potentially avoid the need for invasive arteriography in large number of clinical situations.

Digital Subtraction Arteriography

Critical details of vascular anatomy may be obscured in an angiogram by overlapping stuctures. Traditionally cut films were used to subtract the background images by a labor-intensive process of superimposing a plain mask film and contrast film and reimaging on a third film. With digital technology and computer enhancement this can be done instantaneously and most arteriograms are performed this way. Arterial injection of contrast means less contrast need to be used. This type of arteriogram still remains the gold standard.

In small children with a small blood volume, sufficient concentration could be achieved through intravenous route [IV-DSA] and this is particularly useful in evaluating *long-term patency* of vascular repair/graft. Still, a rapid bolus is required to achieve the concentration and hence a peripherally inserted longline to reach a large central vein or even right atrium is required. To avoid movement artefacts most children need sedation. Intravenous DSA can miss intimal disruptions < 1 mm. On the balance these difficulties are to be weighed against the possibility of avoiding second arterial injury due to an arterial access and significantly less radiation. Parker PM and associates employed IV-DSA to guide management of acute arterial injuries in 9 children. They avoided unnecessary exploration in 4 patients by excluding arterial injuries, identified 1 pseudoaneurysm for ligation and abandoned a planned skin flap since there was no blood supply to the flap. They contend that IV-DSA can be the definite diagnostic procedure in the acute phase.[3]

IATROGENIC INJURIES

Umbilical Artery Catheters

Umbilical artery catheters (UAC) are used in neonatal practice to give a convenient access to the arterial system for blood pressure monitoring and frequent blood gas sampling. They have revolutionized the care of extremely sick premature babies; yet, there is attendant morbidity and mortality attributable to them. The most common complications include thrombosis, infection, hemorrhage and hypertension.

Thrombosis is a result of endothelial damage produced by indwelling UAC catheters thus exposing the highly thrombogenic subintimal smooth muscle layer. Rajani et al studied the effect of low-dose heparin (1 mg/ml) in neonates with umbilical artery catheters. They established by a randomized controlled double-blind study that heparin infusion at this dose through UAC prolonged the duration of catheter patency and did not alter the partial thromboplastin time.[4] Mokrohisky et al. demonstrated that low positioning of umbilical-artery catheters could increase the incidence of associated complications in newborn infants. They recommended thoracic positioning of catheter-tip.[5] Previous studies have established that catheters with an end-hole are safer than catheters with side holes. There is evidence that heparin may be effective in doses as low as 0.25 U/ml as a continuous infusion. Boluses did not have the same effect. Heparin infusion did not alter the incidence of aortic thrombosis. Whereas it can be said that low-dose heparin infusion does not increase the incidence of intra-ventricular hemorrhage in general, whether the same is true in cases of extremely premature babies (< 31 weeks) who are at the highest risk to develop this complication is not known yet.[6] With the implementation of these changes and the availability of small sized catheters, there is an apparent reduction in the morbidity associated with UAC in recent years and further progress needs to be made in the prevention of aortic thrombosis.

Small catheter related thrombi may respond to simple withdrawal of catheter. Minor ischemic complications including transient ischemia of limbs may resolve conservatively. Major aortic thrombosis could present in various ways – severe cardiac failure, hypertension especially in cases with aortorenal thrombosis, impaired renal function and bilateral lower limb ischemia.

Angiography still remains the gold standard for the diagnosis of aortic thrombosis. Non-invasive diagnostic modalities like ultrasound, color-flow doppler are obviously preferable and have been employed by some authors. Radionuclide studies [DTPA] may be useful. The reported incidence of thrombosis varies with the sensitivity of screening method used and may exist even in asymptomatic patients. For monitoring clot lysis and resolution ultrasound is the method of choice.

The treatment of established aortic thrombosis remains controversial. Krueger and colleagues (vide supra) advocated early and aggressive surgical thrombectomy. On the contrary there are isolated reports of spontaneous clot resolution in cases with infrarenal aortic thrombosis treated only with supportive care.[7]

The results of thrombolytic therapy seem to be promising. Streptokinase, urokinase and recombinant tissue plasminogen activator (r-tPA) have all been used with apparent success. Thrombolytic agents act by directly or indirectly activating plasminogen and the resultant proteolytic factor 'plasmin' lyses fibrin. Plasminogen exists in plasma as a free form and in thrombus as a fibrin-specific form. Streptokinase (indirectly) and urokinase (directly) activate both the plasma and the tissue plasminogen. Hence, they produce a systemic 'lytic' state. This is particularly disadvantageous in premature neonates who are at increased risk hemorrhagic complications including intraventricular hemorrhage. Streptokinase is antigenic in nature and has a long half-life of 30-60 min and hence, is not currently recommended. As r-tPA is 'fibrin-specific' maximum activity is generated on the surface of the thrombus providing the least chance of provoking systemic bleeding. However, its superiority over urokinase for this purpose is not established by direct comparative trials in neonates.

In adults r-tPA is the most used thrombolytic agent. Watkins S et al have recently reported their experience in a neonate with bilateral lower limb ischemia caused by thrombotic occlusion as a result of twin-twin transfusion.[8] This neonate had a severe left leg ischemia necessitating fasciotomy below the knee shortly after birth. Subsequently the baby developed bilateral lower limb ischemia with multiple emboli. At the dose of 50 mg/kg/hr, tPA was administered through an umbilical arterial catheter over 13 days. The entire right leg survived and the left foot survived with residual deformity (Figs 25.1A to C). Despite the prolonged duration of administration there was no bleeding complications and the cranial ultrasound remained normal.

Similar results are reported in a retrospective series Hartmann J et al who treated 14 neonates with catheter related thrombosis over six years. They recommend an initial bolus of tPA [0.7mg/kg over 30 min] followed by 0.2 mg/kg/hr as a continuous infusion with a low dose heparin prophylaxis of 2-6 IU/kg/hr.[9] This protocol was derived from adults. There was no incidence of severe bleeding or intraventricular hemorrhage in their series. Dillon et al successfully employed even lower doses. They also suggested that fibrinogen level should be maintained greater than 100 mg/dl.[10] Further multicentered trials are needed to establish a safe and effective protocol for thrombolysis in neonates.

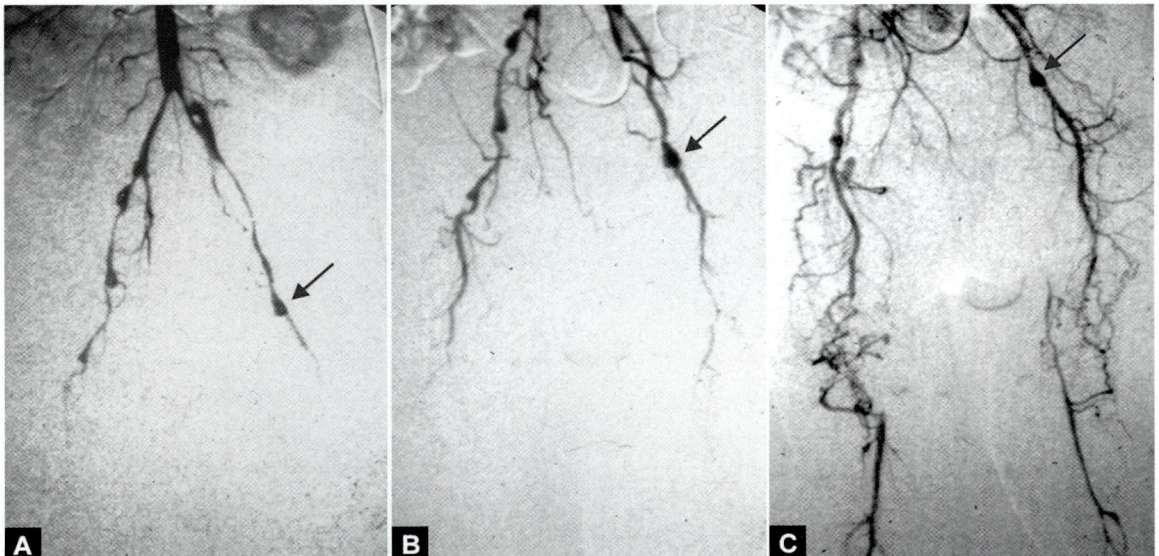

Figs 25.1A to C: Serial angiography in a neonate with bilateral iliac occlusion performed before t-PA infusion **A.** and at 3 days **B.** and 9 days **C.** after commencement of the infusion. Arrows point to the site of thrombosis. The occlusion can be seen to reverse effectively. (Reprinted with permission from Dr S Watkins– previously published in journal of Pediatric Surgery 2001;36 (4):654-656)

Peripheral Vascular Access

Arterial lines are useful for access in sick neonates for continuous blood pressure monitoring, arteriography and cardiac catheterization. Radial, dorsalis pedis, posterior tibial, ulnar, axillary and femoral arteries have been utilized for this purpose.

Common complications associated with intra-arterial catheters include vasospasm, intimal disruptions and flap formation, thrombosis and intramural hematoma. Unless recognised early, limb salvage might be impossible when the complications involve major vessels of the limb. Prevention of injuries is the key. Radial artery is by far the safest. Nevertheless Allen's test should be performed to ascertain satisfactory collateral circulation prior to selection. Percutaneous access, using the shortest length of catheter required, avoiding high pressure boluses, continuous heparin infusion, firm skin fixation and wrist immobilization – all help to minimize complication rates. In a multivariate analysis Franken et al established that catheter size is *the* principal factor in determining the incidence of vasospasm based on radiographic evidence. A large catheter to arterial size ratio should be avoided.[11]

Wardlea SP and colleagues have used 65 femoral arterial and venous catheterization in 53 neonates with a median gestational age of 29 weeks after all the other vascular accesses were exhausted.[12] Transient ischemic episodes occurred in 17%, catheter related sepsis occurred in 19% necessitating removal, but there were no major catheter related complications. This success is obviously due to thin walled pliable catheters of size 3F or 4F tapered over a guidewire inserted using a standard Seldinger's technique by experienced personnel.[12]

Factors influencing occurrence of vascular injury during angiocardiography include multiple previous entries and multiple catheter exchanges. In addition to the above-mentioned measures – accessing left heart through patent foramen ovale whenever possible, shortening catheter indwelling time by rapid execution of procedure and removal as soon as possible – minimize injury. After removal of catheter, firm finger pressure should be applied cephalad to site of skin entry, where the entry into the artery itself is likely to be. Distal pulses and limb perfusion should be carefully monitored after the procedure. In the rare instances when pulse loss occurs, heparin infusion should be commenced.

There are other factors which can affect the potential for injury as well. Epithelial disruption of any kind, hematological abnormalities (hypercoagulability) and hypovolemia at the time of intervention can affect the microcirculation and thus predispose patients to injury. Sadly, when this happens ischemia could result in peripheral gangrene necessitating amputation. In the presence of dry gangrene adequate time should be allowed for collaterals to form and line of demarcation to evolve before deciding the level of amputation (Figs 25.2A and B). Early recognition, aggressive investigation and

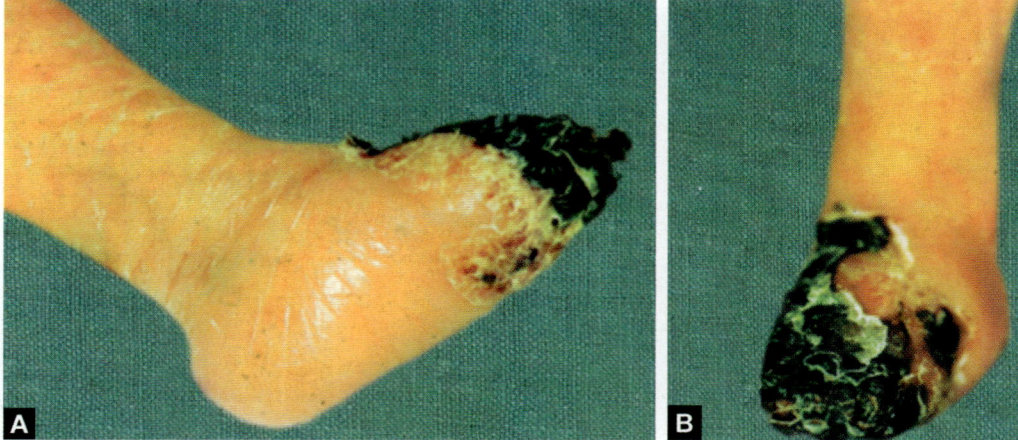

Figs 25.2A and B: Peripheral gangrene in a preterm neonate as a result of indwelling arterial line positioned in dorsalis pedis artery. The line of demarcation was allowed to mature and three weeks later a mid-tarsal amputation was performed

prompt intervention are vital in preventing such a formidable outcome.

The choice of therapy in patients with viable limbs and demonstrable pulse deficits seems to be controversial. Since limb-length discrepancies could occur in this group of patients some authors advocate *aggressive surgical approach* with thrombectomy and/or microvascular reconstruction.[13] The small caliber of the vessels poses distinct surgical difficulties and hence risk of restenosis is high. Moreover, many of these injuries occur in children who are extremely sick due to their primary medical condition. These factors have led others to recommend a conservative policy. A *delayed repair* could be performed if exercise intolerance or limb length discrepancies develop. A delayed repair has been shown to reverse the growth disparity if adequate time period exists before growth potential ceases.[14] Hence, it is obvious that whichever choice is made prolonged follow-up is necessary with particular attention to history of exercise induced claudication and radiological assessment of limb length in doubtful cases.

TRAUMATIC INJURIES

Unlike iatrogenic injuries, trauma – blunt or penetrating – usually occurs in children over 2 years of age who are larger and are generally fit to undergo operative correction. The outcome is optimal if surgery is performed within 6 hours of injury.[14] One cannot overemphasize the fact that a *'high index of suspicion'* is essential especially in a country like India where delays to reach such a surgical facility might be considerable.[15]

Peripheral arterial injuries are often due to blunt injuries accompanying skeletal fractures or penetrating injuries causing direct vascular damage. Pain, pallor, paresthesia, pulselessness, paralysis and poikilothermia (coolness) are indications that obvious arterial occlusion exist. Other 'hard' *signs* of arterial injury are active bleeding, expanding or pulsatile hematoma and bruit/thrill. Their presence indicates that direct exploration should be performed in theatre and that time-delays to perform angiograms are to be avoided. However, in cases of multiple penetrating injuries of the same extremity an angiogram to ascertain the level of injury may be justifiable.

The *'soft' signs* of arterial injuries include history of bleeding, small non-expanding hematoma, unexplained hypotension, injury to anatomically related nerve (sensory/motor deficit), and proximity to a major vessel. In these occasions an angiogram should be considered. One shot angiogram performed by surgeons when single hand-held injection of contrast (10-35 ml of diatrizoate) into the arterial system is made in antegrade or retrograde fashion and this is manually timed to obtain a single plain film. This concept is now being used in the United States as Emergency Center angiogram in patients suspected to have peripheral injuries with soft signs.[16] Alternatively color-doppler along with clinical examination is felt to be very sensitive in excluding vascular injuries. Angiogram performed in radiology suite remains the gold standard.

Penetrating Injuries

In patients with penetrating injury near a major vessel and in cases of gunshot injuries where distant injuries are possible, major vascular trauma should be considered. Bleeding should be temporarily controlled by direct pressure. Blind attempts to control bleeding using clamps and use of tourniquet could be harmful. In theatre, both proximal and distal control should be obtained at a distance from the actual site of injury if possible before hematoma is opened. Small vascular clamps should be used. The anatomy of injury should be defined. Lateral repair is possible in large arteries with tangential injuries. In complete transections contused ends should be resected. Fogarty catheter should be used to remove clots from proximal and distal ends. Spatulation of both ends has been shown to be the key to success. End to end anastomosis is achieved using interrupted 6.0 or 7.0 monofilament sutures placed as widely possible as is consistent with hemostasis. In contradistinction to the continuous suturing technique preferred in adults, interrupted suturing allows subsequent growth in children and minimizes the potential for stenosis. If tension-free anastomosis is not possible, reversed autogenous saphenous vein grafts are preferred. Brisk backbleeding indicates adequate collateral flow and generally predicts good outcome. Intraoperative doppler can assist in making a judgement about flow in distal vessels. Where uncertainty persists a completion angiogram may be useful in excluding the presence of distal emboli.

Major venous injuries should be preferably repaired before arterial reconstrucion. Minor distal veins could be ligated safely. Fasciotomy should be performed if necessary. Nerve injuries could also be repaired during the same time. Routine antibiotic prophylaxis is not required though other factors like possible contamination and time since injury should be taken into consideration before making this decision. Suitable tetanus prophylaxis measures should be taken.

Blunt Injuries

Arterial injuries could accompany major blunt impact trauma and these patients could have multiple system injuries. Assessment of neurological deficit might be difficult. Arteriography should be performed when there is any suspicion.

Upto 3% of patients with long bone fractures or limb joint dislocations could sustain associated arterial injuries. Involvement of superficial femoral artery in fractures of distal femur, popliteal artery in dislocation of knee joint and brachial artery in supracondylar fracture of humerus are typical examples of such injuries. Associated disabling nerve injuries are common.

Priority should be given to early reduction and stabilization of the fracture. If there is severe ischemia or if the procedure will take more than 30 minutes a temporary vascular shunt should be considered to sustain distal blood flow during orthopedic manipulation. Post-reduction vascular assessment is to be performed using palpation of pulse, clinical assessment of perfusion and registration of Doppler signals. It is prudent to perform open explorations if this is not satisfactory. If arteriography is desired it is best performed on-table under same anesthesia.

Compartment Syndrome

Volkmann, in 1881, described paralytic contractures following periods of arterial insufficiency of even few hours. This is due ischemia of muscle causing edema and elevated pressures a closed limb compartment. When the compartmental pressure supercedes venous pressure, outflow gets cut off further aggravating edema and this causes further ischemia. Massive crush, bony fractures, bleeding, orthopedic manipulation, Bier's block, associated venous injuries and infection can all aggravate the vicious cycle. If not promptly interrupted, this cycle leads to permanent contractures as a result of ischemic myonecrosis and the resultant fibrosis. Clinical features during the acute setting include edema, attitude of flexion, hard feeling and tenderness to touch and passive stretch. Monitoring can be done using a wick-catheter technique to assess compartmental pressures. Pressures > 30 mm Hg indicate fasciotomy. It is a safe policy to perform fasciotomy when in doubt. Fasciotomy should include the entire length of the compartment – in the forearm it should extend from the antecubital fossa to the carpal tunnel, in the leg four compartment decompression is effected through two incisions. Though some authors advocate fibulectomy as a method of decompression, this could lead to valgus deformity in children.

It is to be noted that most series on peripheral vascular injuries have a 3-5% incidence of amputation. In cases with massive crush injuries sometimes a primary amputation could be lifesaving. Some patients with combined musculoskeletal, vascular and neural injuries may be better served by amputation and early rehabilitation.

TRUNCAL INJURIES

Cervicothoracic Injuries

Although thoracic great vessel injuries are rare in children, they are attendant with high mortality rate. With a rapid acceleration-deceleration type injury aortic disruption occurs at the junction of fixed and mobile part. Thus, in both vertical and linear high speed impacts junction of aortic arch and descending aorta just distal to ligamentum arteriosum is the most vulnerable site. Patients with penetrating injury to ascending aorta rapidly die of tamponade and those with aortic arch injuries die of rapid exsanguination. When descending aortic injuries are contained by adventitia a pseudoanerysm results. These patients reach hospital safely but if not identified and treated have a 30% mortality rate. Some of the warning features would include dyspnea, back pain, diminished femoral pulses and upper limb hypertension. Even if they are asymptomatic, a widened mediastinum on chest X-ray should prompt arch aortography. Emergency thoracotomy and repair, possibly under bypass is required. For isolated injuries of descending aorta a 'clamp-sew' technique without bypass might be justifiable but prolonged aortic clamping has inherent increased risk of cerebral hypertension, paraplegia due to spinal cord ischemia, distal thrombosis and renal failure. Dacron graft repair has been successfully employed for repair of aortic arch.

Penetrating neck injuries in children are rare. Consequently current practice is based largely on the experience gained in adults. Controversy exists in identifying the type of injuries which require mandatory exploration and those that need selective exploration based on clinical or radiological criteria. Neck is divided into three zones for this purpose. Zone I includes structures below the cricoid cartilage upto clavicle, Zone II comprises of structures between cricoid cartilage upward upto the angle of mandible and Zone III extends above angle of mandible upto the base of skull. Injuries to Zone I and Zone III are investigated using a combination of angiography, esophagogram, esophagoscopy and bronchoscopy. Traditionally violation of platysma was considered to be an indication for mandatory exploration for Zone II injuries.

With improvements in imaging technique obviously fewer patients will need mandatory exploration. Cox CS and colleagues employed a selective policy whereby hemodynamically *unstable* patients underwent emergency explorations and *stable* patients underwent abovementioned investigations and explored only if an obvious injury which needed operative correction. Asymptomatic patients were kept under observation only.[17]

Abdominal Injuries

Penetrating injuries, severe blunt injury or iatrogenic trauma (e.g. tumor resection or Veress needle for laparoscopy) could cause abdominal vascular injuries and they may be associated with visceral injuries. Emergency laparotomy for uncontrollable hemorrhage is the rule. In stable patients renal vascular injury should be excluded using contrast enhanced CT scan or a one shot IVP where facilities are limited. Aortic injuries could be treated with direct repair, vein graft or prosthetic graft. The *Infrarenal* IVC can be ligated. Successful ligation of even the *pararenal* IVC, performed as a life saving measure in seat-belt injury, has been reported.[18] If needed, direct venous repair could be performed under finger pressure control.

Retrohepatic IVC injuries are particularly difficult to manage. The suggested strategy is to pack, resuscitate and then to obtain intrapericardial and suprarenal caval controls. Pringle maneuver completes hepatic isolation to facilitate repair.[14] Venovenous extracorporeal bypass (femoral - right atrial circuit) has been successfully employed as well in tackling these difficult injuries.

RECENT ADVANCES

Microsurgical Techniques

The usefulness of powerful operating microscopes with magnifications as much as X30 and X40, 9-0 to 11-0 monofilament sutures and team approach has helped the emergence of microsurgical techniques and almost all vascular grafts performed in adults can be now performed in children including neonates although this still borders on the experimental. It is to be noted the principles of vascular surgery remains the same but microsurgery helps to implement these principles accurately in the tiny blood vessels as small as 0.5 mm.[19] In addition to saphenous veins, dorsal veins of the foot which possess thick muscularis have been employed by these authors. The types of vascular reconstructions described in the pediatric literature are summarised in Table 25.2.

Long-term follow-up of patients who had autogenous saphenous vein grafts by Cadneau JD and associates, has established that these grafts are effective and durable. They also found that limb–length discrepancy can be reversed and symptoms of claudication relieved using appropriate revascularization techniques.[20] Aneurysmal and non-

Table 25.2: Vascular reconstructions described in children

1. Direct repair (Arteriorrhaphy/Venorrhaphy)
2. Vein patch angioplasty
3. Reversed saphenous vein interposition graft
4. Femoral—Femoral interposition graft (extra-anatomic bypass)
5. Digital vessel reimplantation
6. Distal bypass (to medial plantar artery)
7. Femoropopliteal bypass
8. Iliofemoral bypass
9. Dacron mesh reinforced iliofemoral bypass graft
10. *In situ* venous bypass (popliteal-posterior tibial).

aneurysmal dilatations, graft stenosis or complete occlusion are some of the complications they encountered.

PREVENTION

The incidence of iatrogenic injuries appears to be decreasing mainly owing to the preventive strategies.[14] The traumatic vascular injuries are to be prevented by precautions against childhood injuries by making home and public places safe for the child. Steps should be intensified to curb child abuse. For the victim of trauma supportive care and rehabilitation should begin in the in-hospital phase and must be followed in the society with particular attention to educational needs.

REFERENCES

1. Tandon JN, Kalra A, Kalra K, et al. Profile of accidents in children. Indian Pediatr 1993;30:765-69.
2. Navarre JR, Cardillo PJ, Gorman JF, et al. Vascular trauma in children and adolescents. Am J Surg 1982;143:229-31.
3. Parker PM, Vinocur CD, Smergel E, et al. Intravenous digital subtraction angiography: Its use in evaluating vascular injuries in children. J Ped Surg. May 1989;24: 423-27.
4. Rajani K, Goetzman BW, Wennberg RP, et al. Effect of Heparinization of Fluids Infused Through an Umbilical Artery Catheter on Catheter Patency and Frequency of Complications. Pediatrics 1979;63:552-56.
5. Mokrohisky ST, Levine RL, Blumhagen JD, et al. Low positioning of umbilical-artery catheters increases associated complications in newborn infants. N Eng J Med 1978;229:561-64.
6. Barrington KJ. Umbilical artery catheters in the newborn: effects of heparin (Cochrane Review) In: The Cochrane Library, Issue 4, 2001. Oxford: Update Software.
7. Krueger TC, Neblett WW, O'Neill JA, et al. Management of aortic thrombosis secondary to umbilical artery catheters in neonates. J Ped Surg 1985;20:328-32.
8. Watkins S, Yunge M, Jones D, et al. Prolonged use of tissue plasminogen activator for bilateral lower limb arterial occlusion in a neonat J Ped Surg 2001;36:654-56.
9. Hartmanna J, Husseina A, Trowitzscha E, et al. Treatment of neonatal thrombus formation with recombinant tissue plasminogen activator: six years experience and review of the literature. Arch Dis Child Fetal Neonatal Ed 2001;85:F18-F22.
10. Dillon PW, Fox PS, Berg CJ, et al. Recombinant tissue plasminogen activator for neonatal and pediatric vascular thrombolytic therapy. J Ped Surg 1993;28:1264-68.
11. Franken EA, Girod D, Sequeira FW, et al. Femoral artery spasm in children: catheter size is the principal cause. American Journal of Roentgenology 1982;138:295-98.
12. Wardlea SP, Kelsallb AWR, Yoxallc CW, et al. Percutaneous femoral arterial and venous catheterisation during neonatal intensive care. Arch Dis Child Fetal Neonatal Ed 2001;85:F119-F22.
13. King DR, Wise WE. Vascular injuries. In: Buntain, William L. (Ed): Management of Pediatric Trauma. Philadelphia, WB Saunders 1994;265-76.
14. Reichard KW, Reyes HM. Vascular trauma and reconstructive approaches. Semin Ped Surg 1994;3:124-32.
15. Chandra A, Dronamraju D, Srinivas K, et al. Delayed Repair of Popliteal Artery Following Blunt Injury. Asian Cardiovasc Thorac Ann 1999;7:247-49.
16. Itani KM, Rothenberg SS, Brandt ML, et al. Emergency center arteriography in the evaluation of suspected peripheral vascular injuries in children. J Ped Surg 1993;28:677-80.
17. Cox Jrabc CS, Blackabc CT, Dukeabc JH, et al. Operative treatment of truncal vascular injuries in children and adolescents. J Ped Surg 1998;33:462-67.
18. DeCou JM, Abrams RS, Gauderer MW. Seat-belt transection of the pararenal vena cava in a 5-year-old child: survival with caval ligation. J Pediatr Surg 1999;34(7): 1074-76. Review.
19. La Quaglia MP, Upton J, May JW. Microvascular reconstruction of major arteries in neonates and small children. J Ped Surg Sep 1991,26:1136-40.
20. Cadneau JD, Henke PK, Upchurch GR, et al. Efficacy and durability of autogenous saphenous vein conduits for lower extremity arterial reconstructions in preadolescent children. J Vasc Surgery 2001;34:34-40.

CHAPTER 26

Pediatric Burns

K Mathingi Ramakrishnan, V Jayaraman

Burns are the most devastating type of trauma that the human beings suffer. The postburn scars leave behind indelible blemishes, and the victims may suffer till the end of their lives. In spite of the modern methods available in burn management and advancing knowledge of the basic pathophysiology of burn injuries, India cannot boast about diminishing mortality and morbidity in burns. The incidence of burn injuries is increasing and mortality is also high. Significant morbidity in terms of long-term sequelae such as functional, cosmetic, social and psychological impairment is also seen. Children are at high risk because of their natural curiosity, their mode of reaction, their impulsiveness and lack of experience in calculating the risk of the situation. Though most of our burns occur in the poorer socioeconomic strata of society, burns in children are also seen in the affluent sectors; careless attitude of the parents, negligence and lack of priorities contribute towards this scenario.

EPIDEMIOLOGY

Children unfortunately are the innocent victims of circumstances that result in major fire accidents. Superficial flame burns rate the highest amongst the etiological factors. Open fire cooking, children playing in the kitchen, where cooking is undertaken at the floor level, rodents toppling on open chimney lamps due to lack of electricity are common causes. Scalds due to hot liquids in the domestic setup ranks next in the etiology. More serious types of scalding occurs when older children (2-4 years) fall into hot water or hot milk kept on the floor for cooling under the fan. Neonates suffer burns due to hot water bottles, which are used as warmers.

Electrical burns are very common in the domestic setup, when children place their fingers into open plug sockets and suffer low voltage burns. Playing near dish antennae on top of multistoried buildings could result in serious high voltage electrical burns in the upper limbs. Contact with live wires is a common type of electrical burn when children play and try to retrieve kites. These could result in major burn injuries with entry and exit wounds.

Acid burns are not very common in children, but corrosive esophageal injury occurs due to accidental ingestion of acid which is kept in kitchen closets for cleaning purposes. Children sometimes are innocent victims of homicidal acid burns.

Incidence

The material included in this chapter relates to the analysis of pediatric burns (0-18 years) treated in a tertiary facility of Kilpauk Medical College Hospital during a period of twenty years and in a well equipped private trust children's hospital. In this study we have analyzed a total 427 patients who were admitted to Kanchi Kamakoti Childs Trust Hospital, Chennai for over a period of nine years. The data (Chart I and II) clearly denotes the occurrence as per age, etiology, percentage of burns and mortality.

Age and Sex

Most of the children belonged to the group below 10 years. Male children predominated.

TYPES OF BURNS

Scalds due to hot liquids topped the list. Next common was flame burn. We did have acid burns and electrical burns. Other studies showed that compared with older children, children younger than 4 years were significantly more likely to be admitted with scalds rather than flame burns, had smaller burn injuries, and were less likely to have an inhalation injury.[1]

TIME OF OCCURRENCE

Children suffered burns more during daytime and there were more flame burns during the festival season (September to November).

MORTALITY

Children tolerated burn injury better than adults if the body surface area (BSA) involved was 10-30%. If the BSA involved was over 30% the mortality was higher. Neonates who suffered accidental burns due to use of hot water bottle as warmer, especially in the villages, usually succumbed to the injuries. In larger series, after adjusting for sex, burn size, inhalation injury, and type of burn (flame versus scald), the risk of mortality was substantially higher for children aged 0-1.9 years and for children aged 2.0-3.9 years as compared with children aged 4 years or older.[1]

Mortality also depended upon the delay in resuscitation due to late presentation and due to the innumerable topical applications used on the burnt area at the time of sustaining the injury. The major cause of death in this study was *Pseudomonas septicemia*.

Retrospective and prospective trials have demonstrated that injury characteristics (lower age, larger burn size, presence of inhalation injury), resuscitation variables (delayed intravenous access, lower admission hematocrit, lower base deficit on admission, higher serum osmolarity at arrival to the hospital) and hospital course events (sepsis, inotropic support requirement, platelet count < 20,000, and ventilator dependency) significantly predict increased mortality.[2]

PATHOPHYSIOLOGY OF BURNS

Problems in the pediatric burns are mainly due to physiological immaturity; this is especially true in infants. The temperature regulating mechanism is labile as the ratio of surface area of the body to weight is more. Rapid shifts in the core temperature occur. Deep burns occur rather rapidly due to the thin skin of the infant that has scant dermal appendages, which are close to the surface, permitting the burn to penetrate into the depths easily. Children are also more susceptible to fluid overload and dehydration. Infants require higher energy and their peripheral circulation is labile. Their metabolic demands are also on the higher side. With all these special problems, the children with burns present a special management issue.

Burn injury is associated with anatomic, physiologic, endocrinologic, and immunologic alterations. Cutaneous injury triggers a reaction at a local and systemic level through the release of multiple inflammatory mediators.[3] When the injury is extensive, this becomes a systemic reaction and the cascade of cellular alterations can lead to generalized inflammation and multiple system organ dysfunction (Fig. 26.1). These problems need to be identified and treated properly to prevent or minimize the extent of the damage.[4]

Burn shock is consequent to the massive fluid shifts that occur soon after burn injury. Direct thermal injury results in changes in the microcirculation and capillary permeability increases. Multiple inflammatory mediators are also secreted which increase the vascular permeability throughout the capillary vascular bed all over the body. This results in the leak of intravascular fluid into the extravascular spaces resulting in burn edema, which is maximum at the end of 12 hours post burn in minor burns and lasts till 24 hours in major burns. Hypovolemia occurs due to the fluid shifts at the expense of circulating blood and plasma. This results in burn shock with reduced cardiac output, increased heart rate, oliguria, acidosis and air hunger. The inflammatory mediators that are responsible are bradykinin, histamine, prostaglandins, leukotrienes and hormones. Products of platelet degradation, and interleukins 1 and 6 also act as mediators of burn shock (Fig. 26.1).

In burnt patients the levels of sodium adenosine triphoshphate are reduced in the tissues, which alters the cell transmembrane potential and the concentration of sodium increases in the extravascular compartment. This also contributes to burn edema.

Severe burns can thus cause increased vascular permeability and edema, altered hemodynamics, immunosuppression, hypermetabolism, decreased renal blood flow and increased gut mucosal permeability.

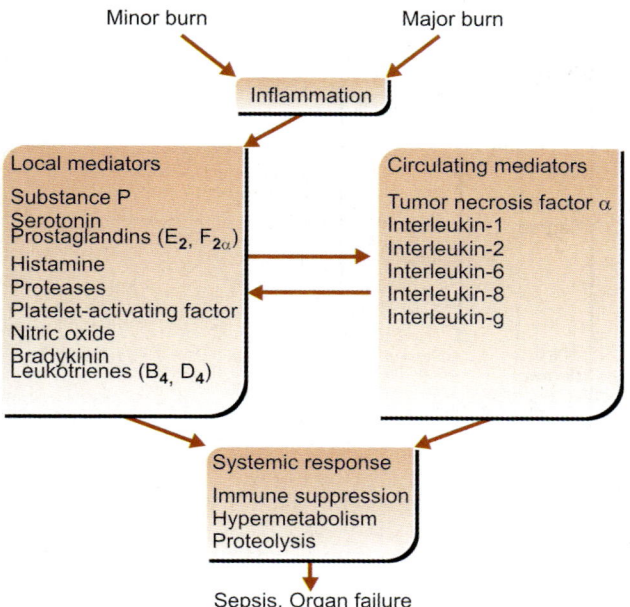

Fig. 26.1: Cascade of cellular alterations that can lead to multiple system organ dysfunction

CLASSIFICATION OF BURNS

Classification of burns can be done according to the agent inducing the injury and according to depth and extent of the total body surface area involved (TBSA).

Agents Causing Burn

- Thermal
  - Scald
  - Contact with hot objects
  - Flame
- Electrical
- Chemical
- Radiation.

Depth

A clear understanding of the depth and structure of the skin is needed to understand the grades of burn (Fig. 26.2).

First Degree Burn (Superficial) (Fig. 26.3)

Only the superficial epithelium is involved. There is always varying degree of erythema and regardless of the type of therapy used, this type of burn heals without scar formation. For about six to ten hours, burn is painful and then gradually it becomes less painful. Sunburns and flame burns are generally of this type.

Second Degree Burn (Partial Thickness) (Fig. 26.4)

Here the entire epidermis and a variable depth of dermis are involved. These are commonly seen due to splashes of hot liquids, flash burns, longer contact with flames and limited exposure to chemicals. Depending upon the extent of dermal involvement it is further divided into superficial and deep partial thickness burn.

The superficial type is painful and has blisters. Since sweat glands and hair follicles are spared the healing is satisfactory and scarring does not occur. These heal in 2-3 weeks time and are painful during healing phase due to regeneration of nerve fibers.

The deeper variety is not very painful and is generally without blisters, but since the reticular layer of the dermis is involved these usually do not heal spontaneously, and when it heals after several weeks, it does so with hypertrophic scarring. The appearance will be almost like third degree burn. A sterile 'pin-prick test' with a hypodermic needle can be very valuable in assessing the depth of the burn.

Third Degree Burn (Full Thickness) (Figs 26.5 and 26.6)

Here the entire thickness of the skin and adnexae are involved. The burn is not very painful and is parchment like in appearance. These do not heal spontaneously and have to be excised and grafted. When the third degree burn is extensive, it gives rise to a systemic response, which may result in shock. If it is allowed to heal by itself, it may result in crippling contractures. These are seen due to prolonged contact with any of the agents causing second-degree burns as seen above.

Fourth Degree Burn (Fig. 26.7)

Involvement of tissues and structures beneath the skin such as muscles and bones signifies a fourth degree burn. These are obviously insensate and a charred appearance is seen. Classically seen due to molten metal, high voltage electrical burns and prolonged contact with flames.

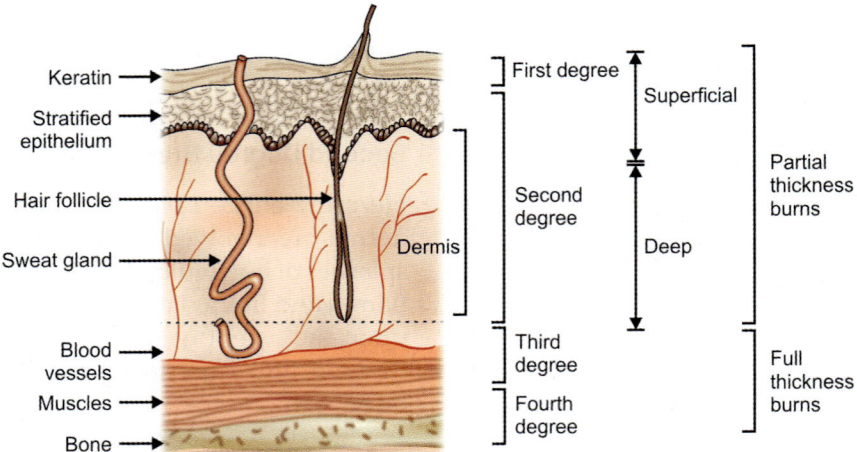

Fig. 26.2: Depth of burn in relation to level of skin

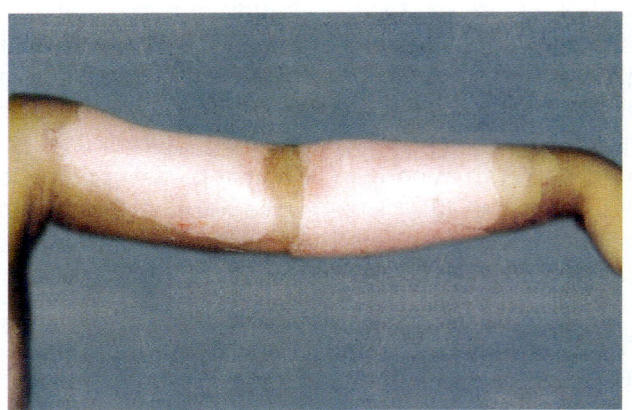

Fig. 26.3: Superficial burns of the arm and forearm

EXTENT OF BURN

TBSA burnt should be quantified early in assessment; it is the single most important factor for management and prognosis. There are various methods to calculate it:

1. **Rule of nines:** According to this algorithm—Head and neck comprise –9% of BSA, front and back of trunk –20% each, each arm–9%, front and back of leg –9% each and the remaining 1% is made up by the genitalia. This rule is quite reliable in patients who are >15 years old but is not suitable for use in children (Fig. 26.8).[5]

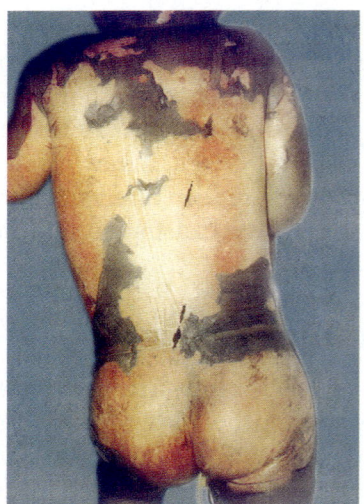

Fig. 26.4: Superficial partial thickness burns of the back of the chest

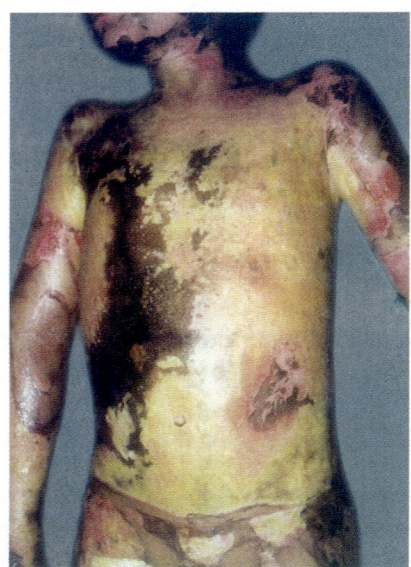

Fig. 26.5: Deep partial thickness burns of the chest

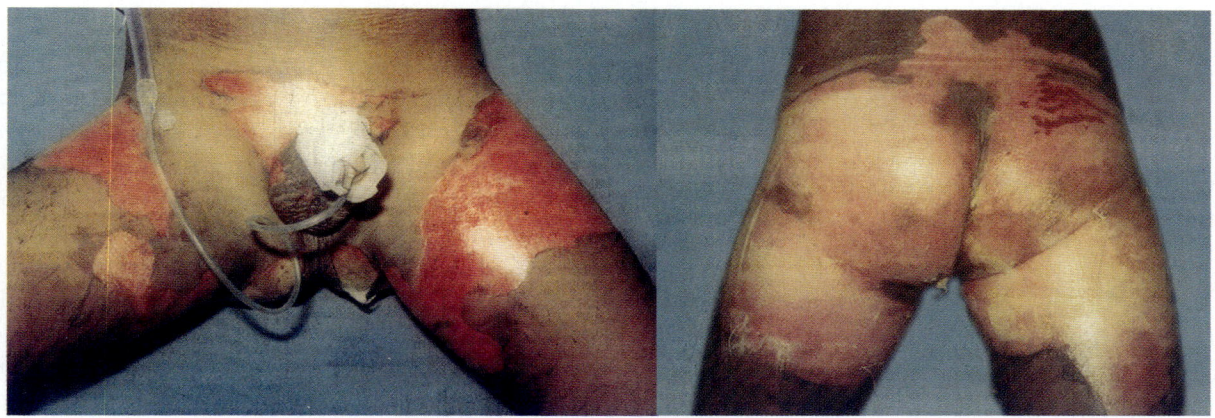

Fig. 26.6: Deep partial thickness burns of the thighs and gluteal region

Table 26.1: Browder chart to calculate TBSA[6]

	Age (in yrs)					
	0	1	5	10	15	Adult
Head	19	17	13	11	9	7
Neck	2	2	2	2	2	2
Antrunk	13	13	13	13	13	13
Post-trunk	13	13	13	13	13	13
Buttock	2.5	2.5	2.5	2.5	2.5	2.5
Genitalia	1	1	1	1	1	1
Upper arm	2.5	2.5	2.5	2.5	2.5	2.5
Lower arm	3	3	3	3	3	3
Hand	2.5	2.5	2.5	2.5	2.5	2.5
Thigh	5.5	6.5	8	8.5	9.0	9.5
Leg	5	5	5.5	6	6.5	7
Foot	3.5	3.5	3.5	3.8	3.5	3.5

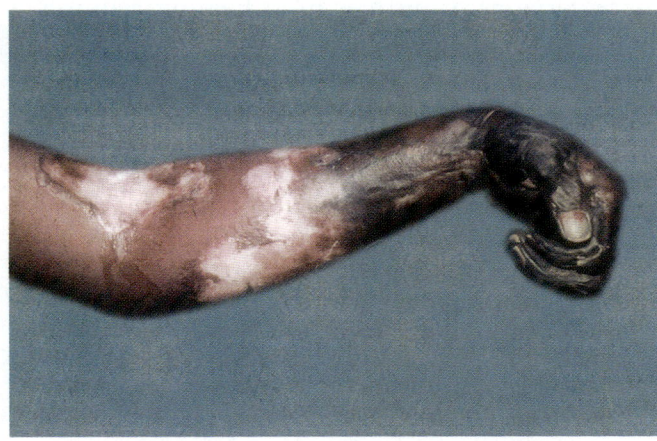

Fig. 26.7: Fourth degree deep burns of the forearm (electrical burns)

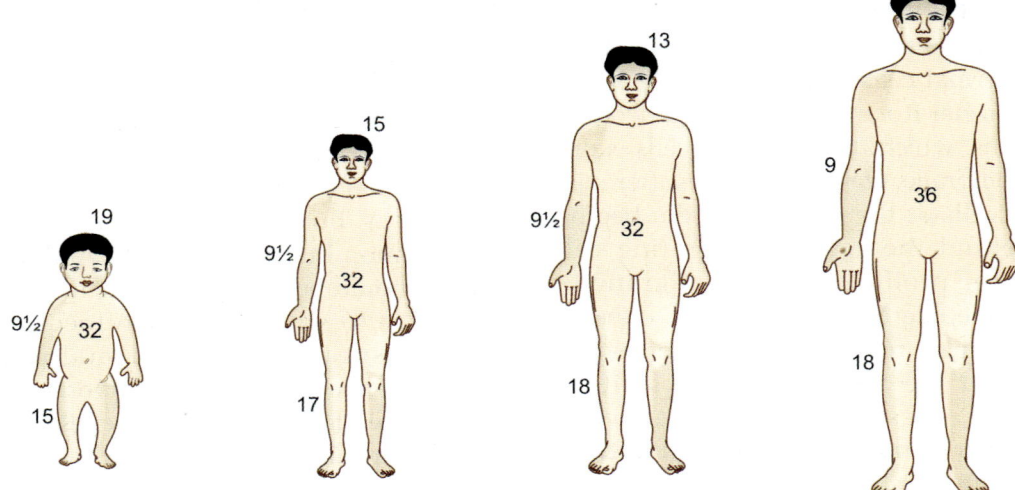

Fig. 26.8: Body surface area to estimate the area of burn

2. **According to palm hands:** A rough estimate of the BSA burnt can be made by the number of palm hands of the patient required to cover the area. Palm surface area roughly equals 1% across all age groups.
3. **Lund-Browder chart:** Allows for precise calculation of the BSA burnt across all age groups (Table 26.1).[6]

BURN WOUND HEALING

Skin is the largest organ in the body, with multi-structural and multi-functional components with regional variations. The ischemic, hypoxic and edematous burn wound takes a very slow course for healing compared to a traumatic wound. Unique characteristics of burn wound healing requires a thorough understanding of normal wound healing which is a very complex and dynamic process consisting of many co-ordinated cellular, biochemical molecular processes. The wound healing goes through phases of angiogenesis, granulation tissue formation, processes of matrix formation, remodeling and epithelialization to the formation of a scar.

Epithelialization

In a regular wound epithelialization begins within hours after injury. In superficial and superficial partial thickness burns epithelialization occurs spontaneously from the dermal remnants of hair follicle and sebaceous glands. In deep partial thickness burns the epidermal cells undergo phenotypic alteration at the margins of the normal skin and loose their adherence to one another and to the basement membrane, which allows for the lateral movement of epidermal cells. The migrating epidermal cells dissect the wound space separating the eschar from viable tissue guided by an array of integrins, which the migrating cells express on their cell membrane. One or two days after injury the epidermal cells at the wound margin begin to proliferate behind the actively migrating cells. The stimulus for proliferation and migration of epidermal cells is epidermal growth factor. If the area of the burn is large, re-epithelialization may not completely cover the raw wound and split skin grafting may be necessary to hasten the wound healing. In smaller burn areas, within ten to twelve days, epithelialization is complete and the burn wound gets closed.

Immunological Response to Burn Injury

Today it has been realized that in massively burnt patients (> 40% TBSA) chaotic cytokine array is responsible for higher mortality rate and not infection as was thought earlier. The appropriate term for the immunological failure that is seen is 'Systemic Inflammatory Response'. As soon as burn injury occurs, macrophage margination and activation occurs. This results in the release of three cytokines ILI, IL6 and TNF-alpha. Macrophages also produce products of lipid peroxidation namely leukotrienes and prostaglandins. All these are very toxic to the patient and these produce T cell failure, inhibit lymphocytes, hemoglobin synthesis and also depress the granulocyte colony formation.

Skin is recognized as the largest immune organ and the effect of heat could well figure in the origin of the pathophysiology encountered. The area of skin burnt quantitatively is related to mortality and cellular functional failure. This immune failure could be the cause of death in children during the shock phase, rather than infection.

EMERGENCY ROOM MANAGEMENT

The initial management of the severely burned patient follows the guidelines established by the Advanced Life Support course of the American College of Surgeons according to which, like any other trauma, airway and breathing assume the highest priority.

Airway and Breathing

Airway management is the first and the foremost priority as there is high incidence (up to 30%) of associated inhalational injury in a severely burnt patient which can be immediately life threatening.[7] Inhalational injury may be present with minimal cutaneous burns and may not be evident at presentation but can develop rapidly. Inhalational injury should be suspected if there is any history of exposure to smoke in a confined space, loss of consciousness, impaired mental status or disorientation and obtundation. Important clinical signs to be looked for are – any hoarseness of voice, stridor (impending airway obstruction), facial burns, singed nasal hair, wheezing and expectoration of black carbonaceous sputum. Affected patients should be given 100% oxygen by mask (to wash out carbon monoxide), oxygen saturation should be monitored and equipment kept ready for intubation. Ideally fibre-optic bronchoscopy should be done on any suspicion and signs such as airway edema, mucosal necrosis, hemorrhages, ulcers and pseudomembranous casts should be looked for. If any of these are present the patient should be intubated and respiratory care protocol established.[8]

The airway injury increases the surface area involved and triggers both local and systemic edema. The direct heat injury to the respiratory mucosa, together with chemical irritation, leads to sloughing of the mucosa and cast formation. The combination of this mechanical obstruction with atelectasis can lead to barotrauma and respiratory insufficiency. If the chest wall has been burned, full inspiratory effort may be restricted.[3]

The final point to be remembered is the fact that the burn patient could also be a victim of associated trauma, hence decreased levels of consciousness or oxygen desaturation should not be blamed only on burn shock or inhalation injury, but could be due to associated head injury.

Circulation and Intravenous Access

It is important to start two intravenous portals, one for infusing fluids and the other for giving drugs through the unburnt skin. Central line though ideal, may invite sepsis and could be disastrous and hence should be inserted only if required urgently. If the child has already gone into shock with falling blood pressure, then a central line must be started.

After appropriate initial stabilization, fluid resuscitation plays the most important role in patient care and survival. The abundance of formulae that have been derived to help the practitioner with management are a testament to this importance. Because of the large open areas of skin and leaky capillaries, the body requires enormous amounts of fluid to maintain adequate organ perfusion. Most practitioners use lactated Ringer's solution for resuscitation. Colloids are usually reserved for the second 24 hours.[3]

A Foley's catheter should be placed and urine output is used as the ultimate objective finding. In an adult, 0.5-1 mL per kilogram per hour of urine is a well-known marker for adequate end-organ perfusion.

In a child, the concentrating capacities of the kidney are less well developed, and 1-2 mL per kilogram per hour is recommended. Inhalation injury dramatically increases the fluid requirements.[3]

A nasogastric tube should be placed to drain the stomach. Stress ulcer prophylaxis with histamine-2 (H_2) receptor blockers and/or antacids is to be started.

Eliciting history for medicolegal purpose: To ensure proper epidemiological documentation and also for medicolegal records, a detailed history should be elicited from the conscious patient and in the case of children from the parents. This would enable implementation of preventive program.

Recording the weight of the patient: Recording of the weight of the burnt child is important for calculating and administering fluids and drugs. Ideally weight is recorded as soon as possible at the emergency room.

Investigations

Consider complete blood count, type and cross-match, carboxyhemoglobin (whenever suspected and feasible), coagulation studies, chemistry panel, arterial blood gases, and chest radiograph (which may not show changes for the first 24-72 hours).

Escharotomy and Fasciotomy

Burn eschar may act an inelastic constricting tourniquet impairing circulation and even respiration. This is seen generally in extremity and chest burns though can occur in neck and abdominal wall burns also. This phenomenon is seen only with deep second and third degree burns only. The constricting effect may not be there initially and develop later on during resuscitation; 8-24 hours period is most critical period. A frequent assessment of the peripheral perfusion can help in early diagnosis. Parameters to be checked are capillary filling time, pulses and oxygen saturation. Doppler can aid the diagnosis in difficult cases. For prevention, extremities with deep burns should be kept elevated and splinted in a functional position. In suspected vascular insufficiency, escharotomy should be performed at the earliest as delay and the subsequent reperfusion injury may have lethal consequences. This procedure involves an incision through the burn eschar to relieve the constriction caused by it. This procedure can be done at the bedside with an electrocautery with the patient under sedation, as the eschar is insensate. A rapid restoration of the circulation suggests a successful procedure; if the blood flow is still not restored then a consideration should be given to fasciotomy, i.e. incision of the deep fascia to alleviate the compartment syndrome.

FLUID RESUSCITATION IN PEDIATRIC BURNS

It is important to bear in mind that a burnt child continues to be a special challenge, since resuscitation therapy must be more precise than that for an adult with a similar burn. Important point to bear in mind is the fact that a burnt child requires intravenous resuscitation for a relatively smaller TBSA (10-20 %) unlike an adult. Primary goal of resuscitation is to support the child throughout the initial 24-48 hours period of hypovolemia that sets in due to extravascular fluid sequestration during postburn shock period.

A delay in fluid resuscitation not surprisingly is a major contributor to mortality in massive burns. Volume contraction due to fluid lost through the burn wound and into normal tissues as a result of increased systemic capillary permeability, when finally resuscitated, contribute to perfusion-reperfusion injury, thus activating neutrophils and releasing free radicals that could contribute to a systemic inflammatory response. The most significant contributor to mortality among the resuscitation measurements is not the amount of fluid given in the first 24 hours, but how soon after the injury fluid was started. The challenge that this represents to the burn community is to provide better communication to emergency care responders, emphasizing institution of resuscitation immediately during the treatment of the thermally injured.[2]

The pertinent questions are:
1. How much fluid should be infused?
2. What type of fluid should be infused?
3. Does the child belong to high-risk burns like inhalation burns, when they may require more fluids, for resuscitation?

Calculation of the Requirements

Cope and Moore in 1947 gave the first rational scheme of fluid resuscitation in burn patients. Though their formula is no longer in use all the modern formulas derive their basic scheme from their formula, i.e. requirements are calculated according to the extent of the burn and the weight of the patient, initially for the first 24 hours. Half of this amount is given in the initial 8 hours and the rest over next 16 hours. Though for adults Parkland's formula is the one that is in most common use, the only formula for calculation in pediatric burn patients is the one devised by Shriners Burn Hospital.[4] According to this formula:

For first 24 hours – Total fluid requirement is 5000 ml/m^2 TBSA burn + 2000 ml/m^2 as maintenance, 50% of this volume is given in initial 8 hours and the rest in ensuing 16 hours. Ringer's lactate is the fluid used for resuscitation.

Thereafter – 3750 ml/m^2 + 1500 ml/m^2 is used for next 24 hours; a part of total of it may be made up by the enteral feeds. Urine output of > 1 ml/kg/hr and stable vitals signify an adequate replacement.

Place of Colloid

There is a controversy regarding the use of colloids in the initial resuscitation scheme. It is known that the plasma proteins are extremely important in the circulation since they generate the inward oncotic force that counteracts the outward capillary hydrostatic force. But protein solutions are not given in the initial 16 hours, as they also leak through the dilated capillaries, and are no more effective than more salt water. After 16 hours, if colloids are added to the crystalloid regimen, the reversal from shock is phenomenal. Either fresh frozen plasma 0.5 - 1 ml/kg TBSA or 5% albumin can be given. A reasonable indication of giving albumin early on, i.e. after 8 hours is serum albumin less than 2 g%.[8]

Place of Whole Blood

In extensive third degree electric burns or in third degree burn over 50% TBSA, actual entrapment of RBC and cell death results in severe hypoxia. This situation can be reversed by whole blood transfusion and preferably fresh blood improves the situation better. Fresh whole blood transfusion is usually given. This can be combined with crystalloids.

Urine Output Monitoring

Measured volume bags are preferably used. Child should void 1 ml/kg/hr of urine if resuscitation is adequate.

Diuretics are generally not indicated during acute resuscitation period. But in children sustaining high voltage electrical burns with myoglobinuria/hemoglobinuria, there is increased risk of renal tubular obstruction. Forced alkaline diuresis is indicated in such situations with urine output as high as 3-5 ml/kg/hr. To alkalinize the urine, sodium bicarbonate is added, while an osmotic diuretic like mannitol achieves a high urine output.

PROBLEMS IN RESUSCITATION

It is important to identify acidosis. Electrolyte estimation must be done periodically and acidosis must be corrected without delay. There is a risk of hyponatremia and hyperkalemia early on.

Thermal injury results not only in massive fluid shifts that cause hypovolemia, but also in release of inflammatory mediators from burn wounds. These mediators deleteriously affect cardiovascular function and lead to burn shock. The end result of a complex chain of events is decreased intravascular volume, increased systemic vascular resistance, decreased cardiac output, end organ ischemic and metabolic acidosis. Without early and full resuscitation therapy these derangements progress to acute renal failure, cardiovascular collapse and death.

Resuscitation in itself is not without complications. Burn edema is worsened with resuscitation, particularly crystalloid solutions. The above given formulae are generalizations only; each child should get individualized treatment to avoid complications.

INFECTION CONTROL

Infection is the most common complication seen in the burn patients. Initially gram-positive organisms are the ones that cause sepsis but as early as 3 days post-burn gram-negative organisms start predominating. Systemic antibiotics are not recommended in burn patients for prevention of burn wound sepsis, as the burn tissue is a poorly perfused tissue. Also this practice leads to the emergence of resistant strains. They are certainly recommended in special circumstances such as:

- Perioperatively— Around the time of burn wound excision to limit the incidence of the bacteriemia. They should be guided by the quantitative burn wound cultures.
- Autografting— At the time of autografting to prevent local loss of the graft and also to prevent infection at the donor site. A first generation oral cephalosporin is good enough till the first dressing change if the cultures are not available.
- Infection elsewhere— In the presence of infection elsewhere such as pneumonitis, thrombophlebitis, urinary tract infection and sepsis, systemic antibiotics are obviously indicated.

Topical therapy is all that is required for most of the burn wounds. Appropriate topical therapy reduces microbial growth and chances of invasive sepsis. It should be soothing in nature, easy to apply and remove and should not have systemic toxicity. Such an ideal antimicrobial probably does not exist. The ones that are most commonly used are given in Table 26.2.[9]

DRESSINGS

Option of closed dressing and open dressing methods are available. In Open method, topical antimicrobials are applied and the wound is left open to warm dry air. *Pseudomonas* infections are rare but this method requires a strict environmental control and is painful. The fluid requirements also increase due to greater evaporative losses. This method is useful for facial and scalp burns. In closed dressings topical antimicrobial creams are applied and then covered with gauze dressings. This method is less painful though more labor intensive. Closed dressings are preferred for the extremities and over the back.

SURGICAL MANAGEMENT OF THE BURN WOUND

A proper assessment of the burn wound guides the choice of the surgical therapy.

First Degree Burn

As there is minimal loss of the barrier function of the skin, the infection and fluid loss are not common. Management aims at providing pain relief and optimal conditions for wound healing. Topical salves and oral analgesics are the only medications required.

Superficial Second Degree Burn

These require daily dressings with topical antimicrobials till spontaneous re-epithelialization

Table 26.2: Topical Antimicrobial Therapy in burns

Agent/Concentration	Application*	Advantages	Limitations
1. Liver sulfadiazine 1%	Twice a day open or closed	• Painless, easy application • Good spectrum • Poor absorption-systemic side • Long lasting action	• Transient leukopenia • Sensitivity reactions • Gram-negative organisms may be resistant • Poor penetration into eschar
2. Mafenide acetate 10%	Twice a day open or minimally closed	• Good penetration into eschar • wide spectrum • Resistance incommon	• Hypersensitivity common. • Metabolic acidosis on occur • Painful • Hemolytic anemia may occur
3. Silver nitrate 5%	Apply 4-8 times/day closed dressing	• Painless • Resistance incommon • No hypersensitivity	• Only surface action • Chances or electrolyte disturbances hyponatremia, hypokalemia • Messy dressings, staging of sheets, leads, floors
4. Cerium nitrate 2.2% + silver sulfadiazine 1%	Twice a day closed	Low systemic toxicity Useful in extensive burns	Same as silver sulfadiazine

* All the agents have a place in comprehensive burn wound management fragment rotation of agents (weekly) decreases the side effects and resistance

occurs in 10-21 days. Alternatively, temporary biological or synthetic dressings can be used.

Deep Second Degree and Third Degree Burns

Early burn wound excision has been shown to be beneficial in these types of burns.[8,10] Advantages are
1. Decrease rates of infection as dead and devitalized tissue is removed.
2. Removal of source of inflammatory mediators.
3. Decreased scarring and more functional rehabilitation.
4. Decreased stay in hospital.
5. Early excision (< 48 hours) is associated with less blood loss.

Two types of burn wound excisions are described
1. *Tangential excision:* Implies sequential excision of burnt skin layers to reach the viable tissue layer. It is more time consuming and is associated with more blood loss and requires a certain experience.
2. *Fascial excision:* This involves removal of all tissue down to the level of deep fascia. This procedure is technically easier and is associated with comparatively less blood loss. As this procedure is cosmetically disfiguring it should be used in only compelling situations such as life-threatening burn wound sepsis.

Blood loss during the surgery can be controlled by use of tourniquets, elevating the limb and local application of thrombin solution or epinephrine soaked pads.

Wound Coverage

After burn wound excision, the tissue bed consists of dermis and the subcutaneous fat. It is necessary to cover this raw area to promote healing and to provide for better cosmetic and functional outcome.

1. *Autograft:* Ideal coverage is the patient's own skin. It is generally possible to get enough split skin autograft in < 40% TBSA burns. Meshing allows more area to be covered and also allows for seepage of the exudates in the postoperative period. Maximum meshing allowed is 4:1. More meshing ultimately leads to more scarring; for this reason the grafts to be used on face and joints should preferably be not meshed.
2. *Autograft with allograft overlay:* If the autograft is inadequate a 4:1 or even 6:1 meshed autograft is used and over it 2:1 meshed allograft is placed. Allograft falls away as the autograft epithelializes

underneath. In massively burnt patients, rejection is not a major issue as there is profound immunosuppression. It is mandatory to screen the donor for HIV, CMV, HBV and HCV before using these grafts.

3. *Allograft:* Allograft can be used for temporary coverage of the wound till the donor sites heal and further grafts can be taken from them. Such situations can arise in massively burnt patients (> 40% TBSA).
4. *Xenograft:* Porcine skin is readily available and it resembles human skin morphologically. It adheres well to the dermis and then is gradually degraded; the main drawback is its inability to prevent infection.
5. *Amniotic membrane:* Amniotic membrane can provide an excellent temporary biological coverage till more autograft is available (Figs 26.9 to 26.11). It is freely available, is non-antigenic and has some infection resisting properties. Cord blood sample should be tested for HIV, CMV, HBV and HCV prior to its use.
6. *Synthetic dressings:* Various biologically engineered membranes such as keratinocyte sheets, silicon mesh with porcine or human collagen and silicon mesh with fetal keratinocytes are available in the west but their cost and availability still precludes common clinical use.[8]

Reasons for the non take-up of grafts:
1. Fluid collections underneath the grafts— Meticulous hemostasis, meshing and good pressure dressings help prevent this complication.
2. Shearing stress on the grafted surfaces— It can be prevented by proper immobilization and splinting.

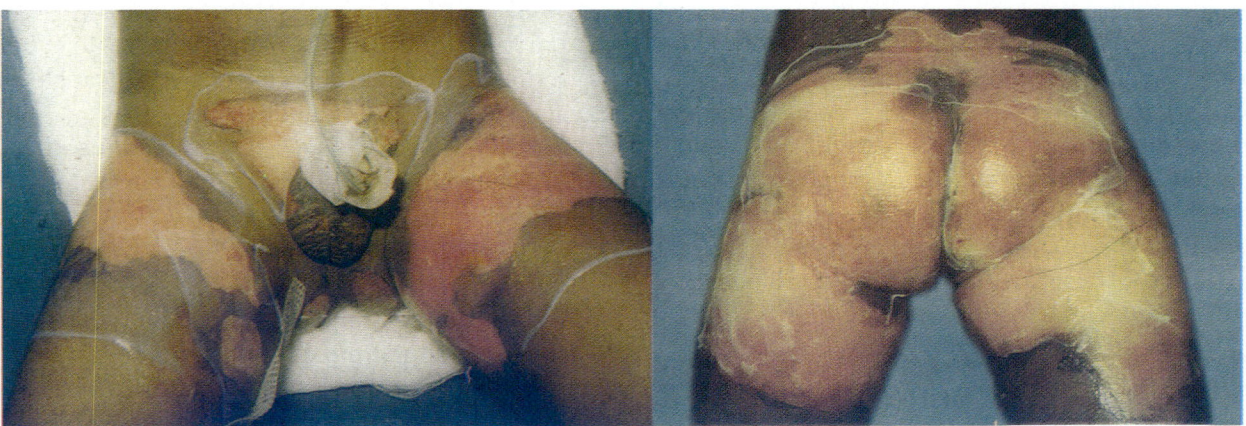

Fig. 26.9: Membrane applied over the areas after cleaning the wound

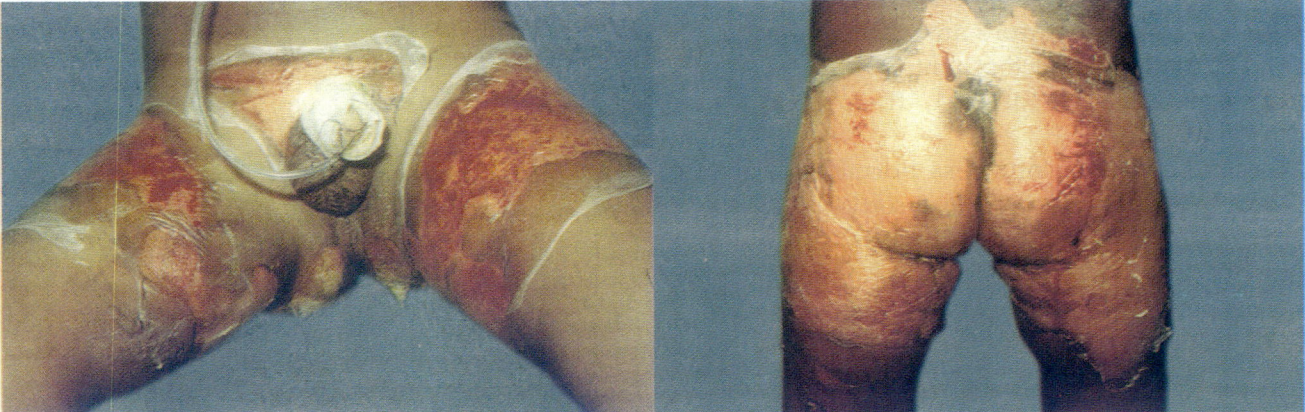

Fig. 26.10: Sixth day after membrane application

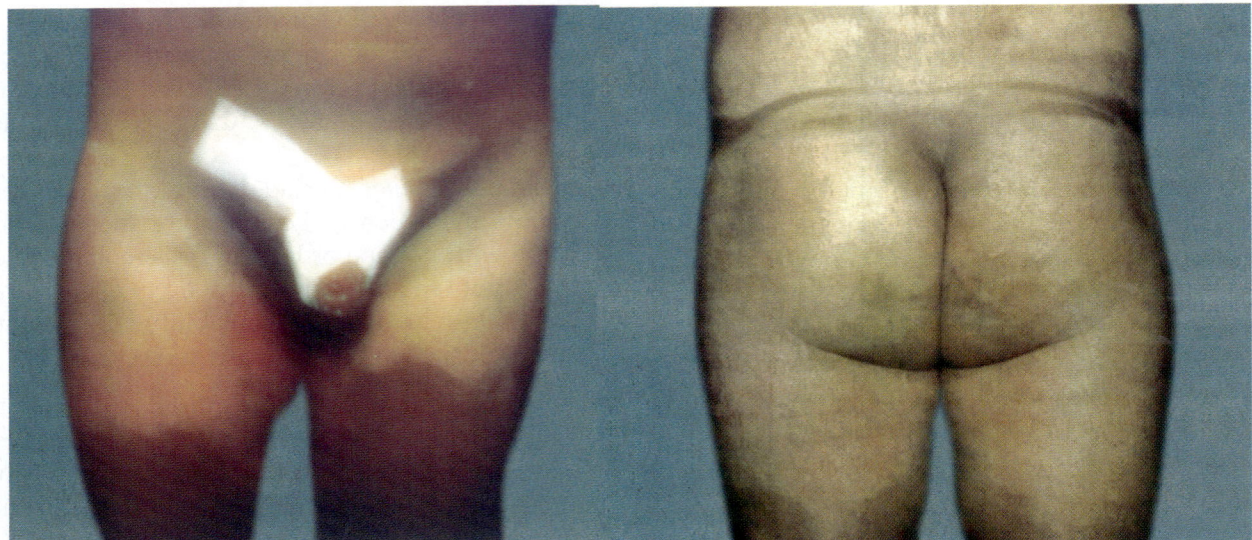

Fig. 26.11: Three weeks after membrane separation and epithelialization

3. Infection— Good perioperative antibiotic cover based on cultures should be used.
4. Residual necrotic tissue in the bed – Adequate excision takes care of this aspect.

Proper care of the donor sites to allow for reuse cannot be overemphasized, as every inch of the skin is precious. Donor area if not properly cared for behaves in the same way as a second degree burn.

HYPERMETABOLIC RESPONSE AND NUTRITION

Hypermetabolic Response

Burns > 40% TBSA cause a tremendous increase in the resting energy expenditure amounting to even 50-100%.[6] The following factors contribute
- Increased release of IL-1, IL-2, TNF-alpha, thromboxanes
- Increased release of stress hormones such as catecholamines, glucagon and cortisol.

All these promote systemic vasoconstriction and may lead to renal and mesenteric ischemia. This hypermetabolic response can be modified to improve the outcome:[8]

1. Ambient temperature should be kept between 28-30 °C.
2. Early enteral nutrition in the postburn period reduces the incidences of bacterial translocation and counters the catabolic state.
3. Beta-blockers can block the deleterious effects of catecholamines to decrease the heart rate and the cardiac output.[11]
4. Growth hormone has also been shown to help in catch up growth by fostering a positive nitrogen balance. It also improves immunity and helps in faster healing at the donor sites.[12]
5. Adequate pain relief also helps in decreasing the stress response. Specially during dressing changes intravenous pethidine can make dressing changes less distressful for these sick children.

Nutrition

Early establishment of enteral feeds as soon as the child is stabilized via a nasogastric tube decreases the metabolic rate, gastric atrophy, stress ulceration and bacterial translocation.[13] Parenteral nutrition leads to more chances of systemic sepsis, thus enteral route with all its advantages is preferred.[14] An adequate calorie intake provided as 40-70% carbohydrates, 10-20% fats and 20-40% protein should be the goal. Calorie requirement is calculated according to the Shriners Burn Institute formulas.[8]

- Infant formula – 1800 kcal/m² maintenance + 1000 kcal/m² area burnt
- For 1-11 years – 1800 kcal/m² maintenance + 1300 kcal/m² area burnt
- > 12 years – 1500 kcal/m² maintenance + 1500 kcal/m² area burnt

COMPLICATIONS AND REHABILITATION

Apart from the myriad acute metabolic and systemic complications the burn patient might experience, the following complications deserve a special mention.

1. **Burn wound sepsis:** Burn wound sepsis is indicated by change of the color to black or dark brown, hemorrhage of the fat underlying the eschar, progression of the partial thickness injury to full thickness, dirty foul smelling exudates, premature separation of eschar or appearance of eruptions. Treatment involves change of topical antibiotics, systemic antibiotics and excision of the burn wound.
2. **Pulmonary complications:** Inhalational injury as such and other conditions like profound immunosuppression, systemic sepsis and ventilation predispose the burnt patient to pneumonia. Management includes judicious use of antibiotics, aggressive physiotherapy and respiratory care.
3. **Gastrointestinal complications:** Hypokalemia in the acute phase, sepsis, hypovolemia all contribute towards ileus in the postburn period. Management includes nasogastric suction and correction of underlying etiology. Gastric ulceration and bleeding- Curling's ulcers are also common due to impaired perfusion and the stress response. Antacids are no longer recommended for prevention as these increase gastric pH and colonization of the stomach. Sucralfate and early enteral feeds are the strategies that are most helpful.
4. **Orthopedic complications:** Osteomyelitis, non-healing fractures, ulcers and heterotrophic calcification are also common.

LONG-TERM COMPLICATIONS

Hypertrophic scar: It is the phase of redness and induration that is seen during the healing phase of deep second degree and third degree burns. Spontaneous resolution occurs in most of the cases. Pruritus associated with these scars can be managed by local application of emollients, 1% hydrocortisone ointment, local triamcinolone injection or systemic anti-histaminics. Pressure garments also help in fast resolution.

Contractures: Burns occuring at the flexor aspects of joints and if deep are especially prone to develop contractures during the healing phase. All scars and split skin grafts have a tendency to shrink, and this tendency is more with thin grafts. Contractures are best prevented by
- Use of thick grafts at the joints.
- Splinting the joints for three months in a functional position after grafting (while keeping in mind that prolonged splinting may cause periarticular fibrosis and joint capsule contractures).
- Pressure garments and silicone gel dressings provide a uniform pressure over the healing area and thus may help in prevention of contractures.

Established contractures require surgical management:
- Local re-arrangement of skin as single or multiple Z-plasties
- Free grafts— A thick free graft can be placed after the excision of the contractures is small. For a large contracture a relaxing incision is given at the site of maximum tension and a free graft is placed in the resulting defect
- Flaps— Full thickness flaps that can be pedicled or myocutaneous flaps can be utilized to release the contractures.
- Tissue expanders— It can be used to expand the nearby normal full thickness skin which can then be used as a rotational flap to release the contracture.

REHABILITATION

Burns produce a severe psychological set back in many individuals and especially in children. Their proper growth and development depends upon their psychological rehabilitation. Nurses and medical staff must be children friendly.

Social rehabilitation also has to be emphasized. They must be accepted by the society at large. Occupational therapy and rehabilitation form an integral part of burn therapy.

REFERENCES

1. Thombs BD, Singh VA, Milner SM. Children under 4 years are at greater risk of mortality following acute burn injury. Shock 2006;26(4):348-52.

2. Wolf SE, Rose JK, Desai MH, Mileski JP, Barrow RE, Herndon DN. Mortality Determinants in Massive Pediatric Burns. Ann Surg 1997;225(5):554-69.
3. Garner WL, Magee W. Acute Burn Injury. Clin Plastic Surg 2005;32:187-93.
4. Monafo WW. Initial management of burns. N Engl J Med 1996;335:1581-86.
5. Lund CC, Browder NC. The estimation of the areas of burns. Surg Gynecol Obstet 1944;79:352.
6. Eichelberger MR. Pediatric trauma. Prevention, acute care, rehabilitation. St Louis 1993, Mosby.
7. Herndon DN, Thompson PB, Traber DL. Pulmonary injury in burned patients. Crit Care Clin 1985;1:79.
8. Herndon DN, Spies M. Modern burn care. Sem Pediatr Surg 2001;10(1):28.
9. Trunkey DD, Lewis FR. Current Therapy of Trauma. ed3, St Louis 1993, Mosby.
10. Thompson P, Herndon DN, Abston S, et al. Effect of early excision on patients with major thermal injury. J Trauma 1986;27:205.
11. Honeycutt D, Barrow RE, Herndon DN. Cold stress response in patients with severe burns after beta-blockage. J Burn Care Rehab 1992;13:181.
12. Ramzy PI, Wolf SE, Herndon DN. Current status of anabolic hormone administration in human burn injury. J Parenter Enteral Nutr 1999;23:S190.
13. Herndon DN, Zieglet ST. Bacterial translocation after thermal injury. Crit Care Med 1993;21:550.
14. Herndon DN. Increased mortality with intravenous supplemental feeding in severely burned patients. J Burn Care Rehab 1989;10:309.

CHAPTER 27

Traumatic Hemobilia in Children

Shilpa Sharma, DK Gupta

Hemorrhage into the gastrointestinal tract due to abnormal communication of blood vessels with intra- or extra-hepatic biliary tract is called hemobilia. In some rare occasions, communication occurs between the branches of cystic artery and the lumen of gallbladder as in necrotising cholecystitis or trauma, leading to hemobilia.

'Bilhemia' is relatively a similar condition where low pressure venous communication leads to flow of bile into the venous circulation leading to a rapidly developing jaundice.

Bleeding into gastrointestinal tract secondary to an enterobiliary fistula is excluded from the definition of hemobilia by Sandblom.[1] Since traumatic hemobilia is not a common entity in the pediatric population, it should be managed in a specialized institution.[2]

Traumatic hemobilia has been described following both blunt and penetrating liver trauma, though the incidence is low in children as compared to adults.[3-13]

Surgical trauma is the commonest cause of hemobilia that includes therapeutic or diagnostic transparenchymal maneuvers (PTC, biopsy, etc.). Non-surgical trauma includes both blunt or penetrating liver injuries and the reported incidence of hemobilia is 1-1.5% of all hepatic traumas (Grade 2-Grade 5). Blunt trauma 1.8% and penetrating trauma accounts for 1%.

PATHOPHYSIOLOGY

Sandblom with his experimental model tried to explain the pathophysiology of post-traumatic hemobilia.[1]
1. Intrahepatic biliary leak causes lysis of clot and erosion of damaged arterial wall.
2. Formation of hepatic artery pseudo-aneurysm that later ruptures into adjacent biliary radical leads to hemobilia.

Surgical closure of liver laceration at initial presentation following trauma may lead to creation of arteriobiliary fistula leading to hemobilia.

CLINICAL PRESENTATION

Traumatic hemobilia is an unusual complication following liver injury characterized by triad of gastrointestinal hemorrhage, biliary colic and jaundice. The biliary colic may present as pain in the right hypochondrium. The gastrointestinal hemorrhage may present as melena or hematemesis. One should always elicit an antecedent history of trauma.

Hemobilia usually manifests by 7-10 days following trauma but a review of literature records hemobilia from 1 day-3.5 years after injury caused by communications between intrahepatic blood vessels and the biliary tree.[14] Thus, one should keep in mind that occasionally hemobilia may present even days or months after the injury.[15,16]

The differential diagnosis includes other causes of enterorrhagia, obstructive jaundice and anemia specially in those cases who have delayed and atypical presentation with jaundice or progressive anemia with or without melena/hematemesis and have doubtful history of antecedent trauma to correlate. In the long-term, patients may present with complications like biliary tract stricture, calculi, sludge or cholangitis.

INVESTIGATIONS

The diagnosis may be suspected on clinical grounds and verified by a combination of various modalities.[2]

Duodenoscopy, CT scan abdomen, USG with Doppler, hepatobiliary scintigraphy, ERCP, MRI and MR angiography and cavitogram have their own specific roles and are very useful for corroborative evidence, comprehensive evaluation and follow-up in the management of hemobilia.

A large number of modalities are required for quick diagnosis and localization of site of hemobilia. Thus, patients of traumatic hemobilia should be treated in a multidisciplinary tertiary care center.

Quick diagnosis is warranted for localization and control of bleed as mortality increases with the delay. Delay also leads to infective complication of intrahepatic bile leak that further aggravates the morbidity.

Ultrasonography and Color Doppler

Ultrasonography with color Doppler study detects any space occupying lesion in liver, aneurysm arising from hepatic arteries/branches, biliary clots and site of liver injury. But fails to visualise site of bleed.

Upper GI Endoscopy

With the advent of side viewing pediatric scopes, it is now possible to visualise active bleed from the papilla. It also rules out other causes of upper GI hemorrhage.

Endoscopic Retrograde Cholangiopancreatography (ERCP)

The role and value of endoscopic retrograde cholangiopancreatography (ERCP) in the pediatric age group is increasing though at a slow pace. Presence of hemobilia is an indication for ERCP.[17] In select group of patients, it can delineate the rent in the biliary radical, posthemobilia clots in CBD and gallbladder and post-traumatic stricture in bitte duct. Endoscopic retrograde cholangiopancreatography (ERCP) revealed biliary leak in right duct in 14 (70%) and in left duct in six (30%) patients in a series.[18] Endoscopic treatment with nasobiliary drainage without sphincterotomy has been reported as the optimal method of management of traumatic hepatobiliary injuries in hemodynamically stable patients from a series of 20 patients out of which 7 were children.[18] Transient mild pancreatitis may occur as a complication of ERCP.[17]

Angiography

Selective hepatic artery angiography is the investigation of choice, as it visualises the site of bleed and offers opportunity to embolise the bleeder and achieve early control of the bleed which otherwise can be life threatening many a times. An intrahepatic false aneurysm in a ten-year-old boy with post-traumatic hemobilia has been successfully embolized during diagnostic angiogram.[19] Selective angiography during episode of active bleeding not only confirms the diagnosis but also localises the site of bleeding and helps controlling it by embolization.[20]

Radionuclide Scans

HIDA scan may show visualization of biliary radicals without tracer pooling and non-excretion to gut due to rapid recycling through vascular communication. Blood pool scan helps in visualizing site of active bleed from GIT and liver, but is inferior to angiography in localisation.

Blood pool scintigraphy of the liver demonstrated accumulation in the central part of the right liver lobe in a 9-year-old girl with severe hemobilia developing one week following surgical evacuation of the subcapsular hematoma due to blunt abdominal trauma.[21] The blood pool scan was also helpful in the post-treatment evaluation as it became normal after embolization of the right hepatic artery.[21]

MRI and MR Angiography

MR angiography has been used to detect active bleeding from the parenchymal injury site and clots.[15] Its useful in identifying the vascular lesions causing hemobilia. MRI angiography has been reported to reveal a ruptured pseudoaneurysm of the ramus dexter of the proper hepatic artery that was successfully treated with embolization.[15]

Contrast Enhanced CT Scan

It is usually done for initial assessment of severity of visceral trauma (Fig. 27.1A). Spiral CT helps in delineating vascular and biliary anatomy, localization of site and any intrahepatic cavity formation.

MANAGEMENT

There is considerable controversy with regard to the management of traumatic hemobilia.

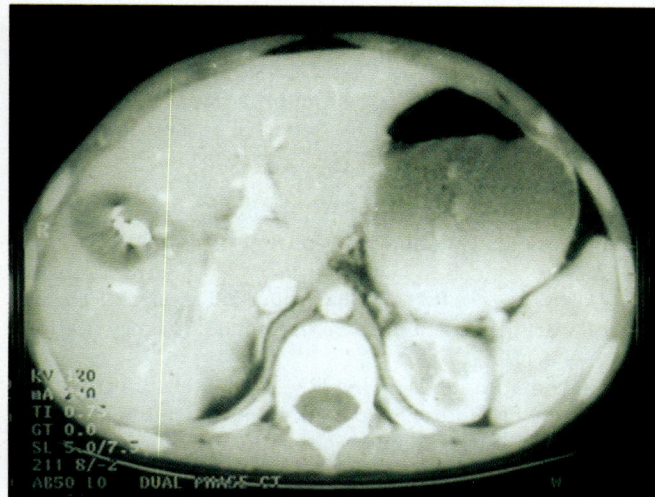

Fig. 27.1A: CT scan of a child with post-traumatic hemobilia demonstrating an intrahepatic cavity

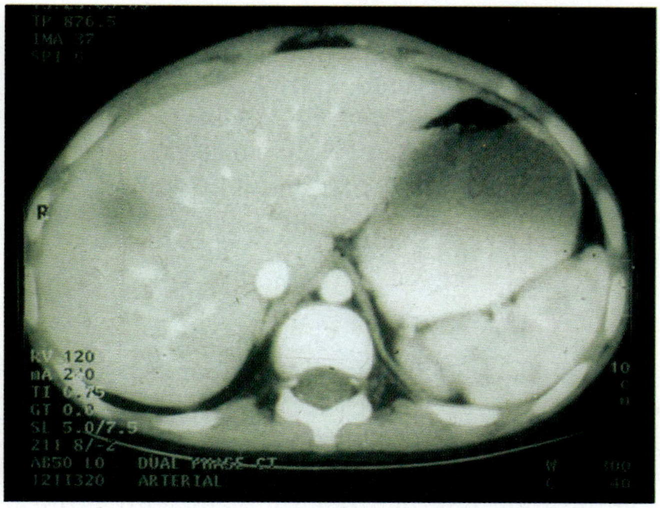

Fig. 27.1B: CT scan of the same child with post-traumatic hemobilia demonstrating a coil embolized into the pseudoaneurysm

Non-surgical Treatment

Non-operative management has become the therapeutic method of choice in hemodynamically stable patients with liver trauma.

There are a few reports of endoscopic management of traumatic hepatobiliary injuries.[18]

Successful non-operative management with repeated angiographic monitoring has been reported in cases in which the bleeding is not massive (< 50% blood volume replacement). However, a mortality of 60-70% has been reported with this approach in literature.[22,23]

Angiographic Embolization

Angiographic embolization has been the preferred treatment in recent years.[24-27] However, 20-30% of cases show recurrences (usually 2-3 weeks postembolization) after an average of two to three attempts.[26]

Arterial embolization is done after placing appropriate catheters as close as possible to the bleeding site (Fig. 27.1B). Embolizing materials used are gelfoam, polyvinyl alcohol particles or steel coils, alone or in combination.[27] Postembolization angiography may be performed to confirm adequacy of embolization. Surgery may be indicated in cases of failed embolization. Angiographic embolization has been reported as an effective treatment with a low complication rate to stop liver hemorrhage.[28] However, few notable complications have been reported like gallbladder infarction.[27]

Surgical Management

Surgical options include hepatotomy with suture ligation of bleeder and repair of biliary rent if feasible, ligation of hepatic artery or its branch, segmentectomy and lobectomy.

Early intervention and direct sulture ligation of bleeding vessels or procedures like lobectomy or segmentectomy have not been reported as encouraging in a immediate post-traumatic situation with high morbidity and recurrence.[16,23] Ligation of common hepatic artery or one of its branches, although a simple procedure, also has a significant morbidity and recurrence rate. Ischemia and sepsis are main complications often requiring formal lobectomy.[29]

Surgical management of traumatic hemobilia by direct ligation of the bleeding vessel has also been done successfully in children without postoperative problems.[4] The authors have had to resort to surgical management in a 10-year-old patient with hemobilia with two failed attempts of angiographic embolization with gelfoam and coils and one attempt of percutaneous embolization of a pseudoaneurysm under ultrasound guidance to control the bleed. Thus failure of embolization techniques with recurrence of massive gastrointestinal bleeding are an indication of early surgical intervention.

Hepatotomy may be done for exact visualization of the rent. Suture ligation of the bleeding vessel and repair of biliary rent may be done under vision. Closure of the hepatic cavity may be done with gelfoam.

FOLLOW-UP

A close follow-up of these children for recurrence or complications, should be kept in practice, so that any recurrence after 2-3 attempts of embolization treatment or development of septic/ischemic complication will be urgently dealt with surgical management. Because these patients carry a higher incidence of morbidity and mortality, further prolongation of conservative methods is not advisable.

Investigations like color doppler ultrasound and contrast-enhanced computed tomography may be done to assess the post-treatment status of the patient. Blood pool scintigraphy of the liver may also be helpful. Long-term observation of cases of traumatic hemobilia for development of post-hemobilia complications like cholelithiasis, stricture, sludge or stone in CBD is recommended.

SUMMARY

Traumatic hemobilia is an unusual but life threatening complication following liver trauma. Any patient with suspected diagnosis of traumatic hemobilia should be managed in a multidisciplinary institutionalized care where facilities of pediatric endoscopy angiography, embolization, hepatobiliary scan and none the less MRI and CT scan should be available. Initial stabilization with blood transfusions if required and angiographic embolization is the initial preferred treatment.

REFERENCES

1. Sandblom P. Hemorrhage into the biliary tract following trauma – 'traumatic hemobilia' Surgery 1948;24:571-86.
2. Giest H, Wolff H, Mau H, et al. Post-traumatic hemobilia in childhood. Zentralbl Chir 1991;116(11):683-90.
3. Gupta LB, Puri AS.Management of traumatic hemobilia with embolization. Indian Pediatr 2006;43(9):825-27.
4. Bajpai M, Bhatnagar V, Mitra DK, Upadhyaya P. Surgical management of traumatic hemobilia in children by direct ligation of the bleeding vessel: J Pediatr Surg 1989;24(5):436-37.
5. Bazzoni-C, Serini-M, Ongari-M, Sguazzini-C, Alleva-M, Lombardi-C. Massive hemobilia caused by necrotic hemorrhagic cholecystitis. Report of a case. Minerva-Chir 1993;48(15-16):887-60.
6. Martin A Croce, Timothy C, Fabian, Jon P Spiers, Kenneth A, Kudsk. Traumatic hepatic artery pseudoaneurysm with hemobilia. The american journal of surgery 1994;168: 235-38.
7. Geis WO. Schultz KA, Gliacchino JL, Freeark RJ. The fate of unruptured hepatic hematomas. Surgery 1981;90: 689-96.
8. Giacomantonio M, Filler RM, Rich RH. Blunt hepatic trauma in children: experience with operative and non-operative management. Journal of Pediatric Surgery 1984;19:519-22.
9. Mac Gillivray DC, Valentine J. Non-operative management of blunt pediatric liver injury–late complications: case report. Journal of Trauma 1989;29:251-54.
10. Stone HH, Ansley JD. Management of liver trauma in children. Journal of Pediatric Surgery 1977;12:3-10.
11. Farron F, Gudinchet F, Genton N. Hepatic Trauma in children: Long-term follow up. Eur J Pediatr Surg 1996;6:347-49.
12. Steiner Z, Brown RA, Jamieson DH, Millar AJ, Cywes S. Management of hemobilia and persistent biliary fistula after blunt liver trauma. J Pediatr Surg 1994;29(12):1575-77.
13. Vallidis E, Paplexandris N. Traumatic hemobilia. Br J Surg 1975,62:234-35.
14. Edward R. Howard. Surgery of liver disease in children Ist ed 1991;220-21.
15. Werner JE, Wijnen RM, Schultze Kool LJ, Rieu PN. A child with traumatic Hemobilia. Ned Tijdschr Geneeskd 2004;26;148(26):1297-300.
16. Fish JC, Nippert RH. Traumatic hemobilia: The dilemma of delay. J Trauma 1969;9:546-53.
17. Issa H, Al-Haddad A, Al-Salem AH. Diagnostic and therapeutic ERCP in the pediatric age group: Pediatr Surg Int 2007;23:111-16.
18. Singh V, Narasimhan KL, Verma GR, et al. Endoscopic management of traumatic hepatobiliary injuries. J Gastroenterol Hepatol 2007;22:1205-1209.
19. Brunelle F, Maurage C, Lacombe A, et al. Emergency embolisation in post traumatic hemobilia in a child. J Pediatr Surg 1985;20:172-74.
20. Hirsch M, Avinoach I, Keynan A, et al. Angiographic diagnosis and treatment of hemobilia. Radiology 1982;144:771-72.
21. Nielsen SL, Mygind T, Miskowiak J. Blood pool scintigraphy and arterial embolization in traumatic hemobilia: Eur J Nucl Med 1982;7(8):389-90.
22. Hendren WH, Warshaw AL, Fleischli DJ, Barlett MK. Traumatic Hemobilia: on operative management with healing documented by serial angiography. Annals of Surgery 1971;174:991-93.

23. Reinhardt GF, Hubay CA. Surgical management of traumatic hemobilia. Am J Surg 1971;121:328-33.
24. Lee M, Himal HS. Hemobilia – Successful treatment by angiographic embolization. Surg Endosc 1992;6(2):75-77.
25. Baumgartner FJ, Moore TC, Klein SR. Angiographic embolization of post-traumatic hemobilia in a six-year-old boy. Dig Dis Sci 1990;35(2):261-62.
26. Hidalgo F, Marvaex JA, Rene M, et al. Treatment of hemobilia with selective hepatic artery embolization. ®J Vasc Interv Radiol 1995;6(5):793-98.
27. Srivastava DN, Sharma S, Pal S, et al. Transcatheter arterial embolization in the management of hemobilia. Abdom Imaging 2006;31(4):439-48.
28. Laopaiboon V, Aphinives C, Pongsuwan P, et al. Hepatic artery embolization to control liver hemorrhages by interventional radiologists: experiences from Khon Kaen University. J Med Assoc Thai 2006;89:384-89.
29. Wiulkinson GM, Mikkelsen WP, Berne CJ. The treatment of post-traumatic hemobilia by ligation of the common hepatic artery. Surg Clin North Am 1968;48:1337-46.

SECTION 3

Thoracic Surgery

Gastroesophageal Reflux in Children

J Boix-Ochoa

"Biography is the only true history;" the history of gastroesophageal reflux borrows from the biographies of many remarkable names, including Bettex, Nissen, Billard, Chevalier Jackson, Allison and Barrett- more of whom later.

In this chapter, the current thinking on gastroesophageal reflux (GER) will be explored, but first it is necessary to describe the condition, to relate its definition to the important parameters, and outline those facets which are particularly significant to patients in the pediatric age-group.

DEFINITION

GER may be a physiological phenomenon, but in clinical practice may well prove to be pathological, (esophagitis, peptic esophagitis, or the more severe erosive esophagitis). From a pediatric point of view, its importance is related to its frequency, and potential for creating serious problems. It is generally agreed that there is a sphincteric mechanism at the lower end of the esophagus. Although its exact nature is unclear, its main function is to prevent gastric contents from passing proximally into the esophagus. Recent studies have shown that the proximal passage of gastric contents is not always pathological but, under certain circumstances, may result in morbidity, even mortality, more often than not resulting from pathological changes in the esophagus itself.

But in addition, there may be an anatomical component, as well as physiological and pathological components (potential or otherwise), and it is therefore relevant to consider problems at the gastroesophageal junction in terms of:[1,2]

1. The physiological problem (GER) which is a direct result of sphincteric incompetence.
2. The anatomical problem. whereby a hiatus hernia is present and the gastroesophageal junction (GEJ) is situated at a level higher than normal.
3. The pathological problem, esophagitis, which is secondary to GER, and this may be erosive or nonerosive, and recent evidence has shown to include both acid and alkaline components.

This concept of division of the problems at the GEJ into these three components is particularly valuable in discussions with the parents of infants with GER, and in all teaching programs.

RELEVANT ANATOMY AND PHYSIOLOGY

It is impossible to understand the mechanisms responsible for gastroesophageal reflux without a knowledge of the relevant anatomy, and this must, whenever possible, be correlated with information on both normal and abnormal physiology.[3]

There are three anatomical components: The esophagus, which acts as the pump; the lower esophageal sphincter, which is effectively the valve: and below this, the stomach, which is the reservoir. The esophagus has an intra-thoracic component and a short, but extremely important, intra-abdominal component. The lower end of the esophagus, where it passes through the hiatus in the diaphragm, is somewhat dilated, and this is referred to as the phrenic ampulla. The very important lower esophageal sphincter is comprised of elements from the muscular mantle of the tubular esophagus, with contributions from the inner layer of the esophagus and the external layer, the latter diverging in a fan-shape leading distally to the high-pressure zone. In addition, there is the gastric sling, which is part of the muscle of the greater curvature of the stomach, helping to build the angle of His (Fig. 28.1).

Boix-Ochoa points out that the high-pressure zone in the lower esophagus is only 0.8 cm at 27 weeks' gestation, but reaches a length of 1.0 cm at term. He stresses the "trinity" of factors responsible for the antireflux mechanism (Fig. 28.2).

1. The length of the intra-abdominal esophagus; (Fig. 28.3)
2. The gastroesophageal angle;
3. The crural fibers of the diaphragm and their pinch-cock action.

As a consequence of these factors, the inspiratory decrease in intra-thoracic pressure and the increase in intra-abdominal pressure are counter-acted.

But there is a fourth factor: The phrenoesophageal membrane, which is not a ligament but a fibroelastic membrane which holds the fundus and lower esophagus in place.

All these factors should be -and usually are -taken into account when surgical measures are adapted to re-establish gastroesophageal competence and combat GER.[4]

Whenever, possible, anatomical factors must be correlated with physiological factors, and here the functional capability of an intact LES is vital (Fig. 28.4). A deficient LES does not allow development of the normal physiological mechanisms designed to prevent GER.

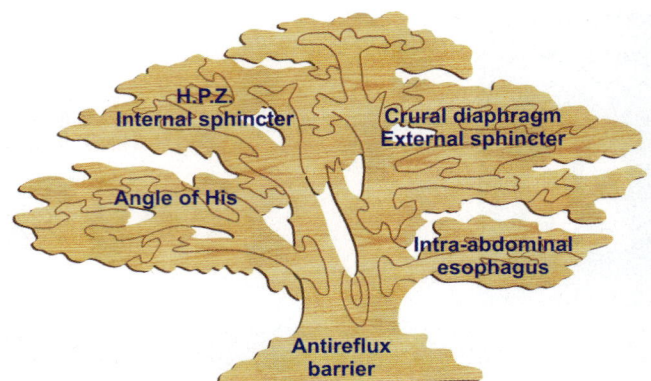

Fig. 28.2: The antireflux barrier is the interaction of different factors. This anatomic and physiologic interplay constitutes the antireflux mechanisms

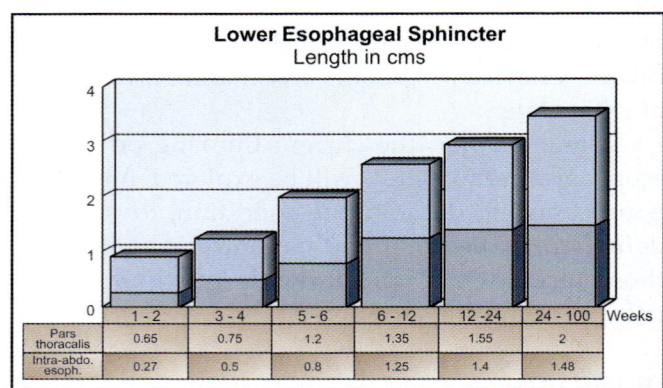

Fig. 28.3: The cornerstone of the GER mechanisms is the lower esophageal sphincter with its intra-abdominal segment, the quality of this segment is balanced with a longer intrathoracic segment to compensate in the some way for its apparent weakness

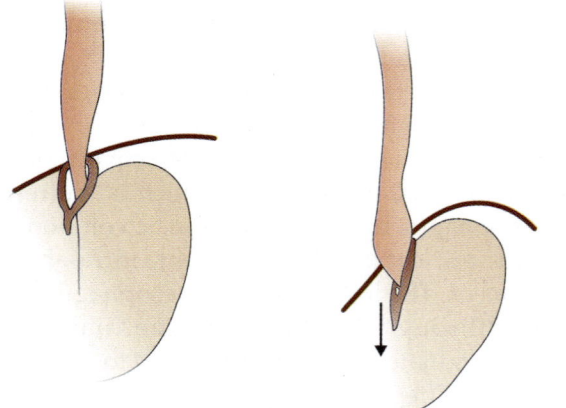

Fig. 28.1: The phrenoesophageal ligament anchors the distal esophagus to the crural diaphragm, therefore contraction of the crural diaphragm (respiration) exerts with the sling fibers of the right crus a pinch-cock-like action on the LES producing a mucosal flap valve preventing the GER

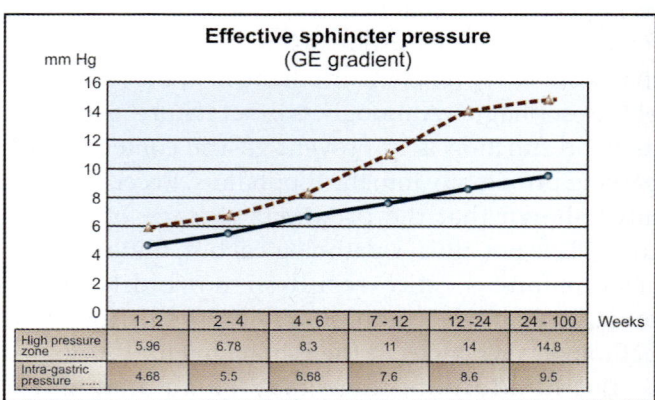

Fig. 28.4: High pressure zone: When the LES barrier is challenged by an increase of intragastric pressure it responds by active contraction exceeding the increase, which shows we are before a dynamic response which increases the tone of the area (HPZ) independently from any other factors

Boix-Ochoa carried out extensive studies on premature babies (4028 cases in all) and found that they have low LES pressure -a fact which correlates well with clinical experience.[4-7]

Of further anatomical significance is the demonstrable asymmetry of the muscular thickness of the GEJ, and the finding that, with an increase in the thickness of the inner circular muscle, this is continuous with the gastric component —thus constituting the gastric SLING and CLASP fibers.

In an important contribution, Mittal draws attention to the dual mechanism, comprising the intrinsic smooth muscle of the esophagus and the extrinsic skeletal muscle of the diaphragmatic hiatus.[8,9] The crural diaphragm is usually 2 cm in length and it follows that part of the LES is intra-abdominal.

An important and normal physiological phenomenon is transient relaxation of the LES (TLESR) which both causes, and fails to prevent, GER. It is interesting, also, that evidence shows the crural diaphragm contracting earlier than the rest of the diaphragm - an important factor in preventing GER (Fig. 28.5).

It is generally recognized that the disturbed anatomical situation when a hiatal hernia is present is associated with hiatal incompetence. From a pathological point of view, one end result of GER is esophagitis, which may be non-erosive or erosive— And referred to as gastroesophageal reflux disease (GERD).

The innervation of the LES must also be taken into account. There are two opposing neuronal systems:
1. Cholinergic; and
2. Non-adrenergic, non-cholinergic; and each may have either stimulating or inhibitory effects. More recently, emphasis has been placed on the role of nitric oxide (NO) and its inhibitory effect on LES relaxation, and on the CAJAL interstitial cells. VIP and CGRA, may also play a role.

The literature on the subject of gastroesopahgeal reflux is now voluminous, and it is only possible to refer to segments of the literature; but nevertheless, the following should be seen in context of the details outlined in the Chapter, in an attempt to correlate the symptomatology and the influence of treatment, which would otherwise be quite incomplete.[10]

1. There are age-related factors, as exemplified by Orenstein's question: "Do infants respond differently to esophageal distention?" An answer is that the baby's prosperity to regurgitate will probably disappear with age.[10-15]
2. Esophageal clearance (Caste") with esophageal peristalsis, and its assessment by radiology and manometry, correlated with the role of saliva, which also plays a role.
3. Esophageal "acidification" and the evidence that the LES pressure falls with this acidification, which no doubt helps establish a vicious circle (Blackshaw).
4. TLESRs, and its impact on "physiological" and "pathological" reflux.
5. The "physiology" of belching.[14,15]
6. Others have commented on the absence of age and gender effects.

Boix-Ochoa summarized the situation, implicating TLESRs, the speed of esophageal clearance and mucosal resistance. and the fact that GER results in chronic esophagitis, aspiration pneumonia. stricture, and at times, the mucosal changes identified as Barrett's esophagus. Thus he demonstrated the clinical correlation, as well as the vicious circle aspect (Figs 28.6 and 28.7).

GERD is now recognized as a chronic condition with associated symptoms, such as heartburn, but endoscopy is only positive in 50% of such cases. Males are affected more than females, but not in the younger age-groups in whom regurgitation is a very common event. Associated features may include weight-deficit, apnea, pneumonia irritability and hematemesis. In

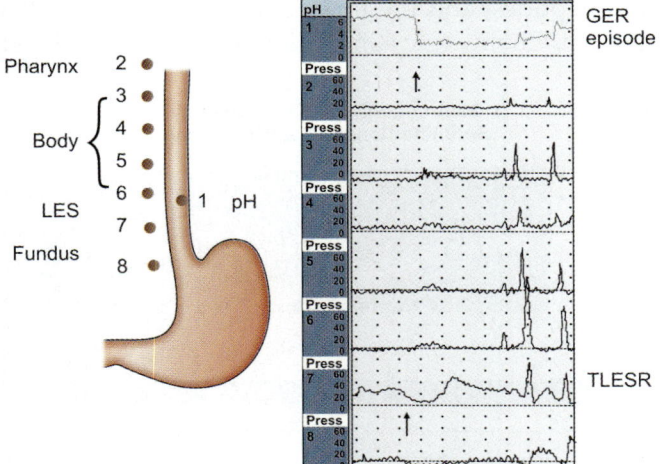

Fig. 28.5: Transient lower esophagus sphincter relaxation: Abrupt relaxation of the LES not preceded by swallowing and fall in esophageal pH due to the gastric reflux

many people there is an essential need for investigation, particularly with pH-metry, barium studies, endoscopy and biopsy. Reflux can be recognized as regurgitant or non-regurgitant, and it is necessary to distinguish reflux from vomiting from other causes and from rumination. The latter is possibly associated with psychosocial factors. GER may lead to GERD which clearly is definitely multifactorial and significant parameters which can be recognized, include age, sex, body-mass index, presence of a hiatus hernia and the number of reflux episodes.

Scintigraphy may be valuable, in particular for demonstrating pulmonary aspiration and decreased esophageal clearance.

Gastric emptying studies are valuable in children, and there is evidence that fundoplication may result in worsening of symptoms if foregut dysmotility is present (Fig. 28.8).

A miscellany of chemical and hormonal factors is involved in these circumstances, including nitric oxide (NO), substance P, carbon monoxide (CO), heme oxygenase, prostaglandins and possibly of more clinical significance—erythromycin.

Other factors include: Calcium channel blockage; the possible role of proton pump inhibitors (PPI) in facilitating the healing of esophagitis the manometric definition of LES -and techniques currently in use, especially the Dent's sleeve technique and more recently. The role of endoscopic measurement of the LES; LES manometry, facilitates recognition of anatomical localization, exact pressure and length and helping in clinical decisions on the roles of medical and/or surgical treatment.[16-22] Electromyography of the esophagus, which is less of a clinical tool than one for research. There has also been a recent increase in interest in duodeno-gastroesophageal reflux and the effect of mucus secreted by the esophagus. Recognising GER and atypical symptoms, including respiratory symptoms such as asthma, laryngitis, apnea, malaise and sudden death is also important. Manometry if available, is of considerable value, including ambulatory manometry. The pepsin factor has also gained importance. Pepsinogen gives rise to pepsin, which in turn acts on protein, breaking it down into peptides, and these are potentiality injurious to mucosa. Cholinergic stimulation may be drug-related

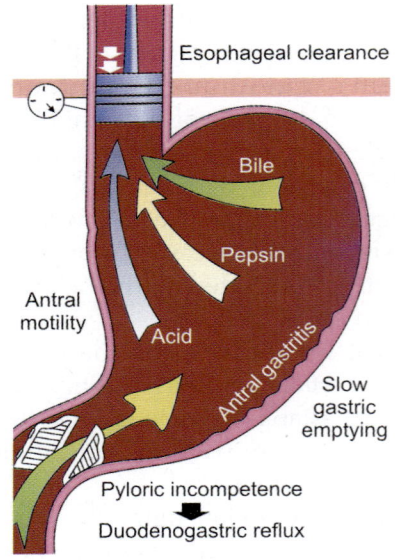

Fig. 28.6: GER aggressivity: The noxiousness of the gastric contents in the esophageal mucosa and the gastroesophageal reflux are the interplay of several factors

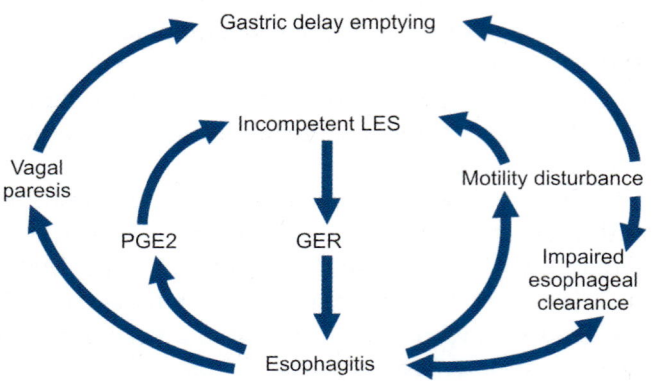

Fig. 28.7: The vicious cycle of GER

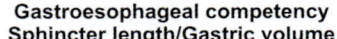

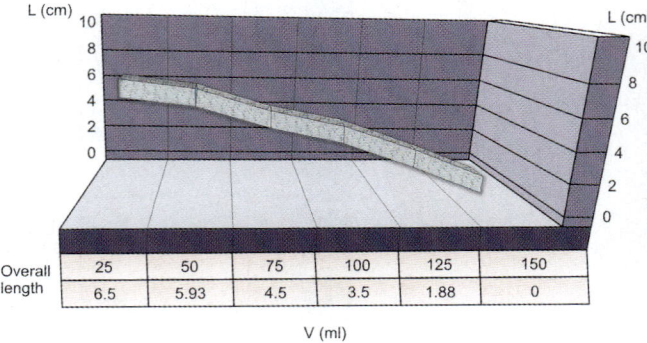

Fig. 28.8: The gastric emptying -delay, produces and increases the gastric volumes, reducing the length of intra-abdominal esophagus and enchancing the risk of GER

with the drugs including Bethanechol, Metaclopramide, Cisapride and Erythromycin. However, recent evidence suggests Cisapride may have potentially dangerous side effects.

HIATUS HERNIA

Recognition of a hiatus hernia is essential, as it results in a reservoir of acid in the supra-diaphragmatic pouch, and also interferes with esophageal clearance and causes a defect in the LES, combined with attenuation of the phreno-esophageal membrane. In the past, the presence of a hiatus hernia was automatically associated with reflux and was an indication for surgery. By definition, hiatus hernia is present when the EGJ and a portion of the stomach are situated above the esophageal hiatus. Today, however, it is appreciated that the situation is more complex, with factors including an inadequate anti-reflux barrier, volume factor and mucosal resistance; esophageal reflux disease (GERD) being associated with a hiatus hernia.

Radiological evaluation is technique - related. This may show an esophageal mucosal ring which can simulate a stricture or incidental changes associated with esophagitis, including erosion and ulceration.

pH-monitoring has, of course, become the gold standard. An early contribution was made by Spencer in 1969, and another some years later by Johnson and de Meester, who stated that 24-hr pH-metry, was necessary to evaluate the total percent of reflux time.

Gastric motility and gastric distension are important factors, but opinions differ regarding the role of fatty foods. Gastric stasis and gastric dysrythmia are also important, and in this context, it must be stressed that gastric stasis is only one factor.

Antroduodenal motility studies as performed by Lorenzo in patients in the pediatric age-group were correlated with the existence of GERD and LES relaxation. Duodenogastroesophageal reflux involves acid, pepsin and bile salts, but it is important to recognize that GERD is only at one end of a spectrum of motility disorders. Perhaps it is relevant to note the role of NO on pyloric tone and gastric emptying.[19,23-26]

Finally, the importance of the LES as a protective barrier cannot be over-estimated. Minimal physiological reflux is permitted, but the role of gastric emptying must always be recognized. If GERD exists with a competent LES, medical treatment is indicated. But if manometry shows a low LES, there is definitely a role for surgery, and the presence or absence of esophagitis, stricture or a Barrett's esophagus, particularly if these persist, leads one toward surgery.[27] Some observers feel that surgical results should be evaluated by manometry, and others have stressed the value of ongoing endoscopic evaluation.

PATHOLOGY AND PATHOGENESIS

The significant pathology in patients with gastroesopahgeal reflux (GER), regardless of age, is esophagitis, part of the GERD complex. This is sometimes referred to as peptic esophagitis, and sometimes squamous esophagitis, the latter term having the advantage of distinguishing the condition from Barrett's esophagus. The process is inflammatory, and affects the squamous lining of the esophagus.

There are several ways to grade the severity of the esophagitis.

The classification introduced by Skinner is particularly useful, having the additional advantage of correlating the changes with the endoscopic findings. Four grades were recognized and described:

Grade 1: Distal esophageal mucosal edema. The may obscure the squamo-columnar epithelial junction.

Grade 2: Mucosal erythema with superficial ulceration, typically linear and vertical and with an overlying fibrinous membrane exudate that is easily wiped, away, leaving a bleeding surface. This is not "scope trauma".

Grade 3: Mucosal erythema with superficial ulceration and associated mucosal fibrosis — A so-called dilatable "early" stricture.

Grade 4: Extensive ulceration with fibrous luminal stenosis. This may indicate irreversible pan-mural fibrosis.

The original classification system proposed by Savary and Miller recognized the following four grades:

Grade 1: Single or isolated erosive lesions, oval or linear, but affecting only one longitudinal fold.

Grade 2: Multiple erosive lesions, non-circumferential, affecting more than one longitudinal fold, with or without confluence.

Grade 3: Circumferential erosive lesions.

Grade 4: Complications: Columnar epithelium, ulcer, stricture and/or short esophagus—alone or associated with Grades 1-3. Later, some observers have separated Grade 4 into 4a and 4b, depending on the presence or absence of acute erosive and/or ulcerative changes.

It is essential that the surgeon understand the grading system, regardless of whether he is the endoscopist assessing the findings, because therapeutic decisions will be influenced by the severity of the esophagitis. Detailed comments on the various grading systems have been made by, among others, Armstrong, Tyagat and Lundel and Boyce.

It is not sufficient, however, to consider only the macroscopic appearances of esopahgitis; it is also important to be familiar with the historical changes which are identifiable. These include lengthening of the papillae so that they occupy more than 2/3 of the thickness of the mucosa. There is also hyperplasia of the basal zone, which may occupy more than 50% of the total thickness of the mucosa. The nuclei of the basal cells are enlarged, and hyperchromatic, but unlike the nuclei of dysplastic cells, they are relatively uniform in size and shape.

Perhaps of greater significance is the finding of intra-epithelial eosinophils, or intra-epithelial neutrophils. This finding is stated to be diagnostic of esophagitis. By contrast, intra-epithelial lymphocytes have little clinical importance because they can be found normally in the esophagus.

This then is the primary pathology, but the pathological process can only be considered alongside the pathogenesis and although peptic esophagitis is essentially the result of refluxate containing acid, the alkaline component of the refluxate may also be significant. Experimental and clinical observations in recent years have drawn attention to duodenogastric-esophageal reflux.

The discussion of pathology also necessitates consideration of what may be referred to as secondary pathological processes, including the development of columnar-lined lower esophagus (Barrett's esophagus).

When GER is associated with aspiration into the respiratory tract, it is inevitable that there will be pathological conditions such as bronchitis and aspiration pneumonia—although these are not the only respiratory manifestations seen in GERD.

THE CLINICAL PICTURE

The symptomatology of gastroesophageal reflux has been described in a wide variety of published articles, and in pediatric surgery and gastroenterology textbooks. Reference to these provide adequate details regarding the clinical details (Fig. 28.7).

It is important, however, to recognize that there are three groups of those patients who present in the pediatric age-group.

GROUP 1

Those with Digestive Symptoms

This is the predominant group in infants and children, and the predominant symptom is vomiting. It is pointed out by Jolley (1998), based on his investigations into the findings with prolonged esophageal pH recording, there are three patient types of GERD, which he refers to as Types 1, 2 and 3. These reflux pattern types correlate with the clinical radiographic and manometric findings, and the prognosis. Thus, in the majority of infants, the symptoms will resolve but this does not necessarily mean that the reflux has ceased and these infants should certainly be kept under observation.

This approach must be born in mind, although it is now well-known, and as Herbst and Meyers 28 stressed, 1981 it is essential to be familiar with the natural history. The evidence has indicated that, in the majority, the symptoms are present by the age of two months, and that 60% have a benign course and are free of symptoms by the age of 18 months.

Some authors have pointed out that about 30% have some persistent symptoms - at least to the age of four - and 5% develop strictures.

This then is the natural history of non-bilious emesis. Appropriate clinical and radiological investigation will enable this group of infants to be distinguished from those with an alternative diagnosis, e.g. pyloric stenosis, urinary-tract infection, etc. however, most babies who "split up" will improve, usually at about the age of 8-9 months, and no doubt that is related to the assumption of a more upright position throughout the day. It follows that the majority who fall into this group will improve, regardless of therapy, and clearly decision-making is largely based on the clinical history and the age of the patient. Although in most instances, vomiting is now associated with failure to thrive, at times it may be forceful and voluminous and vomiting of this nature may not necessarily dispute the possibility that the basic problem is reflux. The age of this group of patients makes it difficult to assess such symptoms as pain and heartburn, which are so common in adults, but it is believed that restlessness and irritability may be on indication that the reflux (GER) is associated with esophagitis (GERD). The pediatric surgeon must be familiarity with the natural history of vomiting in infancy due to reflux, and recognize the fact that he may well see a specific group of patients whose symptoms have not resolved, as would be expected in the majority of infant refluxers.

GROUP 2

Those who Fail to Thrive

Babies who have GER may fail to thrive, even presenting with acute dehydration with electrolyte imbalance. As expected, there will be a correlation between failure to thrive and the degree of vomiting, but it is definitely less than 100%. When electrolyte imbalance is present, which is certainly unusually, there my be difficulties in differentiating GER from pyloric stenosis.

GROUP 3

Respiratory Symptoms

In recent years, it has become clear that various respiratory symptoms may occur as a consequence of GER, including episodes of apnea, choking, respiratory arrest and apparent life-threatening events.[28] Other respiratory features include recurrent aspiration pneumonia, recurrent wheezing, chronic cough, stridor and chronic lung disease. Patients presenting with any of these symptoms may need opt be investigated to determine whether GER is present.

Numerous article's have appeared on this subject, and many authorities have stressed the fact that the casual relationship is not always clear: Reflux may lead to respiratory-tract involvement; or respiratory disease may result in reflux; or their relationship may be coincidental. It is in this group of patients that a complete investigatory profile is required and two investigations which are most likely to be of value here are 24-hour pH metry and scintography. Herbst (1981) summarized the situation as follows: "Once the reflux material gets to the level of the pharynx it may be aspirated and cause pulmonary problems. This is a major problem in children; pulmonary symptoms were present in 47% of patients in our center who had surgical repair. These pulmonary problems may mimic those of recurrent obstructive bronchitis or recurrent aspiration pneumonia. In older patients and adults, usually the lower lobe is involved. Because infants spend a large portion of their time recumbent, there is a predilection for the upper lobes, especially the right. Choking and apnoea may be a major problem, especially in the first year of life. Usually it occurs during or just after feeding and may be associated with bronchospasm".

GROUP 4

Other Associated Conditions and Syndromes

It is particularly important to recognize the Sandifer syndrome, in which there is intermittent head-cocking. Although the mechanism is not clear, clinical evidence indicates that the symptoms are quite definitely related to GER.

Down's syndrome is also associated with GER, as are other neurological abnormalities. Later in the chapter, reference is made to GER in association with various neurological abnormalities and following repair of esophageal atresia.

INVESTIGATIONS

At the outset, it is important to stress that investigations may have clinical implications or may represent the fruits of a wide variety of research activities. Many of these later may eventually become standard clinical investigations, but at present must be considered experimental, e.g. the measurement and assessment of significance of bile salts and bile acids in the refluxate.

To the clinician involved in the care of patients with gastroesophageal reflux, in children and adults, a wide variety of investigative modalities is now available, respiratory one of the most exciting developments in the whole area of GER. At the same time, the pediatric surgeon must recognize that in the vast majority of cases, as outlined in the section of symptoms, investigation will not be required. Even if investigation is considered necessary, it may well be possible to limit it to a radiographic study, provided this study is carried out by an experienced radiologist and, if possible, he clinician in change of the patient is present when the study is performed. The presence of clinician has advantages for both radiologist and surgeon.

The two broad objectives of investigation are:
1. To confirm or deny the presence of GER- recognizing of course that some tests are not 100% sensitive. However, the "gold standard" in this group is recognized to be 24-hr pH-monitoring.
2. To provide information regarding the severity of GER and whether this has proceeded to GERD. The classic and most useful investigation in this group is again 24 hr pH monitoring, but this will frequently need to be supplemented by endoscopy and biopsy.

With these facts firmly in mind, the surgeon of today will know that the following investigations are possible, although not all may be available in this institution.

Radiography

This will certainly not be necessary in all cases. In most infants with non-bilious vomiting. It is usually possible to make a confident diagnosis of GER, along with the prediction of a good prognosis with resolution of symptoms. A barium swallow and limited barium meal is designed to diagnose GER and provide information regarding esophageal function, the presence of absence of an anatomical abnormality (hiatal hernia) and the presence of a stricture in the esophagus. It is best to remember that the narrowing diagnosed as a stricture may be the result of spasm or edema, and is not necessarily an indication of esophageal fibrosis. If a hiatal hernia is present, due notice must be taken of its size, but also it is important to distinguish this from the normal dilatation of the lower end of the esophagus, which is referred to as a phrenic ampulla.

pH Monitoring

This has evolved and been modified since the original description by Tuttle, but in this context attention should also be drawn to the Bernstein test, which was designed to distinguish pain the chest due to reflux from the other causes of chest pain. Today, however, the gold standard investigation is 24 hr pH monitoring, which may be combined with manometric findings.

The contribution of Skinner remains relevant today, although it dates back to 1970. He reviewed the role of esophageal function tests, specifically directing our attention to four tests: manometry, acid perfusion, pH-reflux and acid-clearing. He also related findings to pre- and postoperative studies, specifically with reference to a wide variety of operations including the Belsey Mark IV, the Nissen fundoplication, the Hill operation, the Collis procedure (with or without vagotomy) and the original Allision repair, to name but a few.[29]

Euler and Ament recommended the Tuttle test be include in the diagnostic evaluation of pediatric patients presenting with GER. But this was twenty years ago, and today it is essential not only to be selective in deciding whether pH metry should be performed, and to recognize that more modern tests have replaced the technique described by Tuttle. Euler and Ament have pointed out that the esophageal intraluminal pH test has proved safe, simple and sensitive, indicating as it does hydrogen ion reflux from the stomach to the esophagus across the LES anti-reflux barrier.

For pediatric patients, Johnson and Jolley made a valuable contribution. Their scoring system for 24 hr pH-monitoring is an adaptation of the adult system published by Johnso and De Meester. The test should be performed by a pediatric gastroenterologist with appropriate laboratory facilities and analysis of the pH recording shows:
– frequency of reflux
– the longest single reflux episode,
– the percentage of time the pH was less than 4.
– The state of wakefulness of the patient

These observers describe three patterns of reflux, and indicate that their findings suggest that those with Types 1 and 3 were less likely to resolve with time. Type 2 was more likely to undergo spontaneous resolution.

Esophageal Manometry

While views differ, there is no doubt that this modality, if available, can provide useful information. The most useful study surrounding pH metry, manometry enables recognition of the site of the LES, permitting accurate placement enabling pH measurements at various levels in the esophagus above the LES.

Manometry also provides information regarding the tonus in the LES, and interestingly enough, this is not always low in patient with GER. Other information can be obtained regarding esophageal clearance and peristaltic waves (primary, secondary or tertiary). As with 24 hr pH monitoring, the information must be correlated with the clinical picture and the results of other studies, to facilitate decision-making regarding treatment and to monitor the individual patient's progress. It must however, be stressed that sophisticated manometry studies should only be performed in selected cases, and by a pediatirician experienced in the technique.[30]

Scintigraphy

Radionucleide studies have a definite role to play, but should only be used in selected cases. Orenstein pointed out in 1993 that scintigraphy "can detect neutral postprandial reflux, identify aspiration, quantify gastric emptying and may avoid esophageal intubation". Her view was that simultaneous pH probe and scintigraphy being most sensitive in the early post-prandial state, whereas the pH probe is most sensitive in the fasting state. As early as 1981, Herbst and Meyers suggested that possibly the gastric scintiscan has a number of theoretical advantages; in particular,, the radiation dose is less than that for a single chest film. Fonkalsrud et al were strong advocates for pyloroplasty when significant delayed gastric emptying has been documented, and their method was to use radioisotope techniques with the inclusion of technetium-99m sulphur colloid with the normal diet and to quantify the magnitude of gastric retention at various time intervals. To summarize, scintigraphy has a role, particularly in those patients where delayed gastric emptying or pulmonary aspiration is suspected. But as many authorities have pointed out (including Spitz and co-workers) it is only a modality which should be invoked for selected cases.

One of the most important contributions in the detection of reflux-associated with pulmonary aspiration was by Arasu and co-workers. who found that a gastroesophageal scintiscan was positive only in 17/30 patients with GE reflux. They concluded that the GE scintiscan was complementary to barium studies but that neither scintigraphy nor radiography approached the accuracy of more sophisticated tests.

Endoscopy and Biopsy

It is very tempting, but unnecessary, to perform esophagoscopy and biopsy in many patients with GER, but again, selection is required. Unnecessary endoscopy can only lead to increasing parental anxiety, which in turn, may be reflected in the behavior of the infant. However, although there may be radiographic evidence of esophagitis certainty of this diagnosis demands endoscopy and biopsy, and the findings have been summarized in this chapter under the heading, Pathology. En passant, the value of endoscopy in assessing the nature of esophageal narrowing is undoubted, as is its ability to facilitate dilatation of the stricture if one is present. This of course may be complementary to various operative procedures and if esophagoscopy permits appropriate dilatation. the more invasive method of gastrotomy and retrograde passage of Hegar's dilators is not required. However, these are relatively minor points and the most important aspect of endoscopy is to enable recognition of two complications of GER: (1) esophagitis; (2) presence of columnar lined esophagus, the so called Barrett epithelium.

Endoscopy should be performed by an experienced endoscopist, and the surgeon will need to decide whether he will do it himself, or rely on an appropriate colleague. But it is essential the surgeon should at least be present at the time of the examination.

Much has been written about the technique and role of esophageal biopsy and the need to document the sites from which the biopsy specimens are taken, and the involvement of an experienced pediatric pathologist is of course essential. The endoscopist must be familiar with appropriate techniques involving rigid or flexible endoscopes, and decisions will need to be made regarding the repeating of endoscopy and ongoing surveillance.

A recent contribution by Auters mentions the use of a proton pump inhibitor in patients with Barrett's esophagus, pointing out that even with considerable improvement of the endoscopic lesions, the esophagus is still exposed to the irritating action of the refluxate. There are many other contributions discussing the findings, prognosis etc, and correlating these with the findings on endoscopy and the equally important findings on biopsy.[31-33]

Thus, the various investigatory modalities available are now well documented, and although the pediatric surgeon should be familiar with them all, he needs also to be selective. For the most part, investigation is more important in the adult population. Fortunately, should operative treatment be required for GER, the results tend to be more satisfactory in the pediatric age-group But nevertheless, should symptoms persist postoperatively, such patients should be re-investigated. And as with preoperative investigation, selection of the appropriate modality is all important.

DIAGNOSIS

Consideration of the symptoms, on the one hand, and the results of investigation on the other, enable the diagnosis of GER to be made with a high degree of certainty. Abnormal physical signs may not exist, but note should be taken of the child's habitus and pulmonary findings. Despite knowledge of the natural history of GER, diagnostic delay is by no means unusual, particularly in those children whose GER leads to failure to thrive, or in the group with respiratory problems. In these two groups in particular, various differential diagnoses must be considered, always bearing in mind that GER frequently co-exists with other conditions. This is particularly true when GER is associated with co-morbidity, as in children with neurological impairment or following esophageal atresia repair (Figs 28.9 and 28.10).

The following diagnoses can be recognised, but there may be overlap from one group to another.

1. The *spitters:* These represent the majority of babies and infants with GER and have been well described by Jolley. A clinical diagnosis can usually be made, but under special circumstances, including parental anxiety, limited investigation may be required—rarely more than a radiographic study. Provided adequate explanation is combined with appropriate communication, there is no reason why this need add to parental anxiety.

Prognostic Factors in GER
- Efficacy of antireflux mechanisms
- Volume of gastric fluid
- Potency of refluxed material
- Efficacy of oesophageal clearance
- Tissue resistance of the oesophageal mucosa

Fig. 28.9: Prognostic factors in GER

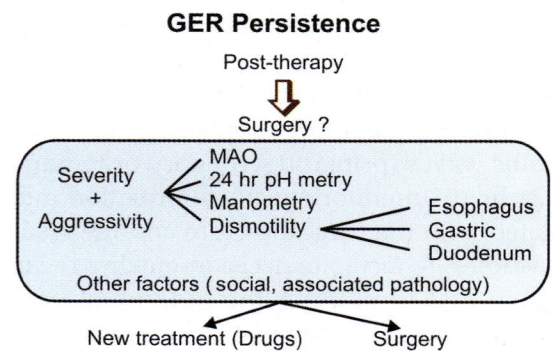

Fig. 28.10: Surgical decision after GER persistence post-medical therapy. To take the surgical decision we have to evaluate several factors by means of more sophisticated diagnostic procedures

2. Where clinical suspicion is high, but the diagnosis may be in doubt. In this group, further investigation is required and this may take the form of 24 hr pH metry or esophagoscopy and biopsy or both.
3. Additional symptoms are present, e.g. irritability and "heart burn" (which is difficult to evaluate in children), and thorough investigation is essential, the nature of which will depend on modalities available. Manometry may be helpful; gastric scintigraphy has a definite role in the final analysis, the pathway to follow is ideally the same as for the second group
4. Clinical suspicion is aroused and investigation reveals an esophageal stricture. Endoscopic examination will usually determine the severity and response to dilatation.
5. When Barrett's esophagus is present, the symptoms are those of GER and/or an associated stricture.
6. Respiratory symptoms dominate the clinical picture—either the GER produces these symptoms, or GER is a result of respiratory tract disease. This group requires a high degree of suspicion, particularly with asthmatic children or following repair of esophageal atresia, which should lead to appropriate investigation.
7. A miscellaneous group, including the Sandifer syndrome, and in the neurologically impaired child.

In summary, therefore, diagnosis of GER should not be difficult, (Fig. 28.11) but difficulties arise, particularly when the symptomatology is atypical.

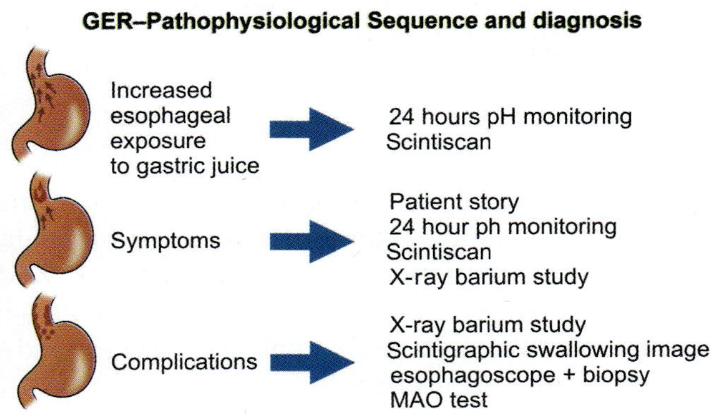

Fig. 28.11: GER: According the symptoms and evolution, the diagnostic measures change

Particular note should be taken of respiratory features because life-threatening episodes may be associated with aspiration into the respiratory tract. To date there is no definite link with sudden infant death syndrome (SIDS) and Campbell (personal communication) has not found evidence of esophagitis in the postmortem examination of babies who have died as a result of SIDS.

TREATMENT

The spectrum of treatment of GER is extremely wide. At one end of the scale, little or no treatment is necessary beyond reassurance of the parents. At the other end however, complex surgical procedures may be required. However, it is too simplistic and unhelpful to divide the therapeutic regimes into two groups—nonoperative and operative. Rather, various treatment groups should be considered, commencing with the infant with an excellent prognosis—which is the large percentage of cases -and concluding with the group requiring complex surgery, e.g. those requiring esophageal resection and replacement, including some patients who have been demonstrated to have a columnar-lined esophagus (Barrett's esophagus) unquestionably more prevalent in adult practice.

Therapeutic Group 1

These latter are this is the group referred to by Jolley as "spitters". Characteristically, the vomiting is frequent but not forceful and the babies continue to thrive. The majority will, in the course of time cease to vomit. This spontaneous improvement is largely related to the beneficial effect of the upright posture, which is a normal development over time. In this group, the appropriate treatment is reassurance for the parents. The problem is essentially a social one: the staining of clothes and furniture, malodor, etc. The parents must be given a complete explanation of their child's problem, because for them there is a real problem.

While most babies in this group are unlikely to be referred to a surgeon, some are, and the surgeon must therefore be familiar with the natural history of reflux in the infant, and the various therapeutic techniques available, including the adoption of the upright posture, possibly more frequent, smaller feedings and thickening of these feedings. A dogmatic approach to these non-operative treatments is to be avoided, but, as many experienced pediatricians have put it, "it's worth a try".

Various agents, including corn flour and rice, have been used to thicken feeds, with Karicare being the product most recently used at the Royal Children's Hospital. Pharmacological therapy is rarely required, although if the vomiting is particularly troublesome, a short course of a prokinetic agent may be indicated. But as stated by Orenstein, pharmacological measures must include drugs which are either prokinetic, e.g. Bethanechol, Metoclopromide or cisipride, or acid-suppressing, viz. hydrogen ion blockers or proton pump inhibitors. In 1992 Reynolds and Putnam provided excellent information regarding prokinetic agents. It needs to be stressed that the vomiting is self-limiting in this group; that the cornerstone of treatment is reassurance and that investigation is either not required at all or limited to a barium meal. Posture is important, but should not include the prone position, as this has been linked to sudden infant death syndrome (SIDS).[33]

Therapeutic Group 2

This is in extension of the first group and differs in the intensity of the vomiting and/or associated symptoms. These babies with GER are irritable, fail to thrive and cause great concern to their parents. Under these circumstances, the presence of GERD (particularly esophagitis) must either be confirmed or excluded. Investigations need to be individualized, the spectrum of severity of symptoms necessitating careful assessment while keeping parental anxiety to a minimum. However, the presence of additional symptoms, i.e. those more serious than the "spitting" type, should lead the clinician in charge to consider investigations over and above the simple radiographic study. The two possible investigations are: (1) 24-hr pH metry; (2) esophagoscopy and biopsy. Wisdom will dictate the management of the individual baby and often a trial of simple measures should precede the more invasive requirements associated with investigation. Many of the babies in this group can be expected to improve spontaneously; but the surgeon must be aware that such symptomatic improvement does not necessarily indicate cessation of reflux, and ongoing clinical surveillance is essential.[34-38]

Therapeutic Group 3

There is a fine line between this and the first two groups, the only thing separating them being the finding on radiology of a hiatus hernia. The identification of such a hernia has to be related to the symptomatology and requires an experienced pediatric radiologist. In simple terms, the measures adopted for the first two groups are indicated for this group too, plus the need to consider operative repair of the hernia if -and the important word is if' -the hernia is large. Thus, note must be taken of its size. The need for individualization of treatment is paramount, and the surgical repair to be performed will vary according to the experience and attitude of the surgeon.

Details regarding appropriate surgical measures will be considered later.[39]

Therapeutic Group 4

It is tempting to list several clinical features which necessitate an antireflux operation be performed, but again the old adage applies: "Neither never nor always are absolute". Nevertheless there are several situations, other than a large hiatus hernia, which usually demand surgical intervention.[40]
1. Failure of a medical regime with persistence of esophagitis.
2. The presence of esophageal stricture.
3. Barrett's esophagus -proven histologically.
4. Respiratory diseases proven to be secondary to GER, including
    - Episodes of apnea, choking, respiratory arrest and apparent life-threatening events;
    - Recurrent aspiration pneumonia
    - Recurrent wheezing
    - Chronic cough
    - Stridor
    - Chronic lung disease.

It is impossible to be dogmatic regarding some patients who should be considered for surgical repair, but all parameters-particularly clinical and investigatory-will need to he evaluated. An occasional indication is hematemesis, but only if it is severe and/or there is ongoing esophagitis.

Therapeutic Group 5

This is an extension of Group 4, and includes surgery in special situations where resolution is unlikely to occur, e.g.
- Following repair of esophageal atresia
- In some neurologically impaired children
- In children with Sandifer's syndrome
- Ongoing failure to thrive secondary to GER.

It is important to recognize these various therapeutic groups but such recognition must be correlated with the total clinical picture and social situation of the patient. Reference to the literature emphasis that there is still and probably always will be some controversy about the indications for, and efficacy of, the various surgical therapeutic regimes available. All options must be considered and related to the findings and the known natural history of GER.

Ten years ago, Boyle pointed out that there had been an evolution in the investigation of refractory respiratory symptoms and the role of "protective" surgery in children with severe neurological impairment or physical handicaps, who require placement of a feeding gastrostomy to provide essential nutrition.

The precise indications vary from center to center.[41-43] Schwagten, in reviewing the experience at the Royal Children's Hospital, Melbourne, found definite trends in the use of fundoplication in children with gastroesophageal reflux. He pointed out that fundoplication was performed there with increased frequency from 1978-1985, and that the years 1984-86 reflected a "catch-up" period with indications for its use extended to patients with severe neurological impairment who had long-standing, uncontrolled reflux. He also looked at fundoplication with gastrostomy, stating that, "whereas in the early 1980's it was standard practice in many institutions to perform a fundoplication with any gastrostomy, current reviews of this practice have reported a high rate of delayed gastric emptying, especially in neurologically impaired patients, with subsequent recurrence of GER and high rates of complications. This has led to increased caution in recommending fundoplication without definite proof of GER in patients requiring gastrostomy."

Schwagten follows with an excellent summary of the dumping syndrome: Pallor, sweating, retching, diarrhea and refusal of feeds which occurs when an abnormally rapid gastric emptying time precipitates initial hyperglycemia and subsequent hypoglycemia. He concludes, management of complicated GER "fundoplication is an accepted part of the Although the overall results of surgery are good with the majority of patients achieving symptom resolution, a significant number have ongoing problems. Our study has limitations and the biases of any descriptive retrospective view, but despite these weaknesses, information is available regarding the main complications."

Indications for fundoplication broadened its use in those with severe neurological impairment and uncontrolled reflux, and changes occurred in the management of patients in the neonatal period. Complications included unwrapping with recurrence of reflux hiatal hernia, adhesive small bowel obstruction, dumping syndrome, post-operative persistence of esophageal stricture, excessively tight wrap, and poor esophageal clearance (mostly in esophageal atresia patients).[44]

This study identified the patients most likely to develop complications. It concluded that the results could assist in the preoperative assessment of the likely benefits of fundoplication in children who often have other complex problems. Stricture was considered the most important indication for fundoplication surgery; all other indications were regarded as relative.

OPERATIVE TECHNIQUES

Nissen Fundoplication

Pride of place is given to the Nissen-Rosetti procedure, in which a 360° wrap stomach around the intra-abdominal esophagus is constructed. There have been many reports of the results following the procedure. Not all have been favorable, but the experience at the Royal Children's Hospital, Melbourne has shown that good to excellent results can be anticipated. No doubt, there is a difference in the results to be expected between children and adults, and this becomes clearer when reports from authorities such as Hill and Nyhus are studied. Clearly, the difference between the beneficial effects of the Nissen procedure relate to the underlying pathology in the two groups, as beautifully pointed out by Boix-Ochoa.

An advocate of the procedure in the pediatric patient is Randolph, who wrote as follows: "The operative technique for Nissen fundoplication has been well described. However, certain features are necessary for success in the infant. The abdominal route is quite simple in infants, and is now our favored approach. The left lobe of the liver is detached from the diaphragm and easily folded to the right of the esophagus. It is useful to pass a mercury sound through the esophagus into the stomach; depending on the age and size of the child, sounds ranging from number 24 to number 30 are used (this is not the routine procedure at the Royal Children's Hospital, Melbourne, where surgeons rely on the passage of a large nasogastric tube).

The phrenicoesophageal ligament is divided completely to reveal the crura and the vagus nerves. The latter are carefully spared and the crura are sutured behind the esophagus. utilizing general bites in the muscle. Non-absorbable sutures are used for this. Several of the short gastric arteries are divided to free the fundus (not all pediatric surgeons believe this is necessary).

Care is taken not to damage the spleen; a window along the lesser curvature is prepared which will permit the fundic wrap to be brought around the cardia without injury to the vagi or the left gastric artery I although at times the left gastric artery may need to be sacrificed. With the fundic wrap in place, sutures are passed through the lateral portion of the fundus, the anterior esophageal wall and the medially placed fundus, using three or four sutures of non-absorbable material. If an adequate amount of fundus is brought around, later dissolution of the repair will be avoided. It is important that the sutures should grasp a significant amount of gastric muscle and be secured without creating tension. The fundus is then sutured to the diaphragm to fix the repair and with the earlier dissection, there is an adequate length of intra-abdominal esophagus provided. Individualization will be necessary regarding the decision whether to perform a gastrostomy. However, it can serve as a convenient vent if gastric decompression is needed in the early postoperative period and is left in place for approximately three months.

Randolph's description highlights the important technical features of the procedure which satisfy the important requirements to provide a functional antireflux barrier. In other descriptions, relatively minor variations are mentioned, including the Toupet procedure in which the wrap is less complete (270° instead of 360°). This procedure was introduced largely to avoid some of the complications of the Nissen fundoplication, particularly gas bloat, dysphagia and dumping syndrome. Fortunately, however, these re relatively rare, and we have been encouraged to continue performing the Nissen fundoplication, even in patients with esophageal motility disturbance, e.g. esophageal atresia or when GER is a complication following cardiomyotomy for achalasia.[45-50]

THAL Fundoplication

This procedure has proved to be very satisfactory is Ashcraft's hands, and the following is his contribution to this alternative option, including some general observations, as well as a description of his surgical technique. With the heading, **THAL Fundoplication**: technique, results, complications and re-operation, Ashcraft has written as follows:

The THAL fundoplication is one of the partial wrap options for the surgical treatment of gastroesophageal reflux (GER). It is created by applying the free wall of the gastric fundus to the anterior aspect of the intra-abdominal esophagus, and is also known as the Dor-Nissen procedure The Boix-Ochoa procedure is quite similar. The same physiological result may be anticipated using the posterior partial wrap fundoplication (Toupet). Proponents of the partial wraps believe that a successful wrap cures the problem of GER, while leaving the patient with ability to vomit and to burp if the need arises. Obviously, in the pediatric patient, the need for one or both of these very physiological functions is more common than in the adult patient population. There are some pediatric patients, particularly those with significant neurological impairment, who are perhaps better served by a complete wrap (Nissen), because there is little hope of any conscious control of the GE junction. Almost always the Nissen will be accompanied by a **STAMM** or other form of gastrostomy used for feeding and/or gastric decompression.

"Our experience with the **THAL** fundoplication has been entirely with open procedures. Because of several features of the operative procedure which we feel are very important, there has been little disturbance of gastrointestinal function, and therefore only a very short hospital stay has been necessary. On an average, my personal experience with over one thousand THAL fundoplication results in the patient not requiring postoperative nasogastric drainage, oral liquids being started within 12 hours of operation, and the patient discharged from hospital within 48 hours. Laparoscopic fundoplication has most commonly been done during the Nissen procedure, because it is far easier to perform than the That or the Toupet. There are several endoscopic surgeons in the United States who have accumulated significant endoscopic experience with the THAL, but whose time to feeding and discharge to feeding is not significantly shorter than ours. The benefit therefore is probably related to the issue of one scar versus several smaller ones. There is no question that the endoscopic procedure requires increased costs of equipment and supplies.

The diagnosis is established most frequently by extended pH-monitoring. We require a barium study in all patients prior to operation to exclude the possibility of achalasia.

Surgical technique: The patient is anesthetised expeditiously and without distending the stomach or the gut. A nasogastric tube of appropriate size is passed by the anesthetist for purposes of intra-operative gastric decompression and to aid in the identification of the gastroesophageal junction. The tube also provides some rigidity for the esophagus during the creation of the fundoplication steps are then carried out: The following steps are then carried out:

1. An upper abdominal transverse incision is made from the left costal margin at the nipple line to the opposite costal margin, dividing both recti. The abdomen is entered cephalad of the transverse colon and the small intestine is protected from handling by the mesocolon. Sufficient relaxation is required to prevent the patient from "bucking" and eviscerating himself.

2. The anterior free wall of the stomach is grasped with a gauze pad and retracted downward. The left lobe of the liver is also grasped and dissected free from the underside of the left diaphragm. It is folded downward and retracted to the right by the second assistant.
3. Incision of the peritoneum at the hiatus is done in a transverse direction and a blunt dissector used to spread areolar tissue on either side of the easily-seen and palpated esophagus. A dissector is passed behind the esophagus from the right to the left, grasping a dacron tape that will be used for traction purposes posterior (right end) vagus nerve has not been included within the tape, the tape is replaced.
4. The G-E junction is adjusted downward while the hiatus is pushed on either side of the esophagus in a cephalad direction. The hiatus is not intentionally enlarged, but the lower 2-4 cm of esophagus is thus mobilised.
5. The distal esophaqus is retracted to the patient's left by the first assistant, exposing both limbs of the crura behind. They are approximated using a figure-of-eight suture of permanent material. It is important to leave a space behind the esophagus so that the hiatus is not narrowed excessively. It is very important not to tie this hiatus-closing suture too tightly, or the muscle will necrose and the hiatus will be larger than it was originally. The suture, having been tied with its needle intact, is now placed and used to anchor the posterior wall of the esophagus to the hiatus, which helps hold the distal esophagus within the abdominal cavity.

The retractor is removed from behind the esophagus and the dacron tape ends are separated. A permanent suture, e.g. 2/0 or 3/0 Gortex is placed and tied at the G-E junction on the left. A fundoplication is created using a continuous suture going up the left side the esophagus suturing stomach to esophagus. The suture line crosses over the front of the esophagus to reach the right side where it is turned downward to the right G-E junction. Thus an inverted "U" is created, holding the anterior free wall of the stomach to the anterior free wall of the intra-abdominal esophagus. It is not necessary to divide any of the short gastric vessels to perform this fundoplication. Its length is assessed by palpating the nasogastric tube through the layers of stomach plied to the esophagus.

Nasogastric tube is removed, the liver replaced in its bed and the wound closed. Boix Ochoa attaches the gastric fundus to the underside of the left hemidiaphragm to exaggerate the angle of His prior to replacing the liver and closure. But we have not found this procedure to be necessary.

Special Situations

When faced with a request for a feeding gastrostomy in a neurologically impaired patient, we nearly always perform a concomitant fundoplication. This is done because most patients when fed by gastrostomy will begin to reflux, even without evidence of GER before. Performing a fundoplication in the presence of an established gastrostomy increases the likelihood of a wound infection and dehiscence. In approximately 50% of patients having repair of esophageal atresia malformations, reflux is a significant problem. In most of these patients, a fundoplication is necessary. It is very important that the fundoplication not obstruct the passage of food or drink, because the motility of the distal esophagus is abnormal in these patients. "We think, therefore, that the partial-wrap fundoplication is certainly the best for these patients."

There can be little doubt that the THAL fundoplication, as practiced by Ashcraft and his colleagues, provides excellent results in infants and children. The surgeon planning to use this procedure would be well advised to pay a visit to Ashcraft and study his technique.

Boix-Ochoa Procedure

Boix-Ochoa (1988) wrote as follows: "All pediatric patients should be treated conservatively before an operation is attempted." Although as a generalization this is true, there are definite exceptions to this rule, as outlined above. Boix-Ochoa goes on to state, "the percentage of patients treated medically or surgically changes enormously from one publication to another, confusing more than a few. The author thinks that this depends on whether the patient has been seen by the surgeon at the onset of symptoms, or whether he had been referred by a pediatrician after therapy has been tried. It is necessary to bear in mind a series of fundamental facts that are derived from the knowledge of the significant physiology. These facts being:[3,4,8,27]

1. Reflux does not necessarily mean sphincter incompetence, and incompetence does not necessarily mean sphincter pathology.
2. During the first stages of life, GOR can be considered as physiological, or the result of a delay in the maturation of the anti-reflux mechanism.
3. A healthy closing mechanism may become incompetent due to displacement or by being overcome by a pathological opening pressure.
4. By reducing esophagitis, the vicious circle can be broken, enabling the possibility of the LES to evolve to maturity.
5. Definite differences exist between children and adults: In the latter, the LES has been subject to years of chronic illness, and it is often impossible to retrieve the situation.
6. Conservative treatment will tend to lessen opening pressures and attacks on the esophageal mucosa, while surgical treatment will only potentiate closing mechanisms.

Operative Treatment

In older children, patients with hiatus hernia, infants with life-threatening apneic spells, severe esophagitis with stenosis, chronic bronchopneumopathy and social problems, are indications for the only appropriate option, which is surgical treatment. Boix Ochoa, like many others, has pointed out that the surgeon has at his disposal a great variety of surgical techniques that offer good results with low mortality and few complications. He also pointed out that, in the beginning, surgical techniques failed because the aim of the early pioneers was only to correct an anatomical abnormality, and thus the operations introduced by Allison (1951) and others fell into disfavor. More recently, interventions have focused on repairing the mechanisms which control reflux and assure a competent LES. Techniques should aim at increasing the high pressure zone, as well as the length of the intra-abdominal esophagus (Fig. 28.12).

With this as a background, and in keeping with the investigatory modalities to be considered, Boix-Ochoa describes a technique which aims at restoring and reinforcing the anatomical relationships (Boix-Ochoa, 1983). He describes the following steps:[42] (Fig. 28.13).

1. Restoration of the length of the intra-abdominal esophagus.

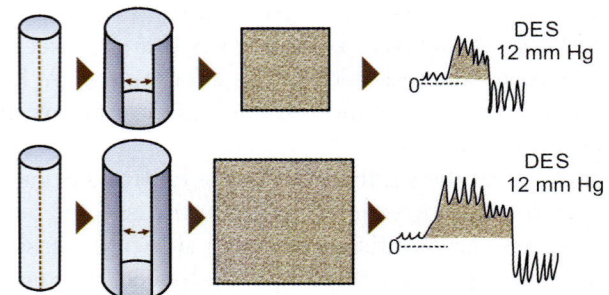

Fig. 28.12: The Boix-Ochoa technique does not increase the pressure in the LES but enchance and enlarge the area of which the closing pressures act. This technique only restores the normal phisiology by increasing the pressure area with the lengthening of the intra-abodminal esophagus and the restoring and sharpening of the His angle

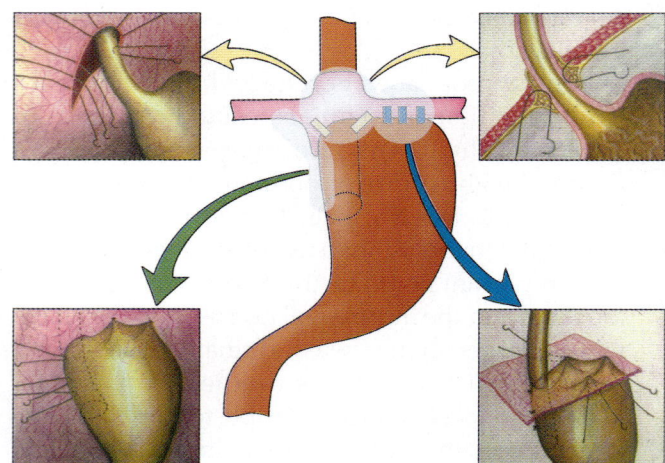

Fig. 28.13: Boix-Ochoa technique for GER in children. The length of intra-abdominal esophagus in restored and anchored to the crura. The crura is tightened. The angle of His restored by a suture taken from the fundus (after sectioning 2-3 short gastric-splenic vessels) to the rim of the right hiatus, and with the reinforcing suture between the fundus and the esophageal wall. Three in a triangle suspending sutures from the fundus to the diaphragm unfolding the fundus like an umbrella

2. Tightening the hiatus and anchoring the esophagus to it.
3. Restoring the angle of HIS by suture from the fundus at the level of the first short gastric artery to the rim of the right hiatus, and in addition, placing a few reinforcing sutures from the fundus to the anterior wall of the stomach.
4. The final step is opening up or unfolding the fundus, much as we would open up an umbrella.

exception to this is to be found in the writings of Orenstein: "Neurologic disease is associated with a high prevalence of GERD which often persists beyond infancy. As many as 15% of institutionalized, severely retarded children have recurrent vomiting, mostly attributed to reflux. An unknown further proportion may have non-regurgitative reflux, responsible for espophagitis or respiratory symptoms. Neurological disease associated with hypertonia and spasticity may provoke reflux episodes by increasing abdominal pressure. Since children with spasticity have a high incidence of hiatal hernia, this rise in abdominal pressure often occurs without a protective increase in crural support of the LES. One study suggests that extensor spasm, air-swallowing and kyphoscoliosis play roles in the development of hiatal hernias found in these children."

Hypotonia may be present in other children with severe neurological disease. Hypotonia leads to supine or stumped postures which are also provocative for reflux episodes. Although Down's syndrome occurs in 1: 660 newborns, 2-10% of infants undergoing fundoplication in various series have had this diagnosis. These children may be somewhat hypotonic, but esophageal manometry also showed a high frequency of simultaneous esophageal contractions in five children studied in detail.

The contrasting normalcy of the LES pressure suggests the possibility that the motility changes may have been primary rather than secondary to esophagitis.

Experience at the Royal Children's Hospital, Melbourne, is in keeping with experience in most other centers. Since 1972, when the first fundoplication was performed there, there have been an increasing number of such anti-reflux procedures being performed, following repair of esophageal atresia, as indicated by Veit et al in discussing trends in recent years. Of particular significance has been the recognition that many anastomotic strictures appear to be reflux-induced and an appropriate anti-reflux operation avoids the necessity for repeated dilatations. To estimate the incidence of reflux in the older patients whose esophageal atresia has been repaired in infancy, a special follow-up clinic as been designed and it is anticipated that study of adult patients in this clinic will facilitate information on postrepair reflux. At the same time, evidence will be accumulated on the incidence of Barrett's esophagus in this group.

In the "early" days, of operations for EA, postoperative emphasis was largely on survival. In recent years, survival has been the norm rather than the exception, in keeping with Meyers, a quarter of a century ago, describing E A as the epitome of modern surgery. With modern advances in anesthesia, antimicrobial therapy and neonatal intensive care, problems other than survival per se have occupied the attention of pediatric surgeons caring for babies born with E A and/or T E F. Thus it has become clear that a most important determinant of survival and subsequent progress has been the progress or otherwise of additional life-threatening anomalies. But another factor assuming increasing importance has been GER. This is so particularly, but not exclusively, in the long-gap group, and it is of particular significance in this group managed by esophago-esophagostomy rather than replacement.

A balanced view is provided by Johnson and Beasley in Chapter 23 of the monograph, esophageal Atresia. They highlighted the possible factors contributing to poor esophageal motility and reflux following esophageal atresia repair (1) inherent esophageal dysmotility; (2) injury to branches of the vagus nerve during surgical procedures; (3) upward displacement with tension of lower esophageal segment with reduction of the length of the intra-abdominal esophagus and alteration of the angle of His for the use of gastrostomy. They addressed the problems of symptoms and complications, highlighting the following: vomiting, respiratory symptoms and peptic esophagitis. They outlined measures to be adopted in management, both non-surgical and surgical, and provided information regarding the indications for operation. In discussing the appropriate surgical objective, they pointed out that this was control of reflux without causing dysphagia, and discussed the role of the various operative procedures available. They concluded that the Nissen fundoplication is probably the most widely used and tested anti-reflux procedure. Because esophageal atresia patients often have esophageal shortening and some will require concomitant gastrostomy to facilitate feeds because gross retardation is present, this combination is not ideally suited to the partial wrap, and the complete wrap of the Nissen fundoplication would seem preferable.

Thus, neurologically impaired children and those who have survived repair of esophageal atresia are the two most important groups of patients where GER complicates a specialized condition, but there are many other anecdotal reports of the association. It is inevitable that the future will bring increasing numbers of contributions relating to GER in both groups, and the well-being of both will be facilitated by further surgical research and closely monitored follow-up studies. Esophageal atresia remains the epitome of modern surgery, but survival is no longer the only determinant. With increasing emphasis on finding the appropriate care for the neurologically impaired child, studies will determine the improved outcome when appropriate investigation and/or medical and surgical treatment is applied to this group.

BARRETT'S ESOPHAGUS (BE)

Although BE is seen predominantly in adult patients with GER, in recent years there have been several reports of its occurrence in children. For this reason alone, the pediatric surgeon must be familiar with the condition, but of even greater importance is the now proven association of BE with adenocarcinoma of the esophagus. The consequent need for the diagnosis to be made and appropriate therapy instituted. Therapy includes the need for continued surveillance should BE persist despite anti-reflux surgery, which is the mainstay of treatment. The early history of BE is highlighted by reference to the contributions of Barrett and Allison. since when there has been an increasing number of reports, particularly detailing aspects of the histopathology. More recently, these reports have highlighted the association with adenocarcinoma of the esophagus. The role of endoscopy and biopsy cannot be overstressed, and the need for cooperation between surgeon, endoscopist and pathologist is paramount.

An excellent summary of BE was given by Cameron and Lomboy (1992), who wrote as follows: "In Barrett's esophagus, the normal squamous lining of the esophagus is replaced by columnar epithelium. Barrett's esophagus is associated gastroesophageal reflux, esophagitis and an increased risk of adenocarcinoma of the esophagus. It is thought to be an acquired condition in which acid resistant columnar epithelium replaced squamous epithelium damaged by acid peptic reflux. The diagnosis of Barrett's esophagus is usually made by endoscopy and biopsy. Little information is available concerning the development and natural history of Barrett's esophagus; however, more information has become available since 1992. Patients with this condition have been followed up to determine their subsequent course and the risk of developing carcinomas. However, when a patient is found to have a Barrett's esophagus, the length of time the disorder has been present is usually unknown. Evaluation of the course of this disorder is difficult because of the large number of undiagnosed cases symptoms are not investigated. Many patients do not have reflux symptoms, or their. We recently estimated that for every known patient with Barrett's esophagus there may be 24 unrecognized cases in the general population.

The diagnosis of Barrett's esophagus has implications for long-term surveillance, and often for longevity, life-insurance and medical insurance. Accurate diagnosis is therefore important, and "the late presentation of a Barrett's esophagus is a problem for all ages, perhaps because Barrett's epithelium exhibits decreased esophageal patient sensitivity".

It is evident that Barrett's esophagus is a much less prevalent condition in children than in adults, and the co-morbidities are virtually all conditions that are congenital or genetic, or arise from perinatal asphyxia. Their association with Barrett's esophagus is explained by their predilection to cause severe chronic GE reflux. One implication of the shortened lifespan is that a regular endoscopic surveillance program for established Barrett's esophagus might not be indicated since the underlying disease is a much more likely cause of mortality than adenocarcinoma arising in Barrett's mucosa. However, of note, is the fact that children with esophageal atresia probably have a normal life expectancy, and ongoing surveillance of these children is now recognized to be all-important.

In summary, recognizing that certain children at high risk with severe reflux may be relatively silent, the clinician should have a high index of suspicion that reflux esophagitis or Barrett's esophagus may be present, and not be hesitant to perform endoscopy with biopsy. Prompt, appropriate treatment of reflux esophagitis or other complications of GE reflux, can significantly improve the quality of life for affected children and their care-givers.

The cornerstone of treatment is undoubtedly anti-reflux surgery, followed by ongoing surveillance. Should BE persist, local therapeutic options include photodynamic therapy, mucosectomy, laser therapy, Argon plasma coagulation, or bipolar electro-coagulation. It is clear that not only will each patient need to be individualized, but the form of therapy advised will be determined by the availability of the various modalities.

Thus, Barrett's esophagus remains an uncommon entity in children. But as time passes, more and more patients with this complication of GER will be recognized and the results of treatment by a wide variety of modalities will be assessed. The final story is yet to be told but until then, all children diagnosed as having BE should be the subject of appropriate reports in the literature.

BIOGRAPHY IS THE ONLY TRUE HISTORY

A myriad of names appear in this chapter and yet they only represent a small number of those who have contributed to our knowledge of the different aspects of GER. A segment of this chapter on GER is designed to pay tribute to the vast number of clinicians, pathologists, radiologists, researchers and others, who have extended our knowledge of this subject. It is inevitable that, although the list is long, it is still incomplete, but nevertheless, and hopefully, it will enable the practicing pediatric surgeon to recognize leaders in the field and be stimulated to further his own knowledge. The importance of history cannot be over-estimated. The list is presented in date order, and when contributions involve multiple-authors, the first author is named and additional details appear in the Bibliography

- 18th Century: Term introduced by John Peter Frank
- 1805: Schmidt—describes ectopic gastric mucosa in the esophagus
- 1807: Bozzini—publishers TER Lichtleitner enabled to inspect upper end of esophagus.
- 1828: Billard—reported esophagitis in children
- 1836: Bright—"account of an remarkable misplacement of the stomach"
- 1853: Bowditch—a treatise on diaphragmatic hernia including some details regarding earlier literature on hiatal hernia.
- 1865: Desormeaux—endoscope to examine the esophagus. Visualized structures.
- 1865: Cruise—suggests esophagoscopy.
- 1867: Voltolini—esophageal spectum with a laryngeal mirror.
- 1868: Kussmaul performs the first esophagoscopy "worthy of the name".
- 1879: Ouincke—penetratinq ulcers of the esophagus.
- 1880: Morell Mackenzie—constructs esophagoscope.
- 1881: von Mikulicz—credited with having devised the technique of esophagoscopy,
    Treatise on esophagoscopy and gastroscopy using platinum wire lamp, water-cooled, as light source.
- 1883: Kronecker—observations on manometer.
- 1884: Morell Mackenzie—defines esophagitis.
- 1891: Gottstein suggests the use of cocaine for esophagoscopy.
- 1896: Roentgen—the important discovery of X-ray, the significance of which cannot be overestimated.
- 1899: Mayo states "Ewald thought that peptic ulceration caused many of the strictures of the esophagus".
- 1906: Tileston defined 12 types of esophageal ulceration.
- 1922: Chevalier Jackson— "the diaphragmatic pinchcock".
- 1929: Jackson writes on peptic ulcer of the esophagus.
- 1935: Winkelstein—peptic esophagitis: a new clinical entity.
- 1942: Negus—described the act of swallowing.
- 1947: Neuhauser and berenberg—cardio-esophageal relaxation as a cause of vomiting in infants.
- 1948: Benedict and Sweet—benign stricture of the esophagus with special reference to esophagitis and hiatus hernia.
- 1948: Allison—peptic ulcer of the esophagus.
    - described reflux esophagitis
- 1950: Barrett—"esophagitis is a blunderbuss term"
- 1950: Barrett—chronic peptic ulcer of the esophagus and esophagitis.
- 1950 : Neurenberg—cardioesophageal relaxation (calasia) as a cause of vomiting in infants.
- 1951: Allison—reflux esophagitis, sliding hiatal hernia and the anatomy of repair.
- 1952 : Sweet—esophageal hiatus hernia of the diaphragm.

- — the anatomical characteristics and technique of repair and results of treatment in 111 consecutive cases.
- 1952: Barrett—chronic peptic ulcer of the esophagus in esophagitis.
- 1955: Harrington—operative repair of hiatus hernia.
- 1956: Nissen—Ein einfache operation zur Beeinffussing der reflux oesophagitus.
- 1956: Fike—the gastroesophageal sphincter in healthy human beings.
- 1957: Barrett—the lower esophagus
- 1958: Bernstein—a clinical test of esophagitis.
- 1958: Botha—mucosal folds of the cardia as a component of the gastroesophageal closing mechanism
- 1958: Tuttle—detection of gastroesophageal reflux by simultaneous measurement of intravenous pressures and pH.
- 1958: Ingelfinger—esophageal motility.
- 1958: Botha.
- 1959: Carre—the natural history of the partial thoracic stomach (hiatus hernia) in children.
- 1959: Nissen and Rosetti—Die behandlung dar Hiatus Hernien und reflux oesophagitis mit gastropexie und fundoplication.
- 1961: Hayward the lower end of the esopahgus.
- 1961: Nissen—gastropexy and fundoplication in surgical treatment of a hiatus hernia.
- 1964: Kinsbourne—hiatus hernia with contortions of the neck.
- 1969: Boerema—hiatus hernia: repair by right-sided sub-hepatic anterior gastropexy.
- 1974: Pieretti—resistant esophageal stenosis associated with reflux after repair of esophageal atresia : a therapeutic approach.
- 1974: Johnson and de Meister—24-hour pH-monitoring of the distal esophagus : a quantiative measure of gastroesophageal reflux.
- 1976: Boix-Ochoa—malturation of the lower esopahgus.
- 1976: Dent—a new technique for continuous pressure measurement.
- 1977: Johnson—evaluation of gastroesophageal reflux surgery in children.
- 1977: Rosetti—fundoplication for the treatment of gastroesophageal reflux and hiatus hernia.
- 1977: Bray—childhood gastroesophageal reflux, neurologic and psychiatric syndromes mimicked.
- 1978: Pellegrini—gastroesophageal reflux.
- 1978: Leibermann—Meffert - muscular equivalent of the lower esophageal sphincter.
- 1979: Angelchik—a new surgical procedure for the treatment of gastroesophageal reflux and hiatal hernia.
- 1979: Sondheimer—gastroesophageal reflux amonst severely retarded children.
- 1981: Ashcraft—treatment of gastroesophageal reflux in children by Thal fundoplication.
- 1982: Spitz—surgical treatment of gastroesophageal reflux in severely mentally retarded children.
- 1984: Jamieson—what is a Nissen fundoplication?
- 1984: Ashcraft—the Thal fundoplication for gastroesophageal reflux.
- 1985: Hassall—Barrett's esophagus in childhood.
- 1986: Boix-Ochoa—a physiological approach to the management of gastroesophageal reflux.
- 1987: Barrett's esophagus in children a histologic and histochemical study in 11 cases.
- 1987: Romeo—disorder of the esophageal motor activity in atresia of the esophagus.
- 1991: Jolley—the risk of sudden infant death from gastroesophageal reflux.
- 1991: Dallemagne—laparoscopic Nissen fundoplication. Preliminary report.
- 1992: Smith—Nissen fundoplication in children with profound neurological disability.
- 1993: Lobe—laparoscopic Nissen fundoplication in childhood.
- 1993: De Cau—feeding Roux-en-Y-jejunostomy.
- 1996: Spechier and Goyal—the columnar - lined esophagus, intestinal metaplasia and Norman Barrett.
- 1998: Watson—the changing face of hiatus hernia and gastroesophageal reflux.

SUMMARY

As philosophised by Steve Jones, "So great is today's knowledge there is no one who has sufficient command of the field to debate it". Jones was referring to the study of evolution, with particular reference to Darwin's magnum opus, 'The Origin of Species". However, the philosophy is also applicable to GER, and although there are many clinicians, researchers, and others who are indisputably experts, their contributions are frequently limited to areas which have interested them most - areas in which their expertise has enabled them to be productive and to provide valuable information for the many who are confronted with day-to-day problems in the field of GER.

This chapter attempts to summaries many of the important aspects of GER, commencing with basic information surrounding its anatomy, physiology and pathology. Without knowledge of these areas, it is impossible for the clinician – be he gastroenterologist, pediatrician or pediatric surgeon – to provide optimal care for his patient. It is just a short step from the basic areas to investigation, diagnosis and treatment. But it soon becomes apparent that different views are expressed reflecting the different eras and authorities, based on research and/or clinical experience. The segment devoted to Barrett's esophagus (BE) in children demonstrates the need to be familiar with this entity, and this segment is followed by a summary of historical events under the heading, "Biography is the only true History" (from Emerson and Carlisle). The importance of a knowledge of the history cannot be over-estimated, and will help the pediatric surgeon in decision-making and communication skills.

It is clear from the many contributions, as well as clinical experience, that GER is somewhat different in infants and children from adult GER. While this is true, it is essential that each case be individualized, and investigated and treated on its merits. Over-investigations is to be avoided; by the same token, under-investigation may have serious consequences for the patient. Although the basic principles of treatment are the same, regardless of age, there are significant differences. For example, spontaneous improvement is the norm in infants, and frequently the only therapeutic requirement is reassurance for the parents. Carre's findings emphasized this fact.

The principles of non-operative or medical therapy are similar, regardless of patient age. But fortunately, in the pediatric age-group, should operation be required, this will usually be a relatively simple procedure, the more complicated operations are usually reserved for complicated GERD in adults. In all age-groups, however, the advent of laparoscopic surgery has changed the pattern of management, and recently the situation was summarized by Walson et al, when they wrote: "Laparoscopy for anti-reflux surgery was first reported in 1991. The development phase allowed instrumentation and techniques to be refined, operating times to be shortened and learning curve problems to be recognized and overcome; laparoscopic surgery for reflux has since becomes commonplace. The published results of laparoscopic antireflux surgery, irrespective of the type of fundoplication, confirm the efficiency of the laparoscopic approach. Furthermore, in comparison with an open approach, laparosocpy controls reflux symptoms well and medium-term outcomes have not been compromised. The length of hospital stay has been shortened to two or three days, and these outcomes have also been confirmed in randomised trials of open versus laparoscopic Nissen fundoplication."

Earlier in their contribution, it is relevant to note that they wrote as follows. "it is paradoxical that recently the number of operations for gastroesophageal reflux and hiatus hernia has increased dramatically, even though extremely effective medication for these conditions is now available in many, if not all, western countries. The traditional indications for antireflux surgery still exist, but they have been impacted upon by cultural factors, cost and associated serious disease."

In conclusion, the pediatric surgeon is required to be selective in his decision to advise operation, and to recognize that the spectrum of GER is such that operation is only indicated in a relatively small percentage of cases.

Two other contributions are relevant to the overall summary, and with this conclusions which can be drawn.

Firstly, that of Carre from Belfast, who summarized the situation as follows: "Of recent years, many investigations in addition to conventional radiology have been devised and used increasingly to study gastroesophageal function and reflux in infants.[70,71] Esophageal manometry, acid reflux tests, 24 hr intraluminal esophageal pH probe monitoring and gastroesophageal scintigraphy. These studies have confirmed that reflux is an exceedingly common event in early infancy. This is not unexpected, since the intra-abdominal section of esophagus is often virtually non-existant at this age, and consequently the important mechanical anti-reflux effect of having the terminal esophagus exposed to intra-abdominal pressure, is lost." Carre also reflected on the relative importance of a partial thoracic stomach in children with reflux, concluding: "the all important recognition of a partial thoracic stomach in infants with reflux will therefore depend not only on an awareness by clinicians and radiologists of its clinical importance, but on the availability of a radiologist with experience of this problem." No doubt the significant word here is "experience", an aspect which is relevant to all facets of the problem of GER.

The other contribution is from Orenstein: [31,33] "Gastroesophageal reflux disease (GERD) is one of the most common motility disorders. Indeed, it is one of the most common pediatric disorders of any sort. During the last few decades, a great deal of progress has been made in understanding its pathophysiology and in defining optimal evaluation and treatment. This progress, however, has also illuminated the complexity of the disease, as well as the limitations of current therapy." The philosophy behind this statement, made in 1994, is still relevant and later in the contribution, the following appeared: "Several issues are indispensable to an understanding of gastroesophageal reflux. Reflux, regurgitation and vomiting are ambiguous terms and are sometimes misused. Another issue that confuses our understanding of reflux is that reflux is a normals and those with severe and obvious GERD."

Orenstein has contributed significantly to the literature on GER and in addition to her own contributions extending over two decades, she has provided an extensive set of references, a study of which facilities our present knowledge of GER. With the passage of time, the many practical and theoretical aspects of the problem have been clarified.

REFERENCES

1. Liebermann D. Anatomie des gastroesphagealen verschlussorgan. In Blumm AlL, Siewert JR, Editors: Refluxtherapie, Berlin 1981.
2. Liebermann D, et al. Muscular equivalent of the lower esophageal sphincter. Gastroenterology 1979;76:31.
3. Boix-Ochoa J, Rowe M. Gastroesophageal reflux. in J. O'Neill, et al in Pediatric Surgery. Mosby Year Book 1998;1:1007-28.
4. Demeester TR, et al. A clinical and *in vitro* analysis of determinants of gastroesophageal competence. A study of the principles of antireflux surgery. Am J Surg 1979;137:39.
5. Boix-Ochoa J, Marhuenda C. Gastroesophageal Reflux in Ashcraft K, et al. Pediatric Surgery. WB Saunders 2000;66:1007-29.
6. Boix-Ochoa J. Gastroesophageal reflux in children. In Jamieson GC, Editor: Surgery of the esophagus. Edinburgh, Churchill Livingstone. 1988.
7. Boix-Ochoa J, Canals J. Maturation of the lower esophagus. J Pediatr Surg 1976;11:749.
8. Mittal RK, Balaban DH. The esophagogastric junction. N Eng. J. Med. 1997;336(13)924-32.
9. Mittal RK, et al. Effect of crural myotomy on the incidence and mechanism of gastroesophageal reflux in cats. Gastroenterology 1993;105:740-47.
10. Cohen S. Development characteristics of lower oesophageal sphinter function: a possible mechanism for infantile chalasia, Gastroenterology 1978;67:252.
11. Omari TI, Dent J. Assessment of oesophageal motor function in children and neonates. J Japan Soc Pediatr Surg 1997;33:25-30.
12. Omari T, et al. Characterization of esophageal body and lower esophageal sphincter motor function in the very premature neonate. J Pediatr 1999;135(4):517-21.
13. Omari T, et al. Measurement of upper esophageal sphincter tone and relaxation during swallowing in premature infants. J Pediatr 1999;135-4:522-25.
14. Newell SJ. Development of the lower oesophageal sphincter in the preterm infant. In Milla J. Editor: Disorders of gastrointestinal motility in children, New York, John Wiley and Sons 1998.
15. Newell SJ, et al. Maturation of the lower oesophageal sphincter in the pre-term neonate. Pediatr Res 1986;20:692.
16. Bonavina L, et al. Length of the distal esophageal sphincter and competency of the cardia. Am J Surg 1986;15:25.
17. O'Sullivan GC, et al. Interaction of lower esophageal sphincter pressure and length of sphincter in the abdomen as determinants of gastroesophageal competence. Am J Surg 1982;143:40.
18. Fyke FE, Code CF, Schlegel JF. The gastroesophageal sphincter in healthy human beings. Gastroenterologia 1956;86:135.
19. Boix-Ochoa J. Gastroesophateal reflux. In Welch K, et al, Editors. Pediatric Surgery, St. Louis, 1986 Mosby-Year Book.
20. O'Sullivan GC, DeMeester TR, Joelsson BE, et al. Interaction of lower esophageal sphincter pressure and length of sphincter in the abdomen as determinants of gastroesophageal competence. Am J Surg 1982;143:40-47.
21. DeMeester TR, Wernly JA, Bryant GH, et al. Clinical and *in vitro* analysis of determinants of gastroesophageal competence. Am J Surg 1979;137:39-46.
22. Winans CS, Harris LD. Quantitation of lower esophageal sphincter competence. Gastroenterology 1967;52:773-78.
23. Johnson HD. The antireflux mechanism in the cardia and hiatus, in Springfield, Ill. 1968, Charles C Thomas.
24. Wernly Md, DeMeester Tr, Bryant GH. Intraabdominal pressure and manometric data of the distal esophageal sphincter, their relationship to gastroesophageal reflux, Arch Surg 1980;115:534.

25. Thor KB, Hill LD, Mercer DD, et al. Reappraisal of the flap valve mechanism in the gastroesophageal junction. Acta Chir Scand 1987;153:25-28.
26. Bardaji C, Boix-Ochoa J. Contribution of the His angle to the gastroesophageal antireflux mechanism. Pediat Surg Int 1986;1:172.
27. Boix-Ochoa J, Casasa JM, Gil-Vernet JM. Une chirurgie physiologique pour les anomalies du secteur cardiohiatal. Chir Pediatr 1983;24:117.
28. Herbst JJ. Gastroesophageal reflux and respiratory disorders. Pediatr Pulmonol 1999;27(4):229-30.
29. Boix-Ochoa J, Lafuente JM, Gil-Vernet JM. 24-Hour esophageal pH monitoring in gastroesophageal reflux. J Pediatr Surg 1980;15:74.
30. Boix-Ochoa J. Diagnosis and management of gastroesophageal reflux in children, Surg Ann 1981;13:123.
31. Orenstein SR. Gastroesophageal reflux. In Wylie R, Hyams JS (Eds): Pediatric Gastrointestinal Disease. Philadelphia, WB Saunders 1993;337-69.
32. Katz PO. Treatment of gastroesophageal reflux disease: use of algorithms to aid in management. Am J Gastroenterol 1999;94 (11Suppl) 3-10.
33. Orenstein SR, Whitington PF, Orestein DM. The infant seat as a treatment for gastroesophageal reflux. N Engl J Med 1983;309:760-63.
34. Vandenplas Y, et al. The role of cisapride in the treatment of pediatric gastroesophageal reflux. The European Society of Pediatric Gastroenterology, Hepatology and Nutrition. J Pediatr Gastroenterol Nutr 1999;28(5):518-28.
35. Gunasekaran TS, Hassall EG. Efficacy and safety of omeprazole for severe gastroesophageal reflux in children. J Pediatr 1993;123:148-54.
36. Cucchiara S, Minella R, Campanozzi A, et al. Effects of omeprazole on mechanisms of gastroesophageal reflux in childhood. Dig Dis Sci 1997;42:293-99.
37. Cohen RC. Cisapride in the control of symptons in infants with gastroesophageal reflux: A Randomized, double-blind, placebo-controlled trial. J Pediatr Gastroenterol Nutr 1996;22:259-69.
38. Cucchiara S. Cisapride therapy for gastrointestinal disease J Pediatr Gastroenterol Nutr 1996;22:259-69.
39. Boix-Ochoa J, Casasa JM. Surgical treatment of gastroesophageal reflux in children. In Nyhus LM, Editor: Surgery annual, New York. Appleton and Lange 1989.
40. Fonkalsrud EW, et al. Surgical treatment of GER: A combined study of 7647 patients. Pediatrics 1998;108:419-22.
41. Boix-Ochoa J. The physiologic approach to the management of gastric esophageal reflux. J Pediatr Surg 1986;21:1032-39.
42. Boix-Ochoa J, Casasa JM. Gastroesophageal reflux: Boix-Ochoa procedure in L. Spitz et al". Pediatric Operative Surgery 5th ed.: 279-86 Champman and Hall.
43. Bardaji C, et al. La plastia de Boix-Ochoa reconvierte al enfermo a la normalidad. Estudio phmetrico de 21 casos. Cir Pediatr 1993;7:14.
44. Hassall E. Antireflux surgery in children: Time for a harder look. Pediatrics 1998;101:467-68.
45. Spitz L. Surgical treatment of gastroesophageal reflux in severely mentally retarded children. J R Soc Med 1982;75:525-29.
46. Vane DW, Harmel RP Jr, King Dr, et al. The effectiveness of Nissen fundoplication in neurologically impaired children with gastroesophageal reflux. Surgery 1985;98:662-66.
47. Wilkinson JD, Dudgeon DL, Sondheimer JM. A comparison of medical and surgical treatment of gastroesophageal reflux in severely retarded children. J Pediatr. 1981;99:202-05.
48. Dalla Vecchia LK, Grosfeld JL, West KW, et al. Reoperation after Nissen fundoplication in children with gastroesophageal reflux. Experience with 130 patients. Ann Surg 1997;226:315-23.
49. Zaloga GP, Chernow B. Prostprandial hypoglucemia after Nissen fundoplication for reflux esophagitis. Gastroenterology 1983;84:840.
50. Van Kempen AAMW, et al. Dumping syndrome after combined pyoroplasty and fundoplication. Eur J Pediatr 1992;151:546.
51. Cohen Z, et al. Nissen fundoplication and Boix-Ochoa antireflux procedure: comparison between two surgical techniques in the treatment of gastroesophageal reflux in children. Eur J Pediatr Surg 1999;9(5):289-93.
52. Dallemagne B, Weerts JM Jehaes C, et al. Techniques and results of endoscopic fundoplication. End Surg 1993;1:72-76.
53. Ferguson CM, Rattner DW. Initial experience with laparoscopic Nissen Fundoplication. Am Surg 1995;61:21-23.
54. Lobe TE. Laparoscopic fundoplication. Semin Pediatr Surg 1993;2:178-81.
55. Peters JH, Heimbucher J, Kauer WK, et al. Clinical and Physiologic comparison of laparoscopic and open Nissen fundoplication (see comments). J Am Coll Surg 1995;180:385-93.
56. Vane DW, Harmel RP Jr, King Dr, et al. The effectiveness of Nissen fundoplication in neurologically impaired children with gastroesophageal reflux. Surgery 1985;98:662-66.
57. Bohmer CJM, Niezen-de Boer MC, Klinkenberg-Knol EC, et al. Gastroesophageal reflux disease in intellectually disabled individuals: Leads for diagnosis and the effect of omeprazole. Am J Gastroenterol 1997;92:1475-79.
58. Wilkinson JD, Dudgeon DL, Sondheimer JM. A comparison of medical and surgical treatment of gastroesophageal reflux in severely retarded children. J Pediatr 1981;99:202-205.
59. Borgstein ES, Heij HA, Beygelaar JD, et al. Risks and benefits of antireflux operations in neurologically impaired children. Eur J Pediatr 1994;153:248-51.
60. Martinez DA, Ginn-Pease ME, Caniano DA. Sequellae of antireflux surgery in profoundly disabled children. J Pediatr Surg 27:267-73.

61. Staiano A, Cuchiara S, et al. Disorders of esophageal motility in children with psychomotor retardation and gastroesophageal reflux. Eur J Pediatr 1991;150:638-41.
62. O'Neill JK, O'Neill PJ, Got-Owens T, et al. Care-giver evaluation of anti-gastroesophageal reflux procedures in neurologically impaired children: What is the real-life outcome. J Pediatr Surg 1996;31:375-80.
63. Dalla Vecchia LK, Grosfeld JL, West KW, et al. Reoperation after Nissen fundoplication in children with gastroesophageal reflux. Experience with 130 patients. Ann Surg 1997;226:315-23.
64. Zaloga GP, Chernow B. Prostprandial hypoglucemia after Nissen fundoplication for reflux esophagitis. Gastroenterology 1983;84:840.
65. Van Kempen AAMW, et al. Dumping syndrome after combined pyoroplasty and fundoplication. Eur J Pediatr 11992;51:546.
66. Caniano DA, Ginn-Pease ME, KIng DR. The failed antireflux procedure: Analysis of risk factors and morbidity. J Pediatr Surg 1990;25:1022-26.
67. Mittal RK. Do we understand how surgery prevents gastroesophageal reflux? Gastroenterology 1994;106:1714-15.
68. Kawahara H, et al. Mechanisms underlying the antireflux effect of Nissen Fundoplication in Children. J Ped Surg 1999;33(11):1618-22.
69. Ireland AC, Holloway RH, Toouli J, et al. Mechanisms underlying the antireflux action of fundoplication. Gut 1993;34:303-308.
70. Carré IJ. Natural history of partial thoracic stomach ("hiatus hernia") in children. Arch Dis Child 1959;34:344.
71. Carré IJ. Postural treatment of children with partial thoracic stomach ("hiatus hernia"). Arch Dis Child 1960;35:569.

CHAPTER 29

Thal Fundoplication

Keith W Ashcraft

RATIONALE

The normal or physiologic function of the lower esophageal sphincter (LES) is to allow the unrestricted passage of food or drink from the esophagus into the stomach. In addition, the normal LES relaxes to allow eructation of swallowed air or to allow vomiting when appropriate. Gastroesophageal reflux (GER) may be defined simply as the inappropriate return of gastric content into the esophagus. GER is an exceedingly common condition both in adults and children (Fig. 29.1). It is primarily an anatomical disorder that becomes much more difficult to manage as the complications of inflammation and scarring progress. Because the pressure gradient between the mediastinum and abdominal cavities is increased by both the patient's weight and activity. The obesity and other activities that result in the increase in the intra-abdominal pressure, will aggravate GER and reduce the chances of successful treatment.

Once hardly considered to be a disease or disorder affecting pediatric patients, GER is now one of the major causes of morbidity in children not due to infections.[1] It has been recognised as a factor in malnutrition, respiratory disorders, otitis and all the manifestations of esophageal mucosal erosion or esophagitis. It may be one of the major causes of "colic" in babies. Both medical and surgical therapy for GER is directed toward symptomatic relief.

The medical therapy for GER is directed toward reducing the production of gastric acid so that continued GER does not result in acid esophagitis or it is directed toward drugs whose function is to enhance prograde emptying of the stomach, reducing the chances for GER to occur. The medications for both of these attacks upon the problem are expensive or carry some significant risks of side effects that have caused some of them to be withdrawn from the market. Arguably the risks of permanent serious side effects may be small but the fact that the medications must be continued ad infinitum is of concern. Because medical therapy for GER provides relief of symptoms only when it is taken, it must be projected over a lifetime. Unrecognised or improperly treated GER may result in esophageal stricture or even sudden death due to laryngospasm. The non-operative treatment of GER may carry a much higher risk than does operative treatment. Many parents are unwilling to accept the risk of medical therapy so surgical treatment of GER

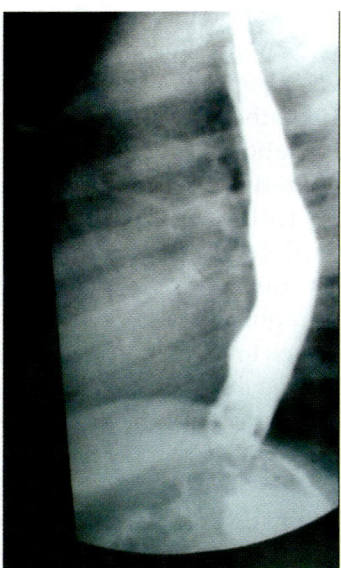

Fig. 29.1: Barium study in a symptomatic child, suggestive of gastroesophageal reflux, absence of angle of His, requiring antireflux surgery

in children has become one of the most commonly performed procedures in pediatric surgery at the time of this writing.

The author feels that a surgical procedure should produce a result that mimics the natural anatomy and function as nearly as possible. In very few areas does the surgeon have a choice of such different procedures as in the surgical treatment of GER. The natural function of the lower esophageal sphincter (LES) is to allow the unobstructed passage of food and drink from the esophagus while also allowing eructation or vomiting of food that is intolerable to the individual. The fact that everybody has some postprandial LES relaxation has been taken into account in the most definitive of tests for GER—the extended esophageal pH monitoring. The episodes of reflux that occur within two hours of ingestion of food are not counted in the scoring of reflux episodes or severity. Given that some reflux is not only normal but also necessary and given that the partial wrap surgical procedures for GER allow "normalcy," may be that the popularity of a fundoplication procedure that does not establish a physiologic state is based upon something other than reason. It is suspected that many of the proponents of the complete wrap simply learned that one procedure and have not considered changing. Many pediatric surgeons can't make the Thal partial-wrap "work" or that the failure rate is excessive. This may be based upon the misconception that any demonstrable reflux by a contrast study in the postoperative Thal patient is interpreted as a sign of failure. This finding would certainly be indicative of failure in the postoperative Nissen fundoplication. Contrast radiographic studies either for preoperative evaluation and diagnosis or for postoperative follow-up are acute studies that generally take place within the postprandial period discounted by the extended pH study. Although contrast radiographs absolutely should precede any operative approach to correction of GER, they are more useful to determine the angle of His and the ability or inability of the gastroesophageal junction to open or relax than they are for diagnosis of GER. The observation of an obtuse angle of His is the best diagnostic sign of GER on a contrast study.

The best test of success for any fundoplication procedure is the assessment of symptomatic relief. If the patient no longer has the GER symptoms he/she had preoperatively, no longer requires medication to counteract acid and does not have obstruction to the passage of food or to eructation and vomiting the procedure may be termed successful.

There has been a recent swing toward minimally invasive surgery performed using multiple incisions, long (and often low-quality instruments) while observing the whole process on a video monitor. Although shortened hospital stay and more rapid return to work have been argumented for the economic feasibility of such techniques, the intraoperative time and costs have often more than wasted the economies gained. Minimally invasive surgery is a relative term.

The author's approach to the Thal fundoplication is a minimally invasive approach that carries with it the distinct advantages of a close personal relationship with the tissues to be rearranged. Using a transverse, upper abdominal incision, only the viscera above the transverse colon are exposed or handled. No incidental procedures such as appendectomy or umbilical herniorrhaphy are added. The rectus muscles are cut rather than stretched as in the usual midline approach and postoperative pain is much reduced as a result. Intestinal motility is not interrupted and the patient does not require nasogastric drainage. The patient may almost always be discharged within 48 hours. Anesthesia time is kept to a minimum. Even "talking" a very junior resident through a Thal procedure results in operative times of less than 40 minutes. Knots are tied the way God intended them to be tied-by hand. Continuous suture techniques distribute tension better than do multiple interrupted sutures. The one disadvantage is that of adhesions between stomach and liver are more intense than with endoscopic techniques.

The Thal fundoplication is created by applying the free wall of the gastric fundus to the anterior aspect of the intra-abdominal esophagus and is also known as the Dor-Nissen procedure or the Boix-Ochoa procedure.[2] Boix-Ochoa in addition produces an umbrella like effect by attaching the fundus of the stomach at three places with the under surface of the diaphragm. The same physiological result as anterior wrapping theoretically may be anticipated using the posterior partial wrap fundoplication (Toupet) but much more dissection is required (Figs 29.2A to D). Additionally, over-distension of the stomach following the Toupet procedure may angulate the intra-

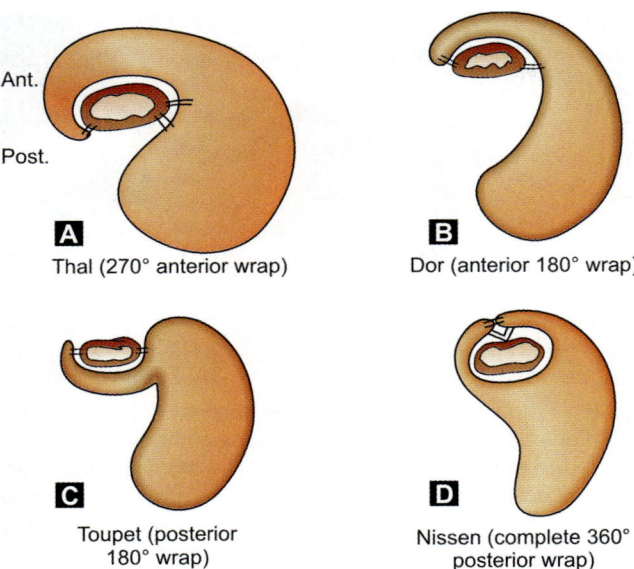

Figs 29.2A to D: Diagrammatic depiction as seen from cranial view of **A.** Thal fundoplication (270 degree anterior wrap), **B.** Dor (180 degree anterior wrap), **C.** Toupet (180 degree posterior wrap) fundoplication and **D.** Nissen fundoplication with a complete (360°) posterior wrap

abdominal esophagus to the point of obstruction. Proponents of the partial wrap believe that a successful wrap cures the problem of GER and yet leaves the patient with the ability to vomit and to burp if the need arises. Obviously, in the pediatric patient the need for one or both of these very physiologic functions is more common than in the adult patient population. There are some pediatric patients, particularly those who have severe neurological impairment, who are perhaps better served by a complete wrap (Nissen) because there is little hope of any conscious control of the GE junction or of significant oral intake (Fig. 29.1). Very commonly in these patients any fundoplicaton is accompanied by a Stamm or some other form of gastrostomy used for feeding and/or gastric decompression.

The author's experience has been entirely with the open procedures in over 1,000 cases with Thal fundoplications. The nasogastric drainage has not been used. The oral liquids are started within 12 hours of operation and the patient is discharged within 48 hours in the vast majority of cases. There are several endoscopic surgeons in the United States that have accumulated significant endoscopic experience with the Thal fundoplication but whose time to feeding and discharge is not significantly shorter than this. The benefit, therefore, is probably related to the issue of one transverse abdominal scar versus several smaller ones. The endoscopic procedure certainly required expertise, increased costs of equipment and the supplies. Also, being the recent development, long-term results with endoscopic procedure are still not known.

All patients required a barium study prior to operation to exclude the possibility of achalasia. About 1% of all the 2000 GER patients in the author's experience had concomitant achalasia and required a distal esophageal myotomy in conjunction with the Thal fundoplication.

SURGICAL TECHNIQUE (FIGS 29.3A TO D)

The patient is best anesthetized expeditiously and without distending the stomach or the gut with nitrous oxide. A nasogastric tube of appropriate size is passed by the anesthesiologist for purposes of intraoperative gastric decompression and to aid in the tactile identification of the gastroesophageal junction The tube also provides some rigidity for the esophagus during the creation of the fundoplication preventing distortion of the gastroesophageal junction during the suturing process.

- An upper abdominal transverse incision is made from the left costal margin at the nipple line to the opposite costal margin, dividing both left and right rectus muscles. The abdomen is entered cephalad of the transverse colon and the small intestine is protected from exposure by the mesocolon. Sufficient relaxation is required to prevent the patient from "bucking" and eviscerating himself.
- The anterior free wall of the stomach is grasped with a gauze pad and retracted downward. The left lobe of the liver is also grasped and dissected free from the underside of the left hemidiaphragm. The liver is folded downward and retracted to the right by the second assistant.
- Incision of the peritoneum at the hiatus is done in a transverse direction and a blunt dissector used to spread the areolar tissue on either side of the easily seen and palpated esophagus. The dissector is passed behind the esophagus from the right to the left, grasping and pulling through a Dacron tape that will be used for traction purposes. Using this tape retractor, the esophagus is lifted and the posterior (right) branch of the vagus nerve

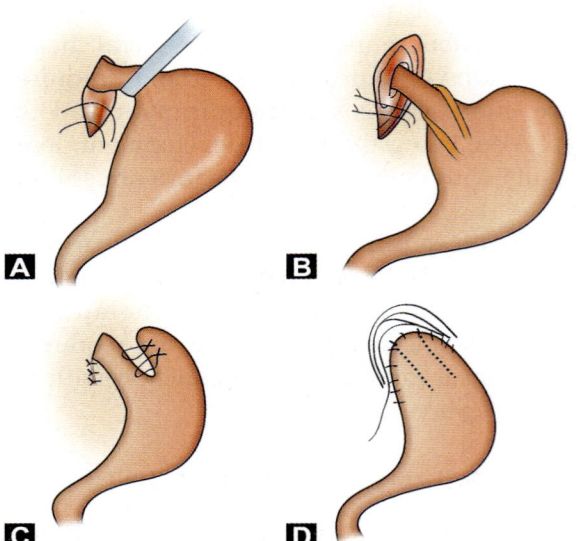

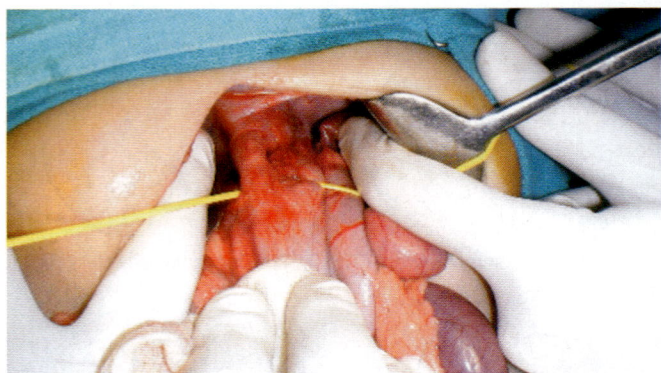

Fig. 29.4: Mobilization of the intra-abdominal segment of the esophagus for 2-4 cm length. The left lobe of the liver has been retracted to the right by the assistant. The stomach has been displaced downward by the gauze pad. The gastroesophageal junction is identified and retracted downward while the hiatus is pushed in a cephalad direction

Figs 29.3A to D: Diagram depicting the surgical technique of the authors' preference for Thal fundoplication. **A.** Mobilization of the gastroesophageal junction, **B.** Approximation of the crura with non-absorbable sutures. Gain of intra-abdominal length of abdominal esophagus and its fixation with the diaphragm **C.** Highest suture from fundus of the stomach is fixed with the esophagus and the diaphragm near the hiatus **D.** Completed Thal's repair (270° wrap)

identified. If the posterior vagus nerve has not been included within the tape, the tape is repositioned.
- Using the tape the GE junction is retracted downward while the hiatus on either side of the esophagus is pushed in a cephalad direction (Fig. 29.4). The hiatus is not intentionally enlarged during the mobilization of the lower 2-4 cm of esophagus.
- Using an "S" or small Richardson retractor, the distal esophagus is retracted to the patient's left by the first assistant, exposing both limbs of the crura behind. The crura are approximated using a figure of eight suture of the nonabsorabale material. It is important to leave a space behind the esophagus so that the hiatus is not narrowed excessively. It is very important not to tie this hiatus closing suture too tightly or muscle necrosis will result in a larger hiatus than was originally present. The hiatus suture is tied with its needle still attached so that it may now be used to anchor the posterior wall of the esophagus to the hiatus. This additional posterior fixation of the distal esophagus within the abdominal cavity adds to the effectiveness of the procedure.
- The retractor is removed from behind the esophagus and the Dacron tape ends are separated. A permanent suture (preferably a 2-0 or 3-0 size) is placed and tied at the GE junction on the left. The fundoplication is created using a continuous suture technique going up the left side of the esophagus, suturing stomach to esophagus. As the suture line crosses over the front of the esophagus to reach the right side the suture line, incorporates the stomach, esophagus and the hiatus. As the right side of the esophagus is reached, the suture line is turned caudally to reach the lesser curvature gastroesophageal junction where it is tied. Thus an inverted "U" suture line is created holding the anterior free wall of the stomach to the anterior free wall of the intra-abdominal esophagus. When complete, the esophagus has been sutured to the anterior half of the esophageal hiatus by the fundoplication suture and to the repaired hiatus posteriorly by the hiatus suture. It is not necessary to divide any of the short gastric vessels to perform this fundoplication.
- The length of the fundoplication is assessed by palpating the nasogastric tube through the layers of stomach applied to the esophagus. The Nasogastric tube is removed, the liver replaced in its bed and the wound closed. Boix-Ochoa attaches the His prior to replacing the liver and closure, a part of the procedure that has not been found necessary. Also, gastrostomy is not performed in routine except for the patient who needs to be fed

by gastrostomy postoperatively. Many younger patients who have a complete-wrap fundoplication require a gastrostomy to prevent gastric bloating, a sometimes serious result of this type of GER procedure.

POSTOPERATIVE CARE

The patient is offered clear liquids six to eight hours after leaving the recovery room and is offered a diet for age the following morning. Once the patient is taking sufficient fluid he is discharged, sometimes as early as 24 hours postoperative. Virtually all patients who are not complicated by other disorders are out of the hospital within 48 hours.

RESULTS

As a group, of the 2078 Thal Fundoplications performed in 1915 patients (1974 and 1999), 78% were neurologically intact and 60% were under one year of age at the time of the initial procedure. Only 4% of these had esophageal atresia and 1% had achalasia.[3]

- Approximately 90% of patients are able to burp and vomit within two weeks following the procedure
- Those patients with severe esophagitis are more likely to suffer transient distal esophageal edema and obstruction requiring a liquid diet for more than a few days
- Only three patients have required reinsertion of the nasogastric tube for the gas-bloat complication that resolved within 24 hours
- There have been two deaths that occurred early in our experience as a result of the surgical procedure- both due to unrecognised small bowel obstruction in severely impaired children
- Seventy five patients required a repeat fundoplication because of recurrent hiatus hernia with herniation of an intact wrap or disruption of the wrap. Three of these patients required a third fundoplication
- One patient had four Thal fundoplications in an attempt to reduce the multiple complications of a failed esophageal atresia repair.

FOLLOW-UP

Initially a repeat barium study used to be performed after four months of surgery to demonstrate that the wrap was intact (Fig. 29.5). Now the barium is done if the patients develop some symptoms.

REOPERATION FOR RECURRENT GER

Recurrence of GER has been due almost equally to disruption of the fundoplication suture line and to recurrence of the hiatus hernia.[4,5] The first 400 patients did not have a mandatory hiatus closure which was called the "limiting stitch" and which is now placed in all patients. The recurrence rate was 7% in those initial 400 patients. Of late, the recurrence rate is 2-3%, mostly because of fundoplication disruption. For some inexplicable reason, it was often found the PTFE suture had been broken and the stomach was found separated from the distal esophagus. No patient was found to have developed adhesions between the stomach and the esophagus sufficient to prevent recurrent GER in face of a suture failure.

Reoperation is often complicated by extensive adhesions between the stomach and the underside of the liver. It is imperative to dissect all the adhesions both for visibility and for the necessary mobility to redo the fundoplication. All steps of the original procedure must be followed if one is to anticipate success. Clearly a thoracic approach for repeat fundoplication would not be feasible because of the gastrohepatic adhesions. Only in cases of extreme neurological dysfunction, Thal procedure may be converted to a Nissen.

SPECIAL SITUATIONS

When faced with the request for a feeding gastrostomy in a **neurologically impaired** patient, a concomitant

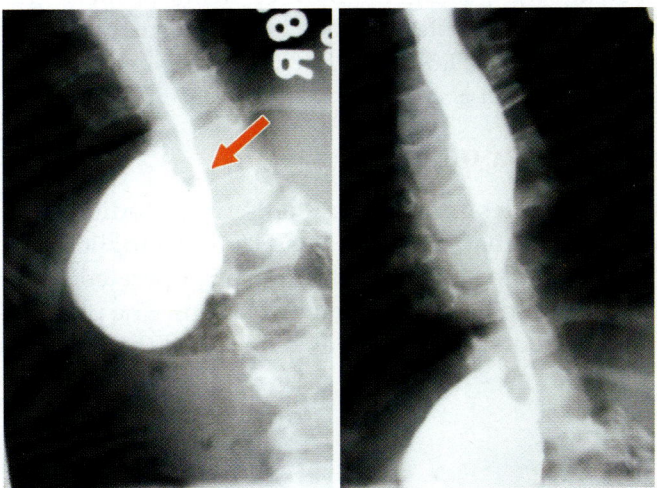

Fig. 29.5: Barium study (AP and lateral view) outlining the Thal fundoplication with the creation of a nice angle of His

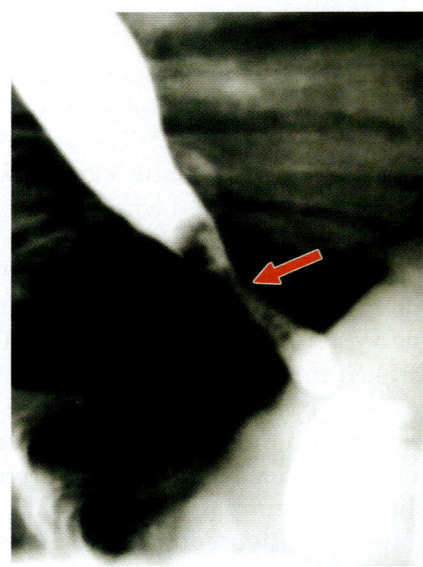

Fig. 29.6: Barium study outlining the filling defect following a food bolus obstruction. The patient had stricture of the lower esophagus and Thal fundoplication had been performed

fundoplication should be performed.[6,7] This is done because most patients when fed by gastrostomy will begin to reflux even without evidence of GER before. To perform a fundoplication in the presence of an established gastrostomy increases the likelihood of a wound infection and dehiscence. In approximately 50% of patients having repair of esophageal atresia malformations, reflux is a significant problem.[8] In most of these patients a fundoplication is necessary. It is very important that the fundoplication should not obstruct the passage of food or drink because the motility of the distal esophagus is abnormal in these patients (Fig. 29.6). It is felt that the partial wrap fundoplication is certainly best for these patients.

LONG-TERM RESULTS

In the author's series, 23 patients were studied who were more than 10 years post-Thal fundoplication. Many of these patients were originally operated upon as babies and had grown into their teens. The patients were selected on the basis of availability and willingness to undergo both a contrast radiographic study and a 24-hour pH study. The selection resulted in data that were not generally reliable for the entire population but approximately one-third of these had a small, presumably "traction" diverticulum at the level of the esophageal hiatus but all had normal pH studies. All were asymptomatic.

SUMMARY

The Thal fundoplication and its related partial-wrap fundoplications have resulted in short and long-term results equal to or better than the published results of the complete wrap. The complications relating to gastric over distension are not seen with the partial wrap procedures and patient/parent satisfaction is quite high.

REFERENCES

1. Jolley SG, Herbst JJ, Johnson DG, et al. Patterns of postcibal gastroesophageal reflux in symptomatic infants. Am J Surg 1979;138:946-50.
2. Boix-Ochoa J, Marhuenda C. Gastroesophageal Reflux, Chapter 28 in Pediatric Surgery, 3E. Ashcraft KW, Murphy JP, Sharp RJ, Sigalet DL, Snyder CL, (Eds). WB Saunders, Philadelphia 2000.
3. Fonkalsrud EW, Ashcraft KW, Coran AG, et al. Surgical treatment of gastroesophageal reflux in children: a combined hospital study of 7467 patients. Pediatrics 1998;101:419-22.
4. Turnage RH, Oldham KT, Coran AG, et al. Late results of fundoplication for gastroesophageal reflux in infants and children. Surgery 1989;105:457-64.
5. Caniano DA, Ginn-Pease ME, King DR. The failed antireflux procedure: analysis of risk factors and morbidity. J Pediatr Surg 1990;25:1022-26.
6. Vane DW, Harmel RP Jr, King DR, et al. The effectiveness of Nissen fundoplication in neurologically impaired children with gastroesophageal reflux surgery 1985;98:662-66.
7. Ramachandran V, Ashcraft KW, Sharp RJ, et al. Thal fundoplication in neurologically impaired children. J Pediatr Surg 1996;31:819-22.
8. Synder CL, Ramachandran V, Kennedy AP, et al. Efficacy of partial wrap fundoplication for gastroesophageal reflux after repair of esophageal atresia. J Pediatr Surg 1997;32:1089-92.

Achalasia Cardia

Shilpa Sharma, DK Gupta

Achalasia comes from a Greek word that means "failure to relax". Cardiospasm is a synonym used to describe the same condition. Achalasia is a primary functional esophageal motility disorder characterized by failure of a hypertensive lower esophageal sphincter (LES) to relax and the absence of esophageal peristalsis.

Achalasia cardia is mainly a disease of young adults with less than 5% cases occurring in children.[1,2] Achalasia cardia is thus a relatively rare problem in children, however, when present it can result in severe disabling symptoms like severe lung disease and growth retardation often requiring surgical intervention.[3] It may occasionally be a cause of mortality due to respiratory complications.

HISTORICAL BACKGROUND

Sir Thomas Willis, in 1672, first described achalasia and treated the problem with a dilation using a whale sponge attached to a whale bone.[4-6] In 1881, Von Mikulicz described the disease as cardiospasm, felt it was a functional problem not a mechanical one. In 1913, Ernest Heller, first successfully performed a esophagomyotomy.[7] In 1929. Hurt and Rake realized that the disease was caused by a failure of the lower esophageal sphincter (LES) to relax. They coined the term achalasia, meaning failure to relax. The first anterior partial fundoplication was reported by Dor in 1962.[8] Toupet reported the first posterior partial fundoplication in 1963.[9]

ETIOPATHOPHYSIOLOGY

The cause of achalasia is unknown.[10] Theories on causation invoke infection, heredity or an abnormality of the immune system that causes the body itself to damage the esophagus (autoimmune disease). The occurrence of achalasia in the first six months of life, the existence of a familial factor, the prevalent possible association with genetic diseases (familial dysautonomia, glucocorticoid insufficiency, Rozycki syndrome) suggest that achalasia in childhood may in certain cases represent a congenital problem, somewhat different from the adult form, which is considered to be an acquired disease.[11]

However, the two main theories that have been developed to explain the onset of this disease are:
1. A primary neurogenic abnormality with a failure of the inhibitory nerves and progressive degeneration of ganglion cells.
2. An acquired deficiency of the myenteric plexus ganglion cells, secondary to GERD, Chagas disease, or viral process.[2,12]

LES pressure and relaxation are regulated by excitatory (e.g. acetylcholine, substance P) and inhibitory (e.g. nitric oxide, vasoactive intestinal peptide) neurotransmitters. Children with achalasia lack nonadrenergic, noncholinergic, inhibitory ganglion cells, causing an imbalance in excitatory and inhibitory neurotransmission. The result is a hypertensive nonrelaxed esophageal sphincter. Microscopically, there is degeneration of ganglion cells in Auerbach's myenteric plexus. This condition is in some ways analogous to megacolon. Normally, there is a lower esophageal high-pressure zone, or lower esophageal sphincter. In achalasia the lower esophageal sphincter is hypertonic, producing resting pressures above normal and relaxing incompletely after swallowing.[13] This produces a functional obstruction, resulting in dilation and elongation of the body of the esophagus with rapid narrowing at the cardia. In vigorous achalasia, simultaneous nonpropagated high-amplitude pressure waves occur throughout the esophageal body.

The irritation caused by the presence of stagnant food in the esophagus may lead to esophagitis and ulcerations. Early in achalasia, inflammation can be seen under the microscope in the muscle of the lower esophagus, especially around the nerves. As the disease progresses, the nerves begin to degenerate and ultimately disappear, particularly the nerves that cause the lower esophageal sphincter to relax. Still later in the progression of the disease, muscle cells begin to degenerate, possibly because of the damage to the nerves. The result of these changes is a lower sphincter that cannot relax and muscle in the lower esophageal body that cannot support peristaltic waves. With time, the body of the esophagus stretches and becomes dilated. Microscopic examination may also show acanthosis.

CLINICAL PRESENTATION

Achalasia is characterized by dysphagia (most common), regurgitation of feeds, chest pain, heartburn and weight loss. There is usually a progressive dysphagia for solid and liquid food. The children learn to compensate for their dysphagia by taking smaller bites, chewing well, and eating slowly. This causes a delay in diagnosis and marked dilation of the esophagus. The dysphagia in achalasia also is different from the dysphagia of esophageal stricture or stenosis. In achalasia, dysphagia occurs with both solid and liquid food, whereas in esophageal stricture or stenosis, the dysphagia typically occurs only with solid food.

Rarely, children may also present with cough and aspiration pneumonitis, as they may be unable to explain the symptoms.

There is no contributory finding in the physical examination. There is no sex predilection, though some have reported a higher incidence in males. A high index of suspicion is required to ask for the contributory investigations.

INVESTIGATIONS

Characteristic chest X-ray findings in achalasia are a widened mediastinum, an air fluid level in the esophagus, an absent gastric air bubble, and aspiration pneumonia.

Barium Swallow

The esophagus appears dilated, and contrast material passes slowly into the stomach as the LES opens intermittently. The distal end of esophagus is usually narrowed and this is known as the bird's beak sign (Fig. 30.1). Cine esophagogram demonstrates aperistalsis in the dilated section and tertiary contractions of the esophageal body may be observed with an air-fluid level.[14] Elongation and dilation of the esophagus produce tortuosity, leading to a sigmoid esophagus in extreme cases.

Stages of achalasia: Achalasia in adults has been categorized by the diameter and length of the esophagus. An esophagus with a diameter of 2-3 cm is normal, grade 1 is < 4 cm, grade 2 is 4-6 cm and bird beak looking, grade 3 is > 6 cm, and grade 4 is a sigmoid esophagus.[15]

Esophageal Manometry

This helps to confirm the findings picked up on a barium swallow and is currently the examination of choice to confirm achalasia. There is incomplete relaxation of the LES in response to swallowing, with a high resting LES pressure and incomplete or absent

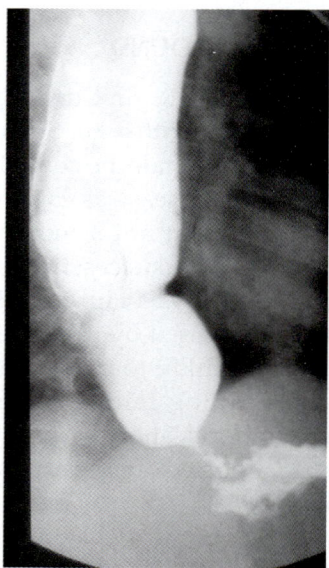

Fig. 30.1: Barium swallow showing the dilated esophagus with narrowed distal end of esophagus known as the Birds beak sign

LES relaxation after deglutition, associated with a lack of peristaltic coordination of the esophageal body during deglutition.[16,17]

24-hour esophageal pH monitoring and scintillographic studies

This may help to rule out gastroesophageal reflux.

CT Scan Chest

If the above findings are not contributory or contradictory to each other, a CT scan chest may be done to rule out a bronchocartilaginous ring at the lower end. However, even a CT scan chest may not pick up the cartilaginous remnant unless planned in smaller sections. The authors have found a bronchocartilaginous ring at the lower end only as a peroperative finding in 3 cases. Thus a high index of suspicion is essential.

MANAGEMENT

The aim of treatment is to relieve symptoms by eliminating the outflow resistance caused by the hypertensive and non-relaxing LES. After the obstruction is relieved, food can pass through the aperistaltic body of the esophagus by gravity. Calcium channel blockers and nitrates have been used in the elderly to decrease the LES pressure, but they have no role in children.

Dilatation

Dilatation with bougies and pneumatic dilatation may provide temporary relief of the symptoms. Pneumatic dilation consists of placing a balloon in the lower esophageal sphincter and inflating it to disrupt the lower circular muscle fibers. There is a definite risk of esophageal perforation bleeding, and gastroesophageal reflux with pneumatic dilatation, and it should be avoided.[18] Gentle dilatation with bougies may be helpful in cachexic patients to build up the nutritional status to make them fit for surgical intervention. The response to dilation is only 20%. Also, if redilatation is needed within 3 weeks, then it should be considered as a failure of the dilatation program and surgical treatment should be considered.

Nasogastric feeding may be given to build up the nutrition of these children. If the nasogastric tube is not negotiable, a gastrostomy may be considered in severely malnourished children.

Esophagoscopy is important to confirm the presence of retained food in a dilated esophagus, esophagitis and esophageal stenosis. During endoscopic examination, resistance may be encountered to the progress of the endoscope.[2,4,14] The lower esophageal sphincter is tight, but the esophagoscope passes with gentle pressure.[19]

The injection of clostridium botulinum toxin into the lower esophageal sphincter is a relatively new procedure.[20,21] It has a high failure rate, offers only a temporary benefit, requires repeated injections, and may produce scarring that can make subsequent surgery more difficult and hazardous.[12,22] This treatment should only be reserved for cases in which there is no possibility of a surgical treatment, and is not recommended in children.

Heller's Cardiomyotomy with Anti-reflux Procedure

Heller cardiomyotomy has been the treatment modality of choice. The classical surgical approach consists of performing myotomy of the esophagus and cardia (Figs 30.2A and B). Some authors have suggested a variation of the technique, removing a strip of muscle tissue (myomectomy). The myotomy/myectomy extends from the LES to 2 or 3 cm above the cardia, is generally associated with anti-reflux procedures, and is done with a view to the fact that

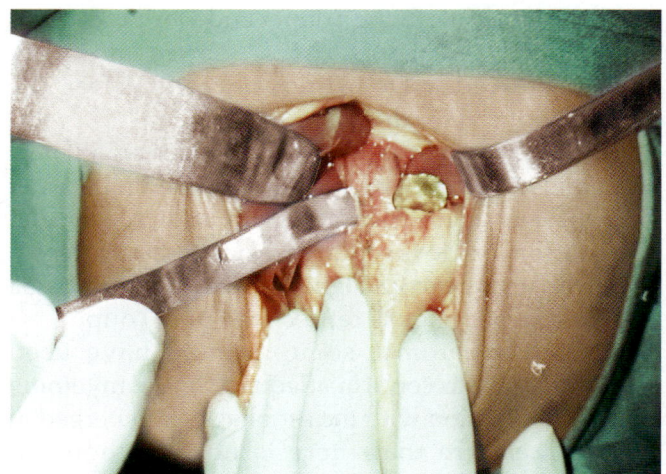

Fig. 30.2A: An operative photograph showing the lower esophageal junction, after mobilization of the peritoneum at the cardioesophageal junction

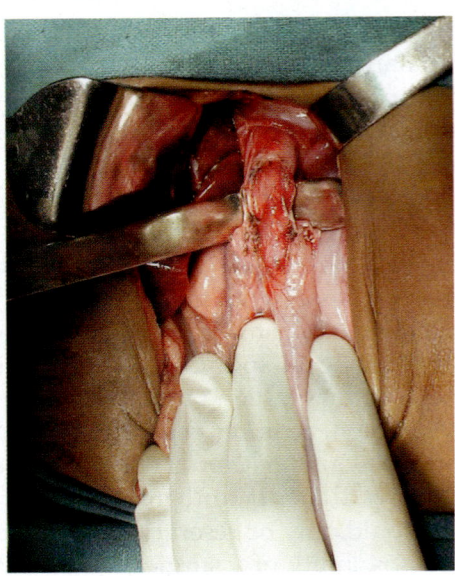

Fig. 30.2B: Operative photograph showing a successful cardioesophageal myotomy with exposure of the mucosa. This was followed by a Thal fundoplication

cardiomyomectomy alone favors gastroesophageal reflux. A long myotomy ensures division of all the lower esophageal high-pressure zone circular muscle fibers and may prevent chest pain from nonpropagated simultaneous contractions or diffuse esophageal spasm.[19] An inadequate myotomy fails to relieve the dysphagia, and one that is too long causes gastroesophageal reflux.[4,19]

An adequate myotomy produces gastroesophageal reflux, so most authors nowadays add a partial fundoplication.[4] Both the Toupet and Dor procedures have their advocates. Most series however have preferred a Dor fundoplication after the myotomy.[3,15,22-25]

Since the Dor partial fundoplication is an anterior wrap and covers a portion of the exposed mucosa, it helps protect against leakage from an unrecognized perforation or devascularization of the mucosa. However, it may carry a higher incidence of dysphagia and gastroesophageal reflux than the Toupet.[22,23] Following myotomy, some authors have used esophagoscopy to confirm adequacy of the myotomy and air insufflation with the esophagus submerged in saline to ensure that there is no unrecognized perforation. If a perforation does occur, suturing can close it safely. A loose partial fundoplication is desirable as the aperistaltic esophagus has negligible propulsive activity.[4] Dissection of the muscular layer for half of the circumference and suturing the cut edges of the myotomy to the fundoplication has been reported to produce traction that keeps the edges apart, lessening the likelihood that the edges will heal together and cause a fibrous stricture producing a recurrence of the high-pressure lower esophageal sphincter.[4]

Laparoscopic/Thoracoscopic Repair

There is an ongoing debate about which approach is better for cardiomyotomy and anti-reflux procedure - open or Laparoscopy.[26]

A laparoscopic Heller myotomy is considered by many to be the appropriate primary treatment of patients with a confirmed diagnosis of Achalasia.[3,27,28] Laparoscopic Heller myotomy has been reported to have excellent results, a short hospital stay, and a fast recovery time. There is excellent exposure of the gastroesophageal junction and the lower two thirds of the thoracic esophagus. The magnification of the operative field allows good visualization of the circular muscle fibers with less disruption and more accuracy. However, expertise is required for a successful outcome. There is definite risk of perforation during the initial learning curve, and one should not hesitate to switch to the open procedure in cases of doubt.

Another ongoing debate is the route for the procedure- thoracoscopically or laparoscopically.[29] A thoracoscopic Heller myotomy and a partial fundoplication has been reported to have a high incidence of gastroesophageal reflux.[3] The fundoplication is better done from the abdominal route.

Some authors have performed a transthoracic limited esophagomyotomy, extending no more than 1 cm onto the stomach, avoiding dissection of the hiatus and preserving the oblique sling muscles of the proximal stomach that form the "collar of Helvitius" without an antireflux procedure.[30] They have reported that their incidence of postoperative dysphagia and gastroesophageal reflux is acceptable.[30] Others have opined that it may be difficult to carry the myotomy far enough onto the stomach without going too far.[4]

Laparoscopic approach is technically easier than thoracoscopy, as the instruments are in line with the long axis of the esophagus instead of being perpendicular to it. Laparoscopy provides easier access to the distal esophagus and proximal stomach, the most difficult and important part of the procedure. Transhiatal laparoscopy provides excellent access.

Rarely, older patients presenting in adulthood with a severely decompensated sigmoid esophagus may require esophagectomy, to prevent severe and frequent chest infections.

However, if the diagnosis is not confirmed and in children less than 5 years, the chances of finding a congenital lesion like bronchocartilaginous ring at the lower end of the esophagus are high and an open laparotomy is advisable. The cartilaginous ring/segment may be palpaple during operation. In such cases, the authors have removed the anterior half of the ring, done a myotomy above the stenosed area and covered with a Thal fundoplication. The cartilage has to be removed very carefully with sharp dissection, taking care not to injure the underlying adherent esophageal mucosa. An inadvertent perforation should be checked with saline or air pushed through a nasoesophageal tube. In case there is a perforation, after closure of the perforation,the procedure should be completed in the same manner with the fundoplication patch so that the wall of the stomach forms a wall of the esophagus. However, the post-operative feeding may be delayed in such cases till a contrast study is done to confirm the sealing of the perforation.

RESULTS

The results are usually good, with relief in symptoms as soon as the patient is able to accept feeds after surgery. A contrast study may be done after 10 days to assess the results. Dilatation may be required in some cases. The most common causes of a poor result following esophagomyotomy are incorrect diagnosis, inadequate myotomy, fibrosis and narrowing of the myotomy and gastroesophageal reflux. In very few cases done in adolescence or adulthood, in those with prior myotomy or those who have developed a gastroesophageal reflux disease stricture, the giant megaesophagus may continue to empty poorly after myotomy and may require esophagectomy.

REFERENCES

1. Meyer's NA, Jolley SG, Taylor R. Achalasia of the cardia in children: A worldwide survey. J Pediatr Surg 199429:1375-79.
2. Hamza AF, Awade HA, Jussein O. Cardiac achalasia in children.Dilatation or surgery? Eur J Pediatr Surg 1999:299-302.
3. Rothenberg SS, Partrick DA, Bealer JF, et al. Evaluation of Minimally Invasive Approaches to Achalasia in Children. J Pediatr Surg 2001; 36:808-810.
4. Vanderpool D, Westmoreland MV. Ericfetner Achalasia: Willis or Heller? BUMC Proceedings 1999;12:227-30.
5. Spiess AE, Kahrilas PJ. Treating achalasia: from whalebone to laparoscope. JAMA 1998;280:638-42.
6. Andreollo NA, Earlam RJ. Heller's myotomy for achalasia: is an added anti-reflux procedure necessary? Br J Surg 1987;74:765-69.
7. Heller E. Extramukose Cardioplastic beim chronishen Cardiospasmus mit Dilatation des esophagus. Mitt Grenzeg Med Chir 1913;27:141.
8. Dor J, Humbert P, Dor V, Figarella J. L'interet de la technique de Nissen modifiee dans la prevention de reflux apres cardiomyotomie extramuqueuse de Heller. Mem Acad Chir (Paris) 1962;88:877-83.
9. Toupet A. Tehnique d'oesophago-gastroplastie avec phrenicogastropexie appliquee dan la cure radicale des hernias hiatales et comme complement de l'operation d'Heller dans les cardiospasmes. Mem Acad Chir (Paris) 1963;89:394-99.
10. Fernandez PM, Lucio LA, Pollachi F. Esophageal achalasia of unknown etiology in children. J Pediatr (Rio J). 2004;80:523-26.
11. Nihoul-Fékété C, Bawab F, Lortat-Jacob S, et al. Achalasia of the esophagus in childhood. Surgical treatment in 35 cases, with special reference to familial cases and glucocorticoid deficiency association Hepatogastroenterology 1991;38:510-3.
12. Patti MG, Albanese CT, Holcomb III GW, et al. Laparoscopic Heller myotomi and Dor fundoplication for esophageal achalasia in children. J Pediatr Surg 2001;36:1248-51.
13. Parrilla Paricio P, Martinez de Haro L, Ortiz A, Aguayo JL. Achalasia of the cardia: long-term results of oesophagomyotomy and posterior partial fundoplication. Br J Surg 1990;77:1371-74.
14. Nakajima K, Wasa M, Kawahara H, et al. Laparoscopic esophagomiotomy with Dor anterior fundoplicacion in a child with achalasia. Surg Laparosc Endosc Percutan Tech 1999;10:236-39.
15. Bonavina L, Nosadini A, Bardini R, Baessato M, Perrachia A. Primary treatment of esophageal achalasia. Long-term results of myotomy and Dor fundoplication. Arch Surg 1992;127:222-26; discussion 227.
16. Chelimsky G, Hupertz V, Blanchard T. Manometric progression of achalasia. J Pediatr Gastroenterol Nutr 2000;31:303-06.

17. Tovar JA, Prieto G, Molina M, Arana J. Esophageal function in achalasia: preoperative and postoperative manometric studies. J Pediatr Surg 1998;33:834-38.
18. Borotto E, Gaudric M, Danel B, et al. Risk factors of oesophageal perforation during pneumatic dilatation for achalasia. Gut 1996;39:9-12.
19. Ferguson MK. Achalasia: current evaluation and therapy. Ann Thorac Surg 1991;52:336-42.
20. Pasricha PJ, Ravich WJ, Hendrix TR, Sostre S, Jones B, Kalloo AN. Treatment of achalasia with intrasphincteric injection of botulinum toxin. Ann Intern Med 1994;121: 590-91.
21. Hurwitz M, Bahar RJ, Ament ME, et al. Evaluation of the use of botulinum toxin in children with achalasia. J Pediatr Gastroenterol Nutr 2000;30:509-14.
22. Hunter JG, Trus TL, Branum GD, Waring JP. Laparoscopic Heller myotomy and fundoplication for achalasia. Ann Surg 1997;225:655-44; discussion 664-65.
23. Oddsdottir M. Laparoscopic management of achalasia. Surg Clin North Am 1996;76:451-58.
24. Paidas C, Cowgill SM, Boyle R, et al. Laparoscopic Heller myotomy with anterior fundoplication ameliorates symptoms of achalasia in pediatric patients. J Am Coll Surg 2007;204:977-83; discussion 983-86.
25. Garzi A, Valla JS, Molinaro F, et al. Minimally invasive surgery for achalasia: combined experience of two European centers J Pediatr Gastroenterol Nutr 2007;44: 587-91.
26. Ancona E, Anselmino M, Zaninotto GE, Constantini M, Rossi M, Bonavina L, Boccu C, Buin F, Peracchia A. Esophageal achalasia: laparoscopic versus conventional open Heller-Dor operation. Am J Surg 1995;170:265-70.
27. Holcomb GW, Richards WO, Riedel BD. Laparoscopic esophagomyotomy for achalasia in children. J Pediatr Surg 1996;31:716-18.
28. Esposito C, Cucchiara S, Borrelli O, et al. Laparoscopic esophagomyotomy for the treatment of achalasia in children. A preliminary report of eight cases. Surg Endosc 2000;14:110-13.
29. Ramacciato G, Mercantini P, Amodio PM, et al. The laparoscopic approach with antireflux surgery is superior to the thoracoscopic approach for the treatment of esophageal achalasia. Experience of a single surgical unit. Surg Endosc 2002;16:1431-37.
30. Ellis FH Jr, Crozier RE, Watkins E Jr. Operation for esophageal achalasia. Results of esophagomyotomy without an antireflux operation. J Thorac Cardiovasc Surg 1984;88:344-51.

CHAPTER 31

Esophageal Strictures

Shailinder J Singh, Leela Kapila

Esophageal stricture can be defined as a narrowing of the esophagus, which requires treatment. esophageal strictures in children are not an uncommon problem but may be difficult to manage. Strictures of the esophagus in pediatric age group are secondary to benign pathology. The common causes of strictures in childhood are: gastroesophageal reflux (GER), corrosive injury and postoperative-secondary to anastomotic scarring (Table 31.1) GER aggravates the strictures that are not primarily due to it. Hence treatment of GER is very important while managing the strictures of esophagus, irrespective of etiology. Anastomotic strictures are localized to the area of operative anastomosis and are amenable to dilatation in majority of circumstances, failure of which leads to limited resection and reconstruction. Corrosive strictures are long and irregular, difficult to manage with dilatation, have a risk of malignancy in the long-run and usually require esophageal substitution. The stricture secondary to GER are localized to lower-third of the esophagus, are short but difficult to treat. Early recognition and prompt appropriate treatment is the second best to prevention.

DEFINITION

There is no universally agreed definition of stricture; many definitions have been used by different authors. Coran in 1989 defined a stricture following esophageal atresia surgery as a narrowing which requires more than 2 dilatations.[1] American Academy of Pediatrics in a survey conducted by it, defined stricture as a narrowing, which requires more than 4 dilatations.[2] In our opinion, a stricture is defined as any compromise to the lumen of the esophagus, which requires dilatation.

INCIDENCE

It is very difficult to give the incidence of stricture in general as different authors have used different criteria and definition for strictures and have applied them to different subgroups of patients. The incidence of anastomotic stricture following the repair of esophageal atresia varies between 8 - 49%, depending upon the criteria for the definition of stricture formation.[3-5] In the experience of Coran, it is present in 19% of the patients following repair of esophageal atresia with or without esophageal fistula.[1] This comes from a series of 224 patients published in 1989 whereas Spitz, from London, in 1987 reported the incidence to be 18% in a series of 145 children. The figures from Melbourne in Australia, quote the incidence to be 30%.[6] In our experience of over 120 cases the stricture rate is approximately 8% and half of these have required

Table 31.1: Etiology of esophageal strictures

1. Postoperative strictures- following repair of esophageal atresia with or without tracheoesophageal fistula (OA ± TOF)
   – Esophageal replacement surgery, surgical correction of gastroesophageal reflux, postsclerotherapy
2. Corrosives strictures—Ingestion of caustic substances
3. Peptic strictures—Gastroesophageal reflux
4. Vascular rings
5. Congenital stenosis of esophagus
6. Esophageal strictures from foreign body impaction
7. Degenerative disorders
8. Achalasia

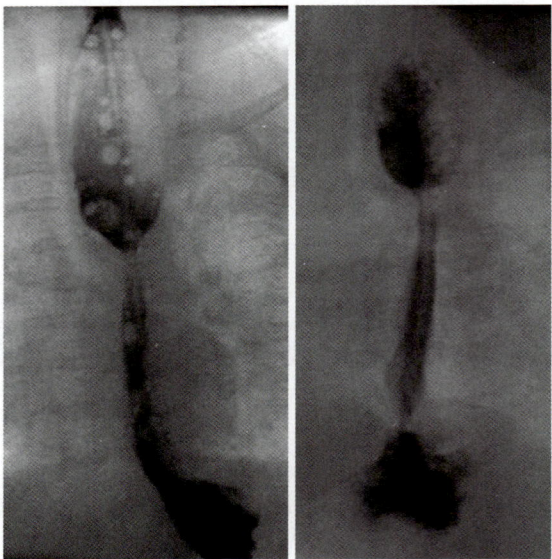

Fig. 31.1: Anastomotic stricture following repair of OA with TEF (neonate weighing 1300 gm, long gap)

Table 31.2: Factors responsible for anastomotic strictures following repair of esophageal atresia with or without tracheoesophageal fistula (OA ± TOF)
1. Tension on the suture line
2. Tenous blood supply
3. Type of anastomosis
4. Anastomotic leakage leading to localized inflammation and infection
5. Gastroesophageal reflux
6. Type of suture material

more than 4 dilatations and one child required resection and reanastomosis.

Esophageal Anastomotic Strictures Following OA Repair with or without TEF

The commonest reason for esophageal anastomosis in pediatric surgery is for esophageal atresia with or without tracheo-esophageal fistula. Anastomotic stricture is the most common reason for further surgery to the esophagus after repair of esophageal atresia (Fig. 31.1).

Various factors implicated in esophageal anastomotic stricture following primary repair of esophageal atresia are: use of silk sutures, two layer anatomises, end to side anastomosis, anastomotic tension gastroesophageal reflux (Table 31.2).[2,7-12] Ischemia and anastomotic leak leading to localised inflammation and infection are also responsible for the stricture.[2,7,13] An esophageal stricture can also occur coincidence ally in association with recurrent fistula, although there is no hard evidence of increased incidences of stricture when a recurrent fistula develops.

The type of esophageal anastomosis has also been thought to be a factor contributing to esophageal stricture. A survey conducted by the American Academy of Pediatrics looked into the incidence of esophageal strictures following double-layered vested anastomosis, the two layered end-to-end anastomosis and single layer end-to-end anastomosis.[2] The stricture was defined as an anastomosis requiring four or more dilatations. The incidence of stricture with his definition was 25 % with Haight anastomosis, 14 percent with two-layered end-to-end anastomosis and 18 percent with single layered end-to-end anastomosis. Interestingly the incidence of anastomotic leak was inversely related to the incidence of stricture following these three types of anastomosis. Coran in 1989, also found a greatly increased incidence of stricture with a 2-layer anastomosis compared with 1 layer anastomosis.[1]

In experience of others also the anastomotic technique has a role to play in the prevention of stricture.[8,11,13] We advocate an end-to-end anastomosis (single layer, interrupted sutures) with careful inversion of mucosa using vicryl sutures. There is minimal forceps handling of the esophageal ends especially the lower pouch. In our opinion extensive mobilization of the lower esophagus is unnecccessary and undesirable. This not only disrupts the segmental blood supply to it but also damages the vagal branches, which supply this segment of the esophagus.[14] The upper esophageal pouch has a longitudinal blood supply and hence can be safely mobilized upto the neck without any risk of vascular compromise. It can have a circular myotomy as well.[15,16]

It is very important to avoid, unnecessary dissection at the site of the fistula, and excessive mobilization of the lower esophagus (Table 31.3). The anastomotic tension should be kept to a minimum. Good blood supply to both the esophageal ends and complete mucosal apposition with inverting sutures (as loose, as few and as far as possible) are the key

Table 31.3: Intraoperative care to prevent strictures following OA ± TOF surgery (author's experience)
• Endoscopic cannulation of TOF before thoracotomy • Flush ligation of TOF • Avoid excessive mobilization and trauma to the distal esophagus • End to end anastomosis — single layer, mucosal inversion • Good hemostasis • Sutures- "as few, as loose, as far as possible" and absorbable.

Table 31.4: Postoperative care to prevent strictures following OA ± TOF surgery (author's experience)

• Elective ventilation and paralysis (If anastomosis under tension)
• Transanastomotic tube
• Routine contrast study
   – Early identification of strictures
   – Diagnosis of GER.

factors to minimize the chances of esophageal strictures.

Children was gastroesophageal reflux certainly have higher incidence of stricture formation. In our experience the neonates, who have anastomosis, performed under tension, leading to iatrogenic hiatus hernia, have higher incidence of stricture. The hiatus hernia leads to GER. In general and especially in these cases we strongly recommend picking up the GER on the first contrast study and institute full medical management (Table 31.4). We do an active follow up on the neonates with GER following OA with or without TEF, all of which are treated with standard medical management of GER: nursing in a special chair with 45° head end up, feed thickeners and H_2 blockers (Ranitidine) or proton pump inhibitors (Omeprazole). At the first clinical suspicion of development of a stricture we undertake esophagoscopy and institute early dilatation. At this procedure the lumen of the esophagus is assessed and depending upon the size, tightness and clinical response to the dilatation the further management is individualized for each patient.

ESOPHAGEAL ANASTOMOTIC STRICTURES FOLLOWING OTHER ESOPHAGEAL ANASTOMOSIS

The other reasons for esophageal anastomosis in pediatric age group are while dealing with a localized stenotic injury to the esophagus secondary to ingestion of corrosive, esophageal replacement procedures (anastomosis of the interposed colon, stomach, gastric tube or jejunum is carried out). In older children with caustic injury inadequate removal of the esophageal cicatrix is an important factor in the development of esophageal stricture following surgery for corrosive strictures. Gastroesophageal reflux is a contributing factor in these cases. It is very important to prevent a stricture when an elective procedure, requiring an esophageal anastomosis, is undertaken by adhering to the basics principles previously mentioned.

CLINICAL PRESENTATIONS OF ESOPHAGEAL STRICTURES

Diagnosis of an esophageal stricture is suspected from a careful history. Feeding difficulties, dysphagia and vomiting are the major symptoms in children with esophageal strictures. In neonatal period or early infancy they manifests as slow feeding and excessive regurgitation with or without cyanotic episodes. Older children often present with foreign body impaction of food in the esophagus. Some older children complain of dysphagia with solids foods, and require the help of oral drinks to push forward the food bolus. Anemia can be the presenting feature in peptic strictures.

DIAGNOSIS

Diagnosis of stricture is confirmed either by endoscopy or contrast swallow. In cases presenting with dysphagia or feeding difficulties a contrast swallow should be done before any endoscopic assessment or intervention. Constant narrowing on swallow is diagnostic of stricture. It also helps in demonstrating the length and severity of stricture. It is a must to look actively for gastroesophageal reflux when the stricture is not too tight and allows the contrast to reach stomach. Once the stricture is demonstrated on contrast swallow, an endoscopy is performed to complete its assessment. At the esophagoscopy a biopsy should be obtained when reflux is suspected. The stricture is dilated. When a child presents with a history of foreign body impaction a plain X-ray of the neck and chest is undertaken followed by endoscopy and removal of foreign body (if possible). A dilatation of the stricture is undertaken if the lumen of the esophagus is visible. In the presence of excessive edema it is preferable to delay the delay the dilatation.

TREATMENT

In patients with mild narrowing of the esophagus and an early diagnosis of the stricture a single or a few dilatations may be all that is required. In patients with associated gastro-esophageal reflux, it is necessary to treat the reflux. Gastroesophageal reflux is documented in about 40% of the patients after repair of esophageal atresia and about half of these develop significant anastomotic stricture.[6] Although in the past such strictures were managed by dilation alone, there is now widespread acceptance that the reflux should be treated surgically.[17] After a successful anti-reflux operation the stricture will usually improve over several weeks but may require one or two further dilatation. In the unlikely event that the stricture fails to resolve or respond easily to dilatation after an anti-reflux operation, the stricture should be resected.[6] In our experience an early diagnosis and aggressive medical management of GER can decrease the incidence for the surgical treatment for the reflux.

METHOD OF DILATATION

Many methods of dilatation have been used over the years (Figs 31.2 to 31.5). They include prograde dilation or retrograde dilation, radial dilation or axial dilatation (Table 31.5). The safest methods of dilatation are: (1) prograde over a guide wire, which is inserted under a direct vision (2) If this fails then a gastrostomy is performed and guide wire is passed under X-ray control (prograde or retrograde). A string is then railroaded via the gastrostomy, across the stricture and brought out through the mouth for retrograde dilatation. After the dilatation the string is brought out transnasaly and left *in situ* till the next dilatation, when it is retrieved orally for further dilatations (Fig. 31.6). This method can be used repeatedly. In the premature child when a stricture develops following the repair of OA, the authors have used syntel biliary and cholangiographic catheter, which is passed via a rigid esophagoscope. The balloon is placed under direct vision across the stricture, the latter is gently dilated with inflation of the balloon.

Prograde dilatation is done with Hurst mercury filled bougie or with more rigid gum elastic bougie. They do not require the presence of a string across the stricture. Retrograde dilatation is achieved using Tucker bougies railroaded through the stricture on a string through a gastrostomy. The method of dilatation

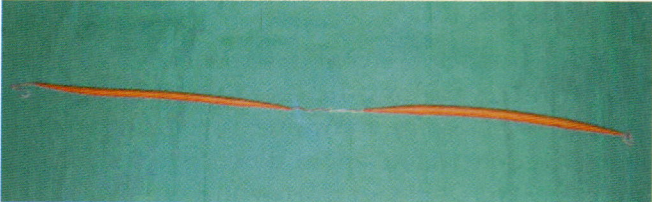

Fig. 31.2: Pilling dilators

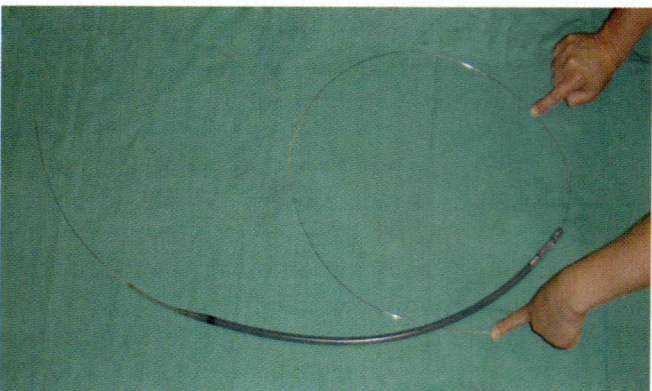

Fig. 31.3: Savary Gilliard dilator

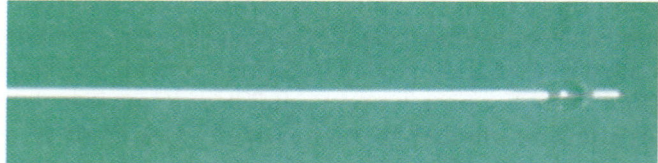

Fig. 31.4: Balloon dilatation catheter

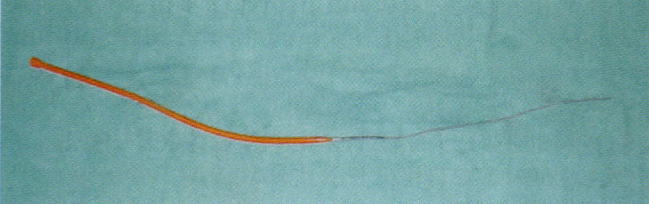

Fig. 31.5: Porges Neoplex dilator

Table 31.5: Types of esophageal dilators used by authors

A. Radial dilators
- Syntel biliary and cholangiography catheters —Balloon dilator

B. Axial dilators
1. Pilling dilator—retrograde or prograde dilatation when there is trans-stricture string
2. Savary Gilliard dilator —Dilators over guide wire
3. Porges neoplex dilator—Filiforms tips with followers

Radiological guidance can be used.
Caution: Dilatation should never be done blindly.

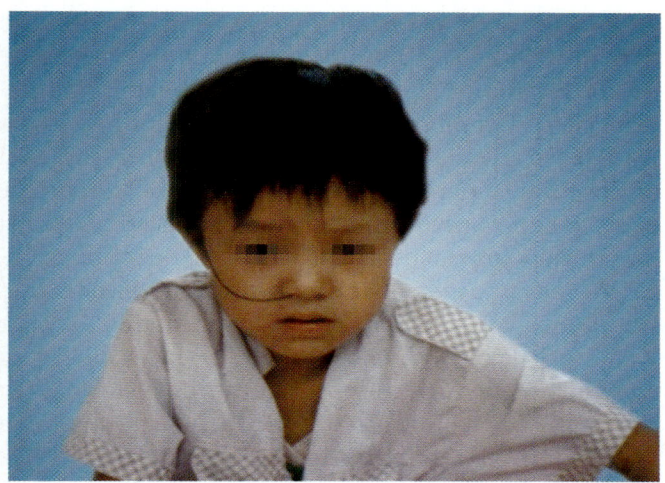

Fig. 31.6: A child with esophageal stricture -dilatation over a string. The string runs across the stricture, comes out transnasaly at one end and via gastrostomy at the other end

involving bougies is called axial dilatation. Ball et al described balloon dilatation under radiological control.[18] The dilatation performed by balloon fall under the category of radial dilatation. The method of balloon dilatation (radial dilatation) has certain characteristic advantages over the bougie dilatation (axial dilatation).[19] In the method of bougienage (retrograde or prograde) an advancing tapered dilator generates axial force, whereas balloon catheter generates radial dilating force. In a series of equivalent esophageal stenosis made by suture plication of esophageal segments in swine, McLean and LeVeen measured shear force and radial force generated by dilation with a Maloney's bougie, a Savary-Gilliard bougie, and an esophageal balloon (Figs 31.3 and 31.4). The mean radial forces generated were similar in all the three techniques. However, the mean shear force with the balloon dilator was significantly lower than that with either bougie. In theory, the reduced shear force associated with balloon dilation might reduce the risk of esophageal perforation. The uses of steroids injected into the strictures have been advocated but is unproven for resistant stricture. It may have a place as a final try before proceeding to resection. A small number of strictures resistant to all forms of dilatation will certainly need resection. In an experience presented from Australia, in the early part of the series involving esophageal atresia with or without tracheo-esophageal fistula, stricture resection was relatively common. Introduction of the Nissen fundoplication decreased the rate of resection of strictures.[6] It was also noticed in the same series that resection of an anastomotic stricture was required most commonly with stage repairs and least commonly with primary one layer, end-to-end anastomosis.[6]

Any method of dilatation carries a risk of septicemia including the formation of brain abscesses.[20] In one series, 4 out of 9 patients had *Staphylococcus aureus* in postoperative blood cultures.[20] These investigators recommend that appropriate antibiotic cover should be provided for patients undergoing esophageal dilatation.

The risk of perforation exists regardless of the method of dilatation and hence the need of postoperative vigilance and observation. In the presence of perforation the early symptoms are restlessness and pain. The pulse rate and the respiratory rate should be monitored regularly. A chest X-ray should be done as and when necessary. The feeds should not be started immediately and the first feed should preferably be a clear fluid in the form of diarolyte.

PREVENTION

Strictures following esophageal atresia with or without tracheoesophageal fistula can be prevented. A single layered end-to-end anastomosis using absorbable sutures, such as polyglycolic acid, gives a low incidence of stricture. The anastomosis should be constructed accurately with good mucosal apposition (with mucosal inversion) with the least possible tension between the ends. Interference of the blood supply of the esophagus (lower pouch) should be kept to the minimum. If these guidelines are followed the incidence of stricture will be reduced considerably. In neonates where anastomosis is under tension a postoperative elective ventilation with paralysis is instituted.

VASCULAR RINGS

The vascular malformations that involve the aortic arch and its major branches are known as vascular rings. They are of two main types: Complete rings and incomplete rings. The complete ring is made of double aortic arch. The incomplete ring is most commonly made of: Right sided aortic arch and the pulmonary artery to the right and anterior side, aberrant subclavian vessels crossing behind the esophagus, and ligamentum arteriosum or ductus arteriosus completing the ring on the left side (Figs 31.7 and 31.8). Compression of the trachea and esophagus by a vascular ring mechanism can occur because of the limited space available for the trachea and esophagus.[21] The incomplete rings are common on oesophagograms but are an unusual cause of dysphagia. These anomalies occur in less than 1% of the population. The most common associated defects are congenital heart disease.[22]

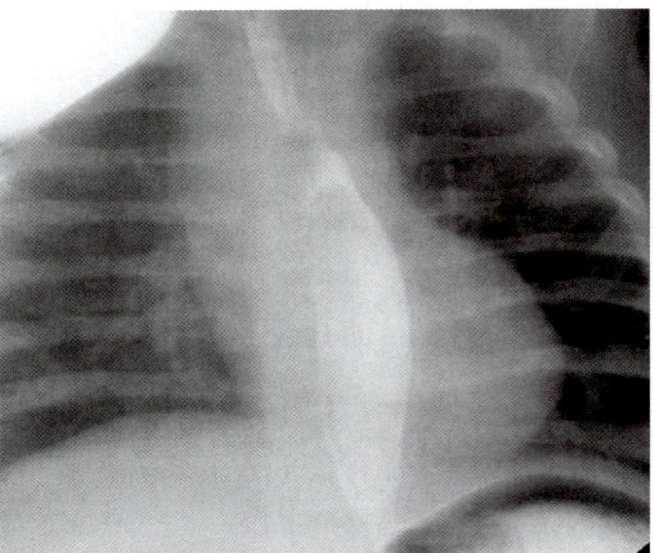

Fig. 31.7: Barium esophagogram revealing indentation on the right side of esophagus consistent with right aortic arch and aberrant subclavian artery complex

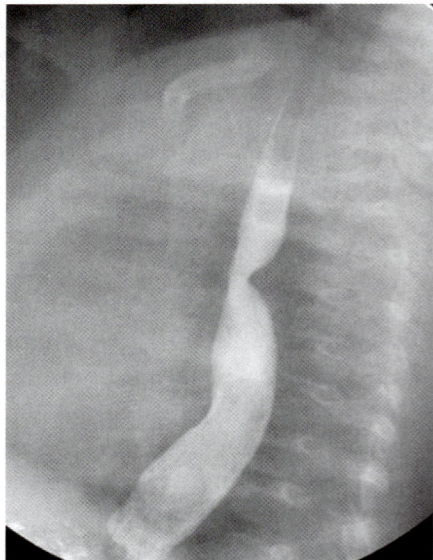

Fig. 31.8: Lateral barium esophagogram showing posterior indentation from aberrant left subclavian artery

Patients with restrictive vascular rings can present with progressive respiratory symptoms or dysphagia-the latter being the commonest. The dysphagia associated with aberrant subclavian artery had been named Dysphagia Lusoria. Stridor or wheezing can be absent in the infant, but these symptoms develop over times because normal growth of the aorta results in symptomatic tracheal compression. The obstruction of the esophagus is incomplete and hence the symptoms of dysphagia are not apparent till the child is eating normal food. Thus children with vascular ring anomalies generally present with the first years of life, but not in the neonatal period. A plain chest radiography can identify a right-sided aortic arch. A contrast esophagogram done while evaluating dysphagia establishes the diagnosis. Thereafter magnetic resonance imaging, echocardiography or digital subtraction angiography further elucidate the anatomy (Figs 31.9 and 31.10).[23-26]

Patients with symptoms require surgical division of this vascular ring.[27-29] The approach is through a left posterior lateral thoracotomy. In complete ring (double aortic arch) the left arch is divided at its narrowest point which is either posterior to the origin of the left subclavian artery or between the ascending aorta and the origin of the left common carotid artery.[27] In incomplete vascular ring it is important to identify the arch and its branches as well as the ligamentous arteriosum. The ligamentum is then doubly ligated and divided, taking care not to injure the recurrent

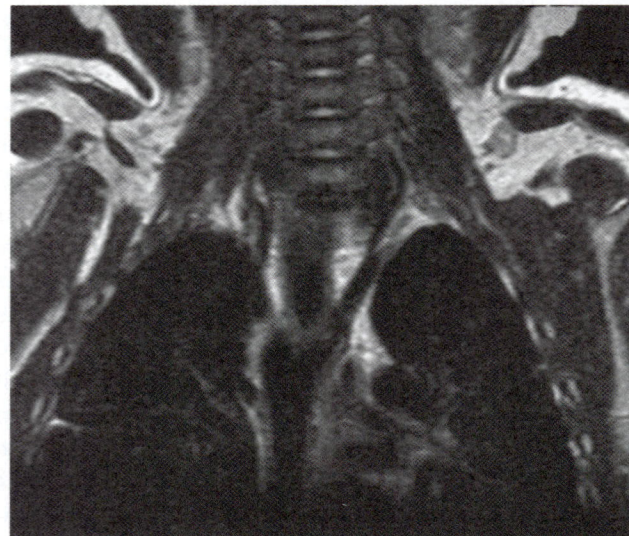

Fig. 31.9: Coronal T2 MRI at the level of posterior mediastinum-demonstrating right aortic arch and aberrant origin of left subclavian artery crossing left of midline

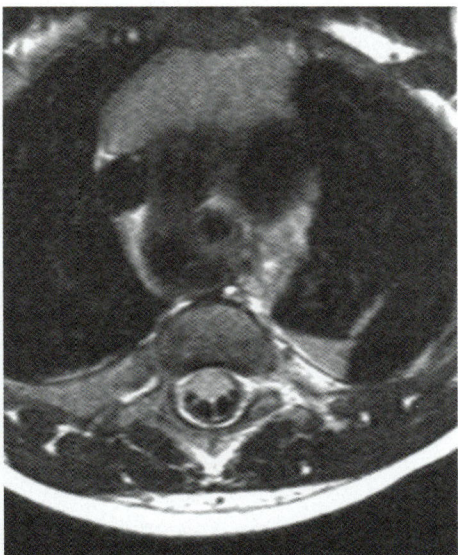

Fig. 31.10: Axial T2 MRI demonstrating right aortic arch, aberrant origin and retrosternal, retro-oesophageal course of left subclavian artery. Obliterated ductus remnant completing the ring

laryngeal nerve. In certain circumstances the aberrant subclavian artery need surgical intervention. Some surgeons detach the retroesophageal aberrant right subclavian artery and reimplant on the aortic arch, while most simply divide this vessel and allow the distal portion to retract across the mediastinum from behind the esophagus.[27]

ESOPHAGEAL STRICTURE SECONDARY TO FOREIGN BODY

Foreign bodies can cause esophageal injury, which can lead to esophageal stricture. These injuries are much more likely from sharper foreign bodies including detachable pop-tops used on aluminium drink cans.[30] These objects are often nearly radiolucent; hence the diagnosis is made late. The usual presentation is with obstructive symptoms. In recent years the ingestion of disc batteries is causing an alarming concern (Table 31.6).[31,32] These batteries may produce esophageal damage by one or all of the three mechanisms: diffusion of alkali from the battery causing caustic injury, low voltage mucosal burns from the electric current generated by the battery that is not fully discharged and/or local pressure necrosis

Table 31.6: Esophageal strictures—battery Ingestion

History
1. Type, size and discharge state of the battery
2. Time since ingestion (duration of contact)
3. Any pre-existing lesions of gastrointestinal tract

Physical Examination

Signs of esophageal perforation:
1. Subcutaneous emphysema
2. Hamman's sign (mediastinal crunch)

General signs and symptoms of sepsis:
1. Tachycardia
2. Increased respiratory rate

Radiographic Identification
- Ap projection— double density shadow (bilaminar structure)
- Lateral projection— step off at junction of anode or cathode
- Both AP and lateral projection views necessary to distinguish it from coin

Complications of Esophageal Impaction
1. Trachea-esophageal fistula
2. Esophageal burn without perforation-esophageal stricture
3. Aorta-esophageal fistula
4. Perforation

Management
- *Emetics:* Emetics are contraindicated as they can cause retrograde impaction in esophagus or airway (the battery already in lower end of esophagus or in the stomach). Esophageal impaction has greater potential for serous outcome because of cumulative effect in localized area (no dilution of chemical and electric effects provided by git secretions)
- *Removal:* Blind removal has high potential for esophageal perforation, also the direct visualization of burns is impossible. Endoscopic removal is best, tight adherence to esophagus requiring considerable care in removal. Subsequent management is on the line of caustic esophageal burn without perforation. Nasogastric stenting and feeding is instituted till another esophagoscopy after 2-3 days. In the waiting period adequate observation should be undertaken looking for signs of esophageal perforation or generalized sepsis.

Esophagoscopic findings
Signs of full thickness esophageal burns:
1. Edema
2. Tight adherence to mucosa
3. Visible mucosal defects
4. Intra-esophageal bubbling on ventilation

Indications for simultaneous bronchoscopy
1. Impaction of more than four hours
2. Full thickness injury to anterior wall of esophagus

(Table 31.5). There is also a risk of systemic toxicity from batteries containing mercury. It is believed that the dead batteries produce less injury.[33] Although there is suggestion that batteries that are 22 mm or larger in size range are dangerous, the potential for injury depends upon the size of the esophagus and the ability of the battery to pass into the stomach.[31] The batteries can some time be mistaken for an ingested coin (Fig. 31.11). A careful look at the anterior-posterior X-ray for a small discontinuity in the outer radius of the image is diagnostic. It is always safer to have a lateral view, which demonstrates a stepping (Fig. 31.12), which confirms the diagnosis. The distinction between a battery and coin is important for the above-mentioned reasons. Greater damage is caused by 3-V lithium batteries than 1.5V alkali battery. Maximal injury occurs on anode side of battery (Fig. 31.13). Esophageal mucosal damage can occur within one hour of the ingestion of the battery and damage to all muscular layers can happen within 4 hours (Fig. 31.14). Batteries in the esophagus for a period of days have produced extensive tracheo-esophageal erosion.[32] This type of injury is reminiscent of a caustic agent, because after removal of the foreign body and presumed interruption of the pathology, progressive injury has continued in severe instances. A catheter or a magnetic device under radiological control can accomplish the removal of battery from the esophagus.

During a 7-year period, 2382 cases of battery ingestion were reported to a national registry set up in USA for battery ingestion.[34] Button cells were ingested by 2320 of these patients; 62 patients ingested cylindrical cells. These cases are analyzed to reassess current therapeutic recommendations, hypotheses

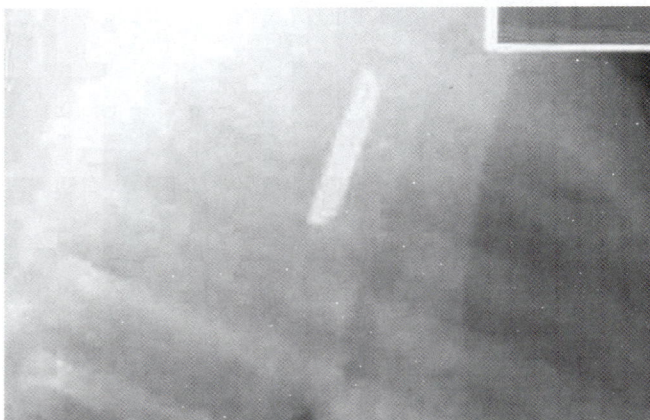

Fig. 31.12: Lateral projection on a child with battery ingestion-Step off at junction of anode and cathode. A lateral projection is sometimes necessary to distinguish it from coin

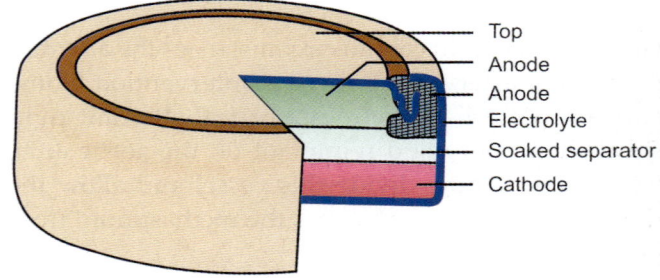

Fig. 31.13: Diagrammatic structure of a button battery

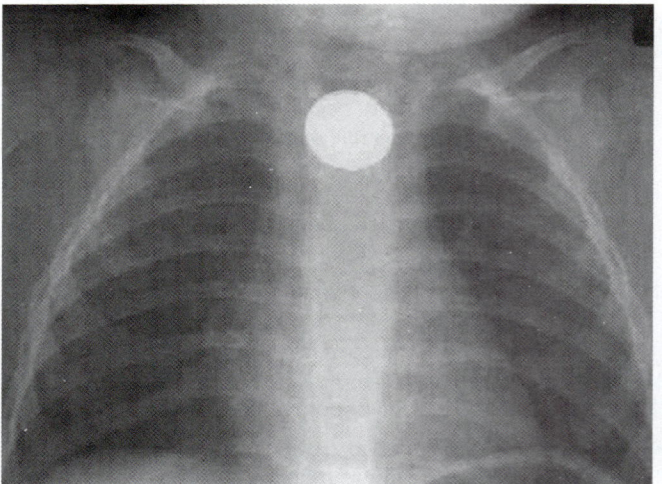

Fig. 31.11: AP radiograph on a child with battery ingestion-Double density shadow (bilaminar structure)

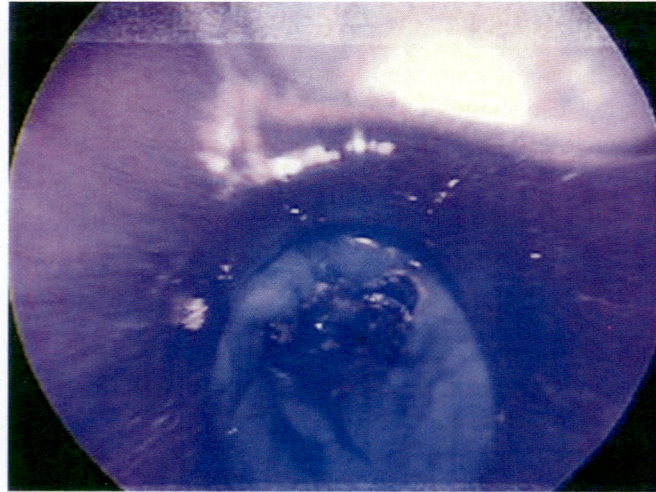

Fig. 31.14: Esophageal damage secondary to battery as seen on esophagoscopy

about battery-induced injury, and strategies for prevention and intervention. Overall, 9.9% of patients were symptomatic. Two children experienced severe esophageal injury following the ingestion of large diameter cells and required repeated dilatation. Outcome was influenced by chemical system. Lithium cells, with their larger diameters and greater voltage, were associated disproportionately with adverse effects. Mercuric oxide cells were substantially more likely to fragment, compared with other chemical constituents of batteries. No clinical evidence of mercury toxicity occurred in this series, although one patient demonstrated minimal elevation of blood mercury levels. A current management protocol is advocated by the registry, advocating a non-invasive approach for most cases of button cell ingestion where an esophageal position is excluded. Manufacturers are urged to provide more securely fastened, child-resistant battery compartments on hearing aids as well as other battery-powered products in household use.

CONGENITAL ESOPHAGEAL STENOSIS

Congenital esophageal stenosis (CES) is a lesion that is difficult to define. The definition and classification given by Nihoul-Fekete et al is the most clear. Congenital esophageal stenosis is defined as an intrinsic stenosis of the esophagus present at birth caused by congenital malformation of esophageal wall architecture.[35] It used to be confused with strictures from other causes like GER. Congenital esophageal stenosis is of three types— (1) Membranous web or diaphragm (2) fibromuscular thickening (3) secondary to tracheobranchial remnants in wall of the esophagus.[35] True CES is a rare condition and is reported to occur in every 25000 - 50000 births.[36] There had been only 500 cases reported in world literature till 1995.[37] There is a higher incidence in Japan as compared to the rest of the world-the reason for which is not known.[38] Congenital membranous web or diaphragm is rarest and represents missed esophageal atresia.[37-39] It is a membrane, which is partially obstructing and is present in middle or lower part of the esophagus. It manifests once the solid food is introduced. The second type of CES is secondary to idiopathic muscular hypertrophy and hence also called fibromuscular stenosis.[35] It resembles hypertrophic pyloric stenosis. The third type of CES is secondary to the presence of remnants of tracheobronchial remnants. It is thought to occur as part of a spectrum of anomalies including OA with or without TOF-related to the separation of the foregut from respiratory tract.[40] CES presents after the introduction of feeds. They can present with symptoms of regurgitation and respiratory distress in newborn.[35] Foreign body impaction can be the first symptom in few.[41] The diagnosis is most often made at the time of resection, these lesions are usually short but are not amenable to repeated dilatation.

FUNCTIONAL ESOPHAGEAL DISORDERS

Diffuse esophageal spasm is an uncommon condition.[42] The original description of this lesion is very complete.[43] A spastic pain usually occurs in the esophagus accompanied by dysphagia. Since this early description, the pathology of diffuse esophageal spasm has been designated as being circular muscle hypertrophy primarily in the lower two thirds of the esophagus. The etiology is unknown.

SCLERODERMA

Scleroderma is an uncommon collagen disorder in children. The distal two thirds of the esophagus, which has smooth muscle, may have its normal peristalsis impaired in the patient with scleroderma. Gastro-esophageal reflux is almost universally present. Esophagitis sometimes progressing to stricture of the esophagus occurs quite commonly in scleroderma.[44,45] Fundoplication has resulted in clinical improvement in many patients despite the fact that the underlying systemic illness and the disordered peristalsis remains unchanged. A scleroderma like disorder of the esophageal motility and poor lower esophageal sphincter pressure has been recently described in breast fed children of mothers who had silicone breast implants. There has, however, been no evidence presented as to the cause and effect.[45]

CORROSIVE STRICTURES

Ingestion of corrosives is a major health problem in children. The tragic consequences of ingestion of corrosive and various treatment schedules have been well summarized by Tucker et al.[46] We will not go into the details of the initial management and diagnosis and restrict the discussion to the treatment of established strictures. Once the stricture is demonstrated on contrast radiography done around day 10-14 after the injury, a program of dilatation is commenced.[47] Various methods can be used ranging from mercury filled bougies, flexible-graded bougie dilatation, guide wire directed systems (Eder-Puestow) or balloon dilatation. Corrosive strictures can be successfully dilated, however the dilatation should be done with great care. The initial dilatation should never be done blindly. In the presence of several strictures and or problem with direct vision, it is much safer to place a transesophageal string. The string is later on used to guide the dilators prograde (through the mouth) or retrograde (through the gastrostomy).[46] The trans-anastomotic string is achieved by first passing a soft tipped flexible guide wire into the distal esophagus via a gastrostomy.[48,49] An endotracheal tube advanced through the gastrostomy up toward the lesser curvature can help in this.[48] A general anesthetic is essential for satisfactory dilatation. It is good to repeat dilatation every week for it to be effective.[50] As a practical tip the dilatation should be commenced with dilator two French size smaller than the estimated size of stricture. It should be stopped at two sizes larger than the size that met initial resistance. Nutritional support is a must during the dilatation and healing phase. This can be achieved by nasogastric feeds, gastrostomy or jejunostomy feedings. In strictures that are resistant to the treatment with dilatation GER should be suspected.[51-53] Gastro-esophageal reflux should be managed surgically if necessary before embarking upon major surgery for these strictures.[54] One study in children has shown that the adjunctive steroid injection into the scar made dilatation treatment more lasting.[55] Localized strictures can be resected with end-to end anastomosis. The fibrotic injury can be more extensive than seen by contrast swallow hence a good endoscopic assessment is a must before undertaking the process of resection with end-to-end anastomosis.[52,53] The problem with this approach to corrosive structure is that if the esophagus continues to be used as a conduit for food during the course of years squamous cell carcinoma develop at the site of injury. Any dysphagia 20-40 years after the dilatation of the caustic strictures should be taken seriously and this fact should be passed to the patient's relatives before discharging them to the care of adult surgeons. Investigation reveals squamous cell carcinoma at the site of the major burn injury usually at the level of the aortic arch.[56] As compared with other patients who have carcinoma of the esophagus, the lesion in this group of patients are more resectable and the patients have a better prognosis probably because dysphagia is apparent earlier because of the esophagus being less distensible. The cicatrix in the esophageal wall may also prevent early local spread of the tumor due to obliterated lymphatics.

ESOPHAGEAL REPLACEMENT

The basic principles of esophageal replacement are:
1. It is generally regarded that the patient's own esophagus is the best conduit but there are exceptions to this.
2. The surgeon must weigh the pros and cons of replacement before undertaking this procedure with informed consent.
3. These patients need long-term follow-up.

PEPTIC STENOSIS

Strictures of the esophagus secondary to GER are severe. They are late complication of GER.[57] These strictures are secondary to severe esophagitis and are accompanied in some instances by Barrett's esophagus. In established strictures the basic tenets of therapy are operative correction of GER (for the oesophagitis to heal) and dilation of the stricture.[44,58-60] In general dilations of strictures secondary to GER are ineffective until the reflux is controlled. After the intraoperative dilation, a standard Nissen fundoplication is performed. Postoperative dilations, using the string-guided technique, are used as and when required. In the overwhelming majority of reflux strictures in children, the use of antireflux operations and dilations are successful. Only in rare instances is resection required. When given a choice between fundoplication and repeated dilatation or a primary esophageal substitution procedure, fundoplication appears to provide better results and fewer long-term complications.[61] Rarely a patient with epidermolysis presents with esophageal stricture. These patients require esophageal substitution because the underlying disease process does not allow dilatation of the esophagus without complete destruction of the mucosa.[62]

A large number of reports confirm the effectiveness of omeprazole in the treatment of esophagitis in children.[63-65] Omeprazole may eventually have a role in managing established reflux strictures, but no reports on its efficacy in this regard have appeared so far. Although its effectiveness in esophagitis is apparent, its success in truly advanced esophagitis in not as impressive; less than half of grade 4 esophagitis healed with omeprazole.[63] Recurrence seems to be inevitable when the drug is stopped.

ESOPHAGEAL ACHALASIA

The etiology of achalasia is unknown. Achalasia is primarily a disease of older people whose symptoms do not begin until adulthood. A congenital etiology is therefore unlikely. Achalasia can occur in a familiar pattern and in such situations pyloric stenosis has been noted.[66] The symptoms can present from childhood. Gastroesophageal reflux can produce spastic reaction in the lower esophagus resembling a clinical and radiological picture of achalasia, hence some surgeons recommend pH monitoring in all the suspected cases of achalasia of the esophagus. A frequent cause of the delayed diagnosis of achalasia is because of its confusion with the symptoms of gastroesophageal reflux.

A barium examination of the esophagus is diagnostic as it reveals a large proximal esophagus with imperfective peristalsis and a bird beak deformity of the distal esophagus. This radiographic picture is classical of achalasia. A manometry can be undertaken to confirm the diagnosis, which reveals non-peristalsis in the body of the esophagus with little or no relaxation of lower esophageal sphincter.[67,68] The treatment is surgical, although calcium channel blockers (Nifedipine) have been shown to reduce the lower esophageal sphincter pressure in children with demonstrated achalasia. The effect is usually transient.[69] Most of the literature dealing with achalasia is found in the adult literature, however the management is similar in children.[70] Bouginage or balloon dilatation sometime produces good symptomatic relief although in adult literature it is associated with a perforation rate of up to 12%.[71] Successful balloon dilatation can result in symptomatic gastroesophageal reflux in a significant number of paediatric patients.[72] The standard accepted surgical treatment for achalasia is esophageal myotomy. This was proposed by Heller 80 years ago. It can be undertaken by thoracic or abdominal approach. The basic principle is to incise both the longitudinal and circular muscle layers of the esophagus down to the submucosa as done in pyloromyotomy. A better resolution of symptoms is reported with abdominal myotomy combined with fundoplication as compared to thoracic myotomy with or without fundoplication.[73] We believe that esophageal myotomy coupled with fundoplication is the ideal procedure for achalasia.

SUMMARY

Esophageal strictures in children are a challenging problem. Prevention is better than cure. An early diagnosis and prompt treatment can save a child's own esophagus. Each case deserves individualized management to prevent complication (Table 31.7).

Table 31.7: Complications of esophageal strictures

Immediate
  Failure to thrive
  Recurrent chest infections
  Perforation— Following dilatation

Long-term
  Malignancy

REFERENCES

1. Coran AG. Current management of esophageal atresia and tracheo-esophageal fistula. Bull. Soc. Sci. Med.Grand-Duche Luxembourg 1989;3:29-51.
2. Holder TM, Cloud DT, Lewis JEJ, Pilling GPI. Esophageal atresia and tracheoesophageal fistula: a survey of its memebers by the Surgical Section of the American Academy of Pediatrics. Pediatrics 1964;34:542.
3. Holder TM, Ashcraft KW, Sharp RJ, Amoury RA. Care of infants with esophageal atresia, tracheoesophageal fistula, and associated anomalies. Journal of Thoracic & Cardiovascular Surgery 1987;94:828-35.
4. Lundertse-Verlop K, Tibboel D, Hazebrock FWJ. Postoperative morbidity in patients with esophageal atresia. Pediatr Surg Int 1987;2:2-5.
5. Holder TM. Esophageal atresia and tracheesophageal fistula. In: Ashcraft KW, Holder TM (Eds). WB Saunder (Philadelphia) Pediatric Esophageal Surgery 1987:29-52.
6. Auldist AW, Beasley SW. Esophageal complications. In: Beasley SW (Eds). Oesophageal atresia (Melbourne) 1990;305-29.

7. Spitz L, Kiely E, Brereton RJ. Esophageal atresia: five year experience with 148 cases. Journal of Pediatric Surgery 1987;22:103-08.
8. Touloukian RJ. Long-term results following repair of esophageal atresia by end ed -to-side anastomosis and ligation of the tracheoesophageal fistula. Journal of Pediatric Surgery 1981;16:983-88.
9. Jolley SG, Johnson DG, Roberts CC, et al. Patterns of gastroesophageal reflux in children following repair of esophageal atresia and distal tracheoesophageal fistula. Journal of Pediatric Surgery 1980;15:857-62.
10. Aprigliano F. Chevalier Jackson Lecture. Esophageal stenosis in children. Annals of Otology, Rhinology and Laryngology 1980;89:391-96.
11. Sharma AK, Wakhlu A. Simple technique for proximal pouch mobilization and circular myotomy in cases of esophageal atresia with tracheoesophageal fistula. Journal of Pediatric Surgery 1994;29:1402-03.
12. Ashcraft KW, Goodwin C, Amoury RA, Holder TM. Early recognition and aggressive treatment of gastroesophageal reflux following repair of esophageal atresia. Journal of Pediatric Surgery 1977;12:317-21.
13. Gough MH. Esophageal atresia--use of an anterior flap in the difficult anastomosis. Journal of Pediatric Surgery 1980;15:310-11.
14. Othersen HB. Pediatric Surgery. Philadelphia: WB Saunders Co, 1980.
15. Livaditis A, Radberg L, Odensjo G. Esophageal end-to-end anastomosis. Reduction of anastomotic tension by circular myotomy. Scandinavian Journal of Thoracic and Cardiovascular Surgery 1972;6:206-14.
16. Starck E, Paolucci V, Onneken M, Herzer M, McDermott J. Conservative treatment of esophageal stenoses with balloon catheters. [German]. Deutsche Medizinische Wochenschrift 1985;110:1025-30.
17. Pieretti R, Shandling B, Stephens CA. Resistant esophageal stenosis associated with reflux after repair of esophageal atresia: a therapeutic approach. Journal of Pediatric Surgery 1974;9:355-57.
18. Ball WS, Strife JL, Rosenkrantz J, Towbin RB, Noseworthy J. Esophageal strictures in children. Treatment by balloon dilatation. Radiology 1984;150:263-64.
19. McLean GK, LeVeen RF. Shear stress in the performance of esophageal dilation: comparison of balloon dilation and bougienage. Radiology 1989;172:983-86.
20. Price JD, Stanciu C, Bennett JR. A safer method of dilating oesophageal strictures. Lancet 1974;1:1141-42.
21. Pegoli Jr W. Pericardium and Great Vessels. In: Oldham KT CPFR, ed. Surgery of Infants and Children, Scientific Principles and practice, 1 ed. New York: Lipincot-Raven, 2000:987-1004.
22. Moutsouris C. The "solid stage" and congenital intestinal atresia. Journal of Pediatric Surgery 1966;1:446-50.
23. Kastler B, Livolsi A, Germain P, Zollner G, Willard D, Wackenheim A. Magnetic resonance imaging in congenital heart disease of newborns: preliminary results in 23 patients. European Journal of Radiology 1990;10:109-17.
24. van Son JA, Julsrud PR, Hagler DJ, et al. Imaging strategies for vascular rings. Annals of Thoracic Surgery 1994;57:604-10.
25. Murdison KA, Andrews BA, Chin AJ. Ultrasonographic display of complex vascular rings. Journal of the American College of Cardiology 1990;15:1645-53.
26. Chernin MM, Pond GD, Bjelland JC, Goldman RL, Sahn DJ, Capp MP. Evaluation of double aortic arch and aortic coarctation by intravenous digital subtraction angiography (IV DSA). Journal of Cardiovascular Surgery 1987;28:581-84.
27. Backer CL, Ilbawi MN, Idriss FS, DeLeon SY. Vascular anomalies causing tracheoesophageal compression. Review of experience in children. [see comments]. Journal of Thoracic and Cardiovascular Surgery 1989;97:725-31.
28. Roberts CS, Othersen HB, Sade RM, Smith CD, Tagge EP, Crawford FA. Tracheoesophageal compression from aortic arch anomalies: analysis of 30 operatively treated children. Journal of Pediatric Surgery 1994;29:334-37.
29. Burke RP, Wernovsky G, van d. V, Hansen D, Castaneda AR. Video-assisted thoracoscopic surgery for congenital heart disease. Journal of Thoracic and Cardiovascular Surgery 1995;109:499-507.
30. Spitz L, Hirsig J. Prolonged foreign body impaction in the oesophagus. Archives of Disease in Childhood 1982;57:551-53.
31. Litovitz TL. Battery ingestions: product accessibility and clinical course. Pediatrics 1985;75:469-76.
32. Votteler TP, Nash JC, Rutledge JC. The hazard of ingested alkaline disk batteries in children. JAMA 1983;249:2504-06.
33. Sigalet D, Lees G. Tracheoesophageal injury secondary to disc battery ingestion. Journal of Pediatric Surgery 1988;23:996-98.
34. Litovitz T, Schmitz BF. Ingestion of cylindrical and button batteries: an analysis of 2382 cases. Pediatrics 1992;89:747-57.
35. Nihoul-Fekete C. Congenital oesophageal stenosis. Pediatr Surg Int 1987;2:86.
36. Valerio D, Jones PF, Stewart AM. Congenital oesophageal stenosis. Archives of Disease in Childhood 1977;52:414-16.
37. Murphy SG, Yazbeck S, Russo P. Isolated congenital esophageal stenosis. Journal of Pediatric Surgery 1995;30:1238-41.
38. Nishina T, Tsuchida Y, Saito S. Congenital esophageal stenosis due to tracheobronchial remnants and its associated anomalies. Journal of Pediatric Surgery 1981;16:190-93.
39. Kluth D. Atlas of esophageal atresia. Journal of Pediatric Surgery 1976;11:901-19.
40. Yeung CK, Spitz L, Brereton RJ, Kiely EM, Leake J. Congenital esophageal stenosis due to tracheobronchial

remnants: a rare but important association with esophageal atresia. Journal of Pediatric Surgery 1992;27:852-55.
41. Bluestone CD, Kerry R, Sieber WK. Congenital esophageal stenosis. Laryngoscope 1969;79:1095-103.
42. Henderson RD, Ho CS, Davidson JW. Primary disordered motor activity of the esophagus (diffuse spasm). Diagnosis and treatment. Annals of Thoracic Surgery 1974;18:327-36.
43. Moersch HJ, Camp, JD. Diffuse spasm of the lower part of the esophagus. Ann Ororhinolaryngol 1934;43:1165-73.
44. Henderson RD, Henderson RF, Marryatt GV. Surgical management of 100 consecutive esophageal strictures. Journal of Thoracic and Cardiovascular Surgery 1990;99:1-7.
45. Levine JJ, Ilowite NT. Sclerodermalike esophageal disease in children breast-fed by mothers with silicone breast implants. JAMA 1994;271:213-16.
46. Tucker JA. Tucker retrograde esophageal dilatation. Ann Otol Rhinol Laryngol 1974;83.
47. Rappert P. Diagnosis and therapeutic management of oesophageal and custic gastric burns in childhood. Eur J Pediatr Surg 1993;3:202.
48. Millar AJ W. Negotiating the "difficult" oesophageal stricture. Pediatr Surg Int 1993;8:445.
49. Tanyel FC, Buyukpamukcu NB, Hicsonmez A. An improved stringing method for retrograde dilatation of caustic oesophageal strictures. Pediatr Surg Int 1987;2:57.
50. Fyfe AH, Auldist AW. Corrosive ingestion in children. Zeitschrift fur Kinderchirurgie 1984;39:229-33.
51. Mutaf O, Genc A, Herek O, Demircan M, Ozcan C, Arikan A. Gastroesophageal reflux: a determinant in the outcome of caustic esophageal burns. Journal of Pediatric Surgery 1996;31:1494-95.
52. Cywes S. Corrosive strictures of oesophagus in children. Pediatr Surg Int 1993;8:8.
53. Mutaf O. Esophagoscopy for caustic esophageal burns in children. Pediatr Surg Int 1992;7:106.
54. Rode H, Millar AJ, Brown RA, Cywes S. Reflux strictures of the esophagus in children. Journal of Pediatric Surgery 1992;27:462-65.
55. Gandhi RP, Cooper A, Barlow BA. Successful management of esophageal strictures without resection or replacement. Journal of Pediatric Surgery 1989;24:745-49.
56. Imre J, Kopp M. Arguments against long-term conservative treatment of oesophageal strictures due to corrosive burns. Thorax 1972;27:594-98.
57. Carre IJ. The natural history of the partial thoracic stomach (hiatus hernia) in children. Arch Dis Child 1959;34:344-53.
58. Boix-Ochoa J, Rehbein A. Oesophageal stenosis due to reflux esophagitis. Arch Dis Child 1965;40:197-99.
59. Little AG, Naunheim KS, Ferguson MK, Skinner DB. Surgical management of esophageal strictures. Annals of Thoracic Surgery 1988;45:144-47.
60. Ohhama Y, Tsunoda A, Nishi T, Yamada R, Yamamoto H. Surgical treatment of reflux stricture of the esophagus. Journal of Pediatric Surgery 1990;25:758-61.
61. Isolauri J, Nordback I, Markkula H. Surgery for reflux stricture of the oesophagus. Annales Chirurgiae et Gynaecologiae 1989;78:120-23.
62. Fonkalsrud EW, Ament ME. Surgical management of esophageal stricture due to recessive dystrophic epidermolysis bullosa. Journal of Pediatric Surgery 1977;12:221-26.
63. Hetzel DJ, Dent J, Reed WD, et al. Healing and relapse of severe peptic esophagitis after treatment with omeprazole. Gastroenterology 1988;95:903-12.
64. Kato S, Ebina K, Fujii K, Chiba H, Nakagawa H. Effect of omeprazole in the treatment of refractory acid-related diseases in childhood: endoscopic healing and twenty-four-hour intragastric acidity. Journal of Pediatrics 1996;128:415-21.
65. De Giacomo C, Bawa P, Franceschi M, Luinetti O, Fiocca R. Omeprazole for severe reflux esophagitis in children. Journal of Pediatric Gastroenterology and Nutrition 1997;24:528-32.
66. Tryhus MR, Davis M, Griffith JK, Ablin DS, Gogel HK. Familial achalasia in two siblings: significance of possible hereditary role. Journal of Pediatric Surgery 1989;24:292-95.
67. Rosenzweig S, Traube M. The diagnosis and misdiagnosis of achalasia. A study of 25 consecutive patients. Journal of Clinical Gastroenterology 1989;11:147-53.
68. Shoenut JP, Trenholm BG, Micflikier AB, Teskey JM. Reflux patterns in patients with achalasia without operation. Annals of Thoracic Surgery 1988;45:303-05.
69. Smith H, Buick R, Booth I, et al. Letter to Editor. J Pediatr Gastroenterol 1988;7:146.
70. Benedict EB. Peptic stenosis of the esophagus. A study of 233 patients treated with bougienage, surgery, or both. American Journal of Digestive Diseases 1966;11:761-70.
71. Sauer L, Pellegrini CA, Way LW. The treatment of achalasia. A current perspective. Archives of Surgery 1989;124:929-31.
72. Ponce J, Garrigues V, Pertejo V, Sala T, Berenguer J. Individual prediction of response to pneumatic dilation in patients with achalasia. Digestive Diseases and Sciences 1996;41:2135-41.
73. Myers NA, Jolley SG, Taylor R. Achalasia of the cardia in children: a worldwide survey. Journal of Pediatric Surgery 1994;29:1375-79.

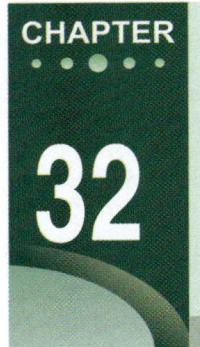

Esophageal Replacement with Colon

D K Gupta, Shilpa Sharma

Esophageal replacement remains a challenging operation to pediatric surgeons and required significant expertise and experience in the field. Various options available for replacing the esophagus are; colon, gastric tube, stomach, jejunum, bridge gastric tube and bridge colonic segment. The choice, however, depends upon the age of the child, the initial pathology and also the surgeon's preference. Though most surgeons would prefer to wait till the child has gained adequate weight, the authors have performed an early replacement even in the newborn period for complicated cases of esophageal atresia.[1,2]

The indications for esophageal substitution are

1. Failed primary anastomosis in esophageal atresia necessitating diversion.
2. Long gap isolated esophageal atresia (EA).
3. Wide gap esophageal atresia and tracheo-esophageal atresia (EATEF).
4. Corrosive esophageal stricture.
5. Severe esophageal trauma.
6. Peptic esophagitis.[3,4]
7. Candidiasis.
8. Scleroderma.
9. Epidermolysis bullosa.[5]

Most esophageal replacements are required either for complicated TEF (wide gap, long gap and major leaks) or the postcorrosive esophageal injuries (alkali and acid ingestions).

Table 32.1 Enumerates the authors' experience in this field.

Criteria for an Ideal Esophageal Substitute are

1. Efficient conduit to supplement the nutritional needs of the child.
2. The conduit should grow with the child and should last for life-long.
3. The surgical technique should be simple, safe and adaptable to small children.
4. Gastric acid reflux into the conduit should be minimal, and if reflux occurs, the substitute should be resistant to acid damage.
5. The presence of the conduit should not impair respiratory or cardiac function.
6. The conduit should not produce any external cosmetic deformity.
7. Postoperative complications if any, should be manageable easily.

TIMING FOR ESOPHAGEAL REPLACEMENT

For the TEF Group

Though the esophageal replacement for esophageal atresia can be performed as a primary procedure in the neonatal period, most of the time it is performed after the diversion (esophagostomy and gastrostomy) has been done, and at a time (6 months to 1 year of age) when the child has gained enough weight and can sit and eat by him/herself.[6]

Table 32.1: Indications for esophageal replacement (1980-2007)	
TEF	46
Postcorrosive (acid and alkali, both)	45
Esophageal perforation	03
Candidiasis	01
Scleroderma	01
Total	96

For the Corrosive Group

The ideal time for operating upon a child with post-corrosive esophageal stricture is at least six months after the insult and after sufficient number of dilatations have been tried and failed (normally at least 6 months of trial). The frequency of dilatation depends upon the length of the stricture, the tightness of the stricture and the pliability of the stricture. The dilatation may be begun 3 weeks after the insult starting at a frequency of twice weekly and then gradually reducing the frequency to fortnightly and then once in 3-4 weeks. If the dilatation is required at an increased frequency than planned and if the size of dilator required is less than the previous size used for dilatation, then there would be a need for esophageal replacement. Some authors have taken the criterion for esophageal replacement as recurrence of the stricture within 3 weeks of the previous dilatation.[4]

ROUTES OF ESOPHAGEAL REPLACEMENT

The common routes for performing esophageal substitution are either retrosternal or the transhiatal mediastinal route (Figs 32.1A to D). Rarely a retrohilar route has been used creating a neohiatus to the left side of the natural esophageal hiatus in the diaphragm along the costal margin to gain access to the thorax. The subcutaneous route was measured as 1.8 cm longer than the retrosternal route that was 1.9 cm longer than the mediastinal (orthotopic) route on autopsy studies.[7] The difference between the subcutaneous and the orthotopic route was 3.7 cm.[7] The subcutaneous route that was used in adults in the past was just in front of the sternum. The advantage was that the food contents could be pushed down manually by the patient himself. However, it was ugly as the movement of the food bolus was visible on the surface. This route has not been used in children, though anecdotal excellent long-term results have been reported using this route.

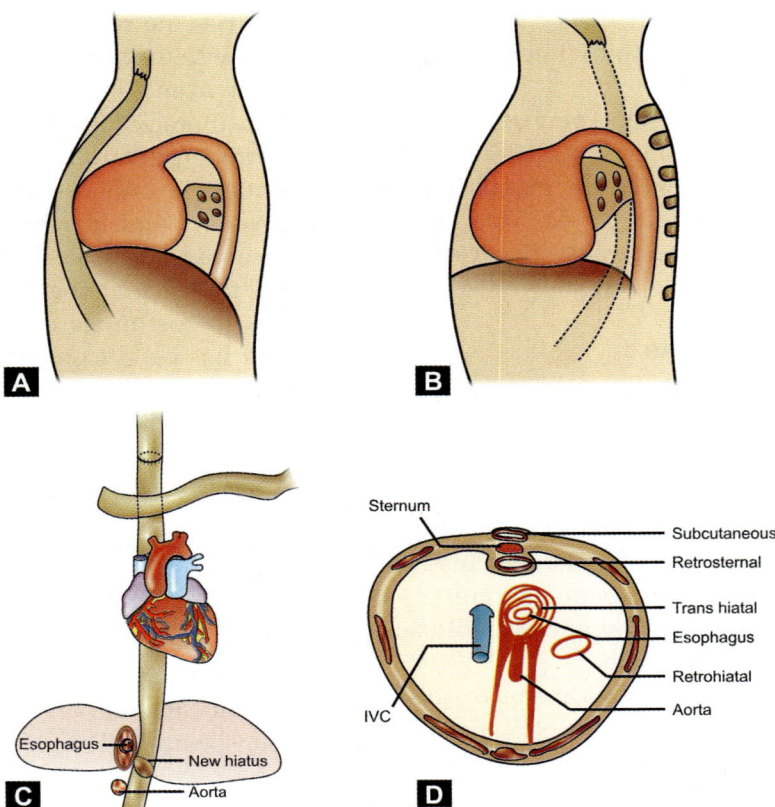

Figs 32. 1A to D: Outlines of the various routes in the chest for esophageal replacement. **A.** Retrosternal **B.** Transhiatal mediastinal, **C.** Retrohilar mediastinal **D.** Various levels of the opening in relation to the diaphragm

Retrosternal (Substernal)

This route is directly behind the posterior sternal surface. It is important to create adequate space for the graft to be housed comfortably at the xiphisternal level, behind the sternum and at the thoracic inlet. The sternal head of the sternomastoid muscle, the sternohyoid and sternothyroid muscles may have to be detached from the bony attachments with the sternum, to prevent compression of the graft and its delicate blood supply specially in the neck region.

Advantages of the retrosternal route are:
1. It is technically simple, safe and very easy to create in children.
2. There is no pulmonary or cardiac compression by the interposed segment.
3. There is less chance of damaging the recurrent laryngeal nerve, trachea and major thoracic vessels, especially in the presence of a scarred mediastinum with old surgery.

Disadvantages:
1. It is the longest route
2. Chances of kinking of the conduit while coursing over the left lobe of the liver.
3. While creating the space, the pleura may be injured causing pneumothorax, unilateral or bilateral.
4. There is a narrow space between the manubrium and clavicle and the scalene muscles. This may compromise vascularity and may also cause obstruction unless mobilized adequately.

Transhiatal (Mediastinal) Route

This is the route, most commonly utilized in newborns, infants and children after the native esophagus has been removed. It is the normal route for esophageal replacement. It uses the normal esophageal hiatus in the posterior mediastinum, thus maintaining the natural route. There is also no risk of kinks and curves using this route. However, the disadvantages are;
– Technically difficult, especially in cases with a scarred posterior mediastinum.
– Chances of damage to the trachea, major vessels and recurrent laryngeal nerve.
– Risk of pulmonary compromise due to compression.
– May need an additional thoracotomy, to remove the esophagus and also to create the enough space for this route.

Retrohilar Route (Waterston operation)

This route initially described by Waterston, is no more used, though it is the shortest of all the three routes.

In this procedure, the colon is used from abdomen to the neck with the transthoracic-retrohilar route. A thoracotomy is performed through the left 6th intercostal space. The diaphragm is incised along its attachment with the costal margin just to the left of the original esophageal hiatus.[8] The middle colic artery is divided on the lower border of the pancreas close to its origin, preserving the ascending branch of left colic artery and inferior mesenteric vein. The isoperistaltic colonic segment is then brought into the chest through a small incision in the diaphragm postero-lateral to the esophageal hiatus and passing behind the tail of the pancreas and stomach. Colon is finally brought in the neck through the retrohilar route and the apex of the pleura, anterior and medial to the left subclavian vessels. In the original Waterston operation, the lower esophageal stump was mobilized and anastomosed to the colon, preserving the gastroesophageal junction.

This carries the risk of injury to the major vessels in the neck with the rare possibility of the catastrophic hemorrhage from subclavian vessels. An inadequate space at the thoracic inlet may also cause compression effect. This operation is now used only very infrequently. The only use may be for a case with left esophagostomy and in which the lower stump has been preserved and also if the mediastinal and the substernal routes are not available. Even with the left sided esophagostomies done earlier, the author's preference has been to mobilize the esophgostomy well and use either the retrosternal or the mediastinal route.

COLON INTERPOSITION

Colonic interposition is the most commonly used procedure to replace the esophagus in the pediatric age group, preferred by most pediatric surgeons around the globe.[6,9] The procedure is reported to have minor complications in the long-term and less of major complications as compared to those seen with the gastric transposition ($P = .001$).[9]

The Advantages of Colonic Interposition Include

1. Reliable vascular pedicle due to the marginal artery of Drummand.

2. Length of the graft is no problem.
3. Can be used as a conduit in any direction—Iso or antiperistaltic.
4. Easy coursing over the liver edge, with due precaution and hitching the liver properly.
5. Relatively safe and easy to perform, even by the beginners.
6. Postoperative complications are infrequent and less serious.

Preoperative Work Up

1. Barium enema for rotational abnormalities of the colon if any and to rule out pouch colon and any intrinsic diseases of the colon like polyposis.
2. Assess cardiac status
3. Build up the nutrition to ensure good healing and endurance of anesthesia
4. If the child is on gastrostomy, ensure sham feeding has being continued to develop taste at least for salt and sweet.
5. If the child is on oral liquids following corrosive stricture, assess the status of the lungs and flow across the pylorus.
6. Good colon preparation using polyethyleneglycol (PEGLEC), rectal washes and oral antibiotics.

Technical Aspects

Colon has rich blood supply supplemented well by various named vessels arising from the ileocolic, middle colic and left colic blood vessels, all making a network in the mesocolon to form the reliable marginal vessels running all along the length of the colon. This arrangement makes it feasible to shape the colon graft for any length so as to reach even the highest point in the neck to be anastomosed even with the pharynx.

The Options while using the Colon Conduit are

1. The right colon and the transverse colon can be used as the conduit, based on the middle colic artery. Though, it would be anti-peristaltic but this is of no significance.
2. The transverse or left colon can also be used as the iso-peristaltic conduit, based on the left colic vessels. It is preferred over the right colon because it is less bulky and the blood supply is also more reliable.[10]

The middle colic is a major vessel and bifurcates in the right and the left branch to anastomose freely with the adjoining vessels to supply the right, transverse and the left colon. Normally, it is the left branch which is more prominent and supplies the larger segment of the transverse colon. However, in about 25% cases, it is the right branch that is more prominent. This is important before deciding as to which branch needs to be preserved so as to maintain a rich blood supply to the colonic graft. Figure 32.2 outlines vascular supply of the colon with implications for using the right or the left colon. A temporary clamp or bulldog may be tried on the proposed branch to be divided, to check the reliability of the vascular supply to the graft so planned.

Any of the isoperistaltic or anti-peristaltic colonic segment may be used. An isoperistaltic orientation is theoretically ideal although this has not been clearly

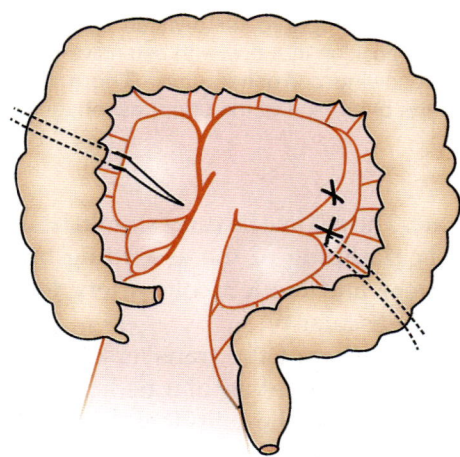

Fig. 32.2A: Antiperistaltic colon graft based on middle colic artery

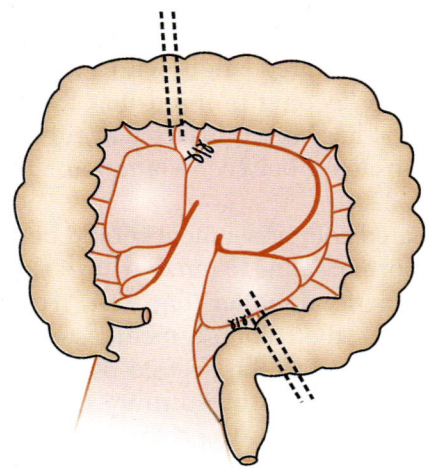

Fig. 32.2B: Isoperistaltic colon graft based on left colic artery

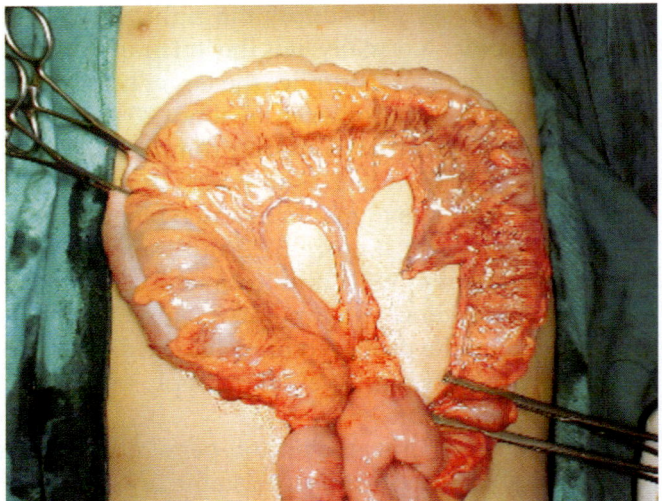

Fig. 32.3: The left colon based on the left branch of the middle colic artery being prepared for division between intestinal clamps for interposition in a boy with extensive stricture of the esophagus following corrosive injury. There were multiple strictures in the pharynx and the upper esophagus

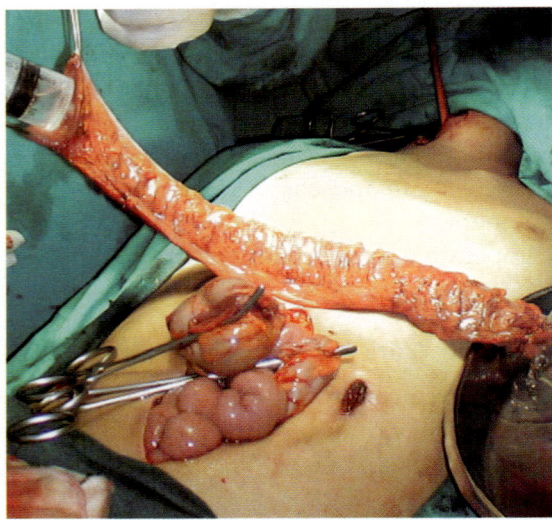

Fig. 32.4: The isolated colonic segment being cleaned on table with normal saline to remove the residual peglec solution / fecal matter

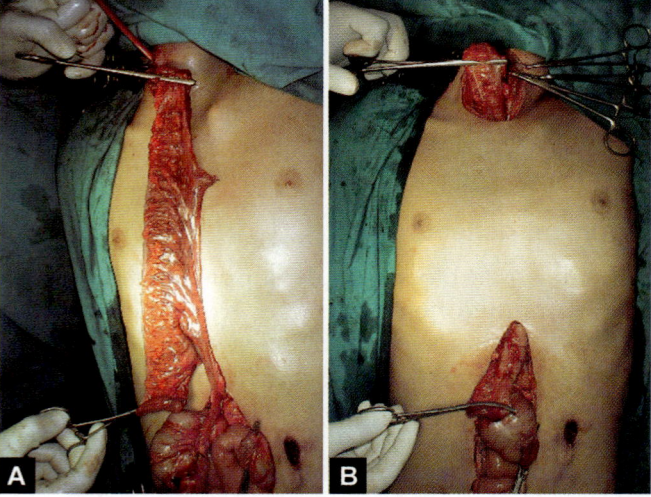

Figs 32.5A and B: A. The length of the colonic segment being assessed by placing the same over the chest wall, **B.** The colonic segment placed in the retrosternal space and found adequate

demonstrate. The colonic flexures should be mobilized, temporarily clamping of the ascending branches of ileocolic artery and the left colic artery to check the adequacy of vascularity.

An interposition of the transverse colon may be maintained by a double vascular pedicle based on the left colic vessels and the marginal paracolic arcade.[9] The omentum is also detached from the transverse colon. Liver is hitched with the cut end of the round ligament behind the xiphisternum so as to allow the graft to have smooth course over the liver edge. The length of the colonic segment should be assessed by measuring the required length with a tape so that it is adequate, also keeping in mind that the colon graft shrinks after it has been transacted at either ends. The colon is transacted between clamps for the desired length (Fig. 32.3).

The isolated colonic segment should be cleaned on table with normal saline to remove the residual peglec solution or the fecal matter (Fig. 32.4). The adequacy of the length of the colon segment is reassessed and the colon is placed in the desired place without any tension or obstruction in its route (Fig. 32.5). Any redundancy is trimmed. The colon graft on its pedicle is passed behind the stomach through the gastro-hepatic ligament to take the desired route; a retrosternal or the mediastinal.

The excess of the pulled colon, if any, is trimmed and the vascularity at the edges is reassessed. A wide and single layer end to end (rarely end to side if the vascularity is in doubt) esophagocolonic anastomosis is performed, using absorbable interrupted sutures. Colon is fixed with the prevertebral or deep cervical facia to prevent its sagging.

The distal end of the graft is anastomosed to the anterior wall of the stomach in the body or near the antrum, in two layers. Few sutures are placed at the

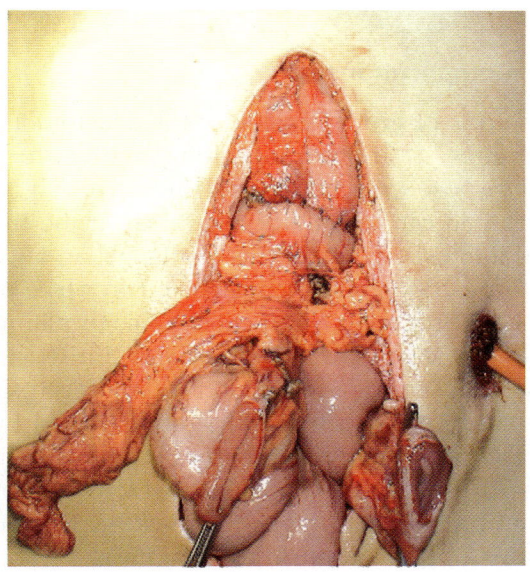

Fig. 32.6: Completed cologastric anastomosis with the gastrostomy tube in place. The proximal and distal ends of colon can be seen, for colocolic anastomosis

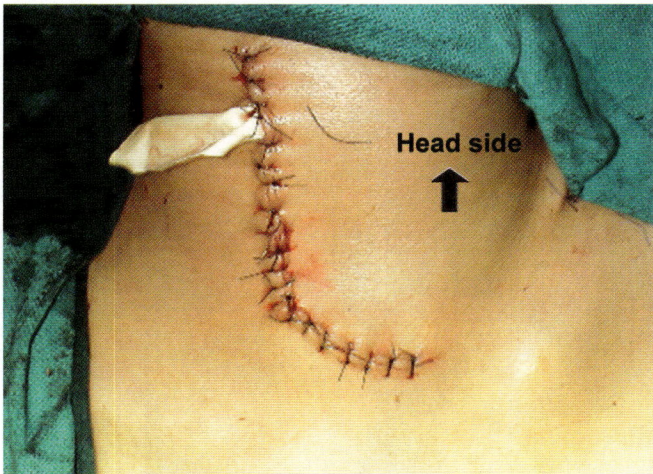

Fig. 32.7: Closure of a neck incision with a glove drain in which the strictured segment was high up in the pharynx. The upper end of the interposed colon was successfully anastomosed to the pharynx

angle of the stomach with the colon to incorporate the antireflux mechanism at the gastrocolic junction.

The ends of the divided colon are approximated and anastomosed in two layers, in front and inferior to the pedicle of the isolated colon graft (Fig. 32.6).

Pyloromyotomy or pyloroplasty is performed only if the vagus has been damaged. Multiple relaxing incisions can be given on the *Taenia coli* to elongate the graft, if the need be to avoid a tension.[11]

Neck wound is closed with a soft drain around the anastomosis (Fig. 32.7). The native diseased and strictured esophagus in patients with corrosive injuries should preferably be removed (Fig. 32.8).

Colon should be decompressed with a nasogastric tube and left open to the atmosphere to avoid acute dilatation and also to drain the swallowed saliva. The retrosternal route is preferred by most authors.[8,12,13] A retrosternal route should however be avoided if the liver is large. Few authors however, perform thoracotomy for doing an esophagectomy under vision. In the authors' experience, it has always been feasible in almost all cases without the need for a formal thoracotomy except in one case with severe periesophagitis following corrosive injury. In another case, the esophageal wall was densely adherent and while mobilizing it, while the esophageal mucosa could be removed completely the muscle wall was left

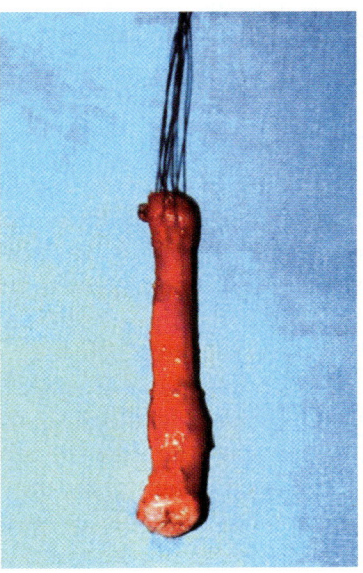

Fig. 32.8: Resected part of strictured esophagus. The authors have been able to resect whole of the native diseased and the strictured esophagus in almost all cases (except in two) without a formal thoracotomy

behind. It is acceptable as it is the diseased esophageal mucosa which is prone to turn malignant and not the muscle. This may be advantageous to utilize the transhiatal approach in children with the past history of major leaks or the scarred mediastinum due to periesophagitis.[14]

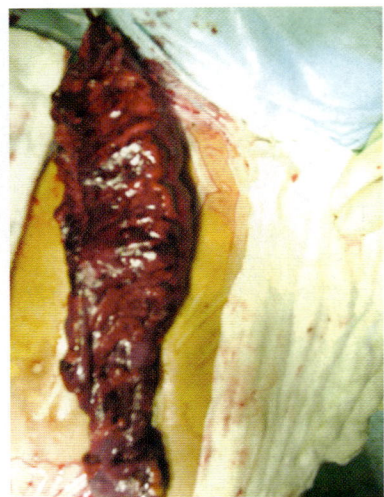

Fig. 32.9: Graft necrosis in a case of colonic interposition. It was a technical fault. The segment selected for interposition was found short and an anastomosis was completed under tension. The result was ischemia of the whole graft. Patient developed blood stained NG aspirate, drop in hemoglobin, and marked tachycardia, with crepitus over the chest wall the next day. Graft was removed in emergency with esophagostomy and gastrostomy

Recent Alterations

Hadidi et al, ligated the trunk of the middle colic artery supplying the transverse colon at the time of doing the gastrostomy operation. This was attempted with an idea to increase the blood supply to the transverse colon through the left upper colic and marginal vessels.[15] They have reported excellent results after colonic interposition based on left colic branch, with only one out of 11 cases, developing stricture in the neck requiring revision. The well thought procedure has however, not been accepted by the most others. Moreover, the colon has a reliable marginal artery and the chances of graft loss are uncommon. Surgeons have achieved equally good results in large series even without the ligation of the middle colic artery.

Contraindications for use of the Colon as an Esophageal Replacement are[6]

i. Incomplete marginal arterial arcade. It may be absent in around 3% of normal individuals.
ii. Associated high anorectal malformation, specially the pouch colon (relative contraindication)
iii. Any other associated colonic disease, polyposis coli, ulcerative colitis.

COMPLICATIONS OF COLON INTERPOSITION

Early Complications

1. Necrosis of graft: Tension at the anastomotic site because of inadequate length of colon can predispose to ischemic graft necrosis (Fig. 32.9). Ischemia can usually be identified at the time of anastomosis. To meet this challenge, an alternate interposition can be constructed in place of the ischemic segment. Short cut can also be planned in the *Taenia coli* if the ischemia is limited to the terminal end for a few cm only. Graft necrosis can be suspected in the postoperative period by the presence of fever, a dark serosanguinous drainage in the NG/mediastinal drain, crepitus, pneumothorax, sepsis or shock. A fibre-optic endoscopy can confirm the diagnosis. Prompt re-exploration with removal of the gangrenous graft is mandatory necessitating diversion in emergency. Subsequently, gastric tube or stomach pull up can be considered to replace the esophagus.[16]
2. Anastomotic leak: Leakage from the proximal esophageal anastomosis is common. This may vary from 20-50%.[17] Leak could be major or minor, with or without symptoms. Ischemia, tension, technically faulty suturing and presence of the esophageal fibrosis at the anastomotic site are the usual reasons for the leak. Majority of the leaks would heal spontaneously provided an adequate drainage has been ensured. Antibiotics and proper nutrition is to be continued. The leak may present as an esophagocutaneous fistula.
3. Gastric outlet obstruction, colonic leak, peritonitis.
4. Mediastinitis, pneumothorax, empyema.
5. Operative mortality ranges from 1-10%.[9]

Late Complications

1. Anastomotic stricture is frequent and is seen in 20-30% cases. The proximal anastomosis is commonly involved. Most strictures respond to dilatation. Lower end strictures are less common and usually require surgical revision, as blind dilatation of the lower anastomosis is hazardous.
2. Obstructive symptoms due the kinking of the lower end of the esophagus over the liver (Figs 10A and B).
3. Redundancy of colon or upper esophageal pouching.[18] Mild redundancy of the colon may

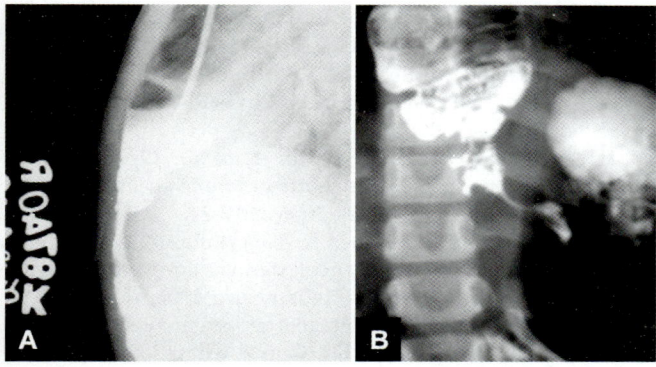

Figs 32.10 A and B: Barium swallow showing partial obstruction in the transposed colon due to kinks and adhesions while coursing over the anterior surface of the liver

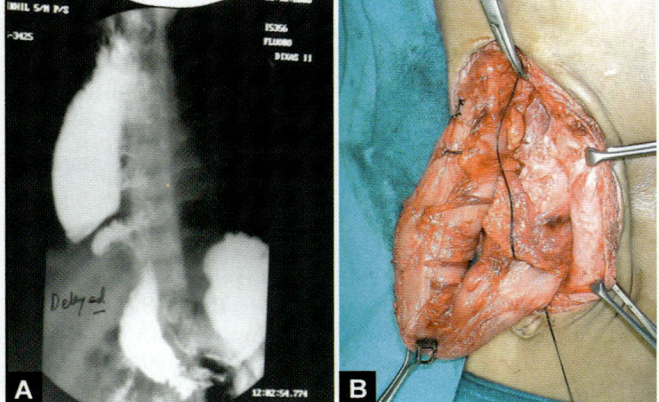

Figs 32.11A and B: A. Follow up case of colonic transposition that presented with recurrent bulky vomiting, due to postoperative cologastric reflux. The barium study showed hold up of the contrast in the transposed colonic segment on delayed film suggestive of obstruction, **B.** Exploration revealed redundant colon in the lower part. The cologastric junction was widely patent. The redundant colon was resected and a re-cologastric anastomosis was made incorporating a valvular mechanism to prevent reflux in the colon

not necessitate revision of the colonic conduit if there is no dysphasia.[14] Redundancy may lead to food stasis, recurrent regurgitation and aspiration. The dilated graft may also cause pulmonary compression. Surgical revision may be required if the patient is symptomatic (Figs 11A and B).
4. Halitosis.
5. Acid reflux: There is no clear difference in the degree of reflux between a direct cologastric anastomosis or if the anastomosis of the colon has been made to the lower esophageal stump.
6. Graft related complications—Colitis.
7. Iron deficiency anemia and transient malabsorption.[19]
8. Inflammatory colonic polyps.
9. Diaphragmatic hernia.
10. Pulmonary symptoms due to chronic acid reflux and aspiration
11. Intestinal obstruction due to adhesions
12. Dumping syndrome.
13. Late graft stenosis.[20]

THE WORLDWIDE EXPERIENCE

Corrosive strictures are common in many countries, e.g. Egypt, Poland, Romania and Turkey, due to the accidental ingestion of washing soda liquid that is used liberally in households (as the milky white fluid kept in drinking water plastic or glass bottles for washing clothes). However, Egyptians possibly have the largest personal and collective experience of over 1200 cases of esophageal replacement using colon. Their postoperative complication rate is also low. Ala Hamza et al reported an experience with more than 850 cases of esophageal replacement over the last 30 years. Complications in the last 475 cases included 10% cervical leakage, 5% proximal strictures, 2% postoperative intestinal obstruction, 1% mortality, and 0.6% late graft stenosis.[20] Colonic replacement of the esophagus was felt as the ideal treatment in cases of caustic esophageal strictures after failure of dilatation. The posterior mediastinal route was preferred as it is shorter, and in long-term follow-up results show improved evacuation and less reflux than with the retrosternal route.[20]

The Factors for this Success could be

1. Referral of most such patients to major centers to be operated upon by the experienced faculty interested in the field.
2. Use of end to side (instead of end to end) and a tension free anastomosis in the neck, reducing the incidence of postoperative leak and the stricture.
3. Exactly measuring the segment of the colon to be used to replace the esophagus.
4. Ensuring good blood supply at either end of the segment of the colon.
5. Removing the native diseased esophagus and placing the colon through the transhiatal route.

6. Using the iso-peristaltic left colon based on the ascending and the descending branches of the left colic artery.
7. Draining the colon in the postoperative period to avoid distension.
8. Incorporation of the valvular mechanism at cologastric junction to prevent reflux.
9. Check endoscopy for early detection of the strictures in the neck and institute dilatation program if the need be.
10. Follow-up with endoscopy to assess for development of any malignancy in the long-term.

FOLLOW-UP

Patients who undergo esophageal replacement should be kept under regular follow up not only for assessing their growth and development status but also to monitor the complications if any. Colonic interposition is one of the safest and best alternatives to the normal esophagus, with minimal short and long-term complications. Patients develop normal eating habits and catch with the height and weight. Postoperative stricture rate is around 10% in experienced hands, mostly managed with dilatations. Half of these may need surgical correction. Moreover, even if the complications develop; these are not serious and easily manageable with the medical or rarely the surgical interventions. Similarly, cologastric reflux and peptic ulcer disease are uncommon. Redundancy may be noted in over 5-10% cases but surgery is indicated only if the patients develop vomiting and dysphasia. In a long-term follow up series of 51 patients reported by Mitchell et al with a mean follow-up of 14 years, reported that almost all the patients were able to eat a normal diet and only 5% had poor results.[12] However, most of these patients were below the 25th percentile for their weight and height. Stone et al reported 86% good results in 37 patients followed up for a mean period of 9.7 years with excellent weight gain and growth development.[21]

REFERENCES

1. Gupta DK, Sharma S, Arora MK, et al. Esophageal replacement in the neonatal period in infants with esophageal atresia and tracheoesophageal fistula J Pediatr Surg 2007;42:1471-77.
2. Gupta DK. Substitution of the esophagus in neonates: an alternative approach. MSR oration delivered at the 32nd Annual Conference of the Indian Association of Pediatric Surgeons, Jaipur Oct 2007;4-7.
3. Aprodu SG, Gavrilescu S, Savu B, et al. Indications for esophageal replacement in children Rev Med Chir Soc Med Nat Iasi. 2004;108:805-8.
4. Ul-Haq A, Tareen F, Bader I, et al. Oesophageal replacement in children with indolent stricture of the oesophagus. Asian J Surg 2006;29:17-21.
5. Demiroayullari B, Sanmez K, Tarkyilmaz Z, et al. Colon interposition for esophageal stenosis in a patient with epidermolysis bullosa. J Pediatr Surg 2001;36:1861-63.
6. Dave S, Gupta DK. Esophageal replacement In Textbook of Neonatal surgery Ed DK Gupta, Chap 2000;55:349-55.
7. Ngan SY, Wong J. Lengths of different routes for esophageal replacement. The Journal of Thoracic and Cardiovascular Surgery 1986;91:790-92.
8. Sherman CD, Waterston DJ. Esophageal reconstruction in children using colon. Arch Dis Child 1957;32:11.
9. Tannuri U, Maksoud-Filho JG, Tannuri AC, et al. Which is better for esophageal substitution in children, esophagocoloplasty or gastric transposition? A 27-year experience of a single center. J Pediatr Surg 2007;42:500-04.
10. West KW, Vave DW, Grosfeld JL. Esophageal replacement in children: experience with 31 cases. Surgery 1986;100:751-57.
11. Lynn HB. Simple method of elongating a colonic segment for esophageal replacement. J Pediatr Surg 1973;8:391-94.
12. Mitchell IM, Goh DW, Roberts KD, et al. Colon interposition in children. Br J Surg 1989;76:681-86.
13. Dickson JAS. Esophageal substitution with colon—The Waterston operation. Pediatric Surg Int 1996;11:224-26.
14. Bassiouny IE, Al-Ramadan SA, Al-Nady A. Long-term functional results of transhiatal oesophagectomy and colonic interposition for caustic oesophageal stricture. Eur J Pediatr Surg 2002;12:243-47.
15. Hadidi AT. A technique to improve vascularity in colon replacement of the esophagus. Eur J Pediatr Surg 2006;16:39-44.
16. Gupta DK. Primary and secondary esophageal replacement by gastric pull up, experience over 27 years. Lecture delivered during the International congress on Long Gap esophageal Atresia and Short Bowel Syndrome, Mannheim, Germany 2007;15-16.
17. Raffensperger JG, Luck SR, Reynolds M, et al. Intestinal bypass of the esophagus. J Pediatr Surg 1996;31:38-47.
18. Glasser JG, Reddy PP, Adkins ES. Treatment of colon conduit redundancy in a child with esophageal atresia. Am Surg 2006;72(3):260-64.
19. Lindahl H, Louhimo I, Virkola K. Colon interposition or gastric tube? Follow-up study of colon-esophagus and gastric tube-esophagus patients. J Pediatr Surg. 1983;18:58-63.
20. Hamza AF, Abdelhay S, Sherif H, et al. Caustic esophageal strictures in children: 30 years' experience. J Pediatr Surg 2003;38(6):828-33.
21. Stone MM, Mahour GH, Weitzmann JJ, et al. Esophageal replacement with colon interposition in children. Ann Surg 1986;316-51.

CHAPTER 33

Gastric Tube Esophageal Replacement

Gabriel O Ionescu

In the last 20-30 years there have been no publications on the topic of esophageal surgery in childhood, without mentioning the well known postulate: "The best esophagus in children is his/her own esophagus".[1-4] Truly a rare operation in childhood, esophageal replacement is still mandatory in cases of extensive damage of the esophagus, mainly due to caustic injuries and in a few cases of long gap esophageal atresia (EALG). Several techniques are commonly used: colonic graft, gastric tube (GT) and gastric transposition are the most popular techniques, depending on the experience and preference of the surgeon. Other options of esophageal replacement or reconstruction have been published, but only small series, with a few cases and lack of long-term follow up: colonic patch, small bowel and sigmoid transposition with microvascular anastomoses, different types of small bowel interposition.[5-12] At present the long-term results and the quality of life in young adults, after esophageal replacement performed in childhood have been published, many with very good results and a normal life.[13-26] This chapter is devoted to the gastric tube esophageal replacement (GTER) in children.

HISTORY

Esophageal replacement by GT is undoubtedly connected with the personality of Prof. Dan Gavriliu, general surgeon in Bucharest, Romania (Fig. 33.1).

He was the first to perform the reversed gastric tube in adults; in 1951, he published his first series of 21 cases.[27] He has positioned the tube initially presternally, then retrosternally and never used the intrathoracic or posterior mediatstinal route. In the original technique he recommended an associated splenectomy to facilitate the tailoring of a tube long enough to easily reach the neck and wrapped the tube with omentum. In 1957 he published a book about surgery of the esophagus and over a long and brilliant carrier he performed close to 1000 GTER and popularized the technique in Romania, Europe and then in North America.[28,29] In an interview he declared performing more than 5000 GTER (!) for all indications, including children with EALG. In the new world the technique is known as Dr.Heimlich's operation. Dr Heimlich from Ohio, without knowing of D Gavriliu's work, described the same technique and published his first short series in 1959.[30] The first GT performed in Canada was by Dr James Fallis, but S Ein has extensively used the GT in Children and published long-term results.[14-21]

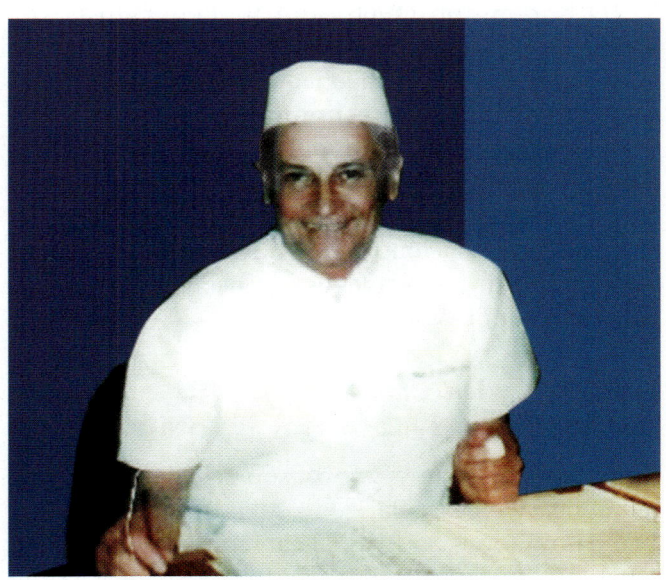

Fig. 33.1: Prof D Gavriliu in his office

In fact, the history of GT is a bit different: Several well known surgeons in Europe and Northern America, at the end of 19th century and beginning of 20th suggested and did experimental work on esophageal replacement with the stomach (D. Biondi 1895, Gosset 1903, Hirsch 1911, Carl Beck and A. Carrel). In 1969 P Orsoni wrote a very comprehensive monograph in French: "Esophagoplasties".[1] In his book, an extensive review of the true history of esophageal reconstruction is presented and he restored the true "paternity" of GTER. Prof Amza Jianu, professor of General Surgery in Bucharest, Romania had been the tutor of Prof D Gavriliu at the beginning of his surgical training. In between 1910-1936 he imagined, proposed and did many experimental works on animals on GTER.[31] He performed the experiments together with Dr D Gavriliu but Amza Jianu never performed his operation on humans; Dr D Gavriliu was the first surgeon using the technique in patients. Over time several modifications of the original technique were published: Transhiatal esophagectomy (Denk, 1913, Turner,1936, Orringer 1978), which later was combined in a one stage operation with colonic graft (B M Rodgers and all 1981).[32-35] In the last decade the most utilized procedure for pediatric esophageal replacement is a combination of transhiatal esophagectomy and the placement of the substitute graft (colon, small bowel or gastric tube) through normal, posterior, mediastinal route, in a one stage operation: For gastric tube it was first published in 1985.[36]

JD Burrington (1968) and JC Pedersen (1996) presented a short series of GTER for EALG performed very early, even in the neonatal period.[37-38]

A very attractive technique has been recently published and experimentally documented, which uses an isolated pediculated gastric tube interposition as esophageal substitute, especially in cases of esophageal atresia long gap.[39-41] The technique claims some interesting advantages but needs bigger series and long-term results.

SURGICAL ANATOMY—PRACTICAL CONSIDERATION FOR GTER TECHNIQUE

When performing any type of esophageal replacement, retaining a well vascularized graft is the main concern. There is no series on esophageal replacement without a few cases of graft failure and necrosis of vascular cause (thrombosis, poor vascular perfusion, compression/twisting of the main pedicle). A few surgeons for improving the graft perfusion, combine vascular grafts (colon, small bowel) with additional blood flow, via micro vascular anastomosis at the level of cervical anastomosis (with facial, internal mammary, or even external carotid artery).

It is unanimously accepted that the stomach has an excellent, rich vascular network, with multiple anastomosis and low septic risk, due to acid secretion. As the vast majority of surgeons use the reversed gastric tube for esophageal replacement (RGTER), the interest is focused on blood supply of the great curvature of the stomach. The great curvature is bordered by the gastroepiploic arcade (gastroomental), resulting from the direct anastomosis of the right (originated from left gastric artery) and left (originated from splenic artery) gastroepiploic vessels. Numerous collateral vessels spread within the great curvature wall where they make large loops with rich anastomosis. In many cases the gastroepiploic arcade is incomplete for 2-7 cm, raising concern in the mind of the surgeon on the quality of blood supply within the gastric tube (30% of cases in my personal series of 107 RGTER). Study on microvascular anatomy has demonstrated an excellent vascularity within the wall of great curvature in all cases, unrelated with a complete or incomplete gastroepiploic arcade. In surgical practice an incomplete arcade is not a contraindication for utilization of GT. Studies published recently on the vascularity of the stomach show that the fundus of the stomach is less well vascularized than the vertical part of the stomach and the antrum; consequently, at least theoretically, an isoperistaltic tube, based on right gastroepiploic artery, will have less perfusion in the end part of the tube than a RGT which is brought up to the neck for anastomosis (Fig. 33.2).

Experimental work of Schilling MK et al 1997 on blood perfusion in different types of GT, based on Doppler flowmetry, proved that the best flow was found in the fundus tube, based on lesser curvature vessels (fundus rotation gastroplasty).[42] They also demonstrate by the same technique that dissection of gastrocolic ligament and vascular disconnection when the tube is made, reduces the blood flow along the great curvature. They recommend intraoperative utilization of Doppler flowmetry which might prevent

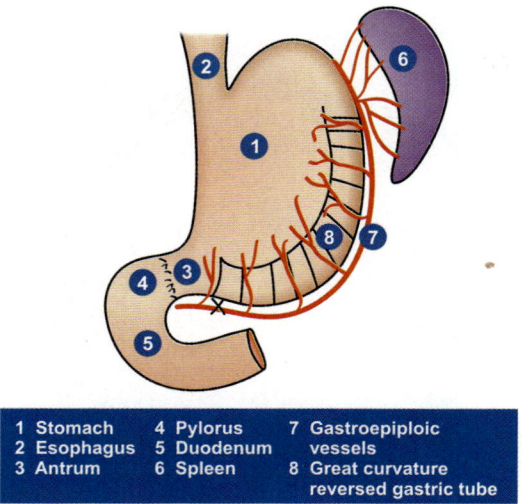

Fig. 33.2: Anatomy of the reversed gastric tube

1. Stomach
2. Esophagus
3. Antrum
4. Pylorus
5. Duodenum
6. Spleen
7. Gastroepiploic vessels
8. Great curvature reversed gastric tube

ischemia-induced anastomotic breakdown.[43] In 2006 Nishikawa K et al.[44] presented their experience with intraoperative thermal imaging in esophageal replacement; they measured the surface temperature of the intact stomach, devascularized stomach and the GT and clearly demonstrated a lower surface temperature in the proximal part of the GT. They conclude that intraoperative thermography is a non invasive, reliable method and recommended to be used when the GT is made. Lazar G et al 2003, in a genuine experimental work, proposed utilization of thoracic epidural anesthesia, to improve the gastric microcirculation when a GT is made.[45] All the above methods to document the satisfactory perfusion of GT are non- invasive procedures, not time consuming and could be used intraoperatively; the author has no personal experience with them.

A previous gastrostomy, incorrectly located on the great curvature and interruption of the gastroepiplooic arcade could be a contraindication for gastric tube; in my series 2 cases presented with gastrostomy on the great curvature and vascular arcade compromised; one case has been converted in colonic graft with excellent result the other had an atypical gastric tube involving the posterior wall of the stomach at the level of the gastrostomy and finally a complete necrosis of the tube occurred.

In conclusion, the great curvature of the stomach offers an excellent, well vascularized structure for esophageal replacement, with a low risk of vascular graft failure, compared to colon interposition or small bowel.

INDICATIONS FOR ESOPHAGEAL REPLACEMENT

Esophageal atresia long gap and extensive esophageal stricture postcaustic ingestion are the most common indications for esophageal replacement in children.[4,20,23,25,38,46-58] The Foker's technique of rapid esophageal elongation, together with various procedures of delayed esophageal anastomosis, almost eliminates the need for replacement in EALG.[59-62] The complete failure of end-to-end anastomosis after primary, delayed or secondary surgery for EALG is a very rare condition which still may require an esophageal replacement.

The correct aggressive treatment of caustic injury with corticoids, early dilatation and eventually endless-loop bougienage in cases of moderate stenosis but resistant to intermittent dilatations significantly reduces the number of cases who need esophageal replacement.[63]

Occasionally, for isolated cases of severe esophageal stricture in patients with epidermolysis bullosa, achalasia, long esophageal duplication, or infectious strictures of the esophagus a replacement of the esophagus could be indicated.[64-67] The choice of the type of replacement mostly depends on surgeon preference. Interestingly Harmel performed esophageal replacement on two siblings with epidermolysis bullosa; his comment was that the GT was easier and performed in shorter time than the colonic graft, but with very good results in both cases.[64] In the past the GT replacement has been used in desperate cases of uncontrollable bleeding due to esophageal varices.[68]

In some cases the GT, colonic graft or gastric transposition have specific indications or cannot be used: In VATER syndrome, esophageal atresia associated malrotation, congenital megacolon, congenital short colon, premature with previous episodes of NEC, multiple intestinal atresias syndrome the colonic graft is contraindicated. Very small stomach as in type I esophageal atresia, gastric scars from caustic ingestion, especially strong acids, inappropriate site of gastrostomy on the great curvature makes the GT unsuitable for replacement.

Gastric transposition, although a very popular and safe operation, should be cautiously used in childhood, only as a last resort, if the other types of replacement are not possible.

Finally it should be mentioned that the GT has occasionally been utilized for other indications such as drainage for the ventricular shunt (ventriculo-gastric shunt), for biliary atresia as gastro-portostomy, via a short isoperistaltic tube (China) and in adult surgery for continent, tubeless gastrostomy in cases of unresectable esophageal cancer.

OPTIMAL TIME FOR ESOPHAGEAL REPLACEMENT

The optimal time for esophageal replacement depends of many factors: primary disease, co-morbid pathology, the level of intensive care unit for safe postoperative care, often an arbitrary decision of the surgeon (i.e. not earlier than 1 yr, 6 or 8 kg). For esophageal atresia there is a general agreement for an early repair/replacement of the esophagus as soon as possible, even in neonatal period, to achieve the oral feeding.[69] All types of replacement (gastric tube, colonic graft and gastric transposition) have been performed successfully in neonatal period or early infancy and can be safely done if the mandatory conditions for a successful GT replacement are achieved (see below).

In case of severe strictures, not responding to dilatations, the replacement should be done after all methods of dilatation have failed. In the author's experience the endless loop dilatations performed over a long time (1-3 years) is an excellent method which, if it is used correctly, could avoid the replacement.[63] The advantages of the method are that it is done daily or twice a day at home, by family (sometimes by the patient if older), no need of anesthesia, very safe, with minimal complications (nasal, choanal, soft palate ulcerations, granuloma, stenosis) and allows concomitant oral feeding. The disadvantages are: presence of the loop, need of a gastrostomy and is difficult to accept by family and patient, mainly for psychological reasons (Fig. 33.3).

Some authors recommend early replacement based on a non-documented idea that the mediastinal fibrosis increases over time and the removal of the damaged esophagus will be difficult and more prone to complications. They recommend the replacement-if needed-at 6 months postingestion of the caustic substance. If the posterior mediastinal route is used, previous mediastinitis from the caustic or iatrogenic perforation, then a long interval is recommended (minimum 1 year) since the complete healing of mediastinitis. In these cases the retrosternal position of GT could be a better option. The damaged esophagus should finally be removed as a separate operation or in one stage. The replacement for esophageal atresia should be performed on baby in good health, with a documented big gastric reservoir, on well accepted "sham feeds"; majority of these cases have their replacement performed between 8-14 months. For caustic strictures the replacement has never been done earlier than 1 year from ingestion in most of the cases (mean 16-24 months).

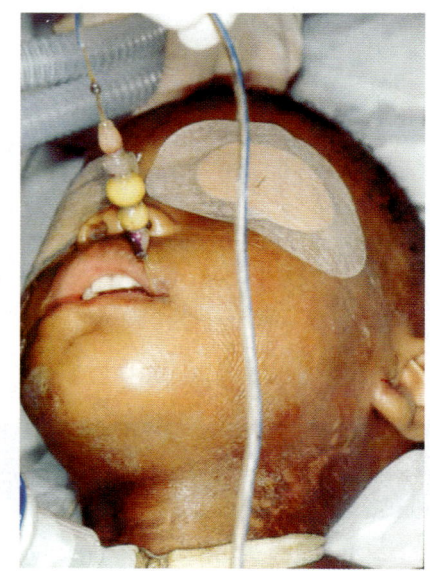

Fig. 33.3: Endless loop dilatation

CHOICE OF ESOPHAGEAL REPLACEMENT: COLONIC GRAFT, GASTRIC TUBE OR TOTAL GASTRIC TRANSPOSITION

The literature regarding the "best esophageal replacement in children" is abundant; almost every year 1 or 2 articles try to answer this question better.[16,70-73] Based on a large series and comparing the long-term results, the first option is equally divided between colonic substitution or gastric tube, followed by total gastric transposition.[4,20-26,36,38,48,49,58,74-84] The other substitution as small bowel, different other gastric tubes from fundus or lesser curvature, Scharli's operation included should be regarded as isolated indications and their utilization should be based on the real contraindications for gastric tube or colonic substitution.[85,86]

PREOPERATIVE PREPARATION FOR GASTRIC TUBE ESOPHAGEAL REPLACEMENT

Esophageal replacement is a major surgery in pediatric patients; postoperative morbidity and even mortality are still recorded in many series. A few cases of failure of any type of esophageal grafts are noticed in most of the series. It is recommended to have implemented a nationally accepted protocol for 1-3 tertiary centers of excellence, with experienced surgeons in esophageal pediatric surgery and high level PICU. In several countries patients who eventually need esophageal replacement are taken over early by a multidisciplinary team to insure best care (pediatric gastroenterologist, nutrition, pneumologist, experienced endoscopist, stoma care, experienced surgeon, anesthesist even psychologist for family or older patient support (teenagers with suicide attempts, interruption of school, stress due to multiple dilatations, etc.).

There are several mandatory conditions that should be fulfilled for a successful GTER:

1. The decision for GTER should be a well planned operation.
2. The best time for safely performing the GT has been discussed. Many of these patients, especially with plurimalformative syndromes or postcaustic injury present with severe malnutrition. Improving the nutritional status is an intimate part of the preoperative preparation; this can take months.
3. Most of the patients who underwent esophageal replacement have a preoperative gastrostomy. The Stamm gastrostomy is most commonly used by pediatric surgeons but often the gastrostomy has been performed elsewhere and could be inappropriate as site or of poor quality (leaking, inflammation, erosions due to gastric juice). In a few cases a new gastrostomy with closure of the old one could be the only option. The surgeon who performs the initial gastrostomy must write detailed notes about the gastric vascularity and if a further gastric tube is possible. Some surgeons prefer a feeding jejunostomy instead of gastrostomy with the reason of having "a stomach free of previous surgery" at the time of replacement. The gastrostomy is a mandatory preliminary step before gastric GTER not only for feeding but for creating a big gastric reservoir. After several months of feeding jejunostomy, the stomach becomes very small and the GT is no longer possible. If the patient is referred with a jejunostomy already in place, before GTER the jejunostomy should be closed and the patient must have a gastrostomy performed. Feeding should be given as large bolus and the gastric capacity should be at 250-750 ml, depending on age (Fig. 33.4).

The big gastric reservoir is a major problem in type I esophageal atresia; in these cases initially the stomach is so small that even placing a gastrostomy tube could be a problem. A well established protocol for gastric enlargement, bu bigger and bigger meals allows the stomach to reach a normal volume in 3-6 months (Figs 33.5 to 33.9).

In cases of EALG a program of "sham feeds" is mandatory. The "sham feeds" should be implemented immediately in neonatal period. For patients with end or lateral esophagostomy it is easy to perform but for patients without esophagostomy, under continuous pharyngeal suction for months, the swallow can still be achieved using an empty bottle.

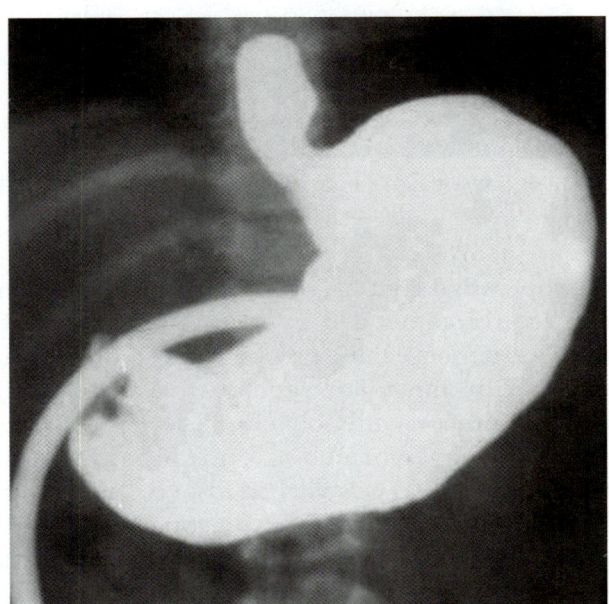

Fig. 33.4: A big gastric reservoir of 1250 ml

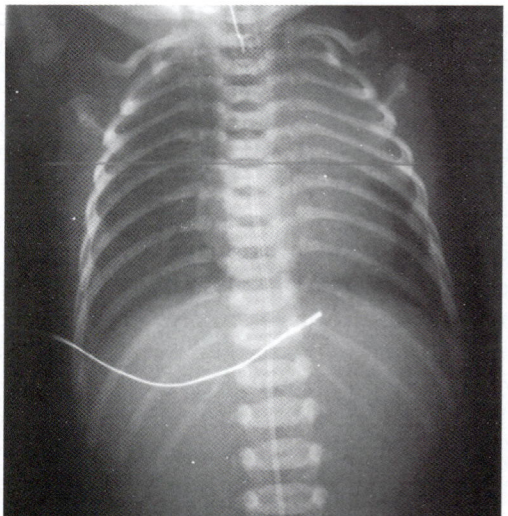

Fig. 33.5: Chest X-ray of Esophageal atresia Type I

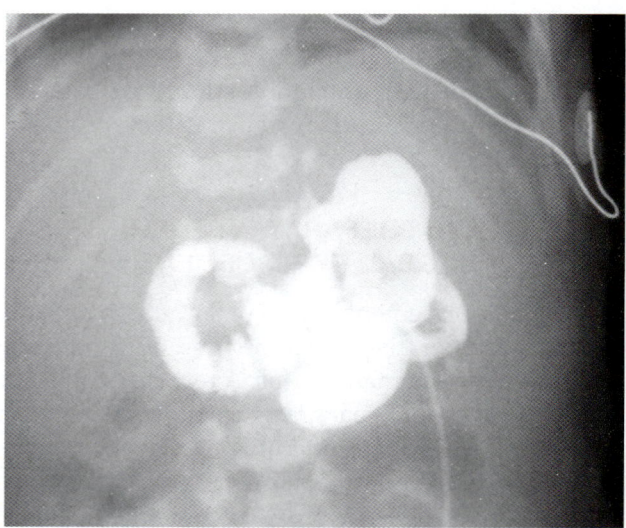

Fig. 33.7: Contrast study 12 days post-gastrostomy: capacity of the stomach was 12 ml

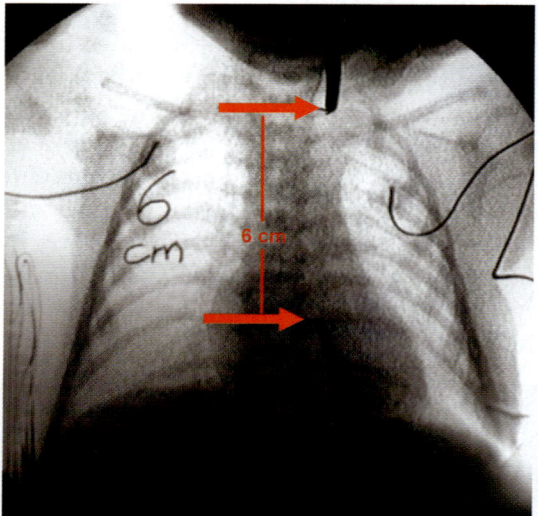

Fig. 33.6: Same case: intraoperative chest X-ray showing a long gap of 6 cm

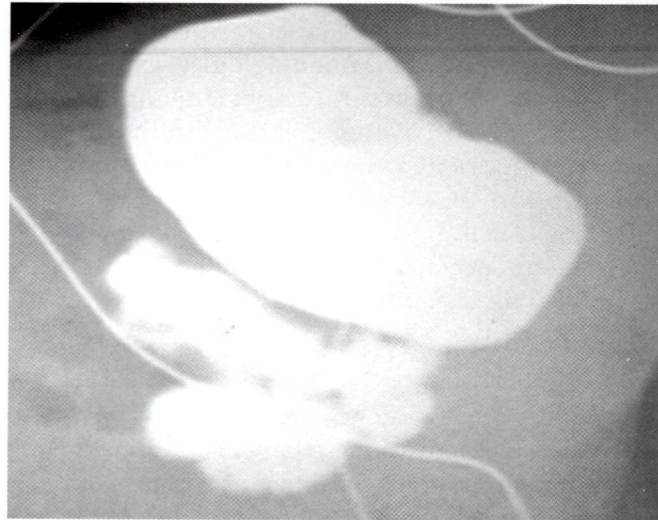

Fig. 33.8: Three weeks later, after bolus feeding the capacity of the stomach was 76 ml

Preoperative contrast study of the stomach and colon are recommended by some surgeons; in the author's experience these preoperative studies are not necessary. In immediate preoperative period, total bowel preparation with Golytely or Clean prep should be carefully performed, if intraoperative the replacement should be switched from colon to gastric tube or vice versa, depending on abnormal vascular findings. The author would also like to mention that the "Informed consent" signed by parents must always include all 3 options of replacement.

OPERATIVE TECHNIQUE OF GTER

Majority of surgeons, including the author routinely use the reversed gastric tube; this technique is presented as: "How do I do the reversed gastric tube esophageal replacement in children?" "There are several differences in between the replacement for EALG and the one for caustic stricture or diseases which require concomitant esophagectomy.

Broad spectrum antibiotic prophylaxis is given 0.5 hr before surgery and an antibiotic treatment is

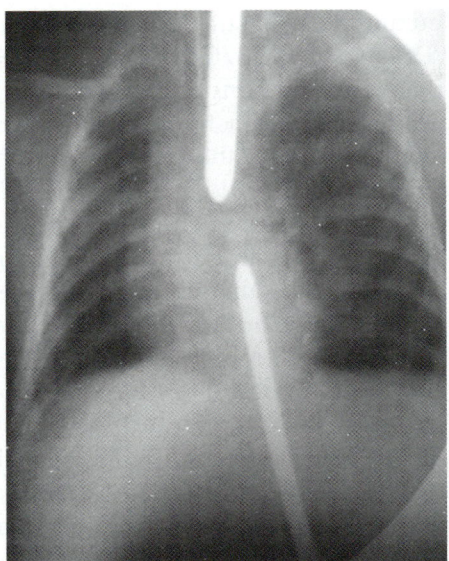

Fig. 33.9: Two months later the gap spontaneously decreased to 1.5 cm

maintained 3-5 days, until any septic complication is ruled out and feeding through gastrostomy is initiated. Good venous access is provided, better by a double lumen central vein line. The left side of the neck from above the angle of the jaw, the whole chest and abdomen are meticulously prepared, sterile and covered with cutting through Opsite. In adult surgery the operation is performed by two surgical teams: one abdominal, building up the tube, another operating on the neck; in children the operation is performed by only one team.

Gastric tube esophageal replacement for Esophageal atresia

The gastrostomy tube is pulled out and the site of gastrostomy is separated from the abdominal wall; this first step could be done before or after laparotomy. The author does the gastrostomy separation as initial maneuver. Through a midline supraumbilical laparotomy, the stomach is approached and inspected. The left triangular liver ligament is divided and the lower esophageal stump prepared as for Nissen fundoplication. The vagus nerves are identified and separated from esophagus; often the posterior nerve is not clearly visible and its identification is abandoned. No upward dissection of lower esophageal stump is performed now, to avoid, an incidental pneumothorax or worse, bleeding from mediastinum, at the beginning of a long operation.

In the original Gavriliu's description of the GT, he recommended mobilization of the splenic angle of the colon "en bloc" with the spleen, even splenectomy. All of these maneuvers are not recommended or necessary. The stomach is inspected, the place where the GT will be created is marked with transfixed sutures and the length of the tube is approximated with a feeding tube which goes from mid part of great curvature till the left mastoid process; that is the necessary length of the further gastric tube. Usually the proximal end of the GT starts 2-5 cm far from the pylorus, on the antral segment. The gastro-epiplooic vessels are identified and followed towards the left but not yet divided; still either tubes, isoperistaltic or reversed could be decided. The gastro-colic ligament is progressively divided from right to left, the great omentum left attached to the colon and the gastro-epiploic arcade to the stomach. The width of the GT is very important; this should be more or less of the same caliber as the native esophagus (Fig. 33.10).[87]

For modeling the GT the author uses a chest drain tube CH 10-14 for babies and 18-22 for older children. The GT is then separated from the great curvature. The reversed or isoperistaltic GT must be decided now and the gastroepiploic vessel ligated and divided at the right or left end of the gastroepiploic arcade (Figs 33.11 and 33.12).

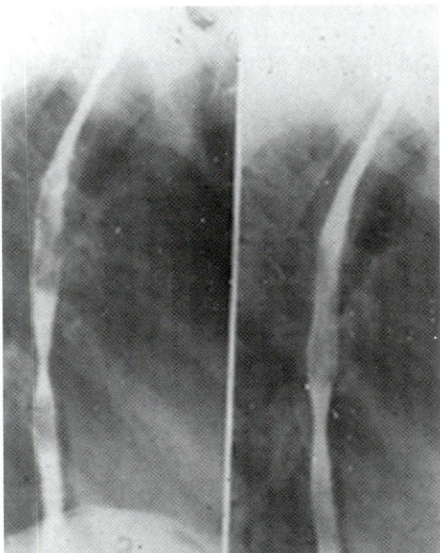

Fig. 33.10: A perfect gastric tube with regard to position, width and uniform caliber

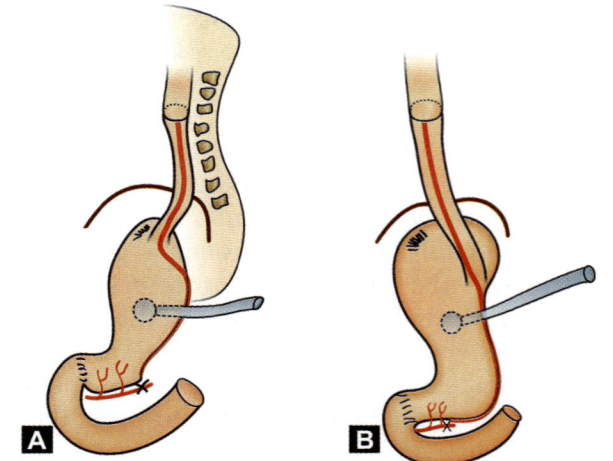

Figs 33.11A and B: Configuration of reversed gastric tube
A. Lateral view of RGTER, **B.** Frontal view of RGTER

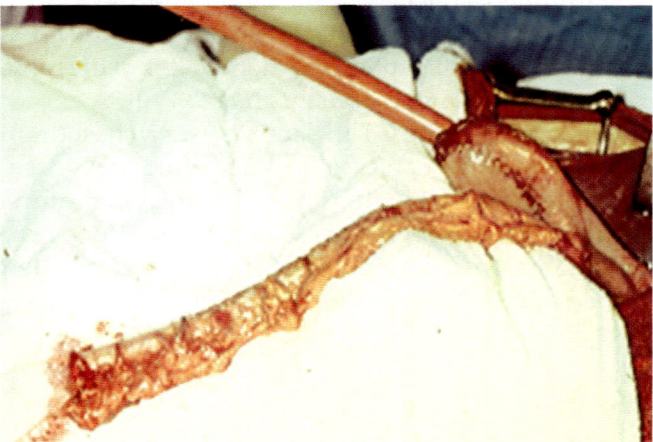

Fig. 33.12: Intraoperative photo of a long reversed gastric tube

The GT could be made in two different manners:
1. Manually, by hand suturing.
2. Mechanically, with staplers suture.

A 2 cm transverse incision is made on the antrum at the chosen level; the chest tube is inserted retrograde within the stomach and placed close the the great curvature. For preventing unnecessary blood loss during separation of the GT, pairs of transfixed sutures are placed over the vessels with a big straight needle. The GT is divided in between the sutures with sewing progressively (P Orsoni's recommendation).[1] The first 3-5 cm of the GT should be larger than the rest of the tube and made funnel shaped, for a good cervical anastomoses.

The initial 97 GT of the authors series were all hand made. The first 3-5 cm of the GT are made with interrupted double layer sutures of resorbable stitches (Vicryl, PDS, Monocryl 3/0-5/0) and the rest of the tube and stomach by continuous, running, double layer sutures. Then the gastrostomy tube is replaced, most commonly through the same site or a new one. Often the gastrostomy could be comfortably included in the long suture line which closes the new great curvature. The GT has to be made water proof and checked by injecting N saline solution under moderate pressure. In babies the author prefers the hand made tube which takes 20-40 min to be done.

The last 10 GT (since 1993) have been done by mechanical suture with staplers (Ethicon, Johnson and Johnson, linear cutter of 55 or 75 mm.) This is a very fast and easy technique, which takes 10 to 15 min. for a very long tube. At the chosen level on the antrum, a complete transverse division is done, the chest tube is inserted in the same manner and the linear cutter is placed as close as possible near the tube. The division is bloodless. In older children the size of the staplers should be quite big (11-14 mm). The risk of a leak due to default staplers could generate life threatening complications (one personal case complicated with mediastinitis). A safe and wise maneuver is to over sew the mechanical suture line with a continuous suture of PDS 3/0-5/0 all along the tube and gastric suture. The water proof should be also checked carefully. At the end of gastric tube suture (manually or by staplers) the long suture line could be sealed with a biological glue (Tisseel or other glues) to decrease the risk of minimal leaking. Without prospective study performed or published the author has used routinely the sealing of the GT with Tisseel, with a real benefit.

After the GT is made, the transhiatal route for the passage of the GT is performed. The technique is well known and common for all types of esophageal replacement in adults and children. By digital dissection the tunnel is progressively made upwards. The dissection should stay at all times strictly in front of the vertebral body. The cervical esophagostomy is mobilized and a retrotracheal digital dissection is gently directed downwards, within the posterior mediastinum. The transhiatal and cervical operator's finger should get together and finalize a wide and comfortable passage. The remnant lower esophageal stump is removed with a cut of the linear cutter. A big Nelaton catheter is passed down through the posterior route and brought to the abdomen. The GT, protected with a finger glove is attached to the catheter and pulled up gently, under direct vision, within the neck. The long suture should be kept in the anterior position. About 2-5 cm of the length of the GT should be left in the abdomen as is the normal anatomy of the esophagus. The intra-abdominal segment of the GT prevents gastro-tube reflux. Together with the GT, a strong no. 1 silk stitch is brought through the posterior mediastinum which will be used to correctly place a long 6-16 mm J-vac drain in the mediastinum. The drain is pulled out by a small separated incision on the neck with its distal end just above the diaphragm.

The cervical anastomoses is the most delicate part of the operation. The GT is trimmed of 1-2 cm and checked for a good vascular supply. Usually there is no problem with the color and the bleeding from the GT. If the GT brought to the neck is blue or with obvious ischemia, the vascularity must be checked all along the tube, identifying the cause (kicking, compression, torsion, damage to the arcade, etc.). In very rare situations a tube with compromised vascularity should be removed and another option of replacement utilized, in the same operation or later (no case in my series). It is crucial to have a long GT; often, after trimming a few cm the GT shows an excellent blood flow. The anastomoses is made end-to-end, one layer, interrupted suture of 5/0 resorbable material. The operation ends by repositioning the gastrostomy in the same place and closure of the abdomen. The duration of the procedure is usually between 1 ½ to 3 ½ hours.

Gastric Tube Esophageal Replacement for Esophageal Stricture and Other Diseases

The removal of damaged esophagus is mandatory. Several cases of malignant transformation of the old esophagus have been published.[88] In Gavriliu's series 3 patients died due to cancer of the remnant esophagus. Peptic ulcer, severe bleeding and cystic transformation of the diseased esophagus—esophageal mucocelle[89] have been reported (one case in my series) (Figs 33.13 and 33.14).

The esophagectomy can be performed as a separate operation, by right or left thoracotomy, or as a transhiatal esophagectomy, by blunt digital dissection or stripping, without thoracotomy, performed concomitantly with the esophageal replacement. The combination of the 2 operations into a one stage operation is today "the golden standard" for the majority of pediatric surgeons.

Preoperative preparations are the same for GTER as for EALG. The operation starts by left cervical approach of the esophagus which is dissected and separated from the trachea. Left recurrent and vagus nerves should be identified and protected. It is recommended to insert a very big intraesophageal

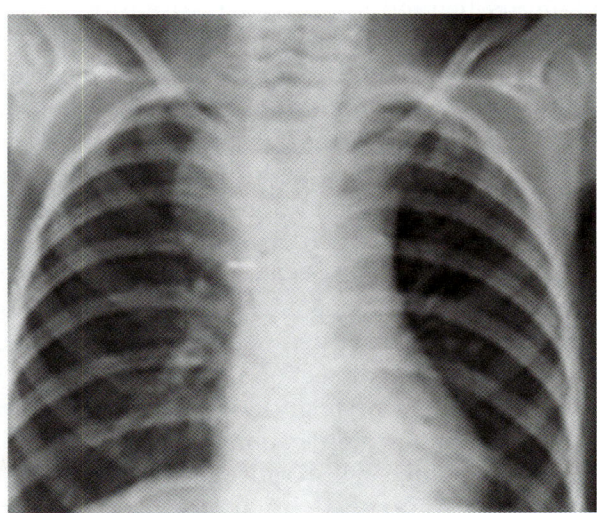

Fig. 33.13: Mucocele of the damaged esophagus left *in situ*. A metallic ring retained within the cystic transformation of the esophagus. The child presented in emergency with life-threatening respiratory distress syndrome due to tracheal compression

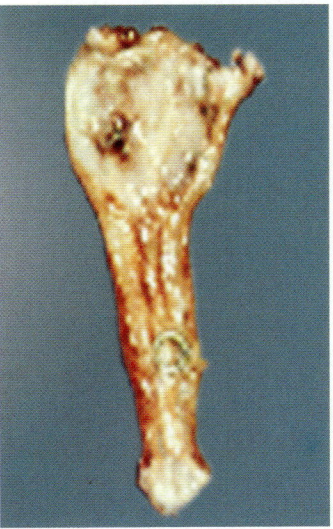

Fig. 33.14: Same case as in Fig.33.13: The damaged esophagus was removed by right thoracotomy. The ring is visible in the lower esophagus

tube, pushed down up to the level of the stricture. By this maneuver the level of esophageal transection is precisely decided with no risk of missing a loose stricture (3 cases in my series, with total gastric transposition performed elsewhere, had the anastomosis with the stomach done below an unrecognized stenosis within the esophagus). Some surgeons prefer to do a preoperative endoscopy on the table. A vascular loop or a soft tube is placed around the esophagus to facilitate the manipulation during dissection. As for the transhiatal esophagectomy, the mediastinal dissection should not be performed initially, to avoid complication at the beginning of a long operation (injury of the trachea, main neck vessels).

The gastric tube is fashioned as previously described. The transhiatal ophagectomy is done by digital dissection upward from the abdomen and downward from the neck. The esophagus is manipulated by the 2 loops surrounding it in the neck and abdomen. Keeping very close to the esophagus, gentle but firm, the dissection is quite uneventful in many cases and surprisingly with minimal bleeding. The most common complication is a pneumothorax– right or left- which will require at the end an ICD. Sporadically injury of the aorta, trachea, main bronchus, main thoracic duct or pericardium, have been reported (none in the author's series of 107 cases). In case of major hemorrhage the surgeon should not hesitate to control the hemorrhage by open thoracotomy. At the end of mobilization the esophagus should move easily up and down. In several cases of teenage patients, the digital dissection is limited, but not complete. In these cases–as in adult surgery–the stripping of the esophagus becomes necessary. The author has performed the stripping in 3 cases with an ordinary varices stripper and the removal of the esophagus has been complete. Then the GT is brought up to the neck through the bed of the removed esophagus and an end-to-end anastomoses is performed (Figs 33.15A and B).

In cases with documented history of severe mediastinitis due to perforation (pleural effusion, empyema, mediastinal drainage for pus collection) the blunt esophagectomy should be avoided. Sophisticated preoperative imaging such as: spiral CT, MRI, MRA cannot predict the risk of catastrophic complications. Two options should be considered:
- One stage operation with esophagectomy performed by open thoracotomy, followed by esophageal replacement via transthoracic or mediastinal route;
- Retrosternal positioning of the gastric tube, followed several months later, by open esophagectomy. This second option is preferred by the author (Fig. 33.16).

Reversed gastric tube vs. isoperistaltic gastric tube

There are still a few surgeons performing the isoperistaltic gastric tube (IGT)[22] based on a false idea

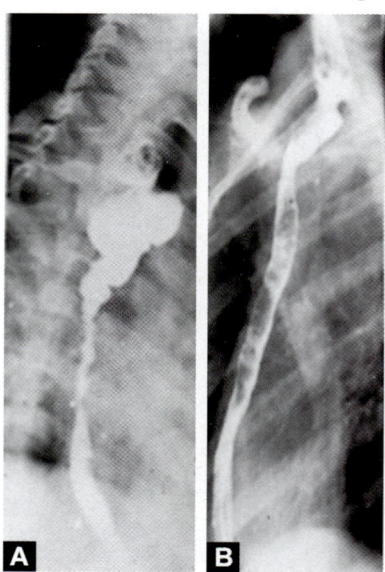

Figs 33.15A and B: A. Severe stricture of the esophagus. During dilatation a perforation with mediastinitis occurred. **B.** Excellent result with GT in retrosternal position

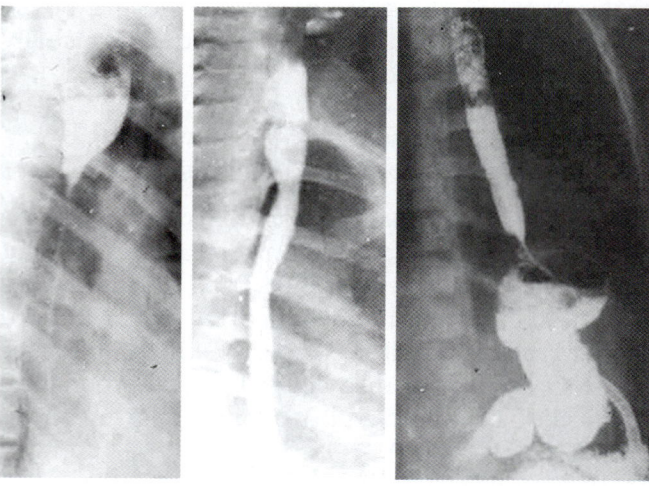

Fig. 33.16: Complete obstruction of the whole esophagus post-caustic injury (left). Result of RGTER with esophagectomy and GT positioned in the posterior mediastinum (middle). General view of GT and the stomach which retains a good capacity (right)

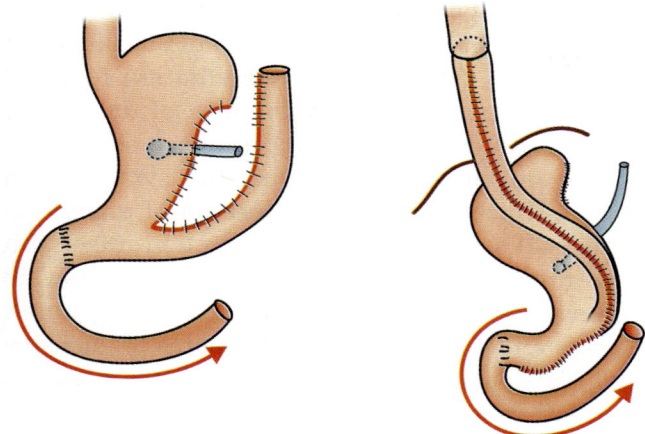

Fig. 33.17: Configuration of an isoperistaltic gastric tube

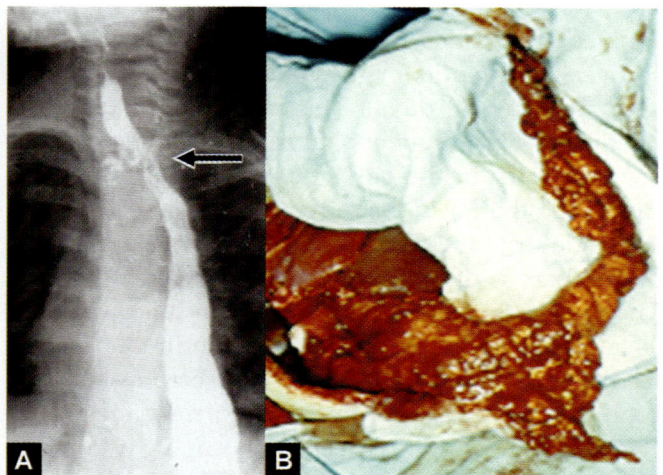

Figs 33.18A and B: A. Isoperistaltic gastric tube with anastomotic fistula. **B.** Intraoperative photo of an isoperistaltic gastric tube (right)

of better passage of the foods through the IGT.[22] Two published series, one in adults, another in children prove the opposite; heavy complications, even mortality; in long-term some patients needed secondary gastro or jejunostomy for feeding (Fig. 33.17).[90,91]

In the author's series 2 cases were performed in the isoperistaltic manner at the beginning of experience with GT, due to apparent better vascularity of the GT. Both cases had anastomotic fistula which closed spontaneously in one case and by redo-anastomoses in the second (Figs 33.18A and B).

In one case severe a dumping syndrome persisted for several years due to rapid passage of the food through the antrum and pylorus. In both cases repeated video recorded barium swallow and follow through did not show any regular peristaltic waves, only some autonomic motility as in the reversed GT. The isoperistaltic GT should be an exceptional indication based on serious anatomic reasons. Otherwise, compared to the RGT has only disadvantages:

1. The IGT is less well irrigated in the distal end which is anastomosed with the cervical esophagus.
2. The IGT should be made much longer than the RGT.
3. To bring up the IGT to the neck, the duodenum and the stomach should be extensively mobilized by a Kocher maneuver, unnecessary in RGT.
4. There is no proof of better motility in the IGT compared with the RGT.
5. In many cases of IGT the stomach is in fact bypassed by food and may generate dumping syndrome.

Pyloroplasty: is it necessary?
Most of the authors who use total gastric transposition associate a true pyloroplasty or just an extra mucosal pyloromyotomy with the reason to avoid delay in gastric emptying.[18,82,83] In the author's experience the drainage procedure is unnecessary in GTER and often can cause negative effects on gastric emptying; none of 107 cases of RGTER had a drainage procedure.

Pharyngo-esophageal replacement with gastric tube and duodenum.

In several cases of extensive esophageal strictures, due to strong caustic agents, the pharynx is also involved or completely destroyed.[92] Most common the hypopharynx, but often the orropharynx are excluded. On video recorded study the contrast material is instantly regurgitated through the nose. All these cases (3 in my series) had concomitant laryngeal injury and a tracheostomy was already in place. The multiple stages of repair of these complicated cases (initial pharyngeal reconstruction with skin flats or free graft of colon or short sigmoid segment, etc.), followed by a type of esophageal reconstruction is not discussed in this chapter. There is a general agreement on very poor results, a few patients being finally able to return to oral feeding.

Concomitant pharyngeal and esophageal reconstruction in such cases can be achieved by an original procedure; one stage pharyngo-esophageal reconstruction with first part of the duodenum (PERDGT)

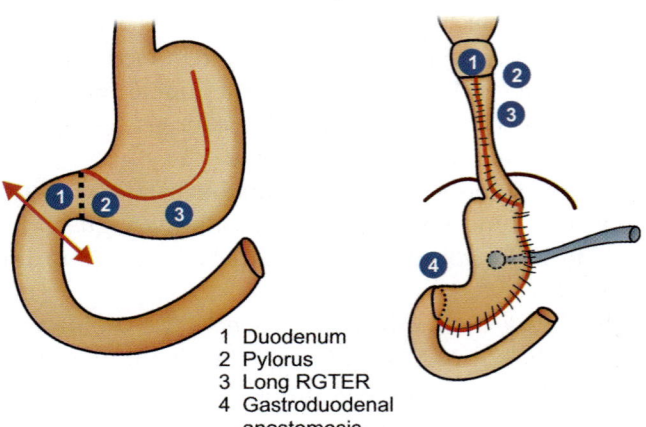

Fig. 33.19: Configuration of pharyngo-esophagoplasty with gastric tube and duodenum

1 Duodenum
2 Pylorus
3 Long RGTER
4 Gastroduodenal anastomosis

and a long gastric tube, associated with transhiatal blunt esophagectomy (Fig. 33.19).

The main steps of the operation are the same with the one stage RGTER for caustic stricture with several modifications. The first approach is on the neck with a long vertical or transverse incision identifying the remnant pharyngeal pouch. Intra-oral maneuver with a finger pushing down the pharynx by an assistant facilitates the preparation of the site for the further anastomoses; if possible, the anastomoses is placed on the posterior and lateral pharyngeal wall and the anastomoses should be as wide as possible. Then the neck is temporarily sutured and the procedure continues intra-abdominal. The first part, mobile of the duodenum is prepared as for a gastric resection. The vascular arcade is meticulously preserved and the duodenum is transected as distal as possible. Through the duodenum, a chest drain tube CH 18-22 is placed and pushed retrograde within the stomach close to the great curvature. On the antrum, 2-3 cm far from the pylorus a linear cutter 75 mm is placed and the first fired for the gastric tube is performed. Often a very long tube is needed to reach the pharynx and the tube goes up to the upper part of the fundus (the longest tube in my series measured 54 cm (21.5 inches). By duodeno-gastric anastomoses the G-I continuity is restored. After the blunt transhiatal esophagectomy, the long tube is pulled through the posterior mediastinum to the neck. Pharyngo-duodenal anastomoses is a real difficult task and can take a long time. As the patients are intubated through the tracheostomy, intraoral maneuver could facilitate the anastomoses. Oral feeding rehabilitation requires patience and time, with involvement of the speech therapist. An amazing finding has been seen in all 3 cases: on video recorded barium swallow the pylorus, which is now in the position of pharyngo-esophageal sphincter keeps its function intact and opens intermittently. All 3 cases achieved impressively good oral feeding for liquid and solid feeding, but in one case rehabilitation lasted 2.5 months of intensive work. Two patients have excellent long-term results; one died in obscure conditions 2.5 years from operation, due to tracheostomy complications.

POSTOPERATIVE CARE

Most of the cases have a smooth postoperative recovery; the ventilatory support is needed for only a short period (1-2 days). There is no need for postoperative TPN. Frequent pharyngeal suctions of saliva are necessary in the early postoperative period. In cases with the GT in the retrosternal position, suction is mandatory for 2-5 days; in the mediastinal position of GT there is often no need for pharyngeal suction. The mediastinal drain is removed in 2-5 days after 24 hours of "nothing coming out". Continuous enteral feeding is initiated through the gastrostomy tube as soon as the bowel movements return to normal. In cases with uneventful course, on day 7 postoperatively the permeability of the GT is checked with a colored cold drink which should flow easily and quickly through the gastrostomy tube. Liquid, then loose and finally soft diet is given progressively. Most of the cases, especially older children are able to eat normally 2-3 weeks postoperatively. The gastrostomy tube is still kept for 1-3 months for safety, in case of eventual stenosis of upper anastomoses.

For GTER performed in early infancy, on babies with serious co morbid problems, oral feeding could be delayed for weeks or months under intensive rehabilitation.

Postoperative dilatation: Yes or No

The GTER has only one important problem which is the risk of progressive narrowing of esophagus-gastric tube anastomoses. Routine postoperative dilatations are not recommended. A strict follow-up by clinical examination, contrast study (better video recorded) and endoscopy should be done monthly (for the first 6 months), for early detection of anastomotic stenosis which requires regular dilatations. In my series, 40% of cases had 1-6 dilatations. The wire guided dilatations are preferable to balloon dilatations which can cause more damage. A long-term follow-up is mandatory in all cases with esophageal replacement in childhood.

COMPLICATIONS OF GTER

Early Postoperative Complications

Except of a pneumothorax or serious bleeding which are immediately recognized and treated, there are several specific complications to GTER.

1. **Anastomotic breakdown or leaking anastomosis** is the most common complication of GTER. The frequency of this complication in large series goes from 66-13% (in author's series) with a mean of 50%.[19,22] The leaking anastomosis presents various degrees of severity, from a minor leak which closes spontaneously in 10-14 days without stenosis, to complete disruption of anastomoses due to limited ischemia of the GT. The fistula of upper anastomoses is significantly more frequent in cases of retrosternal position of the GT than for posterior mediastinal route. In the author's series of 107 cases of RGTER, 9/19 (37%) of cases performed through retrosternal route vs. 7/88 (6%) cases performed through mediastinal route developed a fistula.

   Most of the cases which develop an anastomotic leak would be candidates for stenosis; all these cases should be strictly followed and require esophageal dilatations. In a few cases a surgical revision of anastomosis was necessary (3 cases in author's series) (Fig. 33.20).

2. **Necrosis of gastric tube:** This is a very rare but possibly lethal complication. The cause is always vascular and in most of the cases is due to the stubborn decision of the surgeon to keep a GT which is blue and with poor bleeding when brought to the neck. The partial or total necrosis of the tube is an early complication and the only treatment is emergency resection of the necrotic graft. For the GT in the mediastinal position, severe mediastinitis is often the cause of death (one case in our series); for GT in the retrosternal position the complication is less serious. All attempts to save a compromised tube end up as a failure and delays the removal of the GT (one case in author's series). Removal of a necrotic graft will be followed by a new substitution, performed months later (colon or small bowel segment) with the graft placed retrosternally. The problems of failed esophagoplasty is the subject of several articles.[65,93]

3. **Mediastinitis without compromised graft:** This is a serious challenge of treatment and the true viability of the graft should be proved early by redo operation. Correct drainage, effective antibiotic-therapy, multiple support could not prevent a high mortality. The most common cause of mediastinitis is a leak from the long suture line; when performed with mechanical staplers the risk is even higher.

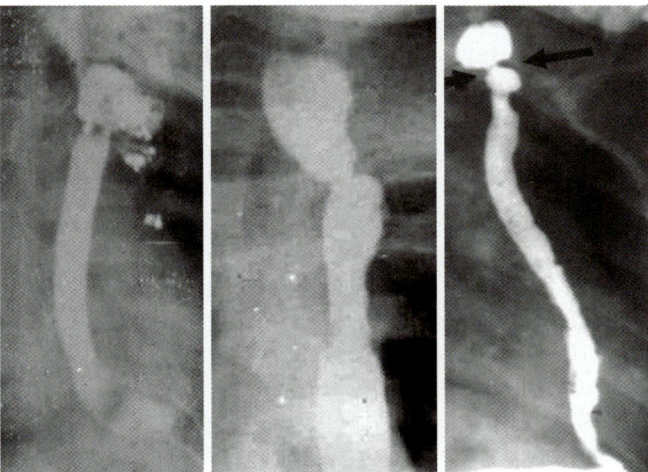

Fig. 33.20: Most common complications of gastric tube. Anastomotic fistula: spontaneous closure (left). Moderate stenosis: several dilatations are necessary (middle). Severe stricture of anastomoses: Short resection with a new anastomoses (right)

Late Complications of GTER

In the literature sporadic cases of rare complications are reported as: broncho-gastric tube fistula, stricture within the tube evolving to complete obstruction, perforation of acquired diverticulum, mucocele on the old esophagus left *in situ* (one case in our series), sporadic cases of peptic ulcer within the GT, majority successfully treated with modern antacid drugs.[18,22,36,89,91,94-97] Gastric reflux within the GT was noticed in many contrast studies but asymptomatic in most of the cases. The reality of the reflux has been demonstrated in author's series by 24 hr pH metry on the GT (10 cases all presenting different grade of reflux). In a few cases (3 cases in author's series) the reflux manifested at night, by unpleasant return in the mouth of gastric content or food. The semi-fowler position partially resolved the symptomatic reflux, which in all cases improved spontaneously over time. Perhaps there is an etiologic relation between the presence of chronic reflux and peptic ulcer within the GT.

H Lindahl and Bornon J have mentioned the presence of "Barrett's esophagus" in mucosal biopsies of the esophagus above the GT esophageal anastomosis.[80,91] If true, a high risk of malignancy is possible early in life.[98] In fact both authors have found gastric cells migrated within the esophagus which is not the known "Barrett's esophagus". In our series 32 patients had endoscopic examinations, with multiple biopsies and none presented with this abnormal histology.

Finally the most common complications of the GT are related to the esophagus-GT anastomoses: fistulae and stenosis. The role of accurate technique, well vascularised GT and utilization of mediatinal route, significantly diminished the rate of these complications (from 37-6% with a mean of 13% in author's series).

DISCUSSION

A comparison between the most popular techniques of esophageal substitution in children is not the purpose of the author. The author's personal experience of 28 years of esophageal replacement (1975-2003) includes: 107 gastric tubes and 6 colonic grafts (transverse and left colon, 2 retrosternally and 4 transmediastinal).

Brief presentation of personal experience. Indications for GTER: 21 cases EALG, 86 caustic strictures. Type I GTER: 19 cases (56): retrosternal route, no concomitant esophagectomy: Rate of fistulae 37% (7 cases). GT dilatation–3 cases; stricture–3 cases (Fig. 33.21).

Type II: 88 cases: posterior mediastinum, transhiatal esophagectomy, no pyloric surgery, mechanical suture 10 cases; rate of fistulae 6% (7 cases). All but 2 cases had reversed gastric tube esophageal replacement.

Comparing the 2 techniques, type II has shown significant advantages:
- Significant decrease of anastomotic fistulae;
- No GT dilatation;

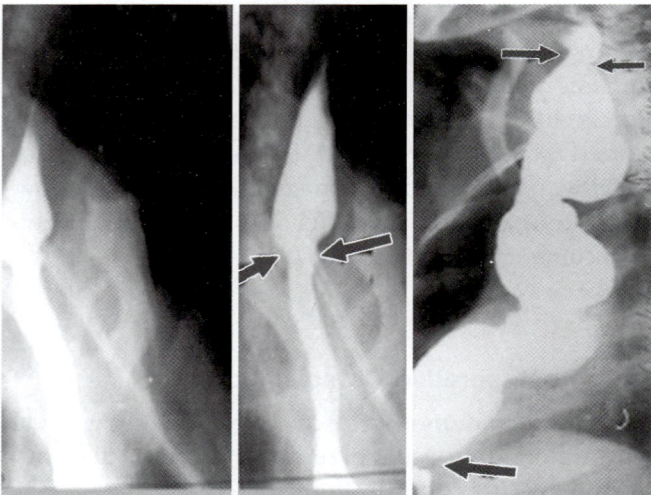

Fig. 33.21: Progressive dilatation of a GT in retrosternal position but without any clinical symptoms

- No stasis within the GT;
- Shorter GT;
- Easy access to postoperative endoscopy.

Most of the complications of the series were already presented. To summarize: gastric graft failure: 2 cases, one death. Anastomotic stricture 5 cases with surgical revision in 2 cases; postoperative bowel obstruction: 5 cases. Peptic ulcer: 2 cases, one Zollinger-Ellison syndrome.

Mortality in the whole series: 7 cases (6.5%) but 5 cases were before 1982 and unrelated with the technique (poor postoperative ventilatory support– 4 cases) and 1 case sudden infant death syndrome. Two deaths were related to GTER: necrosis of the graft 1 and mediastinitus 1. The series has a very good follow-up: 88 patients have been reviewed periodically in 1991, 1996, 2001 and 2003. In 2007, 35 cases of adults with GTER done in childhood were assessed for quality of life.[99] Majority of them have a normal professional, social and familial life; 8 of the work outside of their native country.

In long-term follow-up sophisticated methods of evaluation could be used, but finally a good history, clinical examination, contrast study and eventually endoscopy allows an objective assessment of patients.

An encouraging fact is that after 6-8 months postoperatively, the GT no longer changes its anatomy as for the colon substitution (redundancy, stasis of the graft, dilatation with enormous loops). An interesting

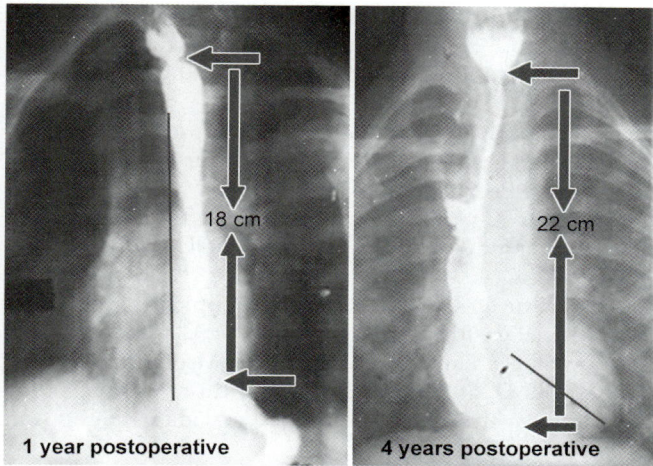

Fig. 33.22: Growth or lengthening? The gastric tube adapts harmoniously to the body growth

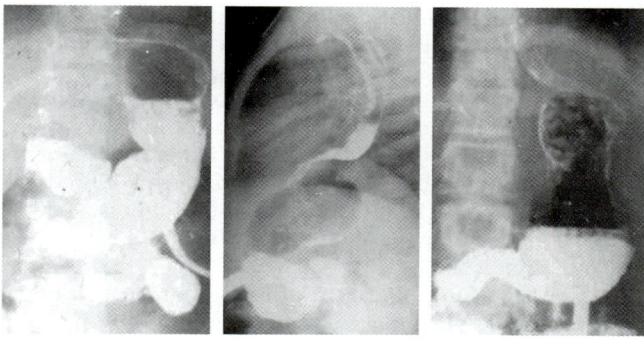

Fig. 33.23: GTER fully preserves the capacity and function of the stomach. The volume of the stomach preoperative (left). Lateral view of the RGTER (middle). The stomach after RGTER (right)

aspect of GTER was the lengthening or "growing" of the tube through teenage and adolescent period: GT "grows" harmoniously with the body growth, about 1 cm per year for both segments thoracic and intra-abdominal (Fig. 33.22).

The advantages of the gastric tube esophageal replacement and esophagectomy in one stage operation, without thoracotomy can be summarized:
1. The gastric tube has an excellent blood supply.
2. The gastric tube presents a very low septic risk due to acid secretion.
3. The gastric tube in most of the cases is an easy operation if performed by an experienced surgeon and utilization of staplers.
4. The gastric reservoir as well as the gastric and pyloric function is fully preserved; this advantage is most probably a crucial advantage of GT and the colonic graft substitution.
5. Performed by an experienced team, in a well equipped tertiary hospital, the operation has a very low rate of morbidity and mortality (Fig. 33.23)

Several critics are formulated for the GT:
1. After GTER the stomach is small and lacks capacity.
2. GTER could have as side effect a megoblastic anemia resistant to treatment.
3. In a few cases "Barrett's esophagus" has been demonstrated within the cervical esophagus with a theoretic risk of malignancy.
4. Some patients complain of "vagotomy-like" symptoms or real dumping syndrome.

In fact most of the disadvantages of GTER were already commented and none were really identified in our series. Complaints of dumping syndrome are mostly related with the isoperistaltic GT.

There is only one problem with the GTER and that is the esophageal anastomoses. With a meticulous good technique, strict follow-up in the early postoperative period, eventually several dilatations, the problem related to the upper anastomoses can be well controlled.

Although a rare operation in childhood, esophageal replacement represents a major procedure which requires expertise, experience, modern technology and a multidisciplinary team at a specialized center. Total gastric transposition is a very safe procedure, very popular in most of the countries but with major long term negative side effects due to complete or partial suppression of the gastric reservoir. The colonic replacement and gastric tube are the only 2 procedures recommended in childhood for preserving the gastric reservoir with all its physiological functions, crucial for further growth.

REFERENCES

1. Orsoni P. Oesophagoplastie. Libraries Malone SA, Paris, 1969.
2. O'Neill Jr JA, Rowe MI, Grosfeld JL, et al. Pediatric Surgery. (5th ed.), Mosby, 1998.
3. Ashcraft KW. Pediatric Surgery. 3rd ed, WB Saunders Comp, 2000.
4. McCollum MO, Rangel SJ, Blair GK, et al. Primary reversed gastric tube reconstruction in long gap esophageal atresia. J Pediatr Surg 2003;38:957-62.

5. Othersen Jr HB, Parker EF, Chandler J, et al. Save the child's esophagus, Part II: colic patch repair. J Pediatr Surg 1997;32:328-33.
6. Hecker W, Hollman G. Correction of long segment esophageal stenoses by a colonic patch. In Rickham PP, Hecker WC, Prevot J (Eds): Progress in Pediatric Surgery, Vol 8, Baltimore, MD, University Park Press 1975;81-85.
7. Spicer RD, Cusick EL. Oesophageal substitution by jejunal free graft: follow-up data and evaluation. Pediatr Surg Int 1996;11:227-29.
8. Chen HC, Tang YB. Microsurgical reconstruction of the esophagus. Semin Surg Oncol, 2000;19:235-45.
9. Cauchi JA, Buick RG, Gornall P, et al. Oesophageal substitution with free and pedicled jejunum: short- and long-term outcomes. Pediatr Surg Int 2007;23:11-19.
10. Prevot J, Lepelley M, Schmitt M. Small bowel esophagoplasty with vascular microanastomoses in the neck for treatment of esophageal burns in childhood. Prog Pediatr Surg 1985;18:108-17.
11. Bax NM, Van Renterghem KM. Ileal pedicle grafting for esophageal replacement in children. Pediatr Surg Int 2005;21:369-72.
12. Heji H, Aronson DC. Long gap esophageal atresia–is jejunal interposition the answer? Long gap esophageal atresia symposium, Mannheim, Germany 2007.
13. Aronson DC. Adults with corrected oesophageal atresia. Long gap esophageal atresia symposium, Mannheim, Germany 2007.
14. Ein SH, Shandling B, Simpson JS, et al. A further look at gastric tube as an esophageal replacement in infants and children. J Pediatr Surg 1973;8:859-68.
15. Ein SH, Shandling B, Simpson JS, et al. Fourteen years of gastric tube. J Pediatr Surg 1978;13:638-42.
16. Wolfstein L, Rabau MY, Avigad I, et al. Esophageal replacement in children: 10 years' experience. Isr J Med Sci 1979;15:742-45.
17. Goon HK, Cohen DH, Middleton AW. Gastric tube oesophagoplasty–a long-term assessment. Z Kinderchir 1985;40:21-25.
18. West KW, Vane DW, Grosfeld JL. Esophageal replacement in children: experience with thirty-one cases. Surgery 1986;100:751-57.
19. Ein SH, Shandling B, Stephens CA. Twenty-one years experience with the pediatric gastric tube. J Pedistr Surg 1987;22:77-81.
20. Ure BM, Slany E, Eypasch EP, et al. Long-term functional results and quality of life after colon interposition for long gap oesophageal atresia. Eur J Pediatr Surg 1995;5:206-10.
21. Ein SH. Gastric tubes in children with caustic injury: a 32-year review. J Pediatr Surg 1998;33:1393-95.
22. Schettini ST, Pinus J. Gastric-tube esophagoplasty in children. Pediatr Surg Int 1998;14:144-50.
23. Avila LF, Encinas JL, Andres AM, et al. Esophageal replacement. 12 years experience. Cir Pediatr 2006;19:217-22.
24. Ionescu G. Gastric tube esophageal replacement in children: a 28 years experience with 107 cases. Long gap esophageal atresia symposium, Mannheim, Germany, 2007.
25. Davenport M, Hosie GP, Tasker RC, et al. Long-term effects of gastric transposition in children: a physiological study. J Pediatr Surg 1996;31:588-93.
26. Ludman L, Spitz L. Quality of life after gastric transposition for oesophageal atresia J Pediatr Surg 2003; 38: 53-57.
27. Gavriliu D, Georgescu L. Esofagoplastie directa cu material gastric. Rev Stiint Med 1951;3:33-36.
28. Gavriliu D. Chirurgia esofagului. Ed Med Bucharest 1957.
29. Gavrilu D. Etat actuel du procede du reconstruction de l'esophage par gastric tube (138 maladaes opere). Ann Chir 1965;19:219-24.
30. Heimlich HJ. Esophageal replacement with a reversed gastric tube. Dis Chest 1959;36:478-93.
31. Jianu A. Gastrostomie und osophagoplastik. Dtsch Z Chir 1912;118:383-90.
32. Orringer MB, Sloan H. Oesophagiectomy without thoracotomy. J Thorac Cardiovasc Surg 1978;76:643-54.
33. Rodgers BM, Ryckman FC, Talbert JL. Blunt transmediatinal total esophagiectomy with simultaneous substernal colon interposition for oesophageal caustic strictures in children. J Pediatr Surg. 1981;16:184-89.
34. Kunath U. Blunt dissection of the esophagus. Chirurg 1980;51:296-302.
35. Adegboye VO, Brimmo A, Adebo OA. Transhiatal esophagectomy in children with corrosive esophageal stricture. Afr L Med Med Sci 2000;29:223-26.
36. Ionescu GO, Tuleasca I. Une nouvelle technique d'oesophagoplasie par tube gastrique chez l'enfant. Chir Pediatr 1985;26:328-30.
37. Burrington JD, Stephens CA. Esophageal replacement with a gastric tube in infants and children. J Pediatr Surg 1968;3:24-52.
38. Pedersen JC, Klein RL, Andrews DA. Gastric tube as the primary procedure for pure esophageal atresia. J Pediatr Surg 1996;31:1233-35.
39. Di Benedetto V, Dessanti A. Experimental technique of esophageal substitution: intrathoracic interposition of a pedunculated gastric tube (PGT) preserving cardiac function. Preliminary results. Hepatogastroenterology 1998;45:2202-05.
40. Samuel M, Burge DM, Moore IE. Gastric tube graft interposition as an oesophageal substitute. ANZ J Surg 2001;71:56-61.
41. Gounot E, Borgnon J, Huet F, et al. Isolated isoperistaltic tube interposition for esophageal replacement in children. J Pediatr Surg 2006;41:592-95.
42. Schilling MK, Mettler D, Redaelli C, et al. Circulatory and anatomic differences among experimental gastric tubes as esophageal replacement. World J Surg 1997;21:992-97.

43. Gastric microcirculatory changes during gastric tube formation: assessment with laser Doppler flowmetry. J Surg Res 1996;62:125-29.
44. Nishikawa K, Matsudaira H, Suzuki H, et al. Intraoperative thermal imaging in esophageal replacement: its use in the assessment of gastric tube viability. Surg Today 2006;36:802-06.
45. Lazar G, Kaszaki J, Abraham S, et al. Thoracic epidural anesthesia improves the gastric microcirculation during experimental gastric tube formation. Surgery 2003; 134:799-805.
46. Ul-Haq A, Tareen F, Bader I, et al. Oesophageal replacement in children with indolent stricture of the oesophagus. Asian J Surg 2006;29:17-21.
47. Tanaka K, Kurobe M, Kanai M, et al. Esophageal replacement using reversed gastric tube for lye stricture in a child: report of a case. Surg Today 2004;34:868-70.
48. Aprodu SG, Gavrilescu S, Savu B, et al: Indications for esophageal replacement in children. Rev Med Chir Soc Med Nat Iasi 2004;108:805-08.
49. Helardot P. Caustic burns of the esophagus, esophagectomy and replacement with gastric tube: comparative study with other procedures. Saudi Med 2003;24:S39.
50. Panieri E, Rode H, Millar AJW, et al. Esophageal replacement in the management of corrosive stricture: when is surgery indicated? Pediatr Surg Int 1998;3: 336-40.
51. Panieri E, Millar AJW, Rode H, et al. Iatrogenic esophageal perforation in children: patterns of injury, presentation, management and outcome. J Pediatr Surg 1996;31: 890-95.
52. Stringer MD: Oesophageal substitution. Editorial comment. Pediatr Surg Int 1996;11:213.
53. Badnassy AF, Bassiouny IE. Esophagocoloplasty for caustic stricture of the esophagus: changing concepts. Pediatr Surg Int. 1993;8:103-08.
54. Pintus C, Manzoni C, Nappo S, et al. Cuastic ingestion in childhood: current treatment possibilities and their complications. Pediatr Surg Int. 1993;8:109-12.
55. Bautista A, Varela R, Villanueva A, Estevez E, TojoR, Cadranel S. Effects of prednisolone and dexamethasone in children with alkali burns of the oesophagus. Eur J pediatric surg 1996;6:198-203.
56. Mutaf O. Esophagoplsty for caustic esophageal burns in children. Pediatr Surg Int 1992;7:106-08.
57. Rappert P, Preier L, Korab W, et al. Diagnostic and therapeutic management of esophageal and gastric burns in childhood. Eur J Pediatr Surg 1993;3:202-05.
58. Ionescu GO, Tuleasca I, Ioan F, et al. L'oesophagoplastie par tube gastrique chez l'enfant. Chir Pediatr 1979;20: 47-51.
59. Khan KM, Foker LE. Use of high-resolution endoscopic ultrasonography to examine the effect of tension on the esophagus during primary repair of long gap esophageal atresia. Pediatr Radiol 2007;37:41-45.
60. Khan KM, Sabati AA, Kendall T, et al. The effect of traction on esophageal structure in children with long-gap esophageal atresia. Dig Dis Sci 2006;51:1917-21.
61. Lopes MF, Reis A, Coutinho S, et al. Very long gap esophageal atresia successfully treated by esophageal lengthening using external traction sutures. J Pediatr Surg 2004;39:1286-87.
62. Foker JE, Linden BC, Boyle EM, et al. Development of a true primary repair for the full spectrum of esophageal atresia. Ann Surg 1997;226:533-41.
63. Okada T, Ohnuma N, Tanabe M, et al. Effective endless-loop bougienage through the oral cavity and esophagus to the gastrostomy in corrosive esophageal strictures in children. Pediatr Surg Int 1998;13:480-86.
64. Harmel RP: Esophageal replacement in two siblings with epidermolysis bullosa. J Pediatr Surg 1986;21:175-76.
65. Dunn JC, Fonkalsrud EW, Applebaum H, et al. Reoperation after esophageal replacement in childhood. J Pediatr Surg 1999;34:1630-32.
66. Pianzola HM, Otino A, Canestri M. Cystic duplication of the esophagus. Acta Gastroenterol Latinoam 2001;31: 333-38.
67. Diaz M, Leal N, Olivares P, et al. Infectious strictures requiring esophageal replacement in children. J Pediatr Gastroenterol Nutr 2001;32:611-13.
68. Sanders GB. Esophageal replacement with reversed gastric tube. Utilisation for bleeding esophageal varices in a four-year-old child. JAMA 1962;181:944-47.
69. Rescorla FJ, West KW, Scherer LR, et al. The complex nature of type A (long-gap) esophageal atresia. Surgery 1994;116:658-64.
70. Lindahl H, Louhimo I, Virkola K. Colon interposition or gastric tube? Follow-up study of colon-esophagus and gastric tube-esophagus patients. J Pediatr Surg 1983;18: 58-63.
71. Aprodu G, Botez C, Munteanu V. Esophagoplasty for esophageal stenosis due to caustic injuries in children: personal experience. J Pediatr Surg Spec 2007;1:12-16.
72. Collard JM, Tinton N, Malaise J, et al. Esophageal replacement: gastric tube or whole stomach? Ann Thorac Surg 1995;60:261-66.
73. Tannuri U, Maksoud-Filho JG, Tannuri AC, et al. Which is better for esophageal substitution in children, esophagocoloplasty or gastric transposition? A 27-year experience of a single center. J Pediatr Surg 2007;42:500-40.
74. Dickson JAS: Esophageal substitution with colon–the Waterston operation. Pediatr Surg Int 1996;11:224-26.
75. Ahmad SA, Sylvester KG, Hebra A, et al. Esophageal replacement using the colon: is it a good choice? J Pediatr Surg 1996;31:1026-31.
76. Reinberg O, Genton N. Esophageal replacement in children: evaluation of the one-stage procedure with colic transplants. Eur J Pediatr Surg 1997;7:216-20.
77. Khan AR, Stiff G, Mohammed AR, et al. Esophageal replacement with colon in children. Pediatr Surg Int 1998;13:79-83.
78. Domini R, Appignani A, Baccarini E, et al. A case of non-functioning antiperistaltic retrosternal colic conduit replaced in situ and substituted with an isoperistaltic segment of ileum-caecum. Eur J Pediatr Surg 1997;7: 301-02.

79. Anderson KD, Randolph JG. The gastric tube for esophageal replacement in children. J Thorac Cardiovasc Surg 1973;66:333-42.
80. Lindahl H, Rintala R., Louhimo I. Results of gastric tube esophagoplasty in esophageal atresia. Pediatr Surg Int 1987;2:282-86.
81. Randolph JG. The reversed gastric tube for esophageal replacement in children. Pediatr Surg Int 1996;11:221-23.
82. Spitz L. Gastric transposition for esophageal replacement. Pediatr Surg Int 1996;11:218-20.
83. Gupta DK, Kataria R, Bajpai M. Gastric transposition for esophageal replacement in children–an Indian experience. Eur J Pediatr Surg 1997;7:143-46.
84. Gupta DK. Primary and secondary esophageal replacement by gastric pull-up, experience over 27 years. Long gap esophageal atresia symposium. Mannheim, Germany, 2007.
85. Scharli AF. Esophageal reconstruction in very long atresias by elongation of lesser curvature. Petiatr Surg Int 1992;7:101-5.
86. Scharli AF. Esophageal reconstruction by elongation of the lesser gastric curvature. Pediatr Surg Int 1996;11:214-17.
87. Barbera L, Kemen M, Wegener M, et al. Effect of site and width of the stomach tube after esophageal resection on gastric emptying. Zentralbl Chir 1994;119:240-44.
88. Schettini ST, Ganc A, Saba L. Esophageal carcinoma secondary to a chemical injury in a child. Pediatr Surg Int 1998;13:519-20.
89. Kamath MV, Ellison RG, Rubin JW, et al. Esophageal mucocelle: a complication of blind loop esophagus. Ann Thocar Surg 1987;43:263-69.
90. Lindecken KD, Kunath U, Janson R. Esophageal replacement by an isiperistaltic gastric tube. Langenbecks Arch Chir 1981;354:265-71.
91. Borgnon J, Tounian P, Auber F, et al. Esophageal replacement in children by an isoperistaltic gastric tube: a 12-year experience. Pediatr Surg Int 2004;20:829-33.
92. Choi RS, Lillehei CW, Lund DP, et al. Esophageal replacement in children who have pharyngoesophageal strictures. J Pediatr Surg 1997;32:1083-87.
93. Andres MA, Burgos AL, Encinas JL, et al. What can we do when an esophagocoloplasty fails? Cir Pediatr 2007; 20:39-43.
94. Stringer DA, Pablot SM. Broncho-gastric tube fistula as a complication of esophageal replacement. J Can Assoc Radiol 1985;36:61-62.
95. Sitges AC, Sanchez-Ortega JM, Sitges AS. Late complications of reversed gastric tube oesoplagoplasty. Thorax 1986;41:61-65.
96. Anderson KD. Gastric tube esophagoplasty. Progr Pediatr Surg 1986;19:55-61.
97. Uchida Y, Tomonari K, Murakami S, et al. Occurrence of peptic ulcer in the gastric tube used for esophageal replacement in adults. Jpn J Surg 1987;17:190-94.
98. Tytgat GNJ, Hammeeteman W. The neoplastic potential of columnar-lined (Barrett's) esophagus. World J Surg 1992;16:308-12.
99. Ionescu GO, Aprodu G, Gavrilescu S. Pediatric gastric tube esophageal replacement: long term results. An adulthood perspective. 2nd World Congress, WCPSA, Buenos Aires, Argentina, 2007.

CHAPTER 34

Gastric Transposition

DK Gupta, Shilpa Sharma

There is no ideal substitute available till date to replace the esophagus. However, the choice revolves around the one which is simple and safe to perform and conforms to the function and anatomy to match the original esophagus. The child should have the ability to swallow and enjoy the taste of the normal food. The operative procedure should have minimal or no short and long-term postoperative complications. In addition, the children should continue enjoying the same for long in their life ahead.

The indications and routes for esophageal replacement have been discussed in the previous chapter of "Esophageal replacement with colon interposition". This chapter entails to gastric transposition.

WHY STOMACH?

Gastric transposition was first done in children only about 3 decades back. Though, organ most commonly used to replace the esophagus in the past has been colon, stomach has been used as gastric pull up in adults with carcinoma esophagus with satisfactory results. The colon interposition was also associated with many complications; like redundancy, reflux, stricture and the graft loss, albeit rarely. This has compelled the surgeons to find an alternate procedure. While colon graft maintained a reasonably good vascular supply on its vascular pedicle, however, the problem was faced if the colon was either not available (polyposis coli, pouch colon, ulcerative colitis) or its vascular arcade was not found satisfactory. Gastric transposition is however, not favored in patients with high pharyngeal strictures.

The authors developed interest in this technique during the past 15 years or so, after having an unpleasant experience with the use of colon in one of their patients who lost graft in the immediate postoperative period. Though, this could actually be considered due to the technical fault as the colon graft had been taken and interposed under tension. This single disaster in our series, prompted us to consider using stomach for the purpose of esophageal replacement. Similarly, the authors had been routinely using the antiperistaltic gastric tube (based on fundus) in children with corrosive injuries. However, the mediastinal leak and the osteomyelitis of the sternum that had followed, from the leak from the suture line of the gastric tube in one of the patients, was very discouraging. Thus, the need for the use of stomach as an alternate to the established procedures of colon interposition and the gastric tube.

The procedure was first performed in few children and our initial results were published in 1997.[1] Subsequently, impressed with the outcome and the ease of the procedure of gastric transposition, the scope and the indications were expanded even in the newborns. Our recent experience with the use of stomach to replace the esophagus not only in children but also in the newborns was published in 2003 and 2007 as an alternative procedure to the colon interposition.[2,3]

Stomach was considered as the best option available in the newborns requiring esophageal replacement. This was because the vascular supply to the colon and the jejunum is very precarious. This not only limits the length of colonic and jejunal segment to reach the neck without tension, but also remained quite risky to use these segments in the neonatal period, specially if there had been major esophageal anastomotic leaks with ongoing infection in the mediastinal region. Also, the size of the stomach in newborns and the infants less than 6 months of age, is too small and unfit for preparing the gastric tube. Moreover, the blood supply to the stomach is rich. The gastric wall is also quite muscular to withstand the mediastinal infection if any. Thus, gastric transposition was considered and it remained the only option to replace the esophagus in the neonatal period. It was tried and also found quite feasible in the newborns who required esophageal replacement following postoperative major leaks and also with the long or wide gap esophageal atresia and tracheoesophageal fistula (EA/TEF) in our set up.[2-4]

Recently, there has been an interest seen with the use of stomach to replace the esophagus. Thus, many surgeons switched over from using colon interpositions to gastric transpositions for esophageal replacement in children.[5,6]

The gastric tube has been preferred by others. However, though the gastric tube has a thick muscular wall and a reliable vascular supply, it has a long suture line and any leak from it may prove very serious. Each procedure for esophageal replacement has its merits and demerits and the choice should be that with which the surgeon is most familiar and most appropriate for age and the indication.[7]

The esophageal lengthening procedures using Scharli's technique of the division of the stomach on the lesser curvature, in which the upper part of the stomach remained in the chest while the lower half remained in the abdomen, has still not become popular. The procedure is associated with high rate of complications like ischemia, leak and even the graft loss.[8,9] The procedure is also considered unphysiological as part of the stomach in the chest and part of in the abdomen, results in paradoxical inflation of the thoracic stomach with the each act of inspiration.[4] The placement of the esophagogastric suture line in the chest may also be risky and any postoperative leak might prove disastrous.

The credit for popularising gastric transposition as the primary procedure for replacing the esophagus goes to Prof. Lewis Spitz, from Institute of Child Health, Great Ormond Street, London, who after noting the unacceptably high complication rate with the use of colon interposition in children, started using stomach, since then, many series have appeared reporting satisfactory and early and long-term results in the newborns, infants and children.[1-4,6,10-16]

AGE FOR GASTRIC TRANSPOSITION

Traditionally, replacement of the esophagus is performed when the child can sit and eat by him/herself. However, with due precaution, the replacement can be done at any time if the condition so demands. Gastric transposition is now generally carried out by most surgeons at around 6-12 months of age, but can be performed even in the newborn period or anytime thereafter when the baby is fit for tolerating the major surgical procedure and the anesthesia. The procedure has been done successfully in childhood and the long-term results including the complications are available.[16,17]

Major postoperative leak following EATEF repair has been correlated with the increased mortality and morbidity in neonates.[18] Colon and jejunum should not be preferred due to delicate arcades. Gastric tube can not be fashioned as the size of the stomach is too tiny. Moreover, the stomach is much smaller in newborns with EA to be housed very well in the mediastinum. However, the smaller sized stomach in EA has never posed a problem for a primary anastomosis to be performed with the esophagus in the neck. The important factor being that in the neonatal stage, the tunnel in the posterior mediastinum is created very easily as compared to that in older children with previous history of thoracotomy and mediastinal leaks. Thus, neonatal gastric transposition has been recognized as the only option of saving the lives of these patients as it can even be performed in the presence of pyothorax and septicemia following the major anastomotic leaks.[1] The advantages of performing the gastric pullup in the newborns are that the procedure of gastric transposition takes only a little more time than performing the diversion procedures (esophagostomy and gastrostomy) in the newborn period. The blood loss is also minimal (10-30 ml only) and the operating time is not much (less than 2 hours). Needless to emphasize that it required expertise and the dependable intensive care facilities for postoperative monitoring, prolonged ventilation, offering the antibiotics, pain relief and central venous access for long-term nutritional support.

ADVANTAGES OF GASTRIC TRANSPOSITION FOR ESOPHAGEAL REPLACEMENT

1. It is a technically easier procedure.
2. The stomach has a thick muscle wall and maintains reliable vascular supply.
3. Adequate length is possible for anastomosis without tension.
4. The fundus being the highest point can reach for the anastomosis in the neck.
5. A single anastomosis is required in the neck.
6. No thoracotomy is required.
7. There is no suture line in the chest, except for the closure of the esophagostomy site and possibly the gastrostomy site also (if the same had been done in the past).
8. It is also an option in patients with pouch colon or where it is risky to use the colon due to precarious blood supply.
9. The gastric transposition procedure has the least short-term morbidity and mortality as compared to the other alternative procedures.

Advantages of Neonatal Gastric Transposition

1. It is the best option available for newborns. Colon and jejunum should not be used due the precarious blood supply especially in the presence of sepsis or pyothorax due to salivary leaks.
2. It avoids the need for a diversion in the neonatal period with the known morbididty and even mortality associated with gastrostomy and esophagostomy.
3. There is no suture line in thorax thus free from the risks of a leak in the chest.
4. Neonatal gastric pullup can be performed even in the presence of sepsis as the stomach being very vascular and muscular, can withstand the sepsis and the local salivary leaks well.
5. This offers the definitive surgery at birth itself and avoids repeated visits to the hospital.
6. Gastric pullup can be performed even in emergency without the need for any preparation.
7. The success rate is quite high even in very sick newborns.

DISADVANTAGES OF GASTRIC TRANSPOSITION

1. Bulk of stomach in mediastinum/thorax can cause respiratory distress and may decrease venous return. It seemed more theoretical rather than seen in practice.
2. Reflux in the bulky stomach is common and can cause aspiration pneumonitis.
3. As vagotomy is part and partial with the procedure, gastric emptying may be delayed despite pyloromyotomy.
4. As the reservoir function of the stomach is lost, there may also be rapid gastric emptying leading to dumping.
5. The loss of gastric reservoir function also effects the growth and development of the patient.

ROUTE FOR TRANSPOSITION

1. Transhiatal route is feasible in most children. It is feasible even in the newborns as there are no mediastinal adhesions in the newborn period. Moreover, the stomach is very small and transhiatal route is quite short.
2. Substernal route is preferred after infancy, though this is little longer than the mediastinal route. Care should also be taken not to prefer this route if liver is large likely to obstruct the stomach during its course.

GASTRIC TRANSPOSITION— SURGICAL PROCEDURE

It may be done as a staged procedure following the initial diversion (with cervical esophagostomy and gastrostomy) that had been done or also as a primary procedure in cases with complicated EA/TEF group (long gap EA without fistula, wide gap EA/TEF not amenable for primary anastomosis and following the major anastomotic leaks after primary anastomosis, if the same is not manageable with other popular methods). The procedure of gastric transposition can be performed either in routine or even in emergency. It does not require any preoperative preparation unlike the colon.

Staged Procedure

With the gastric transposition or even gastric tube in mind in future, the gastrostomy should be sited at the anterior stomach surface well away from the greater curvature with the aim to preserve the gastroepiploic arcade. Sham feeding should be encouraged to develop taste for sweet and sour and also to avoid feeding problems later on.

Operative Technique

The patient in the supine, a folded towel is placed under the shoulders of the patient to extend the neck and expose the esophagostomy site (Fig. 34.1). The cervical esophagostomy is mobilized placing an elliptical incision around it in the neck, detaching it carefully from the sternocleidomastoid muscle. Care is also taken not to injure the esophagus wall and preserve the recurrent laryngeal nerve during its mobilization. Esophagus is mobilized for 2-3 cm and the terminal few mm of its wall are freshened to resect the skin edges. The blood supply to this part of the esophagus is submucosal and does not pose any ischemic threat even after its extensive mobilization in the neck.

An adequate space is created at thoracic inlet with sharp and blunt dissection which would accommodate the fundus of the stomach easily. Cervical facia and sternohyoid muscles may have to be detached from their bony attachments with the manubrium or the clavicle to create enough space at the thoracic inlet. In the authors view, this is one of the most important aspects of the successful surgery to avoid any vascular compression on the major vessels once the stomach is pulled up and housed in the neck.

The abdomen is opened with a supraumbilical midline incision that may extend upto few cms below the umbilicus if the need be. The gastrostomy, if present, is taken down. Invariably, there are dense adhesions between the stomach and the liver. These are separated carefully with sharp and blunt dissection. The left lobe of the liver is freed from its attachment with the left hemidiaphragm, folded on itself and retracted to the right side by an assistant. An access is gained to the gastroesophageal junction. The peritoneum is incised transversely in front of the abdominal esophagus and the lower esophageal segment is freed from all around. With a ribbon tape around the gastroesophageal junction, the esophagus is mobilized. It comes out easily without any blood loss and is usually 3-5 cm long (Fig. 34.2). Both, the anterior and the posterior vagus nerves have to be invariably sacrificed while delivering the esophagus in the abdomen.

The operative steps have been shown in Figures 34.3A to F.

The stomach is mobilized, starting through the gastrocolic ligament. The right gastroepiploic vessel, the gastroepiploic arcade and the right gastric vessels are preserved. The 4-5 short gastric vessels running between the stomach and the spleen are either cauterized or ligated. Authors prefer to ligate these individually to avoid any vessel spasm or even thrombosis. With the use of the diathermy while handling these vessels, the authors have noted that

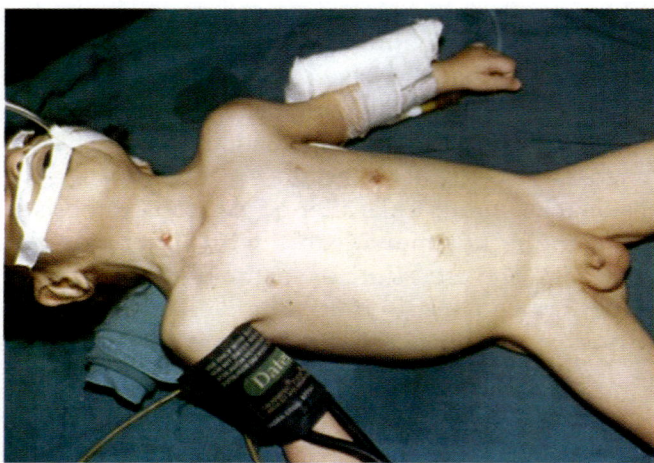

Fig. 34.1: A follow-up case of esophageal atresia, now 1 year of age. The esophagostomy and gastrostomy had been performed in the neonatal period

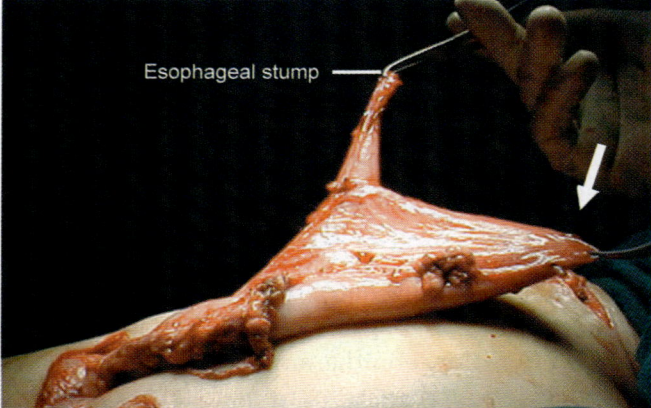

Fig. 34.2: The mobilized stomach with the gastrostomy site. Fundus is shown with a white arrow marking the highest point for anastomosis in the neck. The lower esophageal stump held in the artery clamp, is excised at gastroesophageal junction and sutured in two layers

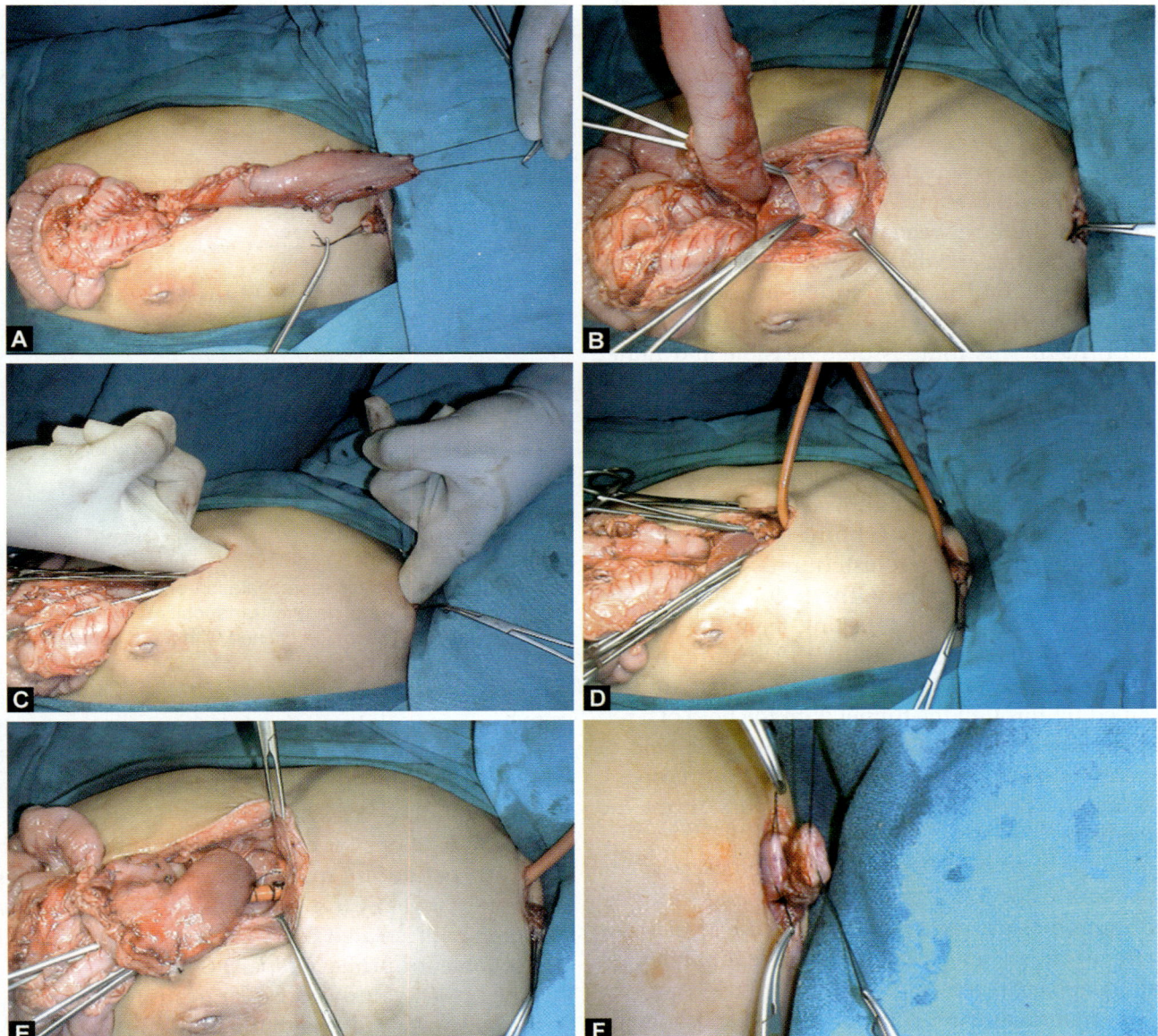

Figs 34.3A to F: Operative steps, **A.** Mobilized stomach placed over chest. **B.** The tunnel is created between the peritoneum and the linea alba, **C.** Finger dissection is being used to create the retrosternal space, **D.** Red rubber catheter is passed through the space, **E.** The lower end of the red rubber catheter is fixed to the fundus of the stomach, **F.** The upper end of the esophagus and the fundus of the stomach are seen through the neck incision, held between the stay sutures. A single layer esophagogastric anastomosis is made in the neck with interrupted sutures

the upper half of the stomach becomes bluish, flaby with comparatively ischemia, possibly due to vascular spasms, hence it is better to avoid the use of diathermy.

The stomach is now pulled toward the left and the left gastric vessels are identified and ligated securely close to their origin. Kocherization of the second part of duodenum is performed to gain length and bring the duodenum and the pylorus in a straight line. Spleen is preserved in all.

The esophageal stump is transected from its junction with the stomach and the defect is closed in 2 layers. The site of the gastrostomy is also closed in two layers. Two stay sutures are applied in the highest point in the stomach, e.g. the fundus, for taking the same up in the neck for the anastomosis

Attention is now given to choose the route. If the mediastinal route is to be used, the feasibility is checked. The esophageal hiatus is stretched and the tunnel is created blindly with the finger in the mediastinal route between the membranous posterior wall of the trachea and the prevertebral facia, reaching upto the neck, and making sure it is adequate and without any obstruction in its path. No thoracotomy is performed. This route is quite feasible and rather preferred in all neonates. If the creation of the tunnel is found difficult due to previous thoracotomy adhesions, the attempt is abandoned and the substernal route is favored. In that case, the hiatus will be closed with a figure 8 suture. The substernal route can be created easily by a blunt finger dissection starting just behind the xiphisternum.

Pyloromyotomy, (rarely, the pyloroplasty if the need be) for about 2 cm, starting from the normal stomach to just proximal to the duodenum is performed as a drainage procedure. Then the stomach is pulled up through the tunnel with the help of a red rubber catheter fixed to the fundus with the help of silk stay sutures marked on right and left corners, ensuring that no torsion of stomach occurs during the procedure.

A single layer esophagogastric anastomosis is made in the neck using 5/0 absorbable interrupted sutures. The anastomosis is constructed above the level of the aortic arch so as to decrease the chances of gastroesophageal reflux.

The pyloric antrum is fixed to the diaphragmatic edges at the hiatus (Fig. 34.4). The stomach is also hitched to the prevertebral fascia to prevent any tension on the anastomosis. A soft glove drain is used to drain the neck wound. The stomach is decompressed with a nasogastric tube the tip of which is carefully placed in the midthoracic region.

A feeding jejunostomy is optional and is reserved for critically ill patients who might take longer time to recover from surgery and require nutritional support. This may also be added later on if the need is felt in the postoperative period due to delay in the institution of normal feeds. Total parenteral nutrition

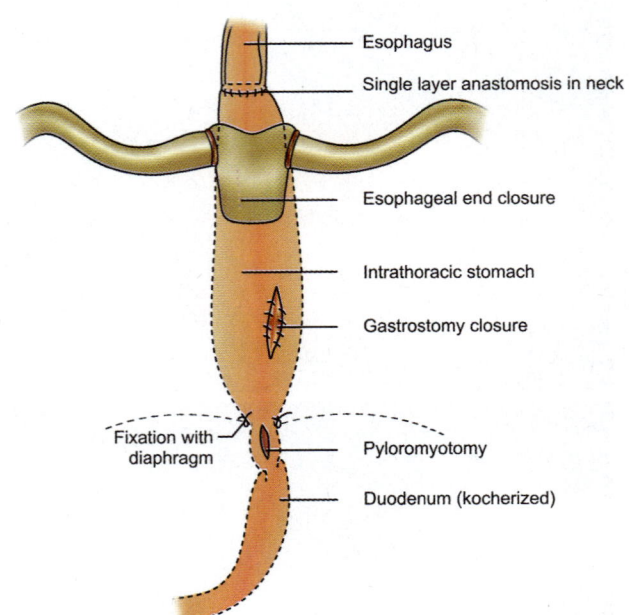

Fig. 34.4: Diagrammatic representation of the final position of the stomach following gastric transposition for esophageal replacement. The pylorus is hitched with the diaphragm

(TPN) is a good alternative but for short-term only. The TPN related cost and the risk of infection, both need serious considerations, especially in developing world providing free services.

The indications for esophageal replacement in the newborn period are mainly due to the complicated cases of EA and TEF (e.g. major leak to avoid diversion, long gap with isolated EA or cases with the wide TEF, not suitable for primary repair) (Fig. 34.5).

The operative procedure for gastric transposition in the newborns are essentially the same (Figs 34.6A - E). However, it requires safe anesthesia for the sick newborns, a close monitoring of vital signs including the insertion of a CVP line. Postoperative elective ventilation is mandatory at least for first few days after surgery. This provides effective oxygenation and stabilizes the patients comfortably. Patients should preferably have an epidural catheter for the morphine infusions for the pain relief. Plasma (and or blood) infusions should be transfused in the first few days to maintain hemodynamic stability and tissue perfusion. A urinary catheter for assessing the urine output is essential.

Gastric Transposition

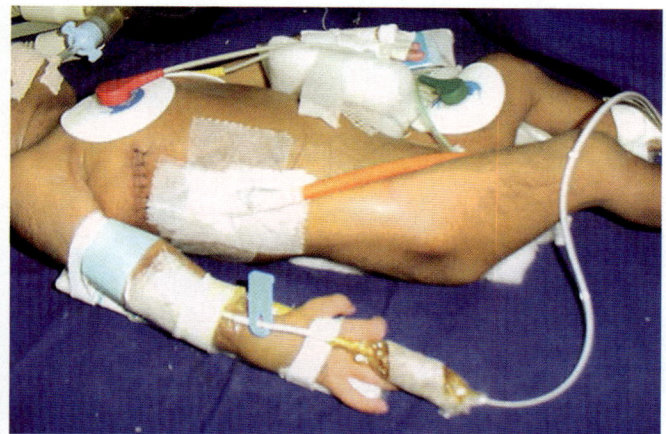

Fig. 34.5: The newborn in the immediate postoperative period who had developed major leak following primary repair for EA and TEF. X-ray chest showed significant pneumothorax and the collapse of the lung on right side. A previous right thoracotomy incision and the chest tube in situ, are seen. Baby on regular neonatal monitoring devices, including ventilatory support, peripheral CVP line and the epidural catheter for morphine infusion for pain relief. To save the baby from further deterioration, a diversion (esophagostomy and abdominal gastrostomy) is usually life saving in the newborn period. With a little added time of anesthesia and surgical risks, gastric transposition offers the definitive procedure in the newborn period itself and avoids the problems associated with the procedure of neonatal diversion

Postoperative care is important and includes

1. Strict monitoring of the respiratory and cardiac status.
2. Elective ventilation with paralysis is helpful.
3. Large bore nasogastric tube to prevent acute gastric dilatation and aspiration.
4. Adequate sedation and relief of postoperative pain by morphine infusion, caudal blocks or epidural catheter. Muscle relaxation may be provided by infusion.
5. A skiagram chest in the immediate postoperative period to look for any pneumothorax or acute gastric dilatation. Insertion of the chest tube in case the pneumothorax is detected.
6. Early institution of drip-in feeds to maintain nutrition. Oral clear liquid feeds are started once the general condition is better or the contrast study performed at postoperative day (POD) 7-10, shows no evidence of anastomotic leak.
7. Small frequent feeds orally and a head up position at an angle of 45 degrees all the time during nursing and sleep.

POSTOPERATIVE COMPLICATIONS (TABLE 34.1)

1. Compression of major vessels in the neck, resulting in decreased venus return. An adequate dissection in the neck would prevent it.
2. Twist of the stomach while pulling the same into the chest. Careful handling and placing the identification sutures on either end of the fundus before pulling the same would avoid the complication.
3. Perforation while performing pyloromyotomy. A proper identification of the same and repair would avoid its consequences.
4. Leak from the closure sites of the native esophagus and the gastrostomy. This is not a common problem with the experienced hands.
5. Bleeding while mobilizing the stomach from the liver surface, short gastric vessels, gastroepiploic vessels. Adhesions with the liver are notorious and may bleed while dissecting the stomach off the liver. With patience and careful sharp and blunt dissection, it can be achieved, though may be time consuming.
6. Ischemia of the fundus of the stomach, if the diathermy has been to divide the short gastric vessels. However, it is never significant enough to cause graft loss. Still, the short gastric vessels should better be ligated to avoid spasm of the vessels.
7. Respiratory and vascular compromise due to the presence of the unusual bulk in the thoracic cavity. As the stomach gets elongated during its pull, the bulk does not cause respiratory compromise. However, it is best to avoid gastric pull up in patients with large and bulky stomach. In such cases, a gastric tube or the colonic interposition may be a better choice.
8. Acute dilatation of the stomach, if the same has not been decompressed well. To have good postoperative gastric decompression, a nasogastric tube must be left in midthorax and allowed to drain freely. It should be checked for patency from time to time.
9. Vomiting, aspiration pneumonia due to stasis of food in the stomach. As vagotomy is invariably performed with gastric transposition, an upright position and avoiding the fatty and large meals just before going to bed may help. An endoscopy

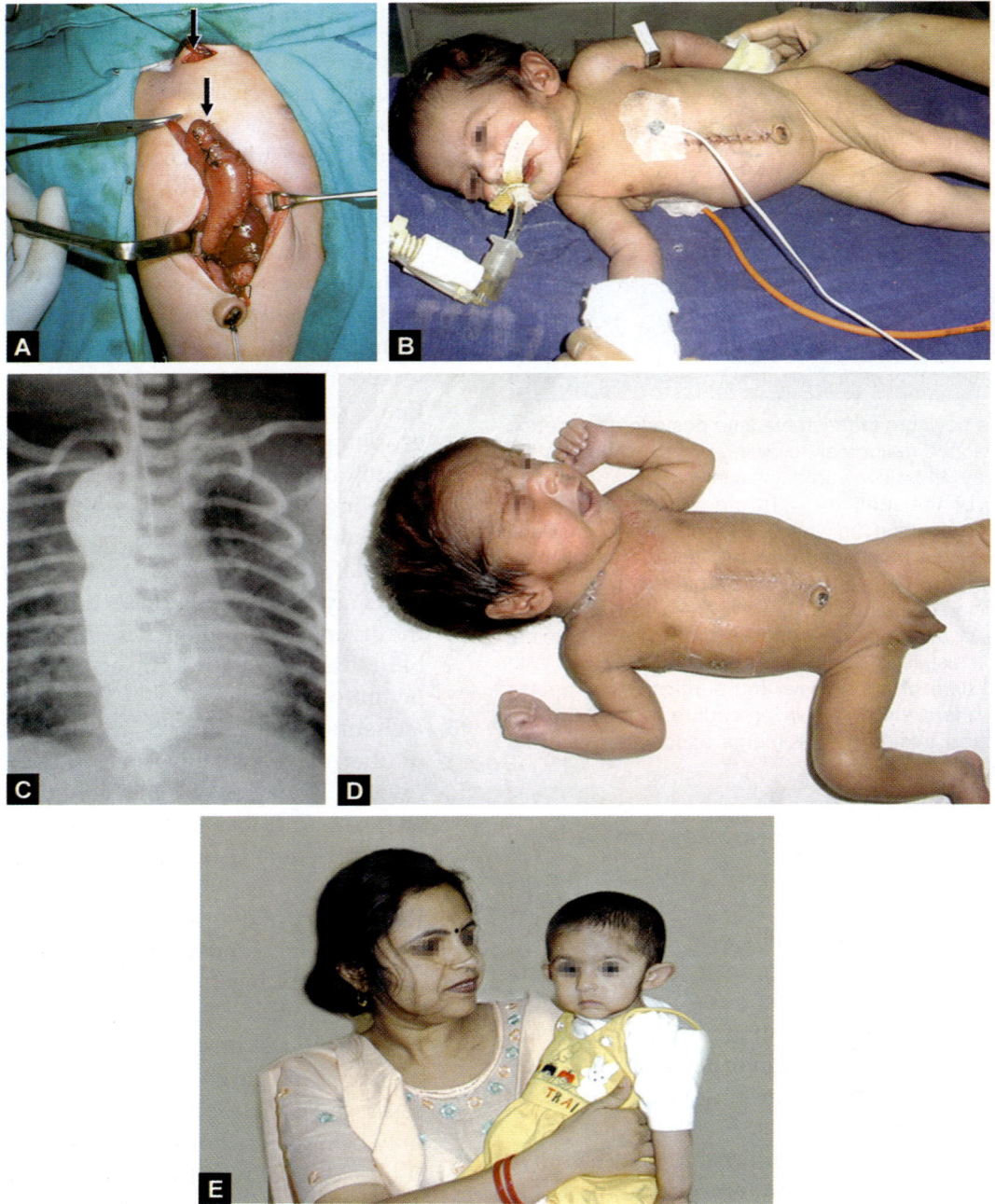

Figs 34.6A to E: Gastric transposition in a newborn following major leak after EA/TEF repair, **A.** The esophagostomy has been mobilized with an elliptical incision in the neck. The stomach has also been mobilized with a midline incision in the abdomen, based on right gastoepiploic vessels and right gastric artery. Thoracotomy incision is not required. The mobilized stump of the lower esophagus seen in the picture, is yet to be resected and suture closed. The fundus of the stomach is the highest point (and not the esophagus stump) and used for making the anastomosis with the esophagus in the neck, **B.** The newborn on postoperative day 3. Abdominal and neck wounds are seen. The chest tube seen in the picture is from the previous thoracotomy while trying an unsuccessful primary repair of the EA and TEF at day 2 of life. Baby is still on elective ventilatory support, **C.** Postoperative barium study on day 9 showing thoracic stomach. No anastomotic leak was detected. Oral feeds resumed slowly the next day, **D.** Same newborn baby on postoperative day 10, is off from all monitoring devices, IV fluids, ventilatory support, CVP line and the epidural catheter. Now only on oral feeds and ready to be discharged once the daily intake is ensured after gastric transposition, **E.** Same baby with the mother at 6 months of age, with normal feeding pattern and catching up with the growth and development

may also be performed to check for the mechanical block.
10. Intestinal obstruction subsequent to laparotomy.
11. Neck or abdominal wound infection.
12. Leaks: Postoperative leaks from the anastomosis in the neck are not uncommon with an incidence of 6-33%. This may result from ischemia, tension on the pulled stomach or due to the technical fault while making the anastomosis. Leaks may be minor, detected only on barium study, or major manifested by salivary or milk leakage from the wound site. Most leaks would close spontaneously without any intervention. The collected material should be drained out freely from under the skin and muscles, removing the skin sutures appropriately.

FOLLOW-UP

The barium study is performed usually on postoperative day 7-10, when the patient has already stabilized, with most catheters and devices are out. The bowel sounds have returned and the wounds are healing (Figs 34.7A to C).

Gastric clearance function tests with the barium swallow and the milk feed mixed with Tc99 colloid scan in the sitting position, and the HIDA scan to evaluate the presence of the duodenogastric reflux (DGR) are performed around day 10 and then at follow up of three months.

Table 34.1: Complications following gastric transposition

Immediate complications
- Vascular compression in the neck
- Chest infection
- Lung collapse
- Ventilation dependency
- Acute gastric dilatation

Early complications
- Anastomotic leak in the neck   6 -33 %
- Delay in feeding   30 %
- Vomiting
- Dumping
- Jejunostomy complications, leak, perforation: 30-50%
- Deaths   6-16%
- Recurrent aspiration
- Pulmonary compression
- Gastroesophageal reflux in the neck
- Duodenogastric reflux in the abdomen

Late complications
- Stricture in the neck   12- 20%
- Intestinal obstruction due to adhesions
- Graft loss - rare
- Loss of reservoir function and poor growth
- In-coordinated swallowing
- Pulmonary function compromise
- Dyspnea
- Anemia
- Reflux gastritis
- Dumping syndrome
- Functional obstruction due to vagotomy

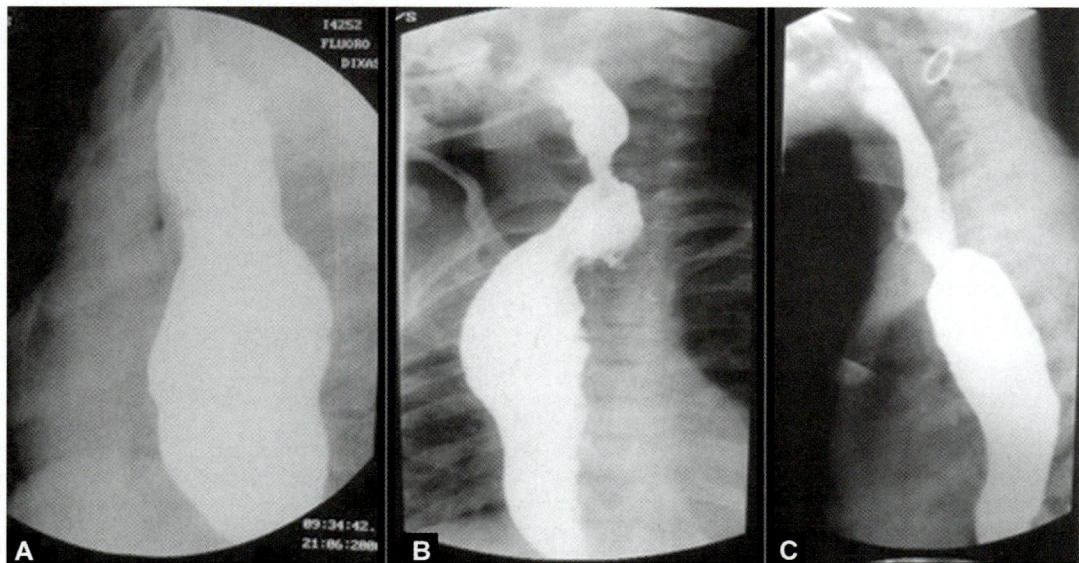

Figs 34.7A to C: Follow up barium studies in different patients showing a near normal contoured thoracic stomach that has adapted as the esophagus in each case

The barium study should be performed first in the lying position and then in the sitting position. The follow up studies show a near normal contour of the thoracic stomach that adapts itself as the esophagus.

PRECAUTIONS

A close watch has to be kept in the immediate postoperative period for pneumothorax and acute gastric dilatation (Fig. 34.8). As neonates demonstrate an accelerated gastric emptying and the presence of the duodenogastric reflux in the immediate postoperative period, a careful feeding and nursing in an upright position (preferably at 45 degree angle from the bed) is essential to prevent aspiration pneumonitis.[4]

Anastomotic leaks in the neck are not uncommon but most of them are minor and resolve within few days.[17,19] Even in the presence of ongoing leak in the neck, the clear water or even milk feed can be initiated. This would help in clearing the tract and provide nutrition. Acidic gastric juice worsens the leak. The pH is monitored. It is usually around 2.5 despite vagotomy. Major leaks result in strictures thus a close watch is needed in the follow up, including the endoscopy at regular intervals. Most of these (50-80 %) respond to dilatation.[17,19] Only rarely is the revision needed.[5] Anastomotic strictures have been reported to be more common in patients having previous caustic esophageal injury.[16]

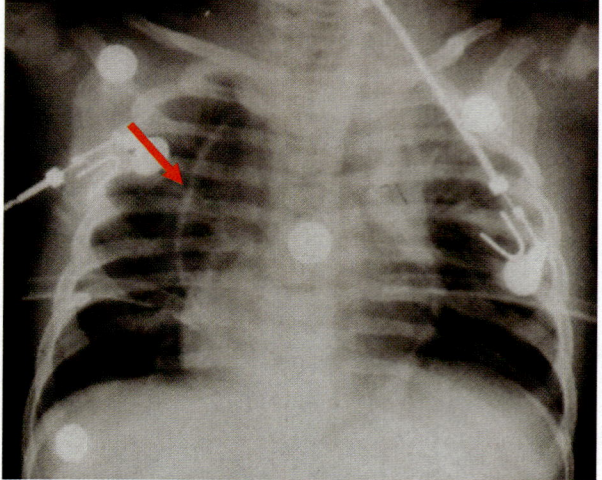

Fig. 34.8: Case of gastric transposition showing acute gastric dilatation in the postoperative period developing respiratory distress. Arrow shows the right boarder of the stomach in the thorax

Gastric transposition for esophageal substitution has been associated with a mortality rate of 5% of patients in the best hands.[16] However, this was the experience reported in higher age group and not that in the neonates, in whom a higher operative mortality is expected. Most of the deaths in children (67%) have been reported in the early postoperative period.[16] The causes of death in the early postoperative period include ongoing sepsis and congenital heart disease besides aspiration that is preventable with close monitoring (Table 34.2).

In the authors' experience with 51 cases of gastric pull ups till date, there has been no graft loss. Other large series have reported similar results.[16] However, in our series, there were 5 deaths of 51 children undergoing gastric transpositions, 31 of these have been done in the neonatal period most of whom were usually very sick and on ventilatory support as well. These deaths were in the neonatal period, due to ongoing lung collapse and sepsis in 2, serious congenital heart disease in 1, and multiple anomalies in another. There was possibly one procedure related death in our series due to vascular compromise at the level of thoracic inlet. This patient had very large liver that bled to touch. He also developed swelling of the face within 3-4 hrs after surgery. Patient collapsed before he could be opened up to relive the possible compression. Since then, the authors are very careful

Table 34.2: The authors experience of neonatal gastric pull up	
N-32, 1998 - 2008*	
• Birth wt	: 1.2 -3 kg
• Preoperative Infection	: 55%
• Complex CHD	: 20 %
• Sick babies	: 22
• Preoperative on ventilator	: 22
• Preoperative Lung collapse	: 07
Immediate Postop. Course	
• Ongoing chest infection	: 8
• Lung collapse	: 3
• Postop. ventilation	: 9.6 days(2- 40)
• Leak in the neck	: 10/32 (33 %)
• TPN for Delay in feeding	: 09/32 (30 %)
• Jejunostomy complications	: 3/7 leak, perforation
Deaths	: 05/32 (15%)
(on day 9, 13,15,16, 29 for ongoing sepsis, CHD)	
• Hospital stay	29 days (9-87)

while making either the tunnel or the space in the neck, before attempting to pull and house the stomach up at the thoracic inlet. Death has been reported a year following the procedure, due to respiratory arrest following aspiration at home.[17]

Difficulty in establishing oral feeds in the early postoperative period is common. Short-term support with total parentral nutrition may be provided. However, jejunostomy may be a better option and should be considered to bye pass the upper gut and provide nutrition. Vomiting and aspiration is also seen frequently.

Redo surgery may be required for the stricture in the neck, mechanical obstruction in its course, jejunostomy related complications besides the intestinal obstruction due to adhesions.[17] A mechanical obstruction may be caused by the compression of the large lobe of the liver on the stomach during its course.

Symptoms mimicking obstruction have been reported due to stasis of food in the thoracic stomach (functional obstruction due to vagotomy) without any evidence of mechanical obstruction.[4] This needs careful assessment for the need of jejunostomy to provide nutrition. It may also lead to aspiration pneumonia during sleep.

POSTOPERATIVE RESULTS

Feeding

Gastric transposition re-establishes effective gastrointestinal continuity with few complications.[5] In a large series of 173 children reported by Spitz et al,[16] the most common indications included failed repair of different varieties of esophageal atresia (127), caustic injury (23), and peptic strictures (8). In more than 90% of these, the outcome was considered good to excellent in terms of absence of swallowing difficulties or other gastrointestinal symptoms. Many, however, preferred to eat small frequent meals. The authors also have similar experience during the follow up studies of patients who had undergone gastric transposition 10 year back or more. Majority of the patients learned the acceptable habit of eating and swallowing in due course of time.[20] There has been no deterioration in the function of the gastric transposition in those patients followed up for more than 10 years. Poor outcome may be associated with multiple previous attempts at esophageal salvage.[16]

Pressure Profile and Manometry Studies

The thoracic stomach does not have peristalsis but responds well to the food bolus. The manometric studies performed after gastric pull up documented mass contractions without any propulsive or peristaltic waves. The baseline pressure was little higher in newborns as compared to that in children. Also, the pressure increased by over 120% both in newborns and children in response to the food bolus.[21] The response was irrespective of the age at surgery and the route adopted (Fig. 34.9).

Growth and Development

It has now been shown that gastric transposition is compatible with normal life, though the growth and development remained subnormal in children followed up for 5-10 years in some series. The height has been calculated as 80-90% of 50th percentile in the authors' series.[21] The average weight was subnormal in most of the patients up to 60-70% of the expected weight. Anemia has been found in 70% of the cases during long-term follow-up.[20]

Quality of Life

In our experience, about two-third patients showed normal gastric clearance on barium or nuclear scanning. One-third of these either showed an obstructed flow (> 20 minutes) or even a rapid clearance (< 2 minutes) from the thoracic stomach. These findings did not change either with the age at surgery or the type of the route used for the gastric transposition. Similarly, a duodenogastric reflux was demonstrated in 67% patients following the gastric transposition in the postoperative period. The values decreased to 40% at 1 year follow up. It was surprising that only a few of them were symptomatic and had bilious vomiting. The significance of positive duodenogastric reflux is yet not clear but may lead to biliary gastritis in the long-term. In our series, a follow up after 10 years with endoscopy and biopsy from the gastric mucosa did not reveal either biliary gastritis or atrophy of the mucosa in the transposed thoracic stomach.[20]

The authors' have noted the decreased functional capacity of the lungs in patients with gastric pull up. This was much more in group of patients who had

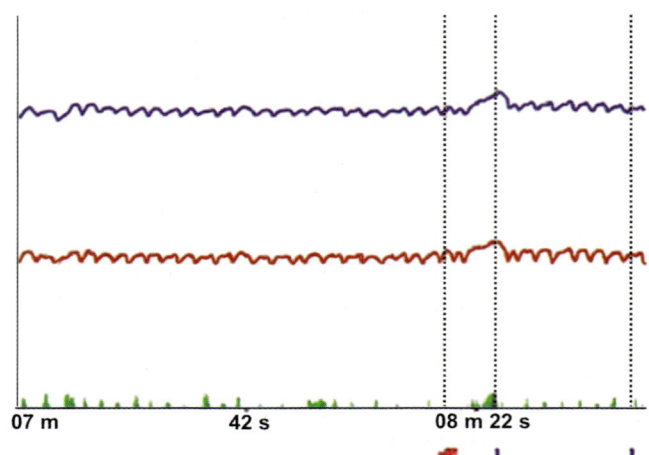

Fig. 34.9: Manometric studies showing mass contraction in response to a swallow

undergone previous thoracotomies. This may be secondary to the pulmonary compression or recurrent aspirations.[20]

The quality of life for patients with esophageal atresia was generally unimpaired by any side effects of gastric transposition.[15] Patients undergoing gastric transposition as a primary procedure experienced fewer disease-specific symptoms in the medium term compared with patients who had undergone previous unsuccessful attempts at reconstruction or replacement of their esophagus.[15]

Colonic interposition is the most commonly used procedure to replace the esophagus in the pediatric age group, preferred by most Pediatric Surgeons around the globe Tannuri et al recently published their 27 years experience with the use of colon as well as stomach, with postoperative merits and demerits of each procedure.[22]

The authors feel that "Gastric transposition is a satisfactory means of esophageal substitution and "probably the best" of all the available options especially for patients with esophageal atresia".[19] Its role in neonates for replacing the esophagus for complicated EA and TEF as an emergency procedure, is unsurpassable with any other procedure.[23] For postcorrosive injuries seen in children above 1 year of age, and leading to extensive stricture formation requiring esophageal replacement, colon maintained a definite place with less serious long-term known complications.

Acidity

Following the vagotomy, which is invariably performed, a rise in the pH is not troublesome even if noticed.[4] Our children, the 24 hr pH study performed during follow up of more than 5 years after the surgery, have shown a pH between 1.7 - 3.6 (Fig. 34.10). Though, it is contrary to the reports mentioning high pH after gastric transposition, it may be a good sign not to have achlorhydria and subsequent chances of malignancy developing later in life.

Intrathoracic stomach apart from facing a vagotomy and elongation, may also have a decreased blood supply to the tune of 20%. The consequences of all these need to be monitored in the long-term.

Rare Serious Complications

Carcinoma: A carcinoma developing at the esophagogastric junction in the neck has been mentioned in an adult who had gastric pull done for the corrosive stricture (Egyptian experience as mentioned by Dr Alla Hamza). However, whether it was due to the abnormal mucosa left in the esophagus, is difficult to assess.

Gastric perforation: A 13-year child who had undergone gastric pull in infancy, presented with scant fresh bleeding by mouth. While undergoing an endoscopic examination in emergency, there was gush of blood in the mouth. An emergency sternotomy was done to locate the site of bleeding. The source was found to be directly from the heart. As the endoscopist was quite a known expert in the field, the iatrogenic injury was ruled out. The bleeding was purported to have resulted from the perforation of the gastric ulcer

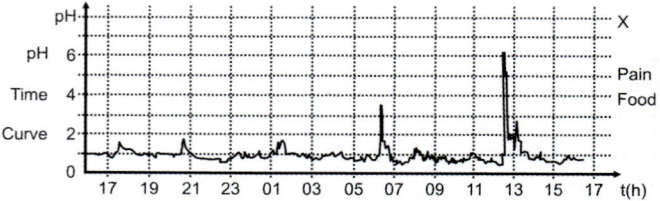

Fig. 34.10: 24 hour pH monitoring showing low pH even during sleep. The high peaks as seen in the diagram show pH levels in response to meals, and are within normal range

in to the heart, leading to the gastrocardiac fistula, severe hemoptysis and death, (personal communication).[24]

In other series with long-term follow-up, such serious problems have not been reported so far.[16,20]

REFERENCES

1. Gupta DK, Kataria R, Bajpai M. Gastric transposition for esophageal replacement in children–an Indian experience. Eur J Pediatr Surg. 1997;7:143-46.
2. Gupta DK, Sharma Shilpa, Arora MK, et al. Esophageal replacement in the neonatal period in infants with esophageal atresia and tracheoesophageal fistula. J Pediatr Surg. 2007;42:1471-77.
3. Gupta D K, Srinivas M, Agarwala S, et al. Neonatal gastric pull up: reality or myth? Pediatr Surg Int. 2003;19:100-03.
4. Gupta DK. Gastric Transposition in neonates. In Textbook of Neonatal Surgery. MBD Publishers, New Delhi. Ed. DK Gupta, 2000;Chap 56:356-60.
5. Hirschl RB, Yardeni D, Oldham K, et al. Gastric transposition for esophageal replacement in children: experience with 41 consecutive cases with special emphasis on esophageal atresia. Ann Surg. 2002;236:531-9; discussion 539-41.
6. Marujo WC, Tannuri U, Maksoud JG. Total gastric transposition: An alternative to esophageal replacement in children. J Pediatr Surg 1991;26:676-81.
7. Othersen HB, Hebra A, Tagge EP. Esophageal replacement for atresia without fistula. Semin Paed Surg 1998;7:134-36.
8. AF Scharli. Esophageal reconstruction in very long atresias by elongation of the lesser curvature Pediatr Surg Int. 1992;7:101-05.
9. Fernandez MS, Gutierrez C, Ibanez V, et al. Long gap esophageal atresia: reconstruction preserving all portions of the esophagus by Scharli's technique. Pediatr Surg Int 1998;14:17-20.
10. Spitz L. Gastric transposition via the mediastinal route for infants with long gap esophageal atresia. J Pediatr Surg1984;19:149-54.
11. Spitz L, Kelly E, Sparnon T. Gastric transposition for esophageal replacement in children. Ann Surg 1987;206:69-73.
12. Spitz L. Gastric transposition for esophageal substitution in children. J Pediatr Surg 1992;27(2):252-59.
13. Spitz L: Gastric transposition for esophageal replacement. Pediatric Surg Int 1996;11:218-20.
14. Spitz L, Ruangtrakool R: Esophageal substitution. Semin Paed Surg 1998;7:130-33.
15. Ludman L, Spitz L. Quality of life after gastric transposition for oesophageal atresia. J Pediatr Surg. 2003;38:53-7; discussion 53-57.
16. Spitz L, Kiely E, Pierro A. Gastric transposition in children--a 21-year experience. J Pediatr Surg. 2004;39:276-81; discussion 276-81.
17. Rygl M, Snajdauf J, Lisa J, et al, Surgical complications following oesophageal replacement by stomach in childhood Rozhl Chir. 2006;85:489-93.
18. Arora M and Gupta DK. Leak related mortality and morbidity in neonates following EATEF repair, A Dissertation for M.Ch degree in Pediatric Surgery, submitted to AIIMS, New Delhi, 1999.
19. Gupta DK. Substitution of the Esophagus in neonates: An alternative approach. MSR Oration delivered at the 32nd Annual Conference of the Indian Association of Pediatric Surgeons, Jaipur Oct 2007;4-7.
20. Jain V, Gupta DK, Sharma S, Kumar R. Long-term evaluation of the intrathoracic stomach in children following gastric transposition. A Dissertation for M.Ch degree in Pediatric Surgery, submitted to AIIMS, New Delhi, 2007.
21. Gupta DK, Charles AR, Srinivas M. Manometric evaluation of the intrathoracic stomach after gastric transposition in children. Pediatr Surg Int. 2004;20(6):415-18.
22. Tannuri U, Maksoud-Filho JG, Tannuri AC, et al. Which is better for esophageal substitution in children, esophagocoloplasty or gastric transposition? A 27-year experience of a single center. J Pediatr Surg. 2007;42:500-04.
23. Gupta DK, Sharma Shilpa, Gupta M. Neonatal Emergency Esophageal Replacement with Gastric Transposition for Esophageal Atresia in Monogram on Esophageal Atresia. Ed. I Sebastian, Bucharest 2008 (in Press).
24. Raboei Enaam. Consultant Pediatric Surgeon, King Fahad Armed Forces Hospital, Jeddah from her personal experience of the case from France.

Jejunal Interposition as a Substitute of Esophagus

Kohei Hashizume, Antonio Dessanti

When the esophagus is congenitally defected or severely damaged after birth because of causative agents or other reasons, substitution of esophagus becomes necessary. It has been controversial what to use as a substitute of the esophagus in infants and children. Organs used as a substitute of the esophagus are stomach, gastric tube, colon, and jejunum.[1-8] Necessary characteristics of the substitute of the esophagus should be, (1) the operation is simple and easy, (2) it should have good peristalsis and good transportation ability, (3) it should not dilate once positioned in the thorax or mediastinum, (4) symptoms caused from the deficit of the organ itself should not severe.

The usage of the jejunum as a substitute of the esophagus is not very popular. It is because the operation is believed to be cumbersome and time-consuming and there is necessity of discarding some length of jejunum to make a sufficient length of vascular pedicle. However, the most important point is not the duration of the operating time but the quality of life of the patient who should live more than 50 years after the operation. So the disadvantage of longer operation time is easily compensated by the better quality of life of the patients, if the function of the jejunum is much better than the other substitutes of the esophagus.[9-11] The authors believe jejunum is the most appropriate substitute of the esophagus in infants and children, and present here the technical points of the operation and also the results of the operation.

TIMING OF OPERATION

It is controversial when the operation of the reconstruction of the esophagus should be done. The point is not the problem of handling the jejunum. Many pediatric surgeons have the experience of operating on the small intestine in babies who weigh less than 1000 grams. However, it is not advisable to perform jejunum interposition in neonates. The severest and disastrous complication of this operation is total necrosis of the interposed jejunum, and it should be prevented at all costs. The main reason of this complication is vascular insufficiency, i.e. arterial thrombosis or venous occlusion. In neonates the mesenteric arteries and veins are very friable, and are liable to be torn, and also the scarceness of mesenteric adipose tissue makes the veins vulnerable to bending and occlusion. So the babies should be grown enough at the time of the operation by enteral feeding through gastrostomy or by parenteral nutrition. The authors think 6 months of age and/or 6 kg of weight is adequate. After 6 months of age, it is rather difficult to start oral feeding even if the resumed continuity of the esophagus is perfect, because the critical period of learning of oral intake is before that time.

TECHNIQUE OF THE OPERATION

The operation needs 2 incisions, right thoracotomy and laparotomy. The patient is placed in semi-left-lateral position and all the upper body is cleaned and draped from axilla to inguinal region (Fig. 35.1). With this positioning, and some rotation of the operation table one can easily perform preparation of jejunal loop through laparotomy and anastomosis of esophagus with jejunum through right thoracotomy. First, the abdomen is opened for the preparation of the jejunal loop. The authors prefer an upper midline incision, as it is much easier to approach the esophageal hiatus with this incision compared to transverse incision.

After opening the abdomen, the intestine is thoroughly inspected for any anomaly such as

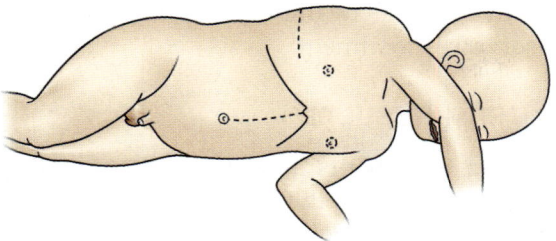

Fig. 35.1: Position of patient during operation—Patient is placed in left semi-lateral position and right arm is raised. Patient is prepared and draped from axilla to inguinal region. The table can be tilted for better exposure according to the place of operation, i.e. intra-abdominal or intrathoracic

malrotation and Meckel's diverticulum. The vasculature of jejunum may be variable, but usually has the configuration shown in the figure. The first jejunal artery with accompanying vein is preserved. The second and third jejunal arteries are usually ligated and cut near their origin, and the fourth artery is preserved and is used as the part of vascular pedicle of the jejunal loop. With these procedures, you can get adequate length of the vascular pedicle, which consists of the fourth jejunal artery and the vascular arcade from the point of the confluence with the first jejunal artery to the point of the confluence with the fourth jejunal artery (Fig. 35.2). The vascular arcade is ligated and divided between the first and the second jejunal artery, and corresponding part of the jejunum is divided. The distal side of divided jejunum is then placed on the anterior chest wall to ensure that this part can be brought to the level of the place designated for the upper anastomosis. Usually one can get adequate length of vascular pedicle and the jejunal loop is easily brought to the upper part of the chest wall (Fig. 35.3). If it is clear that the length of the vascular pedicle is adequate, the arcade is ligated and divided just distal to the point of the confluence with the fourth jejunal artery. The length of the jejunal loop prepared is usually too long for the interposition between the proximal and distal esophagus, and there will be a possibility of interposed jejunum becoming redundant and tortuous in the thorax. So the redundant part of the jejunum, i.e. the distal part should be resected. However, one must be very careful not to resect too much length of the jejunum, it may jeopardize the later anastomosis. The continuity of the jejunum is restored by the anastomosis between the

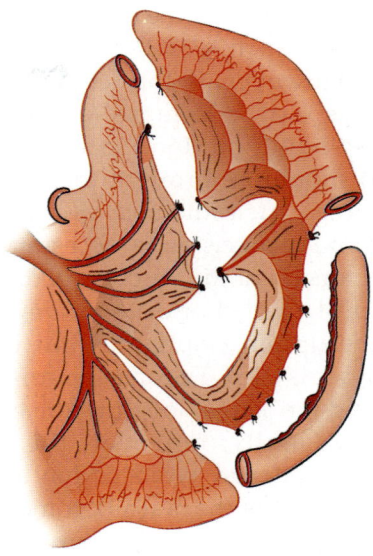

Fig. 35.2: Preparation of jejunum to be transposed—The first jejunal artery is preserved for the circulation of oral part of jejunum and the second and third jejunal arteries are cut to make adequate length of the vascular pedicle. The circulation of the jejunum to be transposed is maintained by the fourth jejunal artery. Redundant part of the jejunum is resected later

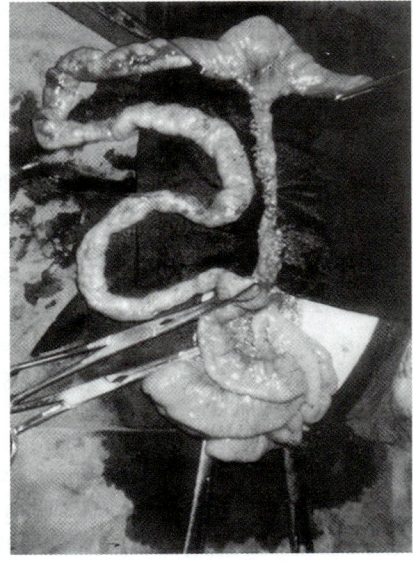

Fig. 35.3: Jejunal loop on chest wall—Prepared jejunal loop is placed on the chest wall to make sure that the length of the vascular pedicle is adequate for the upper anastomosis

oral and anal ends of the jejunum. The jejunal loop prepared is brought to the upper abdomen through a small hole in the mesocolon. Concerning the route to the thoracic cavity, if the length of the lower esophagus is long enough to permit the lower anastomosis done in the right thoracic cavity, the loop should be brought anterior the stomach and through a hole in the diaphragm. However, if the length of the lower esophagus is not adequate enough and the anastomosis should be done in the abdomen, the jejunal loop should be brought to the right thorax thorough retrogastric route and through esophageal hiatus. Maximum precision is necessary to avoid a kinking and torsion of the vascular pedicle.

The level of right thoracotomy depends on the length of the upper esophagus, but usually fifth intercostal space is used. The anastomosis of the upper esophagus and the jejunal loop may be end-to-end or end-to-side. Usually, however, the end-to-side anastomosis is better to avoid undue tension to the vascular pedicle. After the oral anastomosis the length of the remaining jejunal loop is estimated, and if it is too long, additional part of the anal end of the jejunal loop should be resected. By this procedure, the interposed jejunum becomes straight and stasis of food in the interposed jejunum is avoided. During this procedure, however meticulous procedure is needed to avoid injury to the vascular pedicle. This can be accomplished if the resection of the redundant jejunum is done as near the jejunum wall as possible. The anastomosis of the interposed jejunum and the lower esophagus is accomplished by end-to-end fashion. If the lower esophagus is very short and the only remnant, the jejunum may be anastomosed to the stomach directly. A drain is inserted in the right thorax and the thoracic wall is closed, and then the abdomen is closed with a penrose drain near the esophageal hiatus.

After operation, thoracic and abdominal drain should be observed carefully for is any drainage of saliva or intestinal contents. When there is small amount of drainage, if the general condition of the patient has not deteriorated and CAP is not very high, wait and watch policy is the best. After one week the patient is brought to the radiology department, and upper GI study is done. If there is no leakage, oral intake should be started. If it is the first oral intake for the patients they cannot cope with oral feeding at first. Usually several weeks or even months are necessary for them to adapt. If there is a leakage, patient should be on parenteral nutrition, enteral feeding through a gastrostomy, or enteral feeding through an enteral tube inserted through a gastrostomy, depending on the size of the patient and the size of the leakage. Usually the leak will heal spontaneously after 2 weeks of conservative treatment.

LONG-TERM RESULTS

Comparing the results after the reconstruction of esophagus using colon, the long-term results of jejunal interposition is extremely good. The reasons for that are as follows: (1) The possibility of stricture formation at the anastomotic site is less probable. (2) The peristalsis of jejunum is much better than that of colon. (3) There is less tendency of dilatation after some years. (4) There are much fewer intrinsic problems compared to colon such as diverticulum formation and development of adenoma. The patients have few problems, and they show normal growth.[12,13] Thus, the influence of resection of redundant part of the jejunum on growth is nil or minimum.

The follow-up upper G-I contrast study films are shown in Figure 35.4. One can notice almost normal sized jejunum in the right thorax and normal mucosal folds. The jejunum is straight or some redundancy with L-shaped configuration is seen in few cases, but the peristalsis is good and the flow of the barium from upper esophagus through interposed jejunum to the lower esophagus is very good.

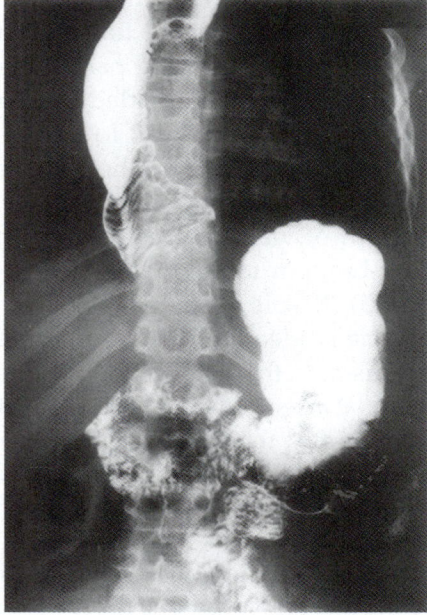

Fig. 35.4: Upper G-I study during follow-up—The interposed jejunum is not tortuous and shows no dilatation. Also peristalsis is normal and transition time is almost normal

REFERENCES

1. Gupta DK, Sharma S, Arora MK, et al. Esophageal replacement in the neonatal period is infants with esophageal atresia and tracheoesophageal fistule. J Pediatr Surg 2007;42:1471-77.
2. Spitz L. Gastric transposition for esophageal substitution in children. J Pediatr Surg 1992;27:252-59.
3. Mitchell IM, Goh DW, Roberts KD, et al. Colon interposition in children. Br J Surg 1989;76:681-86.
4. Ein SH, Standling B, Stephens CA. Twenty- one year experience with the pediatric gastric tube. J Pediatr Surg 1987;22:77-81.
5. Wright C, Cuschieri A. Jejunal interposition for benign esophageal disease: Technical considerations and long-term results. Ann Surg 1987;205:54-60.
6. Nishihira T, Oe H, Sugawara K, et al. Esophageal reconstruction: Rconstruction of the thoracic esophagus with jejunal pedicled segments for cancer of the thoracic esophagus. Dis Esoph 1995;8:30-39.
7. Keller RJ, Sicular A. Jejunal interposition. Gastrointest Radiol 1989;14:9-14.
8. Cusick EL, Batchelor AA, Spicer AD. Development of a technique for jejunal interposition in long-gap esophageal atresia. J Pediatr Surg 1993;28:990-94.
9. Foker JE, Ring SA, Varco RL. Technique of jejunal interposition for esophageal replacement. J Thorc Cardiovasc Surg 1982;83:928-33.
10. Ring WS, Varco RL,L'Heureux PR, et al. Esophageal replacement with jejunum in children: An 18 to 33 year follow-up. J Thorac Cardiovas Surg 1982;83:918-27.
11. Pasch AR, Putnam T. Jejunal interposition for recurrent gastroesophageal reflux in children. Am J Surg 1985;150: 248-51.
12. Fonkalsrud EW, Bustorff-Silva J. Interposition of a jejunal segment between esophagus and pylorus for treatment of multirecurrent gastroesophageal reflux. J pediatr Surg 1999;34:1563-66.
13. Altorjay A, Pászti I, Kiss J, Tasnádi G. Gastrojejunal interposition for esophageal replacement. Pediatr Surg Int 1999;15:132-34.

Colon Patch Esophagoplasty

Enaam Raboei

Early in this century ingestion of caustics was common and resulted in dense strictures for which methods of dilation were advised. As obstructions usually recurred, bypass operations were common with conduits of skin or segments of the gastrointestinal tract. Recently when intensive steroid therapy were used, usually it prevented all but localized areas of stricture. In case of short stricture, different kind of procedures has been advocated for treatment. If the stricture is longer or resistant to dilation, it can be managed by incision and insertion of a colonic patch with excellent long-term results.

Extensive review of the medical literature disclosed the original description of colon patch by Hecker, Hollmann, Biemann Othersen and others in the pediatric series.[1-8] The concept of incision of an esophageal stricture and insertion of a patch was originally reported for the cervical and also the terminal esophagus. Not until Hecker and Hollmann's work was applied even to the thoracic esophagus.

In 1986, Biemann Othersen reported a 10-year experience with the use of the vascularized colic patch in the management of esophageal strictures in children to overcome redundancy and stagnation in the interposed colon often associated with marked growth retardation, with satisfactory long-term results.[1] Biemann Othersen extended his work and demonstrated the effectiveness of this technique in a series of children in 1997.[6]

ADVANTAGES

- Retains continuity of esophagus
- Less injury to vagus nerves
- Permits re-epithelialization and scar regression in the surrounding esophagus
- Preserves the lower esophageal sphincter in most cases.

DISADVANTAGES

- Formation of pseudodiverticulum, if redundant
- Long intrathoracic suture line
- Difficult access to approach the abdomen and the chest simultaneously to carry the colon patch anastomosis in the neck
- Risk of the retained strictured mucosa of the esophagus with the possibility of development of malignancy later.

PREOPERATIVE PREPARATION OF THE PATIENT FOR COLON PATCH

- Programmed esophageal dilatation is accomplished through the use of Savary bougie dilators. Stricture is dilated under general anesthesia with no fluoroscopy control. The dilatation is guided by visual monitoring of the guide wire to confirm its presence in the stomach. This type of dilation was continued for at least one year before considering failure.
- Bowel preparation with cololyte started 24 hours prior to surgery and continued hourly until clear out put obtained.
- The patients are covered by Gentamicin in combination with second generation cephalosporin and Metronidazole.

SURGICAL TECHNIQUE

Many surgical techniques developed for esophageal replacement are still in use. The technique of colon patch as described by Drs. Hecker and Hollmann with a few modifications was used in our institute.[4,8]

The patient is placed in semilateral position so as to have an adequate access to the upper abdomen and also to the right side of the thorax. Two separate incisions were used in all but one child. A midline upper abdominal incision and another on the right side through the 5th intercostal space, exposes the stomach, colon, diaphragm, and the entire length of the esophagus in the chest. We have used transpleural approach. The segment of colon used is based on the middle colic or the left colic artery. Careful measurements determine the length of the colon segment needed. The esophageal stricture is incised longitudinally until the normal esophagus is reached at either end of the stricture.

A template of the patch size required is then made. The colic segment is selected so as to have enough length of the pedicle on the marginal arcade. The colon is cleaned and opened on its anti-mesenteric border. The colon patch is fashioned while still in the abdomen. If the segment of colon is first brought into the chest and then trimmed, its location deep in the thoracic cavity makes control of hemorrhage more difficult. The colic segment is more accessible in the abdomen. The colo-colic anstomosis is made of the remaining colon.

When the patch has been fashioned, it is passed behind the stomach and through a hole in the right diaphragm. The patch should fit without tension or the redundancy and is sewed into place using the continuous sutures. The excess of the colon is excised leaving only a patch (adjoining the mesentery) necessary to bridge the elliptical defect so created in the longitudinal wall of the strictured esophagus.

Instead of passing the patch through the hiatus, we pass it through a small cut in the diaphragm to the right side of the chest. Boix-Ochoa fundoplication was our procedure of choice in the four patients and a Nissen type fundoplication had already been done in another institute. Two chest drains, one anterior and one posterior are used.

Postoperative Care

- Total parenteral nutrition is started 24 hrs postoperative.
- Opacification of the new esophagus is done 5th - 7th day postoperative using non-ionic dye.
- Feeding is started after bowel function has started and the patient's condition gets stabilized.
- The follow up visit is usually every month for a few months and then 6 monthly for the first 2 years.

THE AUTHOR'S SERIES (TABLE 36.1)

Total of five patients have had colon patch performed in our institute. Four patients had extensive caustic strictures and one had a stricture after a failed esophageal atresia repair in the past. All the five patients were males. The age of patients at surgery was around 4 years for the caustic injury patients and 13 years for the one with stricture post-tracheo-esophageal fistula. The site of the stricture was mid esophagus in three, upper two-third in one and lower esophagus in one. The length of stricture varied from 5 -12 cm. Three patients developed anastomotic leaks which were treated conservatively. It subsided in two

Table 36.1: Summary of colon patch esophagoplasty (Author's series)								
#/ Sex	Diagnosis	Age	Site	Length	Postoperative course	Antireflux	Extra-surgery	Follow-up
1/♂	Caustic injury	2.5 yrs	Mid	5 cm	Diverticulum	Preoperative	Resection of diverticulum	20 yrs
2/♂	Caustic injury	3 yrs	Mid	8 cm	Leak	10 days postoperative		14 yrs
3/♂	Post TEF repair	13 yrs	Mid	5 cm	Leak	6 years preoperative		5 yrs
4/♂	Caustic injury	3 yrs	Lower	10 cm	Leak	Intraoperative		4 yrs
5/♂	Caustic injury	3 yrs	Upper 2/3	12 cm	Wound dehiscence Intestinal obstruction	Intraoperative	Wound closure and gastric bypass	2 months

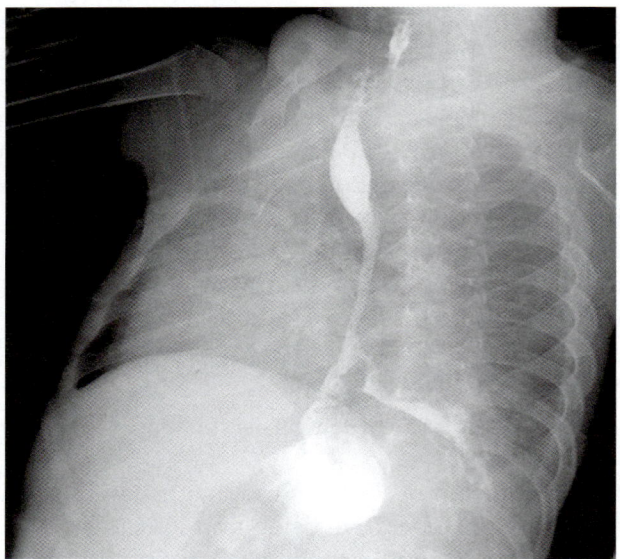

Fig. 36.1: Postoperative contrast study demonstrating an anastomotic leak

and one was managed by a postoperative fundoplication 10 days postcolon patch esophagoplasty (Fig. 36.1). The first patient operated in this series developed patch diverticulum, which was resected 12 years after colon patch esophagoplasty with no intra or postoperative problem regarding the vascularity of the patch. All had pre-, intra- or post-colon patch fundoplication.

The follow-up period ranged from one month to 20 years. All the patients are eating and growing normally after surgery. None have developed respiratory symptoms and there is no malignant change in the older patient.

DISCUSSION

The colic patch currently offers advantages that outweigh any disadvantages. When the patch is perfectly tailored to the defect, no bulging or redundancy is found. It is easily constructed and, with a good marginal artery, can be carried high into the chest. The patients do not require close postoperative follow-up.

The only problem has been that a considerable amount of colon must be discarded to obtain adequate length of the pedicle, but the same amount of bowel would be used as well if the colon interposition is planned.

Our second case with partial anastomotic disruption and prolonged postoperative course, make us suggest that fundoplication should be done simultaneously with the colon patch if it has not been done pre-operatively. The need of fundoplication has also been clearly shown by others.[5,9]

The third case in our series with post TEF repair stricture, the leak stayed long but in our opinion that was because he has been left with severe stricture for 13 years with many trials of dilatation and including the laser therapy in another institute. He was living on liquid and semi liquid diet only. His weight was 17 kg at the time of surgery. The upper pouch pre operatively was filled with turbid fluid which was coming out of his chest drain postoperatively. He was eating for the first time in his life after colon patch procedure (Fig. 36.2).

The current alternative operations for the esophageal strictures are either esophageal replacement using colon, stomach or the small intestine. The entire stomach, when brought up to the proximal esophagus, refluxes and occupies a large space in a small chest.

The gastric tube also allows reflux of acid secretions and may not easily reach high enough. The reconstructed gastric tube is adjacent to the major vessels and organs such as the heart, aorta and trachea, and ulcers if any, occurring in the tube, carry the risk of perforation into these structures. Though the incidence is low, the development of such perforations can cause serious, life-threatening complications.[10]

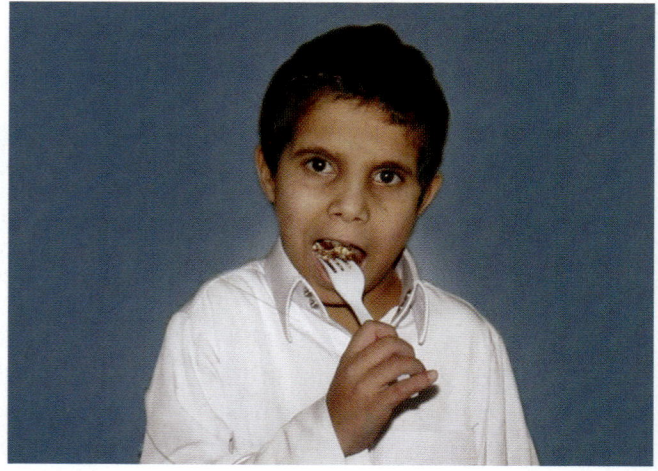

Fig. 36.2: A 13 years old boy eating solids for the first time in his life after colon path esophagoplasty

Small intestine lacks a marginal artery and has a tendency to be redundant. Swallowing is a slow process when food must traverse an interposed piece of small intestine. If the scared esophagus is bypassed, it may accumulate secretions and eventually perforate or carcinoma may develop in the retained scar.

There have been reports of carcinoma developing years after a chemical burn but the average time from injury to carcinoma is 30-40 years with a frequency of 1.2-2.6%.[8] Carcinoma has also been reported in anterothoracic dermatoesophagoplasties. In our patients who have had interposition of a colic patch, the scar in the esophagus has become much more pliable as the tension is relieved after insertion of the patch. Portions of the esophagus, which prior to the patch contain scar epithelium and granulation tissue, eventually become covered with esophageal mucosa. Endoscopic evaluation after patching showed good epithelial covering of the area of previous stricture with improved pliability of the esophageal wall. The patch is easily identified on endoscopy.[4,6] The possibility of carcinoma developing in some of our patients does exist but the risk is presumably minimal.

Originally, it was thought that the length of the stricture may limit the use of the patch technique. We performed colon patch esophagoplasty to more than four inches strictures with good outcome. The gastroesophageal junction was included in one of cases with very good result (Fig. 36.3). None of the patients have had any respiratory or growth problem.

These good results were published by others as shown in Table 36.2. Immediate postoperative leak and the late stricture can be managed conservatively. Tendency of the patch to bulge, producing a pseudo-diverticulum might need a second thoracotomy and repair by plication or excision.[8] The postoperative functional results were good.

Biemann Othersen used a free patch of small intestine anastomosed by microsurgical techniques to the vessels in the neck because the neck anastomosis was thought to be difficult to be treated with a colon vascularised patch.

Recently, we have used the colon patch in one of our cases with very long stricture extending from the neck to the lower-third of the esophagus. The patient had a very short esophagus with a pulled intrathoracic stomach (Fig. 36.4). The colon patch was interposed on its vascular pedicle in front of the stomach and the duodenum, into the cervical esophagus extending to almost the whole of the esophagus with some tension. Repair of hiatus hernia was more accessible through the thoracoabdominal approach. The free patch worked well (Fig. 36.5) though the patient developed significant wound disruption on the fifth day, requiring re-closure of the main abdominal and the thoracic wound.

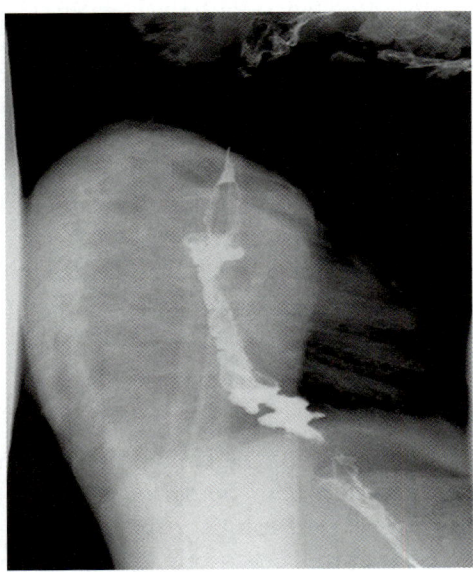

Fig. 36.3: Colon patch involving gastroesophageal junction

Table 36.2: Outcome of colon patch esophagoplasty by different authors						
Literature review	Stricture	Diverticulum	Leak	Secondary operations	Death	No. of cases #
Kennedy	1	1	0	1	0	2
Itgerseb H	3	1	2	3	1	15
Hourang	4	2	1	2	0	16
Raboe	0	1	3	3	0	4
Total	8(21.6%)	5(14%)	6(16%)	9(24%)	1(3%)	37

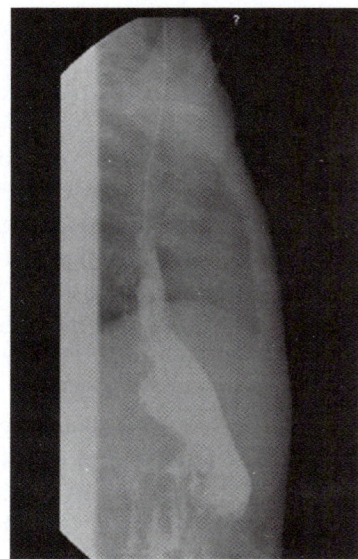

Fig. 36.4: Contrast study demonstrating a scared esophagus with pulled intrathoracic stomach

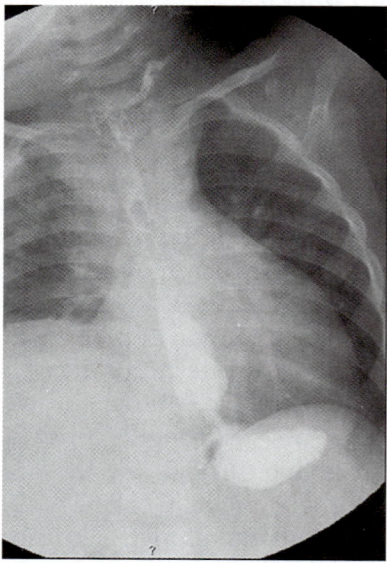

Fig. 36.5: Postoperative contrast study demonstrating a successful colon patch esophagoplasty

This patient continued with bile stained high gastrostomy output and the dye study confirmed the obstruction at the last part of the duodenum. This required abdominal exploration. The pedicle of the colon patch was found traversing in front of the duodenum and the stomach causing obstruction. A gastrojejunostomy with jejuno-jejunostomy was found necessary to bypass the obstruction and avoid any injury to the pedicle supplying the patch. The graft in this case had been passed to the thorax through the hiatus and this might have contributed to the tension on the vascular pedicle. This was possibly avoidable, had an enough length of the pedicle been planned.

CONCLUSION

Colon patch esophagoplasty for short and long esophageal stricture has been used in the past.[11] In the aurhor's series, the immediate postoperative leak from the long suture line has been managed conservatively with good outcome. Our second case with partial anastomotic disruption and prolonged postoperative course make us suggest that fundoplication should be done simultaneously with the colon patch if it has not been done preoperatively. The need of fundoplication has been clearly shown by others in the patients with poor colon patch result. In the third case in our series with esophageal stricture post-tracheoesophageal repair, the leak stayed for long although he has had antireflux surgery. This was possibly due to the fact that he had been left with esophageal stricture for 13 years with many trials of dilatation and laser therapy in another institute. He was living on liquid and semiliquid diet only. The upper pouch was filled with turbid fluid which was coming out of his chest drain postoperatively. He was eating for the first time in his life after the colon patch esophagoplasty.

SUMMARY

The surgical treatment of strictures has been greatly facilitated by the use of the colic patch in which the interposed segment can be tailored to match the gaping defect after a longitudinal esophagotomy through the stricture. The esophagus is not resected from its bed and its nerve supply is not interrupted.

Colon patch esophagoplasty is prone to complications, which can be overcome. Fundoplication should be done simultaneously. Colon patch esophagoplasty is worth considering in benign esophageal strictures, including long gap ones. Our result is encouraging to use colon patch as an alternative to esophageal replacement even for the entire scared esophagus.

There is admittedly no substitute for the damaged and scared esophagus, but of the available conduits, the colic patch has been most satisfactory in our limited experience. We believe it will become the preferred method of treatment of esophageal strictures especially for patients who are difficult to be followed closely in the postoperative period.

ACKNOWLEDGEMENT

The author's would like to acknowledge Dr Reijo Luoma who introduced colon patch esophagoplasty technique in the author's institute.

REFERENCES

1. Bieman Othersen Jr, Smith CD. Colon-patch esophagoplasty in children: an alternative to esophageal replacement. J Pediatr Surg 1986;21:224-26.
2. Hecker WC, Hollmann G. Correction of long segment oesophageal stenoses by a colonic patch. In Rickham PP, Hecker WC, Prevot J (Eds). Progress in Pediatric Surgery. Baltimore: University Park Press 1975;8:81-85.
3. Kennedy AP, Cameron BH, McGill CW. Colon patch esophagoplasty for caustic esophageal stricture. J Pediatr Surg 1995;30:1242-45.
4. Luoma R, Raboei E. Colon-patch oesophagoplasty. Eur J Pediatr Surg 2000;10:194-96.
5. Mehrabi V, Nezakatgoo N, Ansari MJ. Further look at colon-patch oesophagoplasty in benign strictures of oesophagus in children. Z Kinderchir 1989;44:221-27.
6. Othersen HB Jr, Parker EF, Chandler J, Smith CD, Tagge EP. Save the child's esophagus, Part II: Colic patch repair. J Pediatr Surg 1997;32:328-33.
7. Othersen HB Jr, Parker EF, Smith CD. The surgical management of esophageal stricture in children. A century of progress. Ann Surg 1988;207:590-97.
8. Raboei E, Luoma R. Colon Patch Esophagoplasty: An Alternative to Total Esophagus Replacement? Eur J Pediatr Surg. Accepted for publication, Feb; 2007.
9. Thal AP, Hatafuku T, Kurtzman R. New operation for distal esophageal stricture. Arch Surg 1965;90:464-72.
10. Mochizuki Y, Akiyama S, Koike M, Kodera Y, Ito K, Nakao A. A peptic ulcer in a reconstructed gastric tube perforating the thoracic aorta after esophageal replacement. Jpn J Thorac Cardiovasc Surg 2003;51(9): 448-51.
11. Kennedy AP, Cameron BH, McGill CW. Colon patch esophagoplasty for caustic esophageal stricture J Pediatric Surg 1995;30(8):1242-45.

CHAPTER 37

Esophageal Perforation

HS Hassan, HB Othersen

Esophageal perforation is one of the alarming emergencies in pediatric surgery. It is the most rapidly fatal and most serious perforation of the gastrointestinal tract.[1] The incidence of esophageal perforation is noted to be rising, probably due to increasing endoscopic manipulations and aggressive neonatal resuscitation. The incidence in adult perforations is also increasing; Sawyers et al report an upward trend from one in 20000 admissions to one in 8000 admissions.[2]

Fifty-sixty years ago, the disease was always deadly; some believe that it had claimed the life of an ancient great warrior: Alexander the great.[3] In 1947, Barret reported the first surgical intervention for this disease, he repaired a spontaneous rupture of the esophagus by simple suture repair; since then, the management of this emergency condition has evolved rapidly.[4] At present, despite improvement in mechanical ventilation, hemodynamic monitoring, total parentral nutrition, interventional radiology and more effective antibiotics. This condition continues to be associated with significant morbidity and mortality.

A collective review of the world literature reveals a mortality rate of 18-29%.[5] Higher incidences were even reported. In a collective review of 50 cases of neonatal esophageal perforation from 15 series Mollitt et al reported a 30% mortality; another author reports a mortality rate of 65%, mortality rate is lower in children; one author reported a rate only 4%.[6-8] Several factors affect the mortality rate. One of the most important is the time elapsed between injury and intervention. A report showed that if treatment was delayed for more than 24 hours, mortality rate jumped from 13-45%; other factors are the age of the patient, the cause and site of perforation.[9,10]

ETIOLOGY

Intraluminal Causes

1. Instrumentation: Endoscopy, dilatation, intubation (nasogastric or sengstaken tube, sclerotherapy.[11-15]
2. Foreign body, particularly alkaline batteries.
3. Caustic ingestion.[16,17]

Extraluminal Causes

Nasogastric tube, penetrating wounds, blunt trauma operative injuries and fracture spine.[13,18-21]
- Spontaneous perforation (Boerhaave syndrome).[22]

Perforation associated with pre-existing esophageal disease as tumor or esophagitis.[23,24]

In a study by Attar et al the most common cause of perforation was due to instrumentation, 37.5%; among those cases, perforation due to endoscopy was the commonest 54.2%.[9]

In neonates, esophageal perforation is relatively rare.[25] It may be spontaneous, but most commonly traumatic resulting from oropharyngeal suction, passage of nasogastric tube or endotracheal intubation.

PATHOLOGY

Perforations occur either as an immediate total breach of the esophageal wall or as a mucosal laceration that is followed by intraluminal abscess formation and subsequent mural rupture. Thus there may be an interval of many hours between the endoscopy and the appearance of the signs and symptoms of overt perforation. Sharp foreign bodies may perforate immediately, but blunt foreign bodies will sometimes cause pressure necrosis and delayed perforation.[26] An immediate chemical then bacterial mediastinitis occurs which may proceed to empyema, sepsis and multiple organ failure. Mediastinal emphysema occurs early and the characteristic sound can be auscultated over the pericardium. This sign is commonly known as Hammond's crunch. The emphysema can be seen on X-ray films in the mediastinum, or when it dissects far enough superiorly, as it commonly does, it may be palpated subcutaneously above the clavicles. Pneumothorax and pleural effusion may occur. Rupture through the pleura occurs, either immediately or later, as a result of the intense inflammatory response. Rupture into the pericardium has also been reported. The pleural fluid will show a significant amylase activity, thus causing possible confusion with another diagnostic possibility, acute pancreatitis; but serum amylase activity is not elevated in patients with perforation.[27]

Incomplete rupture may occur in some cases; the tear may affect the mucosa only as in Mallory-Weiss syndrome. Continued vomiting and retching may cause the mucosa to become lacerated and a small false lumen of the esophagus to be formed; the lumen may dissect for some distance or remain localized.[28] After sever vomiting, intramural hematoma may result and may dissect and encase the entire esophagus.[29]

CLINICAL FEATURES

In neonates, the most common sign is difficulty in passing a nasogastric tube; the differential diagnosis would be other causes of obstruction as esophageal atresia.[30] The most common symptom is respiratory distress due to pneumothorax, and the presence of increased oral secretion or drooling;. There are also difficulties with feeding: vomiting, cyanosis, coughing and/or choking.[31-34]

In neonatal Boerhaave syndrome, the predilection is to present as a right pneumothorax as opposed to rupture into the left pleural cavity most commonly found in adults, this difference is explained by the close adherence of the aorta to the left side of the esophagus. Dyspnea followed by cyanosis may occur shortly after birth, but usually delayed to six-thirty hours; both are relate to tension pneumothorax. If perforation remains undiagnosed, respiratory distress worsen with the first feeding. Vomiting, coughing, choking episodes and mild hematemesis have been observed. Thoracocentesis may reveal serosanguineous or grossly bloody pleural fluid as well as the contents of the previous feeding. If a chest tube is placed for reduction of the tension pneumothorax hydropneumothorax, formula may reappear immediately following feeding. times, pleural fluid may contain fibrin.[35-41]

In older children there is pain in the neck, chest or epigastrium, depending on the site of perforation. Pain is increased by movement of the head or by swallowing when the perforation is cervical. There is also dysphagia and odynophagia. Palpable subcutaneous emphysema in the neck, due to migration of air upward, may be present.[42] The air trapped in the mediastinum causes a crunching sound on chest auscultation (Hammond's sign). However, these are not frequent in children as they are in adults.[43] Tachycardia, fever, leucocytosis, shock and sepsis may be also present.[33,34]

Perforation of abdominal esophagus from operation or instrumentation may present with both generalized peritonitis and mediastinitis with transit of contaminants through the esophageal hiatus into the mediastinum. If perforation is due to external trauma, the nature and extent of associated injuries to the blood vessels, other mediastinal organs or intra-abdominal contents will determine the presentation. Thus, clinical manifestations of the esophageal injury may be obscured by the concomitant injuries.[43]

INVESTIGATIONS

Plain X-ray

Pneumomediastinum is the abnormality seen most often on plain films and loss of the contour of the descending thoracic aorta due to density seen in the left cardiophrenic angle. In cases with delayed intervention, pleural effusion, pneumothorax, hydropneumothorax mediastinal abscess, mediastinal widening sometimes associated with fluid levels and subcutaneous emphysema might be seen.[45-47]

In cases with suspected perforation in which plain X-ray is negative, a contrast study using diatrizoate meglumine (gastrograffin; Schering Health Care) or iopamidole (Gastromiro; E Merck Pharmaceuticals), which may show a leak; if there is no leak detected, a major perforation is not usually present; and if perforation is still highly suspected, then a barium study could be done safely.[48] Barium is more likely to detect small perforations due to its greater radiographic density and better mucosal adherence.[49]

CT Scan

The study may reveal loculated mediastinal fluid collections, loculated pleural fluid collections. pneumothorax and pneumomediastinum and pulmonary infiltrates. The exact site of perforation can not be assessed by CT, but it may: (1) Determine the presence and extent of mediastinal and pleural involvement initially, and maps the area of surgical drainage, (2) Enables good evaluation of the efficacy of surgical drainage, (3) Gives excellent information about the position of the drainage tube. (4) Shows lesions not seen on the chest X-rays, such as anterior pneumothorax, lung perforation by chest tube, pleural effusion, and pulmonary infiltrates.[50]

TREATMENT

Conservative Management

Mediastinal tissue seems more resistant and esophageal perforation appears more contained in children than adults. When the perforation is restricted to the mediastinum with adequate drainage into the esophageal lumen, only local esophageal suction drainage is necessary. If perforation extends into the pleural cavity, usually on the right side. a thoracic drain is introduced. In case of delayed treatment with formation of intrathoracic abscess, thoracotomy is performed with drainage of the abscess, and when a prolonged period of esophageal obstruction is expected, gastrostomy is performed. Esophagograms are repeated after 10 days. If no perforation can be detected any longer, oral feeding is resumed. Otherwise, drainage is continued for another 10-day period until perforation has disappeared. Suture repair is indicated only in the case of large tear, in which spontaneous healing can not be expected.[51]

Cameron et al[6] made four criteria for conservative management: (1) Esophageal disruption should be well contained within the mediastinum or between the nediastinum and visceral lung pleura, (2) the cavity should be well drained back into the esophagus, (3) minimal symptoms should be present and (4) minimal evidence of clinical sepsis.

Other authors restrict conservative management: consisting of broad-spectrum antibiotics and nasogastric tube for feeding; only to infants with submucosal perforation. Intrapleural perforation can be treated with tube thoracostomy.

Operative management is indicated for massive intrapleural spillage and/or inability to control leakage or pneumothorax with tube drainage and for deterioration of clinical condition or development of complications that warrant surgical exploration.[52]

Operative Intervention

Large tears and massive uncontained perforations require surgical intervention. Many authors prefer to intervene surgically in almost all perforations when diagnosed early, within 24 hours of injury , as the success rate of such interventions is high.[9,53]

Primary Closure and Drainage

This modality is indicated in early cases of perforation, before infection sets in. The perforation is closed with single layer of running absorbable suture (5/0 vicryl). Silk should be avoided as it is thought to excite inflammatory reaction and persists in tissues as a nidus for infection; monofilament sutures are less reactive, but is difficult to handle and the knot may not be secured. A swaged-on needle with suture material that is smooth and thick enough to avoid tearing through tissues is used. Stitches are meant to coapt the edges of the tear without the tension, which may cause necrosis of the suture line and a leak.[54] When repaired early, success rate is 81-87%.[9,53]

Primary Closure with a Buttress

Buttressing the closure with a graft strengthen the suture line and act to minimize the probability of leak, particularly if repair was delayed. Several methods were suggested: pleural patch overlay or intercostal muscle flaps; or pedicled pericardial flap.[55,56]

Debridement and Drainage

In late intervention, tissues which have been bathed with saliva and possibly gastric juice becomes very friable and can't hold sutures. Instead of immediate primary repair, local drainage coupled with feeding gastrostomy or insertion of a total parentral nutrition line niay be necessary, forgoing primary suture repair.[42]

Esophageal Diversion and Exclusion

In late diagnosis, there is usually an intense inflammatory reaction and tissues become very friable, preventing any direct dealing. In such cases, the esophagus is ligated at the gastroesophageal junction using a polypropilene suture snared over a sialastic band and a cervical esophagectomy and a feeding jejunostomy are done.[57] The area bearing the infection is thus excluded from function and is given a chance for healing, after which esophagectomy and esophageal replacement are done. Hopefully, this approach is rarely used.

Esophagectomy and Replacement

In cases of perforation associated with severe damage to the esophagus, as occures in extensive bums after corrosive ingestion; esophagectomy and replacement with stomach, colon or jejunum are done.

REFERENCES

1. Sealy WC. Rupture of the esophagus. Am J Surg 1963;105:505-10.
2. Sawyers JL, Lane CE, Foster JH, et al. Esophageal perforation an increasing challenge. Ann Thorac Surg 1975;19:233.
3. Cirocco WC. Alexander the Great may have died of postemetic esophageal perforation (Boerhaave's syndrome). Jour Clin Gastroenter 1998;26(1):93-94.
4. Barret NR. Report of a case of spontaneous perforation of the esophagus successfully treated by operation. Br J Surg 1947;35:216.
5. Goldstien LA, Thompson WR. Esophageal perforations: a 15 years experience. Am J Surg 1982;143:495-503.
6. Cameron JL, Kieffer RF, Hendrix TR, et al. Selective nonoperative management of contained intra-thoracic esophageal disruption. Ann Thorac Surg 1979;27:404.
7. Banks GJ, Bancerwicz J. Perforation of the esophagus: experience in a general hospital. Br J Surg 1981;68:580-84.
8. Engurn SA, Grosfeld Jl, West KW, et al. Improved survival in children with esophageal perforation. Arch Surg 1996;131(6):604.
9. Attar S, Hakins JR, Suter CM, et al. Esopahgeal perforation: a therapeutic challenge. Ann Thorac Surg 1990;50:45.
10. Bladergroen MR, Lowe JE, Postlethwait RW. Diagnosis and recommended management of esophageal perforation and rupture. Ann Thorac Surg 1986;42:235.
11. Tezel A, Sabin T, Kosar Y, Oguz D, Sahin B, Cumhur T. Esophageal perforation due to endoscopic retrograde cholangiopancreatography. Endoscopy 1998;30(1):S2-3.
12. Hernandez LJ, Jacobson JW. Harris MS. Comparison among the perforation rates of Maloney, balloon, and savary dilation of esophageal strictures. Gastrointestinal Endoscopy 2000;51:460-62.
13. Robinson P, Thomas NB. Intra-abdominal esophageal perforation following naso- gastric tube insertion [letter]. European Radiology 1999;9(8):1697-98.
14. Hou MC, Lin HC, Chang FY, Lee FY, Chen TS, Lee SD. Esophageal perforation following endoscopic variceal ligation and balloon tamponade. Jour Gastroenter and Hepatol 1994;9(6):659-62.
15. Attipou K, Sodji M, Durand-Fontanier S, Laclause BP, Descottes B. [Esophageal perforation, a complication of endoscopic sclerotherapy for esophageal varices]. [French] Sante 1999;9(5):287-88.
16. Turken A, Tanyel FC, Hicsonmez A. Respiratory distress due to esophageal perforation caused by ball point ingestion. Turk Jour Pediatr 1999;41(3):391-93.
17. Samad L, Ali M, Ramzi H. Button battery ingestion: hazards of esophageal impaction. Jour Ped Surg 1999; 34(10):1527-31.
18. Pass LJ, LeNarz LA, Schreiber JT, Estrera AS. Management of esophageal gunshot wounds. Ann Thor Surg 1987; 44(3):253-56.
19. Sartorelli KH, McBride WJ, Vane DW. Perforation of the intrathoracic esophagus from blunt trauma in a child: case report and review of the literature. [Review] Jour Ped Surg 1999;34(3):495-97.
20. Venuta F, Rendina EA, De Giacomo T, Ciccone AM, Mercadante E, Coloni GF. Esophageal perforation after sequential double-lung transplantation. Chest 2000;117(1): 285-87.
21. Brouwers MA, Veldhuis EF, Zimmerman KW. Fracture of the thoracic spine with paralysis and esophageal perforation. European Spine Journal 1997;6(3):211-13.
22. Kuo YC, Wu CS. Spontaneous intramural perforation of the esophagus: case report and review of the literature, Endoscopy 1989;21(3):153-54.
23. Morgan RA, Ellul JP, Denton ER, Glynos M, Mason RC, Adam A. Malignant esophageal fistulas and perforations: management with plastic-covered metallic endoprostheses. Radiology 1997;204(2):527-32.
24. Cappell MS, Sciales C, Biempica L. Esophageal perforation at a Barrett's ulcer Jour Clin Gastroenter 1989;11(6): 663-66.
25. Lee SB, Kuhn JP. Esophageal perforation in neonates. A review of the literature. Am J Dis Child 1976;130:325.
26. Stanley C. Fell' esophageal perforation, in Pearson FG, Deslauries J, Ginsberg RJ, et al. (Eds.), Esophageal surgery. Churchill Livingstone, New York 1995;495.
27. Anonymous. Complications of vomiting the Boerhaave and the Mallory-Weiss syndrome. Western J Med 1974;121(I):50-54.
28. Marks IN, Keet AD. Intramural rupture of the esophagus. Br med J 1968;3:536.
29. Thompson NW, Ernst CB, Fry WJ. The spectrum of emetogenic injury to the esophagus and stomach. Am J Surg 1967;113:13.
30. Pumberger W, Bader T, Golej J, et al. Traumatic pharyngoesophageal perforation in the newborn' a condition mimicking esophageal atresia. Pediatr anaesth 2000; 10(2):201.

31. Lee SB, Kuhn JP. Esophageal perforation in neonates. A review of the literature. Am J Dis Child 1976;130:325.
32. Kransa IH, Rosenfeld D, Benjamin BG, et al. Esophageal perforation in the neonate: an emerging problem in the newborn nursery. J Ped Surg 1987;22(8): 784.
33. Weber TR. Esophageal rupture and perforation. In Welch KJ, Randolph J, Ravitch MM, et al. (Eds): Pediatric surgery, 4th edition. Year Book Medical Publishers, Inc. Chicago 1986;726.
34. Aaronson IA, Cywes S, Louw JH. Spontaneous esophageal rupture in the newborn. J ped surg 1975;10(4):459.
35. Harrel G, Friedland GW, Daily WJ, et al. Neonatal Boerhaave syndrome. Radiol 1970;95:665.
36. Chunn VD, Geppert U. Spontaneous rupture of the esophagus in the newborn. J perdiatr 1962;60:404.
37. Dorsey JM, Hohf RP, Lynn TE. Relationship of peptic esophagitis to the spontaneous rupture of the esophagus, Arch surg 1959;78:878.
38. Fryfogle JD. Discussion of Anderson RL' rupture of the esophagus. J Thorac surg 1992;24:369.
39. Hohf RP, Kimball ER, Ballenger. Rupture of the esophagus in the neonate. JAMA 1962;181:939.
40. Tolstedt GE, Tudor RB. Esophagopleural fistula in a newborn infant. Arch surg 1968;97:780.
41. Fleming PJ, Venugopal S, Lewins MJ, et al. Esophageal perforation into the right pleural cavity in a neonate. J Ped Surg 1980;15(3);335.
42. Holder TM, Ashcraft KW. Esophagus in Welch KJ (Ed): complications of pediatric surgery. Prevention and management. W B Saunders Co. Philadelphia 1982;199.
43. Mercer CID, Hill LID. Perforation, rupture and injury of the esophagus. In Hill Ld, Kozarek R, McCallum R, et al. (Eds). The esophagus. Medical and surgical management. WB Saunders Co. Philadelphia 1988;211.
44. Kimura K, Kubo M, Okasora T, et al. Esophageal perforation in a neonate associated with gastrointestinal reflux. J Ped Surg 1984;19(2):191.
45. Panzini L, Burrell MI, Traube M. Instrumental esophageal perforation: chest film findings. Am J Gastroent 1994;89(3):367.
46. Flynn A, Verrier ED, Way LW. Esophageal perforation. Arch surg 1989;124:1211.
47. Radmark T, Sandberg N, Pattersson G. Instrumental perforation os the esophagus. A ten-year study from two ENT clinics. J Laryngol oto 1986;1100:461.
48. Goh GJ, Pilbrow WJ. Youngs GR. The use of gastrografin for esophageal perforation [letter; comment] Gastroenterology 1995;108(2):618.
49. Phillips LG, Cunningham J. Esophageal perforation. Radiol Clin North America 1984;22(3):607.
50. Ben-Ami T, Rozenman J, Yahav J. Computed tomography in children with esophageal and airway trauma. J ped Surg 1988;23(10):919.
51. Van der Zee DC, Festen, Severijnen SVM, et al. Management of pediatric esophageal perforation. J Thorac Cardiovasc 1988;95:692.
52. Mollitt DL, Schullinger IN, Santulli TV. Selective management of iatrogenic esophageal perforation in the newborn. J Ped Surg 1981;16(6)989.
53. Nesbitt JC, Sawyers JL. Surgical management of esophageal perforation. Am surg 1987;53:183.
54. De Limier AA, Harrison MR. Complications in surgery of the esophagus in de Vries PA, Shapiro SR (Eds.): complications of pediatric surgery. John Wiley and Sons, New York 1982;115.
55. Chavin, Field G, Chandler J, et al. Save the child's esophagus: management of major disruption after repair of esophageal atresia. J Ped Surg 1996;31:48.
56. Wheatley M, Coran AG. Pericardial flap interposition for the definitive management of recurrent tracheoesophageal fistula. J Ped Surg 1992;27:1122.
57. Urschel HC. Discussion of Gouge TH, Depan HJ, Spencer FC: Experience with the Grillo pleural wrap procedure in 18 patients with perforation of the thoracic esophagus. Ann Surg 1989;209:612.

CHAPTER 38

Principles of Lung Resection

DK Gupta, Shilpa Sharma

The surgical management of lung abnormalities requires a thorough knowledge of the surgical anatomy of the lung.[1,2] Though thoracoscopic resections have been attempted by the experts, the principles of surgical resection of the lung remain the same and require experience to deal with the various conditions that may vary from case to case.[3,4] A thorough planning is essential for a successful outcome. The surgeon should be aware of all the possible common and rare anomalies that may form the differential diagnosis of a particular case before planning surgery. The ray of imaging modalities available today makes it essential to choose the most appropriate modality for a particular case without increasing the risk of radiation exposure to the baby (Figs 38.1 and 38.2). The recent introduction of multidetector row computed tomography scanners has altered the approach to image the pediatric thorax but would be more relevant in cases with malignancy or some other rare diseases.[5] Bronchoscopy and spiral computed tomography with multiplanar reconstruction is especially useful to identify rare lesions like stenosis of the bronchus.[6]

ANATOMY OF THE LUNGS

A knowledge of the normal lobar and segmental anatomy of lungs and some key anatomic relations to adjacent structures are important for performing a smooth lung resection without inviting any trouble (Figs 38.3A and B).[7,8]

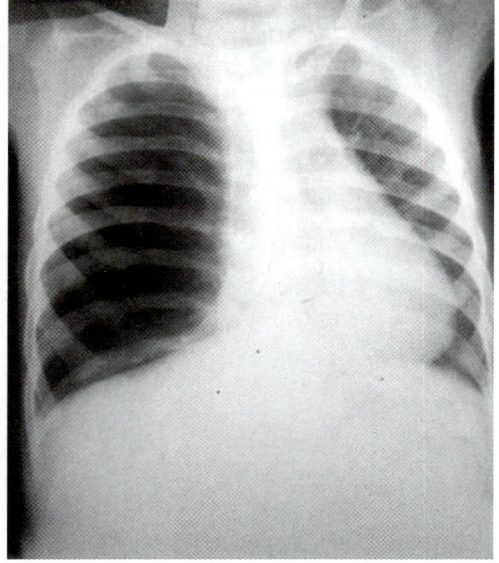

Fig. 38.1: Skiagram chest suggestive of right cystic congenital adenomatoid malformation

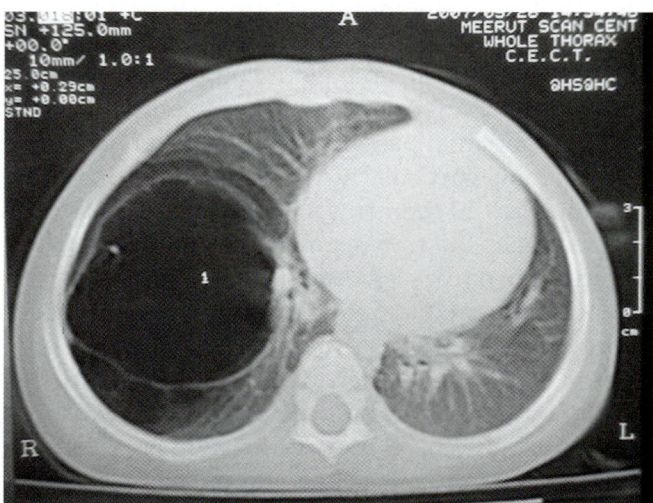

Fig. 38.2: CECT chest suggestive of right cystic congenital adenomatoid malformation with herniation of the right lung towards the left

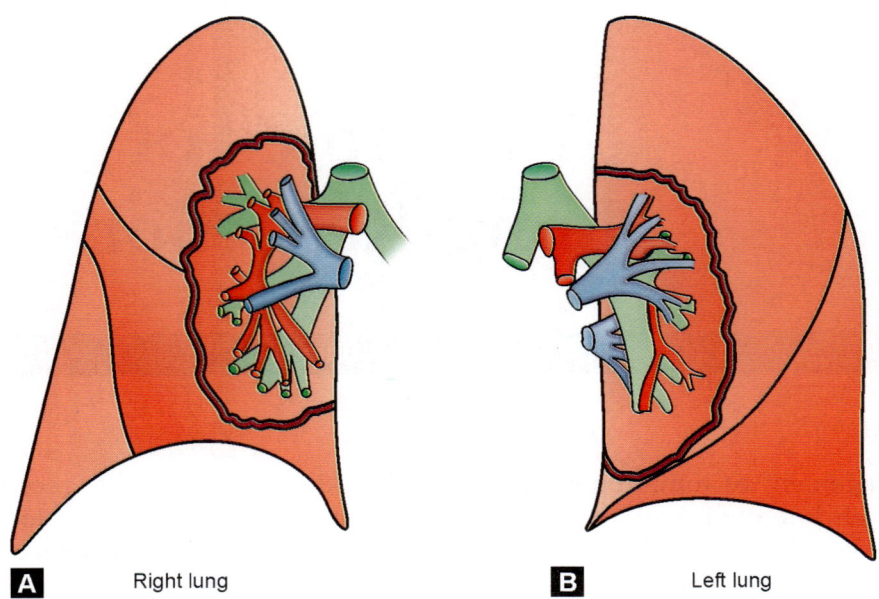

Figs 38.3A and B: A. Diagrammatic representation of the hilum of the right lung, **B.** Diagrammatic representation of the hilum of the left lung

Each lung is divided into lobes by the oblique fissures on both sides and an additional horizontal fissure on the right side (Fig. 38.3). The right lung is normally larger than the left, with an upper, middle, and lower lobe. The left lung is composed of upper and lower lobes similarly situated, and the lingula is analogous to the right middle lobe. The tracheal bifurcation is at the fourth or fifth vertebral body at the time of birth. The right main stem bronchus is larger, more vertical, and about half the length of the left main bronchus (Fig. 38.4). These features account for the preferential passage of the foreign bodies into the right lung, particularly to the right lower lobe. The right lung has 10 segments and the left lung has only 8 segments as the four segments on the left side are fused into two (Figs 38.5A and B).

Each segment is supplied by one or more branches of the pulmonary artery and is drained by its own veins. The bronchus with its branches is central in location (Fig. 38.6). The arteries tend to occupy a position nearer the center of the segments and the veins lie along the intersegmental planes.

The epithelium of the bronchus is ciliated, pseudostratified, columnar epithelium. Smooth muscle demarcates the basal extent of the mucosa. Mucus-producing glands are apparent in the submucosa. Parasympathetic ganglion cells are abundant. Cartilage is an essential structural element for maintaining expiratory patency of the major conducting airways. Proceeding distally in the tracheobronchial tree, luminal size diminishes, and certain features are lost. In particular, as the bronchus becomes a bronchiole, cartilage is lost, the glands disappear, and the epithelium becomes simple,

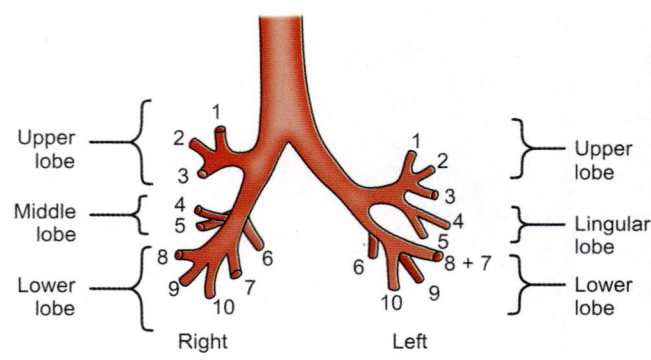

Fig. 38.4: The anatomy of the bronchial tree

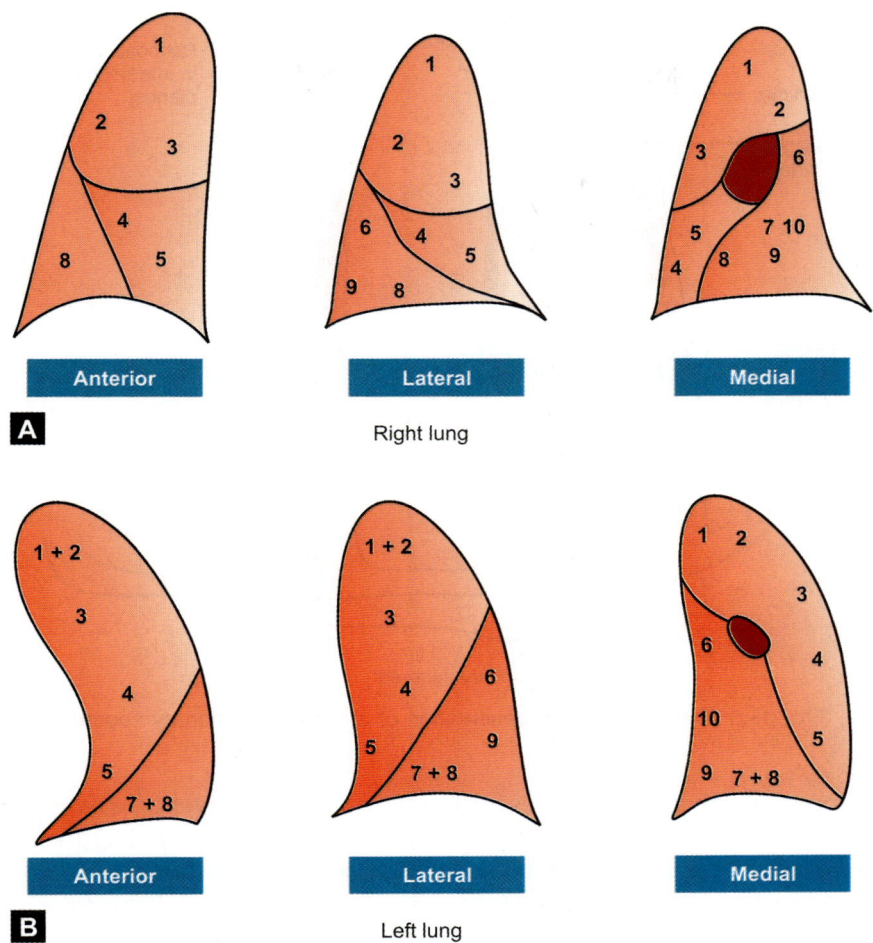

Figs 38.5A and B: Segmental anatomy of the lungs
A. Right lung **B.** Left lung

columnar, and ciliated. Smooth muscle and elastic tissues remain. More distally, these elements drop out of the terminal bronchiole as the need to conduct large volumes of air diminishes. At the level of the respiratory bronchiole and alveoli, where gas exchange occurs, capillaries and epithelial cells are juxtaposed intimately. Most gas exchange occurs by diffusion across a membrane composed of thin cytoplasmic extensions of the Type 1 epithelial cell and the capillary endothelial cell bound by a common basement membrane that is only nanometers in thickness.

PULMONARY VESSELS

The circulation on which respiratory gas exchange depends is derived from the pulmonary artery and its branches. The circulation that provides nutritive support for the lung parenchyma and the bronchi, however, is systemic. Intramural collateral flow from the trachea to the bronchi is derived from the inferior thyroid arteries, which are supplied by the thyrocervical trunks of the subclavian arteries. Venous bronchial drainage is into the azygous and hemiazygous systems. Generally, both arteries and veins follow the segmental and lobar architecture of the bronchi.

Right Pulmonary Artery

It courses transversely for a short distance in front of the right main bronchus and reaches the anterior aspect of the upper lobe bronchus where it supplies

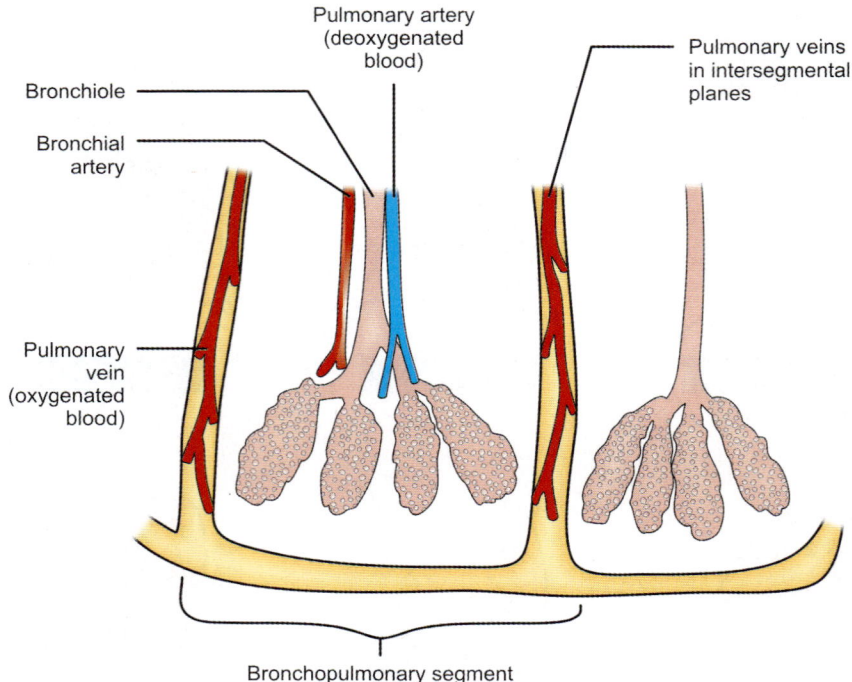

Fig. 38.6: Diagrammatic representation of a bronchopulmonary segment

its first branch to the upper lobe that soon divides into an apical and an anterior vessel. The main pulmonary artery continues downwards, lying in a groove on the anterior surface to the bronchus below its upper-lobe branch and gives off the posterior segmental branch to the upper lobe. The vessel can be found only by dissection in the depths of the fissure as it enters the lobe beneath the fissure.[7]

The middle lobe is supplied by two branches of the pulmonary artery, that arise at the base of the confluence of the fissure distal to the posterior segmental branch to the upper lobe and enter the middle lobe - lower lobe segments. The vessel to the superior segment arises after passing downwards and backwards. A spray of vessels then supplies the remaining four basal segments.

Left Pulmonary Artery

This is longer than that on the right side. The artery curves upwards and over the main bronchus then gives off the first branch which supplies the apical and posterior segments.[7] The vessel then arches behind the upper lobe bronchus, gives off branches to the upper three segments of the lobe. In the interlobar fissure the main vessel gives off a single lingular artery which may be one or may divide into a vessel to each segments of the lingula. The left lower-lobe arteries come from the interlobar part of the main vessel, much as on the right. They come off, more distally, arising close to the bronchi of their segments of supply.

Pulmonary Veins

The venous system is similar on both sides. The veins draining the segments converge to form large trunks and end as the superior and inferior pulmonary veins at the hilum of the lung.[7] The superior pulmonary vein receives the apical, posterior and anterior segmental veins from the upper lobe and two or more veins from the middle lobe. The inferior pulmonary vein receives the veins from the lower lobe segments. The pulmonary veins are most anterior at the hilum.

BRONCHIAL VESSELS

The small bronchial arteries supply nutrition to the lungs. There is usually one main artery to each lung. These arteries (one or two) arise from the aorta just beyond the origin of the left subclavian or they may come from one of the upper aortic intercostals or from the thoracic aorta. On the left side, the main-stem bronchus and its dependent airways are supplied by two bronchial arteries that arise from the anterior surface of the descending thoracic aorta. On the right side, usually there is a single bronchial artery present and it arises from either the third right intercostal artery or the superior left bronchial artery.

Numerous anastomoses between the bronchial and pulmonary arterial systems are of significance in inflammatory lung disease. Early in the course of inflammatory disease, thrombosis of the bronchial artery branches occurs leading to the progressive enlargement of the bronchial arterial system. Massive hemoptysis is always from enlarged bronchial vessels. Bronchial artery embolization techniques to control catastrophic tracheobronchial hemorrhage require a thorough knowledge of the bronchial arterial supply to each lung and its variations. The intercostals bronchial—vascular interplay supplies reticular branches to the midthoracic section of the spinal cord. It is thus vital to know that paraplegia has occurred following embolization of important spinal branches from the bronchial system.

POSTEROLATERAL THORACOTOMY

This is usually planned through the fifth intercostal space as this gives direct access to the hilum of the lung. For lesions in the lower lobe, the 6th intercostal space may also be used, specially in older children. The skin incision is curved with the posterior part being at least 1.5 cm (one finger breadth) below the inferior angle of the scapula. The skin is incised. The subcutaneous tissue is cut and the muscles are incised in the line of incision. The muscles encountered are latissimus dorsi posteriorly and serratus anterior anteriorly. The fifth intercostal space is counted. It is usually just below the space at the tip of the scapula. The intercostal muscles are incised with a cautery along the upper border of the rib below, until the pleura is reached. The pleura is opened and a Finochietto rib retractor is placed and opened slowly to expose the chest cavity (Fig. 38.7). This gives a direct access to the fissures of the lung. The rest of the procedure depends on the affected lobe and the disease. The lobes of the lung are examined for the extent of the disease. In cases of congenital lobar emphysema, the rounded edges of the affected lung may be appreciated in contrast with the sharp edges of the normal lung (Fig. 38.8A to C). The affected lung is held with the help of a lung holding forceps (Fig. 38.9). The congenital anomalies are usually limited to a particular lobe (Figs 38.10A to C). However, the disease may involve the adjacent segments of the other lobes. Thus, after resection of the affected area, the other areas should also be examined for any residual disease and the further decision is taken accordingly.

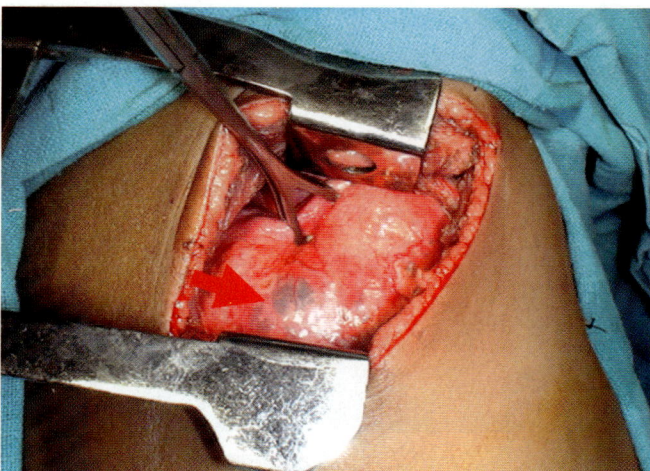

Fig. 38.7: The congenital cystic adenomatoid malformation (CCAM) of the whole of the right lower lobe. The large air filled cyst with transparent wall is marked with the arrow. The self retaining Finochietto rib retractor in place

PULMONARY RESECTION IN CHILDREN

The most common resection performed in infants and children is lobectomy. The pulmonary vessels are large, delicate and thin-walled. These require a different technique than applied to the systemic vessels. Dissection is carried out in a perivascular plane and each vessel should be dissected for a sufficient length, before an attempt is made to pass a right angle clamp behind the vessel. It is preferable to grasp only the adventitia of the vessel. Some surgeons advocate to begin the dissection by encircling the main pulmonary artery proximally with a vessel loop or a blunt angled artery forceps before the more hazardous dissection is started, so that if injury occurs, control is assured. The authors however, do not follow this and feel that a meticulous dissection around the thin walled vessels will prevent any untoward hazard.

442 *Pediatric Surgery—Diagnosis and Management*

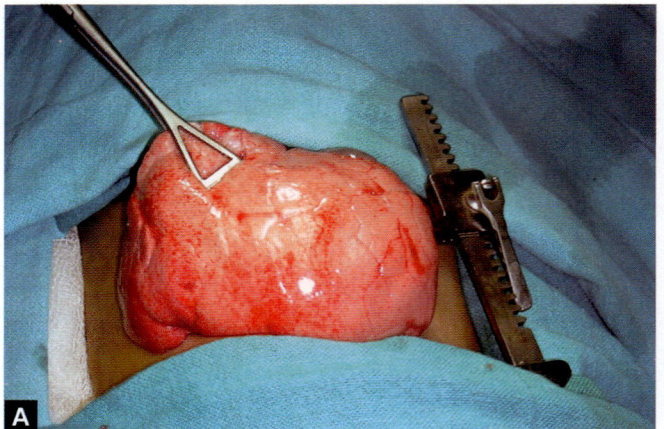
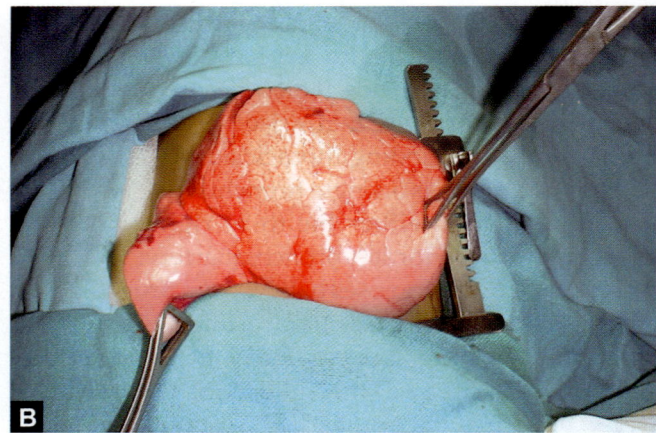
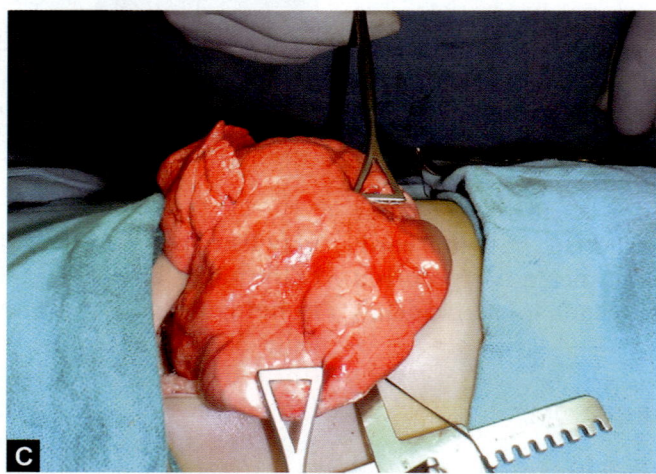

Figs 38.8A to C: A. Rounded edges of the affected lung in a case of congenital lobar emphysema **B.** These are well appreciated in contrast with the sharp edges of the normal lung **C.** An emphysematous bulla may be well appreciated in the affected lobe with congenital lobar emphysema

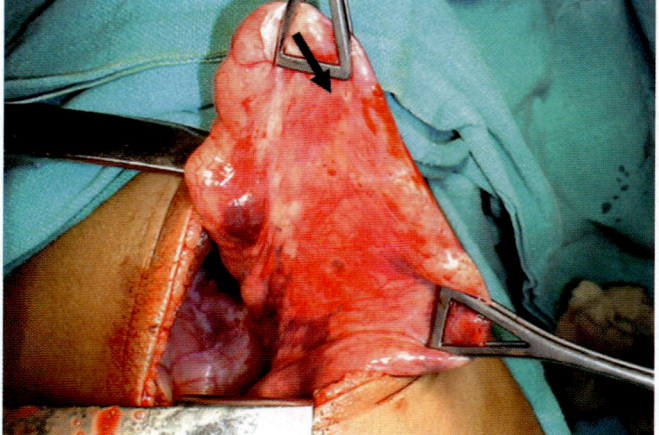

Fig. 38.9: The Congenital Cystic Adenomatoid Malformation (CCAM) of the lung involving the right lower lobe. The abnormal Lobe has been pulled out of the chest cavity. The large cyst has been decompressed, as marked with arrow. Lung is being held by Duval's lung holding forceps

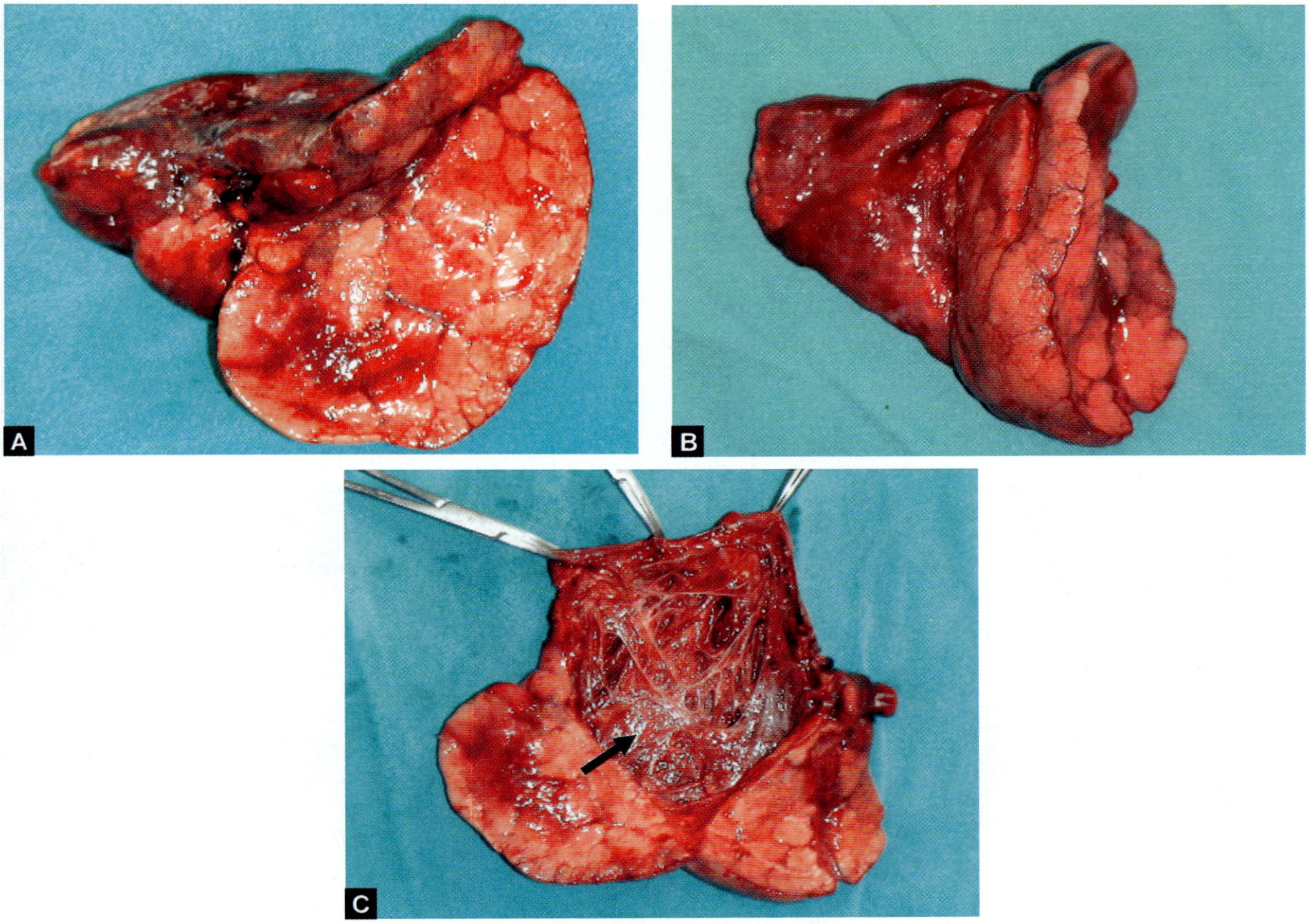

Figs 38.10A to C: The resected specimen of Congenital Cystic Adenomatoid Malformation (CCAM). **A.** Medial view **B.** lateral view **C.** Cut open section, showing the large cyst (marked with arrow) with many other adjoining multiple smaller cysts

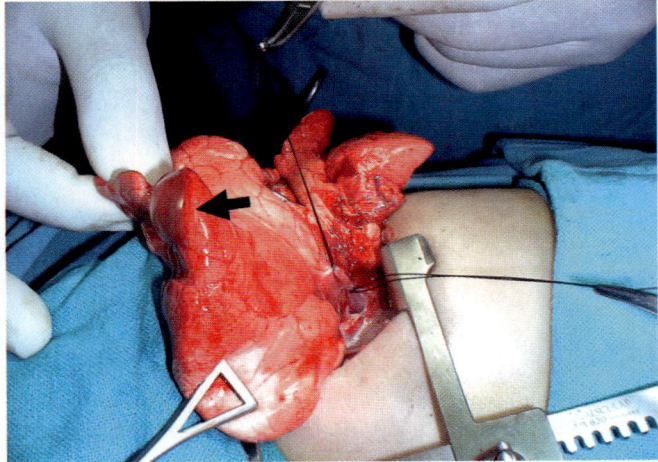

Fig. 38.11: The superior pulmonary vein dissected and held between ligatures. An emphysematous bulla (arrow) can be well appreciated

There are several techniques for ligating the pulmonary vessels. Most commonly, the pulmonary vessels are ligated in continuity and then divided (Fig. 38.11). The technique of triple ligation with division of the vessel, leaving two proximal ligatures separated from each other with an adequate vascular stump is commonly employed. Else a transfixation suture may be applied to the proximal vessel after dividing the vessel between the two simple ligatures. The technique of ligating the main vessel proximal to the bifurcation, and severing the vessel distal to the bifurcation, to produce a large cuff from which the ligature is unlikely to escape, is also safe. The authors also feel it safe and wise to ligate the distal end of the vessel including the lung tissue with it, as this would provides enough strength to the vessel for a secure ligation. It is also important to know that the vessels are very thin and are being tackled while the lung hilum has been stretched, so there are high chances of slippage of a simple suture if ample care is not taken. The role of the assistants is also important to provide a stable environment for meticulous suturing.

Thus, the key points for tacking vessels are
- Vessels should be dissected gently and freed from the investing sheath.
- All vessels should preferably be transfixed and ligated, especially on the proximal side, to avoid slippage of the suture.

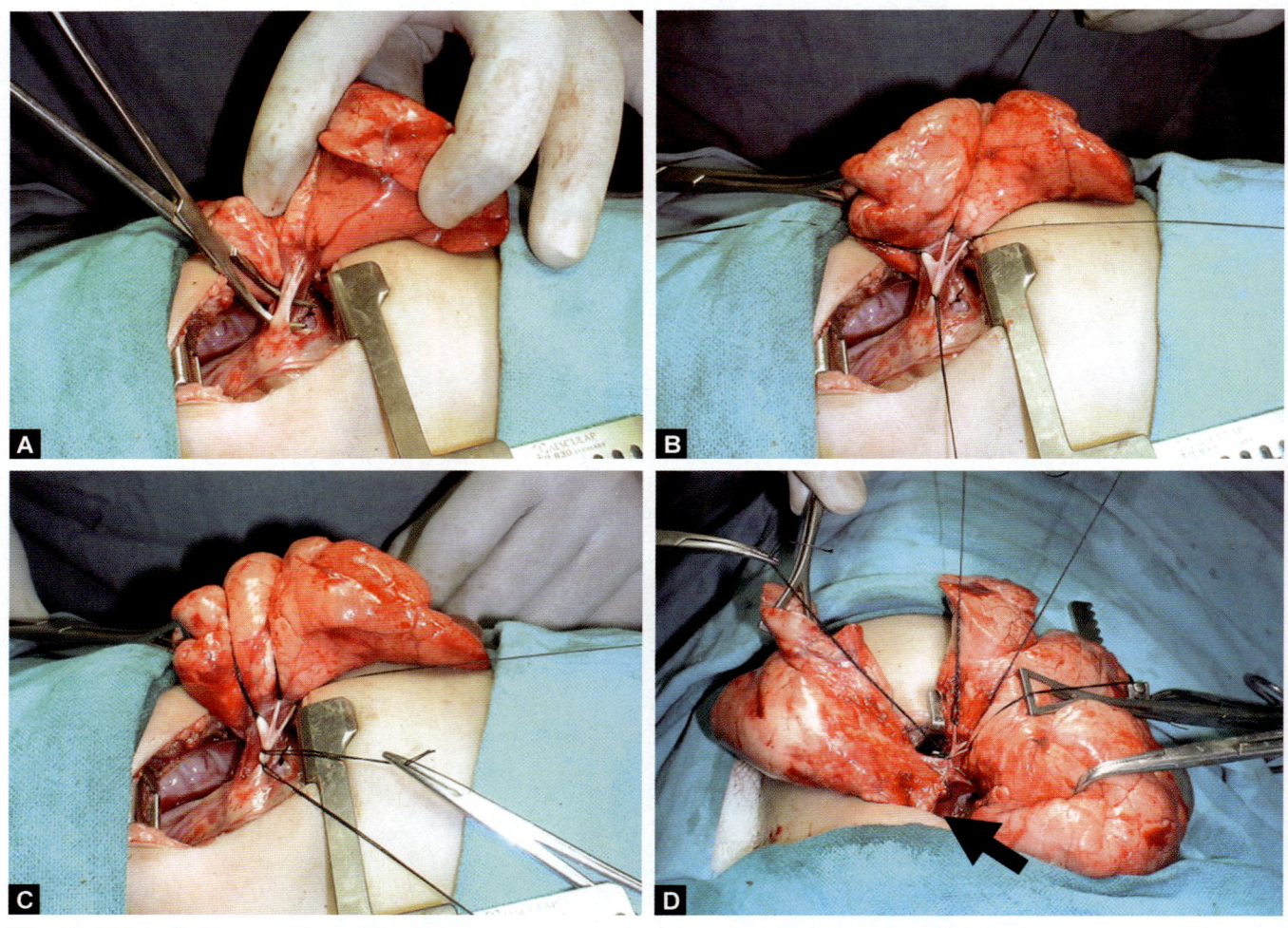

Figs 38.12A to D: The branches of the pulmonary artery to the left upper lobe being dissected **A.** The main branch of the left pulmonary artery to the left upper dissected for a distance. **B.** The distal branches dissected and ligated individually. **C.** The proximal end of the branch secured with double ligatures. **D.** The branches of the left pulmonary artery to the lingular lobe dissected for a distance and held between ligatures. Care should be taken at this step to preserve the main branch to the lower lobe (arrow)

- The vessel should be dissected for a sufficient distance, before being divided.
- Ligation on the distal side may be performed beyond the division of the vessels and this may include even the lung parenchyma (Fig. 38.12A to D).

Bronchial stump closure is easily and reliably done in adults and older children with commercial surgical stapling devices and this technique has the advantage of minimizing potential contamination of the field by an open bronchus technique. In infants and small children, this is undesirable because the size of the instrument may not allow its safe application. When working with small airways, the difference between an acceptable and compromised residual bronchus can be exceedingly small. In addition, some staples may be too large for the secure closure of an infant bronchus. For these reasons, a carefully hand-sewn bronchial closure is preferable in infants and small children (Fig. 38.13). The bronchus should be sucked clean before suturing, while requesting the anesthesiologist to maintain positive ventilation. The inflation of the residual lung should be checked before cutting the desired bronchus. The bronchus stump is closed by using the non-absorbable interrupted sutures (prolene) of the appropriate size. It should finally be checked for any leak while maintaining a positive airway pressure. The residual lobe should be examined for any evidence of abnormality (Figs 38.14A and B).

Right Upper Lobectomy

To access the right upper lobe, the approach is from the anterior side of the hilum.

Two branches of the pulmonary artery and three branches of the pulmonary vein are ligated. The third dorsal branch of the pulmonary artery is ligated.[8] The three bronchial branches and the upper lobe bronchus are then closed.

Right Middle Lobectomy

This is usually combined with a right upper lobectomy or a right lower lobectomy. To access the right middle

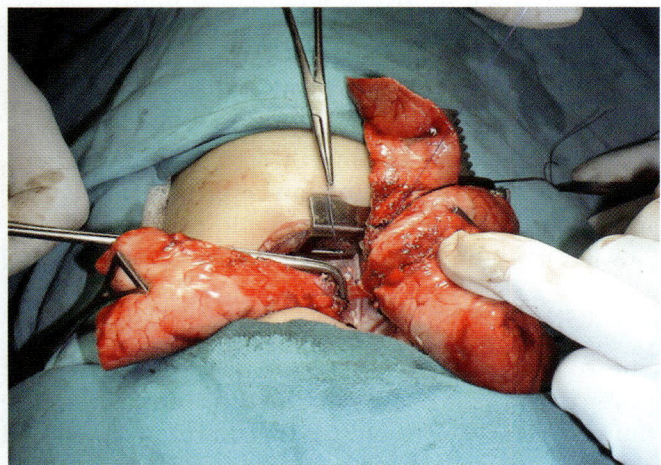

Fig. 38.13: The upper lobe bronchus held with a clamp. The bronchus is divided and then suture closed with interrupted non absorbable sutures (polypropylene)

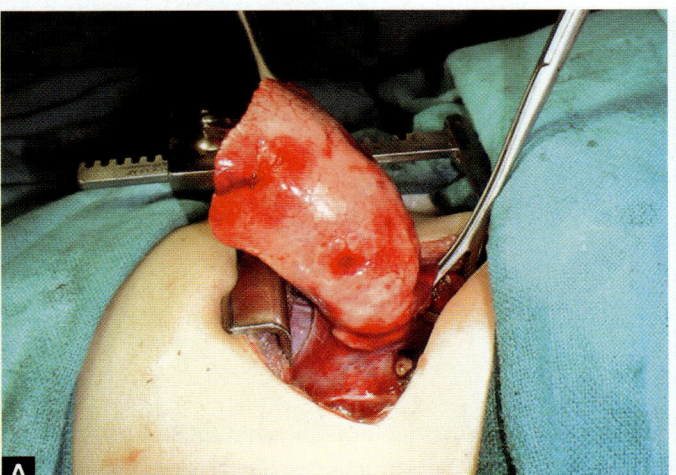
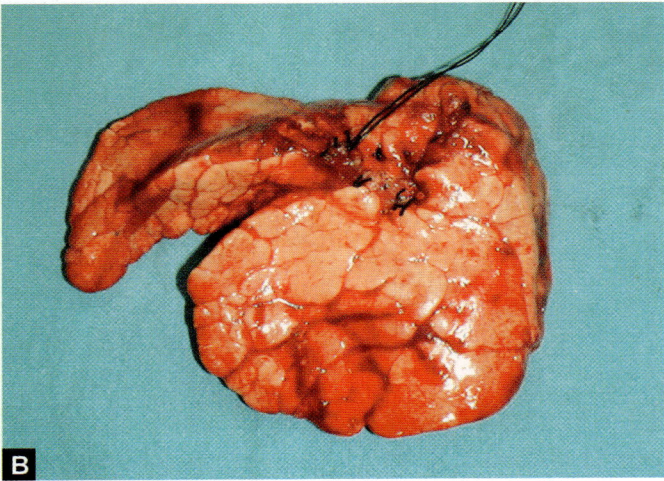

Figs 38.14A and B: A. The residual left lower lobe with intact vascular supply and bronchial connection after upper lobectomy. This will expand in due course of time and occupy the whole hemithorax. **B.** Resected specimen of upper lobe and lingular lobe affected with congenital lobar emphysema

lobe, the approach is from the anterior side of the hilum.

The distal branch of the upper pulmonary artery is ligated. The middle lobe bronchus with its two bronchial branches are then encountered that may be clamped and sewn later. The middle lobe artery is then ligated.

Right Lower Lobectomy

To access the right lower lobe, the inferior pulmonary ligament is first divided. Two branches of the pulmonary artery and the lower pulmonary vein with its two branches are ligated. The two bronchial branches that are visible after ligation of the pulmonary artery branches are then tackled and closed.

Left Upper Lobectomy

To access the left upper lobe, the approach is first the anterior side of the hilum to tackle the vessels one by one. Two proximal branches and two distal segmental branches of the pulmonary artery are ligated. The superior pulmonary vein is then ligated. The upper lobe bronchus is then closed by gaining access through the posterior side of the hilum.

Left Lower Lobectomy

To access the left lower lobe, the inferior pulmonary ligament is first divided. The approach starts from the dorsal hilum and the inferior pulmonary vein is ligated. Two branches of the pulmonary artery are ligated between the upper and lower lobe. The lower lobe bronchus is then closed.

Pneumonectomy

For right pneumonectomy, the azygous is ligated first as it crosses below the bifurcation of the right main bronchus. The right pulmonary artery is found just below the right bronchus and ligated at three places and divided between ligatures. The upper pulmonary vein and then the lower pulmonary vein are ligated. The right main bronchus is then suture closed using interrupted sutures.

For left pneumonectomy, the left pulmonary artery, upper pulmonary vein and lower pulmonary vein are ligated in that order from cranial to caudal direction. The left main bronchus is then suture closed.

MALIGNANCY

The role of thoracotomy and surgical resection of pulmonary metastasis remains uncertain.[9] A large multicenter review suggested that thoracotomy should

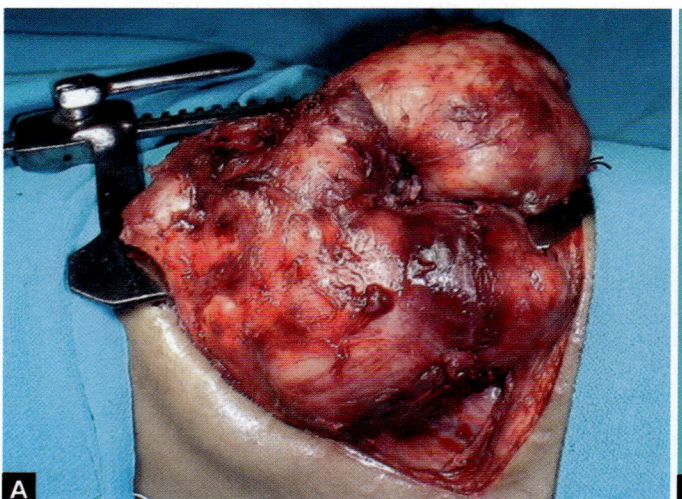 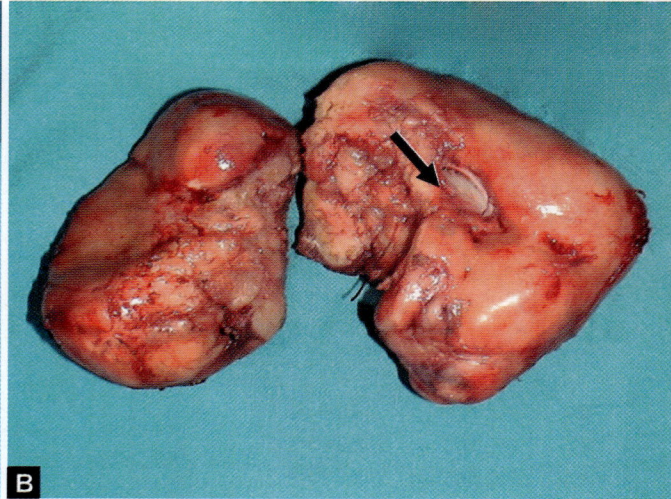

Figs 38.15A and B: A. Vascular pseudotumor of the lingular lobe of left lung lying in the inter lobar fissure displacing surrounding lung that was densely adherent to the chest wall, diaphragm, ribs, intercostal muscles, upper and lower lobe **B.** The mass was densely adherent to the adjoining pericardium that required excision (arrow)

be used cautiously in the management of pulmonary relapse. However, thoracotomy is more appropriate in the management of metastases present at diagnosis that persist after neoadjuvant chemotherapy.[9] Children suffering from cancer are prone to develop systemic fungal infections secondary to the severe immunosuppression caused by the disease itself and the antineoplastic therapy.[10] Intravenous antifungal medications and, when feasible, surgery are used for the treatment of pulmonary aspergillosis.[10] Thoracoscopic resection of metastatic lesions is reasonable for nephroblastoma, but a thoracotomy is suggested for other metastases.[11]

INFLAMMATORY MYOFIBROBLASTIC (PSEUDO) TUMOR OF THE CHEST

Inflammatory myofibroblastic tumors are very rare. These require surgical resection for confirming the diagnosis and providing the only possible effective treatment. A complete resection of the tumor from the chest achieving negative margins, leads to excellent outcome. However, this may not always be possible in all cases as the disease may be fulminant and involve the chest wall and the diaphragm (Fig. 38.15). Various operations performed for this lesion include lobectomy, wedge resections, tracheal/bronchial resections with end-to-end anastomosis and the chest wall resection.[12]

REFERENCES

1. Gupta DK. Management of surgical correctable bronchopulmonary malformations in 3rd World congress on Paediatric Thoracic Disciplines, Izmir, Turkey 2000;20-22.
2. Gupta DK. Oration on Respiratory Distress - Surgery of the Born and the Unborn Child, KGMC, Lucknow, in honor of Retd. Prof AK Wakhlu 2000.
3. Rothenberg SS. Thoracoscopic pulmonary surgery Semin Pediatr Surg 2007;16(4):231-37.
4. Rothenberg SS. First decade's experience with thoracoscopic lobectomy in infants and children. J Pediatr Surg 2008;43(1):40-44; discussion 45.
5. Papaioannou G, Young C, Owens CM. Multidetector row CT for imaging the paediatric tracheobronchial tree. Pediatr Radiol 2007;37:515-29; quiz 612-13. Epub 2007 Apr 25.
6. Anton-Pacheco JL, Galletti L, Cabezali D, et al. Management of bilateral congenital bronchial stenosis in an infant. J Pediatr Surg 2007;42(11):E1-3.
7. Decker GAG, Plessis DJD. The Chest wall, lungs and mediastinum. Lee McGregor's synopsis of Surgical Anatomy Decker GAG, Plessis DJD.Editors Chapter 11.137-52.
8. Willital G H. Lung Resection In Atlas of Children's Surgery (1st edn) 1st Edition. G H Willital, E Kielly, Amin Gohary, Devendra K Gupta, Minju Li, Y.Tsuchida, PABST Publishers, Germany 2005;38-42.
9. Meyers RL, Katzenstein HM, Krailo M, et al. Surgical resection of pulmonary metastatic lesions in children with hepatoblastoma. J Pediatr Surg 2007;42(12):2050-56.
10. Doganis D, Baka M, Pourtsidis A, et al. Successful combination of antifungal agents and surgical resection for pulmonary aspergillosis in a child with Hodgkin disease: review of the literature. Pediatr Hematol Oncol 2007;24:631-38.
11. Guye E, Lardy H, Piolat C, et al. Thoracoscopy and solid tumors in children: a multicenter study. J Laparoendosc Adv Surg Tech A 2007;17:825-30.
12. Lee HJ, Kim JS, Choi YS, et al. Treatment of inflammatory myofibroblastic tumor of the chest: the extent of resection: Ann Thorac Surg. 2007;84:221-24.

Lung Anomalies

John Aiken

Infants and children manifest an extraordinary diversity of congenital and acquired abnormalities of the lung, and collectively these lesions have become increasingly important indications for pulmonary resection in childhood. Although the spectrum of lung abnormalities in children encompasses lesions with diverse etiologies, there is considerable overlap in presentation, anatomic variation, and radiographic appearance of chest lesions.[1] The widespread use of prenatal ultrasound in the past two decades, even in uncomplicated pregnancies, in concert with technological advances in imaging technology has resulted in a dramatic increase in identification of these chest lesions and a better understanding of their natural history. Furthermore, this period has also seen the development of the field of advanced fetal interventions.

Surgical treatment was first used in the 1930's and 1940's, with Reinhoff successfully excising a unilocular cyst from the right upper lobe in 1933, and Fischer reporting the removal of the right upper and middle lobes for cystic disease in a 1-month-old infant a decade later.

Patients with these chest lesions may be asymptomatic, or critically ill with respiratory insufficiency. Great progress has been made toward a better understanding of the natural history with regard to diagnostic and therapeutic possibilities. An efficient and organized approach for the evaluation of these patients should lead to excellent outcomes, although a definitive diagnosis may not be made until surgery. Recent advances in thoracoscopy and video-assisted thoracoscopic surgery have changed practice and decreased morbidity.

EMBRYOLOGY

Lung growth and development begin at approximately 3 weeks' of gestation and proceed until about 8 years of age. Early in prenatal life, developing of the conducting airways (i.e. trachea through to terminal bronchioles) occurs, while in the late prenatal period (after about 16 weeks gestation), the gas exchange units (i.e. respiratory bronchioles, alveolar ducts and alveoli) form. Early childhood experiences the growth of the lung and the continued formation of alveoli. By approximately 8 years of life, lung development is complete and no new alveoli are formed.

The traditional understanding is that the tracheobronchial tree and proximal gastrointestinal tract arise from common foregut anlagen and thus, the term *bronchopulmonary foregut malformation* is often used to describe congenital lung cysts.

At the end of the third week of gestation, the larygotracheal groove can be seen arising as a ventral diverticulum in the embryonic foregut. The laryngotracheal grove elongates caudally to form the primordium of the trachea, which develops two lateral outgrowths, the lung buds. Next, the lateral walls of the foregut, called longitudinal ridges, begin to approximate in the midline, forming the tracheoesophageal septum, which separates the dorsal esophagus from the more ventral tracheobronchial tree. Separation should be complete by the end of the sixth week of gestation. In parallel, the more dorsal aspect of the foregut develops into the primitive esophagus. Also by the end of the sixth week of gestation, the trachea has undergone symmetric distal division into the left and right mainstem bronchi. Progressive bronchial branching continues and by the end of 7 weeks' gestation, the primitive lung is formed with 5 major lobes and three to five orders of bronchi. Mesenchymal proliferation follows in the adjacent mediastinum and gives rise to the lung supporting structures, such as pleura, smooth muscle, cartilage, collagen, and blood vessels. All major bronchial beds are present by 8 to 9 weeks gestation, when closure of the pleural peritoneal canal completes formation of the diaphragm. This process is of profound importance in understanding the physiologic consequences of mass lesions in the fetal thorax.

Recent investigation into the embryology of the foregut in chick embryos has called into question this traditional description. These studies, using scanning electron electron microscopy, have described a paired caudal "lung bud" with no identifiable tracheal primordium. Even more elusive is the developmental program of the lung primordial after separation from the foregut anlagen.

NORMAL ANATOMY

The right lung has upper, middle, and lower lobes and is normally larger than the left lung. The left lung has upper and lower lobes and the lingua is analogous to the right middle lobe. The tracheal bifurcation is at the level of the fourth or fifth vertebral body by the time of birth. The right mainstem bronchus is normally larger, more vertical, and about one-half the length of the left. These anatomic features account for the preferential drainage of endobronchial material or foreign bodies into the right lung, particularly the right lower lobe.

The circulation on which respiratory gas exchange depends is derived from the pulmonary artery and its branches. In contrast, the circulation that provides nutritive support for the lung parenchyma is systemic. The main left bronchus and its dependent airways is supplied by two bronchial arteries arising from the descending thoracic aorta and on the right, a single bronchial artery is typically present from the third intercostals artery or the more superior of the left bronchial arteries. Intramural collateral flow from the trachea to the bronchi is derived from the inferior thyroid arteries. Venous bronchial drainage is to the azygous and hemiazygous systems.

In large airways, respiratory epithelium is ciliated, pseudostratified, columnar epithelium. Smooth muscle demarcates the basal extent of the mucosa. Mucus-producing glands are evident in the submucosa. Parasympathetic ganglion cells are abundant, and cartilage is present. Cartilage is an essential structural element for maintaining expiratory patency of the major conducting airways. Proceeding distally in the tracheobronchial tree, luminal size diminishes, and certain features are lost. In particular, as the bronchus becomes a bronchiole, cartilage is lost and the glands disappear. More distally, smooth muscle and elastic tissue drop out of the terminal bronchiole as the need to conduct large volumes of air diminishes. At the level of the respiratory bronchiole and alveoli, where gas exchange occurs, capillaries and epithelial cells are juxtaposed intimately. Most oxygen and carbon dioxide diffusion occurs across a membrane composed only of thin cytoplasmic extensions of the type I epithelial cell and the capillary endothelial cell, bound by a common basement membrane. This is only nanometers in thickness.

Mass Lesions in the Fetal Thorax

Increased use of prenatal ultrasound in even routine pregnancies, along with high resolution ultrasonography, has lead to a dramatic increase in the antenatal identification of developmental chest malformations, but definitive diagnosis is not possible.[2] The natural history of developmental lung cysts discovered prenatally demonstrates that some decrease in size, some actually resolve, and some enlarge.[3] All developmental lung cysts may act as a mass in the fetal chest with potential important physiologic consequences both before and after birth. The presence of a mass in the fetal thorax can result in mediastinal shift, hydrothorax, and polyhydramnios. In severe cases, *in utero* mediastinal compression and displacement can lead to cardiac failure, nonimmune fetal hydrops, and death of the fetus. The mass lesion in the fetal chest may also result in maldevelopment of the lung with the consequence a hypoplastic lung prone to pulmonary hypertension and respiratory insufficiency at parturition. Although the fetal lung mass is typically unilateral, the pulmonary hypoplasia can be seen bilaterally because often associated mediastinal shift affects development of the contralateral lung.

Fetal hydrops is characterized by signs of congestive heart failure, pleural and pericardial effusions, and anasarca. The development of fetal hydrops secondary to a developmental lung cyst is believed to be the result of several factors including; increased intrathoracic pressure, obstruction of the vena cava with decreased venous return and marked central venous hypertension, increased lymphatic transudate across the lung due to anomalous arterial supply with systemic pressure, and congestive heart failure from compression, mediastinal shift, and arterial venous fistulae. In this setting, the mortality of a fetus that develops hydrops is reported to approach 100% and selected fetuses may be appropriate for *in utero* intervention.[2] Furthermore, polyhydramnios and mediastinal shift *in utero* may induce preterm delivery.

Prenatal intervention is controversial and the potential benefits to the fetus must be balanced against the risks to the mother and of preterm labor and prematurity to the infant. *In utero* interventions include; aspiration, placement of thoraco-amniotic shunts and the EXIT procedure. Generally aspiration is associated with rapid re-accumulation of the pleural fluid requiring serial procedures. Thoraco-amniotic shunts have been demonstrated to reverse fetal hydrops but complications include; occlusion, displacement or being pulled out by the fetus, and induction of preterm labor. Delivery should be planned in a tertiary care environment able to provide both prompt thoracotomy and multidisciplinary critical care for a newborn or preterm infant.

Physiologic problems after birth fall into two general patterns of presentation; respiratory insufficiency secondary to pulmonary hypoplasia and pulmonary hypertension in infants and recurrent pulmonary infections and persistent radiographic abnormalities in older children.

CONGENITAL DISORDERS

Congenital Cystic Adenomatoid Malformation (CCAM)

Congenital cystic adenomatoid malformation (CCAM) is a term applied to a cystic, solid or mixed intra-pulmonary mass that communicates with the normal tracheobronchial tree. These lesions are characterized on pathologic examination by excessive proliferation of terminal respiratory structures (usually bronchioles) forming intercommunicating cysts of various sizes, with an associated suppression of development of the corresponding alveoli. The bronchial (adenomatoid) and alveolar components within the mass can vary considerably, resulting in differences in the ratio of solid and cystic components of a CCAM. The presumed etiology is failure of the bronchial buds to connect to the developing alveolar mesenchyme around 16 to 20 weeks gestation leading to overgrowth of the bronchioles.[4] The cysts are lined by cuboidal or columnar ciliated epithelium and demonstrate a focal increase in elastic tissue. In addition, there is typically an absence of cartilage which may explain the tendency for air-trapping in these cysts. These lesions typically have a normal arterial supply and involvement is generally unilobar, with a predilection for the lower lobes. They are equally distributed between the right and left lobes. There is a slight male predominance, and no racial predilection.

Stocker and colleagues, using pathologic examination, described three subtypes based primarily on cyst size and whether they contained mainly cystic or adenomatoid (glandular) structures.[5] In the Stocker classification, Type I lesions had cysts > 2 cm, Type II lesions had cysts < 1 cm in diameter, and Type III lesions were solid lesions with no cystic spaces. Mucus-producing cells are unique to Type I CCAM. Interestingly, Type II lesions were commonly associated with other severe anomalies including; renal agenesis or dysplastic kidney, syringomyelia, prunebelly syndrome and pectus excavatum.

The increased identification of these lesions prenatally and follow-up with serial ultrasound examinations throughout gestation, has enabled a better understanding of the natural history of CCAMs in utero. Prenatally diagnosed lesions may increase in size, decrease in size, and complete resolution has been reported to occur in about 10-15% of cases. Adzick and colleagues, using prenatal ultrasound, classified these lesions as either macrocystic (> 5 mm cyst diameter) or microcystic (solid or cysts < 5 mm cyst diameter).[6] The characterization is clinically relevant because the natural history for the two subtypes is different. The microcystic lesions are currently believed to be more frequently associated with other developmental abnormalities, and therefore the patients have a poorer prognosis. Associated anomalies, including congenital heart disease, pectus excavatum, renal agensis, skeletal abnormalities, jejunal atresia and others, have been reported, but the incidence is low. The micocystic CCAMs may be seen in association with developmental airway obstruction due to bronchial atresia or stenosis. The pathologic features are consistent and demonstrate focal areas of increased bronchiolar proliferation, variable alveolar development and regional displacement of the unaffected lung parenchyma. Lesions of great size, particularly those that are microcystic or solid in composition, are potentially associated with *in utero* mediastinal, hydrops fetalis, and fetal death.[7] In less dramatic cases, the microcystic lesions are associated with lung maldevelopment resulting in pulmonary hypoplasia and respiratory distress at the time of delivery. In contrast, macrocystic lesions are rarely associated with the development of pulmonary hypoplasia or fetal hydrops. They are often asymptomatic at birth and generally have a favorable prognosis.

Adzick and colleagues suggested that the appearance of anasarca or fetal hydrops in fetuses with microcystic CCAMs is an indication of impending fetal demise; they have reported neonatal survival after fetal lobectomy in a small number of highly selected patients.[2,8] The natural history of *in utero* macrocystic lesions appears less threatening, and although some have been managed with prenatal thoracoamniotic shunting or aspiration, most of these infants can be successfully treated after delivery at term. In addition, it appears that as many as one-third of macrocystic lesions diminish in size during fetal development.[9] This is an important area of active investigation, with lung volume compared to thoracic volume as a ratio emerging as a potentially quantifiable measure to identify fetuses at high risk.[10]

Most CCAMs are easily identified on plain chest radiographs. Larger lesions typically appear as sharply outlined, irregularly shaped, radiolucent areas of multiple sizes. Other consistent findings on plain chest radiographs are atelectasis in the surrounding adjacent lung, mediastinal shift, depression of the ipsilateral hemidiaphragm. In older infants and children, who have infectious complications, air-fluid levels may be present. Microcystic CCAM lesions appear more homogeneous and solid on radiographic imaging. It may be difficult to distinguish CCAM from other chest lesions, particularly pneumothorax or CDH, on plain film. Passage of a nasogastric tube into the stomach or an upper or lower gastrointestinal study may be definitive to diagnose congenital diaphragmatic hernia.

Clinical presentation for CCAM lesions, similar to other congenital lung malformations, is variable. One important factor dictating the mode and time of presentation is the degree to which communication with the tracheobronchial tree leads to air-trapping, progressive lung hyperinflation, and respiratory distress. The majority of CCAMs not diagnosed prenatally are diagnosed in early infancy and respiratory distress is the most common presenting symptom. The severity of symptoms is variable ranging from mild dyspnea and tachypnea to severe repiratory insufficiency. Occasionally, severely affected infants may have all the ventilatory instability of newborns with congenital diaphragmatic hernia. This includes the potential need for conventional mechanical ventilation, high-frequency or jet ventilation, or extracorporeal life support.

Smaller lesions followed antenatally are often asymptomatic at birth and frequently undetectable on plain chest radiograph. A CT scan should be performed at about 3 weeks of age and will almost always demonstrate the lesion.[11] In older infants and children, infectious complications of these lesions secondary to inadequate clearance mechanisms predominate and presentation is typically due to acute or chronic recurring pneumonia.

The principal goal of treatment for CCAM is to resect the area of abnormal lung promptly. Operative management is typically lobectomy. In asymptomatic infants the procedure is generally performed between 3 and 6 months of age. Rarely, cases of multilobar involvement or infectious complications may require pneumonectomy. CT scans are generally obtained to provide anatomic detail and plan resection (Fig. 39.1). Rarely, ventilation-perfusion scan may provide helpful information in planning parenchymal-conserving operations in complicated cases such as multilobar or bilateral involvement. Segmental resection may be appropriate for smaller lesions and has been reported, but data suggest that complications may be higher with no demonstrable long-term benefit with this approach. Pneumonectomy is required in as many as 15-20% of affected patients to achieve complete resection of a complex, multilobar CCAM.[12,13]

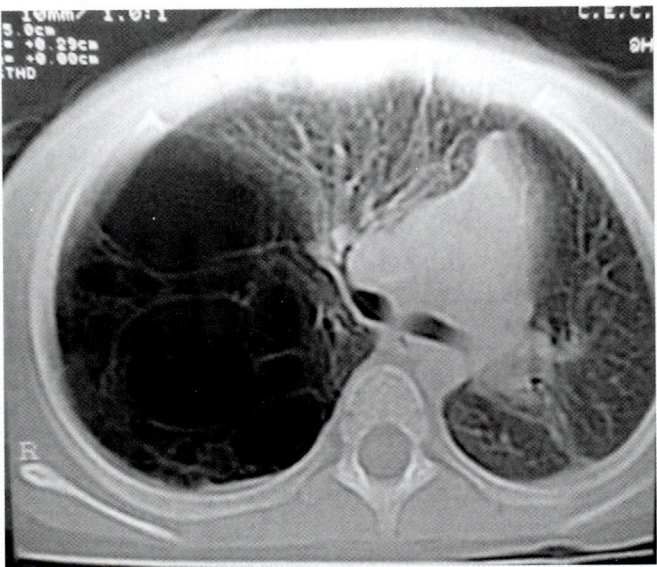

Fig. 39.1: CT scan showing CCAM of the right lobe with mediastinal shift

Thoracoscopic and minimally invasive techniques are currently being used for wedge resection, segmental resection, and lobectomy in selected patients depending on the experience and skill of the surgeon. The use of stapling devices has improved the ability to perform lung segmental and wedge resections without increased risk of postoperative air leak.

Outcome after surgical resection for infants and children is good with survival between 80-100% in modern series.[14] Adzick and colleagues reported survival in four of 6 selected fetuses with microcystic CCAM after *in utero* thoracotomy and lobectomy between 24 and 32 weeks' gestation.[8] The potential complications of lobectomy are similar in incidence as for other lesions and long-term pulmonary function is excellent.

Malignancy in CCAM

There are over two hundred reported cases of malignancy identified in association with developmental lung lesions.[15] Bronchoalveolar carcinoma of the lung has been reported both many years after lobectomy and within a CCAM. In addition, embryonal rhabdomyosarcoma and squamous cell carcinoma have also been demonstrated in association with these lesions.[16]

Congenital Lobar Emphysema

Congenital lobar emphysema (CLE) refers to the abnormal postnatal collection of air within a lobe of the lung that is otherwise anatomically normal. There are a many etiologies which can result in CLE; the unifying theme is partial bronchial obstruction. Mechanisms resulting in CLE include; bronchomalacia due to a developmental defect resulting in the absence of cartilage from a bronchus, intraluminal bronchial obstruction (secretions, mucus plugging), infection damaging alveoli, developmental abnormalities of alveoli, and pulmonary alveolar hyperplasia or polyalveolar lobe. In the classic form, the lobar overinflation is a form of bronchomalacia secondary to a developmental deficiency of cartilage within the bronchial wall that causes focal bronchial collapse during expiration. The cartilaginous deficiency presumably causes the affected bronchus to act as a ball-valve mechanism that permits inflation and expansion of the lobe but not deflation. This specific defect can be demonstrated in about one-half of surgically resected lobes.[17] Endobronchial lesions that may cause CLE include viscid secretions, mucous plugs, or granulation tissue. CLE can also result from external compression of the bronchus including; enlarged heart chambers associated with congenital heart disease, anomalous pulmonary vessels or a large ductus arteriosus, mediastinal lymphadenopathy, vascular rings, and mediastinal bronchogenic cysts. CLE is associated with congenital heart disease or abnormalities of the great vessels in approximately 15% of infants.[18] For this reason, screening echocardiography prior to surgery is appropriate in all affected infants.

CLE is an uncommon lesion and demonstrates an approximately 3:1 male predominance. Interestingly, almost all infants are white and CLE is generally a disease of early infancy. Typically a single lobe is involved. The left upper lobe is most frequently affected (40-50%), followed by the right middle lobe (30-40%), and the right upper lobe (20%). Involvement of the lower lobes or multiple sites is rare.[13] The clinical course of congenital lobar emphysema is as varied as the numerous etiologies, with some infants having mild symptoms that remain stable and others demonstrating rapidly progressive respiratory failure. Respiratory symptoms are nonspecific; tachypnea, dyspnea, wheezing, and cyanosis. The normal responses in infants to respiratory distress and hypoxemia (agitation, crying, tachypnea) exacerbates the process and a vicious cycle ensues. While more than half of patients become symptomatic in the first few days of life, others do not become symptomatic until 1 to 4 months late and some remain asymptomatic. In general, the earlier the onset of symptoms, the more likely the progression of disease with deteriorating lung function and a worsening of respiratory symptoms.

This lesion has significant potential for dramatic and rapid physiologic decompensation in the newborn infant. The lobar overdistension causes compression of adjacent normal lung tissue and mediastinal displacement with herniation of the emphysematous lobe to the contralateral chest (Fig. 39.2). Predictably, the problem may be escalated by intubation and positive-pressure ventilation. In these cases, emergency thoracotomy is necessary and life-saving. This challenging clinical scenario can also occur during preoperative endoscopic evaluation, necessary to eliminate reversible obstructing endobronchial lesions as an etiology for the lobar emphysema, and the surgeon and OR personnel must be prepared to decompress the thorax by emergent thoracotomy and then proceed to definitive lobar resection.

Physical findings in CLE may include an asymmetric thorax, a shift in the apical cardiac impulse to the contralateral side, and focal hyperesonance and diminished breath sounds on the involved side. The plain chest radiograph findings in CLE typically include; lobar hyperinflation, contralateral shift of the mediastinum and trachea, compression and atelectasis of adjacent lung, and flattening of the ipsilateral hemidiaphragm (Fig. 39.3). The differential diagnosis includes pneumothorax, giant cystic adenomatoid malformation, and a pneumatocele. The clinical and radiographic appearance can mimic that of tension pneumothorax, and differentiating CLE from this condition is essential: a tension pneumothorax is characterized by a collapse of the entire affected lung into the hilum; in contrast, in CLE, the adjacent compressed lung can almost always be seen on radiography. In stable patients, computed tomography (CT) and magnetic resonance (MR) imaging can provide helpful anatomic detail, particularly to identify thoracic mass lesions that may be causing extrinsic bronchial compression.[19]

The classic congenital form of CLE is rare in preterm infants; however, an acquired form of the disease has been identified. This acquired form of pulmonary emphysema is more recently described, in the 1970's by Cooney, and is characteristically seen in preterm infants in association with bronchopulmonary dysplasia.[20] The presumed etiology is a combination of barotrauma from positive-pressure ventilation in

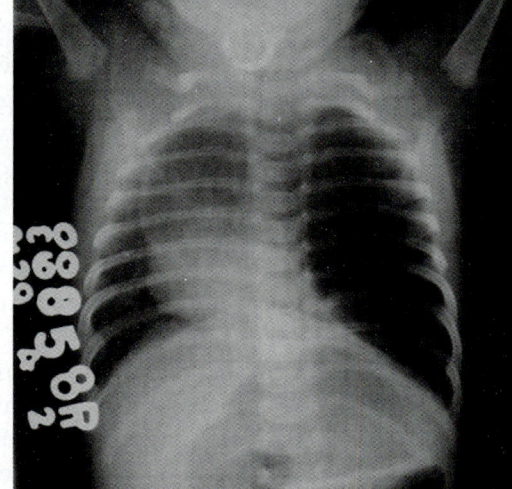

Fig. 39.2: Skiagram of a 5/12 month baby with recurrent URI. The baby had congenital lobes emphyseme of the right upper lobe

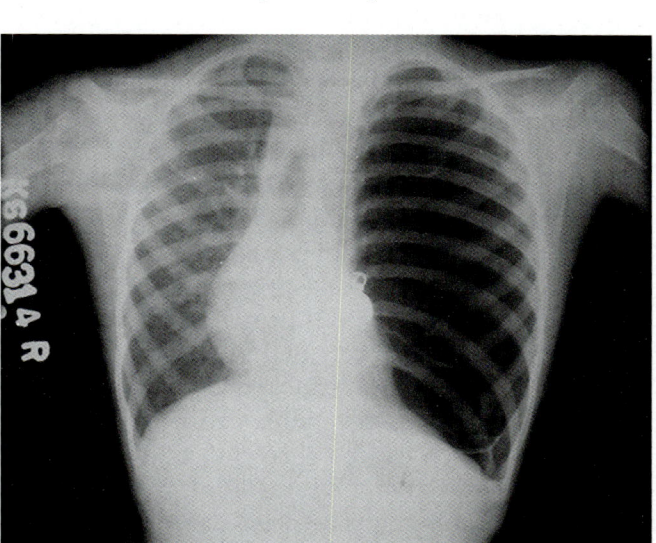

Fig. 39.3: Skiagram chest showing imphysemetous left lobe with flottening of the diaphragm and mediastinal shift

the noncompliant immature lung and oxygen toxicity. In contrast to the congenital form of CLE, the acquired form is seen in older infants because it develops in a time-dependent manner on mechanical ventilation. The hallmark pattern is not unilobar in distribution, but rather, multiple areas of focal hyperinflation and interstitial emphysema and the middle and lower lobes are most commonly involved. Many of these lesions will resolve spontaneously. Occasionally, if a mass effect persists and produces some of the same clinical symptoms of compression of the normal lung and mediastinum seen with other chest lesions, surgical intervention may be indicated. In this setting, outcomes following resection are predictably less optimal than with resection for other lung cysts because often there is little residual normal lung for gas exchange.

Another form of neonatal pulmonary emphysema is focal pulmonary hypoplasia or polyalveolar lobe.[21] This term describes a condition in which a 3 to 5 fold increase in the number of alveoli present results in lobar or segmental emphysema. This condition represents about one-third of cases of congenital lobar emphysema.

The treatment of CLE is lobar resection. Because the causes of CLE are structural, improvement is rarely seen with supportive treatments such as oxygen inhalation, airway humidification, suctioning or antibiotic administration. Medical therapy alone is associated with an early mortality rate of > 50% and 75% of survivors had persistent lobar emphysema.[22] A period of expectant management is acceptable for the largely asymptomatic lesion, however, complete resolution of the radiographic findings is rare, and for this reason surgical resection is indicated.

Surgical resection enables complete expansion of the normal lung and eliminates concerns for potential interference with compensatory lung growth and chronic infection from retained secretions. As noted previously, pre-resection endobronchial evaluation is important to identify reversible causes of bronchial obstruction which can be corrected without parenchymal lung resection. CLE resulting from extrinsic bronchial compression is associated generally with a focal cartilaginous defect of the affected bronchus that is not adequately relieved by simple decompression without lobectomy.

Clinical results of lobectomy in infants and children for this lesion are generally excellent.[23,24] Poor results with reconstructive procedures, such as bronchoplasty and segmental bronchial resection and anastomosis, make these procedures inadvisable. Outcomes after thoracotomy and lobectomy for symptomatic infants are excellent and not different than for lobectomy for other lesions discussed in this chapter. Older children without respiratory symptoms severe enough to warrant pulmonary resection demonstrate normal pulmonary function results in long-term follow-up. In addition, adults who underwent neonatal lobectomy for CLE were demonstrated to have equal ipsilateral and contralateral lung volumes despite the previous lobectomy and this appeared to be related to compensatory tissue growth rather than distension of residual lung parenchyma.[25]

Pulmonary Sequestration

Pulmonary sequestration is a mass of nonfunctioning lung tissue which lacks normal communication with the tracheobronchial tree and has an anomalous systemic arterial supply. Two forms of pulmonary sequestration have been described; extralobar sequestration (ELS) lies outside the normal lung tissue and is invested with its own visceral pleura, and intralobar sequestration (ILS), in which the abnormal pulmonary tissue is incorporated within the visceral pleura of the normal lung.[14]

The precise etiology of the embryologic origin of pulmonary sequestration is unknown. Several theories exist including; formation of an accessory lung bud that becomes an accessory lung mass, embryonic adhesions between the pulmonary bed and the adjoining tissue separates the sequestration from the primary developing lung bud, and persistence of the early embryonic splanchnic blood vessels producing traction on tips of the bronchial tree resulting in separation of the tissue from its "parent lobe". The most widely accepted theory is failure of the pulmonary artery to develop fast enough to supply the whole of the growing lung leading to formation or persistence of systemic arterial supply from the aorta.

Sequestrations represent about one-third of congenital lung lesions in most reported series and the male predominance is as high as 3:1, particularly for extralobar sequestration. Although there is wide variation in reported series, ILS appears to be more common with a ratio of 3 to1. Extralobar sequestrations demonstrate a more variable occurrence pattern in the chest or beneath the diaphragm, but most frequently are basilar, located on the left side at the costophrenic sulcus in the posterior mediastinum, adjacent to the esophagus. Other rare locations for ELS include within the diaphragm and even within the pericardium. ILS is most common within the posterior and basal segments of the lower lobes and more often on the left side.[26] Upper lobe involvement is seen in only 10% to 15% of pulmonary sequestrations and bilateral involvement is rare. None of the postulated embryologic origins for pulmonary sequestration can explain the predilection of ELS for the left side.

On pathological examination, sequestrations tend to be more solid than cystic and demonstrate parenchymal abnormalities similar to microcystic (type II) CCAMs. In extralobar sequestration, the arterial blood supply typically arises directly from the aorta (lower thoracic) and an infradiaphragmatic source is demonstrated in up to 20% of the patients, often passing within the inferior pulmonary ligament. In some large intralobar sequestrations, hemodynamically significant arteriovenous fistulas can be formed and congestive heart failure has been reported. In addition, the abundant blood supply within an intralobar sequestration can occasionally lead to recurrent or massive hemoptysis, spontaneous intrapleural hemorrhage, or massive hemothorax. Venous drainage is variable, but typically is through the pulmonary veins to the left atrium for intralobar lesions and the azygous or hemiazygous system for extralobar lesions. Venous drainage through esophageal or subclavian intercostals and infradiaphragmatic connections to the adrenal or portal vein are reported. As with other congenital lung lesions, many variations in arterial supply and venous drainage combinations have been described.[27]

Coexisting congenital anomalies are common with extralobar sequestrations (> 50%), particularly congenital diaphragmatic hernia, but rarely seen with intralobar sequestrations. Other anomalies seen in association with extralobar sequestrations include; chest wall and vertebral deformities, hindgut duplications, tracheoesophageal fistula and esophageal duplication and congenital heart diseas.[12,13]

Pulmonary sequestrations, similar to other congenital lung lesions, demonstrate a broad spectrum of clinical presentation. Prenatal diagnosis is common, particularly for ELS, and the characteristic appearance is a posterior mediastinal or infradiaphragmatic solid mass. The anomalous arterial blood supply is pathopneumonic on color-flow Doppler ultrasound. Large lesions can be associated with the same physiologic problems described for other mass lesions in the chest. ELS has been associated with severe hydrothorax and fetal hydrops. Because these are often small lesions not typically associated with mediastinal shift and cardiac compression, other etiologies include obstruction of the vena cava or increased lymphatic transudate from abnormal lymphatics within the sequestration in association with systemic pressures.

After parturition, many sequestrations are asymptomatic. The pattern of clinical discovery is different for ELS compared to ILS. Extralobar sequestrations are recognized most often in infancy as incidental finings on chest roentgenograms, particularly in association with diaphragmatic hernia. Other presentations include; respiratory distress, pneumonia, feeding intolerance, hemorrhage, and arterial-venous shunting leading to congestive heart failure.

In contrast, the primary symptoms for ILS are chronic, recurrent respiratory infections with cough, fever, and pleuritic chest pain. The nonspecific nature of the complaints with ILS frequently leads to a delay in diagnosis. The pulmonary infection is introduced through communication with the adjacent lung through alveolar spaces and poor ventilation and inadequate clearing mechanisms facilitate progression of the infection. Because the infectious complications typical of ILS evolve in a time-dependent manner, < 10% of cases are diagnosed in children under one year and only one-third are diagnosed before 10 years of age. The classic presentation of ILS is recurrent pneumonia in the same bronchopulmonary segment, usually lower lobe, in a child > 2 years of age. Recurrent or persistent focal pneumonias, lung abscess, chest pain and hemoptysis are all common.[28]

The radiographic appearance for pulmonary sequestration is nonspecific. Common findings on plain film include; an incidental posterior mediastinal mass low in the chest, lobar atelectasis and pneumonia, and occasionally an air-fluid level. Ultrasound with

Doppler blood flow imaging, contrast enhanced CT, and MR imaging and MR angiography are all helpful diagnostic adjuncts that provide excellent anatomic detail in select patients.[19] Contrast enhanced CT scan and MR angiography has replaced angiography for the evaluation of the arterial supply to pulmonary sequestrations because they provide equally reliable anatomic detail with less potential morbidity than angiography.

The anomalous arterial supply in pulmonary sequestration is elastic and these vessels undergo early cystic or fibrous degeneration. These characteristics in conjunction with inflammatory changes can make control of major vessels challenging during resection. Because of the foregut derivation, occasional communication with the esophagus or stomach occurs and this possibility should be investigated either intraoperatively or preoperatively by axial imaging or contrast studies of the gastrointestinal tract. In particular, an ELS that presents as pulmonary infection should raise suspicion for possible communication with the GI tract.

The standard treatment for both intralobar and extralobar sequestrations is surgical resection. Preoperative imaging typically is CT or MRI. The standard procedure is lobectomy through a traditional thoracotomy incision. For extralobar sequestrations, preoperative imaging is critical to evaluate for possible lesions located below the diaphragm. With extralobar sequestrations, resection does not involve removal of normal lung parenchyma. Although extralobar resections are frequently asymptomatic, resection is recommended for definitive diagnosis and to avoid the risk of hemorrhage, infection, and malignancy. Squamous cell carcinoma, adenocarcinoma, and embyonal rhabdomyosarcoma have all been reported in pulmonary sequestrations.[16] Many surgeons now use thoracoscopy and video-assisted minimally invasive techniques and report equivalent results to open thoracotomy, while avoiding the morbidity associated with thoracotomy.[29] Thoracoscopic series to date have been limited. Patients with intralobar sequestrations often require preoperative treatment with systemic antibiotics prior to resection. The infectious/inflammatory process characteristic of intralobar sequestrations progressively obliterates the normal segmental architectural planes within the lobe, making segmental resection only occasionally possible.

In both intralobar and extralobar forms, a careful search of the thorax must be undertaken prior to resection to identify and control the aberrant systemic arterial blood supply. The aberrant arteries are elastic in type and frequently have atherosclerotic changes, making them extraordinarily friable. The systemic arterial inflow to the pulmonary malformation is multiple in 15% of cases.

As with other pulmonary resections in infants and children, outcomes following resection of pulmonary sequestrations are excellent and survival approaches 100% in the absence of serious co-morbid conditions. In cases of extralobar sequestration, no functioning lung tissue is resected. Morbidity and postoperative complications should be minimal and are not different than for other pulmonary resections. Long-term pulmonary function is expected to be excellent.

Bronchogenic Cysts and Lung Cysts

Bronchogenic cyst is a term which collectively describes congenital cysts located along the tracheobronchial tree or within the lung parenchyma.[4,23] These cysts are believed to arise as a result of abnormal budding of epithelial cells from the primitive tracheobronchial tree. Other malformations included with bronchogenic cysts due to their shared embryology include enteric duplication cysts and neuroenteric cysts. Maier and colleagues classified bronchogenic cysts into five groups based on location: paratracheal, carinal, paraesophageal, hilar, and miscellaneous (pericardial, cervical subcutaneous, and abdominal). About two-thirds of bronchogenic cysts are located peripherally in association with the intraparenchymal bronchi.

Bronchogenic cysts are typically solitary, spherical, unilocular cystic structures that are filled with mucus or fluid (Figs 39.4A and B). They are often attached to but do not communicate with the tracheobronchial tree. Histologically these lesions demonstrate elements consistent with their airway origin including; cartilage, smooth muscle, mucous glands, and respiratory epithelium. Hyaline cartilage plates must be present for this diagnosis and bronchial-type glands generally are present. They typically have a normal bronchial arterial blood supply.

Cystic lung lesions that result from abnormal development of the more distal airways, alveoli, or pleural or lymphatic tissue are termed true lung cysts

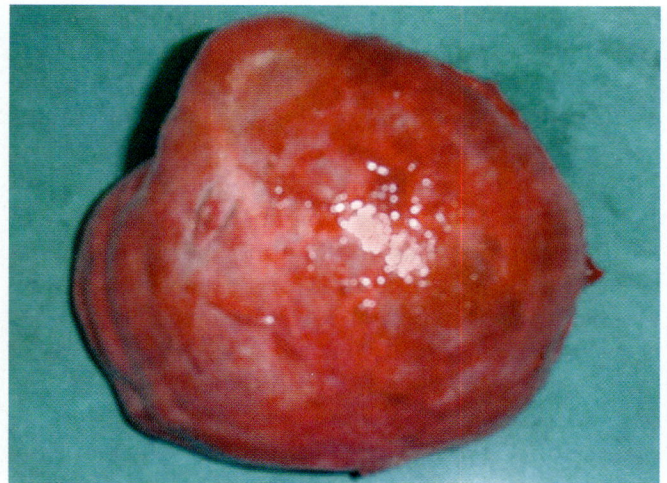

Fig. 39.4A: Excised specimen of a case of bronchogenic cyst containing mucus

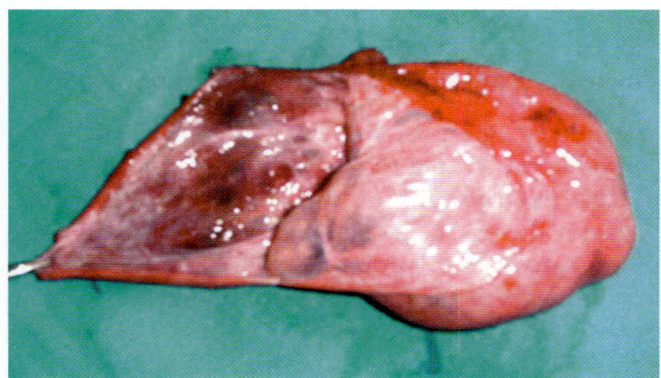

Fig. 39.4B: Cut open specimen of the cyst and the adjoining lung this tissue

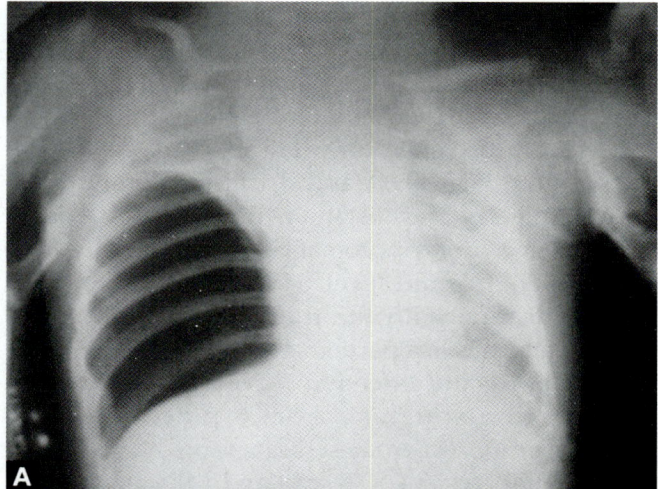

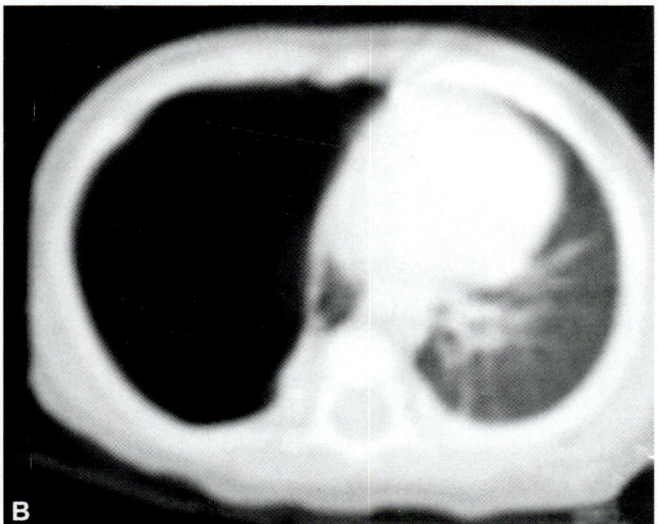

Figs 39.5A and B: A. Skiagram chest of 2½ yr baby who presented with tachypnea. An intercostal tube was placed outside for pneumothorax **B.** CT scan of the same baby showing hypoluscency. On exploration the baby had a peripheral lung cyst and a right lower lobectomy (RLL, cystectomy only) was done

(Figs 39.5A and B). They constitute a heterogenous group of parenchymal lung cystic lesions that even collectively are rare. Differentiation of the tissue of origin is of pathologic interest but generally does not affect presentation or clinical management. One important exception is when the lesion is lymphatic in origin and the result is pulmonary lymphangiectasis. This malformation is typically characterized by diffuse bilateral pulmonary cystic disease, and the outcome is often lethal.

Bronchogenic cysts, similar to essentially all congenital lung cysts, may be discovered incidentally on plain chest radiographs or present with symptoms. The majority of bronchogenic cysts remain asymptomatic and many are first recognized in adults. An exception are bronchogenic cysts in a parabronchial location which often result in progressive air-trapping from partial bronchial obstruction.

Symptomatic presentation is also analogous to other chest cysts including; compression of adjacent hollow viscera, such as the airway or esophagus, or with infection from inadequate drainage of secretions. The most consistent presentation is infection or nonspecific respiratory symptoms in early childhood, such as cough, stridor, or wheezing from airway compression. Symptomatic presentation in infancy is uncommon; however, with mediastinal cysts, partial bronchial obstruction with air-trapping can produce radiographic findings identical to CLE with the potential for acute respiratory distress.

The classic appearance on a plain radiograph of a bronchogenic cyst is that of a smooth, roughly spherical, pratracheal or hilar solid mass without calcification (Figs 39.6A and B). Displacement of the adjacent airway and distal air-trapping are frequent findings, even in asymptomatic patients. The presence of air or an air-fluid level within the cyst suggests communication with the tracheobronchial tree or foregut, and this is a particularly likely finding in the presence of acute infection. Larger lesions can be difficult to distinguish from a lung abscess or macrocystic CCAM on chest radiograph. As with other thoracic mass lesions, CT scan and MR imaging can often provide helpful anatomic detail. Compression of the trachea or esophagus may also be demonstrated on endoscopy or esophogram.

Resection is the standard treatment for virtually all bronchogenic and lung cysts, even in asymptomatic patients because of the risk of infection. This scenario can lead to presentation indistinguishable from a cavitating pneumonia or lung abscess. Persistence of the intraparenchymal cystic abnormality following resolution of the inflammatory process is characteristic. Resection of these well-circumscribed lesions is generally straightforward and in the case of mediastinal cysts, does not require parenchymal lung resection. Occasionally, limited local lung resection or rarely lobectomy may be required. Preoperative antibiotic treatment is necessary for infected lesions. As with many thoracic lesions, thoracoscopic resection of bronchogenic and lung cysts is emerging as a popular approach in selected patients.

Pulmonary Agenesis, Aplasia and Hypoplasia

Pulmonary agenesis, aplasia, and hypoplasia are a constellation of lung malformations characterized by underdevelopment of the lung. In pulmonary agenesis, there is no development of the bronchial tree, pulmonary tissue, or pulmonary vasculature, whereas in pulmonary aplasia, there is a rudimentary bronchial pouch.[13,30] In pulmonary hypoplasia, there is a decrease in the number and size of the bronchial airways, pulmonary alveoli, and pulmonary vasculature. Other congenital malformations are frequently associated with these conditions.

Pulmonary agenesis is the complete failure of development of both the lung parenchyma and tracheobronchial tree. Bilateral pulmonary agenesis is exceedingly rare and incompatible with survival; there are several hundred cases of unilateral pulmonary agenesis reported in the world literature. The embryologic defect is failure of bronchial budding from the trachea in early organogenesis resulting in absence of one or both mainstem bronchi. In the absence of bronchial development, the lung also fails to form. Unilateral pulmonary agenesis is frequently (> 50%) associated with other severe developmental anomalies. Most commonly, these include elements of the VACTERL association (e.g. vertebral, anorectal, cardiac, tracheoesophageal, renal and limb), with cardiac lesions predominant. Pulmonary aplasia is

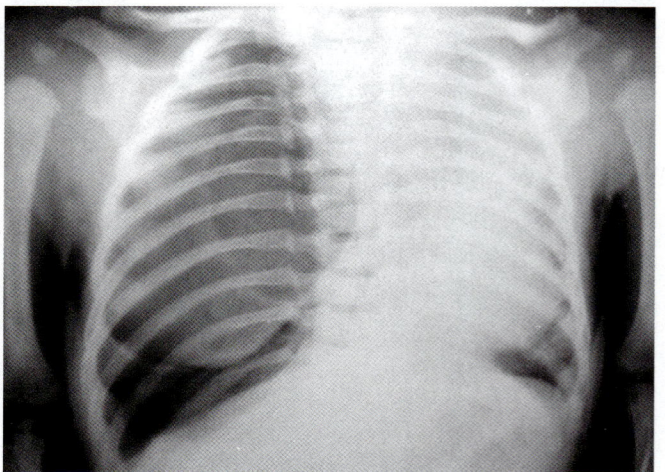

Fig. 39.6A: Skiagram chest outlining a bronchogenic cyst in the right hemithorax

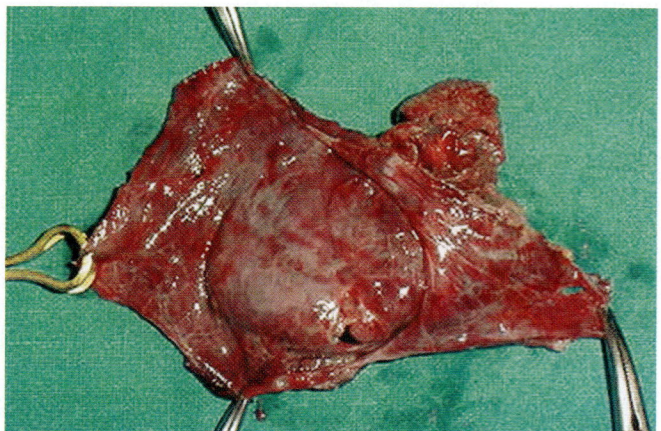

Fig. 39.6B: Excised specimen of the same showing the thickened lining of the cyst

similar with one normal bronchus and a small, blind-ending nub on the opposite side with no or incomplete lung on the affected side.[31,32]

There are several patterns of discovery for patients with pulmonary agenesis; patients without symptoms for whom the finding is incidental, patients with specific respiratory symptoms, or patients with associated anomalies. Respiratory symptoms are nonspecific and include, dyspnea, tachypnea, cough, wheezing, and failure to thrive. Recurrent pneumonia and bronchitis are the most common clinical problems. Infection in the single lung must always be considered a life-threatening problem and aggressive non-operative management is indicated.

On physical examination, the chest may initially appear symmetric, but as the patient ages, there can be a lack of growth on the affected side. Breadth sounds are typically bilateral because the solitary lung expands and crosses into the contralateral chest, but typically only anteriorly, none are heard in the axilla or the base. Heart sounds may be shifted.

The plain radiograph in unilateral pulmonary agenesis is abnormal but nonspecific. Typically one can see a homogeneous density on the affected side with total absence of normal, aerated lung. Herniation of the contralateral lung is best visualized on the lateral film, where it appears in the anterior mediastinum, directly beneath the sternum. On AP film, the ipsilateral diaphragm is elevated and the mediastinum is shifted towards the affected side. On careful inspection, one can see a closer approximation of the ribs on the side of the agenesis versus the normal side. Chest CT scan can be useful in showing the absence of pulmonary parenchyma and tracheobronchial tree. The definitive diagnosis is made by bronchoscopy and the findings are a normal trachea and contralateral mainstem bronchus with complete absence of the ipsilateral bronchus. In children with congenital heart disease, angiography or echocardiography demonstrating absence of the ipsilateral pulmonary artery is pathognomonic. Contrast bronchography is not recommended because it has significant risk to the single normal lung.

The standard treatment for unilateral pulmonary agenesis is nonoperative supportive measures, particularly aggressive antibiotic treatment for recurrent infections. Historically, the prognosis for these patients was poor, and only about one-half of patients with unilateral pulmonary agenesis survived to age 5 years.[13] Most of this mortality is related to perinatal death, problems of associated anomalies, or recurrent pulmonary infections. In more recent years, the prognosis for these patients appears to be improving.

Pulmonary hypoplasia refers to the reduction in size of an entire lung and its individual components. In contrast to pulmonary agenesis and pulmonary aplasia, lung tissue is present, but it is hypoplastic. This condition is characterized by small lung size and low ratio of lung weight to body weight. The mainstem and proximal bronchi are normal, but there are decreased distal bronchial generations and alveoli. Critical factors for normal lung growth include; secretion of lung fluid, distension of air spaces by glottic closing, and space to expand. The embryologic origin is thought to relate to "crowding" in the thorax during organogenesis; therefore any fetal intrathoracic mass lesion can result in pulmonary hypoplasia. Primary pulmonary hypoplasia is rare, with the majority of cases being secondary to some associated abnormality.

The most common cause of secondary pulmonary hypoplasia is a decrease in the volume of the affected hemithorax. There are several causative etiologies including; congenital diaphragmatic hernia (the most common lesion), giant abdominal wall defects (giant omphalocele), pleural effusion (as in hydrops fetalis), or to a small thoracic cage, as in asphyxiating thoracic dystrophy (Jeune syndrome). The next most common cause is oligohydramnios, possibly related to compression of the fetal thorax by the uterus, preventing the lung from growing. Another theory is that the internal stint of fluid that keeps the lung expanded in utero is diminished in oligohydramnios, causing the lung to underdevelop. A third cause of pulmonary hypoplasia results from a decrease in pulmonary vascular perfusion, associated with cardiovascular malformations, such as Tetralogy of Fallot, hypoplastic right heart, or pulmonary artery agenesis. A less common cause is a decrease in fetal respirations which are required to expand the fetal thoracic cage. This decrease in fetal breathing might possibly cause a loss of fetal lung fluid, with resultant pulmonary hypoplasia. Finally, miscellaneous causes include the trisomies 13, 18 and 21. Pulmonary hypoplasia is also seen in Werdig-Hoffman disease or phrenic nerve agenesis.

The newborn clinical presentation varies and depends on the amount of functioning lung tissue and associated congenital malformations. In severe cases, infants demonstrate pulmonary hypertension, persistent fetal circulation, and respiratory failure. For affected infants with respiratory insufficiency, supportive strategies include; standard mechanical ventilation, high frequency oscillatory ventilation, and in carefully selected cases extracorporeal membrane oxygenation (ECMO).

ACQUIRED LUNG ABNORMALITIES

Lung Abscess

A lung abscess is a necrotic, infected cavity within the lung parenchyma caused by pyogenic, toxin-producing bacterial organisms. Lung abscesses are uncommon and most often occur in patients with physiologic vulnerability due to an immunocompromised state. Predictable settings include; (1) post-pneumonic, (2) aspiration of oropharyngeal or gastrointestinal contents, (3) hematogenous seeding, (4) direct spread from the abdomen or from trauma or surgery. Abnormal areas of lung parenchyma with inadequate clearing mechanisms are particularly susceptible. Lung abscesses are considered *primary* if they occur in an otherwise healthy child, and *secondary* when seen in association with pre-existing conditions. Typically a lung abscess communicates with the normal tracheobronchial tree.[33]

There are many risk factors that increase the risk of lung abscess including; altered mental states associated with swallowing dysfunction, hematologic or oncologic disorders, primary or acquired immunodeficiency states, suppressed cough reflex secondary to anesthesia, head injury, or medications, and conditions associated with bronchial obstruction. Aspirated foreign bodies can also lead to pulmonary abscess, as can esophageal functional disorders (achalasia) because they frequently lead to recurrent aspiration. Institutionalized children with periodontal and dental disease and patients treated with chronic antibiotics may also be at increased risk because of development of a large proximal reservoir of potentially pathogenic bacteria. The lung tissue surrounding the abscess typically demonstrates atelectasis and pneumonia. A chronic lung abscess occurs when a surrounding rim of circumferential fibrosis develops.

The inflammatory response associated with a lung abscess recruits phagocytic cells that generate cytotoxic oxidants and proteases that can rapidly destroy adjacent lung parenchyma. The destructive process involves both cellular lung elements and extracellular lung matrix and the result is cavitation.[34]

Lung abscess are typically polymicrobial and reflect oral flora, with both aerobic and anaerobic bacteria. Predominant organisms include; *Bacteroides sp*, Group B hemolytic *Streptococci*, *Escherichia coli*, *Pseudomonas sp*, and Aerobacter aerogenes. *Staphylococcus aureus* and *Klebsiella pneumoniae* are also common and associated with aggressive parenchymal destruction. Fungal infection may also lead to primary or secondary lung abscesses, particularly in immunocompromised patients. Aspergillis, Actinomycoses, and Nocardia sp are most common.[35]

The clinical presentation of a patient with a lung abscess is characterized by fever, cough, chills, night sweats, anorexia, and weight loss. With progression of the destructive process, cavitation and bronchial erosion are heralded by productive cough, purulent sputum, and possibly hemoptysis. Chest radiographs typically show an air-fluid level within a thick-walled cavity in a dependent location, most frequently the right lung; the superior segment of the lower lobe and the posterior segment of the upper lobe. In patients with a lung abscess, consideration should be given to the possibility of an underlying congenital cystic lesion. Definitive evaluation for this possibility is often impossible in the acute setting. Generally, sequential films demonstrate resolution of pneumonia or an abscess, while congenital cystic lesions persist and become more evident.[36]

The medical therapy for a lung abscess requires aggressive antibiotic administration and, as with any abscess, drainage. Drainage commonly occurs spontaneously into the tracheobronchial; thus producing large amounts of purulent sputum. Bronchoscopy may at time be necessary to obtain cultures. Chest physiotherapy, postural drainage, and suctioning are all fundamental elements of care for patients with a lung abscess. This approach should lead to resolution of the abscess in the majority of cases; although a six to twelve week course of antibiotics is generally necessary. Infants, small children, and others who do not expectorate sputum effectively may require more aggressive endoscopic and surgical measures.

Drainage of a lung abscess can be accomplished by a variety of interventional procedures. Endoscopic drainage into the tracheobronchial is possible using needles or catheters passed through a rigid or flexible bronchoscope. The significant risk of these procedures is contamination of an adjacent bronchus or the contralateral lung. Techniques used to lower this risk include; selective intubation of the affected lung, balloon exclusion of the opposite mainstem bronchus, and positioning the involved lung dependently. These risks make general anesthesia required in most cases.

Transpleural diagnostic aspiration and both open and closed external drainage are appropriate for selected patients. The risks of generalized pleural contamination and empyema, however, make these approaches desirable only in circumstances in which the abscess is peripheral in location and chronic enough that there is symphysis between the visceral and parietal pleura. These approaches are best reserved for specific indications in complex abscesses after failure of initial drainage and antibiotics and often performed using CT or ultrasound guidance. Regardless of the drainage technique selected, microbiologic evaluation of the abscess contents is important to guide antibiotic therapy.

Initial empiric antibiotic therapy for patients without risk factors should cover anaerobic organisms as well as gram negative bacteria and *Staphaureus*. Clindamycin rather than penicillin G is recommended due to increasing numbers of resistant oral anaerobes and resistant *Staphaureus* organisms. Ampicillin-sulbactam and Ticarcillin-clavulonate are combinations that also provide excellent broad spectrum empiric coverage. Patients with risk factors such as chronic aspiration or immunodeficiency states should also have coverage for gram-negative bacterial organisms. Long-term antibiotic therapy is the standard for management of lung abscesses, typically 6 to 12 weeks, although the duration of therapy is adjusted based on clinical response (fevers, leukocytosis) and clearing of the chest radiograph.[34]

In addition, immunodeficiency states that can be corrected or modified should have this done. Modulation of immunosuppressive drugs in transplant patients, delay in chemotherapy for oncology patients, treatment with granulocyte colony-stimulating factor for neutropenic patients, and other similar approaches are appropriate when possible.

Operative management of a lung abscess is reserved for patients who fail nonoperative management and demonstrate signs and symptoms of persistent or recurrent infection, and those who develop specific related complications including; massive or recurrent hemoptysis, bronchopleural fistula, and a persistent cavitary lesion. In these settings, operative resection of the involved lung may be necessary. The most common procedure is lobectomy because of the destruction of segmental architecture from infection and inflammation and concern for persistent air leak with wedge or segmental resection. A formidable technical challenge for pulmonary resection in the setting of infection is secure closure of the bronchial stump to prevent bronchopleural fistula and persistent air leak. The use of standard GIA or endoscopic stapling devices has contributed to lowering the mordidity for these resections, and in particular, for wedge and segmental resection.

Bullous Lung Disease

Bullae or blebs are saccular collections of subpleural air within the lung that are thought to result from an air leak from an adjacent alveolus. Generally, the term bleb refers to a smaller air collection within the layers of the visceral pleura and bulla to an emphysematous space greater than 1 cm in diameter. An important functional difference is that bullae are generally associated with the loss of adjacent lung parenchyma, while this is not true for blebs. Blebs and bullae are not associated with normal alveoli or capillaries; hence, no gas exchange occurs within them, although they do communicate with the tracheobronchial tree.[37]

Bullae and blebs may be congenital or acquired. Congenital lesions presumably represent a developmental abnormality of the alveoli and terminal airways during organogenesis. Acquired lesions are believed to result from lung changes related to chronic infection. The process begins with destruction of lung parenchyma leading to loss of elasticity in association with inflammatory changes in the terminal bronchioles producing expiratory obstruction. Consequently, progressive trapping of air, derived from bronchial airflow and/or collateral interalveolar ventilation, occurs in the airway distal to the obstructed bronchus during expiration. The increased pressure that develops with this protracted air trapping causes secondary distension and finally disruption of alveolar walls, producing a bulla. Acquired bullous disease is typically seen in association with conditions associated with chronic or recurrent pulmonary infections such as cystic fibrosis or α-1 antityrypsin deficiency.[38]

Congenital blebs classically present in the teen-age years as spontaneous pneumothorax from rupture into the pleural space. Acquired bullous disease is most often seen in patients with chronic lung disease and therefore the presentation is related to progressive respiratory insufficiency. A common scenario leading to discovery is exercise intolerance from diminished lung volumes and inadequate respiratory reserve.

The standard evaluation of these patients includes plain chest radiographs and contrast-enhanced thin-cut CT scan. Congenital bleb disease is typically located in the lung apices and is frequently bilateral. Acquired bullous disease generally correlates with the underlying parenchymal disease. α-1 antitrypsin deficiency is unique in its propensity to form basal blebs.

The management of blebs and bullae is dependent on several factors including; clinical presentation, degree of symptomatology, and associated underlying lung disease. The classic patient with congenital bleb disease is a tall, thin, athletic teen-aged child who presents with a spontaneous pneumothorax and otherwise normal lungs. Initial management in symptomatic patients is placement of a tube thoracostomy to re-expand the lung and appose the visceral and parietal pleura. After stabilization, CT scan with "thin cuts", particularly in the apical areas, provides excellent evaluation for blebs. Video-assisted thoracoscopic surgery (VATS) has become the standard approach for definitive operative treatment and the procedure involves resection of the apical blebs using an endoscopic stapling device and pleurodesis, generally using mechanical abrasion, talc, or a combination of both. The thoracoscopic approach has lowered morbidity and complications compared to traditional thoracotomy and suture closure of the lung resection margin. Without bleb resection, most series report recurrent pneumothorax in 20-50% of patients after an initial pneumothorax and the recurrence rate approaches 80% after a second pneumothorax.[39] Patients may elect for nonoperative management with the initial presentation based on their ability to tolerate a recurrent pneumothorax. This less aggressive approach is reasonable provided they have complete re-expansion of the affected lung and resolution of any air-leak. Nonoperative management is ill advised if the initial presentation was associated with tension pneumothorax, hemothorax, or hemodynamic instability. The outcome after bleb resection is predictably excellent because parenchymal resection is minimal and the underlying lung is normal.

Surgical management of bullous disease associated with chronic lung disease and infection is more complex and outcomes less good. Bullous disease may affect adjacent normal lung parenchyma by causing compression atelectasis. In these patients with associated lung disease, preoperative planning is essential to correlate areas of disease with physiologic dysfunction and to assess expected tolerance for the procedure and lung resection. This evaluation would typically include ventilation-perfusion scan and pulmonary function tests and is not different than the planning of resectional surgery in any patient with chronic lung disease. In this setting, if preoperative evaluation shows that the bullae occupy more than one-third of the ipsilateral thorax, if ventilation-perfusion scan shows little or no function in the area of the bullae, and if pulmonary function studies indicate tolerance for thoracotomy and lung resection, the outcome is potentially favorable.

Bronchiectasis

Bronchiectasis refers to the structural and functional destruction of the bronchi by chronic and recurrent infection. The most common etiologies in childhood are cystic fibrosis and the chronic lung disease seen in patients with gastroesophageal reflux and recurrent aspiration. The destructive process involves pyogenic bacterial infection that injures and then destroys the structural elements of the airways including; elastin, cartilage, and smooth muscle, and leads to marked collagen deposition and epithelial metaplasia, with replacement of the normal ciliated respiratory epithelium by squamous epithelium. Loss of the normal ciliary transport mechanism further impairs bronchial clearing and perpetuates the infectious process.

Several genetic abnormalities are associated with recurrent pulmonary infections and bronchiectasis in children including; cystic fibrosis, α-1 antitrypsin deficiency, immotile cilia syndrome, and certain immunodeficiency states. Congenital deficiencies of the pulmonary supporting tissues such as bronchomalacia, Williams-Campbell syndrome and Kartagener's syndrome are uncommon associated causes of bronchiectasis. In addition, occasionally endobronchial tumors can result in chronic infection and eventually bronchiectasis distal to the obstruction.

Bronchiectasis can also develop following acute pulmonary infection in an otherwise normal individual, and measles and adenovirus are the most common pathogens. Tuberculosis and pertussis are also important causes in certain susceptible populations. Aspiration of foreign objects that is unrecognized and leads to chronic inflammation and infection is another well recognized cause of bronchiectasis in childhood, particularly in neurologically impaired children.

Bronchiectasis tends to occur in specific lobar distributions, with the lower lobes most frequently involved. Generally the problem occurs in older children and adolescents because the bronchial destruction evolves from chronic infection in a time-dependent manner that typically involves a number of years.

The symptoms of bronchiectasis are a persistent, productive cough and purulent sputum. Because young children often swallow sputum rather than expectorate, the large volumes may be unrecognized. Failure to thrive and poor growth and weight gain are found frequently in association with bronchiectasis with as many as one-half of patients being less than 10th percentile for height and weight. Hemoptysis is rare.

The hallmark of bronchiectasis on plain chest radiographs is persistent findings of focal pneumonia and dilated bronchi associated with hyperinflation in the surrounding lung. Plain radiographs are nonspecific and generally insufficient to adequately evaluate the disease process. Chest CT scan with intravenous contrast and MR imaging have become the standard to assess the extent of involvement and have replaced contrast bronchography and bronchoscopy for evaluation (Fig. 39.7).

Medical therapy consists of antibiotic therapy, including aerosolized antibiotics, when acute pulmonary exacerbations occur and vigorous pulmonary physiotherapy to facilitate bronchial drainage. Bronchoscopy is occasionally needed to assist in clearance of secretions and acquisition of adequate cultures.

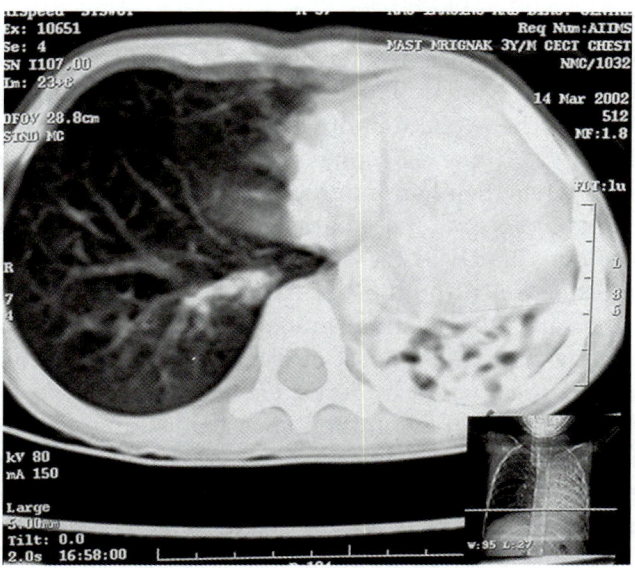

Fig. 39.7: CT scan showing bronchiectatic changes in the left hemithorax

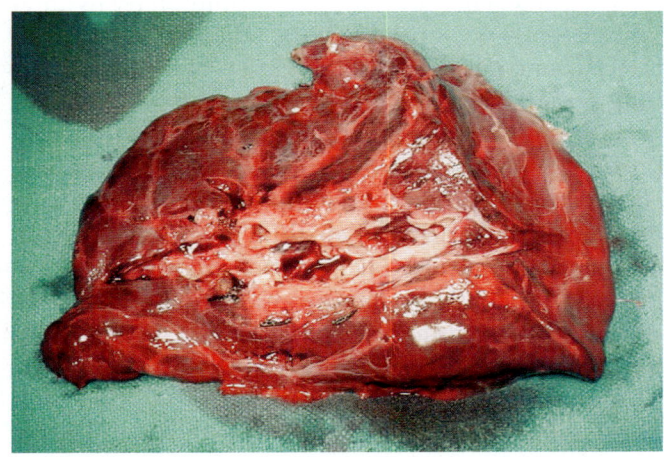

Fig. 39.8: Excised pneumonectomy specimen of a lung with bronchiectatic changes

Surgical Excision (Fig. 39.8)

The surgical aspects have been discussed in chapter 38.

Echinococcal Lung Disease

Echinococcus granulosus and *Echinococcus multilocularis* are parasites responsible for hydatid (watery) cystic lung disease in children. Echinococcus or hydatid cystic disease is endemic in sheep- and cattle-raising areas of the world such as the Middle East, Australia, India, and the Mediterranean countries. The incidence in Turkey has been reported as high as between 1 and

5 per 10,000 inhabitants. Echinococcal infection is endemic but rare among native populations of the Southwest United States, Northwestern Canada, and Alaska. The predominant vector in North America is the dog. Humans become infected as intermediate hosts when their hands or food becomes contaminated by the scoleces of these parasites, which are ingested. The eggs hatch in the stomach and proximal small intestine, releasing the embryos (larval stage), which penetrate the intestinal mucosa to enter the portal venous circulation. Most of the embryos are filtered out in the liver, but some escape the liver to be disseminated, the common sites being lungs, brain, and bone; however, any organ may be involved.[40] The embedded embryos that survive phagocytosis develop into hydatid cysts. In adults, liver involvement is most common, followed by lung, brain, spleen, and other organs. In children, pulmonary echinococcal cysts are more common than liver cysts.[41]

The clinical manifestations of a pulmonary hydatid cyst depends on several factors; whether it is complicated or uncomplicated, the location of the cyst in the lung (central versus peripheral), and the size of the cyst. Some patients demonstrate nonspecific respiratory symptoms such as cough, dyspnea, fever, and chest pain, and others are asymptomatic. Solitary lung cysts are often large, and air-fluid levels may be seen on chest radiograph. Calcifications are rare. Rarely, a large peripheral cyst may produce acute respiratory distress by intrapleural rupture with hydropneumothorax. A central pulmonary hydatid cyst may produce symptoms of bronchial compression with cough, minor hemoptysis, and dull, aching chest pain. Rupture of the hydatid cyst into the bronchus manifests by vigorous coughing up of salty-tasting sputum; hypersensitivity reaction with urticaria, pruritis, severe bronchospasm, and anaphylactic shock; asphyxiation; and secondary infection of the cyst.

Diagnosis of pulmonary hydatid cyst should be suspected in any patient, above the age of 3 years in an endemic area, presenting with single or multiple opacities on the chest radiograph. Uncomplicated hydatid cyst has a sharp outline but is seldom completely circular because it is so soft that it is dented and configured by adjacent structures. Peripheral blood eosinophilia occurs in about one-third of patients with echinococcus. The diagnosis can be confirmed with an accuracy of > 80% with one or more of the following serologic tests; indirect hemagglutination, complement fixation, dot immunobinding, or enzyme-linked immunosorbent assay. Transpleural aspiration is also diagnostic, demonstrating *Echinococcus* sp hooklets and protoscoleces.

The diagnosis of a pulmonary hydatid cyst is an indication for surgery. Antibiotic treatment alone is unlikely to resolve the cyst and surgical resection eliminates the potential for secondary bacterial infection of the cyst. Patients should be treated with periopeartive mebendazole and prompt surgical resection of the thick-walled cyst, with care taken to avoid pleural contamination. The risks of anaphylaxis and local implantation of scoloces appear low with lung disease, but most surgeons experienced with this disease take precautions to avoid spillage whether at the time of diagnosis or treatment.

Removal of the cyst by enucleation without needle aspiration is preferred. At times, wedge or segmental resection is necessary, and even lobectomy if the surrounding lung tissue has been destroyed by prolonged compression or infestion. Agents such as hypertonic saline or ethyl alcohol have been used in conjunction with resection, but the risk is substantial if drainage of these agents into the tracheobronchial tree occurs.

Opportunistic Lung Infections

The number of infants and children who develop opportunistic pulmonary infections (mycobacterial, protozoan, viral, fungal, and bacterial pathogens) is increasing as aggressive treatment regimens for childhood cancer create more immunocompromised hosts. Children at greatest risk include; transplant recipients, oncology patients, patients with human immunodeficiency virus infection, and others. Typically, at risk patients develop diffuse interstitial pneumonitis with a broad range of clinical symptoms from cough and fever to life-threatening respiratory distress. Depending on the underlying disease, many receive empiric antibiotic therapy with trimethoprim-sulfamethoxazole to treat suspected *Pneumocystis carinii* or other possible pathogens. A definitive tissue diagnosis becomes necessary for progressive or refractory disease. The most common surgical requirement for these immunosuppressed patients with interstitial pulmonary disease is to provide tissue samples for histopathology and microbiologic analysis to direct specific therapy. A fundamental principle in the care of these patients is to employ minimally invasive techniques as possible, particularly in neutropenic patients, because of their compromised wound healing ability. Bronchoalveolar lavage may be helpful in identifying some pathogens in immunosuppressed children with pneumonia. Both transbronchial biopsy and percutaneous lung biopsy yield small tissue samples that may be helpful in differentiating among infectious, rejection-related, and inflammatory lung processes. Formal lung biopsy, however, whether by limited open thoracotomy or thoracoscopic techniques, is often preferred because the larger specimens obtainable are more likely to be definitive. Although the surgical procedure is generally well-tolerated, its combination with the underlying disease process yields substantial perioperative morbidity and mortality. In one review of open lung biopsies among childhood bone marrow transplant recipients with interstitial lung disease, the 30-day mortality rate was 45% and the overall mortality rate was 74%.[42] A definitive diagnosis results from open lung biopsy in between 50% and 90% of immunosuppressed patients with interstitial lung disease, although the incidence of treatable disease is substantially lower.[43] The thoacoscopic approach with use of a stapled wedge resection has rapidly gained acceptance in children who are sufficient size to use the commercially available stapling devices the thorax (about 15 kg). Smaller children may also have thoracoscopic lung biopsy, although suture closure of the lung is likely necessary. Conventional open lung using a limited incision biopsy remains an appropriate alternative in selected patients such as those with focal, central disease or prior thoracotomies.

LUNG TUMORS

Primary Lung Tumors

Primary lung tumors are exceedingly rare in children. In a comprehensive review of the world literature in 1983, Hartman and Shocat reported 230 primary tumors, of which approximately two-thirds were malignant.[15] Distinctions between malignant and benign forms of pediatric primary lung tumors are often subtle.

Malignant Tumors

Bronchial adenoma: The most common primary lung tumors in children are a heterogeneous group of low-grade ademcarcinomas termed *bronchial adenomas*. They constitute about 35% of all primary pulmonary neoplasms in children. Patterns of histology in these tumors have given rise to descriptive names: *carcinoid*, *mucpepidermoid carcinoma*, and *adenoid cystic carcinoma (cylindroma)*. The term adenoma is misleading because all are neoplasms with the potential for malignant spread, although the incidence of metastases is low, ranging from 5-10%.[15]

Bronchial carcinoid tumors are the most common, representing approximately 85% in most reported series. These lesions, like other carcinoid tumors, are derived from neural crest stem cells and retain their potential for serotonin and peptide hormone synthesis. Plasma serotonin and urine 5-hydroxyindoleacetic acid levels may be elevated in these patients, and they are therefore potentially useful tumor markers.[44]

Bronchial carcinoids most often arise in a primary or secondary bronchus and the most frequent presenting signs are hemoptysis, cough, and partial bronchial obstruction with recurrent or persistent pneumonia. The duration of symptoms ranges from 1 month to 12 years, with a mean of just over 1 year. These tumors generally involve major bronchi; which explains the fact that the symptoms and physical signs are those of bronchial obstruction. Because of the critical anatomic location, these tumors generally become symptomatic while relatively small, although it appears that the rate of growth is slow. The right lung is affected approximately twice as often as the left.

Bronchial carcinoid tumors generally occur in one of two patterns: (1) as endobronchial polypoid masses that produce segmental bronchial obstruction followed by atelectasis and infection and (2) as "iceberg" lesions with predominantly extrabronchial growth-the small intrabronchial extent of which gives rise to mucosal ulceration and hemoptysis. The carcinoid syndrome has been reported in a single child with an endobronchial carcinoid tumor.

Radiographic imaging is most often nonspecific and nondiagnostic. Bronchoscopic findings are, however, unique and compelling. The lesion is best described as a pink, friable mulberry. Biopsy is not recommended for several reasons: (1) hemorrhage can be substantial or even life-threatening, (2) the histopathology is difficult to evaluate with a small specimen and frozen section techniques, (3) the gross appearance is predictable from a diagnostic point of view and (4) obstructing bronchial adenomas require resection, the nature of which is determined by anatomic rather than pathologic features.

Careful endoscopic mapping under direct vision is essential to planning operative management Endoscopy and video systems have evolved rapidly and offer substantial improvement in this aspect of evaluation. Although endoscopic resection has been reported, it is not recommended because of the risks of hemorrhage, bronchial stenosis, local recurrence, and the inability to examine regional lymph nodes.

In older children and those with small tumors without lymphatic spread, successful segmental bronchial resection has been done. Most patients with endobronchial carcinoid tumors, however, require lobectomy or pneumonectomy, depending on the precise location of the tumor. Regional lymph node sampling, particularly of clinically suspicious nodes, is also appropriate.

Endobronchial carcinoid tumors are radiosensitive, and this may be an appropriate therapy for non-resectable disease, although there are no guidelines due to lack of sufficient data. The 10-year survival rate in children after surgical resection for endobronchial carcinoid tumors is about 90%.[15]

Endobronchial mucoepidermoid carcinomas represent 10-20% of bronchial adenomas. These are typically pedunculated endobronchial tumors that arise most often from the travhea or mainstem bronchi. The presentation and approach for diagnosis and surgical management is essentially identical to that described for endobronchial carcinoid tumors. The principal difference relates to the histopathology; these lesions have both mucus-secreting glandular and epidermoid cells. The incidence of malignancy reported for children with this tumor appears to be extremely low. Only one child is reported to have had malignant spread of this lesion, and in this case the tumor was described to have a predominance of epidermoid cellular elements. The postoperative survival rate approaches 100%.

Adenoid cystic carcinomas (cylindromas) are the least common form of bronchial adenoma in childhood. These are most commonly found in the trachea and are made up of cuboidal or flattened epithelial cells arranged in two layers. The important distinction for this tumor is the observation that it is an indolent malignancy with a propensity for submucosal spread and late recurrence. Clinical presentation, physical signs, and diagnostic approach are similar to those in patients with catcinoids. Intraoperative frozen-section analysis is, therefore, recommended when resecting a bronchial adenoma.

Bronchogenic carcinoma: Primary bronchogenic carcinoma is extremely rare in children, with only about 50 reported cases. Among these rare tumors, most pediatric cases of bronchogenic carcinoma are adenocarcinomas and undifferentiated carcinomas and only 10% are squamous cell carcinomas. These tumors may occur in children of any age, but they are most commonly found during adolescence. The significant risk factor in adults is cigarette smoking; in children papillomatosis is a common antecedent. Most patients are symptomatic with cough, recurrent pneumonia, pleural effusion, or hemoptysis. The disease is typically widespread at diagnosis with mediastinal and distant metastases. Findings suggestive of metastatic disease, such as anemia, weight loss, and bone pain are also common. Although rare, persistent case reports suggest an important etiologic association with pre-existing cystic bronchopulmonary foregut malformations. The experience with bronchogenic carcinoma in children is dismal. The average survival from the time of diagnosis is 7 months.

Childhood bronchogenic carcinoma should be managed according to reasonable adult guidelines, with resection of operable tumors. The limited experience with these tumors precludes meaningful statistical analysis of adjuvant therapy; and treatment is generally individualized. For children with localized disease who undergo complete resection, a small Japanese experience suggests that about one-half have long-term survival.[45]

Pleuropulmonary blastoma: Pleuropulmonary blastoma (PPB) is an embryonal tumor of the lung that appears to arise during organ development, much like Wilm' tumor in the kidney, hepatoblastoma in the liver, and rhabdomyosarcoma and neuroblastoma in soft tissue and sympathetic nervous system sites, respectively.

PPB primarily affects young children; 95% are less than 6 years of age at diagnosis.

Histologically, pleuropulmonary blastoma of childhood differs from adult pulmonary blastoma because of its primitive and embryonic stroma, absence of carcinomatous component, and potential for sarcomatous differentiation.[46] Dehner and colleagues have defined three subtypes of pleuropulmonary blastoma of childhood: type I is exclusively cystic, type II exhibits both cystic and solid components, and type III is a solid tumor without cystic spaces lined by epithelium. Patients with type I tumors appear to have a better probability of survival; however, the evidence for clinical and pathological progression from type I to type III is strong. The embryonic origin of this tumor is uncertain but the tumor resembles fetal lung and is thought to be an expression of the somatopleural mesoderm or the thoracic splanchnopleura. Chromosomal abnormalities, including trisomy of chromosome 8 and abnormalities of chromosome 2q, have been reported and confirmed by comparative genomic hybridization studies. The profile of this tumor bears similarities to that of embryonal rhabdomyosarcoma. Mutations of *p53* and *MYCN* amplification have also been reported in a few cases. Patients with alterations of *p53* appear to have a poor prognosis, raising the possibility that inactivation of *p53* could be a valuable predictor of outcome in these patients.

Approximately 25% of patients registered in the pleuropulmonary blastoma registry have a constitutional or familial association with other neoplasias or dysplasias. Lung cysts are identified radiographically in one-third of affected patients. Cystic nephroma has also been reported in association with this tumor. Neoplastic conditions reported in family members of patients with pleuropulmonary blastoma include; germ cell and brain tumors, lymphoma, leukemia, sarcomas, histiocytosis, Wilms' tumor, thyroid tumors, neuroblastoma, and Sertoli-Leydig tumor. These observations suggest that pleuropulmonary blastoma is a strong marker for familial disease.

The median age at presentation of pleuropulmonary blastoma is 34 months, but those with type I tumors present at a younger age (10 months). Presenting symptoms are nonspecific and commonly include respiratory distress, fever, chest or abdominal pain, pulmonary infections, pneumothorax, cough, anorexia, and malaise.

The lesion generally can be recognized on plain chest radiograph. These are generally peripheral lesions and lobar resection is the most common surgical procedure. Chemotherapy with sarcoma-targeted agents (vincristine, dactinomycin, and cyclophosphamide) has also been used. The overall prognosis is poor with less than 50% survival at two years. Patients with mediastinal or pleural involvement have a significantly poorer clinical outcome.

Other malignant neoplasms: The inventory of other rare primary lung malignancies in children is categorized.

Neurofibrosarcoma, fibrosarcoma, mesothelioma, endothelial sarcoma and others have case reports. The general approach is the same as for the lesions previously discussed; resection of all gross disease and maximal preservation of normal lung tissue. Radiographic imaging is best obtained for all primary lung neoplasms with either CT or MR imaging. Lobectomy or pneumonectomy are appropriate for these lesions if the disease is localized at the time of diagnosis. The limited experience for these rare lesions precludes meaningful statistical analysis of adjuvant therapy, and treatment is generally individualized.

Benign Lung Tumors

Inflammatory pseudotumor: Inflammatory pseudotumor is a rare lesion that presents as a solitary lung nodule in children. As the term suggests, it is not malignant, nor is it truly neoplastic. The lesion is comprised of proliferating spindle cells (fibroblasts and myoblasts) with mitotic figures and inflammatory cells, particularly plasma cells. The histopathology also shows lymphocytes, fat-laden macrophages, as well as other lung parenchymal cell types. The spectrum of histopathology for this lesion has given rise to an abundance of descriptive names; *plasma cell granuloma*, *histiocytoma*, *xanthrofibroma*, and *lung adenoma*. The pathogenesis of this unique local inflammatory process is unknown.

Inflammatory pseudotumor is the most common benign lung mass in infants and children. Seventy-five percent of the children are older than 5 years of age, as this process takes time to develop. Only a small percentage, (20%) have a history of previous pulmonary infection and the lesion may be an incidental finding on chest radiograph. Other presentations include cough, fever, chest pain, hemoptysis, and airway obstruction. Pneumonia is diagnosed in about 10% of these children. Large inflammatory pseudotumors have resulted in esophageal obstruction and death from extrinsic compression of mediastinal structures.

The imaging approach is not different than for other mass lesions in the thorax. Plain chest radiographs are followed by either CT or MR imaging. The lesions appear as solid parenchymal nodules or larger masses and may be indistinguishable from neoplasms. Calcification is common and may be dramatic.

The natural history of these lesions is generally one of either slow growth or spontaneous resolution. Metastatic spread has not been observed. Although a benign lesion, definitive diagnosis is often not possible on intraoperative biopsy. Formal lobectomy or local resection is appropriate, depending on the degree of diagnostic uncertainty and the anatomic relations involved. In large lesions where resection would require a morbid procedure such as pneumonectomy, it would be appropriate to await permanent pathology before proceding with resection.

Hamartomas: Hamartomatous lung nodules are rare in children. They may occur in either endobronchial or parenchymal sites and are characterized by the presence of cartilage, respiratory epithelium, and collagen. Because peripheral lesions are more common, hamartomas are frequently asymptomatic. Predictably, endobronchial lesions are likely to cause clinical symptoms at a relatively small size. Parenchymal lesions may be large and can produce symptoms of respiratory distress or mediastinal compression. Death in the neonatal period has been reported. Surgical indication is the need to establish a diagnosis and the majority can be managed with wedge resection. The results after local resection are expectedly excellent for these benign lesions.

Metastatic Lung Tumors

The approach to children with metastatic lung tumors is considerably different than for adults with similar lesions because patient survival is much better in children. The most common causes of metastatic lung tumors in children are Wilm's tumor and osteogenic sarcoma. Approximately 50% of children with Wilms' tumor will demonstrate pulmonary metastases. The initial approach in the child who presents with Wilm's tumor with pulmonary metastases involves standard surgical management by radical nephrectomy with regional lymphadenectomy and abdominal lymph node sampling and systemic chemotherapy. Pulmonary metastatic lesions which persist after initial chemotherapy or which develop on therapy are resected. These patients are also treated with bilateral whole lung irradiation. About one-half of patients with pulmonary metastases from Wilm's tumor can be saved with this approach.

Adjuvant chemotherapy in the management of patients with osteogenic sarcoma has reduced the incidence of metastatic lung lesions from about 80-30% during the past two decades.[47] Protocols in the United States include an aggressive surgical approach to pulmonary metastases after adequate chemotherapy and appropriate resection of the primary tumor. With a combination of chemotherapy and sometimes multiple (sequential) or bilateral pulmonary resections, approximately 40% of patients with metastatic lung disease from osteogenic sarcoma can be saved. Lung metastases in osteogenic sarcoma are typically small, subpleural nodules that may be numerous. The operative surgical principal is to carefully evaluate the lung at the time of resection and resect all nodules with limited wedge resections and maximize preservation of lung parenchyma. It is common that operative exploration and bimanual palpation reveal lesions not detected on preoperative imaging studies. This is a compelling argument for open thoracotomy rather than thoracoscopy in these patients because the open approach allows bimanual palpation of the lung for detection of small metastatic nodules.

A host of other metastatic lung tumors have been treated surgically in children. The general principles are that the lesions must be stable, the primary disease controlled, the metastatic disease isolated to the lungs, and an aggressive approach supported by oncologists, surgeons, and the patient and family. Generally, these patients first require adjuvant chemotherapy and receive irradiation for radiosensitive tumors.

REFERENCES

1. Langston C. New concepts in the pathology of congenital lung malformations. Semin Pediatr Surg 2003;12:17-37.
2. Adzick NS, Harrison MR, Crombleholme TM, et al. Fetal lung lesions: management and outcome. Am J Obs Gynecol 1998;179:884-89.

3. Roggin KK, Breuer CK, Carr SR, et al. The unpredictable character of congenital cystic lung lesions. J Pediatr Surg 2000;35:801-05.
4. Buntain WL, Isaacs H Jr, Payne VC Jr, et al. Lobar emphysema, cystic adenomatoid malformation, pulmonary sequestration, and bronchogenic cyst in infancy and childhood: A clinical group. J Pediatr Surg 1974;9:85-93.
5. Stocker JT, Madewell JE, Drake RM. Congenital cystic adenomatoid malformation of the lung. Hum Pathol 1977;8:155-71.
6. Adzick NS, Harrison MR, Glick PL, et al. Fetal cystic adenomatoid malformation: prenatal diagnosis and natural history. J Pediatr Surg 1985;20:483.
7. Rice HE, Estes Jm, Hedrick MH, et al. Congenital cystic adenomatoid malformation: A sheep model of fetal hydrops. J Pediatr Surg 1994;29:692-96.
8. Adzick NS, Harrison MR, Flake AW, et al. Fetal surgery for cystic adenomatoid malformation of the lung. J Pediatr Surg 1993;28:806.
9. Budorick NE, Pretorius DH, Leopold GR, et al. Spontaneous improvement of intrathoracic masses diagnosed in utero. J Ultrasound Med 1992;11:653.
10. Comblehomme TM, Coleman B, Hedrick H, et al. Cystic adenomatoid malformation volume ratio predicts outcome in prenatally diagnosed cystic adenomatoid malformation of the lung. J Pediatr Surg 202;37:331.
11. Shackelford GD, Siegel MJ. CT appearance of cystic adenomatoid malformation. J Comput Assist Tomogr 1989;13:612-16.
12. Ryckman FC, Rosenkrantz JG. Thoracic surgical problems in infancy and childhood. Surg Clin North Am 1985;65:1423-54.
13. DeLorimer AA. Congenital malformations and neonatal problems of the respiratory tract. In: Welch KJ, Randolph, JG, Ravitch, MM, et al. Pediatric Surgery; 4th ed. Chicago: Year Book Medical 1986:631.
14. Oldham KT, Colombani PM, Foglia RP, Skinner MA. Principles and practice of pediatric surgery. Lippincott Williams and Wilkins. Philadelphia 2005;2:951-82.
15. Hartman GE, Shochat SJ. Primary pulmonary neoplasms in childhood: a review. Ann Thorac Surg 1983;36:108.
16. Horak E, Bodner J, Gassner I, et al. Congenital cystic lung disease: diagnostic and therapeutic considerations. Clin Pediatr 2003;42:251.
17. Murray GF. Congenital lobar emphysema. Surg Gynecol Obstet 1967;124:611.
18. Jones JC, Almond CH, Snyder HM, et al. Lobar emphysema and congenital heart disease in infancy. J Thoracic and Cardiovasc Surg 1965;49:1.
19. Stein SM, Cox JL, Hernanz-Schulman M, et al. Pediatric chest disease: evaluation by computerized tomography, magnetic resonance imaging, and ultrasonography. South Med J 1992;85:735.
20. Cooney DR, Menke JA, Allen JE. "Acquired lobar emphysema: a complication of respiratory distresss in premature infants. J Pediatr Surg 1977;12:897-904.
21. Tapper D, Schuster S, McBride J, et al. Polyalveolar lobe: anatomic and physiologic parameters and their relationship to congenital lobar emphysema. J Pediatr Surg 1980;15:931-37.
22. Tapper D, Azizkhan RG. Congenital and acquired lobar emphysema. Chapter 38 in Zeigler MM, Aziz Khan RG, Weber TRC (Eds). Operative Pediatric Surgery, McGraw Hill, New York 2003;439-44.
23. Wesley JR, Heidelberger KP, DiPietro MA, et al. Diagnosis and management of congenital cystic disease of the lung in children. J Pediatr Surgery 1986;21:202.
24. McBride JT, Wohl MEB, Strieder DL, et al. Lung growth and airway function after lobectomy in infancy for congenital lobar emphysema. J Clin Invest 1980;66:962.
25. Frenckner B, Freyschuss U. Pulmonary function after lobectomy for congenital lobar emphysema and congenital cystic adenomatoid : a follow-up study. Scand Jour Thorac and Cardiovasc Surg 1982;16:293.
26. Kent M. Intralobar pulmonary spectrum in prog. Pediatric Surg 1991;27;84-91.
27. Stocker JT. Sequestrations of the lung. Sem Diag Path 1986;3:106-21.
28. Buntain WL, Woolley MM, Mahour GH, et al. Pulmonary sequestration in children: a 25-year experience. Surgery 1977;81:413.
29. Mezzeti M, Dell'Agnola CA, Bedoni M, et al. Video-assisted thoracoscopic resection of pulmonary sequestration in an infant. Ann Thorac Surgery 1996;61:1836-37.
30. Gray SW, Skandalakis JE. The trachea and lungs. In Embryology for surgeons: The embryological basis for the treatment of congenital defects. Philadelphia: WB Saunders 1972:293.
31. Hoffmann MA, Superina R, Wesson DE. Unilateral pulmonary agenesis with esophageal atresia and distal tracheoesophageal fistula: report of two cases. J Pediatr Surg 1989;10:1084.
32. Osborne J, Masel J, McCredie J. A spectrum of skeletal anomalies associated with pulmonary agenesis: possible neural crest injuries. Pediatr Radiol 1989;19:425.
33. Grewal H, Smith SD. Lung infections: Lung biopsy, lung abscess, bronchiectasis and empyema. Chap 40 in Zeigler MM, Aziz Khan RG and Waber TR (Eds). Operative Pediatric Surgery, McGraw Hill, New York 2003;455-64.
34. Kosloske A. Infections of the lungs, pleura and mediastinum. In: Welch KJ, Randolph JG, Ravitch MM, et al (Eds). Pediatric Surgery 4th (Ed) Chicago: Year Book Medical1986;657.
35. Alexander JC, Wolfe WG. Lung abscess and empyema of the thorax. Surg CLin North Am 1980;60:835.
36. Cowles RA, Lelli JL Jr, Takayasu J, et al. Lung resection in infants and children with pulmonary infections refractory to medical therapy. J Pediatr Surg 2002;37:643.
37. Miller WS. A study of the human pleura pulmonalis: its relation to the blebs and bullae of emphysema. AJR;1926;15:399.

38. Fitzgerald MX, Keelan PJ, Cugell DW, et al. Long-term results of surgery for bullous emphysema. J Thorac Cardiovasc Surg 1974;68:566.
39. Nathanson LK, Shimi SM, Wood RA, et al. Videothoacoscopic ligation of bulla and pleurectomy for spontaneous pneumothorax. Ann Thorac Surg 1991;52:316.
40. Lucy MR. Hepatic infection. In: Greenfield LJ, Mulholland MW, Oldham KT, et al. (Eds). Surgery: Scientific principles and practice. Philadelphia: JB Lippincott 1993:867.
41. Topcu S, Kurul IC, Tastepe I, et al. Surgical treatment of pulmonary hydatid cysts in children. J Thorac Cardiovasc Surg 2000;120:1097.
42. Snyder CL, Ramsay NK, McGlave PB, et al. Diagnostic open lung biopsy after bone marrow transplantation. J Pediatr Surg 1990;25:871.
43. Bonfils-Roberts EA, Nickodem A, Nealon TF Jr. Retrospective analysis of the efficacy of open lung biopsy in acquired immunodeficiency syndrome. Ann Thorac Surg 1990;49:115.
44. Lack EE, Harris GB, Erakalis AJ, et al. Primary bronchial tumors in childhood. Cancer 1983;51:492.
45. Niitu Y, Kubota H, Hasegawa S, et al. Lung cancer (squamous cell carcinoma) in adolescence. Am J Dis Child 1974;127:108.
46. Hill DA, Jarzembowski JA, Priest JR, Williams GB, et al. Type I Pleuropulmonary blastoma; Pathology and biology study of 51 cases from the international pleuropulmonary blastoma registry. The Am J of Surg Pathology 2008; 32(2):282.
47. Schaller RT, Haas J, Schaller J, et al. Improved survival in children with osteosarcoma following resection of pulmonary metastases. J Pediatr Surg 1975;10:545.

Bronchiectasis and Lung Abscess

Shilpa Sharma, DK Gupta

BRONCHIECTASIS

The incidence of childhood bronchiectasis has declined in the recent past with the widespread use of antibiotics, improved general awareness, better hygiene, better nutrition and childhood immunization against the diseases like pertusis, influenza, pneumococci and measles. Yet, it does remain as an indication for lobectomy in children, especially in the developing world.[1]

DEFINITION

Bronchiectasis is defined as an irreversible focal bronchial dilation, usually accompanied by chronic infection. The bronchial tubes become enlarged and distended forming pockets harboring infection. The damaged bronchial walls impair the complex mechanism of the cilia lining the bronchial tubes, resulting in accumulation of dust, mucus and bacteria.

ETIOLOGY AND PATHOGENESIS

Bronchiectasis may occur in both, the congenital and the acquired forms.

In congenital bronchiectasis, the periphery of the lung fails to develop, resulting in cystic dilation of developed bronchi.

Acquired bronchiectasis develops later in life and may be due to:
1. Direct bronchial wall destruction as a result of infection, noxious chemicals, immunologic reactions, or vascular abnormalities
2. Mechanical alterations due to atelectasis with increased traction on airways, leading to bronchial dilatation and secondary infection.

Predisposing Factors

1. Congenital anomalies — Cystic fibrosis, immune deficiencies, α_1-antitrypsin deficiency, congenital abnormalities of cartilage and connective tissue, e.g. Mounier-Kuhn syndrome, Williams-Campbell syndrome, yellow nail syndrome.
2. Inherited primary ciliary abnormality.
3. Severe pneumonia — following measles, pertussis, adenovirus by weakening bronchial walls and causing pockets of infection to form.
4. Necrotizing pulmonary infections: *Klebsiella* sp, staphylococci, influenza virus, fungi, mycobacteria, mycoplasmas.
5. Bronchial obstruction — Intrinsic or extrinsic - foreign body, enlarged lymph nodes, mucus plug or lung tumor. In childhood this most commonly results from choking on food. When this happens the wall of the tube is injured and air is prevented from passing out beyond the obstruction. The bronchial tube, distal to the obstruction balloons out, to form a pocket for harboring infection and pus.
6. Chronic fibrosing lung diseases—aspiration pneumonia.
7. Immunologic deficiencies—AIDS.
8. Kartagener's syndrome. In 1933, Manes Kartagener, a Zurich pulmonary physician, reported four patients with the triad of sinusitis, bronchiectasis, and situs inversus.[2]

Bronchiectasis may be focal, limited to a single segment/lobe, or widespread affecting multiple lobes in one or both lungs. It most often affects the lower lobes, although the right middle lobe and lingular portion of the left upper lobe are often affected.

Bronchial wall damage may be mediated by bacterial endotoxins and proteases, superoxide radicals and antigen-antibody complexes.[3] On histological examination, the bronchial walls show extensive destruction, chronic inflammation, increased mucus, and loss of cilia with tissue reorganization and fibrosis.

Extensive anastomoses develop between the bronchial and pulmonary vessels with vascular engorgement in cases presenting late. The resultant increased blood flow, right-to-left shunts, and hypoxemia lead to pulmonary hypertension and cor pulmonale in the late phase of the disease.

CLINICAL FEATURES

Bronchiectasis can develop at any age but most often begins in early childhood, though the symptoms may appear much later. The cases presenting late usually have a long history of chronic cough with large quantities of green or yellow sputum that may be foul smelling. Typically, the bout of cough occurs in the early morning when the patient wakes up. The symptoms may occur after an attack of respiratory infection but tend to worsen gradually over the months and the years. Occasionally, although chronic infection exists, the patient may be asymptomatic.

Hemoptysis may result from erosion of the capillaries near the surface of the thinned walls of the bronchial tubes that are prone to rupture easily or from the anastomoses between the bronchial and pulmonary arterial systems. The bleeding is generally minor and self-limiting and may be the first and the only complaint. Occasionally the patient may present with massive hemoptysis as a major emergency. Coughing up blood indicates an added infection.

Recurrent fever or pleuritic pain, wheezing, shortness of breath and cor pulmonale may occur in advanced cases with associated chronic bronchitis and emphysema.

In Williams-Campbell syndrome, there is total or partial absence of cartilage beyond the main segmental bronchi. This produces wheezing and dyspnea early in infancy and imaging modalities may show inspiratory ballooning and expiratory collapse of the affected bronchi.

In yellow nail syndrome, there is congenital hypoplasia of the lymphatic system associated with primary lymphedema, exudative pleural effusion and bronchiectasis. The children presenting late generally have chronic malaise, poor weight gain with decreased appetite.[4]

About 60% cases of foreign body aspiration may present with pneumonia, bronchiectasis and bronchoesophageal fistula. Sterile foreign bodies may remain embedded for months without much respiratory distress symptoms. Skiagram chest may be helpful in the diagnosis of a radioopaque foreign body. CT scan may pick up the radiolucent foreign bodies. However, the undiagnosed organic foreign bodies are troublesome resulting in not only ipsilateral but the risk of contralateral chronic infection also.

The physical findings are usually nonspecific, but persistent crackles over any part of the lungs suggest bronchiectasis. Signs of airflow obstruction like decreased breath sounds, prolonged expiration, or wheezing may be picked up. Finger clubbing may be identified with extensive disease and persistent chronic infection (Fig. 40.1). In very late cases, chest wall defects may be visible due to underlying unhealthy lung and acquired postural changes to counteract the force of chronic coughing.

INVESTIGATIONS

Routine Blood Tests

The hemoglobin level may be reduced in patients presenting with hemoptysis. The total and differential leucocyte count may help to identify the presence of

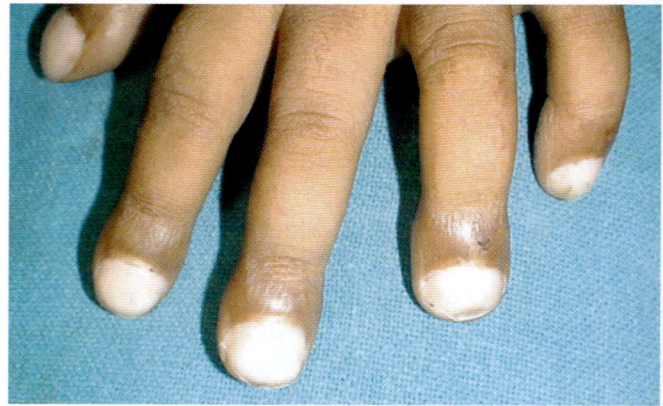

Fig. 40.1: Clubbing in a patient with chronic bronchiectasis

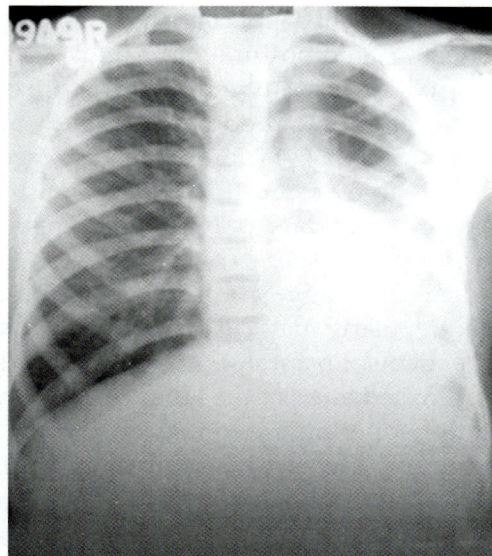

Fig. 40.2: Skiagram chest showing diseased left lower lobe with crowding of ribs and collapse

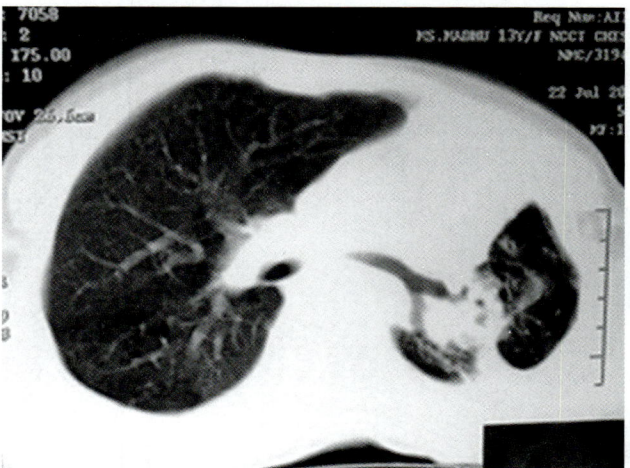

Fig. 40.3A: CT scan chest showing bronchiectatic changes in the lung

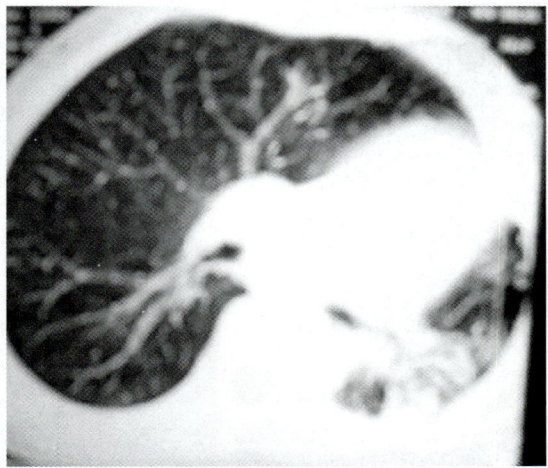

Fig. 40.3B: CT scan chest depicting an atelectatic left lower lobe with multiple fibrocystic lesions replacing lung parenchyma with compensatory hyperinflation of right lung

infection. ESR may be raised in patients chronic underlying disease especially the tuberculosis.

Skiagram Chest

It may show increased bronchovascular markings due to peribronchial fibrosis and intrabronchial secretions, crowding from an atelectatic lung, tram lines (parallel lines outlining dilated bronchi due to peribronchial inflammation and fibrosis), areas of honeycombing, or cystic areas with or without fluid levels (Fig. 40.2). Cystic fibrosis may be suspected in areas where it is common, if the X-ray abnormalities are mostly in the apices or upper lobes. Congenital abnormalities of tracheal or bronchial cartilage and connective tissue are usually detected on X-ray.

CT Scan

High-resolution CT scans of chest has largely replaced bronchography (Figs 40.3A and B). Characteristic findings are dilated airways, indicated by tram lines, by a signet ring appearance with a luminal diameter more than 1.5 times that of the adjacent vessel in cross-section, bronchial wall thickening, airway obstruction, consolidation or the grapelike clusters (Figs. 40.4A and B). Dilated medium-sized bronchi may extend to the pleura due to destruction of lung parenchyma. Helical CT may be superior for knowing the extent of bronchiectasis and its distribution within a given segment, but it has an additional radiation exposure.

Bronchoscopy

Fiberoptic bronchoscopy may be useful to localize endobronchial tumor or foreign body. Abnormal cilia may be found in children with chronic respiratory disease. Ultrastructure and motility examination of cilia obtained on bronchial biopsy or brushing may be done. The nasal ciliary clearance time may be measured. Sputum cultures, bronchial washings, fungal serologic studies and tissue biopsy may be indicated.

474 Pediatric Surgery—Diagnosis and Management

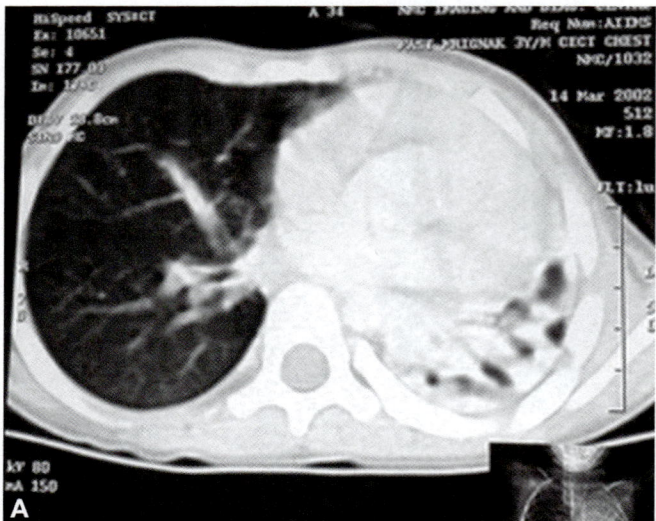

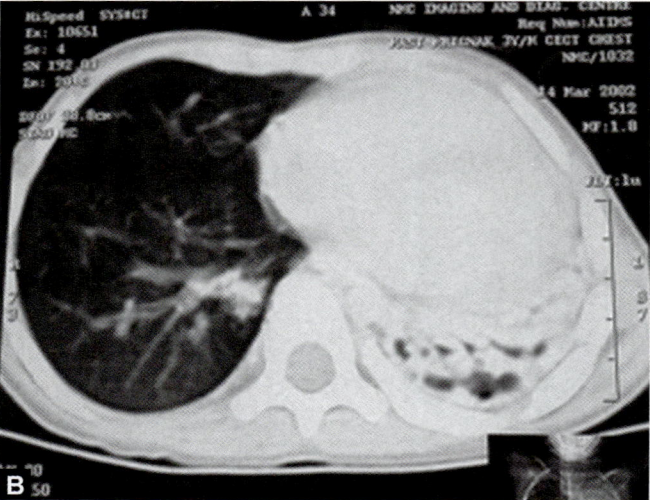

Figs 40.4A and B: CECT with evidence of bronchial wall thickening, consolidation and grapelike clusters suggestive of bronchiectasis. Collapse of the ipsilateral lung with compensatory emphysema of the contralateral lung is also noted

MANAGEMENT

Rationale and timely use of appropriate antibiotics in respiratory infections has a great role in prevention of the damage that leads to bronchiectasis.

Identification of congenital and hereditary conditions that predispose to aspiration and bronchiectasis, immunoglobin replacement in deficiency states, the early detection and removal of foreign bodies and the treatment of recurrent sinusitis, aid in prevention of bronchiectasis.

The treatment revolves around prevention of complications of pneumonia.

Medical treatment of infection includes antibiotics, bronchodilators, and postural drainage.

Hemoptysis may subside after appropriate antibiotic treatment. Blood transfusion may be required if there is massive loss of blood. Oxygen may be required for chronic hypoxemia, pulmonary hypertension, secondary polycythemia, respiratory failure or cor pulmonale.

Postural drainage, clapping, and vibration performed regularly may facilitate sputum clearance in some patients. Postural drainage is important to drain the affected areas of the lungs by gravity. Early treatment of superimposed infection causing fever, chest pain and a change in sputum quality and quantity can prevent complications. Bronchiectasis limited to a very small isolated part of the lung causing recurrent pneumonia can be removed surgically (Fig. 40.5). Surgical resection is rarely necessary but should be considered when conservative management yields to recurrent pneumonia, disabling bronchial infections and frequent hemoptysis. Surgical treatment of bronchiectasis is more effective in patients with localized disease and is usually not advisable if it is a widespread disease. The principles of surgical resection have been discussed in a separate chapter. Anatomic localization of the disease should be mapped by radiologic and scintigraphic investigations. The operative mortality rate varies from 2-6% and the morbidity rate varies from 10-20%.[5,6] Complete resection results in significantly better clinical outcome

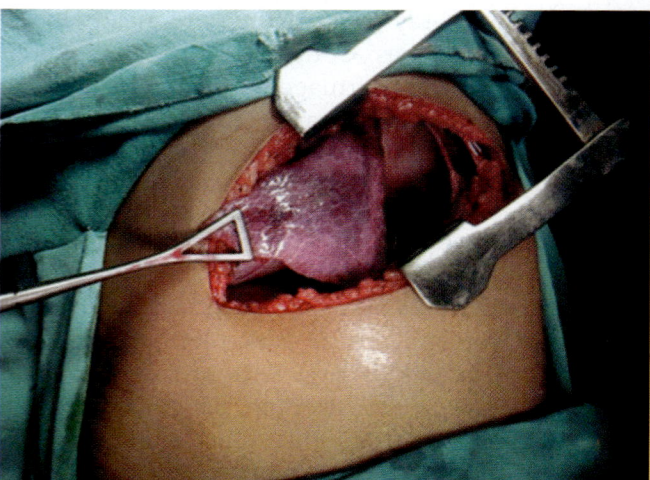

Fig. 40.5: Operative photograph showing the bronchiectatic lobe

than incomplete resection. Pneumonectomy is well tolerated in children without an increase in morbidity and mortality and thus preferred instead of leaving residual disease when bronchiectasis is unilateral.[6]

Mediastinal shift and lung overinflation may occur after pneumonectomy. Pulmonary resection does not alter respiratory function since the resected segments do not contribute much to ventilation.[1]

In case of massive pulmonary hemorrhage, an emergency resection or embolization of the bleeding vessel may be lifesaving. Kartagener's syndrome is an autosomal recessive disorder characterized by the clinical triad of bronchiectasis, sinusitis and dextrocardia (situs inversus). Lobectomy may be required for symptomatic cases (Fig. 40.6).[7] Lung transplantation can be performed in patients with advanced cystic fibrosis and bronchiectasis.

Case Report—Congenital Bronchiectasis

A ten-year-old female presented with cough since 3-4 yrs of age. There was no fever, hemoptysis, respiratory distress or pneumonia. On examination, the air entry was decreased in the left lower region with presence of crepitations. The CT scan chest depicted an atelectatic left lower lobe with multiple fibrocystic lesions replacing lung parenchyma, traction bronchiectasis of the left upper and lower lobe segmental bronchi. There was mediastinal shift to the left with the compensatory hyperinflation of the right lung (see Figs 40.3A and B).

On left sided thoracotomy, the lower lobe and lingula and more than half of the upper lobe, were found solid in consistency. The lower lobe bronchus was filled with purulent material. Left lower lobectomy was done. The cut section showed features of congenital bronchiectasis with absence of bronchial cartilage and abnormal parenchyma within the area of involvement that was confirmed histologically (Figs 40.7A and B).

CHRONIC LUNG ABSCESS

Pediatric lung abscess usually follows an episode of aspiration or bacterial pneumonia. Associated

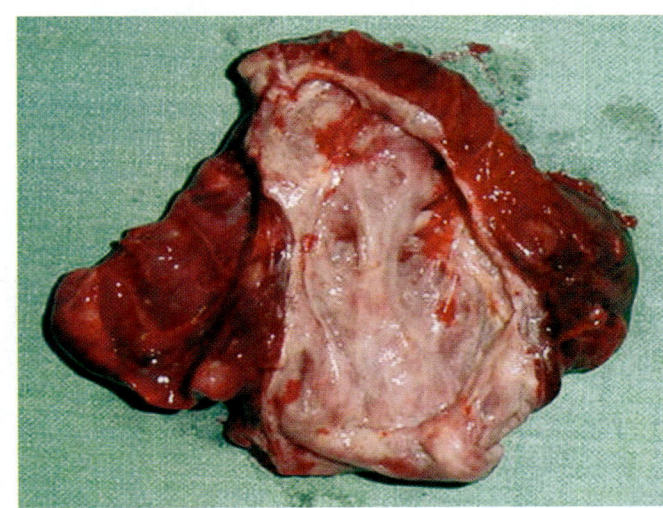

Fig. 40.6: Excised specimen following lobectomy of a bronchiectatic lobe

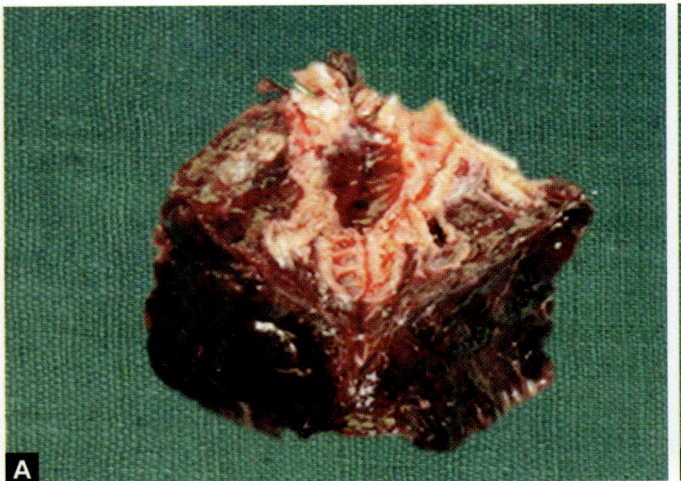
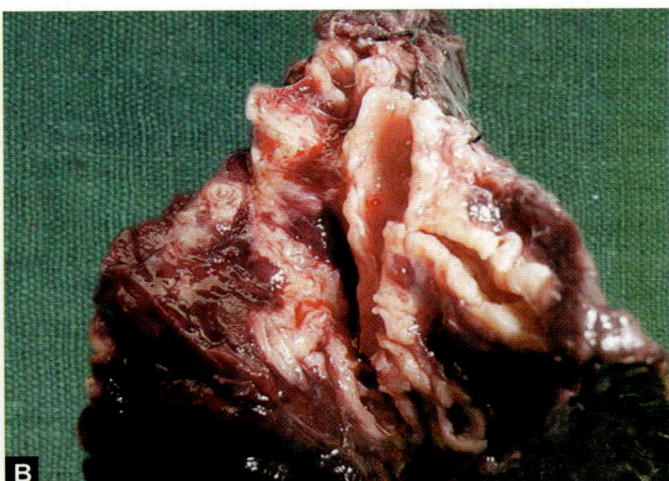

Figs 40.7A and B: A. The cut section of lobectomy specimen showing dilated bronchial tree, **B.** Close up view showing the thickened bronchial wall, with non-aerated lung at periphery

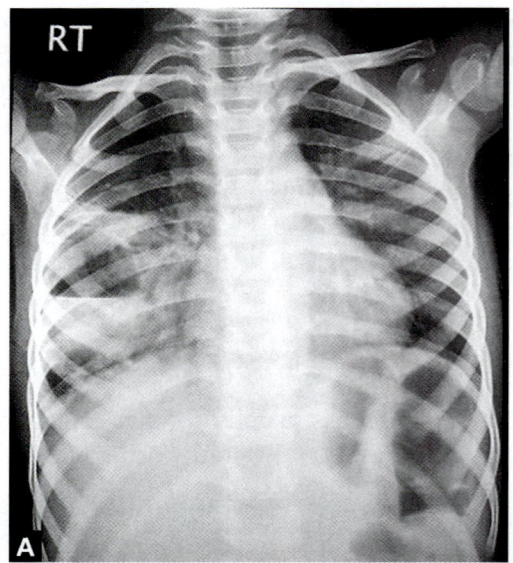

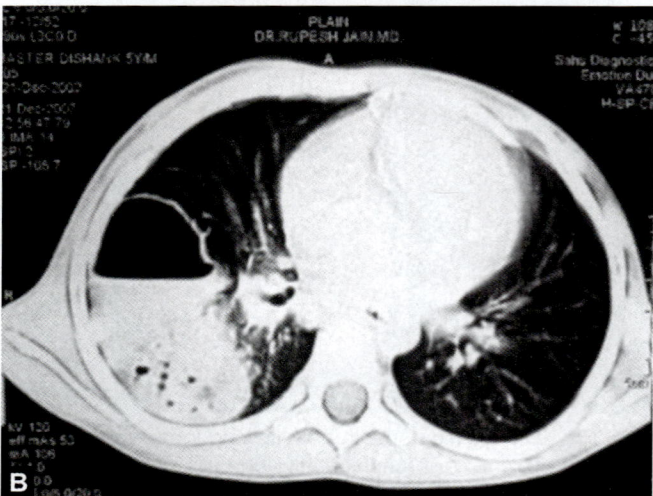

Figs 40.8A and B: A three-year-old child presented with fever, cough and chest pain, **A.** The Skiagram chest showing an air fluid level in the right middle lobe, **B.** The CECT showing the lesion along with the bronchiectatic surrounding lung. Right lower lobectomy was done, the histopathology was inconclusive

conditions include leukemia, congenital immune deficiency, endocarditis, cerebral palsy, and prematurity.[8] Most children have polymicrobial infections, usually containing both aerobic and anaerobic bacteria. The success of medical treatment has been found to be age related; with children below 7 years, requiring chest tube drainage or resection of the involved lobe for cure and adolescents recovering on antibiotics and chest physiotherapy.[8] The chest tube drainage may be performed for solitary peripheral bacterial abscesses. Wedge resection is required for multiple, central, or fungal abscesses.[8] Lung abscesses are now uncommon but are seen in immunocompromised children who are vulnerable to fatal infections. Medical failures can be identified within the first week of treatment. Early and aggressive surgical treatment is indicated in such children, and may be lifesaving.

When medical therapy for lung abscess fails, tube drainage may be considered.[9] Chronic lung abscesses are usually associated with severe sepsis or complicated by a bronchopleural fistula that may not respond to medical treatment and the chest tube thoracostomy. Lobectomy should be considered in patients who have major life-threatening bleeding or massive pulmonary necrosis. The required surgical procedures include decortication, lung debridement, bronchial closure, lobectomy or segmentectomy.[4,10] Few cases may have persistent air leakage due to poor healing amidst infection requiring treatment by repeated bronchial closure.[11] Adequate treatment with follow up is essential as secondary lung abscesses due to inadequate response to medical therapy may require lobectomy.[12]

Hydatidosis of lung may rarely be diagnosed in children only after complications like empyema, lung abscess and bronchiectasis ensue. A lung abscess may cause bronchiectasis of the adjoining lung tissue due to compression effect (Fig. 40.8).

The diagnosis may be missed on initial appearance due to overshadowing by the complications. However, a high degree of suspicion may help in timely diagnosis and needful precautions as the disease needs special handling due to the antigenicity of the fluid. Chest radiographs and thoraco-abdominal ultrasound are very useful for the diagnosis of pulmonary hydatidosis. Immunological tests for hydatidosis may supplement the diagnosis. In a series of 232 cases of pulmonary hydatid cyst in children, bronchiectasis was observed in seven cases.[13] CT is useful for diagnosis of atypical or complicated lesions and to detect associated bronchiectasis.

REFERENCES

1. Ayed AK, Al-Rowayeh. A Lung resection in children for infectious pulmonary diseases. Pediatr Surg Int. 2005;21: 604-08. Epub 2005.

2. Berdon WE, Willi U. Situs inversus, bronchiectasis, and sinusitis and its relation to immotile cilia: history of the diseases and their discoverers-Manes Kartagener and Bjorn Afzelius. Pediatr Radiol 2004; 34:38-42. Epub 2003 Oct 10. Comment in:Pediatr Radiol 2004;34:585-86.
3. Lindskog GE. Bronchiectasis revisited. Yale J Biol Med 1986;59:41-53.
4. Gupta DK, Sharma Shilpa. Late infections of Lung and Pleura in Pediatric Thoracic Surgery, Ed. D H Parikh, David C G Crabbe, S Rothenberg and AW Auldist 2006 Ist edition, Springer, UK [In press].
5. Haciibrahimoglu G, Fazlioglu M, Olcmen A, et al. Surgical management of childhood bronchiectasis due to infectious disease. J Thorac Cardiovasc Surg. 2004;127:1361-65.
6. Otgun I, Karnak I, Tanyel FC, et al. Surgical treatment of bronchiectasis in children. J Pediatr Surg. 2004;39:1532-36.
7. Sahajananda H, Sanjay OP, Thomas J, et al. General anaesthesia for lobectomy in an 8-year-old child with Kartagener's syndrome. Paediatr Anaesth. 2003;13:714-17.
8. Kosloske AM, Ball WS Jr, Butler C, et al. Drainage of pediatric lung abscess by cough, catheter, or complete resection. J Pediatr Surg. 1986;21:596-600.
9. Weissberg D. Percutaneous drainage of lung abscess. J Thorac Cardiovasc Surg. 1984;87:308-12.
10. Sharma S, Gupta DK. Empyema thoracis—Tubercular and Nontubercular In: Swati Bhave Ed. Textbook of Adolescent Medicine. New Delhi Jaypee Brothers. Chap 20,2006;8: 678-84.
11. Wu MH, Tseng YL, Lin MY, et al. Surgical treatment of pediatric lung abscess. Pediatr Surg Int. 1997;12:293-95.
12. Emanuel B, Shulman ST. Lung abscess in infants and children. Clin Pediatr (Phila) 1995;34:2-6.
13. Hafsa C, Belguith M, Golli M, et al. Imaging of pulmonary hydatid cyst in children J Radiol. 2005;86:405-10.

CHAPTER 41

Pulmonary Tuberculosis in Children

Shilpa Sharma, DK Gupta

Thoracic surgery owes its inception to the high incidence of pulmonary tuberculosis and its complications seen in the pre-antibiotic era. However, with the introduction of Rifampicin in the 1960's, the role of surgery has decreased considerably. In recent years, the emergence of multidrug resistant strains of *M. tuberculosis* coupled with an increase in atypical mycobacterial infections has led to the increase in surgical interventions for pulmonary tuberculosis.

The World Health Organization (WHO) declared tuberculosis (TB) to be a global public health emergency in 1993. Today, 19-43.5% of the world's population is infected with *Mycobacterium tuberculosis* with more than 8 million new cases of TB occurring each year. Tuberculosis is one of the major causes of morbidity in developing countries.[1,2] According to WHO, developing countries including India, China, Pakistan, Philippines, Thailand, Indonesia, Bangladesh, and the Democratic Republic of Congo account for nearly 75% of all cases of TB, accounting for about 0.5 million deaths every year by this disease, worldwide.[3] The incidence and severity of pulmonary infections due to tuberculosis are expected to increase with the increasing incidence of HIV infection.[4] The highest TB incidence and HIV infection prevalence are recorded in sub-Saharan Africa, and, as a consequence, children in this region bear the greatest burden of TB/HIV infections.[5]

WHO's new Global Plan to Stop TB 2006-2015 advises countries with a high burden of tuberculosis (TB) to expand case-finding in the private sector as well as services to the patients with HIV and multidrug-resistant TB (MDR-TB).[6] Tuberculosis control program is a balance between accurate diagnosis of the disease and effective treatment of cases to eliminate the disease in the community. Thus, undiagnosed cases resulting from inadequate diagnostic facilities contribute an impediment to TB control efforts in the community.[7] Hence, there is an urgent need to have more accurate, affordable tools that would be available for use at all levels of health care to achieve total eradication of TB in the community.[7]

The need of applying science to the diseases of poverty has been felt and considered essential also.[8,9] Collaboration between national TB and HIV programs and some degree of integration of services at the local level have been advocated by World Health Organization and other International bodies. There has been a decrease in mortality in cases with pulmonary tuberculosis without HIV infection, attributed to improved health care and prompt initiation of therapy.

Diagnosis of tuberculosis in children is difficult as children are less likely to have obvious symptoms of tuberculosis. Tuberculosis in infants and children younger than four years of age is much more likely to spread throughout the body through the bloodstream. Thus, children are at much greater risk of developing miliary tuberculosis. Hence, the need for the prompt diagnosis and treatment of tuberculosis.

CHILDREN AT RISK

1. Children living in a household with an adult who has active tuberculosis
2. Children infected with HIV or with an immunocompromised state following chemotherapy or prolonged steroid use.
3. Children living in high endemic regions
4. Poor socioeconomic status. It is common in children residing in rural areas.[2]

5. Undernourished children.
6. Children living in small enclosed areas and in areas with poor ventilation.
7. Infections like measles, varicella, and pertussis, may activate quiescent TB.
8. Hereditary factors. Children with certain human leukocyte antigen (HLA) types have a predisposition to TB. Presence of a Bcg gene has been implicated in sensitivity to acquisition of TB.

TUBERCULAR BACILLI

Mycobacterium tuberculosis is the most common cause of TB. Other rare causes are *Mycobacterium bovis* (bovine source) and *Mycobacterium avium* (from birds). *M. bovis* infection has been traced to the use of cheese made from unpasteurized milk.

M. tuberculosis is an aerobic, non-spore-forming, non-motile slow-growing bacillus with a curved and beaded rod-shaped morphology. It can survive under adverse environmental conditions. The acid-fast characteristic of the mycobacteria is its unique feature. Humans are the only known reservoirs for *M. tuberculosis*.

PATHOPHYSIOLOGY

The route of infection is inhalation of the aerosolized bacteria. The small size of the droplets allows them to remain suspended in the air for a prolonged period of time. The organism is slow growing and tolerates the intracellular environment, where it may remain metabolically inert for years before reactivation and causing disease. The main determinant of the pathogenicity of TB is its ability to escape host defence mechanisms, including macrophages and delayed hypersensitivity responses.

Although a single organism may cause disease, 5-200 inhaled bacilli are usually necessary for infection. Primary infection of the respiratory tract, thus occurs as a result of inhalation of these aerosols.

After inhalation, the bacilli are deposited, usually in the midlung zone, into the subpleural distal respiratory bronchioles or the alveoli. The alveolar macrophages then phagocytose the inhaled bacilli but are unable to kill them, thus the bacilli continue to multiply unimpeded. The infected macrophages are then transported to the regional lymph nodes. The initial pulmonary site of infection and its adjacent lymph nodes is known as the primary complex or Ghon focus.

Progression of the primary complex may lead to enlargement of hilar and mediastinal nodes with resultant bronchial collapse. The primary focus may progress when it cavitates and the organisms spread through contiguous bronchi.

Lymphohematogenous dissemination of the mycobacteria may occur to other lymph nodes and distant regions in the body like kidney, epiphyses of long bones, vertebral bodies, meninges and occasionally, to the apical posterior areas of the lungs. A widespread miliary TB may occur when caseous material reaches the bloodstream from a primary focus or a caseating metastatic focus breaks in the wall of a pulmonary vein (Weigert focus). Bacilli may remain dormant in the apical posterior areas of the lung for several months or years, with progression of disease later on.

A cell-mediated immune response terminates the unimpeded growth of the *M. tuberculosis* 2-3 weeks after initial infection. The CD4 helper T cells activate the macrophages to kill the intracellular bacteria with resultant epithelioid granuloma formation. The CD8 suppressor T cells lyse the macrophages infected with the mycobacteria, resulting in the formation of caseating granulomas. Mycobacteria cannot continue to grow in the acidic extracellular environment, thus most infections are controlled. The only evidence of infection is a positive tuberculin skin (Mantoux) test result.

CLINICAL FEATURES

Children with asymptomatic infection may be identified on a routine examination, or they may be identified subsequent to tuberculosis diagnosis in a close contact.

Primary Pulmonary Tuberculosis

Tuberculosis may present with generalized symptoms like fever of unknown origin, failure to thrive, night sweats, anorexia, significant weight loss, nonproductive cough, or unexplained lymphadenopathy.

Pulmonary TB may manifest as endobronchial TB with focal lymphadenopathy, progressive pulmonary disease, pleural involvement, and reactivated pulmonary disease.

Endobronchial TB with enlargement of lymph nodes is the most common form of pulmonary TB.

Symptoms result from pressure on various structures by the enlarged lymph nodes. Persistent cough may be indicative of bronchial obstruction, while difficulty in swallowing may result from esophageal compression. Vocal cord paralysis may be suggested by hoarseness or difficulty in breathing.

Progression of the pulmonary parenchymal infection leads to enlargement of the caseous area and may lead to pneumonia, atelectasis and air trapping in young children. The child usually appears ill with symptoms of fever, cough, malaise, and weight loss.

Tubercular pleural effusion may present with acute onset of fever, chest pain that increases in intensity on deep inspiration, and shortness of breath. Fever usually persists for 14-21 days.

Reactivation TB usually has a subacute presentation with weight loss, fever, cough, and rarely, the hemoptysis. Reactivation TB typically occurs in older children and adolescents.

Tuberculosis can present in any form and has been reported even in infants presenting as a superior mediastinal mass extending into the right chest.[10] Extrapulmonary TB includes peripheral lymphadenopathy, tubercular meningitis, miliary TB, skeletal TB, and other organ involvement.

Any child with pneumonia, pleural effusion, a cavitary or mass lesion in the lung that does not improve with standard antibacterial therapy should be evaluated for tuberculosis.

PHYSICAL EXAMINATION

Primary TB is characterized by the absence of any signs on clinical evaluation. Tuberculin hypersensitivity may be associated with erythema nodosum and phlyctenular conjunctivitis. The classic signs of pneumonia include tachypnea, nasal flaring, grunting, dullness to percussion, egophony, decreased breath sounds, and crackles. Mediastinal shift may be present with massive pleural effusion. There may be post-tussive crackles.

INVESTIGATIONS

Definitive diagnosis of TB depends upon isolation of *M. tuberculosis* from secretions or biopsy specimens. Newer diagnostic modalities have been developed including nucleic acid detection (NAD) and gamma-interferon assays.[11]

Erythrocyte Sedimentation Rate (ESR)

This is a non-specific marker for chronic infection. It is however, useful to monitor the progression of the disease while the child is being investigated. It is also useful to follow the course of the disease after the initiation of anti tubercular treatment. In cases where no positive finding is available for documentary evidence, a trial of anti tubercular treatment may be started on the basis of clinical findings amidst a raised ESR. The fall in ESR will then be supportive in favour of a diagnosis of tuberculosis.

It has been reported that there is a rise in serum zinc levels in various age groups of children after antitubercular therapy (mean 61.89 +/- 3.21-65.24 +/- 3.60 microg/dl) and significant fall in serum copper levels in different age groups of children (mean 129.96 +/- 3.18 to 124.91 +/- 3.48 microg/dl).[3] The Cu/Zn ratio also changed significantly from 2.11 +/- 0.12 to 1.92 +/- 0.12.[3]

Specimens for bacteriologic examination—Sputum, gastric lavage, bronchoalveolar lavage, lung tissue and lymph node.

Gastric aspirate may be used in place of sputum in children less than 6 years as they may not be able to cough out sputum. An early morning sample should be obtained for undiluted bronchial secretions accumulated during the night. Initially, the stomach contents should be aspirated, and then a small amount of sterile water injected through the orogastric tube, should also be aspirated. As gastric acidity is poorly tolerated by the tubercle bacilli, neutralization of the specimen should be done immediately with 10% sodium carbonate or 40% anhydrous sodium phosphate. Even with utmost care, the tubercle bacilli can be detected in only 70% of infants and in 30-40% of children with disease. Sputum specimens and bronchoalveolar lavage may be used in older children. Nasopharyngeal secretions and saliva are not acceptable.

Acid Fast Bacilli (AFB) Staining

This provides preliminary confirmation of the diagnosis. It also can give a quantitative assessment of the number of bacilli being excreted (e.g. 1+, 2+, 3+).

For a reliable positive result, smears require approximately 10,000 organisms per millilitre.

Therefore, the results may be negative in early stages of the disease or with sparse bacilli. A single organism on a slide is highly suggestive and warrants further investigation. Ziehl-Neelsen staining method is used. However, AFB smear cannot be used to differentiate *M. tuberculosis* from other acid-fast organisms such as other mycobacterial organisms or *Nocardia* species.

Mycobacterium Culture

This is the definitive method to detect bacilli and more sensitive than examination of the smear. Approximately 10 AFB per millimetre of a digested concentrated specimen are sufficient to detect the organisms by culture. A culture also allows identification of specific species and testing for drug sensitivity. Due to the emergence of MDR organisms, determination of the drug sensitivity panel of an isolate is important so that appropriate treatment can be ensured.

However, since *M. tuberculosis* is a slow-growing organism, a period of 6-8 weeks is required for colonies to appear on conventional culture media. Conventional solid media include the Löwenstein-Jensen medium (an egg-based medium) and the Middlebrook 7H10 and the 7H11 media (which are agar-based media). Liquid media (e.g. Dubos oleic-albumin media) also are available, and they require incubation in 5-10% carbon dioxide for 3-8 weeks.

Modern automated radiometric culture methods (e.g. BACTEC) have enabled rapid growth of mycobacteria. The methodology employs a liquid Middlebrook 7H12 medium containing radiometric palmitic acid labelled with radioactive carbon-14 (^{14}C). Several antimicrobial agents are added to this medium to prevent the growth of nonmycobacterial contaminants. Production of $^{14}CO_2$ by the metabolizing organisms provides a growth index for the mycobacteria. Growth is generally detected within 9-16 days.

Mycobacterial growth indicator tubes (MGITs), with round-bottom tubes with oxygen-sensitive sensors at the bottom indicate microbial growth and provide a quantitative index of *M. tuberculosis* growth.

Nucleic Acid Techniques

These include nucleic acid probes and polymerase chain reaction (PCR). Although their sensitivity and specificity in smear-positive cases exceed 95%, the sensitivity of smear-negative cases varies from 40-70%.

Nucleic acid probes help advance identification of the M tuberculosis complex. Sensitivity and specificity approach 100% when at least 100,000 organisms are present.

Polymerase chain reaction (PCR). Nucleic acid amplification tests allow direct identification of *M. tuberculosis* in clinical specimens, unlike the nucleic acid probes, which require substantial time for bacterial accumulation in broth culture.

The US Food and Drug Administration has approved 2 tests, the amplified *M. tuberculosis* direct test that targets RNA and the AMPLICOR *M. tuberculosis* test that targets the DNA. The most commonly used target sequence for the detection of *M. tuberculosis* has been the insertion sequence IS6110. The amplified M. tuberculosis direct test is an isothermal transcription-mediated amplification.

Enzyme-linked Immunoassay (ELISA) Test

A new test, Quantiferon (QFT-g), has recently been approved (May, 2005) by the US Food and Drug Administration (FDA). The test basically detects the presence of interferon gamma release protein (IFN-g) from the blood of sensitized patients, when the blood is incubated with the early secretory antigenic target-6 (ESAT6) and culture filtrate protein 10 (CFP10) peptides. The test is as sensitive as, and more specific than, the tuberculin skin test and has been recommended as a screening tool for diagnosing the disease as well as infection.

No available serodiagnostic test for TB has adequate sensitivity and specificity for routine use in diagnosing TB in children.

Mantoux Test

Although the sensitivity and the specificity are less than 100%, it is still widely used.

The dosage of 0.1 mL or 5 TU purified protein derivative (PPD) is injected intradermally into the volar aspect of the forearm using a 27-gauge needle. A detergent called Tween 80 to prevent loss of efficacy on contact and adsorption by glass stabilizes the PPD. A wheal should be raised and should measure approximately 6-10 mm in diameter. The test is read 48-72 hours after administration. The amount of induration and not erythema is measured transverse to the long axis of the forearm.

The test is interpreted on the basis of rule of 5, 10, and 15 mm.

Induration of 5 mm or more is considered positive in i. children having close contact with known or suspected contagious cases of the disease, ii. children with immunosuppressive conditions (e.g. HIV).

Children who have an abnormal CXR finding consistent with active TB, previously active TB, or clinical evidence of the disease.

Induration of 10 mm or more is considered positive in; children who are at a higher risk of dissemination of tuberculous disease, including those younger than 5 years or those who are immunosuppressed because of conditions such as lymphoma, Hodgkin disease, diabetes mellitus, and malnutrition; children with increased exposure to the disease.

Induration of 15 mm or more is considered positive in children aged 5 years or older without any risk factors for the disease.

False-positive reactions often are attributed to asymptomatic infection by environmental nontuberculous mycobacteria (due to cross-reactivity). The Mantoux test may be positive in children who have immigrated or been adopted from areas where tuberculosis is rampant.[12,13] This does not mean that they are infected. It only indicates that they have been exposed to the bacilli. About 90-95% of the population in endemic areas is supposed to be MT positive.

False-negative results may be due to vaccination with live-attenuated virus, anergy, immunosuppression, immune deficiency, malnutrition, improper administration, improper storage, and contamination.

Not all children exposed to the bacilli become infected, and it may take 3 months for the Mantoux test to become positive. Unfortunately, children younger than 5 years may develop disseminated TB in the form of miliary disease or tubercular meningitis before the Mantoux test result becomes positive. Thus, a very high index of suspicion is required when a young patient has a history of contact.

Children may have asymptomatic infection with a positive Mantoux test without any clinical or radiographic manifestations.

Imaging Studies

Chest radiograph is the most important diagnostic tool for evaluating pulmonary TB (Fig. 41.1 and 41.2).

Computed tomographic scan and magnetic resonance imaging. These are not routinely indicated when CXR findings are unremarkable. However, in the presence of pulmonary TB, these imaging studies can help demonstrate the hilar lymphadenopathy,

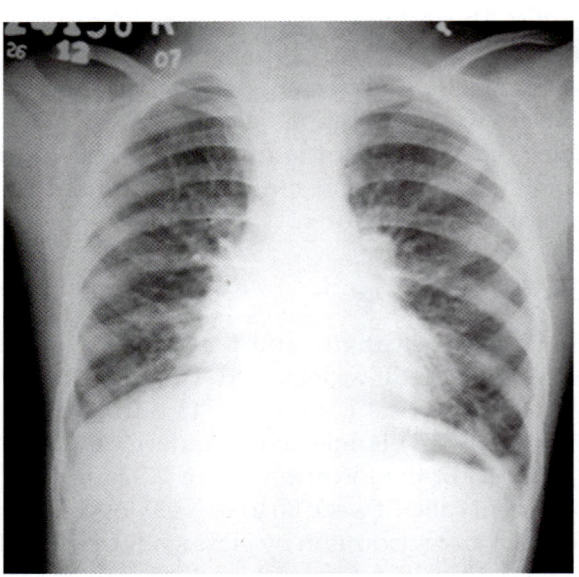

Fig. 41.1: Skiagram chest PA view with multiple heterogenous opacities suggestive of Kochs

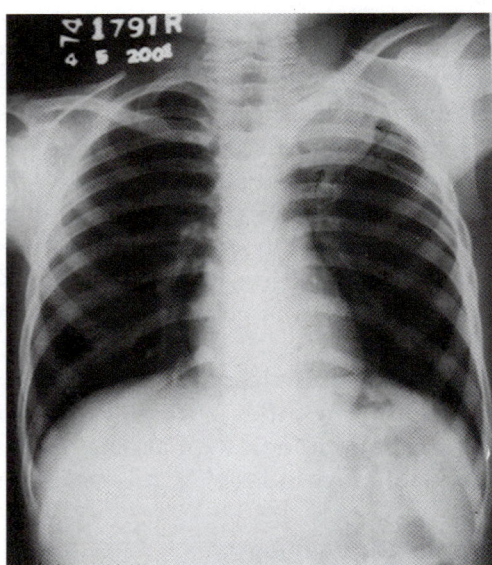

Fig. 41.2: Skiagram chest PA view with mass left upper lobe, that was excised. The histopathology was suggestive of tuberculosis

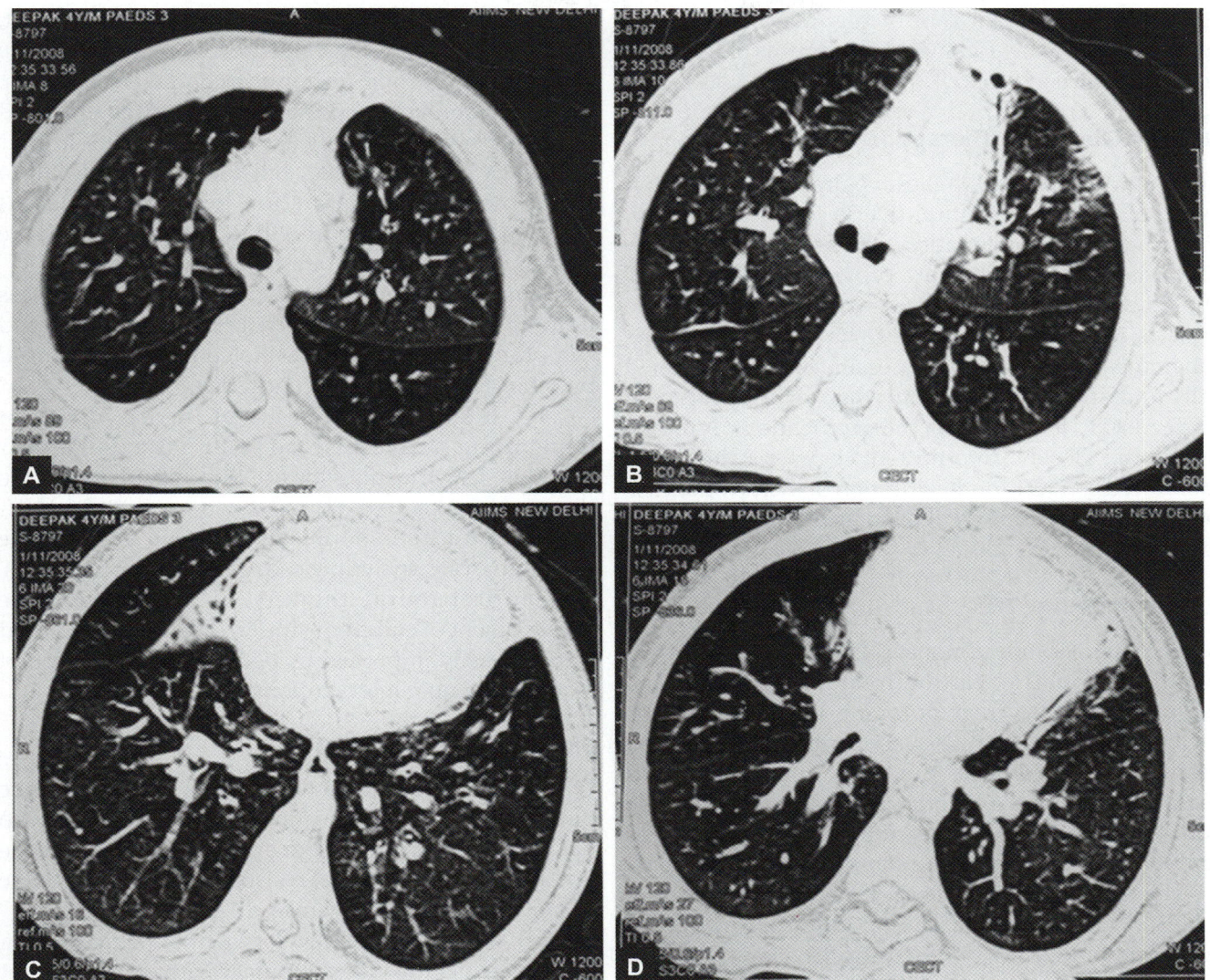

Figs 41.3A to D: CECT chest with evidence of airspace opacities of the left upper lobe, collapse consolidation of left upper lobe, medial segment right middle lobe and lingual lobe

endobronchial TB, pericardial invasion, and early cavitations or bronchiectasis (Figs 41.3A-D to 41.5).[4,5]

MEDICAL TREATMENT

Current recommendations for the treatment of pulmonary TB include a 6-month course of INH and rifampin, supplemented during the first 2 months with pyrazinamide.

Ethambutol is not routinely recommended for children less then five years age as one of its side effects is impaired vision and that is difficult to monitor in younger children. Streptomycin may be added if the infection is massive or drug resistance is suspected.

Drug sensitivity studies may not be required if the risk of drug resistance is not significant. Significant risk factors include residence in areas with greater than 4% primary resistance to INH, history of previous treatment with anti-tubercular drugs and history of exposure to a drug-resistant case. The purpose is to decrease the development of MDR-TB in areas where primary INH resistance is high.

Another treatment option is a 2-month regimen of INH, rifampin, and pyrazinamide daily, followed by 4 months of INH and rifampin twice a week. Effective treatment for the hilar adenopathy (when susceptible organisms) includes a 9-month regimen of INH and rifampin daily or a 1-month regimen of INH and rifampin once a day followed by 8 months of INH and rifampin twice a week.

Directly Observed Therapy (DOT)

Since non-compliance to these regimens is a common cause of treatment failure, (DOT) is recommended. This involves administration of the medication under supervision by a health care provider or nurse. DOT should be used for all children with tuberculosis. The lack of pediatric dosage forms of most anti-tuberculosis medications necessitates using crushed pills and suspensions. Even when drugs are given under DOT, tolerance of the medications must be monitored closely. Intermittent regimens should be monitored by DOT for the duration of therapy because poor compliance may result in inadequate drug delivery.

Extrapulmonary TB

Most cases of extrapulmonary TB, including cervical lymphadenopathy, can be treated with the same regimens used to treat pulmonary TB. Exceptions include bone and joint disease, miliary disease and meningitis. For these, the recommendation is a regimen of 2 months of INH, rifampin, pyrazinamide and streptomycin once a day, followed by 7-10 months of INH and rifampin once a day.

The other recommended regimen is 2 months of 4 drugs; INH, rifampin, pyrazinamide, and streptomycin, followed by 7-10 months of INH and rifampin twice a week.

Capreomycin or kanamycin may be given instead of streptomycin in areas where resistance to streptomycin is common.

Tuberculosis and HIV

The use of a regimen that uses rifabutin instead of rifampin has been advised when treating HIV disease and TB simultaneously.

The treatment regimen for TB initially should include at least 3 drugs and should be continued for at least 9 months. INH, rifampin, and pyrazinamide with or without ethambutol or streptomycin should be administered for the first 2 months. Treatment of disseminated disease or drug-resistant TB may require the addition of a fourth drug.

The tuberculin skin test (TST) or the Mantoux test, which is the standard marker of *Mycobacterium tuberculosis* infection in immunocompetent children, has poor sensitivity when used in HIV-infected children.[5] Novel T cell assays may offer higher sensitivity and specificity, but these tests still fail to make the crucial distinction between the latent *M. tuberculosis* infection and the active disease and are limited by cost considerations.[5]

Symptom-based diagnostic approaches are less helpful in HIV-infected children, as TB-related symptoms can not be differentiated from those caused by other HIV-associated conditions.

HIV-infected children are at increased risk of developing active disease after TB exposure or infection, which justifies the use of isoniazid preventive therapy once active TB has been excluded.[5] HIV-infected children should also receive appropriate supportive care, including co-trimoxazole prophylaxis, and antiretroviral therapy, if indicated.[5] The management of children with TB/HIV infection could thus be vastly improved by better implementation of readily available interventions.

Multidrug Resistant TB

Primary resistance is defined as the resistance developing to anti-TB treatment in an individual who has no history of prior treatment. Secondary resistance involves the emergence of resistance during the course of ineffective anti-TB therapy.

Risk factors for the development of primary drug resistance include patient contact with drug-resistant contagious TB, residence in areas with a high prevalence of drug-resistant *M. tuberculosis*, HIV infection, and the use of intravenous drugs. Secondary drug resistance reflects non-compliance to the regimen, inappropriate drug regimens, and/or interference with absorption of the drug.

According to the current guidelines, the child who is at risk or the one who has the disease resistant to INH, at least 2 drugs (to which the isolate is sensitive on culture) should be administered. Another principle is not to add only a single drug to an already failing regimen. The pattern of drug resistance, toxicities of the drugs, and patients' responses to treatment, all determine the duration and the regimen selected.

The initial treatment regimen for patients with MDR-TB should include 4 drugs, e.g. at least 2

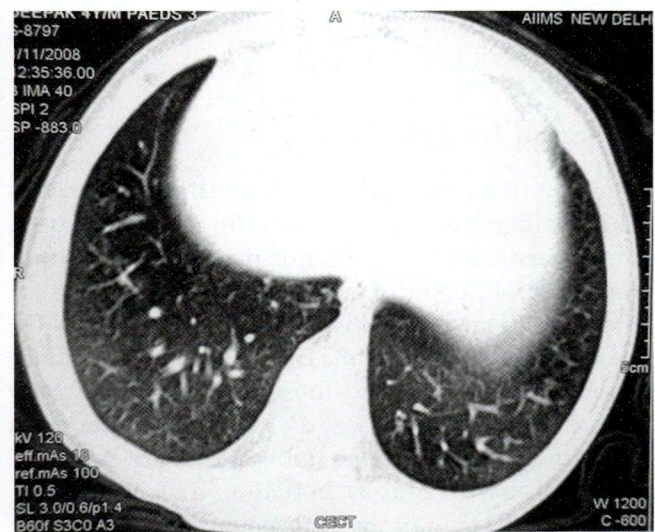

Fig. 41.4: CECT chest with evidence of patchy ground glass densities in bilateral lung fields

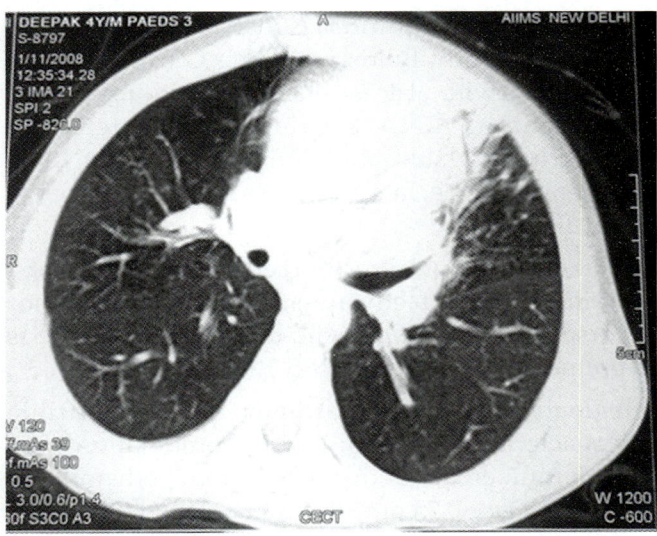

Fig. 41.5: CECT chest with evidence of small (R) paratracheal precarinal, subcarinal and left hilar lymph nodes suggestive of infective etiology

bactericidal drugs (e.g. INH, rifampin), a pyrazinamide, and either the streptomycin or another aminoglycoside (also bactericidal) or high-dose ethambutol (25 mg/kg/d) should be incorporated into the regimen.

Six-month treatment regimens and intermittent therapy are not advocated for patients with strains resistant to INH or rifampin. In isolated INH resistance, the 4-drug, 6-month regimen should be started initially for the treatment of pulmonary TB. INH should be discontinued when resistance is documented. Pyrazinamide should be continued for the entire 6-month course of treatment.

In the 9-month regimen, INH should be discontinued upon the documentation of isolated INH resistance. If ethambutol was included in the initial regimen, continue treatment with rifampin and ethambutol for a minimum of 12 months. If ethambutol was not included, then sensitivity tests are repeated, INH is discontinued and 2 new drugs are added (e.g. ethambutol and pyrazinamide).

Resistance to both INH and rifampin is a complicated issue. The initial drug regimen is continued (with 2 drugs to which the organism is susceptible) until bacteriologic sputum conversion is documented; followed by at least 12 months of 2-drug therapy. The role of new agents such as quinolone derivatives and amikacin in MDR cases remains unclear.

Antitubercular Drugs

Antimycobacterial agents against *Mycobacterium* species are used to treat TB, leprosy, and other mycobacterial infections. These are classified as first-line and second-line drugs. First-line agents include rifampin, isoniazid (INH), pyrazinamide, ethambutol, and streptomycin. First-line drugs have less toxicity with greater efficacy than second-line drugs. All first-line agents are bactericidal with the exception of ethambutol.

Second-line agents are capreomycin, ciprofloxacin, cycloserine, ethionamide, kanamycin, ofloxacin, levofloxacin, and para-aminosalicylic acid.

INH and rifampin are effective against bacilli in necrotic foci and intracellular populations of mycobacteria. Streptomycin, aminoglycosides, and capreomycin have poor intracellular penetration. MDR-TB is defined as resistance to at least INH and rifampin. The emergence of drug-resistant strains has necessitated use of second-line agents.

There is a promising pipeline of more than 20 new anti-tuberculosis agents at various stages of development, and several are already entering early clinical trials. Donald PR.

Childhood tuberculosis (TB) comprises a significant part of the TB caseload, particularly in developing communities. It is essential that the pharmacokinetics and toxicity of any new agent should be assessed in a population of children over a range of ages.[14]

Rifampin: Bactericidal for M. tuberculosis. Penetrates well into all body fluids including CSF. For use in combination with at least one other antituberculous drug. Inhibits RNA synthesis in bacteria by binding to beta subunit of DNA-dependent RNA polymerase, which, in turn, blocks RNA transcription. Dose - 10 mg/kg.

Isoniazid: Commonly referred to as INH. Best combination of effectiveness, low cost, and minor adverse effects. Prophylactic dose of pyridoxine is recommended with it. Dose- 5-10 mg/kg.

Streptomycin: For treatment of susceptible mycobacterial infections. Use in combination with other antituberculous drugs (e.g. INH, ethambutol, rifampin). Dose 0.75 gm - 1 gm/day IM.

Pyrazinamide: Pyrazine analog of nicotinamide that may be bacteriostatic or bactericidal against *M tuberculosis*, depending on concentration of drug attained at site of infection. Dose -15-30 mg/kg.

Ethambutol: Diffuses into actively growing mycobacterial cells, such as tubercle bacilli. Impairs cell metabolism by inhibiting synthesis of one or more metabolites, which in turn causes cell death. Not given in younger children. In children more than 12 years if no previous antituberculous therapy has been taken, then 15 mg/kg PO, otherwise -25 mg/kg.

Ethionamide: Bacteriostatic against *M tuberculosis*. Recommended when treatment with first-line drugs (INH, rifampin) has failed. Treats any form of active TB. However, only should be used with other effective antituberculous agents. 15-20 mg/kg/d divided tid/qid; not to exceed 1 gm/d; concomitant administration of pyridoxine recommended.

Para-aminosalicylic acid: Bacteriostatic agent useful against *M tuberculosis*. Inhibits onset of bacterial resistance to streptomycin and INH. 150 mg/kg/d PO divided tid/qid; not to exceed 12 gm/d.

Kanamycin: Aminoglycoside antibiotic produced by Streptomyces kanamyceticus. May be used as second-line agent in treatment of TB. 15-30 mg/kg/d IM.

Rifabutin: Ansamycin antibiotic derived from rifamycin S. Inhibits DNA-dependent RNA polymerase, preventing chain initiation, in susceptible strains of *Escherichia coli* and *Bacillus subtilis* but not in mammalian cells. If GI upset occurs, administer dose bid with food. 10-20 mg/kg/d orally.

Fluoroquinolones have not been approved for use in patients less than 18 years.

Monitoring for Side Effects

Adverse effects of INH (e.g. hepatitis) are rare in children; therefore, routine determination of serum aminotransferase levels is not necessary. Monthly monitoring of hepatic function tests may be done for patients with severe or disseminated TB, miliary TB, concurrent or recent hepatic disease, clinical evidence of hepatotoxic effects and those receiving high daily doses of INH (10 mg/kg/d) in combination with rifampin, pyrazinamide, or both. In the rare event the patient has symptoms of hepatitis, discontinue the regimen and evaluate liver function. If the tests are normal or return to normal, then a decision to restart the medications may be made. Re-introduce the drugs one by one.

FOLLOW-UP

A regular follow-up in every 4-8 weeks should be done to ensure compliance and to monitor the adverse effects of and response to the medications administered. The weight of the child should be measured at each visit. The sclera should be examined for any evidence of jaundice.

Follow-up ESR and CXR may be obtained after 2-3 months of therapy to observe the response to treatment in patients with pulmonary TB. However, hilar lymphadenopathy may take several years to resolve. Thus, a normal CXR is not required for termination of therapy.

COMPLICATIONS

1. Miliary tuberculosis
2. Tubercular meningitis
3. Pleural effusion
4. Pneumothorax
5. Complete obstruction of a bronchus - if caseous material extrudes into the lumen
6. Atelectasis
7. Bronchiectasis
8. Stenosis of the airways
9. Bronchoesophageal fistula
10. Endobronchial disease.

ROLE OF SURGERY

It must be emphasized that medical therapy remains the mainstay of treatment in pulmonary tuberculosis and surgical treatment is primarily used to handle complications and hasten recovery.

In children, the primary complex is usually directly or indirectly the primary etiologic factor for surgical intervention. The indications for surgical intervention are limited in children and the challenge lies in determining the timing and nature of intervention. Table 41.1 lists the indication for surgery in pediatric pulmonary tuberculosis.[15-18]

Pre-operative Management

Tuberculosis is cured by effective antitubercular therapy and all surgical candidates must have preferably completed at least 3 months of appropriate antitubercular treatment before any surgical intervention. The probable exception to this principle are children with acute airway obstruction, drug resistant organisms, children with evidence of progressive disease while on treatment and other complications like massive hemoptysis and bronchopleural fistula. The preoperative assessment includes a pulmonary function test, room air ABCJ analysis and nutritional assessment. Total parenteral nutrition or Ryle's tube feeding may be initiated to counter the chronic debilitating effects of tuberculosis. The serum albumin level is maintained above 3 gm/dl and anaemia is treated prior to surgery. Rigorous chest physiotherapy, incentive spirometry and deep breathing exercises are instituted prior to surgery. Patient counseling is important and the child is motivated to adopt the above measures with a view to continue in the postoperative period. These measures are absolutely vital to decrease morbidity and ensure success after surgery.

Endobronchial Tuberculosis

Primary tuberculosis lymphadenopathy of the subcarinal and paratracheal nodes can result in airway obstruction and secondary damage due to atelectasis, obstructive emphysema and pulmonary infection. A "node compression syndrome" has been described in infants and children.[19] The narrow, compliant pediatric airway may be compressed between the subcarinal and paratracheal lymph node groups. The lymph nodes may erode into the bronchus causing bronchial ulcerations and intraluminal obstruction.

In the review by Hewitson et al, 64 of the 168 (38%) children who required surgical intervention for pulmonary tuberculosis presented with acute or chronic major airway obstruction.[15] Almost half of the children who require hospitalization for complications of pulmonary tuberculosis have radiological evidence of mediastinal lymphadenopathy.[20]

The diagnosis of major airway obstruction can be suspected on an over penetrated chest radiograph or a high Kilovolt radiograph. A chest computed tomography (CT) scan is the definitive modality to diagnose airway compression and identify the enlarged mediastinal nodes. The lung parenchyma can be evaluated to see the extent of obstructive emphysematous or atelectatic changes.

Steroid therapy is widely used to relieve the airway obstruction and acts by reducing mucosal edema and perilymphatic inflammation. However, the response to corticosteroids is only transient and surgical decompression is the definitive treatment for this complication.

Table 41.1: Indications of surgery in pediatric pulmonary tuberculosis

A. *Complications of Primary Tuberculosis*
1. Airway obstruction-extrinsic lymph node compression or intraluminal obstruction
2. Progressive primary infection- cavity formation.

B. *Sequelae*
1. Post-tuberculous pulmonary obstruction, bronchiectasis
2. Bronchial stenosis/stricture
3. Phrenic nerve entrapment.

C. *Other Indications*
1. Drainage of lung abscess
2. Bronchopleural fistula, bronchoesophageal fistula
3. Massive hemoptysis
4. Chest wall sinus
5. Post-tubular constrictive pericarditis
6. Pulmonary aspergilloma
7. Fibrothorax / Trapped lung
8. Suspicion of malignancy
9. Pulmonary resection for multidrug-resistant tuberculosis
10. Tubercular rib osteomyelitis
11. Tubercular empyema
 [Discussed in detail in Chapter 43]

Surgery should always be preceded by rigid bronchoscopy to evaluate the site of airway compression and also assess any intraluminal erosion or involvement. The surgical procedure advocated in lymph node compression syndrome is incision and curettage of the node with partial preservation of the capsule which is usually adherent to the hilar structures.[21] Evacuation of nodes is easily achieved in cases of caseous degeneration. Lymph node excision should never be attempted as it can lead to damage of the airway wall or other vital structures. A reduced hospital stay and faster recovery following surgical decompression of mediastinal adenopathy causing airway obstruction has been reported.[19] The subcarinal nodes are more easily accessible and decompression of these nodes can relieve obstruction to both the main bronchi.

The treatment of chronic airway compromise is medical therapy, but some authors recommend early surgery.[22] Long-term compression can lead to bronchial stenosis and the obstructed lung segment may be permanently damaged due to secondary bacterial infection. Surgery is however, more hazardous in these patients with chronic obstruction due to dense adhesions and fibrosis seen in these patients. In some patients, despite node decompression, airway narrowing may persist due to the fibrous scarring associated with the lesion.

Intraluminal obstruction can occur secondary to the endobronchial tuberculosis or due to granulomatous tissue obstructing the airway. Bronchoscopic removal of the caseous material or granulation tissue can lead to re-inflation of the distal atelectatic segment. Hemorrhage and damage to the bronchial wall are potential complications.

Post-tuberculosis Pulmonary Destruction

In cases with poor response to medical therapy or multi-drug resistance, the lung may be extensively damaged. The decision about pulmonary resection is based primarily an symptomatology and the risk of contralateral lung damage. In contrast to adult patients, children with post-tuberculous pulmonary destruction usually have chronic bronchiectatic disease of the lower lobes. The probable etiology for this lesion is usually untreated nodal compression. Hence, most authors recommend aggressive and early surgical management of nodal compression to prevent subsequent damage.[23] The bronchiectatic lesions in pulmonary tuberculosis are usually peripheral and are of the cylindrical type. The middle lobe syndrome is an atelectasis persisting for more than 1 month. The large Iymph nodes, the relatively narrow lumen and peculiar angle of take off, all lead to middle lobe atelectasis and secondary infection. The indications for pulmonary resection in tuberculosis are listed in Table 41.2. Lobectomy is the first surgical option, but in extensive lesions, with completely damaged lung tissue, pneumonectomy may be indicated.

Preoperative physiotherapy and broad spectrum (including anaerobic) antibiotics are used routinely to decrease sputum production. Overholt et al described the use of the posterior thoracotomy in a prone position to avoid contralateral lung contamination.[23] Single lung ventilation is used routinely to prevent contamination. Rib resection is usually required for a contracted hemithorax. The latissimus dorsi muscle may be preserved as a flap, based on the thoracodorsal artery and can be used to cover the bronchial stump. An extrapleural approach for pneumonectomy is advocated to minimize iatrogenic trauma and blood loss.[24] Postoperatively, bronchopleural fistulae are the most common complication. Covering the bronchial stump with latissmus dorsi, intercostal muscle, biological glue or omentum has been described to decrease the incidence of bronchopleural fistulae.[25,26] Extensive skeletonization of the bronchial stump should be avoided to ensure good vascularity and healing.

Table 41.2: Indications for pulmonary resection in cases of tuberculosis

1. Persistently positive sputum cultures with cavitation after 6 months of continuous optimal chemotherapy with 2 or more drugs.
2. Symptomatic bronchiectasis not controlled with conservative measures
3. Advanced disease with extensive caseation necrosis.
4. Massive life- threatening hemoptysis or recurrent severe hemoptysis.
5. Trapped lung
6. Localized disease (encompassing 1-2 segments of the lung) with resistant organisms.
7. A mass lesion of the lung in an area of tubercular involvement (Fig. 41.2).

Role of Pulmonary Resection for Multi-drug Resistant TB

The goal of surgical treatment in multidrug resistant tuberculosis is to eliminate the predominant bacterial foci in the lungs. Atypical mycobacterial infections often require surgical resection to decrease the incidence of complications and progressive damage. In adult patients, Pomerantz et al have reported selective left lung destruction twice more commonly in cases with multidrug resistant tuberculosis.[27,28] This has been termed as the left bronchial syndrome. The typical left lung affliction has not been noted in atypical infections. Lobectomy or segmental resections are preferred in such cases.

Miscellaneous Indications

Tuberculous pleural disease may need surgical intervention in the acute phase or in the chronic phase of pleural fibrosis. Pleural fibrosis regresses with time and therefore, the indication for decortication is primarily based on sympotomatology or postural problems (like scoliosis). During primary tubercular infection, pleural effusions are seen in 8-10% cases and may require tube thoracostomy for drainage.[29]

Peribronchial lymph nodes may cause circumferential bronchial constriction which will heal with scarring and lead to bronchial stenosis.[30] Endobronchial tuberculosis can also result due to direct inoculation prior to effective antitubercular therapy. A 10-15% patients with active pulmonary disease have evidence of endobronchial tuberculosis. The left main bronchus is more commonly involved as it is more prone for extrinsic lymph node compression and is also anatomically compromised by the aortic arch. Surgery is indicated to prevent the complications of obstructive emphysema, bronchiectasis and infection. In the presence of damage to the distal lung parenchyma, a lobectomy is indicated. Bronchoplastic procedures or stenting are options in bronchial stenosis with preserved lung parenchyma.

Phrenic nerve palsy and eventration can occur due to nerve entrapment. Debulking of the nodes with or without diaphragmatic plication may be indicated in these patients.

Massive hemoptysis is rarely seen in children and can result due to erosion of a bronchial artery or secondary to *Aspergillus* superinfection.[25] The site of bleeding is localized by angiography or bronchoscopy. Bronchial blockage (to prevent flooding of the contralateral lung) and embolization are the immediate measures. Failure to respond to conservative measures necessitates surgical excision of the involved lobe.

Bronchopleural fistulae are rare but pose difficult problems, seen in pulmonary tuberculosis. The immediate management includes an intercostal drainage of the pneumothorax. Surgical management is indicated for unresponsive bronchopleural fistulae. Pulmonary resection is usually required to eliminate the involved lobe and its bronchus.

In conclusion, surgical management of pulmonary tuberculosis has a definite role. The indications for surgical intervention are not well defined and the decision should be based on symptomatology and the risk of ongoing damage. Preoperative physiotherapy and optimization of lung function is vital for good postoperative results. In children, aggressive surgical treatment of the tuberculous adenopathy is indicated to prevent pulmonary damage. Pulmonary resections during childhood are required for the sequelae of airway obstruction and chronic tuberculous secondary infection. Morbidity after surgical intervention is common but mortality in most series is less than 2 %.

PREVENTION

BCG vaccine is usually given at birth to all newborns in developing countries where the disease is endemic.

The best method to prevent cases of pediatric tuberculosis is to find, diagnose, and treat cases of active tuberculosis among adults. Children do not usually contract tuberculosis from other children or transmit it themselves. Adults pass tuberculosis on to the children. Improved contact investigations and use of directly observed therapy should increase the success rate of finding and treating the adult cases of tuberculosis, therefore reducing the number of cases of pediatric tuberculosis.

Mothers infected with tuberculosis should remain away from their babies till their sputum is negative. This is usually after 2 months of a 4 drug regimen given to adults.

PROGNOSIS

Prognosis varies according to the clinical manifestation. Poor prognosis is associated with disseminated TB, miliary disease, and tubercular meningitis. Higher mortality rates occur in children younger than 5 years (20%).

The new WHO Stop TB Strategy, released in 2006 has identified six principal components to reduce the global burden of TB by 2015. They are
1. Pursuing high quality DOTS expansion and enhancement.
2. Addressing Tb/HIV, MDR-TB and other challenges.
3. Contributing to health system strengthening.
4. Engaging all care providers.
5. Empowering patients and communities; and
6. Enabling the promoting research.

REFERENCES

1. Gupta DK, Rohatgi M, Misra D. Abdominal tuberculosis in children; edited by Seth V. A publication of Indian Pediatrics, the official Journal of Indian Academy of Pediatrics, New Delhi.1991, chapter 10;188-94.
2. Gupta DK, Sharma Shilpa. Abdominal Tuberculosis in Adolescence in Textbook of Adolescent Medicine. Ed Swati Bhave. Jaypee Brothers New Delhi 2006; Chapter 20.5:663-69.
3. Mohan G, Kulshreshtha S, Dayal R, et al. Effect of therapy on serum zinc and copper in primary complex of children. Biol Trace Elem Res 2007;118:184-90.
4. Brockmann VP, Viviani ST, Peña DA. Pulmonary complications in children with human immunodeficiency virus infection. Rev Chilena Infectol 2007;24(4):301-5. Epub 2007 Aug 20.
5. Marais BJ, Graham SM, Cotton MF, Beyers N. Diagnostic and management challenges for childhood tuberculosis in the era of HIV. J Infect Dis 2007;196 (Suppl 1):S76-85.
6. Varma JK, Wiriyakitjar D, Nateniyom S, et al. Evaluating the potential impact of the new Global Plan to Stop TB: Thailand, 2004-2005 Bull World Health Organ 2007;85(8):586-92.
7. Kehinde AO, Ige OM, Dada-Adegbola HO, et al. Pulmonary tuberculosis in Ibadan: a ten-year review of laboratory reports (1996-2005). Afr J Med Med Sci 2006;35(4):475-78.
8. Ridley R. Applying science to the diseases of poverty Bull World Health Organ 2007;85(7):509-10.
9. Friedland G, Harries A, Coetzee D. Implementation issues in tuberculosis/HIV program collaboration and integration: 3 case studies J Infect Dis 2007;196 (Suppl 1):S114-23.
10. Gillies MJ, Farrugia MK, Lakhoo K. An unusual cause of a superior mediastinal mass in an infant. Pediatr Surg Int. 2007;[Epub ahead of print].
11. Andresen D. Microbiological diagnostic procedures in respiratory infections: mycobacterial infections. Paediatr Respir Rev 2007;8(3):221-30.
12. Fortin K, Carceller A, Robert M, et al. Prevalence of positive tuberculin skin tests in foreign-born children. J Paediatr Child Health 2007;43(11):768-72.
13. Mandalakas AM, Kirchner HL, Iverson S, et al. Predictors of Mycobacterium tuberculosis infection in international adoptees Pediatrics 2007;120(3):e610-16.
14. Donald PR. The assessment of new anti-tuberculosis drugs for a paediatric indication. Int J Tuberc Lung Dis 2007;11(11):1162-65.
15. Hewitson IP, Yon Oppell Yo. Role of thoracic surgery for childhood. World I Surg 1997;21:468-74.
16. Lees WM, Fox RT, Shields TW. Pulmonary surgery for tuberculosis in children. Am Thorac Surg 1967;4:327-30.
17. Lowe IE, et al. Pulmonary tuberculosis in children. J Thorac Cardiovac Surg 1980;80:221.
18. Tuberculosis in Surgical lung diseases in childhood, (Eds). Poradowska W, Reszke S, Kulicz S pp, Polish Medical publishers, Warsaio 1972:163-88.
19. Malatinszky I, Sashegyi B. Broncho-pulmonary lesions associated with lymph node compression -the 'node compression syndrome'. Tuberdl 1970;51:412.
20. Worthington MG, Brink JG, Odell J A, et al. Surgical relief of acute airway obstruction due to primary tuberculosis. Am Thorac Surg 1993;56:1054-62.
21. Nokvi AJ, Nohl-Oser HC. Surgical treatment of bronchial obstruction in primary tuberculosis report of seven cases. Thorax 1979;34:464-69.
22. Freixinet J, Yarela A, Lopez L, et al. Surgical treatment of childhood mediastinal tuberculous lymphadenitis. Am thorac Surg 1995;59:644.
23. Overhold RH, Woods FM. The prone position in thoracic surgery. J Int Coll Surg 1947;10:216.
24. Brown J, Pomerantz M. Extrapleural pneumonectomy for tuberculosis. Chest surg Clin North Am 1995;5:289.
25. Rizzi A, Rocco G, Robustellini M, et al. Results of surgical management of tuberculosis experience in 206 patients undergoing operation. Ann thorac surg 1995;59:896.
26. Reed CE. Pneumonectomy for chronic infection fraught with danger? J Am thorac surg 1995;59:408-11.
27. Pomerantz M, Madsen L, Globel M, et al. Surgical management of resistant mycobacterial, tuberculosis and other mycobacterial pulmonary infection. Am thorac surg 1991;52:1108.
28. Pomerantz M, Brown JM. Surgery of pulmonary mycobacterial disease: In: Mastery of cardiothoracic surgery, (Eds). LRKaiser, IL Kron, TL Spray, Lippincott-Roven publishers Philadelphia 1988:266-71.
29. Mouroux J, et al. Surgical management of pleuro-pulmonary tuberculosis. J Thorac Cardovasc Surg 1996;111:662.
30. Watanabe J, et al. Endobronchial tuberculosis. World J Surg 1997;21:482-87.

Chylothorax

Spencer W Beasley

Chylothorax refers to an accumulation of lymphatic fluid in the pleural cavity, and has a variety of causes (Table 42.1) of which the most common is idiopathic chylothorax of infancy. Chylothorax may occur in up to 1% of children following thoracic surgery and is a less frequent complication of central line placement.[1-4] In iatrogenic cases, it is usually caused by direct injury to the thoracic duct.[1]

ANTENATAL CHYLOTHORAX

Congenital chylothorax may be diagnosed on antenatal ultrasonography, but fetal thoracentesis to measure the lymphocyte count in the pleural effusion does not establish its cause with certainty.[5,6]

Table 42.1: Causes of chylothorax in children	
Cause	Comment
Idiopathic chylothorax of infancy	Most common congenital defect of thoracic lymphatics, or from birth trauma
Pulmonary lymphangiectasis/lymphangiomatosis	Congenital abnormality of pulmonary lymphatics
Trauma	Usually iatrogenic from operative injury, e.g. during cardiac surgical procedures - most resolve spontaneously
Malignancy	Obstruction of the thoracic duct by lymphoma, usually affects older children
Miscellaneous disease	Benign tumors, superior vena cava thrombosis

Antenatal pleuroamniotic shunting may improve the prognosis of congenital chylothorax with hydrops[7] and allow the chylothorax to resolve before birth, with delivery at term and no ongoing respiratory disease. In other fetuses, the chylothorax persists, may require premature delivery and intensive respiratory support including mechanical ventilation and prompt thoracocentesis, although the optimal timing of delivery of chylothorax diagnosed in the third trimester is yet to be determined. Intrapartum thoracocentesis in four fetuses with severe bilateral chylothoraces under ultrasonographic guidance prior to cesarean delivery at 31-34 weeks has been described.[7] All four infants were born in relatively good condition, but all eventually required intubation, ventilation and chest tubes. Two of these survived.

About 50% of fetuses with pulmonary lymphangiectasia abort between 19 and 24 weeks gestation with multiple malformations or anencephaly.[8]

POSTNATAL CHYLOTHORAX

Spontaneous chylothorax in the neonatal period has a 2:1 male predominance.[9] Several cases of congenital chylothorax in siblings have been described, with a pattern consistent with autosomal recessive inheritance.[9-11] Reports of recurrent congenital chylothorax in male offspring have led to the suggestion of a possible X-linked recessive inheritance pattern in some families.[12,13]

Chylothorax may develop after repair of congenital diaphragmatic hernia, perhaps more frequently than generally appreciated.[14,15] It has been described also in older children with unexplained rib and other fractures, and failure to thrive, in which situation it is suggestive of child abuse.[16,17]

Traumatic causes include operative trauma and also during the hyperextension of the spine, with the rupture of the duct from stretching as occurs during diving and wrestling.

Lymphoma may cause chylothorax. Less commonly, it is seen in association with neuroblastoma.[18] In one infant with a mediastinal neuroblastoma it resolved following ligation of the thoracic duct after multiple thoracentesis and chest tube drainage had failed. Congenital chylothorax has been reported in fetal (neonatal) thyrotoxicosis secondary to maternal Graves' disease, and with congenital hypothyroidism.[19,20]

When chylothorax occurs with multiple cutaneous lymphangiomas it tends to have favorable course, with complete regression of the cutaneous lymphangiomas.[21] Primary congenital pulmonary lymphangiectasis (CPL) is a relatively rare and poorly understood condition that produces chylous pleural effusions and pulmonary hypoplasia and is assumed to be due to a developmental error of the lymphatic system that results in pulmonary lymphatic obstruction.[8] Most cases are sporadic, but CPL can occur in siblings, or as part of a multiple congenital anomalies syndrome such Noonan, Ullrich-Turner and Down's syndromes.[8,22-24]

INVESTIGATIONS

A plain X-ray of the chest is usually the first radiological investigation performed. Computerised tomography of the chest and nuclear lymphangiography may assist in identification of the origin of the pleural effusion, but are usually unable to demonstrate a congenital fistula or other pathology of the thoracic duct. Localisation of the site of lymphatic leakage has been demonstrated by scintigraphy after oral administration of a ^{123}I labelled long-chain fatty acid derivative iodophenyl pentadecanoic acid (IPPA).[25] The full extent of disseminated lymphangiomatosis that presents with chylothorax (including bone lesions and other visceral involvement) is best demonstrated on T2-weighted MR images.[26]

Evaluation of the content of the pleural fluid confirms the diagnosis of chylothorax (Table 42.2). Chyle is usually opaque ("milky"), but if the infant is

Table 42.2: Characteristics of chyle*

Parameter	Characteristic of chyle
Fat content	> 400 mg/dL
Triglycerides	> 22 mg/dL
Protein	50% of plasma protein
Specific gravity	> 1.012
Gram's stain	> 90% lymphocytes
Sudan red stain	Chylomicrons[27,35] +

* Modified from Rodgers and McGahren[11]

not being fed orally the low fat content may make it appear serosanguinous or straw-colored.

MEDICAL TREATMENT

Non-operative treatment of chylothorax is effective in up to 80%.[1,27] Total parenteral nutrition (TPN) may be more effective than oral medium chain triglyceride (MCT) in the treatment of spontaneous congenital chylothorax.[28] A medium chain triglyceride (MCT) diet reduces lymphatic flow through the thoracic duct, and is primarily indicated in the treatment of postoperative chylothorax of the newborn. Intermittent thoracentesis under echo-guidance to drain the chyle from the chest may be effective, although the thoracentesis may need to be performed several times. The development of superior vena cava thrombosis or obstruction indicates that conservative management is less likely to be successful.[1]

The combination of ventilatory support, repeated thoracentesis, thoracotomy tube drainage, total parenteral nutrition (TPN) and MCT feeds would be expected to result in resolution of the chylothorax in the majority of patients (Fig. 42.1). One report suggests that high-frequency ventilation (HFV) may have a role where conventional mechanical ventilation has failed.[29] Continuous somatostatin infusion for 14 days for chylothorax after cardiac surgery has been employed.[30] Most effusions resolve within six weeks.[9] The thoracic duct carries a large number of T-lymphocytes and the continuous loss of lymph may lead to the setting of immuno-deficiency.

SURGICAL TREATMENT

Surgical intervention for congenital chylothorax is recommended if medical treatment (including MCT diet, TPN and chyle drainage) is unsuccessful

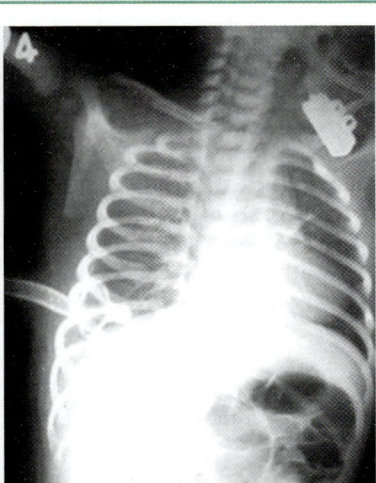

Fig. 42.1: Skiagram chest of a newborn who had chylothorax in the rigth thoracic cavity. The patient improved after intercostal tube drainage and total parenteral nutrition therapy for 2 weeks

(Table 42.3).[28] Surgery is more likely to be required in congenital chylothorax than in chylothorax that occurs following cardiothoracic surgery.[1]

Early surgical intervention should be considered where the child has an elevated right heart pressure or central venous thrombosis, as non-operative treatment is less likely to be successful.[27,31] Surgical intervention tends to be earlier if the less invasive procedures of thoracoscopy or insertion of a pleuro-peritoneal shunt are used.[31,32] Overall, surgical intervention reduces hospital stay.[9] Thorascopic techniques have now been adapted to allow identification of the leak site, application of surgical clips or fibrin glue to control it, and to assist in the accurate placement of pleuro-peritoneal shunt tubing.[33]

The usual purpose of surgical intervention is to occlude the thoracic duct, by identifying the point of chyle leakage and under-running it. Where the exact source of chyle cannot be identified, surgery is directed at limiting the accumulation of chyle by obliterating the pleural cavity: For example, partial pleurodesis may be used where there is difficulty identifying the exact leakage point at thoracotomy or thorascopy. Alternatively, fibrin glue can be applied to the general area of leakage.[11]

Pleuro-peritoneal shunt may be helpful where repeated thoracentesis has failed and may be effective in 75-95%.[11,31] The shunt is best placed subcutaneously. In a series where the pump chamber was externalised, shunt malfunction and infection were recognised as complications.[34] The most common indication for the procedure has been refractory chylothorax following surgical correction of congenital heart disease. In a series of seven patients in whom Denver double-valued shunts were implanted under general anesthesia, the shunts were required for an average of 44 days.[6]

REFERENCES

1. Beghetti M, La Scala G, Belli D, et al. Etiology and management of pediatric chylothorax. J. of Pediatrics 2000;136(5):653-58.
2. Allen EM, Van Heeckeren DW, Spector ML, et al. Management of nutritional and infection complications of postoperative chylothorax in children. J. Pediatr Surg 1991;26:1169.

Table 42.3: Therapeutic modalities available	
1. Decrease lymphatic flow through thoracic duct	• Medium chain triglyceride diet • Nil orally, total parenteral nutrition
2. Drain chyle from pleural space	• Needle thoracentesis • Tube thoracentesis
3. Obliteration of thoracic duct or area of leakage	• Surgical occlusion (via thoracotomy or thoracoscopy) • Pleurodesis
4. Supportive treatment	• Ventilatory assistance • TPN
5. Monitor protein levels and lymphocyte numbers	• Drainage of chyle also includes protein and lymphocytes

3. Kurekci E, Kaye R, Koehler M. Chylothorax and chylopericardium: a complication of a central venous catheter. J. Pediatrics 1998;132(6):1064-66.
4. Moadel-Sernick RM, Crooke GA, Freeman LM. Lymphoscintigraphy demonstrating thoracic duct injury in an infant with hypoplastic left heart syndrome. Clinical Nuclear Medicine 2000;25(5):335-66.
5. Mohan H, Paes ML, Haynes S. Use of intravenous immunoglobins as an adjunct in the conservative management of chylothorax. Pediatric Anesthesia 1999;9(1):89-92.
6. Engum SA, Rescorla FJ, West KW, Scherer LR 3rd, Grosfield JL. The use of pleuroperitoneal shunts in the management of persistent chylothorax in infants. J Pediatr Surgery 1999;34(2):286-90.
7. Gonen R, Degani S, Kugelman A, Abend M, Bader D. Intrapartum drainage of fetal pleural effusion. Prenatal Diagnosis 1999;19(12):1124-26.
8. Bouchard D, Di Lorenzo M, Youssef S, Simard P, Lapierre JG. Pulmonary lymphangiectasia revisited. J Pediatr Surgery 2000;35(5):796-800.
9. Buttiker V, Fanconi S, Burger R. Chylothorax in children: guidelines for diagnosis and management. Chest 1999;116(3):682-87.
10. Fox GF, Challis D, O'Brien KK, Kelly EN, Ryan G. Congenital chylothorax in siblings.
11. Rodgers BM, McGahren ED, "Mediatinum and Pleura". Surgery of infants and children: scientific principles and practice. Oldham KT, Colombani PM, Foglia RP, Lippincott-Raven, Philadelphia 1997;924-26.
12. Defoort P, Thiery M. Antenatal diagnosis of congenital chylothorax by gray scale sonography. J Clin Ultrasound 1978;6:47-48.
13. King PA, Ghosh A, Tang MH, Lam SK. Recurrent congenital chylothorax. Prenat Diagn. 1991;11:809-11.
14. Kavvadia V, Greenough A, Davenport M, Karani J, Nicolaides KH. Chylothorax after repair of congenital diaphragmatic hernia - risk factors and morbidity. J Pediatr Surgery 1998;33(2):500-02.
15. Naik S, Greenough, A, Zhant YX, Davenport M. Predication of morbidity during infancy after repair of congenital diaphragmatic hernia. J Pediatr Surgery 1996;31(12):1651-54.
16. Geisman SL, Tilelli JA, Campbell JB, Chiaro JJ. Chylothorax as a manifestation of child abuse. Pediatric Emergency Care 1997;13(6):386-89.
17. Guleserian KJ, Gilchrist BF, Luks FI, Wesselhoeft CW, DeLuca FG. Child abuse as a cause of traumatic chylothorax. J Pediatr Surgery 1996;31(12):1696-97.
18. Ease D, Balaraman V, Ash K, et al. Congenital chylothorax and mediastinal neuroblastoma. J Pediatr Surg 1991;26:96.
19. Ibrahim H, Asamoah A, Krouskop RW, Lewis D, Webster P, Pramanik AK. Congenital chylothorax in neonatal thyrotoxicosis. J Perinatology 1999;19(1)68-71.
20. Kessel I, Makhoul IR, Sujov P. Congenital hypothyroidism and non-immune hydrops fetalis: associated? Pediatrics 1999;103(1):E9.
21. Dutheil P, Leraillez J, Fuillemette J, Wallach D. Generalized lymphangiomatosis with chylothorax and skin lymphangiomas in a neonate. Pediatric Dermatology 1998;15(4):296-98.
22. Yamamoto T, Koeda T, Tamura A, Sawada H, Nagata I, Nagata N, Ito T, Mio Y. Congenital chylothorax in a patient with 21 trisomy syndrome. Acta Paediatrica Japonica 1996;38(6):689-91.
23. Takeuchi K, Moriyama T, Oomori S, Masuko K, Maruo T. Management of acute chylothorax with hydrops fetalis diagnosed in the third trimester of pregnancy. Fetal Diagnosis and Therapy 1999;14(5):264-65.
24. Puddy V, Lam BC, Tang M, Wong KY, Lam YH, Wong K, Yeung CY. Variable levels of mosaicism for trisomy 21 in non-immune hydropic infant with chylothorax. Prenatal Diagnosis 1999;19(8):764-66.
25. Kettner BI, Aurisch R, Ruckert JC, Sandrock D, Munz DL. Scintigraphanic localisation of lymphatic leakage site after oral administration of iodine-123-IPPA. J Nuclear Medicine 1998;39(12):2141-44.
26. Konex O, Vyas PK, Goyal M. Disseminated lymphangiomatosis presenting with massive chylothorax. Pediatric Radiology 2000;30(1):35-37.
27. Bond SJ, Guzzetta PC, Snyder ML, et al. Management of pediatric postoperative chylothorax. Ann Thorac Surg 1993;56:469.
28. Fernando Alvarez JR, Kalache KD, Grauel EL. Management of spontaneous congenital chylothorax: oral medium-chain triglycerides versus total parenteral nutrition. American J Perinatology 1999;16(8):415-20.
29. Kugelman A, Gonen R, Bader D. Potential role of high frequency ventilation in the treatment of severe congenital pleural effusion. Pediatric Pulmonology 2000;29(5):404-08.
30. Rimensberger PC, Muller-Schenker B, Kalangos A, Beghetti M. Treatment of persistent postoperative chylothorax with somatostatin. Ann. Thorac Surg 1998;66(1):253-54.
31. Rheubau KS, Kron RL, Carpenter MA, et al. Pleuroperitoneal shunts for refractory chylothorax after operation for congenital heart disease. Ann Thorac Surg 1992;53:85.
32. Graham DD, McGahren ED, Tribble CG, et al. Use of video-assisted thoracic surgery in the treatment of chylothorax. Ann Thorac Surg 1994;57:1507.
33. Reynolds M. Disorders of the thoracic cavity and pleura and infections of the lung, pleura and mediastinum. Ins: Pediatric Surgery 5th edn. O'Neill, JA, Rowe MI, Grosfeld JL, Fonkalsrud EW and Coran AG (Eds). Mosby St Louis, 1998 pp 913-14.
34. Wolff AB, Silen Ml, Kokoska ER, Rodgers BM. Treatment of refractory chylothorax with externalized pleuroperitoneal shunts in children. Ann Thorac Surg 1999;68(3):1053-57.

CHAPTER 43

Empyema Thoracis

Shilpa Sharma, DK Gupta

Thoracic empyema is a life-threatening condition in pediatric surgical practice.

Empyema thoracis in children has been dealt since ages by pediatricians initially who then refer the case to the pediatric surgeon when they feel the need. It is thus vital for every pediatric surgeon to be well versed with the etiology, stages of empyema and its natural course. Empyema thoracis forms about 5-15% of the cases seen by a pediatrician. Empyema is usually a post-pneumonia sequelae. *Staphylococcus aureus* is the commonest etiological agent (77%); with clustering seen during hot and humid months. Community acquired methicillin resistant *S aureus* (MRSA) is showing an increasing trend. Most children are treated with parenteral cloxacillin and an aminoglycoside. Culture positivity has decreased significantly over the years due to the availability of broad spectrum antibiotics which the patients receive before presentation. Tube drainage is used in 80-90% of fibropurulent cases and is successful in 70-80% cases.[1,2] At a referral center, upto 3-5% of the cases may require decortication. Early diagnosis and appropriate treatment may prevent the need for any surgical intervention. Surgery is mainly required by children with persistent pleural sepsis after 10 days of Tube drainage. Delaying surgery has a significantly higher potential of requiring decortication.

HISTORICAL BACKGROUND

Empyema has been recognized since ancient times. Around 500 BC, 2500 years ago, Hippocrates made the first recorded description of empyema and advocated the concept of open drainage and irrigation.[3]

Aristotle identified the increased morbidity and mortality associated with empyema and described drainage of empyema fluid with incision. In 1876, Hewitt described a method of closed drainage of the chest in which a rubber tube was placed into the empyema cavity and drained via a water seal drainage.

Decortication for treating empyema was popularized by George Farber in the late 19th Century. The US Army empyema commission recommended closed drainage in the 1920's to decrease the mortality associated with open drainage. In the early 20th century, surgical therapies for empyema (thoracoplasty, decortication) were introduced. However, the greatest impact on the history of treatment of empyema has been the introduction of broad spectrum antibiotics that decreased the morbidity and mortality.

The practice of surgical drainage as part of therapy for empyema has continued into the era of modern medicine with an ongoing debate regarding timing and indications.[4-7]

DEFINITION

Empyema is defined as a collection of purulent material in the pleural space as a result of combination of pleural dead space, culture medium of pleural fluid and inoculation of bacteria.[2] Empyema is an advanced parapneumonic effusion.

Though parapneumonic effusions may be noted in 50-90% of childhood pneumonias, the progression to empyema is rare. In a study with 3248 children with pneumonia, 1 in 155 cases progressed to empyema.[8]

ETIOLOGY

The etiology of empyema may arise from any source of infection in close viscinity to the pleura.
1. Pneumonia- Viral, Bacterial, Tubercular, Mycotic
2. Postoperative infection
3. Lung abscess
4. Trauma
5. Subphrenic abscess
6. Generalized sepsis
7. Adjacent infections—retropharyngeal or mediastinal abscess
8. Esophageal perforation
9. Retained tracheobronchial foreign bodies
10. Cystic fibrosis
11. Endotracheal tumor
12. Instrumentation
13. Congenital anomalies[9]
14. Malignancy[10]
15. Immunocompromised, disseminated infections.

Empyema is a well-recognized complication of pneumonia and its prevalence is increasing in the childhood population.[11] Bacterial pneumonia is the most common of pleural empyema. Pulmonary infections of these patients extend into the pleural space.

Empyemas may result due to—
1. Direct extension of infection to the pleural space from the lung. Subpleural pneumatoceles seen in *Staphylococcus pneumonia* may rupture spontaneously and transmit the infection to the pleural space. Empyemas can result from rupture of a lung abscess into the pleural into the pleural space.
2. Contiguous infections of the esophagus, mediastinum, or sub-diaphragmatic region may extend to involve the pleura. Similarly, retropharyngeal, retroperitoneal, or paravertebral processes may extend to adjacent structures and involve the pleura as well.
3. Obstruction of pulmonary lymphatics may lead to seeding of the pleural fluid and lead to empyema
4. Increased pleural permeability may be associated with lung abscesses.
5. Hematogenous spread may be responsible for secondary infection of a sterile parapneumonic effusion.
6. Host factors that contribute to alterations in pleural permeability, such as inflammatory diseases, infection, trauma, or malignancy, may allow accumulation of fluid in the pleural space, which becomes secondarily infected.[12]

BACTERIOLOGY

The bacteriology of parapneumonic empyemas has changed over the years.[13] The most common bacteria implicated for empyema are *Staphylococcus aureus*, *Pneumococci*, *E. coli*, *pseudomonas*, *Klebsiella* and anaerobes (Table 43.1).

The cultures are sterile in 30-50% of the cases due to antibiotics.

Ravitch et al had reported that *staphylococcus aureus* was the most common pathogen (92% cases) associated with empyema in children below 2 years of age.[14] The presence of associated superficial skin lesions, osteomyelitis and cystic fibrosis is associated with *Staph.aureus* empyema. In a study by Hardie et al in 1996 of community acquired pneumonias complicated by empyema, *Streptococcus pneumonial* was the most common pathogen seen in 40% cases.[15]

Hoff et al noted 44% of patients had negative cultures and none of the empyemas were associated with *Staph.aureus* or *Haemophilus influenzae*.[6]

In adolescents, the most commonly implicated organisms are *Staphylococcus aureus*, *Streptococcus pneumoniae*, and group *A streptococci*.[13]

Group A *streptococci* may be observed as a complication of an infected skin disorder, such as

Table 43.1: Causative organisms in pediatric post-pneumonic empyema

A. Aerobic
- Staphylococcus aureus
- Streptococcus pneumoniae
- Haemophilus influenzae
- *Less common*
  - Diplococcus
  - E. Coli
  - Klebsiella
  - Pseudomonas
- Mycobacterium tuberculosis

B. Anaerobic
- Microaerophilic Streptococcus
- Fusobacterium
- Bacteroides
- Peptostreptococcus

varicella, impetigo, or infected eczema. Historically, *Streptococcus pneumoniae* was the most common organism but with the routine use of *pneumococcal vaccine, Staphylococcus aureus* is now the most commonly retrieved organism.[16,17]

There has been an increasing incidence of methicillin resistant staphylococci infections.[18-20] *Haemophilus influenzae* is rarely encountered since the advent of the *H. influenzae* B vaccine.

Pseudomonas is a common organism, which is frequently isolated in sick, ventilator dependent children. Anaerobic organisms have emerged as important pathogens in sick, hospitalized children and in empyemas resulting from underlying aspiration pneumonia or lung abscess. Anaerobes have also been recognised as important cause of childhood and adolescent empyema.[21]

Tuberculosis being rampant in developing countries may present as acute empyema. In cases of late diagnosis, noncompliance with antitubercular treatment and resistant strains of mycobacterium, it is usually a chronic disease with underlying parenchymal involvement.[2] Rare organisms like *Serratia marcescens* have also been implicated.[22]

Mycoplasma pneumoniae and viruses can rarely result in exudative pleural effusions.

PATHOPHYSIOLOGY

The development of parapneumonic effusions is a slow process.[23]

The pleural space is a potential space lined by mesothelial membrane, containing only small volumes of transudative fluid, with a protein content less than 1.5 gm/dL. The pleural fluid normally is composed of lymphocytes, macrophages, and mesothelial cells, with an absence of neutrophils. Interaction of the mesothelium with the invading bacteria, polymorphonuclear leukocyte and inflammatory mediators can increase the pleural permeability. Further recruitment results in the increased neutrophil chemotactic mediators and thus pleocytosis

The American Thoracic Society (1962) described three stages of empyema that continue to be applied in the classification of the disease. The progression of pleural fluid collection evolves from stage 1-3 (Table 43.2).

1. *Exudative (Acute) stage:* The pleural inflammatory reaction results in increased permeability and a small fluid collection. The fluid contains mostly neutrophils, and often is sterile. At this stage, the effusion is thin with few cellular elements and amenable to thoracentesis. The exudative pleural fluid is a nutritionally rich culture media for bacterial pathogens. Host defenses are inhibited because phagocytosis is prevented by a lack of surface for adhesions. The pleura and lung are mobile and the pleural fluid pH, glucose and LDH levels are normal. This stage lasts only 24-72 hours and then progresses to the fibrinopurulent stage if the infection is not controlled at this stage with appropriate antibiotics.

2. *Fibrinopurulent (Transitional) stage:* This stage is characterized by invasion of the organism into the pleural space, progressive inflammation and polymorphonuclear (PMN) leukocyte invasion. Protein and fibrinous material accumulate with formation of fibrin membranes, which forms partitions or loculations within the pleural space. Inflammation is characterized by progressive decreases in the pleural fluid glucose and pH and increased protein and lactate dehydrogenase. White blood cells are present within the fluid, and the Gram's stain is usually positive. The pH and glucose values show a fall with increase in LDH levels. This consolidation of the infected pleural fluid also leads to loss of lung mobility Loculation in the fibrinopurulent stage walls of the infection and prevents resolution. This stage lasts for 7-10 days and often requires more aggressive treatment like tube thoracostomy.

3. *Organizing (Chronic) stage:* A thick pleural peel is formed by resorption of fluid and as a result of fibroblast proliferation and fibrin resorption. The organized collagen on the pleural surface is called

Table 43.2: Important parameters of the pleural fluid in various stages of empyema

	Acute exudative	Transitional fibrinopurulent	Chronic organizing
Viscosity	+	++	+++
WBC	+	++	+++
Lactate dehydrogenase	+	++	+++
pH	+++	++	+
Glucose	+++	++	+
Lung expansion	+++	++	+

the peel. The lung parenchyma becomes entrapped, forming a fibrothorax, capillary proliferation extends from the fibrinous peel into the visceral pleura. This stage usually occurs within 2-4 weeks after the initial presentation.

The pleural inflammatory response thus leads to an increased procoagulant activity and depressed fibrinolytic activity, causing fibrin deposition. Loculations are formed with fibrin strands covered by fibroblasts that proliferate and deposit basement membrane proteins over the pleura. These proteins prevent the separation of the visceral and parietal pleura and lead to the formation of a pleural peel.

Following timely initiation of proper antibiotic therapy, the inflammatory process resolves. Re-epithelialization of the pleura occurs with migration of pleural mesothelial cells into areas of denudation. However, inappropriate or delayed treatment leads to exuberant pleural inflammation resulting in pleural fibrosis and restrictive lung disease.

The bacteriology of the pleural fluid has an impact on the progression of the empyema. It is established that anaerobic organisms lead to early loculation, which impairs closed drainage. The pleural peel is thicker in *Strepococcus* and *Hemophilus empyemas* as compared to staphylococcus empyemas. Empyema may be localized (encapsulated) or may involve the entire pleural cavity.

CLINICAL PRESENTATION

The clinical features of acute empyema in childen are usually a manifestation of the primary underlying infection. Most acute cases present with symptoms of bacterial pneumonia like fever, dull chest pain, cough, dyspnea, and possibly cyanosis. Children are also likely to have respiratory distress, headache, febrile seizures and abdominal distension secondary to paralytic ileus. The clinical picture of empyema can be blunted due to the use of antibiotics. Pleuritis may cause abdominal pain and vomiting.

Tubercular empyema is usually chronic and presents with malaise, low-grade fever, weight loss and anorexia. Immunocompromised patients may be afebrile.

PHYSICAL EXAMINATION

The general physical examination may reveal anemia, malnutrition, clubbing and occasionally cyanosis in chronic cases.

Inspection may reveal shrinkage of chest wall, decreased mobility of chest wall on respiration and tracheal/mediastinal shift. A cystic swelling may be seen over the chest wall which may have a positive cough impulse in cases of empyema neccessitans. Breath sounds may not be abdominal in very young children.

Palpation findings include decreased mobility of chest wall, crowding of ribs and mediastinal shift. Stony dullness, vocal fremitus and tenderness may be elicited on percussion.

Auscultation reveals crackles, decreased or absent breath sounds, and possibly a pleural rub if the process is recognized before a large amount of fluid accumulates. However, all these physical findings may vary depending on the organism and the duration of the illness. Chronic empyema in delbilated patients shows significant chest wall abnormalities like decreased hemithorax volume and obliteration of the intercostal space with scoliosis.

In a multivariate analysis, a history of prolonged fever, tachypnea and pain on abdominal palpation on admission were the most significant clinical predictors for empyema.[24]

Empyema necessitans that usually occurs near the fifth costochondrial junction and results due to the erosion of the chest wall may present with a swelling on the chest wall. The empyema can erode into a bronchus, forming a bronchopleural fistula, which presents with cough and copious purulent sputum. Extension of the infection to neighboring structures and metastatic abscess can also occur.

DIFFERENTIAL DIAGNOSIS

The differential diagnosis include lung abscess, hemothorax, pleural effusion, pulmonary infarction, pulmonary sequestration and rarely cases of congenital diaphragmatic hernia with delayed presentation and post-traumatic diaphragmatic rupture. Inadvertent placement of chest tube in the latter two cases has been shown to increase morbidity due to intestinal injury.

INVESTIGATIONS

Blood Investigations

Hemoglobin: It may be decreased.

WBC Count: An elevated WBC count and a predominance of polymorphonuclear leukocytes is seen in acute cases.

Erythrocyte sedimentation rate: It may be raised.

Serum C-reactive protein levels: These have been reported to be higher among children with empyema than among those with uncomplicated pneumonia (234 mg/L vs. 178 mg/L; p = 0.037).[24]

Blood culture: It may be obtained to assist in the identification of the offending organism.

HIV screening: It may be advised in emaciated children with chronic illness and pyrexia.[25]

Sputum: if present may be sent for AFB culture if there is suspicion of tuberculosis.

Mantoux test: A strongly positive mantoux test may aid in the diagnosis of tubercular etiology though it may be negative in immunocompromised individuals.

Radiologic Evaluation

Standard Chest Skiagram

Postero-anterior and lateral view in upright position is essential to assess the diaphragmatic margins for pleural fluid, which are obliterated with pleural fluid collections (Fig. 43.1). Upto 400 ml may be required before these costophrenic angles are obscured in older children and adolescents, therefore further diagnostic imaging may be needed. In the presence of posterior cost-phrenic angle obliteration, a decubitus CXR is mandatory to assess the degree of fluid collection. Parapneumonic effusions more than 10 mm thick on decubitus view are considered significant and thoracentesis must be carried out. Air fluid levels and early loculation suggests anaerobic infection. The other potential causes of air-fluid levels include bronchopleural fistula, ruptured lung abscess, or esophageal perforation. The presence of pneumatoceles suggests staphylococcal infection. In cases of tuberculosis, associated underlying lung pathology may be identified. With moderate effusion, the radiograph may demonstrate displacement of the mediastinum to the contralateral hemithorax as well as scoliosis.

Lateral decubitus views are required for indistinct diaphragmatic contours. Free-flowing pleural effusions suggest less complicated parapneumonic processes, which may not require extensive diagnostic and therapeutic interventions.

Ultrasonography

Ultrasonography may be helpful in few cases to distinguish between fibrinous septations or presence of consolidated lung.

CT Scan

CT imaging has emerged as the study of choice in patients with complex fluid collections (Figs 43.2 to 43.5).

Chest CT imaging can be used to detect and define pleural fluid and image the airways, precisely define the loculations guide interventional procedures, and discriminate between pleural fluid and chest consolidation. The amount of pleural thickening is well appreciated on a CT scan image (Fig. 43.2). The mediastinal window is very helpful to study the extent of the pleural fluid and also so identify loculated lesions (Figs 43.3A to C). Split pleura sign and lenticular collection in a case of empyema may be identified on CT scan. A CT scan is mandatory in an opacified chest (white-out). Computed tomogram (CT) scan with intravenous (IV) contrast in preoperative evaluation of childhood empyema is also helpful to identify pediatric intrathoracic tumors that can mimic childhood post-pneumonic empyema.[10]

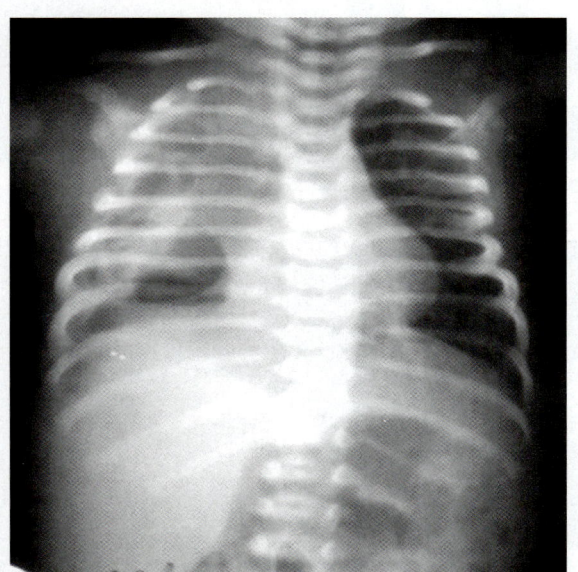

Fig. 43.1: Skiagram chest depicting obscured right costophrenic angle and air fluid level suggestive of fluid collection

The associated underlying lung pathology may also be studied in detail especially in cases of tuberculosis. The degree of lung trapping can be assessed that is particularly important in the child because hampered lung growth can effect subsequent function. A lung abscess is depicted as a intrapulmonary fluid pocket while an extrapulmonary fluid pocket is suggestive of an empyema on cut sections of CT scan.

CT or US guided thoracentesis helps in diagnosis as well as treatment.[26,27] It is also important to remember that the radiological picture may lag behind the clinical stage. Radiographic evidence of pleural thickening may persist for several months following empyema treatment. A CT image is also helpful to follow the progress of the disease and see if the chest tube is at the appropriate place in cases of loculated collections (Figs 43.4A to C).

Examination of the Pleural Fluid

Detailed examination of the aspirated fluid is essential for identifying the causative organism and the stage of the empyema to institute proper therapy accordingly. Cell count and differential is done. The fluid is turbid and contains > 15,000/dL white blood cells. Gram's stain may reveal gram-positive or negative organisms. The aspirated pleural fluid may

Fig. 43.2: CT scan showing thickened pleura on the right side due to empyema

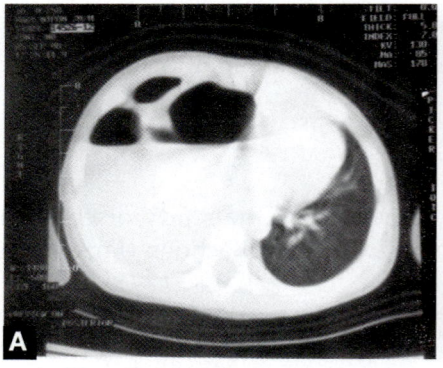
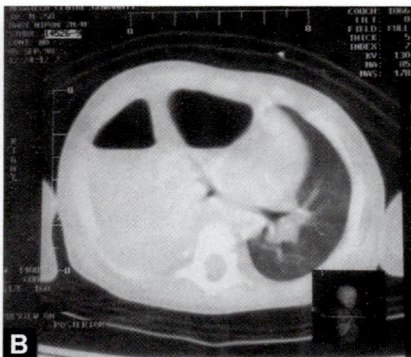
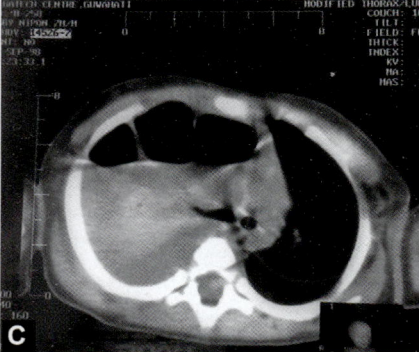

Figs 43.3A to C: Mediastinal window images of CT scan chest depicting the levels of loculated fluid collections

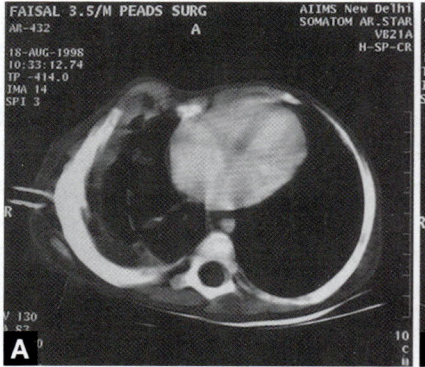
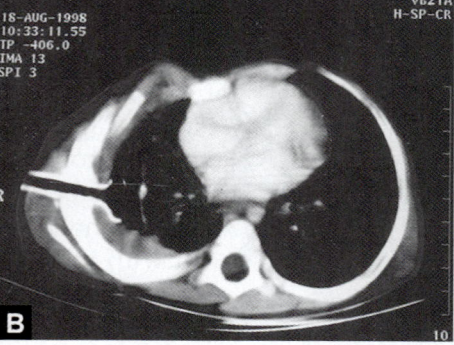
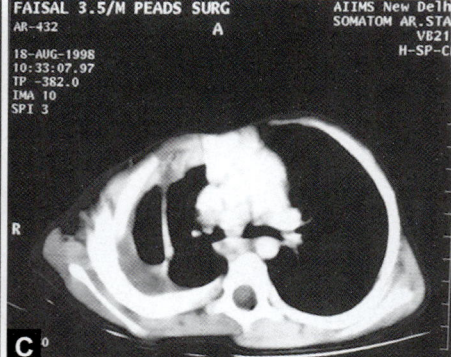

Figs 43.4A to C: Various axial sections of CT scan of a patient showing the
A. Point of insertion of the chest tube **B.** Tract occupied by the chest tube **C.** Loculated empyema

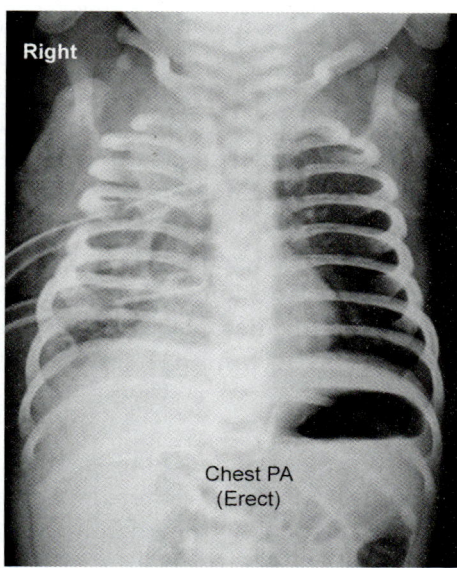

Fig. 43.5: Skiagram chest showing two chest tubes inserted in a case of right sided empyema with adequate drainage and lung expansion during the course of treatment

Table 43.3: Biochemical features of a simple parapneumonic effusion and an empyema

Character	Parapneumonic effusion	Empyema
	Clear/straw colored	Purulent/foul smelling
pH	> 7.2	< 7.0
Glucose	> 40 mg/dL	< 40 mg/dL
LDH	< 100 IU/L	> 1000 IU/L
Pleural fluid Protein/serum protein	< 0.5	> 0.5
Pleural fluid LDH	< 0.6	LDH/serum > 0.6

be investigated for glucose, Lactic dehydrogenase, pH, specific gravity, protein, amylase, Lipid stain or triglycerides and Serologic studies. A pH of less than 7, glucose estimation of < 40 mg/dL and LDH levels of > 100 iµ/L is suggestive of empyema (Table 43.3).[28,29] Others however, do not rely completely on these criteria in isolation as they have low sensitivity (18-53%).[30] Pleural fluid assessment is helpful in planning drainage and instituting antibiotic therapy.

It is important to note that pleural fluid pH measurements are not valid if the patient is acidotic with a low serum pH.

Bacterial, mycobacterial, and fungal cultures of the fluid may be sent but the treatment should be initiated based on the clinical course. Community-acquired methicillin-resistant S.aureus is a substantial and increasing proportion of S.aureus infections in previously healthy neonates most commonly in male infants 7 - 12 days of age.[31] In a series of 304 patients, a total of 292 microorganisms were cultured from the pleural fluid samples of 207 patients (to yield a positive microbiological culture rate of 68%).[32] Isolated bacteria included aerobic gram-negative bacteria (n = 129), aerobic gram-positive bacteria (n = 105), anaerobic bacteria (n = 51) and M. tuberculosis (n = 7).[32] Of these aerobic bacterial infections, gram-negative bacteria were isolated more frequently from the older population and involved a significantly higher mortality rate and longer stay, compared to those with other bacteria (p = 0.001 and p < 0.001 respectively).[32]

Pleural fluid latex agglutination (or counter immuno electrophoresis [CIE] for specific bacteria) may be helpful if the cause of the infection cannot be ascertained from culture results.

TREATMENT

The therapy in pediatric empyema is directed to save life, eliminate the empyema, ensure lung re-expansion, restore mobility of the chest wall and diaphragm, restore respiratory function to normal and reduce hospital stay. The treatment is based on the stage of disease at presentation, the type of bacteria involved, the response to initial therapy and the degree of lung trapping.

The objectives of treatment are:
1. Control of the infection.
2. Drainage of the purulent pleural fluid and eradication of the sac to prevent chronicity.
3. Re-expansion of the affected lung to restore function.

Complicated cases require tube thoracostomy or surgery for their resolution.

The therapy instituted depends on the causative factor, stage of empyema, state of the lung, presence of bronchopleural fistula, ability to obliterate the space and the patients condition.

The therapeutic decision depends on available clinical, radiologic, and laboratory evidence and host factors with individualization for each case. General measures include increase in the protein and fluid intake. Physiotherapy and breathing exercises will help in early re-expansion of the lung following evacuation of the fluid.

THORACENTESIS

Aspiration of pus from the pleural space establishes the diagnosis of empyema. Small or loculated collections may require radiologically guided aspiration. The aspirated fluid should be collected anaerobically and placed on ice.

It can provide both significant diagnostic information and therapeutic relief for parapneumonic effusions. The presence of pus establishes the presence of an empyema, and the determination of the Gram's stain, cell differential, and biochemical analysis helps to guide therapy. In cases of streptococcal infection, the pus is very thin with pH above 7.2, glucose above 40 mg/dL and LDH below 1000 IU per litre. In such cases, only a diagnostic needle aspiration suffices.

Performing thoracentesis before the initiation of antibiotics increases the diagnostic yield of the fluid cultures and allows more specific antimicrobial therapy.

In cases of tubercular etiology, antitubercular chemotherapy should be started immediately, and the pus in the pleural space aspirated through a wide-bore needle till it ceases to reaccumulate. In many cases no other treatment is necessary.

ANTIBIOTIC THERAPY

Appropriate antibiotic should be based on the Gram's stain and culture of the pleural fluid. However, because many patients may have already received antibiotics at the time of thoracentesis, an empiric selection of the most appropriate antibiotics is done based on the most common pathogens causing pneumonia for the patient's age and geographic location.[16]

When the organism is identified, change of antibiotics to the most specific cover for the pathogen is done.

The response to therapy determines the duration of treatment. The patient receives 10-14 days of intravenous antibiotics followed by oral antibiotics for 1-3 weeks.

Antitubercular treatment is mandatory for tubercular empyema. A 6 month course with 4+2 drugs or a 9 month course with 3 drugs is recommended. The treatment may be required for a longer time in cases with associated Pott's spine. Compliance with the treatment is essential.

It is believed that effective antibiotics usually ensure sterility of even loculated collections. But the lysis of bacteria leads to interleukin production and other inflammatory mediators which cause persistent fever and other symptoms. Therefore, adequate drainage is vital to ensure the cessation of this inflammatory cascade.

The most controversial area in the management of parapneumonic effusions is the identification of patients who would benefit from pleural drainage and the selection of the appropriate drainage intervention.[33,34] However, long-term follow-up studies show no differences in pulmonary function or exercise capacity between groups managed by antibiotics drainage and those who underwent drainage procedures in the early stages of empyema.

TUBE THORACOSTOMY

Chest tube drainage with an underwater seal is done for cases in stage 2. Diagnostic thoracentesis and chest tube drainage are effective therapy in more than 50% of patients. Prompt drainage of a free-flowing effusion prevents the development of loculations and a fibrous peel. Most children with nontubercular empyema heal well in the long run, even without immediate surgical intervention.

A large bore intercostal drainage tube is placed in the most dependent area of the cavity. The most dependent site can be determined by previous thoracentesis or radiography. The chest tube is connected to a underwater seal with mild to moderate negative suction (-10 to -15 cm H_2O). It is important to ensure patency of the chest tube by regular milking and keep the water column low.

Studies which have shown good results with just drainage and antibiotics have usually predominant *Staph. aureus* infection. Anaerobic infections are known to loculate early and a more aggressive surgical drainage is warranted.[6] Response to initial therapy is the most important factor which determines subsequent treatment. Cessation of fever, decrease in leucocytosis and lung re-expansion should be noted in 24-48 hours after chest drainage. When inserted in early stages of empyema, ICD may be sufficient if kept for 5-7 days or till drainage decreases to less than 30 ml/day and the patient is afebrile. Antibiotic therapy is continued till 3-4 weeks. The degree of lung trapping as defined by CT scan/CXR is an important factor that decides mode of treatment in pediatric empyemas. Significant lung trapping in children required a more aggressive approach. Sometimes two intercostals tubes are needed for adequate decompression, one for the air and one for the fluid that is in the dependent position (Fig. 43.6).

The tube is removed when the lung re-expands and drainage ceases. If the fluid is not free flowing, further radiologic imaging are undertaken to better define the pleural space disorder.

INTERVENTIONAL RADIOLOGY

The placement of small-bore catheters, specifically localized to loculated pleural fluid collections, has helped to facilitate drainage. Smaller diameter tubes are better tolerated with less morbidity. Radiologists can lyse adhesions directly using imaging during the tube placement.

Interventional radiologists have used fibrinolytics in complicated empyema with loculations and ameliorated fibrous peel formation and fibrin deposition.

Intrapleural fibrinolytics like urokinase, streptokinase and tissue plasminogen activator (TPA) have been used to treat obstructed thoracostomy tubes, increase drainage in multiloculated effusions, and to lyse adhesions.[35-38] Intrapleural urokinase treatment in children with complicated parapneumonic effusion has been reported as an effective and safe therapy.[39] The mean fluid drained during the first 24 hours and the first 72 hours after urokinase instillation were significantly greater than those during 24 hours before instillation, p = 0.002 and p < 0.001, respectively.[39] The total volume of fluid drained was also greater in the urokinase group than that in the control group (p < 0.001). The mean duration of chest tube drainage was significantly shorter in the urokinase group (8.7 +/− 2.8 days vs. 14.7 +/− 6.1 days, p < 0.02).[39] The mean length of hospitalization was also significantly shorter in the urokinase group.[39]

Streptokinase 1-2 lacs u/Kg/dose) is diluted to 50 ml with saline and instilled through the chest tube; the chest tube is clamped for 2 hours and the patient is rotated at 15 minute intervals. The irrigation if carried out for 5 days has shown good results.

Bronchopleural fistula BPF, bleeding diathesis and hypersensitivity to fibrinolytic agents formation of anti streptokinase antibody are contraindications to this form of therapy.

SURGICAL TREATMENT

There is a difference in surgical approaches for empyema in adults and children.

Early decortication and fibrinolytic treatment are sufficient for pediatric patients, while a variety of techniques including open drainage, rib resection and thoracomyoplasty are required in adult patients with empyema.[40]

Since the 1990s two new treatment modalities have been described; fibrinolysis and early VATS (video-assisted thoracoscopic surgery). Both these treatments have now been used as a first-line therapy resulting in a shorter hospital stay and fewer complications than the conservative approach.[41]

Surgical treatment is required for chronic empyema which may be caused by delayed medical attention, inadequate antibiotic therapy, inadequate drainage, presence of foreign body, infliction of postresectional space and chronic pulmonary infection like mismanaged tuberculosis. Other causes of ICD failure include improper positioning of tube, improper selection of tube size, inadequate physiotherapy, presence of BPF and underlying pleural thickening. The pleural thickening is akin to scar formation after any inflammation. Thickened parietal pleura restrict chest wall movement while thickened visceral pleura immobilizes lung and prevent it from expanding. Multiloculated empyema or persistently symptomatic effusion is likely to require surgical intervention.

Rib Resection

Resection of a short segment of rib is necessary if the pus is thick and loculated or if the patient remains toxic after intercostals tube drainage. This provides adequate exposure, allows one to evacuate the pus, break up loculations and adhesions, and assess the need for decortication. After cleaning the cavity thoroughly, a tube may be placed in its most dependent portion and attached to underwater seal drainage.

Open Drainage

In chronic cases with thick pus, a wide bore tube may be left in place, open to atmospheric pressure. This is helpful in adolescents with chronic tubercular empyema after a 3-5 weeks period closed intercostal tube drainage when the amount of 24 hour draining pus has decreased to less than 25 ml. Open drainage prevents the intercostal tube from getting blocked by flakes of pus at the bottom of the underwater seal bag and allows the empyema cavity to heal from inside outwards. The antitubercular chemotherapy prevents formation of further purulent fluid. With a small polythene bag attached to the tube, the adolescent can carry on with his daily chores and not having to carry a heavy underwater seal bag.

Eloesser had described the open 'U' shaped flap procedure in 1935 for open drainage. It was originally described for tuberculous empyema, combines some of the virtues of open and closed drainage and eliminates the need for wide-bore tubes open to the air.[42] It is rarely required now due to improved diagnostic modalities and effective antibiotics.

Decortication

Thoracotomy is done to remove the pleural peel and lyse the adhesions if the patient does not respond promptly to treatment. The term decortication refers to the removal of the thick fibrotic visceral pleural peel. Infact, the acutal procedure, which is usually performed, is pleural debridement and breaking up of the loculations which ensures drainage. A mini thoracotomy procedure for treating pediatric empyemas has also been described.[43] A 5 cm incision is centered over the empyema and the underlying rib is resected. The purulent debris is evacuated and the loculations are broken. An early decision to perform thoracotomy and pleural debridement is also advantageous because the peel is thinner and loculations can be lysed with less blood loss. A mini thoracotomy and pleural toilet/decortication definitely ensures complete adhesiolysis and effective drainage.

Decortication is indicated in encased lung, lung adherent in twisted positions, crowding of ribs, scoliosis and pneumothorax in radiographs without column movement in ICD indicating rigid immobile collapsed lung. Decortication comprises removal of the organized inflammatory membrane. It comprises of two types of procedures:
1. Removal of the visceral peel alone and
2. Empyectomy comprising of extrapleural dissection outside the parietal pleura and removal of the complete cavity (Fig. 43.6).

Striping the parietal pleura may be done by extrapleural dissection before opening the pleural cavity. Length of hospital stay, duration of antibiotics and long-term morbidity are reduced by this more aggressive approach with rapid resolution of symptoms, but it is a major operative procedure with increased cost and short-term morbidity.[44] Early decortication has been reported as a safe and curative treatment in childhood empyema thoracis with low morbidity.[45]

Thoracotomy and decortication is very effective, with a reported 95% success rate for patients with fibrinopurulent effusions and is likely to remain a treatment of choice for advanced empyema.

Video-assisted Thoracoscopic Surgery (VATS)

Preoperative CT scan will help to assess the location and thickness of pleural peels and enable to site thoracoscopic ports more effectively. VAT has proved to be an effective and less-invasive replacement for the limited decortication procedure.[46-48]

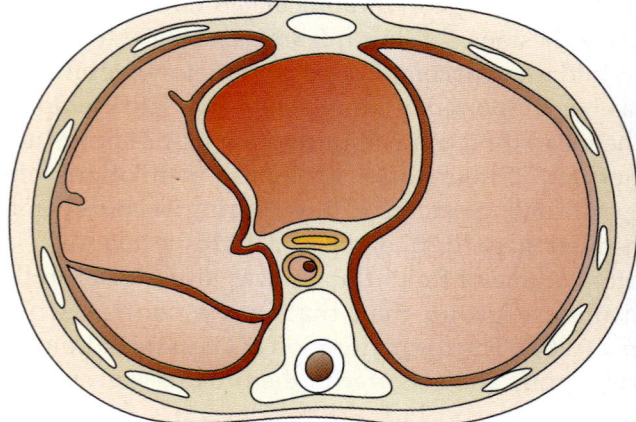

Fig. 43.6: Schematic diagram showing the line of dissection for empyemectomy

Video-assisted thoracoscopic surgery has been safely and effectively performed for neonatal empyema in a 1-month-old infant with staphylococcal pneumonia complicated with multiloculated empyema.[49]

Thoracoscopic debridement closely imitates open thoracotomy and drainage. Mechanical removal of purulent material and the breakdown of adhesions loculi can be accomplished easily with no attempt to peel away the thickened pleura. Thoracoscopic debridement alone is inadequate in very late stages where the encasing thick pleura need to be removed.

Thoracoscopic decortication has also been done by few enthusiastic surgeons. The drawbacks include suboptimal decortication of parietal pleura in the presence of bleeding and inadvertent lung injuries causing incidental air leaks which in turn obscures endoscopic vision. It may, thus, not be beneficial for very thick pleura of stage 3 was noted in 8 of 9 patients and no patients required a second surgical intervention.

Thoracoscopy has to be performed early in the course of the disease while the peel is pliable and can be removed.

The main prognostic factor for thoracoscopic treatment of pleural empyema is the interval between diagnosis and surgery.[50] A 4-day limit, corresponding to the natural process of empyema organization, is significant. The assessment of loculations by ultrasonography alone is not sufficient to predict the postoperative course.[50]

VATS results in more rapid relief of symptoms, earlier hospital discharge, and significantly less discomfort and morbidity.

About 90% of TS patients can be discharged within 5-7 days and all by 3 weeks. Normal skiagrams of the chest have been reported by 1 month follow up.[51]

Recent studies support the early application of video-assisted thoracic debridement in children with empyema compared with traditional therapy, as it decreases the number of procedures and studies performed and the duration of chest tube drainage and is associated with less pain and shorter recovery period than open thoracotomy.[52]

Despite the benefits, a small percentage of patients still progress to require thoracotomy VATS is most effective in the slightly less affected patients in whom early and potentially more aggressive treatment has been initiated. However, some authors feel that there is no evidence to support a better clinical outcome from VATS compared to a chest drain with intrapleural fibrinolytic in children with empyema.[53]

A balloon-assisted single-port thoracoscopic debridement in children with thoracic empyema has been described.[54]

A balloon connected to a 12 F feeding tube is inserted into the thoracic cavity and inflated with air before the entrance of the thoracoscope. By this maneuver, a cavity is formed just under the entrance point following which a routine debridement and chest irrigation are performed by thoracoscopy.

A balloon inflated in the thoracic cavity may achieve a wider field of vision for thoracoscopic surgery, and single-port thoracoscopy has been reported as sufficient and safe for the dissection.

Lobectomy and Pneumonectomy

Surgical excision of a lobe or the whole lung though not described frequently by many in the west, remains an important component of the management in our country where tuberculosis is rampant. In a minority of patients even after adequate decortication the lung does not expand due to necrosis of the underlying lung. In such cases, resection of the affected lung segment will be prudent. The author's large Institutional experience shows that the lung excision (complete or in part) of Empyema Thoracis patients, is required not only to excise the diseased lung but also to prevent the other lung from being flooded with the secretions from the diseased lung. Also, rib excision may have to be done to have a good access to thorax in the advanced cases with deformed chest. Rarely, the cases may be so difficult that even a second look thoracotomy may be required before a lobectomy could be performed. In the West, patients are seen much early in the course of disease so that the pleural thickening seldom exceeds 1-2 mm. In contrast, Indian patients are seen in advanced stage of disease so that the pleural thickening may reach even 2-3 cm.

Indication for pulmonary resection in cases of tubercular empyema include
1. Persistently positive sputum cultures with cavitation after 6 months of continuous optimal chemotherapy with 2 or more drugs. Resistant tuberculosis should be ruled out. Relative

indications for surgical intervention like severe cavitation, bronchiectasis, or bronchial stenosis may contribute to failure of chemotherapy in some patients.
2. Localized pulmonary disease caused by atypical mycobacterium or *M.tuberculosis* with broad resistance to chemotherapy.[55] Localized disease is defined as that encompassing 1-2 segments of the lung.
3. A mass lesion of the lung in an area of tubercular involvement. This helps for simultaneous diagnosis of the mass lesion and treatment of tuberculosis.[56]
4. Massive life- threatening hemoptysis or recurrent severe hemoptysis. Massive hemoptysis is defined as more than 600 ml in 24 hours and severe hemoptysis is more than 200 ml in 24 hours. Asphyxiation is the usual cause of mortality from hemoptysis. Bleeding arises from abundant bronchial arterial circulation to the cavitated portion of the lung. Bronchoscopy is performed to determine the lobe from which bleeding arises, as frequently bilateral cavitary changes may be present. In stabilized patients with localized site of bleeding, lobectomy is the most definitive form of therapy for severe hemoptysis.[57]
5. A broncho pleural fistula secondary to mycobacterial infection that does not respond to tube thoracostomy.

COMPLICATIONS

The complications have been listed in Table 43.4.

Empyema Necessitans

A swelling appears over the chest wall which is in communication with the underlying empyema. It has a positive cough impulse. It usually does not require any additional treatment and heals spontaneously with adequate treatment of the underlying empyema.

Fibrothorax, is a rare complication seen in adolescents who have presented very late.

Bronchopleural Fistula (BPF)

BPF is a troublesome complication of ET and it delays discharge from hospital. BPF prevents expansion of lung by creating positive intrapleural pressure and in turn rigid encased and splinted lung around the fistulous opening prevents spontaneous closure of BPF. To break this vicious cycle decortication is essential. Most of the BPF will spontaneously close within 48 hours of satisfactory lung expansion. Formal suturing of BPF will often fail due to the friability of underlying diseased lung. The usual options are either to apply a stapler more medial to BPF or to resect the affected lung segment. Vascularized latissimus dorsi flap is a viable option for closing BPF. Hence surgeons should avoid damage to this muscle during open thoracotomy. Some surgeons claim that BPF will most often close by conservative ICD. According to one surgeon only one out of five BPF require thoracoscopic intervention. Although PTFE is used to suture BPF in adults, it is not known whether it has ever been used in pediatric cases. BPF should not be confused with post decortication air leaks as the later will settle promptly within 10 days.

Streptococcus pneumoniae is an uncommon etiological organism in children with hemolytic uremic syndrome (HUS). Patients with *S. pneumoniae*-associated HUS commonly have a pneumonia or meningitis. Historically, *S. pneumoniae*-associated HUS usually has a poor clinical outcome. Patients with empyema complicating pneumococcal pneumonia have been reported to develop renal failure with oliguria requiring peritoneal dialysis for a period of 9 to 26 days.[58]

S. pneumoniae-associated HUS remains a rare but severe complication of invasive pneumococcal infection in children.[58] It is important for pediatricians to note that children with pneumococcal pneumonia with severe hematologic and renal dysfunction should be investigated for evidence of *S. pneumoniae*-associated HUS.[58]

The mortality in pediatric empyemas is less than 10% in most series.[6-8]

Table 43.4: Complications of empyema

- Empyema necessitans
- Bronchopleural fistula
- Anemia
- Osteomyelitis of ribs/vertebrae
- Pericarditis
- Pulmonary esophageal fistula
- Metastatic abscess—Mediastinal, vertebral, other sites
- Wound infection
- Empyema relapse
- Persistent atelectasia

LONG-TERM EFFECTS

Despite the variability in presentation, most patients recover without sequelae.

A number of studies have demonstrated resolution of the radiographic abnormalities by 3-6 months following therapy, with little to no symptoms reported at follow-up examination of 122 children (median age 4.3 years), 103 (84%) required chest drains of whom 83/103 (81%) received urokinase; 5 (4%) required surgical decortication. On admission, 56 (46%) had a scoliosis, 68 (62%) on the 2nd radiograph, and 68 (59%) at discharge; overall 87 (71%) had a scoliosis at some stage.[59] In all cases, there was a single thoracic curve with the direction towards the side of the effusion.

There was no association between scoliosis and size or type of effusion, nor inflammatory markers. There was a statistically significant but small effect from duration of illness prior to admission. At follow-up, 6 (5%) had a mild residual scoliosis but all subsequently resolved. Intraobserver variability for measurement of Cobb angles was +/− 4.6° and interobserver variability was +/− 5.8°. Scoliosis was common but always resolved so therapy is unnecessary; follow up is recommended to exclude coincidental idiopathic scoliosis.[59]

Pulmonary function testing performed following hospitalization has not shown marked abnormalities, regardless of clinical course. The only abnormality observed may be slight expiratory flow limitation. Mild obstructive abnormalities were the only findings observed in patients evaluated 12 years (± 5) following recovery from empyema. In advanced stages of Empyema, few patients silently suffer restrictive lung disease and abnormal spirometry. Some increased bronchial reactivity has been reported at later follow-up examinations; however, lung function and exercise response return to normal for most patients.

Early recognition of pneumonia with parapneumonic effusion, effective intervention to identify the causative organism, and initiation of definitive therapy reduce morbidity and complications associated with this process.

Mild airway obstruction was noted with reduced EFV values in nearly 50% of the children.[60] None of the children had any restrictive features on spirometry and these was no difference noted between children treated with or without chest drainage.

REFERENCES

1. Gupta DK, Sharma S. Management of empyema - Role of a surgeon. J Indian Assoc Pediatr Surg 2005;10:142-46.
2. Sharma Shilpa, Gupta DK. Empyema Thoracis -Tubercular And Nontubercular in Textbook of Adolescent Medicine. Ed Swati Bhave. Jaypee Brothers, Delhi Chapter 20,2006;8: 678-84.
3. Paget S. Empyema In: Paget 5th ed. The surgery of the chest. New York. EB Treat. 1897:204-29.
4. Foglia RP, Randolph J. Current indications for decortication in treatment of empyema in children. J Pediatr Surg 1987;22:28-33.
5. Kosloske AM, Cartwright KC. The controversial role of decortication in the management of pediatric empyema. J Thorac cardiovasc Surg 1988,96:166-70.
6. Hoff SJ, Noble HIII WW, Heller RM, et al. Postpneumonic empyema in childhood: Selecting appropriate therapy. J Pediatr Surg 1989;24:659-64.
7. Kosloske AM, Cushing AH, Shuck JM. Early decortication for anaerobic empyema in children. J Pediatr Surg 1980;15:422-29.
8. Chonmaitree T, Bwell KR. Parapneumonic Pleural effusion and empyema. Review of a 19 year experience, 1962-1980. Clin Pediatr 1983;72:414-19.
9. Gezer S, Tastepe I, Sirmali M, et al. Pulmonary sequestration: a single-institutional series composed of 27 cases. J Thorac Cardiovasc Surg 2007;133:955-59.
10. Sharif K, Alton H, Clarke J, et al. Paediatric thoracic tumours presenting as empyema. Pediatr Surg Int 2006;22:1009-14.
11. Cremonesini D, Thomson AH. How should we manage empyema: antibiotics alone, fibrinolytics, or primary video-assisted thoracoscopic surgery (VATS)? Semin Respir Crit Care Med 2007;28:322-32.
12. Hoth JJ, Burch PT, Bullock TK, et al. Pathogenesis of post-traumatic empyema: the impact of pneumonia on pleural space infections. Surg Infect 2003;4:29-35.
13. Schultz KD, Fan LL, Pinsky J, Ochoa L, Brian Smith E, Kaplan SL, Brandt ML. The Changing Face of Pleural Empyemas in Children: Epidemiology and Management Pediatrics 2004;113:1735-40.
14. Ravitch M, Fein R. The changing picture of pneumonia and empyema in infants and children : a review of the experience at the Haviett lane Home from 1944 through 1958. JAMA 1961;175:1039-43.
15. Hardie W, et al. Pneumococcal pleural empyemas in children. Clin Infect Dis 1996,22:1057-59.
16. Baranwal AK, Singh M, Marwaha RK, Kumar L. Empyema thoracis: a 10-year comparative review of hospitalised children from south Asia. Arch Dis Child 2003;88:1009-14.
17. Ghosh S, Chakraborty CK, Chatterjee BD. Clinico-bacteriological study of empyema thoracis in infants and children. J Indian Med Assoc 1990;88:189-90.

18. Gorak EJ, Yamada SM, Brow JD. Community-acquired methicillin-resistant Staphylococcus aureus in hospitalised adults and children without known risk factors. Clin Infect Dis 1999;29:797-800.
19. Verma S, Joshi S, Chitnis V, et al. Growing problem of methicillin resistant staphylococci-Indian scenario. Indian J Med Sci 2000;54:535-40.
20. Fortunov RM, Hulten KG, Hammerman WA, et al. Community-acquired Staphylococcus aureus infections in term and near-term previously healthy neonates Pediatrics 2006;118(3):874-81.
21. Brook I. Microbiology of empyema in children and adolescents. Pediatrics 1990;85:722-26.
22. Sharma R, Sharma B, Sinha P, Rishi S. Empyema thoracis caused by Serratia marcescens in a 2-year-old child. Indian J Med Sci 2006 Sep;60(9):387-88.
23. Antony VB, Mohammed KA. Pathophysiology of pleural space infections. Semin Respir Infect 1999;14:9-17.
24. Lahti E, Peltola V, Virkki R, et al. Development of parapneumonic empyema in children. Acta Paediatr 2007;96:1686-92.
25. Hernandez Borge J, Alfageme Michavila I, Munoz Mendez J, Campos Rodriguez F, Pena Grinan N, Villagomez Cerrato R. Thoracic empyema in HIV-infected patients: microbiology, management, and outcome. Chest 1998;113:732-38.
26. Ravin CE. Thoracentesis of loculated pleural effusion using-scale ultra sonic guidance chest 1977;71:666-68.
27. Stark DD, Federle MD, Goodman PC. Radiographic assessment of CT and tube thoracostomy. Am J Radiol 1983;141:253-58.
28. Light RW, Griard WM, Jurkinson SG. Para pneumanic effusions. Am J Med 1980; 69:507-12.
29. Light RW. Parapneumonic effusions and empyema. Clin Chest Med 1985;6:55-59.
30. Poe RH, Marin MG, Israel RH, et al. Utility of pleural fluid analysis in predicting tube thoracostomy/decortication in parapneumonic effusions chest 1991;100:963-67.
31. Fortunov RM, Hulten KG, Hammerman WA, et al. Community-acquired Staphylococcus aureus infections in term and near-term previously healthy neonates Pediatrics 2006;118:874-81.
32. Lin YC, Tu CY, Chen W, et al. An urgent problem of aerobic gram-negative pathogen infection in complicated parapneumonic effusions or empyemas. Intern Med 2007;46(15):1173-78.
33. Ozel SK, Kazez A, Kilic M, Koseogullari AA, Yilmaz E, Aygun AD. Conservative treatment of postpneumonic thoracic empyema in children. Surg Today 2004;34: 1002-05.
34. Sonnappa S, Jaffe A. Treatment approaches for empyema in children. Paediatr Respir Rev. 2007;8:164-70.
35. Bouros D, Schiza S, Siafakas N. Fibrinolytics in the treatment of parapneumonic effusions. Monaldi Arch Chest Dis 1999;54:258-63.
36. Thomson AH, Hull J, Kumar MR, et al. Randomised trial of intrapleural urokinase in the treatment of childhood empyema. Thorax 2002;57:343-47.
37. Bouros D, Schiza S, Tzanakis N. Intrapleural urokinase versus normal saline in the treatment of complicated parapneumonic effusions and empyema. A randomized, double-blind study. Am J Respir Crit Care Med 1999;159:37-42.
38. Fernández A, Larraz G, Fernández G, et al. Intrapleural streptokinase in the treatment of complicated parapneumonic empyema An Pediatr (Barc) 2007;66: 585-90.
39. Chen JP, Lue KH, Liu SC, et al. Intrapleural urokinase treatment in children with complicated parapneumonic effusion. Acta Paediatr Taiwan 2006;47:61-66.
40. Nadir A, Kaptanoglu M, Gonlugur U, et al. Empyema in adults and children: difference in surgical approaches, report of 139 cases. Acta Chir Belg 2007;107:187-91.
41. Cremonesini D, Thomson AH. How should we manage empyema: antibiotics alone, fibrinolytics, or primary video-assisted thoracoscopic surgery (VATS)? Semin Respir Crit Care Med 2007;28:322-32.
42. Eloesser L. An operation for tuberculous empyema. Surg Gynecol Obstet 1935;60:1096.
43. Raffensperger JG, Suck SR, Shkolnik A, et al. Mini-thoracotomy and chest tube insertion for children with empyema. J Thorac cardiovasc Surg 1982; 84:497-504.
44. Avansino JR, Goldman B, Sawin RS, Flum DR. Primary Operative Versus Nonoperative Therapy for Pediatric Empyema: A Meta-analysis. Pediatrics 2005;115:1652-59.
45. Gün F, Salman T, Abbasoglu L, et al. Early decortication in childhood empyema thoracis. Acta Chir Belg 2007;107:225-27.
46. Grewal H, Jackson RJ, Wagner CW, et al. Early video-assisted thoracic surgery in the management of empyema. Pediatrics 1999;103:63.
47. Stovroff M, Teague G, Heiss KF, Parker P, Ricketts RR. Thoracoscopy in the management of pediatric empyema. J Pediatr Surg 1995;30:1211-15.
48. Liu HP, Hsieh MJ, Lu HI, Liu YH, Wu YC, Lin PJ. Thoracoscopic-assisted management of postpneumonic empyema in children refractory to medical response. Surg Endosc 2002;16:1612-14.
49. Leung C, Chang YC. Video-assisted thoracoscopic surgery in a 1-month-old infant with pleural empyema. J Formos Med Assoc 2006;105(11):936-40.
50. Kalfa N, Allal H, Lopez M, et al. Thoracoscopy in pediatric pleural empyema: a prospective study of prognostic factors J Pediatr Surg 2006;41(10):1732-37.
51. Rothenberg SS. Thoracoscopy in infants and children. Semin Paed Surg 1994;3.277-82.
52. Fuller MK, Helmrath MA. Thoracic empyema, application of video-assisted thoracic surgery and its current management. Curr Opin Pediatr 2007;19(3):328-32.
53. Kerek O, Hilliard T, Henderson J. What is the best treatment for empyema? Arch Dis Child 2008;93:173-74.

54. Tander B, Ustun L, Ariturk E, et al. Balloon-assisted single-port thoracoscopic debridement in children with thoracic empyema. J Laparoendosc Adv Surg Tech A 2007;17: 504-08.
55. Iseman MD. Treatment of multi-drug resistant tuberculosis. N Engl J Med 1993;329:784.
56. Whyte RI, Deegan SP, Kaplan DK, Evans CC, Donelly RJ. Recent surgical experience for pulmonary tuberculosis. Respir Med 1989;83:357.
57. Cahill BC, Ingbar DH. Massive hemoptysis, assessment and management. Clin Chest Med 1994;15:147.
58. Lee CF, Liu SC, Lue KH, et al. Pneumococcal pneumonia with empyema and hemolytic uremic syndrome in children: report of three cases. J Microbiol Immunol Infect 2006;39:348-52.
59. Mukherjee S, Langroudi B, Rosenthal M, et al. Incidence and outcome of scoliosis in children with pleural infection. Pediatr Pulmonol 2007;42(3):221-24.
60. Redding GJ, Walund L, Walund D, et al. Lung function in children following empyema. Am J Dis Child 1990;144:1337-42.

Chapter 44

Chest Wall Deformities

Amulya K Saxena, Günter H Willital

Congenital thoracic wall deformities represent a spectrum of musculoskeletal disorders of the anterior chest wall. Most of these deformities fortunately are not life-threatening and do not manifest in severe functional pathophysiology of the thoracic organs. The management of these deformities, however, have gained more importance in the past decade because of the increased participation in competitive school sports as well as athletics, and the changing trends in the world of fashion which expose more of the chest to the public view. It is important to note that, although thoracic wall deformities do not arouse the sympathy generated by limb or cranial anomalies, children with such deformities are viewed with curiosity by their classmates and are often confronted by teasing remarks.

Except for severe chest wall deformities, it is generally extremely difficult to predict the course of progression after the deformities have been discovered in early infancy. Therefore, mild forms of abnormalities warrant the wait- and-watch approach during the first 4-5 years before operative management could be considered. In mild cases, the dormant deformity sometimes becomes accentuated during adolescent growth. Since, the deformities can also manifest frequently primarily during the pubertal spurt often with rapid progression, operative correction in young adults is more favorable in mild cases. The wait-and-watch approach much consider the vertebral anomalies such as scoliosis that may significantly result or affect the secondary deformities of the thoracic cage.

CARDIOPULMONARY EFFECTS

Chest wall depression is better tolerated in infancy, however many older children report subjective complaints such as dyspnea, cardiac dysthesia and limited work performance. Chest wall depression results in a variable displacement of the heart to the left and could be associated with significant rotation. This is well documented by CT scans of the thorax that demonstrate the degree of cardiac compression resulting from the sternum and costal cartilages. Although, surgical correction has been performed in many centers mainly for esthetic and psychological reasons, however, compression and secondary changes of the intrathroracic organs have been indications for surgery[1] (Fig. 44.1). Many individual patients reported with specific cardiac problems, such as supraventricular tachycardias and recurrent heart failure, were relieved by correction of the depressed sternum.

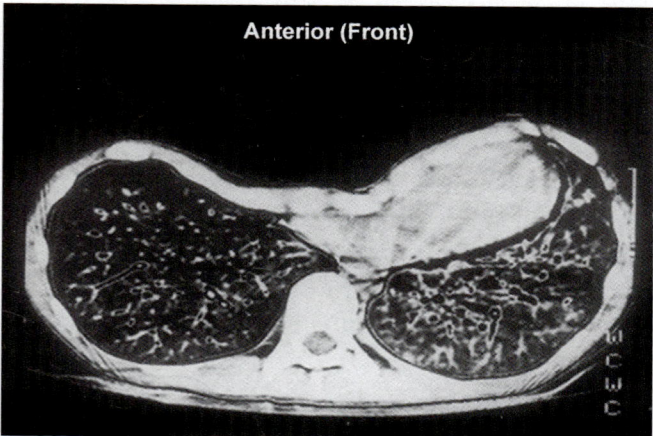

Fig. 44.1: Magnetic resonance image showing the degree of cardiac compression in a mild form of funnel chest deformity

Mechanical factors such as cardiac displacement due to the deformity are furthermore responsible for the functional disturbances of the right and left sides of the heart in systole and diastole. This has been attributed to be more a disorder of compliance of the right side of the heart than the output of the ventricle. Decreased right ventricle filling due to impaired function of the right atrium is also responsible for the reduced stroke volume during exercise.[2] Preoperative echocardiographic and Doppler's findings have also correlated well with the extent of cardiac displacement.[3] A significant increase in the cardiac index after operation is evident when patients performed exercises in sitting position, presumably on the basis of an increased stroke volume. A decrease in the heart rate at any given work performance after operation, evident as the improvement in exercise capacity, is due to the result of an increase in cardiac stroke volume and could explain the subjective circulatory stabilization experienced by the patients.

Restrictive impairment of pulmonary function, expressed by reduced total lung capacity and inspiratory vital capacity is found in patients with funnel chest although normal functions have also been observed.[4-8] Even after surgical correction of the deformity there is a significant reduction in the total capacity and inspiratory vital capacity of the lungs, probably a result of the decreased compliance of the chest wall.[9,10] However, the efficiency of breathing (ratio of tidal volume/inspiratory vital capacity) at maximal exercise improves significantly after operation.[2]

CLASSIFICATION

Patients with chest wall deformities are best graded according to the Willital's classification, which is based on morphologic findings of the thorax (Fig. 44.2). This classification divides congenital chest wall deformities into 11 types - funnel chest (4 types), pigeon chest (4 types), combination of funnel and pigeon chest, chest wall aplasia and cleft sternum (Table 44.1).[11] Since most of the centers today employ metal struts for the correction of this deformity, this classification allows assessment of the operation technique with regards to the location of implantation of the metal struts, as well as the determination of the number of struts to be used for internal stabilization of the chest wall.[12] Records of patients with thoracic wall deformities at our medical center have shown 86%

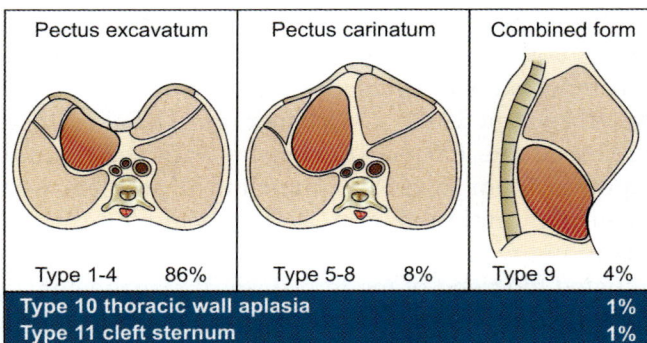

Fig. 44.2: Schematic representation of Willital classification of chest wall deformities and percentile distribution of 902 patients, operated at the Pediatric Surgical University Clinic, Münster from 1984-97

Table 44.1: Willital's classification of congenital chest wall deformities	
Type	Description
i.	Symmetric pectus excavatum within a normal configured thorax.
ii.	Asymmetric pectus excavatum within a normal configured thorax.
iii.	Symmetric pectus excavatum associated with platythorax.
iv.	Asymmetric pectus excavatum associated with platythorax.
v.	Symmetric pectus carinatum within a normal configured thorax.
vi.	Asymmetric pectus carinatum within a normal configured thorax.
vii.	Symmetric pectus carinatum associated with platythorax.
viii.	Asymmetric pectus carinatum associated with platythorax.
ix.	Combination of pectus excavatum and pectus carinatum.
x.	Thoracic wall aplasia/hypoplasia.
xi.	Cleft sternum defects.

with depression deformities, 8% with protrusion deformities, 4% with combined depression-protrusion deformities, and 2% with other forms.

PECTUS EXCAVATUM

Historical Background of Surgical Repair

Pectus excavatum (funnel chest), a depression deformity of the chest wall was first reported by Bauhinus 1594 case published by Schenck. The deformity was however first described by Eggel in 1870.[13,14] The earliest surgical repair of this deformity was reported by Meyers in 1911 and subsequently by Sauerbruch in 1913.[15,16] Ochsner and DeBakey then reviewed the early experiences with repair and reported them in 1938.[17] The clinical problem was carefully analyzed and a simplified operative technique was described by Brown in 1939 which initiated the trend of modern surgical management.[18] Later on, in 1949 Ravitch's report on a technique involving the excision of all deformed cartilages with anterior fixation of the sternum using Kirschner's wires and silk sutures in, and Hegemann's report on surgical management with metal struts to stabilize the sternum in 1965, laid the foundation for the present techniques practiced worldwide.[19,20] Since the 1960's a variety of techniques are presently being used for the correction of funnel chest, however no procedure is universally accepted as a the optimal procedure. It is very important that the primary correction of the deformity is successful since secondary repair of recurrent funnel chest is technically more challenging and difficult to perform.

Clinical Relevance

The incidence of funnel chest is 1 in 1000 live births with a 3:1 male-female predominance (Fig. 44.3).[21] Although it appears that the vast majority of instances

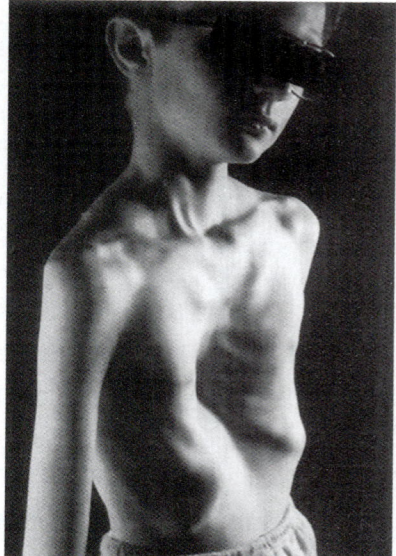

Fig. 44.3: A 9-year-old boy with an asymmetric funnel chest deformity (Type 2) preoperatively

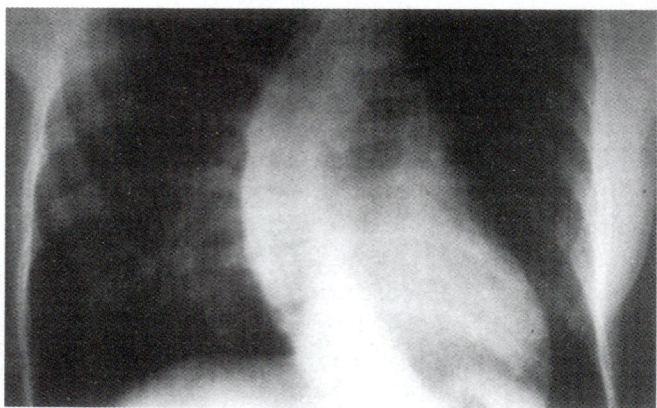

Fig. 44.4: Roentgenograms of the thorax in a 9-year patient showing extensive scoliosis

are sporadic, familial incidences have been frequently documented.[22] An autosomal dominant inheritance accounts for the genetic predisposition of this deformity.[23] However, acquired chest depression deformities secondary to cardiac surgery has been observed at our center. Pectus excavatum is more severe in patients with an associated Marfans's syndrome. It is also important to consider Marfan's syndrome in all patients with this deformity that have scoliosis (Fig. 44.4). Opthalmologic evaluation to identify subluxation of the lens, and echocardiographic examinations to identify the dilatation of the aortic root or mitral valve regurgitation, must be carried out preoperatively to support the diagnosis of Marfan's syndrome, if present. Musculoskeletal abnormalities, most frequently scoliosis, are associated with pectus excavatum, and may not require surgical evaluation. Our method of repair is shown and explained under the surgical technique section.

PECTUS CARINATUM

Historical Background of Surgical Repair

Pectus carinatum (pigeon chest), a protrusion deformity is the second most common malformation of the anterior chest wall. Ravitch in 1952 was the first to suggest that surgical correction was the only effective method for the treatment of this deformity. He surgically corrected the chondromanubrial prominence by resecting the multiple deformed costal cartilages and performing a double osteotomy.[24] Later on, Lester in 1953 performed a repair involving resection of the anterior part of the sternum, but abandoned this approach due to unsatisfactory results. He then reported a second less radical technique which involved subperiosteal resection of the lower body of the sternum and sternal ends of the costal cartilages.[25] Chin in 1957 and Brodkin in 1958 employed an operative procedure which used the traction effect of the rectus muscles to relocate and maintain the sternum in a corrected position.[26,27] This method was further modified by Howard who preferred the radical resection of cartilages and a sternal osteotomy.[28] Later, in 1960, Ravitch reported another surgical procedure that left the sternum alone, and involved the resection of the affected costal cartilages along with the shortening of perichondrial strips with reefing sutures.[29] In 1963, Ramsay utilized a rectal muscle flap to fill the lateral defects resulting from the protrusion without altering the position of the sternum or resecting the deformed costal cartilages.[30] Also in 1963, Robicsek reported a technique that involved subperichondrial resection of the deformed lateral asymmetric costal cartilages, transverse sternal displacement, and resection of the protruding lower portion of the sternum along with the reattachment of the xiphoid and rectus muscles to the new lower margin of the sternum.[31] Welch in 1973 and Pickard in 1979 reported techniques which were similar and involved costal cartilage resection and sternal osteotomy.[32,33]

Clinical Relevance

Pectus carinatum represents an array of abnormal development of the anterior chest wall. In our single center surgical experience it constitutes 12% patients operated upon with anterior chest wall deformities with a 2:1 male-female predominance. Although the pathogenesis of pigeon chest is not exactly defined, excessive overgrowth of costal cartilages has been implicated in the etiology of both, pectus excavatum as well as pectus carinatum.[34] The delayed clinical presentation of pectus carinatum when compared to pectus excavatum, may be due to the fact that the protruding infantile abdomen accentuates pectus excavatum in early childhood and recession of the abdominal contour which occurs in the later years emphasizes the protrusion defect in early adolescence. Musculoskeletal abnormalities, most frequently scoliosis, are associated with pectus carinatum, and

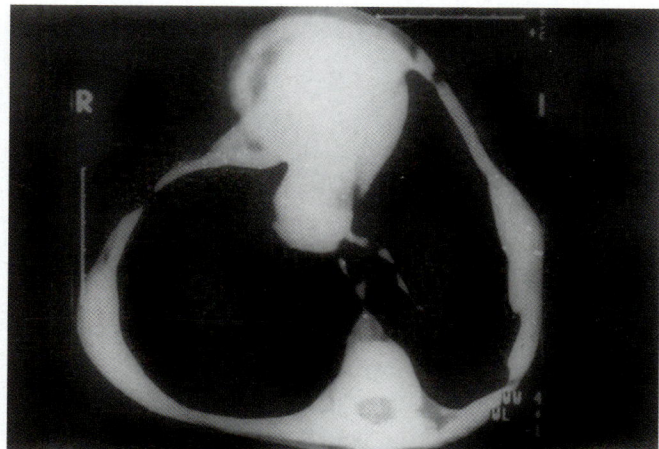

Fig. 44.5: Computer tomography scan of a 17-year-old patient with pectus carinatum demonstrating the extent of cardiac displacement

may not require surgical correction.[35] The severity of the deformity is extremely variable. Surgical correction has been performed mainly for esthetic and psychological reasons, however, displacement and secondary changes of the intrathroracic organs have been indications for surgery (Fig. 44.5).

SURGICAL TECHNIQUE FOR PECTUS EXCAVATUM AND PECTUS CARINATUM

The Willital technique has been the standard technique for the correction of pectus excavatum, pectus carinatum and other combined forms of protrusion-depression combined deformities at our center with excellent long-term results. Using this technique, repair is performed using a standard method of double bilateral chondrotomy parasternally and at points of transition to normal ribs. This is followed by detorsion of the sternum, retrosternal mobilization, correction of the inverted ribs and stabilization of the displaced sternum with one trans-sternal and two bilateral parasternal metal struts. The technical steps have been elaborated below to explain this surgical procedure.

A vertical midline incision is made in boys; otherwise in girls, a submammary incision that is curved upward at the midpoint (over the deepest point of the sternal defect) is preferred, thus avoiding the complication of breast deformity and impaired breast development (Fig. 44.6).[36] In the incision, skin, fat and pectoral muscles are reflected in a single flap and the entire dissection is performed with a needle-tipped

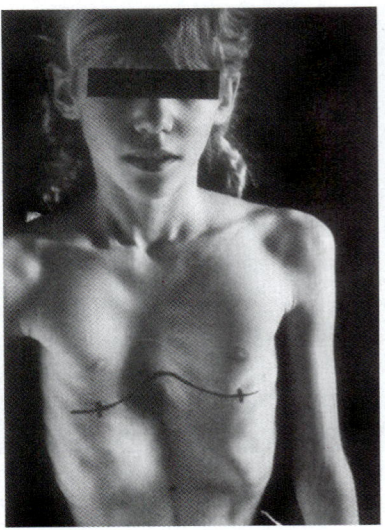

Fig. 44.6: Preferred line of incision for female patients with chest wall deformities

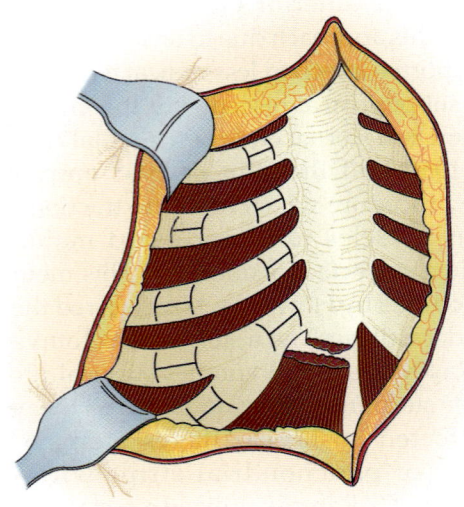

Fig. 44.8: "H" form incision of the perichondrium parasternally and at points of transition to normal ribs.

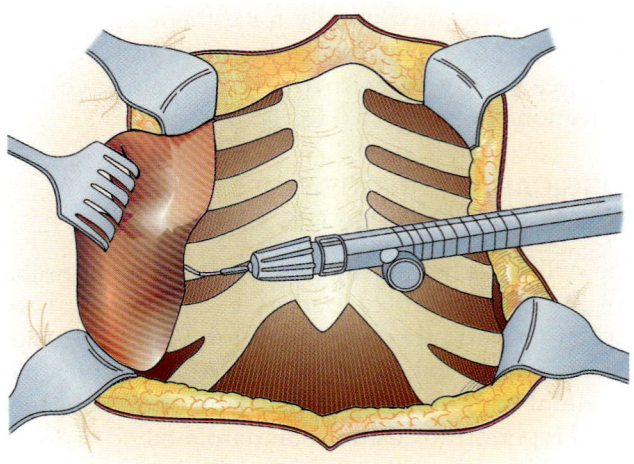

Fig. 44.7: En bloc dissection of the area of depression using electrocautery

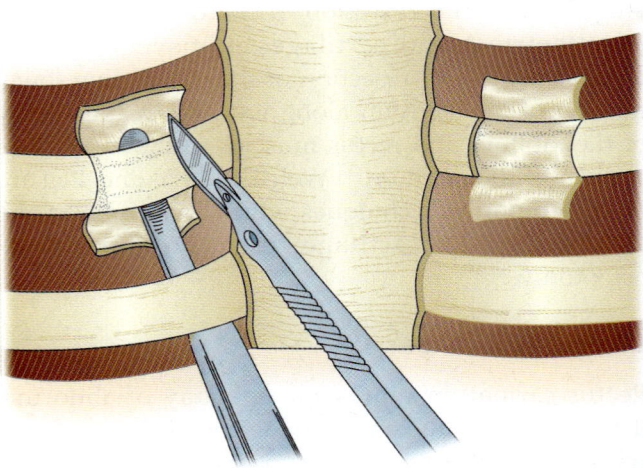

Fig. 44.9: Resection of cartilages after pealing the pericondrial sheath using a scalpel

electrocautery (Fig. 44.7). The pectoral muscles are severed from its insertion at the edge of the sternum and costal cartilages to expose the entire impression of the deformity, generally formed by 5-8 pairs of ribs (third to tenth rib). When the deformed costal cartilages have been completely exposed, the perichondrium is incised with the needle-tip cautery in form of an H (Fig. 44.8). The subperichondrial dissection is carried out with small, sharp periosteal elevators and the perichondrium is scraped away from the underlying cartilage (Fig. 44.9). The deformed costal cartilages are resected parasternally from their junction with the rib to within 1 cm of the sternum as well as at the level of transition to the normal ribs, leaving the uppermost normal cartilages intact (Fig. 44.10). The attachment of the rectus muscle to the sternum is severed, and the sternum is elevated with a Kocher clamp and dissected free from the anterior mediastinal tissue after retrosternal mobilization. A partial transverse sternal wedge osteotomy is

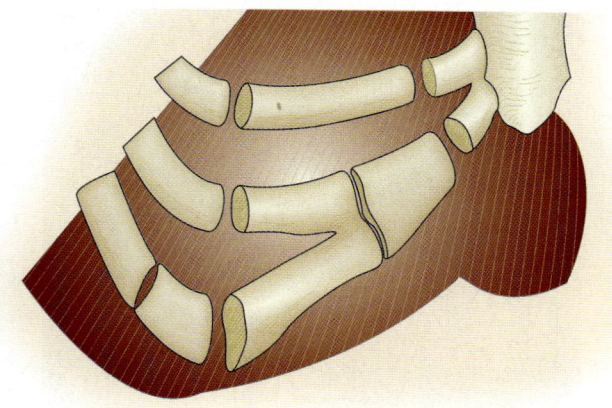

Fig. 44.10: Multiple incisions and resections of deformed lower costal cartilages

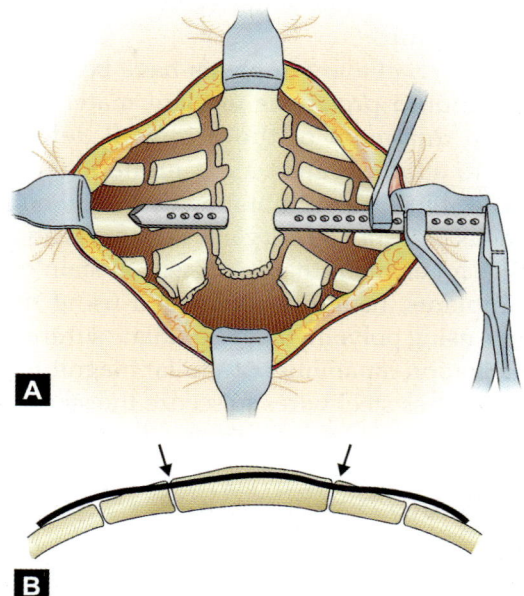

Figs 44.11A and B: A. Intraoperative placement of the transverse strut through the sternum **B.** The strut is bent at the points indicated by arrows to fit the newly constructed thoracic contours

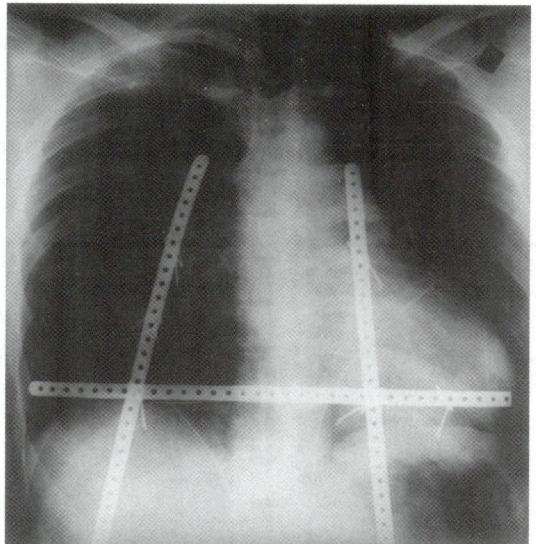

Fig. 44.12: Roentgenogram demonstrating an overview of strut placement for the correction of chest wall deformities

performed at the Angle of Ludovici. Once the sternum is dissected free as described, a perforated steel strut is then passed trans-sternally, with its edges resting anteriorly on the ribs. The strut must be bent in such a way so that it fits the thorax wall perfectly at the edge of the impression. Two parasternal metal struts are also employed, with the points of fixation being the second rib and the lowest end of the rib cage (Figs 44.11A and B). The trans-sternal strut is fixed to the two parasternal struts with stainless steel wires for additional support. The two parasternal struts also provide anchorage to the completely mobile chest segments, which were formed as a result of double bilateral chondrotomy (Fig. 44.12). Heavy resorbable suture material is then used to close the sternal osteotomy as well as to secure the struts to the chest wall. Two single limb chest tubes are placed in parasternal positions at the level of the highest costal cartilage resection. The pectoral muscle flaps and the severed rectus muscles are then sutured and fixed to the sternum. The overlying subcutaneous and cutaneous structures are finally united in the conventional manner to restore the normal chest wall anatomy.

Perioperative antibiotic therapy is administered; with ceftriaxon being the drug of choice. All patients are also administered strong analgetics for first 24-72 hours. The chest tubes are generally removed on the third day or when the drainage is < 25 ml for a twelve-hour shift. Wound infections are rare and the patients are mobilized after chest tube removal. On the fourth day pulmonary exercises are commenced and are continued for a period of three weeks. At the time of discharge patients are advised to avoid body contact sports until the struts have been removed. The struts are removed after a period of 12 months in patients >12 years, but are retained for 15-24 months in younger children, so as to stabilize the thorax that is still under the growth spurt.

Stainless steel alloy implants have been accepted as the standard prosthetic implant material for the operative treatment of thoracic wall deformities. Allergy to stainless steel alloy implants is seldom experienced in patients, but may have fatal outcomes if not detected prior to surgery. Patients with allergy to nickel, an element that is present in stainless steel alloy implants, have been managed using titanium implants using polyethyleneterphtalate sutures which exhibit fixation capabilities of similar magnitude to 20-gauge stainless steel wires to secure the sternum and ribs.[37]

RESULTS AND COMPLICATIONS

Repairs are generally completed with an extremely limited number of mild complications like pneumothorax, pleura effusions or wound infections. Cardiopulmonary injuries are rare and blood transfusions are seldom required. Good long-term results have been reported worldwide after the surgical correction of funnel chest deformities with a relatively low recurrence rate of 2-5%. Lower rates of recurrence have been observed also in many long-term studies after the correction of funnel chest[1,38-41] (Figs 44.13A and B) Irrespective of the technique, we consider the main reasons for recurrence are

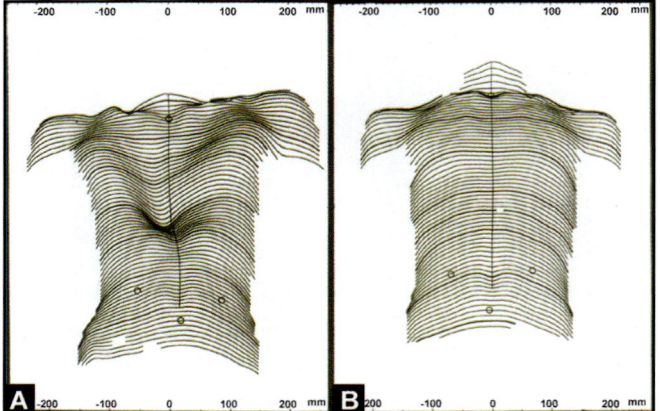

Figs 44.13A and B: Chest wall video raster stereographs are performed on all the patients to document the extent of the deformity and the success of operative repair using our technique. Video raster stereograph performed on a 17-year-old patient, **A.** preoperatively (left) and **B.** postoperatively 5-years later (right)

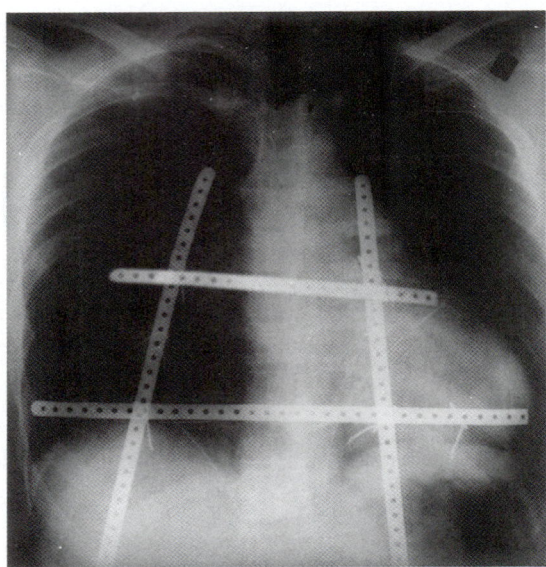

Fig. 44.14: Roentgenogram demonstrating the utilization of a second trans-sternal strut for additional support in severely deformed chest wall deformities

(a) inadequate mobilization of the depressed chest wall (b) unstable fixation of the mobilized chest wall and (c) no or inadequate remodeling of the lowest parts of the deformed ribs.[42] Complete exposure of sternum and ribs is necessary for satisfactory results as it allows complete intraoperative assessment of the deformity and is of significant importance in patients >15 years of age who may require an additional trans-sternal strut because of the extensive area of sternal depression (Fig. 44.14). This also allows placement of struts and stainless steel wires under complete vision and avoids serious complications such as cardiac perforation.[43]

POLAND'S SYNDROME

Poland's syndrome is a spectrum of anomalies that include the absence of the pectoralis major and minor muscles along with a complex of hand anomalies including syndactyly, brachydactyly or ectrodactyly, deformed or absent ribs, absence of axillary hair and decreased amount of subcutaneous fat (Fig. 44.15) Lallemand in 1826 and Froriep in 1839 initially descried this syndrome, however it was Poland, an English medical student, in 1841 who published a partial description observed during his anatomic dissection.[44-46] It was however Thomson in 1895 who elaborately described the full spectrum of the deformity.[47]

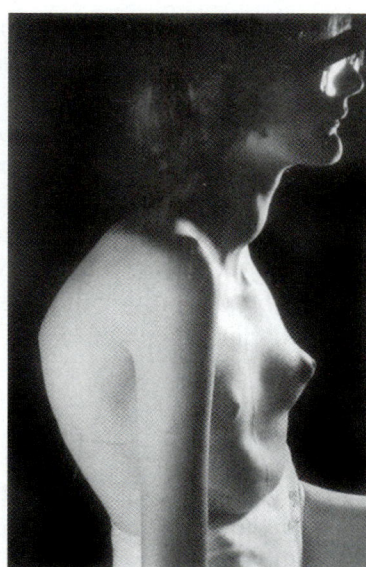

Fig. 44.15: A 10-year-old girl with Poland's syndrome and multiple rib hypoplasia of the right thoracic wall after successful surgical correction using the Willital technique. The girl was operated previously for a ventricular septum defect and therefore has a sagittal thoracic wall incision. The patient also demonstrated an extensive kyphosis and scoliosis of the vertebral column. The degree of hypoplastic breast development is still evident when compared to the normal contralateral breast

The extent and the severity of involvement of the anomalies is variable and its presentation can differ in the affected patients. Poland's syndrome is seldom familial and is associated with a sporadic occurrence in approximately 1:30000 live births.[48,49] The exact etiology of Poland's syndrome is however not yet established. It is however though that abnormal migration of the embryonic tissue forming the pectus muscle, hypoplasia of the subclavian artery or intrauterine injuries may be responsible. Surgical correction for patients with Poland's syndrome is reserved for patients with severe aplasia of the ribs with a major depression deformity. Several techniques such as split rib grafts with Teflon felt and latissimus dorsi muscle flaps with placement of rib grafts have been employed for the correction of the deformed ribs.[50-52] We prefer to use the surgical technique described previously, for the correction of the partially hypoplastic thoracic cage with excellent results. Breast reconstruction is required in most girls but it is best delayed until late puberty to achieve optimal reconstructive results compared to the growth of the contralateral breast. Most of the surgeons prefer the reconstruction with latissimus dori flaps, however atrophy of flaps with time has been observed. Prosthetic implants have also been employed with mixed results as to their complete success reported. It is of paramount importance to discuss the expectations of the patients and the parents prior to the onset of surgical management to achieve acceptable results.

STERNAL DEFECTS

These defects constitute a broad spectrum of rather rare deformities of the sternum and heart. While the specific cause is yet unexplained, a partial or complete failure of fusion is responsible the defects that occur. Cardiac pulsations are quite prominent with each type of cleft sternum, suggesting that the heart is partially outside the chest wall (ectopia cordis) in true cases. Associated cardiac defects and multiple anomalies in other body regions usually preclude survival. In 1818 Weese provide the first anatomic classification of the defects. Later on Roth in 1939, Shaotsu in 1957 and Cantrell in 1958 provided further classifications of sternal defects. Review of the medical literature on this topic provides four types of sternal defects which are largely based on the tissue coverage of the heart.

1. Thoracic Ectopia Cordis

This type of sternal defect constitutes a completely open heart with no overlying somatic structures. There open heart is found to be associated with intrinsic cardiac anomalies. The sternum is generally fused cranially however entire split sternum is rare. The pathology is further associated with a lack of midline somatic tissues and a smaller than normal thoracic cavity in the affected infants. Upper abdominal defects such as rectus diastases or omphalocele are frequent but are rarely associated with the eventration of the abdominal viscera.

The first attempted repair of ectopia cordis was performed in 1925 by Cutler and Wilens, however, in 1975 it was Knoop who performed the first successful repair.[53,54] Skin flap coverage had been since used in a two stage reconstruction for the management of thoracic ectopia cordis. However, successful one staged correction has been reported by Amato who performed a construction of the partial anterior thoracic cavity surrounding the heart, but however avoided the return of the heart to its orthotopic location.[55]

The successful repair of such anomalies are dictated by the presence and the severity of the intrinsic cardiac anomalies rather than the type of surgical approach itself. There have been no recent advancements or successes reported in the management from the surgical point of view, however advances in fetal ultrasound techniques have aided in the early recognition of the deformity and termination of the fetus in pregnancy.

2. Cervical Ectopia Cordis

Cervical ectopia cordis occurs rather infrequently when compared to thoracic ectopia cordis. The patients present with cranial displacement of the heart and the fusion of the apex of the heart and the mouth of the cleft. Several craniofacial anomalies frequently accompany cervical ectopia cordis. Unfortunately this group of patients face the same fate of morbidity and mortality as those with thoracic ectopia cordis. No successful management or survivors with this anomaly have been reported to date.

3. Thoracoabdominal Ectopia Cordis

Syndrome of cardiac and parietal anomalies are generally a part of the defect in the distal closure of the sternum. This syndrome is referred commonly to as a pentology with the following associated anomalies: (a) distal cleft sternum, (b) ventral defect of the anterior abdominal wall that may be a true omphalocele, (c) pericardiopleural communication through an inferior pericardial defect, (d) anterior diaphragmatic defect, and (e) congenital cardiac defect generally in the form of tetralogy of Fallot. It is important to note that these clefts may also occur without the full syndrome. In this defect the heart lacks the severe anterior rotation as seen in thoracic ectopia cordis and is covered by a thin membrane or skin overlying the distal cleft sternum. The position of the heart may also vary from lying in the thoracic cavity to an extreme localization entirely within the abdominal cavity. An interesting finding in this anomaly is the diverticula of the left ventricle which quite frequently protrudes through the diaphragmatic and pericardial defect into the abdominal cavity.

The operative correction of the cleft sternum and associated defects require a staged approach, with priority given to the management of the severe defects.

The general approach however would most likely mandate primary correction of the omphalocele with a delayed approach to the treatment of the cardiac defect. Advances and experience gained in pediatric cardiac surgery have decreased the morbidity and mortality of these anomalies. Early repair of the defect provides a better opportunity for the direct closure of the sternal defect with the attachment of the diaphragm. Successful operative outcomes and long-term survival are better when compared to thoracic ectopia cordis.

4. Cleft or Bifid Sternum

This is the least severe of the anomaly of the sternum represented by a partial or complete sternal cleft. Most cases however involve the upper part of the sternum and manubrium with an intact xiphoid or intact lower-third of the body of the sternum. The heart in these patients is orthotopically located with an intact pericardium along with an intact skin covering. Intrinsic cardiac defects are generally extremely rare. Also, clinically, the patients are asymptomatic and the surgical repair is directed to render protection to the heart. Surgical repair is recommended in infancy within the first 3 months of life when the chest wall is most flexible and primary closure is accomplished without difficulty. Modifications of techniques, with the basic principle of bilateral oblique incision through the costal cartilages to produce greater length to allow midline approximation of the longitudinal sternal ends, lateral cartilage division and medial relocation to close the defect as well as the utilization of prosthetic materials, have been successfully employed for the closure of this defect.

REFERENCES

1. Saxena AK, Schaarschmidt K, Schleef J, et al. Surgical correction of pectus excavatum: the Munster experience. Langenbeck's Arch Surg 1999;384:187-93.
2. Morshius WJ, Folgering HT, Barentz JO, et al. Exercise cardiorespiratory function before and one year after operation for pectus excavatum. J Thorac Cardiovasc Surg 1994;107(6):1403-09.
3. Clausner A, Clausner G, Basche S, et al. Importance of morphological findings in the progress and treatment of chest wall deformities with special reference to the value of computer tomography, echocardiography and stereophotogrammetry. Eur J Pediatr Surg 1991;1:291-97.

4. Wynn SR, Driscoll DJ, Ostrom NK, et al. Exercise cardiorespiratory function in adolescents with pectus excavatum. J Thorac Cardiovasc Surg 1990;99:41-47.
5. Cahill JL, Lees GM, Robertson HT: A summary of preoperative and postoperative cardiorespiratory performance in patients undergoing pectus excavatum and carinatum repair. J Pediatr Surg 1984;19:430-33.
6. Castille RG, Staats BA, Westbrook PR: Symptomatic pectus deformities of the chest. Am Rev Respir Dis 1982;126:564-69.
7. Derveaux L, Ivanoff I, Rochette F, et al. Mechanism of pulmonary function changes after surgical correction for funnel chest. Eur Respir J 1988;1:382-85.
8. Kaguraoka H, Ohnuki T, Itaoka T, et al. Degree of severity of pectus excavatum and pulmonary function in preoperative and postopertive periods. J Thorac Cardiovasc Surg 1992;104:1483-88.
9. Derveaux L, Clarysse I, Ivanoff I, et al. Preoperative and postoperative abnormalities in the chest X-ray indices and in the lung function in pectus deformities. Chest 1989;95:850-56.
10. Glimeno F, Eijgelaar A, Peset R. Lung function changes after operation for pectus excavatum and carinatum. Bull Bur Physiopath Respir 1984;20:17A.
11. Willital GH, Maragakis MM, Schaarschmidt K, et al. Indikation zur Behandlung der Trichterbrust. Dtsch Krankenpfleger Zeitsch 1991;6:418-23.
12. Willtal GH: Operationsindikation-Operationstechnik bei Brustdeformierung. Z Kinderchir 1981;33:244-52.
13. Bauhinius J. Schenck von Grafenberg, Johannes: Observationum medicarum, rararum, novarum, admirabilium, et montrosarum, liber secundus. De partibus vitalibus, thorace contentis. Observation 1594:264:516.
14. Eggel. Eine seltene Missbildung des Thorax. Virchow's Arch 1870;49:230.
15. Meyer L. Zur chirurgischen Behandlung der angeborenen Trichterbrust. Verh Berliner Med 1911;42:364-73.
16. Sauerbruch F: Die Chirurgie der Brustorgane. Berlin, Verlag Springer 1920;440-44.
17. Ochsner A, DeBakey M. Chone-chondrosteron: Report of a case and review of the literature. J Thorax Surg 1938;8:469-511.
18. Brown AL: Pectus excavatum (funnel chest). J Thorac Surg 1939;9:164.
19. Ravitch MM. The operative treatment of pectus excavatum. Ann Surg 1949;129:429-44.
20. Hegemann G, Leutschaft R: Die operative Behandlung der Trichterbrust. Thoraxchirurgie 1965;13:281-87.
21. Clausner A, Hoffmann-v Kapp-herr S: Gegenwartiger Stand der Trichterbrust. Dtsch Med Wschr 1995;120:881-83.
22. Ravitch MM: Congenital deformities of the chest wall and their operative correction. Philadelphia, WB Saunders, 1977;78-205.
23. Leung AKC, Hoo JJ: Familial congenital funnel chest. Am J Med Genetics 1987;26:887-90.
24. Ravitch MM: Unusual sternal deformity with cardiac symptoms—Operative correction. J Thorac Surg 1952;23:138-44.
25. Lester CW: Pigeon breast (pectus carinatum) and other protrusion deformities of the chest of developmental origin. Ann Surg 1953;137:482-89.
26. Chin EF: Surgery of the funnel chest and congenital sternal prominence. Br J Surg 1957;186:360-76.
27. Brodkin HA: Pigeon breast—congenital chondrosternal prominence. Etiology and surgical treatment by xyphosternopexy. Arch Surg 1958;77:261-70.
28. Howard R. Pigeon chest (protrusion deformity of the sternum). Med J Aus 1958;2:664-66.
29. Ravitch MM: The operative correction of pectus carinatum (pigeon breast). Ann Surg 1960;151:705-14.
30. Ramsay BH: Transplantation of the rectus abdominis muscle in the surgical correction of a pectus carinatum deformity with associated parasternal depressions. Surg Gynecol Obstet 1963;116:507-8.
31. Robicsek F, Sanger PW, Taylor FH, et al. The surgical treatment of chondrosternal prominence (pectus carinatum). J Thorac Cardiovasc Surg 1963;45:691-701.
32. Welch KJ, Vos A: Surgical correction of pectus carinatum (pigeon breast). J Pediatr Surg 1973;8:659-67.
33. Pickard LR, Tepas JJ, Shermeta DW, et al: Pectus carinatum: Results of surgical therapy. J Pediatr Surg 1979;14:228-30.
34. Humberd CD. Giantism of the infantilism type and its disclosure of the pathogenesis of pigeon breast and funnel chest. Med Rec 1938;147:444-49.
35. Waters P, Welch K, Micheli LJ, Shamberger R, et al. Scoliosis in children with pectus excavatum and pectus carinatum. J Pediatr Orthop 1989;9(5):551-56.
36. Hougaard K, Arendrup H: Deformities of the female breasts after surgery for funnel chest. Scand J Cardiovasc Surg 1983;17:171-74.
37. Saxena AK, Willital GH: Surgical correction of funnel chest using titanium struts. Surg Childh Intern 1998;6(4):230-32.
38. Shamberger RC, Welch KJ: Surgical repair of pectus excavatum . J Pediatr Surg 1988;23(7):615-22.
39. Hecker WC, Happ M, Soder C, et al. Klinik und Problematik der Kiel- und Trichterbrust. Z Kinderchir 1988;43:15-22.
40. Haller JA, Scherer LR, Turner CS, et al. Evolving management of pectus excavatum based on a single institutional experience of 664 patients. Ann Surg 1989;209:578-83.
41. Saxena AK, Willital GH: Surgical repair of pectus carinatum. Int Surg 1999;84:326-30.
42. Willital GH, Meier H: Cause of funnel chest recurrences-operative treatment and long-term results. Progr Pediatr Surg 1977;10:253-56.
43. Pircova A, Sekarski-Hunkeler N, Jeanrenaud X, et al. Cardiac perforation after surgical repair of pectus excavatum. J Pediatr Surg 1995;30(10): 1506-8.

44. Lallemand LM: Èphermérides Médicales de Montpellier 1826;1:144-47.
45. Froriep R: Beobachtung eines Falles von Mangel der Brustdrüse. Notizen aus dem Gebiete der Natur- und Heilkunde 1939;10:9-14.
46. Poland A: Deficiency of the pectoralis muscles. Guys Hosp Rep 1841;6:191-93.
47. Thomson J: On a form of congenital thoracic deformity. Teratologia 1895;2:1-12.
48. Friere-Maia N, Chautard EA, Opitz JM, et al. The Poland syndrome- Clinical and genealogical data, dermatoglyphic analysis, and incidence. Hum Hered 1973;23:97-104.
49. McGillivray BC, Lowry RB: Poland syndrome in British Columbia: Incidence and reproductive experience of affected persons. Am J Med Genet 1977;1:65-74
50. Ravitch MM: Atypical deformities of the chest wall - absence and deformities of the ribs and costal cartilages. Surgery 1966;59:438-49.
51. Urschel HC Jr, Byrd HS, Sethi SM, et al. Poland's syndrome: Improved surgical management. Ann Thorac Surg 1984;37:204-11.
52. Halller JA Jr, Colombani PM, Miller D, et al. Early reconstruction of Poland's syndrome using autologous rib grafts combined with a latissimus muscle flap. J Pediatr Surg 1984;19:423-29.
53. Cultler GD, Wilens G: Ectopia cordis: a report of a case. Am J Dis Child 1925;30:76-80.
54. Saxena NC: Ectopia cordis child surviving: prostheis fails. Pediatr News 1976;10:3.
55. Amato JT, Cotroneo JV, Gladiere R: Repair of complex ectopia cordis. Meeting of the American College of Sugeons, Chicago, 1988.

SECTION 4

Gastrointestinal Surgery

Disorders of the Umbilicus

Sudipta Sen

The most exhaustive work on the umbilicus is the classic text by Cullen, published in 1916. The umbilicus is of vital importance for intrauterine survival of the fetus, but has no physiological significance after birth, though it retains its cosmetic and emotional appeal. This structure is also of importance to the pediatric surgeon, who is often the first to be consulted regarding any umbilical disorder in the child. Moreover, in this modern age of near scarless surgery, this natural scar is being put to novel uses to improve cosmesis.

EMBRYOLOGY

Embryological events of pediatric surgical importance are as follows:

1. The yolk sac is divided into an intracoelomic portion and an extracoelomic portion by the infolding and flexion of the developing body wall of the embryo. The intracoelomic portion becomes the primitive alimentary canal and maintains a connection with the extracoelomic portion through the vitelline or omphalomesenteric duct. This connection is normally lost by the fifth to seventh week of gestation. Persistence of this alimentary connection or its accompanying vessels can cause abnormalities, viz. persistence of whole or part of the omphalomesenteric duct results in Meckel's diverticulum, patent omphalomesenteric duct, sinus, cyst and umbilical polyp. Omphalomesenteric arterial remnants can cause a fibrous band to the umbilicus, and is also the artery to a Meckel's diverticulum. Portions of the omphalomesenteric vein can result in preduodenal portal vein.
2. The allantois is connected by the urachus to the developing bladder. The urachus normally gives rise to the median umbilical ligament but may persist in several abnormal forms, viz. fully patent urachus, umbilical urachal sinus or urachal cyst.
3. After the return of the midgut into the abdomen, the fibromuscular umbilical ring contracts and continues to do so after birth if not closed already. Persistence of the fascial opening results in umbilical hernia.

CLINICAL DISORDERS OF THE UMBILICUS

Umbilical Granuloma

It is a small mass of granulation tissue, developing at the base of the cord after the cord separates and ranges in size from 1-10 mm (Fig. 45.1). This is treated by one or more application of silver nitrate till the area epithelialises. If this is not successful an umbilical polyp is suspected (Figs 45.2A and B).

Umbilical Infections

Acute

Although modern perinatal care has reduced the incidence of omphalitis, life threatening infection can still occur. Common pathogens are *Staphylococcus aureus*, *Streptococcus pyogenes* and *gram-negative* bacilli. Infections can be polymicrobial. Clinical's features include purulent umbilical discharge, periumbilical skin discoloration and cellulitis, sometimes progressing to fascitis and gangrene of abdominal

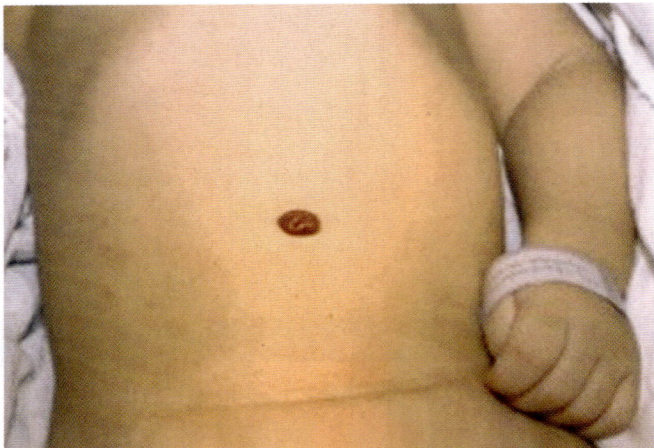

Fig. 45.1: Umbilical granuloma

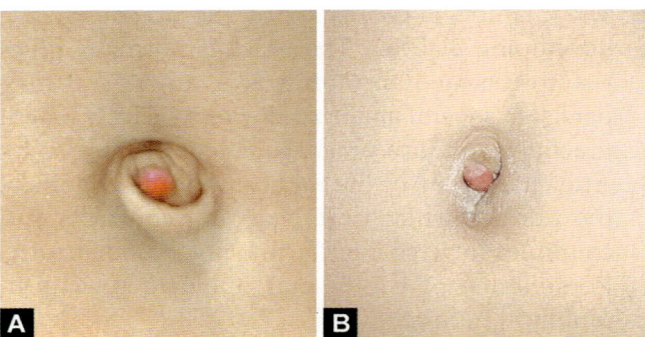

Figs 45.2A and B: Umbilical polyps may be identified by careful inspection

wall. Signs of systemic sepsis are often present. Breakdown of umbilical stump and spontaneous evisceration has been described. Portal venous thrombosis and subsequent extrahepatic portal hypertension can occur. Treatment in early stages is antibiotic therapy, but in cases of necrotising fasciitis debridement will be needed.

Chronic

Chronic umbilical discharge is common and can result from infection in umbilical remnants, e.g. umbilical artery. Excision of umbilical remnants is curative.

Delayed separation of umbilical cord has been associated with heritable neutrophil mobility defects. However, normal variation in cord separation is wide (3-67 days mean 14-15 days).

Omphalomesenteric Remnants

There is a broad range of possibilities. Complete patency of the omphalomesenteric duct from the ileum to the umbilicus presents with fecal discharge and occasionally with prolapse of the proximal and distal ileum via the omphalomesenteric duct (Fig. 45.3). The patent duct can be excised via an umbilical or inferior circum-umbilical incision, the duct traced to the ileum, divided and the ileal opening closed. Care must be taken to ligate a vitelline vessel if present along the duct.

Small duct mucosal remnants and sinuses present with nonfecal discharge and surgical exploration is indicated. It is important that a full exploration of all umbilical structures is performed, including the intraperitoneal undersurface of the umbilicus, to identify and remove any bands to the ileum, including a Meckel's diverticulum if attached to such a band. Cystic remnant of the omphalomesenteric duct may become infected and require preliminary drainage and subsequent excision.

Omphalomesenteric duct remnants or associated vessels may present with mechanical intestinal obstruction or gangrene caused by angulation, volvulus or internal herniation.[1]

Urachal Remnants

A fully patent urachus presents with urinary discharge from the umbilicus, which can be suspected from the

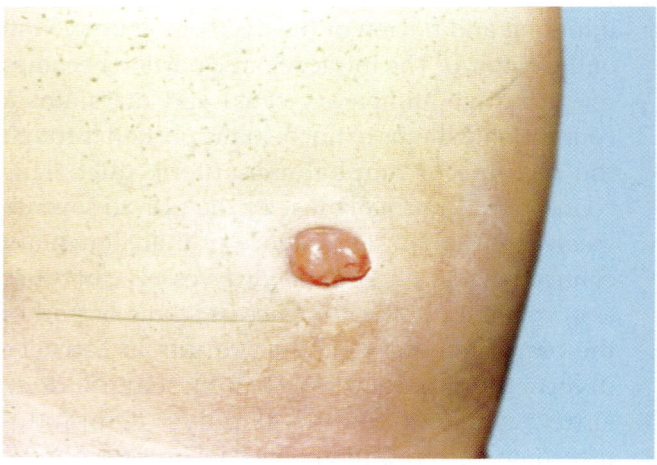

Fig. 45.3: A patent vitello intestinal duct

clear nature of the discharge and associated ammoniacal rash. Frank drainage of urine from the umbilicus requires an investigation of the urinary tract to look for bladder outflow obstruction. Urachal sinus presents with discharge while urachal cysts often present as an infected painful mass between the umbilicus and the suprapubic area. Characteristic CT findings of pyourachus have been described as midline location deep to the rectus abdominis, conical shape extending from a tip at the umbilicus and base over the bladder dome, inflammatory changes in the surrounding tissues including intraperitoneal fluid or abscess if perforation has occurred.[2]

Urachal remnants are generally excised via an umbilical or infraumbilical incision. The patent urachus is transected and ligated at the level of the bladder with absorbable suture. An infected urachal cyst requires drainage and subsequent removal at laparotomy.

Umbilical Hernia

At birth, the umbilicus is surrounded by a dense fascial ring that represents a defect in the linea alba. When the supporting fascia of the umbilical defect is weak or absent, a hernia will result (Figs 45.4A and B). The umbilical hernia in children is surrounded by the dense fascia of the umbilical ring through which a peritoneally lined sac attached to the overlying skin protrudes. The umbilical ring continues to close over time and the fascia of the umbilical defect strengthens, accounting for the spontaneous resolution of this defect in most children.

An "indirect" umbilical hernia with its defect superior to umbilical ring causing a proboscoid hernia has also been described. In this defect the umbilical cicatrix is displaced progressively in an inferior direction as the hernia enlarges.

The umbilical hernia of childhood is different from a 'hernia of the umbilical cord". The latter is a small omphalocoele, covered with amnion and not with skin.

Childhood umbilical hernias are equally common in boys and girls. The exact incidence is unknown, but is possibly higher in African infants. It is commonly found in premature infants of which most will resolve. Umbilical hernia with small ring diameter (< 1.0 cm) are more likely to close then those with ring diameter >1.5 cm. The hernia tends to disappear

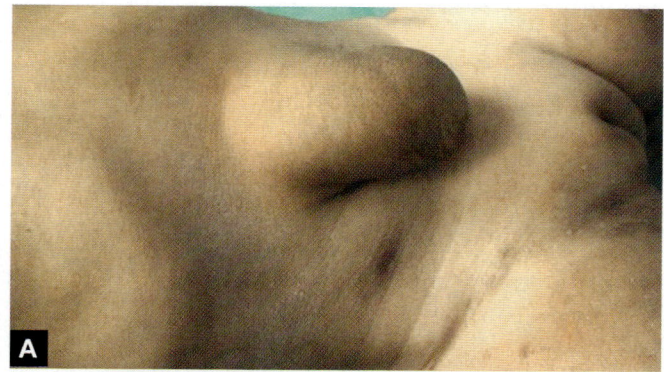

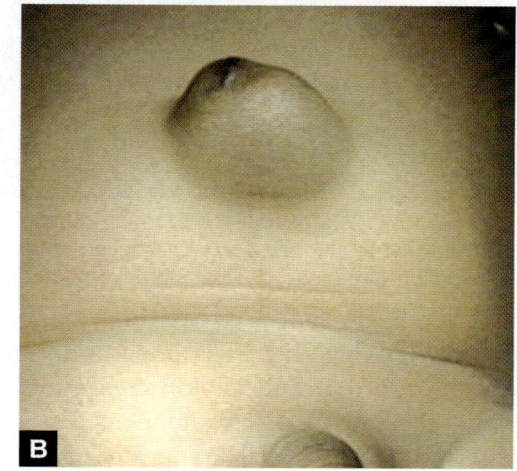

Figs 45.4A and B: Umbilical hernia **A.** Large **B.** Moderate sized

abruptly when the fascial ring closes with the child's growth. Umbilical herniae generally remain uncomplicated but an occasional child presents with strangulation. Incidence of strangulation in umbilical hernia is estimated to be one in 1500 umbilical herniae in childhood.[3] Strangulation is not an uncommon mode of presentation in African children, though the actual risk of strangulation in the individual case is still very small.[4,5] Umbilical hernia is commonly observed in Down's syndrome, trisomy 18, trisomy 13, mucopolysaccharidosis, congenital hypothyroidism and Beckwith Wiedemann's syndrome.

Events such as incarceration are definite but rare indication for surgery. Persistence to school age is a relative indication, specially for defect > 1.5 cm, though the repair can well be postponed to later childhood. When operating in infancy for a concomitant inguinal hernia, it is tempting to operate on the umbilical hernia, but it is better left alone.

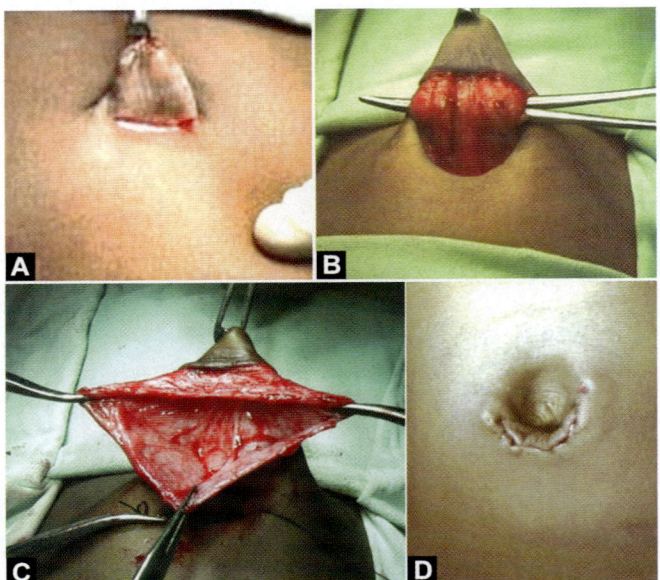

Figs 45.5A to D: Operative steps of repair of umbilical hernia **A.** Infraumbilical incision **B.** Dissection of the sac **C.** Examination of the sac **D.** Postoperative photograph

Repair of umbilical hernia is done under general anesthesia. An infraumbilical skin crease incision is made (Figs 45.5A to D). A subcutaneous dissection is performed to circumscribe the sac. The sac is transected and may be dissected from the under surface of the umbilical skin, but this step is unnecessary. Leaving a remnant of peritoneal sac under the skin causes no complication. Suturing good facial edges in one layer is sufficient. Inversion of umbilical skin is maintained with fine absorbable dermal suture between the underside of the umbilicus and the midportion of the facial closure. The skin is closed with intradermal absorbable suture and pressure dressing applied.

SURGICAL USES OF THE UMBILICUS

The umbilicus can be used in postnatal life in several ways – cannulation of the umbilical arteries and vein in neonates for vascular access and monitoring, as a port for placement of laparoscopy, to make a "scarless" entry to the children for pyloromyotomy, for placing a intestinal or urinary stoma, and for placing a stoma for Mitrofanoff port.[6]

RECONSTRUCTION OF THE UMBILICUS

Patients of exstrophy of the bladder lack a normal umbilicus and reconstruction of an umbilicus is a part of the cosmetic rehabilitation of these children. The umbilicus may be preserved and transposed more cephalad at the time of bladder closure.[7] Otherwise an "umbilicus" may be created very simply by bringing out catheters via a skin opening made in the position of a normal umbilicus during the bladder closure operation in childhood. More sophisticated techniques have also been described for umbilical reconstruction.[8,9] The "kangaroo pouch" technique involves making a small cutaneous pouch by folding a vertical, superiorly based rectangular skin flap and anchoring this pouch deeply to the rectus fascia.

REFERENCES

1. Cilley RE, Krummel TM, In Pediatric Surgery (Eds). O"Neill JA, Rowe MI, Grosfeld Jl, et al. 5th edition, Masby St. Louis 1998;1029-43.
2. Herman TE, Shackelford GD. Pyourachus: CT manifestations. J Comput Assist Tomogr 1995;19(3):440-43.
3. Papagrigoriadis S, Browse DJ, Howard ER. Incerceration of umbilical hernias in children: a rare but important complication. Pediatr Surg Int 1998;14:231-32.
4. Mawera G, Muguti GI. Umbilical Hernia in Bulawayo: some observations from a hospital based study. Cent Afr J Med 1994;40(11):319-23.
5. Meier DE, Olaolorun DA, Omodele RA, et al. incidence of umbilical hernia in African children: redifinition of "normal" and reevaluation of indications for repair. World J Surg 2001;25(5):645-48.
6. Khoury AE, Van Savage JG, McLorie GA, et al. Minimizing stomal stenosis in appendico vesicostomy using the modified umbilical stoma J Urol 1996 155(6):2050-51.
7. Hanna MK. Reconstruction of umbilicus during functional closure of bladder exstrophy. Urology 1986;27:340.
8. Shinohara H, Matsuo K, Kikuchi N. Umbilical reconstruction with an inverted C-V flap Plastic Reconstr Surg 2000;105(2):703-05.
9. Feyaerts A, Mure PY, Jules JA, et al. Umbilical reconstruction in patients with exstrophy: the kangaroo pouch technique. J Urol 2001;165:2026-27.

CHAPTER 46

Inguinal Hernia and Hydrocele

AR Williams, SJ Singh, L Kapila

Hernial repair in childhood was originally described in the 1st century AD with transcrotal excision of the testis together with the hernial sac. However, an accurate description of hernial anatomy was made in 1756 by Pott, with ligation of the hernial sac described in 1877 by Czerny. Turner, in 1912, documented that high ligation alone of the hernial sac was the procedure of choice.

Inguinal herniae in children are almost exclusively indirect. Hydroceles commonly coexist with inguinal herniae, and the common surgical management of both conditions, namely division of the sac (herniotomy) or the patent processus vaginalis (PPV), is based on the explanation that they have the same embryological basis.

Treatment of inguinal hernia in childhood aims to avoid the complications of this condition. For reducible herniae it is reasonable to undertake surgery as soon as convenient. A hernia presenting acutely incarcerated but then reduced subsequently at presentation should be dealt with as a 'planned emergency'. The frankly irreducible hernia should be treated operatively, immediately after fluid resuscitation, especially if there is intestinal obstruction or evidence of peritonitis.

Management of hydrocele alone may be more conservative since hydroceles may resolve spontaneously, although division of the PPV is generally undertaken after the first two years of life to prevent unremitting swelling of the testicle which can be unsightly and may become painful. 'Adult-type' hydroceles in children are rare, and trans-scrotal operations to address the tunica vaginalis are undertaken after an underlying PPV has been excluded.

EPIDEMIOLOGY

Inguinal herniae are much commoner in boys than girls (up to 9:1), commoner with increasing degrees of prematurity, and commoner on the right side (60%). Hydroceles, as stated above, commonly co-exist with herniae since peritoneal fluid is in communication with the scrotal portion of peritoneum as a consequence of PPV. Spontaneous resolution (probably in up to 90% of cases) is the rule. Rowe reported patency of the processus vaginalis as 60% during the first year of life, 40% in the second year.[1] However, a PPV need not necessarily lead to a symptomatic hydrocele as demonstrated by adult postmortem studies.[2]

Approximately 15% of inguinal herniae are bilateral. The issue of bilaterality has been the source of recent controversy, as it has been standard practice since the mid-1950s in some centers to explore the contralateral groin. The early descriptions of contralateral herniae reported incidence of contralateral hernia of up to 75%. More recent data have been at odds with this, and in two recent reports contralateral operation was required in 5.7% and 7.7% of cases.[3,4] The likelihood of bilateral hernia increases with lower gestational age. A recent report asserts that in order to prevent one contralateral childhood hernia, 30 contralateral groins would require exploration, although for children born at 29 weeks gestation or less, that figure drops to 13.[5] Based on this, many centers (including the authors') no longer advocate the 'routine' exploration of the contralateral groin. Some authors have described the use of ultrasound, plain radiology with pneumoperitoneum at operation on one side, and laparoscopy (discussed later) to address diagnosis of an asymptomatic contralateral hernia.[6,7]

Inguinal herniae are also associated with testicular maldescent, intersex conditions, and with more complex anomalies such as the exstrophy-epispadias complex.[8]

EMBRYOLOGY AND ANATOMY

The development and descent of the testis is inextricably linked to the development of herniae and hydroceles developing consequent on abnormalities of the processus vaginalis.[9, 10] The descent of the testis can be considered a multistaged process under complex neurohormonal control; an enlarging gubernaculum first anchors the embryonic testis near the groin as the abdominal cavity grows. A peritoneal diverticulum (which evolves into the processus vaginalis) develops within the gubernaculum, and this complex migrates into the scrotum. Following the completion of testicular descent by the 38th week of gestation, the processus vaginalis obliterates between deep ring and upper pole of testis, leaving the testis clothed by a peritoneal layer then called tunica vaginalis. In girls, the processus vaginalis extends into the groin and thus into the labium majus as the 'canal of Nuck' in association with the round ligament of the uterus. The canal of Nuck seems to become obliterated earlier in the female than the processus vaginalis in the male (around the 7th month of gestation).

Incomplete obliteration (*i.e.* a PPV) allows communication of peritoneal fluid, as in a hydrocele, or visceral herniation. A schema considering this spectrum of problems is well described, and in summary is:[10]

- Wide open PPV throughout its length, allowing visceral herniation
- 'Congenital' hernia (Fig. 46.1A)
- PPV only in its proximal portion ('funicular process'), lower end obliterated
- 'Acquired' hernia, which presents later (Fig. 46.1B)
- Narrow PPV throughout its length
- 'Communicating' hydrocele (Fig. 46.1C)
- Closed processus vaginalis above and below an encysted remnant
- Encysted hydrocele of the spermatic cord (Fig. 46.1D).

The hernial sac may be associated with viscera (the so-called 'sliding' hernia), and commonly this involves cecum (right), sigmoid colon (left) and bladder (both sides). Rarely, inguinal herniae do not involve the processus vaginalis, as in direct herniae. The etiology of these is less clear cut although at operation a deficient posterior inguinal canal wall may be identified.

Hydroceles likewise may occur as secondary events, usually due to intrascrotal pathology. Torsions of testes or testicular appendages, intrascrotal infection, and tumor all commonly give rise to hydroceles. It is also well recognized that acute systemic illnesses (which may, like Henoch-Schonlein purpura, cause orchitis) may give rise to acute hydrocele.

CLINICAL PRESENTATION

The key clinical difference between hernia and hydrocele is the ability to 'get above' a hydrocele. Classically the symptoms of a hernia are retold by the parents of the presence of a bulge arising in the groin, when the child cries or strains, descending into the

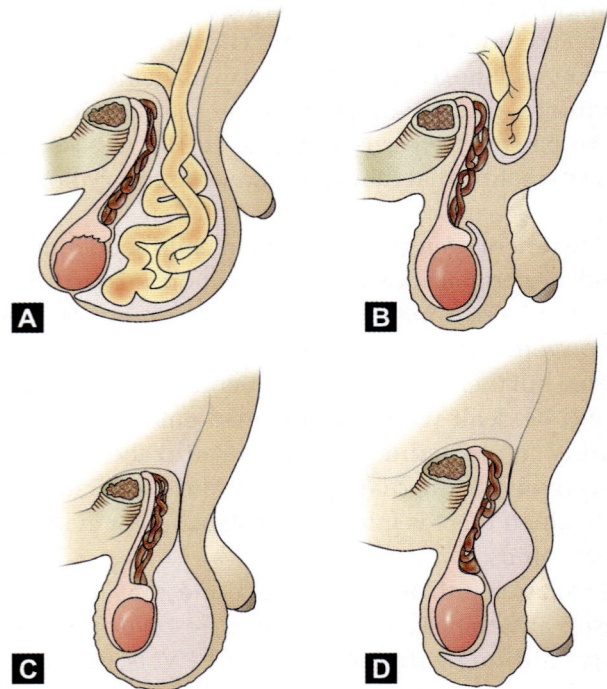

Figs 46.1 A to D: A. Wide open PPV throughout its length, allowing visceral herniation 'Congenital' hernia **B.** PPV only in funicular process, lower end obliterated, 'Acquired' hernia **C.** Narrow PPV throughout its length 'Communicating' hydrocele **D.** Encysted hydrocele of the spermatic cord

scrotum, reducing spontaneously or with manual assistance. A hydrocele is described as a testicular swelling that may not be related to the activities of the child but frequently waxing and waning over the course of the day. It may be bluish in color. A hernia may cause pain in various guises ('ache', 'drag', 'burn') whereas a hydrocele is rarely symptomatic.

On examination, the presence (or absence) of a testis is noted. A hernia if present is usually reducible with ease (with a characteristic palpable 'squelch'), whereas a hydrocele generally is not. In girls, a gonad can descend into a hernial sac akin to a 'lobster in a pot'. It may then present as a lump that the examiner can get above. A hydrocele generally transilluminates brilliantly, but it is worthwhile remembering, especially in infants, that the entire scrotum can be made to transilluminate, therefore this sign may not in itself be diagnostic.

Frequently, the signs are not obvious. A consistent history of a lump from child or parents may be the only clinical features of an inguinal hernia. The spermatic cord may be palpably thicker, with the peritoneal layers of a hernial sac felt to slide over each other in the 'silk' sign. A cough impulse is very difficult to elicit in younger children, and one maneuver is to rest (or 'dangle') the child, abdomen over a hand or arm to increase intrabdominal pressure and declare the hernia (Gornall's sign).

Under the age of 1 year, the incarceration rate of an inguinal hernia is up to 30%, dropping to under 15% by the age of 18 months.[11] An incarcerated hernia typically presents with a history of an unsettled crying child, sometimes with a history of vomiting, whence a lump in groin is then noted. The overlying skin may be reddened, edematous, and may be tender. Rarely, there may be frank evidence of intestinal obstruction with abdominal distension and bile stained vomiting, or there may be evidence of peritonitis.

A large inguinoscrotal hydrocele (or abdominoscrotal hydrocele) may rarely be mistaken for an irreducible hernia, since it may not be possible to identify its upper limit. Symptomatically however, it is rarely painful or tender (unless there have been repeated forceful futile attempts at reduction). Sometimes, the only means of differentiating between this and hernial incarceration is operatively.

In the neonate with meconium peritonitis, the scrotum may take on a black tinge, colored by the free meconium having passed via a PPV into the scrotum. In infants and children with a PPV, which need not have been symptomatic, intrabdominal sepsis (such as acute purulent appendicitis) may cause an acute pyoscrotum. As mentioned above, intrascrotal pathology may cause a hydrocele *de novo*, in which case the history and examination findings are dictated by the underlying condition. In the setting of the acute scrotum, the underlying pathology will be demonstrated at scrotal exploration. Painless hydroceles, especially when associated with a palpably abnormal testis, must be imaged with ultrasound, since there may be an underlying tumor. A hydrocele in the absence of PPV or intrascrotal pathology is very rare indeed in children.

MANAGEMENT

Any reducible inguinal hernia, which presents in an outpatient setting, may be listed for elective repair. Infant herniae should be repair expediently because of the increased risk of incarceration. Herniae presenting in children on the neonatal intensive care unit should ideally be repaired prior to the child's discharge, so that lung and other system maturation will have been optimized.

The inguinal hernia that presents incarcerated should be reduced with analgesia and (if required) sedation. Generally, gentle pressure ('taxis') in the direction of the neck of the hernia will bring about a successful reduction in the majority of cases. These herniae will generally have associated edema and it is probably best to allow this to settle for 24-48 hours prior to inguinal herniotomy. When a child presents with an acute abdomen, scrupulous attention to fluid resuscitation is necessary, even if the hernia is reduced successfully. The general state of the child is all the more crucial if operative reduction is required.

Surgical Management

Consent

The authors routinely explain the risk of vas and vessel damage with subsequent testicular atrophy, especially when a hernia has presented incarcerated. Other issues include risks of general anesthesia, wound infection, recurrent hernia, contralateral hernia, and ascending testis.

Anesthesia and Analgesia

It is usual to perform groin exploration for inguinal herniotomy under general anesthesia, although in ex-premature neonates with significant chronic lung disease, spinal anesthetic may be the modality of choice. At the authors' institution, the use of caudal spinal anesthetic is routine, although some larger children undergo ilioinguinal nerve blockade as an adjunct to general anesthesia.

Operative Procedure

Approach through the Inguinal Canal

The prepared and draped groin in incised preferably along an appropriate crease. Care is taken to site the incision lateral to the pubic tubercle away from the fatty tissue of the mons pubis as this interferes with exposure. A convenient way of siting the incision appropriately is to palpate the course of the spermatic cord containing the hernial sac as it traverses the inguinal canal. The fatty layer of Camper's fascia and fibrous Scarpas are divided along the line of the incision so that the underlying fibers of the external oblique aponeurosis are visible. Inguinal ligament and external inguinal ring are then identified.

The inguinal canal is entered either via a window created by a stab incision over the canal, widened to allow delivery of the cord, or by extending that incision to lay open the canal to the level of the external ring. The ilio-inguinal nerve can be identified and preserved. The cremasteric fibres running along the line of the canal must be split to reveal the shiny surface of the hernial sac associated with its spermatic cord. The cord is delivered, and holding the glistening sac cephalad along the line of the inguinal canal with a pair of forceps, the remainder of the cord contents are swept away gently from the sac (Fig. 46.2). It is usual to walk along the sac (perpendicular to its direction) whilst sweeping away vas and vessels until it has been defined circumferentially. Care should be taken to avoid picking up vas or vessels so as to lower the risk of crush-type injury to these structures.

When the sac has been isolated with confidence from vas and vessels, it should be dissected along its path to the internal ring, taking care not to loop or kink vas or vessel pedicle, and taking care not to tear what is frequently a very flimsy mesothelial layer: thin sacs in small babies which are edematous as a result

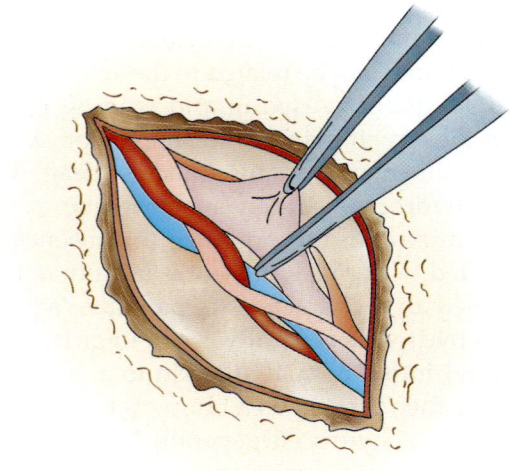

Fig. 46.2: The hernial sac is grasped whilst vas and vessels are swept away

of incarceration are especially easy to damage. The usual landmark to announce the peritoneal limit of this dissection is the appearance of extraperitoneal fat. The sac then needs to be sutureligated: it is the authors' policy to use an absorbable suture such as vicryl, as nonabsorbable sutures have been seen rarely to cause chronic suppuration and suture granulomata.

A sac that is clearly empty may be merely twisted before transfixion. Any suspicion of hernial contents demands the sac be opened to inspect the contents and then reduce. Rarely, one aspect of the sac may comprise a visceral element (the so-called sliding hernia), commonly bladder or mobile bowel. It is safer to fashion a purse-string transfixion taking care not to catch the visceral component of a sliding hernia that can then be reduced. In girls, it is common to open the hernial sac in order to positively identify female internal genitalia, especially if the hernia is bilateral.

The deep ring and posterior wall in infants and children seldom need attention since the etiology is the processus vaginalis. However, with the presence of a very large hernia, the internal ring may become very large and the posterior wall lax. The benefit of plication of internal ring and posterior inguinal canal wall is contentious, but may be undertaken to guard against the risk of a potential direct recurrence. In girls, the internal ring is frequently closed as a matter of course, but in boys it is important not to jeopardise the vas and vessels as they traverse it.

The external oblique aponeurosis, Scarpas and Campers fasciae may be closed in layers, with a subcuticular layer under the skin.

It is imperative after the procedure to document the position of the gonads, since secondary maldescent or ascent of the testis is well described.

Extracanalicular Approach

The cord with its coverings may be identified easily, particularly in infants, as it emerges from the external inguinal ring. The sac may be dissected free of vas and vessels without opening the inguinal canal, although it must be remembered that more cord coverings will be encountered on the approach.

The Preperitoneal Approach

A hernia may be approached in this manner by incising external oblique above the inguinal canal and dissecting downwards to the internal inguinal ring. It may be a useful approach when dealing with an irreducible or obstructed hernia, allowing access to perform a laparotomy and, if necessary, intestinal resection. Some surgeons use this approach to perform reduction and laparotomy prior to a standard inguinal herniotomy performed through the inguinal canal.

The Recurrent Inguinal Hernia

This is a challenging problem, since the inguinal canal may well be encased in scar tissue. A useful approach through the old skin incision is to begin the dissection laterally onto the external oblique aponeurosis where the tissues are virgin. Careful dissection into the inguinal canal and subsequent identification of the sac, vas and vessels should be undertaken prior to completing the herniotomy as described. When taking consent it is important to reiterate the increased risk of vas and vessel damage during the dissection.

HYDROCELE

Operatively, a patent processus vaginalis causing hydrocele is approached identically to an inguinal hernia, since its anatomy is identical. Occasionally encysted hydroceles may be excised from the spermatic cord. The distal hydrocele should be drained through the PPV if possible, although direct needle aspiration is easy. Occasionally, a hydrocele may reaccumulate. A pre-emptive approach during herniotomy or division of the PPV is to extend the opening in the distal sac down as far as safely possible. Very rarely, a hydrocele may recur because of recanalisation or incomplete division of the processus vaginalis and requires re-exploration of the groin. Local procedure such as eversion, excision, or plication of the tunica vaginalis may be employed additionally.

COMPLICATIONS

Inguinal herniae require operation, since they risk incarceration. As stated above under the age of 1 year, the incarceration rate of an inguinal hernia is up to 30%, dropping to under 15% by the age of 18 months.[11] Incarceration jeopardises the testis and the incarcerated contents of the hernial sac.

Testicular atrophy is described to occur in around 2% of boys who present with an incarcerated hernia. Visceral injury is less common. At operation for an irreducible hernia one must suspect intestinal compromise and carry out a laparotomy if needed. Scrupulus attention must be paid to preoperative resuscitation of a child with an irreducible hernia requiring surgery. Reduction of an incarcerated hernia is achieved preoperatively much more frequently in children than in adults, in whom *'reduction en masse'* is a concern. This entity is rare in children, but may be considered in a child whose symptoms and signs fail to settle after reduction.[12] In the female 'lobster in a pot' hernia whereby an ovary becomes incarcerated in the groin, the trapped gonad is said to be at increased risk of torsion.

Anesthetic-related complications are now rare with more specialisation in pediatric and neonatal anesthesia. There remains a significant risk of postoperative apnea in infants however, especially the ex-premature population.[13] For this reason it is usual to observe the 'at risk' group of babies overnight after an inguinal herniotomy. Other postoperative complications of inguinal herniotomy include wound infection, scrotal hematoma, injury to the vas and vessels, recurrent hernia, and iatrogenic ascent of the testis.

Generally wound infection rates are of the order of 1-2%. Prophylactic antibiotics are probably not beneficial and their use is not routine at the authors' institution. Bleeding at the time of operation is uncommon, and is usually caused from cremasteric fibers. Rarely it can be from vessel puncture (inferior epigastric or femoral vessels) at the time of plication of the posterior wall or the floor of the inguinal canal. The distal (transected) aspect of the hernial sac, which is usually left *in situ*, may ooze to contribute to a scrotal hematoma, especially if the hernial sac is inflamed and friable after incarceration. Hemostasis with bipolar diathermy is effective, but vigilance for bleeding and scrupulous technique is also important.

Injury to the vas and vessels is rare (less than 1%). In case of division of the vas, interrupted 7/0 or 8/0 monofilament sutures are placed circumferentially to fashion an end-to-end vasovasostomy. Microvascular anastomosis, when the vessels are divided, is a precise and demanding procedure requiring optical magnification for satisfactory results and is therefore, best undertaken by appropriately trained surgeons.

Recurrent hernia is uncommon, overall rate around 1% or less. The rate of recurrence for neonatal repair is higher.[14,15] When recurrences occur, they are generally seen within the first postoperative year. Important causes are missed or torn hernial sacs (thus attention to dissection of the sac in its entirety is important), injury to the floor or posterior wall of the inguinal canal (direct hernia), bleeding and infection. Rarer causes such as connective tissue disease should be borne in mind.

Subsequent abnormalities of the testis are well recognised. Atrophy may be seen as a result of incarceration as described above, but decrease in testicular volume has been noted in some patients:[16] the significance of this is unclear. Iatrogenic ascent of the testis has also been recognised in about 1% after inguinal herniotomy.[17] Occasionally a hydrocele develops after herniotomy: it usually settles without intervention but sometimes requires a scrotal procedure or rarely re-exploration of the groin to exclude a 'recurrent' PPV.

Rarer complications include suture granulomata, which may present years after operation, and direct visceral (*e.g.* bladder and bowel when involved in sliding herniae) or vascular injury.[18]

In infant age group, complications of inguinal herniae or herniotomy are commoner than in older children. This probably has implications for more rigorous follow-up of infants undergoing inguinal herniotomy.

NOVEL APPROACHES

Laparoscopy is becoming increasingly popular in its applications in most aspects of pediatric surgery. In adults, laparoscopy has become established as a reliable means of inguinal herniorrhaphy using a mesh placed at the internal inguinal ring by either trans- or pre-peritoneal approach. Some authors have described laparoscopy in inguinal hernia in children for diagnostic and/or therapeutic means.[19,20] An angled telescopy can be passed with ease through an open hernial sac, although the more traditionally placed paraumbilical port allows both sides to be visualized.[19] Laparoscopic assessment is crucial if there is associated impalpable testis. Laparoscopic herniotomy with purse-string sutures placed at the inguinal ring has been described.[20]

Finally, there are evolving possibilities of manipulating the mechanisms, which normally cause obliteration of the processus vaginalis. *In vitro*, calcitonin-gene-related peptide (CGRP) has been demonstrated to cause cellular fusion within the processus.[21] Together with hepatocyte growth factor (HGF), it contributes to transformation of peritoneal mesothelium into mobile mesenchymal cells. The role of CGRP in testicular descent in other species has been characterised, its source probably being the genitofemoral nerve. The work on basic biology of the processus vaginalis raises exciting future possibilities for the nonsurgical treatment of herniae and hydroceles.

ACKNOWLEDGEMENT

The authors are grateful to Miss Katie Midwinter, FRCS, for the illustrations.

REFERENCES

1. Rowe MI, Copelson LW, Clatsworthy HW. The patent processus vaginalis and the inguinal hernia. J. Pediatr. Surg 1969;4:102.
2. Golka T, Holschneider AM, Fischer R, Blessing MH. Zur Frage der Pathogenitat des offenen processus vaginalis peritonei. Z. Kinderchir 1989;44:88-90.
3. Schwobel MG, Schramm H, Gitzelmann CA. The infantile inguinal hernia–a bilateral disease? Pediatr Surg Int 1999;15:115-18.
4. Ballantyne A, Jawaheer G, Munro FD. Contralateral groin exploration is not justified in infants with a unilateral inguinal hernia. Brit. J. Surg 2001;88(5):720-23.

5. Lander AD, Paranjothy R, Parashar K. How many contralateral groin explorations are needed to avoid one contralateral inguinal hernia? Presented at BAPS 1999, Liverpool.
6. Erez I, Rathaus V, Werner M, et al. Preoperative sonography of the inguinal canal prevents unnecessary contralateral exploration. Pediatr Surg Int 1996;11: 487-89.
7. Kervancioglu R, Bayram MM, Ertaskin I, Ozkur A. Ultrasonographic evaluation of bilateral groins in children with unilateral inguinal hernia. Acta Radiologica 2000;41(6):653-57.
8. Nicholls G, Duffy PG. Anatomical correction of the exstrophy-epispadias complex: analysis of 34 patients. Brit J Urol 1998;82(6):865-69.
9. Hutson JM. Inguinoscrotal Swellings in the Newborn. Textbook of Neonatal Surgery Ed. Gupta DK. 2000 Modern Publishers, New Delhi 110002, India 118-20.
10. Skandalakis JE, Gray SW. Embryology for Surgeons, Baltimore, Williams and Wilkins, 2nd ed, 1984;578-84.
11. Grosfeld JL. Hernias in children. Rob and SmithÕs Operative Surgery: Pediatric Surgery Eds. Spitz L, Coran AG. Chapman and Hall, London 1995;222-38.
12. Olguner M, Agartan C, Akgur FM, Aktug T. Pediatric case of hernia reduction en masse. Pediatr Int 2000;42(2): 181-82.
13. Allen GS, Cox CS Jr., White N, et al. Postoperative respiratory complications in ex-premature infants after inguinal herniorrhaphy. J Ped Surg 1998;33(7):1095-98.
14. Moss RL, Hatch EI Jr. Inguinal hernia repair in early infancy. Am J Surg 1991;161(5):596-99.
15. Phelps S, Agrawal M. Morbidity after neonatal inguinal herniotomy. J Pediatr Surg 1997;32(3):445-47.
16. Leung WY, Poon M, Fan TW, et al. Testicular volume of boys after inguinal herniotomy: combined clinical and radiological follow-up. Pediatr Surg Int 1999;15(1):40-41.
17. Surana R, Puri P. Iatrogenic ascent of the testis: an under-recognized complication of inguinal hernia operation in children Brit J Urol 1994;73(5):580-81.
18. Nagar H. Stitch granulomas following inguinal herniotomy: a 10-year review. J Pediatr Surg 1993; 28(11): 1505-07.
19. Rescorla FJ, West KW, Engum SA, et al. The "other side" of pediatric hernias: The role of laparoscopy. Am Surgeon 1997;63(8):690-93.
20. Montupet P, Esposito C. Laparoscopic treatment of congenital inguinal hernia in children. J Pediatr Surg 1999; 34(3):420-23.
21. Hutson JM, Albano FR, Paxton G, et al. In vitro fusion of human inguinal hernia with associated epithelial transformation. Cells Tissues Organs 2000;166(3): 249-58.

Rare Pediatric Hernias

DK Gupta, Shilpa Sharma, Kamlesh Pal

All pediatric surgeons are well versed with the repair of congenital inguinal hernias. However, there are times when they are confronted with rare hernias. Rare forms of the inguinal hernia are encountered more frequently when approached by the laparoscopic technique than during the open approach.[1] Routine video recording during laparoscopy provided an objective and absolute picture of the true incidence of these unusual forms of the hernia. On retrospective evaluation of these videos, direct hernias were found in 2.2%, femoral hernias in 1.1%, hernias en pantaloon in 0.7% and a combination of indirect, direct, and femoral hernia in 0.4% cases.[1]

FEMORAL HERNIA

Femoral hernia is very rare in children and its diagnosis remains a challenging problem in childhood.[2] The incidence is 0.5-1% of all cases of pediatric groin hernias.[2-4] Femoral hernias are seen more frequently in girls.

In case of the femoral hernia, the defect is through an anatomic triangle surrounded by the inguinal ligament above, the lower border of the pubic bone medially and the femoral vein laterally. The hernia follows the space below the inguinal ligament through the femoral canal. The canal lies medial to the femoral vein and lateral to the lacunar ligament. A femoral hernia is more prone to incarceration or strangulation as it protrudes through a narrow neck.

The swelling during its last part of reduction may be seen to reduce through a defect inferior to the inguinal ligament. The diagnosis is confirmed during operation.

Femoral hernias occur at any age, but are extremely rare in infancy.[5] The hernia is more common on the right side. The duration of symptoms may range from a few days to many years. A correct diagnosis can only be made preoperatively in only 12-70% of the cases, in different series.[2,4-7] Childhood femoral hernia is often missed clinically because of difficulty in eliciting their clinical signs.[8]

The most common mode of presentation is a recurrent painless lump in the upper part of the groin on the medial side of the thigh. The swelling reduces with manual compression. If the swelling persists even after the repair of the inguinal hernia, the diagnosis should be revised and the possibility of femoral hernia should be kept in mind. The femoral hernias may be diagnosed during surgery at a negative exploration for a clinically diagnosed inguinal hernia. During an operation for inguinal hernia, it is essential to think of the presence of the femoral hernia when a non-obliterated processus vaginalis is not found.[4,8] Rarely, the child may present with an incarceration. The rate of irreducible femoral hernia may be quite high (48%).[7]

The differential diagnosis is either an inguinal hernia or a recurrent inguinal hernia. An irreducible femoral hernia needs to be differentiated from the inguinal lymph nodes.

The sensitivity of high resolution ultrasonographic (USG) study in the diagnosis of inguinocrural hernias has been reported to be higher (87.5%) than that of the clinical examination (72%).[9] Similarly, the sensitivity in the diagnosis of complications in these hernias was reported to be significantly high on high resolution USG (85%) as compared to clinical examination (36%).[9] A femoral hernia should positively be excluded if the operative findings at inguinal exploration are inconsistent with the preoperative signs and in any child with a suspected recurrent inguinal hernia.

Repair

Femoral hernia has been treated using a variety of techniques such as classic tissue-based and prosthetic mesh repairs. In children, an excision of the sac and repair of the femoral canal is curative.[3] The operation can be done from above or below the inguinal ligament. The author's approach is to repair the femoral hernia with a transverse incision placed below the inguinal ligament. As the sac carries with it a good amount of femoral fat, the sac needs to be separated well and identified from the fatty tissue before closed securely.

In McVay's tissue-based repair, the Cooper's ligament is approximated with the conjoined tendon, through an inguinal incision placed just above the medial side of the inguinal ligament. This type of hernia repair results in an unwanted tension.[10] The Cooper's ligament is though strong yet it lacks the elasticity. Therefore, sutures may cut through the tissues in the postoperative period. McVay's Cooper ligament repair with the advantage of covering all potential hernia sites in the myopectineal orifice has been used to repair the femoral hernias in children. Authors have not experienced any recurrence after surgical repair of the femoral hernia with the approach below the inguinal ligament.

The well-known advantages of tension-free hernia repair led to the development of new techniques for femoral hernia repair using prosthetic material. In 1974, Lichtenstein and colleagues have described 'plug' technique for femoral hernia repair with a recurrence rate less than 2%.[11]

Recently, femoral defect has been repaired successfully in children using a mesh plug. There were no complications after a follow-up period for 2 years.[12] In a series of 712 inguinal hernias in 542 children, repaired laparoscopically, direct hernias were found in 2.3%, femoral hernias in 1%, hernias en pantalon in 0.7%, and a combination of indirect and femoral hernia in 0.2%.[13]

Laparoscopic groin exploration and femoral hernia repair has some distinct advantages. The procedure is safe and effective even in the pediatric patients.[14] The advantages of the laparoscopic approach include its technical ease, feasibility as an outpatient procedure, cord structures remaining untouched, the superior diagnostic ability, simultaneous repair of the bilateral hernias and clear visualization of the anatomy.[13]

The incidence of postoperative recurrence varies from 0-13% in different series.[5,6] A correct preoperative diagnosis will lead to appropriate surgical approach and management, thus avoiding the unnecessary morbidity and preventing unnecessary re-operations.[6]

RICHTER'S HERNIA

A richter is hernia is defined as a herniation of the antimesenteric border of the bowel through a fascial defect.

As only a portion of the circumference of the bowel is involved, the bowel may not be obstructed, even if the hernia is incarcerated or strangulated, and the patient may not present with obstructive symptoms. Richter's hernia can occur with any of the various abdominal hernias and is particularly dangerous, as a portion of strangulated bowel may be reduced unknowingly into the abdominal cavity, leading to perforation and peritonitis. The patient may complain of pain or have tachycardia and fever due to the strangulation.

LITTRE'S HERNIA

This term is given to herniation of the Meckle's diverticulum through an inguinal hernia. It is extremely rare to happen. A Littre's hernia is defined as any hernial sac which contains a Meckel's Diverticulum.[15] It has been reported in association with inguinal, umbilical, femoral, sciatic, ventral, and lumbar hernias.[15] This hernia is rare, particularly in children, in whom the umbilical hernia is reported to be the most common variety. Littre's hernia is difficult to diagnose, but should be suspected in patients with gastrointestinal bleeding, incompletely reducible hernias, and hernias with fecal fistulae.[15] It may be confused with cryptorchidism when Meckel's diverticulum adheres to and envelops the testicle making palpation of the gonad difficult.

The recommended treatment is resection of the Meckel's diverticulum from within the opened hernial sac followed by herniorrhaphy.[15]

VENTRAL HERNIA

This is commonly seen in children as follow-up of conservatively managed abdominal wall defects. The hernia size may be small or large, with a narrow or wide neck (Fig. 47.1). The contents are small bowel loops but liver may also be projecting out in the sac if the size of the hernia is more than 5 cm in diameter. The contents are usually not reducible completely as there are dense adhesions between the under surface of the skin and liver or the intestine. The rectus muscles are wide apart, thinned out and weak, forming the neck of the hernia. All ventral hernias should be repaired, preferably before 1 year of age so that the contents can be reduced and the rectus muscles can be approximated in the midline. With this, the abdominal cavity also gets a chance to grow with the age of the patient. Various options available to repair the ventral hernia include:

Primary Repair of the Defect

after reducing the hernial contents inside the abdominal cavity (Fig. 47.1). In case of difficulty in bringing the muscles together in the midline, additional techniques may be adapted and these include; stretching or the mobilization of the abdominal wall from lateral sides, raising of the anterior rectus sheath vertical flaps on one or both sides and suturing these together in front of the intestine. In cases of anticipated difficulty in closing the hernia, a slow pneumoperitoneum may be introduced to increase the size of the abdominal cavity well in advance.

Moderate Sized Defects

Prolene mesh prosthesis may be used to fill the gap between the rectus muscles if these can not be approximated. The available skin is used to cover the mesh. If the same is not sufficient to cover the defect, alternate materials like dura, pericardium, cultured skin are used till the complete healing of the wound takes place. The mesh is removed after many months or years when the abdominal cavity has grown in size and the rectus muscles can be brought together in the midline.

Phantom Hernia

The size of the ventral hernias may be so huge that the abdominal cavity never got a chance to grow, and all the abdominal contents remained in the sac and grew outside the abdomen. It is thus impossible to reduce the hernial contents into the abdominal cavity due to lack of space (Figs 47.2A and B). Such cases should first be investigated for evaluating the position of great vessels, the kidneys and the liver by CT/MRI and nuclear scans. The management should be staged; first allowing the skin from lateral abdominal wall to enlarge in size with the use of tissue expanders, then the hernia is repaired with or without the mesh to bridge the gap between the rectus muscles.

In neglected cases, a severe lumbar lordosis may well become an alternative factor to produce visceroabdominal disproportion observed before surgery, and its correction after surgery may well induce the abdominal cavity to rapidly enlarge.[16] It may be speculated that the dehiscence of abdominal rectus muscles associated with omphalocele causes the tension of ventral muscles to decline and then, imbalance in tension between ventral (abdominal) and dorsal (back) muscles causes the lumbar lordosis to increase. Thus, during the staged procedure, the prosthetic sheet should be attached under moderate tension, and its plication should be carried out at regular intervals to maintain the tension of abdominal rectus muscles.[16]

INCISIONAL HERNIA

Iatrogenic hernia in general, occurs in 2-10% of all abdominal operations secondary to breakdown of the

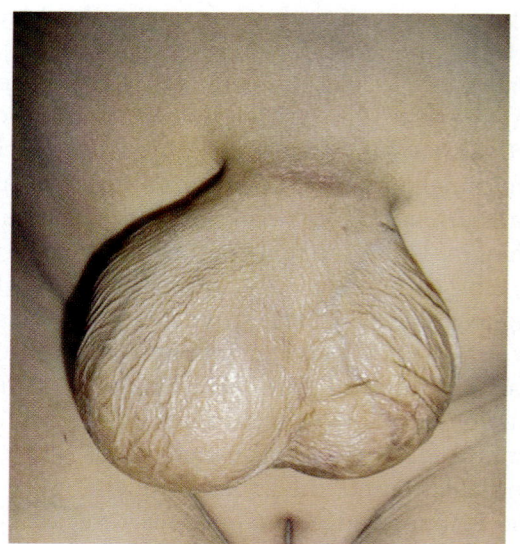

Fig. 47.1: A small ventral hernia in a girl that can be repaired primarily

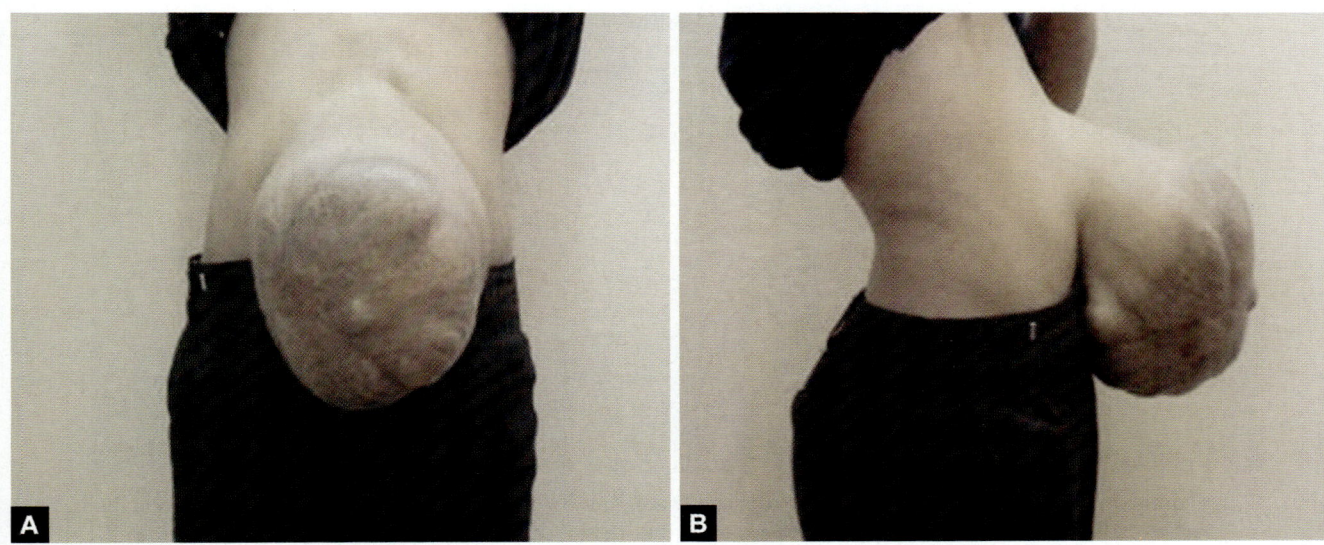

Figs 47.2A and B: A ten-year-old boy presenting with postomphalocele large ventral hernia with a narrow neck and severe lumbar lordosis. The CT scan showed presence of most intestinal loops and the liver in the sac outside the abdomen. The vertebral spine, the aorta and the inferior vena cava were found displaced anteriorly to the level of the anterior abdominal wall

fascial closure of wound to the prior surgery. Even after repair, recurrence rates approach 20-45%. However, its incidence of incisional hernia in children is much lower due to good muscle strength, better wound healing ability and the routine practice of skin crease incisions.

While having an access to the kidneys, the intercostal nerve which lies posteriorly immediately below the last rib in between the internal oblique and the transverse abdominal muscles, an effort should be made to spare this nerve by dissecting both proximally and distally, enabling careful padding and traction of the nerve out of the operative field. The division of the nerve leads to muscle denervation and lumbar hernia. Postoperatively, the muscle denervation leading to the flank bulge must be differentiated from the flank incisional hernia, which is rare. In the later instance, a fascial defect is usually palpable. Most importantly, wound infection accounts for the majority of incisional hernias.

SPIGELIAN HERNIA

This rare form of abdominal wall hernia occurs through a defect in the spigelian fascia, which is defined by the lateral edge of the rectus muscle at the semilunar line (from costal arch to the pubic tubercle).

LUMBAR HERNIA

Lumbar hernias are also known as posterior body wall hernias (Figs 47.3 and 47.4). Congenital lumbar hernia is a rare anomaly with only 45 cases reported in the English-language literature.[17] Hernias in the lumbar region are classified as; (1) Those through the superior lumbar triangle (of Grynfelt-Lesshaft) and (2) Those through the inferior lumbar triangle (of Petit). Superior lumbar hernias are more commonly reported.[18] However, some series have reported a relatively high incidence of inferior lumbar hernia.[17]

Hernia through the Superior Lumbar Triangle (of Grynfelt-Lesshaft)

It is an inverted triangle, larger in size, more constant, most common site of lumbar hernia, contains T12 and L1 nerves and is avascular. A superior lumbar hernia is a protrusion of preperitoneal fat or peritoneum with sac formation or a viscus through the lumbar area just below the 12th rib.

The base of the triangle is the 12th rib and serratus posterior inferior muscle. The anterior boundary is the posterior border of the internal oblique muscle, posterior boundary is the anterior border of the sacrospinalis muscle. The floor of the triangle is formed

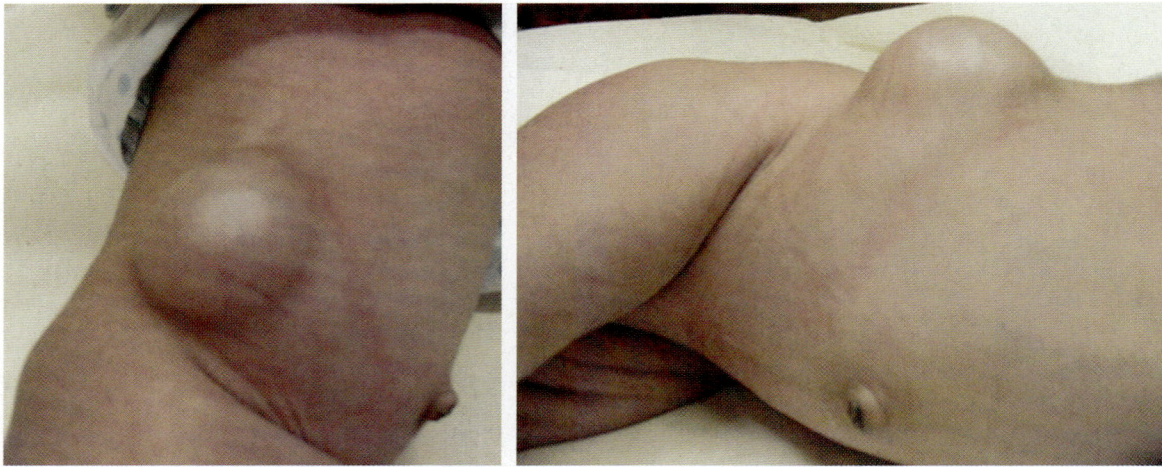

Fig. 47.3: Right side lumbar hernia in a 1-month-old child. There was a well defined circular defect in the abdominal wall muscles. With adequate mobilization, the defect could be closed primarily

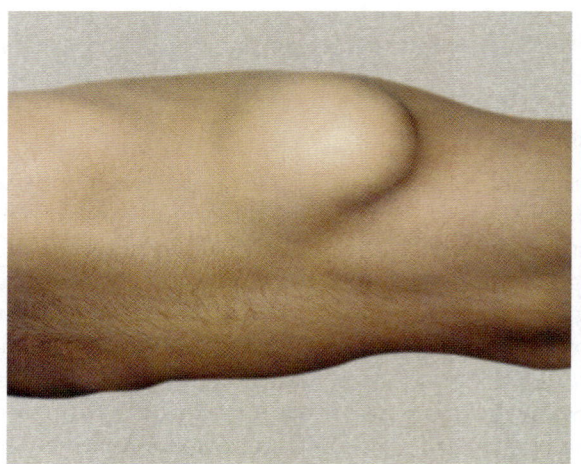

Fig. 47.4: The lumbar hernia in a child, with a circular defect in the abdominal wall muscles. The defect was repaired primarily with success

by the aponeurosis of the transversus abdominis muscle arising by fusion of the layers of the thoracolumbar fascia formed by the external oblique and latissimus dorsi muscles.

Hernia through the Inferior Lumbar Triangle (of Petit)

The base of the triangle is the iliac crest. The anterior (abdominal) boundary is the posterior border of the external oblique muscle. The posterior (lumbar) boundary is the anterior border of the latissimus dorsi muscle. The floor of the triangle is formed by the internal oblique muscle with contributions from the transversus abdominis muscle and posterior lamina of the thoracolumbar fascia and the internal oblique muscle. The triangle is covered by superficial fascia and skin. This is smaller in size, least common site of lumbar hernia, contains no nerves but is vascular. If the hernia through this triangle is small the ring is formed by the thoracolumbar fascia and fibers of internal oblique muscles. If it is large, the ring may include the boundaries of the whole inferior triangle. Enlargement of the ring is by section of the fascia.

Associated Anomalies

Congenital variants have been described, frequently associated with musculofascial and skeletal abnormalities, specifically "lumbocostovertebral syndrome" and/or meningomyelocele (Figs 47.5A and B).[19] The defect results from a single somatic defect occurring during the third to fifth week of embryonal development. As there are various reports on its association with the lumbocostovertebral syndrome, a spinal X-ray and/CT scan may be done to rule out the additional defects.[20-22]

Meningomyelocele may predispose to lumbar herniation secondary to abnormalities in muscular innervation related to nerve entrapment in the spinal dysraphism.[19]

The lumbar hernias may also be associated with the defects in the thoracic cage. The associated anomalies of the ribs and the vertebrae may be extensive and large enough for the liver, lungs, kidney and spleen (left sided) to herniate outside. There may

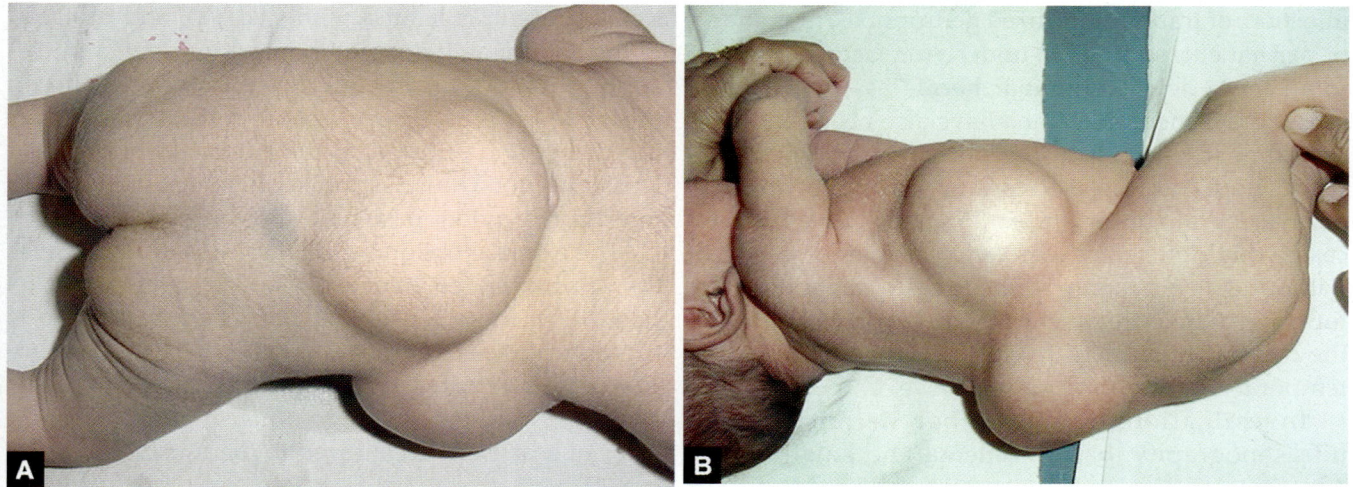

Figs 47.5A and B: Right side lumbar hernia in a newborn baby associated with meningomyelocele

be paradoxical breathing resulting in respiratory distress, especially in the newborns (Figs 47.6A and B). The large defects involve absence, deficiency, twisting, widening, deformity and the fusion of the remaining ribs. On the right side, the defect may be covered with a large right lobe of the liver and may remain asymptomatic. However, as the important structures in the hernia sac remain unprotected and remain at risk to trauma, a surgical repair at an appropriate time is warranted. The closure of the defect involves approximation of ribs and the muscles as much as possible it could be done comfortably. The remain defect should be closed with a mesh. If the defect is small and less than 5 cm in diameter, there is no problem with the paradoxical breathing and no stabilization is required. However, large defects, more than 5 cm in size require stabilization of the chest. This could be accomplished by utilizing the available deformed, flat and/fused ribs to shape them appropriately by splitting, twisting or angulating them to support the mesh graft.

The hernia may be an isolated defect in the lumbar region, well circumscribed or it may be associated with hydrometrocolpos, meningomyelocele, anorectal malformation, undescended testis and multiple other anomalies.[17,18,20] The diagnosis of the hernia may be delayed due to its juxtaposition to a posterior meningomyelocele and may result in incarceration.[20] Acquired lumbar hernia generally can be attributed to surgery,

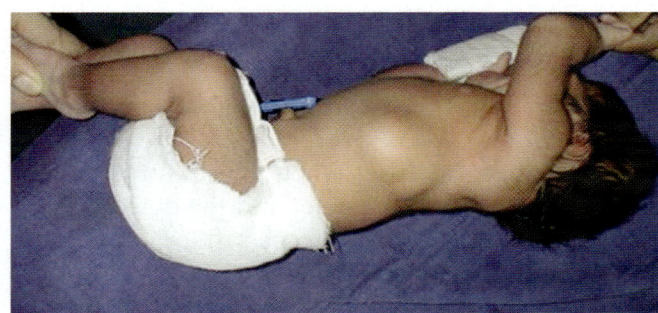

Fig. 47.6A: Thoracolumbar hernia in a newborn presenting with respiratory distress

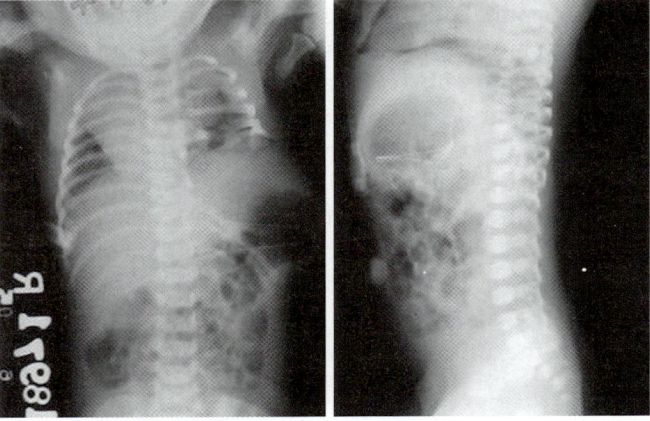

Fig. 47.6B: Skiagram showing defect in the rib cage on the left side of the chest. There was herniation of left lung, left lobe of the liver, left kidney and the spleen through the defect. The diaphragm was thin and amuscular. The hernial defect was repaired and the gap was covered using ribs from the lower thoracic cage

infection, or trauma. Localized neuropraxis, temporary or permanent, may be the underlying factor, common to all these defects. Lumbar hernia associated with intrathoracic neuroblastoma have also been reported. The lumbar hernia is also reported to have resulted from neuropraxis secondary to intrathoracic paravertebral tumor and its management. In both cases, this deficiency was temporary and resolved without specific therapy. These cases suggest a role for conservative treatment for the hernia itself, when the neural impairment resulting in the defect is of a temporary nature.[19]

Investigations for a lumbar hernia include ultrasonography, barium enema and small bowel contrast studies to rule out hydronephrosis or renal lump; bowel content, etc. A dorsal and lumbosacral X-rays may be done to rule out vertebral pathology.

REPAIR

Early operation is the treatment of choice, and repair with local tissues is preferable.[17] The need for prosthetic material arises when the size of the defect is more than 5 cm in diameter and the defect cant be closed primarily.[17] A successful operation by mobilization and approximation of the muscle edges offers a good quality of life.[17] Operative repair is recommended for these patients before 12 months of age.[18]

The repair is done with the patient in the lateral kidney position with the hernia side up. The affected flank is extended by extension of the ipsilateral lower extremity and flexion of the opposite extremity at the knee. The choice of the repair material depends upon the size of the defect. For small defects, the defect in the thoracolumbar fascia and muscles is repaired with nylon. For large hernias, a flap graft or a mesh (single or double) or both may be used. The authors have rotated the distal ends of the 10th and 11th ribs to support the thin muscular repair in a case of large defects.

Dowd-Ponka Repair of Lumbar Hernia[23]

An oblique or vertical incision is given over the hernia site. In superior hernia, the sac lies beneath skin, superficial fascia, and latissimus dorsi muscle. In inferior hernia, there is no layer of muscle. The hernial sac, if present, is ligated with silk (3-0) and replaced in the abdomen. If a large lipoma is present, a purse-spring suture or several interrupted sutures will keep the fat down. A Marlex or Prolene patch is placed over the defect and sutured to the external oblique and latissimus dorsi muscles and lumbar periosteum using interrupted nylon/prolene.

The external oblique and latissimus dorsi muscles are approximated over the Marlex patch as far as possible without tension. A flap of gluteal fascia is turned upto to cover the remaining defect and secure it with interrupted nylon sutures to the muscles present. A large hernial ring may require a second layer of Marlex mesh sutured to the muscles.

INTERNAL HERNIAS IN THE ABDOMEN

Internal abdominal hernias are uncommon varieties of hernias. These are difficult to detect and also remain mostly asymptomic. They have confusing anatomy and obscure etiology. They account for about one percent of all cases of intestinal obstruction.

Two types of internal hernias may be encountered:
1. The passage of a viscus through a defect either in a mesentery or the omentum.
2. Protrusion of a viscus through an opening formed by a fold of peritoneum.

Hernias through Mesenteric or Omental Defect

These have been called 'false hernias' as there is no hernial sac. All mesenteries in the abdominal cavity are subject to defects through which herniation may take place. These defects may be developmental or as the result of trauma. The chief locations are through the mesentery, greater omentum, sigmoid mesocolon, broad ligament of the uterus or the falciform ligament. Paraduodenal herniation is the most common.[24] These hernias are asymptomatic unless incarcerated. The frequency of internal herniation is given in Table 47.1.

Table 47.1: The frequency of internal herniation	
Paraduodenal	42-53%
Paracecal	13%
Through the epiploic foramen	8%
Transmesenteric	8%
In the sigmoid region	6%
Other congenital and acquired hernias	12%

The hernia may start in the relatively avascular areas of the mesentery. The defect then enlarges until at least one free edge is formed by an important artery. It is usually a branch of the superior or the inferior mesenteric artery. In many cases, an intestinal loop may pass freely through the defect without any strangulation. However, adhesions may develop between the hernial ring and the herniated intestinal loop, making it vulnerable to symptoms due to strangulation.

Omental herniation can occur between arc of Barkow and any of the descending arteries. For the repair, the ring is enlarged between clamps. The omentum is incised and the bowel is freed. The hernia is reduced and the clamped tissue is suture ligated. The defect in the omentum must be closed with continuous or interrupted sutures to prevent recurrences. Decompression of the proximal intestine without incising the ring may also permit reduction of the herniated loop and closure of the omental defect.

Rarely the loops of the small bowel, appendix, cecum, and the ascending colon may be placed within the anterior and posterior leaves of the un-fused greater omentum. Appendectomy and the resection of the sac should be performed to achieve successful outcome. Embryologically, anatomically and clinically, the intra-mesenteric hernias may take place in any part of mesentery that has congenital openings or pouches. Hernia at the terminal ileum (pouch of Treves') is one such example. It may enlarge to house the intestinal loops in the pouch.

Mesenteric herniation takes place through defect in mesentery of small intestine, transverse mesocolon and most commonly the sigmoid mesocolon. At least one free edge of the ring is usually formed by a branch of the superior mesenteric or the inferior mesenteric artery. Since there is no sac, the obstructed loops are clearly visible. Any injury to the vessel at the edge of the defect must be avoided. The dilated loop needs to be decompressed first before reducing the hernia. The vascular injury must be avoided.

Hernias beneath a Mesenteric or Peritoneal Fold

In this second group of internal hernias there is no break in the peritoneum, the herniated viscus enters and enlarge a naturally occurring fold or pocket of peritoneum. A sac is always present.

A. *Hernia through the epiploic foramen of Winslow:* For unknown reasons, this hernia is extremely uncommon in children despite of the fact that the epiploic foramen is normally open. The boundaries of the foramen are; superiorly the caudate process, anteriorly the hepatoduodenal ligament containing portal triad, posteriorly the inferior vena cava and inferiorly the first part of the duodenum and the transverse part of the hepatic artery. The neck of the ring should not be incised under any circumstances. To reduce the hernia, the hepatogastric ligament is opened and the incarcerated intestine is decompressed carefully taking all care not to allow contamination. After the decompression of the bowel has been achieved, the aspiration site is closed with a purse string suture. The hernia is reduced and the defect in the hepatogastric ligament is closed. Fixation of an abnormally mobile cecum or right colon may be helpful to avoid recurrences.

B. *Hernia through the transverse mesocolon:* The herniated loop enters lesser sac to the left of the middle colic vessels called space of Riolan.

C. *Paraduodenal hernias:* Abdominal cavity is full of pouches and fossae. Moynihan in 1889 described nine fossae or peritoneal pockets which form potential spaces for internal herniations.[25] Only five of these fossae are constant enough to be of clinical importance and have been outlined below in Table 47.2. These hernias, though rare, have been reported in children.[26]

Paraduodenal hernias are formed during the period of fixation of colon (by 5th month of the fetal life). They are known by the direction of the herniated loop, if the loop passes to the right, it is a right paraduodenal hernia; without reference to the midline of the body or to the specific fossae concerned. Paraduodenal sacs usually contain

Table 47.2: The five paraduodenal fossae		
Fossa	Direction of Hernia	Incidence (%)
1. Superior duodenal fossa of Treitz	Right	30-50
2. Paraduodenal fossa of Landzert	Left	2
3. Inferior duodenal fossa of Treitz	Right	50-70
4. Intermesocolic fossa of Broesike	Right	Rare
5. Mesentericoparietal fossa of Waldeyer	Right	01

small intestine, though rarely may contain cecum, ascending colon or sigmoid colon. The surgical treatment of strangulated paraduodenal hernia includes the reduction of the hernia and the eradication of the fossa. This may be performed either by closing the neck of the fossa or by enlarging the orifice so that there are no chances of the pouch formation. Injury to major blood vessels must be avoided. Enterostomy may be required for decompression of the contents of the hernia. The herniated contents should be looked carefully for the viability and an appropriate action should be taken if the need be.

D. *The paracecal hernias:* Six fossae are related to the cecum.
   1. Superior ileocecal fossa
   2. Inferior ileocacal fossa
   3. Retrocecal or retrocolic fossa
   4. Hartmann's fossa
   5. Paracolic fossa
   6. Iliaco-subfascialis.

Out of these, first two are important. Superior ileocecal fossa is formed by supeior ileocecal fold of ileocolic mesentery and contains the anterior branch of the ileocolic artery. The inferior ileocecal fossa has an anterior prominent ileoappendicular fold which occasionally contains the ileoappendicular artery. The hernial sac may be found under the cecum.

COMPLICATIONS

Rare hernias through narrow necks like femoral hernia and internal hernias are prone to complications if not identified and treated in time once the symptoms appear. The reason being rarity of the lesion, the abnormal sites and the difficulty in making the diagnosis without surgery. Hernias visible outside the abdominal cavity may be examined for risk of complications. Reducible hernia refers to the ability to return the contents of the hernia into the abdominal cavity, either spontaneously or manually. An incarcerated hernia is no longer reducible. The vascular supply of the bowel is still not compromised, though the symptoms due to bowel obstruction are common. A strangulated hernia when the vascular supply of the bowel is compromised secondary to incarceration of hernia contents, poses a serious challenge.

Complications following repair of the hernia are many and most are avoidable. These include;

1. Vascular complications like seroma or hematoma formation though uncommon in children, still can happen rarely. Main vessel may also be injured if it is included in the clamp while widening the necl of the sac.
2. Neurological injury of the nerves may occur in the close proximity, e.g. T12 or L1 nerves during repair of a lumbar hernia through the superior lumbar triangle.
3. Injury of the hollow viscus (most likely the colon) is likely to happen if the hernia is incarcerated or is of a sliding type. This is likely to happen during the opening of the sac, or by taking deep bites of the protruding fats.
4. Recurrence of the hernia is likely to occur if the anatomical details have not been kept in mind while making a diagnosis or repairing the defect.
5. Infection of the wound or even peritonitis, is a serious threat if the bowel gets injured during surgery.

REFERENCES

1. Schier F, Klizaite J. Rare inguinal hernia forms in children. Pediatr Surg Int 2004;20:748-52.
2. Shonubi AM, Musa AA, Salami BA, et al. Femoral hernias in children at the Olabisi Onabanjo University Teaching Hospital, Sagamu, Nigeria. East Afr Med J 2004;81: 447-49.
3. Radcliffe G, Stringer MD. Reappraisal of femoral hernia in children. Br J Surg 1997;84:58-60.
4. Al-Shanafey S, Giacomantonio M. Femoral hernia in children. J Pediatr Surg 1999;34:1104-06.
5. Ollero Fresno JC, Alvarez M, Sanchez M, et al. Femoral hernia in childhood: review of 38 cases. Pediatr Surg Int 1997;12:520-21.
6. De Caluwac D, Chertin B, Puri P. Childhood femoral hernia: a commonly misdiagnosed condition. Pediatr Surg Int 2003;19:608-9.
7. Asai A, Takehara H, Okada A, et al. A case of femoral hernia in a child. Tokushima J Exp Med 1992;39: 145-47.
8. Fonzone Caccese A, Caccioppoli U, Aliotta A, et al. Femoral hernia in childhood: a rare entity. Pediatr Med Chir 1999;21:145-48.
9. Dattola P, Alberti A, Dattola A, et al. Inguino-crural hernias: preoperative diagnosis and postoperative follow-up by high-resolution ultrasonography. A personal experience. Ann Ital Chir 2002;73:65-68.
10. McVay CB, Savage LE. Etiology of femoral hernia. Ann Surg 1961; 154:25-32.
11. Lichtenstein IL, Shore JM. Simplified repair of femoral and recurrent inguinal hernias by a 'plug' technique. Am J Surg 1974;128:439-44.

12. Ceran C, Kaylaoaylu G, Sanmez K. Femoral hernia repair with mesh-plug in children. J Pediatr Surg 2002;37: 1456-58.
13. Schier F. Laparoscopic inguinal hernia repair-a prospective personal series of 542 children. J Pediatr Surg 2006 June;41(6):1081-84.
14. Lee SL, DuBois JJ. Laparoscopic diagnosis and repair of pediatric femoral hernia. Initial experience of four cases. Surg Endosc. 2000 Dec;14(12):1110-13. Comment in: Surg Endosc 2000 Dec;14(12):1097.
15. Mishalany HG, Pereyra R, Longerbean JK. Littre's hernia in infancy presenting as undescended testicle. J Pediatr Surg 1982;17:67-69.
16. Nagaya M, Kato J, Niimi N, Tanaka S. Lordosis of lumbar vertebrae in omphalocele: an important factor in regulating abdominal cavity capacity. J Pediatr Surg 2000;35:1782-85.
17. Wakhlu A, Wakhlu AK. Congenital lumbar hernia. Pediatr Surg Int 2000;16:146-48.
18. Pul M, Pul N, Garses N. Congenital lumbar (Grynfelt-Lesshaft) hernia. Eur J Pediatr Surg 1991;1:115-17.
19. Lafer DJ. Neuroblastoma and lumbar hernia: a causal relationship? J Pediatr Surg 1994;29(7):926-29.
20. Hancock BJ, Wiseman NE. Incarcerated congenital lumbar hernia associated with the lumbocostovertebral syndrome J Pediatr Surg 1988;23(8):782-83.
21. Somuncu S, Bernay F, Rizalar R, Aritürk E, Günaydin M, Gürses N. Congenital lumbar hernia associated with the lumbocostovertebral syndrome: two cases. Eur J Pediatr Surg 1997;7(2):122-24.
22. Akçora B, Temiz A, Babayigit C. A different type of congenital lumbar hernia associated with the lumbocostovertebral syndrome. J Pediatr Surg 2008; 43(1):e21-23.
23. Ponka JL. Hernias of the abdominal wall. WB Saunders. Philadelphia 1980;532-53.
24. Skandalakis LJ, Gadaez R Thomas, Mansberger RA, Mitchell EW. Modern Hernia Repair. The embryological and anatomical basis of surgery 1996;388.
25. Moynihan BGA. Retro-peritoneal Hernia, Balliere, London 1889.
26. Gomez-Fraile A, Cuadros J, Matute JA, et al. Paraduodenal hernia in childhood. Pediatric surgery International 1989; 4:286-87.

CHAPTER 48

Peritonitis in Children

Rajiv Chadha

Intra-abdominal infections have been well recognized throughout the history of medicine and are very commonly encountered in pediatric surgical practice. This is especially so in developing countries like India where the incidence of infective gastrointestinal diseases and their sequelae is very high. Improvement in outcome and reduction in mortality to 10-20% today is largely due to better supportive care, improved and effective antibiotics, widespread application of ultrasonography and computed tomography to localize intraperitoneal collections and improved interventional techniques. However, mortality persists with patients succumbing to the effects of sepsis and eventual multisystem organ failure (MSOF). The single most influential factor in successful treatment of intra-abdominal infections is early prompt diagnosis and effective treatment, and for this, a thorough knowledge of the pathophysiology of peritonitis and the application of the various diagnostic and therapeutic options available is essential.

ANATOMY AND FUNCTION OF THE PERITONEAL CAVITY

The peritoneal cavity consists of the greater and lesser sacs, which communicate via the foramen of Winslow. Within the greater sac, compartmentalization by various ligaments and retroperitoneal attachments creates sites of fluid accumulation and subsequently, abscess formation. These include the right subhepatic space, the right and left subphrenic spaces, the paracolic gutters, and the pelvis (Fig. 48.1). Posteriorly, the right subhepatic space opens into the Morrison's pouch, one of the most dependent spaces in the peritoneal cavity, making it a likely site of fluid accumulation and abscess formation.

The peritoneum consists of a single layer of mesothelial cells, with a basement membrane supported by an underlying layer of highly vascularized connective tissue. The total area of the peritoneum is approximately 1.8 m² in the adult; proportionately lower in the child.[1] The mesothelial cells contain microvilli 1.5 - 3.0 μm in length, which greatly increase the surface area of the mesothelial cells. A 1 mm increase in thickness of the peritoneum by fluid can result in sequestration of large volumes of fluid, explaining the massive fluid shifts associated with diffuse peritonitis.[2] The peritoneal membrane can be divided into two parts: *visceral*, surrounding and lining the viscera and *parietal* which lines the posterior

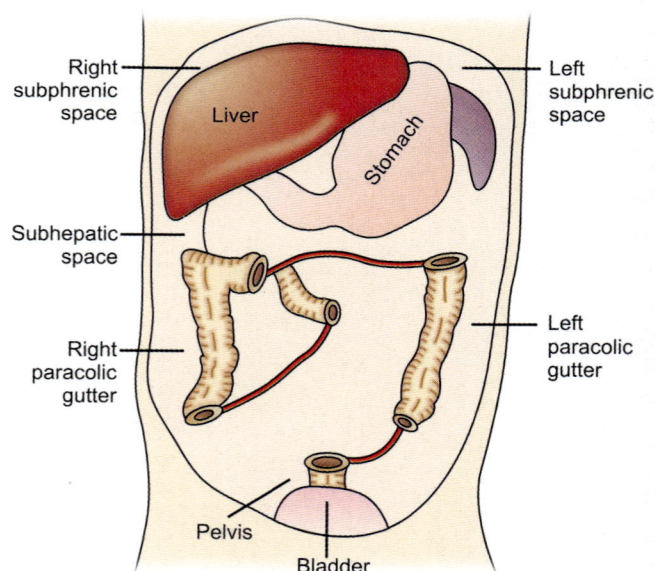

Fig. 48.1: The intraperitoneal spaces which may be sites of abscess formation following peritonitis

aspect of the anterior abdominal musculature and also lies superficial to the retroperitoneal viscera, including the aorta, vena cava, ureters and kidneys. The parietal portion is richly supplied with nerves and when irritated, causes severe pain localized to the affected area. The visceral peritoneum in contrast is poorly supplied with nerves and its irritation causes vague pain which is usually located to the midline.

One half of the peritoneum, about 1 m^2, functions as a passive semipermeable membrane to the diffusion of water, electrolytes and macromolecules.[1] Under normal circumstances, the peritoneal cavity is largely a potential space, as only a thin film of lubricating fluid separates the parietal and visceral layers.[3] This fluid itself closely resembles lymph fluid and has a low specific gravity, protein content of about 3g/dL and < 3000 cells/cu mm. This fluid is circulated through the peritoneal cavity and this movement of fluid is largely produced by the creation of a negative pressure area in the subphrenic space by diaphragmatic motion. This upward movement of peritoneal fluids is responsible for the occurrence of many subphrenic abscesses. Most of the peritoneal fluid is absorbed into the lymphatic circulation via the mesothelial lining of the parietal peritoneal surfaces, with the remainder absorbed through diaphragmatic lymphatics.[1] Mesothelial cells also absorb solutes by the continuing process of endocytosis. Exchange of solutes across the peritoneal lining is the basis for peritoneal dialysis.[3] The clearance of particulate matter, cells and microorganisms contained in peritoneal fluid may however be largely dependent upon diaphragmatic lymphatics.[1] In the peritoneum overlying the muscular portion of the diaphragmatic surface, intercellular gaps or *stomata* are present between peritoneal mesothelial cells. The diameter of these stomata varies from 4 - 12 μm depending on diaphragmatic stretching and contraction.[4,5] Fluid as well as particulate and other substances are channeled via the stomata through fenestrations in the basement membrane and carried to specialized diaphragmatic lymphatics called *lacunae*. During the respiratory cycle, relaxation of the diaphragm in expiration opens the stomata and promotes rapid filling of the lacunae.[1] At inspiration, contraction of the diaphragm empties the lacunae into efferent lymphatic channels and ultimately to the central circulation via the thoracic duct. As shown by animal experiments, this process of fluid movement and particulate clearance via the diaphragmatic lymphatics is rapid.[6]

Several factors can influence the diaphragmatic clearance mechanism or "pump". Animal experiments show that introduction of platelets or other agents into the peritoneal cavity can occlude the stomata.[7,8] Body positioning can also influence the effectiveness of diaphragmatic clearance and the head-up position has been found to delay the appearance of bacteria in the circulation after intraperitoneal injection.[6] Reducing spontaneous respiration by the application of muscular paralysis and mechanical ventilation has been observed to decrease particulate clearance from the peritoneal cavity and lower the incidence of bacteremia.[9,10] These effects result from chemical paralysis of the diaphragm and elimination of the "pumping mechanism", as well as the application of positive intrathoracic pressure that impairs thoracic lymphatic flow. Although this diaphragmatic "pump" mechanism is an effective local defense mechanism, its benefit in terms of host survival is uncertain. Both animal and human studies have shown that the incidence of bacteremia and mortality were reduced when the diaphragmatic clearance of bacteria was impaired.[9,11] It is possible that the local clearance and carriage of bacteria into the systemic circulation may overwhelm systemic defenses and paradoxically increase mortality.

LOCAL RESPONSE TO PERITONEAL INJURY OR INFECTION

The objective of the local response to infection is the removal or containment of microorganisms from the peritoneal cavity. This response however, can be initiated by any noxious stimulus that causes mesothelial or vascular endothelial cell injury. It has been shown that similar local physiological effects can be produced by endotoxin as well as by organisms such as gram-positive bacteria, *Bacteroides* species, and yeasts that have no endotoxin, or only biologically inactive forms of endotoxin.[12] It is likely that the overall inflammatory response, both local and systemic is a general one, and not specific for any single infective agent. The systemic response is mediated by cytokines such as tumor necrosis factor (TNF) and interleukin-1 (IL-1).[13,14] A similar *sterile* peritonitis can in fact, be initiated by noninfective agents such as gastric juice, pancreatic juice, bile salts or meconium.

In addition to mechanical clearance of bacteria via lymphatics, the local peritoneal inflammatory process consists of (i) changes in blood flow and vascular permeability with influx of fluid, (ii) cellular immune response, and (iii) fibrin deposition and mechanical sequestration.

Changes in Blood Flow and Vascular Permeability

The earliest physiological changes are an increase in blood flow and an influx of fluid to the foci of inflammation. These are mediated by histamine released from tissue mast cells and basophils, and later by bradykinin.[1] Both histamine and bradykinin cause pain, vasodilatation and increased permeability of the small peritoneal blood vessels. Other vasoactive substances such as prostaglandin E2α (PGE2α) and leukotriene C4 (LTC4) also contribute to the observed vascular changes. The initial fluid that accumulates is a transudate with low protein content. Later however, with increasing vascular permeability, there is exudation of large volumes of fluid rich in immunoglobulins, complement factors, coagulation factors and cytokines.[1] This massive third space fluid-shifts and loss of plasma proteins can lead to hypovolemic shock and in addition, may impair bacterial phagocytosis by diluting opsonins and impeding neutrophil mobility and migration.[15]

Cellular Response

Several major cell types play key roles in the inflammatory response. These include resident and recruited macrophages, mesothelial cells, adjacent capillary endothelial cells, and recruited neutrophils.[16] Several humoral mediators are involved in activating both macrophages and neutrophils, modulating leukocyte metabolic activity, chemotaxis, and opsonization of bacteria.[1] The first step in the response to contamination is probably induced by a host response to microbial cell products. In the case of gram-negative organisms, this is most likely lipopolysaccharide (LPS).[3] For gram-positive organisms, the cell wall product teichoic acid and specific cell wall glycans induce a macrophage response.[3] Macrophages serve as an early line of cellular defense and coordinate the inflammatory response. Macrophage products include IL-1, IL-6, IL-8, IL-10, IL-12, TNF-α, GM-CSF, granulocyte colony-stimulating factor (G-CSF), monocyte chemoattractant protein-1 (MCP-1), monocyte inflammatory protein a (MIP-a), and several eicosanoids. These molecules recruit and activate mesothelial cells as well as mediate macrophage microbicidal activity.[3,17] Mesothelial cells produce a variety of inflammatory molecules that recruit additional cells to the peritoneal cavity and activate them there. These cells also secrete IL-8, a neutrophil chemoattractant and activator as well as various adhesion molecules.[3]

Neutrophils are the key effector cells in the inflammatory response and possess an array of granular enzymes that are capable of digesting basement and interstitial proteins, facilitating directed migration and allowing for digestion of injured tissue.[3] Although C5a anaphylotoxin possesses the most potent neutrophil chemoattractant properties, C3a, C567 complex, kallikrein, IL-1, IL-8, and platelet aggregation factors (PAF) also have chemotactic effect.[1] By 4 to 6 hours following injury, significant neutrophil influx has occurred and is peaked at about 8 hours.[11] Several substances influence leukocyte metabolism and the production and release of lysosomal enzymes. These include anaphylotoxins, and kallikrein, which induces superoxide anion generation and lysosomal enzyme release in neutrophils.

Capillary cells adjacent to the site of injury can be activated by the injury or humoral mediators and produce a variety of adhesion molecules as well as IL-8 and platelet-activating factor (PAF). Thus, activation of vascular endothelium is a key mechanism of inflammation.[3] Activated PAF also stimulates platelet aggregation, which may play a role in the platelet sequestration and thrombocytopenia observed in septic shock.[1]

Fibrin Deposition and Mechanical Sequestration

Normally, intact mesothelial cells maintain fibrinolytic activity within the peritoneal cavity by the secretion of tissue plasminogen activator (t-PA).[18] With mesothelial cell injury and inflammation, local fibrinolytic activity is suppressed due to the loss of plasminogen activator.[19] As high concentrations of fibrinogen are present, fibrin deposition readily occurs by activation of the intrinsic pathway.[20]

The role of fibrin deposition in the local inflammatory response is to isolate or contain contamination and thereby prevent widespread dissemination. Fibrinous adhesions cause the adherence of loops of intestine and omentum to one another as well as the parietal peritoneal surface, thus creating physical barriers against the spread of bacterial contamination.[1] Fully developed fibrous adhesions are seen at 10 days and become maximal 2-3 weeks after peritoneal injury.[3] It is worthwhile to remember that small children have a poorly developed omentum, and thus, there are more chances of rapid progression to diffuse peritonitis.

In some patients, the development of an intraperitoneal abscess is the culmination of the sequestration process described above.[1] Within the adhered mass of viscera, fibrin and bacteria, liquefaction develops from the release of proteolytic enzymes from perishing leukocytes and the action of bacterial exozymes. The resultant tissue damage and liquefaction results in abscess formation.

Peritoneal Healing

The peritoneum appears to heal rapidly after injury. It appears that the replacement of the injured mesothelium occurs over the entire wound simultaneously and the rate of healing is independent of the size of the peritoneal wound. Within 3 days after injury, the wound is covered by connective tissue cells, and by day 5, these new cells resemble normal mesothelium.[21] However, as noted above, peritoneal injury in the presence of inflammation and infection results in adhesion formation. With time, fibrous adhesions undergo remodeling and usually become progressively attenuated. However, in the setting of severe peritoneal injury or persistent infection, filmy fibrinous adhesions are transformed into dense fibrous adhesions by the ingrowth of fibroblasts, capillaries and the deposition of collagen.[1]

FACTORS INFLUENCING PERITONEAL INFLAMMATION AND INFECTION

There are several factors, both local and systemic, which influence the outcome after peritoneal injury and inflammation. These are especially important with regard to peritonitis secondary to gastrointestinal perforation.

Bacterial Virulence

Although more than 500 species of bacteria are normally present in the colon where there are between $10^{10} - 10^{12}$ bacteria/mm^3, the vast majority of these are anaerobic species which contribute little to clinical intra-abdominal infection.[3] Despite the massive contamination and complexity of the microbial spectrum that occurs with fecal contamination, within 48 hours, only a few isolates are recovered in peritoneal fluid culture.[22] The most common facultative gram-negative bacteria isolated in clinical infections are species of *Escherichia coli*, *Klebsiella*, *Proteus*, *Pseudomonas* and *Enterobacter*, which make up less than 0.1% of the normal colonic flora.[3] Even the most common obligatory anaerobic pathogen, *Bacteroides fragilis*, accounts for only 1% of the colonic flora.[3] Commonly isolated gram-positive species include Enterococci and *Staphylococci* and *Streptococci* species. This indicates that only a few pathogenic bacteria survive to propagate the infection.

Innate virulence factors also play a role in the pathogenesis of infection. It has been shown in experimental models that *E. coli* and *Enterococcus* were the predominant organisms during the peritonitis phase, while *B. fragilis* predominated during the abscess phase.[23] The presence of capsular polysaccharide in the case of *B. fragilis* is strongly associated with abscess formation. Extracellular products such as coagulase and catalase secreted by *Staphylococcus aureus* enhance its virulence.[3] The size of the bacterial inoculum also influences the virulence, both the ability to produce infection as well as the severity of the disease. The ability to adhere to the mesothelial surface may also enhance the virulence of organisms such as *Enterobacteriaceae* (in the early phase), and *Bacteroides fragilis* (8 hours or more after infection).[3,24] Such organisms are resistant to mechanical removal by saline lavage.

Bacterial *synergism* also potentiates the virulence of a single organism. Polymicrobial infections, specifically combinations of aerobic and anaerobic species, exhibit significantly greater lethality than comparable infections involving a single species of pathogenic bacteria.

Adjuvant Factors

The simultaneous presence of various adjuvant substances increases bacterial virulence and/or

Table 48.1: Adjuvant substances for peritoneal infection
Endogenous factors
Blood, ferrous iron
Platelets
Fibrin
Intraperitoneal fluid
Necrotic tissue
Gastric juice, pancreatic juice, urine, meconium, chyle
Bile, bile salts
Foreign material
Macroscopic foreign material
Suture material, surgical clips
Prosthetic implants
Sponges
Hemostatic pads/powders
Surgical drains
Microscopic foreign material
Barium sulfate
Talc powder, other glove powder
Clothing fibers

interferes with host defenses. Such adjuvant substances are invariably present following gastrointestinal perforation, trauma or a surgical procedure (Table 48.1). These adjuvant substances may be endogenous or foreign materials.

Blood is the most important adjuvant substance. The lethality of *E. coli* is enhanced *in vitro* by hemoglobin.[25] Although it is not clear whether it is due to the liberation of iron, an essential growth factor for *E. coli*, or depression of neutrophil migration and phagocytic function.[26-28] The presence of both fibrin and platelets within the peritoneal cavity also may impair physical bacterial clearance by blockage of the diaphragmatic lymphatics.[8] Other substances originating from the gastrointestinal tract itself like bile salts, gastric mucin, pancreatic secretions as well as chyle and urine have been shown to have adjuvant activity.[1,3]

Foreign materials such as barium sulfate, talc or cellulose probably also impair phagocytosis by causing the premature activation of neutrophils and release of lysosomal enzymes.[29,30] Retained suture materials and drains may have a similar effect. It is therefore important that during surgical intervention, attention should be paid to meticulous hemostasis, copious lavage to remove adjuvant material, the thorough evacuation of intraperitoneal fluid, and minimizing the use of foreign material such as hemostatic agents and suture material.[1]

SYSTEMIC RESPONSE TO PERITONEAL INJURY OR INFECTION

The systemic response to peritoneal infection is similar to the response of the body to other forms of injury and includes the release of catecholamines, glucocorticoids, aldosterone and antidiuretic hormone.[3] The systemic response is best studied under three broad headings, namely hypovolemia and its consequences, pulmonary complications, and effects on tissue metabolism.

Hypovolemia and Hemodynamic Changes

The development of hypovolemia is central to the systemic response and is largely due to the fluid influx, often copious, occurring in the peritoneal cavity. The reduction in intravascular volume reduces venous return and cardiac output. Systemic hypotension may also be the result of secretion of TNF, IL-1, platelet activating factors, and nitric oxide, which have vasodilatory effects and may reduce systemic vascular resistance.[13,14] Diminished urine flow develops as a result of the effects of increased aldosterone and antidiuretic hormone secretion. Thus, a clinical setting of hyperdynamic or "warm" septic shock may be created, characterized by tachycardia, fever, oliguria, hypotension, and warm extremities. There is increased cardiac output, low peripheral vascular resistance, low arteriovenous oxygen difference, and high mixed-venous oxygen content.[1]

Effects on Pulmonary Function

Abdominal distension secondary to fluid accumulation within the peritoneal cavity as well as within the bowel reduces diaphragmatic mobility and decreases ventilatory volume, producing eventual atelectasis.[1] Beta-adrenergic stimulation leads to intrapulmonary shunting while increased pulmonary vascular permeability also develops as a result of a number of inflammatory mediators.[1] Fluid accumulates in the pulmonary interstitium and decreases pulmonary compliance. Early manifestations of these changes include hyperventilation and the development of respiratory alkalosis. With worsening pulmonary edema and alveolar collapse, severe hypoxemia can develop, leading to respiratory distress syndrome (RDS).

Effects on Tissue Metabolism

During the response to peritonitis, the metabolic rate is increased. However, hypovolemia reduces cardiac output. There is tissue hypoxia with increasing anaerobic glycolysis and subsequent metabolic acidosis. As glycogen stores are depleted at an early stage, protein catabolism is augmented to release amino acids for use as an energy source. This can lead to severe loss in lean body mass.

PERITONITIS

A variety of etiologic agents including bacteria, viruses, fungi, chemical agents as well as trauma and foreign bodies can cause inflammation of the peritoneum. Peritonitis can be categorized into three main divisions. *Primary peritonitis* refers to an infection of the peritoneal cavity that has no intrabdominal source. *Secondary peritonitis*, the most common in clinical practice, is defined as peritonitis resulting from an intra-abdominal source, most commonly, the perforation of a hollow viscus. *Tertiary peritonitis* develops following the treatment of secondary peritonitis and represents either a failure of the host inflammatory response, or a superinfection.

CLINICAL PRESENTATION OF PERITONITIS

The clinical presentation of peritonitis is fairly similar in the various pediatric age groups, although the diagnosis is considerably more difficult to make in the newborn and small infant as will be discussed later.

The history and physical examination are pivotal in deciding the need and urgency for intervention and the use of diagnostic techniques. A brief history of the duration of illness, the presence of fever and its nature, as well as previous hospitalizations and surgery is important. Especially in the older child, abdominal pain is usually the predominant presenting symptom. The pain of fully established peritonitis is constant, burning and aggravated by motion or movement.[1] The extent of pain may be localized or diffuse depending upon the area of parietal peritoneum that is inflamed. Visceral peritoneal irritation, usually from distension of a hollow viscus, causes dull, poorly localized, often periumbilical crampy pain.[3] Anorexia, nausea and possibly vomiting, as well as thirst and oliguria are frequently present.[1]

Physical Examination

Important physical signs include fever, tachycardia and tachypnea or labored breathing. If septic shock is present, there may be tachycardia, hypotension, and warm, pink extremities. Patients prefer to remain still and supine, so that there is minimal exacerbation of pain. Gentle percussion followed by direct palpation will show as well as localize tenderness. With generalized peritonitis, abdominal tenderness is diffuse and is often maximal at the site overlying the region where the peritonitis originated. Bowel sounds are usually markedly diminished or absent. Abdominal wall rigidity due to voluntary guarding and reflex muscle spasm can be extensive.[1] In localized peritonitis, tenderness is focal, and the remainder of the abdomen may be relatively soft and nontender.[1] A rectal or vaginal examination may also be performed in order to localize pelvic tenderness or intrapelvic collections.[3]

Physical signs may be minimal or absent in patients receiving corticosteroids, or with altered consciousness from head injury or encephalopathy. In these cases, the diagnosis may rest upon other diagnostic modalities.

Clinical Presentation in Infants and Small Children

It is considerably more difficult to make a diagnosis of peritonitis in infants, including newborns, as well as in small children. A small infant with far advanced peritoneal inflammation may only wince or draw up the legs in response to abdominal palpation, whereas an older child will respond more decisively to the resultant pain.[31] Bowel sounds are also difficult to assess in newborns or small infants.

A newborn with spontaneous gastrointestinal perforation and peritonitis may present at an early stage with refusal of feeds and evidence of physiological instability. This includes lethargy, temperature instability, recurrent apnea, episodes of bradycardia and evidence of poor capillary circulation, such as delayed capillary fill.[32] Gastric retention and vomiting may be marked and the progress of abdominal distension is often very rapid. A history of rectal bleeding and diarrhea may be present, especially where the perforation follows inflammatory bowel disease.[32] Metabolic acidosis and oliguria may develop very rapidly. Edema and erythema of the abdominal wall is a cardinal sign of underlying peritonitis in the newborn and small infant, and is often accompanied by scrotal edema. Purulent fluid may sometimes track down a patent processus vaginalis and present with unilateral or bilateral scrotal abscess or collection.

LABORATORY AND RADIOGRAPHIC INVESTIGATIONS

In general, laboratory tests may not be very specific. Leukocytosis, with a predominance of immature neutrophil forms is almost always present. It should be remembered however, that newborns with abdominal sepsis and peritonitis usually have neutropenia, thrombocytopenia, and metabolic acidosis. A neutrophil count of less than 6000 cells/mm^3 is most commonly associated with gram-negative neonatal septicemia.[33] Thrombocytopenia is nearly universally present and levels of C- reactive protein may be elevated. It is essential in newborns, and probably also in small infants, to take specimens of blood, both peripheral and from indwelling cannulas, urine, and if necessary, cerebrospinal fluid, for culture studies.

Plain radiographs of the abdomen may reveal obliteration of the peritoneal fat lines and the psoas shadow indicating the presence of peritoneal edema (Fig. 48.2). Fluid in the peritoneal cavity along with fluid-filled bowel loops may result in the abdomen appearing almost completely opaque on a plain skiagram (Fig. 48.3). Free air may be visible on an upright abdominal film. The erect radiograph should be obtained with the beam centered at the level of the diaphragm and a waiting period of at least 5 minutes. As little as 3 - 5 ml of subdiaphragmatic air can be detected in this fashion in a small child.[31] In neonates with gastrointestinal perforation, a massive hydropneumoperitoneum or pyopneumoperitoneum may be recognized by the presence of an air-fluid level, which is too great in length for even an obstructed segment of colon (Fig. 48.4). If the child is unable to assume the erect position, a lateral decubitus film with the patient's left side down should be requested. Air-

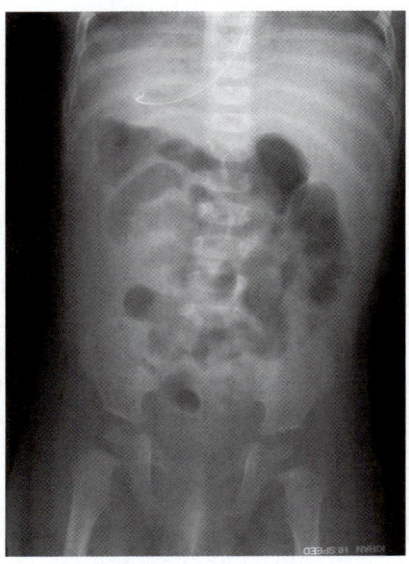

Fig. 48.2: Abdominal skiagram in a patient with primary peritonitis showing peritoneal edema with thickened abdominal wall and central displacement of bowel loops

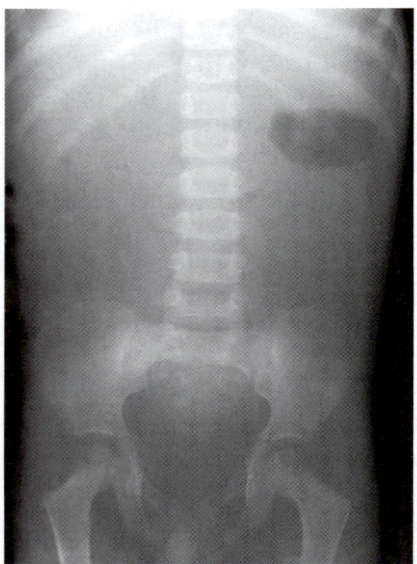

Fig. 48.3: An opaque appearance of the abdomen due to fluid filled bowel loops and intraperitoneal fluid in a child with jejunal perforation and peritonitis

filled loops of bowel, with thickened opaque walls may be found when bowel edema and paralytic ileus is present. Other findings that support the diagnosis of intra-abdominal infection include pneumatosis intestinalis, air in the portal vein, a mass effect or extraluminal gas collections suggestive of an abscess. These findings are more characteristic of neonatal

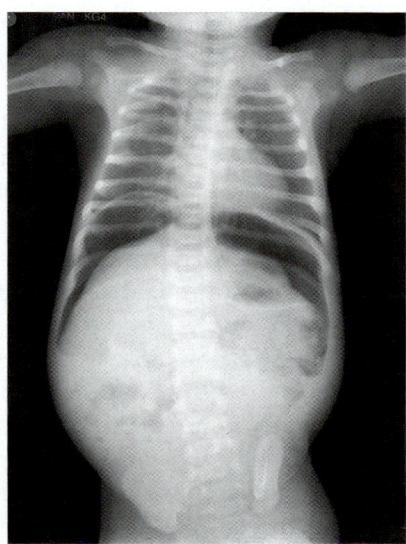

Fig. 48.4: Massive pyopneumoperitoneum with a huge air-fluid level in a 1 ½ month old child with ileal perforation

necrotizing enterocolitis (NEC),[33] a topic that is covered elsewhere.

The role of more elaborate diagnostic studies in peritonitis is limited to those patients presenting with abdominal pain who have no immediate compelling indication for abdominal exploration and in whom the diagnosis may be in doubt.[1] In general, ultrasonography, computed tomography (CT) and especially magnetic resonance imaging (MRI) should not be routinely used in patients with acute peritonitis. However, imaging experience has shown that many of the morphological changes of peritonitis, such as thickening of the visceral and parietal peritoneum, inflammatory changes in the omentum and mesentery, and free or loculated fluid collections often with higher density than bland ascites are well shown with CT. The source of the peritonitis, such as a perforation of bowel, is often apparent as well.

PRIMARY PERITONITIS

Primary peritonitis, also known as idiopathic peritonitis, represents peritonitis occurring without any intra-abdominal source of infection.[34,35] According to the Western literature, the incidence of primary peritonitis has decreased in recent decades, and at present represents less than 1% of all cases of peritonitis.[36] This condition is primarily treated without surgery. Although previous studies suggested that the incidence of primary peritonitis is highest in girls 4 to 6 years of age, recent studies suggest that there is an equal distribution between boys and girls.[37] Most commonly, primary peritonitis is seen in children with nephrotic syndrome, systemic lupus erythematosus, or hepatic dysfunction with cirrhosis and ascites, or in those undergoing peritoneal dialysis.[38-41]

Apart from the open ends of the fallopian tubes, the peritoneal cavity is a closed space. Therefore, the means by which bacteria gain access to the peritoneal cavity is difficult to understand. At present, the most likely explanation is the hematogenous route as in some series; the organism cultured from the peritoneal fluid has also been found in other sites, such as the mouth or the urinary system.[34] Lymphatic spread as well as ascending genitourinary routes has been implicated.[34,42] It is possible that ascending infection from the genitalia may occur in girls as the fallopian tubes open into the peritoneal cavity. The theory of translocation of enteric bacteria is less favored now, although the predominant pathogens in primary peritonitis, at least in adults today, are coliform bacteria.[1]

Clinical History and Investigations

The history in children is usually acute with acute abdominal pain, fever, nausea, vomiting and lethargy.[43] Abdominal distension may be present and there is usually diffuse tenderness and "rebound" tenderness. The most important differential diagnosis is perforated acute appendicitis, although with primary peritonitis, the disease usually develops faster and presentation and pain is more acute.[35] The total leukocytic count is raised, with relative neutrophilia. Plain abdominal radiographs should be obtained in order to rule out the presence of pneumoperitoneum.

Diagnostic paracentesis is of value if ascites is present, for example in nephritic syndrome and cirrhosis with ascites. In primary peritonitis, > than 500 WBCs/mm^3 are present, and granulocytes predominate.[43] The pH is less than 7.35 and lactate levels more than 5 mg/dL.[44] If the gram stain or culture yields a mixed flora of both gram-positive and gram-negative organisms, or else the presence of gross feces, bile or blood, it is more likely that intestinal perforation is the cause of peritonitis.[1] In these cases, immediate exploratory laparotomy is indicated. In cases where

Table 48.2: Classification of primary peritonitis in childhood
Peritonitis in otherwise normal children
Peritonitis associated with other conditions such as: • Nephrotic syndrome • Hepatic dysfunction with cirrhosis and ascites • Peritoneal dialysis for renal failure • Presence of ventriculoperitoneal shunt for hydrocephalus • Conditions requiring long-term steroid administration • Cystic fibrosis

differentiation from perforated acute appendicitis is difficult, computed tomography (CT) scan may be of help.

A classification of primary peritonitis in children is shown in Table 48.2.

In the case of primary peritonitis occurring in children who are otherwise normal, the incidence has shown a marked reduction over the past few decades, perhaps related to the widespread availability and early use of oral antibiotics for a variety of respiratory tract infections, dental diseases or urinary tract infections.[42,45] Since then, however, sporadic reports of Group A streptococcal peritonitis with an association with simultaneous positive cultures from the trachea, pharynx or tonsils in otherwise healthy patients have been noted.[46] Similar infection due to *Streptococcus pneumoniae*, often penicillin resistant, has also been reported.[47,48] Blood cultures should therefore always be obtained and may also be positive for *Strep. pneumoniae*.[48] If the peritoneal fluid examination confirms the diagnosis of primary peritonitis, antibiotic treatment, usually with a sulfbactam-ampicillin and gentamicin combination or a third-generation cephalosporin is usually effective. Laparoscopy or laparotomy is indicated only if the peritoneal fluid is not accessible or the patient does not improve with intravenous antibiotics.[43] Following surgery, intravenous antibiotics and nasogastric aspiration is continued until the white cell count is normal and the ileus resolves.[43]

Peritonitis in Children with Nephrotic Syndrome and Hepatic Cirrhosis with Ascites

Peritonitis is a known complication of nephrotic syndrome (NS) in childhood. Increased susceptibility to peritonitis in these patients may be related to reduced cellular immunity and chemotaxis, impaired opsonization, and decreased levels of immunoglobulins.[43] Loss of complement proteins I and B of the alternative complement pathway in urine in patients with NS may also be responsible for the increased susceptibility.[49] The most commonly documented causative organism is *Streptococcus pneumoniae*, although gram-negative organisms have also been reported.[40,50] In 79% of cases, steroids were being used to treat the NS or relapse was diagnosed.[50-52] The most common presenting symptoms are diffuse abdominal pain, fever, rebound tenderness, nausea and vomiting.[43] Fifteen to twenty-seven percent of children may experience more than one episode of peritonitis during the course of NS.[50] Treatment is directed towards antibiotic coverage to include both gram-positive and gram-negative organisms until the results of peritoneal, blood and urine cultures are available.

In children with hepatic dysfunction and cirrhosis with ascites, primary peritonitis is more frequently due to the gram-negative organisms that colonize the intestinal tract, such as *E. coli* or *Klebsiella pneumoniae*.[43] This is probably because of reduced hepatic clearance of bacteria from the blood as well as the lymphatic system, thus increasing the opportunity for bacteria to persist in ascitic fluid.[41] In addition, patients with cirrhosis and ascites have reduced amount of protein in ascitic fluid, correlating with decreased levels of opsonin and complement.[53,54]

Peritonitis in Children Undergoing Peritoneal Dialysis

Peritonitis is a major complication of peritoneal dialysis in patients of end-stage renal disease and is more often seen in patients undergoing continuous ambulatory peritoneal dialysis (CAPD) rather than in patients undergoing intermittent peritoneal dialysis.[3] Most cases are caused by catheter contamination. The incidence is an average of 1.3 episodes per patient per year.[3] It has been shown that rates are lowest with use of a double-cuffed catheter with a downward directed tunnel.[55] Use of exit-site mupirocin and antibiotic prophylaxis during catheter insertion and other invasive procedures also lowers the risk.[55] Usually the infection is monomicrobial and fungal infections are more common. The most common infecting organism is a gram-positive coccus, usually *Staphylococcus aureus* or *Streptococcus epidermidis*. Occasionally, *Pseudomonas*, yeast and atypical tubercle bacilli may be recovered.[3] The clinical presentation includes abdominal pain, fever, and a high neutrophil count in the cloudy dialysate fluid. The fluid should be cultured and intravenous or intraperitoneal antibiotic therapy started. The options include ceftazidime and vancomycin or aminoglycosides.[1,43] A recent report suggests that a combination of intraperitoneal ceftazidime and cefazolin is very effective and avoids the renal toxicity, which may be seen with use of aminoglycosides.[56] Clinical improvement is usually seen after 24 to 36 hours. Removal of the catheter is indicated only if there is no improvement after 4 to 5 days of antibiotic therapy, the presence of fungal or tubercular peritonitis, or a severe skin infection at the catheter site.[3] The increased risk of intraperitoneal hypercoagulation and hypofibrinolysis in these patients may also explain the blockage of the peritoneal catheter, which may be seen in some patients.[57]

A similar form of peritonitis may also be seen in patients who have a ventriculoperitoneal shunt. Shunt-induced peritonitis should be suspected in any child who has a ventriculoperitoneal shunt and abdominal symptoms.

TUBERCULOUS PERITONITIS

Abdominal tuberculosis and tuberculous peritonitis are extremely common in developing countries like India. In recent years however, an upsurge in incidence has also been reported in the West.[1,3] Typically, tuberculous peritonitis is believed to be caused by hematogenous spread, although the primary source of infection (lungs, intestine) may no longer be clinically apparent.[1] Some cases may be the result of reactivation of latent peritoneal tuberculosis established by hematogenous spread from a pulmonary focus during an earlier episode of acute disease.[3] Otherwise infection could result from spread from tuberculous mesenteric lymph nodes, transmurally from tuberculosis of the ileocecal region, or a tuberculous pyosalpinx.

Clinical Manifestations

In the early phase, the manifestation may be acute with rapid development of increasing abdominal distension and pain. Usually however, the symptoms consist of progressive abdominal distension and ascites (100%), fever (27%), and loss of weight (18%).[58] A "doughy" feel of the abdomen may be present and rolled-up omentum may be palpable. Ascites may sometimes be loculated. The tuberculin test is usually positive.[3,59] Pulmonary tuberculosis is concomitantly present in 50% cases.[60] Concomitant tuberculosis involving other organ sites, e.g. meningitis may sometimes be present.[58,61]

The "dry" or *chronic* form of peritoneal tuberculosis may also be seen when there is resolution of ascites and formation of dense adhesions and matting of bowel loops. Acute or subacute intestinal obstruction may be present. Clinical manifestations of generalized tuberculosis may be present in at least a third of these patients, and consist of anorexia, weight loss and night sweats.[3] Occasionally, a "purulent" form of peritoneal tuberculosis may be seen where a mass of omentum, bowel and caseating lymph nodes form an abscess which may occasionally burst leading to a spontaneous fecal fistula. Peritonitis may also occur in patients with primary intestinal tuberculosis in whom a bowel perforation may occur proximal to a tubercular stricture of the intestines.

In the ascitic stage, the diagnosis of peritoneal tuberculosis can be made by paracentesis, which would yield fluid with elevated protein content, lymphocyte pleocytosis and glucose concentration below 30 mg/dL. Acid-fast bacilli (AFB) are detected in the peritoneal fluid cultured conventionally in 80% cases,[60] although according to other sources,[59] the yield may not be so good. Mycobacterium tuberculosis may also be detected in ascitic fluid by the polymerase chain reaction method,[58] or by the finding of high interferon gamma and adenosine deaminase activity.[60] Recently, ultrasonography (US) and computed tomography (CT) scan of the abdomen have been reported to be effective in the diagnosis of peritoneal tuberculosis.[58,62,63] According to Demirkazik et al[63] peritoneal and omental thickening detected by CT and ascites with fine mobile septations shown by US strongly suggest the ascitic type of peritoneal tuberculosis. The two modalities should be used together for accurate diagnosis of tuberculous peritonitis.[63] Ozates et al[58] also found that US and CT findings of high density ascites contributed well to the diagnosis of peritoneal tuberculosis.

Diagnostic laparoscopy, using the open technique of trochar insertion is recommended if diagnosis cannot be made by paracentesis or other diagnostic modalities.[1,59,60,62] Laparoscopic findings include complete studding of the visceral and parietal peritoneal surfaces as well as the omentum with small, whitish tubercles.[1] Stalactite-like fibrinous masses hanging from the parietal peritoneum may be present. Other findings include dense adhesions between abdominal viscera and inflamed hemorrhagic areas on the peritoneum.[64] Laparoscopy combined with peritoneal biopsy or biopsy of nodules gives the diagnosis in 75 to 85% of cases.[60] As a last resort, open laparotomy with peritoneal biopsy may be performed; the placement of drains or bowel exteriorization is best avoided.[3]

Treatment

The mainstay of treatment is aggressive multiagent antitubercular chemotherapy for a period of 6-9 months.[58,59] Surgery is reserved for patients in whom it is essential to make a diagnosis, or for complications such as intestinal obstruction, intestinal perforation with peritonitis intraperitoneal abscess or enterocutaneous fistula. Wherever possible, surgery should be performed after at least 6 weeks of antitubercular chemotherapy.

SECONDARY PERITONITIS

Secondary peritonitis results from contamination from an organ within the peritoneal cavity. The majority of these cases result from primary lesions involving the gastrointestinal tract. Some cases are a consequence of blunt or penetrating abdominal trauma, while approximately 10% of cases represent postoperative peritonitis caused by complications of abdominal surgery.[1] As secondary peritonitis can be caused by a wide range of diseases, the morbidity and mortality depends upon a whole range of factors including the organ of involvement, the specific disease process, the age of the child, the delay before presentation as well as the presence of disease involving other organ systems. Postoperative peritonitis associated with a leaking anastomosis is associated with a substantial mortality, perhaps approaching 30%.[1,2]

Management

It is essential that as soon as secondary peritonitis is diagnosed, aggressive preoperative resuscitation and antibiotic therapy is instituted. The primary principles in the management of secondary peritonitis are: (i) resuscitation, (ii) initiation of antibiotic therapy, (iii) surgical management, and (iv) continued postoperative metabolic support.

Resuscitation

All cases of secondary peritonitis are accompanied by significant " third space" losses of extracellular fluid, which can at times be immense. This includes fluid accumulating in the peritoneal cavity, fluid exuding from the surface of the abdominal viscera as well as fluid that may collect inside the lumen of dilated intestinal loops in the presence of ileus. Hypovolemia, which often develops rapidly, can have serious consequences in neonates and infants. Major fluid deficits and metabolic derangements should be corrected before surgery, although surgery for acute perforations of the gastrointestinal tract should not be inordinately delayed on this account. In these cases, resuscitation should continue during surgery.[3] The type of fluid used for resuscitation depends upon the level of gastrointestinal perforation. In general however, in cases of intestinal perforation and peritonitis, replacement with adequate volumes of lactated Ringer's solution is necessary and should be accompanied by transfusion of plasma or salt-free albumin to restore both intravascular volume and colloid osmotic pressure. Infusing low doses of dopamine may help in patients with significant hypotension as it improves blood flow and reduces the incidence of acute renal failure.[3] Vital signs- temperature, blood pressure, pulse rate, respiration rate are continuously recorded. The effectiveness of fluid resuscitation efforts can be judged by the restoration of pulse rate and arterial blood pressure to normal levels. Placement of a urinary catheter is essential since restoration of urine output to levels of at least 1 - 1.5 ml/kg/hour is a reliable indicator of adequate restoration of intravascular volume. Insertion of a central venous pressure (CVP) line and the use of invasive peripheral arterial and central cardiac pressure-monitoring lines may help provide more precise estimation of intravascular volume and cardiac output.[1] However, these invasive monitoring techniques are often difficult to install and maintain in infants and small children.

Supplemental oxygen is essential, especially in the newborn or small infant with gross abdominal distension and in more extreme situations, endotracheal intubation and mechanical ventilation may be needed to preserve oxygenation.

Nasogastric intubation is essential and serves to reduce abdominal distension and prevent pulmonary aspiration. H-2 blocking agents such as ranitidine or famotidine should be administered to prevent stress-related gastric ulceration.

Antibiotic Therapy

Antibiotic therapy is begun along with the initial resuscitation, and the initial selection of antibiotics is empiric. It has recently been reported that 76% of patients with peritonitis had peritoneal fluid cultures with mixed aerobic and anaerobic bacteria, with *Escherichia coli* and *Bacteroides fragilis* the most common combination.[65] Presumptive antibiotic therapy should therefore include coverage for both aerobic gram-negative rods and anaerobic organisms. For most cases of secondary bacterial peritonitis, a single antibiotic agent with both aerobic and anaerobic activity is preferred. Second or third-generation cephalosporins or beta-lactamase inhibitor combinations are satisfactory. Alternatively, a combination of a monobactam and metronidazole yields cure rates of 80-90%.[66] However, for cases of hospital-acquired or severe secondary peritonitis, potent broad-spectrum agents should be selected. Effective regimens include carbapenem, or a combination of an aminoglycoside with metronidazole (or clindamycin) and ampicillin.[1] The selection of antibiotics should definitively be influenced by consideration of institutional antibiotic-resistance patterns when treating complex bacterial peritonitis.

Once antibiotic therapy is begun, changes in the antibiotic regime should be based primarily on the clinical progress. As a general rule, infections should show definite evidence of response within 72 hours of initiation of treatment. The duration of antibiotic therapy is determined by the clinical circumstances. The judgement of stopping antibiotic therapy should be made based on the indicators of temperature, white blood cell count (WBC) and the differential leukocytic count.[67,68] It should also be realized that the absence of response is not an automatic indication that the wrong antibiotic was selected. In most cases, the same antibiotic should be continued and a search made for a localized septic anatomic focus requiring drainage, debridement or excision.[3]

Surgical Management

The mainstay of surgical treatment consists of source control, peritoneal toilet and prevention of recurrent infection.[69] Control of the source of infection involves resecting, excluding or patching the diseased viscera at laparotomy, or more recently, laparoscopic methods in selected case.[69] It is essential to evacuate all purulent collections, with particular attention to subphrenic, subhepatic, interloop and pelvic collections.[3]

The second goal is to minimize the risk of recurrent sepsis. Standard intraoperative techniques to achieve this goal include intraoperative debridement with removal of fibrin, blood and necrotic material, and copious irrigation of the peritoneal cavity with saline. Addition of antiseptics or antibiotics to the irrigating fluid is of doubtful help in reducing mortality, but may help reduce the incidence of postoperative wound infection.

Certain nonstandard surgical techniques have been described to prevent recurrent sepsis but there benefit remains controversial. These include radical peritoneal debridement, continuous postoperative lavage, and planned repeat laparotomy. *Radical peritoneal debridement* implies the removal of all fibrin and necrotic tissue including abscess cavity walls, which may act as foci and media for bacterial growth. However, this technique may itself cause significant bleeding and fibrin deposition and at present is not recommended.[1] *Continuous postoperative irrigation of the peritoneal cavity* with large volumes of crystalloid solution via multiple catheters placed in the peritoneal cavity at the time of surgery has not conclusively been proved to be of significant benefit. *Planned repeated laparotomy* is a technique developed to prevent recurrent sepsis by repetitive abdominal exploration to debride necrotic material and drain abscesses. Several studies conducted in adults have shown encouraging results with this technique.[70,71] However, in a study of peritonitis in childhood, Haecker et al[72] found that radical adjuvant surgical measures were not necessary and hypothesized that during peritonitis, compartmentalization of the focus of infection prevents further systemic reactions and ultimately leads to removal of the infectious agents by endogenous mechanisms.

Postoperative Peritonitis

Postoperative peritonitis is usually the result of anastomotic leakage and is often discovered on the fifth to seventh postoperative day. Early diagnosis is essential as delay contributes greatly to increase in mortality. This is especially true for most centers in India where intensive care facilities or facilities for administering total parenteral nutrition may be lacking. In the newborn who develops an anastomotic leak following a bowel anastomosis, the first signs may be reduced spontaneous activity, lethargy, temperature instability, increased gastric aspirate and abdominal distension. An erect radiograph of the abdomen may be very helpful in diagnosing an anastomotic leak in these situations (Fig. 48.5). Drainage, controlled fistula formation, exteriorization, repair or resection and reanastomosis are performed as indicated.[3]

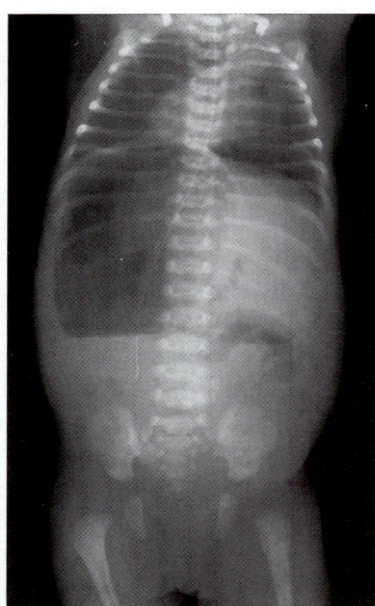

Fig. 48.5: Gas under the diaphragm and a large air-fluid level in a neonate with an anastomotic leak following surgery for ileal stenosis

MECONIUM PERITONITIS

Meconium peritonitis occurs due to contamination of the peritoneal cavity in utero or in the immediate perinatal period and usually results in severe peritonitis, often with intraperitoneal calcification. Meconium is first formed in the 3rd month of intrauterine life and consists primarily of amniotic fluid, squamous cells, bile salts and pigments, and pancreatic and intestinal enzymes.[73,74] Sterile meconium in the peritoneal cavity excites a strong fibroblastic response. This has been shown to be due to a marked proinflammatory response in the peritoneal macrophage with elevation of both procoagulant activity (PCA) and tumor necrosis factor alpha (TNF-alpha).[75] Foreign body granulomas and calcification due to deposition of calcium salts develops by the fourth day.[76] In most cases, the perforation seals spontaneously.

According to the Western literature, this condition is usually due to perforation of the obstructed bowel in complicated meconium ileus.[76,77] However, in Asian countries like India, meconium ileus is uncommon. Intestinal atresia or stenosis, volvulus, internal hernia, congenital peritoneal bands, ruptured Meckel's diverticulum or appendicitis may also lead to perforation and meconium peritonitis.[76] In a review of 32 cases of meconium peritonitis, Niramis et al found that the obvious causes were ileal atresia in 4, jejunal atresia in 3 and appendiceal perforation in 1. In the other 23 patients, no apparent cause of perforation was noted.[78]

The clinical presentation of meconium peritonitis in the newborn has been classified into four types[76]:

1. *A meconium pseudocyst* is formed by meconium leakage over an extended period. There may be a calcified fibrous cyst wall, which may be formed entirely from neighboring loops of intestine.
2. *Adhesive meconium peritonitis* with numerous inflammatory adhesion bands and matted bowel loops. This results from widespread peritoneal contamination and may be associated with bowel obstruction.
3. *Meconium ascites* results from bowel perforation occurring at term or immediately after birth. Meconium-stained ascitic fluid fills the peritoneal cavity. Intraperitoneal calcification may be absent or of the fine, stippled variety.

4. *Infected meconium peritonitis* results from a perforation that as not sealed before birth, allowing bacterial contamination of the peritoneal cavity. This is the most serious form of meconium peritonitis.

Antenatal diagnosis may be made during maternal ultrasound examination.[76,79] Clinical presentation of meconium peritonitis includes gross abdominal distension, an edematous, erythematous abdominal wall, a palpable abdominal mass, and features of bowel obstruction. Niramis et al found plain abdominal X-rays to show abnormal calcification and mass lesion in the peritoneal cavity in 71.9 and 46.9% respectively (Fig. 48.6).[78] Scrotal calcifications due to calcification of meconium tracking down the processus vaginalis may be noted, and in one report, abdominal, scrotal and thoracic calcifications due to healed meconium peritonitis were noted.[80] Rarely, disseminated intravascular meconium may complicate meconium peritonitis and have devastating consequences.[81]

Patients who have an incidental finding of abdominal or scrotal calcifications do not require surgery. Surgery is primarily required for intestinal obstruction or persistent bowel leak.[76] Surgical options include resection of the pseudocyst and devitalized intestine with either a primary anastomosis or a temporary enterostomy. Surgery is often very difficult due to the presence of dense vascular adhesions and matting of the bowel loops. A large series[78] showed that partial resection of the cyst and bowel exteriorization yielded better survival figures than primary anastomosis after resection of all diseased bowel. Simple drainage, bowel rest, total parenteral nutrition and administration of antibiotics followed by definitive surgery after 2 to 3 weeks has also been shown to be successful.[82] Recent studies show that with proper management, survival should be expected in virtually every case.[83]

TERTIARY PERITONITIS

Tertiary peritonitis, also known as persistent diffuse peritonitis (PDP) is a condition that may follow initial successful, usually operative, treatment of secondary peritonitis. This may represent both a failure of host response, as well as superinfection.[1]

The clinical picture mimics that of occult sepsis, consisting of low grade fever, leucocytosis, elevated cardiac output and general hypermetabolism. Both CT and laparotomy usually fail to identify a focal source of infection. In adults, if superinfection is present, culture data may yield two distinct categories of microorganisms: (i) highly virulent gram-negative aerobic bacteria such as *Pseudomonas* or *Serratia* species which have extensive resistance to antibiotics, and (ii) low virulence organisms such as *Staphylococci epidermidis* and *Candida* species which are resistant to the initial antibiotic therapy.[1] Treatment is based on sensitivity information and operative management has very little role.

A study of peritonitis in children found that PDP is a distinct form of peritonitis even in children, accounting for approximately 25% of cases.[84] The authors emphasized that rates of host defence affecting disease, extra-appendicular origin, and mortality were markedly higher in children with PDP, and that survival could be improved by the choice of more conservative treatment options, avoiding unnecessary operations in some instances.[84]

PERITONITIS IN CHILDHOOD: AN INDIAN PERSPECTIVE

In developing countries like India, the causes, epidemiology and presentation of peritonitis are quite

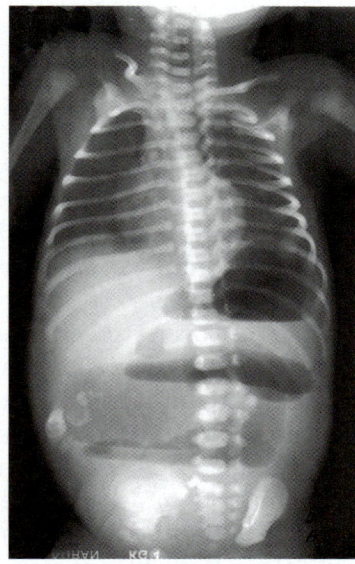

Fig. 48.6: Calcified meconium seen on the abdominal skiagram of a patient of ileal atresia with perforation and localized meconium peritonitis

different from those described in the Western literature. This is true, both for newborns and infants as well as older children. This is largely because a very large percentage of the population lives in poor socio-economic conditions, with very little access to proper sanitation and hygiene. In this scenario, diarrheal diseases and other infections of the gastrointestinal tract are very common, increasing the risk of secondary peritonitis due to perforations of the gastrointestinal tract. There is often a substantial delay before patients are brought for treatment and often, the child has been inadequately treated by several local doctors before finally being referred to a tertiary care center in a precarious condition. In addition, diseases like abdominal tuberculosis, enteric (typhoid) fever with its sequelae, amebic colitis, and helminthic diseases like roundworm infestation are extremely common. The following section briefly describes our recent experience with peritonitis in newborns and older children at the Department of Pediatric Surgery, Lady Hardinge Medical College and associated Kalawati Saran Children's Hospital, New Delhi. Kalawati Saran Children's Hospital (KSCH) is a very busy children's hospital catering to a large population derived from Delhi and neighboring North Indian states. The vast majority of patients belong to the poor socio-economic strata of society.

Peritonitis in Newborns—the KSCH Experience

During a study carried out from March 1998 to October 2000 (2 ½ years), 85 newborns with peritonitis were admitted to the Pediatric Surgery ward of Kalawati Saran Children's Hospital, New Delhi. Fifty-nine were males and 26 were females. The largest number was made up of patients with necrotizing enterocolitis (NEC) of the small and/or large bowel, comprising 43 patients (50.6%); there were 11 patients with spontaneous gastrointestinal perforation without gangrene (SIP) (13%), and 9 patients with meconium peritonitis (9.5%). The etiology of peritonitis in these 85 patients is shown in Table 48.3, and the various features that these patients presented with and their demographic characteristics are summarized below.

Of the 85 patients, 8 were brought on the first day of life, 41 between 2-7 days after birth, and 36 neonates were 8-30 days old at presentation. Four patients weighed less than 1000 g at admission, 38 patients weighed between 1000-2000 g, 34 patients between 2000-2500 g, and 9 patients weighed more than 2500 g at admission.

Table 48.3 Peritonitis in newborns: etiology–KSCH experience (March 1998–Oct 2000)

Diagnosis	Number of Patients
Necrotizing enterocolitis (NEC)	43
Non-NEC perforation	11
Jejuno-ileal atresia with perforation	5
Meconium peritonitis	9
Hirschprung's disease with perforation	1
Malrotation with gangrene	5
Iatrogenic rectal perforation	1
Bowel injury at unrelated procedure	1
Primary peritonitis	1
Anastomotic dehiscence	5
Post-NEC limited leak (cecal perforation)	1
Sealed bowel perforation	2

The most commonly seen clinical signs and symptoms were abdominal distension in 82 patients (96% of patients), bilious vomiting/nasogastric aspirate in 81 patients (95%), constipation 76 (89%), abdominal wall erythema 32 (37.6%), an abdominal mass 10 (12%), gastrointestinal bleeding 12 (14%), and overt neonatal sepsis in 45 patients (53%). Abdominal guarding and tenderness was seen in 30 patients (35%). Significantly, in 33 patients, there was a history of diarrheal disease preceding the abdominal distension. Thirty-eight patients (45%) had been receiving top-feeds while the remaining 47 patients were on breast-feeds alone.

A study of the data tabulated above reveals certain interesting facts. 43 patients had NEC with perforation and 11 patients had spontaneous intestinal perforation (SIP), i.e. intestinal perforation in the absence of gross intestinal gangrene or necrosis. The etiopathogenesis of NEC in newborns has been studied extensively and is the subject of numerous articles in the literature. Spontaneous gastrointestinal perforations in the newborn have also been studied and are thought to be due to the undesirable side effects of an asphyxial defense mechanism, known as selective circulatory ischemia which is activated by perinatal stress, hypoxia or shock.[85-87] Redistribution of blood flow during hypoxia, hypovolemia, or other stress states, with shunting away from mesenteric vascular beds, is thought to result in microvascular injury, and subsequent loss of mucosal integrity.[88-90] The ultimate result may therefore be extension of microvascular thrombosis with transmural necrosis and intestinal perforation. As with NEC, multiple factors are responsible, including bacterial colonization of the gut, presence of a hyperosmolar luminal substrate such as carbohydrate, and immaturity of the immune system.[85] The neonate also has an immature immune system, and prematurity is associated with deficiencies in complement, opsonization, phagocyte function, immunoglobulin A (IgA) and immunoglobulin M (Ig M), and the function of T lymphocytes.[85]

In the West, SIP is predominantly seen in premature infants 4-5 days old, with a perinatal history of stress and asphyxia.[85] In contrast however, our data shows that most newborns with NEC or SIP are of normal birthweight or of borderline low birthweight. Most of these children are born at home and have been doing well for anywhere from 2-20 days when they develop abdominal symptoms. Many of these children also have a prior history of infective diarrheal disease and/or 'ghutti' intake. Ghutti is an indigenous substance containing opioids and is often given by poor working women to their infants to keep them quiet. Excess administration of ghutti causes a form of paralytic ileus due to the overdose of opioids and predisposes to infective gastrointestinal diseases. One fact that is almost universal is the poor socio-economic status of our patients and the poor hygiene in which these newborns are nurtured indicating that morbidity and mortality is largely preventable. It is likely that the pathogenesis of NEC and SIP in these patients is two-fold: (i) As a consequence of poor hygiene and sanitation, these vulnerable newborns are very prone to developing gastroenteritis or enterocolitis of viral (often with secondary bacterial infection) or bacterial origin. A contributory factor is that many of these newborns are not being breast-fed but are on top-feeds which may well be infected. In the presence of severe gastroenterocolitis, transmural extension of mucosal inflammation and ulceration may lead to intestinal perforation and peritonitis. In cases where the disease process is even more severe or extensive, it may result in NEC with gross gangrene or necrosis of the bowel. (ii) Several other infectious diseases like respiratory tract illnesses, or febrile illnesses due to a variety of infecting agents including exanthemata are also very common in developing countries like India. These diseases often result in dehydration and hypovolemia due to a combination of fever, reduced oral intake, and delayed and ineffective treatment. In addition, many of these patients also have diminished resistance to infection due to general malnutrition as well as the systemic effects of the illness. The net result is the creation of a stress state and the possibility of shunting of blood away from the mesenteric vascular beds with its consequences as described above. It is obvious that a stress state with hypovolemia, hypotension and diminished resistance to infection is also an additional contributing factor in patients with infective diarrheal diseases who develop NEC or SIP.

A variety of operative procedures were performed on the patients in our series, including resection and primary anastomosis or primary closure of perforations in 54 patients. There were 47 deaths, overall a mortality of 55.2%. These included 13 out of 15 patients who were admitted in very poor general condition and often were premature or of low birthweight. Many of these newborns had evidence of severe neonatal sepsis. These patients were thought to be in too poor a general condition to withstand major surgery and intraperitoneal drains were inserted under local anesthesia. Overall, most deaths were due to the consequences of severe overwhelming neonatal sepsis.

Peritonitis in Children Aged 1 Month to 12 Years

During the period from February 1999 to March 2001, 90 patients in the age group of 1 month to 12 years were admitted with peritonitis in the pediatric surgery ward of Kalawati Saran Children's Hospital, New Delhi. The etiology of peritonitis in these 90 patients is shown in Table 48.4. There were 55 male and 35 female patients, (a male: female ratio 1.57:1). Of the 12 patients with primary peritonitis however, 7 were girls and 5 were boys.

A study of Table 48.4 reveals certain interesting facts. According to the Western literature, the majority of cases of childhood peritonitis are due to perforated appendicitis.[91] In contrast, in our series, tuberculous peritonitis, peritonitis due to non-specific perforation(s) of the intestine with/without bowel gangrene, enteric (typhoid) perforations, and roundworm infestation with intestinal perforation were frequent causes of peritonitis (Fig. 48.7).

Table 48.4 Peritonitis in children (1 month to 12 years age): etiology–KSCH experience (Feb 1999- March 2001)

Diagnosis	Number of Patients
1. Primary peritonitis	12
2. Tuberculous peritonitis	18 (Total)
a. Primary tuberculous peritonitis	16
b. Stricture with proximal perforation	2
3. Secondary peritonitis	48 (Total)
a. Non-specific intestinal perforation with/without associated bowel gangrene	
1 month to 1 year age	10
1 year to 12 years age	10
b. Enteric (typhoid) perforation	7
c. Appendicular perforation with peritonitis:	5
Local peritonitis	(3)
Generalized peritonitis	(2)
d. Round worm infestation with intestinal perforation	3
e. Perforated Meckel's diverticulum	6
f. Postoperative peritonitis after anastomotic leak	7
4. Miscellaneous causes	12

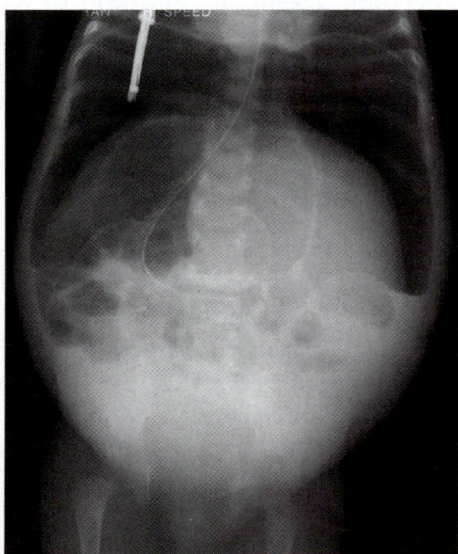

Fig. 48.7: Skiagram abdomen in errect posture of a case with enteric perforation leading to generalized peritonitis

Tuberculous peritonitis was seen in as many as 18 patients (20% of the total). In 2 of these patients, primary peritoneal tuberculosis was absent, the peritonitis being secondary to intestinal tuberculosis with a bowel perforation proximal to a stricture. The early or ascitic form of tuberculosis was seen in only 3 patients, the remaining patients presenting with the chronic form of peritoneal tuberculosis with matted bowel loops and features of intestinal obstruction. 4 patients presented with an umbilical fecal fistula secondary to perforation of matted, edematous intestinal loops. This is likely to be a consequence of delayed presentation and/or inadequate primary treatment.

In 20 patients, peritonitis was due to a single or multiple perforation(s) of the small or large intestine with/without the presence of associated gangrene of the bowel. Significantly, out of these 20 children, 10 were in the age group of 1 month to 1year. In this particular group, 6 children (60%) had a history of gastroenteritis with vomiting and diarrhea or diarrhea alone, immediately preceding the presentation with peritonitis. In 2 patients, there was a history of respiratory tract illness, and in 1 child a history of high-grade fever for a few days prior to the development of peritonitis. Four patients (40%) were malnourished with weight less than the 50th percentile of normal for the age. Thus, in a large percentage of these small infants, predisposing factors and stress in the form of infective gastroenteritis/enterocolitis, other infectious diseases and malnutrition were present. It is likely that in these infants, the etiopathogenesis of intestinal perforation, gangrene, and peritonitis is similar to that described earlier for the majority of newborns presenting with SIP/NEC and peritonitis at our institution. Postoperative mortality in this group was high, as many as 6 infants (60%) succumbing to varying combinations of severe sepsis, persistent peritonitis, dyselectrolytemia, poor general condition and malnutrition.

There were 17 older children (age group 1 year to 12 years) in whom peritonitis was due to intestinal perforation with/without gangrene of the bowel. In 7 of these children, the clinical history, investigations and operative findings suggested that intestinal perforation was due to typhoid enteritis, while in the remaining 10 patients, no specific cause of bowel perforation or gangrene could be found.

Miscellaneous causes of peritonitis included blunt abdominal trauma with jejunal perforation (2 patients), perforated ileal duplication cyst (1), ileal volvulus around a chylolymphatic cyst with proximal perforation (1), acid ingestion with intestinal perforation (1), perforation of the gall bladder (1), foreign body perforation (1), ruptured liver abscess (1), ruptured perinephric abscess (1) and a trichophytobezoar with jejunal perforation in 1 patient.

The overall mortality in this series of 90 patients was 10% (9 patients). Significantly, all the 9 patients who died had peritonitis as a consequence of SIP or NEC with gangrene and bowel perforation, 6 in the age group of 1 month to 1 year, and 3 who were 1-12 years old at presentation. It is clear therefore, that peritonitis and its consequences are more severe in this vulnerable group of patients. The illness often pursues a very fulminant course and morbidity and mortality may be very high.

REFERENCES

1. Hiyama DT, Bennion RS. Peritonitis and Intraperitoneal Abscess, in Zinner MJ, Schwartz SI, Ellis H (Eds): Maingot's Abdominal Operations (ed 10), chap 17. Stamford CT, Appleton and Lange 1997;633-53.
2. Wittman DH, Walker AP, Condon RE. Peritonitis and intraabdominal infection, in Schwartz S, Shires G, Spencer F (Eds): Principles of Surgery (ed 6). New York, NY, McGraw-Hill 1991;1449-83.
3. Solomkin JS, Wittman DW, West MA, Barie PS. Intraabdominal Infections, in Schwartz SI, Tom Shires G, Spencer FC, Daly JM, Galloway AC (Eds): Principles of Surgery (ed 7), chap 32. New York, NY, Mc-Graw Hill 1999;1515-50.
4. Wang NS. The preformed stomas connecting the pleural cavity and the lymphatics in the parietal pleura. Am Rev Respir Dis 1975;111:12-20.
5. Leak LV, Just EE. Permeability of peritoneal mesothelium: a TEM and SEM study. J Cell Biol 1976;70:423a.
6. Steinberg B. Infections of the Peritoneum. New York, NY, Hoeber 1944.
7. Dumont AE, Robbins E, Martelli A, et al. Platelet blockade of particle absorption from the peritoneal surface of the diaphragm. Proc Soc Exp Biol Med 1981;167:137-42.
8. Dumont AE, Maas WK, Iliescu H, et al. Increased survival from peritonitis after blockade of transdiaphragmatic absorption of bacteria. Surg Gynecol Obstet 1986;162: 248-52.
9. Skau T, Nystrom PO, Ohman L. Bacterial clearance and granulocyte response in experimental peritonitis. J Surg Res 1986;40:13-20.
10. Last M, Kurtz L, Stein TA, et al. Effect of PEEP on the rate of thoracic lymph duct flow and clearance of bacteria from the peritoneal cavity. Am J Surg 1983;145:126-30.
11. Maddaus MA, Ahrenholz D, Simmons RL. The biology of peritonitis and implications for treatment. Surg Clin North Am 1988;68:431-43.
12. Wiles JB, Cerra FB, Siegel JH, et al. The systemic response: does the organism matter? Crit Care Med 1980;2:55-60.
13. Tracey KJ, Beutler B, Lowry SF, et al. Shock and tissue injury induced by recombinant human cachectin. Science 1986;234:470-74.
14. Dinarello CA. Interleukin-1. Rev Infect Dis 1984;6:51-95.
15. Dunn DL, Barke RA, Ahrenholz DH, et al. The adjuvant effect of peritoneal fluid in experimental peritonitis. Ann Surg 1984;199:37-43.
16. Dunn DL, Barke RA, Knight NB, et al. Role of resident macrophages, peripheral neutrophils, and translymphatic absorption in bacterial clearance from peritoneal cavity. Infect Immunol 1985;49:257-64.
17. Ertel W, Morrison MH, et al. The complex pattern of cytokines in sepsis: Association between prostaglandins, cachectin, and interleukins. Ann Surg 1991;214:141-48.
18. Hau T, Payne WD, Simmons RL. Fibrinolytic activity of the peritoneum. Surg Gynecol Obstet 1979;148:415-18.
19. Raftery AT. Effect of peritoneal trauma on peritoneal fibrinolytic activity and intraperitoneal adhesion formation. Eur Surg Res 1981;13:397-401.
20. Vipond MN, Whawell SA, Thompson JN, et al. Peritoneal fibrinolytic activity and intra-abdominal adhesions. Lancet 1990;335:1120-22.
21. Raftery AT. Regeneration of parietal and visceral peritoneum: An electron microscopic study. J Anat 1973;115:375-92.
22. Sawyer MD, Dunn DL. Antimicrobial therapy of intraabdominal sepsis. Infect Dis Clin North Am 1992;6:545-70.
23. Weinstein WM, Onderdonk AB, Bartlett JG, et al. Experimental intra-abdominal abscesses in rats: Development of an experimental model. Infect Immun 1974;10:1250-55.
24. Zaleznik DF, Kasper DL. The role of anaerobic bacteria in abscess formation. Ann Rev Med 1982;33: 217-29.
25. Yull AB, Abrams JS, Davis JH. The peritoneal fluid in strangulation obstruction: The role of the red blood cell and E.coli bacteria in producing toxicity. J Surg Res 1962;2:223.
26. Hau T, Hoffman R, Simmons RL. Mechanisms of the adjuvant effect of hemoglobin in experimental peritonitis, I. in vivo inhibition of peritoneal leukocytosis. Surgery 1978;83:223-29.
27. Pruett TL, Rotstein OD, Fiegel VD, et al. Mechanism of the adjuvant effect of hemoglobin in experimental peritonitis, VIII. A leukotoxin is produced by Escherichia coli metabolism in hemoglobin. Surgery 1984;96:375-83.
28. Ward CG. Influence of iron on infection. Am J Surg 1986;151:291-95.
29. Zimmerli W, Waldvogel FA, Vaudaux P, et al. Pathogenesis of foreign body infection: Description and characteristics of an animal model. J Infect Dis 1982;146:487-97.
30. Zimmerli W, Lew PD, Waldvogel FA. Pathogenesis of foreign body infection: evidence for a local granulocyte defect. J Clin Invest 1984;73:1191-200.

31. Raffensperger JG. Peritonitis in infancy, in Raffensperger JG (Ed). Swenson's Pediatric Surgery (ed 5), section 7. Norwalk CT, Appleton and Lange 1990;626.
32. Rowe MI. Necrotizing enterocolitis, in Welch KJ, Randolph JG, Ravitch MM, O'Neill, Jr. JA, Rowe MM (Eds): Pediatric Surgery (ed 4), chap 99. Chicago, Year Book Medical Publishers 1986;944-57.
33. Albanese CT, Rowe MI. Necrotizing enterocolitis, in O'Neill, Jr JA, Rowe MI, Grosfeld JL, Fonkalsrud EW, Coran AG (Eds): Pediatric Surgery (Ed 5), chap 87. St. Louis, MO, Mosby- Year Book Inc 1998;1297-320.
34. Clark JH, Fitzgerald JF, Kleiman MB. Spontaneous bacterial peritonitis. J Pediatr 1984;104:495-500.
35. Ein SH. Primary peritonitis, in Welch KJ, Randolph JG (Eds); Pediatric Surgery (Ed 4), chap 102. Chicago, Year Book Medical Publishers 1986;976-77.
36. Fowler R. Primary peritonitis: changing aspects 1956-1970. Aust Paediatr J 1971;7:73-83.
37. McDougal WS, Izant RJ, Zollinger RM. Primary peritonitis in infancy and childhood. Ann Surg 1974;181:310-13.
38. Speck WT, Dresdale SS, McMillan RW. Primary peritonitis and the nephrotic syndrome. Am J Surg 1974;127:267-69.
39. Hoefs JC, Runyon BA. Spontaneous bacterial peritonitis. Dis Mon 1985;31:1-48.
40. Krensky AM, Ingelfinger JR, Grupe WE. Peritonitis in childhood nephrotic syndrome. Am J Dis Child 1982;136:732-36.
41. Larchev VF, et al. Spontaneous bacterial peritonitis in children with chronic liver disease: Clinical features and etiologic factors. J Pediatr 1985;106:907.
42. Harken AH, Shochat SJ. Gram positive peritonitis in children. Am J Surg 1973;125:769-72.
43. West KW. Primary peritonitis, in O'Neill, Jr. JA, Rowe MI, Grosfeld JL, Fonkalsrud EW, Coran AG (Eds). Pediatric Surgery (ed 5), chap 90. St. Louis MO, Mosby-Year Book Inc 1998;1345-48.
44. Garcia-Tsao G, Conn HO, Werner E. The diagnosis of bacterial peritonitis: Comparisons of pH lactate concentration and leukocyte count. Hepatology 1985;5:91-96.
45. Marshall R, Teele DW, Klein JO. Unsuspected bacteremia due to Haemophilus influenzae; outcome in children not initially admitted to hospital. J Pediatr 1979;95:690-95.
46. Graham JC, Moss PJ, McKendrick MW. Primary group A streptococcal peritonitis. Scand J Infect Dis 1995;27:171-72.
47. Ma JS, Chen PY, Chi CS, et al. Invasive Streptococcus pneumoniae infections of children in central Taiwan. J Microbiol Immunol Infect 2000;33:169-75.
48. van Houten MA, Ab E, Zwierstra RP, et al. Primary peritonitis due to Streptococcus pneumoniae in childhood. Ned Tijdschr Geneeskd 1998;142(14):793-96.
49. Matsell DG, Wyatt RJ. The role of I and B in peritonitis associated with the nephrotic syndrome of childhood. Pediatr Res 1993;34:84-88.
50. Gorensek MJ, Lebel MH, Nelson JD. Peritonitis in children with nephrotic syndrome. Pediatrics 1988;81:849-56.
51. Tapaneya-Olarn C, Tapaneya-Olarn W. Primary peritonitis in childhood nephrotic syndrome: A changing trend in causative organisms. J Med Assoc Thailand 1991;74:502-06.
52. Tsau YK, Chen CH, Tsai WS, et al. Complications of nephrotic syndrome in children. J Formosan Med Assoc 1991;90:555-59.
53. Runyon BA. Patients with deficient ascitic fluid opsonic activity are predisposed to spontaneous bacterial peritonitis. Hepatology 1980;8:632-35.
54. Runyon BA, Unland ET, Merlin T. Inoculation of blood cultures bottles with ascitic fluid: improved detection of spontaneous bacterial peritonitis. Arch Intern Med 1987;147:73-75.
55. Verrina E, Honda M, Warady BA, et al. Prevention of peritonitis in children on peritoneal dialysis. Perit Dial Int 2000;20(6):625-30.
56. Rusthoven E, Monnens LA, Schroder CH. Effective treatment of peritoneal dialysis- associated peritonitis with cefazolin and ceftazidime in children. Perit Dial Int 2001;21(4):386-89.
57. De Boer AW, Levi M, Reddingius RE, et al. Intraperitoneal hypercoagulation and hypofibrinolysis is present in childhood peritonitis. Pediatr Nephrol 1999;13:284-87.
58. Gurkan F, Ozates M, Bosnak M, et al. Tuberculous peritonitis in 11 children: clinical features and diagnostic approach. Pediatr Int 1999;41:510-13.
59. Demir K, Okten A, Kaymakoglu S, et al. Tuberculous peritonitis-reports of 26 cases, detailing diagnostic and therapeutic problems. Eur J Gastroenterol Hepatol 2001;13(5):581-85.
60. Verspyck E, Struder C, Wendum D, et al. Peritoneal tuberculosis. Ann Chir 1997;51(4):375-78.
61. Manohar A, Simjee AE, Haffejee AA, et al. Symptoms and investigative findings in 145 patients with tuberculous peritonitis diagnosed by peritoneoscopy and biopsy over a five year period. Gut 1991;32(4):457-58.
62. Lam KN, Rajasoorya C, Mah PK, et al. Diagnosis of tuberculous peritonitis. Singapore Med J 1999;40(9):601-04.
63. Demirkazik FB, Akhan O, Ozmen MN, et al. US and CT findings in the diagnosis of tuberculous peritonitis. Acta Radiol 1996;37(4):517-20.
64. Apaydin B, Paksoy M, Bilir M, et al. Value of diagnostic laparoscopy in tuberculous peritonitis. Eur J Surg 1999;165(2):158-63.
65. Brook I. A 12-year study of aerobic and anaerobic bacteria in intra-abdominal and postsurgical abdominal wound infections. Surg Gynecol Obstet 1989;169:387-92.
66. Sawyer MD, Dunn DL. Antimicrobial therapy of intraabdominal sepsis. Surg Infect 1992;6:545-70.
67. Stone HH, Bourneuf AA, Stinson LD. Reliability of criteria for predicting persistent or recurrent sepsis. Arch Surg 1985;120:17-20.

68. Lennard ES, Dellinger EP, Wertz MJ, et al. Implications of leukocytosis and fever at conclusion of therapy for intra-abdominal sepsis. Ann Surg 1982;195:19-24.
69. Nathens AB, Rotstein OD. Therapeutic options in peritonitis. Surg Clin North Am 1994;74(3):677-92.
70. Penninckx FM, Kerremans RP, Lauwers PM. Planned relaparotomies in the surgical treatment of severe generalized peritonitis from intestinal origins. World J Surg 1983;7:762-66.
71. Wittman DH, Aprahamian C, Bergstein JM. Etappenlavage: advanced diffuse peritonitis managed by planned multiple laparotomies utilizing zippers, slide fastener, and Velcro analogue for temporary abdominal closure. World J Surg 1990;14:218-26.
72. Haecker FM, Berger D, Schumacher U, et al. Peritonitis in childhood. aspects of pathogenesis and therapy. Pediatr Surg Int 2000;16:182-88.
73. Forouhar F. Meconium peritonitis- pathology, evolution and diagnosis. Am J Clin Pathol 1982;78:208-13.
74. Marchildon MB. Meconium peritonitis and spontaneous gastric perforations. Clin Perinatol 1978;5:79-91.
75. Lally KP, Mehall JR, Xue H, et al. Meconium stimulates a pro-inflammatory response in peritoneal macrophages: implications for meconium peritonitis. J Pediatr Surg 1999;34(1):214-17.
76. Wiener ES. Meconium peritonitis, in Welch KJ, Randolph JG, Ravitch MM, O'Neill, Jr. JA, Rowe MI (eds), Pediatric Surgery (ed 4), chap 97. Chicago, Year Book Medical Publishers 1986;929-31.
77. Groff DB. Meconium disease, in Ashcraft KW (ed): Pediatric Surgery (ed3), chap 32. Philadelphia, WB Saunders 2000;435-42.
78. Niramis R, Watanatittan S, Anuntakosol M, et al. Meconium peritonitis. J Med Assoc Thai 1999;82(11):1063-70.
79. Konje JC, de Chazal R, Mac Fadyen U, et al. Antenatal diagnosis and management of meconium peritonitis: A case report and review of the literature. Ultrasound Obstet Gynecol 1995;6(1):66-69.
80. Salman AB, Karaoglanoglu N, Suma S. Abdominal, scrotal, and thoracic calcifications owing to healed meconium peritonitis. J Pediatr Surg 1999;34(9):1415-16.
81. Kolker SE, Ferrel LD, Bollen AW, et al. Disseminated intravascular meconium in a newborn with meconium peritonitis. Hum Pathol 1999;30(5):592-94.
82. Tanaka K, Hashizume K, Kawarasaki H. Elective surgery for cystic meconium peritonitis: Report of two cases. J Pediatr Surg 1993;28:960-61.
83. Caresky JM, Grosfeld JL, Weber TL, et al. Giant cystic meconium peritonitis (GCMP): Improved management based on clinical and laboratory observations. J Pediatr Surg 1982;17:482-89.
84. Karaguzel G, Tanyel FC, Senocak ME, et al. Persistent diffuse peritonitis in children. Turk J Pediatr 1998;40(2):151-58.
85. Scherer III, LR. Peptic ulcer and other conditions of the stomach, in O'Neill, Jr. JA, Rowe MI, Grosfeld JL, Fonkalsrud EW, Coran AG (eds): Pediatric Surgery (ed 5), chap90. St. Louis MO, Mosby-Year Book Inc, 1998; 1119-33.
86. Barlow B, Santulli TV. Importance of multiple episodes of hypoxia or cold stress on the development of enterocolitis in an animal model. Surgery 1975;77:687-90.
87. Touloukian RJ. Gastric ischemia: The primary factor in neonatal perforation. Clin Pediatr 1973;12:219-25.
88. Tououkian RJ, Posch JN, Spencer R. The pathogenesis of ischemic gastroenterocolitis of the neonate: selective gut mucosal ischemia in asphyxiated neonatal piglets. J Pediatr Surg 1972;7:194-205.
89. Harrison MW, Connell RS, Campbell JR, et al. Microcirculatory changes in the gastrointestinal tract of the hypoxic puppy: An electron microscopy study. J Pediatr Surg 1975;10:599-608.
90. Harrison MW, Connell RS, Campbell JR, et al. Fine structural changes in the gastrointestinal tract of the hypoxic puppy: A study of the natural history. J Pediatr Surg 1977;12:403-08.
91. Estel S, Festge OA, Stenger D. Etiology and therapy of peritonitis in childhood. Zentralbl Chir 1988;113(4):241-48.

Infantile Hypertrophic Pyloric Stenosis

Sengamalai Manoharan, Azad B Mathur

HISTORY

Hildanus in 1627, was the first author who described what was thought to be a case of infantile hypertrophic pyloric stenosis (IHPS).[1] However, the history does not fit with the usual evolution of the IHPS, as the child recovered spontaneously, and no pathological proof is provided with the case. It is likely that it was a case of overfeeding.

Patrick Blair in 1717, described a more typical clinical and postmortem finding of IHPS, and presented it to the Royal Society in London.[2] The first complete description was by Harald Hirschsprung, a Pediatrician from Copenhagen, in 1888, and established the clinical and postmortem findings as a new, specific entity, and named it Angeborener Pylorusstenose (congenital pyloric stenosis) because he believed that this pathology was congenital, by failure of the involution of the fetal pylorus.[3]

Use of atropine remained at the center of the medical management, till the surgical treatment was established. Cordua performed jejunostomy in 1892, Lobker attempted gastroenterostomy in 1898 and, 1899 Nicoll tried pyloric dilatation via gastrostomy. Pyloroplasty and extramucousal pyloroplasty was then described by Dent, Nicoll, Fredet, and Weber.[4]

On 23 August 1911, Wilhem Conrad Ramsted first performed his pyloromyotomy without transversal suture.[5] On 18 June 1912, he successfully repeated his new technique on another male patient; and reported these two cases to the Natural Science Assembly at Munster. The Ramsted operation is nowadays a standard surgical technique for the IHPS.

ANATOMY

There is a pyloric obstruction caused by hypertrophy of the muscle, involving the internal circular layer on gastric side.

The enlarged pylorus has an olive shape measuring usually 2-2.5 cm in length and 1-1.5 cm in diameter. The "olive" is pale, contrasting with the pink color of the duodenal cul-de-sac.

Histologically, the mucosa and adventitia are normal. The edematous mucosa is seen as a longitudinal fold at the contrast study. The stomach is distended and frequently hyperkinetic.

ETIOLOGY

Etiology is unknown. Whether the condition is congenital or acquired is debated. Thompson Benson in 1897, described it as a neurologic dysfunction at the stomach and pyloric level leading to uncoordinated and sometimes antagonistic contractions. Therefore, the hypertrophy is a consequence of this hyperactivity.

There has been lot of research on this subject and various factors associated with this pathology namely are:decrease in ganglion cells in hypertrophic pyloric muscle, immature ganglion cells; pyloric ulcer leading to antropyloric spasm and muscular hypertrophy; hypergastrinemia; substance P causing chronic pylorospasm followed by a hypertrophy of the pyloric muscle.[6-11]

Studies investigating the role of encephalin, neuropeptide Y, vasoactive intestinal polypeptide and gastrin releasing peptide shows reduction of immunoreactivity in intramuscular nerve supporting cells and lack of nitric oxide synthase have been suggested as a factor in the pathogenesis of IHPS.[12-13]

Ultrastructural abnormalities of enteric nerves and the interstitial cells of Cajal have been implicated.[14] Increased insulin-like growth factor and platelet derived growth factor system in the pyloric muscle in IHPS have also been noted. The Neuronal cell adhesion molecule (NCAM) plays an essential role in the development and function of the peripheral nervous system. It has been reported that NCAM, NADPH diaphorase and neurofilament immunoreactive fibers were absent or markedly reduced within the hypertrophied circular and longitudinal musculature.[16] It suggests that this condition may be a consequence of a developmental deficiency preventing the proper innervation of the pyloric muscle layer. Genetic mutations involving the production of nitric oxide may be responsible for many cases of IHPS.[17,18] An association between systemic erythromycin in infants and subsequent IHPS, with the highest risk in the first 2 weeks of age, has been reported.[19]

ASSOCIATED ANOMALIES

Some associations are genetically X-linked described by Spicer,[4] including esophageal atresia, and neuronal dysfunction. Other non-genetic malformations are: inguinoscrotal pathology, encephalocele, hydrocephalus, cardiac malformations, gastroesophageal reflux, and hiatus hernia are well known.

Jaundice, described with IHPS, usually resolves after pyloromyotomy.[20]

INCIDENCE

It is 1.5-4 in 1000 live births amongst whites but is less in Africans and Asians.

The highest incidence is in the north of Europe, and incidence is increasing with an increased number in the spring and autumn.[4]

It has been observed that there is male predominance with familial predisposition. If mother had the pathology then 19% of the male and 7% of the female offspring are likely to be afflicted. Only 5% of the male and 2.5% of the female offspring of a father with pyloric stenosis will develop the disease;[18] environmental and seasonal variations have been described.

DIAGNOSIS

The infant with hypertrophic pyloric stenosis often starts vomiting at 3-4 weeks of life, and sometimes earlier. The vomit contains milk or curds and is non bilious; it can have a brownish discoloration or have coffee-ground appearance, caused by chronic gastritis. The vomiting is always forceful and may be abrupt or insidious in onset. The vomiting occurs shortly after feeding, and the infant remains hungry. A delay in the diagnosis may result in pronounced malnutrition and severe electrolyte imbalance.

IHPS has been diagnosed in premature debilitated infants; at birth, and even in utero.[21-23]

The diagnosis of IHPS is made by physical examination in 75%; it should start by a feeding of formula if the infant state allows it (infant alert, active). This makes visible gastric peristaltic waves that progress successively from the upper left to the mid right of the abdomen.

The examiner should stay on the left of the patient while baby is supine in mother's arms, relaxed, warm and reassured. The left hand is placed at the epigastrium with the mid-finger tip just above and to the right of the umbilicus. The right hand is beneath the infant for support, giving a slight extension to the back in order to ease the palpation of the "olive" which is pushed forward by the vertebrae. If it is not palpated, then the test is repeated just after an episode of vomiting.

Some may suggest surgery after confirming the presence of pyloric "tumor" by test feed but authors recommend ultrasound confirmation of the pathology to avoid negative laparotomy. Demonstration of pyloric muscle thickness of 4 mm or more by ultrasound and pyloric channel length of 16 mm or more increases the specificity of the test to 100% (Fig. 49.1).[24] Earlier, an upper gastrointestinal examination with the barium was recommended, which is replaced by ultrasound examination to confirm the diagnosis.

DIFFERENTIAL DIAGNOSIS

This includes primary medical and surgical conditions that result in projectile non-bilious vomiting such as pylorospasm, gastroesophageal reflux, gastric atony, metabolic disorders and increased intracranial pressure. Other surgical causes of non-bilious emesis

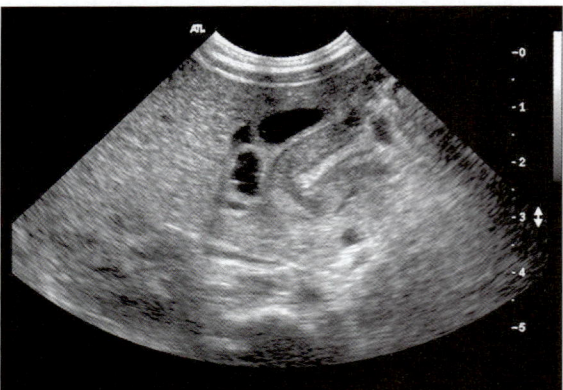

Fig. 49.1: Longitudinal section of the pylorus in an infant of IHPS as shown by ultrasound

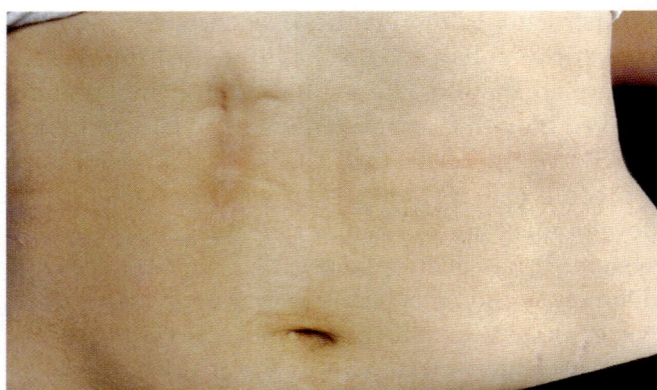

Fig. 49.2: Postoperative scar after surgery for IHPS during infancy

include gastric antral web, pyloric atresia, pyloric duplication cyst and ectopic pyloric pancreas.

PREOPERATIVE MANAGEMENT

The longer duration prior to presentation to a hospital and the frequent vomiting can lead to severe dehydration with electrolyte imbalance. Vomiting of gastric contents leads to depletion of sodium, potassium and hydrochloric acid, resulting in hypokalemic, hypochloremic metabolic alkalosis. The kidneys conserve sodium at the expense of hydrogen ions, leading to paradoxical aciduria. In more severe dehydration, in an attempt to retain fluid and sodium, renal potassium losses worsen. The renal and the gastric loss of K^+, will not be reflected in the serum level until the intracellular K^+ is severely depleted.

The hypokalemia and acid urine are late signs of metabolic alkalosis.

Preoperative Fluid Resuscitation

- Type of fluid: 5% Dextrose with 0.45% Saline. Add 2 mmol of KCl in each 100 ml of fluid.
- Volume: 150 ml per kg of body weight per 24 hours.
- Investigation: Serum electrolytes every 12 hours.
- Nasogastric loss: Replace ml for ml by normal saline.
- The most important factor is serum HCO_3 level, 25-28 mEq/l denoting a safe correction of alkalosis before proceeding to surgery.

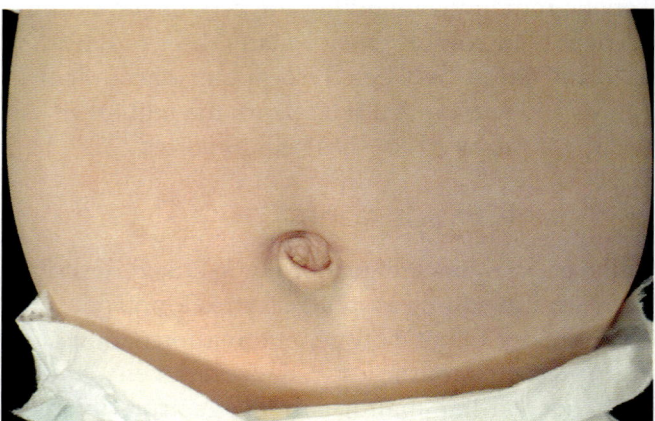

Fig. 49.3: Picture of healed supraumbilical scar after pyloromyotomy

OPERATIVE MANAGEMENT

Patient is operated after correction of fluid and electrolytes, under general anesthesia in a warm theatre.

Since the initial description of pyloromyotomy as the curative procedure for infantile hypertrophic pyloric stenosis, it has been achieved through diverse upper abdominal approaches to pylorus. The supraumbilical incision was described by Tan and Bianchi in 1986 with the intention of achieving an unscarred abdomen (Figs 49.2 and 49.3).[25] Since the original publication various authors have described some modifications. We have described a modification and have used our approach successfully in more than forty patients with no complication of perforation, wound dehiscence or conversion to right hypochondrial incision.[26,27]

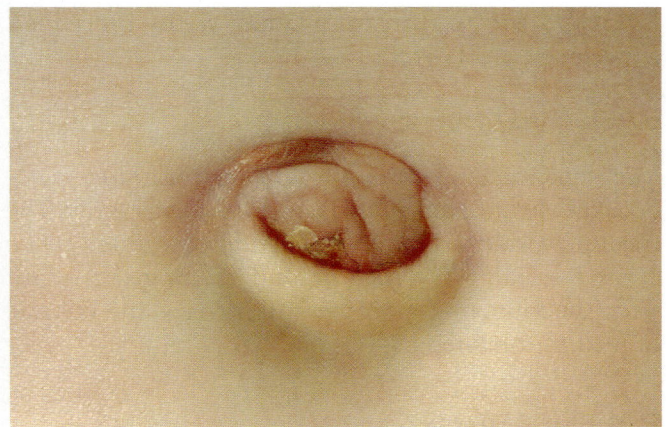

Fig. 49.4: Picture shows a skin incision as semilunar supraumbilical incision

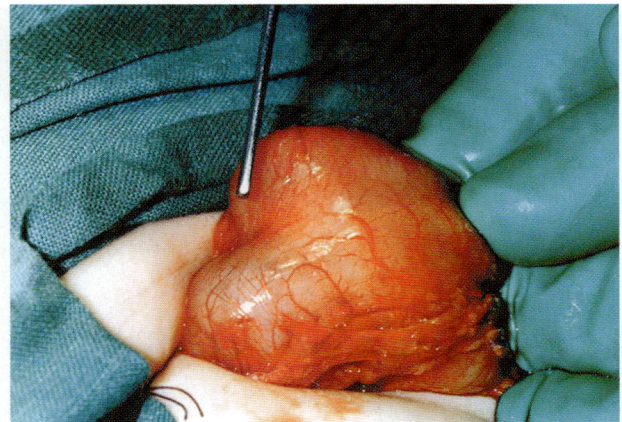

Fig. 49.5: Delivering of pyloric tumor through supraumbilical wound

SURGICAL TECHNIQUE

All patients are fully resuscitated pre-operatively. Separate gentle cleaning of umbilicus is performed followed by standard preoperative cleaning. A supraumbilical skin incision is made around one-half of the umbilicus and carried down to the abdominal wall fascia with sharp dissection as shown in Figure 49.4.

The incision is modified at the level of the rectus sheath. A midline vertical incision is made up to the tip of the xiphisternum and a 4/0 vicryl (ethicon) stitch is placed at the cephalic end of the incision as a landmark. At the umbilical end the incision is converted in the shape of an inverted T. The transverse incision through the sheath needs to be longer on the right side of the midline, approximately double the size as compared to its arm on the left side. Two stay sutures are placed at the corners of the transverse incision.

The pylorus is delivered easily and pyloromyotomy performed (Figs 49.5 and 49.6). We use the back of the scalpel handle to split pyloric muscle after making a very superficial incision on pyloric swelling.

Before returning the pylorus to the peritoneal cavity, a perforation should be carefully looked for, and if there is one, it should be closed with an omental patch. A meticulous closure of the fascial wound is done by 4/0 vicryl (ethicon) stitch. Hemostasis is achieved before skin closure and a sterile dental roll is used for pressure dressing for forty-eight hours.

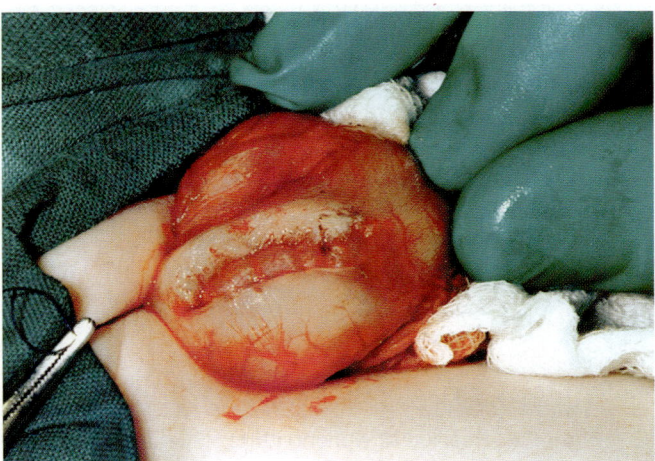

Fig. 49.6: Ramsted's pyloromyotomy performed through supraumbilical wound

Laparoscopic Pyloromyotomy

Alain et al first described Extramucosal pyloromyotomy by laparoscopy in 1991.[28] This has gained popularity in recent years. A 5 mm port is placed in the umbilicus under direct vision (Fig. 49.7) and the abdomen is insufflated with carbon dioxide. Two 3 mm stab incisions using a No.11 scalpel blade, are made, 1 in the epigastrium and another in the right mid-abdomen (Fig. 49.8). The grasper inserted through the right mid-abdomen incision, stabilizes the pylorus and the serosal surface of the hypertrophied pylorus is incised using a pylorotome, inserted through the epigastric incision. The pylorotome is then removed and pyloromyotomy completed using a pyloric spreader.

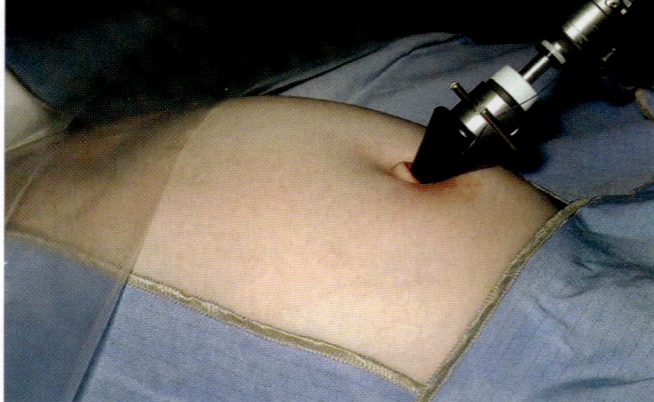

Fig. 49.7: Umbilical telescopic port for laparoscopic pyloromyotomy

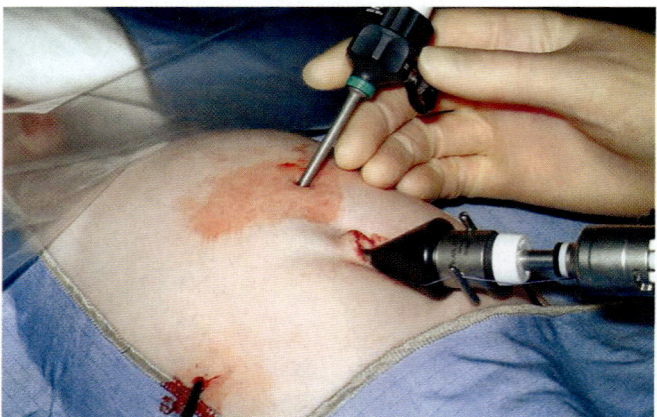

Fig. 49.8: Position of working ports for laparoscopic pyloromyotomy

A meta-analysis of studies comparing laparoscopic versus open pyloromyotomy found 8 studies comparing the 2 methods from 1966-2002 and included 595 patients (355 open and 240 laparoscopic).[29] Four studies were retrospective reviews, 3 were prospective and only 1 study was a randomized controlled trial. Mucosal perforations and incomplete pyloromyotomy were both more common with laparoscopic pyloromyotomy, although not significantly so. Compared with open procedure, laparoscopic pyloromyotomy is associated with similar operating time, shorter time to full feeds and shorter postoperative length of stay. A retrospective review in 2004, comparing 232 laparoscopic pyloromyotomies with 225 open procedures, showed no significant difference in rate of complications.[30] Van Der Bilt JDW et al, has reported decreased complication rates from laparoscopic pyloromyotomy with increased experience.[31]

POSTOPERATIVE CARE

Maintenance intravenous fluids are continued postoperatively until the infant is feeding satisfactorily. The timing of reintroduction of feeds continues to be controversial.[32] We recommend feeding the infant from the following morning and increase the volume of feed as tolerated.

COMPLICATIONS

Pyloromyotomy is associated with a low incidence of morbidity and mortality.

Mucosal perforation is usually because of excessive dissection on the side of duodenum. It should be recognized and closed with one or two sutures and a patch of omentum tied over it. Other complications include incomplete pyloromyotomy, hemorrhage, wound infection and dehiscence. Postoperative vomiting usually improve with time.

OTHER TECHNIQUES AND NONOPERATIVE TREATMENT

Balloon dilatation of pylorus has been tried with discouraging results.[33]

It has been described to perform pyloromyotomy with exteriorization of the pylorus.

Non-surgical treatment by frequent small feeding has been described. Medical treatment involving intravenous and oral atropine in addition to fluid and electrolyte replacement has also been reported. However, these are not preferred approaches in most countries.

REFERENCES

1. Fabry (Willhem) von Holden. (Hildanus) Opera Quae Extant Ominia. Frankfort. Beyerus, 1646:541.
2. Blair P. On the dissection of a child much emaciated. Phil. Trans 1717;30:631-32.
3. Hirschsprung. H. Falle von angeborener pylorus stenose. JB Kinderheilk 1888;27:61.
4. Spicer RD. Infantile hypertrophic pyloric stenosis: a review. Br J Surg 1982;69:128-35.
5. Pollock WF, Norris WJ. Dr Conrad Ramstedt and pyloromyotomy. Surgery 1957;42:966-70.

6. Belding HD, Kernohan JW. A morphologic study of the myenteric changes plexus and musculature of the pylorus with special reference to the hypertrophic pyloric stenosis, Surg Gynecol Obstet 97:3255.
7. Friesen SR, Boley JO, Miller DR. The myenteric plexus of the pylorus: it's early normal development and its changes in hypertrophic pyloric stenosis, Surgery 1956;39:21.
8. Marcowitz RJ, Wolfson BJ, Huff DS, Capitanio MA. Infantile hypertrophic stenosis - congenital or acquird? J Clin Gastroenterol 1982;4:39-44.
9. Dodge JA. Production of duodenal ulcers and hypertrophic pyloric stenosis by administration of pentagastrin to pregnant and newborn dogs. Nature 1970;225:284-85.
10. Spitz L. Zail SS. Serum gastrin levels in congenital hypertrophic pyloric stenosis, J Pediatr Surg. 1976;11:33.
11. Tam PK. Observation and perspectives of the pathology and possible aetiology of infantile hypertrophic pyloric stenosis: a histological, biochemical, histochemical and immunocytochemical study, Ann Acad Med Singapore 1985;14:523.
12. Kobayashi H, O'Brian DS, Puri P. Selective reduction in intramuscular nerve supporting cells in infantile hypertrophic pyloric stenosis. J. Pediatr. Surg. 1994;29: 651-54.
13. Vanderwinden JM, M, Maileux P, Schiffman SN. Nitric oxide synthetase activity in hypertrophic pyloric stenosis. N. Engl. J Med 1992;327:511-15.
14. Langer JC, Berezin I, Daniel EE. Hypertrophic pyloric stenosis: ultrastructural abnormalities of enteric nerves and the interstitial cells of Cajal. J Pediatr Surg 1995;30:1535-43.
15. Ohshiro K, Puri P. Increased insulin-like growth factor and platelet derived growth factor system in the pyloric muscle in infantile hypertrophic pyloric stenosis. J Pediatr Surg 1998;33:378-81.
16. Kobayashi H, O'Brian DS, Puri P. Immunochemical characterisation of neural cell adhesion molecule (NCAM), nitric oxide synthase and neurofilament protein expression in pyloric muscle of patients with hypertrophic pyloric stenosis. J. Pediatr. Gastroenterol. Nutr. 1995;20:319-25.
17. Mitchell LE, Risch N. The genetics of infantile hypertrophic pyloric stenosis, Am J Dis Child 1993;147:1203.
18. Saur D, Vanderwinden JM, Seidler B, et al. Single-nucleotide promoter polymorphism alters transcription of neuronal nitric oxide synthase exon 1c in infantile hypertrophic pyloric stenosis. Proc Natl Acad Sci U S A 2004; 101:1662-67.
19. Mahon BE, Rosenman MB, Kleiman MB. Maternal and infant use of erythromycin and other macrolide antibiotics as risk factors for infantile hypertrophic pyloric stenosis. J Pediatr. 2001;139(3):380-84.
20. Carter CO, Evans KA. Inheritance of congenital pyloric stenosis. J Med Genet 1969;6:233-39.
21. Tack ED. Perlman JM, Bower RJ, et al. Pyloric stenosis in the sick premature infant: Clinical and radiologic findings. Am J Dis Child 1988;14:68-70.
22. Zenn MR, Redo SF: Hypertrophic pyloric stenosis in the newborn, J Pediatr Surg 1993;28:1577.
23. Katz S, Basel D, Brabski D. Prenatal gastric dilatation and infantile hypertrophic pyloric stenosis, J Pediatr Surg 1988;23:1021.
24. Keller H, Waldermann D, Greiner P. Comparison of pre-operative sonography with intraoperative findings in congenital hypertrophic pyloric stenosis. J Pediatr Surg 1987;22:950-52.
25. Tan K X, Bianchi A. Circumumbilical incision for pyloromyotomy. Br J Surg 1986;73:399.
26. Mathur AB, Moncreiff M, Clark S. Pyloric stenosis; Modified supraumbilical incision. Presented at the 14th annual meeting of the Asian Association of Pediatric Surgeons, Mumbai, Nov 1997.
27. Karri V, Bouhadiba N, Mathur AB. Pyloromyotomy through circumbilical incision with fascial extension. Pediatr Surg Int 2003;19:695-96.
28. Alain JL, Grousseau D, Terrier G. Extramucosal pyloromyotomy by laparoscopy. J Pediatr Surg 1991;25:1191-92.
29. Hall NJ, Van Der Zee J, Tan HL, et al. Meta-analysis of laparoscopic versus open pyloromyotomy. Ann Surg 2004; 240:774-78.
30. Yagmurlu A, Barnhart DC, Vernon A, et al. Comparison of the incidence of complications in open and laparoscopic pyloromyotomy: a concurrent single institution series. J Pediatr Surg 2004;39:292-96.
31. Van Der Bilt JDW, Kramer WL, Van Der Zee DC, et al. Laparoscopic pyloromyotomy for hypertrophic pyloric stenosis. Surg Endosc 2004;18:907-09.
32. A Wheeler, S Najmaldin, N Stoodley, D M Griffiths, D M Burge, J D Atwell. Feeding regimens after pyloromyotomy. Br J Surg 1990;77:1018-19.
33. Hayachi AH, Giacomantonio JM, Lau HY, et al. Balloon catheter dilatation for hypertrophic pyloric stenosis. J. Pediatr. Surg 1990;25:1119-21.

Gastric Volvulus

Shilpa Sharma, D K Gupta

Volvulus is derived from the latin word volvere, that means 'to roll'. Gastric volvulus is usually a disease occurring in adults with only about 10-20% of cases occur in children, usually before age 1 year, but cases have been reported in children up to 12 years age.

Though the number of cases reported was only just over 300 cases till 1991, yet a high index of suspicion has helped to identify more cases recently.[1-5] Gastric volvulus in children is thus a rare surgical emergency. However, it may be an important cause for mortality if diagnosis is delayed and gastric perforation occurs. Chronic gastric volvulus could also be responsible for many incidences of apparent life-threatening event in infancy.[6]

Berti first described gastric volvulus in 1866.[7] Berg performed the first successful operation on a patient with gastric volvulus in 1896. Borchardt described the classic triad of severe epigastric pain, retching without vomiting, and inability to pass a nasogastric tube in 1904.[8]

DEFINITION

Gastric volvulus is an abnormal degree of rotation of one part of the stomach around another varying from 180 degrees to 360 degrees.[9] The abnormal rotation creates a closed loop obstruction that can result in incarceration and strangulation.

According to the axis of rotation of the stomach, 3 types of gastric volvulus have been described:
   i. *Organoaxial volvulus:* Stomach rotates about its longitudinal axis.[9,10] The antrum rotates in opposite direction to the fundus of the stomach. This is the most common type in both children and adults and is usually associated with diaphragmatic defects. Strangulation and necrosis commonly occur with this type and have been reported in 5-28% of cases.
   ii. *Mesenteroaxial volvulus:* Stomach rotates about a line perpendicular to the cardiopyloric line. The rotation is usually incomplete and occurs intermittently. Vascular compromise is uncommon. Patients usually have chronic symptoms. It is more often seen in young children than in adults and is associated with ligamentous laxity but not with diaphragmatic defects.
   iii. *Combined form:* Stomach rotates on both its long and short axes This form is usually observed in patients with chronic volvulus.

PREDISPOSING FACTORS

Gastric volvulus may be primary (idiopathic) or secondary depending upon the absence or presence of associated anomalies.

Type 1—Primary Gastric Volvulus

The stomach is anchored at the esophageal hiatus by the peritoneal reflection, gastrophrenic, gastrocolic, gastrosplenic and gastrohepatic ligaments (Fig. 50.1). In neonates, absence or attenuation of these ligaments predisposes to gastric volvulus. Acute idiopathic gastric volvulus is relatively rare in children.[3,11]

Type 2—Secondary Gastric Volvulus in Presence of Associated Anomalies

Associated anomalies include ;
1. Congenital diaphragmatic hernia,[3,12,13]
2. Traumatic diaphragmatic hernia[14]

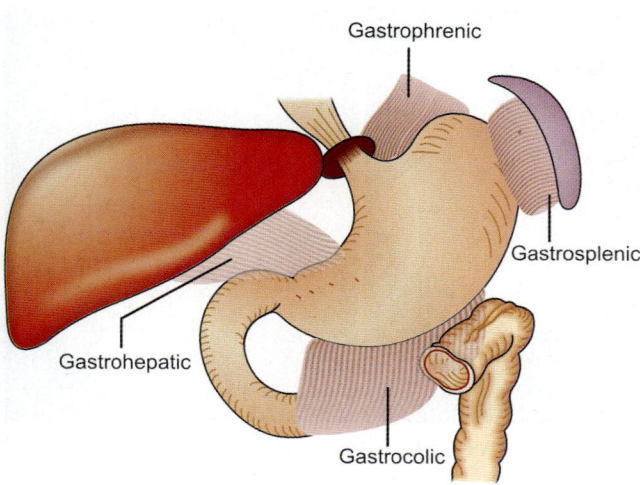

Fig. 50.1: Normal ligamentous attachments of the stomach

3. Eventration of the diaphragm[15]
4. Wandering spleen[12,16]
5. Asplenia-polysplenia syndromes[17]
6. Parahiatal hernia[18,19]
7. Morgagni hernia[20]
8. Hypertrophic pyloric stenosis in an infant.[21,22]

Miller et al reviewed the anatomic defects associated with this type of gastric volvulus, as diaphragmatic defects - 43% Gastric ligaments - 32% Abnormal attachments, adhesions, or bands - 9% Asplenism - 5% small and large bowel malformations - 4% Pyloric stenosis - 2% Colonic distension - 1% Rectal atresia - 1%.[1] There may be a combination of associated anomalies.[12]

CLINICAL PRESENTATION

Gastric volvulus has been described as acute or chronic depending upon the mode of presentation. The symptoms depend on the degree and rapidity of twisting. Symptoms may range from mild abdominal pain and vomiting, when no or partial outlet obstruction is present, to severe pain and retching, when there is complete obstruction and ischemia. Chronic gastric volvulus is more common than acute gastric volvulus.[4]

The gastric volvulus in children is usually associated with other anomalies and is thus secondary.[23] The most common association is with diaphragmatic hernia and thus the volvulus is intrathoracic. Intrathoracic gastric volvulus usually presents in infancy.[24] Intrathoracic gastric volvulus may present as an acute case or as a chronic case.[25]

In chronic cases, the patient may complain of non-specific symptoms, intermittent episodes of abdominal pain, abdominal fullness following meals and dysphagia. The child with chronic type of gastric volvulus may present with recurrent chest infections and weight loss There are few abdominal signs because the stomach is in the thorax. Chronic volvulus may be detected incidentally on plain chest radiographs or on upper gastrointestinal (GI) series.

Acute Intrathoracic gastric volvulus manifests as sharp chest pain radiating to the back and rarely dyspnea. Occasionally, some patients present with hematemesis secondary to mucosal ischemia and sloughing. This can rapidly progress to hypovolemic shock from loss of blood and fluids. Acute intra-abdominal gastric volvulus presents as the sudden onset of severe epigastric or left upper quadrant pain. In acute cases, the child may present with symptoms of acute intestinal obstruction.[1] A case of perforated stomach may present with pyoperitoneum.[1] In a series, 8 cases with organoaxial volvulus had presented with acute apnea associated with pallor, cyanosis, and hypotonia.[5]

The typical features described in adults include Borchardt's triad of epigastric pain, retching with no vomiting, and difficulty or failure to pass a nasogastric tube as an acute presentation.[26,27] These are however not seen frequently in children. None of the patients in a series of 18 patients had Borchardt's triad.[4] When acute GV in children fails to exhibit the full gamut of Borchardt's triad, the diagnosis may be delayed.[4] Upper GI series can be diagnostic during an acute attack.

COMPLICATIONS

Gastric volvulus may be complicated with ulceration, perforation, hemorrhage, pancreatic necrosis, omental avulsion and rarely splenic rupture.[28]

Organoaxial volvulus is more commonly associated with strangulation. Because of the rich vascular supply of the stomach, strangulation occurs in only 5-28% of cases Increased pressure within the hernia sac associated with gastric distension can lead to the ischemia, necrosis and perforation.[29] Gastric perforation can result in sepsis and cardiovascular collapse.

INVESTIGATIONS

Plain Radiograph

Plain radiograph may suggest the diagnosis of gastric volvulus which can be confirmed with a contrast study. A single large air-fluid level or a single bubble without additional bowel gas seen on plain abdominal radiography may indicate gastric volvulus.[30] A retrocardiac gas-filled viscus in cases of intrathoracic stomach confirms the diagnosis. The diaphragm should be seen for evidence of any herniation or eventration. Bilateral eventration of the diaphragm with perforated gastric volvulus in an adolescent has been reported.[15] Pneumoperitoneum should be looked for as an evidence of perforation. If a nasogastric tube is passed, it may be seen to coil at the esophagogastric junction that may be inferior to its normal location.[1] Plain radiographic findings that are suggestive of gastric volvulus should be confirmed with a barium study.

Ultrasonography

The ultrasonographic features consist of a constricted segment of stomach, with 2 dilated segments located above and below the constricted part, akin to a peanut. However, most report normal findings on ultrasonography, thus an upper GI series should be used to confirm the diagnosis if suspected.

Contrast Studies

If barium moves past the esophagogastric junction, the upside-down configuration of the stomach and the degree of obstruction can be documented organoaxial volvulus is demonstrated as reversal of greater and lesser curvatures with two air fluid levels.[31] In mesentericoaxial volvulus, the stomach may be seen in inverted position with pyloroantral obstruction showing a beaked appearance.

The combination of an abdominal radiograph and upper gastrointestinal contrast study usually allows an unequivocal diagnosis in all cases.[32] The barium study is highly sensitive and specific for gastric volvulus (Figs 50.2A and B). However, the diagnosis

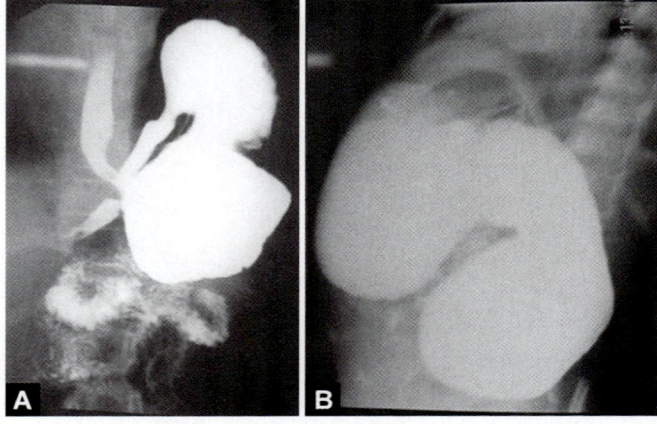

Figs 50.2A and B: Barium meal swallow depicting gastric volvulus

may be missed in cases of intermittent torsion. The upper GI series may show only a paraesophageal hernia or eventration of the diaphragm during a symptom-free interval, leading to a false-negative diagnosisA study has demonstrated the peanut sign on ultrasonography in a case of chronic gastric volvulus.

Other Investigations

The computed tomography (CT) scanning and magnetic resonance imaging (MRI) appearance of gastric volvulus can be variable. The extent of diaphragmatic herniation, the points of torsion, and the final position of the stomach determine the appearance (Figs 50.3A and B).

Gastric volvulus may be discovered during scintigraphic examination for chronic GI bleeding, sometimes incidentally, as an intrathoracic stomach with the greater curvature superior to the lesser curvature. Similarly angiography for massive or refractory GI hemorrhage has shown displaced gastroepiploic arteries are high beneath the left hemidiaphragm in gastric volvulus. The angiographic appearance is sensitive and specific during an acute episode.

Fiberoptic endoscopy has a limited role in the diagnosis of gastric volvulus because the twist precludes passage of the endoscope. Laboratory studies are generally unrewarding, although levels of amylase and alkaline phosphatase may be increased.

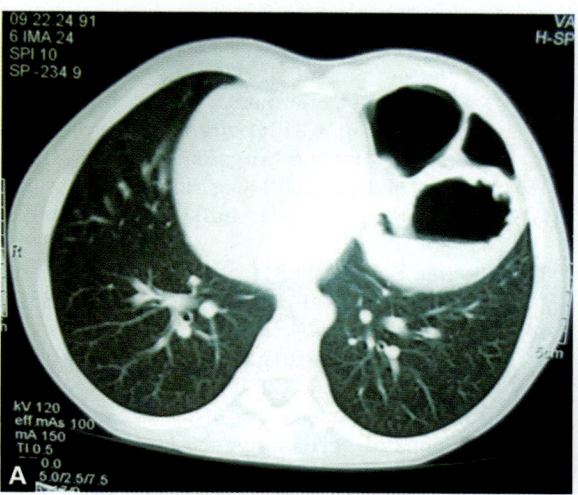 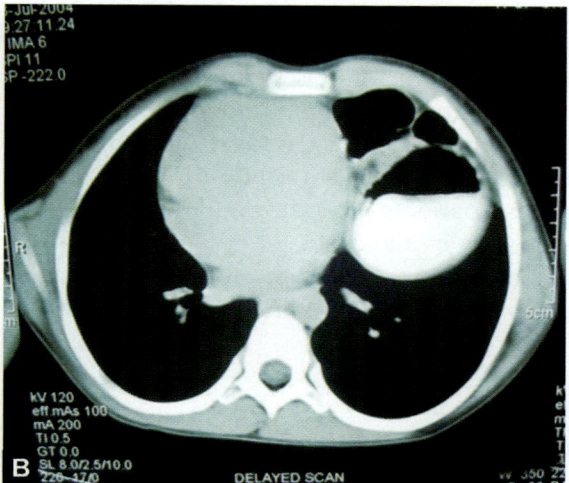

Figs 50.3A and B: **A.** CT scan chest **B.** abdomen, depictive of gastric volvulus with air fluid level and stomach shadow in the chest

DIFFERENTIAL DIAGNOSIS

In acute gastric volvulus, the differential diagnosis includes acute gastric dilatation, gastric outlet obstruction like prepyloric mass and pyloric web, perforated peptic ulcer, ruptured gallbladder.[33]

MANAGEMENT

Reduction of acute gastric volvulus may be attempted with nasogastric decompression though it is often unsuccessful. Nonsurgical treatment has been described for primary gastric volvulus by few authors but secondary gastric volvulus needs immediate surgical intervention to minimize the risk of infection and perforation which may lead to mortality.[28] The treatment for chronic idiopathic gastric volvulus may be based on the age at diagnosis, the severity of symptoms, and how patients are expected to comply with conservative measures.[4]

Emergent surgical intervention is indicated for acute gastric volvulus. With chronic gastric volvulus, surgery is performed to prevent complications.

Although the treatment of gastric volvulus is surgical, endoscopic reduction can be attempted in selected patients of acute and chronic cases with multiple comorbid conditions who are poor candidates for surgery. The scope is advanced beyond the point of torsion, then rotated to untwist the stomach. However, there is a risk of gastric perforation and should not be attempted in patients who appear to have vascular compromise. Failure to reduce the twist necessitates surgery. Percutaneous endoscopic gastrostomy can be performed after reduction of the volvulus to reduce the incidence of recurrence. Some authors argue that surgical intervention is necessary in these cases only when endoscopic management fails or when the volvulus recurs.

Surgical goals of treatment include:
1. Reduction of the volvulus
2. Prevention of recurrence
3. Repair of predisposing factors.

Most cases of acute and chronic gastric volvulus can now be approached laparoscopically. A combined laparoscopic and endoscopic approach has also been used to better assess the intraluminal and intra-abdominal status of the stomach as well as its position before, during, and after fixation.

Laparoscopy assisted anterior gastropexy may be performed to fix the stomach in its anatomically correct position.[5,34] Some authors feel that routine gastropexy for all patients with a radiologic diagnosis of gastric volvulus is not mandatory.[32] Prophylactic gastropexy should be mandatory in patients developmental anomalies of the ligamentous connections.[16]

Gastrostomy may be done in older children with adequate stomach size to prevent recurrence, help in decompression and for feeding later on.[1] An anterior gastropexy with associated antireflux fundoplication may be performed.[5] Diaphragmatic defects may be repaired. Plication of the diaphragm and gastropexy is needed for cases associated with eventration of the diaphragm.[15]

Patients with signs of acute peritonitis are better explored through a midline laparotomy incision. Partial or total gastrectomy is required in the setting of necrosis. Peritoneal lavage is done for cases with gastric perforation after gastrectomy of the involved segment or repair of the perforation. The healing is poor in these patients after strangulation and a re-exploration may be required.

Gastric decompression with either a nasogastric tube or gastrostomy is maintained until the return of bowel function.

MORTALITY

The mortality rate for acute gastric volvulus is reportedly 42-56% in general with a nonoperative mortality as high as 80%. The patients have a higher mortality if gastric perforation has occurred. Almost the whole stomach is ischaemic with poor healing after gastrectomy.[1] The mortality rate for chronic gastric volvulus is 10-13%.

REFERENCES

1. Sharma S, Gopal SC. Gastric volvulus with perforation in association with congenital diaphragmatic hernia. Indian J Pediatr 2004;71:948-48.
2. Miller DC, Pasquale MD, Seneca RP, et al. Gastric volvulus in the pediatric population. Arch Surg 1991;126:1146-49.
3. Honna T, Kamii Y, Tsuchiada Y. Idiopathic gastric volvulus in infancy and childhood. J Pediatr Surg 1991;25:707-10.
4. Chang SW, Lee HC, Yeung CY, et al. Gastric volvulus in children. Acta Paediatr Taiwan 2006;47(1):18-24.
5. Darani A, Mendoza-Sagaon M, Reinberg O. Gastric volvulus in children. J Pediatr Surg 2005;40:855-58.
6. Okada K, Miyako M, Honma S, et al. Discharge diagnoses in infants with apparent life-threatening event. Pediatr Int 2003;45:560-63.
7. Berti A. Singulare attortigliamento dele' esofago col duodeno seguita da rapida morte. Gazz Med Ital 1866;9:139.
8. Borchardt M. Aus Pathologie und therapie des magenvolvulus. Arch klin Chir 1904;74:243.
9. Cameron AEP, Howard ER. Gastric volvulus in childhood. J Pediatr Surg 1987;22:944-47.
10. Cole B, Dickinson SJ. Acute volvulus of the stomach in infants. Surgery 1971;70:707-17.
11. Ratan SK, Grover SB. Acute idiopathic mesenteroaxial gastric volvulus in a child. Trop Gastroenterol 2000;21:133-34.
12. Pelizzo G, Lembo MA, Fvanchalla A, et al. Gastric volvulus associated with congenital diaphragmatic hernia, wandering spleen abdomino-thoracic left kidney: CT findings. Abdom Imaging 2001;26:306-68.
13. Kotobi H, Auber F, Otta E, et al. Acute mesenteroaxial gastric volvulus and congenital diaphragmatic hernia. Pediatr Surg Int 2005;21(8):674-76. Epub 2005 Jul 9.
14. Kohli A, Vij A, Azad T. Inrathoracic gastric volvulus - acute and chronic presentation. J Indian Med Assoc 1997;95:522-23.
15. Oh A, Gulati G, Sherman ML, et al. Bilateral eventration of the diaphragm with perforated gastric volvulus in an adolescent. J Pediatr Surg 2000;35(12):1824-26.
16. Spector JM, Chappell J. Gastric volvulus associated with wandering spleen in a child. J Pediatr Surg 2000;35(4):641-42.
17. Aoyama K, Tateishi K. Gastric volvulus in three children with asplenic syndrome. J Pediatr Surg 1986;21:307-10.
18. Chattopadhyay A, Prakash B, Vijayakumar, et al. Parahiatal hernia with gastric obstruction in a child. Indian J Gastroenterol 2003;22:107-08.
19. Samujh R, Kumar D, Rao KL. Paraesophageal hernia in the neonatal period: suspicion on chest X-ray. Indian Pediatr 2004;41(2):189-91.
20. Estevão-Costa J, Soares-Oliveira M, Correia-Pinto J, et al. Acute gastric volvulus secondary to a Morgagni hernia Pediatr Surg Int 2000;16(1-2):107-08.
21. Anagnostara A, Koumanidou C, Vakaki M, et al. Chronic gastric volvulus and hypertrophic pyloric stenosis in an infant. J Clin Ultrasound 2003;31(7):383-86.
22. OÄŸuzkurt P, Senocak ME, HiÃ§sÃ¶nmez A. A rare coexistence of two gastric outlet obstructive lesions: infantile hypertrophic pyloric stenosis and organoaxial gastric volvulus. Turk J Pediatr 2000 Jan-Mar;42(1):87-89.
23. Youssef SA, Di Lorenzo M, Yazbeck S, et al. Gastric volvulus in children. Chir Pediatr 1987;28:39-42.
24. Al Salem AH. Intrathoracic gastric volvulus in infancy. Pediatric Radiology 2000;30(12):842-45.
25. Kohli A, Vij A, Azad T. Inrathoracic gastric volvulus-acute and chronic presentation. J Indian Med Assoc 1997;95:522-23.
26. Carter R, Brewer 3rd LA, Hinshaw DB. Acute gastric volvulus. A study of 25 cases. Am J Surg 1980;140:99-106.
27. Llaneza PP, Salt WB 2nd. Gastric volvulus. More common than previously thought? Postgrad Med 1986;80(5):279-83, 287-88.
28. Talukder BC. Gastric volvulus with perforation of stomach in congenital diaphragmatic hernia in an infant. J Indian Med Assoc 1979;73:219-21.
29. Farag S, Fiallo V, Nash S, Navab F. Gastric perforation in a case of gastric volvulus. Am J Gastroenterol 1996;91:1863-84.
30. Andiran F, Tanyel FC, Balkanci F, et al. Acute abdomen due to gastric volvulus: diagnostic value of a single plain radiograph. Pediatr Radiol 1995;25 Suppl 1:S240.
31. Park W, Choi S, Suh S. Pediatric gastric volvulus - Experience with 7 cases. J Kor Med Sci 1992;7:258-63.
32. Elhalaby EA, Mashaly EM. Infants with radiologic diagnosis of gastric volvulus: are they over-treated? Pediatr Surg Int 2001;17(8):596-600.
33. Yen JB, Kong MS. Gastric outlet obstruction in pediatric patients. Chang Gung Med J 2006;29(4):401-05.
34. Schleef J, von Bismarck S. An easy method for laparoscopic-assisted percutaneous anterior gastropexy. Surg Endosc 2000;14:964-65.

CHAPTER 51

Gastrointestinal Bleeding

A K Basu, D Basak

Gastrointestinal bleeding (GI bleeding) is a common condition encountered in children. Sometimes it occurs in patients undergoing treatment for other disease. Others present with gastrointestinal bleeding as the first manifestation of an underlying disease. The patient may be vomiting of blood (site of bleeding is usually above the ligament of Treitz) or may be passing blood per anus (site of bleeding is below the duodeno-jejunal flexure). In either situation the blood passed may be fresh or altered. The bleeding may be severe enough to necessitate admission and treatment of hemorrhagic shock before initiating investigations toward a specific etiology and its subsequent treatment. Fortunately in most children the bleeding ceases spontaneously, giving us ample time to investigate and home in on an accurate diagnosis. The search for an etiology is however considerably influenced by the age of the child as is evident from the list of conditions in Table 51.1.[1] For the benefit of readers an empirical approach to diagnosis has however been included in Table 51.2.

GI BLEEDING IN THE PEDIATRIC POPULATION—AN OVERVIEW

As stressed above, the approach to children with GI bleeding is distinct in different age groups. Certain underlying similarities however can not be overlooked. Questioning the parents on the amount of blood loss, assessing the vital parameters and hemoglobin estimation are essential in gauging the hemodynamic status of the child. If bleeding is severe and is estimated to be greater than 15% of the blood volume then resuscitation must precede investigation for specific diagnosis. A patient in shock is initially treated with crystalloids like Lactated Ringer's solution followed by blood or packed cell transfusion depending on the hemoglobin level and the hematocrit. Once the patient's hemodynamics gets stabilized, investigations are initiated toward a specific etiology (Table 51.2) and the treatment started.

In a newborn, assessment of the coagulation status for bleeding disorders, Roentgenogram of the abdomen for NEC or volvulus neonatorum, examination of the perineum for anal fissure and examination of stool to exclude infective diarrhea are useful.

In infants and older children upper or lower GI endoscopy, Roentgenogram of the abdomen for intestinal abstruction or isotope tagged RBC scans are useful. Angiography becomes imperative in patients where the site of bleeding remains elusive in spite of the usual imaging investigations. In some patients, endoscopy of the upper or lower GI is performed on the operation table and sometimes passage of the endoscope through the enterotomy wound becomes necessary.

GI BLEEDING IN NEONATES

A newborn with GI bleeding having history of perinatal stress may be suffering from *erosive gastritis*. A newborn being treated for septicemia may develop GI bleeding as a consequence of *consumptive coagulopathy* (or DIC). Bleeding from the GI tract along with bleeding from sites in an otherwise normal newborn may be due to *hemorrhagic disease of the newborn.*[2] It is impotant to enquire about administration of vitamin K to the newborn. *Maternal*

Table 51.1: Etiology of GI bleeding in the pediatric population

I. Neonates
   A. Upper GI
      - Erosive gastritis
      - Hemorrhagic disorders
      - Swallowed maternal blood
      - Trauma during nasogastric tube insertion
   B. Lower GI
      - Necrotising enterocolitis (NEC)
      - Anal Fissure
      - Malrotation with volvulus
      - Infective diarrhea
      - Following P/R examination

II. Infants
   A. Upper GI
      - Esophagitis
      - Gastritis
      - Infantile Hypertrophic Pyloric Stenosis (IHPS)
   B. Lower GI
      - Anal fissure
      - Intussusception
      - Gangrene of bowel
      - Infective diarrhea
      - Intestinal duplication
      - Intestinal polyps (rarely)

III. Older Children
   A. Upper GI
      - Peptic ulcer disease
      - Portal hypertension
      - Arterio-venous malformation
      - Tropical jejunitis
      - Drug induced
   B. Lower GI
      - Meckel's diverticulum or duplication
      - Polyps
      - Juvenile polyposis coli
      - Peutz-Jeghers syndrome
      - Familial adenomatous polyposis
      - Helminthiasis
      - Trauma
      - Infective diarrhea
      - Tuberculosis, amebiasis
      - Henoch-Schonlein purpura
      - Angiomatous malformations
      - Tumors

Table 51.2: Approach to a child with gastrointestinal bleeding

- Nasogastric tube
- Examination of abdomen for features of peritonitis or lump anorectal examination
- Platelet count, bleeding time, coagulation profile (P time, aPT time), (Ap test to detect maternal blood in gut of newborn)
- Plain abdominal roentgenogram
- Upper GI contrast study (barium or soluble contrast),
- Upper GI endoscopy
- Tc 99m isotope tagged RBC Scan (Fig. 51.1)
- Lower GI contrast study (barium or soluble contrast),
- Lower GI endoscopy (Figs 51.2 and 51.3)
- Selective angiography
- Laparoscopy/Laparotomy
- Per operative endoscopy

intake of drugs like sulphonamides may interfere with vitamin K absorption in newborn or cause derangement of livere function and lead to bleeding in newborn. When coagulopathy is suspected in a newborn assessment of the bleeding time and coagulation profile (prothrombin time and activated partial thromboplastin time) is advised. Ap. test is performed to detect *maternal blood in the newborn's vomitus*. A change in the color of a sample of vomitus following treatment with sodium hydroxide, confirms the presence of maternal blood.

Saline lavage (a cold saline lavage may cause hypothermia) antacid, H_2 receptor antagonists (1-3 mg/kg/day over 4 days), coating agents like sucralfate usually cures erosive gastritis. If continuous bleeding lowers the hemoglobin level to below 12 g/dL fresh blood should be transfused immediately. In patient with septicemia, a proper microbiological screen is instituted and appropriate antibiotic administered.

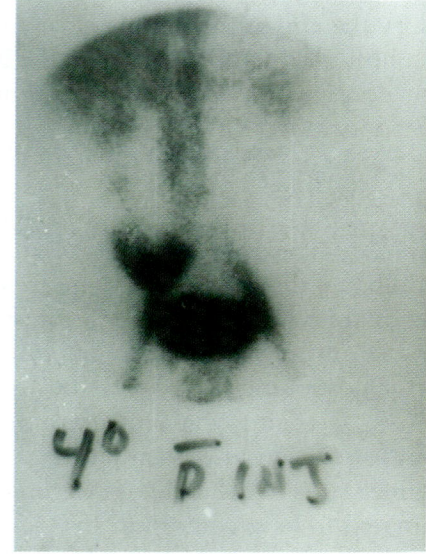

Fig. 51.1: Technetium scan showing ectopic gastric mucosa

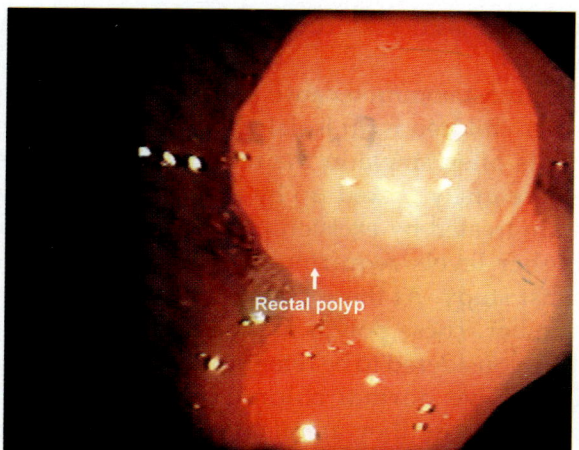

Fig. 51.2: Pedunculated rectal polyp

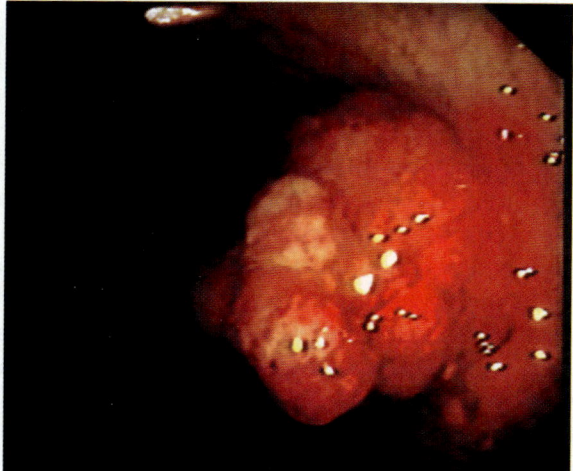

Fig. 51.3: Sessile adenomatous polyp of colon

An upper GI bleed of more than 20 ml of blood is sufficient for the appearance of altered blood in stool. A patient *with malrotation of gut with volvulus* will have bilious vomiting with altered blood per anum. The vomitus may also contain blood. A straight radiogram of the abdomen will show a paucity of gas in the bowels. Treatment of midgut volvulus requires urgent resuscitation and prompt laparotomy for division of the Ladd's bands (the Ladd's procedure). Contrary to popular belief anal fissures can result following either losse motion or constipation. Stools are streaked with blood. Nappies may be spotted. The treatment includes regulation of stool to normal soft consistency and local application of anesthetics.[3]

In **NEC** the sool is mixed with blood, which may be altered or bright red. There is more often than not, a history of perinatal stress. Features of septicemia may be obvious. Early in the disease the abdomen will be tender. As the disease progresses, features of peritonitis appear. Investigations include full septic screening and straight radiogram fo the abdomen to detect the presence of gas in the bowel wall (pneumatosis intestinalis), gas in the protal vein or pneumoperitonium appear.

GI BLEEDING IN INFANTS

Infants with **IHPS** rarely present with blood tinged vomiting.[4] They usually present with nonbilious vomiting, show visible gastric peristalsis and may have a palpable pyloric tumor. Ultrasonography has been very helpful in the diagnosis of pyloric tumors, which are not clinically palpable. Straight radiogram of the abdomen or contrast study of the upper gastrointestinal tract are rarely necessary to demonstrate gastric hold up or string hold up or string sign at the pylorus. The treatment is surgery following resuscitation.

Another cause of nonbilious vomiting mixed with streaks of blood is *Reflux esophagitis*. Upper GI contrast study, esophageal pH monitoring, esophageal manometry, technetium milk scanning and perhaps endoscopy help in reaching a diagnosis. Treatment consists of antacids, thickening of feeds, maintenance of upright posture, small frequent feeds and prokinetic agents. Rarely antireflux surgery is necessary.[5,6]

An important cause of lower GI bleeding between 2 months and 2 years is *intussusception*. Prior to bleeding which is classically described as "red current jelly", the child has episodic abdominal pain. A sausage shaped lump in the abdomen is easily palpable. Ultrasonography examination is of great help in the diagnosis of a lump in the restless child. Single or double contrast enema study also helps in diagnosis and treatment of the condition. Cases in which hydrostatic reduction fails, surgery is necessary.[5]

In tropical countries infants often present with *infective dysentery*. In such cases, stool is mixed with blood and mucus. Such a patient will have no feature of intestinal obstruction. Stool examination and culture will help in diagnosis and treatment.

GI BLEEDING IN OLDER CHILDREN

Peptic ulcers: in older children can develop acutely following burns (Curling's ulcer) head injury

(Cushing's ulcer), malignancy and sepsis. They are promptly diagnosed by endoscopy and treated with cold saline lavage, antacid, H_2 receptor antagonists and treatment of the primary disease. They rarely require surgery.[1]

Erosive gastritis: following ingestion of drugs is another cause of massive upper GI bleeding in children. Such bleeds may be fatal. Prompt diagnosis is possible by eliciting a history of drug intake and performing endoscopy. Treatment follows the principles of peptic ulcer management. The offending drug must be identified and withdrawn.

Portal hypertension: in children can cause alarming upper GI bleeding in children. The common causes of portal hypertension in our country are extrahepatic portal obstruction, non-cirrhotic portal fibrosis and biliary or postnecrotic cirrhosis. Patients usually present with massive bleeds and have a palpable spleen. Upper GI endoscopy will confirm the diagnosis. Ultrasonography, Doppler study of portal circulation and splenoportovenogram help in diagnosing the site of obstruction and size of the portal vein. Present day therapy include variceal sclerotherapy, banding or injection of gel foam. Rarely, surgery for devascularization or shunting the portal blood into the systemic circulation is performed.

Arterio-venous malformation: in the stomach or in the intestine can give rise to alarming bleeding. Diagnosis may be made by isotope tagged RBC scan or by angiography. At operation the mesentery adjacent to the malformation is usually abnormal.[7,8]

Tropical jejunitis: is a disease of tropical countries. Patients of tropical jejunitis present with features of intestinal obstruction and GI bleeding. At laparotomy segments of small intestine are found to be in various stages of necrosis.

Patients with *Meckel's diverticulum:* have episodic, maroon colored massive bleeding. The diverticulum is lined by ectopic gastric mucosa. Acid secreted from the ectopic mucosa cause peptic ulcer on the adjacent alkaline mucosa. Similar bleeding can occur in patients or tubular duplication containing ectopic gastric mucosa. Such patients are usually older. At times a tender spot can be found in the abdomen. In 90% of cases the diverticulum can be picked up by Tc 99m Pertechnitate scan.[9,10] Wedge resection of the diverticulum is performed if the adjacent ileum is healthy. Resection and anastomosis with adjacent ileum becomes necessary when the adjacent bowel is abnormal.

The most common cause (80%) of rectal bleeding in older children is an isolated rectal polyp. A rectal polyp is often single in the rectum in 40% of cases. They are easily picked up by per rectal examination and are treated by excision. Some polyps may occur at higher levels requiring colonoscopy or double contrast study. At these polyps may be two or three in number. These polyps are inflammatory in origin and are considered to be retention polyps. Since, these polyps have normal colonic tissue arranged in haphazard way they are also regarded as hamartomatus polyps.[11] Polyps can easily be removed during sigmoidoscopy or colonscopy. If the polyps are more than five in number, periodic colonoscopic surveillance is mandatory.

Juvenile polyposis syndrome is an uncommon condition and can occur in infancy or in older children. These patients present with features of rectal bleeding and protein loosing enteropathy. Morphologically these polyps resemble juvenile polyps but are multiple in number and can involve the entire GI tract. In older children the involvement may be limited to varying portions of the colon and rectum. In localized disease, limited resection of the colorectum and regular colonoscopic surveillance is an option. Some authors recommend prophylactic colectomy, mucosal resection of the rectum and ileoanal anastomosis.[12]

Patients of *Peutz-Jeghers syndrome* have hamartomatous (hamartoma of muscularis mucosae) polyps in the intestine along with pigmentations around buccal mucosa, conjunctiva and rectal mucosa (Fig. 51.4).[13] They are most commonly found in the small intestine (Fig. 51.5).[14] It has an autosomal dominant inheritance. Patients may present with colicky abdominal pain, features of intestinal obstruction or anemia. Patients with this syndrome may develop intestinal and extra-intestinal malignancies. Such patients need regular follow-up to detect signs of early malignancy. If a laprotomy is performed, conservative surgery for intestinal obstruction along with intraoperative endoscopic removal of larger polyps is the preferred mode of treatment.[1] Rarely a *lymphoid polyp* in young children present with recurrent severe bleeding. They are usually diagnosed by colonoscopy and require surgery.

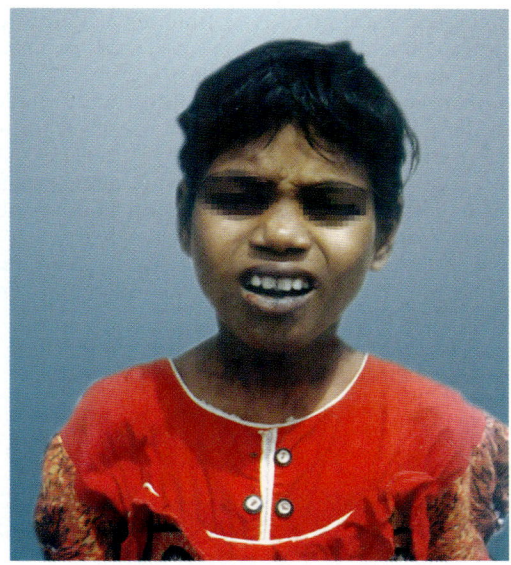

Fig. 51.4: Perioral pigmentation in a patient of Peutz-Jeghers syndrome

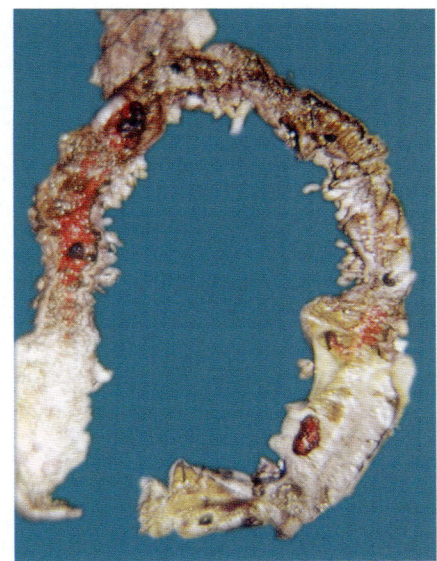

Fig. 51.5: Jejunal polyps in the patient in Fig. 51.4

Familial adenomatous polyps usually involve colon and rectum of patients in their teens. It has autosomal dominant transmission and the patients develop cancer of colon at an early age. There is a deletion in the long arm of chromosome.[5] The polyps can occur anywhere from stomach to anus.[15] Patients present with diarrhea, bleeding per rectum and anemia. Many patients are diagnosed during surveillance of relatives of diagnosed patients. The investigations are the same as for juvenile polyposis syndrome. Total colectomy with rectal mucosectomy and ileoanal pull though with or without a reservoir is the preferred method of treatment in all symptomatic patients. All these patients need regular endoscopic follow-up.[16]

Some recent publications mention *hookworm infestation* as a cause of massive gastrointestinal bleeding.[17] In tropical countries *amoebic colitis and tuberculosis* of large gut may present with recurrent severe bleeding. Repeated stool examination for parasites and acid fast bacillus is necessary to arrive at a correct diagnosis. Colonscopic biopsy also helps in the diagnosis. Medical treatment with anthelmenthics, antiamoebic and anti tubercular drugs is usually sufficient to control the bleeding.

REFERENCES

1. Aresman RM. gastrointestinal Bleeding in Pediatric Surgery 5th ed. O Neill JA, Roww MI, Grosfeld JL (Eds), Mosby 1998;1253-56.
2. Lulseged S. Hemorrhagic disease of the newborn: overview of 127 cases. Ann Trop Pediatr 1993;13:331.
3. Berman W, Holtzapple P. Gastrointestinal hemorrhage. Pediatr Clin North Am 1975;23:885.
4. Spitz L, Batcup G. Haematemesis in infantile hypertrophic polyric stenosis: the source of bleeding. Br J Surg 1979;66:827.
5. Forkalsrud E, et al. A combined hospital experience with fundoplication and gatric emptying procedure for gastro-esophageal reflux in children. J Am Coll Surg 1995;180:445.
6. Raffensprger J, Luck S. Gastrointestinal bleeding in children. Surg. Clin North Am 1976;56:413.
7. Mitra SK, et al. Side to side splenorenal shunt without splenectomy in noneirrhotic portal hypertension in children. J Pediatr Surg 1993;28:398.
8. Orloff MJ, Orlaff MS, Rambotti M. Treatment of Bleeding oesphagogastric various due to extrahepatic hypertension: results of portal-systemic shunts during 35 years. J Pediatr Surg 1994;29:142.
9. Duszynski D. Jewett T, Alba J. 99 mTc Na partechnetate scanning of the abdomen with particular reference to small bowel pathology. Am J Roentgenol Radium Ther Nucel Med 1971;113:258.
10. Sfakinanakis C, Conway J. Detection of ectopic gastric mucosa in Meckel's Divarticulum and in other aberrations

by scintigraphy. II Indication and methods – a – 10 year experience. J Nucl Med 1981;22:732.
11. Morson BC. Some peculiarities in the histology of intestinal polyps. Dis colon Rectum 1962;5:337.
12. Jass JR. Juvenile polyposis. In Philips RKS, et al. Editors: Familial adenomatous poyposis and other polyposis syndrome, Boston, 1994, Little Brown.
13. Jeghers H, McCusicx VA, Katz KH. Generalized intestinal polyposis and melanin spots of the oral mucosa, lips and digits: a syndrome of diagnostic significance. N Engl J Med 1949;241:1031.
14. Trovar JA, Eizaguirre AA, Jimenez J. Peutz-Jeghers syndrome in children: report of two cases and review of the literature. J Pediatr Surg 1983;18:1.
15. Domizio P, et al. Upper gastrointestinal pathology in familial adenomatous polyposis: results from a prospective study of 102 pateints. J Clin Pathol 1990;43:738.
16. Berger A, et al. Excision of rectum with colonic J pouchanal anastomision for adenocarcinoma of the low and mid-rectum. World J Surg 1992;16:470.
17. Kumar J, Jiwane AV, Kathari P. Massive gastrointestinal bleeding in an infant: A diagnostic dilemma. J Ind Ass Pediatr Surg 2001;6: 112-14.

Idiopathic Primary Intussusception

Essam El-Sahwi

DEFINITION

Intussusception means telescoping of one segment of the gastrointestinal track into the other, usually the proximal segment goes into the distal.

Intussusception is the most common cause of intestinal obstruction in children under the age of two. The most frequent occurrence of intussusception is in midsummer and midwinter. The ratio of males to females is 3:1. The peak is seen in an infant 5-9 months of age and 80% of patients are under the age of two.[1,2]

TYPES

The terminal ileum usually telescopes into the right colon producing the following types of intussusception:

Ileocolic, ileo-ileocolic, or colocolic, may occur if the right colon goes into the transverse colon, or cecocolic if the cecum invaginates in the ascending colon.[3]

ETIOLOGY

Primary Intussusception

In 95% of infants and children, primary intussusception has no obvious cause. Some factors incriminated include
A- Disordered peristalsis due to weaning.
B- Preceding attack of gastroenteritis.
C- Adenovirus infections leading to hypertrophy of the Peyer's patches which act as a leading point in intussusception.
D- Mobile ileocecal junction.
E- Long bloodless fold of Treves.

Secondary Intussusception

- In a minority of cases, intussusception is secondary to an obvious cause such as Meckel's diverticulum, submucons lipoma. Inverted appendix or polyps, intramural hematoma (Henoch-Schoenlein purpura), or intestinal lymphoma.[3]

PATHOLOGY

The mass of intussusception is composed of the following layers: entering layer and returning layer which constitute the (intussusceptum), and the receiving layer (the intussuscipiens). Early in the disease, the intestine is viable, but if the case is neglected, the bowel becomes gangrenous due to composition of the blood supply in the squeezed mesentery between the layers of intussuscipiens leading to perforation and peritonitis.[1]

CLINICAL PICTURE

It is imperative to differentiate intussusception into early and late cases, as this will have clinical, and therapeutic implications.[1] Intussusception may present as an emergency or even in postoperative cases.[4,5]

Symptoms

Early Cases

Intermittent colicky pain in a previously healthy robust active baby. The exception is a child with cystic fibrosis, Henoch-Schonlein purpura who may fail to thrive. Pain may cause the baby to draw his legs up to the Abdomen. Pallor and sweating are seen during the attack of pain. Reflex vomiting (nonbilious) is a

582 Pediatric Surgery—Diagnosis and Management

frequent early sign and is due to traction on the mesentery dragged by intussusception. Passage of blood or mucus unmixed with stools per rectum is a common symptom.

Neglected Cases

In neglected cases prolonged ischemia produce infarction of the bowel with subsequent peritonitis, and abdominal distension absolute constipation, and cessation of passage of blood per rectum. Vomiting is copious and might be feculent.

Signs

Early Cases

Pallor and sweating are common signs during the attack of colicky pains palpable sausage shape mass many be felt in the different quadrant of the abdomen palpation of the right iliac fossa palpation feels empty (sign D'ance). Rectal examination will reveal the passage of blood and mucus on withdrawal of the finger.

Neglected Cases

On physical examination, the abdomen is often distended, the right lower quadrant may feel empty, and a sausage -shaped mass may be palpable in the upper right to midabdomen (65%). The apex intussusception can sometimes be palpated on rectal examination (Figs 52.1A and B). The child is often febrile, and the blood count may show a leukocytosis. (A diagnostic barium enema may demonstrate the intussusception with a coil-spring sign at the point of bowel invagination).

The general condition deteriorates due to electrolyte imbalance and peritonitis.

INVESTIGATIONS

In early cases, sonography is helpful in the diagnosis of intussusception 75% of the cases (Target sign) (Figs 52.2A to D).

In doubtful cases, barium enema will show obstruction of the flow of the barium and the typical meniscus sign or cobra head sign (Figs 52.3A and B). Only in late cases plain X-ray anteroposterior and decubitus radiographs of the abdomen may demonstrate dilated loops of small intestine, air-fluid levels, or a soft tissue mass in the right upper quadrant.

Plan X-ray anteroposterior and decubitus films will show absence of intestinal gases from the ileocoecal junction, also it may visualize the soft tissue shadow of the mass of the intussusception.

TREATMENT

An infant with intussusception is managed by insertion of a nasogastric tube, intravenous fluid resuscitation, and antibiotics. After rehydration, the child is taken to the radiology suit for an attempted hydrostatic reduction of the intussusception under sonographic guidance.[6]

A sedative should be administered prior to the examination once hypovolemia has been corrected. The surgical staff should be in attendance for the attempted reduction, with the anesthesiologist and

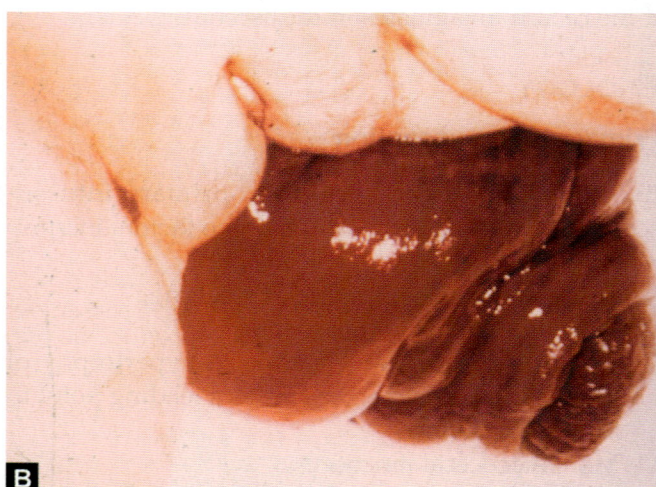

Figs 52.1A and B: Intussusception presenting as mass protruding from the rectum

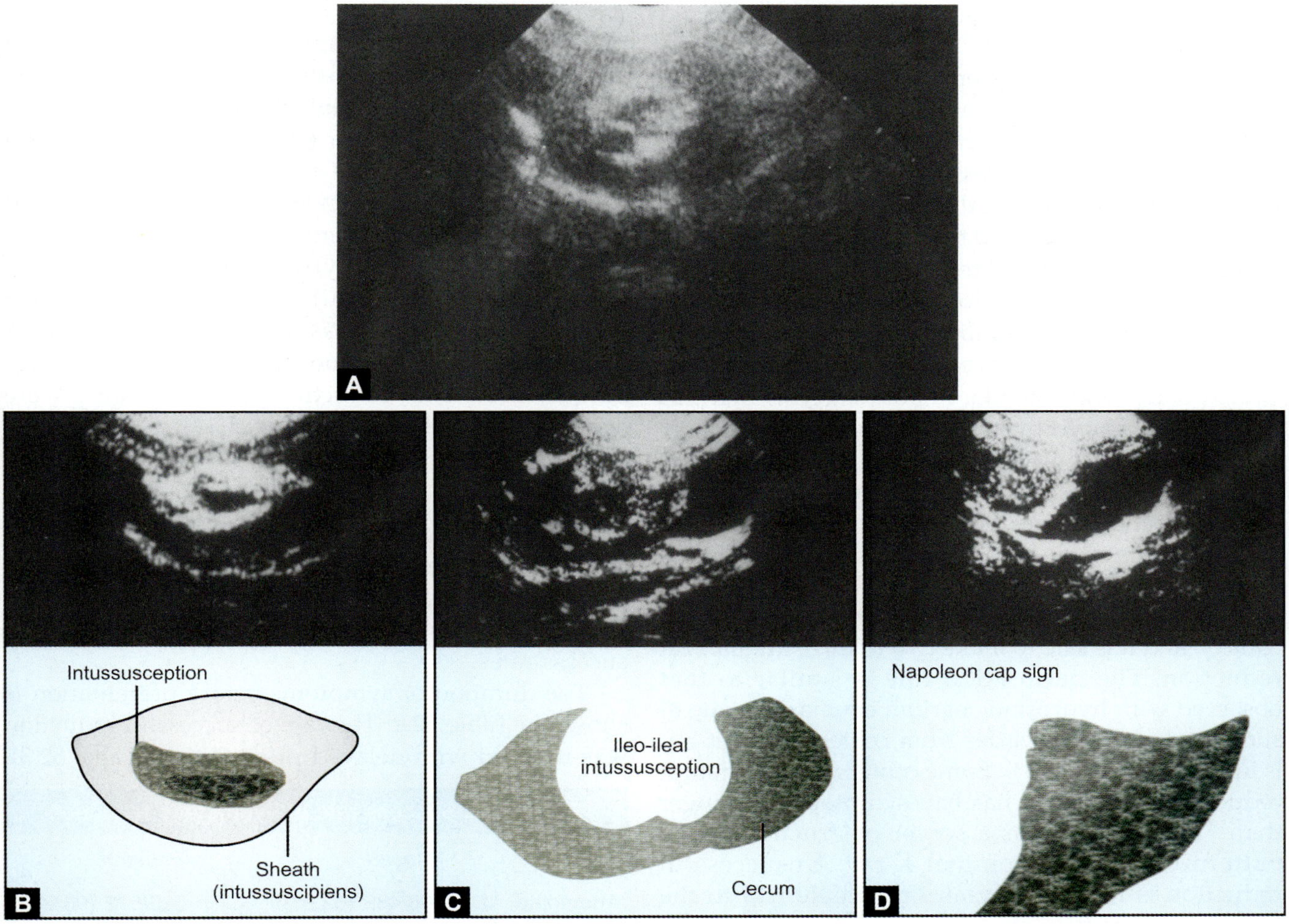

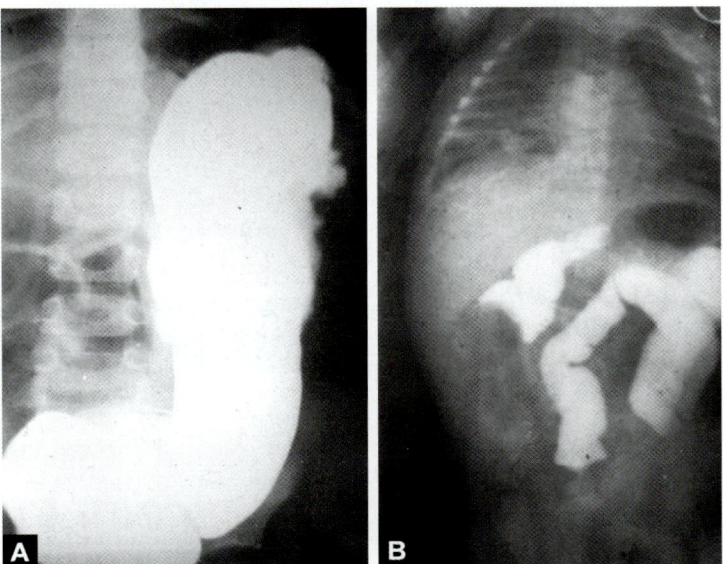

Figs 52.2A to D: A. Ultrasonography depicting the typical target sign suggestive of intussusception, **B to D.** Ultrasonographic findings in intussusception with their diagrammatic representations

Figs 52.3A and B: Barium studies showing the cut-off sign suggestive of intussusception

operation room staff alerted and standing by should reduction be unsuccessful.

Hydrostatic barium enema reduction has been the main stay of non-operative treatment.[7] The enema is performed with 13-foot column and limitation of continuous hydrostatic pressure 5-minute time frames. Reduction is considered satisfactory when the intussusceptum is reduced through the ileocecal valve and the contrast material refluxes into multiple small bowel loops. Air reduction of intussuscption was introduced in a large number of cases in China.

This technique is now commonly performed in the United States and Canada. Report suggests that this technique is as effective as barium enema reduction. The air pressure must be monitored, with a maximum of 110 mm Hg in children and 80 mm Hg in infants. This perforation occurs more commonly in babies less than 6 months of age with symptoms present for more than 3 days.[2]

The procedure is performed under fluoroscopic control, and it is safe to make two to three attempts at reduction. The perforation rate is similar to that observed with hydrostatic barium enema. The rate of successful reduction varies from center to center but is in the range of 50-75%. Some centers do not attempt reduction if the infant has had symptoms for longer than 72 hours and has a server obstructive bowel pattern on plain abdominal X-ray. Unsuccessful reduction is followed by an immediate trip to the operating room.[2]

The Alexandria University Experiment in Hydrostatic Reduction of Intussusception

The study was divided into two 8-years phases for comparison: phase I from 1983 through 1990 and phase II from 1991 through 1998.

During phase I, we started HR under US guidance in 1984 with a small number of cases and generally increased after gaining confidence and experience with the technique. Exclusion criteria from a trial with HR included any of the following :tender abdomen, bilious vomiting , abdominal distension, fluid levels on X-rays films, and age less than 3 months.

Diagnosis and reduction were initially done by the first author- subsequently the technique was taught to pediatric surgical residents routinely. We do not have access to a 24-hour service for barium reduction, however's we had 50 cases during phase I that had undergone a trial of reduction with barium under flouroscopy. The diagnosis was made by finding the typical target appearance in transverse section and the pseudokidney in longitudinal scans. In phase II, in suspicious cases a diagnostic saline enema was given to provide contrast and enhance diagnostic accuracy.

HR was done using a worm saline reservoir at a height of 1 mm above the level of the patient, introduced through a 10-18 Fr Foley catheter after strapping the buttocks, monitoring progress by US (Aloka SSD- 650, Tokyo) with a 5 MHz sector transducer. Cases initially reduced on US (disappearance of the mass) were re-examined after 1 and 4 h for confirmation of reduction. Cases for surgery. Details of reduction and/or surgery were accurately recorded and analyzed.

Results

A total of 489 cases were studied in phase II. The diagnostic accuracy of US in detecting intussusception was 474/489 (96.9 %) in phase I and 572/572 (100%). Table 52.1 shows the details of trials of reduction and success rates.

The duration of symptoms before presentation is shown in Table 52.2. The rate of successful reduction was reduced with delayed presentation (Table 52.3).

Table 52.1: Success rate of hydrostatic reduction

	Phase I	Phase II
Attempted	308/489 (62.9%)	532/572 (93%)
Success	221/308 (71.7%)	457/532 (85.9%)
Unreduced	87	75

Table 52.2: Duration of symptoms

	Phase I	Phase II
<1 day	160 (32.7%)	268 (46.8%)
1-2 days	200 (40.8%)	263 (45.9%)
> days	129 (26.3%)	41 (7%)
Total	489	572

Table 52.3: Relation of reducibility of duration of symptoms

	Phase I	Phase II
<1 day	87/101 (86.1%)	195/205 (95.1%)
1-2 days	97/123 (78.8%)	211/239 (88.2%)
> days	37/84 (44%)	51/88 (57.9%)
Total	221/308 (71.7%)	457/532 (85.9%)

Table 52.4: Analysis of unreduced cases

	Phase I	Phase II
Negative exploration	8 (9%)	3 (4%)
Ileocolic	25 (28.7%)	15 (20%)
Ileo-ileocolic	51 (58.6%)	52 (69.3%)
Total	87	75

Table 52.5: Management of unreduced primary intussusception

	Phase I	Phase II
Difficult simple reduction	57/76 (75%)	46/67 (68.6%)
Ileocolic	19/76 (25%)	21/67 (31.3%)
Resection anastomosis	76	67
Total	489	572

Table 52.6: Complications of hydrostatic reduction

	Phase I	Phase II
Recurrence	19/221 (8.5%)	28/457 (6.1%)
Perforation	3/308 (0.9%)	4/532 (0.7%)
Negative exploration	8/87 (9%)	3/75 (4%)

Unreduced cases were admitted for emergency surgery; the findings ad exploration were recorded in operative records. These ranged between negative explorations where a reduced intussusception was found, indicated by a congested ileum and cecum, primary intussusception, either ileo-colic or ileo-ileocolic, and secondary intussusception, and the cause was reported (Table 52.4) shows the details of findings at operation for unreduced cases.

Cases of primary intussusception found at surgical exploration were treated by simple reduction with milking; when irreducible or gangrenous, resection anastomosis was performed. Table 52.5 shows the incidence of resection: 25% in phase 30.4% and I in phase II. The complications encountered included recurrence, perforation, and negative exploration. Table 52.6 shows the details of complications encountered during HR.

Among 50 cases that underwent barium reduction, 31 were reduced (62%) with recurrence in 3 and perforation in 2. Perforation resulted in barium peritonitis, the patients had a stormy postoperative course, and one of them eventually died.

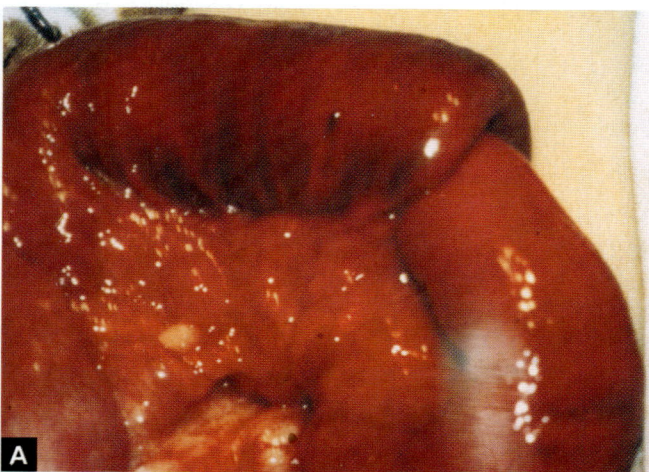
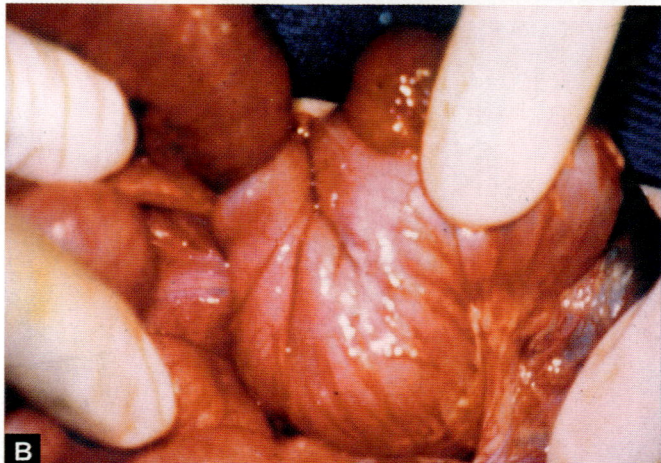

Figs 52.4A and B: A. Operative photograph of an intussusception **B.** Manual reduction of the intussusception

Operative Intervention

In cases of failed hydrostatic reduction or in the presence of peritonitis or if the duration has been for more than 24 hours, an operative intervention is indicated with initial resuscitation. The various surgical techniques range from the manual reduction to the resection of the gangrenous bowel with end-to-end anastomosis (Figs 52.4A to 52.5C). Warm compression of the intestinal segment involved intussusception is helpful not only in reduction of the intussusception but also prevent further damage of the intestine by reducing the edema. It also helps to identify the area of demarcation between the healthy and unhealthy segment of the intestine. After reduction the intestine, it is vital to look for any.

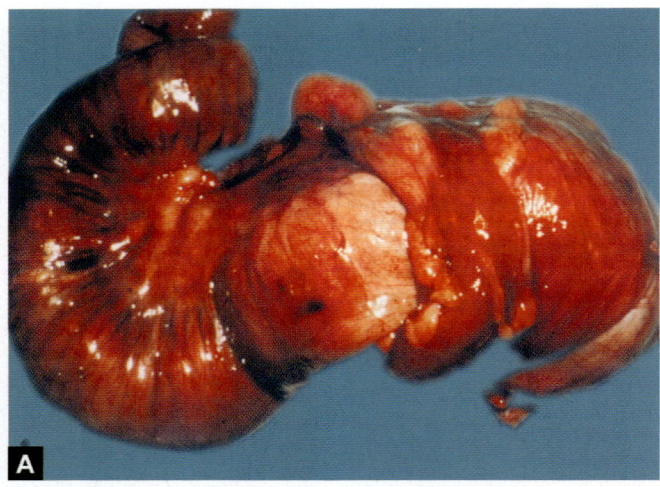

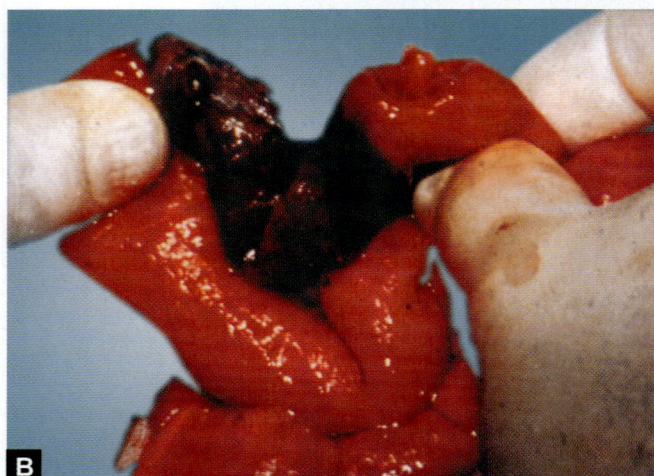
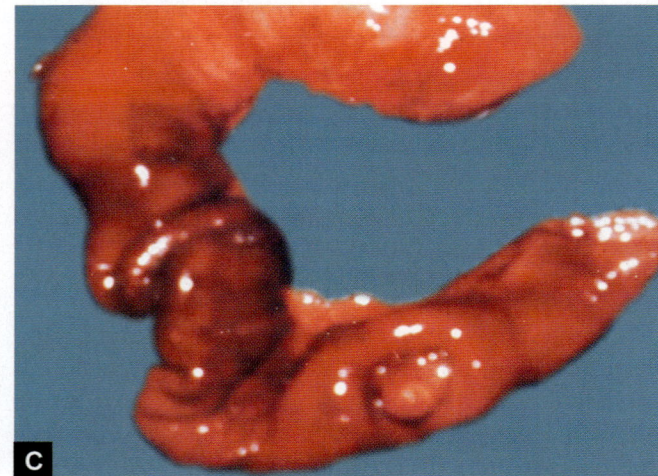

Figs 52.5A to C: A. Operative photograph of an intussusception **B.** Gangrenous segment of intestine seen after reduction **C.** Resected specimen of intestine

Neglected Cases

Resection of the gangrenous bowel is required in neglected cases that might even amount to right hemicolectomy or subtotal colectomy and restoration of the bowel continuity by an end-to-end anastomosis in 2 layers.

PROGNOSIS

In the hands of an experienced surgeon the mortality rate should approach zero. Deaths do occur if treatment is delayed. This shows the importance of early diagnosis of intussusception and it is always safer for the practitioner to refer any case of bleeding per rectum in the suspected age group to a pediatric surgical center.[4]

REFERENCES

1. El-Sahwi E. Intussusception, in El-Sahwi Textbook of Surgery, Chapter 6, Alexandria University Press, 1996;504.
2. Rattan KN. Intestinal intussusception in children: a review of 70 cases. Indian J Gastroenterol 2000;19(2):92.
3. Peh WC. Reduction of intussusception in children using sonographic guidance. AJR Am J Roentgend 1999;173(4): 985-88.
4. Roeyen G. Intussusception in infants: an emergency in diagnosis and treatment. Evr J Emerg Med 1999;6(1): 73-76.
5. DeVaries S. Postoperative intussusception in children. Br J Surg 1999;86(1):81-83.
6. Kuyama H. Is barium enema reduction safe and effective in patients with a long duration of intussusception? Paediatr Surg Int 1999;15(2):501-07.
7. Hadidi AT. Childhood intussusception: a comparative study of nonsurgical management. J Pediatr Surg 1999;34(2):304-07.

CHAPTER 53

Meckel's Diverticulum

M Gregor Walker, F Carl Davis

HISTORY AND INCIDENCE

In 1809, in the fifth volume of *Beiträge zur vergleichenden Anatomie*, John Friedrich Meckel identified the omphalomesenteric duct as the origin of the small bowel diverticulum that was later to bear his name.[1] The first documented report of this anomaly was over 200 years earlier by Fabricus Hildanus and Littre reported its appearance in a hernia in 1745.[2,3] Salzer is credited for first identifying heterotopic mucosa within the diverticulum.[4]

Although it is widely accepted that Meckel's diverticulum is the most common congenital anomaly of the gastrointestinal tract, the incidence is unclear. Traditional teaching has concentrated on the much-quoted "rule of two's" (2% incidence, located within 2 feet of the ileocecal valve, 2 inches in length and usually symptomatic before 2 years of age). There is much evidence that this adage, albeit useful for teaching purposes, is outdated. All reports quoting incidence are confined to either autopsies or incidental finding at laparotomy, neither being representative of an otherwise healthy population. The incidence quoted in the literature varies from 3-4%.[5-10] In asymptomatic patients the male to female ratio is nearly equal (1.3:1) but males are more likely to suffer complications (3.3:1).[5]

An increased incidence of Meckel's diverticulum is seen in association with other conditions including esophageal atresia, anorectal malformations and exomphalos.[11,12] There also appears to be an estimated three-fold increase in incidence in Crohn's disease.[13]

EMBRYOLOGY

In early embryonic life the yolk sac is connected to the midpoint of the primitive gut by the vitelline (omphalomesenteric) duct. Between the fifth and seventh week of development this connection involutes. It is not known why failure of involution can occur but a variety of anomalies result, of which Meckel's diverticulum is the most surgically significant. The duct may remain patent throughout its length resulting in an omphaloileal (umbilical-intestinal) fistula. A variety of mucosa-lined cysts are also seen.

ANATOMY

Meckel's diverticulum is an example of a true diverticulum in which all normal intestinal layers are present. It is, by definition, situated on the antimesenteric border of the ileum, usually within 100 cm (rather than 2 feet) of the ileocecal junction and length varies between 1-8 cm. The blood supply to the Meckel's diverticulum is characteristic. During development of the embryo, the paired vitelline arteries pass on either side of the mesentery to ramify over the yolk sac. The left vitelline artery normally disappears and the proximal section of the right persists as the superior mesenteric artery. The Meckel's diverticulum is supplied by the distal section of the right vitelline artery, which persists as an end-artery branch of the superior mesenteric artery. Occasionally remnants of the vitelline vessels can result in bands connecting the diverticulum to the anterior abdominal wall or the mesentery, both scenarios potentially causing intestinal obstruction.

The Meckel's diverticulum can invert and in this form is more likely to cause an intussusception.[14,15] A rare anatomical variant is the so-called "giant" Meckel's diverticulum. There is controversy regarding the distinction between this lesion and segmental dilatation of the ileum and ileal dysgenesis. However, as with all vitellointestinal remnants (Fig. 53.1), the identification of the vitelline artery supplying the lesion is characteristic.[16]

HISTOLOGY

Heterotopic Mucosa

Heterotopic mucosa (Fig. 53.2) of gastric, pancreatic and duodenal origin can be present within a Meckel's diverticulum and the presence of such mucosa is more likely in symptomatic cases.[5,17-23] There is great debate as to the incidence of heterotopic mucosa with widely varying figures quoted in the literature (Table 53.1). However, there is unanimous agreement that in cases with heterotopic gastric mucosa *Helicobacter pylori* has no part to play in the symptomatology.[19-21]

Tumors

Various series have reported malignant change within a Meckel's diverticulum. Given the different heterotopic mucosa that can be found, it is not surprising that a wide range of malignancies have been reported in adults including carcinoid tumors, leiomyosarcoma and adenocarcinoma.[24-27] Tumors reported in children include lymphoma, adenomyoma and nesidioblastosis.[23,28,29]

Like carcinoid tumors found in the appendix, those found in a Meckel's diverticulum are usually small, solitary and asymptomatic. However, they have a greater potential to metastasize than appendiceal carcinoids but there have been no cases reporting carcinoid tumors arising from a Meckel's diverticulum in children.[25]

CLINICAL PRESENTATION

Most published series have reported that approximately half of children with a symptomatic Meckel's diverticulum present under the age of 2 years though that has not been our experience in Glasgow. Between 1946 and 1991, 281 Meckel's diverticula were resected and less than one-third were in children less than 2 years of age (Fig. 53.3).

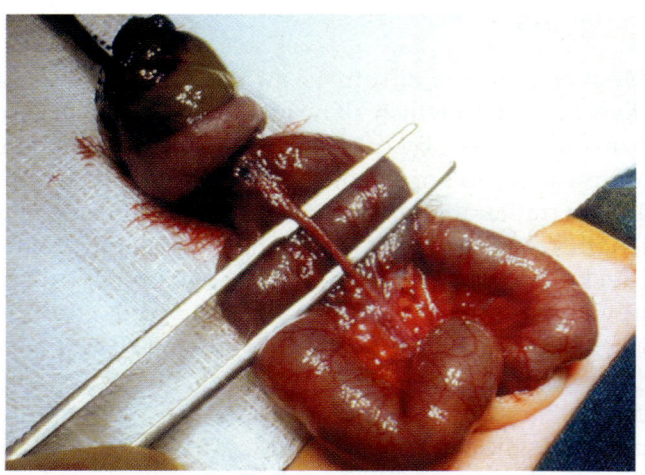

Fig. 53.1: Vitellointestinal remnants demonstrating the characteristic blood supply

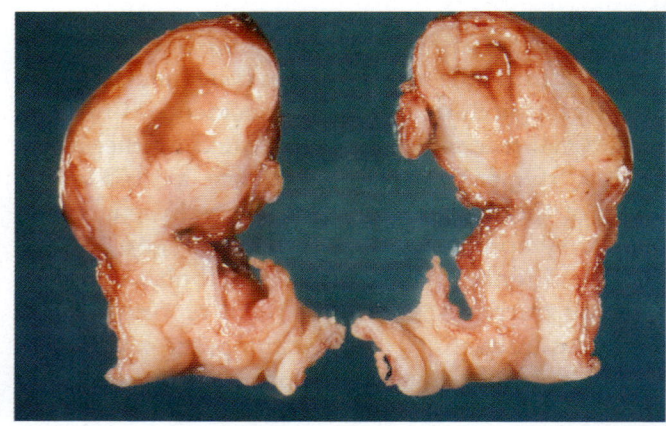

Fig. 53.2: Meckel's diverticulum opened showing the macroscopic differences between the gastric mucosa (above) and the ileal mucosa (below)

Table 53.1: Relationship between heterotopic mucosa and symptomatology				
Authors	Years of study	Total cases	Heterotopic mucosa in symptomatic patients	Heterotopic mucosa in asymptomatic patients
Matsagas et al[9]	1978-1993	62	8/15 (53%)	4/47 (8.5%)
DeBartolo et al[17]	1920-1971	151	21/51 (41%)	19/100 (19%)
Arnold et al[5]	1984-1994	58	4/13 (31%)	7/45 (16%)
St Vil et al[7]	1970-1989	142	71/117 (61%)	7/25 (28%)

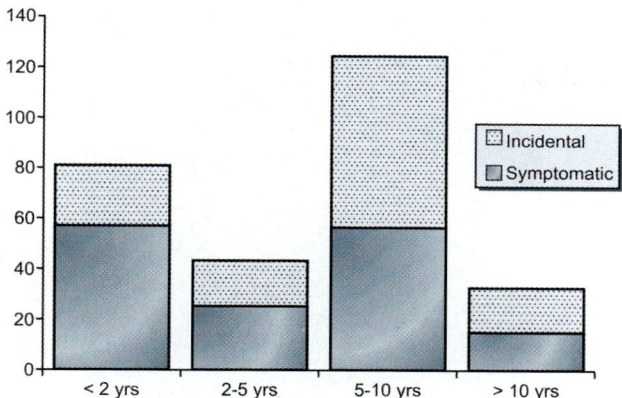

Fig. 53.3: Age distribution of 281 resected Meckel's diverticula in Glasgow (1946-1991)

Meckel's diverticulum can present with gastrointestinal bleeding, intestinal obstruction, perforation or inflammation. A Meckel's diverticulum can also be found incidentally during laparotomy or laparoscopy. Each method of presentation will be discussed and the management options explored.

Gastrointestinal Bleeding

Painless gastrointestinal bleeding is the commonest presenting complaint in most reported studies of Meckel's diverticulum. It usually occurs in children less than 5 years of age and can present with melena (black, tarry stools) or hematochezia (fresh red blood per rectum). The blood loss can vary from chronic insidious bleeding leading to anemia to acute massive blood loss presenting with shock.

On presentation, if there has been significant blood loss, the patient may require fluid resuscitation. The volume required should be estimated on the basis of the examination and should not be delayed until laboratory data are available. Intravenous access should be obtained early, and blood can be sent to establish the full blood count, hematocrit, platelet count, coagulation studies and for cross-match. Initial resuscitation with crystalloid or colloid is appropriate until blood is available (if indicated). Salient points in the history are previous episodes of bleeding, family history of bleeding disorders, and medications that may alter hemostasis. An accurate history taken from the parents or carer can usually distinguish between upper and lower GI bleeding although, due to the cathartic action of blood, vigorous upper GI bleeding can produce bright red blood per rectum. In such a situation the child is likely to have had a major bleed and is likely to be profoundly shocked. Examination should be directed toward estimating blood loss and establishing a diagnosis. A nasogastric tube should be passed; the aspirate should clarify whether the bleeding point is pre- or post-pyloric in origin. In the pediatric patient these steps are nearly always possible before planning surgery, and it is unwise to rush an unstable, hypovolemic child to the operating room (OR).

Investigations of the child with lower GI hemorrhage should not delay resuscitation. Stable patients with resolution of symptoms who have a positive 99m Technetium-pertechnetate scan (Meckel's scan) should be prepared for resection of the diverticulum on a semiurgent basis. In patients where the Meckel's scan is negative but have evidence of repeated hemorrhage, further investigation is indicated. 99mTechnetium-labelled red cell scans can detect bleeding at a rate of over 0.1 ml/min.[30] Angiography requires a bleeding rate of over 0.5 ml/min.[31] A child who presents with ongoing bleeding or presents with repeated episodes sufficient to drop the hemoglobin concentration to less than 9 g/dl should be explored by laparoscopy or laparotomy. Endoscopy does not often show bleeding points in children, although it is often performed to exclude other causes before laparotomy is performed.

Obstruction

Meckel's diverticulum can precipitate intestinal obstruction in a number of ways, the most common being intussusception and volvulus. These will be discussed in turn, followed by some more unusual examples reported in the literature.

Intussusception

Most cases of intussusception are idiopathic. In older children and adults it is more common for a lead point to cause the intussusception.[32] In our 17-year series of intussusceptions, which included 255 cases undergoing laparotomy, there were 21 cases with lead points identified of which the commonest was a Meckel's diverticulum (Table 53.2). In our experience, as with other series, intussusceptions caused by a Meckel's

Table 53.2: Lead points in a series of 255 cases of intussusception requiring surgery at RHSC, Glasgow	
Lead points	Number
Meckel's diverticulum	13
Intestinal duplication	4
Polyp	3
Lymphoma	1

diverticulum were not successfully reduced by contrast enema.[33,34]

The ultrasound appearance of the inverted Meckel's diverticulum causing an intussusception is characteristic (Fig. 53.4). A Meckel's diverticulum can rarely be identified during attempted air enema reduction (Fig. 53.5).[15,34]

Children with a Meckel's diverticulum acting as the lead point of an intussusception are likely to be in need of urgent fluid resuscitation. Following an unsuccessful attempt to reduce the intussusception by contrast medium or air enema, the child should be taken to the OR. Access to the abdomen is through a right-sided transverse incision. Making the incision above the level of the umbilicus offers better exposure. The Meckel's diverticulum should be excised. It is likely that a more extensive resection will be necessary to ensure both ends of the anastomosis are healthy and well perfused. Primary anastomosis should be possible even in cases of perforation.

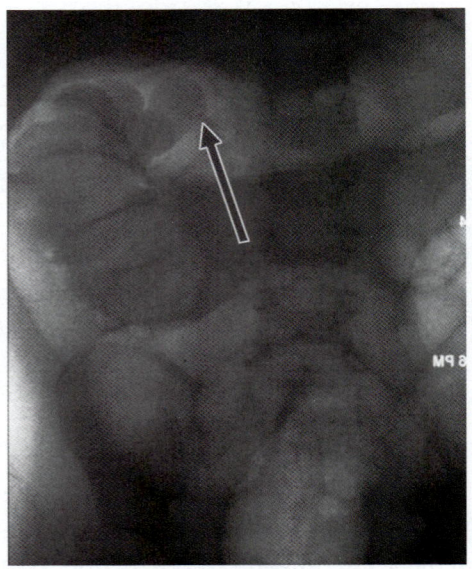

Fig. 53.5: Attempted air reduction of intussusception with a lead-point (arrow) which was found at laparotomy to be a Meckel's diverticulum

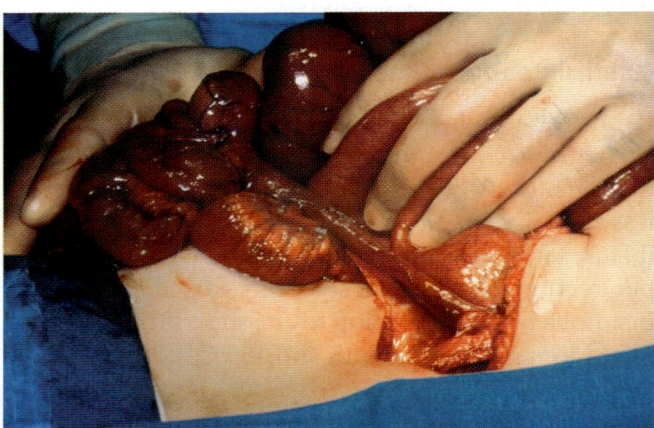

Fig. 53.6: Internal hernia around a patent vitellointestinal duct

Volvulus and Other Causes of Obstruction

Congenital bands can attach the Meckel's diverticulum to the umbilicus. This attachment can act a pivot point for axial rotation and resulting volvulus.[35] Although this is an uncommon complication the results can be devastating if urgent surgery to untwist the volvulus is not undertaken. Bands that run from the Meckel's diverticulum to the mesentery can cause obstruction of the small bowel. These bands are also a potential site for internal herniae (Fig. 53.6).[36] A long Meckel's diverticulum can cause obstruction or ischemia by wrapping around adjacent bowel.[37]

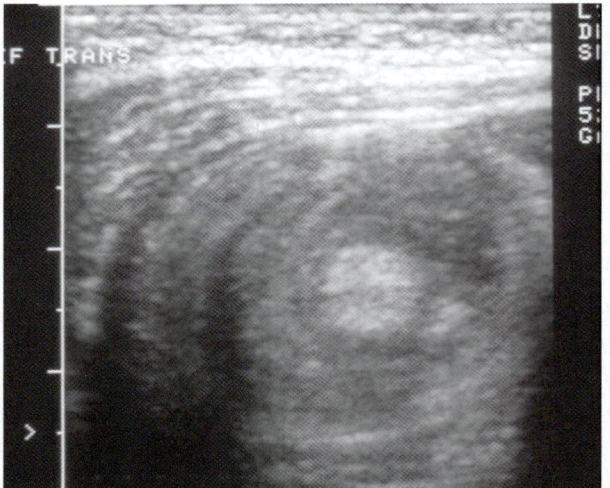

Fig. 53.4: Echogenic appearance on ultrasound scan of an inverted Meckel's diverticulum acting as a lead-point for an intussusception

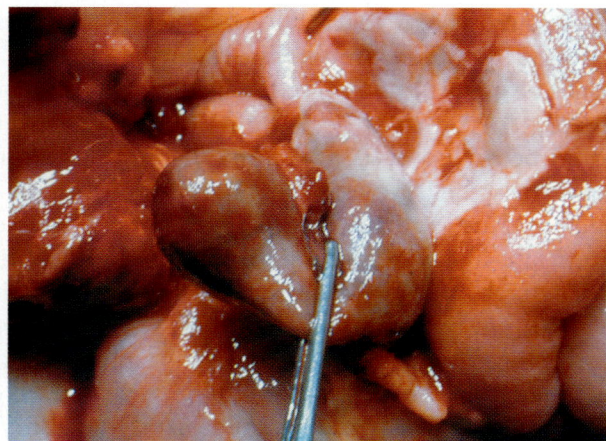

Fig. 53.7: Inflamed, gangrenous Meckel's diverticulum with free pus

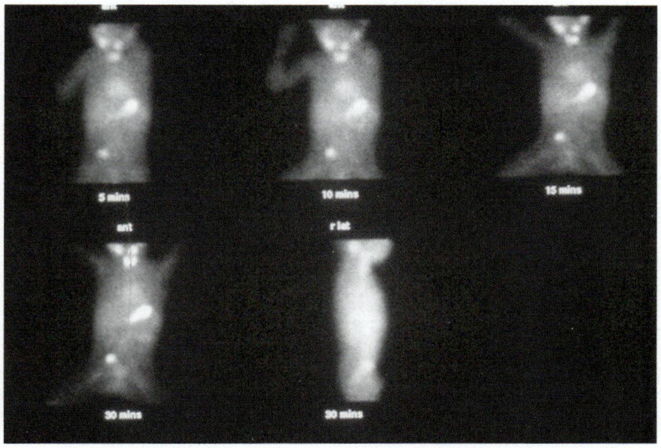

Fig. 53.8: Positive 99m Technetium-pertechnetate scan with heterotopic gastric mucosa visible in the right lower quadrant

Inflammation

Meckel's diverticulitis can be difficult to distinguish clinically from appendicitis. In cases of suspected appendicitis where the macroscopic appearance of the appendix does not correlate with the clinical picture or intraperitoneal findings, the ileum should be followed to at least 100 cm from the ileocecal junction. If an inflamed Meckel's diverticulum is found (Fig. 53.7), resection should be undertaken.

Perforation can result from diverticulitis and the child may present with generalized peritonitis. Rarely this can mimic necrotizing enterocolitis in neonates.[38] Ulceration can be within the diverticulum or in the adjacent ileal mucosa.[39] At laparotomy the perforation should be sought and the resection margins should include the ulcer. Perforation has also been reported as a result of impaction of a fish-bone in a Meckel's diverticulum.[40]

INVESTIGATIONS

Technetium Scanning

^{99m}Technetium-pertechnetate (Tc^{99}) scanning was first clinically reported in 1970 by Jewett, Duszynski, and Allen.[41] This technique is useful in identifying heterotopic gastric mucosa and uses the principle that superficial mucous secreting cells of functional gastric mucosa store and secrete intravenously administered pertechnetate ions carrying the ^{99m}technetium isotope.[42] Meckel's diverticula that do not contain gastric mucosa will not be detected. It is less likely these will be symptomatic. Other abnormalities of the small intestine containing gastric mucosa, for example duplications, will give positive scans.[43]

For the first 15 minutes after IV injection of the isotope, anterior views of the abdomen are acquired every minute. Lateral and posterior views are taken 15 minutes postinjection. Repeat delayed views at 30 minutes may be useful. The bladder should be emptied both prior to and at 30 minutes into the study, as renal excretion of pertechnetate into the bladder can obscure a Meckel's diverticulum. Uptake of radionucleotide is usually less dense than in the stomach, but a Meckel's diverticulum will be seen most often in the right lower quadrant (Fig. 53.8) although it can change position during the examination.

There are a number of recommendations to optimize the accuracy of this test. The patient should be fasted and the stomach and bladder can be emptied with a nasogastric tube and urethral catheter respectively. Glucagon, pentagastrin, and H$_2$-blockers have been given to augment the sensitivity of the study.[44,45] Glucagon inhibits intestinal peristalsis and therefore, prevents spillage of gastric contents into the bowel. Pentagastrin increases the uptake of the radionucleotide. Cimetidine, an H$_2$ receptor antagonist that inhibits the secretion of pertechnetate into the gastric lumen can be given orally for 2 days prior to the study. In patients who present as emergencies with gastrointestinal bleeding cimetidine can be given intravenously as a slow bolus 20 minutes prior to the scan.

Despite these measures there is still a considerable error associated with this test. False-positives may have heterotopic gastric mucosa in an alternative lesion as mentioned previously. Cooney et al reported 5 out of 26 patients (19%) who underwent laparotomy following a positive scan with no identifiable pathology.[46] In patients who present with gastrointestinal bleeding, the sensitivity of this test can be as low as 60%.[47,48] If faced with a patient with recurrent bleeding and a negative scan, surgical exploration is indicated.

Other Investigations

Ultrasonography can be useful in detecting the complicated Meckel's diverticulum.[34,49] Angiography can detect the vitelline artery and can be useful even in the absence of active bleeding although the "noise" from surrounding vasculature can make the identification of this artery difficult.[50] Superselective catheterization of distal ileal arteries can overcome this problem.

Laparoscopy has the advantage of offering the opportunity to proceed with diverticulectomy at the time of the diagnostic examination.

SURGICAL MANAGEMENT (DIVERTICULECTOMY)

A Meckel's diverticulum can be excised at laparotomy, by a laparoscopic-assisted method or by laparoscopy alone. For open excision, access is obtained through a right transverse incision and the ileum is followed proximally from the ileocecal junction. The contents of this segment of bowel may appear dark due to recent hemorrhage. Once the Meckel's diverticulum has been identified the vitelline artery supplying it should be ligated and divided. The lumen of the small intestine 10 cm to either side of the diverticulum should be occluded using a non-crushing technique. Resection of the ileal segment containing the Meckel's diverticulum should be performed in all cases (Fig. 53.9). In cases presenting with gastrointestinal hemorrhage, the bleeding may originate from the diverticulum but it is more commonly from an ulcer of the adjacent ileal mucosa (Fig. 53.10). Once resection is performed an inspection of the mucosal surface of the adjacent ileum should be undertaken to identify a bleeding point. More often than not such a lesion is not visible, although if one is seen the resection margin should be extended to include this rather than oversewing the lesion.

Closure of the ileum is performed by an end-to-end anastomosis. Single-layer anastomosis with 4/0 or 5/0 vicryl or PDS on a non-traumatic needle is appropriate. The resected sample should be sent for histological examination. If a resection of the ileal segment is performed it is unusual for there to be extension of heterotopic gastric mucosa beyond the resection margins. If this is found it should be accurately documented and the patient should be made aware, as this may be a potential site for further bleeding in the future.

Laparoscopy is being used more frequently with some success.[51-54] The advantages of laparoscopic diagnosis include the ability to perform resection at

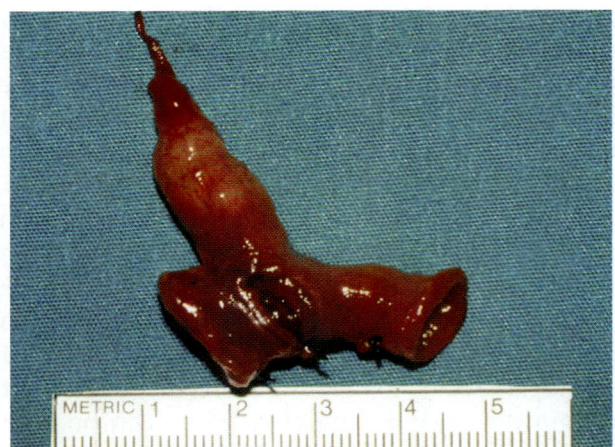

Fig. 53.9: Resected ileal segment containing a Meckel's diverticulum

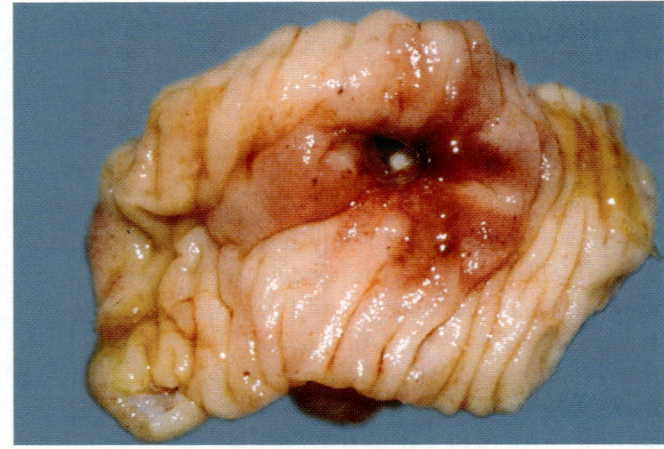

Fig. 53.10: Peptic ulcer situated at the neck of a Meckel's diverticulum

the time of diagnosis. This can be performed extracorporeally by exteriorization of the bowel through the umbilical port, or in the larger patient a total laparoscopic method can be employed utilizing the endo GIA stapling device.[52,53] Some authors have reported excision of the Meckel's diverticulum using an "endoloop" in a similar manner to removal of the appendix.[54]

MANAGEMENT OF INCIDENTAL MECKEL'S DIVERTICULUM

The management of the incidentally discovered Meckel's diverticulum has been a source of great debate over the years and there have been no guidelines to aid the surgeon in deciding whether or not to resect. The deciding factor is the estimated lifetime risk of complications arising from a Meckel's diverticulum. Meckel estimated the lifetime risk of complications to be 25% although more recent reports place it at between 4 and 6%.[8,9,55] These reports assume an incidence of 2% in the general population. However, if the incidence were lower than this, the rate of complications would be accordingly higher.

Some authors suggest a selective approach, advocating resection of a Meckel's diverticulum with a narrow neck or macroscopic evidence of heterotopic mucosa. However, the macroscopic appearance is not a good indicator of the potential for future complications.[56,57] The morbidity associated with resection of the lesion is low, particularly in children.[58] We recommend excision of incidentally discovered Meckel's diverticula in all patients if the resection can be carried out safely. The very ill patient who would benefit from expeditious surgery, or the neonate where resection and anastomosis can be challenging are not candidates for incidental excision. It is important however to clearly document the presence of the Meckel's diverticulum for future reference.

OUTCOME

The commonest long-term complication following Meckel's diverticulectomy is bowel obstruction secondary to adhesions, which is estimated to have an incidence of 5-10%. A large study looking at both children and adults quoted a worse outcome in symptomatic cases with an incidence of postoperative complications of 12% and long-term complications of 7%[8]. The figures for asymptomatic cases were 2% for both groups. In our series of 281 patients over 45 years mortality and complication rates were higher in the symptomatic group. Improvements in intensive care management of the sick infant and child should ensure that mortality in children with a Meckel's diverticulum is close to zero.

REFERENCES

1. Meckel JF. Beiträge zur vergleichenden Anatomie. Leipzig, Germany. Carl Heinrich Reclam 1908:91-93.
2. Lichtenstein M. Meckel's Diverticulum. Quarterly Bulletin of Northwestern University Medical School 1941;15:296.
3. Littre A. Observation sur une nouvelle espece de hernia. Hist Acad Roy de Sci 1745:300.
4. Salzer H. Uber das offerne meckelesche divertikel. Wein Klein Wochenenschr 1904:17;614.
5. Arnold JF, Pellicane JV. Meckel's diverticulum: a ten-year experience. American Surgeon 1997;63(4):354-55.
6. Moore TC. Omphalomesenteric duct malformations. Seminars in Pediatric Surgery 1996;5(2):116-23.
7. St-Vil D, Brandt ML, Panic S, et al. Meckel's diverticulum in children: a 20-year review. Journal of Pediatric Surgery 1991;26(11):1289-92.
8. Cullen JJ, Kelly KA, Moir CR, et al. Surgical Management of Meckel's diverticulum. An epidemiologic, population-based study. Annals of Surgery 1994;220:564-69.
9. Matsagas MI, Fatouros M, Koulouras B, et al. Incidence, complications, and management of Meckel's diverticulum. Archives of Surgery 1995;130(2):143-46.
10. Aktan AO, Gulluoglu BM, Cingi A, et al. Short note: Incidence of Meckel's diverticulum in Turkey. British Journal of Surgery 1997:84(5);683.
11. Simms MH, Corkery JJ. Meckel's diverticulum: its association with congenital malformation and the significance of atypical morphology. British Journal of Surgery 1980;67:216-19.
12. Nicol JW, MacKinlay GA. Meckel's diverticulum in exomphalos minor. Journal of the Royal College of Surgeons of Edinburgh 1994;39(1):6-7.
13. Andreyev HJ, Owen RA, Thompson I, Forbes A. Association between Meckel's diverticulum and Crohn's disease: a retrospective review. Gut 1994;35(6):788-90.
14. James GK, Berean KW, Nagy AG, et al. Inverted Meckel's diverticulum: an entity simulating an ileal polyp. American Journal of Gastroenterology 1998;93(9):1554-55.
15. Kim G, Daneman A, Alton DJ, et al. The appearance of inverted Meckel's diverticulum with intussusception on air enema. Pediatric Radiology 1997;27(8):647-50.
16. Koudelka J, Kralova M, Preis J. Giant Meckel's diverticulum. Journal of Pediatric Surgery 1992;27(2):1589-90.
17. DeBartolo HM Jr, van Heerden JA. Meckel's diverticulum. Annals of Surgery 1976;183(1):30-33.

18. Csemmi G. Gastric pathology in Meckel's diverticulum. Review of cases resected between 1965 and 1995. American Journal of Clinical Pathology 1996;106(6):782-85.
19. Bemelman WA, Bosam A, Wiersma PH, et al. Role of Helicobacter pylori in the pathogenesis of complications of Meckel's diverticula. European Journal of Surgery 1993;159(3):171-75.
20. Parikh SS, Ranganathan S, Prabu SR, et al. Heterotopic gastric mucosa and Helicobacter pylori infection in Meckel's diverticulum in Indian subjects. Journal of the Association of Physicians of India 1993;41(10):647-48.
21. Chan GS, Yuen ST, Chu KM, et al. Helicobacter pylori in Meckel's diverticulum with heterotopic gastric mucosa in a population with relatively high *H. pylori* prevalence rate. Journal of Gastroenterology and Hepatology 1999;14(4):313-16.
22. Taylor RH, Owen DA. Acute inflammation of pancreatic tissue in a Meckel's diverticulum. Canadian Journal of Surgery 1982;25(6):656-57.
23. Schrier F, Saubrery A, Kosmehl H. A Meckel's diverticulum containing pancreatic tissue and nesidioblastosis in a patient with Beckwith-Wiedemann syndrome. Pediatric Surgery International 2000;16(1-2):124-27.
24. Silk YN, Douglass HO, Penetrante R. Carcinoid tumours in Meckel's diverticulum. American Surgeon 1998;54(11):664-67.
25. Moyana TN. Carcinoid tumours arising from Meckel's diverticulum. A clinical, morphologic and immunohistochemical study. American Journal of Clinical Pathology 1989;91(1):52-56.
26. Tan JC, Wong KS, Teh CH, et al. Perforated leiomyosarcoma of Meckel's diverticulum. Singapore Medical Journal 1997;38(10):442-43.
27. Kusumoto H, Yoshitake H, Mochida K, et al. Adenocarcinoma in Meckel's diverticulum: report of a case and review of 30 cases in the English and Japanese literature. American Journal of Gastroenterology 1992;87(7):910-13.
28. Al-Dabbagh AI, Salih SA. Primary lymphoma of Meckel's diverticulum: a case report. Journal of Surgical Oncology 1985;28(1):19-20.
29. Yao JL, Zhou H, Roche K, et al. Adenomyoma arising in a Meckel's diverticulum: case report and review of the literature. Pediatric and Developmental Pathology 2000;3(5):497-500.
30. Smith R, Copely DJ, Bolen FH. 99mTc RGC scintigraphy: correlation of gastrointestinal bleeding rates and scintigraphic findings. American Journal of Roentgenology 1987;148:869-74.
31. Afshani E, Berger PE. Gastrointestinal tract angiography in infants and children. Journal of Pediatric Gastroenterology and Nutrition 1986;5:173-86.
32. Bhisitkul DM, Todd KM, Listernick R. Adenovirus infection and childhood intussusception. American Journal of Diseases in Childhood 1992;146:1331-33.
33. Ein SH. Leading points in childhood intussusception. Journal of Pediatric Surgery 1976;11(2):209-11.
34. Daneman A, Myers M, Shuckett B, et al. Sonographic appearances of inverted Meckel's diverticulum with intussusception. Pediatric Radiology 1997;27(4):295-98.
35. D'Souza CR, Kilam S, Prokopishyn H. Axial volvulus of the small bowel caused by Meckel's diverticulum. Surgery 1993;114(5):984-87.
36. Hawkins HB, Slavin JD Jr, Levin R, et al. Meckel's diverticulum. Internal hernia and adhesions without gastrointestinal bleeding – ultrasound and scintigraphic findings. Clinical Nuclear Medicine 1996;21(12):938-40.
37. Matthews P, Tredget MW, Balsitis M. Small bowel strangulation and infarction: an unusual complication of Meckel's diverticulum. Journal of the Royal College of Surgeons of Edinburgh 1996;41(1):55-56.
38. Gandy J, Byrne P, Lees G. Neonatal Meckel's diverticular inflammation with perforation. Journal of Pediatric Surgery 1997;32(5):750-51.
39. Canty T, Meguid MM, Eraklis. Perforation of Meckel's diverticulum in infancy. Journal of Pediatric Surgery 1975;10:189-93.
40. Christensen H. Fishbone perforation through a Meckel's diverticulum: a rare Laparoscopic diagnosis in acute abdominal pain. Journal of Laparoendoscopic and Advanced Surgical Techniques. Part A 1999;9(4):351-52.
41. Jewett TC Jr, Duszynski DO, Allen JE. The visualization of Meckel's diverticulum with 99mTc-pertechnetate. Surgery 1970;68:567.
42. Williams JG. Pertechnetate and the stomach – a continuing controversy. Journal of Nuclear Medicine 1983;24:633-36.
43. Rosenthall L, Henry JN, Murphy DA, et al. Radiopertechnetate imaging of the Meckel's diverticulum. Radiology 1972;105(2):371-73.
44. Baum S. Pertechnate imaging following cimetidine administration in Meckel's diverticulum of the ileum. American Journal of Gastroenterology 1981;76(5):464-65.
45. Yeker D, Buyukunal C, Benli M, et al. Radionuclide imaging of Meckel's diverticulum: cimetidine versus Pentagastrin plus glucagon. European Journal of Nuclear Medicine 1984;9(7):316-19.
46. Cooney DR, Duszynski DO, Camboa E, et al. The abdominal technetium scan (a decade of experience). Journal of Pediatric Surgery 1982;17(5):611-19.
47. Poulsen KA, Qvist N. Sodium pertechnetate scintigraphy in detection of Meckel's diverticulum: is it usable? European Journal of Pediatric Surgery 2000;10(4):228-31.
48. Swaniker F, Soldes O, Hirschl RB. The utility of technetium 99m pertechnetate scintigraphy in the evaluation of patients with Meckel's diverticulum. Journal of Pediatric Surgery 1999;34(5):760-64.
49. Daneman A, Lobo E, Alton DJ, et al. The value of sonography, CT and air enema for detection of complicated Meckel diverticulum in children with nonspecific clinical presentation. Pediatric Radiology 1998;28(12):928-32.
50. Mitchell AW, Spencer J, Allison DJ, et al. Meckel's diverticulum: angiographic findings in 16 patients. American Journal of Roentgenology 1998;170(5):1329-33.

51. Lee KH, Yeung CK, Tam YH, et al. Laparascopy for definitive diagnosis and treatment of gastrointestinal bleeding of obscure origin in children. Journal of Pediatric Surgery 2000;35(9):1291-93.
52. Schmid SW, Schafer M, Krahenbuhl L, et al. The role of laparoscopy in symptomatic Meckel's diverticulum. Surgical Endoscopy 1999;13(10):1047-49.
53. Valla JS, Steyaert H, Leculee R, et al. Meckel's diverticulum and laparoscopy in children. What's new? European Journal of Pediatric Surgery 1998;8(1):26-28.
54. Schier F, Hoffmann K, Waldschmidt J. Laparoscopic removal of Meckel's diverticula in children. European Journal of Pediatric Surgery 1996;6(1):38-39.
55. Soltero MJ, Bill AH. The natural history of Meckel's diverticulum and its relation to incidental removal. American Journal of Surgery 1976;132(2):168-73.
56. Michas CA, Cohen SE, Wolfman EF Jr. Meckel's diverticulum: should it be excised incidentally at operation? American Journal of Surgery 1975;129(6):682-85.
57. Aubrey DA. Meckel's diverticulum. A review of the sixty-six emergency Meckel's diverticulectomies. Archives of Surgery 1970;100(2):144-46.
58. Vane DW, West KW, Grosfeld JL. Vitelline duct anomalies. Experience with 217 childhood cases. Archives of Surgery 1987;122(5):542-47.

Appendicitis

Kurosh Paya

Although Leonardo da Vinci has already illustrated the appendix in his anatomic drawings in 1492, a first anatomic description of a vermiform appendix was not done before 1521 by Berengario DaCarpi.[1]

Certainly much more older are descriptions of an appendicitis of an Egyptian mummy from Byzanz. Reports on an appendicitis were first published by Jean Fernel 1544 and von Hilden 1652. These were followed by impressive reports on perforations of the appendix by L Heister, Mestivier and J Hunter in the 18th century. The first appendectomy was performed 1735 by C Amyand on an eleven-year old boy who developed appendicitis in the region of a scrotal hernia. In 1827, F Melier proposed the surgical treatment of appendicitis as standard therapy but was stubbornly ignored. For a long time the treatment of appendicitis remained a domain of internists who treated the patients with opium and bed rest as well as with drainage in case of abscesses. In 1886, Reginald Heber Fitz from Boston, for a short period a scholar also of the famous R Virchow in Vienna, imprinted the term "appendicitis" and also demanded an early surgical treatment and resection of the appendix, respectively. At that time chloroformism as well as Lister's principles of asepsis have met with approval.

Since it was clear at the end of the 19th century that vermiform appendix was responsible for two-thirds of all cases of fatal peritonitis, a basis for diagnosis and treatment of this disease was rapidly found. Already in 1889, numerous reports on the surgical therapy of appendicitis were published among others also by McBurney. In 1894, he reported on a new surgical method which he had taken over from his colleague JB Murphy and published for the first time, the gridiron.[2] This method made it's way worldwide and is now accepted as standard. Already ten years later Murphy was able to report on 2,000 accomplished appendectomies in the American Journal of Medical Sciences.[3] But not till the era of antibiotics in the fifties of our century appendicitis could loose the nimbus of an extremely dangerous disease. In 1910 the operative mortality, for a country like Switzerland, lay in the range of 6.2% compared to a cumulative mortality of 5.7 %.[4] Appendectomy now represents one of the most important abdominal teaching operations for young surgeons.[1,5] Today appendicitis is the most frequent indication for operation in the childhood and in general appendectomy presents the third-most operation worldwide.

EPIDEMIOLOGICAL FACTS

In the USA, about half a million appendectomies are performed every year which accords with an incidence of 260/100,000 inhabitants. There are similar numbers in Europe. For instance, in Austria approximately 20,000 in 1998 and in France about 200,000 appendectomies were performed in 1996 (Table 54.1). Table 54.2 outlines the morbidity and mortality in India.

ANATOMIC AND HISTOLOGIC BASICS

The vermiform appendix develops from a common gemma with the cecum in the distal part of the primitive intestinal loop between the 6th and 8th embryonic week, and exists in this type only in primates. It becomes visible from the 8th week of development; at this time in the child, the appendix has a length of about 10 cm. The appendix is an about

Table 54.1: Appendectomies/100,000 inhabitants in different countries[6]

- Less than the half of these patients do really have appendicitis (110/100,000). Therefore, nearly 50% are so-called "negative" appendectomies - appendectomies without an inflamed vermiform appendix. Especially in young women this rate can be 2.5 times higher than in the respective male population. This can be explained by the insecure diagnostic demarcation to other causes of pain in the right hypogastric zone in women, and by the known increased morbidity and mortality in cases of an overlooked appendicitis. In general the incidence of newly diagnosed appendicitis is slightly but steadily retrograde. This process cannot be explained by now but in the last decades, for some regions there is reported upon a decrease of up to 46%.[7] Apparently also genetic factors seem to play an important role in the disease process. The highest rate of appendicitis is found within the white population, while Black Africans and Asians only suffer half as much from appendicitis. In Africa the incidence of appendicitis is particularly low. To what extent only predisposition or other habits of life are responsible for that cannot be answered yet. A higher frequency of appendicitis has also been described within families. Children whose parents have been appendectomized early during childhood, are also frequently appendectomized early. Whether this is caused by an increased sensibility of parents or by genetic factors is still unclear.[8] There exists a sex-specific distribution, in consequence of, males do have a 1.1-1.7 times higher risk to develop appendicitis. These data comply with a whole life-span risk for men of 8.6-6.7% for women to suffer from appendicitis. On the other hand, women do have a much higher risk to get appendectomized (23.1% of women, 12% of men).

Age shows a distribution with a peak in the age group of 14-19 years. In this group there is a relative disease frequency of 230/100,000 whereas frequency is decreasing to 50/100,000 at the age of 45 and to about 13/1000,000 at the age of 80.[9,10,11] These data underline the enormous importance of this disease, especially for pediatric surgery.

Table 54.2: Morbidity and mortality in developing contries

Incidence: 110/100,000 year
Maximum in the age group of 14-19 years: 230/100,000/year

Whole lifespan risk to
suffer from appendicitis: Men   8.6%
                            Women   6.7%

Incidence for surgical interventions is 2.5 times higher in women
   Morbidity : 5.1-33%
   Mortality : 0.001-0.5%[12]

[12]Seiler ChA. Standard open surgical procedure in appendicitis: From the past to the present. In Krähenbühl L, Frei E, Klaiber Ch., Büchler MW. Acute Appendicitis: Standard Treatment or Laparoscopic surgery? Prog Surg, Verlag Karger, Basel 1998;25:59-69

2.5-24 cm long (in adulthood about 9 cm) and about 0.5 cm thick, at the beginning of the cecum caudal departing, blind-ending, worm-shaped enteral compartment. In the correct way, one has to say that the cecum departs cranially from the appendix, because the appendix represents the start of the large bowel. But it is—as an blind-ending structure with a comparably narrow lumen (1-2 mm)—turned off for the passage of the bowel movement (feces), and is therefore functionally and anatomically considered an "appendix" of the cecum. The observation that the cecum is only partly and the appendix is not filled with meconium (therefore no growth stimulus is given) explains why the vermiform appendix is so thin in contrast to the colon/cecum.[13] Although the appendix belongs to the colon, it does not form *Taenias*, because the outer lengthwise-muscle layer of the Muscularis propria builds an even plate at the passage to the appendix, and possibly has a pretty peristaltic movement. This runs in the direction from the tip to the base. At the point at which the *Taenias* of the cecum converge, one can most easily find the base of the appendix. Histologically it corresponds to the colon. However, the appendix exhibits a high content of defending cells, and several lymphoid follicles lying tightly against one another in the mucosa and submucosa, respectively, underlining its immunological importance. Noteworthy, the number and density of mucosal lymphoid follicles increases during adolescence. This period of enhanced development of lymphoid follicles corresponds exactly with the age range showing the highest incidence of appendicitis.

Blood supply is through the mesenteriolum (mesoappendix) by the appendicular artery originating from the ileocecalic artery which in its turn generally originate from the inferior right colic artery coming from the superior mesenteric artery.

The mesenteriolum is an expansion of the iliac mesenterium and passes under the ileum to the appendix. The appendicular artery takes its course along the free edge and works as a functional end artery. Its branches break through the wall until they reach the mucosa. In the luminal area arterioles build a fine reticulum. The base of the appendix may be supplied by small branches of the anterior and posterior cecal artery. The venous drainage runs and parallel to the arteries, whereby again a basket-like reticulum is formed in the area of the lymphoid follicles. The lymphatic drainage of the cecum passes to the ileocecal lymph nodes along the superior mesenteric artery into the cysterna chyli. There are anastomoses to retroperitoneal lymph nodes. The appendix in its turn does not have an own lymphatic drainage but as a whole is considered, similar to the tonsils, a lymphatic organ. Thereby the often observed contemporarily inflammatory response of tonsils and appendix can be explained. Malformations of the appendix are very rare. Generally, it is a question of either an agenesis or a reflection whereby the cecum can also be involved. While the frequency of this congenital malformation lies in the range of a thousandth part, the diverticulum as acquired dysplasia is more frequent. Diverticula are evaginations of the mucosa through the muscularis propria. A congenital "diverticulum", also an evagination affecting the entire wall, is added to the rudimentary reflections.

The posteromedial passage about 2-3 cm below the ileac opening into the cecum conforms to the McBurney point at the outer belly. This point lies at the junction between the lateral and the middle third of a line thought of between the anterior superior iliac spine and the bellybutton (Fig. 54.1).

The position of the vermiform appendix lies shortly medial or under the McBurney point in about 59%. In considerable 25% of all cases the appendix is positioned between the anterior superior iliac spine and the bellybutton. 27-65% have a retrocecal position (Figs 54.2 A to D).[14-16]

This position particularly raises difficulties for diagnosis and surgery. Retroileal or only partly retrocecal (transverse) inflamed appendices usually follow a typical clinical pattern while the symptomatology of strictly retrocecal, cranially directed appendices is rather unspecific. Even with ultrasonography, retrocecal appendicitis is only visible for skilled people and the operation is technically difficult for beginners in the operating room.

CLINICAL SYMPTOMS AND DIAGNOSIS

Abdominal pain is a frequent symptom and the cause of up to 20% of all visits. With every fifteenth child there underlies a serious disease. This among others can be an appendicitis. The other diseases with urgent necessity for surgical interventions are rather rare. The appendicitis is clinically recognized by a typical tenderness to pressure, Blumberg's sign, and the most frequent accompanying symptoms, vomiting and loss of appetite. However, diagnosis is still extremely difficult and only ultrasonography, in the hands of an

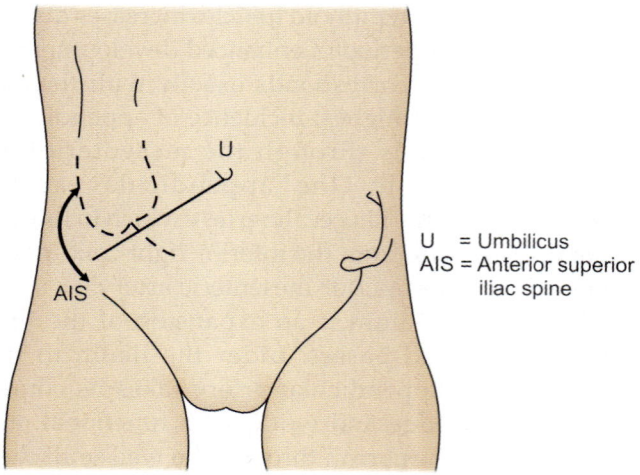

Fig. 54.1: McBurney point

U = Umbilicus
AIS = Anterior superior iliac spine

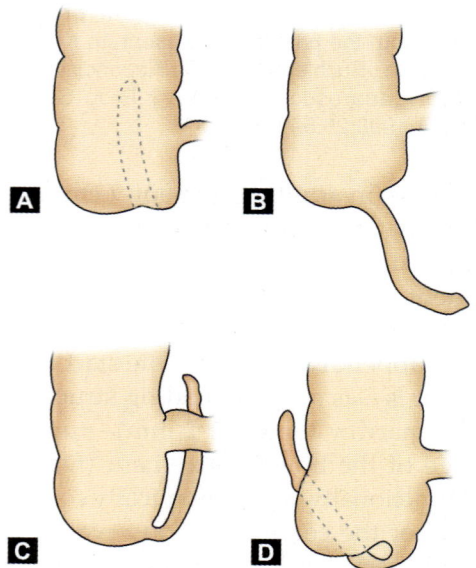

Figs 54.2A to D: A. Retrocecal, **B.** Mediocaudal (Pelvic) **C.** Retroileal, **D.** Lateral (Paracecal) position of the appendix

experienced physician, is a reliable remedy.[17] In daily practice new examination methods like MRI, nuclear-medical examinations (autologously marked leukocytes), or CT are, because of their poor availability, only of academic interest.

Appendicitis is a very rare event under an age of 4 and seldom up to 6 years, but if, rather less symptomatic and painful. Unfortunately, just the nearly obligatory perforation with all the signs of a peritonitis leads to the doctor and therefore to a diagnosis in this age group. Peritonitis is still the main cause of the very high morbidity. According to results from great studies the morbidity lies in a range between 5-33%. Principal causes of a perforated appendix with localized or already generalized peritonitis are local infections especially with adipose children, the occurrence of a paralytic ileus caused by a peritonitis, or an intra-abdominal abscess. Also late complications like adhesions and an adhesive strangulation of intestines are typical consequences of a peritonitis. On the other hand, not surgically treatable diseases like enteritis are – as a differential diagnosis—only difficult to distinguish from an appendicitis. An often similar symptomatology, above all a tenderness to pressure in the hypogastric zone and the, for not skilled persons, complicated examination under the difficult circumstances with children make diagnosis extremely hard. Due to the fear of an overlooked appendicitis a low specificity is tolerated in favor of a high sensitivity. This means that already in case of an insignificant suspicion for appendicitis, the patient is attributed to a surgical department and often also operated. The generally accepted rates for appendectomies in case of a wrong positive preoperative diagnosis are 20-25%. For the year 1997, large studies within surgical quality-assurance programs state childhood appendectomy-rates with a negative histological finding between 18.6-21.2%.[18] In the past years enlarged attention has been drawn to the increase of specificity to say of unerring aim without accepting a low sensitivity, that is an increased overlooked appendicitis-rate and therefore an increased rate of perforation.[19,20] In addition there are intensive efforts to develop a simple strategy to clarify acute abdominal pain in childhood. In a long-term prospective study together with other hospitals those criteria were proved that usually are referred to for diagnosis and that are also feasible in a consulting room or in basic-care providing hospitals. In contrast to the acute abdominal pain of grown-ups, fewer diseases are of question as differential-diagnostic causes. Thereby the diagnostic pathway is vastly uncomplicated.

In the author's series collective unspecific abdominal pain and functional discomforts were 40%, infectious enteropathies 25%, appendicitis 12%, and urogenital infections are remarkable 4%. All other noteworthy diseases were reported in less than 1% of all cases. From this is experience the following schemes could be deduced.

The two main criteria are the clinical examination and the ultrasonic examination by a physician who is especially experienced in abdominal ultrasonography in childhood and particularly in ultrasonic diagnostics of the appendicitis. In addition, the typical history and the results from laboratory experiments (Table 54.3) are observed. These criteria are assessed individually. If one or both main criteria (clinics, sonography) and at least one accessory criterion (history, laboratory) are met the patient is suspected of having an appendicitis, and will need hospitalization. If no other cause of disease is found and an appendicitis cannot reliably be excluded, the hospitalization either leads to an immediate surgery or to an re-evaluation after two to six hours intervals without food intake and parenteral fluid supply until verification or exclusion of an appendicitis. This is recognizable with a relatively high probability during the further course. If only one main criterion, clinical or sonography, is typical for an appendicitis and the second main criterion as well as both accessory criteria are negative, the child can be discharged under adequate care. Within 24 hours an ambulatory control has to follow. If history and laboratory investigations are positive and both main criteria—clinics and ultrasound are negative, the patient is hospitalized but is allowed to drink clear liquid. IV fluid in these cases is not necessary.

If laboratory or history alone is positive, patient is referred back to the practitioner/pediatrician for further control. This procedure is in a more or less structured manner applied in many pediatric clinics, whereas the importance of ultrasonography is definitely greater in European countries in contrast to Asian countries and the United States. This method has especially proved when the pediatric surgeon is

> **Table 54.3: Main and accessory criteria**
>
> *Main criteria*
>
> The following clinical symptoms ("clinical picture") were, based on large investigations of the OMGE and also on own observations, determined as positive and are listed with decreasing frequency.
> - Vomiting
> - Anorexia
> - Tenderness and rebound pain of the right side of abdomen
> - Local or diffuse abdominal guarding
>
> The sonographic criteria ("sonography") were determined by Puylaert in 1986; the following are considered as positive:[21]
> - Presentation of appendix
> - Wall stiffness, missing compressibility
> - Diameter > 6 mm is suspicious, > 9 mm corresponds with an inflammation
> - Perifocal edema
> - Wall thickening and net-cap
> - Fecolith
>
> *Accessory Criteria*
>
> The history is difficult to define but special points, e.g. duration of pain > 6 hr, start of pain within the last 24 hr, pain shifting to the right side of abdomen, proved typically positive. The positive related to criteria "history" are:
> - Start of pains without further common symptoms in the region of the bellybutton
> - The duration paint between the 6 to 24 hr, if no guarding exists
> - No intestinal infections in the near surroundings, with healthy brothers and sisters
> - Diarrhea, acute rhinitis, cough, and start of fever before start of pain are negative signs
>
> Laboratory—chemistry criteria ("laboratory") which support an appendicitis are:
> - Leukocytosis between 10,000 and 20,000/mm^3
> - CRP at start of pain at least 8 hours before: > 0.5[22]
>
> The combination of ultrasonography and clinical finding reach a specificity of 99% a sensitivity of 91%, and therefore a positive predictive power of nearly 100% (own observation).[23,24]

trained and experienced in abdominal sonography because the valuation of a nevertheless dynamic examination in combination with the own experience in clinical examination turns out significantly better in contrast to that of a radiologist who does perform this examination without special background. In the USA, the value of sonography is more inferior. In USA and in Asian countries clinic symptomatology and laboratory investigation are the most important criteria. Especially in countries with many children and less good medical care the greater experience of the physician does successfully replace missing technical devices like sonography, laboratory investigation and radiography. On the other hand, in the USA, there exists a more profit-orientated health system where examination methods like ultrasonography are difficult to establish.

Formerly practiced examinations, like the rectal-axillary temperature difference are obsolete for the diagnosis of appendicitis due to the unreliability of the measurement.

The typical symptoms of appendicitis are also apparent abdominal pain, guarding, relaxation-position, nausea or vomiting. These are, especially in childhood, very common symptoms which could appear with various distinctions in many other abdominal and also systemic diseases, and in connection with enteritis. In childhood, abdominal pain along with appendicitis first develop in the region of the bellybutton and then within hours shift to the right lower quadrant where they steadily increase. A primary examination in this early stage makes diagnosis very difficult. Because a high rate of wrong positive diagnoses still leads to numerous unnecessary appendectomies and therefore also to enormous costs, many institutions try to establish clear diagnostic criteria. These criteria should – also without technical resources—enable a prompt (that means before perforation occurs) diagnosis on the one hand and also to prophylactically operate as few as possible children on the other hand. All these efforts have shown that the clinical experience of the examiner is the most important instrument. Also computer-based decision-making systems could not improve diagnosis of appendicitis.[25-27]

The diagnostic accuracy in fact could be increased through forms which were necessary for the computer presentation but this was mainly due to the forced precision of the surgical examination. All attempts, for instance by entering into scoring systems, to establish standardized diagnostics, following objectively measurable criteria were disappointing (Table 54.4).[28]

The experience of the surgeon is presently and will also be in the 21st century the most important and safest diagnostic criterion.[29] The so called "wait and see" policy has proved helpful. Most hospitals in Europe hospitalize a child with a well-founded

Table 54.4: MANTREL's Score (Alvarado)[29]	
Migration of pain from central area to right lower quadrant	1 point
Anorexia or acetonuria	1 point
Nausea with vomiting	1 point
Tenderness in the right lower quadrant	2 point
Rebound tenderness	1 point
Elevated temperature ³ 38°C (100.4 °F)	1 point
Leukocytosis (>10,4000 cells/mm^3)	2 point
Shifted WBC count (> 5% neutrophils)	1 point
Total possible points	10 points

Fundamentally it can be written down that diagnosis is based on clinical examination, laboratory analysis and ultrasonography. The algorithm for the management of appendicitis is given in Figure 54.3.

Clinical Examination

A history of abdominal pain for last 12-24 hours without fever or diarrhea migrating from the central area to the right lower quadrant, typical tenderness to pressure above the McBurney Point, and rebound tenderness are frequent. The patient is anorectic and frequently vomits in a relatively early stage. In most cases the last defecation is still normal. The often mentioned rectal-axillary temperature difference of more than one centigrade celsius is unreliable. With children it is often not carried out exactly and moreover only appears in advanced stages. In later stages abdominal guarding is added to distinct pain existing in the right lower quadrant and tenderness to touch. The tongue is coated in nearly all cases and perioral paleness is found. In case of an existing Douglas' abscess frequent, highly liquid bowel

suspicion of appendicitis but without clear diagnosis and will re-examine the child after some hours without food intake and perhaps with parenteral fluid supply. As mentioned above, in Europe ultrasonography has been additionally established as the most valuable diagnostic resource. Thereby the rate of unnecessary appendectomies could be, in large series, reduced to 13% and less. In the USA, computed tomography (CT) is used instead of ultrasonography due to organizing and cost-technical assumptions.

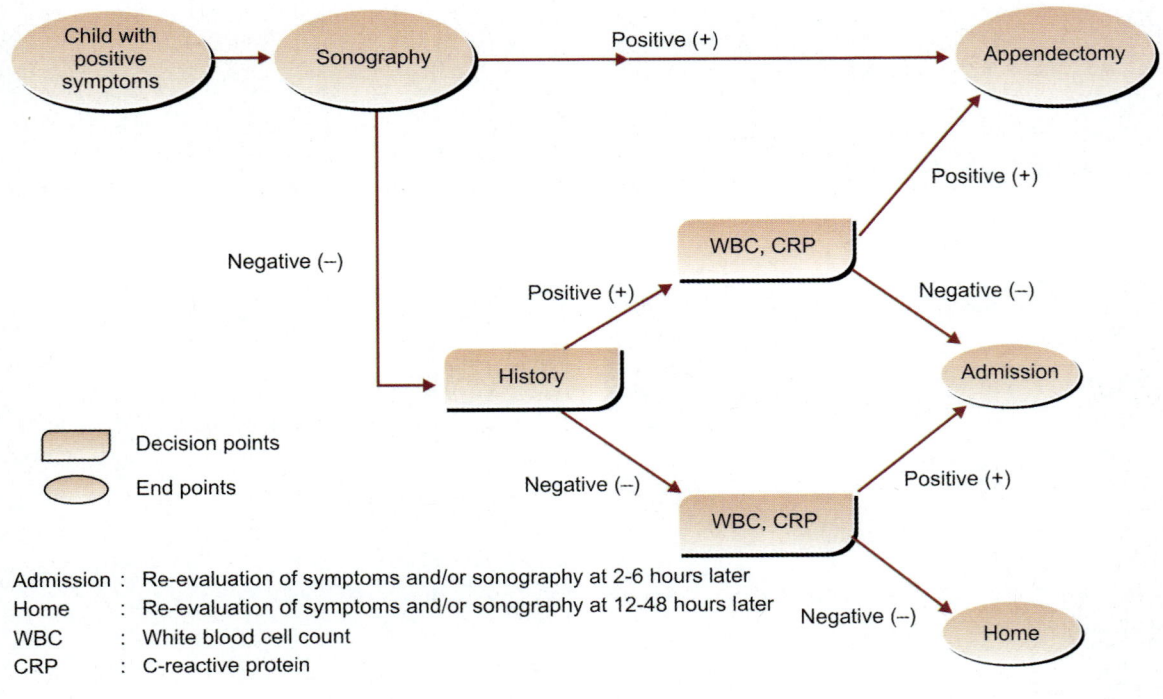

Admission : Re-evaluation of symptoms and/or sonography at 2-6 hours later
Home : Re-evaluation of symptoms and/or sonography at 12-48 hours later
WBC : White blood cell count
CRP : C-reactive protein

Fig. 54.3: Algorithm for the management of appendicitis

movement can often simulate enteritis. Besides the obligatory anorexia, a blown abdomen is the most frequent symptom in children under the age of three.

Laboratory—Chemical Analysis

If appendicitis is the presumptive diagnosis, an analysis of the urine is obligatory. Usually, the determination of leukocytes, nitrate as well as erythrocytes is sufficient to recognize an urinary tract infection as differential diagnosis. Further helpful information about the hydrational condition of the child is offered by the specific weight and the determination of ketone in the urine (acetonuria).

Blood examination for the red blood count and differential white blood count, and the analysis of the C-reactive protein (CRP) together with the clinical findings reach a high sensitivity and specificity. The laboratory finding is positive, if leukocytosis is of more than 10,000/mm^3 or a CRP-level higher than 0.5 mg/dl exists.

Ultrasonography

Appendicitis-criteria according to Puylaert (Table 54.3): The special power of sonography lies in the plain presentation of typical and important differential diagnoses(Figs 54.4A to D). Ileus, intussusception, enlarged lymph nodes, ovarian cysts, renal and liver affections, tumors, and others cause symptoms mimicking an appendicitis and can be distinguished safely (Figs 54.5A to D). Ultrasonography offers a

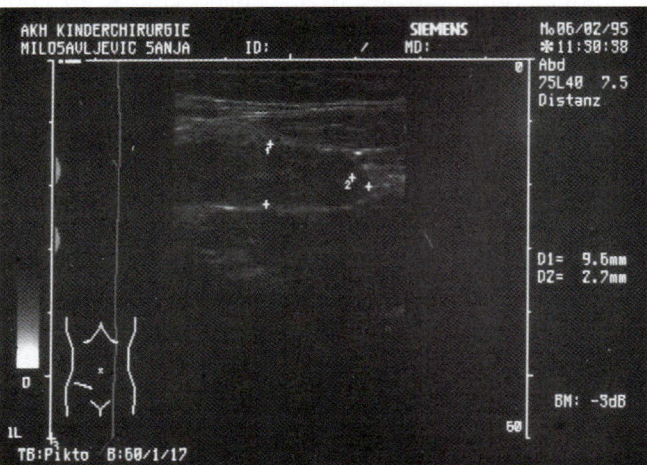

Fig. 54.4A: Sonographic view of appendicitis seen in longitudinal view

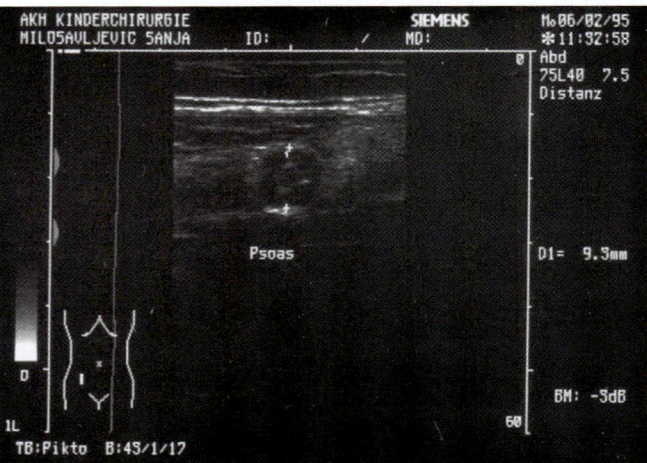

Fig. 54.4B: Sonographic view of appendicitis in transverse section

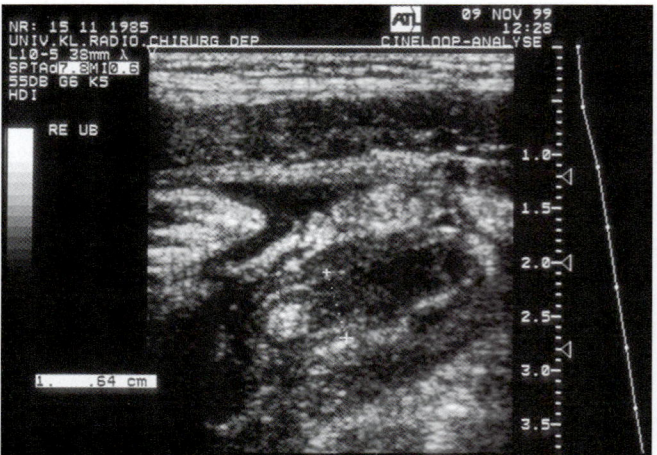

Fig. 54.4C: Sonographic view of fecalith in longitudinal section

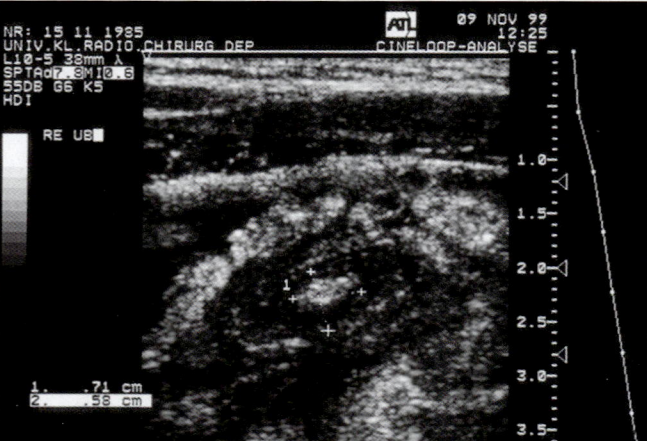

Fig. 54.4D: Sonographic view of fecalith in transverse section

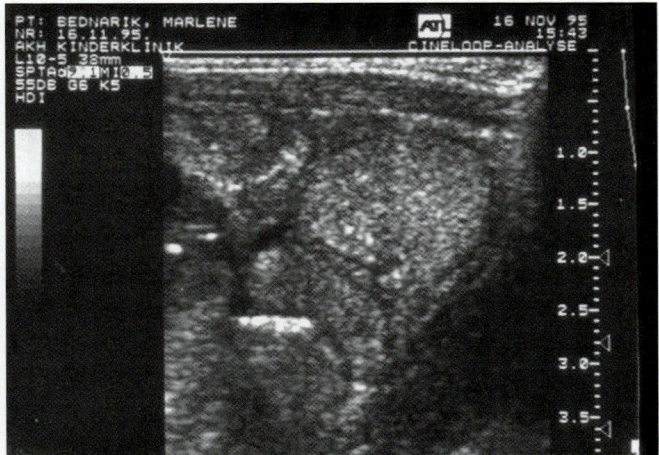

Fig. 54.5A: Sonographic view of ileus

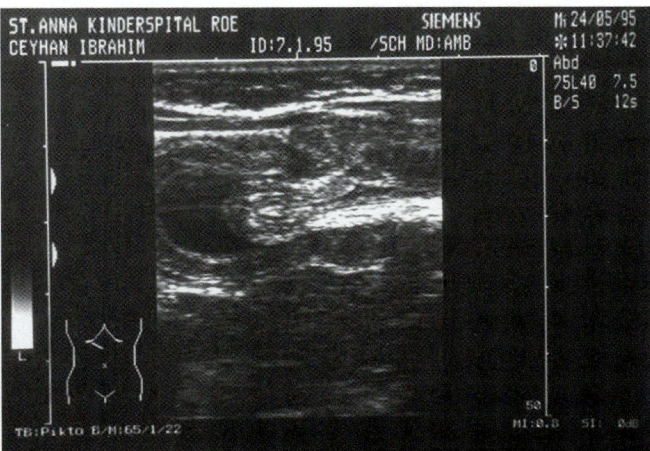

Fig. 54.5B: Sonographic view of intussusception in longitudinal section

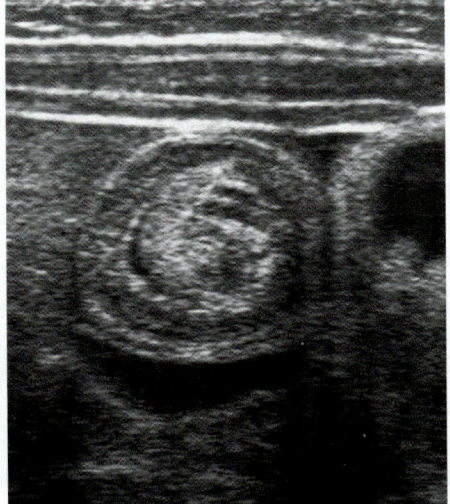

Fig. 54.5C: Sonographic view of transverse (intussusception section)

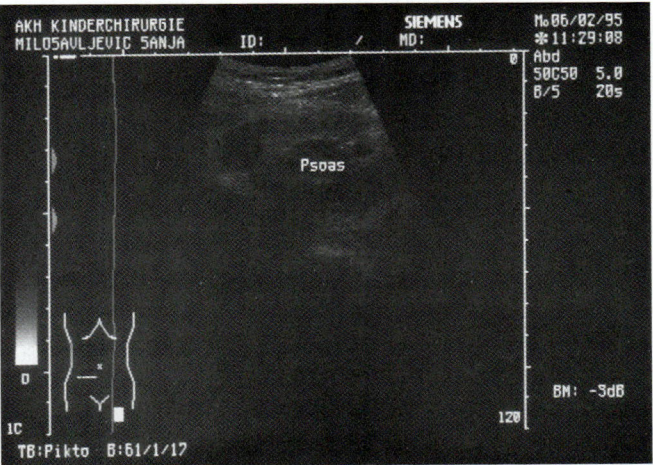

Fig. 54.5D: Sonographic view of mesenteric lymph nodes

sensitivity around 90% and a specificity of nearly 100% for the detection or exclusion of an acute appendicitis.[31] There is a positive predictive value of 92%, the negative predictive value is 99%.

MRI

On T2-weighted ultra turbo spin-echo images, acute appendicitis appears with a markedly hyperintense center, a slightly hyperintense thickened wall, and a markedly hyperintense periappendiceal tissue. Unenhanced axial T2-weighted spin-echo imaging is the most sensitive sequence for. MR imaging seems to be a valuable technique for depiction of acute appendicitis (Fig. 54.6).[32] Yet MR, as diagnostic remedy, is not sufficiently evaluated to be able to give a general judgement, but in the future it seems to be able to replace ultrasonography as well as CT as diagnostic resource because of the reproducible presentation of pictures and the missing roentgen burden.

CT Scan

Rarely used in Europe and Asia, more frequently applied in the USA, CT together with contrast medium is able to describe the inflammatory altered vermiform appendix (Fig. 54.7).[33] But one has to consider that such

604 Pediatric Surgery—Diagnosis and Management

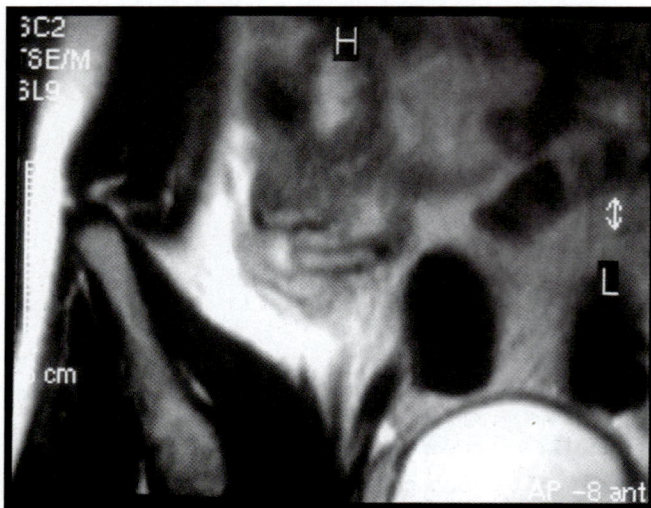

Fig. 54.6: MRI depicting appendicitis

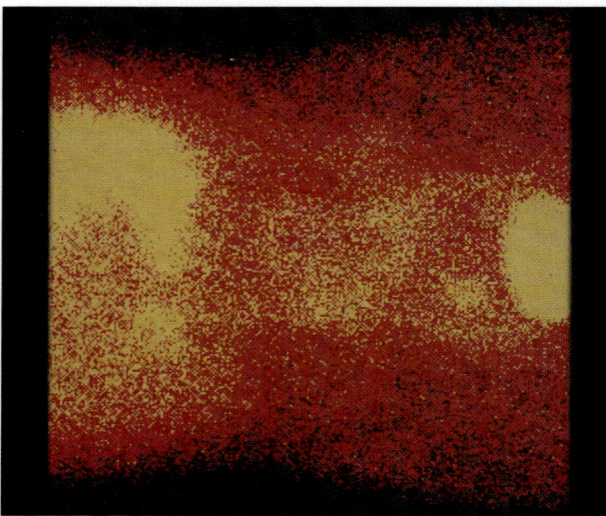

Fig. 54.8: Scintigraphy Meckel's diverticulum

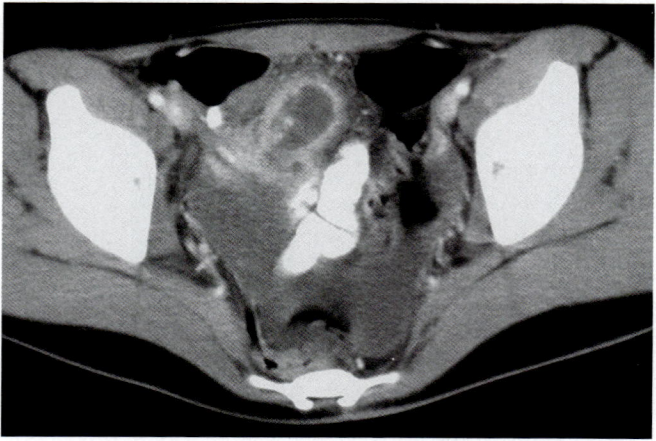

Fig. 54.7: CT scan depicting appendicitis

an examination is expensive and complex and also includes burden with X-rays. Its efficacy in childhood is lower than in connection with adults. Due to the above mentioned reasons, CT is generally seen as second choice after ultrasonography.[34]

Nuclear Medicine

During the past years studies have been published dealing with the detection of inflammation by labeled, autologous leukocytes. With this method a sensitivity of 27-97% and a specificity between 38-94% can be reached. Like for CT, radioactive substances are necessary and an experienced ultrasound-examiner is able to gain the same information without any burden for the young patient. But for the detection of a Meckel's diverticulum radionuclide imaging can be a very helpful tool (Fig. 54.8).

Diagnostic Laparoscopy

In contrast to adults the diagnostic laparoscopy has only a minor importance for the diagnosis of acute appendicitis in childhood. Exceptions are prepubertal and pubertal girls, for these laparoscopy is an important diagnostic tool.[35,36] Otherwise it is reserved to the clarification of chronically recurrent abdominal pain also in connection with a simultaneously planned, concomittant appendectomy (Figs 54.9A and B).[37]

For this purpose it is an ideal instrument.[38]

DIFFERENTIAL DIAGNOSIS

Functional discomfort generally manifests within a few hours in a chronic course with a self-limiting character of the single episode. The kind of pain is not leading and the absence of a more exact specification in young children is also unreliable. Often cyclic vomiting is accompanying. Typically, children report upon more pain during examination than objectively can be observed. Attention intensifies symptomatology. The general condition is barely reduced. Also appetite is not reduced. Enteritis as one of the most important differential diagnoses in childhood is most easily recognized by an exact clinical history and

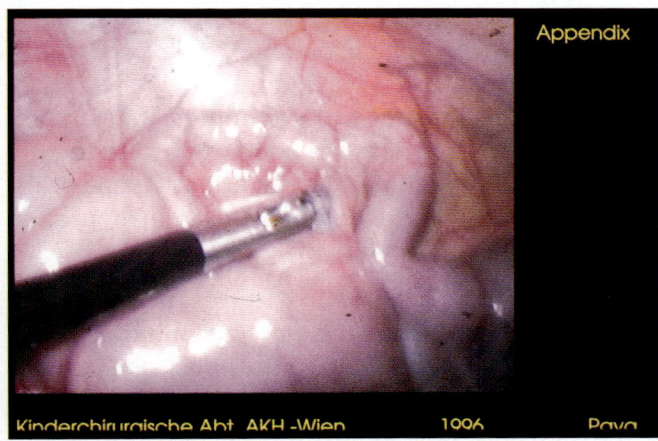

Fig. 54.9A: Appendix seen in laparoscopy

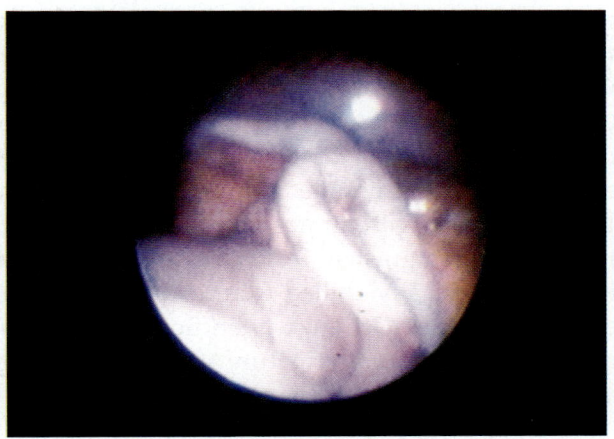

Fig. 54.9B: Laparoscopic view with 2 mm scope

observation. Mainly virally caused, children are suffering from cough or cold, headache, fever and fatigue in the days before abdominal pain appear. Abdominal pain itself is diffuse, cramping and at the beginning associated with episodes of diarrhea. Such episodes occur in advanced stages of an appendicitis only. Nevertheless, a careful observation is important then, because viruses preferentially attack-with (Paramyxoviridae-mumps, enteric viruses-Coxsackie B) or without (Adenovirus) viremia-lymphatic organs, to which also the appendix belong. Particularly the intestinal types of the adenovirus group which do not attack the respiratory organs are able to cause swelling of mesenteric lymph nodes for months and can be a trigger for appendicitis. With abdominal ultrasonography, the picture of a mesenteric lymphadenitis is observed which is a frequent finding together with ear-ache and simultaneously appearing abdominal pain in the right upper quadrant. The blood count is rather indicating a leukopenia than a leukocytosis, the CRP level is low. In the differential blood count a lymphocytosis would appear. Bacterial enteritis is mainly caused by *Campylobacter, Yersinia*, and *Salmonella*. Typically diarrhea, in most cases connected with subfebrile or febrile temperatures, is in the foreground whereas abdominal pain is appearing late and seems to be diffuse. Often also family members, friends, or playmates are afflicted. The blood sample shows a strongly increased number of leukocytes, in particular a leftward shift is existing, and the CRP is increased.[39] Bacterial enteritis are also able to initiate appendicitis and the following three germs *Campylobacter jejuni, Yersinia pseudotuberculotica* and *enterocolitica* are the most frequent inducers of a bacterial appendicitis.[40] Especially appearing in childhood up to the age of four, an inflamed Meckel's diverticulum is barely to distinguish from an acute appendicitis. But in general this is only a rare event. The probability that a Meckel's diverticulum becomes symptomatic is about 2%. Of this percentage only a small part appears as inflammation, another part manifests as bleeding or ileus.

In young women during puberty, diseases of the internal genitalia are more common causes of discomfort. Functional ovarian cysts are very frequent. These typically disappear with start of menses but can also persist for months and therefore cause pain. They are ultrasonographically easy to identify. The treatment, if necessary, is only conservative. If the cysts are larger than 5-8 cm, a laparoscopic enucleation is possible. These, including many small cysts, may lead to a torsion of the ovary and therefore to intensive acute abdominal pain. The torsion of an ovarian cyst is, in any case, an indication for immediate surgery. This is only limitedly valid during neonatal period. At that age, the necrotic ovary may possibly be resorbed. Also without torsion or bleeding, ovarian cysts, predominantly in puberty, are the cause of deep-seated rather chronic, cyclically relapsing abdominal pain. Teratoma, dysgerminoma, and other germ cell tumors but also malformations of the uterus or the vagina (Mayer-Rokitansky-Küster-Hauser syndrome, Uterus dimetria with one-sided vaginal atresia) may cause symptoms of appendicitis. Laparoscopy represents for all of these diseases an essential part of diagnostics.[41]

Also sexual transmitted diseases like PID (pelvic inflammatory disease) are possible differential diagnoses. This disease almost only appears in sexual active girls. The inverted conclusion that an appearance of PID is coupled with a loss of virginity however is not admissible. In most cases the right-sided salpingitis with an abscess in the small pelvis can only be distinguished from an appendicitis by an ultrasonographically skilled examiner, and can also be in connection with an appendicitis *ab externis*. Furthermore, in sexually mature young women one has to think of pregnancy or ectopic pregnancy.

If the pain is appearing periodically and menarche fails to come, the cause may be a congenital malformation like the Mayer-Rokitansky-Küster-Hauser syndrome (Rokitansky sequence).[42] This syndrome represents a congenital combination of malformations which is characterized by a normal female chromosome complement (46XX), normal secondary sex characters, vaginal atresia, and uterus malformation (bicornuate or bipartite). The vaginal atresia leads to an obstruction of menstrual blood, which increases in consequence of every period and therefore causes pain. During this stage of development, also an endometriosis can get symptomatic although, this is typically causing dysmenorrhea and dyspareunia in young women.

In pre-school children of both gender pneumonias, in particular lobular pneumonias on the right in connection with peritoneal symptoms may simulate an appendicitis. There is a typical retraction of the intercostal space during inspiration, cough, and hyperpyrexia. Sonographically, free fluid is copiously found in the abdomen together with a pleural Winkel's effusion but there is no indication for an inflammatory event in the right lower quadrant. A pulmonal radiography leads to the right diagnosis.

Urinary tract infection is a frequent, spastic, and painful event in preschool children, can be accompanied by fever and may correspond to the first symptoms of a vesicoureteral reflux. In school-age children, dysuria appears as an accompanying symptom of appendicitis in up to 20%.

A bacterial meningitis starting with abdominal pain and cramps is extremely dangerous. However, in most cases headache, visual disturbance, hyperpyrexia, neck stiffness, diffuse peritoneal guarding, and foudroyant worsening of the general condition of the child exist. In such cases, the lumbar puncture is favored above other diagnostics.

Otitis media may too cause abdominal pain in pre-school children. Abdominal sonography frequently reveals an accompanying mesenteric lymphadenitis. These findings are, in case of a hasty examination, often misinterpreted as appendicitis.

Pseudoappendicitis diabetica: In diabetes mellitus right-sided abdominal pain can occur which impose colicly, chronically, and heavily. An unnecessary operation as well as an actual appendicitis recognized too late, lead to the high morbidity among these children. In case of known diabetes and especially of an existing diabetic decompensation, ultrasonography is an helpful instrument.

The idiopathic net torsion as well as the idiopathic segmental infarct of the greater omentum are clinically similar to an appendicitis, in particular if the maximal point lies on the right side. Both events can be diagnosed laparoscopically and treated accordingly.[43] Abdominal lymphangiomas are also sometimes operated as a misdiagnosed appendicitis. With ultrasonographic help, this presumptive diagnosis should be detected preoperatively and therefore, a transverse laparotomy should be chosen. Typhlitis in connection with an acute leukemia is hardly to distinguish from appendicitis. This is a fatal prognosis due to the frequently associated, uncontrollable sepsis.

Furthermore, other differential diagnosis of abdominal pain include clinical history, pancreatitis, cholelithiasis, urolithiasis, peptic ulcer, dyspepsia, amebic abscess, hepatitis, and injuries through anal foreign bodies. These are promptly to distinguish only with a careful clinical history and examination.

In general the following standard is valid: the younger a child is and the more anxious the mother is, the sooner the patient should be hospitalized.

Most Frequent Misdiagnosis[44]

- Gastroenteritis
- Upper respiratory tract infection
- Sepsis of other origin
- Urinary tract infection
- Encephalitis
- Febrile seizure
- Blunt abdominal trauma.

ETIOLOGY

The etiology of appendicitis is not clarified until now, although two facts are supported by some studies. On the one hand, genetic differences in the development of immunologic protection-factors could be responsible for, on the other hand also environmental and dietary factors seem to play an important role. Striking are variations of sexual distribution, of different populations, and between towns and rural districts. An explanation for the latter distinction could be the higher socio-economic status of the white population in countries like the USA and Europe, or that of inhabitants of large towns. There are also existing seasonal differences with the greatest accumulation of appendicitis during summer season and the lowest appearance in winter.[45]

Most authors consider the fiber-deficient nutrition of the industrial countries and large towns as the most important etiologic factor. This is supported by the fact that fecoliths, which often occur in consequence of constipation, are also the most frequent starting-point of appendicitis. The association between fecoliths and appendicitis is proved.[46] The fecolith leads to a occlusion of the lumen, therefore to a local obstruction, to ischemia, and finally to a local inflammation. The so called appendicitic primary lesion is generated. From these foci granulocytes start migration through all wall layers.

As immunohistochemical investigations have shown, the previously common saying that the vermiform appendix is nothing than a useless, rudimentary organ, is not right. The appendix morphologically and topographically correspond to a GALT (gut associated lymphoid tissue).[47] The appendix together with the tonsils, the Peyer's plaques, and the mesenteric lymph nodes appears responsible for immunoregulatory mechanisms in the lymphatic system. Therein, partial causes of inflammation could be found. Possibly the first step of inflammation, the focal infiltration of the lamina propria, is demonstrably associated with an increase of T lymphocytes (CD3) and plasma cells concerning the whole organ.[48] Meanwhile it is known that during inflammations of the appendix different cytokine levels (IL-2, IL-6, TNF-alpha) are increased. These are also used for the detection and proof of chronically relapsing appendicitis.[49]

The germs which are found with appendicitis generally correspond with the intestinal flora. About 20% are aerobic germs, 20% are anaerobic, and in about 60% aerobic as well as anaerobic germs are found in smears taken during appendicitis.[50]

The most common germ is *E. coli* followed by *Bacteroides fragilis*, *Peptostreptococcus* and *Pseudomonas sp*. Viral infections with mumps virus, Coxsackie type B, and adenoviruses are frequently seen in appendicitis. The real significance of this observation is still not verified, although in general, the meaning is distributed that, based on a lymphoid hyperplasia appendicitis can evolve. Occasionally, in immuno-suppressed patients (e.g. AIDS patients, patients under chemotherapy) a viral infection with cytomegalovirus (CMV) or Epstein-Barr viruses can act as primary promoter of inflammation. Uncommon causes include yersiniosis, parasites (oxyures), Crohn´s disease, foreign bodies, tuberculosis, volvulus of appendix, intussusception, septa, tumors, and diverticula.[51] Necrotizing enterocolitis seems to be responsible for the very rare appendicitis in the neonatal period.[52]

Eating habits: Absence of dietary fiber.

Fecolith: Occlusion of the lumen – local obstruction – ischemia – local inflammation – migration of granulocytes through all layers.

Yersiniosis: The infection with *Yersinia pseudo-tuberculotica* and *enterocolitica*, *Campylobacter jejuni*, *Salmonella typhi*, and also the very rare infection with Mycobacterium tuberculosis are considered as trigger of appendicitis. The bacterial colonization with *E. coli* is rather a part of an already commenced inflammation than a possible primary cause.

Viral infection or lymphoid hyperplasia: Under chemotherapy, immunosuppression, AIDS

Worms, especially oxyures (*Enterobius vermicularis*) and ascarides are by far the most frequently seen parasites. They are able to induce a lymphoid reaction or cause appendicitis through obstruction. Helminthic diseases are a common incidental finding in histologically not-inflammatory altered appendices. The incidence is, with about 4%, highest in childhood (between the age of 6 and 15).[53]

Chronic inflammatory diseases (Crohn´s disease): Also Crohn´s disease is able to primarily or secondarily manifest in the appendix and causes an inflammation there. In these cases an ileocecal resection is necessary.

Foreign bodies: Ingested foreign bodies in the lumen like screws, plastic parts, or kernels are inducing an inflamed appendix. But in general it cannot be deduced from these events that swallowing of foreign bodies leads with a higher probability to appendicitis.

Tuberculosis may be the cause of an appendicitis, but is rather simulating one, e.g. with mesenteric expansion (sometimes observed as primary manifestation in pre-school children). Typically, there are multiple, enlarged mesenteric lymph nodes and caseating granulomas in the peritoneum.

Volvulus of the appendix and appendiceal intussusception:

A volvulus of the vermiform appendix is a rare event in childhood. In the literature only a small number of cases are described.[54-56] It presents itself as an intermittently occurring abdominal pain which acutely exacerbates. Mucoceles, fecoliths (Bonnoud), and idiopathic forms are described as the main causes.

In these situations the color-coded Doppler ultrasonography is useful. Also the intussusception of the appendix into the cecum is a very rare event and is promptly revealed by ultrasonography (beside this, intussusception represents an indirect proof of peristaltic movement). There also exists a congenital form of an inverse appendix.

Septa and atresia are extremely rare, duplications are seen more frequently. They lead to a mucous retention. A septum at the base of the appendix can be simulated by a mucous fold (Gerlach's valve).

APPENDICEAL NEOPLASMS

Most frequent neoplasms are carcinoids with a frequency of 0.02-1.5% in all histological preparations. In principle, carcinoids are malignant tumors. The appendiceal carcinoid exhibits less DNA-aneuploidy than carcinoids of the ileum and therefore, more frequently shows a benign course.[57] Due to the risk of metastasis mainly in mesenteric lymph nodes and liver, all carcinoids with an unsteady behavior, those above a diameter of 1 cm, positive lymph nodes, infiltration of the serosa or the mesenteriolum, or a position at the basis should be considered for hemicolectomy or at least for further clarification with indium[111]-labeled octreotid. At a size < 1cm no further therapy is necessary, if appendectomy was carried out and the base lies in the uneffected region. If the tumor is larger than 2 cm, a right-sided hemicolectomy is indicated. Appendiceal carcinoids emerge from neuroendocrine, subepithelial cells. In contrast to jejunoileal carcinoids, the staining with S-100 for appendiceal carcinoids is positive. Rarely, also adenocarcinomas or adenomas are possible. In these cases one has to look for familiar polyposis which is an indication for prepubertal, subtotal colectomy. But adenocarcinomas of the appendix are an extreme rarity in childhood. The age-peak lies in the 6th decade. Rarely lymphoma may also involve the appendix (Fig. 54.10). Benign tumors are mainly asymptomatic mucosal hyperplasias, metaplasias, or adenomas, which, for instance as cystadenomas are producing mucine and can become sypmtomatic therefore. They form mucoceles which may rupture and cause a peritoneal pseudomyxoma. All, benign as well as malignant tumors of the appendix may, to a significantly higher rate be associated with synchronous or metachronous, gastrointestinal tumors with another localization.[58]

PATHOGENESIS

In most cases appendicitis follows a cascadic pattern. Fecoliths, helminthes, viral lymphadenitis, or foreign bodies cause an obstruction of the lumen whereby pressure arise to the mucosa and the wall of the appendix which subsequently leads to a venous congestion and arterial hypoperfusion of the distal part of the vermiform appendix. Meanwhile, pathogenic bacteria start to overgrow this area and migrate through the underlying mucosa. The intraluminal increase in pressure develops very rapidly because the

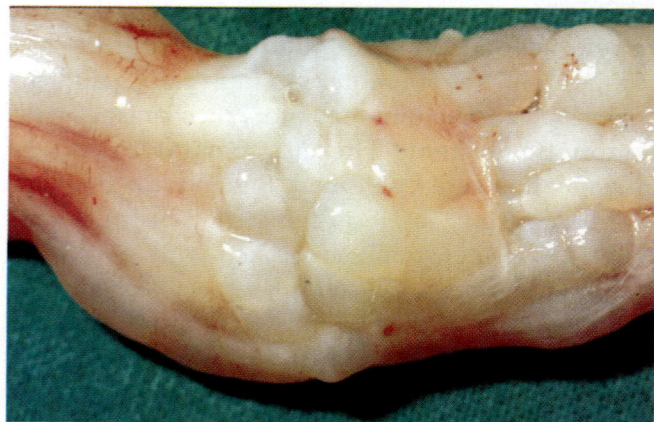

Fig. 54.10: Lymphoma appendix

vermiform appendix is not expansible due to its structural design.[59] Granulocytes migrate through the mucosa, submucosa, muscularis, and finally also through the serosa. Aschoff's primary complexes are formed which are aggregations of neutrophil granulocytes. On the serosa fibrin is built up and the whole wall slowly becomes necrotic. The base of the vermiform appendix is generally free from inflammation. This may be due to an additional blood supply via branches of the cecal artery at the base, whereas the appendicular artery as an terminal branch is not able to sufficiently ensure the peripheral blood supply during an inflammation. If this process cannot be stopped, perhaps a necrosis develops followed by open ulceration and then perforations results. Unlimited, this may first of all result in local and then in a generalized peritonitis, sepsis and death, or a perityphlitic abscess is formed which breaks through and drains, building a fistula. Whether an arising inflammation always and absolutely leads to the end point gangrene or perforation is questionable. Autotherapy or curing by conservative treatment is also possible. Several studies and investigation indicate that chronically relapsing abdominal pain in the right lower quadrant may be due to afflictions of the appendix.[60] By studying the cytokine expression of the vermiform appendix, nearly identically increased values were found in acute appendicitis and in appendectomies due to chronic recurrent abdominal pain, whereas in elective appendectomies due to other causes expression patterns comparable to those of unaffected appendices were found.[61]

Also the fact that many patients are free from pain after appendectomy supports the hypothesis of a recurrently appearing appendicitis.[62]

Histopathologic Classification (According to Zimmermann, Bern)

I	II
Acute appendicitis	Chronic appendicitis
Appendicitis due to specific infections and infestations	Appendicitis in inflammatory bowel disease
Idiopathic granulomatous appendicitis	Eosinophilic appendicitis
Appendicitis in arteritis and collagen vascular disorders	Neurogenic appendicitis/ appendicopathy (Masson´s pseudoappendicitis)
Other types	

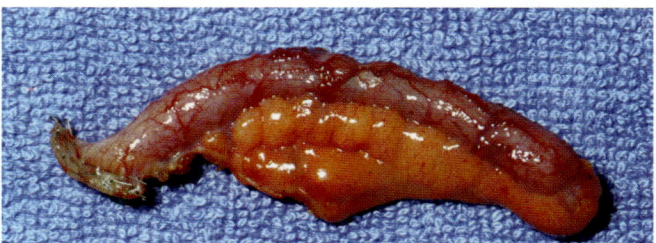

Fig. 54.11: Resected specimen of acute appendicitis

CURRENT CLASSIFICATION OF APPENDICITIS ACCORDING TO HISTOLOGICAL BASIS

Acute appendicitis (Fig. 54.11): Thickened, rigidity of wall, injected; mucous membrane defect, neutrophil granulocytes in the mucosa and submucosa/disorder of mucosal epithelium, granulocyte accumulation, extravascular granulocytes, leukocytes in the lumen.

Phlegmenous and ulcerophlegmenous appendicitis (Figs 54.12A and B): Fibrinously purulently coated, surrounding (mesenteric) phlegmonas; passing through all wall layers, including serosa; fibrinous appositions, defects of the superficial wall layers up to the serosa. After 10–14 hours: transmural granulocytic infiltration; phlegmonous inflammation. After 24 hours ulcers = ulcerophlegmonous inflammation.

Gangrenous appendicitis: Necrotic wall areas without opening; gangrene of the whole wall without perforation.

Perforating appendicitis: (Figs 54.13A and B) Perforation and outflow of fecal content through defects of the abdominal cavity; defects of the whole wall.

Neurogenic appendicitis: Macroscopically nearly not remarkable, obliteration; intramucous or submucous proliferation of nervefibers, possibly with central neurinoma at the peak in case of obliteration.

Focal appendicits: Macroscopically normal; histologically, in case of an extensive incision, inflammation restricted to one area is detectable – if only few incisions are carried out, not visible "normal" histology.

Recurrent appendicitis: Macroscopically, frequently thickened, partly whitish glittering, or totally normal. Increased fat tissue. Frequently coproliths in the lumen. Histologically rare lymphocytic infiltration, extensively multiplied reactive lymph nodes, lymphoid hyperplasia. Sometimes fibrotic reconstruction.

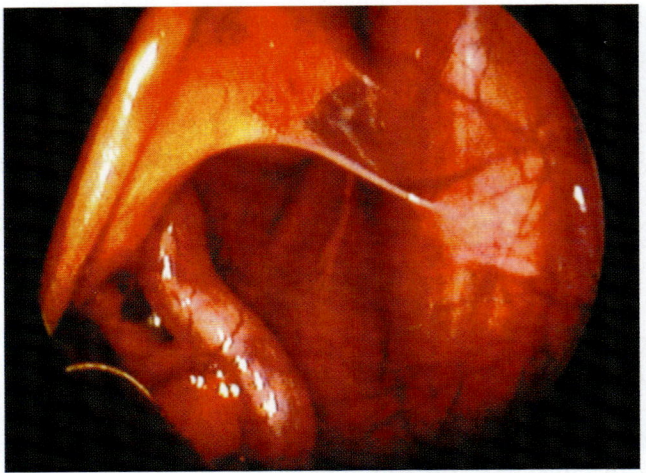

Fig. 54.12A: Phlegmonous appendicitis seen laparoscopically

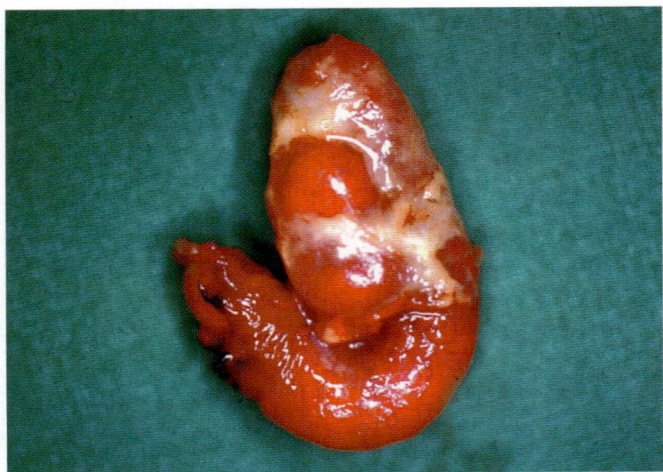

Fig. 54.12B: Phlegmonous appendicitis

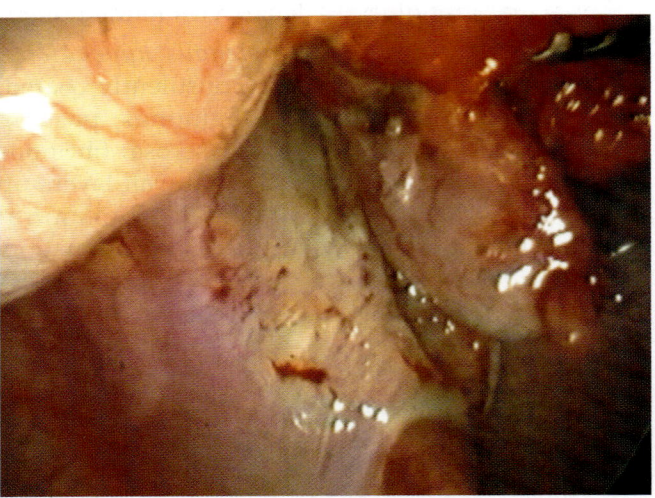

Fig. 54.13A: Perforated appendicitis

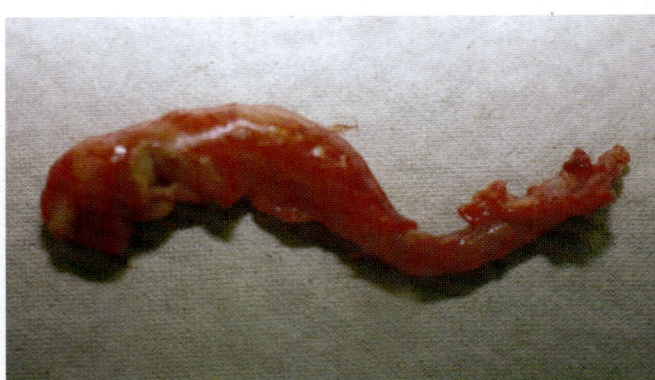

Fig. 54.13B: Resected specimen of perforated appendicitis

COMPLICATIONS OF APPENDICITIS

1. Diffuse peritonitis.
2. Perforation with stercoral abscess, covered with the greater omentum or ileal loops, in case of a retrocecal position through the cecum or open with Douglas' abscess and diffuse peritonitis, respectively. At an age of 0-4 the frequency of perforations is at least 40%.
3. Thrombophlebitis of the appendicular vein with propagation and septic liver abscesses.
4. Healing with scar formation and relapsing appendicitis at the base of scar obliteration.
5. Adhesive strangulation of the intestines.
6. Appendicular mucocele: Obstruction of secretion in case of an over-wounded appendicitis and allantoid distension of the thinned appendix distally from the obliteration (scar, coprolith, foreign body, etc.) with recurrent pain symptomatology.

THERAPY

Surgical Therapy

The surgical excision of the inflamed vermiform appendix is the commonly accepted treatment. The McBurney's incision (gridiron incision) as it was introduced by McBurney and Murphy 1894, is the method of choice. Since 1983 the first laparoscopic appendectomy was reported by K Semm, a Munich gynecologist, this surgical method has developed into an accepted alternative.[63]

Gridiron incision: This operation method starts from an access in the right lower quadrant, which crosses the McBurney point in the main cleavage line. After discission of the subcutis, the external oblique aponeurosis is cleaved along the strands, the underlying musculature is extensively bluntly separated, and finally the peritoneum is incised following the craniocaudal direction. By luxating the cecum, the base of the appendix can be presented. The vascular supply is interrupted by clinging ligations of the mesenteriolum. A contusion mark is set at the base, where the appendix will be ligated and above be abscised. After disinfection with iodine the stump is sent to the bottom of a cecal purse string suture. Originally, this was also covered by serous tunic fixed with suture. In France, it is not usual to sink the stump. Also in case of a laparoscopic surgery no stump-sinking is performed. Some centers prefer a drainage in case of a perforation or an intra-abdominal abscess.

MINIMAL INVASIVE TECHNIQUES

The Laparoscopic Appendectomy

The minimal invasive surgery has helped to reduce the complication rate in cholecystectomy (the second in frequency operation after appendectomy), the stay in hospital, and the duration of pain. In 1893 Semm, for the first time, has also successfully described appendectomy via laparoscopy. In some pediatric surgery centres, nearly all cases of appendicitis are endoscopically operated (e.g. University hospital Jena, Germany; university hospital Utrecht, Netherlands). Today, 80% of all appendectomies are performed conventionally, 20% laparoscopically (laparoscopic appendectomies in 1996: in Switzerland about 30%, in France and Austria about 7-9%, in the Netherlands 4%, and about 20% in the USA). This is, even though several studies not only have shown no disadvantages of the minimal invasive technique but more or less significant advantages.[64] But, a final, statistically really unobjectionable comparison does not exist yet. In the author's series there were advantages in favor of the laparoscopic technique in inflamed appendicitis and especially in the group of perforating appendicitis.[65]

The causes of the delayed popularity of the laparoscopic appendectomy are various. The gridiron incision is not only an established technique, but also the most frequent teaching operation. In addition, the laparoscopic operation is technically much more pretentious and therefore the learning process is slower and the fear of complication higher. Also for the non-medical staff, the expenditure in the operation room is much higher. The minimal invasive technique is especially device-depending and therefore much more expensive. Considering the epidemiologic importance of the appendicitis, this cost factor may be crucial.[66] In general, a better diagnostic view, a lower wound-infection rate, a shorter postoperative pain phase, a shorter duration of hospitalization, and a better cosmetic result are the stated advantages of the minimal invasive technique in contrast to an open appendectomy (Fig. 54.14A and B).[67] But in fact, there are no prospectively randomized studies in childhood and only a small number in adults which statistically

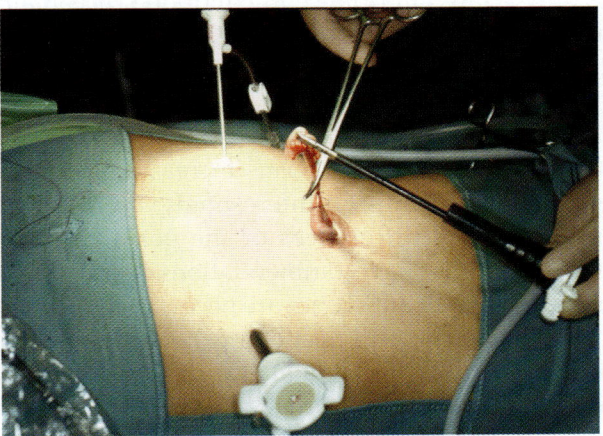

Fig. 54.14A: Laparoscopically assisted appendectomy

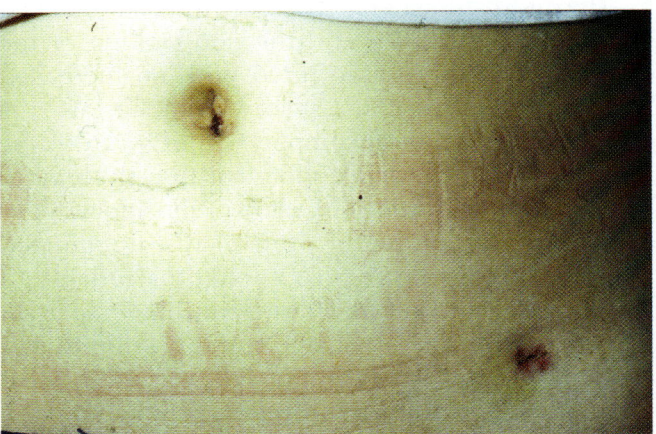

Fig. 54.14B: Wound after 2 trocar technique

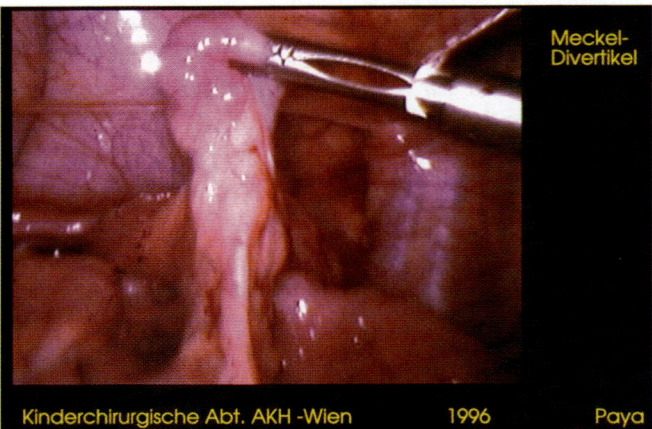

Fig. 54.15: Laparoscopic dissection of Meckle's diverticulum

unobjectionably investigate the benefit of both methods for the patients.[68] Other differential diagnosis can easily be identified and tackled (Fig. 54.15).

In acute appendicitis a very small skin incision in case of a conventional appendectomy is, in general only possible with a loss of view and with an increase in risk. Especially in case of generous indications in the conventional technique and therefore a high percentage of appendectomies with a histologically unaffected appendix, the portion of very small skin incisions is high. As a result, the difference to minimal invasive surgery is not so clear considering the postoperative recovery period and the cosmetic result. But in case of a histologically verified appendicitis, there is a significant difference in favor of the laparoscopy considering the dimension of the skin incision (particularly, if devices of the new generation with 1.2-5 mm optics and instruments are used).

The disadvantages of laparoscopy are a prolonged duration of operation and the non-sinking of the appendiceal stump associated with an increased incidence of abscesses. Meanwhile, the latter is considered as a typical complication of laparoscopic appendectomy. The endoabdominal abscess seems to be caused by an unclean excision of the appendix or by a local distribution of previously encapsulated abscesses, respectively. To avoid this reliably, a mechanical clamp-suture instrument should be used. A further technical advantage is the possibility of a carefully directed aspiration of pus with the help of an endobag (plastic recovery-bag) whereby the appendix can be removed from the abdomen without contamination of the abdominal wall. In principle, the removal of the appendix is easier because it can be worked *in situ* and the basis is hardly affected from the inflammatory process.[69] In particular in case of a perforation, the noticeable advantages are a shorter, postoperative duration of pain and a shorter resting period.

Delayed Resection

In case of an existing perforation with local peritonitis or perityphlitic abscesses, a drainage with antibiotic protection as initial treatment, alone can make cure possible. Some weeks later the elective stump appendectomy follows.[70] Thereby, the morbidity of peritonitis and abscess formation could be decreased.[71]

The drainage is performed under ultrasonographic control or CT directed and therefore is often carried out in the interventional center of the radiologic department. But this can, in no case prevent the patient from being appendectomized.

NON-SURGICAL THERAPY

Antibiotic Therapy in Appendicitis

The antibiotic therapy ranks high in the treatment of appendicitis.[72] An antibiotic therapy without surgery is only suggestive in case of insufficient possibilities for surgery or perforation in combination with drainage (delayed surgery). In such cases, drainage is performed under ultrasound- or CT-directed control. If the acute inflammation is abated and the drainage is removed, resection of appendix via laparoscopy or gridiron incision is necessary. But this treatment option has only a rare importance in childhood. It is mainly important for the treatment of appendicitis in adults.

The germ-spectrum in appendicitis which is found in the lumen primarily shows *E. coli*, *Bacteroides fragilis*, *Enterobacter*, and *Pseudomonas*. In the course of inflammation anaerobic germs increasingly colonize appendix and ileum.[73,74] Interestingly, there are also found seasonal differences of the germ-spectrum. There are numerous recommendations concerning the question whether antibiotics are necessary in principle as well as the correct selection of the right antibiotic. From all these studies, it finally can be concluded that the administration of a broad-spectrum antibiotic at least half an hour before skin incision leads to best results. Whether the postoperative antibiosis has to be continued, depends on the surgical finding, local circumstances, and additional risk factors like diabetes mellitus as concomitant disease.

Recommendation

Perioperative prophylaxis: Single dose of cephalosporin, e.g. Cefoxitim, amoxicillin + clavulanic acid, piperacillin, or clindamycin/gentamicin; also metronidazole alone is an possible alternative.

Postoperative treatment: Gangrenous or perforation: broad-spectrum antibiotic for 3-5 days.

Peritonitis: Broad-spectrum antibiotic + metronidazole for 5-10 days.

POSTOPERATIVE CARE

Postoperative care is confronted with two fundamental problems. Cure shall proceed without further infections and normal feeding shall quickly be possible. Both aims are not difficult to reach in childhood because in case of a technically troublefree appendectomy – no matter which technique is used – a rapid cure (within one or three days) is the rule. Especially the degree of inflammation and to a minor extent age and the anesthetic procedure are crucial for cure.[75] The duration of hospitalization are strongly reflecting cultural and health-political circumstances. So in Europe, the patient with a common health insurance is generally nursed in the unit for one week and is then discharged in healthy condition. In America, the patients is often discharged on the same day because the costs are extremely high for the family and not always covered by the insurance company. Despite this, the complication rates are comparable. These facts show that not the postoperative care in an unit but the perioperative and operative care are the most crucial components for a rapid recovery. In case of an appendicitis without complications the patients is already allowed to drink water after 6-8 hours, and if this is tolerated well it is started with a pasty diet. In most cases the patients are allowed to take regular food after three days. During the first days sufficient fluid intake is important, but fresh fruits and vegetables, sweets, and flatulent food should be avoided for at least 10-14 days. In case of peritonitis or an intensive manipulation of the cecum (perhaps with intramural hematoma) a paralytic ileus may occur postoperatively. In these cases, it is better to adhere to food withdrawal and parenteral fluid supply, as well as electrolyte substitution. A temporary stomach tube often simplifies the situation. Fever can persist for some days but is not always associated with the need for antibiotic therapy. But if the fever reappears several days after surgery, one has to think of a subcutaneous or intra-abdominal abscess. If there is no bowel evacuation after three to four days, stimulation with a small clyster, in case of preschool children with the help of an intestinal tube, has a relieving effect. But it is always to think of a fluid deficit which has to be corrected. Bed rest is only necessary as long as the patient himself wants to stay there. Also younger children are able to walk without pain after surgery. The pain situation itself is very individual. In general in young patients a single dose of a nonsteroid antirheumatic like paracetamol or metamizole (in most cases given as suppository on the operating table or on the first postoperative day) is sufficient for pain relief. All complicated cases with median laparotomy, intraperitoneal or subcutaneous drainage, or generalized peritonitis are, of course exceptions. For these cases an additional intravenous dose of opiates with fewer side-effects (e.g. tramadol or nubain) is often necessary.

POSTOPERATIVE COMPLICATIONS

The complication rates after appendectomy are still lying between 5.1-33%, whereby the highest proportion is found in the group of the perforating appendices. In spite of a drastic improvement after the introduction of antibiotic therapy, the mortality rate lies, mainly due to multimorbid patients, still between 0.001-0.5%. Complications can be classified into early, that means immediately occurring after surgery, and late complication. Early complications are first of all peritonitis, the intra-abdominal abscess, the disturbance of wound healing, and the paralytic ileus. They nearly always occur due to a perforating appendicitis. The causes of perforation are first of all associated with a delayed start of treatment and a history anamnesis of more than 36 hours (in > 65% of all perforations).[76] Precautions to avoid these complications are a perioperative antibiotic prophylaxis, clean and fast surgery, lowest possible contamination of the abdominal wall, adequate preoperative fluid replacement, and careful lavage with normal saline. Drainages, which are not unusual in adults, are very controversial in children.[77]

Most hospitals also refuse drainage in case of a multiquadrant peritonitis. One exceptions might be the primary drainage without resection of the appendix in case of an extremely progressive appendicitis. Appendectomy is performed as described above, after the abatement of inflammation. If an intra-abdominal abscess is existing, there are again two treatment options. In most cases, a complete resolution of the abscess can be achieved and therefore a relaparotomy be avoided by intravenous administration of antibiotics and temporary food withdrawal.[78] The second option is surgery. Either a relaparotomy is performed or a laparotomy is carried out to clear or drain the abscesses. The process can be followed by ultrasonography.[79]

Late complications are ileus, caused by adhesions, and stump appendicitis. Also chronic pain may occur as a consequence of nerve lesions, consecutive development of neurinomas, or scar pain. The adhesive strangulation of intestines is typically taking place after a peritonitis and nearly always requires relaparotomy or laparoscopy.

Perioperative complications are a rupture of the appendix, possibly a cecal lesion, a erroneous opening of the bladder, or bleeding due to an insufficient ligation of the appendicular artery. In case of minimal invasive surgery technical complication are added. These are injuries of blood vessels with severe bleeding due to the first trocar or the Veress' needle, and injuries of abdominal organs also due to trocar insertion or through monopolar coagulation, resulting in a leakage current. Perforations of intestinal loops, liver, spleen and bladder as well as thermic damages of cecum or ileum are occurring.

PROGNOSIS

The operative treated appendicitis is considered as cured after wound healing. A relapse is only possible, if a residual stump was left. Indigestions or immunological deficiencies in cases of a premature appendectomy were not observed till now. Although, all possible functions of the appendix are only partly clarified.

Since the notion appendicitis exists, also the conception of chronic appendicitis is known. Although, the existence of such a chronic course is denied by the vast majority of surgeons. On the other hand, the recurrent appendicitis is accepted and proved by several studies.[80] It has been shown that patients who are again and again suffering from more or less typical discomforts are not operated until the clinically clear picture of an acute appendicitis is observed. The diagnosis is objectively verified by adequate studies. That means that there exists a milder course of the disease which sooner or later ends up in a complicated appendicitis in most cases. In these cases the early appendectomy is an advantage and often the diagnostic laparoscopy is the better operative access.

FUTURE ASPECTS AND RESEARCH

The vermiform appendix is increasingly confronted with new scopes for instance as conduit or replacement in operations of the lower urinary tract. There are also new indications like PFIC (progressive familial intrahepatic cholestasis), where the appendix is needed as diversification between gallbladder and skin. Therefore, the indication for appendectomy has to be more precisely in the future. Due to the better diagnostic situation today, fewer false positively diagnosed patients are appendectomized.[81]

Appendicitis is one of the most discussed topics of surgical research. Clinical investigation about diagnostic criteria, especially the attempt to establish computer-based systems, are supported by the OMGE. Until now these efforts were disappointing. Clinical history and examination should be structurally recorded. Therefore, large prospective studies are necessary to answer the questions whether it shall be operated early or only actively be observed, or whether technical developments like ultrasonography are able to replace the active observation. Due to these and other studies, progress has been made in the establishment of objective parameters for the recognition of appendicitis which are now a part of our evidence-based medicine. Immunocytochemical and immunohistological investigations are carried out in many centers. The role of cytokines for the development of appendicitis is a large chapter of the surgical research. The key-words are among others Pgp 9.5, nerve growth factor, and growth-associated protein 43. One part of research is dealing with neuroimmunological processes within the appendix. Thereby specific neuropeptides like SP are investigated referring to their importance for the immune system and the appendicitis, respectively. It is postulated that up to a fourth of all appendectomies, in which a histologically unaffected appendix was found, are cases of neuroimmunoappendicitis, which are based on an increased density of nerve fibers sensitive to two neuropeptides.[82] Currently, a meta-analysis has revealed that appendectomized patients less frequently fall sick with ulcerative colitis. Also nothing is known about the responsible immunological processes.[83]

REFERENCES

1. Williams GR. Presidential address: A history of appendicitis. Annals of Surgery 1983;197(5):495-506.
2. McBurney C. The incision made in the abdominal wall in cases of appendicitis, with a description of a new method of operating. Ann Surg 1894;20:38-43.
3. Murphy JB. Two thousand operations for appendicitis, with deductions from his personal experience. Am J Med Sci 1904;128:187-211.
4. de Quervain F. Die Behandlung der akuten Apendicitis, auf Grund einer schweizerischen Sammelstatistik. Corr Blatt Schweiz Aerzte 1913;43:1609-24.
5. Broschung U. History of "right iliac fossa pain": From internal to surgical treatment– with special reference to the evolution in Switzerland. Progress in Surgery 1998;25:1-9.
6. Eriksson St. Acute appendicitis – ways to improve diagnostic accuracy. Eur J Surg 1996;162:435-42.
7. Henderson J, Goldacre MJ, Fairweather JM, Marcovitch H. Conditions accounting for substantial time spent in hospital in children aged 1-14 years. Arch Dis Child 1992;67:83.
8. Brender JD, Marcuse EK, Weiss NS, Koepsell TD. Is childhood appendicitis familial? Am J Dis Child 1985;139: 338.
9. Addiss DG, Shaffer N, Fowler BS, Tauxe RV. The epidemiology of appendicitis and appendectomy in the United States. Am J Epidemiol 1990;132(5):910-25.
10. Luckmann R. Incidence and case fatality rates for acute appendicitis in California. A population-based study of the effects of age. Am J Epidemiol 1989;129(5):905-18.
11. Treutner KH, Schumpelick V. Epidemiologie der Appendicitis. Chirurg 1997;68:1-5.
12. Seiler ChA. Standard open surgical procedure in appendicitis: From the past to the present. In Krähenbühl L, Frei E, Klaiber Ch, Büchler MW. Acute Appendicitis: Standard Treatment or Laparoscopic surgery? Prog Surg, Verlag Karger, Basel 1998;25:59-69.
13. Broman I. Entwicklung des Darmes. In Broman I: Die Entwicklung des Menschen vor der Geburt; Bergmann JF, München 1927.
14. Ramsden WH, Mannion REJ, Simpkins KC, deDombal FT. Is the appendix where you think it is-and if not, does it matter? Clinical Radiology 1993;47:100-103.
15. Wakely CPG. The position of the vermiform appendix as ascertained by an analysis of 10,000 cases. J of Anatomy 1933;67:277-83.
16. Schumpelick V, Dreuw B, Ophoff K, Prescher A. Appendix and Caecum. Embryology, anatomy, and surgical applications. Surgical Clinics of North America 2000;80(1):295-318.
17. Hahn J, Höpner F, v Kalle T, Mac Donald E, Prantl F, Spitzer I, Färber D. Appendizitis im Kindesalter. Der Radiologie 1997;37:454-58.
18. Collopy BT, Rodgers L, Woodruff P, Williams J. Early experience with clinical indicators in surgery. Australian and New Zealand Journal of Surgery 2000;70(6):448-51.
19. Berr Jr J, Malt RA. Appendicitis near its centenary. Ann Surg 1984;2000:567-75.
20. Sola JE, McBride W, Rachadell J. Current diagnosis and management of appendicitis in children. International pediatrics 2000;15(1):30-32.
21. Puylaert JB. Acute appendicitis: US evaluation using graded compression. Radiology 1986;158(2):355-60.
22. Eskelinen M, Ikonen J, Lipponenen P, Alhava E. A computer-based diagnostic score to aid in diagnosis of acute appendicitis. A prospective study of 1333 patients with acute abdominal pain. Theoretical Surgery 1992;7: 86-90.
23. Peltola H, Ahlqvist J, Rapola J, Rasanen J, Louhimo I, Saarinen M, Eskola J. C-reactive protein compared with white blood cell count and erythrocyte sedimentation rate in the diagnosis of acute appendicitis in children. Acta Chir Scand 1986;152:55-58.
24. Schwerk WB, Wichtrup B, Rothmund M, Ruschoff J. Ultrasonography in the diagnosis of acute appendicitis: a prospective study. Gastroenterology 1989;97(3): 630-39.
25. Dickson JA, Edwards N, Jones AP. Computer-assisted diagnosis of acute abdominal pain in childhood. Lancet 1985;1(8442):1389-90.
26. Eskelinen M, Ikonen J, Lipponen P. The value of history and clinical examination in the diagnosis of acute appendicitis in childhood, with special reference to computer-based decision making. Theor Surg 1993;8: 203-09.
27. Ohmann C, Kreamer M, Jäger S, Sitter H, Pohl C, Stadelmayer B, Vietmeier P. Akuter Bauschmerz – standardisierte Befundung als Diagnoseunterstützung. Chirurg 1992;63:113-23.
28. Alvarado A. A practical score for the early diagnosis of acute appendicitis. Annals of Emergency Medicine 1986;15:557-64.
29. Graff L, Mucci D, Radford MJ. Decision to hospitalize. Objective diagnosis-related group criteria versus clinical judgement. Annals of Emergency Medicine 1988;17(9): 943-52.

30. Alvarado A. A practical score for the early diagnosis of acute appendicitis. Annals of Emergency Medicine 1986;15:557-64.
31. Rice HE, Arbesman M, Martin DJ, Brown RL, Gollin G, Gilbert JC, Caty MG, Glick PL, Azizkhan RG. J Does early ultrasonography affect management of pediatric appendicitis? A prospective analysis. Pediatr Surg 1999;34(5):754-59.
32. Hormann M, Paya K, Eibenberger K, Dorffner R, Lang S, Kreuzer S, Metz VM. MR imaging in children with nonperforated acute appendicitis: value of unenhanced MR imaging in sonographically selected cases. Am J Roentgenol 1998;171(2):467-70.
33. Balthazar EJ, Rofsky NM, Zucker R. Appendicitis: the impact of computed tomography imaging on negative appendectomy and perforation rates. Am J Gastroenterol 1998;93(5):768-71.
34. Rothrock SG, Pagane J. Acute appendicitis in children: Emergency Department Diagnosis and Management. Annals of Emergency Medicine 2000; 36(1): 39-51.
35. Lee KH, Yeung CK, Tam YH, Liu KKW. The use of laparoscopy in the management of adnexal pathologies in children. Australian and New Zealand Journal of Surgery 2000;70(3):192-95.
36. OU CS, Rowbotham R. Laparoscopic diagnosis and treatment of nontraumatic acute abdominal pain in women. J of Laparoendoscopic and advanced Surgical Techniques – Part A 2000;10(1):41-45.
37. Paya K, Rebhandl W, Urbania A, Leberl K, Glaser CH, Mittlböck M, Horcher E. Is diagnostic laparoscopy justified in children with recurrent abdominal pain? Acta Chir Austriaca 1998; 30 (6): 344-48.
38. Decadt B, Sussmann L, Lewis MPN, Secker A, Cohen L, Rogers C, Patel A, Rhodes M. Randomized clinical trial of early laparoscopy in the management of acute non-specific abdominal pain. British J of Surgery 1999;86: 1383-86.
39. Eriksson ST. Acute appendicitis – ways to improve diagnostic accuracy. Eur J Surg 1996;162:435-42.
40. Sue K, Nishimi T, Yamada T, Kamimura T, Matsuo Y, Tanaka N. A right lower abdominal mass due to Yersinia mesenteric lymphadenitis. Pediatr Radiol 1994;24:70-71.
41. Lee KH, Yeung CK, Tam YH, Liu KKW. The use of laparoscopy in the management of adnexal pathologies in children. Australian and New Zealand Journal of Surgery 2000;70(3):192-95.
42. Rokitansky K. Über sogenannte Verdoppelung des Uterus. Medizinisches Jahrbuch des Österreichischen Staates 1938;26-39.
43. Plannelss-Roig MV, Jabaloyas Fernandez J, Barcia-Espinosa, Pous Serrano S, Moya Fernandez A, Rodero-Rodero D. Idiopathic segmental infarct of the epiploon. Apropos a new case and a review of the literature. Rev Esp Enferm Dig 1991;79(3):209-10.
44. Rothrock SG, Pagane J. Acute appendicitis in children: Emergency Department, Diagnosis and Management. Annals of Emergency Medicine 2000;36(1):39-51.
45. Addiss DG, Shaffer N, Fowler BS, Tauxe RV. The epidemiology of appendicitis and appendectomy in the United States. Am J Epidemiol 1990;132(5):910-25.
46. Nitecki S, Karmeli R, Sarr MG. Appendiceal calculi and fecaliths as indications for appendectomy. Surg Gynecol Obstet 1990;171(3):185-88.
47. Bjerke K, Brandtzaeg P, Rognum TO. Distribution of immunoglobulin producing cells is different in normal human appendix and colon mucosa. Gut 1986;27:667-74.
48. Tsuji M, Puri P, Reen DJ. Characterisation of the local inflammatory response in appendicitis. J Pediatr Gastroenterol and Nutr 1993;16:43-48.
49. Wang Y, Reen DJ, Puri P. Is a histologically normal appendix following emergency appendicectomy always normal? Lancet 1996;347:1076-79.
50. Kokoska ER, Silen ML, Tracy TF Jr, Dillon PA, Kennedy DJ, Cradock TV, Weber TR. The impact of intraoperative culture on treatment and outcome in children with perforated appendicitis. J Pediatr Surg 1999;34(5):749-53.
51. Altermatt S, Meuli M, Sacher P. Incidence of yersiniosis in children with suspected acute appendictis. A prospective study. Pediatr Surg Int 1994;9:55-56.
52. Bax NMA, Pearse RG, Dommering N, Molenaar JC. Perforation of the appendix in the neonatal period. J of Pediatr Surg 1980;15(2):200-02.
53. Wiebe BM. Appendicitis and Enterobius vermicularis. Scand J Gastroenterology 1991;26(3):336-38.
54. Abdullaev M. [Volvulus of the vermiform process]. Khirurgiia-Mosk 1979;89.
55. Akers D, Hendrickson M, Markowitz I, Kerstein M. Volvulus of an appendiceal mucocele presenting as a small bowel obstruction. J LA State Med Soc 1988;140:29-33.
56. Paya K, Saadi S, Hörmann M, Rebhandl W, Horcher E. [Isolated volvulus of the appendix-a diagnostic problem] Zentralblatt für Kinderchirurgie 1999;8(1):34-36.
57. Goolsby CL, Punyarit P, Mehl PJ, Rao MS. Flow cytometric DNA analysis of carcinoid tumors of the ileum and appendix. Hum-Pathol 1992;23(12):1340-43.
58. Connor SJ, Hanna GB, Frizelle FA. Appendiceal tumors: retrospective clinicopathologic analysis of appendiceal tumors from 7,970 appendectomies. Dis Colon Rectum 1998;41(1):75-80.
59. Papadopoulos StA, Nikolaou CCh, Manouras AI, Apostolidis NS, Golematis BCH. The effect of obstruction of the appendiceal lumen on ist aerobic and anaerobic flora – an experimental study in rabbits. IJSS 1998;5.
60. Falk S, Schutze U, Guth H, Stutte HJ. Chronic recurrent appendicitis. A clinicopathologic study of 47 cases. Eur J Pediatr Surg 1991;1(5):277-81.
61. Wang Y, Reen DJ, Puri P. Is a histologically normal appendix following emergency appendicectomy always normal? Lancet 1996; 347: 1076-79.
62. Stevenson RJ. Chronic Right-Lower-Quadrant Abdominal Pain: Is there a Role for Elective Appendectomy? J Ped Surg 1999;34(6):950-54.
63. Semm K. Endoscopic appendectomy. Endoscopy 1983;15:59-64.

64. Sauerland ST, Lefering R, Holthausen U, Neugebauer EAM. Laparoscopic vs conventional appendectomy – a meta analysis of randomised controlled trials. Langenbecks's Arch Surg 1998;383:289-95.
65. Paya K, Rauhofer U, Rebhandl W, Deluggi St, Horcher E. Perforating appendicitis: an indication for laparoscopy? Surg Endosc 2000;14:182-84.
66. Paya K, Rebhandl W, Horcher E. [Minimal invasive techniques in childhood: laparoscopy] Pädiatrie and Pädologie 1998;3:42-48.
67. Blakely ML, Spurbeck WW, Laksman S, Hanna K, Schropp KP, Lobe TE. Laparoscopic appendectomy in children. Seminars in Laparoscopic Surgery 1998;5(1):14-18.
68. Golub R, Siddiqui F, Pohl D. Laparoscopic versus open appendectomy: a metaanalysis. J Am Coll Surg 1998;186(5):545-53.
69. Paya K, Fakhari M, Rauhofer U, Felberbauer FX, Rebhandl W, Horcher E. Open versus Laparoscopic Appendectomy in Children: A Comparison of Complications. Journal of the Society of Laparoendoscopic Surgeons 2000;4:121-24.
70. Vargas HI, Averbook A, Stamos MJ. Appendiceal mass: Conservative therapy followed by interval laparoscopic appendectomy. The American Surgeon 1994;60:753-58.
71. Elmore JR, Dibbins AW, Curci MR. The treatment of complicated appendicitis in children. What is the gold standard? Arch Surg 1987;122:424-27.
72. Eriksson S, Granstrom L. Randomized controlled trial of appendicectomy versus antibiotic therapy for acute appendicitis. Br J Surg 1995;82(2):166-69.
73. Thadepalli H, Mandal AK, Chuah SK, Lou MA. Bacteriology of the appendix and the ileum in health and in appendicitis. Am Surg 1991;57:317-22.
74. Papadopoulos StA, Nikolaou CCh, Manouras AI, Apostolidis NS, Golematis BCH. The effect of obstruction of the appendiceal lumen on its aerobic and anaerobic flora – an experimental study in rabbits. IJSS 1998;5.
75. Foulds KA, Beasly SW, Maoate K. Factors that influence length of stay after appendectomy in children. Australian and New Zealand J of Surgery 2000;70(1):43-46.
76. Brender JD, Marcuse EK, Koepsell ThD, Hatch EI. Childhood appendicitis: Factors associated with perforation. Pediatrics 1985;76(2):301-06.
77. Lund DP, Murphy EU. Management of perforated appendicitis in children: a decade of aggressive treatment. J of Ped Surg 1994; 29(8): 1130-34.
78. Okoye BO, Rampersad B, Marantos A, Abernethy LJ, Losty PD, Lloyd Da. Abscess after appendectomy in children: the role of conservative management. British J of Surgery 1998;85(8):1111-13.
79. Eriksson S, Tisell A, Granstrom L. Ultrasonographic findings after conservative treatment of acute appendicitis and open appendicectomy. Acta Radiol 1995;36(2):173-77.
80. Barber MD, McLaren J, Rainey JB. Recurrent Appendicitis. British J of Surgery 1997;84:110-12.
81. Richter M, Laffer U, Ayer G, Blessing H, Biaggi J, Bruttin JM, Brugger JJ, Liechti J, Konig W. Wird tatsächlich zu häufig appendektomiert? Resultate der prospektiven Multicenterstudie der Schweizerischen Gesellschaft für Allgemeinchirurgie. Swiss Surgery 2000;3:101-07.
82. Di Sebastiano P, Fink T, di Mola FF, Weihe E, Innocenti P, Friess H, Buchler MW. Neuroimmune appendicitis. Lancet 1999;354:461-66.
83. Vlachonikolis IG, Koutroubakis IE. Am J Gastroenterology 2000;95:171-76.

CHAPTER 55

Short Bowel Syndrome

DK Gupta, Shilpa Sharma

Short bowel syndrome (SBS) continues to be one of the most challenging problems in pediatric surgery. SBS is a state in which small intestine length is inadequate to digest and absorb nutrients for normal growth and development. Though various forms of treatment have been experimented with, yet there is none ideal. Patients with short bowel syndrome present with diverse derangements in the initial disease with a complex array of secondary problems. Conscientious decision making and judicious planning right in the beginning can go a long way in improving the quality and quantity of life in children suffering from this formidable disorder. Though an intestinal transplant may be the best form of treatment for this pathology, the majority feel it is much more expensive than the present scheme of treatment.[1]

ETIOLOGY

The causes of SBS may be divided into congenital and acquired (Table 55.1). The most common causes in order of frequency of occurrence are; Necrotising enterocolitis, Intestinal atresia, Midgut volvulus, Gastroschisis and Long segment Hirschsprung's disease.[2]

Congenital short bowel syndrome is a very rare condition of the newborn with total length of small bowel being short, with several reports demonstrating high mortality.[3,4] This is always associated with malrotation. The baby may present with chronic diarrhea and failure to thrive. An upper gastrointestinal endoscopy will show a straight duodenum.[4] The small bowel biopsies are histologically normal parenteral nutrition is recommended. Enteral feeding with an amino acid-based formula containing long-chain fatty acids may be introduced early and gradually advanced.[4] The follow-up reported at 24 months is a regular diet, with normal growth and development of the child. The introduction of early enteral feeds promotes intestinal adaptation, with subsequent weaning off parenteral nutrition.[4]

Table 55.1: Causes of short bowel syndrome		
Congenital	*Acquired*	*Functional short gut physiology*
Necrotizing enterocolitis	Mesenteric vascular accidents	Proximal diverting stoma
Intestinal atresia	Trauma – loss of intestinal vascularity	Enteropathies
Midgut volvulus	Post-traumatic mesenteric thrombosis	Lymphangiectasis
Gastroschisis	Regional enteritis	Pseudo-obstruction
Long segment Hirschsprung's disease	Postoperative complications *(proximal ostomy for ulcerative colitis and familial polyposis)*	Radiation enteritis
Meconium ileus		
True congenital short gut	Malignancy	

Short bowel syndrome can also result from Continence-preserving operations like proximal ostomy performed for either ulcerative colitis or familial polyposis.[5] The postoperative complications of these procedures include obstruction or mesenteric ischemia requiring resections. These are prone to form desmoid tumors and adenocarcinoma.[5] SBS related to desmoid tumors has been reported to have a poor prognosis in patients undergoing resection alone. A more aggressive approach to intestinal transplantation in these patients may thus be warranted.[5]

CLINICAL SEQUELAE OF SBS

Loss of a significant length of the small bowel results in interrelated physiologic events as a result of decreased small intestinal mucosal absorptive cell mass. Nutritional and metabolic effects ensue from diminished intraluminal digestive capacity and rapid intestinal transit leading to an excessive loss of fluids, nutrients, electrolytes and bile salts. The loss of a significant bowel length also affects enteroendocrine system profoundly impairing local hormonal reflex loops.

The following clinical sequelae are seen:

1. *Malnutrition:* This results following grossly impaired absorption of all nutrients. The child becomes cachexic with time.

2. *Diarrhea:* The inadequate absorptive surface leads to a lesser fraction of ingested food and intestinal secretions getting absorbed thus causing an excessive volume loss and diarrhea. There is a rapid intestinal transit across a shortened intestinal length. Gastric hypersecretion, a transient phenomenon, most commonly seen with proximal and midgut resections complicates the initial phase in SBS.[6,7] Increased gastric secretions and excessive salt load thus secreted compounds the diarrhea. The pH in the proximal small intestine is lowered leading to inactivation of digestive enzymes and reduced digestive capability. Thus, a beneficial effect of histamine receptor blockers has been seen in controlling the diarrhea. Loss of cholecystokinin and secretin secondary to loss of enteroendocrine cell mass leads to impaired gallbladder motility, decreased bile secretion and decreased pancreatic secretions.

3. *Malabsorption:* This is a key finding in patients with short-bowel syndrome. Malabsorption of nonessential and essential nutrients, fluids, and electrolytes, if not compensated for by increased intake, leads to diminished body stores and subclinical and (eventually) clinical deficiencies. After intestinal resection, adaptation (a spontaneous progressive recovery from the malabsorptive disorder) may be evident.[8] Growth hormone and glucagon-like peptide-2 have been reported to facilitate a condition of hyperadaptation in short-bowel patients.[8] Decreased output of brush border disaccharidases results in carbohydrate malabsorption producing reducing substances in stools.[9] Malabsorbed fats and carbohydrates pass into colon and are fermented by colonic bacteria into volatile short chain and hydroxylated fatty acids which also contribute to diarrhea. Malabsorption of proteins also accompanies bile salt malabsorption resulting from extensive ileal resections produces diarrhea, steatorrhea and loss of fat soluble vitamins. Loss of enterohepatic circulation resulting from deceased ileal absorptive surface area leads to depletion of bile acid pool which can't be compensated even with increased hepatic synthesis. Bacterial overgrowth is also a contributing factor towards diarrhea. Malabsorptive diarrhea due to short bowel syndrome results in nutrition compromise, often requiring parenteral nutrition. Crohn's disease was the most common cause of SBS in a series.[10] Most subjects with Crohn's disease undergo surgeries, resulting in loss of the ileocecal valve.[10] Loss of ileocecal valve permits reflux of colonic bacteria into small bowel and increased bacterial counts in small bowel lumen. Adaptive processes may lead to dilated dysfunctional loops with poor motility susceptible to bacterial overgrowth. The endotoxins of these bacteria damage mucosa, affect motility, deconjugation of bile salts and aggravate stasis Bacterial translocation can further enhance endotoxic shock, septicemia and bowel necrosis.[11,12]

4. *Vitamin deficiencies:* Impaired fat absorption leads to deficiency of fat soluble vitamins. Rickets can occur due to impaired vitamin D absorption.[13] Vitamin deficiency states can be potentiated by

cholestyramine if it is used to bind the bile salts to decrease the secretory diarrhea associated with bile salt malabsorption. Vitamin B_{12} deficiency can result due to loss of ileal absorptive surface as well as due to excessive consumption by bacterial overgrowth.

5. *Cholelithiasis and renal stones:* Massive ileal resection disrupts the enterohepatic cycling of bile salts and depletes the bile pool rendering the bile lithotropic.[14] Deficiency of taurine also predisposes to cholelithiasis. Decreased secretion of cholecystokinin interferes with the gallbladder contractility adding an element of stasis. These factors predispose the patients to gallstone formation. Children with short bowel syndrome have a propensity to develop hyperoxaluria and oxalate renal stones. This is a result of metabolism of increased carbohydrate load that generates excess of oxalate and unabsorbed fatty acids binding calcium more avidly than oxalate, leaving oxalate free for absorption into circulation leading to hyperoxaluria.[15]

6. *D-lactic acidosis:* D-lactic acidosis is a rare and severe complication of short bowel syndrome in children. Some children with SBS develop recurrent episodes of metabolic acidosis associated with altered sensorium sometimes even progressing to coma resulting from the colonization of bowel with lactobacilli that converts excess carbohydrate to D-Lactate via enzyme D-lactate dehydrogenase. This enzyme is not present in the human beings. D-lactate is then absorbed but it can't be metabolized leading to severe metabolic acidosis.[16] Intestinal flora (Lactobacilli) is responsible for the production of d-lactic acid after fermentation of food carbohydrates. The patient may present with acute neurological symptoms including dysarthria and disorientation.[17] Biological analysis may reveal metabolic acidosis, increased plasma d-lactic acid assessed by organic acid chromatography analysis and a very important increase in expired hydrogen during glucose breath test. Lactobacillus fermentum may be isolated in the gastric liquid and rectal swabs. The treatment consists of intravenous sodium bicarbonate, antibiotic therapy and interruption of enteral nutrition. d-lactic acidosis should be suspected when neurological symptoms occur in a child with short bowel syndrome. They can be prevented by treating intestinal bacterial overgrowth.[17]

7. *Complications:* All patients with true short bowel syndrome will require total parenteral nutrition (TPN) is associated with a host of acute and long-term complications. The overall morbidity and mortality is extremely high with complications like sepsis; hydroelectrolyte imbalances secondary to loose stools; thrombosis or infection of the catheter; TPN-related cholestasis, weight/age deficit greater than 40%, rickets and malabsorption syndromes.[1] Multiple central venous accesses need to be performed in these patients. The use of catheters in patients requiring short/medium- term parenteral nutrition has less complications than patients on home long-term parenteral nutrition.[18] TPN related complications especially CVP line related sepsis and cholestasis are the leading causes of morbidity and mortality in children with short bowel syndrome. CVP line sepsis episodes are more common in patients with a shorter bowel length supporting the general principle that bacteriemia leading from increased intestinal permeability is a causative factor. TPN associated cholestasis is defined as a cholestatic state associated with a prolonged course of TPN. A conjugated bilirubin level greater than 2.0 mg/dl may be the criteria after other causes have been ruled out.[19] The exact etiology of TPN associated cholestasis has not been definitely established. The clinical implications of TPN associated cholestasis include increased rates of sepsis, cirrhosis and increased mortality.[19]

PHYSIOLOGICAL CHANGES

Adaptation

Adaptation is a compensatory response by the residual small bowel after a sudden reduction in mucosal surface area characterized by increased cell turn over, and enhanced digestive and enzymatic activity of the remnant bowel. The adaptive response begins with an increase in the crypt cell proliferation rate, which results in an increased villus height and an overall increase in the functioning surface area for nutrient absorption.[20] In some situations, the actual length of the residual bowel increases; in almost all instances the diameter increases significantly.[20] If the resection or the loss is extensive or the adaptive response insufficient then lifelong dependence on TPN with its risk for associated complications is to be anticipated.

The remaining intestine lengthens to a greater degree after a resection of the proximal small bowel when compared with that after resection of the distal portion.[21] Ileum is more adept to adaptation then jejunum.[22] After resection of the jejunum, residual ileum adopts many of the morphologic features of the jejunum.[23] The age at the time of small bowel loss also influences the adaptation - neonates have greater chances of having a successful adaptation as remnant intestine of neonates can increase in length substantially.[24] The length of the residual bowel is the prime determinant of the adaptive response. The adaptive process is effective enough to allow full enteral nutrition even after 70 - 80% of the small bowel mass has been removed.[25] The best results occur when the ileocecal valve remains intact as it helps to prolong the intestinal transit, thereby promoting absorption. Loss of ileocecal valve almost doubles the minimum length of residual bowel required for successful adaptation. Minimum length required for eventual successful adaptation has been reported to be 40 cm without an intact ileocecal valve and 25 cm in the presence of an intact ileocecal valve.[25] But the minimum length required depends on the age, status of the residual bowel and type of residual bowel as seen above. If the underlying disease is necrotising enterocolitis, then SBS can occur even with adequate bowel length as the residual bowel may also have widespread mucosal damage.[26]

Mechanisms and Mediators that Propagate the Adaptive Response

1. *Intraluminal nutrients*: The reversal of gut mucosal atrophy associated with prolonged TPN and starvation has been observed with initiation of enteral feeds.[27] Thus enteral nutrients act as stimulators of intestinal mucosal maintenance. Apart from the direct trophic effects, multiple factors such as hormones, secretions, peristalsis increased mucosal blood flow contribute to the indirect effect of enteral feeds in adaptive response. Complex nutrients that need more metabolic energy to absorb and digest trigger a better adaptive response, the so-called functional workload hypothesis.[28] Long chain and unsaturated fatty acids are specially trophic to intestinal mucosa.[29] Glutamine has been reported as vital for the proliferative effects of endogenous growth factors like epidermal growth factor and insulin like growth factor.[30]

2. *Gastrointestinal secretions*: Endogenous pancreaticobiliary secretions have been found to be trophic to gut mucosa. Transposition of ampulla of vater to distal ileum leads to villous hyperplasia beyond the ampulla. Bile alone has been shown to stimulate RNA and DNA synthesis in bowel mucosa, an effect that is potentiated in conjunction with pancreatic secretions. Somatostatin sometimes used to decrease the fecal volume loss in SBS, acts by diminishing the output of pancreatic secretions, also blunts the adaptive response and this effect is reversible with growth factor administration in vivo.[31]

3. *Humoral factors*: Many hormones have been implicated to participate in the adaptive response. The role of hormonal component has been shown by crossed circulation or vascular parabiosis experiments in animals. Enteroglucagon blood levels increase after intestinal resection and remain elevated and have been proposed to foster an adaptive response.[32] Peptide YY has been shown to slow intestinal motility (acts as an ileal brake) and increase the time of contact between enteral nutrients and mucosa thereby helping in adaptation.[33] Most convincing evidence has been gathered so far for epidermal growth factor and its receptor.[34] Increased expression of EGF mRNA and protein, ileal EGF receptor during adaptation and blunted adaptation following decrease in endogenous EGF production and its restoration by exogenous EGF administration are the evidences for its role in adaptation.[30] Other factors implicated in mediating adaptation include glucagon like peptide-2 and hepatocyte growth factor.

MANAGEMENT

Over the last few decades, survival of these children has dramatically improved largely attributable to early diagnosis and more facilities for imparting proper care.

The development and refinement of TPN has revolutionized the management of these cases. The management may be medical or surgical.

MEDICAL MANAGEMENT

With appropriate medical management a large fraction of children with SBS may adapt progressively to a full enteral feeding regimen.

The medical management comprises of the following:
1. Acute phase management
2. Nutritional support
3. Control of diarrhea
4. Management of metabolic complications.

Acute Phase Management

In the acute phase, the treatment focuses on the replacement of fluid and electrolytes as the patient is at risk for dehydration, sodium imbalance and metabolic acidosis. Fluid losses are monitored and replaced adequately, electrolytes are monitored frequently and a constant vigil is kept for any abnormalities. Ringer's lactate solution is preferred because of its lower chloride content and given the propensity of these children to develop acidosis.

Nutritional Support

This should begin promptly, either by the parenteral route or the enteral route. Central venous lines are placed after sepsis is cleared. If there is evidence of infection, peripheral parenteral nutritional support is established. Ongoing fluid losses are calculated and can be either added in TPN solution or given by a second line so that the TPN formulation is stable and does not require daily adjustment. After a stable state is reached, TPN is cycled so that the patient has significant periods of each day off the line. This allows for mobility and appears to reduce the incidence and severity of TPN associated cholestasis.[35] Adequate quantities of micronutrients and fat soluble vitamins should be added to the daily TPN solution.

Enteral feeds should be started as soon as the bowel function returns. This also depends on the etiology of SBS, as patients with necrotising enterocolitis may take up to 3 weeks to resume normal bowel function. Enteral nutrition stimulates the adaptation and decreases the incidence of cholestasis associated with TPN. Gradual introduction of the enteral feeds is done as rapid introduction may exacerbate the secretory diarrhea with its attendant fluid losses. Elemental formulas are used initially to facilitate digestion and absorption and also to decrease the incidence of allergic reactions. Many such hypoallergenic formulas are available such as the protein hydrolysate formulas (pregestimil,vivonex) and even amino acid formulas (neocate). The proteins in these formulas are hydrolysed extensively through an enzymatic process and have very low antigenicity. Consequently, they are well tolerated by most children with SBS.[36] In contrast to adults, tolerance of small infants to fat based formulas is more and they do not do well on calorically dense high carbohydrate formulas. So pediatric formulas generally have 40-50% of calories as fats. The composition of long chain and medium chain fatty acids varies in different formulas. Long chain fats have a higher calorie density and are better stimulators of adaptation but medium chain fats are more easily absorbed in a patient with SBS.[29]

The carbohydrates present in enteral formulas are generally well absorbed except for lactose. Ratio of carbohydrates to fats ultimately determines the osmotic load presented to the intestine. Carbohydrates are digested rapidly, producing a high osmotic load, so a formula with only a modest carbohydrate content is preferred. Small children have more difficulty with carbohydrate rich formulas as they have greater propensity for bacterial overgrowth when fed these formulas, while in older children excess carbohydrates are converted to short chain fatty acids in colon, which are then absorbed, thus providing additional calories.[36] Proteins in the formulas are better provided in hydrolysed partially digested forms. But even complex proteins may be well absorbed and protein absorption is rarely a problem in SBS.

Feeds are initiated as a dilute infusion in a continuous tube feeding pattern. Initially, concentration is advanced at low volume rates reaching to a full concentration of 0.67 cal/ml for small children and 1 cal/ml for bigger children. Once the final concentration is reached in low volumes, enteral feeding rates are advanced, and parenteral rates are decreased isocalorically every 1-3 days as tolerated. Tolerance to enteral feeds is determined by testing for reducing substances in stools and monitoring volume and consistency of stools. As fat malabsorption is not osmotically significant and protein malabsorption rarely seen, advancement of feeding is based on above criteria which monitor carbohydrate malabsorption only. Deficiency of fat soluble vitamins A, D, E and K, heavy metal deficiency such as of zinc, calcium, magnesium should be looked for and adequate replacement should be done.

Appropriate enteral feeding devices are selected based upon the duration of expected adaptation interval, etiology of SBS and motility of the residual bowel. Nasogastric tube feeding is indicated when the expected duration of tube feeds will be less than 3-4 months, when the child does not require continuous enteral feeds or when the child may be able to place his or her own nasogastric tube . Gastrostomy feedings are usually ideal for the long-term feeds and for continous drip in feeds. These can be placed surgically or percutaneously with endoscopic guidance, with proper care and new generation of gastrostomy devices, the peristomal and other complications are minimal. Jejunostomy tubes are indicated in children with poor GI motility or those who do not tolerate gastrostomy feeds. Bolus feeds cannot be given and blockage with administration of complex formulas are the common problems. Given the advantages of continuous feeds in SBS patients, availability of new generation of infusion pumps have facilitated the administration of continuous feeds even in home settings. After the patient is stabilized and the acute phase is over, therapies targeted at promoting adaptation may be started. Most important is the early initiation of enteral feedings. Potential candidates are epidermal growth factor, insulin growth factor-1, glucagon like peptide -2 and hepatocyte growth factor.

Control of Diarrhea

Diarrhea in a patient with SBS results from multiple causes, the causative factor should be identified and therapy instituted accordingly. Early secretory diarrhea is controlled with careful dietary modifications guided by pH , volume and consistency of stools. Gastric hypersecretion complicates the acute phase of adaptation by augmenting diarrhea. Histamine-2 receptor blockers are useful in reducing water and sodium losses related to hypergastrinemia.[37] If a more potent agent is required, proton pump inhibitors can be utilized such as omeprazole.[38] Medications to slow peristalsis are used to prolong the intestinal transit time thereby allowing a longer contact time for absorption. Loperamide hydrochloride is a synthetic opiod derivative that inhibits motility in small bowel and colon. It is frequently used to slow the intestinal transit in the SBS, dose is 1 - 2 mg three times daily. If a second agent is required specially as the feedings are gradually advanced, then codeine in a dose of 0.5-1 mg/kg/dose 3-4 times a day is added.[39] Use of antimotility agents, especially in children without an ileocecal valve, increases the risk of bacterial overgrowth . Bacterial overgrowth causes pain, fever, sudden increase in diarrhea with foul smelling stools and can retard the process of adaptation. When suspected , a specimen of stools and a gastric aspirate is taken for culture sensitivity, oral feeds are discontinued, antimotility agents are stopped, oral antibiotics usually metronidazole and intravenous fluids are instituted . Cholestyramine exchanges chloride ions and bind bile salts forming nonabsorbable complexes. The dose is 100-250 mg/kg/day in 3 divided doses.[39] Use of cholestyramine may exacerbate fat malabsorption by diminishing bile acid pool leading to steatorrhea, hence it is not recommended for long-term use. Somatostatin and its synthetic analogues have been used in SBS. They act by reducing gastric acid secretion, gallbladder contraction, pancreatic exocrine output, bowel motility and small intestinal secretions. Increasing intestinal transit time and reducing secretions can result in improved fluid, electrolyte and substrate absorption, and is thought to be the mechanism by which somatostatin is beneficial.[40] The net effect of somatostatin analogues on the process of intestinal adaptation is not clear yet. Other issues regarding their use is the side effect profile - abdominal pain, nausea, increased incidence of gallstones, facial flushing and headache.

Addition of 2% pectin to the diet improves the consistency of the stools and prolongs the intestinal transit and thus helps in adaptation. Management of diarrhea entails the prevention and treatment of troublesome perineal rash that develops in these children. Emollient oils such as coconut oil and zinc oxide paste can be used in early stage while 10% mixture of cholestyramine powder in a suspension of aquaphor base helps bind the excess bile acids which potentiate the rash. Vagotomy has been reported as a possible procedure for the treatment of diarrhea, although this occurrence has no clear explanation.[41]

Management of Complications

Most devastating and frequent complication is the sepsis that is associated with central venous lines. The catheter related sepsis is more common in children with SBS as compared to other conditions requiring prolonged CVP lines placement. The incidence of enteric organisms causing CVP line sepsis is more in SBS patients.[42]

For these reasons, care of the central catheters should be meticulous. Regular dressings in proper aseptic manner, frequent cultures, flushings with urokinase and antibiotic installation (the so called antibiotic lock technique) can all be helpful in preventing CVP line related sepsis.

Bacterial overgrowth predisposes to episodes of gram-negative sepsis. Management includes stopping oral feeds, oral and/or intravenous antibiotics, assessment of motility and finding out dilated, dysmotile segments. Contrast radiographs with 24 hour and 48 hour films help in delineating problematic loops. Small dysmotile and dilated segments should be excised and longer ones can be tapered or used for intestinal lengthening procedures. Selective enteric decontamination with nonabsorbable oral antibiotics can also be helpful in reducing attacks of sepsis. Malabsorption results in deficiency of fat soluble vitamins and trace metal deficiencies. Adequate supplement doses of vitamin A, D and E should be added to diet. Vitamin K should be administered intravenously every week. Vitamin B_{12} supplementation may be required after ileal resections as ileum is the sole site for its absorption. Vitamin B_{12} can be administered parenterally or intranasally every one to 3 months. Zinc and calcium can be replaced orally while magnesium may be required to be administered parenterally as oral magnesium salts incite osmotic diarrhea. Cholelithiasis is seen in almost 10% of children with SBS. Cholecystectomy is recommended if gallstones are identified at any time. Some authors even recommend prophylactic cholecystectomy after major ileal resections.[43] Oxalate renal stones are best prevented. Avoidance of steatorrhea, selective use of cholestyramine and frequent lookout for this problem are the currently recommended strategies.

D lactic–acidosis occurs due to enteric overgrowth with lactobacilli. Acute management consists of intravenous fluids, bicarbonate replacement and appropriate antibiotic therapy. Ultimately, therapy consists of decreasing carbohydrate intake, preventing bacterial overgrowth and treatment of GI tract with antibiotics to eliminate lactobacilli.

TPN associated cholestasis is one of the major complication leading to morbidity and mortality in the setting of SBS. Preventive strategies include early initiation of enteral feeds, prevention of sepsis, preventing overfeeding (hepatic steatosis), early cycling of TPN, removal or reduction of copper and manganese in TPN solutions and use of taurine supplemented PN.[19] Use of ursodeoxycholic acid and cholecystokinin has shown some promise in the management of TPN associated cholestasis. Administration of oral antibiotics may cause of reduction of the intraluminal bacteria and this decrease the incidence of translocation and indirectly decrease the incidence of cholestasis.[19]

SURGICAL THERAPY

Failing medical management, a trial of surgical intervention may be justified in some cases. undertaken. Surgical management may be done to achieve:

1. Institution of enteral tube feeding
2. Restoration of gastrointestinal continuity
3. Correction of obstruction
4. Resection of stagnant segments
5. Prolonging intestinal transit
6. Small bowel lengthening procedures
7. Intestinal transplantation.

Institution of Enteral Tube Feeding

Children with short bowel syndrome and concomitant intestinal failure have insufficient functional capacity to absorb sufficient nutrients, electrolytes, and/or fluid to sustain independent life. Although parenteral nutrition is often necessary, at least initially, the therapeutic goal should be to enhance intestinal adaption and enteral nutrient assimilation, and thereby reduce parenteral nutrition requirements. The induction of hyperphagia is critical. Enteral intake can be enhanced through enteric tube feeding like gastrostomy or jejunostomy that may be done by open surgery or percutaneous endoscopically.[44]

Restoration of Gastrointestinal Continuity

The foremost goal of surgical therapy in these cases is to restore the gastrointestinal continuity. Intestinal adaptation is facilitated after restoration of continuity like after closing on ileostomy or colostomy. The distal ileum, ileocecal valve and colon slow intestinal transit and add absorptive mucosa.

Correction of Obstruction

Any stricture and adhesive obstructions in the bowel should be treated early as these delay the process of adaptation.

Resection of Stagnant Segments

Dilated segments of bowel resulting from adaptation or ischemia lead to dysmotility, bacterial overgrowth, bacterial translocation, enteritis and malabsorption should be resected if the remaining bowel is of adequate length and the dilated segment is short. Other options include tapering, plication and intestinal lengthening procedures. Tapering removes valuable mucosal surface area so should not be performed in patients with already borderline short small intestine. Intestinal plication, which uses an inversion of the bowel wall, salvages absorptive mucosa and at the same time narrows the dysfunctional lumen. Plication may cause obstruction and dysmotility, also breakdown of plication can occur leading to recurrence of symptoms. Patients with critical small bowel length associated with dilated segments are best treated by performing a lengthening procedure.

Prolonging Intestinal Transit

Many procedures to prolong intestinal transit time have been tried in the past like pacing, denervation, recirculating bowel loops and vagotomy and gastric resection. However, only construction of intestinal valves and interposition of bowel segments have been found to be clinically useful.

Intestinal Valves

The purpose of creating intestinal valves surgically is to simulate ileocecal valve function, to slow intestinal transit and to prevent bacterial back wash into proximal bowel. Intestinal valves cause dilatation and hypertrophy of the proximal intestine and this may serve as the first step to subsequent bowel lengthening procedures.[45]

Intussuscepted nipple valves are the most commonly used valves. The valve is constructed like a Brooke ileostomy and preferably at the ileocolonic junction with about 8 cm of intestine (Fig. 55.1).

A prosthetic valve made of polytetraflouroethylene requires only 3 cm of native intestine for its construction.[45] It is made by placing a prosthetic band 1 cm wide around the intestine and then intussuscepting the intestine retrogradely over the band (Figs 55.2A to C).

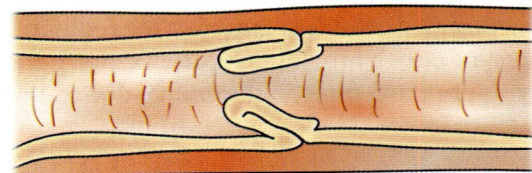

Fig. 55.1: Intussuscepted nipple valve

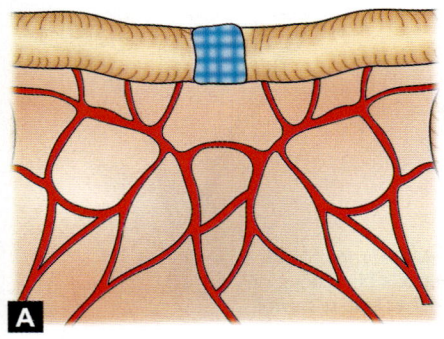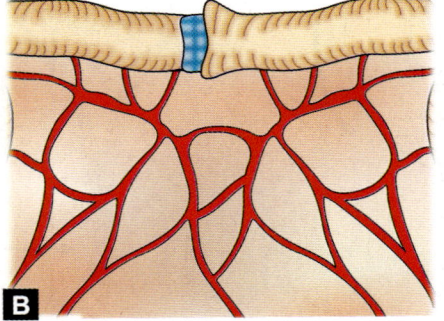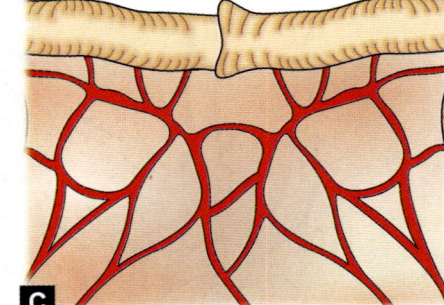

Figs 55.2A to C: Prosthetic valve

Construction of the appropriate diameter and length of the valve is difficult as these vary with patient age, growth rate, diameter of the intestine and motility. The results of these valves have been variable. Potential complications include obstruction due to construction of too tight a valve, no benefit due to too loose a valve, erosion of the prosthetic into the lumen of small intestine and obstruction due to dislodgment and tissue reaction. Other valves like mucosal flap valve and ileocolonic valves have also been described but are not in much clinical use.

Interposition of Bowel Segments

This has been done by placing reversed intestinal segments or using colonic segments for interposition. Reversed intestinal segments induce retrograde peristalsis and slow the intestinal transit (Fig. 55.3). In addition, disruption of the nerve plexuses slows the myoelectrical activity. An alteration of the hormonal milieu has also been reported . Clinical improvement has been noted in upto 80% of the patients in whom an antiperistaltic segment has been used.[46] The complications noted are transient obstructive symptoms and anastomotic leakage. There is a doubt about the long-term efficacy also. Optimal length for antiperistaltic segment is almost 10 cm in adults and 3-4 cm in children.[46] In children, the interposed segment grows along with the rest of the intestine, so consistent results cannot be achieved.

Interposing a colonic segment in the remnant small intestine in either an isoperistaltic or antiperistaltic fashion will retard intestinal motility due to inherent slow peristaltic activity of the large bowel. By interposing a slower isoperistaltic segment proximally, the rate at which nutrients are delivered to the small intestine is slowed. The antiperistaltic segments of colon are placed in a more distal location like small intestinal segments. Interposed colonic segments absorb water, electrolytes and nutrients in addition to increasing the transit time.[46] The effects are inconsistent but many patients have been reported to have a successful outcome. Stasis is a necessary side effect of these procedures that leads to bacterial overgrowth. Eosinophilic colitis presenting with bleeding can occur in interposed colonic segments.[47] It may even necessitate excision of the interposed segment.

Small Bowel Lengthening Procedures

Longitudinal Intestinal Lengthening Procedure (Bianchi Procedure)

The procedure is based on the anatomical observation of peculiar blood supply of small intestine. The intestinal vasculature divides within the two mesenteric leaves into end arteries which alternate to each side of intestine. By dividing the bowel longitudinally between the two mesenteric leaves at a relatively avascular plane midway between the mesenteric vessels passing to each hemisegment., two parallel vascularized loops of half the diameter as the original one can be obtained (Fig. 55.4). The hemisegments are rolled into tubes either by manual suturing or by stapler and are anastomosed isoperistaltically to each other. In effect , a vascularized

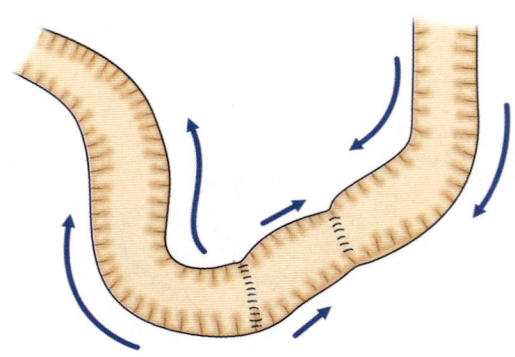

Fig. 55.3: Reversed intestinal segment

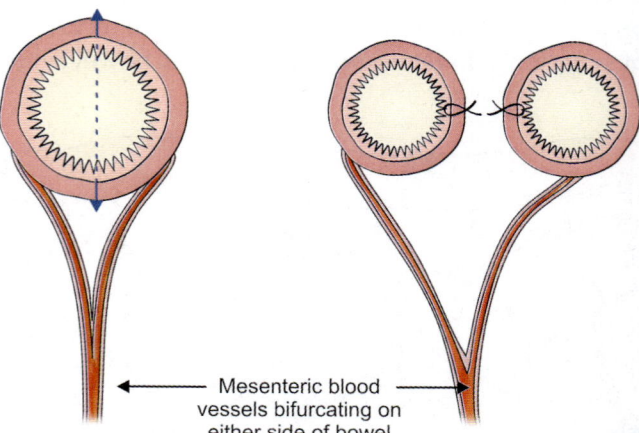

Fig. 55.4: Longitudinal intestinal lengthening

loop of half the diameter and double the length is produced without loss of any valuable mucosa. The reduction in bowel diameter removes the problems of ineffective peristalsis and stasis (atrophy and bacterial translocation) while an increased bowel length prolongs transit and mucosal contact time. Disruption of peristalsis due to the division of circular muscle also helps by prolonging the transit time specially in the early postoperative period.[48]

This procedure is recommended in refractory short bowel syndrome with dilated small bowel loops. However, this procedure may not prolong survival in the setting of liver dysfunction.[48] Thus the trial of medical management should not be too prolonged. Children with an obviously short length who may not adapt on medical management should be offered longitudinal intestinal lengthening procedure early when liver dysfunction has not yet set in. This procedure is not recommended in conditions like inflammatory bowel disease, chronic vascular occlusions and chronic infections, as all these conditions lead to an abnormal and unreliable vascularity. Similarly, segments like duodenum having essentially no mesentery are not suitable for longitudinal lengthening.

Successful adaptation to full enteral feeds has been reported in 45-70% of the children who underwent this procedure for refractory SBS.[49,50] Factors associated with better outcome were more than 40 cm of residual small intestine, presence of ileocecal valve, presence of colon and treatable liver dysfunction.

Complications include leakage, fistula formation, stenosis due to inadequate vascularity. Loss of hemiloop due to vascular insult has also been seen but all these complications have been infrequent.[48] Most of the mortality and morbidity was due to liver dysfunction (Figs 55.5A to F).[49]

Transverse Bowel Lengthening (Kimura's Procedure)

This technique consists of creation of an alternative blood supply on the antimesenteric surface of the small intestine and then dividing intestine into two parallel loops in the transverse place, isolating one loop on the new blood supply.[51,52] The procedure is performed in 2 stages. In first stage a strip of serosa is removed from the antimesenteric bowel wall and this loop is anastomosed to a portion of the abdominal wall or liver that has been stripped off its peritoneal covering. With time collaterals develop and at 8-12 weeks the bowel is transversely divided into 2 loops. This technique may be used in circumstances where conventional LILT can't be done like in duodenum.[48] Random nature of the blood supply from vascular adhesions portends an increased risk of ishemic bowel loss in this surgical procedure. Further intra-abdominal surgery is very difficult after this procedure, so this procedure is generally recommended as the final lengthening option and cholecystectomy may be added at the same time given the propensity of the patients with SBS for developing gallstones (Fig. 55.6).[45]

Sequential Intestinal Lengthening

A combination of transverse and longitudinal bowel lengthening has been proposed to achieve increased bowel length. Initially a nipple valve was used to dilate the bowel, then dilated loop was divided horizontally and vertically at the same time into 3 segments which were rolled into tubes. The nipple valve was resected and isoperistaltic anastomosis was done.[53]

Serial Transverse Enteroplasty Procedure (STEP)

The serial transverse enteroplasty procedure (STEP) procedure is a successful and safe approach to lengthen small bowel in patients with short bowel syndrome.[54] However, postlengthening dilatation may occur, which can lead to bacterial overgrowth and malabsorption. Some authors have reported success with a 2 STEP procedure to address this problem.[55] Reapplication of the procedure requires careful stapling and a removal of small blind-ending segments to avoid further stasis.[55]

Intestinal Transplantation

Due to high incidence of associated complications this is usually the last option. Results are not as good as solid organ transplantation. Vascular anastomoses should be performed according to the state of graft and the recipient. The portal route is the first choice when possible. A two-stage gut reconstruction could decrease the incidence of complications, and offer a useful method in living-related small bowel transplantation.[56] Generally, a cadaveric graft is used

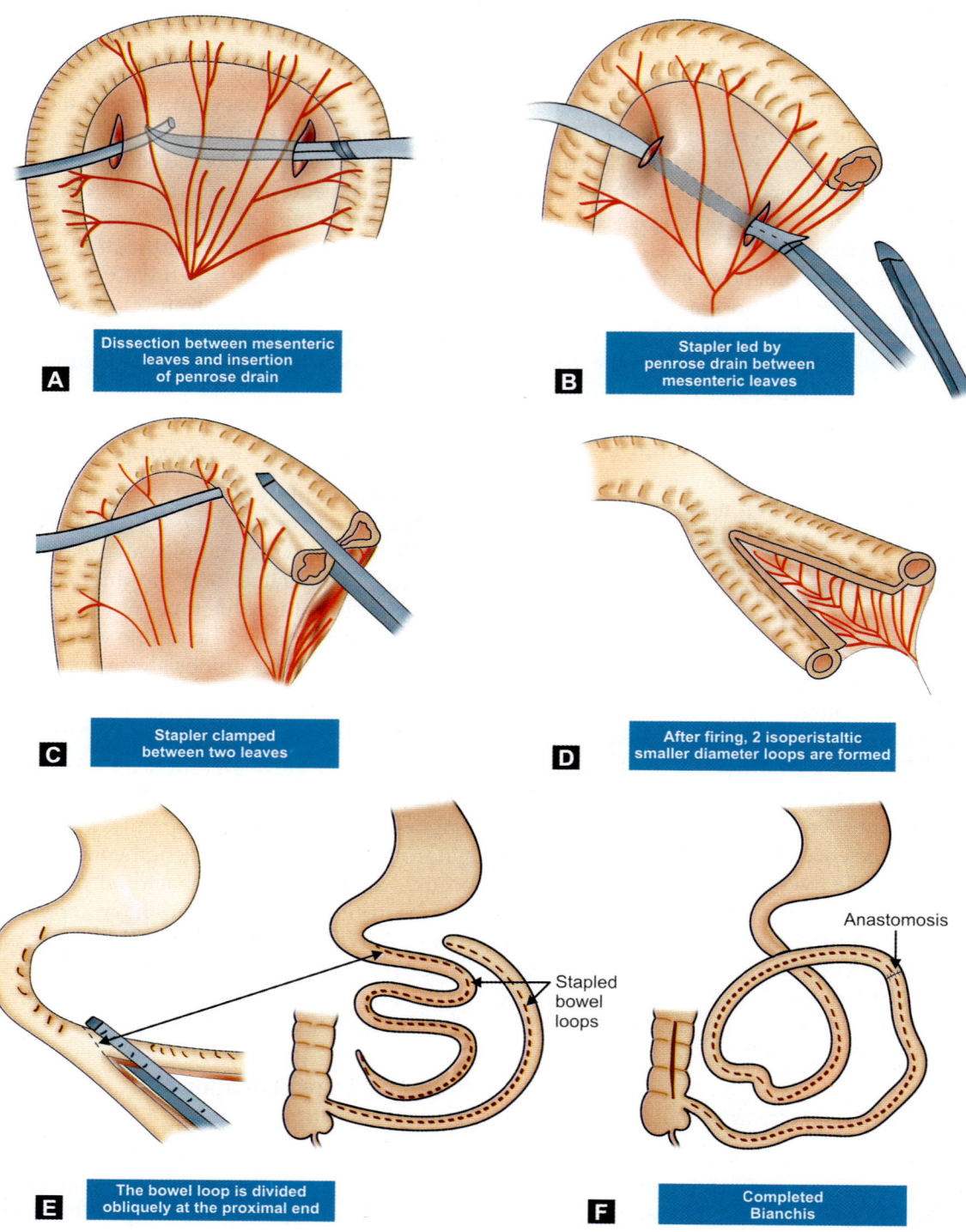

Figs 55.5A to F: Steps of Bianchi's procedure

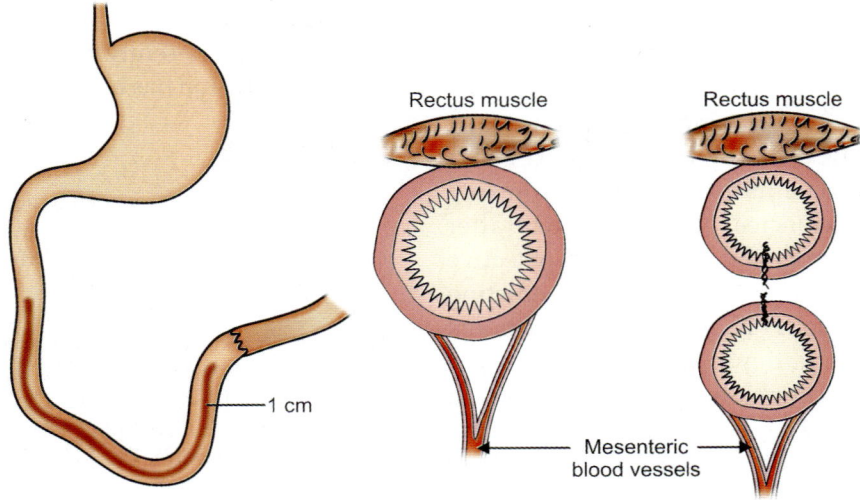

Fig. 55.6: Transverse intestinal lengthening Kimura's procedure

after ABO matching and a screening for cytomegalovirus. In the face of associated end stage liver disease, combined liver and small bowel transplant can be attempted but survival rates are less. Postoperative immunosuppression is mainly based on tacrolimus (FK506) and steroids, while azathioprine, cyclophosphamide and mycophenolate mofetil are useful in episodes of rejection. The lack of biochemical markers (like creatinine in renal transplant, bilirubin in liver transplant) makes it difficult to assess the post-transplant function. Assessment is based on clinical findings of stool frequency, volume, consistency and repeated endoscopies and mucosal biopsies. Rejection is very common due to abundance of gut associated lymphoid tissue. Sepsis, dysmotility, and post-operative gastrointestinal lymphoproliferative disease are the other commonly seen complications.

MORBIDITY AND MORTALITY

The overall morbidity and mortality is extremely high. Several complications have been encountered, the most common ones being sepsis,; hydroelectrolyte imbalances secondary to loose stools; thrombosis or infection of the catheter; TPN-related cholestasis, and malabsorption syndromes.[1]

Sepsis is related to central venous line and episodes of bacterial overgrowth. An early consideration for bowel lengthening procedures and intestinal transplantation in a child whom a trial of medical management is not successful, should be given. Waiting till the liver disease is clearly end stage gives poor results with intestinal transplantation which must be then combined with liver transplant.[2]

Stomas constructed in most congenital malformations that lead to the short bowel syndrome like state or are a result of it have their own inherent complications. Patients with ileostomies are at risk for severe metabolic disturbances. The small intestine essentially manages the balance of water and electrolytes and the absorption of nutrition.[57] In short-bowel syndrome, dangerous consequences like kidney disorders may arise.[57] In general the mortality rate for SBS has remained stable after a substantial decrease was seen with the introduction of TPN in early 80's. Mortality rates range from 17-22% and the most common causes are sepsis and hepatic failure.[2]

LONG-TERM OUTCOME

Majority of the children with SBS do well from a cognitive and development point of view.[58,59] 10-15% of patients have some developmental delay.[58] Most of the patients grow well, although they may remain small than their peers. The presence or absence of ileocecal valve affects the stool consistency and frequency.[59] Surgical lengthening with both Bianchi and STEP procedures results in improvement in enteral nutrition, reverses complications of TPN and avoids intestinal transplantation in the majority with few surgical complications. Intestinal transplantation can salvage most patients who later develop life-threatening complications or fail to wean TPN.[60] Children with SBS are still at risk for different nutrient malabsorption even after weaning off TPN for a long time. Therefore, they need long-term, regular monitoring and intensive nutritional care to prevent various nutrient deficiencies.[61] Bowel growth after massive small bowel resection provides an objective parameter of adaptation and a means of predicting ability to be weaned from TPN. Aggressive nutritional support makes even patients whose disease was previously considered hopeless, likely candidates to achieve freedom from TPN.[62] The treatment is very expensive, more for developing countries where there is very little support from the government. The shorter the segment of the retained bowel and the longer the survival, the higher the cost.

RECENT ADVANCES

Multidisciplinary Pediatric Intestinal Rehabilitation Programs

A multidisciplinary approach to intestinal rehabilitation allows for fully integrated care of inpatients and outpatients with SBS by fostering coordination of surgical, medical and nutritional management.[63] A multidisciplinary intestinal rehabilitation team has been found to decrease the liver failure related mortality due to early referral and increased survival to transplant.[64]

Analysis of the preliminary outcomes of the Group for the Improvement of Intestinal Function and Treatment [GIFT] program suggests that the natural history of neonatal short bowel syndrome remains unaltered to date despite a coordinated approach to care.[64] However, improved communication and integration with the transplant service have resulted in earlier assessment, increased rates of transplantation, and decreased mortality from liver failure.[64] Another multidisciplinary approach team has been reported to be associated with improved survival.[63]

New Developments

Medicine is an ever changing field with research going on to develop better agents. Research is on for inducing neomucosal growth and further refinement of composite bowel tubes aimed at increasing actual enterocyte mass. Recently growth hormone and omega 3 fatty acid infusion has been tried in these patients.[65,66]

REFERENCES

1. Varela-Fascinetto G, Greenawalt SR, Villegas-Alvarez F. Short bowel syndrome in patients studied at the National Institute of Pediatrics in Mexico. Care, cost and perspectives. Arch Med Res. 1998 Winter; 29:337-40. Erratum in: Arch Med Res 1999;30:159.
2. Sigalet DL. Short bowel syndrome in infants and children: An overview. Sem Ped Surg 2001;10: 49.
3. Schalamon J, Schoeber PH, Gallippi P, Matthyssens L, Hollwarth ME. Congenital short bowel: a case study and review of literature. Eur J Ped Surg 1999;9:248.
4. Hasosah M, Lemberg DA, Skarsgard E, Schreiber R. Congenital short bowel syndrome: A case report and review of the literature. Can J Gastroenterol 2008;22:71-74.
5. Thompson JS, Gilroy R, Sudan D. Short bowel syndrome after continence-preserving procedures. J Gastrointest Surg 2008;12:73-76.
6. Straus E, Gerson CD, Yalow RS. Hyper secretion of gastrin associated with the short bowel syndrome. Gastroenterol 1974;66:175.
7. Bohane TD, Haka-Ikse K, Biggar WD, et al. A clinical study of young infants after small intestinal resection. J Pediatr 1979;94:552.
8. Jeppesen PB. Growth factors in short-bowel syndrome patients. Gastroenterol Clin North Am 2007;36(1):109-21.
9. Dudrick SJ, Latifi R, Fosnocht DE. Management of the short bowel syndrome. Surg Clin North Am 1991;71:625.
10. Keswani RN, Neven K, Semrad CE. Screening for celiac disease in short bowel syndrome Nutr Clin Pract 2008; 23:72-75.
11. Deitch EA, Ma W, Ma L, et al. Endotoxin induced bacterial translocation: A study of mechanisms. Surgery 1989;106:292.
12. Deitch SA, Berg R, Specian R. Endotoxin promotes the translocation of the bacteria from the gut. Arch Surg 1987;122:185.
13. Touloukien RJ, Gertner JM. Vitamin D deficiency rickets as a late complication of short gut syndrome during infancy. J Ped Surg 1981;16:230.
14. Pellerin D, Bertin P, Nihoul-Fekete CL, et al. Cholelithiasis and ileal pathology in childhood. J Ped Surg 1975;10:35.
15. Earnest DL, et al. Hyperoxaluria in patients with ileal resection : an abnormality in dietary oxalate absorption. Gastroenterology 1974;66:1114.
16. Mayne AJ, Handy DJ, Preece MA, et al. Dietary management of D-Lactic acidosis in short bowel syndrome. Arch Dis Child 1990;65:229.
17. Dahhak S, Uhlen S, Mention K, et al. [D-lactic acidosis in a child with short bowel syndrome.] Arch Pediatr 2008 Feb;15(2):145-48. Epub 2008 Feb 1.

18. Gamba PG, Orzali A, De Coppi P. Vascular access in patients affected by short bowel syndrome. J Vasc Access 2000;1(1):33-35.
19. Teitelbaum DH, Tracy T. Parenteral nutrition associated cholestasis. Sem Ped Surg 2001;10:72.
20. Wolvekamp MCJ, Heineman E, Taylor RG. Towards understanding the process of intestinal adaptation. Dig Dis 1996;14:59.
21. Thomson JS, Quigley EM, Adrian TE. Factors affecting outcome following proximal and distal intestinal resection in dog : An examination of the relative roles of mucosal adaptation, motility, luminal factors and enteric peptides. Dig Dis Sci 1999;44:63.
22. Dowling RH. Small bowel adaptation and its regulation. Scand J Gasteroenterol Suppl 1982;74:53.
23. Weaver LT, Austin S, Cole TJ. Small intestinal length: A factor essential for gut adaptation. Gut 1991;32:1321.
24. Gambarara M, Ferretti F, Papadatou B, et al. Intestinal adaptation in short bowel syndrome. Transplant Proc 1997;29:1862.
25. Georgeson KE, Breaux CW. Outcome and intestinal adaptation in neonatal short bowel syndrome. J Ped Surg 1992;27:344.
26. Cooper A, Floyd TF, Ross AJ, et al. Morbidity and mortality of short bowel syndrome acquired in infancy : An update. J Ped Surg 1984;19:711.
27. Dworkin LD, Levine GM, Farber NJ, et al. Small intestinal mass of the rat is partially determined by the indirect effect of the intraluminal nutrition. Gastroenterology 1976; 71: 626.
28. Warner BW, Vanderhoof JA, Reyes JD. What's new in the management of short gut syndrome in children . J Am Coll Surg 2000;190:725.
29. Booth IW. Enteral nutrition as primary therapy in short bowel syndrome. Gut 1994;35:S69.
30. O'Brien DP, Nelson LA, Huang FS, Warner BW. Intestinal adaptation: Structure, function and regulation. Sem Ped Surg 2001;10(2):56.
31. Liu CD, Rongiore AJ, Richardson C, et al. EGF improves intestinal adaptation during somatostatin administration in vivo. J Surg Res 1996;63:163.
32. Bloom S, Polak JM. The hormonal pattern of intestinal adaptation. Scand J Gastroenterol (Suppl) 1982;74:93.
33. Savage A, Adrian TE, Carolan G. Effects of peptide YY on mouth to cecum intestinal transit time and on the rate of gastric emptying in healthy volunteers. Gut 1987;28:166.
34. Warner BW, Vanderkolk WE, Can G, et al. Epidermal growth factor receptor expression following small bowel resection. J Surg Res 1997;70:171.
35. Zeigler MM. Short bowel syndrome in infancy: Etiology and management. Clin Perinat 1986;13:163.
36. Vanderhoof JA, Young RA. Enteral nutrition in short bowel syndrome. Sem Ped Surg 2001;10(2)65.
37. Hyman PE, Garrey TQ, Harada T. Effect of ranitidine on gastric acid hypersecretion in an infant with short bowel syndrome . J Ped Gastroenterol Nutr 1985;4:316.
38. Nightingale JM, Walker ER, Farthing M, et al. Effect of omeprazole on intestinal output in the short bowel syndrome. Aliment Pharmacol Ther 1991;5:405.
39. Schwartz MZ, Kuenzler KA. Pharmacotherapy and growth factors in the treatment of short bowel syndrome. Sem Ped Surg 2001;10(2): 81.
40. Rosen GH. Somatostatin and its analogues in the short bowel syndrome. Nutr Clin Pract 1992;7:81.
41. Safioleas M, Stamatakos M, Safioleas P, et al. Short bowel syndrome: Amelioration of diarrhea after vagotomy and pyloroplasty for peptic hemorrhage. Tohoku J Exp Med 2008;214(1):7-10.
42. Kurkchubasche AG, Smith SD, Rowe MI. Catheter Sepsis in short bowel syndrome. Arch Surg 1992;127:21.
43. Goulet OJ, Revillon Y, Dominique Y, et al. Neonatal short bowel syndrome. J Pediatr 1991;119:18.
44. Buchman AL. Use of percutaneous endoscopic gastrostomy or percutaneous endoscopic jejunostomy in short bowel syndrome. Gastrointest Endosc Clin N Am 2007;17(4):787-94.
45. Collins JB, Georgeson KE, Vicente Y, Kelly DR, Figueroa R. Short bowel syndrome : Sem Ped Surg 1995; 4(1):60.
46. Thompson JS. Surgical approach to the short bowel syndrome: Procedures to slow intestinal transit . Eur J Ped Surg 1999;9:263.
47. Glick PL, de Lorimier AA, Adzick NS, Harrison MR. Colon interposition: An adjuvant operation for short gut syndrome. J Ped Surg 1984;19:719.
48. Bianchi A. Autologous gastrointestinal reconstruction. Sem Ped Surg 1995;4(1):54.
49. Bianchi A. Experience with longitudinal intestinal lengthening and tailoring. Eur J Ped Surg 1999;9:256.
50. Waag KL , Hosie S , Wessel L. What do children look like after longitudinal intestinal lengthening . Eur J Ped Surg 1999;9:260.
51. Kimura K, Soper RT. Isolated bowel segment (model D: creation by myoenteropexy). J Ped Surg 1990; 25: 512.
52. Kimura K, Soper RT. A new bowel elongation technique for the short bowel syndrome using isolated bowel segment Iowa models. J Ped Surg 1993;28:792.
53. Georgeson KE, Halpin D, Figueroa R, et al. Sequential intestinal lengthening procedures for refractory short bowel syndrome. J Ped Surg 1992;27:344.
54. Dutta S. The STEP procedure: defining its role in the management of pediatric short bowel syndrome J Pediatr Gastroenterol Nutr 2007 Aug;45(2):174-75. Comment on: J Pediatr Gastroenterol Nutr 2007;45:257-60.
55. Ehrlich PF, Mychaliska GB, Teitelbaum DH. The 2 STEP: An approach to repeating a serial transvers enteroplasty. J Pediatr Surg 2007;42:819-22.
56. Qian SK, Gao LH, He HS, Zhu XF. Vascular anastomosis and two-stage reconstruction of the gut in a living-related small bowel transplant recipient: a case report. Transplant Proc 2007;39:3547-50.

57. Brüwer M, Utech M, Senninger N, et al. Metabolic consequences in patients with intestinal stoma. Ther Umsch 2007;64:529-35.
58. Beers SR, Yaworski JA, Stilley C, et al. Cognitive defects in school age children with severe short bowel syndrome. J Ped Surg 2000;35:865.
59. Rickham PP, Irving I, Shmerling DH. Long-term results following extensive small intestinal resection in the neonatal period. Prog Ped Surg 1977;10:65.
60. Sudan D, Thompson J, Botha J, et al. Comparison of intestinal lengthening procedures for patients with short bowel syndrome. Ann Surg 2007;246:593-601; discussion 601-04.
61. Wu J, Tang Q, Feng Y, et al. Nutrition assessment in children with short bowel syndrome weaned off parenteral nutrition: a long-term follow-up study. J Pediatr Surg 2007;42:1372-76.
62. Rossi L, Kadamba P, Hugosson C, et al. Pediatric short bowel syndrome: adaptation after massive small bowel resection. J Pediatr Gastroenterol Nutr 2007;45:213-21.
63. Modi BP, Langer M, Ching YA, et al. Improved survival in a multidisciplinary short bowel syndrome program J Pediatr Surg 2008;43:20-24.
64. Diamond IR, de Silva N, Pencharz PB, et al. Neonatal short bowel syndrome outcomes after the establishment of the first Canadian multidisciplinary intestinal rehabilitation program: preliminary experience. J Pediatr Surg 2007;42:806-11.
65. Krysiak R, Gdula-Dymek A, Bednarska-Czerwińska A, Okopień B. Growth hormone therapy in children and adults. Pharmacol Rep 2007;59:500-16.
66. Jain SK, Pahwa M. Management of short gut syndrome by omega 3 fatty acid infusion. Clin Nutr 2007;26:810.

Intestinal Obstruction

Alpana Prasad, Rajiv Chadha

Intestinal obstruction is defined as an interference with the normal aboral transit of intestinal contents. It is probably the most common reason for emergency surgery in infants and children.[1] Depending on the degree of obstruction to the flow of intestinal contents, intestinal obstruction may be defined as *partial* or *complete*. This distinction is important, since the prognosis and treatment are different. Intestinal obstruction may be further characterized as *simple* or *strangulated*, depending on the integrity of the blood supply to the involved bowel. Strangulation obstruction is an important, but also, one of the most difficult acute abdominal conditions to recognize, and may be life-threatening if the diagnosis is delayed.

HISTORICAL ASPECTS

The first recorded surgical procedure for an intestinal obstruction was performed by Praxagoras in 350 BC when he created an enterocutaneous fistula to relieve an obstruction. Non-operative management was the general rule until the nineteenth century, when surgical procedures became more frequent for intestinal obstruction. Most significant advances occurred in the early twentieth century when parenteral administration of saline solution was observed to be important in the management of intestinal obstruction and the radiographic techniques for its diagnosis were developed. Intestinal decompression by tubes in 1930s and the use of antibiotics in 1940s and 1950s were further important additions to the management of bowel obstruction.[2]

ETIOLOGY

Intestinal obstruction may either be due to an actual physical barrier known as *mechanical* or *dynamic* obstruction, or due to a functional failure of progressive intestinal transit called *paralytic ileus* or *adynamic* obstruction.[3] Mechanical obstructions may have congenital or acquired causes. Congenital causes may present in the neonatal period, as in intestinal atresia, or later, as in malrotation, duodenal web, or Hirschsprung's disease. The various causes of pediatric intestinal obstruction have been classified in Table 56.1.

Table 56.1: Etiology of Intestinal obstruction in children

A. Mechanical obstruction of the lumen / Dynamic obstruction

   I. **Obturation of the lumen (Intraluminal)**
   - Intussusception
   - Impactions– bezoar, roundworms, foreign body, feces, polyp, tumor.

   II. **Intrinsic lesions of the bowel (Intramural)**
   - Congenital– atresia/stenosis, duplication, Meckel's diverticulum
   - Inflammatory – tubercular, regional enteritis, NEC
   - Traumatic, e.g. duodenal hematoma
   - Neoplastic – tumor, malignant stricture
   - Latrogenic– anastomotic stricture, radiation stricture.

   III. **Extrinsic lesions of the bowel**
   - Adhesions (postoperative, postinfectious)
   - Bands – congenital, inflammatory
   - Hernia – external hernia – inguinal, femoral, umbilical, incisional internal hernia – due to congenital/ surgical defect in the mesentery
   - Extrinsic mass – abscess, hematoma, tumor, annular pancreas, anomalous vessel
   - Volvulus – gastric, midgut, colonic.

B. Inadequate propulsive activity / Adynamic obstruction

   I. Neuromuscular defect – megacolon, paralytic ileus
   II. Vascular occlusion – arterial, venous.

Paralytic Ileus

It is characterized clinically by the failure of aboral passage of intestinal contents in the absence of a mechanical obstruction. In ileus, the normal peristaltic motor function of the small intestine fails to occur. It is seen in most patients undergoing abdominal operations and is caused by several neural, humoral and metabolic factors. It may be caused by local factors such as peritonitis, ischemia or surgical manipulation of the bowel, retroperitoneal hemorrhage, operation or inflammation. Neuromuscular inhibition of intestinal motility also occurs due to prolonged intestinal distension, distension of other organs like the ureter, fractures of the spine or ribs, basal pneumonia or occult/systemic sepsis, uremia, diabetic ketoacidosis, and myxedema. Electrolyte imbalance, particularly hypokalemia, hyponatremia and hypomagnesemia, contribute to ileus. Drugs such as narcotics, antacids, anticoagulants, phenothiazines and ganglion-blocking agents, are other important causes of ileus. It is an acute, usually self-limiting condition.

Idiopathic Intestinal Pseudo-obstruction

It is characterized by symptomatic recurrent intestinal obstruction, like cramping abdominal pain, vomiting, distension and diarrhea or steatorrhea, without demonstrable radiographic findings of mechanical obstruction. The pathophysiologic effects are similar to those of mechanical obstruction, except that strangulation is rare. Heredity plays a role in this disorder. The main feature of chronic idiopathic intestinal pseudo-obstruction (CIIP) in older children is a hypotonic duodenum. It is suggested that this condition may result from ischemic injury to the peristaltic control mechanism.[4]

PATHOPHYSIOLOGY OF INTESTINAL OBSTRUCTION

Simple Mechanical Intestinal Obstruction

In simple mechanical obstruction, the blood supply of the gut is intact. An obstructed gut dilates proximal to the obstruction due to accumulation of large volumes of fluid and gas, and this presents with abdominal distension. Initially, the peristaltic activity of the dilating gut increases to overcome the obstruction, causing rushes of hyperperistaltic bowel sounds, or high pitched tinkling sounds, or both. Later, as ileus develops, the obstructed gut becomes silent. Intestinal distension causes reflex vomiting. Water and electrolyte absorption is impaired and intestinal secretion is increased in the obstructed bowel. Inadequate fluid intake combined with the loss of fluid, by repeated vomiting and into the lumen of the obstructed gut, depletes the extracellular fluid, so that the child becomes dehydrated, hypovolemic, acidotic and may go into shock. Metabolic effects of fluid loss in simple mechanical obstruction depend on the site and duration of the obstruction. Proximal obstruction, causing relatively greater vomiting and less intestinal distension, results in the losses of water, Na^+, Cl^-, H^+ and K^+, producing dehydration with hypochloremia, hypokalemia and metabolic alkalosis. In distal obstruction with relatively greater intestinal distension, the serum electrolyte abnormalities are usually less dramatic. Intestinal distension also leads to increased intra-abdominal pressure, decreased venous return from the lower limbs and splinting of the diaphragm with impairment of ventilation.

During intestinal obstruction, whatever the cause, there is stasis and rapid proliferation of intestinal bacteria, which leads to the small intestinal contents becoming feculent. Bacterial translocation in the distended, obstructed intestine may be responsible for the systemic infections and septic consequences associated with intestinal obstruction.

Strangulation Obstruction

This occurs when the blood supply to the obstructed gut becomes impaired, which may be due to significantly increased intraluminal pressure, or due to a closed loop obstruction. A *closed loop obstruction* refers to a mechanical obstruction in which both the afferent and the efferent segments of the involved bowel are occluded, and hence, children with this condition are at high risk of developing strangulation, necrosis, and perforation. Pressure necrosis can develop if unyielding adhesive bands or hernial rings hold the obstructed distending gut. The deformity or twisting of the mesentery, as in volvulus or intussusception, can cause mesenteric vascular occlusion, which is a very dangerous condition and demands early treatment before gangrene of the bowel arises. Mesenteric vascular occlusion alone may give rise to gangrene without mechanical obstruction. In addition to the effects of strangulation, the child has all the ill effects of simple obstruction. The loss of blood and plasma in strangulation obstruction is greater in predominant venous vascular obstruction than in predominant arterial vascular obstruction, and it can lead to shock in an already dehydrated child. Besides the loss of blood and plasma, another important factor in strangulation obstruction is the toxic material in the lumen of the strangulated bowel, which is formed due to the presence of bacteria and necrotic tissue. The ischemic gut mucosa readily permits the transudation of bacteria and toxins prior to perforation, producing systemic effects. As the strangulated gut becomes gangrenous, it may perforate into the peritoneal cavity, causing generalized peritonitis and septic shock. If it perforates into a hernial sac, the transudate containing lethal toxins and bacteria is more localized.

Colonic Obstruction

It generally follows a slower course producing less fluid and electrolyte disturbances than small bowel obstruction. There being more gut to dilate, the resulting abdominal distension may be so severe as to interfere with the child's respiration by pushing up the diaphragm. Initially, only the colon dilates, but in the presence of incompetent ileocecal valves (seen more commonly), the dilatation progresses proximally involving the small bowel. The symptoms of dehydration are less severe as the colon can still absorb fluid above the obstruction. When the ileocecal valve is competent (which is uncommon), the obstructed colon behaves like a closed loop and the massively distended colon may perforate; the cecum being a likely site of perforation. Some of the common causes of colonic obstruction in children are acquired colonic stricture or stenosis following necrotizing enterocolitis, and Hirschsprung's disease.

DIAGNOSIS OF INTESTINAL OBSTRUCTION

Intestinal obstruction should be suspected in any child presenting with abdominal pain of acute onset, vomiting, absolute constipation (obstipation) and abdominal distension with or without abdominal tenderness.

Abdominal pain is typically crampy, occurring in paroxysms at 4-5 minute intervals in proximal obstruction and less frequently in distal obstruction. As the bowel distends, its motility is inhibited and the crampy pain may subside. When crampy abdominal pain is replaced by continuous severe abdominal pain, strangulation or peritonitis should be suspected. Closed loop obstructions are associated with sudden onset of severe unremitting abdominal pain, out of proportion to the physical findings.

In high intestinal obstructions like those in the duodenum or upper jejunum, the vomiting appears almost simultaneously with pain, even before the onset of any significant distension and it may be constant, frequent and profuse. In contrast, in low small bowel obstructions, vomiting occurs a few hours after the onset of pain by which time there is significant abdominal distension with or without visible peristalsis. In distal intestinal obstruction, the vomiting is less frequent, but it is feculent because of the large bacterial population of intestinal contents. Vomiting is effortless in paralytic ileus. Obstipation indicates complete intestinal obstruction, after the bowel distal to the obstruction has emptied. In partial intestinal obstruction, the child may continue to pass loose stools, but abdominal distension and vomiting may still be present.

Physical examination should confirm the diagnosis, determine the level and degree of obstruction, exclude peritonitis, and estimate physiologic compromise and the influence of intercurrent illness. The most common systemic manifestations of intestinal obstruction are related to hypovolemia (e.g. tachycardia, tachypnea, altered mental status, oliguria, and hypotension). The presence of features of hypovolemia unresponsive to volume repletion, along with fever and leukocytosis, suggests the presence of strangulated bowel.

The abdomen is usually distended and hyperresonant and visible peristalsis may be present. The distension is central in small bowel obstruction and peripheral in large bowel obstruction, but this classic distribution of distension may not be so evident in infants and children. Peristaltic activity is more likely to be seen in children with chronic subacute intestinal obstruction as in tubercular involvement, or Hirschsprung's disease. Presence of a visible hernia or a previous laparotomy scar should be noted.

Abdominal tenderness is unusual in uncomplicated obstruction. However, localized tenderness, rebound tenderness and guarding suggest peritonitis and strangulation. Palpation may reveal distended loops of bowel, a hernia, or a mass (intussusception, feces, or tumor being the most common). The classic sausage shaped lump, hardening under the palpating finger synchronously with the bout of pain, is that of an intussusception. A "doughy" feel of the abdomen on palpation may suggest that the obstruction is probably due to abdominal tuberculosis.

On auscultation, the bowel sounds in intestinal obstruction are usually frequent, high-pitched, tinkling or musical, but in prolonged obstruction the bowel sounds disappear as intestinal motility decreases. In contrast, the abdomen is silent in diffuse peritonitis or in obstruction due to paralytic ileus. A rectal examination should never be omitted as it may reveal impacted stool, occult or frank blood, or an intraluminal mass such as a polyp or intussusceptum. During rectal examination, the presence of mucus and blood (red "currant jelly") with absence of stool on the finger stall, suggests intussusception, whereas, a tense tender fluctuant mass in the pouch of Douglas indicates a pelvic abscess.

INVESTIGATIONS

Investigations are usually done to confirm the clinical suspicion and assess the general condition of the child. The results of the investigations do help in establishing the diagnosis but cannot and should not replace clinical judgement.

Laboratory Evaluation

The laboratory tests include hemoglobin estimation with a complete blood count; serum sodium, chloride, potassium, bicarbonate and creatinine; blood urea and urinalysis. These tests do not verify the presence of intestinal obstruction; rather, they give some evidence of the severity of the physiologic derangement or indicate the presence of ischemic bowel. The white blood cell count may be normal or mildly elevated in simple mechanical obstruction; but higher white blood cell counts arouse the suspicion of ischemic bowel. An elevated hematocrit and blood urea nitrogen reflect the degree of third space fluid losses and dehydration. Serum electrolytes are generally normal in distal obstruction; however, a pattern of metabolic alkalosis with hypokalemia and hypochloremia is seen in proximal bowel obstruction.

Radiologic Investigations

Radiographs usually confirm the clinical diagnosis and define more accurately the site of obstruction.[5] Four X-ray views of the abdomen, including an upright chest, upright abdomen, supine abdomen and a left lateral decubitus view, are advisable in all patients with intestinal obstruction. The abdominal X-rays may reveal abnormally large quantities of gas in the bowel. In supine views, the distended small bowel is identified by the presence of valvulae conniventes (Fig. 56.1), whereas, the presence of haustral markings indicate colonic distension. The pattern of air-fluid levels in the upright views, in conjunction with the clinical history can help differentiate between a proximal small bowel or a distal intestinal obstruction. In complete mechanical small bowel obstruction, there is usually no gas visible distal to the level of the obstruction or in the pelvis, a "cut-off" sign which is almost pathognomonic of the condition (Fig. 56.2). The presence of significant amounts of colonic gas should raise the suspicion of a large bowel rather than a small bowel obstruction. Plain films may fail to distinguish

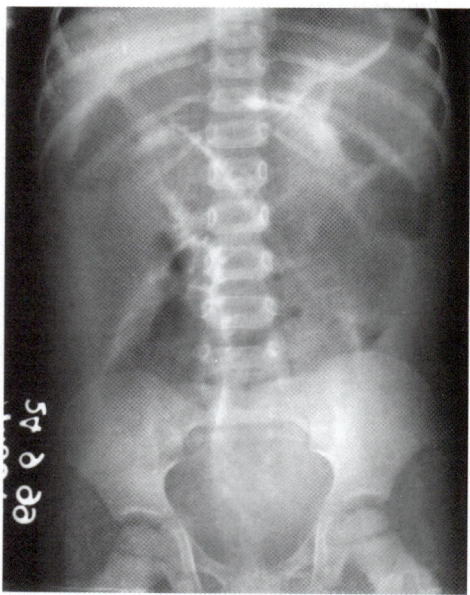

Fig. 56.1: Plain abdominal skiagram (supine view) in a child with jejunal obstruction, showing valvulae conniventes with "concertina" effect

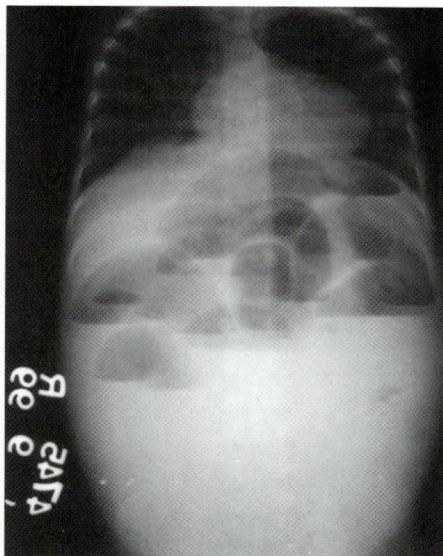

Fig. 56.2: Complete ileal obstruction due to ileocolic intussusception. Note complete absence of gas distal to the obstruction ("cut off" sign)

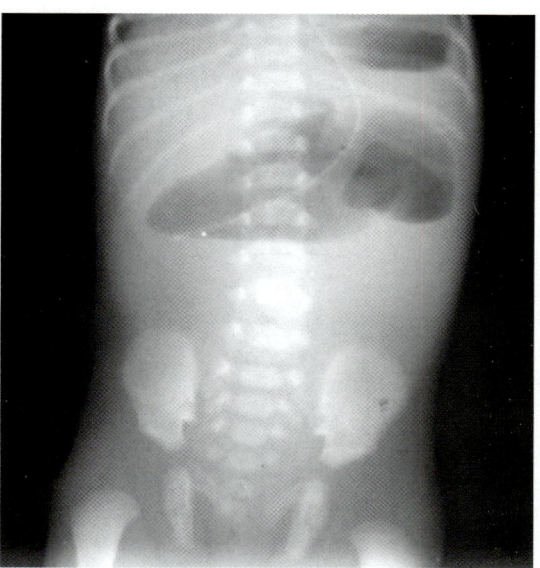

Fig. 56.4: Neonatal mid-jejunal atresia. The larger air-fluid level represents the loop just proximal to the site of atresia

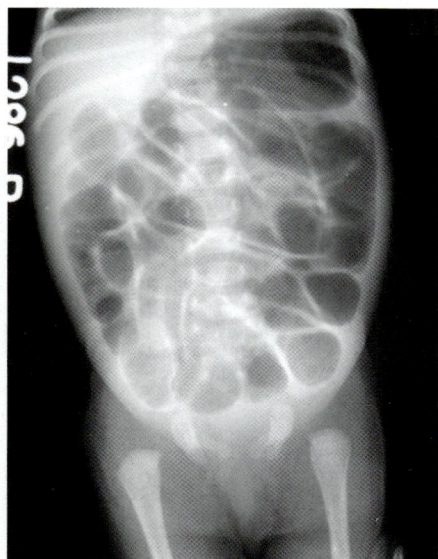

Fig. 56.3: X-ray of the abdomen in a child with drug-induced paralytic ileus. Gas is present throughout the gastrointestinal tract

paralytic ileus from mechanical obstruction, as gas-fluid levels are seen in both the conditions. In ileus however, the uniform presence of gas throughout the gastrointestinal (GI) tract including the stomach, small intestine and colon is more common (Fig. 56.3). When clinical symptoms indicate intestinal obstruction, the clinical findings supersede X-rays, as such films may appear normal despite the presence of strangulation obstruction.[6]

In newborns, thumb-sized intestinal loops (rule of thumb) and air-fluid levels are highly suggestive of neonatal intestinal obstruction.[7] The more distal the level of intestinal atresia, the greater the number of distended intestinal loops and air-fluid levels observed on the abdominal radiographs. The site of atresia may appear as a larger loop with a significant air-fluid level[7] (Fig. 56.4).

It is essential to realize however, that in newborns and small infants, it is very difficult to differentiate between dilated loops of small and large intestine on a plain abdominal skiagram as the colonic haustral markings are usually lacking.[7,8] Therefore, differentiation between distal small bowel and colonic obstruction may be very difficult. Often however, despite the absence of haustral markings, neonatal colonic obstruction may be suggested by the presence of a large dilated loop or air-fluid level at the periphery of the abdominal field (Figs 56.5A and B). A grossly increased transverse diameter of the abdomen may be apparent on the abdominal radiograph in such patients (Figs 56.5A and B). It has also been suggested that a barium enema is essential in newborns with suspected low intestinal obstruction to differentiate between colonic obstruction (colonic atresia, neonatal Hirschsprung's disease, meconium plug syndrome,

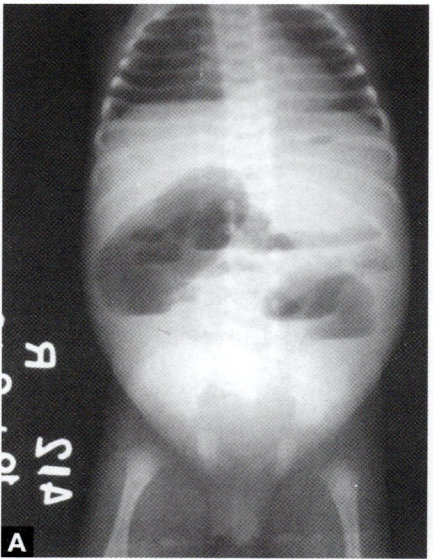
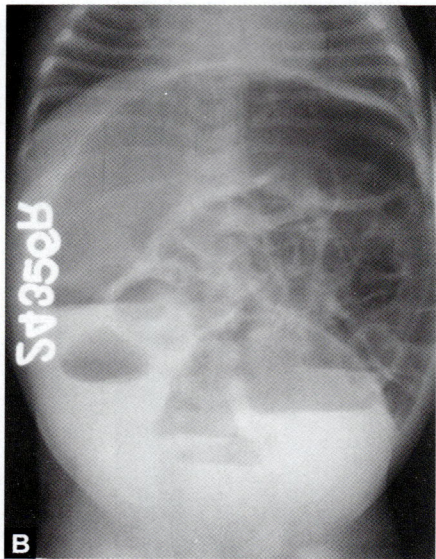

Figs 56.5A and B: Neonatal colonic obstruction seen in **A.** Colonic atresia at the level of the descending colon and **B.** Classic Hirschsprung's disease (errect views). Note large distended colonic loop, lacking haustral markings, at the periphery of the abdominal field with increased transverse diameter of the abdomen

small left colon syndrome), and low ileal obstruction (distal ileal atresia, meconium ileus, total colonic aganglionosis).[7,9,10] In the case of small bowel obstruction, a "microcolon" is characteristically seen on the barium enema (Fig. 56.6). Omission of a barium enema may also result in failure to identify an associated colonic or rectal atresia in patients with a more proximal bowel atresia.[11,12] The contrast enema may also locate the position of the cecum in regard to intestinal rotation and fixation.[10] A gastrografin enema may be both diagnostic and therapeutic in cases of meconium ileus and meconium plug syndrome.[13,14] Barium studies of the upper gastrointestinal (GI) tract are also often required for the diagnosis of malrotation and associated conditions.[15]

The role of radiologic contrast studies in suspected intestinal obstruction in older children is more controversial. Although contraindicated in high grade or complete obstruction, contrast examinations may still be helpful in selected cases, for example in suspected cases of intussusception or Hirschsprung's disease. Barium enema is both diagnostic and therapeutic in intussusception where hydrostatic reduction is a well-established procedure for management. The characteristic "beak" of volvulus at the cecum or terminal ileum and medial deviation of the cecum on contrast enema examination, suggests

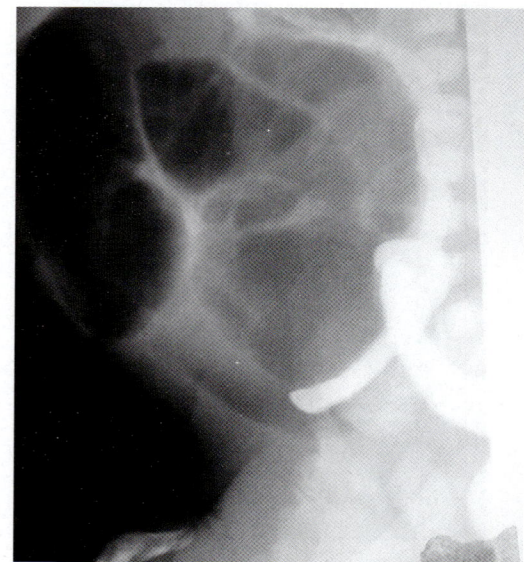

Fig. 56.6: Barium enema in a newborn with jejunal atresia showing "microcolon"

the persistence of an omphalomesenteric duct remnant as the etiology of obstruction.[16] Upper GI and follow-through contrast studies are not routinely advised in suspected intestinal obstruction, especially in children, and may provide misleading information.[17] However, for upper GI contrast studies, metrizamide is highly useful because it is nearly isotonic, is not absorbed or

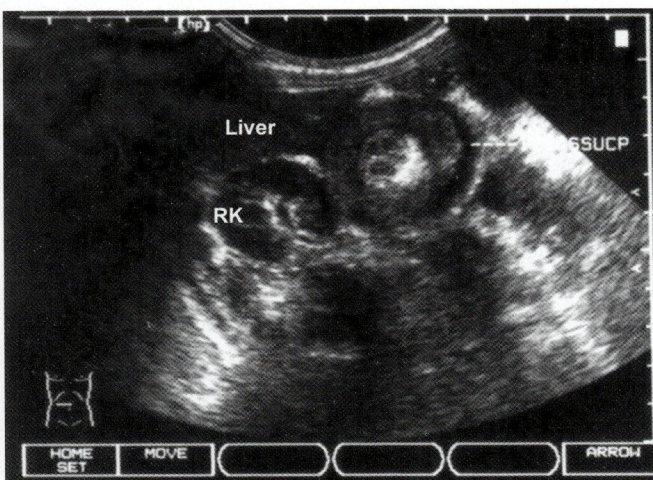

Fig. 56.7: Abdominal ultrasonogram in a child with ileocolic intussusception showing "target lesion" of the intussusceptum

diluted significantly in the gut, is not toxic, and is quickly absorbed if it escapes into the peritoneum through a perforation. In difficult diagnostic cases of partial or intermittent small bowel obstruction, small intestinal transit with radiopaque, non-digestible markers, has also been done to challenge and localize the site of obstruction.[18]

Abdominal ultrasonography has been shown to be useful in the diagnosis of small bowel and colonic obstruction and can help in determining the location and cause of obstruction.[19,20] It is the most useful investigation in defining the character of an abdominal mass, the only limitation being the presence of excessive bowel gas. It can delineate the mass of an intussusception, which is characteristically seen as a "target lesion" (Fig. 56.7). An ultrasound is the investigation of choice for pelvic pathology especially in adolescent girls. Roundworm infestation, which is a relatively common cause of intestinal obstruction in children in developing countries, has been shown to have a typical ultrasonographic appearance. In longitudinal section, the ascaris worm presented as a linear intraluminal mass with 3 or 4 linear echogenic interfaces; in the cross-section, it is round, sometimes appearing as a target sign; and some worms also showed serpentine movement.[21] Abdominal sonography has been suggested as a successful basic diagnostic technique in early postoperative intestinal obstruction when it can separate mechanical causes, such as intussusception, from paralytic ileus.[22] Okada et al have analyzed hemodynamics in the superior mesenteric artery using pulsed Doppler sonography (PDS) and have found it useful in differentiating strangulating obstruction from simple obstruction.[23]

Contrast enhanced CT scans or MRI may occasionally be needed to assist in the diagnosis of intestinal obstruction. CT is sensitive for diagnosing complete obstruction of the small bowel and for determining the location and cause of obstruction.[24] On CT, the criteria for small bowel obstruction included a discrepancy in caliber between the proximal dilated and the more distal collapsed small bowel loops, or generalized small-bowel dilatation (> 2.5 cm) in the presence of a collapsed colon.[25]

TREATMENT OF INTESTINAL OBSTRUCTION

The overlapping sequence of events in the management of children with intestinal obstruction should be investigation, resuscitation and operation. Active preoperative management is needed to stabilize the child hemodynamically so as to minimize the intraoperative morbidity and mortality. This involves establishing an intravenous line and replacing fluid and electrolyte deficits and continuing losses; ensuring adequate urine output; and typing and cross-matching blood, if surgery is anticipated. In addition to the fluid therapy, withholding of all oral intake and intestinal decompression are other important supportive measures in these patients. A good caliber nasogastric tube should be placed and hourly aspiration is done along with continuous drainage. There is no advantage in the use of long intestinal tubes over the standard nasogastric tube.[26] The use of antibiotics in simple mechanical intestinal obstruction, during the period of non-operative management, is controversial. Since the non-ischemic but distended small intestine may allow the passage of bacteria and toxins into the portal circulation and peritoneal cavity, broad-spectrum antibiotics that include coverage of gram-negative aerobes and anaerobes, should be administered during resuscitation, particularly if strangulation is suspected.

Surgery is usually necessary in most patients with suspected complete small bowel obstruction. The presence of fever, tachycardia, localized tenderness and leukocytosis indicates that surgery is mandatory in these patients, including those with no history of previous abdominal surgery and those with incarcerated external hernias.[27,28] Conservative or non-operative therapy can be attempted for 6-12 hours in early simple mechanical obstructions, especially partial or early postoperative obstructions (within 3 weeks of a previous laparotomy), and in children with recurrent small bowel obstructions. Most of the patients successfully treated non-operatively will show definite clinical improvement within 24 hours, and nearly all will improve by 48 hours, and so this is the maximum period of observation prior to proceeding for surgery.[26] The consequences of delay include necrosis and perforation and may necessitate a massive bowel resection and lead to local or systemic sepsis.

The decision to operate is based on clinical judgement. The timing of surgery depends on three factors: Duration of obstruction, reflected in the severity of fluid, electrolyte and acid-base abnormalities; the opportunity to improve vital organ function; and consideration of the risk of strangulation.[3] Except in very exceptional cases, surgical intervention should only be undertaken when the child is adequately hydrated and has an adequate urine output and normal serum electrolytes, and this should be achieved as soon as possible, preferably within 6-8 hours of presentation and admission.

Operative Treatment

All children with intestinal obstruction undergo surgery under general anesthesia, administered with an endotracheal tube in place. Vomiting and tracheobronchial aspiration of the feculent vomitus is a serious risk during induction in these children.

In general, the nature of the problem determines the approach to the operative management in these children. Surgery involves relieving the obstruction with, if present, resection of gangrenous bowel. In incarcerated inguinal hernia, operative reduction and herniotomy is usually sufficient. Lysis of adhesions or division of band(s) relieves obstruction due to adhesions or bands. Excision of a lesion with restoration of intestinal continuity is a frequently used approach, as in non-reducible intussusception, intestinal duplications or strictures and stenosis. The placement of a cutaneous fistula, such as a colostomy, proximal to the obstruction is also a recommended surgical alternative. Laparotomy, enterotomy and removal of foreign body, bezoar and roundworms, is the treatment in obturation obstruction of small bowel due to these causes. If technically possible, the distended bowel should be emptied of its luminal contents, so as to improve the blood supply of the bowel and facilitate abdominal closure.[29] Creating an intestinal bypass is rarely done in pediatric patients.

The determination of bowel viability may sometimes be extremely difficult. The color of bowel, presence of motility and arterial pulsations are reassuring indicators of viable bowel. If intestinal viability is questionable, it should be placed in warm packs for 15-20 minutes and then re-examined. If there is still a reasonable doubt regarding its viability, the bowel should be resected.

Intestinal Obstruction in Childhood—Experience at Kalawati Saran Children's Hospital (KSCH)

At Kalawati Saran Children's Hospital, New Delhi, in the two-year period from February 1999-March 2001, there were a total of 279 admissions in the Pediatric Surgery department with the diagnosis of intestinal obstruction. Of these, 108 (39%) were newborns, while 171 patients (61%) were infants and children more than 1 month of age. The various causes of neonatal intestinal obstruction are shown in Table 56.2, while the etiology of intestinal obstruction in children more than 1 month of age is depicted in Table 56.3. The topic of neonatal intestinal obstruction is discussed in detail elsewhere and will not be covered in this chapter.

In our series, the common causes of intestinal obstruction were intussusception, postoperative obstruction due to adhesions, Hirschsprung's disease, obstruction due to roundworms, tuberculous intestinal obstruction, and non-specific acute jejunoileitis (Table 56.3).

Table 56.2 Neonatal intestinal obstruction—the KSCH experience- February 1999-March 2001 (n= 108)

Diagnosis	Number (%)
Duodenal atresia/stenosis	20 (18.5%)
Jejunoileal atresia	42 (39%)
Colonic atresia	5 (4.6%)
Malrotation with/without volvulus	13 (12%)
Neonatal Hirschsprung's disease	8 (7.4%)
Meconium ileus	6 (5.5%)
Meconium plug syndrome	2 (1.8%)
Mesenteric cyst with obstruction	1 (1%)
Obstructed inguinal hernia	1 (1%)
Obstructed hernia of umbilical cord	1 (1%)
Neonatal sepsis and ileus	9 (8.3%)

Table 56.3: Causes of intestinal obstruction in children 1 month-12 years old- KSCH experience—February 1999- March 2001 (n= 171)			
Disorder	Total (%) (n = 171)	Infants 1 month to 1 year (n = 93)	Children > 1 year (n = 78)
Intussusception	33 (19.3%)	28	5
Adhesive obstruction	21 (12.3%)	6	15
Hirschsprung's disease	20 (11.7%)	16	4
Obstruction d/t worms	19 (11.1%)	0	19
Tubercular obstruction	14 (8.2%)	0	14
Jejunoileitis	14 (8.2%)	1	13
Meckel's diverticulum	13 (7.6%)	5	8
Malrotation	11 (6.4%)	6	5
Incarcerated hernia	7 (4.1%)	7	0
Other causes	19 (11.1%)	9	10

The majority (28/33) of patients presenting with obstruction due to intussusception were infants between 3 months to one year, and all underwent either operative reduction (14/33) or resection of non-viable segment of the intestine and primary anastomosis (19/33). All those who presented with incarcerated inguinal (n = 5) or umbilical (n = 2) hernia were also infants less than 6 months age and all underwent operative reduction.

The infrequent causes of intestinal obstruction in our series were congenital or inflammatory bands (n = 5); non-specific intestinal strictures (n = 3); paralytic ileus (n = 3); intraperitoneal abscesses with adhesive obstruction, duplication cyst and chylolymphatic mesenteric cyst in two cases each; and a bezoar and intestinal lymphoma in one case each.

The common causes of pediatric intestinal obstruction such as congenital atresia or stenosis, intussusception, anomalies of rotation and necrotizing enterocolitis have been discussed in detail elsewhere in this book. Some of the remaining causes will be discussed here especially those disease entities which are commonly seen in developing countries like India.

PARALYTIC ILEUS

Usually resolves spontaneously on conservative therapy, which includes nasogastric decompression, administration of intravenous fluids for the maintenance of intravascular volume, and correction of electrolyte imbalance, especially hypokalemia. When ileus persists or occurs without an obvious etiology, a laparotomy may sometimes be necessary to confidently rule out mechanical obstruction or intra-abdominal sepsis.

Mortality from obstruction with intestinal gangrene ranges from 4.5-31%, whereas with simple mechanical obstruction relieved within 24 hours, the mortality is about 1%.[3,28] Because no test reliably detects strangulation preoperatively, operation should be performed as soon as is reasonable.

ACUTE JEJUNOILEITIS

Acute necrotizing inflammation of the small intestine or acute necrotizing jejunoileitis has been frequently reported from South Asian countries.[30] The etiology of the condition is still obscure. In children, this condition has been described in only a few reports, although Parvathy and Varma found it to be a common disorder in children.[31-34] In a detailed study, Chandrasekharam et al reported 18 patients in whom the diagnosis was confirmed at laparotomy, and found that abdominal pain, fever and blood in stools were the most frequent presenting features.[30] X-rays features and other investigations including bacteriological studies were non-specific. All patients presented in the period from May to October. Other authors have also reported similar findings.[31,33] In 12 of the 18 patients reported by Chandrasekharam et al, bowel resection was performed, and in those patients in whom complete resection of the involved bowel was possible, the postoperative course was very smooth.[30] An interesting finding noted by the authors was the presence of extensive neovascularization in the resected bowel with evidence of Type I and Type III hypersensitivity reactions in 4 patients.[35] An immune mediated etiology was suggested.[30,35]

In our series of 14 patients, the age ranged from 3 months to 12 years, although the majority of patients were 6 years to 12 years old at presentation. Somewhat similar to the findings of Chandrasekharam et al, 12 of the 15 patients presented between May and October.[30] The common presenting symptoms included abdominal pain, fever, abdominal distension and obstipation. Three patients had a history of diarrhea preceding the presentation with features of jejunoileitis. Abdominal distension and tenderness,

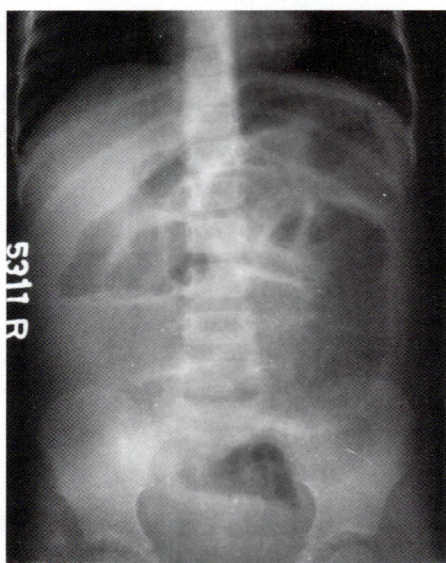

Fig. 56.8: Plain abdominal skiagram (errect view) in a 3-year-old child with jejunoileitis showing dilated jejunal loops with thickened walls and paucity of distal gas

visible bowel loops and features of toxemia were commonly seen. Blood in the stools was reported by only 4 patients (29%). We found that abdominal X-rays were quite helpful in diagnosing this condition. Characteristic findings included dilated jejunal and proximal ileal loops, thickened bowel wall, and paucity of gas in the distal bowel (Fig. 56.8). In 3 patients, ultrasonography (US) showed the presence of free fluid in the abdomen. Four patients were managed conservatively with nasogastric suction, intravenous fluids and observation. Significantly, in these 4 patients, clinical improvement was very gradual, occurring over a period of 5-12 days. One of these patients was readmitted 12 days after discharge with recurrence of symptoms and signs and underwent laparotomy. A total of 11 patients underwent laparotomy. Laparotomy showed congestion, inflammation, and varying degrees of necrosis of the small intestine, usually extending from the mid-jejunum to proximal or mid-ileum. Flimsy bowel adhesions were seen frequently, and in 3 patients, inflamed omentum with hemmorhagic areas was seen adherent to the bowel loops. Enlarged mesenteric lymph nodes were common. In 10 patients, the surgical procedure consisted of proximal decompression of the bowel, adhesionolysis, and peritoneal lavage as the condition of the bowel was not severe enough to warrant bowel resection. Postoperatively, the time-interval before resolution of signs and symptoms varied from 5-14 days. One boy, aged 4 ½ months had extensive jejunal and ileal necrosis and underwent resection of two long segments of intestine with anastomosis of viable bowel. This child died in the early postoperative period as a consequence of sepsis and multi-organ failure. It is noticeable, that as compared to other reports, bowel resection was performed in only one patient, reflecting perhaps that most of our patients presented with disease at an early stage.[30,31,33] In addition, probably because in 10 out of the 11 patients who underwent laparotomy, diseased bowel was not removed, the postoperative course was usually stormy and prolonged. Histopathological examination of resected bowel and omentum showed evidence of non-specific hemmorhagic necrotizing inflammation.

OBSTRUCTION DUE TO ROUNDWORM INFESTATION

Roundworm (ascaris lumbricoides) infestation, usually of the ileum, is common in children in tropical and sub-tropical countries like India. It is a frequent cause of abdominal pain and partial small intestinal obstruction in children. In our experience, roundworm boluses were the fourth most common cause of intestinal obstruction and all these children were more than 2 years of age. Those children presenting with subacute obstruction are initially managed conservatively with intravenous fluids, nasogastric suction, antispasmodics and antihelminthics. In our series of 19 children presenting with roundworm obstruction over a period of two years, two-thirds (13/19; 68%) were managed conservatively. In the remaining 6 children presenting with acute intestinal obstruction, surgical exploration was done. There were no deaths in our series, although postoperative morbidity and mortality in these children is not uncommon.[36,37] Surgery is reserved for those presenting with acute intestinal obstruction and those who fail to improve on conservative treatment. Factors such as bands or adhesions contribute to failure of medical therapy. Early recognition of the condition would avoid serious complications and morbidity.[36]

ADHESIVE INTESTINAL OBSTRUCTION

Intraperitoneal adhesions are a common cause of postoperative and recurrent obstruction in infants and children. The incidence of obstruction caused by postoperative adhesions in children, has been reported as 2.2-8%.[29,38,39] In children, adhesions ranked seventh as the cause of intestinal obstruction in the series of Janik et al, but if neonatal intestinal obstruction and pyloric stenosis were to be excluded, then adhesions would be the fourth commonest cause in this series.[38] In our experience, adhesions were the second most common cause of intestinal obstruction in infants and children (excluding neonatal causes and pyloric stenosis). Intra-abdominal adhesions form after almost any laparotomy, especially for inflammatory conditions, intussusception, Meckel's diverticulum, malrotation, congenital diaphragmatic hernia and gastroschisis.[38,39] Majority of adhesive obstruction, 80-90%, occurs within the initial two years of the previous laparotomy.[38,39] Adhesions occur in the areas of ischemia or serosal damage. Rough tissue handling, presence of foreign material such as glove powder, excessively long suture ends, residual blood in the peritoneal cavity, mass ligatures of omentum or mesentery, and excessive use of dry pads or sponges, are some of the factors that significantly increase the likelihood of adhesion formation.

Sudden onset of crampy abdominal pain followed by loss of appetite, nausea and bilious vomiting in a child with history of abdominal surgery should suggest the diagnosis of adhesive intestinal obstruction. The clinical manifestations vary with the site (proximal or distal) and the stage of obstruction at the time of presentation and have been detailed earlier in this chapter. Mostly, the diagnosis of adhesive intestinal obstruction is clinical, but it needs to be confirmed by plain supine and erect abdominal radiographs. Rarely, contrast studies may be required in selected cases.

The initial treatment of adhesive intestinal obstruction is resuscitation as outlined above, and administration of broad-spectrum antibiotics to suppress bacterial translocation and help prolong the viability of ischemic intestine.

In the management of adhesive intestinal obstruction, the most difficult part is to decide if and when the child is to undergo surgery. When incomplete obstruction is suggested on clinical and radiographic findings, the child may be kept on conservative trial. In the series of Akgur et al, by conservative approach in selected patients with adhesive intestinal obstruction, overall 40% were spared operation, without any adverse occurrence.[40] It must be kept in mind that bowel perforation can occur even with incomplete intestinal obstruction and hence, surgery should be considered if the child does not improve significantly in 6-12 hours of conservative trial. As a general rule, the presence of fever, tachycardia, leucocytosis, and/or abdominal tenderness, or complete obstruction, warrants immediate surgical exploration.[40] At the time of surgery, it is advisable to enter the peritoneal cavity through a new incision or a fresh extension of the previous one, as the bowel may be adhered to the old scar and thereby be at risk of injury during laparotomy. The operations performed are adhesionolysis alone or combined with decompressive enterotomy, resection-anastomosis of bowel of doubtful viability, or repair of intestinal perforation(s). It should be kept in mind that during the first six weeks after an initial surgery, if the child presents with adhesive obstruction and undergoes surgical exploration, the risk for iatrogenic injury to the bowel is greatest, because the adhesions are highly vascular and heavily collagenized during this interval. Therefore, careful sharp dissection of adhesions with gentle handling of the intestine is a must in these patients. Janik et al have reported that delaying adhesiotomy and entering the gastro-intestinal tract during adhesiotomy are associated with significantly increased morbidity.[38] In their experience, the rate of wound infection in these children ranged from 4-50%, being lowest for those children who had lysis of adhesions only, and highest for those who had lysis and decompressive enterotomy or perforation repair.[38]

POSTOPERATIVE INTUSSUSCEPTION

Postoperative small bowel intussusception occurs spontaneously and is an uncommon cause of intestinal obstruction. It usually involves the small bowel alone and occurs within two weeks of a previous laparotomy. It has been seen in the upper jejunum after routine herniotomy (without opening the sac) in an infant, and in the midileum after endorectal pull-through surgery for Hirschsprung's disease.[1] Typically, the child does well for several days and may even resume oral intake. Thereafter, the child may present with abdominal cramps, anorexia, bilious vomiting, abdominal distension, and irritability, suggesting a mechanical obstruction. The diagnosis of this condition is difficult, as it needs to be differentiated from the postoperative paralytic ileus. Abdominal radiographs show an obstructive pattern. A barium enema is usually not helpful, because most of these lesions are located in the ileum or jejunum.[41] Abdominal ultrasonography may help in the diagnosis of postoperative intussusception. However, the best diagnostic procedure is an upper GI contrast examination. In general, most postoperative small bowel intussusceptions require surgery for correction. In most cases, the intussusception can be reduced manually and strangulation is uncommon.

REFERENCES

1. Filston HC. Other causes of intestinal obstruction, in O'Neill, Jr JA, Rowe MI, Grosfeld JL, Fonkalsrud EW, Coran AG (Eds): Pediatric Surgery, (ed 5) chap 79, St. Louis MO, Mosby Year Book, 1998;1215-22.
2. Wangensteen OH. Historical aspects of the management of acute intestinal obstruction. Surgery 1969;65:363-83.
3. Jones RS. Intestinal Obstruction, in Sabiston, Jr. DC, Lyerly HK (Eds): Textbook of Surgery: The biological basis of modern surgical practice (ed 5), Baltimore, WB Saunders, 1997;915-23.
4. Shaw A, Schaffer H, Tejak K, et al. A perspective for pediatric surgeons: chronic idiopathic intestinal pseudo-obstruction. J Pediatr Surg 1979;14:719-27.
5. Frimann-Dahl J. The acute abdomen, in Margulis AR, Burhenne JJ (Eds): Alimentary Tract Roentgenology, St. Louis, Mosby, 1967;1:141.
6. Mucha, Jr P Small intestinal obstruction. Surg Clin North Am 1987;67:597-20.
7. Grosfeld JL. Jejunoileal atresia and stenosis, in O'Neill,Jr. JA, Rowe MI, Grosfeld JL, Fonkalsrud EW, Coran AG (Eds): Pediatric Surgery (ed 5) St. Louis, MO, Mosby Year-Book. 1998;1145-58.
8. Kassner EG, Kottmeier PK. Absence and retention of small bowel gas in infants with midgut volvulus: mechanisms and significance. Pediatr Radiol 1975;4: 28-30.
9. Grosfeld JL. Jejunoileal atresia and stenosis, in Welch KJ, Randolph JG, Ravitch MM, O'Neill, Jr. JA, Rowe MI (Eds): Pediatric Surgery (ed 4). Chicago, Year-Book 1986; 838-48.
10. Grosfeld JL. Alimentary tract obstruction in the newborn. Curr Prob Pediatr 1975;5:3-47.
11. Benson CD, Lofti MW, Brough AJ. Congenital atresia and stenosis of the colon. J Pediatr Surg 1968;3:253-57.
12. Jackman S, Brereton RJ. A lesson in intestinal atresias. J Pediatr Surg 1988;23:852-53.
13. Noblett HR. Treatment of uncomplicated meconium ileus by Gastrografin enema: a preliminary report. J Pediatr Surg 1969;4:190-97.
14. Rescorla FJ. Meconium Ileus, in O'Neill,Jr. JA, Rowe MI, Grosfeld JL, Fonkalsrud EW, Coran AG (Eds): Pediatric Surgery (ed 5). St. Louis, MO, Mosby Year-Book; 1998;1159-71.
15. Toulouikian RJ, Ide Smith E. Disorders of rotation and fixation, in O'Neill,Jr. JA, Rowe MI, Grosfeld JL, Fonkalsrud EW, Coran AG (Eds): Pediatric Surgery (ed 5) St. Louis, MO, Mosby Year-Book 1998;1199-214.
16. Fenton LZ, Buonomo C, Share JC, et al. Small intestinal obstruction by remnants of the omphalomesenteric duct: findings on contrast enema. Pediatr Radiol 2000;30(3): 165-67.
17. Dunn JT, Halls JM, Berne TV. Roentgenographic contrast studies in small bowel obstruction. Arch Surg 1984;119:1305-8.
18. Hennigs S, Jager H, Gissler M, et al. Small intestinal transit with radioopaque markers to localize intermittent small bowel obstruction. (article in German) Rofo Fortschr Geb Rontgenstr Neuen Bildgeb Verfahr 2000;172(12): 1000-05.
19. Ko YT, Lim JH, Lee DH, et al. Small bowel obstruction: sonographic evaluation. Radiology 1993;188(3):649-53.
20. Lim JH, Ko YT, Lee DH, et al. Determining the site and causes of colonic obstruction with sonography. Am J Roentgenol 1994;163(5):1113-17.
21. Mahmood T, Mansoor N, Quraishy S, et al. Ultrasono-graphic appearance of Ascaris lumbricoides in the small bowel. J Ultrasound Med 2001;20(3):269-74.
22. Meiser G, Meissner K. Ileus and intestinal obstruction – ultrasonographic findings as a guideline to therapy. Hepatogastroenterology 1987;34:194-99.
23. Okada T, Yoshida H, Iwai J, et al. Pulsed doppler sonography for the diagnosis of strangulation in small bowel obstruction. J Pediatr Surg 2001;36(3):430-35.
24. Gazelle GS, Goldberg MA, Wittenberg J, et al. Efficacy of CT in distinguishing small-bowel obstruction from other causes of small-bowel dilatation. Am J Roentgenol 1994;162:43-47.
25. Jabra AA, Eng J, Zaleski CG, et al. CT of small-bowel obstruction in children: sensitivity and specificity. Am J Roentgenol 2001;177(2):431-36.
26. Pickleman J. Small bowel obstruction, in: Zinner MJ, Schwartz SI, Ellis H, et al (Eds): Maingot's Abdominal Operations, (ed 10). Appleton and Lange 1997;1159-72.
27. Asbun HJ, Pempinello C, Halasz NA. Small bowel obstruction and its management. Int Surg 1989;74:23-27.
28. Stewardson RH, Bombeck CT, Nyhus LM. Critical operative management of small bowel obstruction. Ann Surg 1978;187:189-93.
29. Festen C. Postoperative small bowel obstruction in infants and children. Ann Surg 1982;196:580-83.
30. Chandrasekharam VVS, Mathur M, Agarwala S, et al. A clinicopathological study of acute necrotising jejunoileitis. Accepted for publication in Pediatric Surgery International. Pediatr Surg Int 2001; (in press).

31. Kalani BP, Shekhawat NS, Sogani KC. Acute segmental necrotising enteritis in children. Am J Dis Child 1985;139:586-88.
32. Gupta SD, D'Silva V, Salelkar AV, et al. Acute ischemic enteritis in Goa. Br J Surg 1977;64:420-23.
33. Parvathy TC, Varma KK. Necrotising enteritis in children-Part I. (A clinical study). Ind Pediatr 1981;18:557-62.
34. Parvathy TC, Varma KK. Necrotising enteritis in children-Part II. Pathology and Pathogenesis. Ind Pediatr 1982;19:525-32.
35. Chandrasekharam VVS, Srivastava DN, Mathur M, et al. Angiographic and immunological studies in acute necrotising jejuno-ileitis. Accepted for publication in Journal of Tropical Pediatrics. J Trop Pediatr 2001; (in press).
36. Surendran N, Paulose MO. Intestinal complications of round worms in children. J Pediatr Surg 1988;23(10):931-35.
37. Sarkar PK, Pan GD, Bhowmick PK. Management of roundworm obstruction in light of pathogenesis. J Indian Med Assoc 1987;85:5-8.
38. Janik JS, Ein SH, Filler RM, et al. An assessment of the surgical treatment of adhesive small bowel obstruction in infants and children. J Pediatr Surg 1981;16(3):225-29.
39. Wilkins BM, Spitz L. Incidence of postoperative adhesion obstruction following neonatal laparotomy. Br J Surg 1986;73:762-64.
40. Akgur FM, Tanyel FC, Buyukpamukcu N, et al. Adhesive small bowel obstruction in children: the place and predictors of success for conservative treatment. J Pediatr Surg 1991;26(1):37-41.
41. West KW, Stephens B, Rescorla FJ, et al. Postoperative intussusception: Experience with 36 cases in children. Surgery 1988;104:781-87.

Abdominal Tuberculosis

Shilpa Sharma, DK Gupta

Abdominal tuberculosis is still a common disease in developing countries. Abdominal tuberculosis is defined as infection of the peritoneum, hollow or solid abdominal organs with Mycobacterium tuberculi.

It can involve any part of the gastrointestinal tract; peritoneum, lymph nodes, and solid viscera like liver, spleen and pancreas.[1] Its clinical presentation is protean thus causing a diagnostic dilemma, frequently mimicking other diseases. The accurate diagnosis of abdominal tuberculosis requires a high index of suspicion, as most of the investigations are non-specific and less sensitive. Abdominal tuberculosis is predominantly a disease of adolescence and young adults. The incidence and severity of abdominal tuberculosis are expected to increase with increasing incidence of HIV infection. Though potentially curable, it is a major cause of morbidity and mortality in developing countries.[2]

INCIDENCE

Some of the largest series of abdominal tuberculosis in the world have been reported from developing countries.[3] The incidence is rising in Western countries due to immigration from Third World countries and rising trend of human immunodeficiency virus infection.[4]

In a series from India, Abdominal tuberculosis accounts for 0.8% of all hospital admissions, 15% of all intestinal obstructions and 5-7% of all gastrointestinal (GI) perforations (excluding appendicular).[5] It is, however, commoner in children, affecting those above 5 years of age and particularly those residing in rural areas.[2] In a study from Madras in India, 3.6% of 1028 hospitalized children had abdominal tuberculosis.[6] Involvement of the chest, meninges or lymph nodes is more common, the overall incidence of tuberculosis being as high as 0.7-2 per 1000 children.[6]

The disease is predominant in females.

The incidence of abdominal involvement in cases with pulmonary Kochs was much higher before the era of antitubercular drugs.[7,8] Extra-pulmonary tuberculosis accounts for 10-15 percent of all cases of tuberculosis and may represent up to 50 percent of patients with AIDS. Other sites of extra-pulmonary tuberculosis more frequent than abdominal Kochs in decreasing order of frequency include lymphatic, genitourinary, bone and joint, miliary and meningeal tuberculosis. Tuberculosis (TB) of the gastrointestinal tract (GIT), is thus the sixth most frequent form of extra-pulmonary site.[9] Abdominal tuberculosis denotes involvement of gastrointestinal tract, peritoneum, lymph nodes, and solid organs, i.e. liver, spleen, and pancreas. Each is further classified into primary (no evidence of past/present pulmonary Tuberculosis) or secondary (complicating pulmonary TB, usually from swallowing of infected sputum, sometimes from hematogenous spread). Additionally, the peritoneum may also be infected by reactivation of latent focus, rupture of mesenteric lymph nodes and from tubercular salpingitis. Hepatosplenic tuberculosis is common as a part of disseminated and military tuberculosis.

Nearly all cases of abdominal TB are due to the human strain of Mycobacterium tuberculosis, although few reports implicate atypical mycobacteria in some cases. Infection due to the bovis species is rare, largely due to the practice of boiling milk. In India, the organism isolated from all intestinal lesions has been *Mycobacterium tuberculosis* and not *M. bovis*.[10]

PATHOGENESIS

The peritoneum and the ileocecal region are the most likely sites of infection. The involvement of the gastrointestinal tract is seen in 65-78% of patients of abdominal Tuberculosis.[2]

The postulated routes of infection into the gastrointestinal tract include hematogenous spread from reactivation of old primary lung focus, ingestion of infected sputum from active pulmonary focus, contiguous spread from adjacent organs and through lymph channels from infected nodes.

The most common site in the intestine is the terminal ileum and ileocecal region due to increased physiological stasis, increased fluid and electrolyte absorption, minimal digestive activity and an abundance of lymphoid tissue at this site. It has been shown that the M cells associated with Peyer's patches can phagocytose BCG bacillis. The frequency of bowel involvement declines as one proceeds both proximally and distally from the ileocecal region. The other sites in order of frequency include colon and jejunum. The perianal region is relatively uncommon site. Tuberculosis may also present as a nonhealing fistula in ano with undermined edges. Rarely, tuberculosis may involve unusual sites like esophagus, stomach, duodenum and appendix.

PATHOLOGY

Tuberculosis is a chronic inflammatory lesion with formation of characteristic tuberculous granulomas of variable size in the mucosa or the Peyer's patches. They are often seen just beneath the ulcer bed, mainly in the submucosal layer. Microscopically, the submucosa is primarily involved with chronic inflammatory cells, epitheloid cell granulomas and Langerhans giant cells (with nuclei at the periphery). Submucosal edema or widening is inconspicuous. These granulomas characteristically tend to be confluent, in contrast to those in Crohn's disease. Caseation necrosis is the absolute differentiating feature from Crohn's disease. Acid fast bacilli (AFB) are found in only 4.6% of cases.[11]

Tubercular ulcers are relatively superficial and usually do not penetrate beyond the muscularis.[12] They may be single or multiple, and the intervening mucosa is usually uninvolved. These ulcers are usually transversely oriented in contrast to Typhoid or Crohn's disease where the ulcers are longitudinal or serpiginous.[13] Cicatrical healing of these circumferential ulcers results in strictures. Occlusive arterial changes may produce ischemia and contribute to the development of strictures.[14] Endarteritis also accounts for the rarity of massive bleeding in cases of intestinal tuberculosis.[15] Angiograms of superior mesenteric arteries have been shown to be abnormal with arterial encasement, stretching and crowding of vessels, and hypervascularity.[15] Patients with strictures had occlusion of the vasa recta, while ulcerated lesions had hypervascularity.

In chronic lesions there may be variable degree of fibrosis of the bowel wall which extends from submucosa into the muscularis. Mesenteric lymph nodes may be enlarged, matted and may caseate. Characteristic granulomas may be seen only in the mesenteric lymph nodes specially after antitubercular treatment has been started.

The initial stage seen in the authors experience is a stage of acute inflammation characterized by neo-vascularization, congestion and edema formation noticed over the serosal surface of the intestine, gonads, uterus. These types of lesions are most commonly seen in the upper jejunum and mid-ileum. The symptoms produced include recurrent acute pain abdomen specially after food intake. Other symptoms are usually missing. There is no fever and no loss of appetite. Hematological tests are normal and so is the serology for tuberculosis. The diagnosis can however, be made on laparoscopy or diagnostic laparotomy.

The chronic intestinal lesions produced by tuberculosis are of three types—ulcerative, hypertrophic, and stricturous. These lesions may occur in combinations, i.e. ulceroconstrictive or ulcero-hypertrophic.

The ulcerative form is more often seen in malnourished patients, while hypertrophic form is classically found in relatively well nourished patients. The bowel wall is thickened and the serosal surface is studded with nodules of variable size. These ulcerative and stricturous lesions are usually seen in the small intestine. Colonic and ileocecal lesions are ulcerohypertrophic. The patient often presents with a right iliac fossa lump constituted by the ileocecal region, mesenteric fat and lymph nodes. The ileocecal angle is distorted and often obtuse. Both sides of the ileocecal valve are usually involved leading to incompetence of the valve, in distinction to Crohn's disease. In tuberculous peritonitis, the peritoneum is studded with multiple whitish or yellow-white tubercles. It is thick and hyperemic with a loss of its shiny luster. The omentum is also thickened, vascular and inflamed.[16]

The gross pathology is characterized by transverse ulcers, fibrosis, thickening and stricturing of the bowel wall, enlarged and matted mesenteric lymph nodes, omental thickening, and peritoneal tubercles. In children, however, involvement of the peritoneum and lymph nodes are more common than GI tuberculosis.

Peritoneal Tuberculosis Occurs in Four forms[1]

1. Wet type with generalized ascites
2. Encysted (loculated) type with a localized abdominal swelling;
3. Dry type with adhesions and
4. Fibrotic type with abdominal masses composed of mesenteric and omental thickening, with matted bowel loops felt as lump(s) in the abdomen.

It is common to find a combination of these types.

The nodal involvement due to tuberculosis is commonly mesenteric or retroperitoneal. The lymph nodes may show evidence of caseation or calcification. Intestinal, peritoneal, and nodal tuberculosis may occur together in varying combinations. The abdominal solid organs may also be affected with tuberculosis namely liver, spleen and pancreas. However, primary tuberculosis of solid organs remains very rare and requires confirmation beyond doubts.

CLINICAL PRESENTATION

The disease is more rampant in malnourished children hailing from rural or lower socioeconomic backgrounds, but it not uncommon to see the disease in higher societies living in an endemic area. It is more commonly seen in adolescent girls. Fifteen percent of the affected children have active pulmonary tuberculosis, and a further 15-20% have an evidence of past tuberculosis.[17] Abdominal tuberculosis in older children may present with varied presentations like Granulomatous hepatitis, Terminal ileitis, mesenteric lymphadenitis, ascites, gastrointestinal symptoms and may mimic Crohn's.[7,8]

The clinical presentation is diverse and a high degree of suspicion is important to guide the array of investigations in the proper direction. The delay in presentation can vary between 1 and 14 months.[18] The clinical presentation of abdominal tuberculosis can be acute, chronic or acute on chronic.[19,20] One-third of patients with abdominal tuberculosis have constitutional symptoms of low- high grade fever (40-70%), weight loss (40-90%), night sweats, anorexia and malaise.[1]

The characteristic abdominal symptom described is alternating constipation and diarrhea. Other symptoms include diarrhea, constipation and pain which can be either colicky due to luminal compromise, or dull and continuous when the mesenteric lymph nodes are involved. On physical examination, the characteristic doughy abdomen may be felt on palpation. There may be features of ascites, lump abdomen, or visible peristalsis with dilated bowel loops. The authors have managed an unusual case of tubercular sigmoid stricture presenting with features suggestive of Hirschsprung's disease. The diagnosis could be established only during laparotomy. Thus, in cases with doubt, a trial of antitubercular treatment or an exploratory laparotomy may be justified depending upon the clinical presentation.

The tubercular peritonitis and nodal forms are more commonly seen in children and adolescents as compared to gastrointestinal form.

Peritoneal Tuberculosis

1. *Wet type peritonitis with generalized ascites.* The abdomen is grossly distended and stands out prominently in a malnourished child, with little muscle mass and subcutaneous fat.

2. *Encysted (loculated) ascites type:* The child may be asymptomatic or present with systemic symptoms. The physical examination may reveal a localized abdominal lump, which may be due to loculated ascites, enlarged lymph node or matted omentum and intestines.

3. *Dry type with adhesions:* This is the usual type seen in a child with relatively good immunity. The child presents with subacute abdominal obstruction or a history of feeling of a moving ball of wind. A high index of suspicion is essential to start a trial of

antitubercular treatment that provides early relief in these cases.

4. Classic "Plastic" form: This is the fibrotic type with abdominal masses composed of mesenteric and omental thickening, with matted bowel loops felt as lump(s) in the abdomen. The child has gastrointestinal symptoms along with a doughy feel of the abdomen. The latter is due to diffuse peritonitis with thickening and adhesions of omentum, mesentery and peritoneum. The symptoms include diarrhea (attributed to malabsorption, which itself is due to reduced absorptive surface, obstruction of lymphatics or blind loops due to stenosis/adhesions) or alternating diarrhea and constipation. The classic presentation is, however, with attacks of subacute intestinal obstruction, most of which resolve on conservative management. A lump is found in 25-33% of cases, most often in the right iliac fossa, in the ileocecal and small bowel tuberculosis.

Mesenteric Lymphadenitis

Nodal involvement can present as a lump abdomen or intestinal obstruction due to kinks and adhesions. Obstruction of bile duct, pancreatic duct, duodenum, inferior vena cava and ureter by a lymph node have all been reported, but are rare.

Gastrointestinal Involvement

Acute Inflammatory Stage
In the inflammatory stage, the child may present with nonspecific symptoms of vague abdominal pain, mild discomfort, anorexia, malaise and fever. After a relay of investigations, if no cause is identified, an exploratory laparotomy is done in view of the persisting symptoms. On laparotomy, only congestion and neovascularization may be appreciated. A serosal biopsy may be done though without any significance as most of the time it is not positive for evidence of tuberculosis. The histopathological report is often nonspecific tuberculosis. It has often been seen that the symptoms subside on starting antitubercular treatment. The ESR if high initially is a good measure to follow the response to therapy.

Esophagogastroduodenal Tuberculosis

The involvement of esophagus is extremely rare.[21] Clinical presentation includes dysphagia, odynophagia and a midesophageal ulcer due to esophageal tuberculosis.

Stomach and duodenal tuberculosis each constitute around 1 percent of cases of abdominal tuberculosis. Gastroduodenal tuberculosis may present with dyspepsia and gastric outlet obstruction. Most patients (73%) in a series of 30 cases of duodenal tuberculosis reported from India had symptoms of duodenal obstruction mostly due to extrinsic compression by tuberculous lymph nodes.[22] Complications include hematemesis, perforation, fistulae (pyeloduodenal, duodenocutaneous, blind), excavating ulcers extending into pancreas and obstructive jaundice by compression of the common bile duct.[22,23] There was no associated pulmonary lesion found in more than 80 percent cases.[23] Segmental narrowing may be seen on barium studies. Duodenal strictures are usually short. CT scan may reveal thickening of the wall and/ or lymphadenopathy. Endoscopy findings are nonspecific, and demonstration of granulomas or acid fact bacilli on endoscopic biopsy material is unusual. Surgical bypass has been required in the majority of cases to relieve obstruction but successful endoscopic balloon dilatation (TTS balloon, Microvasive) of duodenal strictures has also been reported.[24]

Jejunoileal Tuberculosis

Though not so common, tubercular involvement of the jejunum and ileum may present with malabsorption and subacute intestinal obstruction. On exploration, there is jejuno-ileitis with nonspecific inflammatory changes on biopsy.

Terminal Ileal and Ileocecal Tuberculosis

Small bowel or ileocecal tuberculosis most commonly presents with obstructive symptoms due to narrowing of the lumen by hyperplastic cecal tuberculosis, strictures of the small intestine or due to adhesions. Adjacent lymph nodal involvement can lead to traction, narrowing and fixity of bowel loops. In India, around 3-20 percent of all cases of bowel obstruction are due to tuberculosis.[2]

Stricturous type of intestinal tuberculosis presents with features of recurrent subacute intestinal obstruction in the form of obstipation, vomiting, abdominal distension, and colicky abdominal pain. This may be associated with gurgling, feeling of ball of wind moving in the abdomen, and visible intestinal loops.

Intestinal perforations due to tubercular etiology are usually single and proximal to a stricture. Tuberculosis accounts for 5-9 percent of all small intestinal perforations in India, and is the second commonest cause after typhoid fever.[25,26]

Ulcerative type of intestinal tuberculosis can present with chronic diarrhea and features suggestive of malabsorption. Malabsorption is a common complication and tuberculosis should be ruled out in every case of malabsorption in India.[2] The cause of malabsorption in intestinal tuberculosis is postulated to be bacterial overgrowth in a stagnant loop, bile salt deconjugation, diminished absorptive surface due to ulceration, and involvement of lymphatics and lymph nodes.

Segmental Colonic Tuberculosis

Segmental colonic tuberculosis refers to involvement of the colon without ileocecal region, and constitutes 9.2 percent of all cases of abdominal tuberculosis. It commonly involves the sigmoid, ascending and transverse colon. Multifocal involvement is seen in one third of patients with colonic tuberculosis.[27] The median duration of symptoms at presentation is less than 1 yr. Lower abdominal pain is the predominant symptom and hematochezia occurs in less than one-third.[27] There may be chronic constipation. Other manifestations of colonic tuberculosis include fever, anorexia, weight loss and change in bowel habits. The diagnosis is suggested by barium enema or colonoscopy. Colonic tuberculosis may simulate late presentation of Hirschsprung's disease, Crohn's disease, ameboma or malignancy.

Rectal and Anal Tuberculosis

Involvement of the rectum with tuberculosis is rare and may present with hematochezia, constitutional symptoms and constipation.[28] The rectal bleeding may be caused by mucosal trauma caused by hard stool traversing the strictured segment. Digital examination may reveal an annular stricture. The stricture is usually tight and of variable length with focal areas of deep ulceration. Anal tuberculosis is not uncommon and may also be seen in pediatric patients.[29] The usual presentation is with anal discharge and multiple fistulae with ragged margins. Perianal swelling may be seen in one-third cases.

Acute Abdomen

Abdominal tuberculosis may rarely present with an 'acute abdomen (14%) which may be due to rupture of a caseous lymph node, intestinal perforation, tubercular peritonitis or ruptured mesenteric abscess.[19] The patient may present with complications like acute obstruction or perforation especially in the presence of stricture. Involvement of the appendix is usually a part of ileocecal involvement. However, unusual cases of isolated acute appendicitis or tubercles seen in an incidental case of appendectomy have been reported.[20]

Varied Presentation

Abdominal tuberculosis may also present with pyrexia of unknown origin. The involvement of the liver presenting as hepatomegaly may be diagnosed on liver biopsy and abnormal liver function tests like reversed AG ratio and disproportionate elevation of ALP.[30] The miliary and local forms of hepatic tuberculosis have quite similar clinical presentations and pathological features. Hepatosplenic tuberculosis is common as a part of disseminated and military tuberculosis. In neglected cases, the child may develop military tuberculosis and appear cachexic.

Children may also present with urinary symptoms in cases of genitourinary tuberculosis. It is not unusual to find children with renal tuberculosis presenting as a nonfunctioning kidney, pyonephrosis or discharging sinus in the lumbar region. Female patients of abdominal tuberculosis may present with menstrual disorders or later with infertility as a result of involvement of the uterus or fallopian tubes.

Tubercular psoas abscess is also common in children presenting with malaise, distension of the abdomen in the lumbar region and altered gait. The diagnosis may be suspected on eliciting the restricted extension movement of ipsilateral hip joint and confirmed on ultrasonography. A cold abscess is sterile on culture.

INVESTIGATIONS

Diagnosis is usually made through a combination of radiologic, endoscopic, microbiologic, histologic and molecular techniques.

Hematological Tests

It is usual to find anemia and hypoalbuminemia. Total leucocyte count is raised in 50% cases. There may be associated lymphocytosis.

Erythrocyte Segmentation Rate (ESR)

A raised ESR, though nonspecific, is a very supportive finding and supplements the clinical finding. Other factors contributing to a raised ESR should be taken into account. It is a good marker to assess the response to treatment.

Mantoux Test

An induration of less than 6 mm diameter indicates either-(a) an uninfected patient, (b) recent infection, (c) anergy due to malnutrition or disease states like measles, or (d) overwhelming tuberculosis infection (50% of autopsy proved cases of severe tuberculosis had been Mantoux negative). Induration in the range of 6-9 mm indicates either past infection or BCG vaccination. It may also be found in some cases of active infection particularly where atypical mycobacteria are involved. Induration of 10-14 mm in a child less than 5 years of age, strongly indicates active infection. Patients with more than 14 mm are four times more likely to have active disease than those with a Mantoux test in the range of 10-14 mm. If the patient has been vaccinated with BCG before, then an induration of more than 15 mm at 1 year, or 12 mm at 2 years after vaccination is considered positive.

Serologic Tests

Soluble antigen fluorescent antibody (SAFA) and ELISA tests have a limited role because of their inability to distinguish between past and present infections.

A positivity rate of 92 for ELISA with 12 percent false positives and a positivity rate of 83 percent with 8 percent false positives for SAFA, has been reported.[31] Using competitive ELISA with monoclonal antibody against 38 kd protein, a sensitivity of 81 percent, specificity of 88 percent and diagnostic accuracy of 84 percent has been reported.[32] However, ELISA remains positive even after therapy, the response to mycobacteria is variable and its reproducibility is poor. Hence the immunological tests can only suggest a probable diagnosis and should not be relied on completely.

Radiology

Chest Skiagram

Evidence of tuberculosis in a chest skiagram supports the diagnosis but a normal chest skiagram does not rule it out. It may show signs of active tuberculosis in 15% of patients.[33] The findings can be—(a) miliary tuberculosis in a sick child without eosinophilia, (b) atelectasis, emphysema, bronchiectasis, parenchymal opacity—any of these when present with pleural effusion or hilar lymphadenopathy, indicates active disease, (c) patchy consolidation or infiltration can be non-specific, but when associated with a positive Mantoux test and cavitation in the apex, it indicates activity. Signs of 'old' tuberculosis are present in 20% of patients, like obliterated costophrenic angle, calcified hilar lymph nodes or a fibrocalcific lesion.[33]

Plain Skiagram Abdomen

Plain skiagram abdomen may show enteroliths proximal to the site of obstruction. A mottled calcification in the mesenteric lymph nodes and any evidence of ascitis may be seen on the plain film. An errect skiagram is also invaluable at the time of abdominal pain in demonstrating dilated jejunal and ileal loops with multiple air fluid levels, with an absence of gas in the colon and fixed bowel loop in cases of obstruction, pneumoperitoneum in cases of perforation and any intussusception. It may be helpful to demonstrate hepatosplenomegaly.

Contrast Studies

The combined modalities of barium meal and enema together are positive in 80-85% cases of gastrointestinal tuberculosis.[33] The former is considered superior in picking up ileocecal involvement, the commonest site

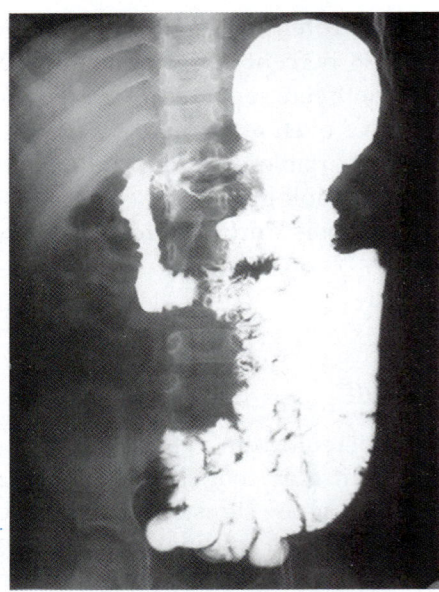

Fig. 57.1: Barium meal follow through in a case of abdominal tuberculosis depicting matted bowel loops displaced on the left side of the abdomen

in GI tuberculosis while the latter is more sensitive for colonic involvement (Fig. 57.1). Small bowel lesions are sometimes missed due to overlapping loops.

Barium Meal Follow Through

The radiologic findings that may be seen on small bowel *barium meal* study are:[1]
1. mucosal irregularity and rapid emptying (ulcerative)
2. flocculation and fragmentation of barium (malabsorption)
3. stiffened and thickened folds
4. luminal stenosis with smooth but stiff contours ("hour glass stenosis")
5. dilated loops and strictures
6. displaced loops (enlarged lymph nodes), and
7. adherent fixed and matted loops (adhesive peritoneal disease).

The mucosal details possible with double contrast barium examination allows visualization of the ulceration in the early stages of the disease. These ulcers are shallow with characteristic elevated margins. With progression, the ulcers may become confluent. Other features include bowel wall thickening, and extrinsic compression by lymph nodes.

Barium Enema

The following characteristics may be seen on a barium enema:[33]
1. Early involvement of the ileocecal region manifests as spasm and edema of the ileocecal valve. Thickening of the ileocecal valve lips and/or wide gaping of the valve with narrowing of the terminal ileum ("Fleischner" or "inverted umbrella sign") are characteristic.
2. "Conical cecum", deformed (irregular, shortened, narrowed) cecum and pulled up due to contraction and fibrosis. The hepatic flexure may also be pulled down due to a shortened ascending colon
3. Increased (obtuse) ileocecal angle and dilated terminal ileum, appearing suspended from a retracted, fibrosed cecum ("goose neck deformity").
4. Deformed and incompetent ileocecal valve
5. "Purse string stenosis"– localized stenosis opposite the ileocecal valve with a rounded off smooth cecum and a dilated terminal ileum.
6. "Stierlin's sign" characterized by lack of barium retention in the inflamed segments of the ileum, cecum and variable length of the ascending colon, with a normal configured column of barium on either side. It appears as a narrowing of the terminal ileum with rapid emptying into a shortened, rigid or obliterated cecum.
7. "String sign" – narrow stream of barium indicating stenosis.

Both stierlin and string signs can also be seen in Crohn's disease and hence are not specific for tuberculosis.

Enteroclysis followed by a barium enema may be the best protocol for evaluation of intestinal tuberculosis.

Ultrasonography

Ultrasonographic examination of the abdomen is helpful in peritoneal and nodal tuberculosis. It may also identify thickened and dilated bowel loops. The findings are however operator dependent. The following features may be seen on ultrasonography.
1. Free or loculated ascites. Fluid collections in the pelvis may have strands, debris and thin septae. These fine mobile strands or septae may be due to high fibrin content of the exudative ascitic fluid.

2. "Club sandwich" or "sliced bread" sign is due to localized fluid between radially oriented bowel loops, due to local exudation from the inflamed bowel (interloop ascites).
3. Lymphadenopathy may be discrete or conglomerated (matted). The echotexture is mixed heterogenous, in contrast to the homogenously hypoechoic nodes of lymphoma. Small discrete anechoic areas representing zones of caseation may be seen within the nodes. Calcification in healing lesions is seen as discrete reflective lines. Both caseation and calcification are highly suggestive of a tubercular etiology, neither being common in malignancy related lymphadenopathy.
4. Bowel wall thickening is best appreciated in the ileocecal region. The thickening is uniform and concentric as opposed to the eccentric thickening at the mesenteric border found in Crohn's disease and the variegated appearance of malignancy. Diseased intestine is recognised as non-specific bowel wall thickening showing as a hypoechoic halo measuring more than 5 mm. Dilated small bowel loops and occasionally, ulceration may be visible.
5. A thickening of the small bowel mesentery of 15 mm or more and an increase in mesenteric echogenicity combined with mesenteric lymphadenopathy may be seen in early abdominal tuberculosis.[34] Pathologically, this mesenteric thickening results from lymphadenopathy, fat deposition, and edema due to lymphatic obstruction which makes it more echogenic.
6. Pseudo-kidney sign – involvement of the ileocecal region which is pulled up to a subhepatic position.

Ultrasonography may also be useful for guiding procedures like ascitic tap and fine needle aspiration cytology or biopsy from the lymph nodes or hypertrophic lesions.[35-37] US-guided fine-needle aspiration biopsy (FNAB) has been used successfully in the diagnosis of abdominal tuberculosis.[36,37]

Computed Tomographic (CT) Scan

Ileocecal tuberculosis is usually hyperplastic and well evaluated on CT scan. Circumferential thickening of cecum and terminal ileum, adherent loops, large regional nodes and mesenteric thickening can together form a mass centered around the ileocecal junction.

CT scan can also pick up ulceration or nodularity within the terminal ileum, along with narrowing and proximal dilatation. Involvement around the hepatic flexure of colon is common. Complications of perforation, abscess, and obstruction are also seen. Tubercular ascitic fluid is of high attenuation value (25-45 HU) due to its high protein content. Thickened peritoneum and enhancing peritoneal nodules may be seen. A smooth peritoneum with minimal thickening and marked enhancement after contrast suggests tuberculous peritonitis whereas nodular and irregular peritoneal thickening suggests the presence of peritoneal carcinomatosis.[38] Omental thickening is well seen often as an omental cake appearance.[39]

Lymph nodes may be interspersed. The contrast enhancement of tuberculous lymph nodes on contrast-enhanced CT (CECT) have been described as (four patterns) – peripheral rim enhancement, non-homogenous enhancement, homogenous enhancement and homogenous non-enhancement, in order of frequency.[40] Different patterns of contrast enhancement could be seen within the same nodal group, possibly related to the different stages of the pathological process. Caseating lymph nodes are seen as having hypodense centers and peripheral rim enhancement. The presence of nodal calcification in the absence of a known primary tumor in patients from endemic areas suggests a tubercular etiology. CT findings can help differentiate it from other inflammatory and neoplastic diseases, particularly lymphoma and Crohn's disease.[41] In tuberculosis the mesenteric, mesenteric root, celiac, porta hepatis and peripancreatic nodes are characteristically involved, reflecting the lymphatic drainage of the small bowel. The retroperitoneal nodes (*i.e.*, the periaortic and pericaval) are relatively spared, and are almost never seen in isolation, unlike lymphoma.

The tuberculous involvement of the pancreas may show as well defined hypoechoic areas on ultrasonography and as hypodense necrotic regions within the enlarged pancreas. CT was more accurate than ultrasound in detecting abnormalities like peri-portal and peripancreatic lymph nodes, and bowel wall thickening. However, bowel wall dilatation was better appreciated on ultrasound than CT scan.

Magnetic Resonance Imaging when compared to CT added no additional information.[42]

Cytology and Biochemistry of Ascitic Fluid

In presence of ascites, the diagnosis can be established with Cytology and Biochemistry. The ascitic fluid in abdominal tuberculosis is clear or straw colored, with glucose concentration less than 30 mg/dl, high protein content greater than protein > 3g/dl, with a total cell count of 150-4000/cu mm, usually more than 1,000/cu mm (consisting predominantly of lymphocytes (> 70%). The ascites to blood glucose ratio is less than 0.96.[43] The serum ascitis albumin gradient is less than 1.1g/dl, and adenosine deaminase levels above 36 U/l.[44] Adenosine deaminase is increased in tuberculous ascitic fluid due to the stimulation of T-cells by mycobacterial antigens. In coinfection with HIV the ADA values can be normal or low. High interferon-?? levels in tubercular ascitis have been reported to be useful diagnostically.[45] Combining both ADA and interferon estimations may further increase sensitivity and specificity. AFB smear and culture are positive in only 10-15% cases but the yield rises dramatically by culturing a litre of fluid concentrated by centrifugation.[46] Fluorescent staining with auramine-O is superior to Ziehl-Neelsen staining with regard to positivity and ease of detection. In children, AFB may be recovered from stomach wash, keeping in mind that scant saprophytic mycobacteria may also be present as normal flora.

Polymerase chain reaction (PCR) conducted with ascites fluid has produced DNA sequences compatible with tuberculosis.[47] PCR can be a rapid and reliable method for identification of peritoneal tuberculosis; acceleration of the diagnostic decision-making process prevents exposure to unnecessary surgery and allows early initiation of anti-tuberculosis treatment.

Percutaneous Peritoneal Biopsy

It is recommended only if there is ascites, and may be positive in 64% cases.[48] An open biopsy or a laparoscopy aided biopsy directed at suspicious looking areas gives better results. Image-guided percutaneous peritoneal biopsy seems to be a sufficient, safe and inexpensive method for diagnosis of peritoneal tuberculosis.[49]

Imaging Bacterial Infection with (99mTc) Tc-ciprofloxacin (Infecton)

A new radioimaging agent, Tc-99m ciprofloxacin (Infecton) has been used to detect deep seated bacterial infections, such as intra-abdominal abscesses. Patients with suspected bacterial infection have been subjected to Infecton imaging and microbiological evaluation reporting an overall sensitivity of 85.4% and a specificity of 81.7% for detecting infective foci.[50] Sensitivity was higher (87.6%) in microbiologically confirmed infections. Infecton may aid in the earlier detection and treatment of deep seated infections and serial imaging with infecton might be useful in monitoring clinical response and optimizing the duration of antimicrobial treatment.

Colonoscopy

Colonoscopy has been used for the diagnosis of colonic or ileocecal tuberculosis. The appearance is non-specific. Most commonly ulcers, strictures, or edematous and polypoid mucosal folds are seen. Mucosal pinkish nonfriable nodules of variable sizes with ulcerations in between the nodules in a discrete segment of colon most often in the cecum, are pathognomic.[1] Areas of strictures, pseudopolypoid edematous folds, and a deformed and edematous ileocecal valve may be seen.

Multiple biopsies should be taken from the edge of the ulcers. The tissue should also be examined for AFB smear and culture as the histology may not be characteristic.

Endoscopic biopsy specimens may be subjected to polymerase chain reaction for detection of AFB.[51] Granulomas have been reported in 8-48 percent of patients and caseation in a third of positive cases. The limitations of colonoscopic biopsy are that previous antitubercular therapy can alter the histology, and the fact that granulomas are often found in the submucosa. Of 82 patients of GI tuberculosis, colonoscopy was diagnostic in 47 patients only.[52]

Laparoscopy

It is a very useful investigation in doubtful cases. Visual appearances have been found to be more helpful (95% accurate) than either histology, culture or guinea pig inoculation (82. 3 and 37.5% sensitivity respectively).[16]

The laparoscopic findings in peritoneal tuberculosis can be grouped into 3 categories:
1. Thickened peritoneum with tubercles: Multiple, yellowish white, uniform sized tubercles (about 4-5 mm), diffusely distributed on the parietal peritoneum. The peritoneum is thickened,

hyperemic and lacks its usual shiny luster. The omentum, liver and spleen can also be studded with tubercles.
2. Thickened peritoneum without tubercles.
3. Fibroadhesive peritonitis with markedly thickened peritoneum and multiple thick adhesions fixing the viscera.

Markers for Treatment Response

ESR

The most common marker used to assess response to antitubercular treatment is ESR that tends to fall with a positive response to antitubercular treatment.

Acute Phase Proteins

Acute phase proteins may be measured in tuberculous patients to form a baseline to measure the response to treatment. A significant decrease in the concentrations of C-reactive protein, ceruloplasmin, haptoglobin and alpha-1-acid glycoprotein has been seen with antitubercular treatment.[53] The proportions of patients with abnormal values on admission and at the end of treatment were 62 and 14% for C-reactive protein, 78% and 50% for ceruloplasmin, 86% and 26% for haptoglobin and 92% and 6% for alpha 1-acid glycoprotein, respectively.

Cancer Antigen–125 Levels (CA–125)

Cancer antigen–125 levels have been measured to be high in cases of abdominal tuberculosis. CA – 125 may thus serve as a potential follow-up marker of disease activity and treatment response in tuberculous peritonitis.[54]

DIFFERENTIAL DIAGNOSIS

In the hypertrophic form of intestinal tuberculosis, the clinical picture may mimic malignant neoplasms such as lymphoma or carcinoma. In the ulcero-hypertrophic form, it may mimic inflammatory bowel disease. The nodal form of abdominal tuberculosis may closely mimic lymphomas. Ascitic form can be difficult to distinguish from malignant peritoneal disease and sometimes ascites due to chronic liver disease. In cases of hepato-splenomegaly, all other causes need to be excluded before considering a tubercular etiology.

Sometimes, when all investigations are negative and TB is strongly suspected, then a laparotomy (or a mini-lap) may be indicated for inspection of peritoneal cavity, taking a biopsy of a lymph node or omental nodule or correction of a stenotic bowel lesion can also be done simultaneously, if found.

TREATMENT

Laparotomy

In circumstances where the clinical suspicion of intra-abdominal disease is strong, but results of investigations are equivocal, a diagnostic laparotomy may be a safer option. Where clinical suspicion is strong and imaging features are suggestive, a therapeutic trial of ATT may be justified. However, laparotomy is definitely indicated where malignancy cannot be ruled out with certainty. In many patients, it may not be possible to rule out malignancy even at laparotomy. A frozen section examination may help in such cases. A mesenteric lymph node should always be removed in such cases as caseation and granulomas are much more likely to be present in lymph nodes than intestinal lesions.[10] An omental nodule may also be taken for biopsy. The correction of a stenotic bowel lesion may be done if found. Rarely cases may present with acute intestinal obstruction and need urgent laparotomy (Figs 57.2A and B).

Medical Treatment

Antimicrobial treatment is the same as for pulmonary tuberculosis. Medical treatment with standard full course of Anti Tubercular Treatment (ATT) is indicated in all patients with abdominal tuberculosis.[1] In peritoneal tuberculosis, only medical treatment is required. Intestinal tuberculosis is a systemic disease. In GI tuberculosis, surgery may be required and preferably should be done 6-8 weeks after starting the antitubercular therapy. Though the use of short course regimens for 6-9 months have been found to be equally effective by few studies, many physicians still extend the treatment duration to 12-18 months according to the conventional regimens in cases of abdominal tuberculosis.[55] This is justified in view of the unpredictable absorption due to the diseased gut and associated symptoms like vomiting and malabsorption.

The main drugs used are Isoniazide, rifampicin, ethambutol, pyrazinamide (PZA) and streptomycin (SM). Thiacetazone and PAS are not recommended for

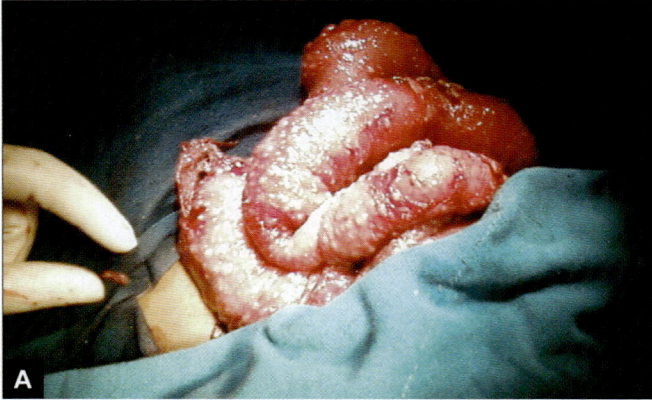
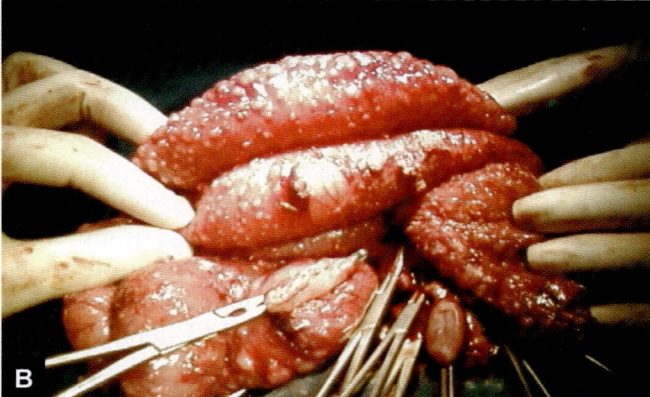

Figs 57.2A and B: A. Operative findings of abdominal tuberculosis in a child showing severely matted bowel loops and tuberculomas. The child had presented with acute intestinal obstruction and required urgent laparotomy. **B.** Resection of the matted loops and ileostomy was done to relieve the obstructive symptoms and give time for antitubercular treatment to act. The anastomosis was performed after an interval of 4 weeks

use for abdominal tuberculosis. In a study of 350 patients with extrapulmonary tuberculosis (including 47 children), a 9 months regime using only INH and rifampicin was successful in 95% cases with 0.7% cases relapsing in a follow-up of 9 years.[56]

Patients with peritoneal, nodal, or ulcerative intestinal disease are usually treated with drugs (ATT). Some authors have recommended the addition of corticosteroids in patients with peritoneal disease in order to reduce subsequent complications of adhesions. No controlled studies have been performed to show their benefit. Patients with intestinal obstruction due to strictures and hypertrophic lesions require surgical treatment. However, some reports have shown successful treatment of obstructing intestinal lesions with ATT alone.[57]

Though patients usually report improvement in systemic symptoms in few weeks, relief of intestinal symptoms may require a much longer duration.

Routine LFT estimations are not necessary, unless the patient has suspected icterus or malaise, anorexia or abdominal pain. INH, rifampicin and pyrazinamide should be discontinued in the presence of icterus or a three-fold rise in transaminases.[15] As the antitubercular therapy causes healing with fibrosis, this may result in further narrowing and intestinal stricture. Therapy can also alter the histopathological picture and may even increase the perforation rate.[9,58]

Surgery

In extra-GI tuberculosis, surgery is not required in all cases, the major role of surgery being biopsy.[1] The abdomen should be closed without drainage even in the presence of ascites or peritonitis. In GI tuberculosis, if symptoms recur after starting drugs, then elective surgery is planned. Emergency surgery may be required in 25-30% cases of abdominal tuberculosis[2] particularly those who present with perforation, acute intestinal obstruction not responding to conservative measures, acute peritonitis and rarely significant hematochezia. Bypassing the stenosed segment was practiced when effective antitubercular drugs were unavailable, as any resectional surgery was considered hazardous in the presence of active disease. This practice however, produced blind loop syndrome, fistulae and recurrent obstruction in the remaining segments. With the advent of antituberculous drugs, more radical procedures became popular in an attempt to eradicate the disease locally. These procedures were often not tolerated well by the malnourished patient. Moreover, the lesions are often widely spaced and not suitable for resection.

The recommended surgical procedures today are conservative. A period of preoperative drug therapy is controversial. Strictures which reduce the lumen by half or more and which cause proximal hypertrophy or dilation are treated by strictureplasty.[59,60] This involves a 5-6 cm long incision along the antimesenteric side which is closed transversely in two layers. A segment of bowel bearing multiple strictures or a single long tubular stricture may merit resection. Resection is segmental with a 5 cm margin. Tubercular perforations are usually ileal and are associated with distal strictures. Resection and anastomosis is preferred as simple closure of the lesions is associated with a high incidence of leak and fistula formation and thus higher mortality.[61] For ileocecal tuberculosis, limited resection of the ileocecal area rather than formal right hemicolectomy, involves lesser dissection and thus less chances of injury to the duodenum or ureter. For colonic lesions, resection is advocated.

Some obstructing intestinal lesions may also relieve with antitubercular drugs alone without surgery.[57] The mean time required for the relief of obstructive symptoms was 6 months.

Emergency surgery for intestinal obstruction is best avoided as it carries 18-24% mortality.[2] Thus, every patient who presents with intestinal obstruction should initially be managed conservatively. Tubercular perforations carry a high mortality despite surgery. In contrast, elective surgery for GI tuberculosis carries only 0.5-2% mortality. Despite the advent of newer antitubercular drugs, abdominal tuberculosis carries a mortality of 4-12% which is largely due to associated problems of malnutrition, anemia, and hypoalbuminemia and due to acute complications.

REFERENCES

1. Gupta DK, Sharma Shilpa. Abdominal Tuberculosis in Adolescence in Textbook of Adolescent Medicine. Ed Swati Bhave. Jaypee Brothers New Delhi Chapter 2006;20(5):663-69.
2. Gupta DK, Rohatgi M, Misra D. Abdominal tuberculosis in children; edited seth V. A publication of Indian Pediatrics, the official Journal of Indian Academy of Pediatrics, New Delhi 1991;chapter 10:188-94.
3. Bhansali SK. Abdominal tuberculosis: Experiences with 300 cases. Am J Gastroenterol 1977;67:324-37.
4. Goldman KP. AIDS and tuberculosis. Tubercle 1988;69:71-72.
5. Bhansali SK, Sethna JR. Intestinal obstruction: a clinical analysis of 348 cases. Indian J Surg 1970;32:57-70.
6. Parthasarthy A, Sumathi N, Manohanan R, et al. Controversies in tubersulosis. Indian J Pediatr 1987;54:779-84.
7. Akcam M, Artan R, Yilmaz A, Cig H, Aksoy NH. Abdominal tuberculosis in adolescents—Difficulties in diagnosis. Saudi Med J 2005;26(1):122-26.
8. Blanc P, Perrin I, Barlet L, Talbotec C, Goulet O, Paupe A, Lenclen R, Carbajal R. Peritoneal tuberculosis in children: report of two cases. Arch Pediatr 2004;11(7):822-25.
9. Sharma MP and Bhatia V. Abdominal tuberculosis Indian J Med Res 120, October 2004;305-15.
10. Vij JC, Malhotra V, Choudhary V, Jain NK, Prasaed G, Choudhary A, et al. A clinicopathological study of abdominal tuberculosis. Indian J Tuberc 1992;39:213-20.
11. Tandon HD. The pathology of intestinal tuberculosis. Trop Gastroenterol 1981;2: 77-93.
12. Tandon HD, Prakash A Pathology of intestinal tuberculosis and its distinction from Crohn's disease. Gut 1972;13:260-69.
13. Anand BS. Distinguishing Crohn's disease from intestinal tuberculosis. Natl Med J India 1989;2:170-75.
14. Kapoor VK. Abdominal tuberculosis. Postgrad Med J 1998;74:459-66.
15. Shah P, Ramakantan R. Role of vasculitis in the natural history of abdominal tuberculosis - evaluation by mesenteric angiography. Indian J Gastroenterol 1991;10:127-30.
16. Bhargava DK, Shriniwas, Chopra P, Nijhawan S, DasarathyS, Kushwaha AK. Peritoneal tuberculosis: laparoscopic patterns and its diagnostic accuracy. Am J Gastroenterol 1992;87:109-12.
17. Sherman SS, Rohwedder MD, Ravikrishnan KP, et al. Tubercular enteritis and peritonitis. Arch Intern Med 1980;140:506-08.
18. Ihekwaba FN.Abdominal tuberculosis: a study of 881 cases. J R Coll Surg Edinb 1993;38(5):293-95.
19. Cheung HY, Siu WT, Yau KK, Ku CF, Li MK. Acute abdomen: an unusual case of ruptured tuberculous mesenteric abscess. Surg Infect (Larchmt) 2005 Summer;6(2):259-61.
20. Waqar SH, Malik ZI, Zahid MA. Isolated appendicular tuberculosis. J Ayub Med Coll Abbottabad 2005;17(2):88-89.
21. Tassios P, Ladas S, Giannopoulos G, Larion K, Katsogridakis J, Chalerelakis G, et al. Tuberculous esophagitis. Report of a case and review of modern approaches to diagnosis and treatment. Hepatogastroenterology 1995;42:185-88.
22. Gupta SK, Jain AK, Gupta JP, Agrawal AK, Berry K. Duodenal tuberculosis. Clin Radiol 1988;39:159-61.
23. Berney T, Badaoui E, Totsch M, Mentha G, Morel P. Duodenal tuberculosis presenting as acute ulcer perforation. Am J Gastroenterol 1998;93:1989-91.
24. Vij JC, Ramesh GN, Choudhary V, Malhotra V. Endoscopic balloon dilation of tuberculous duodenal strictures. Gastrointest Endosc 1992;38:510-11.
25. Dorairajan LN, Gupta S, Deo SV, Chumber S, Sharma L. Peritonitis in India – a decade's experience. Trop Gastroenterol 1995;16:33-38.
26. Kapoor VK. Abdominal tuberculosis: the Indian contribution. Indian J Gastroenterol 1998;17:141-47.
27. Arya TVS, Jain AK, Kumar M, Agarwal AK, Gupta JP. Colonic tuberculosis : a clinical and colonoscopic profile. Indian J Gastroenterol 1994;13 (Suppl) A 116.
28. Puri AS, Vij JC, Chaudhary A, Kumar N, Sachdev A, Malhotra V, et al. Diagnosis and outcome of isolated rectal tuberculosis. Dis Colon Rectum 1996;39:1126-29.
29. Wadhwa N, Agarwal S, Mishra K. Reappraisal of abdominal tuberculosis. J Indian Med Assoc 2004;102:31-32.
30. Chien RN, Lin PY, Liaw YF. Hepatic tuberculosis: comparison of miliary and local form. Infection. 1995;23(1):5-8.

31. Chawla TC, Sharma A, Kiran U, Bhargava DK, Tandon BN. Serodiagnosis of intestinal tuberculosis by enzyme immunoassay and soluble antigen fluorescent antibody tests using a saline extracted antigen. Tubercle 1986;67: 55-60.
32. Bhargava DK, Dasarathy S, Shriniwas, et al. Evaluation of enzyme-linked immunosorbent assay using mycobacterial saline-extracted antigen for the serodiagnosis of abdominal tuberculosis. Am J Gastroenterol 1992;87:105-08.
33. Kapoor VK, Chatterjee TK, Sharma LK. Radiology of abdominal tuberculosis. Aust Radiol 1988;32: 365-67.
34. Jain R, Sawhney S, Bhargava DK, Berry M. Diagnosis of abdominal tuberculosis: sonographic findings in patients with early disease. AJR 1995;165:1391-95.
35. Radhika S, Rajwanshi A, Kochhar R, Kochhar S, Dey P, Roy P. Abdominal tuberculosis. Diagnosis by fine needle aspiration cytology. Acta Cytol 1993 Sep-Oct;37(5):673-8. Comment in: Acta Cytol 1995 Sep-Oct;39(5):1075. Acta Cytol 1996 Mar-Apr;40(2):389-90.
36. Gupta S, Rajak CL, Sood BP, Gulati M, Rajwanshi A, Suri S. Sonographically guided fine needle aspiration biopsy of abdominal lymph nodes: experience in 102 patients. J Ultrasound Med 1999;18(2):135-39.
37. Malik A, Saxena NC. Ultrasound in abdominal tuberculosis. Abdom Imaging 2003;28(4):574-79.
38. Rodriguez E, Pombo F. Peritoneal tuberculosis versus peritoneal carcinomatosis: Distinction based on CT findings. JCAT 1996; 20: 269-72. Journal, Indian Academy of Clinical Medicine _ Vol. 2, No. 3 _ July-September 2001 177.
39. Sood R. Diagnosis of Abdominal Tuberculosis: Role of Imaging Journal, Indian Academy of Clinical Medicine. 2001;2:169-77.
40. Pombo F, Rodriguez E, Mato J, et al. Patterns of contrast enhancement of tuberculous lymph nodes demonstrated by computed tomography. Clinical Radiology 1992;46: 13-17.
41. Pereira JM, Madureira AJ, Vieira A, Ramos I. Abdominal tuberculosis: imaging features. Eur J Radiol. 2005;55(2): 173-80.
42. Zirinsky K, Auh YH, Kneeland JB, et al. Computed tomography, sonography and MR imaging of abdominal tuberculosis. JCAT 1985; 9: 961-63.
43. Wilkins EGL. Tuberculous peritonitis : diagnostic value of the ascitic/blood glucose ratio. Tubercle 1984;65:47-52.
44. Bhargava DK, Gupta M, Nijhawan S, Dasarathy S, Kushwaha AKS. Adenosine deaminase (ADA) in peritoneal tuberculosis : diagnostic value in ascites fluid and serum. Tubercle 1990;71:121-26.
45. Sathar MA, Simjer AE, Coovadia YM, Soni PN, Moola SA, Insam B, et al. Ascitic fluid gamma interferon concentrations and adenosine deaminase activity in tuberculous peritonitis. Gut 1995;36:419-21.
46. Singh MM, Bhargava AN, Jain KP. Tubercular peritonitis. N Engl. J Med 1969;281:1091-94.
47. Wang YC, Lu JJ, Chen CH, Peng YJ, Yu MH. Peritoneal tuberculosis mimicking ovarian cancer can be diagnosed by polymerase chain reaction: a case report. Gynecol Oncol 2005;97(3):961-63.
48. Shukla HS, Bhatia S, Nathani YP, et al. Peritoneal biopsy for diagnosis of abdominal tuberculosis. Postgrad Med J 1982;58:226-28.
49. Vardareli E, Kebapci M, Saricam T, Pasaoglu O, Acikalin M. Tuberculous peritonitis of the wet ascitic type: clinical features and diagnostic value of image-guided peritoneal biopsy. Dig Liver Dis. 2004 Mar;36(3):199-204. Comment in: Dig Liver Dis. 2004 Mar;36(3):175-77.
50. Britton KE, Wareham DW, Das SS, Solanki KK, Amaral H, Bhatnagar A, Katamihardja AH, Malamitsi J, Moustafa HM, Soroa VE, Sundram FX, Padhy AK. Imaging bacterial infection with (99m)Tc-ciprofloxacin (Infecton). J Clin Pathol 2002;55(11):817-23.
51. Anand BS, Schneider FE, EI-Zaatari FA, et al. Diagnosis of intestinal tuberculosis by polymerase chain reaction on endoscopic biopsy specimens. Am J Gastroenterol 1994;89:2248-49.
52. Kalvaria I, Kottler RE, Max IN. The role of colonoscopy in the diagnosis of tuberculosis. J Clin Gastroenterol 1988;10:516-23.
53. Immanuel C, Acharyulu GS, Kannapiran M, Segaran R, Sarma GR. Acute phase proteins in tuberculous patients. Indian J Chest Dis Allied Sci. 1990;32:15-23.
54. Wu JF, Li HJ, Lee PI, Ni YH, Yu SC, Chang MH. Tuberculous peritonitis mimicking peritonitis carcinomatosis: a case report. Eur J Pediatr. 2003;162:853-55. Epub 2003 Oct 8.
55. Balasubramanian R, Nagarajan M, Balambal R, Tripathy SP, Sundararaman R, Venkatesan P. Randomised controlled clinical trial of short course chemotherapy in abdominal tuberculosis: a five-year report. Int J Tuberc Lung Dis 1997;1:44-51.
56. Lorin MT, Katharine HKM, Jacob SC. Treatment of tuberculosis in children. Pediatr Clin North Am 1983;30: 333-48.
57. Anand BS, Nanda R, Sachdev K. Response of tuberculous strictures to antituberculous treatment. Gut 1988;29: 62-69.
58. Mohd Behari HM. Perforation of tuberculous enteritis. Med J Malays 1978;32:282-84.
59. Pujari BD. Modified surgical procedures in intestinal tuberculosis. Br J Surg 1979;66:180-81.
60. Katariya RN, Sood S, Rao PG, et al. Stricturoplasty for tubercular strictures of the gastrointestinal tract. Br J Surg 1977;64:496-98.
61. Ara C, Sogutlu G, Yildiz R, Kocak O, Isik B, Yilmaz S, Kirimlioglu V. Spontaneous small bowel perforations due to intestinal tuberculosis should not be repaired by simple closure. J Gastrointest Surg 2005;9:514-17.

CHAPTER 58

Alimentary Tract Duplications

Richard G Azizkhan

Congenital alimentary tract anomalies are rare developmental errors that have historically been known by a number of different names, including enterocystomas, enterogenous cysts, supernumerary accessory organs, ileum duplex, giant diverticula, and unusual Meckel's diverticulum. The term *duplication* in relation to the intestinal tract was first used by Fitz in 1884. In 1937, Ladd suggested that such anomalies be collectively designated as alimentary tract duplications. In the 1950s, Gross further defined the clinical and pathologic features of these anomalies and recommended that the term duplication be used to describe all such lesions in diverse locations from the mouth to the anus. As proposed by Gross, current nomenclature reflects the anatomic location of the duplication rather than the histologic features of its mucosal lining.

Duplication anomalies are found throughout the alimentary tract. Approximately 80% are located within the abdominal cavity, while the remaining are intrathoracic or cervical (Fig. 58.1).[1] These anomalies vary widely in size and are either spherical or tubular. Seventy-five percent are considered cystic, with no communication to adjacent intestine; 25% are cylindrical structures that may or may not have one or more direct communications across a common septum. All intestinal duplications have a well-developed layer of smooth muscle and are lined with various types of gastrointestinal mucosa; multiple mucosal types are frequently found in the same lesion. Most intestinal duplications share a common wall with a segment of normal intestine. Thoracic duplications may or may not share a muscular wall with the esophagus, whereas duplications in the abdomen generally share a muscular wall and lie in the mesentery of the gastrointestinal (GI) tract. Because multiple duplications are found in 10-20% of cases, the diagnosis of one duplication mandates the search for another duplication elsewhere in the GI tract.

One-third of intestinal duplications typically present within the newborn period, approximately two thirds present within the first two years of life, and others present later in childhood or in adulthood. Some duplications (e.g. esophageal, colonic and rectal) are often associated with other congenital anomalies. Although duplication anomalies are sometimes diagnosed incidentally, most patients present with pain and/or obstructive symptoms resulting from the

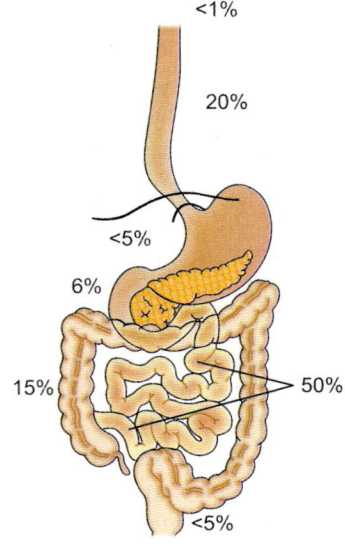

Fig. 58.1: Distribution of alimentary tract duplications

effects of distention of the duplication or compression of adjacent organs. Additionally, abrupt hemorrhage with hemodynamic instability can occur if a cyst lined with gastric mucosa ulcerates and later erodes into adjacent organs and/or vessels. Preoperative diagnosis can be difficult because symptoms are often confused with other more common surgical diagnoses.

Although duplications in the pediatric population are benign, duplications that remain undiagnosed into adulthood may present as malignancies later in life. Although rare, malignant tumors can occur in various gastrointestinal sites.[2-5] Resection or other surgical procedures are thus required to eliminate symptoms and prevent recurrence. For the most part, the choice of operative approach is determined by the anatomy of the duplication and the extent to which it integrates with normal anatomic structures. Attention to vital structures and vessels is of paramount importance in preserving function without significant compromise.

In this chapter, I will expand the general information presented in my overview by briefly discussing various embryological theories and by focusing on relevant anatomy, clinical presentation, diagnostic guidelines, and diverse surgical approaches for the wide spectrum of alimentary tract duplication anomalies.

EMBRYOLOGY

Since the early 1900s, a number of different theories attempting to explain the embryologic events that culminate in intestinal duplication have been proposed, but no single theory adequately explains duplications in all alimentary tract locations. It is thus likely that some combination of theories is correct or that these anomalies occur through some as yet undefined mechanism.

The *split notochord theory* relates alimentary tract duplications to the neurenteric canal, and provides an explanation for the 15% of enteric duplications associated with vertebral defects.[6] Before the formation of the mesoderm, the embryo consists of two layers (endoderm and ectoderm) that are in direct contact. These layers remain in contact for a short while at the primitive pit until mesoderm forms between them. A transient opening (the neurenteric canal) develops, connecting the neural ectoderm with the gastrointestinal endoderm. The notochord forms in the mesoderm, just caudal to the neurenteric canal. In the pathologic state, the migrating notochord is split by the persistent neurenteric canal, resulting in the development of vertebral anomalies. Enteric duplications are among the possible abnormalities related to failure of regression of the neurenteric canal. The *diverticular theory* suggests that there is a failure of the normal regression of embryonic diverticula, which are common in the developing human GI tract.[7] Their presence at numerous sites around the gut wall offers an explanation for small cystic duplications in the intestinal wall and for enteric cysts located in the presacral space. This theory does not explain the preponderance of enteric cysts in the bowel mesentery, or the finding of multiple types of mucosa lining the wall of these duplications. Another theory postulates that *errors of epithelial recanalization* result in formation of cysts located intramurally.[8] This could explain the presence of small submucosal duplications. For the interested reader, in-depth information pertaining to the embryogenesis of duplications can be found in a comprehensive embryology text for surgeons edited by Skandalakis and Gray.[9]

ORAL AND LINGUAL DUPLICATIONS

Oral and lingual duplications are extremely rare. They may affect the lips, tongue and the pharynx and may present as small asymptomatic lesions or as complete and obvious duplications of the mouth and tongue, sometimes containing ectopic gastric mucosa. Treatment consists of excision or repair with closure of the remaining mucosa.

CERVICAL AND THORACIC DUPLICATIONS

Though relatively uncommon, esophageal duplications are a well-recognized entity in pediatric surgery, and meta-analysis of reported findings indicates that they comprise approximately 20% of alimentary tract duplications.[1] They are part of the spectrum of pulmonary foregut anomalies that includes neurenteric and bronchogenic cysts, esophageal atresia, and tracheoesophageal fistula. These anomalies originate from the primitive foregut prior to its separation into the trachea and esophagus. Early in embryogenesis, there is a single primitive foregut tube. During the first three to four weeks of development, a ridge divides this tube into two lumina. Abnormal budding or division can leave rests of cells that form cysts anywhere along the tracheobronchial tree or esophagus. The fact that some cysts are remote from the source of origin implies their migration during embryogenesis. Because the foregut has cells that have both gastrointestinal and respiratory potential, embryologically derived cysts can have either or both types of epithelial lining.

Esophageal duplications are primarily cystic, but can be tubular, and 10% of tubular duplications connect to the esophageal lumen (Figs 58.2A to F). Most cystic duplications are simple and unilocular and contain thick, mucinous material, however, complex multiloculated cysts also occur. Multiple cystic duplications occur as either separate intrathoracic cysts or multiple intramural esophageal cysts. The mucosal lining of esophageal duplications contains gastric mucosa in up to 40% of cases, but may contain pseudostratified columnar, small intestinal, or large intestinal mucosa.[10]

Duplications can occur anywhere along the esophagus and two thirds of duplications occur on the right side of the esophagus. Distal esophageal

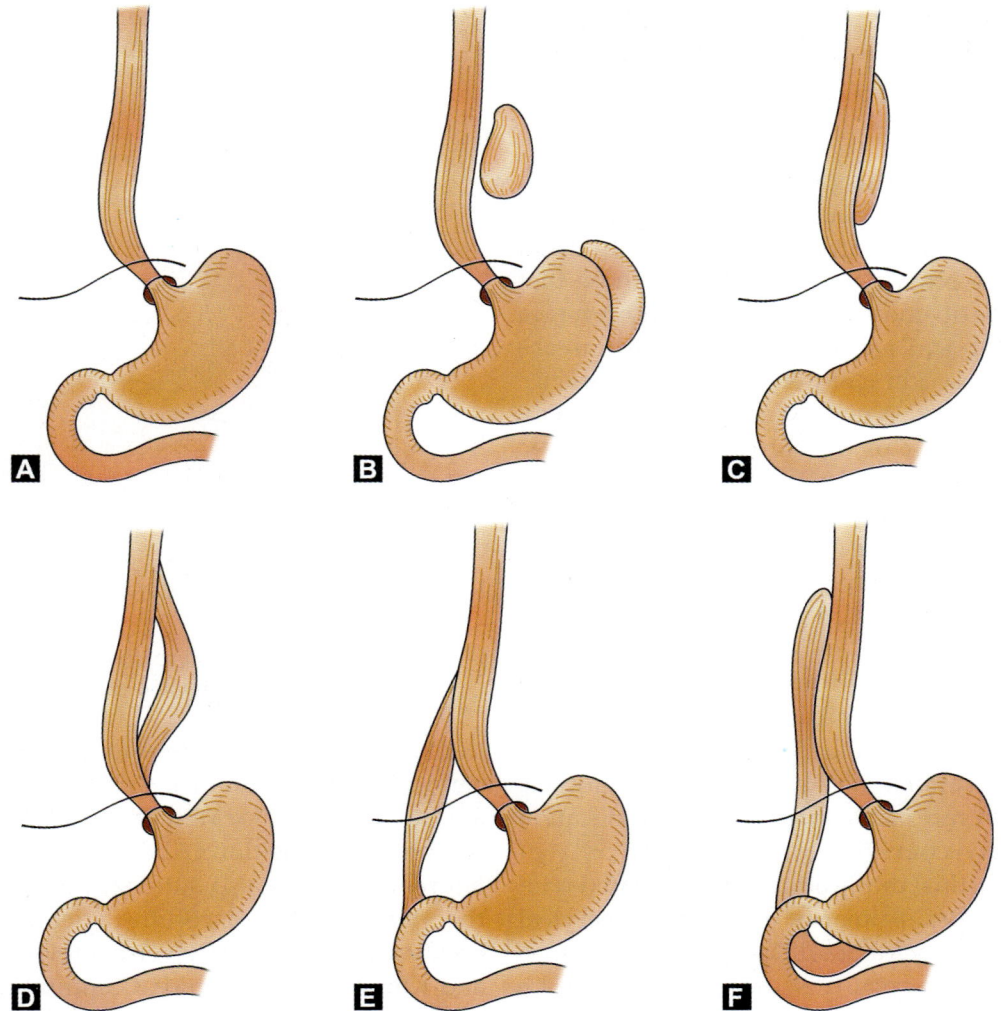

Figs 58.2A to F: A. Schematic of normal esophagus, stomach and duodeum, **B.** Esophageal cystic duplication, **C.** Esophageal duplication (intramural cystic), **D.** Tubular esophageal duplication, **E.** Tubular esophageal duplication emptying into the duodenum, **F.** Tubular esophageal duplication emptying into the posterior gastric region

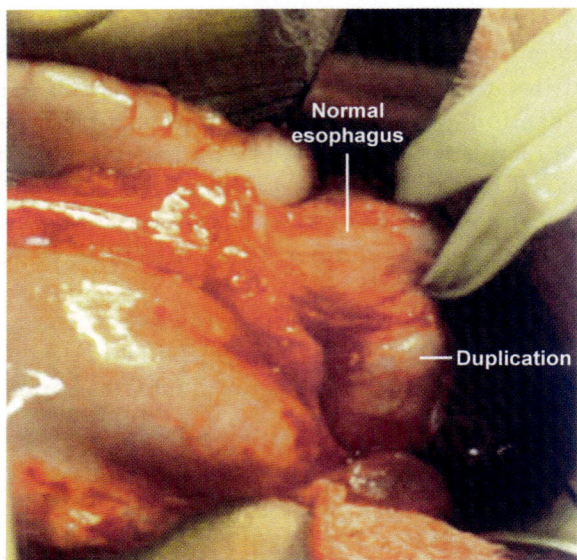

Fig. 58.3: Operative view of distal esophageal duplication

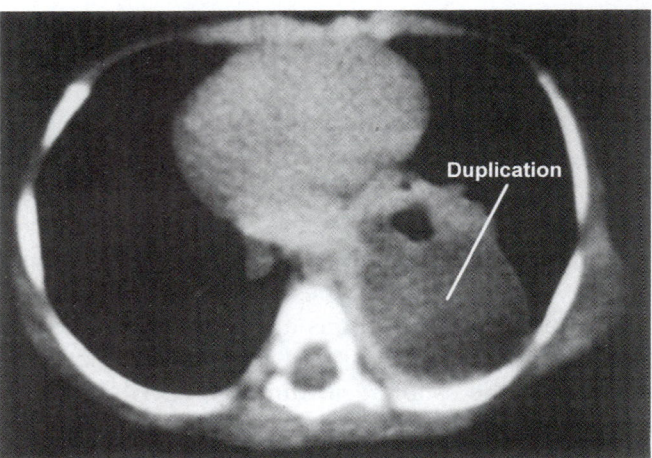

Fig. 58.4: CT scan of chest demonstrating large cystic duplication of the esophagus

duplications are the most common, occurring in 60% of cases; 23% of cases occur in the upper esophagus, and 17% in the middle portion.[11] Patients with distal duplications are often asymptomatic, but those that are symptomatic may present with dysphagia (Fig. 58.3). Cervical esophageal duplications are generally diagnosed in children due to the presence of a neck mass or symptoms of upper airway obstruction. They can be confused with cystic hygromas, thyroglossal duct cysts, branchial cleft cysts, or other solid tumors such as teratomas. Duplications of the middle esophageal portion usually present with compression of the trachea at a young age, and can also be confused with bronchogenic cysts (Fig. 58.4).

Esophageal duplications can traverse the diaphragm and communicate with the stomach, duodenum, or jejunum (Fig. 58.5). As well, separate intestinal duplications may coexist with a thoracic duplication.[12] In rare cases, three or more duplication anomalies may coexist. Approximately 50% of posterior mediastinal duplications are associated with vertebral anomalies, primarily of the lower cervical and upper thoracic vertebrae. These duplications, as well as neurenteric cysts (discussed below) can be explained by the previously cited split notochord theory.

Foregut duplications that communicate with the spinal canal are called *neurenteric cysts*. These

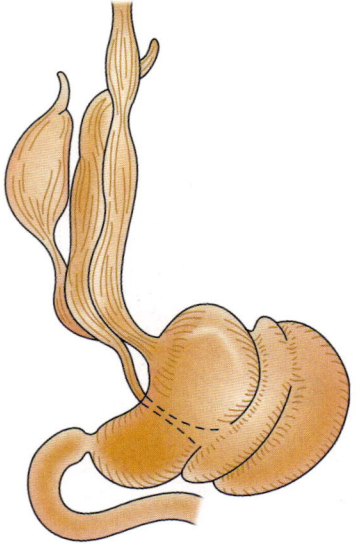

Fig. 58.5: Multiple complete tubular esophagogastric duplications

duplications are most often found adjacent to lower cervical or upper thoracic vertebral anomalies; they are only rarely located intracranially or in the lumbosacral position. About half of patients with neurenteric cysts also suffer from malformations of the spinal cord and column such as spina bifida, hemivertebrae, butterfly vertebrae spondylolisthesis, and Klippel-Feil deformity. Communication with the spinal canal may exist through a fistula or a fibrous tract. It is not unusual to find coexisting intraspinal and mediastinal lesions, and they reportedly occur in 25-75% of cases; coexisting intestinal duplications have also been reported. Additionally, there have been reports of other coexisting esophageal anomalies, such as esophageal web and esophageal atresia, both pure and with a tracheoesophageal fistula. Though coexisting pulmonary abnormalities such as bronchiectasis, intrapulmonary bronchogenic cysts, bronchial atresia, and extralobar sequestration have been reported, they are rare.[13-15] Such reports nevertheless reflect the wide spectrum of embryology-related abnormalities that can occur.

Prenatal ultrasound may suggest the presence of a thoracic duplication, but it generally cannot differentiate various types of echogenic masses. A plain chest radiograph may reveal a posterior mediastinal mass and related vertebral anomalies. A barium esophagogram can be helpful by revealing extrinsic compression of the esophagus by the duplication, but it rarely shows a connection between the esophagus and duplication, and does not distinguish an esophageal duplication from a bronchogenic cyst. When tubular duplications communicate with the esophageal lumen, they can be revealed on a barium esophagogram (Fig. 58.6). While many vascular rings show esophageal distortion, they too are usually recognizable; tracheoscopy and esophagoscopy can, however, be useful in differentiating them from duplications. A computed tomography (CT) scan is extremely helpful in providing information that differentiates a cystic mass from solid neurogenic tumors and vascular structures, thus providing specific anatomic details of the relationship of the lesion to other thoracic and mediastinal structures; it does not differentiate between epithelial and nonepithelial lined cysts (Fig. 58.4). Technetium-99m pertechnetate scintigraphy is used to determine if there is secreting gastric mucosa.

Virtually all recognized esophageal duplications should be excised. The surgical approach depends on the location and extent of the duplication(s) as well as adjacent structures involved. Simple cystic duplications adjacent to the normal esophagus can be readily excised. Intramural esophageal duplications that share a common muscular wall are best removed by excising the mucosa of the duplication and preserving the lumenal integrity of the normal esophagus. In some patients, especially those with distal esophageal duplications, esophageal motility may remain abnormal post-resection. Thoracoabdominal incisions may be required to remove large tubular duplications that traverse the diaphragm and communicate with the gastric or intestinal lumen. These lesions are particularly notorious for causing peptic ulceration and gastrointestinal hemorrhage. Once resected the long-term prognosis is generally excellent.

GASTRIC DUPLICATIONS

Duplications of the stomach are the least common of the abdominal duplications. Nearly twice as many females as males are affected. Most cases are identified in the first year of life, but many are not diagnosed until maturity. Gastric duplications vary in size, ranging from small asymptomatic lesions to very large palpable cystic masses that displace adjacent structures. These lesions are generally located on the greater curve or posterior wall of the stomach, but can be located on the lesser curve, the anterior wall, or in the pylorus (Figs 58.7A and B). Pyloric duplications are quite rare, and imitate pyloric stenosis by compressing the lumen of the pylorus, causing projectile vomiting with accompanying electrolyte disturbances and malnutrition. Only rarely are gastric duplications completely separate form the stomach and located in the retroperitoneum. Although case reports of imperforate anus and vertebral anomalies do appear in the literature, specific anomalies are not typically associated with gastric duplications.

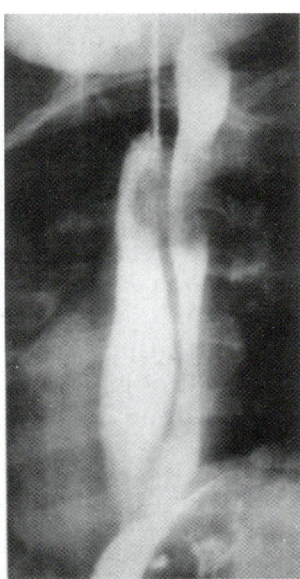

Fig. 58.6: Barium esophagogram demonstrating tubular esophageal duplication

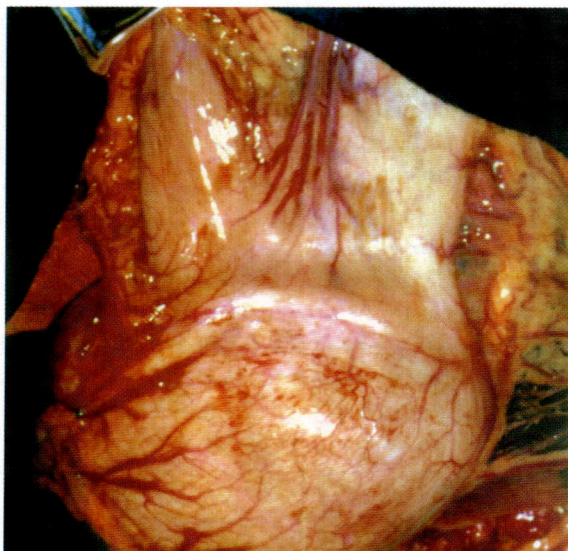

Fig. 58.7A: Operative view of cystic gastric duplication situated on the greater curvature of the normal stomach

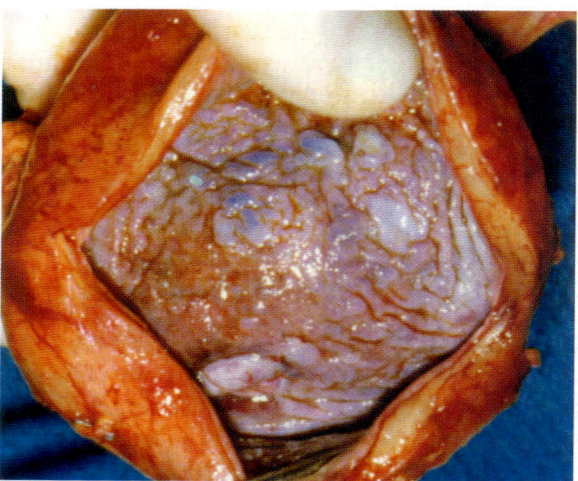

Fig. 58.7B: Resected specimen opened

These duplications are cystic and generally do not communicate with the lumen of the stomach. Penetrating ulcerations of the cyst wall and erosion into the stomach, pancreas or colon or through the abdominal wall have, however, been reported. Gastric duplications are commonly present in infants with abdominal distention and non-bilious vomiting; weight loss is frequently present as a result of volume depletion and malnutrition from protracted vomiting. Gastrointestinal hemorrhage is also frequently seen, either as melena or hematemesis. Pain is secondary to distention of the cyst or peptic ulceration.

Complications associated with gastric duplications occur frequently, with gastrointestinal bleeding and perforation with peritonitis being the most common.

Prenatal ultrasound may suggest the diagnosis, but an upper GI series or postnatal ultrasound is generally required to confirm it. CT delineates the dimensions and anatomic boundaries of the lesion. Contrast in the GI tract helps determine whether a connection to the stomach is present. Because pancreatic pseudocysts are the most common cysts in the lesser sac, mistaking a gastric duplication for a pancreatic pseudocyst is a common error.

Although removal of the entire duplication is the ideal treatment, the presence of a common muscular wall between the diverticulum and the normal stomach may render this impossible. If so, surgeons must be familiar with alternatives. When the area of common gastric wall is small, the entire duplication, together with a portion of normal gastric wall, may be removed. When the defect is large, a partial gastrectomy or stripping of the mucosa as described by White may be indicated.[16] With this procedure, the duplication is first aspirated to prevent spillage and is then opened along its entire length, creating two flaps that have their base on the common wall. Each of these flaps is resected back to the common wall, with the surgeon taking care to protect the gastroepiploic vessels. The small remaining mucosal strip at the base is then removed. Although White's technique originally entailed suturing the transverse colon to the bed of the cyst, Lembert's sutures may be used to invert the raw area if it is not too large. A third option is removing the entire common wall between the duplication and the normal stomach and reconstructing the stomach. These latter two options are best for lesions that are difficult to separate from the stomach.

As cited earlier, pyloric duplications are rare. The surgical treatment of choice is complete extramucosal excision of the duplication. More complicated procedures such as gastrojejunostomy and mucosal stripping have been done, but these are rarely indicated.

DUODENAL DUPLICATIONS

Duplications of the duodenum are also rare, comprising about 6% of enteric cysts of the alimentary tract.[1] At least half present in the first few months of

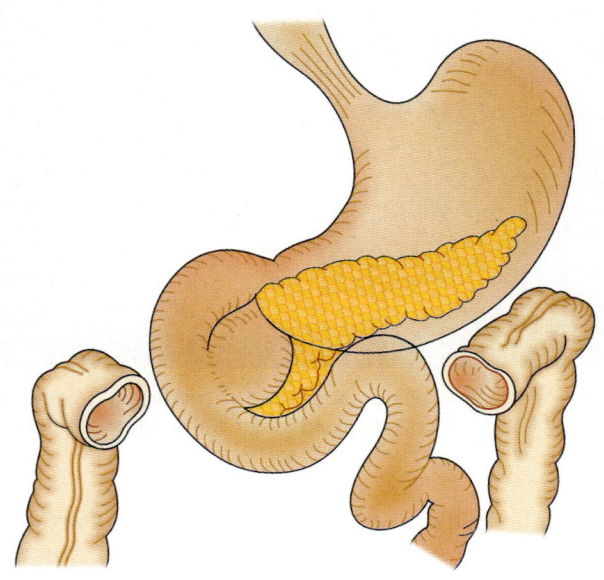

Fig. 58.8: Cystic duplication of the duodenum

life and most usually present before age 10, but some patients are not diagnosed until later in life. Duodenal duplications vary in size and are commonly cystic. These lesions are usually lined with duodenal mucosa, but ectopic gastric mucosa is sometimes (15-20%) present.[17,18] Duodenal duplications occur in the first and second portions of the duodenum and usually (75%) do not connect to the duodenum. They are most often located posteromedially, sharing a common wall with the true duodenum and often partially embedded in the head of the pancreas (Fig. 58.8). Duodenal duplications generally occur singly, but they have been reported to occur in association with Meckel's diverticulum and other duodenal, gastric, thoracic, and ileal duplications.

Obstruction of the duodenum is the usual clinical presentation. Other presenting symptoms include vomiting, gastrointestinal bleeding and perforation from ectopic gastric mucosa, and jaundice or pancreatitis from ampullary obstruction. A palpable mass is also sometimes noted. In many patients, however, symptoms may be vague and difficult to localize, making duplications quite difficult to diagnose and prolonging the course of illness.

Diagnosis is generally made after an upper GI series. These studies demonstrate complete obstruction or narrowing of the duodenal lumen, a widened C-loop, or an intraluminal-filling defect of the duodenum. Ultrasound and CT are also valuable in that they define the anatomy of the duplication in relation to surrounding organs and vascular structures. The presence of a cyst with motility in its wall, as revealed by ultrasound, is highly suggestive of a duplication. Since some lesions connect to the pancreatic duct, an endoscopic retrograde cholangio-pancreatography (ERCP) may be helpful. Additionally, a technetium-99m iminodiacetic acid scan can rule out a choledochal cyst.

Treatment options include resection of the cyst with or without a segment of the duodenum, or partial excision of the cyst and total mucosal excision. These options are particularly attractive for those patients who have ectopic gastric mucosa within the cyst; leaving this mucosa increases the risk of postoperative peptic complications.

Duplications Associated with Pancreatitis

Some duodenal duplications appear to connect to a pancreatic duct.[19] These anomalies largely occur in the head of the pancreas and may be associated with nausea, vomiting, weight loss and abdominal pain. Most patients experience multiple episodes of pancreatis and have a history of multiple hospitalizations with undiagnosed abdominal pain. Diagnosis is extremely difficult, but ERCP is particularly helpful in delineating the anatomy of the duplication and its connection to the pancreas. In addition to resection, some patients may require a Whipple procedure or a Roux-en-Y jejunal drainage of the cyst. Since the best procedure for any one lesion is dependent upon the anatomy of the cyst and its connection to the pancreatic duct, operations for this problem must be individualized.

ILEAL AND JEJUNAL DUPLICATIONS

The small intestine is the most common location of enteric duplications, accounting for about half of all lesions in large published series. Of these, two thirds are located in the ileum and one third is located in the jejunum. These duplications are present in both cystic and tubular forms. Noncommunicating spherical cystic lesions of varying sizes are the most common. They are frequently located at the ileocecal junction and share a common blood supply and wall with the

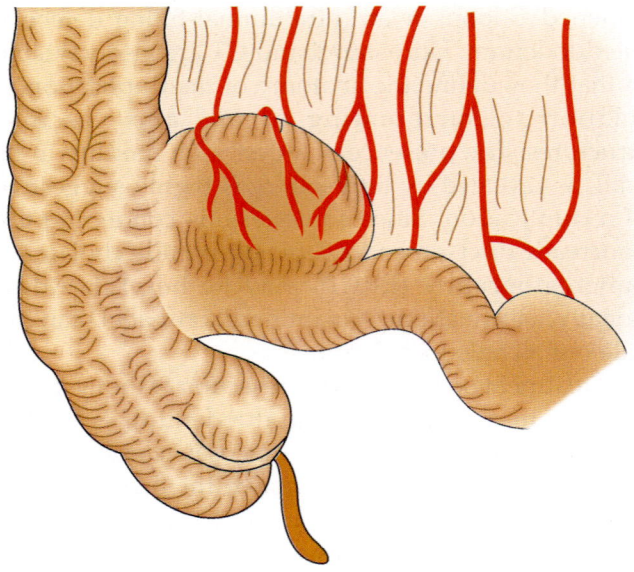

Fig. 58.9: Cystic ileocecal duplication

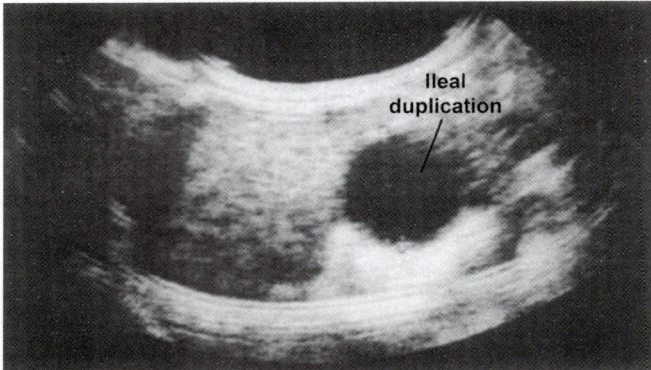

Fig. 58.10: Abdominal ultrasound demonstrating ileocecal duplication in a 3-year-old infant with abdominal pain

ileum (Fig. 58.9). Tubular duplications may be separate from the bowel, have a separate but attached wall, or may share a common wall. They are typically found within the mesentery and generally share a common blood supply and a common muscular wall with the adjacent bowel. Communication with the normal intestine is uncommon, but when present, it may lie at one or several points along the common wall. If the communication is located distally, the lesion may drain into the small bowel and remain asymptomatic. If, however, the lesion is proximal, the distal end of the duplication dilates, causing obstruction, perforation or volvulus. Gastric mucosa occurs in 33% of ileal and 50% of jejunal duplications, and is more likely to occur in tubular duplications (80%) than in cystic duplications (20%).[18] This point is important to keep in mind because tubular duplications are more difficult to resect and if the ectopic gastric mucosa is not removed, complications are likely to occur.

Fifty percent of small bowel duplications present during the neonatal period and 50% present between 1 month and 2 years of age; seventy five percent present by age 2. These duplications are mobile and thus are often difficult to palpate. Because of the high incidence of gastric mucosa in jejunal duplications, peptic ulceration with hemorrhage occurs frequently, and complications from ulceration (e.g. melena and perforation) are more commonly seen with these duplications than with those in any other part of the GI tract. Other complications include intestinal obstruction and volvulus. In children older than 2 years of age, rectal bleeding and intussusception are common presentations. Small bowel duplications tend to occur either as an acute event in the perinatal period, or with a puzzling clinical picture after a long asymptomatic period. Ileal duplications are frequently diagnosed as appendicitis, Hirschsprung's disease, or intussusception; jejunal duplications are sometimes confused with Meckel's diverticulum, peptic ulcer disease, malrotation, or atresia when presentation occurs in the newborn period. Ultrasound can be helpful in revealing cystic duplications and a Meckel scan performed for bleeding occasionally reveals ectopic mucosa (Fig. 58.10). Generally, however, diagnosis is made at laparotomy for intestinal obstruction rather than preoperatively.

Operative approach varies, depending upon the anatomy of the duplication and its adjacent intestine, which may share a common blood supply. Cystic duplications and short tubular duplications are most easily treated with resection of the duplication alone or resection of the duplication and the involved wall (Fig. 58.11A). The latter procedure requires intestinal reconstruction with an end-to-end anastomosis (Fig. 58.11B). By contrast, long tubular duplications are far more difficult to treat and present the surgeon with a clinical challenge. When resection of the intestine is not an option because of the length of normal bowel that would have to be sacrificed, other approaches must be used. Long tubular duplications that are not amenable to complete resection may

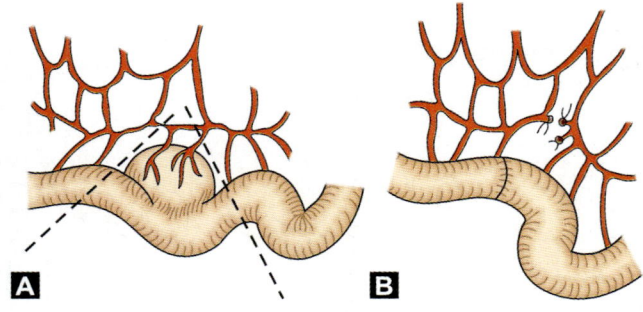

Figs 58.11A and B: A. Ileal cystic duplication, **B.** Duplication was resected and an ileoileostomy performed

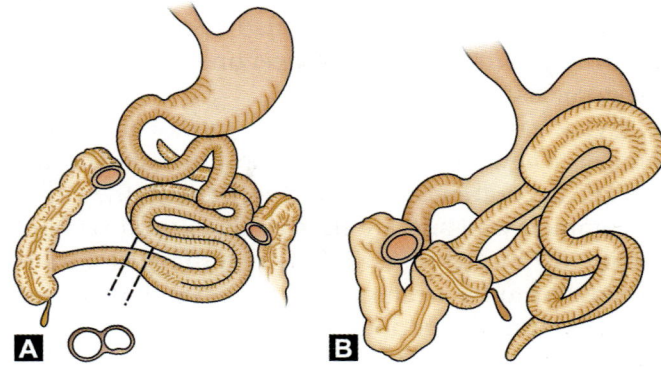

Figs 58.13A and B: A. Long tubular duplication of jejunoileal region with a shared blood supply and common wall, **B.** Gastroduplication procedure. Distal end of the ileal duplication is anastomosed to the stomach. The distal ileal continuity is maintained

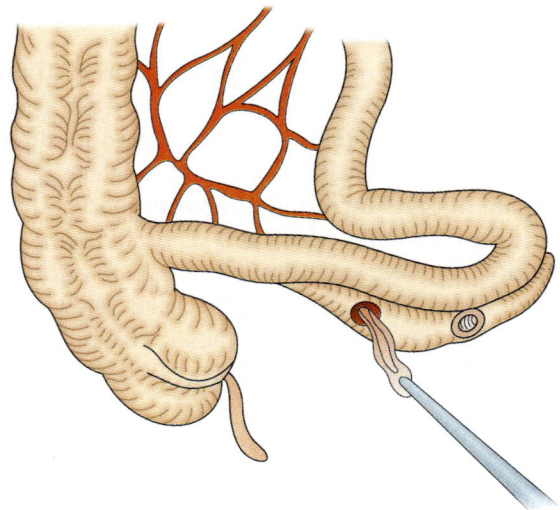

Fig. 58.12: Mucosal stripping of long tubular ileal duplication

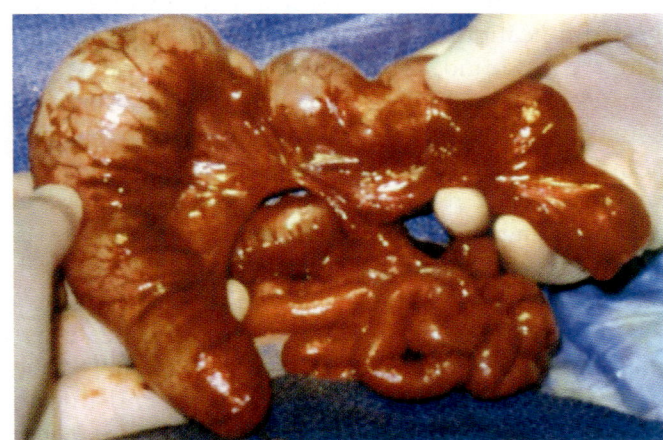

Fig. 58.14: Long cystic colonic duplication with separate blood supply from the normal colon

require stripping the mucosa of the duplication as described by Wrenn (Fig. 58.12).[20] Ischemia of the adjacent small intestine after this operation has, however, been reported. A unique method of treatment that is worthy of consideration is gastroduplication. Described by Jewett and colleagues in 1958, this procedure involved connecting the distal end of the lumen of the duplication to the gastric lumen. The treatment included resection of the connection between the ileum and the duplication with reconstruction of the normal ileum by end-to-end anastomosis. The distal end of the long duplication was then anastomosed to the stomach, leaving the long duplication draining into it (Figs 58.13A and B). A 25-year follow-up of the patient on whom this procedure was performed revealed no complications.[21]

COLONIC DUPLICATIONS

Review of available cases suggests that there are three types of enteric duplications associated with the hindgut.[22,23] These include midline duplications, cystic remnants of the tailgut, and bilateral duplications of the colon and rectum (Fig. 58.14). Midline duplications are almost always cystic and as such, have the characteristics of other cystic enteric duplications. They lie posterior to the rectum and usually share a common wall with it. Signs of bowel obstruction are frequently present, but volvulus, urinary retention, and colonic perforation are also seen. Treatment generally entails colonic reconstruction and anastomosis.

Cystic tailgut duplications are more common in females. They are located between the anus and the sacrum. In contrast to midline duplications, they have no common wall and are thus easily excised without sacrificing the rectum wall. The cystic structure is considered to be a remnant of the opening between the ectoderm and endoderm at the posterior end of the neural tube, and hence represents the persistence of a normal embryonic structure. Gastric mucosa is present in about 10% of these duplications. Presenting signs and symptoms include an asymptomatic mass, rectal bleeding, rectal prolapse and constipation caused by rectal recompression; some children also present as fistula in ano. Twenty percent to 45% of these duplications have a fistula to the rectum or the skin.[24] Ultrasound, CT scan, and barium enema are thus useful in evaluating these anomalies. CT or MRI is used to rule out anterior meningomyelocele. Treatment consists of resection of the entire duplication or its mucosa, using a transanal or posterior sagittal approach. In light of reports of adenocarcinoma in untreated rectal duplications, at least a mucosal resection should be performed.[25,26]

In contrast to midline and tailgut duplications, bilateral duplications are primarily tubular, and exist as a side-by-side rather than an over-and-under doubling. Such pairing often is accompanied by pairing of other midline structures of the posterior part of the body, but most cases show less than complete doubling. Review of reported cases of bilateral duplications[23] reveals a wide spectrum of anorectal duplication anomalies, including double rectum that may empty into the genitourinary tract, vagina, or perineum (Figs 58.15A to C). Patients with colorectal duplications also have a high incidence of complete duplications of the bladder, uteri, and external genitalia (bifid penis and scrotum). Patients with hindgut duplications have a high incidence of skeletal abnormalities, which may manifest in vertebral, pelvic and sacral anomalies — an example being a patient with a hindgut duplication and cloacal exstrophy. The mucosal lining of these duplication anomalies is usually normal colonic mucosa.

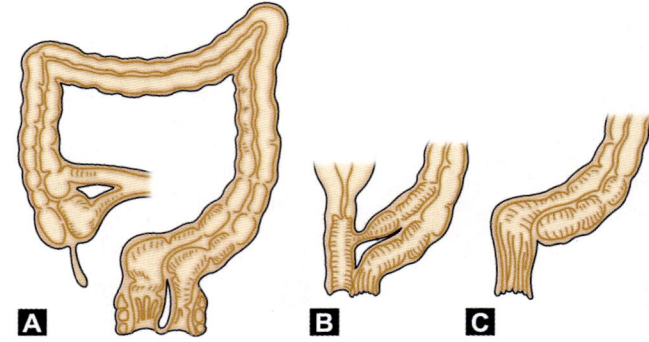

Figs 58.15A to C: Variation of tubular colonic duplication including: **A.** complete duplication from ileocecal valve to anus, **B.** colonic duplication with rectovaginal fistula, **C.** blind-ending colonic duplication

As revealed in a review of 57 patients with tubular colonic duplications (1876-1981) conducted by Yousefzadeh and colleagues, associated anomalies are common.[27] Gastrointestinal anomalies were seen in 49% of patients, and included double appendix, double ileum, omphalocele, Meckel's diverticulum, and malrotation. Eighty percent of patients had anomalies involving at least one system other than the GI tract, and 55% of patients had anomalies involving at least three systems; urologic, genital, and spinal anomalies were common.

Tubular colonic duplications are often observed at birth together with duplications of the genitals or bladder. Patients also may present with acute or chronic lower intestinal obstruction, rectovaginal fistula, rectal prolapse, and urinary tract infections. Diagnosis is generally made by urinary tract evaluation, perineal inspection, and contrast studies of the colons. Due to the high incidence of coexisting anomalies, meticulous clinical and diagnostic evaluation of patients is essential.

Symptoms are caused when the distal obstructed pouch of the duplication that usually connects to the normal colon proximally fills with feces, thereby causing compression of the normal colon (Figs 58.16A and B). Although each case must be individualized, treatment generally involves either of two surgical approaches. In the first approach, the distal part of the duplicated colon is connected to the normal colon with a linear stapler, the connection being distal enough to ensure that the duplication does not fill with

Alimentary Tract Duplications

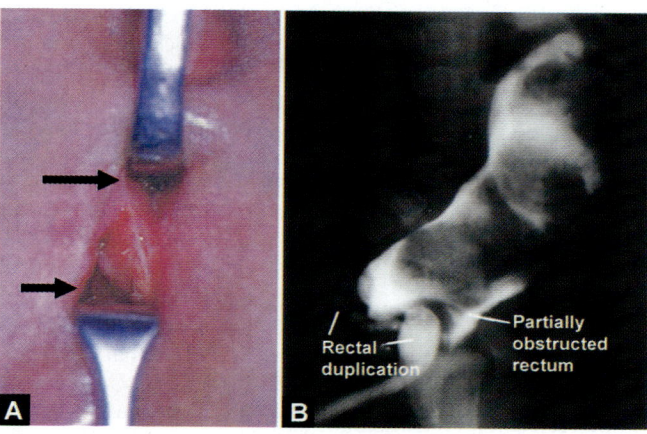

Figs 58.16A and B: A. Duplicated anal opening in a 9-month-old female with anorectal duplication, **B.** Contrast enema in this same patient demonstrating partially obstructed rectosigmoid colon from tubular duplication

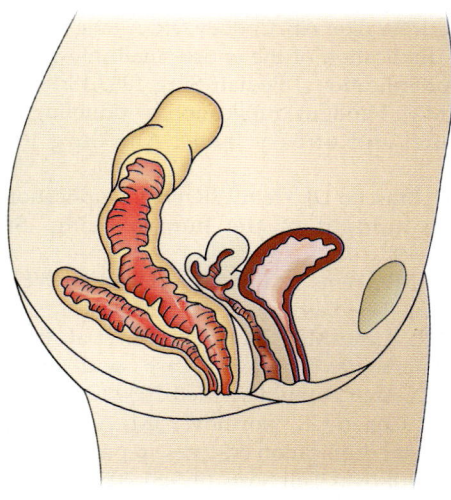

Fig. 58.17A: Tubular rectal duplication with separate anal opening

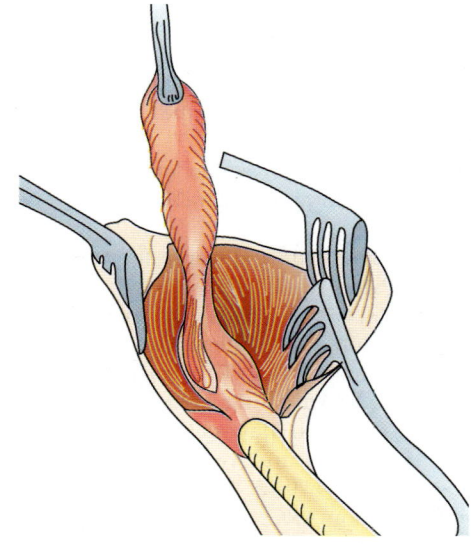

Fig. 58.17B: Posterior sagittal excision of rectal duplication. A Hegar dilator is placed in the normal rectal lumen to facilitate dissection

feces. In cases where the normal rectum and the duplication are separated, the distal part of the duplication can alternatively be resected (Figs 58.17A and B). When the duplicated colon connects to the urinary tract or vagina, the second surgical approach is generally used. With this approach, the duplication is divided and an endorectal mucosectomy of the distal duplication is performed. The muscular cuff is then closed and an end-to-side anastomosis connecting the remaining distal end of the duplication to the normal colon is performed. Since tubular duplications do not usually have ectopic gastric mucosa, resection of the duplicated segment is rarely necessary. Although malignancy has been reported in untreated cases of colonic duplication, these reports do not exist in cases treated with distal diversion.

SUMMARY

Duplications of the alimentary tract comprise a rare, but interesting constellation of anomalies. The clinical presentation and symptoms of patients are variable, often making an accurate diagnosis quite difficult and prolonging the course of illness. Both diagnosis and treatment require a methodical, individualized approach.

REFERENCES

1. Heiss K. Intestinal duplications. In: Oldham KT, Colombani PM, Foglia RP (Eds). Surgery of Infants and Children: Scientific Principles and Practice. Lippincott-Raven 1997:1265-74.
2. Orr MM, Edwards AJ. Neoplastic change in duplications of the alimentary tract. Br J Surg 1975;62:269-74.
3. Hickey FW, Corson JM. Squamous cell carcinoma arising in a duplication of the colon. Cancer 1981;47:602-09.
4. Fletcher DJ, Goodfellow PB, Bardsley D. Metastatic adenocarcinoma arising from a small bowel duplication cyst. Europ J Surg Oncol 2002;28:93-94.
5. Downing R, Thompson H, Alexander-Williams J. Adenocarcinoma arising in a duplication of the rectum. Br J Surg 1978;65:572-74.
6. Bentley JFR, Smith JR. Developmental posterior enteric remnants and spinal malformation. Arch Dis Child 1960;35:76-86.
7. Lewis FT, Thyng FW. Regular occurrence of intestinal diverticula in embryos of pig, rabbit, and man. Am J Anat 1908;7:505-19.
8. Bremer JL. Diverticula and duplications of the intestinal tract. Arch Pathol 1944;38:132-40.
9. Skandalakis JE, Gray SW (Eds). Embryology for Surgeons. 2nd ed. Baltimore, Md: Williams and Wilkins;1994.
10. Ware GW, Conrad HA. Thoracic duplication of the alimentary tract. Am J Surg 1953;86:264-72.
11. Arbona JL, Fazzi JG, Mayoral J. Congenital esophageal cysts: case report and review of literature. Am J Gastroenterol 1984;79:177-82.
12. Fallon M, Gordon ARG, Lendrum AC. Mediastinal cysts of foregut origin associated with vertebral abnormalities. Br J Surg 1954;41:520-33.
13. Fowler CL, Pokorny WJ, Wagner ML, Kessler MS. Review of bronchopulmonary foregut malformations. J Pediatr Surg 1988;23:793-97.
14. Nobuhara KK, Gorski YC, LaQuaglia MP, Shamberger RC. Bronchogenic cysts and esophageal duplications: common origins and treatment. J Pediatr Surg 1997;32:1408-13.
15. Gerle RD, Jaretzki A III, Ashley CA, et al. Congenital bronchopulmonary foregut malformation. New Engl J Med 1968;278:1413-19.
16. White JJ, Morgan WW. Improved operative technique for gastric duplication. Surgery 1970;67: 522-26.
17. Dickinson WE, Weinberg SM, Vellios F. Perforating ulcer in a duodenal duplication. Am J Surg 1971;122:418-20.
18. Brown MF. Duplications of the intestinal tract. In:Ziegler M, Azizkhan RG, Weber T (Eds). Operative Pediatric Surgery. New York, NY: McGraw Hill 2002:855-66.
19. Ogura Y, Kawarada Y, Mizumoto R. Duodenal duplication cyst communicating with an accessory pancreatic duct of Santorini. Hepato-Gastroenterol 1998;45:1613-18.
20. Wrenn EL. Tubular duplication of the small intestine. Surgery 1962; 52:494-98.
21. Jewett TC Jr, Walker AB, Cooney DR. A long-term follow-up on a duplication of the entire small intestine treated by gastroduplication. J Pediatr Surg 1983;18:185-88.
22. Ravitch MM. Hindgut duplication — doubling of colon and genital and urinary tracts. Ann Surg 1953;137: 588-601.
23. Beach PD, Brascho DJ, Hein WR, et al. Duplication of the primitive hindgut of the human being. Surgery 1961;49:779-93.
24. LaQuaglia MP, Feins N, Eraklis A, Hendren WH. Rectal duplications. J Pediatr Surg 1990;25:980-84.
25. Prasad AR, Amin MB, Randolph TL, et al. Retrorectal cystic hamartoma: report of 5 cases with malignancy arising in 2. Arch Pathol Lab Med 2000;124:725-29.
26. Michael D, Cohen CR, Northover JM. Adenocarcinoma within a rectal duplication cyst: case report and literature review. Ann Royal Coll Surg 1999;81:205-06.
27. Yousefzadeh DK, Bickers GH, Jackson JH Jr, Benton C. Tubular colonic duplication – review of 1876-81 literature. Pediatr Radiol 1983;13:65-71.

CHAPTER 59

Bezoars in Children

Shilpa Sharma, DK Gupta

Bezoars, today, known as an uncommon cause for gastrointestinal symptoms, have been mysteries since ancient times and are known to propound diagnostic and therapeutic challenges. The incidence has decreased dramatically in the recent times, and most of the residents now see it as a museum specimen. The diagnosis depends on a high index of suspicion. The most common type is Trichobezoar (hair) that is usually found in adolescent psychiatric females. Some patients have bezoars that fill their entire stomach, while others are able to loosen them with ingestion of cellulase enzyme especially in cases of phytobezoars (vegetable matter). Treatment of the causative factor is essential to prevent recurrence.

TERMINOLOGY

The word "bezoar" has been derived from the arabic word "bazahr", Persian word 'Padzahr' or Turkish word 'Panzehir', all meaning antidote or counter-poison.[1] Animal bezoars were widely used in medicine until the 18th century.[2] Bezoars are concretions of foreign materials that are created in the intestinal tract of various animals and humans.[3] Bezoars have built up a reputation as being talismans of luck, power, or health, to ward off the evil spirits for the last couple of thousand years. Bezoars have been said to cure animals and people of rabies by attaching the bezoar to the wound to suck out the poison. Bezoars were used as antidotes to some poisons and were considered so precious that a gold-framed bezoar was included in the inventory of Queen Elizabeth's crown jewels in 1962. The term trichobezoar was first described by Baudemant in 1779 while the term phytobezoar is attributed to Quain since 1854.

DEFINITION

Bezoars are masses of solidified concretions of organic or non-biological foreign material commonly found in the stomach or small bowel. A bezoar is a concretion (*tightly packed collection*) of a *partially digested or undigested* foreign substance in the stomach or intestine. It has a tendency to remain there indefinitely unless removed.

CLASSIFICATION[1]

1. *Trichobezoars:* An agglomeration of hair.[4,5] Trichobezoars take the shape of the stomach, its surface is slimy and it has a foul odour due to putrefaction of food. These are the most common types of bezoars encountered.
2. *Phytobezoars:* These consist of partially digested agglomeration of vegetable matter such as leaves or undigested foods. Phytobezoar is made of fibrous food stuff, most commonly due to unripened persimmons.[6] A persimmon bezoar is also known as diospyrobezoar. The phytobezoar is a compact mass of fibers, skins, seeds, leaves, roots, or stems of plants.
3. *Lactobezoars:* These are milk coagulums seen in small babies who are artificially fed. It is grayish white in color, shaped like the stomach and has slimy surface. The presence of casein as the predominant protein is necessary for the development of a lactobezoar.[7] It has even been reported in an eight year old girl.[8]
4. *Pharmacobezoars:* These are concretions of medication (sucralfate, aluminum hydroxide gel), shellac.

5. *Iniobezoars (coirbezoars):* Concretions due to coconut cover fibers or rope.[9]
6. *Pseudobezoars:* These include loose aggregation of pits, seeds, citrus pith, or even bubblegum may mimic true bezoars. Jungle banana seeds and sunflower seeds have also been implicated.[10,11]
7. *Rare forms:* These include cloth ingestion, Paper ingestion, plastic ingestion, Vinyl glove ingestion, Sponge bezoar and Polystyrene bezoar.[12-16] Children have been reported to swallow plastic toys.[17] Combination forms like trichophytobezoars may also be found.

ETIOLOGY

Neuropsychiatric Disorders

This is the most common cause in children with bezoar formation. These are usually adolescent females who in a rage of temper or unsound mind pluck their long hair and swallow it.[4,5] Huge trichobezoars have been reported in these patients. In a series of 24 children with trichotillomania attending psychiatry outpatient department, the majority were females (66.7%).[18] Most belonged to age group 6-10 years (54.2%) and nuclear family (68.5%). Nail-biting (25.0%) was the commonest associated neurotic trait, followed by enuresis (20.9%) and temper-tantrum (12.5%).[18] A past history of hysterical fits and neurotic depression was found in 3 cases (12.5%) and 2 cases (8.3%) respectively. Family history of neurosis was seen in mothers and fathers of 20.9% and 12.5% cases respectively. Trichobezoars and trichophytobezoars were found in 6 cases (25.0%) and 3 cases (12.5%) respectively. Upto 22.2% cases of trichobezoar were asymptomatic and detected only on screening psychiatric patients.[18]

The other types of bezoars reported in mentally retarded patients include, "polystyrenomania" from ingestion of styrofoam cups and vinyl glove bezoar.[15,16] A girl with aicardi syndrome has been reported to lose 10 pounds weight due to the development of a lactobezoar.[8]

Associated Partial Congenital Obstructions

Associated partial congenital obstructions like duodenal web, operated case of ileal atresia, serious digestive antecedents, corrosive esophagogastritis and follow up case of esophageal atresia.[2]

Intraluminal Obstruction

Phytobezoars as a cause of small bowel obstruction has been associated with a carcinoid tumor of the ileocecal area.[19]

Postpartial Gastrectomy

Phytobezoars may occur in patients after partial gastrectomy, especially when accompanied by vagotomy. Hypochlorhydria, diminished antral motility, and incomplete mastication are the main predisposing factors. Unpeeled persimmon, orange or grapefruit pulp are the usual offenders, thus postgastrectomy patient must be warned of ingesting citrus fruits as a prophylactic measure.[20]

Postgastroplasty

The vertical banded gastroplasty used in the treatment of morbid obesity has been associated with gastric bezoars. This may be a predisposing factor in obese older children.

Diabetic Gastroparesis

Causes a loss of normal pyloric function and decreased gastric acidity, thus predisposing to formation of phytobezoars.[21]

Uremia

Uremic patients frequently present predisposing conditions such as autonomic neuropathy, diabetes mellitus and delayed gastric emptying.[22]. Gastric bezoars cause anorexia. Thus the possibility of a gastric bezoar should be considered during evaluation of anorexic uremic patients.

Trichotillomania and Trichophagia

Some people may have a bad habit of plucking their hair (trichotillomania) and chewing it constantly. It also has been reported in adolescent girls with a normal frame of mind.[23] Such patients are cured after surgical removal of the bezoars and not prone to recurrence.

PATHOGENESIS

Trichobezoars are concretions of hair casts in the stomach. The hair strands get retained in the folds of the gastric mucosa because the friction surface is insufficient for peristalsis propulsion. In about 5% of patients there are separate hair masses in the stomach.[5,24]

The phytobezoar is a compact mass of plant products that collects in the stomach or small intestine. Other food particles, such as fats, crystals, granules, fibers, and residues of salts, are incorporated into the mass and contribute to the growth of the bezoar.[25]

Persimmon is a fruit grown mainly in Japan and Asia that contains large amount of 'shibuol' a phlobatanin, that is coagulated by gastric acid into a compound that efficiently bonds vegetable fibers, seeds, and pieces of skin together.[1] Ingestion of unripe persimmons, especially on an empty stomach with or no food matter to interfere with the contact and aggregation of the seeds and fragments of skin, predisposes to development of this type of bezoar. Patients that have undergone surgical procedures for peptic ulcer disease or any procedure on the stomach or who for other reasons, such as diabetic gastroparesis, have a loss of normal pyloric function and decreased gastric acidity are prone to form phytobezoars Persimmon peels or pits, orange or grapefruit pulp are the usual offenders.

Non-persimmon phytobezoars have tannin monomers, which are polymerized in the stomach to form the necessary glue for bonding the vegetables. Another factor may be mechanical and dependent on the insoluble and indigestible fibre content. Although firm and compact when freshly removed phytobezoars tend to be friable and crumble early after drying. On section they are found to be composed of an amorphous gummy material interspersed with cellulose fibers and occasionally seeds and skin.

SITES

The most common site for bezoar formation is the stomach followed by the small intestine. Rarely, esophageal bezoars have also been reported.[26]

The trichobezoars may extend from the stomach to the small intestine or even the colon in continuity, this entity is known as Rapunzel syndrome.[27] The name is driven from the name of a princess in a fairy tale who had very long hair, thus the trichobezoar with a tail extending into the intestinal lumen simulate very long hair. Recently, synchronous bezoars have also been reported in the stomach and the small intestine, one in stomach and the other either in jejunum or ileum.[28,29]

CLINICAL PRESENTATION

Trichobezoar are classically seen in an adolescent female with mental retardation who presents with alopecia and an upper abdominal mass which on moving can cause intermittent gastric outlet obstruction.[4,5] In a comprehensive review of 303 cases upto 1938, about 80% of the cases were less than 30 years and more than 90% were females.[30]

The history of ingestion of hair or any material like plants, seeds or even plastic is important.

Most bezoars are generally asymptomatic but may present with bloating, vague upper gastrointestinal discomfort, malabsorption, and postprandial fullness. There may be appreciable loss of appetite, weight-loss, vomiting, loose stools, pancreatitis, pain abdomen, jaundice, anemia and hypoalbuminemia.[5,31]

When the size increases, symptoms due to mass effect like abdominal pain, compression or intestinal obstruction are produced. It often occurs in adolescent girls with psychiatric disorders.[32] The patient may present with only a short history of mild abdominal pain despite having a trichobezoar weighting 700 g and measuring 24 × 16 × 10 cm.[33] Complicated cases may present with Gastroenteritis, GI bleeding, intestinal obstruction, peritonitis or perforation chronic irritation of the gastric antral mucosa may also lead to formation of hyperplastic polyps.[17,27]

Early diagnosis and treatment is important to avoid later fatal complications such as gastric perforation and intestinal necrosis.[34,35]

A firm, nontender, freely mobile epigastric mass may be seen and palpated in uncomplicated cases. One may appreciate the crepitus on palpation. A rare case of sunflower-seed bezoar impacted at the anal verge has also been reported.[11] It is not unusual for children to have rectal impactions with seeds of some fruits in some parts of the world. A per rectal palpation is essential to rule out this cause in children presenting with constipation.

INVESTIGATIONS

A plain abdominal skiagram may pick up a bezoar as a space occupying lesion. In cases presenting with small bowel obstruction, the erect abdominal film may show multiple air-fluid levels. A barium swallow may delineate a filling defect in the stomach of the same shape, with partial penetration of the barium into the mass causing an irregular outline. Renal excretion of oral gastrografin has been seen on an abdominal film in a patient with incomplete intestinal obstruction due to multiple bezoars.[36] Ultrasonography may depict an intraluminal mass presenting as an arc-like surface echo casting clear posterior acoustic shadow within the lumen of the dilated small bowel. Compression of the mass with a transducer may induce fluid shift around the mass.[37] Ultrasound might thus suggest the diagnosis, though not confirm it.[5]

CT scan of a trichobezoar occupying the entire lumen of the stomach may appear as a concentric inhomogeneous mass with entrapped air, surrounded by contrast material.[38] A mottled appearance with variable proximal dilatation of the small bowel may be seen in cases with the bezoar confined to the small intestine.[38] Beside conventional radiology and sonography, the diagnostic procedure of choice is endoscopy.[25] On endoscopy, bezoars have an unmistakable irregular surface and may range in color from yellow-green to gray-black. An endoscopic biopsy that yields hair or plant material is diagnostic.

NON-OPERATIVE TREATMENT

With-holding Feeding

Treatment of lactobezoars has been done by with-holding feeding for 24 hours. There was no recurrence of symptoms following resumption of feeding.[39]

Dissolution with Enzymatic Digestion

Dissolution of the undigested bolus by ingestion of cellulase and proteolytic enzymes such as papain have been proved effective in the management of phytobezoars. 1.2 L of dissolved cellulase (0.5 g/dL water) can be given orally over 24 hours for 2 days. Parenteral Metoclopramide for several days may increase peristalsis by accelerating gastric emptying.

Complete dissolution of the gastric phytobezoar with cellulase was achieved in all 7 patients in a series with no side effects or recurrences during follow-up.[40]

In a series of 36 patients with phytobezoars, Papain was successful in treating 87% (13 of 15) and cellulase in 100% (19 of 19) of the patients. Adverse effects reported in the papain group were gastric ulcer, esophageal perforation, and hypernatremia; the cellulase group did not report any adverse effects.[41] Enzymatic dissolution is ineffective for large bezoars.[4]

Suction and Lavage

A food bolus requires no treatment. A liquid diet, gastric suction and lavage may be beneficial. Gastric lavage with 1% sodium bicarbonate has also been reported

Solution following partial gastroscopic bezoar crumbling.[42]

The dissolution of large gastric phytobezoars with cola nasogastric lavage has been reported to be effective following failed attempt at endoscopic fragmentation and removal.[21,43] Patients were treated with 3 liters of Cocacola nasogastric lavage over 12 hour period. Nasogastric lavage was very well tolerated and complete phytobezoar dissolution was achieved all cases without any procedure-related complications. With this safe, rapid and effective method, patients may be treated in the medical ward, avoiding therapeutic endoscopy or surgery.[21] Serial water-soluble contrast enemas have been used in the treatment of sodium poly styrene sulfonate bezoars.[44]

Endoscopic Retrieval

After the first gastroscopic removal of a bezoar by McKechne in 1972, different endoscopic methods have been reported including a water jet, forceps, snare, and basket.[45]

Saeed banding device has been used to remove food impaction in patients with eosinophilic esophagitis.[46]

Mechanical endoscopic fragmentation of the bezoar followed by removal of residual bezoar in one or more sittings has been done. In a series using a modified needle-knife (bezotome) and a modified mechanical lithotriptor (bezotriptor), 18 bezoars upto 10 × 8 × 8 cm in size, were successfully fragmented and complete clearance was achieved with no complications.[37,47] The disadvantages of gastroscopic removal include failure in huge and solid bezoars and risks of perforation and intestinal obstruction.[4]

Gastroscopy with Laparoscopically Assisted Fragmentation

A two channel method using gastroscopy with laparoscopically assisted fragmentation for retrieval of large gastric bezoar has been reported.[48]

ESWL Fragmentation

Fragmentation with extracorporeal shock wave lithotripsy has also been described.[49]

OPERATIVE REMOVAL

Gastrotomy

Gastrostomy is the treatment of choice for trichobezoars. Endoscopic removal of trichobezoar usually fails and open surgery is required.[4,5] The rocklike concretions usually require only surgical removal. Gastrostomy is done and all the contents are evacuated. The bezoar has the shape of the stomach, is foul smelling and has slimy surface. Trichobezoars have an unmistakable irregular surface and may range in color from yellow-green to gray-black and is coated with food particles. Phytobezoar is greenish brown in colour and lactobezoar is grayish white.

Vinyl glove bezoars require surgical removal as endoscopic removal is impossible because the gloves become hardened and matted.[15] Surgical removal has also been required for polystyrene bezoar.[16] Pathological and biochemical examination reveals the composition of the mass.

Rapunzel Syndrome

The diagnosis of Rapunzel syndrome is usually made during laparotomy when during extraction of the bezoar, the tail keeps coming from the pyrolic end and may even be as long as 100 meters long. Surgical extraction is the therapy of choice in Rapunzel syndrome. It has been seen that endoscopic removal fails due to the large extension in these cases.

Milking of Bezoars into Caecum

Ileum is the most commonly reported site of obstruction in persimmon phytobezoars. At laparotomy, milking of the bezoars into caecum is successful in most of the cases.[6]

This treatment has also been recommended for total jungle banana obstruction.[10] As recurrence and presentation at multiple sites are possible, all of the gastrointestinal tract should be thoroughly examined intraoperatively.[10]

Enterotomy and Direct Extraction

If milking of the contents beyond the ileocaecal junction in small bowel obstruction due to phytobezoars is not possible, enterotomy and direct extraction of the contents is done.[6] Psychotherapy, behavior modification, and antipsychotic treatment are essential to prevent recurrence. Clomipramine may be of benefit in such cases.

COMPLICATIONS

Bezoars when present for a long time induce changes in the stomach and the intestine. In children, the most devastating effect is due to the space they occupy in the stomach. This causes malnutrition, repeated vomiting and bloating sensation. During childhood good nutrition is mandatory for health. Other common complications include ulceration, bleeding, obstruction, perforation, and so also the intussusception may also occur with small bezoars.[4,20,50] Mortality rate may be as high as 30% in untreated cases, mainly due to gastrointestinal bleeding, obstruction or perforation.[4] Multiple ulcers secondary to extensive pressure in the antrum were observed in a case with recurrent bezoar formation.[32] A case intestinal obstruction associated with the superior mesenteric artery blocking the duodenum has also been reported.[51]

Fatal massive gastrointestinal bleeding from a large gastric ulcer caused by a vinyl glove bezoar while awaiting surgical consultation has been reported.[15] The most common cause for mortality is gastric perforation. In cases with a history of trichophagia and signs of peritonitis, urgent surgical exploration is mandatory.

Complications can also occur during attempted removal. Copious pooling of fluid and solid food particulate was noted in the posterior oropharynx, interfering with immediate intubation and then bronchial aspiration have been repoted in a boy during Endoscopic attempted removal of an esophageal bezoar.[26]

FOLLOW-UP

Treatment should also focus on prevention of recurrence, since elimination of the mass will not alter the conditions contributing to their formation.[5]

Psychiatric follow-up is needed to prevent this complication in children with serious digestive antecedents and to reduce the risk of recurrences.[4] A subsequent psychiatric consultation in a girl operated twice for trichobezoar at an interval of seven years revealed depressive personality disorder.[32]

High-fiber diets are being recommended by government agencies, cancer institutes, and manufacturers of high-fiber foods. Patients who have undergone surgical procedures for peptic ulcer disease or stomach cancer or have a loss of normal pyloric function and decreased gastric acidity are prone to form phytobezoars. Such patients should avoid identified foods that lead to phytobezoar formation—oranges, persimmons, coconuts, berries, green beans, figs, apples, sauerkraut, brussels sprouts, and potato peel.[25] The feeding habits of children should be supervised with adults and any abnormal feeding habit of swallowing non edible substances should be kept on a check.

REFERENCES

1. Gupta D K, Sharma Shilpa. Bezoars in Textbook of Adolescent Medicine. Ed Swati Bhave. Jaypee Brothers, Delhi 2006 Chapter 20;4: 659-62.
2. Williams RS. The fascinating history of bezoars. Med J Aust 1986;145:613-14.
3. Meltzer E, Steinlauf S. Bezoars: from ancient talismans to modern disease. Harefuah 2002;141:142-44,223.
4. Dumonceaux A, Michaud L, Bonnevalle M, Debeugny P, Gottrand F, Turck D Arch. Trichobezoars in children and adolescents. Pediatr 1998;5:996-99.
5. Barzilai M, Peled N, Soudack M, Siplovich L. Trichobezoars Harefuah 1998;135:97-101,167.
6. Zafar A, Ahmad S, Ghafoor A, Turabi MR. Small bowel obstruction in children due to persimmon phytobezoars. J Coll Physicians Surg Pak 2003;13:443-45.
7. Schreiner RL, Brady MS, Ernst JA, Lemons JA Lack of lactobezoars in infants given predominantly whey protein formulas. Am J Dis Child 1982;136:437-39.
8. Smith BJ, Bachrach SJ. An unexpected finding in an eight-year-old child with cerebral palsy and weight loss. J Natl Med Assoc 2006 Feb;98(2):280-83.
9. Somani AK, Malpani NK, Vardhan V. Multiple iniobezoars causing acute intestinal obstruction. Indian J Gastroenterol 1998;17:30-31.
10. Schoeffl V, Varatorn R, Blinnikov O, Vidamaly V. Intestinal obstruction due to phytobezoars of banana seeds: a case report. Asian J Surg 2004;27:348-51.
11. Sawnani H, McFarlane-Ferreira Y. Proctological crunch: sunflower-seed bezoar. J La State Med Soc 2003;155:163-64.
12. Uretsky BF. Letter: Paper bezoar causing intestinal obstruction. Arch Surg 1974;109:123.
13. Battin M, Kennedy J, Singh S. A case of plastikophagia. Postgrad Med J 1997;73(858):243-44.
14. McAlinden MG, Potts SR. Sponge bezoar: a rare cause of abdominal pain. Ulster Med J 1999;68:36-37.
15. Kamal I, Thompson J, Paquette DM. The hazards of vinyl glove ingestion in the mentally retarded patient with pica: new implications for surgical management. Can J Surg 1999;42:201-204.
16. Finley CR Jr, Hellmuth EW, Schubert TT. Polystyrene bezoar in a patient with polystyrenomania. Am J Gastroenterol 1988 ;83:74-76.
17. Misra SP, Dwivedi M, Misra V. Endoscopic management of a new entity-plastobezoar: a case report and review of literature. World J Gastroenterol 2006;12(41):6730-33.
18. Bhatia MS, Singhal PK, Rastogi V, et al. Clinical profile of trichotillomania. J Indian Med Assoc 1991;89:137-39.
19. Pitiakoudis M, Koukourakis M, Giatromanolaki A, Tsaroucha AK, Polychronidis A, Simopoulos C. Phytobezoars as a cause of small bowel obstruction associated with a carcinoid tumor of the ileocecal area. Acta Chir Iugosl 2003;50:131-33.
20. Cavusoglu Z, Olcay E, Dagoglu T, Akgun E, Vural S, Ates R. Occlusion of the gastric outlet caused by a trichobezoar Kinderarztl Prax 1990;58:531-34.
21. Ladas SD, Triantafyllou K, Tzathas C, Tassios P, Rokkas T, Raptis SA. Gastric phytobezoars may be treated by nasogastric Cocacola lavage. Eur J Gastroenterol Hepatol 2002 ;14:801-803.
22. Catalano C, Leone L, Fabbian F, Conz PA. Stomach phytobezoars in two uremic anorexic patients. Nephron 2002 ;90:352-54.
23. Candelotti P, Tulli M, Pasquini R, Carlucci A, Tomassini N, Tosti M. Obstructive syndrome caused by trichobezoars: historical disease or disease still current? Description of a case in adolescence. Minerva Pediatr 2000;52:739-42.
24. Santiago Sanchez CA, Garau Diaz P, Lugo Vicente HL. Trichobezoar in a 11-year old girl: a case report. Bol Asoc Med P R 1996;88:8-11.
25. Emerson AP. Foods high in fiber and phytobezoar formation. J Am Diet Assoc 1987;87:1675-77.
26. Macksey L. Aspirated bezoar in a pediatric patient: A case report. AANA J 2006 ;74:295-98.
27. Kaspar A, Deeg KH, Schmidt K, Meister R.Rapunzel syndrome, an rare form of intestinal trichobezoars. Klin Padiatr 1999;211:420-22.
28. Hoover K, Piotrowski J, St Pierre K, Katz A, Goldstein AM. Simultaneous gastric and small intestinal trichobezoars—a hairy problem. J Pediatr Surg 2006;41(8): 1495-97.

29. Palanivelu C, Rangarajan M, Senthilkumar R, Madankumar MV Trichobezoars in the stomach and ileum and their laparoscopy-assisted removal: a bizarre case. Singapore Med J 2007;48(2):e37-39.
30. Debakey M, Ochsner A. Bezoars and Concretions- A Comprehensive Review of the Literature with an Analysis of 303 Collected Cases and a Presentation of 8 additional cases. Surgery 1938; 4:934-63; 1939; 5:132-160.
31. Stein-Wexler R, Wootton-Gorges SL, Shakibai S, et al. Trichobezoar: an unusual cause for pancreatitis in a patient with sickle cell anemia. Clin Adv Hematol Oncol. 2006;4(6):471-73.
32. Eryilmaz R, Sahin M, Alimoglu O, Yildiz MK. A case of Rapunzel syndrome Ulus Travma Derg 2004;10:260-63.
33. Rouskova B, Kalousova J, Vyhnanek M, Szitanyi P.Trichobezoar-Rapunzel syndrome—case report Rozhl Chir 2004;83:460-62.
34. Gockel I, Gaedertz C, Hain HJ, Winckelmann U, Albani M, Lorenz The Rapunzel syndrome: rare manifestation of a trichobezoar of the uppergastrointestinal tract. D Chirurg 2003;74:753-56.
35. Pul N, Pul M. The Rapunzel syndrome (trichobezoar) causing gastric perforation in a child: A case report. Eur J Pediatr 1996;155:18-19.
36. Zissin R, Oscadchy A, Shapiro-Feinberg M. Renal excretion of oral gastrografin seen on an abdominal film in a patient with incomplete intestinal obstruction due to multiple bezoars. Isr Med Assoc J 1999;1:200-201.
37. Ko YT, Lim JH, Lee DH, Yoon Y. Small intestinal phytobezoars: sonographic detection. Abdom Imaging 1993;18:271-73.
38. Gayer G, Jonas T, Apter S, Zissin R, Katz M, Katz R, Amitai M, Hertz M.Clin Bezoars in the stomach and small bowel - CT appearance. Radiol 1999;54:228-32.
39. Erenberg A, Shaw RD, Yousefzadeh D. Lactobezoar in the low-birth-weight infant. Pediatrics 1979;63:642-46.
40. Bonilla F, Mirete J, Cuesta A, Sillero C, Gonzalez M. Treatment of gastric phytobezoars with cellulase. Rev Esp Enferm Dig. 1999 ;91:809-14. Comment in: Rev Esp Enferm Dig 1999;91:806-808.
41. Walker-Renard P. Update on the medicinal management of phytobezoars. Am J Gastroenterol 1993;88:1663-66.
42. Sikorski T. A case of phyto-mucous bezoar of the stomach. Pol Tyg Lek 1992;47(20-27):92-94.
43. Kato H, Nakamura M, Orito E, Ueda R, Mizokami M. The first report of successful nasogastric Cocacola lavage treatment for bitter persimmon phytobezoars in Japan. Am J Gastroenterol 2003;98:1662-63.
44. Koneru P, Kaufman RA, Talati AJ, Jenkins MB, Korones SB. Successful treatment of Sodium PolyStyrene Sulfonate bezoars with serial water-soluble contrast enemas. J Perinatol 2003;23:431-33.
45. McKechnie JC. Gastroscopic Removal of a Phytobezoar. Gatroenterol 1972;62:1047-50.
46. Smith CR, Miranda A, Rudolph CD, Sood MR. Removal of impacted food in children with eosinophilic esophagitis using Saeed banding device. J Pediatr Gastroenterol Nutr 2007;44(4):521-23.
47. Wang YG, Seitz U, Li ZL, Soehendra N, Qiao XA. Endoscopic management of huge bezoars. Endoscopy 1998;30:371-74.
48. Kanetaka K, Azuma T, Ito S, Matsuo S, Yamaguchi S, Shirono K, Kanematsu T. Two-channel method for retrieval of gastric trichobezoar: report of a case. J Pediatr Surg 2003;38:e7.
49. Benes T, Chmel J, Jodl J, et al. Treatment of a Gastric Bezoar by Extracorporeal Shock Wave Lithotripsy. Endoscopy 1991;23:346-48.
50. Hani MA, Guesmi F, Bouasker I, Zoghlami A, Najah N. Stomach perforation: an unusual complication of gastric bezoars. Tunis Med 2003;81:351-53.
51. Wadlington WB, Rose M, Holcomb GW Jr. Complications of trichobezoars: a 30-year experience. South Med J 1992; 85:1020-22.

Ascariasis Lumbricoides

Essam El-Sawhi

Helminthic infestation is widely prevalent in developing countries. Patients are usually malnourished, present with features of acute intestinal obstruction either due to massive infestation of the intestine by round worms or sometimes following inadequate anthelminthic therapy. These worms form a ball causing mechanical obstruction. Occasionally, this round worm mass could be palpated per abdomen. If it persists for a long period they can cause intestinal ischemia, perforation and peritonitis. Uncomplicated round worm obstruction can be treated conservatively, but if it becomes persistent or develops complication, a laparotomy is indicated.

ETIOLOGY

The infective stage of ascariasis lumbricoides is the mature larvae containing egg.[1,2] It is broadly oval, has a thick shell with an outer mamillated covering, and measures approximately 40 × 60 mm eggs are passed in the faeces of infected individuals and mature in 5-10 days under favorable environmental conditions to become infective.

Each female has a life span of 1-2 year and is capable of producing 200,000 eggs/24 hour.

PATHOGENESIS

After a human host ingests the eggs, larvae are released from the eggs and penetrate the intestinal wall before migrating to the lungs via the venous circulation. They then break through the pulmonary tissues into the alveolar spaces, ascend the bronchial tree and trachea, and are reswallowed. On their arrival in the small intestine, the larvae develop into mature adult worms. Males measure 15-25 cm × 3 mm, and females measure 25-35 cm × 4 mm.[2] The pathogenesis of pulmonary ascariasis is not known, although a hypersensitivity phenomenon may be involved. Adult worms may cause gastrointestinal disease by obstructing the gut or biliary tree, or pancreatic duct or the appendix or goes to the peritoneum.

CLINICAL MANIFESTATIONS

No specific gastrointestinal symptoms occur in some patients, but the frequency is unknown. During the larval migratory phase, an acute transient pneumonitis (Loffler's syndrome) associated with fever and marked eosinophilia may occur. Acute intestinal obstruction may develop in patients with heavy infections. Children are more prone to this complication because they have smaller diameters of the intestinal lumen and often have large numbers of worms. Worm migration can cause peritonitis, secondary to intestinal wall penetration, and common bile duct obstruction resulting in acute obstructive jaundice.[2] The adult worms can be stimulated to migrate by stressful conditions (e.g. fever, illness, or anesthesia) and by some antihelminthic drugs. Ascaris lumbricoides has been found in the appendiceal lumen in acute appendicitis, but a causal relationship is uncertain.

Intestinal Ascariasis

Ascaris induced intestinal obstruction is a frequent complication in children with heavy worm loads in endemic areas.[3] It constitutes 5 to 35% of all cases of bowel obstruction in such regions. It is caused by an aggregated mass of worms blocking the bowel lumen especially in the terminal ileum. The obstruction is usually partial.

However, when prolonged, it can become complete. Prolonged obstruction may be complicated by intussusception, volvulus, hemorrhagic infarction of the bowel, and perforation.[1]

The symptoms start with colicky abdominal pain, vomiting, and constipation. Vomiting of worms is a frequent occurrence and often gives a clue to the cause. Physical findings include abdominal distention, increased bowel sounds, and a characteristic lump, usually felt in the right lower quadrant.

Complicated obstruction is suspected when the child is febrile, is toxic, and has physical signs of peritonitis. Plain abdominal films reveal air-fluid levels and multiple linear images of ascaris in dilated bowel loops. Filling defects may be identified in contrast studies (Figs 60.1A and B). Ultrasonography of the abdomen can demonstrate dilated bowel with thickened wall and worm mass causing bowel obstruction. The worms are identified as curved echogenic structures, depicting active mobility on real -time scanner.[3]

The echogenic structures may reveal central anchoic tube, representing digestive canal of the worm. Treatment is primarily conservative and includes adequate fluid and electrolyte replacement, nasogastric suction, specific antihelminitics therapy, and antibiotics. Grastrografin (Squibb; diatrizoate meglumine 66% and diatrizoatre sodium 10%) 15 to 30 ml introduced into the stomach through a nasogastric tube has been advocated for partial bowel obstruction .

Gastrografin is a hyperosmolar substance and causes excess fluid in the vicinity of and around the worm mass causing their separation . Laparotomy is indicated in the following situations: persistence of mass in the same site for more than 24 hours; persistent abdominal pain and tender mass; toxemia and rising pulse rate with disappearance of the mass.

The most common surgical procedure is to express and advance the parasite bundle manually toward the colon. If this maneuver is unsuccessful, worms can be delivered through enterotomy. Intestinal resection is warranted if the bowel shows evidence of gangrene or infarction (Figs 60.2A to D).

Prognosis is good if the patients present early or have partial bowel obstruction. However, often patients present late in their illness, with complicated obstruction and underlying malnutrition.

They tolerate surgical procedures poorly. Mortality rate is high in patients needing bowel resection for complicated obstruction

Appendicular Ascariasis

In endemic areas with high parasite load, the moving adult worm may enter the appendicular lumen and reach its tip. As a result, acute appendicular colic and even gangrenous appendicitis may occur and the worms may reach the peritoneal cavity adjacent to the appendix The diagnosis is usually made at laparotomy and management has been surgical.[4] If the disease presents early, colonoscopic removal of the worms has also been described.

Pancreatic Biliary Involvement

Ascaris is an important cause of pancreatic biliary disease in countries with a high rate of infection. The magnitude of the problem can be judged by the fact that in endemic areas, ascariasis is equal to gallstones as a cause of biliary tract disease (37% Vs 35%). In another study, Ascaris was the cause of pancereatitis in 59 of 256 patients (23%) compared with 112 subjects (44%) with gallstone – induced pancreatitis.

Although diagnosed predominantly in tropical countries, roundworms are seen worldwide, including the United States. An increase awareness of pancreatic biliary Ascaris is important in view of the recent mass migration of people from endemic countries of the Far East and frequent travel to such countries. Despite the small lumen of the ampulla, roundworm invasion is not uncommon, perhaps because the duodenum and upper jejunum are the natural habitat of the parasite . From the ampulla, the worms migrate into the bile duct, gallbladder, and the intrahepatic biliary tree, resulting in biliary colic, pyogenic cholangitis, and hepatic abscess. Another mechanism of biliary obstruction is when fragments

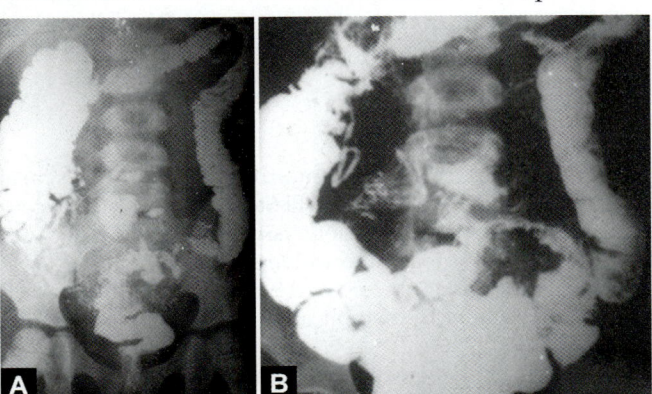

Figs 60.1A and B: Contrast studies demonstrating filling defects

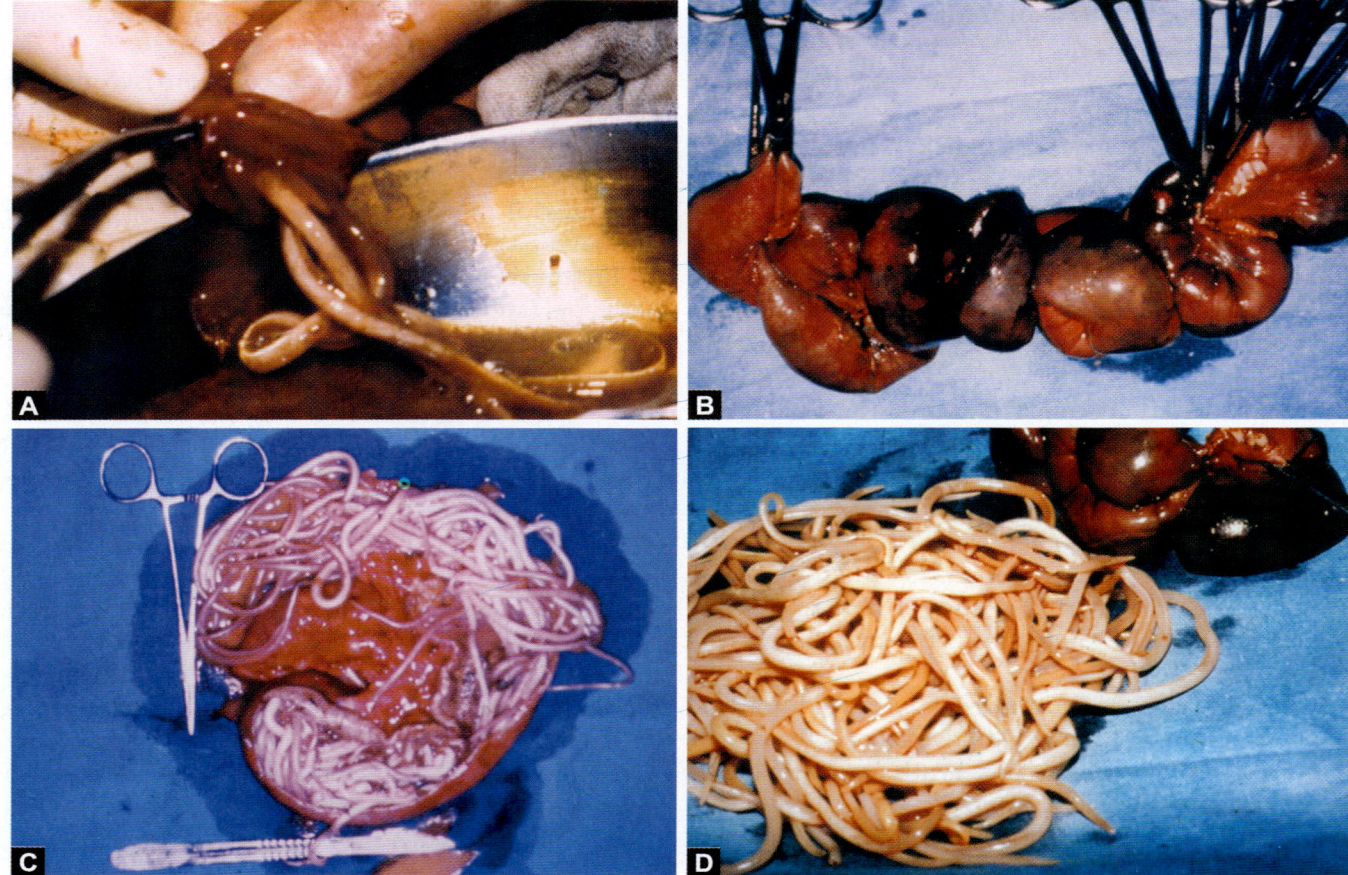

Figs 60.2A to D: Operative photographs of laparotomy for Ascariasis. **A.** Ascaris causing obstruction of the small intestine. **B.** Resected gangrenous Intestine **C.** Cut open section of the intestine. **D.** Evacuated ascaris

of the adult worms serve as a nidus for gallstone formation. Ascaris-related biliary stones are usually of the pigment type, and are aided in their formation by factors such as bile stasis and ascending bacterial infection.

It is estimated that in endemic countries, ascaries ova or an immature worm is the cause of stone formation in 10 to 66% of patients. As in the biliary tree, presence of roundworms in the pancreatic ducts may cause acute pancreatitis or the calcified remnants of the worm may result in recurrent episodes of pancreatitis.

Peritoneal Ascariasis

Ascaris may enter the peritoneal cavity through a gangrenous bowel filled to the bursting point with ascarides or through a perforation caused by typhoid, amebic, or tubercular ulcer. In a small percentage, the worms may be seen wandering in the peritoneum with intact bowel. In either of these conditions, patients present with fatal peritonitis.

If patients survive, wandering peritoneal ascaris disintegrate, and a granulomatous reaction is elicited around the disintegrated worm and ascaris eggs. A chronic granulomatous peritonitis with adhesions simulating tubercular peritonitis occurs.[3]

REFERENCES

1. El-Sahwi E. Surgical manifestations of Ascaris Lumbricoides Infestation, in El-Sahwi Textbook of Surgery Chapter 6, Alexandria University Press 1996;524.
2. Kazura R. Ascaris Lumbricoides in Nelson's Textbook of Paediatrics Chapter 245, W B Saunders 1996;292.
3. Ochoa B. Surgical complications of Ascariasis. World J Surg 1991; 222.
4. Sandouk F. Pancreatic-Biliary Ascariasis: Experience of 300 cases. Am J Gastroenterol 1997;92:2264-68.

CHAPTER 61

Hirschsprung's Disease

Edward Kiely

Hirschsprung's disease has probably existed from antiquity. The earliest recognisable description was by Frederick Ruysch in 1691. He described a five year old child who had died and who had gross dilatation of the sigmoid colon at postmortem.[1]

Other case reports of patients who had severe constipation and gross distension from the neonatal period were reported in the literature prior to Hirschsprung's landmark description.[2,3] In 1886, at a pediatric conference in Berlin, Hirschsprung describes the course of two male infants who had died aged 7 and 11 months of age respectively. Autopsies had shown marked dilatation and hypertrophy of the colon with no apparent obstruction distally.[3]

Further reports followed and by 1908 Finney had collected 206 cases from the literature. At that stage the disease was known as Hirschsprung's disease.[2]

Various theories regarding the aetiology were proposed but none found lasting acceptance. Most attention was paid to the megacolon which attained a size and thickness rarely seen by present day surgeons. A colonic diameter of greater than 15 cm with a wall thickness of 3 cm has been described.[2] In the absence of a visible obstruction and given the normal appearance of the distal bowel, the physicians of the day were unable to explain the condition.

A disorder of neuromuscular function was considered a likely cause of the condition. In 1908, Finney was aware of suggestions that the intramural plexuses were absent in Hirschsprung's disease.[2] He was unable to find any literature on the subject. When such evidence did arrive in the form of two papers from Dalla Valle the surgical world seemed unaware.[4,5] Dalla Valle described the autopsy features of two brothers who had died of Hirschsprung's disease. He documented the absence of ganglion cells in the distal normal calibre colon.

These findings were confirmed in a further two cases by Cameron in 1928.[6] However, the cause of Hirschsprung's disease remained controversial until 1948 when Whitehouse and Kernohan from the Mayo Clinic described aganglionosis in 11 patients with Hirschsprung's disease.[7] In the same year Zuelzer and Wilson reported similar findings in a further 11 patients.[8] It is notable that, of these 22 patients, only three were alive at the time of writing.

In Zuelzer and Wilson's paper there are a few other notable features.[8] Five of their patients belonged to one family. In two children with colostomies, studies on the distal bowel showed an absence of peristalsis. Finally, one of their children became unwell, collapsed and died within an hour in a manner which might in retrospect be attributed to the enterocolitis of Hirschsprung's disease.

Finally, in 1949, Bodian et al confirmed that the aganglionic segment extended to and included the rectum.[9]

In the absence of a defined aetiology treatment was unsatisfactory. Nonoperative treatment was shown to be unsatisfactory. In Finney's review he noted that two thirds of those treated with medication subsequently died.[2] The comparable surgical mortality was 48%. Colostomy was often followed by return of normal health but symptoms returned with stoma closure.[8] Excision of dilated bowel with anastomosis was followed by a return of symptoms.

Somewhat better results were achieved by colectomy and ileorectal anastomosis but there are no follow up details.[10] Similarly, sympathectomy was employed to produce colonic relaxation and some success was reported.[11,12] No follow up is provided and the lack of subsequent reports suggests that failure was the rule.

All changed in 1948 when Swenson and Bill from the Children's Hospital in Boston produced the first report of a successful treatment for Hirschsprung's disease.[13] In this report the authors undertook rectosigmoidectomy to remove the 'spastic' portion of the bowel in three patients and had good results. The second report[14] noted that 23 patients had now undergone surgery. The extent of resection was determined by the appearance of the bowel on a barium enema. At this time the authors seemed unaware of the histological features of Hirschsprung's disease.

The following year a further report from Dr Swenson noted the absence of peristalsis in the affected bowel and suggested that aganglionosis was responsible for the clinical features of Hirschsprung's disease.[15]

By 1955 the importance of rectal biopsy as an aid to diagnosis was understood.[16] This last refinement ushers in the modern era of management of this disorder. All variations in biopsy technique, laboratory diagnosis and surgical management are based on the original descriptions of aganglionosis and rectosigmoidectomy.

ETIOLOGY AND PATHOGENESIS

The etiology of Hirschsprung's disease is unknown. It is clear that enteric ganglion cells migrate from the neural crest, along the course of the vagus nerves, to the intestine.[17] In the human fetus the rectum is innervated by the twelfth week of gestation.[18] The passive migration and neuronal differentiation appears to depend on the intercellular matrix.[19]

The conventional theory to explain the presence of an aganglionic segment in Hirschsprung's disease is that migration was incomplete. Failure of ganglion cell precursors to differentiate and mature would result in similar findings. The distal aganglionic bowel remains tonically contracted and does not exhibit normal peristalsis. The reason for the increased muscle tone is not clear. Study of the aganglionic bowel shows abnormalities of neuropeptides and reduced levels of nitric oxide synthase in the enteric nervous system.[20,21] A number of the ganglion cells are part of an inhibitory system of neurones that facilitate intestinal relaxation.[22] Their absence probably accounts for the tonic contraction that results.

MOLECULAR GENETICS

At present two genes have been implicated in strongly increasing the susceptibility to Hirschsprung's disease, and doubtless others will come to light in the near future. Mutations of the RET proto-oncogene have been intensively studied.[23,24] This gene has been located to the long arm of chromosome -10q11.2.[25,26] The RET gene encodes a tyrosine kinase transmembrane receptor whose ligand is a neurotrophic factor.[27] The manner in which the gene abnormality contributes to aganglionosis is unclear. Mutations of the RET proto-oncogene have been found in 50% of those with familial Hirschsprung's disease but were not related to the length of the aganglionic segment.[28,29] In sporadic Hirschsprung's disease mutations of this gene are found in 10-30% of patients.[28,30]

The second gene which has been implicated is termed the endothelin-B receptor gene (EDNRB). This gene has been localised to chromosome 13q22.[31] Mutations of this gene carry a risk of Hirschsprung's disease in heterozygotes and homozygotes together with sex dependent variable penetrance. In homozygotes the risk of Hirschsprung's disease was 74% compared to 21% in heterozygotes.

Apart from the genetic factors affecting the growth and development of the enteric nervous system, the role of the intercellular matrix has also received attention. Deficiency in the microenvironment may inhibit or prevent migration of neural cells in the distal intestine.[32,33]

At present there is no unifying concept to explain how these factors interact to produce the clinical picture of Hirschsprung's disease.

INCIDENCE

The incidence of Hirschsprung's disease is 1 in 4,500 to 1 in 5,000.[34-36] The male/female ratio is about 4 to 1 overall, but this disparity diminishes to 1.5 to 2:1 with total colonic disease.[36,37]

The pattern of inheritance is unclear but with longer segment disease (beyond the sigmoid colon) inheritance is compatible with a dominant gene with incomplete penetrance.[37]

In studies of RET gene mutation, similar mutations showed greater penetrance in males than in females and resulted in differing lengths of aganglionic bowel within the same family.[28,29]

The risk to siblings also varies. For disease confined to the distal half of the large bowel the risk for a male sibling is 5%, regardless of the sex of the index case.[37] The risk to a female sibling is 1% if the index case is male and 3% if the index case is female.

For longer segment disease (proximal colon with or without small bowel) an affected male results in risks of 17 and 13% to future male and female siblings respectively.

For longer segment disease, when the index case is female, the risk is 33% for a subsequent male sibling and 9% for a subsequent female sibling. Finally, in a single hospital review from Boston, a definite history of Hirschsprung's disease was reported in 5% of patient's families.[38]

For offspring of affected patients the exact risk is not clear but is raised above that of the general population. Parker et al considered that those with short segment disease had perhaps a 2% risk of having affected children, with a higher risk for those with long segment disease.[39]

ASSOCIATED ANOMALIES

The literature suggests that a substantial number of these children will have other abnormalities. In a birth cohort of about 700,000 infants in British Columbia, Spouge and Bard found other anomalies in almost 30% of infants with Hirschsprung's disease.[34] These included urological anomalies (2.2%), anorectal malformations and colonic atresia (4.5%), small bowel atresia (1%), deafness (2.2%) and cardiovascular anomalies (5.6%). Also included was Down's syndrome (2.8%).

A more recent review from Denmark showed that 5% of patients with Hirschsprung's disease had Down's syndrome.[40] The Boston review showed a higher proportion of patients with Down's syndrome (8%) and an overall incidence of 22% for associated anomalies in these children.[38] This figure is in keeping with other reports in the literature. It is clear therefore that a systematic effort should be undertaken to establish the presence or absence of other anomalies in these children.

The recognition of other GI anomalies such as pyloric stenosis and small bowel atresia (both about 1%) may be delayed by the presence of Hirschsprung's disease.[34,41] Equally, the recognition of Hirschsprung's disease may be delayed by prior treatment of these problems.

There is also an association with other disorders of the neural crest. These are sometimes referred to as neurocristopathies.[42] These have received detailed attention because of the possible insight that might be provided into the molecular basis for Hirschsprung's disease. Included in this group of conditions are Ondine's Curse (congenital central hypoventilation syndrome), Waardenburgh's syndrome (sensori neural deafness and disorders of pigmentation), multiple endocrine neoplasia (MEN2A) and familial medullary thyroid carcinoma.

MEN2A includes medullary thyroid cancer, hyperparathyroidism and phaeochromocytoma. Association of all these conditions with Hirschsprung's disease have been recorded. The association of Ondine's Curse appears to be ominous in terms of survival.[43,44]

The link with Waardenburgh's syndrome has been clear for over 20 years and has recently been attributed to mutation in the gene encoding endothelin 3.[45-46]

Mutations in the RET proto-oncogene are known to account for all MEN2 variants and these mutations occur at sites known to be linked with Hirschsprung's disease.[47] A link with neuroblastoma and ganglio-neuroblastoma has also been established but the mechanism is not understood.[48,49]

Patients with two or more neural crest abnormalities are rare. The author has not encountered Hirschsprung's disease in over 200 children with neuroblastoma, nor indeed any of the other neurocristopathies in over 150 patients with Hirschsprung's disease.

PATHOLOGY

An absence of ganglion cells in the intermuscular (Auerbach's) and submucosal (Meissner's) plexuses is the hallmark of Hirschsprung's disease. In association with this feature, thickened nerve trunks are seen in the intermuscular plane and in the submucosa.

The length of the aganglionic segment varies. Two large multicentre reviews from the United States and Japan show that disease confined to the rectum, with or without the sigmoid colon, constitutes 75-80% of the total.[50,51] In a further 7-15% the left colon and splenic flexure are involved and about 8% have total colonic aganglionosis. A small number of this group of children have extensive or even total small bowel aganglionosis.

The standard histological technique for examining tissue is by hematoxylin and eosin staining of formalin fixed tissue. Reliable diagnoses can be produced by pathologists who have sufficient interest and experience. Diagnosis is reliable even on very small biopsy specimens. An added refinement is to have accurate intraoperative results based on frozen section histology. However, such expertise is not present in all hospitals and surgeons, of necessity, have to adapt their approach to make the best use of local facilities.

Acetylcholinesterase (AChE) staining is also popular but not universally available.[52] Meier-Ruge considers this histochemical technique to be more reliable and easier to use in practice.[53] This histochemical stain shows the absence of ganglion cells and heavy staining of coarse nerve fibres in the bowel wall, including the muscularis mucosae and lamina propria. The heaviest staining of nerve fibres is in the distal bowel, with fewer nerves being seen more proximally. Lake et al from Great Ormond Street reported no false positive or false negative diagnoses in dealing with 458 suction rectal biopsies.[55] They considered that acetylcholinesterase histochemistry provided the most reliable means of diagnosing Hirschsprung's disease.

Others have reported less encouraging results with a 29% false negative rate.[56] For the present, in most centres, hematoxylin and eosin staining may be the most practical means of diagnosis.

The junction between ganglionic and aganglionic bowel is called the transition zone and usually corresponds to the area of tapering or coning between dilated and non-dilated bowel seen on X-ray or at laparotomy. With long segment disease however, false cones are known to occur so the gross appearance is not a reliable guide to the presence or absence of ganglion cells.

Histologically the transition zone is considered to show reduced numbers of ganglion cells and an increase in nerve fibres. The length of the transition zone varies from a few millimetres to many centimetres. The level at which ganglion cells terminate in Auerbach's and Meissner's plexuses are similar at each point in the circumference.[57] Gross irregularities of the associated nerve fibres are also seen in the transitional zone with increasing abnormality and thickening of the extrinsic nerves towards the distal aganglionic bowel.[58] It is also clear that the ganglion cells are not evenly distributed around the circumference of the bowel. At different points of the circumference the bowel may be ganglionic or aganglionic.[57,59] At this hospital we have seen many children who have transitional zone changes extending over long lengths of colon.

CLINICAL PRESENTATION

About 94-98% of normal full term newborn infants will pass meconium within the first 24 hours of life.[60,61] It is exceptional for a normal baby not to have opened its bowels by 48 hours. A history of delayed passing of meconium is considered a common feature of Hirschsprung's disease. At least 40% of my own patients with Hirschsprung's disease had passed meconium within the first 24 hours of life. A failure to pass meconium in this time is not a reliable indicator on its own.

The presence of abdominal distension is usual unless the baby has had a rectal examination or rectal washout. Bilious vomiting and poor feeding are also common.

The majority of infants who present within the neonatal period have signs of low intestinal obstruction—distension, bilious vomiting and little or no passage of stool.

Examination will reveal generalised distension, active bowel sounds and a narrow empty rectum on rectal examination. Withdrawal of the finger may be followed by passage of gas and meconium.

Plain abdominal X-ray will show many loops of distended gas filled bowel with typically, an absence of gas in the rectum (Fig. 61.1). The differential diagnosis will include causes of low intestinal obstruction in addition to Hirschsprung's disease such as intestinal atresia, meconium ileus, small left colon and meconium plug syndromes.[62,63]

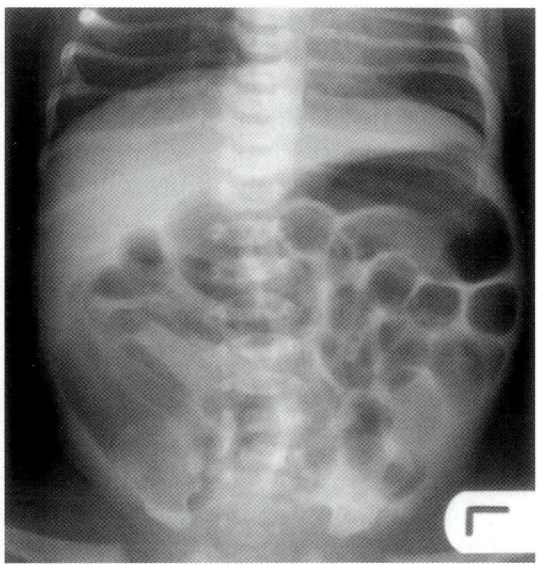

Fig. 61.1: Longitudinal section of rectum showing the level of mucosal incision in relation to columns of morgagni and dentate line (level of incision of internal sphincter)

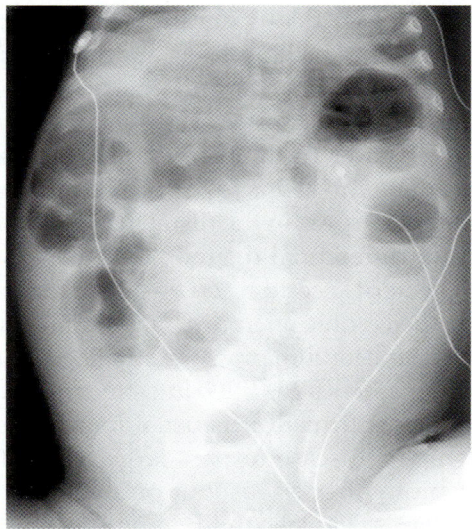

Fig. 61.2: Drawing of completed operation with broken line indicating amount of aganglionic colon which is excised

The second type of acute presentation is with enterocolitis. Hirschsprung's two index patients died after a diarrhoeal illness associated with mucosal ulceration.[3] Bill and Chapman wrote the first clear description of Hirschsprung's enterocolitis.[64] They described a syndrome of fever, distension and explosive diarrhea, progressing rapidly in some patients to hypovolemia and death. The mortality at that time was 32%. They related the occurrence of enterocolitis to mechanical obstruction and recommended decompression. X-rays show gross distension with thickened bowel wall (Fig. 61.2).

There is now an extensive and contradictory literature on the subject. The etiology remains obscure. Some have noted a relationship to the presence of Clostridium difficile and its toxins in the stool to the development of enterocolitis.[65] Others have not confirmed this.[66] Our own figures suggest an increased risk with Down's syndrome, female gender and a family history of Hirschsprung's disease.[67] Diagnosis within the first week of life appears to lessen the risk of enterocolitis.[68] Bill and Chapman noted that enterocolitis tends to recur and this has been confirmed by Elhalaby et al, who noted a mean number of 2.2 episodes in those who developed this complication.[68]

The third and least common acute mode of presentation is with intestinal perforation. The risk of perforation is higher with total colonic disease and in these children, the perforation is usually in the aganglionic bowel. With short segment disease, the perforation is proximal to the aganglionic zone.[69]

In older infants and children the history is of long standing constipation and distension, sometimes associated with failure to thrive. The clinical picture of massive abdominal distension and marasmus that was frequently seen 60 years ago, is not often encountered today. These children would have been managed with a combination of laxatives, suppositories and enemas but with only partial success.

Thus far I have not personally encountered a child who was entirely asymptomatic for the first 12 months of life. Such patients have been described but this must be quite rare. I have encountered one patient with total colonic aganglionosis who was entirely asymptomatic for the first four months of life and this is the longest period of lack of symptoms I have encountered in a child with Hirschsprung's disease. It is not clear why children with similar lengths of aganglionic bowel have such differing clinical presentations.

INITIAL MANAGEMENT

The management for those presenting with neonatal intestinal obstruction is the same as for any other form of obstruction—intravenous fluids, nasogastric decompression and consideration of antibiotics. If rectal examination produces gas and meconium then causes of complete mechanical obstruction, such as atresia, have been out-ruled. If no gas or meconium are produced after rectal examination then a single rectal washout with saline is performed. The aim is to establish if there is gas in the distal intestine to narrow the range of differential diagnoses. If there is no gas after the washout, a contrast enema is performed. This will show the colonic anatomy, may demonstrate the presence of a meconium plug or a small left colon, and if the contrast reaches gas filled intestine then intestinal continuity is confirmed. It is usual for children with Hirschsprung's disease to pass large amount of gas and meconium after a washout or a contrast enema and the infant's clinical condition will then improve.

If the presentation is with enterocolitis then urgent decompression is necessary. A rectal examination and rectal washouts are employed and are usually successful. Failure to decompress under these circumstances will indicate a need for surgery. If decompression is successful then surgery should be deferred until a time of greater physiological stability. All these children should receive oral Vancomycin as well as broad spectrum intravenous cover.

For those infants and children presenting with a history of constipation, the need for urgent investigation is less pressing. Recourse to enemas and washouts will alter the appearance of the bowel on a contrast enema. This is perhaps less relevant a concern at the present time than was previously the case when diagnosis was predominantly based on the enema appearance.

DIAGNOSIS

There is no substitute for a tissue diagnosis. Reliance on contrast enemas or manometry is less secure and less accurate.

Rectal suction biopsy has been proved satisfactory and reliable in the hands of expert pathologists.[70] All surgeons do not have access to such expertise and may need to provide larger or full thickness biopsies.[16] Regardless of the method used, the biopsies should be taken from the posterior rectal wall, at least 25 mm above the dentate line. The bowel below this level is hypoganglionic and the failure to see ganglion cells may not be pathological.[71]

Various methods of obtaining biopsies have been described. Suction biopsy instruments are widely used in young infants but we have found the use of punch biopsy forceps to be preferable in older children.[72,73] Inevitably, rectal biopsy is followed by a small but inevitable number of complications which include bleeding, perforation and occasional fatality.[74]

The use of anorectal manometry has largely been confined to specialist centres. This technique assesses the relaxation of the internal anal sphincter in response to rectal distension. A failure of the sphincter to relax, or indeed an increase in tone, is a feature of Hirschsprung's disease.[75] Although the instrumentation and technique are straightforward, the method has not found widespread use. In some centres manometry is used as a screening test to more clearly define those who need to undergo biopsy.

Contrast enemas are widely used, both to make the diagnosis and to establish the position of the transition zone. Not infrequently contrast enemas are requested in the presence of intestinal obstruction in newborns to more clearly define large bowel anatomy. Subsequent to the enema marked decompression may be achieved and the infant's condition improved.

When specifically looking for Hirschsprung's disease the recommendation is to use 50% dilute barium sulphate. The fluid is injected slowly and the least possible amount of contrast is used.[40,76] The irregular contracted rectum and distal sigmoid colon with a transition cone into dilate proximal bowel will be seen. With standard length Hirschsprung's disease the contrast enema appearance will usually correspond with the histological findings. With long segment or total colonic disease the appearance on the enema may not be reliable and false cones are known to occur.

A delayed X-ray film taken at 24-48 hours may demonstrate retention of contrast, lending support to a diagnosis of Hirschsprung's disease (Fig. 61.3).[76] Little has changed in the radiological diagnosis of Hirschsprung's disease since Hope et al in 1965 suggested that the cardinal features included a transition cone, irregular bizarre contractions of the aganglionic zone and barium retention.[76] However, the reliability of barium enema in this context is questionable. The experience of Smith and Cass is fairly typical—in a series of 24 infants, mostly neonates, the false negative rate for barium enema was 24%.[76] In addition the error rate was 53% in judging

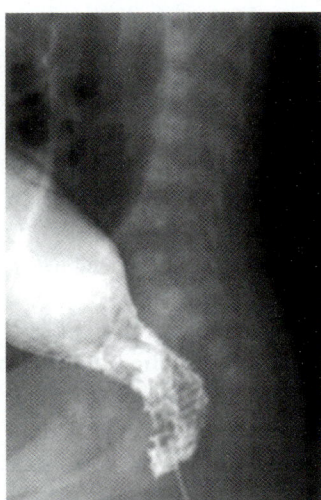

Fig. 61.3: Longitudinal section of rectum showing triangle of posterior rectal wall and opposing anterior wall of ileum to be ecised with GIA stapler

the position of the transition zone. Others have reported substantial - up to 43% - false positive rates of diagnosing Hirschsprung's disease by barium enema in infancy.[78,79]

In this hospital we no longer utilise barium enema when Hirschsprung's disease is suspected. The diagnosis is made only by rectal biopsy and the level of transition is made on the basis of operative frozen section biopsy.

TREATMENT

Once the diagnosis has been established there are many options for treatment. The first decision is whether or not to bring out a stoma. Many infants can be managed for a period of weeks or months by means of daily saline rectal washouts. However, a proportion of children will not achieve satisfactory decompression by this means. Some of these children will have extensive disease but in some with standard length Hirschsprung's cannot be managed in this way. Equally, some families cannot tolerate this type of intervention. Whatever the circumstances, if washouts are unsatisfactory then a stoma will be necessary.

The next consideration is where to site the stoma. For many years in this hospital the approach to Hirschsprung's disease was a three stage reconstruction—right transverse colostomy, pull-through at 6-9 months of age and colostomy closure some weeks later. Others have used a two stage procedure—fashioning the stoma above the transition zone and then using the stoma as the apex of the pull-through. It is clear however that in many, a single stage reconstruction is safe and effective.

A multiplicity of procedures is available, some of which may be performed laparoscopically. Regardless of the method used the aim is to relieve symptoms and achieve optimal bowel control with a minimum of complications.

The decision to perform a single or multi stage procedure should be based on local facilities and expertise. It will also depend on the characteristics of the patient population. If delayed presentation is a feature of the local population then primary pull-through of very dilated bowel may be inadvisable.

Single stage procedures can only be accomplished if reliable frozen section histology is available. Incorrect information from intraoperative frozen sections will result in abnormal bowel being pulled through or normal bowel being discarded. This concern is not purely theoretical and it seems likely that only laboratories dealing with large numbers of such biopsies will be able to produce acceptable results.[80]

In the absence of such expertise, biopsies taken at the time of stoma formation may be examined prior to the definitive procedure.

In attempting to define the length of the aganglionic bowel, biopsies may be sent from the apex of the sigmoid colon, distal descending colon, splenic or hepatic flexures and appendix of terminal ileum. Given the unpredictable anatomy of the transition zone it is unwise to take biopsies closer than at these intervals. In addition, each of these sites can be brought to the anus.

Three pull-through operations and their variants are in common use throughout the world and will be described here. These are the Swenson, Duhamel and Soave procedures.[13,81-84] All are modified from the original descriptions but in each case the original concept is valid.

The Rehbein State and endorectal transanal pull-throughs are not described here.[85-87] These operations have not gained widespread acceptance and, to this author at least, the concept in each case is unsound.

When performed by open operation the initial approach is similar for each operation. The patient is placed in semi-lithotomy position and a bladder catheter is inserted. Various incisions are used but it is essential to be in a position to dissect deep in the pelvis and this can only be achieved if the incision is close to the symphysis. A lower mid line incision is the most adaptable. The site chosen for the pull-through is chosen on the basis of histological evaluation either by frozen section or standard formalin-fixed tissue histology.

There are three phases to each of the operations— a colonic, rectal and anal phase. The colonic phase consists of mobilising the sigmoid and descending colon up to and including the splenic flexure. The meso-colic vessels are then divided in order to allow the site of the proposed pull-through to extend at least 7cm over the symphysis. Great care is necessary to achieve the required bowel length with an adequate blood supply. Once the proximal bowel has been prepared for the pull-through, attention is turned to the rectal phase of the operation.

In each case the use of a fixed table mounted retractor is of great value at this phase of the procedure. The Swenson operation entails dissection of the rectum from its attachments in a plane on the rectal muscle wall. Although many advocate commencing this phase with ligation of the inferior mesenteric vessels, this is unnecessary. The dissection may be commenced on the wall of the distal sigmoid or upper rectum. The use of fine right angled artery forceps and bipolar diathermy makes this a rapid and relatively trouble free dissection. It was an extremely tedious dissection when the vessels required individual ligation. Bipolar diathermy is satisfactory for all but larger adolescents.

The dissection advances distally, dissecting the full circumference of the rectum. Deep in the pelvis it is important to remain close to the rectum on its anterior aspect. When the dissection has reached to within 2 cm of the dentate line anteriorly and 1 cm posteriorly this phase is complete. The distal extent of the dissection is judged by inserting a finger in the anus. At this stage the bowel is divided at the level chosen for the pull-through and the two ends sutured closed.

The anal phase of the dissection then commences. The apex of the dissected rectum is drawn out through the anus, everting the rectum. If the dissection has been adequate the anus may be partially everted. An incision is made from 9 to 3 o'clock anteriorly through the rectal wall, 1-2 cm above the dentate line. Only the bottom of the dentate line can be identified with any certainty and this is the point from where measurements are made.

Through this opening in the rectum the ganglionic colon is pull through with care to avoid torsion. The colon is opened at its apex and sutured full thickness to the cut edge of anorectum with interrupted absorbable 4/O sutures.

The incision of the rectum is then completed in stages, as is the anastomosis.

Posteriorly in the 6 o'clock position the suture line should be about 1 cm from the dentate line. The rectum is now free and should be sent for histological examination.

The commencement of the Duhamel procedure is identical. The early phase of rectal dissection is also the same. The dissection proceeds circumperentially until within 3-4 cm of the dentate line. This level is well below the pelvic peritoneum.

The anal phase then commences. It is best to partially evert the anus for this phase. This is easily accomplished by using tissue forceps at the 3 and 9 o'clock positions. An incision is then made along the dentate line from 4 to 8 o'clock and a retrorectal tunnel developed initially with scissors and then with a long clamp. This tunnel should quickly reach the level of the abdominal dissection. The tunnel is then widened to accommodate the pull-through bowel.

The previously divided and sutured bowel is then pulled through with care to avoid torsion. The open end is sutured to the anal incision with interrupted absorbable 4/O sutures. Finally, the double wall between rectum and colon is stapled and divided with a linear stapler. Alternatively, a crushing clamp can be left attached.

Within the abdomen the rectum is transected a few millimetres beyond the apex of the staple line. The open end of rectum is then closed with a running extramucosal 4/O suture. As this suturing takes place deep in the pelvis great care is necessary to ensure accurate placement of the sutures.

The early stages of an endorectal pull-through are as outlined above. There is no phase of perirectal dissection however. The tendency is to commence the endorectal resection as low as is convenient. This usually occurs close to the peritoneum of the pelvic floor. Infiltration of fluid into the submucosa is often mentioned as an aid to dissection. In practice it seems to obscure the anatomy and is probably rarely performed.

At the level chosen the muscle coat is divided with scissors circumferentially to enter the submucosal plane. This plane is then dissected with gauze pledgets or with artery forceps. The dissection is easier in young infants. The submucosal dissection progresses to a level about 1cm above the dentate line and the mucosal tube is then everted.

Some surgeons opt to perform the distal part of the anorectal resection from below, but it may be difficult in practice to have the rectal and anal planes of dissection coincide.

Once the dissection has been completed the mucosal tube is divided 1-2 cm above the dentate line and the ganglionic bowel is pulled through and sutured at this level. There seems little reason to perform the original Soave operation which left the pull through bowel outside the anus and most now perform the Boley modification.[88]

The catheter is usually removed after 24 hours and enteral feeding resumed once intestinal function is established.

When these operations have been performed as single stage procedures, an EUA performed 2-3 weeks after operation is recommended. This allows assessment of healing and of any tendency to stenosis or septum formation.

In the presence of a defunctioning stoma a contrast study should be performed after two weeks. If the appearances are satisfactory the stoma may then be closed.

Management of Patients with Total Colonic Aganglionosis

Total colonic aganglionosis, with or without small bowel involvement is reported in 7-8% of children with Hirschsprung's disease in large series.[50,51] The author's own incidence is 14%.[89]

Presentation is similar to other children with Hirschsprung's disease but there is an impression that many infants with total colonic disease have delayed onset of symptoms. As noted above, one of my own patients was entirely symptom free for the first four months of life while being breast fed.

On occasion the clinical features may be indistinguishable from meconium ileus or necrotising enterocolitis.[90,91] Perforation when it occurs in these infants is usually in the aganglionic bowel.[69,89,91] Only an awareness of the possibility will lead to a timely diagnosis. The author's experience suggests that recognition of total colonic disease is frequently delayed and several ineffective operations may be performed as a result. In common with others we have found that a short rectal pouch, as for recto sigmoid disease, is preferable to the long side to side Martin modification.[89,92,93] Neither have we attempted single stage procedures in these children. They have very loose stools initially and are more easily managed with an ileostomy. Otherwise, severe and distressing perianal excoriation may result.

Mortality in this group of patients has diminished markedly. Between 1978 and 1982 the mortality in our patients was 30%. In the years 1980-1996 this figure had dropped to 6%.[89,91] The improvement in survival is related to improved central venous catheters for intravenous feeding, the use of loperamide to prolong bowel transit and routine monitoring of urinary sodium. The last of these we have found to be of great benefit.[91] On spot urines, the urinary sodium should be greater than 10 mmols/L. Twenty four hour collection of urine allows more accurate estimation of sodium balance but in practical terms repeated spot checks are entirely satisfactory.[94]

For infants with total or near total intestinal aganglionosis we are not clear that there is a surgical solution. Others have reported extended myotomy/myectomy under these circumstances combined with a stoma. Ziegler et al reported on a heterogenous group of 16 patients with very extensive disease.[95] They were treated in eight different centres. Twelve had 10 cm or less of ganglionic intestine and the remainder had up to 40 cm of small bowel.

Of 10 survivors, two were on full enteral feeds, both of whom had less than 10 cm of ganglionic intestine. It was not clear whether a simple myotomy was more or less affective than a myectomy. The evidence therefore is that in desperate circumstances this may be an option worth trying. The variability of presentation with Hirschsprung's disease and the unpredictable nature of severe short bowel make it difficult to make informed decisions under these circumstances. Nixon noted that he had one patient who had 19 cm of jejunum who had undergone a standard Duhamel procedure and who had survived into adult life prior to the advent of home intravenous feeding.[96]

EARLY COMPLICATIONS

Surgery for Hirschsprung's disease is associated with all the usual complications that may follow major intestinal surgery. In a review of major series, Fonkalsrud suggested that postoperative bleeding is uncommon (less than 2%).[97] Wound infection was reported in about 7% but this was probably an underestimate, as most infections present after discharge from hospital. Other wound complications such as dehiscence also occur but are relatively uncommon.

Procedure specific complications such as leakage have received considerable attention. If there are systemic signs of leakage after a single stage pull-through, a proximal defunctioning stoma should be fashioned and left in place for about three months. This is sufficient time for healing to occur. The incidence of leakage varies widely in different series. Swenson et al reviewing 483 patients, reported anastomotic leakage in 5%.[98] Subsequently, 6.2% of patients had an anastomotic stricture. The early mortality was 3.3%.

Leakage after a Duhamel procedure is unusual. A radiological leak was seen in two of my own patients from the apex of the rectal pouch—a rate of 1.3%. Reviewing the experience in Indianapolis, Engum and Grosfeld reported one enterocutaneous fistula in 235 children after a Duhamel operation.[99] Formation of a faecal bolus in the neorectum was reported in 11%. There were no operative deaths in this series.

Complications specific to the endorectal procedure and its modifications include cuff abscesses and anastomotic strictures. Cuff abscesses seem to be relatively uncommon. Polley et al reported a 2% incidence of cuff abscesses in their patients.[100] Langer et al reported that almost 50% of their patients undergoing endorectal pull-through required subsequent dilatation.[101]

Reviewing a personal series of 57 patients, Wright and Cord Udy reported similar rates of complication - 5 and 43% for cuff abscess and the need for dilatation.[102] The mortality in this latter series was 3%.

It is clear that staged reconstruction is associated with an incidence of stoma related problems.[101] However, it seems that in terms of early complications, primary pull-through is as safe as a staged procedure even in the newborn.[103]

LONG-TERM COMPLICATIONS

The difference in outcome between published series is so great as to make one doubt that the same condition is being treated. A significant paper in this regard was published by Mishalany and Woolley in 1987.[104] They studied a group of 62 patients who had agreed to attend up to 30 years after surgery. In this selected group of patients, three were totally incontinent (4.8%) and half the patients has varying degrees of fecal incontinence. The end result in terms of continence did not seem to be related to the type of pull-through performed.

It is difficult to reconcile this figure with, for example, Swenson's own series which quoted 90% of patients with a normal bowel habit and 3.5% of patients who had soiling.[98] Swenson further noted that no patient followed for more than 11 years had permanent soiling.

Others have reported similarly encouraging results in terms of bowel control. Polley reported 0% incontinence amongst 67 patients over three years of age.[100] Sixteen of these patients had long segment or total colonic disease.

Rescorla et al noted that patient satisfaction improved with increased length of follow-up—from 58% being very satisfied at five years to 88% at 15 years.[104] Whether this reflects improved functioning or improved acceptance is unclear but this feature has been noted in many series. Probably both factors are of importance. Rescorla et al further mentioned that up to 9% of patients had episodes of soiling at 5-10 years follow up but those followed for 15-20 years had no soiling. A more recent review from the same centre noted that at 15 years follow-up, 28% had constipation. Clearly therefore a number of patients have unsatisfactory bowel habits after surgery and these problems are, almost certainly, under-reported. From Melbourne Catto-Smith et al reported on a group of 60 patients with Hirschsprung's disease, 8.9 years after reconstructive surgery.[106] This was a study based on questionnaires, personal diaries and structured interviews and was not performed by the operating surgeons. Almost all had undergone an endorectal pull-through. Just over 50% had significant soiling. In great distinction to other reports, there was little tendency to improve with age.

Conversely, in a retrospective review, Yanchar and Soucy reported that in those under 15 years of age continence was poor in 50% but this figure had dropped to 8% over the age of 15 years.[107] The exact number who had symptoms of constipation with a need for medical treatment is unclear although many series report substantial numbers of patients who required sphincterotomy. Figures vary widely from 9 to 29%.[104,105] Presumably these children were the more severely affected. There is therefore evidence of seriously disordered bowel function in substantial numbers of children after surgery for Hirschsprung's disease. These facts need to be understood by the family before embarking on treatment.

Management of Major Complications

Recurrent entrocolitis is usually associated with persisting obstruction. This may be the result of an anastomosis which is too proximal or abnormal innervation of the pull-through bowel. The treatment for this complication, as well as for intractable strictures and fistulae, is a repeat pull-through.

My own experience is that sphincterotomy is usually unhelpful—in the words of one parent 'an operation usually followed by another operation'. This author would agree with Swenson et al and Wright and Cord-Udy that the results of sphincterotomy are disappointing.[98,99] It is not clear to me that this operation has any part to play in the management of persisting constipation or recurrent enterocolitis in these patients.

Several patients from elsewhere have been encountered when sphincterotomy was performed through a posterior sagittal approach. All developed fistulae and none were relieved of their symptoms.

In those whose symptoms are not controlled by simple measures, a three stage approach is recommended—ileostomy, pull-through and later stoma closure. The results of this approach have been fairly satisfactory. The most satisfactory results were achieved when surgery was undertaken for structural/anatomical problems.[108] The results from these patients were comparable to those expected after a first pull-through.

In a few patients, surgery was undertaken because of persisting incontinence after initial pull-through. No improvement was achieved in these patients and this is no longer regarded a valid indication for surgery.

Coran and colleagues from Ann Arbor have reported similarly encouraging results after repeat pull-through.[109]

It is not clear that aganglionosis ever recurs. West, Grosfeld et al have reported on five children with what they considered to be acquired aganglionosis.[110] Reviewing the literature, they considered that ischemia was the etiology behind the disappearance of the ganglion cells. In discussion on this paper, Molenaar noted that experimentally, ganglion cells were resistant to ischemia. Others have never encountered recurrent Hirschsprung's disease despite seeing substantial numbers of such patients (Mahour in discussion of the same paper). It is not clear that full circumferential examination of the apex of the pull-through bowel was undertaken in these children and an alternative explanation is that of a transitional zone pull-through.[59] Similarly, a long transitional zone with irregular distribution of ganglion cells may be responsible for some of what are termed 'skip lesions'.

ULTRASHORT SEGMENT HIRSCHSPRUNG'S DISEASE

This is usually defined as a condition when manometry shows a Hirschsprung's trace in the presence of normal histology. It is sometimes termed anal sphincter achalasia. Consequently, only those with access to anorectal manometry are in a position to diagnose this condition. Detailed immunohistochemical examinations have shown abnormalities of neuronal markers.[111] Once diagnosed, the condition has been treated with sphincterotomy with variable success.

For those without the requisite technology the condition cannot be diagnosed and the patients must be treated symptomatically.

STAGED VERSUS PRIMARY PULL-THROUGH

Primary pull-through has been performed for many years. Swenson et al reported that, of their 470 patients, 50% had undergone a primary pull-through without protective stoma.[98] Furthermore, the incidence of anastomotic leakage was not diminished by the presence of a stoma. In the event of leakage however, formation of a stoma was considered life saving. Their recommendation was that surgery be deferred until after the age of six months.

Much has changed in the care of young infants since that publication in 1975. It is clear that major surgery may be safely undertaken soon after birth. It is obvious that single stage reconstruction is dependent on accurate frozen section histology or histochemistry. As noted above, frozen section histology is not completely reliable under all circumstances.

In addition, a successful outcome after a primary pull-through presumes that the enteric nervous system is stable at birth and undergoes no further change. This may not be the case.

We have been performing single stage pull-throughs for some years and have reported no excess of surgical complications.[112] With the passage of time however, we have a concern that these children have an increase in disorders of bowel habit requiring treatment. These patients are under ongoing review and at present we are not clear that a single stage procedure may in the end be the best option.

OPEN VERSUS LAPAROSCOPIC PULL-THROUGH

We have no experience with the transanal endorectal pull-through performed solely from the perineum.[87,113,114] As only a very limited view of the mesocolon is possible with this approach there is clearly the possibility of performing an ischemic pull-through. Reported results are good but to this author at least, the technique has an in-built flaw—the inability to see and dissect the mesocolon.[114]

All three procedures may be performed laparoscopically and early results are encouraging.[115] In our experience, this probably represents the next advance in the treatment of Hirschsprung's disease. The same operation may be performed laparoscopically as would be carried out at open surgery but without the trauma of access. Our preference again is for the Duhamel procedure. We have sited the camera port in the right upper quadrant and the working ports in the right iliac fossa, left upper quadrant and occasionally left iliac fossa as well. At this early stage, with fewer than 30 patients undergoing surgery, the results appear similar to the open procedure.

INTESTINAL NEURONAL DYSPLASIA

This disorder has been diagnosed primarily in Europe and its existence as a distinct entity is a subject of debate. Described initially in 1971 by Meier-Ruge its existence and relevance have been contested ever since.[116] The pathological features include hypoplasia of nerve plexuses, increased Acht activity, heterotopic ganglion cells in the lamina propria and muscle coats, together with aplasia or hypoplasia of the sympathetic innervation of the myenteric plexus. From the literature there seems little correlation between symptoms and histological features and this will obviously impair surgical decision-making.[117] The subject has been recently reviewed but remains confusing.[118] In this hospital, the pathologists are not convinced of the existence of this condition. Nonetheless, it seems likely that there are other disorders of the enteric nervous system which remain to be defined.

REFERENCES

1. Leenders E, Sieber WK. Congenital megacolon observation by Frederick Ruysch—1691. J Pediatr Surg 1970;5:1-3.
2. Finney JMT. Congenital idiopathic dilatation of the colon (Hirschsprung's disease) Surg Gynecol Obstetr 1908;6: 624-43.
3. Hirschsprung, Stuhltragheit Neugeborener in Folge von Dilatatior, und Hypertrophie des Colons Jahrb F Kinderh 1887;27:1- 7.
4. Dalla Valle A, Ricerche istologiche su di un caso di Megacolon congenito. Pediatria 1920;28:740-52.
5. Dalla Valle A. Contributo alIa conoscenza della forma famigliare del megacolon congenito. Pediatria 1924;32: 569-99.
6. Cameron JAM. On the etiology of Hirschsprung's disease. Arch Dis Child 1928;3:210-11.
7. Whitehouse FA, Kernohan JW. Myenteric plexus in congenital megacolon, Arch Int Med 1948;82:75-111.
8. Zuelzer WW, Wilson JL. Functional intestinal obstruction on a congenital neurogenic basis in infancy. Am J Dig Child 1948;75:40-64.
9. Bodian M, Stephens FD, Ward BCH. Lancet 1949;1:6-11.
10. Barrington~Ward LE. Enlargement of colon and rectum, Br J Surg 1914;1:345-60.
11. Wade ABf Royle ND. The operative treatment of Hirschsprung's disease: A new method, Med J Austr 1927;1: 137-41.
12. Scott WJM, Morton JJ. Sympathetic inhibition of the large intestine in Hirschsprung's disease. J Clin Invest 1930;9:247-61.
13. Swenson 0, Bill AH. Resection of rectum and rectosigmoid with preservation of the sphincter for benign spastic lesions producing megacolon, Surgery '948;24:212-20.
14. Swenson Of Neuhauser EBD, Pickett LK. New concepts of the etiology, diagnosis and treatment of congenital megacolon (Hirschsprung's disease). Pediatrics 1948;4: 201-09.

15. Swenson O, Rheinlander HF, Diamond I. Hirschsprung's disease: A new concept of the etiology. Operative results in thirty four patients. N Engl J Med 1949; 241:551-56.
16. Swenson O, Fisher JH, MacMahon HE. Rectal biopsy as an aid in the diagnosis of Hirschsprung's disease. N Engl J Med 1955;253:632-35.
17. Yntema CL, Hammond WS. The origin of intrinsic ganglia of trunk viscera from vagal neural crest in the chick embryo. J Comp Neurol 1954;101:515-41.
18. Okamoto E, Ueda T. Embryogenesis of intramural ganglia of the gut and its relation to Hirschsprung's disease. J Pediatr Surg 1967;2:437-43.
19. Le Douarin NM, Teillet M-A M. Experimental analysis of the migration and differentiation of neuroblasts of the autonomic nervous system and of neuroectoderma: mesenchymal derivatives, using a biological cell marking technique. Dev Bioi 1974;41:162-84.
20. De Laet MH, Dassonville M, Stetaert H, et al. Decrease of vasoactive intestinal polypeptide, methionine-enkephaline, substance p and increase of neuropeptide Y immunoreactive nerve fibers in aganglionic colon of Hirschsprung's disease, Neurochem Int 1989;14:135-41.
21. Vanderwinden JM, De Laet M-H, Schiffmann SN, et al. Nitric oxide synthase distribution in the enteric nervous system of Hirschsprung's disease, Gastroenterology 1993;105:969-73.
22. Crema A, Del Tacca M, Frigo GM, Lecchini S. Presence of a non-adrenergic inhibitory system in the human colon. Gut 1968;9:633-37.
23. Romeo G, Ronchetto P, Luo Y, et al. Point mutations affecting the tyrosine kinase domain of the RET proto-oncogene in Hirschsprung's disease. Nature 1994;367:377-78.
24. Edery P, Lyonnet S, Mulligan LM, et al. Mutations of the RET proto-oncogene in Hirschsprung's disease. Nature 1994;367:378-80.
25. Lyonnet S, Bolino A, Pelet A, et al. A gene for Hirschsprung's disease maps to the proximal long arm of chromosome 10. Nature Genetics 1993;4:346-50.
26. Yin L, Ceccherini I, Pasini 8, et al. Close linkage with the RET protooncogene and deletion mutations in autosomal dominant Hirschsprung disease. Hum Mol Genet 1993;2:1803-08.
27. Martucciello G, Tam P, RET protein in human fetal development and in Hirschsprung's disease in Hlrschsprung's disease and allied disorders 2nd Edition (2000) p 81-88 (Eds) Holschneider AM, Puri P Harwood Academic Publishers, Singapore.
28. Attie T, Pelet At Edery P, et al. Divorcity of RET proto-oncogone mutations in familial and sporadic Hirschsprung's disease. Hum Mol Gen 1995;4:1381-86.
29. Edery P, Pelet A, Mulligan LM, et al. Long segment and short segment familial Hirschsprung's disease: variable clinical expression at the R ET locus.
30. Angrist M, Bolk S, Thiel B, et al. Mutation analysis of the RET receptor tyrosine kinase in Hirschsprung's disease, Hum Mol Gen 1995;4:821-30.
31. Puffenberger EG, Hosoda K, Washington SS, et al. A missense mutation of the Endothelin-B receptor gene in multigenic Hirschsprung's disease. Cell 1994;79:1257-66.
32. Pomeranz HO, Sherman DL. Smalheiser NR, et al. Expression of a neurally related Laminin binding protein by neural crestwderived cells that colonize the gut: Relationship to the foramtion of enteric ganglia. J Compar Neurol 1991;313:625-42.
33. Shimotake T, Iwai N, Vanagihara J, et al. Impaired proliferative activity of mesenchymal cells affects the migratory pathway for neural crest cells in the developing gut of mutant murine embryos. J Pediatr Surg 1995;30: 445-47.
34. Spouge D, Baird PA, Hirschsprung disease in a large birth cohort. Teratology 1985;32:171-77.
35. Passarge E. The genetics of Hirschsprung's disease. Evidence for heterogeneous etiology and a study of sixty-three families. N Engl J Med 1967;276:138-43.
36. Orr JD, Scobie WG. Presentation and incidence of Hirschsprung's disease. Br Med J 1983;287:1671.
37. Badner JA, Sieber WK, Garver KL, Chakravarti A. A genetic study of Hirschsprung disease, Am J Hum Genet 1990;46:568-80.
38. Ryan ET, Ecker JL. Christakis NA, Folkman J. Hirschsprung's disease: Associated abnormalities and demography. J Pediatr Surg 1992;27:76-81.
39. Carter CO, Evans K, Hickman V. J Med Genet 1981;18:87-90.
40. Russell MB, Russell CA, Niebuhr E. An epidemiological study of Hirschsprung's disease and additional anomalies. Acta Pediatr 1994;83:68-71.
41. Bodian M. Carter CO. A family study of Hirschsprung's disease, Ann Hum Genet 1963;26:261-71.
42. Bolande RP. The neurocristopathies. A unifying concept of disease arising in neural crest maldevelopment, Hum Pathol 1973;5:409-29.
43. Haddad GG, Mazza NM, Defendini R, et al. Congenital failure of automatic control of ventilation, gastrointestinal motility and heart rate. Medicine 1978;57:517-26
44. O'Dell K, Staren E. Sassuk A. Total colonic aganglionosis (Zeulzer-Wilson syndrome) and congenital failure of automatic control of ventilation (Ondine's curse). J Pediatr Surg 1987; 22: 1019-20
45. Omenn GS, McKusick V A. The association of Waardenburg syndrome and Hirschsprung megacolon. Am J Med Gonot 1070; 3: 217-223
46. Pingault V, Bondurand N, Lemort N, et al. A heterozygous endothelin 3 mutation in Waardenburg.Hirschsprung disease: is there a dosage effect of EDN3/EDNRS gene mutations on neurocristopathy phenotypes? J Med Genet 2001;38:205-08.
47. Eng C, Clayton D, Schuffenecker I, et al. The relationship between specific RET proto-oncogene mutations and disease phenotype in multiple endocrine neoplasia type 2. International AET Mutation Consortium Analysis. JAMA 1996;276:1575-79.

48. Chatten J, Voorhess ML. Familial neuroblastoma. Report of a kindred with multiple disorders including neuroblastomas in four siblings, N Engl J Med 1967; 277:1230-36.
49. Michna SA, McWilljams NS, Krummel TM, et al. Multifocal ganglioneuroblastoma coexistent with total colonic aganglionosis. J Pediatr Surg 1988;23:57-59
50. Kleinhaus S, Boley SJ, Sheran M, Sieber WK, Hirschsprung's disease: A survey of the members of the Surgical Section of the America' Academy of Pediatrics. J Pediatr Surg 1979;14:588-97.
51. Ikeda K, Goto S. Diagnosis and treatment of Hirschsprung's disease. An analysis of 1628 patients Ann Surg 1984;199:400-05.
52. Kamijo K, Hiatt AB, Koelle GB. Congenital megacolon. A comparison of the spastic and hypertrophied segments with respect to cholinesterase activities and sensitivities to acetyl-choline, DFP and the barium Ion. Gastroenterology 1953;24:173-85.
53. Meier-Auge W. Histological diagnosis and differential diagnosis in: Hirschsprung's disease and allied disorders (2000) 2nd Edition p 252-265 Eds. Holschneider AM, Puri P, Harwood Academic Publishers, Singapore.
54. Garrett JR, Howard EA. Nixon HH. Autonomic nerves in rectum and colon in Hirschsprung's disease. A cholinesterase and catecholamine histochemical study, Arch Dis Child 1969;44:406-17.
55. Lake BD, Puri P, Nixon HH, Claireaux AE. Hirschsprung's disease. An appraisal of histochemically demonstrated acetylcholinesterase activity in suction rectal biopsy specimens as an aid to diagnosis, Arch Pathol Lab Med 1978;102:244-47.
56. Hamoudi AB, Reiner CB, Boles ET, et al. Acetylcholinesterase staining activity of rectal mucosa. Its use in the diagnosis of Hirschsprung's disease. Arch Pathol Lab Med 1982;106:670-72.
57. Gherardi G. Pathology of the gangtionic-aganglionic junction in congenital megacolon. AMA Arch Pathol 1960;69:520-23.
58. Miura H, Ohi R, Tseng 8W, Takahashi T. The structure of the transitional and aganglionic zones of Auerbach's plexus in patients with Hirschsprun's disease: A computer assisted three-dimensional reconstruction study. J Pediatr Surg 1996;31:420-26.
59. Ghose 81, Spuire BA, Stringer MD, et al. Hirschsprung's disease: Problems with trarlsition-zone pull-through. J Pediatr Surg 2000;35:1805-59.
60. Sherry SN, Kramer I. The time of passage of the first stool and first urine by the newborn infant. J Pediatr 1955;46: 158-59.
61. Clark DA. Times of first void and first stool in 500 newborns. Pediatrics 1977;60:457-59.
62. Davis W8, Allen RP I Favara BE, Slovis TL. Neonatal small left colon syndrome. Am J Roentgenol A ad Ther Nucl Med 1974;120:322-29.
63. Clatworthy HW, Howard WHR, Lloyd J. The meconium plug syndrome, Surgery 1956;39:131-42.
64. Bill AH, Chapman ND. The enterocolitis of Hirschsprung's disease. Its natural history and treatment. Am J Surg 1962;103:70-74.
65. Thomas DFM, Fernie DS, Bayston R, et al. Enterocolitis in Hirschsprung's .disease: A controlled study of the etiologic role of Clostridium difficile. J Pediatr Surg 1986;21:22-25.
66. Wilson-Storey D. Microbial studies of enterocolitis in Hirschsprung's disease. Pediatr Surg Int 1994;9:248-50.
67. Carneiro PMA. Brereton RJ, Drake DP, et al. Enterocolitis in Hirschsprung's disease. Pediatr Surg Int 1992;7:356-60.
68. Elhalaby EA, Coran AG, Blane CE, et al. Enterocolitis associated with Hirschsprung's disease: A clinical radiological characterization based on 168 patients. J Pediatr Surg 1995;30:76-83.
69. Newman B, Nussbaum A, Kirkpatrick JA. Bowel perforation in Hirschsprung's disease. Am J Roentgenol 1987;148:1195-97.
70. Dobbins WO. Bill AH. Diagnosis or Hlrscncnsprung's diseases excluded by rectal suction biopsy. N Engl J Med 1965;272:990-93.
71. Aldridge AT, Campbell PE, Ganglion cell distribution in the normal rectum and anal canal. A basis for the diagnosis of Hirschsprung's disease by anorectal biopsy. J Pediatr Surg 1968;3:475-90.
72. Noblett HA. A rectal suction biopsy tube for use in the diagnosis of Hirschsprung's disease. J Pediatr Surg 1969;4:406-09.
73. Shandling B, Auldist AW. Punch biopsy of the rectum for the diagnosis of Hirschsprung's disease. J Pediatr Surg 1972;7:546-51.
74. Aees 81, Azmy A, Nigam M, Lake BD. Complications of rectal suction biopsy. J Pediatr Surg 1983;18:273-75.
75. Lawson JON, Nixon HH. Anal canal pressures in the diagnosis of Hirschsprung's disease. J Pediatr Surg 1967;2:544-52.
76. Hope JW, Borns PF, Berg PK. Roentgenologic manifestations of Hirschsprung's disease in infancy. Am J Roentgenol 1965;95:217-29.
77. Smith GHH, Cass D. Infantile Hirschsprung's disease -is a barium enema useful? Pediatr Surg Int 1991;6:318-21.
78. Taxman TL, Yulish BS, Rothstein FC. How useful is the barium enema in the diagnosis of infantile Hirschsprung's disease? Am J Dis Child 1986;140:881-84.
79. Rosenfield NS. Ablow RC. Markowitz RI, et al. Hirschsprung disease: Accuracy of the barium enema examination, Radiology 1984;150:393-400.
80. Maia DM, The reliability of frozen-section diagnosis in the pathologic evaluation of Hirschsprung's disease. Am J Surg Pathol 2000;24:1675-77.
81. Duhamel B. Une nouvelle operation pour le megacolon congenitale: L'abaissement retro-rectal et trans-anal du colon at son application possible au traitement de qualques autres malformations, Presse Med 1956;64:2249-51.
82. Duhamel B. A new operation for the treatment of Hirschsprung's disease, Arch Dis Child 1960;35:36-39.

83. Soave F. Eine neue Methode zur chirurgischen Behandlung des Morbus Hirschsprung. Zentralb f Chir 1963;31:1241-49.
84. Soave F. A new surgical technique for treatment of Hirschsprung's disease Surgery, 1964;56:1007-14.
85. Rehbein F in Kinderchirurgische Operationen, Hippokrates, Stuttgart 1976;309.
86. State D. Surgical treatment for idiopathic congenital megacolon (Hirschsprung's disease). Surg Gynecol Obstetr 1952;9:201-12.
87. De la Torre-Mondragon L, Ortega-Salgado JA. Transanal endorectal pull-through for Hirschsprung's disease. J Pediatr Surg 1998;33:1283-86.
88. Boley SJ. New modification of the surgical treatment of Hirschsprung's disease, Surgery 1964;56:1015-17.
89. Tsuji H, Spitz L, Kiely EM, et al. Management and long-term follow-up of infants with total colonic aganglionosis. J Pediatr Surg 1999;34:158-62.
90. Stringer MD, Brereton RJB, Drake DP, et al. Meconium ileus due to extensive intestinal aganglionosis. J Pediatr Surg 1994;29:501-03.
91. Ratta BS, Kjely EM, Spitz L, Brereton RJ. Improvements in the management to total colonic aganglionosis, Pediatr Surg Int 1990;5:30-36.
92. Nihoul-Fekete C, Ricour Q, Martelli H, et al. Total colonic aganglionosis (with of without ileal involvement): A review of 27 cases J Pediatr Surg 1986;21:251-54.
93. Martin LW. Surgical management of Hirschsprung's disease involving the small intestine Arch Surg 1968;97:183-90.
94. Schwarz KB, Ternberg JL, Bell MJ, Keating JP. Sodium needs of infants and children with ileostomy. J Pediatr 1983;102:509-13.
95. Ziegler MM, Royal RE, Brandt J, et al. Extended myectomy-myotomy. A therapeutic alternative for total intestinal aganglionosis. Ann Surg 1993;218:504-11.
96. Nixon HH. Personal communication.
97. Fonkalsrud EW. Early post-operative complications following treatment of Hirschsprung's disease and allied disorders in: Hirschsprung's disease and allied disorders (2000) 2nd Edition p425-431 Eds. Holschneider H, Puri P. Harwood Academic Publishers, Singapore.
98. Swenson O, Sherman JO, Fisher JH, Cohen E. The treatment and postoperative complications of congenital megacolon: A 25 year follow-up, Ann Surg 1975;182: 266-73.
99. Engum SA, Grosfeld JL. Hirschsprung's disease: Duhamel pull-through in: Pediatric surgery and urology: Long-term outcomes Eds. Stringer MD, 01dham KT, Mouriquand PDE, Howard ER, WB Saunders, London 1998;329-39.
100. Polley TZ, Coran AG, Wesley JR, A ten year experience with ninety two cases of Hirschsprung's disease. Including sixty-seven consecutive endorectal pull through procedures. Ann Surg 1985;202:349-55.
101. Langer JC, Fitzgerald PG, Winthrop AL, et al. One stage versus two stage Soave pull through for Hirschsprung's disease in the first year of life. J Pediatr Surg 1996;31: 33-37.
102. Wright V, Cord Udy C. Hirschsprung's disease: Endorectal pull through in: Pediatric Surgery and Urology (2000) 2nd Edition p. 340-8. Eds. Holschneider AM, Puri P. Harwood Academic Publishers, Singapore.
103. Teitelbaum OH, Cilley RE, Sherman NJ, et al. A decade of experience with the primary pull-through for Hirschsprung's disease in the newborn period. A multicenter analysis of outcomes. Ann Surg 2000;232:372-80.
104. Mishalany HG, Woolley MM. Postoperative functional and manometric evaluation of patients with Hirschsprung's disease. J Pediatr Surg 1987;22:443-46.
105. Rescorla FJ, Morrison AM, Engles D, et al. Hirschsprung's disease. Evaluation of mortality and long-term function in 260 cases, Arch Surg 1992;127:934-42.
106. Catto-Smith AG, Coffey CMM, Nolan TM, Hutson JM. Fecal incontinence after the surgical treatment of Hirschsprung disease. J Pediatr 1995;127:954-57.
107. Yanchar NL, Soucy P. Long term oucome after Hirschsprung's disease: patients' perspectives. J Pediatr Surg 1999;34:1152-60.
108. Wilcox DT I Kiely EM. Repeat pull-through for Hirschsprung's disease J Pediatr Surg 1998:33:1507-09.
109. van Leeuwen K, Teitelbaum OH, Elhalaby EA, Coran AG, Long-term follow-up of redo pull-through procedures for Hirschsprung's disease: efficacy of the endorectal pull-through, J Pediatr Surg 2000;35:829-33.
110. West KW, Grosfeld JL, Rescorla FJ, Vane OW. Acquired aganglionosis: A rare occurrence following pull-through procedures for Hirschsprung's disease. J Pediatr Surg 1990;25:104-09.
111. De Caluwe D, Yoneda A, Akl U, Puri P. Internal anal sphincter achalasia: outcome after internal sphincter myectomy. J Pediatr Surg 2001;36:736-38.
112. Pierro A, Fasoli L, Kiely EM, et al. Staged pull-through for rectosigmoid Hirschsprung's disease is not safer than primary pull-through. J Pediatr Surg 1997;32:505-09.
113. Albanese CT, Jennings RW, Smith B, et al. Perineal one-stage pull-through for Hirschsprung's disease J Pediatr Surg 1999;34:377-80.
114. Langer JC, Seifert M, Minkes RK. One-stage Soave pull-through for Hirschsprung's disease: A comparison of the transanal and open approaches. J Pediatr Surg 2000;35: 820-22.
115. Georgeson KE, Cohen AD, Hebra A, et al. Primary laparoscopic-assisted endorectal colon pull-through for Hirschsprung's disease: A new gold standard. Ann Surg 1999;229:678-83.
116. Meier-Ruge W. Uber ein Erkrankengshild des Colon mit Hirschsprung-Symptomatik Verh Dtsch Ges Pathol 1971;55:506-09.
117. Csury L, Pena A. Intestinal neuronal dysplasia. Myth or reality? Literature review. Pediatr Surg Int 1995;10: 441-46.
118. Holschneider AM, Puri P. Intestinal neuronal dysplasia in: Hirschsprung's disease and allied disorders (2000) 2nd Edition, p. 147-154 Eds. Holschneider AM, Puri P. Harwood Academic Publishers, Singapore.

Total Colonic Aganglionosis

Lester W Martin

The author's personal experience with total colon aganglionosis includes a total of 45 patients seen over a period of 40 years. Since the first patient in 1959, the author has struggled both clinically and in the laboratory with several methods of preserving and utilizing a portion of the colon for the dual purposes of acting as a storage reservoir and at the same time, reabsorption of liquid in order to decrease stool frequency. A number of other investigators have contributed significantly to the pool of knowledge, reporting their experience and suggestions for modifications of the surgical approach.[1-13] A side-to-side anastomosis of the entire colon to the ileum at one time appeared to be a satisfactory solution, but after several years persistent colonic distention proved to be a problem.[14] Side-to-side anastomosis of the entire left colon and rectum to the distal ileum as an extended Duhamel procedure has been the authors standard operation for a number of years, but occasional problems with incomplete evacuation and recurrent enterocolitis prompted further modifications.[2,9,15-18] In our current method, the author has decreased the length of the reservoir and placed it entirely within the pelvis in an extraperitoneal location which affords more effective evacuation. The author also excises more of the posterior portion of the internal anal sphincter because of the frequency of the tight internal sphincter syndrome if the entire sphincter is retained.[19,20]

DIAGNOSIS

The diagnosis must be considered in any child with suspected Hirschsprung's disease.[8,21,22] Radiographic examination with contrast enema demonstrating retention of contrast within a nondilated colon for 24 hours is further suggestive, but the diagnosis is confirmed by rectal biopsy. The proximal extent of the aganglionosis is determined at the time of operation by serial extramucosal seromuscular biopsies obtained at progressively more proximal levels from the colon wall. Appendiceal aganglionosis may occur in the presence of normal ganglia in the ascending and transverse colon and therefore cannot be relied upon when establishing the level of the transition zone.

ILEOSTOMY

The author prefers a 3-stage operative approach. The first operation confirms the diagnosis, determines the extent of the aganglionosis, and creates an end ileostomy. The author prefers a midline incision above the umbilicus. Seromuscular extramucosal biopsies are obtained from the sigmoid colon, then from progressively higher levels until dilated, ganglionated bowel is encountered. Each biopsy is carefully labeled and examined by frozen section technique. When ganglionated bowel is confirmed, which is generally at the level of the dilated bowel and within 10-25 cm proximal to the ileocecal junction, this point is selected for the ileostomy. The small bowel is transected and the ileostomy established through a separate incision to the right of the working incision. The stoma is immediately matured by full thickness turnback and is located so as to most readily accommodate an appliance. The distal end of the ileum is exteriorized as a mucous fistula through the upper end of the working incision. This non-functioning stoma affords a convenient port for colonic irrigations and instillation of topical agents in preparation of this aperistaltic bowel for subsequent surgery. It also provides a vent for decompression to help prevent fulminant diversion colitis which can develop in the totally diverted aganglionic colon and result in complete obliteration of the lumen or even loss of the entire full thickness of colon.

DEFINITIVE OPERATION

The author prefers to defer the definitive operation until the infant is near one year of age and weighs approximately 20 pounds (9 kg). The pelvis at this age, is of sufficient size to accommodate the mechanical GIA stapler for the pelvic anastomosis. Also, the author has found the rectal anastomosis (described below) which is the critical part of the operation, can be performed much more acurately and with superior results in the one- year- old as compared to doing the procedure on the newborn infant since the one-year-old is quadruple the size of a newborn. The elected age of one year allows ample time after the completed surgery for toilet training. During the interim period, before the definitive operation, enteral feedings are supplemented, if necessary, with parenteral alimentation.

To minimize gross contamination of the operative field, mechanical cleansing of the gut lumen is essential. Oral Go-Lytley*, or one of its variants, provides excellent preoperative mechanical cleansing of the functional small bowel, but cannot be depended upon to cleanse the distal defunctioned aganglionic bowel.

Preoperative mechanical cleansing of the aganglionic defunctioned distal ileum and colon is difficult to achieve because of the absence of peristalsis. Rectal irrigations, irrigations through the distal ileal mucous fistula, and installation of topical antibiotics are all employed; but after vigorous attempts at bowel cleansing, it may still be found upon opening the abdomen, that there is considerable residual stool within the aganglionic colon. Consequently, the surgeon must resort to intraoperative measures of mechanical irrigation as described below.

The patient is placed in the lithotomy position with the operating table in 10-12° Trendelenburg with the buttocks protruding 2-3 inches beyond the end of the table and elevated on one or two folded towels. The patient is prevented from slipping cephalad on the table with either shoulder straps or adhesive strapping over the shoulders behind the patient's back, and attached to the foot end of the table. An indwelling Foley catheter is placed in the bladder and a nasogastric tube placed to empty the stomach and is either left in place postoperatively or replaced by a gastrostomy tube at the end of the procedure. We avoid using nitrous oxide anesthesia because of its association with uncontrollable intestinal distention. A #28 or #30 French size catheter is inserted into the rectum and taped in position. The antiseptic preparation of the skin of the abdomen includes the stoma in a widely draped operative field.

The abdomen is opened through the old midline scar, extending the incision around the umbilicus and distally as far as necessary to provide adequate exposure. Any residual inspissated stool found in the aganglionic colon must be removed without contamination of the operative field. To accomplish this, an assistant from outside the sterile operative field, instills physiologic saline solution through the indwelling rectal tube. The surgeon then manipulates the colon to detach the particles of stool and force them out through and around the tube. This procedure is repeated until the returns are clear and the colon is free of palpable stool. This is then followed by an irrigation once with an antiseptic solution then irrigate once with an antiseptic solution and the rectal tube is left open to drainage. The ileostomy is detached from the abdominal wall, and in order to provide sufficient length for the end of the ileum to reach the anus without tension, the mucosa of the ileostomy, which had previously been turned back for maturation is carefully unfolded. The mesentery of the terminal ileum is lengthened by incision, carefully preserving its blood supply. An opening is then created in the pelvic peritoneum posterior to, but immediately adjacent to the rectal wall. Blunt dissection is continued distally to the level of the levator muscles.

The surgeon then moves to the perineal portion of the operation. The rectum is further irrigated and the perineum is prepared and draped as a separate sterile field. Retraction sutures are placed to provide exposure. With electrocautery an incision is made through the mucosa only, at the level of the top of the columns of Morgagnii and extended around the posterior 180° of the anorectal circumference (Fig. 62.1). The transitional epithelium overlying the columns can be rolled downward by gentle gauze

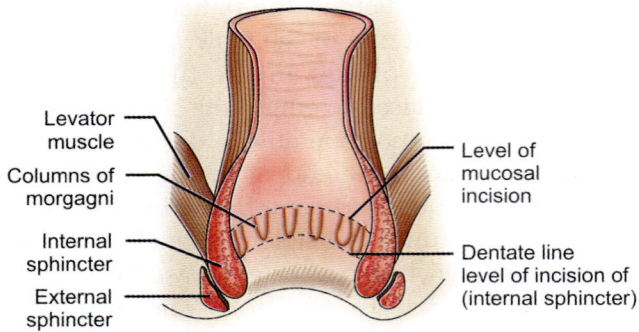

Fig. 62.1: Longitudinal section of rectum showing the level of mucosal incision in relation to columns of Morgagni and dentate line (level of incision of internal sphincter)

traction with the left hand while the right hand dissects the mucosa from the underlying muscle layer, which is the internal sphincter. Dissection is continued distally as far as the level of the dentate line (distal extent of the anal columns). At the level of the dentate line, the muscle layer (internal sphincter) is incised transversely for the entire 180°; then the plane of dissection is directed upwards between the posterior rectal wall and the puborectalis sling to connect to the presacral dissection plane previously established from above. The objective is to remove the portion of the internal sphincter located above the dentate line throughout the entire posterior 180°. The overlying transitional epithelium is preserved in order to preserve sensation for autonomic, involuntary continence of liquid ileal stool. The author's experience with the continence-preserving operation for over 200 patients with ulcerative colitis with liquid ileal stool has convinced us of the necessity for preserving this transitional epithelium which contains the sensory fibers of the autonomic reflex arc controlling involuntary night-time continence.[23] The author's experience also strongly suggests that removal of the portion of the internal sphincter above the level of the dentate line is necessary to minimize the problem of the tight postoperative sphincter associated with colonic distention with dilatation and postoperative enterocolitis. Removal of the portion of the internal sphincter above the dentate line has not interfered with continence in the author's patients.[19] The fibers located distal to the dentate line are adequate for control.[20] In fact, postoperative manual dilatations are still sometimes required.

The end of the ganglionated ileum (ileostomy site) is then withdrawn through the pelvis with its mesentery directed posteriorly towards the sacrum. The posterior 180° of the open end of the ileum is anastomosed to the preserved transitional anal mucosa with interrupted absorbable sutures. Since this is a one-layer mucosal anastomosis, it is imperative that there be no tension on the suture line. The GIA stapler is then applied twice to cut out a triangular segment of the opposing walls of the rectum and ileum (Fig. 62.2). The base of the triangle includes the posterior 180° of the rectum and anterior 180° of ileum. The apex of the triangle is at the tip of the stapler. Because of the potential for septal regrowth and to further assure hemostasis, the author then oversews the staple line on each side with a continuous lock stitch of absorbable suture starting at the lower end. The suture line is easily retracted downwards by traction applied to the suture in order to provide exposure for progressively higher placement of each stitch and the suture line is continued upwards to within 1 cm of the apex.

The surgeon then returns to the abdominal field and with electrocautery a longitudinal incision is made in the adjacent (opposing) anti-mesenteric walls of the ileum and rectum, thus entering the lumen of each, extending the incisions distally to where the ileum and rectum are stapled together. A right angle clamp can then be inserted into one opening and passed beneath the septum represented by the apex of the triangle of

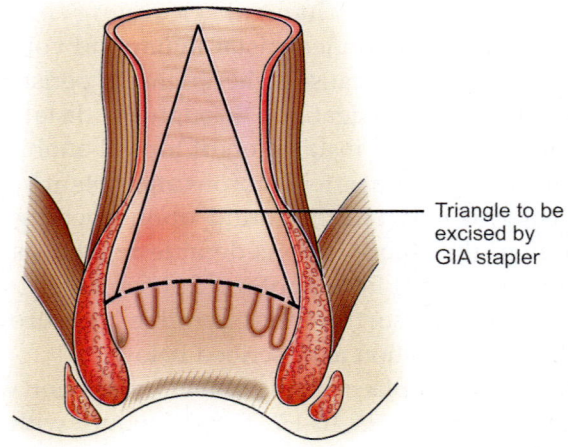

Fig. 62.2: Longitudinal section of rectum showing triangle of posterior rectal wall and opposing anterior wall of ileum to be excised with GIA stapler

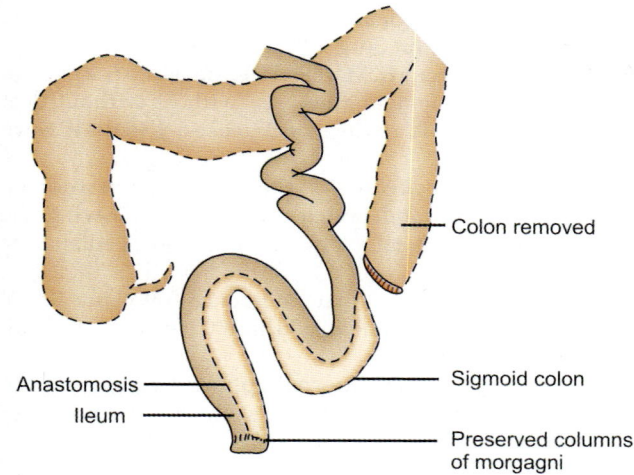

Fig. 62.3: Drawing of completed operation with broken line indicating amount of aganglionic colon which is excised

rectal and ileal wall previously excised from below. This residual septum is divided with electrocautery and the surgeon can then continue the suture lines (which were started from below) proximally on each side to complete the long side-to-side anastomosis by either hand suturing or with multiple applications of the GIA stapler. The small bowel and colon can be intussuscepted through the enterotomy by traction for each subsequent application of the clamp. When the anastomosis has been completed as far as the junction of the sigmoid and the descending colon, the colon proximal to the completed anastomosis is resected, along with the attached segment aganglionic of ileum (Fig. 62.3). The aganglionic colon has defective peristalsis and if left in place, can fill with stool, which can inspissate, then calcify and cause ulceration and perforation of the colon.

The author's usual postoperative routine has included a proximal diverting, divided ileostomy to divert the fecal stream and avoid any possibility of leakage of the long extraperitoneal anastomotic suture line. The ileostomy is closed after three months. A contrast enema is obtained to confirm the integrity of the anastomotic suture line prior to ileostomy closure. A digital rectal examination is also performed to confirm healing with pliable tissues and no bleeding and to determine that there has been no septal regrowth.

On three occasions when the remaining small bowel was short and the author was confident of the integrity of the anastomosis, the author has as an alternative to diversion, elected instead to utilize 10 days of total parenteral feedings and strict nothing by mouth with satisfactory results. The author feels more secure; however, with a temporary totally diverting proximal ileostomy, which is subsequently closed by resection and end-to-end anastomosis.

RESULTS

The operation as described above has evolved over a period of 40 years based on the author's personal experience with 45 patients. In addition, the numerous reports, comments, and suggestions from friends and colleagues from around the world have been of great value in modification of the technique and improving the results.[24,25]

Numerous complications were encountered in our earlier experience but all patients recovered and are now leading essentially normal lives. In our more recent patients, the only problems encountered have been related to a tight sphincter in 25% of the patients. This has usually been easily overcome by insertion of a #38 French rectal tube at home by the parent and has occurred only during the first year.

For the first year or two following operation, bowel habits are often irregular, sometimes occurring only at night during sleep. By the age of approximately 5 years, however, all have complete control with movements two or three times daily. There have been no deaths related to the operation.

REFERENCES

1. Boley SJ. A new operative approach to total colonic aganglionosis. Surg Gynecol Obstet 1984;159:481-84.
2. Burrington JD, Wayne ER. Modified Duhamel procedure for treatment of total aganglionic colon in children. J Pediatr Surg 1976;11:391-92.
3. Dorman G. Universal aganglionosis of the colon. Arch Surg 1957;75:906-09.
4. Endo M, Watanabe K, Fuchimoto Y, Ikawa H, Yokoyama J. Long-term results of surgical treatment in infants with total colonic anganglionosis. J Pediatr Surg 1994;29: 13101-04.
5. Goto S, Gunter M, Scherer LR, Bloch T, Grosfeld J. Surgical treatment of total colonic aganglionosis: efficacy of aganglionic patch enteroplasty in the rat. J Pediatr Surg 1986;21:601-07.
6. Ikeda K., Goto S. Total colonic aganglionosis with or without small bowel involvement: an analysis of 137 patients. J Pediatr Surg 1986;21:319-22.

7. Kimura K, Nishijima E, Muraji T, Tsugawa C, Matsutmo Y. Extensive aganglionosis: further experience with the colonic patch graft procedure and long-term results. J Pediatr Surg 1988;23:52-56.
8. Kleinhaus S, Boley SJ, Sheran M, Sieber WK. Hirschsprung's disease. A survey of the members of the surgical section of the American Academy of Pediatrics. J Pediatr Surg 1979;14:588-97.
9. Martin LW. Surgical management of Hirschsprung's disease involving the small intestine. Arch Surg 1968;97:183-89.
10. Pellerin D, Nihoul-Fekete C, Bertin P. An extensive form of Hirschsprung's disease treated by Lester Martin's ileocoloplasty. Ann Chir Infant 12:71 Abstract. J Pediatr Surg 1971;23:725-27.
11. Prevot J, Joly A, Babut J. La technique de Lester Martin dans le traitement de la maladie de Hirschsprung a forme colique totale. Annals de Chirurgie Infantile Paris 1976;17:103-12.
12. Ross MN, Chang JHT, Burrington JD, Janik JS, Wagner ER, Clevenger P. Complications of the Martin procedure for total colonic aganglionosis. J Pediatr Surg 1988;23:725-27.
13. Ziegler MM, Ross AL, Bishop HC. Total intestinal aganglionosis: a new technique for prolonged survival. J Pediatr Surg 1987;22:82-88.
14. Martin LW. Total colon aganglionosis: preservation and utilization of entire colon. J Pediatr Surg 1982;17:635-37.
15. Duhamel B. A new operation for the treatment of Hirschsprung's disease. Arch Dis Child 1960;85:38-39.
16. Martin LW. Surgical management of total colonic aganglionosis. Ann Surg 1972;176:343-46.
17. N-Fekete C, Ricour C, Martelli H, Lortat Jacob S, Zpellerin D. Total colonic aganglionosis (with or without ileal involvement): A review of 27 cases. J Pediatr Surg 1986;21:251-54.
18. Perrault J, Stockwell M, Stephens C, Forstner G. Malabsorption and pouch ulcerations following the Martin repair for total colonic aganglionosis. J Pediatr Surg 1979;14:458-61.
19. Martin L, Fischer J. Anal continence following Soave procedure: analysis and results in 100 patients. Ann Surg 1986;203:525-30.
20. Swenson O. Partial internal sphincterectomy in the treatment of Hirschsprung's disease. Ann Surg 1964;160:540-45.
21. Bodian M. Chronic constipation in children with particular reference to Hirschsprung's disease. Practitioner 1952;169:517-21.
22. Sieber WK. Hirschsprung's disease. Chapter 106. Pediatric Surgery 4th Edition. Year Book Medical Publishers, Chicago 1986;995-1016.
23. Martin L, Torres A, Fischer J, Alexander F. The critical level for preservation of continence in the ileoanal anastomosis. J Pediatr Surg 1985;20:664-67.
24. Coran AG, Bjordal R, Eck S. Surgical management of total colonic and partial small intestine aganglionosis. J Pediatr Surg 1969;4:531-37.
25. Passarge E. Genetics of Hirschsprung's disease. Clin Gastroenterol 1973;2:507-13.

Variant Hirschsprung's Disease

Prem Puri

The typical patient with Hirschsprung's disease is a newborn presenting with delayed passage of meconium and abdominal distension or a young child presenting with severe chronic constipation. The diagnosis is confirmed by the histological and histochemical evaluation of suction rectal biopsies which demonstrate absence of ganglion cells in the submucosa and increased acetylcholinesterase (AChE) activity in the lamina propria. However, there are a number of patients who clinically resemble Hirschsprung's disease despite the presence of ganglion cells in rectal biopsy. Various terms have been used to describe these conditions such as "chronic idiopathic intestinal pseudoobstruction", "pseudo-Hirschsprung's disease", "neonatal intestinal pseudo-obstruction" and "intestinal hypoperistalsis syndrome". There is a growing interest to further investigate these relatively rare functional bowel disorders, since the diagnosis and management of these patients continues to be a challenge for clinicians. Over the past two decades our group has focused its research interest into delineating variant Hirschsprung's disease based on specific histochemical, immunohistochemical and electronmicroscopic studies.

Since 1981, it has been the author's policy to obtain suction rectal biopsy specimens from patients who have severe chronic constipation or are suspected to have functional intestinal obstruction. The suction rectal biopsy specimens are obtained at 3, 5 and 7 cm from the pectinate line and examined by conventional hematoxylin and eosin (HandE) staining, histochemistry and immunocytochemical staining. If the results of suction rectal biopsy show normal AChE activity in lamina propria and muscularis mucosae with normally appearing ganglion cells or without ganglion cells, and the patient continues to have signs and symptoms of obstruction or severe constipation, we perform a full-thickness rectal biopsy. Immediately after the biopsy specimen is obtained, the tissue is divided into four parts and processed for HandE staining, AChE histochemistry, NADPH-diaphorase histochemistry, immunohistochemistry (PGP9.5, peripherin, nNOS, NCAM, NGFR and c-kit) and electronmicroscopic studies. If necessary further full-thickness bowel biopsies or seromuscular bowel biopsies are obtained for additional investigations using whole-mount preparation technique.

Between 1981 and 2003, full-thickness bowel biopsy or resected surgical specimens from 151 patients (61 boys and 90 girls) with clinical symptoms suggesting HD, were examined in our research laboratory. Their ages ranged from 1 day to 9 years. One hundred and three patients had onset of symptoms in the neonatal period. Eighty-three patients were from Ireland and in 68 patients, biopsy material was sent to our laboratory from other countries. Table 63.1 shows various functional bowel disorders diagnosed using different histological techniques.

Table 63.1: Variant Hirschsprung's disease (1981-2007)	
Intestinal neuronal dysplasia	73
Hypoganglionosis	17
Immature ganglia	9
Internal sphincter achalasia	41
Smooth muscle disorders	22
Total	**162**

INTESTINAL NEURONAL DYSPLASIA

Intestinal neuronal dysplasia (IND), a clinical condition that resembles Hirschsprung's disease (HD), was first described by Meier-Ruge in 1971 as a malformation of the enteric plexus.[1] In 1983, Fadda et al subclassified IND into two clinically and histologically distinct subtypes.[2] Type A occurs in less than 5% of cases, is characterized by congenital aplasia or hypoplasia of the sympathetic innervation, and presents acutely in the neonatal period with episodes of intestinal obstruction, diarrhea and bloody stools. The clinical picture of Type B resembles HD and is characterized by malformation of the parasympathetic submucous and myenteric plexuses and accounts for over 95% of cases of isolated IND. IND occurring in association with HD is of Type B. The characteristic histologic features of IND B include hyperganglionosis of the submucous and myenteric plexuses, giant ganglia, ectopic ganglion cells, and increased acetylcholinesterase (AChE) activity in the lamina propria and around submucosal blood vessels.[3,4]

The incidence of isolated IND has varied from 0.3 to 40% of all suction rectal biopsies in different centers.[5-8] IND immediately proximal to a segment of aganglionosis is not uncommon and often presents as persistent obstructive symptoms after a pull-through operation for HD.[9] Some investigators have reported that 25 to 35% of patients with HD have associated IND.[2,3,9] However, others have rarely encountered IND in association with HD.[10] The uncertainty regarding the incidence of IND has resulted from the considerable confusion regarding the essential diagnostic criteria.[11] The diagnostic difficulty is centered on a wide variability encountered in the literature, not only in terms of age of the patient, the type of specimen examined and the stains performed, but also the diagnostic criteria used.[11] Many investigators have raised doubts about the existence of IND as a distinct histopathologic entity.[12-14] It has been suggested that the pathologic changes seen in IND may be part of normal development or may be a secondary phenomenon induced by congenital obstruction and inflammatory disease.[14,15] One strong piece of evidence that IND is a real entity stems from animal models. Recently, two different *Hox11L1* knockout mouse models have been generated. In both cases, homozygous mutant mice were viable, but megacolon developed at the age of 3 to 5 weeks. Histological and immunohistochemical analyses showed hyperplasia of myenteric ganglia, a phenotype similar to that observed in IND.[16-18] However, the mutation screening of this gene in 48 patients with IND did not show any sequence variant, either causative missense mutation, or neutral substitution.[19] More recently Von Boyen et al reported abnormalities of the enteric nervous system in heterozygous endothelin B receptor (EDNRB)-deficient rats resembling IND in humans.[20] They showed that a heterozygous 301-bp deletion of the EDNRB gene led to abnormalities of the submucous plexus, such as giant ganglia, hyperganglionosis and hypertrophy of the nerve fiber strands. These findings support the concept that IND may be linked to a genetic defect.

Since the first description in 1971, most controversy surrounding IND has been regarding which histologic diagnostic criteria are required for definitive diagnosis. The presently recognized diagnostic criteria, previously reported by our group and supported by others, are hyperganglionosis and giant ganglia, in addition to the presence of at least 1 of the following on suction rectal biopsy: ectopic ganglia in the lamina propria, increased AChE-positive nerve fibers around submucosal blood vessels and in the lamina propria.[3,4,11,21,22] However, Lumb and Moore feel that giant ganglia can be a normal feature in normal bowel having identified them in segments of adult bowel removed during surgery for colorectal carcinoma.[23] To overcome the confusion in diagnostic criteria, Borchard et al, produced guidelines for identifying IND in mucosal rectal biopsies.[24] These comprised two obligatory criteria (hyperplasia of the submucous plexus and an increase in AChE-positive nerve fibers around submucosal blood vessels) and 2 additional criteria (neuronal heterotopia and increased AChE activity in the lamina propria). In the author's experience, hyperganglionosis and giant ganglia are the most important features for the diagnosis of IND in suction rectal biopsies, except in the newborn, where hyperganglionosis is a normal finding.[4]

Another controversial area surrounding IND is whether the histologic findings are age-related. The recent description of hyperganglionosis, considered to be one of the most important criteria of IND, as an age-dependent finding, has caused further confusion. Recent studies have found that the enteric nervous system continues to develop in the postnatal period.

Wester et al investigated the number of ganglion cells per ganglion and ganglion cell density in whole-mount preparations of the submucous plexus of normal distal colon and found a marked decrease of ganglion cells density with increasing age, but the number of ganglion cells per ganglion remained constant.[25,26] Knowledge of the ganglion cell density of the normal human enteric nervous system is scantly, apparent by the huge variation among reports of the normal neuron density in the myenteric plexus. The reported density varies more than 200 times among the different studies.[27-30] This results in difficulties defining conditions such as hyperganglionosis. Schofield and Yunis reported that 8.3% of 456 investigated cases had features of IND, using increased AChE activity in the lamina propria and hyperganglionosis (defined as more than 5 ganglia per high-power field in the submucosa) as diagnostic criteria.[31,32] These patients had a high incidence of prematurity, indicating that some histological features of IND may be related to age and development. Age-related alterations of the enteric ganglia were discussed further by Smith, who described a significantly higher number of submucous ganglia in children under 4 weeks of age compared with older children.[10] It would be desirable with better knowledge of the enteric nervous system and also with quantitative diagnostic criteria of IND to distinguish normal variation from pathological conditions. Moore et al introduced a morphological scoring system based on the findings of hyperganglionosis, giant ganglia, maturity of neurons, heterotopic neuronal cells and AChE activity in the lamina propria, muscularis mucosa or adventitia of submucosal blood vessels.[33] Hyperganglionosis and increased AChE activity of nerve fibers in the lamina propria were of major importance in this scoring system.

Suction rectal biopsy is the principal method for the diagnosis of disorders of intestinal innervation. It is necessary to include a sufficient amount of submucosa in the suction biopsy specimens. Traditionally, hematoxylin and eosin staining and AChE histochemistry (Figs 63.1A to C) in suction rectal biopsy specimens have provided the basis for the diagnostic evaluation of IND. However, there has been discussion about whether AChE histochemistry is sufficient for the accurate diagnosis of IND and other additional staining techniques have been proposed. Meier-Ruge et al suggest lactate-dehydrogenase histochemistry.[34,35] In the author's laboratory, newer neuronal markers currently are being used, such as reduced nicotinamide-adenine dinuleotide phosphate (NADPH) diaphorase histochemistry and immunohistochemistry using antibodies raised against neural cell adhesion molecule, Protein Gene Product 9.5 (PGP9.5), S-100, Peripherin and Synaptophysin. Ganglion-cell counting can be difficult. Standard Immunohistochemical techniques, using antibodies raised against neuron specific enolase or PGP 9.5, which are commonly used to display the enteric nervous system, are less suitable for cell counting because they stain not only the cell bodies but also the

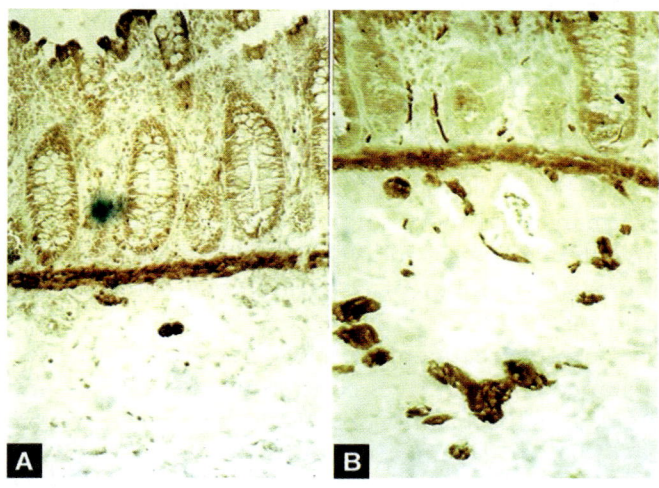
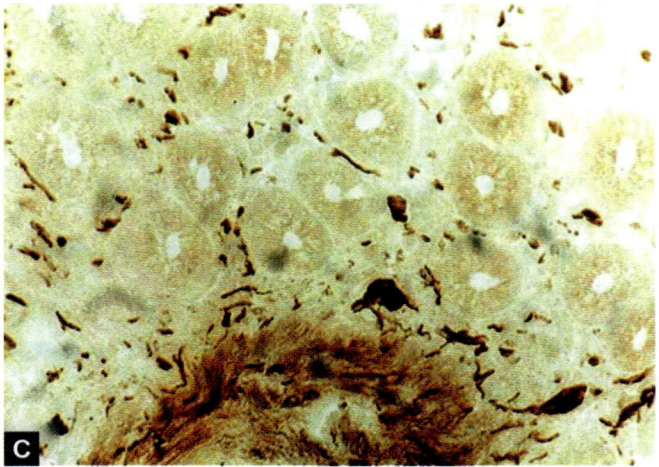

Figs 63.1A to C: AChE staining **A.** Normal rectal suction biopsy **B.** Rectal suction biopsy from a patient with IND showing hyperganglionosis, giant ganglia and increased AChE activity in the lamina propria **C.** ganglia cells in the lamina propria in IND (original magnification x125)

axonal processes. Recently, cuprolinic blue staining has been proposed as the method that stains the largest number of ganglion cells.[26] Furthermore, this method stains only the cell bodies and not the axons, which makes it relatively easy to distinguish the individual cells. The whole-mount preparation elegantly shows 3-dimensional morphology of the submucous and myenteric plexuses in IND, demonstrating markedly increased number of ganglion cells compared to controls.

Current treatment of IND Type B is in the first instance conservative, consisting of laxatives and enemas. In the majority of patients the clinical problem resolves or is manageable in this way. If bowel symptoms persist after at least 6 months of treatment, internal sphincter myectomy should be considered. Recently Gillick et al reported results of treatment in 33 patients with IND followed-up for periods ranging from 1 to 8 years (mean, 2.4 years).[36] Twenty-one (64%) patients had a good response to conservative management and currently had normal bowel habits. Twelve patients (36%) underwent internal sphincter myectomy after failed conservative management. Seven of these patients now had normal bowel habits. Two patients were able to stay clean with regular enemas. Three patients who continued to have persistent constipation after myectomy and underwent resection of redundant and dilated sigmoid colon now have normal bowel habits. Scharli reported that 13 of the 22 cases required internal sphincter myectomy, which resulted in satisfactory results in 90% of the patients within 3 months. Resection and pull-through operation is rarely indicated in IND. The indication for surgery should not be determined on the basis of histopathological findings alone: rather the decision must be based on the individual patient's clinical symptoms.

HYPOGANGLIONOSIS

Isolated hypoganglionosis is rare. Clinically, it resembles HD.[5,37,38] Failure to pass meconium may be the first symptom in the neonatal period, whereas infants and older children present with chronic constipation. The diagnosis of hypoganglionosis by means of suction biopsy is difficult. Rectal suction biopsy results with absent or low level of AChE activity in the lamina propria and absence or reduction of submucosal ganglion cells may raise suspicion of hypoganglionosis. A full-thickness rectal biopsy allows the inspection of the myenteric plexus and is essential for the diagnosis of hypoganglionosis. The characteristic histologic features of hypoganglionosis include sparse and small myenteric ganglia, absent or low AChE activity in the lamina propria, hypertrophy of muscularis mucosae and circular muscle.[39] Meier-Ruge et al performed morphometric measurements in resected bowel specimens from patients with hypoganglionosis and found a dramatic decrease in plexus area and nerve cell number in the myenteric plexus and an increase in distance between ganglia.[40]

Gut innervation has a complex, 3-dimensional structure, which is difficult to appreciate on thin sections. The whole-mount preparation technique produces a 3-dimensional picture to better show the structure of neuronal networks and their relationship of branching and inter-connecting nerve fibers to each other and to the neighbouring tissues.[21] This technique therefore is especially useful for the investigation of pathologic changes in the submucosal and myenteric plexuses such as hypoganglionosis.[41] The great advantages for the histologic evaluation become obvious when whole-mount preparations are compared with sections.

Recently, a marked reduction in myenteric and muscular c-kit positive interstitial cells of Cajal (ICCS) in the large bowel of patients with isolated hypoganglionosis has been suggested to contribute to motility dysfunction.[42] Furthermore abnormality of the neuromuscular junction has been reported in hypoganglionosis which may further contribute to disturbances in gut motility.[43]

There is little information regarding the genetic basis of isolated hypoganglionosis. Inoue and coworkers performed mutation screening of RET and GDNF gene in children with hypoganglionosis but found no sequence variants, either causative missense mutation or neutral substitution.[44]

Treatment of hypoganglionosis is similar to Hirschsprung's disease involving resection of the affected segment and pull-through operation.

IMMATURE GANGLIA

Immature ganglia are usually seen in the biopsy results from premature infants presenting with functional intestinal obstruction. Acetylcholinesterase staining of suction rectal biopsy specimens show small ganglia and ganglion cells. However, AChE histochemical technique usually fails to distinguish small ganglia from nerve supporting cells (enteric glia). NCAM and NADPH-diaphorase staining methods can usually clearly show small ganglion cells that are same size as enteric glial cells. Cathepsin D has been further used to show the maturation of enteric ganglion cells.[45] The histological proof of maturation of ganglion cells in the myenteric plexus of young infants was accompanied by the improvement of the bowel function, i.e. peristalsis. The treatment of patients with immature ganglia is conservative consisting of laxative and enemas.

INTERNAL SPHINCTER ACHALASIA

The internal anal sphincter (IAS), which is a specialized smooth muscle continuation of the circular muscle layer of the rectum, plays an important role in the maintenance of anorectal continence and in the pathophysiology of incontinence and constipation.[46] The IAS relaxes in response to rectal distension, a phenomenon called the rectosphincteric inhibitory reflex, which is mediated by intramural nerves descending from the rectum to the IAS. The IAS receives adrenergic, cholinergic and nonadrenergic, noncholinergic (NANC) innervation. Several investigators have reported that IAS relaxation is brought about by the activation of intramural NANC nerves. Recently, it has been shown that nitrix oxide (NO) is the NANC neurotransmitter mediating neurogenic relaxation of the human internal sphincter.

Internal anal sphincter achalasia (IASA) is a clinical condition with presentation similar to Hirschsprung's disease but with the presence of ganglion cells on suction rectal biopsy. The diagnosis of IASA is made on anorectal manometry, which shows the absence of rectosphincteric reflex on rectal balloon inflation. Previously, IASA has been referred to as ultrashort segment Hirschsprung's disease (HD).[47] The ultrashort segment Hirschsprung's disease, which is a rare condition, is characterized by an aganglionic segment of 1 to 3 cm long and normal acetylcholinesterase (AChE) activity in the lamina propria and increased AChE activity in the muscularis mucosae.[48] Many patients who are considered to have ultrashort HD on abnormal anorectal manometric findings show presence of ganglion cells and normal acetylcholinesterase (AChE) activity in suction rectal biopsies.

Many investigators have therefore suggested that the term IASA is more suitable because it reflects more accurately failure of relaxation of the internal sphincter, which is the causative factor in this condition.[47,49] The exact pathogenesis and pathophysiology of IASA is not understood fully. Altered intramuscular innervation has been reported in IASA and this is believed to be responsible for the motility dysfunction seen in these patients. Hirakawa et al reported absence of nitrergic innervation within the IAS muscle in patients with IASA and suggested that nitrergic nerve depletion may play an important role in the development of IASA.[46] More recently, Oue and Puri reported defective innervation of the neuromuscular junction (NMJ) of the IAS in patients with IASA.[50] If the NMJ is abnormal, the neurotransmitter chemicals synthesizing neurons cannot be transmitted to muscle cells, thereby causing motility dysfunction. Altered distribution of c-kit positive interstitial cells of Cajal (ICCs) has been reported in the internal sphincter of patients with internal sphincter achalasia which may further contribute to motility dysfunction in these patients.[51]

Posterior internal sphincter myectomy has been recommended as the treatment of choice for patients with internal sphincter achalasia. De Caluwe et al reported bowel function in 15 consecutive patients with IASA 2 to 6 years after posterior internal sphincter myectomy.[52] At the time of follow-up, 7 patients had regular bowel motions and were not on any laxatives. Six patients had normal bowel habits but were on small doses of laxatives. One patient was able to stay clean with regular enema regimen. One patient required resection of dilated and redundant sigmoid colon and now had normal bowel habits with laxatives.

Recently, intra-anal injection of botulinum toxin has been used to treat patients with IASA.[53] This treatment modality has been found to be safe and effective but only short-term treatment in these children.

SMOOTH MUSCLE CELL DISORDERS

These patients who show no apparent innervation abnormalities in the pathologic specimens demonstrate abnormalities of smooth muscle cells on electron-microscopy. The outcome of smooth muscle disorders is usually poor. There are two main types of smooth muscle cell abnormalities (1) perinuclear vacuolation and (2) "central core" degeneration. All total 22 patients in the latter group had Megacystis-microcolon intestinal hypoperistalsis syndrome (MMIHS).

Perinuclear Vacuolation

All 10 patients assessed in this group showed identical findings in the smooth muscle cells such as perinuclear vacuolation with well-preserved mitochondria and an increase in collagen, whereas neuronal components appeared quite normal ultrastructurally. Six of the 10 patients had marked lipofuscin deposition in smooth muscle cells. These patients usually have no peristaltic contractions in the bowel. Nine of the 10 patients in the author's series have died.

Megacystis-microcolon-intestinal Hypoperistalsis Syndrome

Megacystis-microcolon-intestinal hypoperistalsis syndrome (MMIHS) is a rare congenital and generally fatal cause of functional intestinal obstruction in the newborn.[54,55] This syndrome is characterized by abdominal distension caused by a distended non-obstructed urinary bladder, microcolon and decreased or absent intestinal peristalsis (Figs 63.2A and B). Usually incomplete intestinal rotation and shortened small bowel are associated. Although more than 100 cases have been reported in the literature, the etiology of this syndrome is not yet fully understood. Puri et al in 1983 reported two newborns with MMIHS in whom light microscopy of the intestine showed thinning of the longitudinal muscle coat and abundant amounts of connective tissue between the muscle fibers.[56] Electron microscopic evaluation of the smooth muscle cells of the ileum and bladder showed disorganization of myofilaments, cytoplasmic central core "vacuolar type" degeneration and abundant interstitial connective tissue proliferation. These smooth muscle abnormalities are seen in all hollow viscera including urinary bladder and uterus. Since their report, a number of other investigators have confirmed the presence of thinning of the longitudinal muscular coat of the bowel and vacuolation and degeneration in smooth muscle cells of bowel and bladder in this syndrome.[57] More recently, Piotrowska et al reported deficiency of contractile and cystoskeletal proteins in

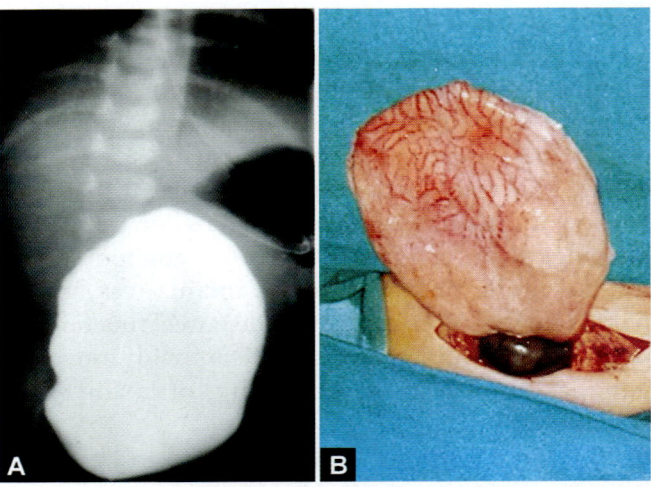

Figs 63.2A and B: A. Voiding cystourethrogram showing massively dilated bladder in a newborn with MMIHS, **B.** Operative photograph of the large urinary bladder in the same patient

smooth muscle cells in MMIHS bowel and Rolle et al reported markedly increased collagen deposits within the bladder wall.[58,59] Furthermore, MMIHS has been reported to be associated with loss or deficiency of interstitial cells of Cajal (ICCs) in the bowel of these patients.[60] ICCs are pacemaker cells which are densely distributed throughout the whole gastrointestinal tract. ICCs have important functions in neurotransmission, generation of slow waves and regulation of mechanical activities in the gastrointestinal tract especially for co-ordinated peristalsis.

The management of patients with MMIHS is frustrating. A number of prokinetic drugs and gastrointestinal hormones have been tried without success. Surgical manipulation of the gastrointestinal tract has generally been unsuccessful. The outcome of this condition is generally fatal. The need for surgical intervention should be made carefully and individualized, in that most explorations have not been helpful and probably are not necessary.

REFERENCES

1. Meier-Ruge W. Ueber ein Erkrankungsbild des Kolon mit Hirschsprung Symptomatik. Ver Deutsch Ges Pathol 1971;55:506-10.
2. Fadda B, Maier WA, Meier-Ruge W, et al. Neuronale intestinale Dysplasie. Eine kritische 2-Jahresanalyse klinischer und bioptischer Diagnose. Z Kinderchir 1983;138:284-87.

3. Schaerli AF. Neuronal intestinal dysplasia. Pediatr Surg Int 1992;7:2-7.
4. Kobayashi H, Hirakawa H, Puri P. What are the diagnostic criteria for intestinal neuronal dysplasia? Pediatr Surg Int 1995;10:459-64.
5. Puri P. Variant Hirschsprung's disease. J Pediatr Surg 1997;32:149-57.
6. Meier-Ruge W. Epidemiology of congenital innervation defects of the distal colon. Virchows Arch V Pathol Anat 1992;420:171-77.
7. Milla PJ, Smith VV. Intestinal neuronal dysplasia. J Pediatr Gastroenterol Nutr 1993;17:367-57.
8. Martuciello G, Caffarena PE, Lerone M, et al. Neuronal intestinal dysplasia: Clinical experience in Italian patients. Eur J Ped Surg 1994;4:287-92.
9. Kobayashi H, Hirakawa H, Surana R, et al. Intestinal neuronal dysplasia is a possible cause of persistent bowel symptoms after pull-through operation for Hirschsprung's disease. J Pediatr Surg 1995;30:253-59.
10. Smith VV. Isolated intestinal neuronal dysplasia: A descriptive histological pattern or a distinct clinicopathological entity? In Hadziselimovic F, Herzog B (Eds): Inflammatory Bowel Disease and Morbus Hirschsprung's Disease. Dordrecht, The Netherlands, Kluwer Academic 1992;203-14.
11. Puri P, Wester T. Intestinal neuronal dysplasia. Semin Pediatr Surg 1998;7:181-86.
12. Csury L, Pena A. Intestinal neuronal dysplasia: Myth or reality? Literature review. Pediatr Surg Int 1995;10: 441-46.
13. Kapur RP. Neuronal dysplasia: a controversial pathological correlate of intestinal pseudoobstruction. Am J Med Genet 2003;122A:287-93.
14. Lake BD. Intestinal neuronal dysplasia. Why does it only occur in parts of Europe? Virchows Arch 1995;426: 537-39.
15. Oguzkurt P, Senocak ME, Akcoren Z, Buyukpamukcu N. Diagnostic difficulties in neuronal intestinal dysplasia and segmental colitis. J Pediatr Surg 2000;35:519-21.
16. Hatano A, Aoki T, Dezawa M, Yusa S, Iitsuka Y, Koseki H, Taniguchi M, Tokuhisa T. A novel pathogenesis of megacolon in Ncx/Hox11L1 deficient mice. J Clin Invest 1997;100:795-801.
17. Shirasawa S, Yunker AMR, Roth KA, Brown GA, Horning S, Korsmeyer SJ. Enx (Hox11L1)-deficient mice develop myenteric neuronal hyperplasia and megacolon. Nat Med 1997;3:646-50.
18. Yamataka A, Hatano M, Kobayashi H, Wang K, Miyahara K, Sueyoshi N, Miyano T. Intestinal neuronal dysplasia-like pathology in Ncx/Hox11L.1 gene-deficient mice. J Pediatr Surg 2001;36:1293-96.
19. Costa M, Fava M, Seri M, Cusano R, Sancandi M, Forabosco P, Lerone M, Martuciello G, Romeo G, Ceccherini I. Evaluation of the Hox11L1 gene as a candidate for congenital disorders of intestinal innervation. J Med Genet 31, 2000.
20. von Boyen GBT, Krammer HJ, Suss A, Dembrowski C, Ehrenreich H, Wedel T. Abnormalities of the enteric nervous system in heterozygous endothelin B receptor deficient (spotting lethal) rats resembling intestinal neuronal dysplasia. Gut 2002;414-19.
21. Rolle U, Nemeth L, Puri P. Nitrergic innervation of the normal gut and in motility disorders of childhood. J Pediatr Surg 2002;37:551-67.
22. Rolle U, Piotrowska AP, Puri P. Abnormal vasculature in intestinal neuronal dysplasia. Ped Surg Int 2003;19: 345-48.
23. Lumb PD, Moore L. Are giant ganglia a reliable marker of intestinal neuronal dysplasia B (IND B). Virchows Arch 1991;432:103-06.
24. Borchard F, Meier-Ruge W, Wiebecke B, Briner J, Muntefering H, Fodisch HJ, Holschneider AM, Schmidt A, Enck P, Stolte M. Innervationsstoerungen des Dickdarms – Klassifikation und Diagnostik. Pathologe 1991;12:171-74.
25. Wester T, O'Briain S, Puri P. Morphometric aspects of the submucous plexus in whole-mount preparations of normal human distal colon. J Pediatr Surg 1998;33(4): 619-22.
26. Wester T, O'Briain S, Puri P. Notable postnatal alterations in the myenteric plexus of normal human bowel. GUT 1999;44;666-74.
27. Smith VV. Intestinal neuronal density in childhood: a baseline for the objective assessment of hypo- and hyperganglionosis. Pediatr Pathol 1993;13:225-37.
28. Ikeda K, Goto S, Nagasaki A, et al. Hypogenesis of intestinal ganglion cells: a rare cause of intestinal obstruction simulating aganglionosis. Z Kinderchir 1988;43:52-53.
29. Meier-Ruge W, Morger R, Rehbein F. Das hypoganglionaere Megakolon als Begleiterkrankung bei Morbus Hirschsprung. Z Kinderchir 1970;8:254-64.
30. Yunis EJ, Schofield DE. Intestinal neuronal dysplasia in a case of sigmoid stenosis. Pediatr Pathol 1992;12:275-80.
31. Schofield DE, Yunis EJ. What is intestinal neuronal dysplasia? Pathol Ann 1992 ;27:249-62.
32. Schofield DE, Yunis EJ. Intestinal neuronal dysplasia. J Pediatr Gastroenterol Nutr 1991;12:182-89.
33. Moore SW, Laing D, Kaschula ROC, et al. A histological grading system for the evaluation of co-existing NID with Hirschsprung's disease. Eur J Pediatr Surg 1994;4:293-97.
34. Meier-Ruge W, Bronnimann PB, Gambazzi F, et al. Histopathological criteria for intestinal neuronal dysplasia of the submucous plexus (type B). Virchows Arch 1995;426:549-56.
35. Meier-Ruge W. Is intestinal neuronal dysplasia really a myth or an invented disease? Pediatr Surg Int 1995;10:439.
36. Gillick J, Tazawa H, Puri P. Intestinal neuronal dysplasia: Results of treatment in 33 patients. J Pediatr Surg 2001;36:777-79.
37. Schaerli AF. Standardization of terminology of dysganglionoses. Pediatr Surg Int 1995;10:440.
38. Kobayashi H, Yamataka A, Lane GJ, Miyano T. Pathophysiology of hypoganglionosis. J Ped Gastroenterol Nutr 2002;34:231-35.

39. Puri P, Fujimoto T. Diagnosis of allied functional bowel disorders using monoclonal antibodies and electron-microscopy. J Pediatr Surg 1988;23:546-54.
40. Meier-Ruge WA, Brunner LA, Engert J, et al. A correlative morphometric and clinical investigation of hypoganglionosis of the colon in children. Eur J Pediatr Surg 1999;9:67-74.
41. Watanabe Y, Ito F, Ando H, Seo T, Kaneko K, Harada T, Iino S. Morphological investigation of the enteric nervous system in Hirschsprung's disease and hypoganglionosis using whole-mount colon preparation. J Pediatr Surg 1999;34(3):445-49.
42. Rolle U, Yoneda A, Solari V, Nemeth L, Puri P. Abnormalities of c-Kit positive cellular network in isolated hypoganglionosis. J Ped Surg 2002;37(5):709-14.
43. Kobayashi H, Li Z, Yamataka A, Lane GJ, Miyano T. Overexpression of neural cell adhesion molecule (NCAM) antigens on intestinal smooth muscles in hypoganglionosis: is hypoganglionosis a disorder of the neuromuscular junction? Pediatr Surg Int 2003;19(3): 190-93.
44. Inoue K, Shimotake T, Tomiyama H, Iwai N. Mutational analysis of the RET and GDNF gene in children with hypoganglionosis. Eur J Pediatr Surg 2001;11(2):120-23.
45. Tatekawa Y, Kanehiro H, Kanokogi H, Nakajima Y, Nishijima E, Muraji T, Imai Y, Tsugawa C, Toyosaka A, Nakano H. The evaluation of meconium disease by distribution of cathepsin D in intestinal ganglion cells. Pediatr Surg Int 2000;16(1-2):53-55.
46. Hirakawa H, Kobayashi H, O'Briain S, et al. Absence of NADPH-diaphorase activity in internal anal sphincter (IAS) achalasia. J Pediatr Gastroenterol Nutr 1995;20: 54-58.
47. Neilson IR, Yazbeck S. Ultrashort Hirschsprung's disease: Myth or reality. J Pediatr Surg 1990;25:1135-38.
48. Meier-Ruge W. Ultrashort segment Hirschsprung's disease: An objective picture of the disease substantiated by biopsy. Z Kinderchir 1985;40:146-50.
49. Lake BD, Puri P, Nixon HH, et al. Hirschsprung's disease – An appraisal of histochemistry demonstrated acetylcholinesterase activity in suction rectal biopsy specimens as an aid to diagnosis. Arch Pathol Lab Med 1978;102;224-47.
50. Oue T, Puri P. Altered intramuscular innervatio and synapse formation in internal sphincter achalasia. Pediatr Surg Int 1999;15:192-94.
51. Piotrowska AP, Solari V, Puri P. Distribution of interstitial cells of Cajal in the internal anal sphincter of patients with internal anal sphincter achalasia and Hirschsprung's disease. Arch Pathol Lab Med 2003;127:1191-95.
52. De Caluwe D, Yoneda A, Akl U, Puri P. Internal anal sphincter achalasia: outcome after internal sphincter myectomy. J Ped Surg 2001;36(5):736-38.
53. Ciamarra P, Nurko S, Barksdale E, Fishman S, Di Lorenzo C. Internal anal sphincter achalasia in children: clinical characteristics and treatment with Clostridium botulinum toxin. J Pediatr Gastroenterol Nutr 2003;37(3):315-19.
54. Berdon WE, Baker DH, Blanc WA, et al. Megacystis-microcolon-intestinal hypoperistalsis syndrome: A new cause of intestinal obstruction in the newborn. Report of radiologic findings in five newborn girls. Am J Roentgenol 1976;126:957-64.
55. Granata C, Puri P. Megacystis microcolon intestinal hypoperistalsis syndrome. J Pediatr Gastr Nutr 1997;25: 12-14.
56. Puri P, Lake BD, Gorman F, et al. Megacystis-microcolon-intestinal hypoperistalsis syndrome: A visceral myopathy. J Pediatr Surg 1983;18:64-69.
57. Rolle U, O'Briain S, Pearl RH, Puri P. Megacystis-microcolon-intestinal hypoperistalsis syndrome: evidence of intestinal myopathy. Ped Surg Int 2002:18:2-5.
58. Piotrowska AP, Rolle U, Chertin B, De Caluwe D, Bianchi A, Puri P. Alterations in smooth muscle contractile and cytoskeleton proteins and interstitial cells of Cajal in megacystis microcolon intestinal hypoperistalsis syndrome. J Ped Surg 2003;38(5):749-55.
59. Rolle U, Puri P. Structural basis of voiding dysfunction in megacystis microcolon intestinal hypoperistalsis syndrome. J Pediatr. Urol 2006:2:277-84.
60. Rolle U, Piotrwska AP, Puri P. Interstitial cells of Cajal in the normal gut and in interstial motility disorders of childhood. Pediatr Surg Int 2007:23:1139-52.

CHAPTER 64

Swenson's Pull-through

DK Gupta, Shilpa Sharma

In 1948, it was Orvar Swenson who recognized the cause of Hirschsprung's disease-based on a series of clinical observations indicating that there was a defective segment of distal colon producing a partial bowel obstruction.[1,2] Till then, people had thought the defect to be in the dilated and thickened bowel rather than in the distal and narrow segment. Swenson showed that peristaltic tracings from the dilated proximal colon were not able enter the more distal narrow segment. He thus devised the operation in which the distal segment was removed and the intestinal continuity was restored by pulling down of the proximal colon and its anastomosis at the anus. After this, the bowel started functioning normally. The Swenson's procedure was thus the first ever pull-through procedure described for treating the Hirschsprung's disease, and later published by Swenson and Bill in 1948.[3]

Prior to 1948, there was no clear understanding of the etiology of the disease.[4-6] It is assumed that the absence of ganglion cells was known even earlier as the accepted cause of Hirschsprung's disease and this had led to the concept of distal colon dysfunction and the basis for the distal colonic resection in the Swenson's pull-through technique. However, Swenson denied this and reported that it played no role whatsoever in devising the successful operation.[4] Since then, Hirschsprung's disease has remained a subject of interest for research with new concepts in etiology, diagnosis and treatment.[7-11]

The surgical principle is to remove the diseased portion of the bowel that is aganglionic distal rectum, and maintain the bowel continuity to allow normal defecation. The aganglionic segment is resected from the sigmoid colon down to the rectum, and an oblique anastomosis is performed between the normal sized (undilated) ganglionic colon and the low rectum.

PREOPERATIVE ASSESSMENT AND PREPARATION

A thorough history dating back to stool pattern at birth should be taken. All previous record of operative findings, procedures done and histopathology reports with emphasis on the area from which the biopsy samples have been taken should be studied. A skiagram abdomen may help to identify any fecaloma and also if the patient is constipated or not especially in cases with a single stage pull-through. A distal cologram to outline the adequacy of the distal bowel for pull-through without the need to mobilize the colostomy is essential. A good bowel preparation is essential before the pull-through procedure, especially if it is to be done as a primary procedure without a diverting colostomy. To achieve this, a mechanical cleaning of the distal colon and rectum is done with washes.

The technique demands meticulous dissection of the rectum down to within 2 cm above the ano-dermal junction. If the dissection moves off of the rectal wall, a significant incidence of injury to genitourinary innervations may occur. The results of a properly performed Swenson's procedure are good; however, it is a technical demanding procedure and the results vary with the surgical expertise. Due to this reason, it is not as popular as the Duhamel or modified Soave (Boley Scott) procedures.

The operation has two components—an abdominal (to mobilize the bowel) and the perineal (to make the anastomosis with the rectum). Initially, the anastomosis used to be completed at the anorectum. This resulted in high incidence of postoperative enterocolitis (early, 16%; late, 27%), and this was attributed to the too much of the aganglionic rectum that had been left behind.[2] The procedure has since been modified by resecting virtually whole of the posterior rectal wall (and the very top most aspect of the internal sphincter), making an oblique anastomosis leaving about 1.5 cm of rectal wall anteriorly and only 0.5 cm of rectal wall posteriorly.[2] This involves a meticulous end to end anastomosis in 2 layers that might be quite time consuming.

Recently, staplers have been used for completing the anastomosis. Following the transabdominal rectosigmoidectomy, the coloanal end to end anastomosis by means of a circular intraluminal stapler has also been reported as a safe and easy technique to treat Hirschsprung's disease, allowing a deep rectal resection which is very difficult to achieve by manual suturing. As the anastomosis is located in an extraperitoneal position, there is minimum risk of peritoneal involvement even if there is anastomotic leakage. The reported outcome was fast recovery, good functional results and minimum complications.[12] However, long term concern about the high rate of anastomotic stricture remains as one third of patients may develop strictures with the use of circular staplers.

Just like a primary transanal endorectal pull-through (TEPT by Boley Scot approach), the entire procedure of Swenson's pull through can also be performed through the transanal approach and the initial results have been quite satisfactory.[13-15]

AGE AT SWENSON'S PROCEDURE

Swenson's pull-through is mostly performed in stages and beyond the neonatal age, in children in whom a diversion has already been done. Though, the procedure can also be performed in the neonatal period as a primary procedure, there is a high risk of damage to the nerves and thus is not routinely advocated in the neonatal age. Carccassonne reported results on 98 infants less than 3 months of age, treated with single stage Swenson's procedure. There were no deaths. There was only one anastomotic leak that also closed promptly under cover of the colostomy.[16] The early definitive procedure in the neonatal period has the advantage of merging the period of incontinence with the normal period of bowel training.[16]

In the series reported by Wilcox et al, 38 out of 51 patients operated with Swenson's procedure were neonates with a mean gestational age of 39.6 +/− 1.7 weeks and weight 3.3 +/− 0.54 kg, at 10.3 +/− 5.8 days of age. The short and long-term results were reported as good.[17] Majority of the surgeons still prefer to stage the procedure in the neonates diagnosed with Hirschsprung's disease rather than doing the one stage procedure in the neonatal period (BAPS survey, 51% versus 41%) with stoma formation in the neonatal period.[18] The three stage Swenson's procedure may be performed salery especially in all those children who present late with thick and dilated bowel. With changing times, the primary Swenson's pull-through is being adopted increasingly by the experienced surgeons preferring this technique.[19]

RELATIVE CONTRAINDICATIONS

Swenson's procedure is not a good choice for a redo procedure (after failed Duhamel's or Soaves procedure) unless compelled. A previous surgery leaves much fibrosis on healing and a further dissection outside the bowel may result in the damage to the nerves and other structures in the pelvis. If it has been decided to do a Swenson's pull-through, then it should preferably be covered with a proximal colostomy as a diverting stoma to protect the neo anastomosis.

SURGICAL PROCEDURE

General anesthesia is used. It may be supplemented with caudal analgesia depending upon the anethetists choice. The baby is placed in lithotomy position. The baby's bottom is brought to the end of the operating table and raised with a towel or a small sand bag to improve the accessibility and the ease of perineal dissection. The abdomen, perineum, and thighs are prepared and draped in case an abdominal incision is needed. Appropriate sized Foley's catheter is inserted into the bladder.

Anal Dilatation

The first step is to perform slow and gentle anal dilatation with one finger at a time and dilating according to the size of the bowel to be anastomosed and the patient's age.

Abdominal Part of the Procedure

The classically described incision for the procedure was a left para-median incision. A modified hockey-stick incision in the left lower quadrant is now preferred by most. The skin, subcutaneous tissue and muscles are divided using diathermy. The peritoneal cavity is opened. The transition zone is identified and the part of the colon to be pulled down is marked with stay sutures. A biopsy is taken for frozen section to ensure the level of the ganglionic bowel. The left colon is dissected from the lateral parietal wall. The peritoneal folds at the peritoneal reflection are opened anterior to the rectum. The dissection may be commenced on the wall of the distal sigmoid or the upper rectum, in a plane close to its wall. The dissection advances distally and around the full circumference of the rectum. It is vital to remain close to the rectum on its anterior aspect to avoid any injury to the urethra.

The dissection may be facilitated by an upward traction applied on the aganglionic rectum and the bladder retracted anteriorly. Multiple blood vessels enter directly into the bowel wall. Each of these vessels must be dissected out and coagulated. Dissection is carried down to within 2 cm of the anal verge anteriorly and 1 cm posteriorly in an oblique fashion to avoid injury to the autonomic nerves.

The extent of the downward dissection is judged by inserting a finger in the anus. The bowel is transected a little above the peritoneal reflection and suture closed. The proximal segment of the redundant aganglionic rectum and the proximal ganglionic colon mobilized, as needed. At this stage the bowel is divided at the level chosen for the pull-through and the two ends suture closed temporarily.

Anal Part of the Procedure

Stay sutures are applied to mark all four quadrants at 3, 6, 9 and 12 o' clock position. The suture at 12 o' clock position is placed with care to remain close to the anal verge so as not to injure the urethra in male patients. The anocutaneous junction (Dentate line) is identified. Narrow right angled retractors, may be used to facilitate the procedure if needed. The closed apex of the dissected rectum is drawn out through the anus with the help of a grasper, everting the rectum (Fig. 64.1). If the dissection has been adequate the anus

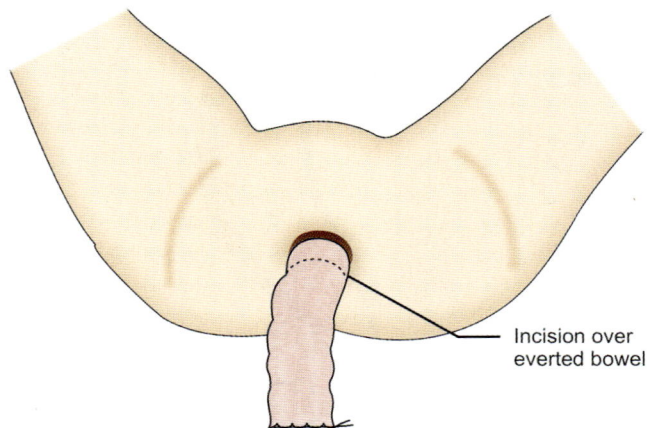

Fig. 64.1: Bowel everted through the anal verge

may be partially everted. An incision is made with the diathermy from 9 to 3 o'clock position anteriorly through the rectal wall, 2 cm above the dentate line.

Through this opening in the rectum, the ganglionic colon is pulled through with care to avoid torsion. The colon is opened at its apex and sutured full thickness to the cut edges of anorectum with interrupted absorbable 4/0 sutures. Classically, silk sutures were used, but nowadays these have been replaced with Vicryl or PDS sutures. The anastomosis is allowed to recede and is gently pulled upward from the abdominal wound. Posteriorly, the suture line should be about 1 cm above from the dentate line (Figs 64.2A and B). A rolled antibiotic ointment soaked paraffin gauze or sofratulle is placed in the anal canal to take care of the dead space between the muscular cuff and the pulled through bowel. The abdomen is closed in layers by the assistant at the abdominal end.

Trans Anal Dissection for Single Stage Swenson's Procedure

A circumferential incision is given about 2 cm proximal to the dentate line anteriorly and 1 cm proximal to the dentate line posteriorly. It is marked with stay sutures all around to facilitate dissection. The stay sutures help to distribute equal tension and prevent the tearing of the rectal wall. Meticulous dissection requires experience and technical skills. The dissection proceeds around the full thickness of the rectal wall. The peritoneal cavity is opened as the dissection proceeds

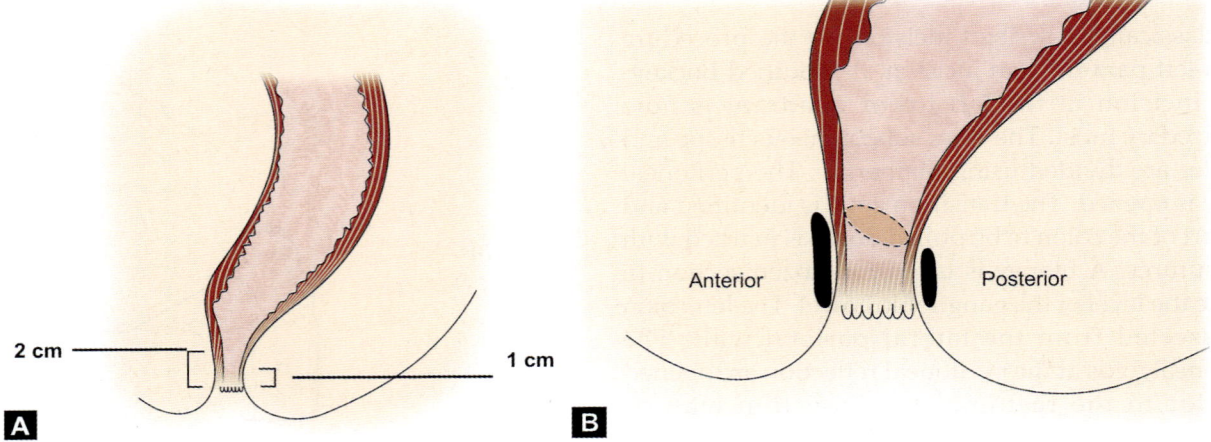

Figs 64.2A and B: Swenson's procedure: the junction of the red and pink shows the oblique line of anastomosis of ganglionic pulled-through-bowel and remaining anoproctodeum

upwards. Attention is focused on the mesenteric attachments and the vessels running in the sigmoid mesocolon. This is continued till the transition zone is appreciated in the bowel hanging out of the anal verge. The bowel proximal to the transitional zone is biopsied and confirmed for the ganglion cells before anastomosing the same at the neo anus using vicryl or PDS interrupted sutures in two layers.

Though it is much easier to mobilize the full thickness bowel (full thickness rectum) from the perineal side, unlike fashioning a mucosal tube during the transanal endorectal pull-through (TEPT) procedure, yet the mobilization of the bowel all around deep in the pelvis has always remained a matter of concern to the surgeons for an inadvertent injury to the nerves, urethra and bladder, with long term sequelae.

COMPLICATIONS

Early Complications

1. Injury to the urethra and the bladder.
2. Bleeding due to the retraction of major vessels
3. Increased frequency of stool
4. Early coloanal stenosis
5. Anastomotic leak
6. Hematuria
7. Transient urinary retention
8. Enterocolitis, though partially preventable, yet can occur even after a technically correct procedure.[20]

Late Complications

1. Enterocolitis.
2. Fecal Incontinence: There has been a concern about the effect of prolonged traction of sphincter muscle in single stage transanal Swenson's procedure. If adequate care is taken to preserve the anal canal, incontinence should not occur. Postoperative soiling may be present without frank incontinence
3. Stenosis at the anastomotic site: This may occur more frequently if the three stage procedures has been adopted. Anal dilatation is helpful.
4. Residual disease due to error in the operative procedure or the histology frozen report.

LAPAROSCOPY

Laparoscopy has been used to complete the abdominal part of the dissection and remove whole of the aganglionic bowel and preparing the same for the anastomosis at the anal verge, using laparoscopic technique.[21] Curran and Raffensperger first tried this technique in dogs to assess its feasibility and then used it successfully in a group of 8 patients, reportedly with a reduced morbidity and no complications.[22,23] Kumar et al, reported the use of laparoscopic Swenson's procedure for one stage primary as well as two stage secondary procedures, with good short-term results, and there was no difference in operating time between the primary and secondary pull-through procedures.[24] George et al also reported the advantages of the

Swenson's laparoscopic approach with shorter lengths of hospital stay and fewer postoperative complications.[25]

OUTCOME

The reported outcome following Swenson's operation varies in different series.[26] Swenson himself had made various observations over the past 6 decades as to why everyone could not reproduce his results.[27,28] One of the most serious complications of a Swenson's pull-through, is a leak at the anastomosis. In a combined series with 880 children from seven centres operated with Swenson's procedure, the leak rate was 5.6%. The postoperative enterocolitis was 11%. There was a need for a secondary re-operation (6%) that stemmed from anastomotic leaks and anal strictures, requiring diverting colostomies.[29] Others have also reported a similar complications with the need for secondary operations. However, there are authors who have been using Swenson's operation without encountering problems that required reoperation.[30-33]

Though, the chances of injury to the pelvic nerves during Swenson's procedure have been high, yet if performed properly by a trained surgeon, there have been no problems with the urinary or the sexual function.[29] Swenson, in 1975 reported the outcome in 80 patients who were married and collectively had 146 children.[34]

The results of postoperative continence also vary in different series. Bai et al, reported a 8 to 16 year follow-up in 45 patients who had undergone Swenson's procedure, 23 patients (51.1%) had bowel dysfunction and 17(37.8%) had fecal soiling.[35] Although, most patients had good or fair quality of life after surgical correction in this series, the long-term outcome was not as good. In another series with Swenson's pull-through procedure, the immediate postoperative recovery and long term anorectal functions have been reported quite satisfactory and compared well with other techniques.[32,36]

Drossman et al, in a study on 800 normal adults who had no gastrointestinal complaints, determined the normal range of bowel movements as; at least 1 movement every three days and no more than 3 movements per day.[37] Using this criterion, upto 96% of the patients were reported to have normal bowel pattern and were continent following Swenson's pull through.[29] The long-term incidence of postoperative constipation has been reported as 54% after the Duhamel, 43% after the Soave, and 4% after the original Swenson's operation.[38] With passage of time, most children with Hirschsprung's disease after pull through procedure significantly improve with respect to fecal continence, but this may not be until later adolescence.[39]

The overall mortality rate after surgery for Hirschsprung's disease, in a series of 880 cases treated with Swenson's operation was 2.5%. However, during the last 20 years the mortality has fallen to 1.25%.[29] Soave in his own series of 271 patients reported 4.5% mortality.[40] The mortality rate in 260 patients treated with the Duhamel modification was 6.2%.[41] Most series lately have reported no mortality with Swenson's procedure.

REOPERATIONS

There is very less need for the reoperations following Swenson's procedure if performed by experienced surgeons. In Pena's series of cases requiring re-operations for Hirschsprung's disease, the initial operations were Soave (20), Duhamel (15), Swenson (5), transanal endorectal (4), myectomy (3), unknown (3), and laparoscopic Swenson (1).[20] The main indications for revisions following the Swenson's procedures are stricture unresponsive to dilatation, post-anastomotic leak and fecal fistula.[42] For a redo following Swenson's procedure, a re-Swenson, Boley Scot or a Duhamel technique may be used.[42] The re-do procedures should be done with proximal diversion of stools with a colostomy. If the anal canal is quite fibrosed and unyielding and there is no anal mucosa left, it is advisable to use the original Soave's pull through technique to avoid postoperative complications due to possible retraction of the bowel. Usually the results following the redo pull-through operations for Hirschsprung's disease may be as effective as primary procedures in terms of continence and stool frequency.[43]

COMPARISON WITH OTHER PROCEDURES

It is not easy to make a precise comparison amongst different types of operative procedures used for pull through in children with Hirschsprung's disease. The complications and the outcome of the patient would depend on the age at presentation and the surgery, degree of thickened bowel, level of the resection of the bowel, level and type of the anastomosis at the anal canal (oblique or circular, staplers or manual), length of the bowel involved with the disease, the experience of the surgeon and the episodes of enterocolitis before and after surgery.

Sarioglu et al compared the results of Swenson's operation with the Duhamel's technique in 138 and 59 patients respectively and found that only the anastomotic stricture rate was significantly higher in patients who had undergone Swenson's procedure. The incidence of other complications like wound infection, dehiscence, anastomotic leak, adhesive intestinal obstruction, pelvic abscess, intra-abdominal abscess, mucosal prolapse, anastomotic stricture and fistulas were found equally common in both procedures. When urinary incontinence, enterocolitis, soiling and constipation were considered, there was no significant difference between these two groups.[44] Yanchar and Soucy found that the Duhamel's procedure was associated with more chances of constipation.[39]

The authors using the Boley Scot principle of soave's technique in 111 children with HD, found the procedure quite good, with stricture (4.5 %), adhesive obstruction (4%) and wound infection (2.5%) as the main complications. The short and the long-term results were excellent for primary as well as for the redo cases. A proper selection of patient for a single or multistage procedure was found to be more important to achieve good results rather than the technique itself.[45] Another series reported from the authors institute showed that the early complications were seen with equal frequency in patients undergoing Swenson and Duhamel operation. However, the late complications were seen less often with the Swenson's procedure.[36] The Boley Scot and the Swenson's procedures do require patience and surgical expertise to master the skills, while the Duhamel operation being surgically simpler is considered a safer method for the beginners.[44,46,47]

In a survey done by the Surgical Section of the American Academy of Pediatrics, the leak rate after Boley Scot was 6.9%.[48] Similar leak rate has also been reported following Duhamel procedure. The Duhamel modification has also been reported to have a rectal pouch problem that ranges from 10-25% consisting of impactions and at times bleeding.[49,50]

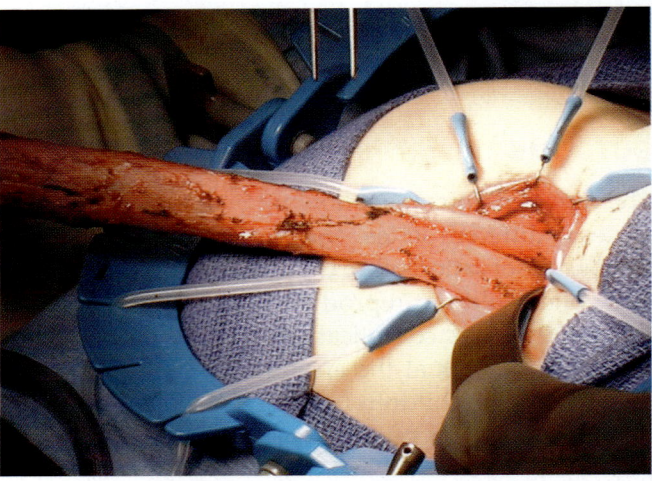

Fig. 64.3: Dr Pena at work performing Swenson's procedure as a single stage in the prone position with the help of specially designed retractors. These incorporate the dentate line within the hooks thus assuring good continence results. According to Dr Pena, "The results of Swenson's procedure are good if performed by a good surgeon"[52] (Courtesy: Dr Alberto Pena for kind permission)

Soave modification has been associated with abscess formation between the retained aganglionic muscular sleeve, retraction of the pulled-through normal colon, and mucosal prolapse even years after the operation. Soaves procedure has been associated with the need for prolonged daily rectal dilatations. In a large review, it was reported that Soave modification had the highest incidence of postoperative enterocolitis followed by that of Duhamel and then the Swenson's procedure.[51]

STAGED VERSUS SINGLE STAGE

The major advances that have occurred in the management of Hirschsprung's disease include the definitive management in a single stage. Recently, Swenson's Pena has been successfully performing Swenson's procedure as a single stage in the prone position with the help of specially designed retractors[52] (Personal communication) (Fig. 64.3). There have been no significant difference in complication rates reported between staged versus primary pull-through. A one-stage Swenson's transanal pull-through has also been reported as a safe alternative with no increased instances of anastomotic leaks, wound infections or postoperative bowel obstructions.[53] Some advocate definitive management in the newborn period.[54] However, others feel it risky to do a primary Swenson's procedure in the newborn period, and other options like a primary Duhamel are more satisfactory.[55] The authors feel a primary trans anal endorectal boley Scot is even safer.[56] It is a matter of surgeons preference and the time of presentation of the baby.[57,58] The bottom line remains, all techniques are as good and safe, with short and long-term satisfactory outcome, provided these are mastered well.

REFERENCES

1. Swenson O, Rheinlander HF, Diamond I. Hirschsprung's disease: a new concept of the etiology. N Engl J Med 1949; 241:551-56.
2. Swenson O. Hirschsprung's Disease: A Review Pediatrics Vol. 109, No. 5 May 2002, 914-18.
3. Swenson O, Bill AH. Resection of the rectum and rectosigmoid with preservation of the sphincter for benign spastic lesions producing megacolon. Surgery 1948;24: 212-20.
4. Swenson O. My early experience with Hirschsprung's disease. J Pediatr Surg 1989 Aug;24(8):839-44; discussion 844-45.
5. Swenson O, Neuhauser EBD, Pickett LK. New concepts of the etiology, diagnosis and treatment of congenital megacolon (Hirschsprung's disease). Pediatrics 1949;4:201-09.
6. Swenson O. How the cause and cure of Hirschsprung's disease were discovered. J Pediatr Surg 1999 Oct; 34(10):1580-81.
7. Swenson O. Treatment of Hirschsprung's disease. J Pediatr Surg 1998 Dec;33(12):1849. Comment on: J Pediatr Surg 1998 Jun;33(6):951.
8. Swenson O. Patients with congenital megacolon that had ganglion cells seen at the line of resection who did not do well and on rectal biopsy were reported to have no or diminished ganglion cells. J Pediatr Surg 2003 Apr;38(4):654-56.
9. Swenson O. Hirschsprung's disease--a complicated therapeutic problem: some thoughts and solutions based on data and personal experience over 56 years. J Pediatr Surg 2004 Oct;39(10):1449-53; discussion 1454-7. Comment in: J Pediatr Surg 2005 May;40(5):888-9; author reply 890.
10. Madonna MB, Luck SR, Reynolds M, et al. Swenson procedure for the treatment of Hirschsprung's disease. Semin Pediatr Surg 1998;7(2):85-88.
11. Fitzgerald CJ. New concepts of the etiology, diagnosis, and treatment of congenital megacolon (Hirschsprung's disease), by Orvar Swenson, MD, et al, Pediatrics, 1949;4:201-9. Pediatrics 1998;102(1 Pt 2):205-07.
12. Gaztambide Casellas J, Sánchez Díaz F, García Soldevilla N, et al. Rectosigmoidectomy and end to end coloanal anastomosis with mechanical stapler for treatment of Hirschsprung disease. Cir Pediatr 2004;17(2):61-64.
13. Podevin G, Lardy H, Azzis O, et al. Technical problems and complications of a transanal pull-through for Hirschsprung's disease. Eur J Pediatr Surg 2006;16(2): 104-08.
14. Skába R, Kalousová J, Simsová M, et al. Transanal resection of the recto-sigmoid--the future in the treatment of classic Hirschsprung's disease? Rozhl Chir 2003;82(12): 620-23.
15. Peterlini FL, Martins JL. Modified transanal rectosigmoidectomy for Hirschsprung's disease: clinical and manometric results in the initial 20 cases. J Pediatr Surg 2003;38(7):1048-50.
16. Carcassonne M, Guys JM, Morrison-Lamcombe G, et al. Management of Hirschsprung's disease: curative surgery before three months of age. J Pediatr Surg 1989;24:1032-34.
17. Wilcox DT, Bruce J, Bowen J, Bianchi A. One-stage neonatal pull-through to treat Hirschsprung's disease. J Pediatr Surg 1997 Feb;32(2):243-5; discussion 245-47.
18. Huddart SN. Hirschsprung's disease: present UK practice. Ann R Coll Surg Engl 1998;80(1):46-48.
19. Santos MC, Giacomantonio JM, Lau HY. Primary Swenson pull-through compared with multiple-stage pull-through in the neonate. J Pediatr Surg 1999;34(7):1079-81.
20. Peña A, Elicevik M, Levitt MA. Reoperations in Hirschsprung disease. J Pediatr Surg 2007;42(6):1008-13; discussion 1013-14.
21. Arany L, Jennings K, Radcliffe K, Ross J. Laparoscopic Swenson pull-through procedure for Hirschsprung's disease. Can Oper Room Nurs J 1998;16:7-13.
22. Curran TJ, Raffensperger JG. The feasibility of laparoscopic swenson pull-through J Pediatr Surg 1994 Sep;29(9): 1273-75.
23. Curran TJ, Raffensperger JG. Laparoscopic Swenson pull-through: a comparison with the open procedure. J Pediatr Surg 1996;31(8):1155-6; discussion 1156-57.
24. Kumar R, Mackay A, Borzi P. Laparoscopic Swenson procedure: an optimal approach for both primary and secondary pull-through for Hirschsprung's disease. J Pediatr Surg 2003 Oct;38(10):1440-43.
25. George C, Hammes M, Schwarz D. Laparoscopic Swenson pull-through procedure for congenital megacolon. AORN J 1995 Nov;62(5):727-8,731-36.
26. Bourdelat D, Vrsansky P, Pages R. Duhamel operation 40 years after: a multicentric study. Eur J Pediatr Surg 1997; 7:70-77.
27. Swenson O, Fisher JH. Treatment of Hirschsprung's disease with entire colon involved in aganglionic defect. Arch Surg 1955;70:535.
28. Swenson O. Early history of the therapy of Hirschsprung's disease: facts and personal observations over 50 years. J Pediatr Surg 1996;31:1003-08.
29. Sherman JO, Snyder ME, Weitzman JJ, et al. A 4-year multinational retrospective study of 880 Swenson procedures. J Pediatr Surg 1989;24:833-38.
30. Weizman JJ, Hanson BA, Brennan LP. Management of Hirschsprung's disease with the Swenson procedure. J Pediatr Surg 1972;7:157-62.

31. Shandhogue LKR, Bianchi A. Experience with primary Swenson resection and pull-through for neonatal Hirschsprung's disease. Pediatr Surg Int 1990;5:446-48.
32. Waldron DJ, O'Donnell B. The Swenson operation for treatment of Hirschsprung's disease. Irs J Medical Sci 1989; 158:175-77.
33. Madonna MB, Luck SR, Reynolds M, Schwarz DK, Arensman, RM. Swenson procedure for the treatment of Hirschsprung's disease. Semin Pediatr Surg 1998;7:85-88.
34. Swenson O, Sherman JO, Fisher JH, Cohen EL. The treatment and postoperative complication of congenital megacolon. Ann Surg 1975;182:266-73.
35. Bai Y, Chen H, Hao J, et al. Long-term outcome and quality of life after the Swenson procedure for Hirschsprung's disease. J Pediatr Surg 2002 Apr;37(4):639-42.
36. Agarwala S, Bhatnagar V, Mitra DK. Long-term follow-up of Hirschsprung's disease: review of early and late complications. Indian Pediatr 1996 May;33(5):382-86.
37. Drossman DA, Sandler RS, McKee DC, et al. Bowel patterns among subjects not seeking health care. Gastroenterology 1982;83:529-34.
38. Quinn FMJ, Fitzgerald RJ, Guiney EJ, O'Donnell B, Puri P. Hirschsprung's disease: a follow-up of three surgical techniques 1979-1988. In: Hadziselmovic F, Herzog B. (Eds). Pediatric Gastroenterology: Inflammatory Bowel Disease and Morbus Hirschsprund. Dordrecht, the Netherlands: Kluwer Academic Publisher 1992;297-301.
39. Yanchar NL, Soucy P. Long-term outcome after Hirschsprung's disease: patients' perspectives. J Pediatr Surg 1999;34(7):1152-60.
40. Soave F. Endorectal pull-through 20 years experience. J Pediatr Surg 1985;20:568-79.
41. Rescorla FJ, Morrison AM, Engles D, West KW, Grosfeld JL. Hirschsprung's disease. Evaluation of mortality and long-term function in 260 cases. Arch Surg 1992;127:934-41.
42. Langer JC. Repeat pull-through surgery for complicated Hirschsprung's disease: indications, techniques, and results. J Pediatr Surg 1999;34(7):1136-41.
43. van Leeuwen K, Teitelbaum DH, Elhalaby EA, Coran AG. Long-term follow-up of redo pull-through procedures for Hirschsprung's disease: efficacy of the endorectal pull-through. J Pediatr Surg 2000;35(6):829-33; discussion 833-34.
44. Sarioglu A, Tanyel FC, Senocak ME, et al. Complications of the two major operations of Hirschsprung's disease: a single center experience. Turk J Pediatr 2001;43(3):219-22.
45. Gupta DK, Sharma S, Bhatnagar V, Bajpai M, Agarwala S. Late presentations of Hirschsprung's disease (HD) - an Indian scenario. Colorectal Club Dublin 2006.
46. Agarwala S, Bhatnagar V, Mitra DK. Long term follow-up of hirschsprungs disease: review of early and late complications. Ind pediatr 1996;33:384-86.
47. Agarwala S, Bhatnagar V, Mitra DK. Stone's enterostomy crushing clamp for modified Duhamel's procedure. Trop gastroenterol 1998;19:164-66.
48. Kleinhaus S, Boley SJ, Sheran M, Sieber WK. Hirschsprung's disease, a survey of the Members of the American Academy of Pediatrics. J Pediatr Surg 1979;14: 588-97.
49. Livaditis A. Hirschsprung's disease: long-term results of the original Duhamel operation. J Pediatr Surg 1981;16:484-86.
50. Grosfeld J, Balantine VN, Csicsko JF. A critical evaluation of the Duhamel operation for Hirschsprung's disease. Arch Surg 1978;113:454-59.
51. Holschneider AM, Borner W, Burman O, et al. Clinical and electromonmetrical investigations of postoperative continence in Hirschsprung's disease. An international workshop. Z Kinderchir 1980;29:39-48.
52. Pena A. Director, Colorectal Centre for children, Cincinnatti children's Hospital, Medical centre, USA. Personal communication.
53. Weidner BC, Waldhausen JH. Swenson revisited: a one-stage, transanal pull-through procedure for Hirschsprung's disease. J Pediatr Surg 2003;38:1208-11.
54. Coran AG, Teitelbaum DH. Recent advances in the management of Hirschsprung's disease. Am J Surg 2000;180:382-87.
55. Pierro A, Fasoli L, Kiely EM, Drake D, Spitz L. Staged pull-through for rectosigmoid Hirschsprung's disease is not safer than primary pull-through. J Pediatr Surg 1997;32(3):505-09.
56. Gupta DK, Sharma Shilpa. Modified Boley Scot technique for Hirschsprung's disease - A twenty-five year experience. 7th Congress of European Paediatric Surgeons Association. Maastricht Netherlands 2006.
57. Gupta DK. Plenary Lecture delivered on Experience with management of patients with Hirschsprung's disease including Total colonic Aganglionosis, during the Symposium on Hirschsprung's disease, University of Cluj-Napoca, Romania, December 2006.
58. Sharma Shilpa, Gupta DK. Functional Constipation and Late Onset Hirschsprung's Disease in Textbook of Adolescent Medicine. Ed Swati Bhave. Jaypee Brothers New Delhi. Chapter 20. 2006;2:648-53.

CHAPTER 65

Duhamel's Pull-through

Sandeep Agarwala

Since the introduction of a definitive corrective procedure for Hirschsprung's disease by Swenson and Bill in 1948, the surgical options have gradually been refined.[1] Swenson's technique consisted of resection of entire aganglionic colon and the proximal ganglionic colon being anastomosed to the rectum in an oblique fashion. The anastomosis is 0.5 cm proximal to the dentate line posteriorly and 1 cm proximal anteriorly. State's operation was a low anterior resection leaving 7-10 cm of aganglionic rectum, while the Rehbein's procedure left about 3-5 cm of aganglionic rectum. Both these procedures have now been abandoned as they resulted in a high incidence of residual symptoms. Bernard Duhamel in 1956 and Soave in 1964 devised procedures which eliminated much of the pelvic dissection.[2,3] Soave performed an endorectal mucosectomy distal to the pelvic peritoneum and pulled down the proximal ganglionic colon through the aganglionic muscular cuff of the rectum.

In the Duhamel's procedure the pelvic dissection distal to the pelvic peritoneum is done retrorectaly, with no dissection anteriorly thereby avoiding any damage to the nerve supply. The rational for Duhamel's procedure included ease of performance, prevention of anastomotic leaks and strictures while eliminating the obstruction and preserving the sensory receptors. The operative principles of his technique included:

1. Minimal pelvic dissection.
2. Retrorectal approach for the pulled-through colon to the anal opening.
3. Partial disruption of the internal anal sphincter posteriorly.
4. Preservation of the anterior wall of the rectum and its nerve supply.
5. Elimination of colo-rectal septum with wide side-to-side anastomosis (stapled or crushed auto-anastomosis) between the anterior aganglionic rectum and the pulled down ganglionic colon.

Several modifications have been described to the original Duhamel's procedure. Most of these pertain to:

1. Level of posterior rectal incision to anastomose the pulled through colon.
   a. *Duhamel I operation:* The original technique in which the anal incision was at the anocutaneous junction.[2] This resulted in a higher incidence of soiling, because of complete disruption of the internal anal sphincter.
   b. *Grob's modification:* The anal incision was above the internal sphincter thereby completely preserving the sphincter.[4] There was no more soiling but fecal impaction due to inert anal sphincter became common.
   c. *Duhamel II operation:* Duhamel recognized the deficiency of his earlier procedure which he corrected by making the anal incision 0.5-1cm proximal to the dentate line thereby partially disrupting the sphincter. This ensured adequate continence to gasses and liquid feces and did not lead to constipation. This is practiced widely today.
2. Various techniques/clamps for the side-to-side anastomosis between the rectal stump and the pulled-through colon.
   a. *Kocher's clamps:* Used in the original procedure.[5,6]

b. *Various other clamps applied a retrograde manner through the anus:* Ochsner, Gross, Zachary, Sulamaa, Ikeda and many others.[7-10]
c. *Stones enterostomy crushing clamps:* These were applied in a prograde manner, through the colotomy in the pulled-through colon.[11]
d. *GIA linear cutter:*[12] This is frequently used nowa days.[12]

3. Methods of obliterating the proximal blind rectal pouch.
   a. Closure of the proximal end of the rectal stump, as described originally by Duhamel, as low as possible leaving no common wall.
   b. Martin's modification: In this modification the entire juxtaposed common wall between the anterior aganglionic rectum and the posterior pulled-through colon is eliminated, either by a long crushing clamp or staplers and the proximal open end of the rectal stump is anastomosed to the colotomy on the pulled-down colon in an end-to-side manner.

The patients with Hirschsprung's disease who are to undergo Hirschsprung's disease can be managed in three ways:

1. *Primary Duhamel's pull-through without a diverting colostomy:* This is suitable in cases where the proximal ganglionic colon is not excessively dilated as in neonates and some infants. When this is attempted in an older child with hugely dilated colon, this entire dilated segment, which is actually normal ganglionic segment, will need to be resected.
2. *Two stage procedure:* The initial colostomy is performed at the junction of the ganglionic and aganglionic colon (leveling colostomy) after proper identification by frozen section biopsy. During the second stage Duhamel's pull-through is done after taking down the stoma and using the proximal end for pull-through. The advantage of a two stage procedure needs to be seen against the following disadvantages:
   a. Need for frozen section biopsy at the time of the leveling colostomy to accurately site the stoma.
   b. The need to handle the stoma at the time of the pull-through procedure.
   c. Absence of a proximal diverting stoma to protect the anastomosis at the time of pull-through.
3. *Three stage procedure:* Initially a proximal diverting stoma is made in the right transverse colon (in the usual short segment Hirschsprung's disease). This is usually sufficiently proximal in most cases to permit its preservation following the definitive operation. During the procedure for colostomy, seromuscular biopsies are obtained from the collapsed aganglionic colon and the distal most end of the dialated ganglionic colon. These sites are marked with silk sutures for easy identification during the definitive pull-through procedure. Second stage Duhamel's procedure is done without touching the colostomy and 4-6 weeks later the colostomy is closed.

A three stage Martin's modification of the Duhamel II procedure using a GIA linear cutter is performed most frequently now.[13] More recently laparoscopy assisted Duhamel's pull-through has been described.[14]

INDICATIONS

All confirmed cases of short segment and long segment Hirschsprung's disease.

All redo pull-through procedures following a failed Swensons's and Soave's pull-through.

PREOPERATIVE EVALUATION

1. *Barium enema:* Initial screening and diagnosis. Also indicates the extent of aganglionosis and the suitability for a primary pull-through. It also helps in deciding the suitable stoma site for diversion.
2. *Rectal biopsy:* This can be either a suction biopsy, a punch biopsy which are obtained from 3 and 5 cm proximal to the ano-cutaneous junction. The open biopsy is a full thickness rectal biopsy obtained under anesthesia. These are processed by routine H and E staining and also acetylcholine esterase stains.
3. Distal most level of ganglionic bowel is ascertained by obtaining a seromuscular biopsy from the colon at the time of the diversion and marking this site with silk sutures. If this has not been done then the level can be ascertained by frozen section biopsy during the pull-through procedure.
4. *Baseline evaluation:* Hemoglobin, serum proteins, renal functions.

PREOPERATIVE PREPARATION FOR PULL-THROUGH

A first generation cepahlosporin or ampicillin + gentamycin + metrogyl is started 24 hours prior to surgery. The mechanical bowel preparation differs slightly depending on the procedure:

1. For Primary pull-through:
   a. Twice daily rectal washes with normal saline starting at least a week or two prior to surgery.
   b. Low residue diet for three days prior to surgery
   c. Gut irrigation using polyethylene glycol solution (70 ml/kg) on the day prior to surgery.
   d. On the morning of the surgery a rectal flatus tube is inserted to ensure complete evacuation of the colon.
2. For two stage procedure in which the leveling stoma has to be brought down:
   a. All the above steps are done except that to the initial rectal washes a distal colostomy washout is also added. This should be done with a flatus tube, positioned in the rectum and fluid instilled through the rectal tube.
   b. On the morning of the surgery a rectal flatus tube is inserted to ensure complete evacuation of the colon.
3. For three stage procedure in which the diverting stoma will remain untouched:
   a. Only rectal washes and distal colostomy washout as described previously for two to three days is adequate.
   b. On the morning of the surgery a rectal flatus tube is inserted to ensure complete evacuation of the colon.

PROCEDURE

General anesthesia supplemented with caudal analgesia is used. A nasograstic tube is inserted at the outset. The child is placed in lithotomy position with a folded towel under the lower back. The head end of the table is slightly lowered. Anal dilatation, appropriate for age is performed. The proximal diverting stoma is covered and excluded. The patient is cleaned and draped and a Foley's catheter is placed into the bladder.

Left lower abdominal curved skin crease incision is made and the muscles and peritoneum divided. A midline or left paramedian incision may be more appropriate in adults and older children or when the disease involves long segment.

Sigmoid colon is identified and delivered into the wound. Silk sutures marking the previous biopsy sites is identified and the proximal level of colonic resection ascertained. If the proximal biopsy was reported as ganglionic then that becomes the level up to which colon is resected. If the proximal biopsy was also reported as aganglionic then more proximal seromuscular biopsies are obtained and sent for frozen section examination to ascertain the level of ganglionosis.

The peritoneum over the mesosigmoid is incised both laterally and medially and then joined anteriorly in the colo-vesical pouch. Both the ureters are identified so as to avoid injury.

Colon is mobilized distally up to the level of pelvic peritoneum. The superior rectal branch of the inferior mesenteric artery is preserved to supply the rectal pouch. Proximal mobilization is done so that the level at which the proximal transection would be done can be brought easily to below the pubic symphysis. This may sometimes need division of the left colic artery so that the colon that will be pulled down will be based on the left branch of the middle colic through the marginal artery of Drumond.

The mobilized colon is retracted anteriorly and cranially so as to expose the retrorectal space. A space is created by blunt finger dissection initially and then with a 'peanut' on a long Kelly's clamp (Fig. 65.1). This is continued till the peanut is able to evert the rectum outwards to expose the posterior half of the dentate line. Care should be taken not to injure the superior rectal artery.

The rectum is transected just above the pelvic peritoneum between two non-crushing intestinal clamps. The proximal end of the colon to be resected, as identified by the presence of ganglion cells previously, is also divided between two non-crushing intestinal clamps and the resected segment is removed. If there are fecalomas, these can be manipulated into the bowel to be resected and removed with it. The distal end of the resected segment should be marked with a silk suture for easy identification by the pathologist.

The distal end of the ganglionic colon which is to be pulled, down is closed with a running silk suture, the ends of which are left long. The mesenteric and

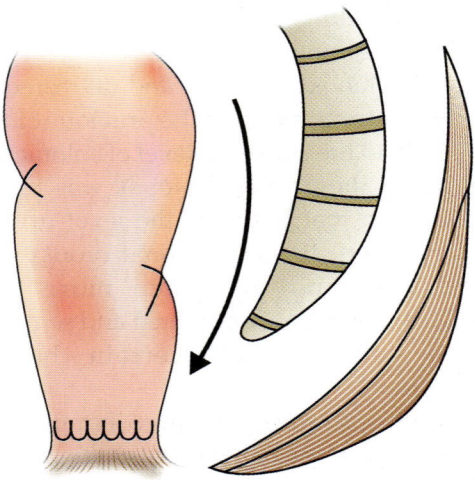

Fig. 65.1: Diagrammatic representation of retrorectal space dissection

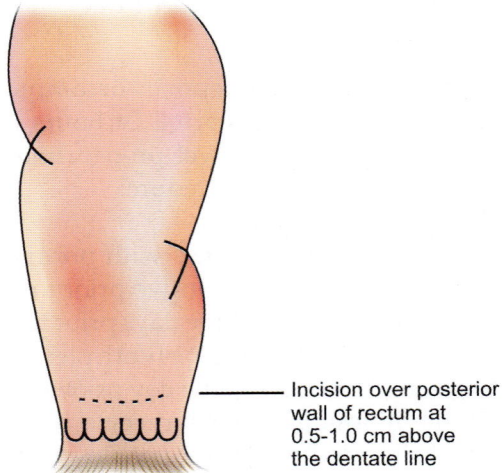

Fig. 65.2: Incision over the posterior rectal wall

antimesenteric ends should be marked with different coloured sutures (e.g. Catgut and silk) to avoid rotation during pull-through.

The intestinal clamp is removed from the proximal end of the rectal stump and the rectum cleaned with povidone iodine solution. Four silk stay suture are taken on this rectal stump at 3, 6, 9 and 12 o'clock positions.

The Kelly's clamp with a 'peanut' is again passed into the retrorectal space so as to evert the dentate line out of the anal canal. Posterior 180° (half circumference) full thickness incision is made on the rectal wall, between silk stay sutures placed at 3, 6 and 9 O'clock positions. The incision should be 0.5-1.0 cm proximal to the dentate line (Fig. 65.2).

Another Kelly's clamp is now used to grasp the protruding 'peanut' and the abdominal Kelly's clamp is then withdrawn, thereby guiding the tip of the rectal Kelly's clamp into the abdomen through the posterior rectal incision and the retrorectal space.

The stay sutures left long on the closed end of the colon to be pulled-down is grasped by this Kelly's clamp and is gradually pulled out of the rectum, gently guiding the colon through the retrorectal space and out through the posterior half circumference rectal incision. During this maneuver the surgeon ensures that there is no twisting of the colon and that the mesentry of the pulled-through colon is posteriorly in the sagittal plane.

Posterior half circumference of the pulled down colon is then incised transversely about 1 cm proximal to the closed end and its proximal lip is sutured to the distal lip of the rectal incision with interrupted vicryl sutures.

The remainder of the half circumference of the pulled-down colon is incised and the tip of the pulled-down colon is removed for histopathological examination. Stay sutures are taken on this anterior half circumference of the pulled down colon along with the anterior lip of the half circumference rectal incision, at 3, 12 and 9 o'clock. At this juncture there are two juxtaposed loops of bowel in the perinium. Anteriorly is the aganglionic rectum and posteriorly the pulled down ganglionic colon. The common wall between the two is the posterior wall of the rectum and the anterior wall of the colon (Fig. 65.3).

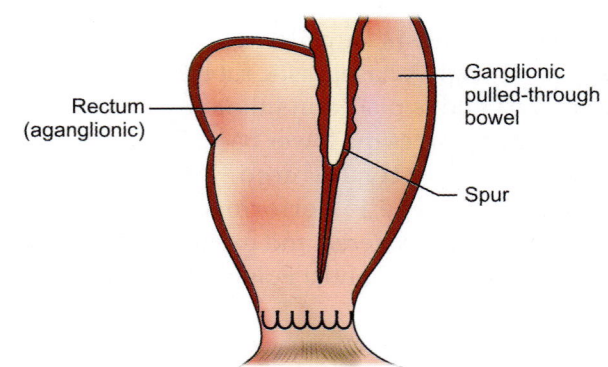

Fig. 65.3: There is a common wall between the posterior wall of the rectum and anterior wall of the colon

Stay sutures are taken on the pulled-through colon, in the abdomen, just opposite the open rectal stump and a longitudinal colotomy on the pulled-down colon is made. The lumen of both the rectum and colon is irrigated and cleaned.

GIA linear cutter 55 or 75 is then inserted through the anus with one blade in the aganglionic rectum and the other in the pulled-down ganglionic colon. Care is taken so that the entire length of the two colon walls is included and the tip of the stapling device is protruding well beyond the rectal stump and the colotomy in the abdomen. The stapler is then fired to complete the longitudinal anastomosis and the division of the common wall. In case the entire common wall is not divided, the same needs to be completed by another firing with the stapler now applied from the abdominal end in a prograde fashion.

The other alternative for dividing the common wall between the rectum and the pull-through bowel is by using the Stone's enterostomy crushing clamp (Fig. 65.4). The clamp has a box junction and two blades of either three inches or four inches in length. This is applied from the abdominal side with one of the blades being positioned into the pull-through bowel through the colostomy as described earlier and the other into the proximal open end of the retained rectal stump with the hinge of the clamp in the colon at the colostomy site. The tips of both the blades is seen from the rectal end and a ring retainer is placed on it and the screw tightened to gently crush the common wall.

The open proximal end of the rectal stump is anastomosed to the colotomy on the pulled-through colon in an end-to-side fashion (the so called Martin's modification). This anastomosis is extraperitonealized after placing a small pelvic drain of corrugated red rubber. The peritoneum on both the medial and the lateral aspects of the pulled-through colon is repaired taking care not to injure the ureters. The abdominal wound is closed in layers with vicryl for the peritoneum, muscles, sheath and the Scarpa's fascia and subcuticular absorbable sutures for the skin.

All stays are removed from the perinium, which is then cleaned and a rectal pack of paraffin gauze inserted. This is to be removed after 24 hours. The abdominal wound is cleaned and dressed. The completed anatomy of the rectum has anteriorly aganglionic bowel and posteriorly pulled-down ganglionic bowel.

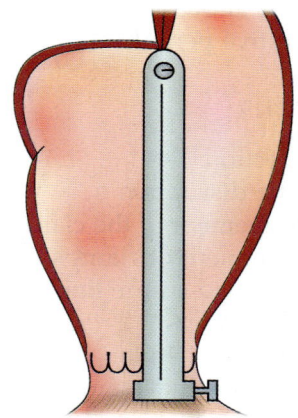

Fig. 65.4: Stone's clamp in place

In cases where the crushing clamp has been applied, on the first postoperative day, the screw on the ring retainer is fully tightened to crush the common wall. Auto-anastomosis between the two walls takes place and the clamp slips out of the rectum in 5-7 days (Fig. 65.5). The completed anatomy is just as when staplers are used. The main disadvantage of using the clamp is that the patent needs to be in the hospital till the clamps slip out. The advantage of using the enterostomy crushing clamp is that the same instrument can be used again and again in many patients. The advantage of using the enterostomy crushing clamp instead of the classically described Kocher's clamp is that its blades are longer and so it can easily crush the entire common wall. Further, just the tip of the blades and the ring retainer protrudes

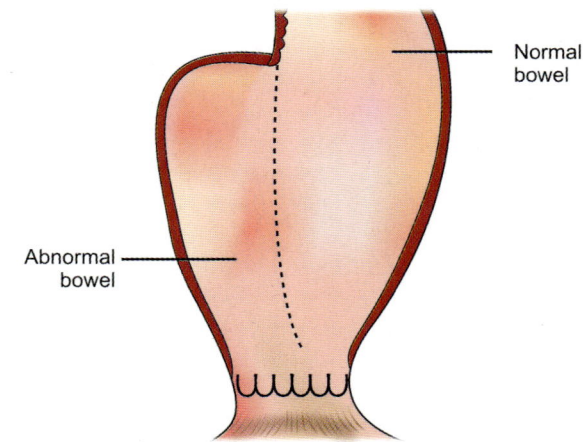

Fig. 65.5: Final result of the completed procedure with the anterior aganglionic bowel and posterior pulled-through ganglionic bowel

out of the rectum, allowing the child to be ambulatory in the postoperative period.

COMPLICATIONS

1. Wound infection
2. Anastomotic disruption
3. Early dislodgement of the clamps
4. Non-dislodgement of clamps
5. Failure of stapled suture line
6. Injury to the ureters
7. Enterocutaneous fistula
8. Recurrent or residual symptoms
9. Fecal soiling or incontinence
10. Enterocolitis
11. Adhesive intestinal obstruction
12. Fecaloma formation especially when Martin's modification is not done.

ACKNOWLEDGEMENT

This chapter is a modified version of article published in GI Surgery Annual, Volume 11, Supplement 1, 2004- reproduced here with the permission of the editor of GI Surgery Annual.[15]

REFERENCES

1. Swenson O, Bill AH. Resection of rectum and rectosigmoid with preservation of sphincter for benign spastic lesion producing megacolon. Surgery 1948;24:212.
2. Duhamel B. Therapies chirurgicale infantile. Paris 1957.
3. Soave F. A new original technique for treatment of Hirschsprung's disease. Surgery 1964;56:1007.
4. Grob M. Intestinal obstruction in the newborn infant. Arch Dis Child 1960;35:40.
5. Duhamel B. A new operation for the treatment of Hirschsprung's disease. Arch Dis Child 1960;35:38-40.
6. Duhamel B. Retrorectal and trans-anal pull-through procedure for the treatment of Hirschsprung's disease. Dis Colon Rectum 1964;7:455.
7. Bill AH, Donald JC. Modified procedure for Hirschsprung's disease to eliminate rectal pouch. Surg Gynecol Obstet 1969;128:831.
8. Zachry BB, Lister J. Crushing instrument for Duhamel's procedure in Hirschsprung's disease. Lancet 1964;1:476.
9. Sulamaa M. Anastomotic clamp for retrorectal transanal pull-through procedure in Hirschsprung's disease- A new modification of Duhamel's operation. Ann Chir Inf 1968;9:63.
10. Ikeda K. New techniques in the surgical treatment of Hirschsprung's disease. Surgery 1967;61:503.
11. Agarwala S, Bhatnagar V, Mitra DK. Stone's enterostomy crushing clamp for modified Duhamel's procedure. Tropical Gastroenterol 1998;19:164.
12. Steichen FM, Spigland NA, Numez D. The modified Duhamel's operation for Hirschsprung's disease performed entirely with mechanical sutures. J Pediatr Surg 1987;22:435.
13. Martin LW, Altemeier WA. Clinical experience with a new operation (modified Duhamel's procedure) for Hirschsprung's disease. Ann Surg 1962;156:678.
14. Bax NMA, van der Zee DC. Laparoscopic removal of aganglionic bowel using the Duhamel's Martin modified in five consecutive infants. Pediatr Surg Int 1995;10:116.
15. Agarwal S. Duhamel's pull-through for Hirschsprungs disease. GI Surgery Annual 2004;11:1-7.

Soave's (Boley Scot) Endorectal Pull-through

DK Gupta, Manish Pathak, Shilpa Sharma

HISTORICAL BACKGROUND

Endorectal pull-through technique was first described by Franco Soave in 1964 for patients with Hirschsprung's disease.[1] He was inspired by the work of Rehbein and Romualdi (1959) on the treatment of cases of High Anorectal Malformation (ARM) with rectourethral fistula. This procedure was based on removing the mucosa and submucosa of the rectum and pulling the ganglionic bowel through the aganglionic muscular cuff, and leaving it hanging beyond the anal verge, till adhesions developed between the two segments of bowel. The excess of the bowel was later excised may be after 2 weeks or so. Thus, there was no formal anastomosis at the anus in this original Soave's procedure. This procedure was considered practical and life saving in critically ill children in that era, especially in those children who were quite sick and the bowel was not healthy. However, Soave in 1964, published another paper with his modification. It consisted of making a circumferential cut, through the muscular coat of the colon at the pelvic peritoneal reflection. Working in an intramural plane, the mucosa was separated from the muscular coat down to the anal canal. The freed mucosa was excised and the proximal normal colon was pulled through this retained viable spastic aganglionic muscular sleeve. A telescoping type of anastomosis was then made that added an extra layer of colon wall at the anastomosis.[2]

The procedure was later modified by Boley Scot and published in 1964 and 1968.[3,4] He performed an extrapelvic anastomosis between the anal canal mucosa and the mucosa of the normal colon. Marks reported cutting the sleeve posteriorly, a practice now widely used.[5]

Further modification was suggested by Coran and Weintraub, with the eversion of the mucosal-submucosal tube on to the perineum to facilitate the performance of anastomosis.[6]

The endorectal pull-through has evolved from a transabdominal dissection to a transanal approach. Transanal mucosal proctectomy was described by Parks for low rectal malignancies (1972).[7] Rintala et al (1993) used this technique for the operative treatment of Hirschsprung's disease (HD).[8] Since then, there have been many modifications. Transanal approach has been used either alone or in combination with the laparotomy in difficult situations.

Endorectal pull-through by complete transanal dissection was described by de la Torre-Mondragon and Ortego-Salgado in 1998.[9] Georgeson et al in 1999 described the laparoscopic assisted mobilization of aganglionic colon, along with trans-anal dissection.[10]

SCIENTIFIC BASIS OF ENDORECTAL PROCEDURE

This procedure is based on the belief that by remaining within the muscular cuff of the aganglionic segment, injury to the nerves is avoided and the integrity of the internal sphincter is preserved.

INDICATIONS OF ENDO-RECTAL PULL-THROUGH

1. All confirmed cases of short-segment and long-segment Hirschsprung's disease.
2. Total colonic aganglionosis with ileoanal endorectal anastomosis.
3. All redo pull-through procedures following a failed Swenson, Duhamel or Endorectal pull-through.

PREOPERATIVE EVALUATION FOR DIAGNOSIS

1. **Baseline investigations:** Hemogram, liver and renal function tests.
2. **Barium enema:** This is used for initial screening and diagnosis of Hirschprung's disease (Fig. 66.1). It also helps in determining the suitability for a primary pull-through procedure. A massively dilated ganglionic bowel will preclude the endorectal pull through procedure and necessitates diversion of stools with a proximal appropriate colostomy. A lateral film and a late film after 24 hours must be the part of barium study to gain maximal information.

   A properly performed barium study also gives information about the level of the transition zone, indicating the extent of aganglionosis and planning for the appropriate type of pull though operative procedure.
3. **Rectal biopsy:** This is the gold-standard test for confirming the diagnosis of HD and all patients must have a proof of diagnosis as far as possible, before undergoing pull-through procedure.
4. **Anorectal manometry:** Absence of recto-sphincteric relaxation reflex suggests Hirschprung's disease. This is not routinely performed in all cases of HD but the study is extremely useful in patients with ultrashort variety of HD, to establish the diagnosis when rectal biopsy has remained unhelpful.

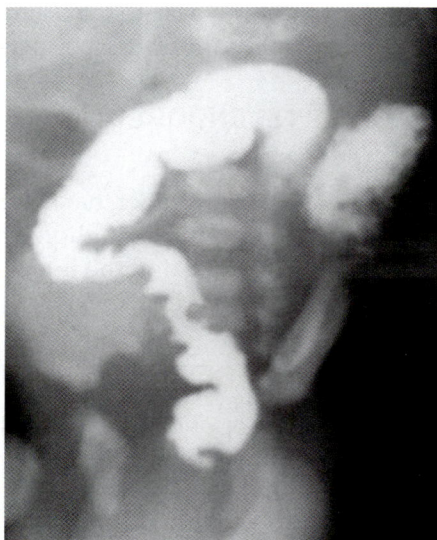

Fig. 66.1: Barium enema suggestive of rectosigmoid Hirschprung's disease

SURGICAL PROCEDURE

The soave's pull-through can be performed as a single stage surgery or it can be staged into two or even three stages, depending on the experen e of the surgeon, extent of the disease, the condition of the baby (anemia, enterocolitis, epsis, fecolomas) and the degree of the dilatation of the bowel.

In the three-stage procedure, first a proximal diversion is done. The site of diversion varies according to the level of aganglionosis found on barium study. The authors prefer a "right transverse colostomy" for the standard type of rectosigmoid HD. The normal bowel distal to colostomy remains out of circulation and decreases in size remarkably in due course of time, may be a few months. For the technical reasons and to avoid any loss of healthy colon during the definitive surgery, a "leveling colostomy" (after confirming with frozen biopsy) is preferred in patients who have the long segment HD, involving the descending colon or the splenic flexure.

In the patients with total colonic aganglionosis (involving not only whole of the colon but also the terminal ileum extending for about 10-25 cm proximally from the ileocaecal valve in 50% cases), a "leveling ileostomy" is performed. A frozen seromuscular biopsy proves quite helpful and should always be done while constructing the stoma as the "Leveling diversion". Also, before discharging the patient, the parents should be taught the technique of distal stomal and rectal washes, to avoid stool deposition and fecoloma formation.

At the time of second admission for pull-through procedure, distal stomal and rectal washes are continued as in-patient to make the bowel absolutely clean for the pull-through. Taking down of the stoma will be required in case of long segment Hirschsprung's disease. If the long segment disease is suspected then child is given low residue diet for 3-4 days. Only clear fluids are allowed the day prior to surgery. Polyethyleneglycol (75-80 ml/kg) orally or through nasogastric tube is also given the day prior to surgery to ensure that the bowel to be pulled down is found absolutely clean during surgery.

The neonates do not require anything other than saline enema to prepare the bowel for pull-through. Intravenous antibiotics should be started 24 hours prior to surgery and continued in the postoperative period.

In older children, a barium enema should be done, preferably after 12 weeks of initial diversion to confirm the resolution of the faecaloma and the decrease in the size of dilated proximal bowel. In case the bowel is found still dilated and unfit for pull through, the definitive surgery is further delayed and the distal wash outs are continued more effectively.

SINGLE-STAGE PROCEDURE (PRIMARY PULL-THROUGH)

Primary pull-through is rapidly gaining acceptance since the successful report by So et al in 1980.[11] The pull through procedure is performed as a single stage without the need for a diversion. This is suitable in cases where the proximal colon is not excessively dilated as in the neonates and also in some infants and children with effectively decompressed bowel. This is discussed in detail in the next chapter.

TWO-STAGE PROCEDURE

Leveling colostomy is done in the first stage. Stoma is made at distal most part of normal ganglionic bowel. Left lower quadrant oblique incision is made, and the transition zone is looked for. Seromuscular frozen section biopsy is taken from the hypertrophied bowel just proximal to the grossly visible transition zone. A seromuscular layer is dissected off the underlying submucosa for about a cm and sent for frozen biopsy. It is important to remember that the transition zone may extend for several centimeters. Along this zone, ganglionic cells may be present on one side of the circumference but may not be on the other. Thus, it is safer to place the stoma at a more proximal distance. Part of the colon used in the colostomy should "contain adequate number of ganglion cells and absence of hypertrophied nerve bundles".

Colostomy can either be loop or divided. Loop colostomy with an adequate spur is preferred by most surgeons. Appropriate sized red rubber catheter (RRC) is passed through small hole in mesentery closer to the wall of the bowel avoiding the injury to the marginal vascular arcade. A spur is made by taking seromuscular stitches between the adjoining ascending and descending limbs of the hooked bowel loop.

Advantages of Spur while Making a Colostomy

1. Helps in complete diversion of stoma.
2. Prevents stomal prolapse.
3. Prevents stomal retraction.

Dismantling of the stoma and the pull-through of ganglionic bowel is done as the second stage definitive surgery.

THREE-STAGE PROCEDURE

Short segment Hirschsprung's is the most common (75-80%) type. The right transverse colon can be used for fashioning the colostomy in all such cases as the first stage. During this procedure, multiple seromuscular biopsies are taken from the suspected aganglionic, ganglionic and the normal colon, proximal to gross transition zone to identify distal most part of the ganglionic bowel. Biopsy sites are closed with silk sutures so as to facilitate identification during the pull-through procedure. In the second stage, the pull-through procedure is completed. The colostomy closure is done as the third stage surgery.

Advantages of Three-stage Procedure

1. Colostomy can be made even when frozen-section facility is not available.
2. Colostomy allows the decompression of the distal bowel, making it fit for pull through procedure.
3. Under the colostomy cover, the child grows well and improves nutritionally.
4. Pull-through procedure is completed without the need to mobilize the colostomy.
5. The anal anastomosis is well protected by the colostomy, in the immediate postoperative period after the second stage.

Disadvantages of Three-stage Procedure

1. Requirement of multiple admissions and operations places a significant burden on both the family and the health care system.
2. The level of the colostomy may not allow the second stage of the pullthrough without mobilization of the colostomy in cases with the long segment disease.
3. The distal segment of the colon may undergo disuse atrophy if left for long or the child is lost for follow-up and thus may not function properly after the colostomy closure in the third stage.

Cuff length– The recommended length of the cuff has progressively shortened. There has been a concern that long cuff may increase the incidence of constipation or enterocolitis. Presently most surgeons prefer to limit the seromuscular cuff length to about 3-5 cm only.

Pull-through– In this chapter the modified Soave or the Boley Scott transabdominal pull through procedure will be discussed.

Determining the part of bowel to be pulled down– If the leveling colostomy had been done at the first stage, then the stoma should be pulled down during the pull-through.

If the right transverse colostomy and sero-muscular biopsy was done in first stage then report of the seromuscular biopsy, proximal to the gross transitional zone is important. If it showed presence of the adequate number of ganglion cells along with the absence of the hypertrophic nerve fibers, then the bowel just proximal to biopsy site can be pulled down safely during the second stage. If the seromuscular biopsy showed the absence of ganglion cell, then a frozen section biopsy will be required intra-operatively. Similarly, during the primary pull-through procedure, the level of the ganglionic bowel should always be confirmed by the frozen section biopsy.

SURGICAL TECHNIQUE

General anesthesia supplemented with caudal analgesia is used. Child is placed in the lithotomy position. It enables the surgeon to achieve abdominal and perineal approach easily. Child's buttock's are brought to the end of the operating table and raised with a small roller or the sand bag to improve the accessibility of the anal region for dissection.

Abdomen, perineum, and thighs are prepared and draped. Appropriate sized Foley's catheter is inserted into the bladder. An adequate hockey-stick or left lower abdominal curved skin-crease incision is made (Fig. 66.2). Incision incorporates the colostomy take down in a two-stage procedure. The abdominal muscles are divided and peritoneum is opened to enter the abdominal cavity. The diagnosis is reconfirmed. The level of the ganglionic bowel is determined.

The lateral peritoneum over the mesosigmoid is incised laterally to mobilize the colon. Both the ureters are identified so as to avoid an inadvertent injury. Colon is mobilized proximally and also distally upto the reflection of the pelvic peritoneum. The vascular supply to the ganglionic bowel is preserved carefully. The bowel is freed and dissected of the pelvic peritoneum from anterior and lateral sides. Traction is applied with the atraumatic clamps on either side of distal bowel. The ganglionic bowel is mobilized proximally, preserving the marginal vessels. Adequacy of mobilization is ascertained by the ability to bring the ganglionic bowel over to the pubis bone easily to have a tension free anastomosis. This usually matches with the length of the bowel sufficient to reach the anal verge. Occasionally, the mesentery is foreshortened and it is necessary to ligate the inferior mesenteric artery and or the left colic artery, so that the vascular supply of the descending colon is based on the left branch of the middle colic artery alone or supplemented by the left colic artery or its ascending branch, through the arcades forming the marginal artery of Drummond. Given an opportunity, the inferior mesenteric artery and its continuation as the superior rectal artery, is preserved to maintain the rich blood supply to the sero-muscular cuff in the pelvis.

Endorectal dissection is then started about 2 cm. below the peritoneal reflection (Figs 66.3A and B). Soave in his original description used the infiltration of local anesthesia into the seromuscular coat of rectosigmoid segment to facilitate the endorectal dissection.[1] Endorectal dissection begins by completely clearing the mesentery and the fat over a 2 cm. length of bowel. The seromuscular layer is incised transversely all around with the diathermy, taking care not to go deep and enter the mucosa. This requires

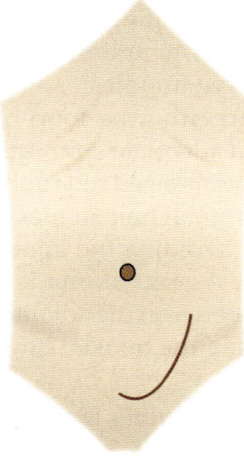

Fig. 66.2: Abdominal incision

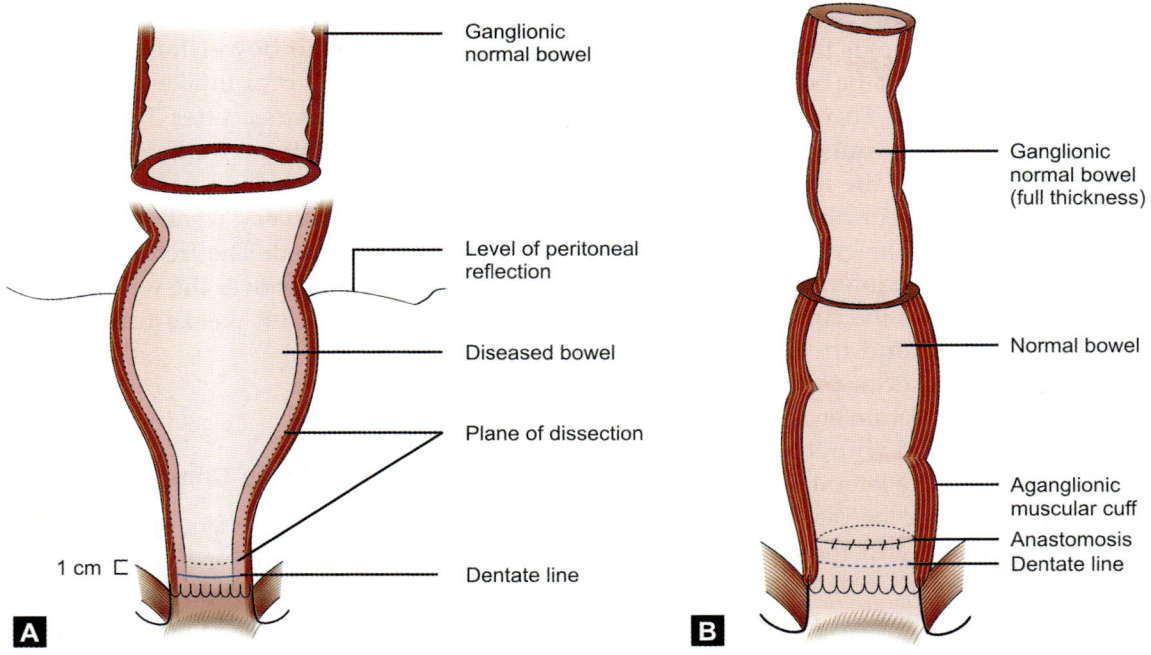

Figs 66.3A and B: A. The submucosal plane of dissection begins 2 cm above the peritoneal reflection **B.** Completed Scot Boley's modified Soave's procedure. The ganglionic bowel is pulled through the aganglionic cuff

experience to get into the submucosal plane of dissection. Once the submucosal layer is reached, the seromuscular layer is dissected down gradually circumferentially. Cotton tip applicator is used to separate the seromuscular layer bluntly from the deeper submucosal layer.

As the muscular cuff begins to develop, a uniform traction is applied to the mucosal tube with right angled clamps. This dissection is facilitated by a well co-ordinated traction and counter-traction to the mucosal and seromucular tube. Communicating vessels in the submucosal plane are picked up individually and cauterized carefully, preferably with the bipolar forceps to avoid mucosal perforations. All bleeding points in the muscular cuff are cauterized. Previous history of enterocolitis and the rectal biopsy cause some difficulty in mucosal tube separation. Dissection is carried from the abdominal side in the pelvis to reach 1-1.5 cm. above the dentate line. As one goes deeper down in the pelvis, the dissection becomes more difficult near the attachment of the anal sphincter with the anal mucosa. At this stage, one may stop the dissection from the abdominal side and plan to complete the final part of the dissection from the perineal route under vision (described as below).

The bowel is transected above the peritoneal reflection in between clamps. The aganglionic bowel is now excised and the edges of the ganglionic bowel are cleaned with povidone iodine and readied to be delivered to the perineum through the seromuscular tube. The posterior wall of the seromuscular cuff is slit open for 3-4 cm in the midline to prevent ring effect.

Perineal Stage

The anal dilatation is done as the first important step. Then the anal mucosa is everted with thick silk sutures and anchored at four corners in position. A circumferential incision is given in the anal mucosa with the diathermy, about a cm from the dentate line. This is just to mark the lower limit of the dissection of the mucosal sleeve and the level of the coloanal anastomosis.

Narrow retractors are placed in the anal canal and the transected end of the mucosal tube is everted out onto the perineum by a Kelly's clamp. The mucosa is separated from the underlying muscle, if any, till the circumferential incision already marked. With a Kelly's clamp, the ganglionic bowel is brought down. The assistant at abdominal end holds the cut edges of the muscular cuff and ensures that the bowel is not twisted while it is being pulled down. To avoid the possibility of retraction, the outer (seromuscular) wall of the pulled colon is sutured with the inner (muscle) wall of the cuff, about half a cm above the coloanal anastomosis at 6-8 places. The coloanal anastomosis is then completed using fine interrupted Vicryl/PDS absorbable sutures between the full thickness of the pulled colon and the cuff and the mucosa junction (Fig. 66.4). The colon is now pulled back in the abdomen to invert the neorectum back into its position. The muscular cuff is sutured with the pulled through colon at the anterior and the lateral edges.

A Penrose drain used to be placed in the past in between the pulled colon and the cuff to avoid an hematoma or the abscess formation. With the availability of better antibiotics and refinement in surgical techniques, it is not practiced now. Similarly, the abdomen wound is closed without any drain, unless the dissection has been difficult resulting in gross contamination.

POSTOPERATIVE CARE

Postoperative monitoring of vital parameters is done. Adequate pain relief is ensured. Postoperative hemoglobin, blood urea, and serum electrolytes are monitored. Patient is kept on maintenance intravenous fluids. Intravenous broad spectrum antibiotics are given as per the institutional protocol. Patient is kept nil per orally and on continuous nasogastric drainage till the return of the bowel movement. Patient is discharged once the oral intake is adequate. Rectal examination is performed after 3 weeks very gently to assess for the anastomosis. The parents are taught to start anal dilation starting twice a day. The size of dilator is increased every week till the appropriate sized dilator is reached. The frequency of dilation is then reduced gradually over the weeks. The diverting colostomy is closed 6-8 weeks following the pull-through procedure.

COMPLICATIONS

Intraoperative and Early Complications

1. *Bleeding*– This may be troublesome if the patient has had enterocolitis or the child is older with good musculature and if there is a faecoloma in the dilated bowel. The authors feel that Xylocaine with Adrenaline may lead to postoperative hemorrhage and derangement of the muscle plane and thus do not recommend its use.
2. *Rotation of bowel*– Stool does not come out, can pass a finger from below. Can be diagnosed with a cutoff sign on Barium.
3. *Inversion of the cuff*– if one is not careful. This may lead to obstructive symptoms. It may be diagnosed as a lump on per rectal examination.
4. Injury to the ureter.
5. Injury to the vas.
6. Intestinal obstruction.
7. Cuff abscess.
8. Wound infection.
9. Early anorectal stenosis.
10. Anastomotic leak.
11. Perineal excoriation/Edema.
12. Frequency of stool.
13. Faecal fistula.
14. *Mucosal prolapse:* This happens if the extension of dissection is done upto the cutaneous ring. It results in visible mucosa and mucosal secretions and wet perineum.
15. *Stricture at the cuff level*– It takes time to develop and may become apparent on per rectal examination performed after 3 weeks or later. It is best avoided by slitting the cuff vertically in the midline posteriorly.

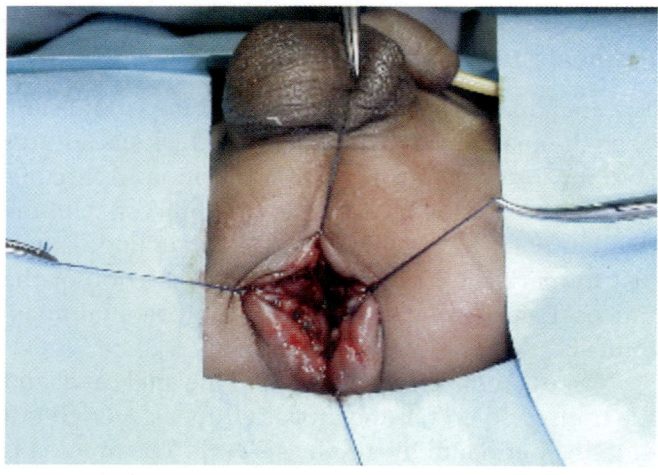

Fig. 66.4: Completed coloanal anastomosis

Complications Specific to Classical Soave

1. Nuisance-bowel is hanging out, requiring redo surgery to excise the redundant bowel. However, the procedure has merit in cases with anticipated risk of retraction.
2. Septicemia.
3. Ischemia.
4. Putrefaction of bowel.

Late Complications

1. Enterocolitis.
2. Incontinence.
3. Constipation.
4. Intestinal obstruction.
5. Urinary and sexual dysfunction.
6. Residual disease.
7. Ischemic aganglionosis.
8. Stricture.

Enterocolitis– The incidence of enterocolitis post pull-through ranges from 2-40% but is typically between 20-30%.[12-18] Most of the episodes occur within the first 2 years after pull-through. Patients with long segment Hirschsprung's disease, trisomy 21 have a higher incidence of enterocolitis. Anastomotic stricture or narrowing of anastomosis also increases the incidence of enterocolitis. Fortuna et al noted 27% incidence of enterocolitis following endorectal pull-through.[19] Agostino Pierro et al did not find any significant difference in the incidence of enterocolitis between staged and primary pull-through patients.[20] Authors found higher incidence of enterocolitis in younger infants, i.e. < 4 months (20%) than that in children. Teitelbaum et al noted a higher (42%) incidence of enterocolitis in primary pull-through patients and was probably due to a very low threshold for making the diagnosis of enterocolitis.[21] The younger age of operation in this series might have been responsible for the higher incidence of enterocolitis. Thirty percent incidence of enterocolitis was noted following transanal endorectal pull-through by Minford et al.[22]

Hackam et al also compared the staged and single stage repair and found that the enterocolitis rate was similar in both the groups.[23] Kvan Leeuwen et al compared the perineal and transabdominal pull-through approaches with the incidence of enterocolitis and did not find any significant difference between the two groups.[24]

Incontinence– A properly performed pull-through procedure in a mentally normal child, should not have complication like incontinence. Still, the incidence of incontinence ranges from 3-8% in various series.[25,26] A higher incidence of postoperative incontinence is noted in mentally retarded patients. Yanchar, et al studied the long-term outcome in Hirschsprung's disease patients undergoing endorectal pull-through in 37 patients.[25] Only 64% patients were interpreted as having normal stooling habits. Most children had significant improvement in fecal continence with time. Fortuna et al also found that though short-term continence was less than 50%, all of them (100%) became continent by 15 years after pull-through surgery.[19] So, et al found that 79% of operated children had normal bowel control following pull-through. There has been a concern about the effect of prolonged traction of sphincter muscle during transanal approach.[27]

Kvan Leeuwen et al did not find any difference in the number of stools per day or manometric findings between perineal and abdominal approach.[24] Other series also suggest reasonably good outcome. In general, the continence improves with age.

Constipation– Incidence of constipation has been reported up to 30% after a pull-through, but most of the patients can be managed by dietary modification and oral medication. Mechanical causes, e.g. stricture, twist of the bowel, ischemia resulting in fibrotic anorectum, should be ruled out in all such cases. The retained muscular cuff may also contribute to obstruction as it might form a ring around the pulled colon.

Sexual and urinary dysfunction– As the endorectal dissection remains mainly inside the muscular cuff, the procedure is not associated with the risk of nerve injury so, the incidence of sexual and urinary dysfunction is almost nil.

OUTCOME AND COMPARISON BETWEEN DIFFERENT PROCEDURES

Fortuna et al analyzed complications and long-term outcome following operative treatment for Hirschsprung's disease and found more complications following the Soave pull-through than the Duhamel pull-through.[19] Minford et al compared the morbidity and medium term functional outcome of the Duhamel operation and the transanal endorectal pull-through.[22]

The functional outcome was similar in both the groups. Klein MD et al published their 30 years experience of Hirschsprung's disease and found highest incidence of post-pull-through enterocolitis with the Duhamel procedure, less with the Swenson, and least with the endorectal pull-through. In contrast, the incidence of complications other than enterocolitis, was highest with the Swenson, and least with the transanal endorectal pull-through.[28] Yanchar et al (1999) did not find significant difference among the types of pull-through procedures except constipation, which was found more following Duhamel pull-through.[22,25]

REDO FOR SOAVE-REDO PULL-THROUGH

Redo pull-through may be required for retained segment of aganglionic bowel, acquired aganglionosis due to ischemia, severe anastomatic stricture, or intestinal neuronal dysplasia. Overall outcome following redo pull-through is not as good as after initial pull-through. If there has not been any incidence of severe enterocolitis then redo endorectal pull-through can be attempted. Otherwise, Duhamel or Swenson procedure is chosen as redo endorectal pull-through. According to Langer JC et al Duhamel procedure is the preferred redo procedure for technical reasons.[29] Gobran et al evaluated the safety and efficacy of transanal endorectal pull-through for patients with persistent symptoms after pull-through for Hirschsprung's disease.[30] There were no anastomotic deaths or anastomotic leakage.

AUTHOR'S EXPERIENCE WITH THE SOAVE'S PROCEDURE FOR HD[31-38]

A total of 128 patients of HD were treated between 1981-2005 by various techniques of Soave's endorectal (Boley Scott) procedure (Table 66.1). The diagnosis was based on barium enema, rectal biopsy and preoperative frozen section. Immunohistochemistry was used only in few selected cases with diagnostic challenge. Anorectal manometry was useful in diagnosis of Ultrashort segment HD, 7 in this series. The age of the patients ranged from 2 days to 24 years. Majority of them (70%) presented beyond infancy and the male to female ratio was 10:1. The rectosigmoid region was involved in 101. rectum in 10, transverse or ascending colon in 3, total colon in 12 and whole gut in 2 cases. Associated anomalies included hypospadias (2), and hydrometerocolpos, undescended testis and colonic atresia in one each. Three children required sigmoid colotomy as the initial procedure to remove the large and hard fecoloma that had failed to be cleaned by all other methods. Of the 128, endorectal pull-through procedures, 7 were post-myemectomy for HD done elsewhere and 12 were cases of total colonic aganglionosis (4 our own and 8 referred from outside). A Martin's modification of ileocolic anastomosis and ileoanal endorectal pull through was done using the only the ileum for the anastomosis at the analverge (Figs 66.5A and B). The classical Soave's procedure was done in the beginning of the series in only 10 patients. Recently, 16 patients were selected for the transanal endorectal pull-through.

Two cases underwent modified technique of ileal loop endorectal pull-through, for the complicated type of rectosigmoid variety of HD. A carefully selected ileal loop based on its pedicle was bridged in between the ascending colon and the anus, as described and published by the authors in 1989. Both these cases had undergone transverse colostomy for rectosigmoid type of HD under 1 year of age. They were then lost for follow-up while still being on colostomy, for 12 and 7 year respectively. Distal cologram showed the colon distal to the colostomy site quite thin, narrow in caliber and shortened. At surgery, the distal unused colon was found atrophied and the blood supply was quite fragile making it unusable for the pull-through procedure, despite being ganglionic. The whole of the atrophied colon was excised. A segment of the ileum, appropriate in length on its vascular supply, was selected and bridged in between the ascending colon (proximal to the transverse colostomy) and the anal verge. The ascending colon stoma was closed later.

Table 66.1: Details of the operative techniques used by the authors in 128 patients with Hirschsprung's disease (1980-2005)

Operative procedure	No.
Classical Soave procedure (in early 1980's)	10
Modified Soave, (Boley Scott) abdomino-perineal pull-through,	72
Martin's modification of ileo-anal endorectal pull-through for total colonic aganglionosis	12
Ileal loop endorectal pull-through for complicated HD	02
Transanal endorectal pull-through	16
Redo cases for HD	16

In the authors' experience, an endorectal (Boley Scot) procedure was always found feasible for all types of failed cases of HD including Duhamel and Swenson, requiring redo procedures.

Average frequency of stools in the initial postoperative period was 5.6 per day which gradually reduced to 2.4 at 3 months. Nine of the patients were treated after the age of 15 years, one of them aged 24 years after marriage. All these were performed as the staged pull-through with an initial proximal transverse colostomy. Incidentally, HD related enterocolitis has not been common in our practice and so also the postoperative incontinence or the constipation.

The authors, the parents and the patients have been quite happy with the procedure and the outcome. However, two patients with total colonic aganglionosis undergoing endorectal pull-through had high frequency of stools, recurrent enterocolitis, perianal skin excoriation and incontinence, requiring many hospital admissions, blood transfusions, antibiotic courses. The life has truly been miserable in both these. They have been advised for permanent diversion.

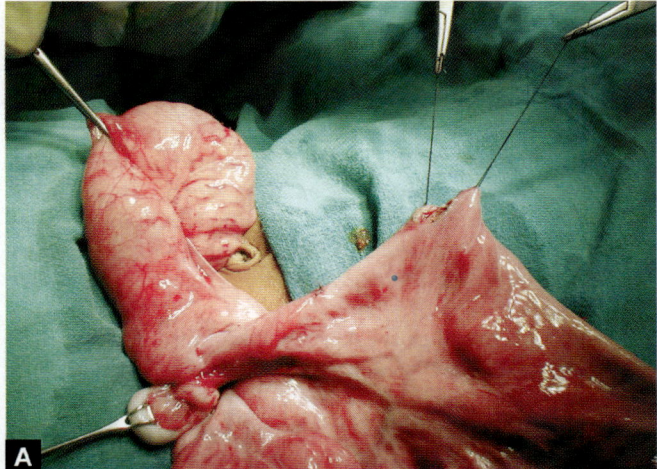
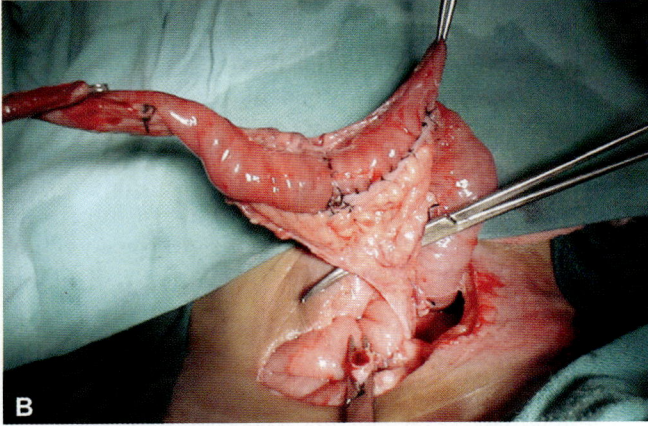

Figs 66.5A and B: A. Operative photograph of a case of total colonic aganglionosis. **B.** Ileum prepared for Soave's pull-through with a left colonic patch

Sixteen of these underwent redo pull-through (12 of these referred from outside to our center with various complications). Anal dilatations were advised in all for about 3 months after surgery. However, surgery related complications included anastomotic stricture in 2, anastomotic stenosis in 1, adhesive obstruction in 3, wound infection in 2, residual disease in 2, fecal fistula in 1, ureteral injury in 1 (case of long segment HD undergoing multiple surgeries), bleeding in 1 requiring a redo laparotomy and the bowel rotation in another who had continued with constipation. In this case, the finger could be negotiated beyond the anal verge. The rectal washout could be performed but there was no return. It was the barium study that showed a twist in the bowel in the pelvis. A de-twist and redo colocolic anastomosis (without dismantling the pulled through anastomosis) was successful.

REFERENCES

1. Soave F. Hirschsprung's disease; a new surgical technique. Arch Dis Child 1964;39:116.
2. Soave F. A new operation for the treatment of Hirschsprung's disease. Surgery 1964;56:1007-14.
3. Boley SJ. New modification of the surgical treatment of Hirschsprung's disease. Surgery 1964;56:1015-17.
4. Boley SJ. An endorectal pull-through operation with primary anastomosis for Hirschsprung's disease. Surg Gynecol Obstet 1968;127(2):353-57.
5. Marks RM. Endorectal split sleeve pull-through procedure for Hirschsprung's disease. Surg Gynecol Obstet. 1973;136:627-28.
6. Coran AG, Weintraub WH. Modification of the endorectal procedure for Hirschsprung's disease. Surg Gynecol Obstet 1976;143(2):277-82.
7. Parks AG. Transanal technique in low rectal anastomosis. Proc R Soc Med 1972;65(11):975-76.
8. Rintala R, Lindahl H. Transanal endorectal coloanal anastomosis for Hirschsprung's disease. Pediatric Surg Int 1993;8:128-31.
9. De la Torre-Mondragon L, Ortega-Salgado JA. Transanal endorectal pull-through for Hirschsprung's disease. J Pediatr Surg 1998;33(8):1283-86.
10. Georgeson KE, Cohen RD, Hebra A, et al. Primary laparoscopic-assisted endorectal colon pull-through for Hirschsprung's disease: a new gold standard. Ann Surg 1999;229(5):678-82; discussion 682-83.

11. So HB, Schwartz DL, Becker JM, Daum F, Schneider KM. Endorectal "pull-through" without preliminary colostomy in neonates with Hirschsprung's disease. J Pediatr Surg 1980;15(4):470-71.
12. Caneiro P, Brereton R, Drake D, et al. Enterocolitis in Hirschsprung's disease. Pediatric Surg Int 1992;7:356-60.
13. Estevao-Costa J, Carvalho JL, Soares-Oliveira M. Enterocolitis risk factors after pull-through for Hirschsprung's disease. J Pediatr Surg 2000;35(1):153.
14. van Leeuwen K, Teitelbaum DH, Elhalaby EA, Coran AG. Long-term follow-up of redo pull-through procedures for Hirschsprung's disease:efficacy of the endorectal pull-through. J Pediatr Surg 2000;35(6):829-33; discussion 833-34.
15. Hackam DJ, Filler RM, Pearl RH. Enterocolitis after the surgical treatment of Hirschsprung's disease: risk factors and financial impact. J Pediatr Surg 1998;33(6):830-33.
16. Langer JC, Durrant AC, de la Torre L, Teitelbaum DH, Minkes RK, Caty MG, Wildhaber BE, Ortega SJ, Hirose S, Albanese CT. One-stage transanal Soave pull-through for Hirschsprung disease: a multicenter experience with 141 children. Ann Surg 2003;238(4):569-83; discussion 583-85.
17. Teitelbaum DH, Caniano DA, Qualman SJ. The pathophysiology of Hirschsprung's-associated enterocolitis: importance of histologic correlates. J Pediatr Surg 1989;24(12):1271-77.
18. Moore SW, Albertyn R, Cywes S. Clinical outcome and long-term quality of life after surgical correction of Hirschsprung's disease. J Pediatr Surg 1996;31(11): 1496-502.
19. Fortuna RS, Weber TR, Tracy TF Jr, Silen ML, Cradock TV. Critical analysis of the operative treatment of Hirschsprung's disease. Arch Surg 1996;131(5):520-24; discussion 524-25.
20. Pierro A, Fasoli L, Kiely EM, Drake D, Spitz L. Staged pull-through for rectosigmoid Hirschsprung's disease is not safer thanprimary pull-through. J Pediatr Surg 1997;32(3):505-09.
21. Teitelbaum DH, Cilley RE, Sherman NJ, et al. A decade of experience with the primary pull-through for Hirschsprung disease in the newborn period: a multicenter analysis of outcomes. Ann Surg 2000;232(3):372-80.
22. Minford JL, Ram A, Turnock RR, et al. Comparison of functional outcomes of Duhamel and transanal endorectal coloanal anastomosis for Hirschsprung's disease. J Pediatr Surg 2004;39(2):161-65.
23. Hackam DJ, Superina RA, Pearl RH. Single-stage repair of Hirschsprung's disease: a comparison of 109 patients over 5 years. J Pediatr Surg 1997;32(7):1028-31; discussion 1031-32.
24. Van Leeuwen K, Geiger JD, Barnett JL, Coran AG, Teitelbaum DH. Stooling and manometric findings after primary pull-throughs in Hirschsprung's disease: Perineal versus abdominal approaches. J Pediatr Surg 2002; 37(9):1321-25.
25. Yanchar NL, Soucy P. Long-term outcome after Hirschsprung's disease: patients' perspectives. J Pediatr Surg 1999;34(7):1152-60.
26. Polley TZ Jr, Coran AG, Wesley JR. A ten-year experience with ninety-two cases of Hirschsprung's disease. Including sixty-seven consecutive endorectal pull-through procedures. Ann Surg 1985;202(3):349-55.
27. So HB, Becker JM, Schwartz DL, Kutin ND. Eighteen years' experience with neonatal Hirschsprung's disease treated by endorectal pull-through without colostomy. J Pediatr Surg 1998;33(5):673-75.
28. Klein MD, Philippart AI. Hirschsprung's disease: three decades' experience at a single institution. J Pediatr Surg 1993;28(10):1291-93; discussion 1293-94.
29. Langer JC, Minkes RK, Mazziotti MV, Skinner MA, Winthrop AL. Transanal one-stage Soave procedure for infants with Hirschsprung's disease. J Pediatr Surg 1999;34(1):148-51;discussion 152.
30. Gobran TA, Ezzat A, Hassan ME, O'Neill J. Redo transanal endorectal pull-through: a preliminary study.Pediatr Surg Int 2007 Feb;23(2):189-93. Epub 2006 Dec 16.
31. Gupta DK. Plenary Lecture delivered on Experience with management of patients with Hirschsprung's disease including Total colonic Aganglionosis, during the Symposium on Hirschsprung's disease, University of Cluj-Napoca, Romania, December 2006.
32. Gupta DK. Late Presentation of Hirschsprung's disease. Lecture delivered during the Colorectal Club Meeting, Dublin, Ireland, July 2006.
33. Sharma Shilpa, Gupta DK. Functional Constipation and Late Onset Hirschsprung's Disease in Textbook of Adolescent Medicine. Ed Swati Bhave. Jaypee Brothers New Delhi Chapter 20, 2006;2:648-53.
34. Lall A, Gupta DK, Bajpai M. Neonatal Hirschsprung's Disease. Ind J Ped 2000;67(8):583-88.
35. Gupta DK, Lama TK, Srinivas M. Association between Hirschsprung's disease and colonic atresia. Jour Ind Assoc Pediatr Surg 1999:4(4);208-12.
36. Gupta DK. Lecture delivered on the Role of Myectomy for Hirschsprung's disease and Management of complicated Hirschsprung's disease, during the Round Table Meet on Hirschsprung's Disease, during the 2nd World Congress of the World Federation of the Association of Pediatric Surgeons, held in Buenos Aires, Argentina, September 2007.
37. Pratap A, Gupta DK, Shakya VC, et al. Analysis of Problems, Complications, Avoidance and Management with Transanal Pull-through for Hirschsprung's Disease Jour Ped Surg 2007;42:1869-76.
38. Rohatgi M, Gupta DK. Isolated Ileal Loop Endorectal Pull Through, "A New Approach in the Management of Complicated Hirschsprung's Disease". J Pediatr Surg 1989;24:177-79.

Transanal Endorectal Pull-through

DK Gupta, Shilpa Sharma

The transanal endorectal pull-through (TEPT) procedure was described by De la Torre and Ortega in 1998.[1] All the components of the pull-through procedure starting from mucosectomy, colectomy, and anorectal anastomosis were performed in five patients with Hirschsprung's disease (HD), only by transanal route. The authors reported their initial results using this approach, all with normal bowel movements. The procedure of doing a primary pull-through in patients with HD, without any diversion, has gained a wide acceptance, since its successful report by So et al in 1980.[2]

INDICATIONS FOR TEPT

1. Classical Short segment Hirschsprung's disease, involving rectosigmoid region.
2. Ultrashort segment Hirschsprung's disease.

There is a selection criterion before the patient could be considered for TEPT

These include:
1. The TEPT procedure can be done at any age, including even in the neonatal stage.[3] However, the operation is most commonly performed in infants as the proximal bowel is still not much dilated.
2. A barium enema study must suggest the diagnosis of HD and also the level of aganglionosis in the A-P, lateral films and the late films. In newborns, the presence of residual barium in the 24 hour delayed film is suggestive of Hirschsprung's disease (Fig. 67.1).
3. The rectal biopsy should confirm the diagnosis of HD should have been confirmed by.
4. The HD disease should be a short segment disease, limited to the rectosigmoid region. Rarely, the HD disease that extends up in the descending colon, can be approached with TEPT but this is not a commonly considered indication for TEPT (Fig. 67.2).
5. The patient with thick and dilated bowel is normally unfit for this procedure. However, most infants with HD should be fit to undergo TEPT, as the bowel is still not much dilated.
6. TEPT can also be performed in children who have dilated bowel, but as a part of three stage procedure. First, a proximal colostomy should be done to decompress the bowel. Then after about 3 months, size of the bowel is assessed by barium study. Once confirmed that the bowel has reduced in size, a TEPT can be performed as the definitive

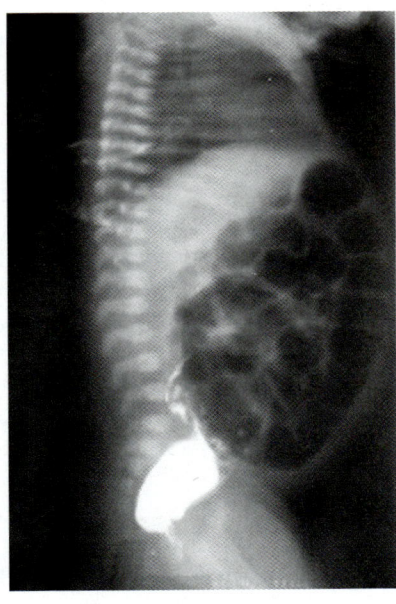

Fig. 67.1: Residual barium in the 24 hour delayed film in a newborn suggestive of Hirschsprung's disease

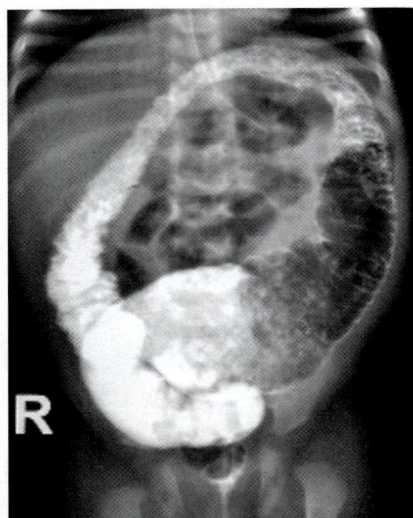

Fig. 67.2: Barium enema showing a case of rectosigmoid Hirschsprung's disease with the bowel dilated upto the splenic flexure of colon

procedure. Then, the colostomy is closed after 6-8 weeks as the final stage.

CONTRAINDICATIONS FOR TEPT

1. Operated case of Hirschsprung's disease with Duhamel or Swenson procedure.
2. Grossly dilated bowel in an older child.
3. Patient without a confirmed diagnosis of HD.
4. Patient with a long segment Hirschsprung's disease.
5. Patients with total colonic aganglionosis (TCA).
6. Any history of bleeding disorders.

Relative Contraindications for TEPT

1. Obese child with fat laden mesentery. It is difficult to manage the thick mesentry by transrectal route.
2. The blood vessels in severely anemic patients with hypoproteinemia, are fragile and easily get torn during manipulations, resulting in bleeding and hematoma formation.
3. Moderately dilated bowel.
4. Disease extending beyond the rectosigmoid upto the descending colon.

PREOPERATIVE ASSESSMENT

1. The diagnosis is confirmed with a rectal biopsy.
2. A barium enema establishes the extent of the disease. TEPT is feasible only for short segment disease and if the proximal colon is not grossly dilated. If the bowel is dilated, bowel washes are given regularly for about a week to allow the dilated bowel to shrink so that the same could be accommodated at the anus for the colorectal anastomosis.
3. If the bowel remains grossly dilated on a repeat Barium performed after adequate preparation for 3-6 months, then it may be worthwhile to perform a three stage procedure and allow the distal bowel to shrink. If the patient has had repeated episodes of enterocolitis, then also a three stage procedure is preferred.
4. Children referred with a colostomy, if the bowel is not too dilated, TEPT may be planned, followed by the colostomy closure after 6-8 weeks.

PREOPERATIVE PREPARATION

1. To remove the fecalomas, if any,
2. To prepare the colon with bowel wash outs.
3. Only clear fluids are allowed the day prior to surgery to keep the colon clean.
4. Polyethylene glycol (Peglec-75-80 ml/kg) orally or through nasogastric tube over 3-4 hours is also given the day prior to surgery to ensure that the bowel is clean during surgery. If the colon is loaded with fecal matter, Polyethylene glycol may be given for two days.
5. In older children, half the dose of Peglec, may be repeated on the same day too. Clear water may be allowed even after the polyethylene glycol so that the remnants are washed off and do not stick to the bowel.
6. Serum electrolytes may be monitored on daily basis and on the morning prior to surgery and corrected accordingly.

The TEPT procedure should preferably be done only by the trained pediatric surgeons with some experience in the field of treating patients with HD. Each step is important, specially the initiation of the formation of the mucosal tube through the transanal route. It requires surgical technique, expertise, patience and acumen for decision making, to perform mucosectomy, colectomy and the endorectal pull through. One should not hesitate to combine with the abdominal approach, if the need be, to avoid complications. To achieve this purpose, Takegawa et al in 2005 developed an experimental model in rabbit, for purposes of training and improving the surgical techniques for TEPT, described by de la Torre and Ortega.[4]

SURGICAL TECHNIQUE

General anesthesia is used. It may be supplemented with caudal analgesia depending upon the anesthesiologist's choice. The baby is placed in jack knife or the lithotomy position, depending on the surgeon preference. However, in babies with the possibility of the additional use of abdominal incision, a lithotomy position is preferred. The baby's bottom is brought to the end of the operating table and raised with a small support or a sand bag to improve the accessibility of the anal region for dissection. The abdomen, perineum, and thighs are prepared and draped, so that in case an abdominal incision is needed, the field is available and easily accessible. Appropriate sized Foley's catheter is inserted into the bladder.

The first step is to assess the cleanliness of the rectum. If in doubt, rectum should be cleaned with savlon or povidone iodine gauze swabs. The next step is to perform a gentle and slow anal dilatation with one finger at a time and dilating according to the patient's age and the bowel size.

Stay sutures are applied to mark all four quadrants at 3, 6, 9 and 12 o' clock position. The suture at 12 o' clock position is placed with care to remain close to the analverge so as not to injure the urethra in male patients. Retractors are placed to show the analmucocutaneous junction. Initiation of dissection at the anal verge to separate the mucosa from the muscle coat is the most difficult part of the TEPT. This requires experience, patience and technical innovative skills.

The Dentate line is identified and the mucosa deep circumferential incision is given about 1-1.5 cm, proximal to the dentate line. Mucosa may be marked with stay sutures all around to facilitate dissection. The stay sutures help to distribute equal tension and prevent the tearing of the mucosa.

The dissection proceeds in the submucosal plane slowly all around tackling the vessels as they come, taking care not to injure the mucosa (Figs 67.3A and B). This is done cephalad upto the level of the peritoneal reflection. When the dissection has reached this level, there is a loose fold of tissue that can be well appreciated at the posterior limit of the dissection. At this point, the muscle cuff is incised transversely in between the stay sutures. Then it is incised all around circumferentially and the peritoneal cavity is entered.

A vertical incision is made in the muscular cuff in the midline posteriorly from above downwards to make it V shaped as the edges of the muscle cuff separate out. It is now stretched with the fingers to achieve adequate space in the pelvic for further dissection of the bowel from now onwards.

The dissection is made full thickness all around the bowel. The attention is focused on dealing with the mesentery of the sigmoid colon and the vessels

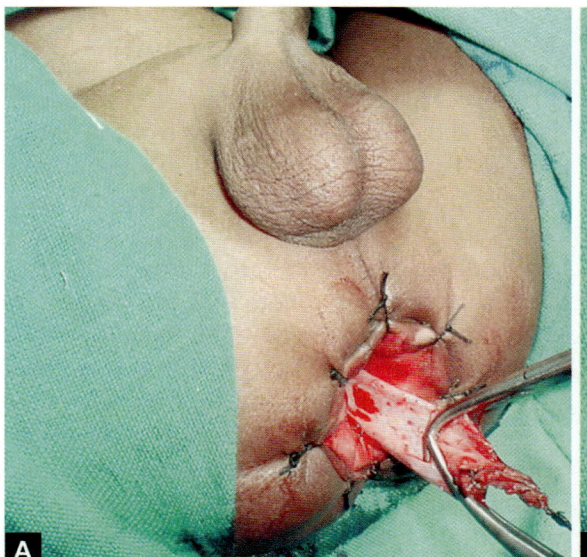
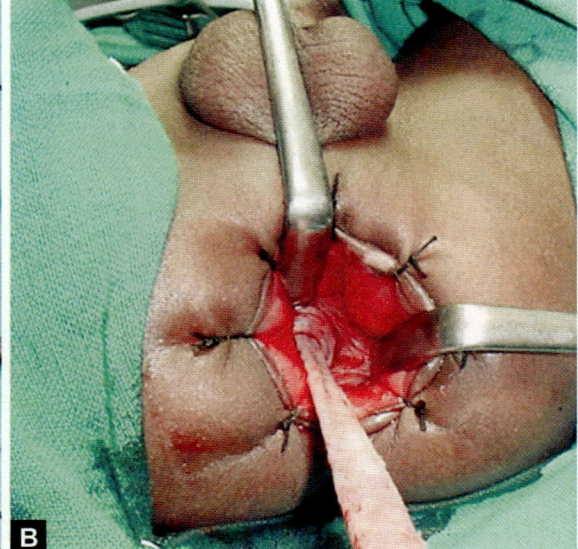

Figs 67.3A and B: Dissection of the mucosal sleeve in process

running in it. With a gentle pull on the bowel, the mesenteric vessels are identified and divided either by ligation or cauterized securely, making sure that the vessels do not get retracted. This is the critical step and is repeated till all the main vessels in the mesentery have been divided, sufficient length of the bowel has been mobilized well above the transition zone, which can be visibly appreciated.

The level of dissection can be assessed clinically as well as confirmed with a frozen biopsy taken from the seromuscular coat proximal to the visible transitional zone. Enough margin of error should be given to the stretching caused during the process of mobilization of the bowel. That is why, when the transanal endorectal pull-through is performed in the neonates, the gross examination and sampling is more accurate, as the dissection and mobilization is much easier (Fig. 67.4). This leads to a clearer pathology report.[3]

The limitation of this process is due to the fixation of the descending colon in the retroperitoneum that does not allow further mobilization of the colon by transanal route.[5] Ideally, TEPT procedure has the advantage of avoiding injury to the pelvic muscles and nerves.[6]

The coloanal anastomosis is begun after ensuring hemostasis inside the muscular cuff. The sutures are placed in one quadrant at a time through the edge of the mucosa of the anal canal and the full thickness of the pulled-through bowel (Fig. 67.5).

A rolled paraffin gauze or sofratulle soaked with povidone iodine or antibiotic ointment is gently placed in the rectum for next 24 hours. This serves as a

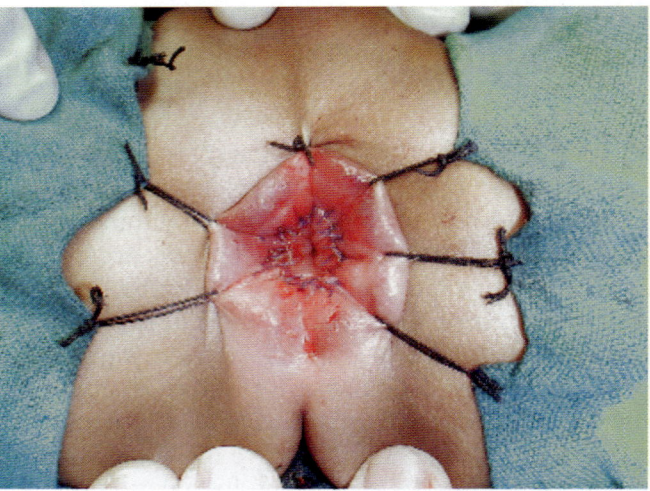

Fig. 67.5: Completed coloanal anastomosis

repellent at the neo-anastomosis, helps in achieving hemostasis and avoiding the dead space in between the muscular cuff and the pulled-through ganglionic bowel.

Postoperative monitoring of vital parameters is done. Adequate pain relief is ensured. The rectal pack is removed 24 hours after surgery. Patient is kept nil orally and on continuous nasogastric drainage till the ileus subsides. This may take 1-3 days. The patient is kept on maintenance intravenous fluids and intravenous broad spectrum antibiotics. Perineal hygiene is maintained. Patient can be discharged once the oral intake is adequate and the bowel has moved satisfactorily.

AIIMS EXPERIENCE ON PRIMARY TEPT

Primary TEPT was performed in 14 cases from the period 2003-2006. The age range of the patients was 1 month to 7 years. The indications were classical rectosigmoid Hirschsprung's disease in 11 cases, ultrashort segment Hirschsprung's disease in 2 cases and a suspected ultrashort segment Hirschsprung's disease in one case. There was no problem in 11 cases apart from the area where the rectal biopsy had been taken previously in 3 cases. There were problems in reaching the transition zone and the abdomen needed to be opened in 3 cases that were of the older age group. The reasons included a thick mesentery due to chronic anemia in 2 and a missed long segment HD and dilated bowel in one case that was initially suspected to be a case of ultrashort segment Hirschsprung's disease.

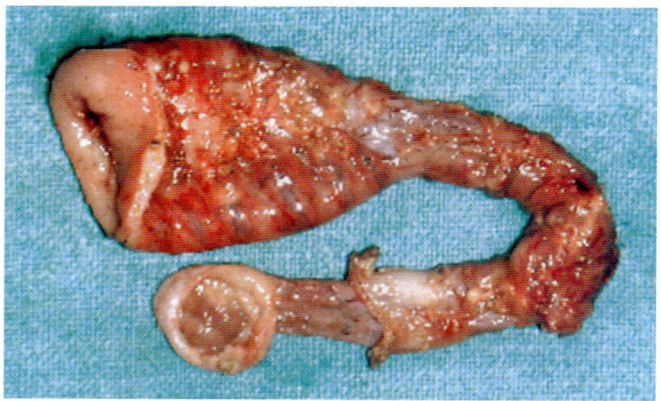

Fig. 67.4: Resected specimen of the pulled-through bowel showing the mucosal sleeve and the full thickness of the bowel. The transition zone can be seen clearly

FOLLOW-UP

The rectal examination is done after 3 weeks and the need for anal dilatation is assessed. Dilatation is usually not needed for single stage TEPT as the anal canal has been dilated adequately during operation and the daily passage of stools act as natural dilator. Moreover, the babies have an increased frequency of stool during the initial postoperative period due to the anal dilatation. A weekly calibration may be required for about 6 weeks to prevent anal stricture.

Anal dilatation program is however, very essential in patients undergoing TEPT for the three stage procedure. The anal calibration is done after 2 weeks and the parents are taught to start anal dilation after 3 weeks. The dilation is first started twice a day. The size of dilator is increased every week till the appropriate size of the dilator is reached. Frequency of dilation is then reduced gradually. The diverting colostomy is closed 6-8 weeks following the pull-through procedure.

COMPLICATIONS

Early Complications

1. Inadvertent mobilization of full thickness of rectal wall.
2. False positive rectal biopsy for ganglion cells.
3. Bleeding per rectum, hemoperitoneum, hematoma formation.
4. Cuff abscess/infection.
5. Increased frequency of stool.
6. Early colo-anal stenosis.
7. Anastomotic leak.
8. Perineal excoriation, redness and Edema.
9. Transient urinary retention.[7]
10. Pneumoperitoneum.[8]
11. Peritonitis.[8]
12. Urethral injury.[8]
13. Enterocolitis.[5]

Late Complications

1. Enterocolitis.
2. *Fecal Incontinence:* There has been a concern about the effect of prolonged traction of sphincter muscle during transanal approach.[9] Fecal incontinence is a preventable complication that is likely because of anal canal damage.[10] If adequate care is taken during TEPT, to preserve the anal canal, incontinence should not occur. Postoperative soiling is not uncommon and may be present without frank incontinence.[11]
3. Constipation if the muscular cuff is longer than 10 cm or not incised in the midline posteriorly. The muscular cuff on healing may form a fibrotic ring encircling the pulled colon. This is manageable with dilatation program either with the finger or with the metal dilators. However, utmost care is needed while doing the dilatations as bowel perforations have resulted. Constipation can be managed by dietary modification and oral medications.
4. Stenosis at the analcolic anastomotic site is more common in patients undergoing three stage pull through procedures. Anal dilatation is helpful.
5. Residual disease may be left if the surgeon has not been careful and has pulled the "normal looking bowel" without confirming the frozen section biopsy report. Sometimes even the frozen biopsy may deceive. The biopsy not only should confirm the ganglion cells but also ensure absence of hypertrophied nerve fibers.

OUTCOME

The anorectal functions after TEPT surgery are reported as normal. The stooling disorders are seen in a few and are probably related to the—(a) decrease or disappearance of the sigmoid loop, (b) dysfunction of the "neo-rectosigmoid", (c) an open and fixed anorectal angle and (d) achalasia of the internal anal sphincter.[7,11] This has also been confirmed on postopertive defecography.[11]

Patients with TEPT also have increased frequency of stool. The postoperative mean total gastrointestinal transit time (TGITT), the left colonic transit time (LCTT) and rectosigmoid colonic transit time (RSTT) measured in 58 patients, have shown to be significantly shorter than the preoperatively values ($P < 0.01$) and similar to the control group. The rectoanal inhibitory reflex is regained in due course of time but only in some patients.[11] A gradual recovery could be noted in the stooling patterns with the passage of time after surgery.[12] The stooling disorders are less common and the recovery is also faster in patients with short segment involvement of the bowel and if the surgery has been done at the younger age.[12] The normal urodynamic studies are reported in children 6 months after single stage transanal endorectal pull through.[7]

The integrity of the anorectal sphincter after TEPT is a poorly understood and controversial issue. Recently, three dimensional, vector manometric studies have been done to assess the same.[9] The computerised 8-channel vector manometry allows a segmental, 360 degrees analysis of muscular defects along the anal canal. It has been reported that TEPT preserves the functional integrity of the anorectal sphincter complex and has a favourable clinical and manometric outcome.[9]

Early results show that primary transanal endorectal pull-through is feasible and safe for the majority of the cases of HD with the rectosigmoid variety.[12-14] Although follow up is still relatively short, the preliminary results seem quite favorable and cost effective.[15] TEPT, no wonder, has become popular and the first choice of the experienced surgeons.

The long-term outcome following TEPT remains obscure. A hidden mortality has been reported during the long-term follow up of patients after this procedure. The possible causes for death are metabolic problems, enterocolitis, severe pneumonia and septic shock of unknown etiology. Some patients have died suddenly without a cause being found.[16] Thus, a close follow-up of all patients is strongly recommended after the one stage transanal endorectal pull-through especially those with general poor health and belonging to the poor socioeconomic region.[16]

Transanal Endorectal Pull-Through (TEPT) is characterized by no scars, shorter operating time, less bleeding, less postoperative pain and less discomfort, shorter hospital stay, less morbidity and earlier recovery than the similar abdomino-perineal pull-through procedures.[14,17] There is also a low incidence of operative and postoperative complications in experienced hands.[14] The hazards and the morbidity associated with laparotomy and diversion colostomy may be avoided with a one-stage technique adopted in majority of children (70-80%) with the rectosigmoid variety of Hirschsprung's disease.[13,17]

REDO TEPT

The TEPT can also be used for the redo procedures and has been reported to be successfully performed in 18 symptomatic patients requiring redo procedures for residual aganglionosis.[18] This TEPT approach may be combined with transabdominal mobilization of the intestine, if the need be depending on the length of the residual aganglionic segment.[18,19] A diversion colostomy should be seriously considered for the redo cases, either as the preliminary procedure or combined with the main pull-through. It makes the procedure safer and complication free.

THE MUSCULAR CUFF

The use of a long muscular cuff of 8-10 cm is not unusual while performing the TEPT procedure. However, it must be slit open posteriorly to give it a V shape. There is a recent trend to use a short muscular cuff for the TEPT. Rintala et al and Langer et al, have used a shorter cuff of only 2-3 cm, without the need for a slit in its posterior wall, and with similar postoperative results.[20] Whether this is important to reduce the postoperative complications, especially the incidence of enterocolitis, is debatable. However, may be that a long rectal muscular cuff might increase the incidence of postoperative enterocolitis and constipation. This may be obviated by a simple modification and perform the transanal pull-through procedure with an oblique mucosectomy and an oblique anastomosis, with a short and split muscular cuff. This has been associated with much less postoperative anastomotic stricture as compared to that with the conventional transanal procedure.[21] Complete bowel continence at one year followup after operation was also better (92.1% v/s 86.6%).[21] An experimental study has been done to compare the results of transanal endorectal pull-through with the laparoscopic assisted transanal pull-through.[22]

Langer et al reported the experience with the use of Laparoscopic assisted TEPT in 1999.[23] The results showed that laparoscope was helpful to confirm the orientation of the bowel and achieve adequate hemostasis. Though, the transanal colectomy can be performed with or without the laparoscopic assistance, the advantages of laparoscopic assistance include: 1) more exact determination of transitional zone; 2) easier separation of peritoneal reflection, 3) better control of final position of the colon; 4) minor traction on the perineal muscles. This procedure also gives excellent clinical results and permitted early postoperative feeding. The hospital stay is also short.

Langer et al compared the results of open versus laparoscopic assisted pull-through and the primary transanal versus laparoscopic assisted procedure. It was found that with the TEPT, the hospital stay was short, treatment cost was less and there was no increased risk of complications. It was also highlighted that the routine use of laparoscopic visualization or mini-laparotomy was not always necessary but should rather be reserved for children who are at higher risk for missing the long segment Hirschsprung's disease.[24]

The short-term results after TEPT are the same as seen after the transanal mucosectomy combined with abdominal approach.[20] When compared with the Duhamel procedure, the TEPT also had similar medium-term functional outcome. TEPT is however, more suitable for single-stage neonatal treatment of HD due to less dilatation of the bowel.[25,26] Al-sawaf et al showed that the stool pattern and enterocolitis scores were somewhat better in the TEPT group as compared to the open group.[27] As TEPT requires more stretching of the anal sphincters, the postoperative continence score has been found better with the use of the abdominal approach.[27] In most series, the overall functional outcome following properly performed TEPT in selected group of patients has been highly satisfactory and comparable with other established procedures.[17,24,28-33]

REFERENCES

1. De la Torre-Mondragon L, Ortega-Salgado JA. Transanal endorectal pull-through for Hirschsprung's disease. J Pediatr Surg 1998;33:1283-86.
2. So HB, Schwartz DL, Becker JM, Daum F, Schneider KM. Endorectal "pull-through" without preliminary colostomy in neonates with Hirschsprung's disease. J Pediatr Surg 1980;15:470-71.
3. Berrebi D, Fouquet V, de Lagausie P, et al. Duhamel operation vs neonatal transanal endorectal pull-through procedure for Hirschsprung disease: which are the changes for pathologists? J Pediatr Surg 2007;42:688-91.
4. Takegawa B, Ortolan EP, Rodrigues AM, et al. Experimental model for transanal endorectal pull-through surgery. Technique of De la Torre and Ortega. J Pediatr Surg 2005;40(10):1539-41.
5. Teeraratkul S. Transanal one-stage endorectal pull-through for Hirschsprung's disease in infants and children J Pediatr Surg 2003;38:184-87.
6. Hadidi A. Transanal endorectal pull-through for Hirschsprung's disease: experience with 68 patients. J Pediatr Surg 2003;38(9):1337-40.
7. Ateay O, Hakgader G, Kart Y, et al. The effect of dilated ganglionic segment on anorectal and urinary functions during 1-stage transanal endorectal pull through for Hirschsprung's disease. J Pediatr Surg 2007;42:1271-75.
8. Podevin G, Lardy H, Azzis O, et al. Technical problems and complications of a transanal pull-through for Hirschsprung's disease. Eur J Pediatr Surg 2006;16(2):104-8.
9. Till H, Heinrich M, Schuster T, V Schweinitz D. Is the anorectal sphincter damaged during a transanal endorectal pull-through (TERPT) for Hirschsprung's disease? A 3-dimensional, vector manometric investigation. Eur J Pediatr Surg 2006 Jun;16(3):188-91.
10. Pena A, Elicevik M, Levitt MA. Reoperations in Hirschsprung disease. J Pediatr Surg 2007;42:1008-13; discussion 1013-14.
11. Zhang SC, Wang WL, Bai YZ, Wang W. Evaluation of anorectal function after transanal one-stage endorectal pull through operation in children with Hirschsprung's disease Zhongguo Dang Dai Er Ke Za Zhi 2007;9:188-92.
12. Zhang SC, Bai YZ, Wang W, Wang WL. Clinical outcome in children after transanal 1-stage endorectal pull-through operation for Hirschsprung disease. J Pediatr Surg 2005;40(8):1307-11.
13. Rehman Y, Emblem R, Björnland K. Transanal resection of colon for Hirschsprung's disease. Tidsskr Nor Laegeforen 2005;125(17):2358-59.
14. Rintala RJ. Transanal coloanal pull-through with a short muscular cuff for classic Hirschsprung's disease. Eur J Pediatr Surg 2003;13(3):181-86.
15. Dasgupta R, Langer JC. Transanal pull-through for Hirschsprung disease Semin Pediatr Surg 2005;14:64-71.
16. Tander B, Rizalar R, Cihan AO, et al. Is there a hidden mortality after one-stage transanal endorectal pull-through for patients with Hirschsprung's disease? Pediatr Surg Int 2007;23:81-86.
17. Hadidi A. Transanal endorectal pull-through for Hirschsprung's disease: a comparison with the open technique. Eur J Pediatr Surg 2003;13:176-80.
18. Hadidi A, Bartoli F, Waag KL. Role of transanal endorectal pull-through in complicated Hirschsprung's disease: experience in 18 patients. J Pediatr Surg 2007;42:544-48.
19. Gobran TA, Ezzat A, Hassan ME, et al. Redo transanal endorectal pull-through: a preliminary study. Pediatr Surg Int 2007;23:189-93.
20. Rintala RJ, Wester T. Transanal endorectal pull-through with short muscular cuff in the treatment of Hirschsprung disease. Preliminary study with 37 patients. Cir Pediatr 2003;16(4):161-65.
21. Li AW, Zhang WT, Li FH, Cui XH, Duan XS. A new modification of transanal Soave pull-through procedure for Hirschsprung's disease. Chin Med J (Engl) 2006;119:37-42.
22. Papandreou E, Baltogiannis N, Cigliano B, et al. Transanal endorectal pull-through with or without laparoscopic assistance? Development of an experimental model. Pediatr Med Chir 2004;26:253-55.

23. Langer JC, Minkes RK, Mazziotti MV, et al. Transanal one-stage Soave procedure for infants with Hirschsprung's disease. J Pediatr Surg 1999;34:148-51.
24. Langer JC, Seifert M, Minkes RK. One-stage Soave pull-through for Hirschsprung's disease: a comparison of the transanal and open approaches. J Pediatr Surg 2000;35:820-22.
25. Minford JL, Ram A, Turnock RR, et al. Comparison of functional outcomes of Duhamel and transanal endorectal coloanal anastomosis for Hirschsprung's disease. J Pediatr Surg 2004;39(2):161-65.
26. Sapin E, Centonze A, Moog R, et al. Transanal coloanal anastomosis for Hirschsprung's disease: comparison between endorectal and perirectal pull-through procedures. Eur J Pediatr Surg 2006;16:312-17.
27. El-Sawaf MI, Drongowski RA, Chamberlain JN, et al. Are the long-term results of the transanal pull-through equal to those of the transabdominal pull-through? A comparison of the 2 approaches for Hirschsprung's disease. J Pediatr Surg 2007;42:41-47.
28. Pratap A, Shakya VC, Biswas BK, et al. Single-stage transanal endorectal pull-through for Hirschsprung's disease: perspective from a developing country. J Pediatr Surg 2007;42(3):532-35.
29. Pratap A, Gupta D K, Shakya VC, et al. Analysis of Problems, Complications, Avoidance and Management with Transanal Pull Through for Hirschsprung's Disease. Jour Ped Surg 2007;42:1869-76.
30. Gupta DK. Plenary Lecture delivered on Experience with management of patients with Hirschsprung's disease including Total colonic Aganglionosis, during the Symposium on Hirschsprung's disease, University of Cluj-Napoca, Romania, December 2006.
31. Gupta DK, Shilpa Sharma. Functional Constipation and Late Onset Hirschsprung's Disease in Textbook of Adolescent Medicine. (Ed) Swati Bhave. Jaypee Brothers New Delhi. Chapter 20. 2006;2:648-53.
32. Lall A, Gupta DK, Bajpai M. Neonatal Hirschsprung's Disease. Ind J Ped 2000;67(8):583-88.
33. Gupta DK. Lecture delivered on the Role of Myectomy for Hirschsprung's disease and Management of complicated Hirschsprung's disease, during the Round Table Meet on Hirschsprung's Disease, during the 2nd World Congress of the World Federation of the Association of Pediatric Surgeons, held in Buenos Aires, Argentina, September 2007.

CHAPTER 68

Crohn's Disease

Robert Cywes, Arnold G Coran

HISTORICAL OVERVIEW

Chronic interstitial enteritis has been documented in the literature since the nineteenth century. Crohn, Ginzberg and Oppenheimer first classified the clinical and pathological manifestations of "regional ileitis" in 1932.[1] Subsequently, the protean intestinal and extra-intestinal manifestations of Crohn's disease (CD), with its inconsistent response to medical therapy and its strong recurrent tendency despite surgical removal of all obvious disease, has been well described. However, etiology remains obscure and directed therapy absent. Treatment remains broadly symptomatic, supportive and suppressive. While mortality rates have decreased, morbidity remains high.

Although there are many similarities with the disease as it occurs in adults, various aspects of diagnosis and management differ in childhood, including the effect and treatment of the disease with regards to growth and development.

EPIDEMIOLOGY

Symptoms of CD begin during childhood or adolescence in 20-25% of all patients, with a peak incidence in the second and third decades of life.[2] Since the original description of CD, its incidence relative to ulcerative colitis (UC) has increased dramatically. In studies of Scottish and Welsh children under 16 years of age, the incidence of CD has risen from 1.3-3.1 per 100,000 with UC remaining stable at 0.7 per 100000.[3,4] The age-specific incidence of CD in North America in 1984 for 10 to 19-year-olds was approximately 3.5 per 100000 and of UC, 2.0 per 100000.[2] In 1993, the prevalence of CD in a British childhood population was 16.6 per 100 000 and of UC. 3.4 per 1000000.[3] There is no evidence that the age of onset of CD is decreasing.[2] Most pediatric cases occur between ages 16 and 20 years, with less than 5% of cases occurring under 5 years of age and with only rare reports of CD in infants.[5] There is an equal incidence of inflammatory bowel disease in males and females.[6]

ETIOLOGY

The etiology of both CD and UC remains obscure. Familial and ethnic predisposition to these diseases has led to an intense investigation of genetic associations. At the time of diagnosis, the likelihood of detecting inflammatory bowel disease in a first-degree relative of a proband is 5-25% and the risk to siblings of patients with CD is 17-35 times greater than the general population.[7,8]

Support for an autoimmune basis for CD comes from reports that bone marrow transplantation following myeloablation appears to cure CD. In a long-term follow-up study, four of five patients with leukemia and CD remain disease-free up to fourteen years after bone marrow transplantation.[9] The one patient who had a relapse of CD two years after transplantation had mixed host/donor hemopoietic chimerism with persistent host immunity An autoimmune etiology would also explain the familial and ethnic preponderance of inflammatory bowel. disease.

Since the recognition of CD, attempts have been made to link its cause to a variety of environmental agents and microorganisms.[10,11] However, to date, no persistent direct link to a multitude of transmissible agents or soluble mediators of inflammation has been established.

It is more likely that CD is a genetically based autoimmune disease that becomes clinically activated by an environmental trigger. Genetic analysis may someday be used to prognosticate the course of an individual's inflammatory bowel disease and provide specialized therapy or avoid ineffectual treatment.[12]

PATHOLOGY

In children and adults, CD may manifest as an acute, subacute or chronic inflammatory condition transmurally affecting the gastrointestinal tract anywhere from mouth to anus. Three general patterns of gross bowel involvement dominate: (a) the terminal ileum with variable segments of right colon is affected in 50-60% of children; (b) approximately 30-35% have small bowel involvement only, mostly in the temlinal ileum; (c) isolated involvement of the colon and rectum is seen in 10-15% of cases.[13] Perianal and perineal involvement occurs in 25% of children, often preceding intestinal symptoms, but occurs less frequently than in adults.[14] Biopsy of macroscopically uninvolved areas frequently reveals evidence of microscopic inflammation.[15] There is a high incidence of upper gastrointestinal tract involvement in children with CD with up to 42% having lesions of the esophagus, stomach and duodenum.[16]

Macroscopically, the mucosa has a cobblestoned appearance interspaced with normal appearing skip segments. Aphthous ulcers may be seen in the mouth. The intestine appears thickened secondary to inflammation with creeping fat. Strictures causing obstruction, fistulas and abscesses may be encountered. Microscopically, the entire bowel wall thickness is involved with a chronic non-caseating granulomatous process that differentiates the disease from UC. Giant cells may be seen.

CLINICAL MANIFESTATIONS

Unlike UC where bloody diarrhea is the initial presenting feature in more than 90% of cases, the onset of CD is often insidious. In 25-35% of children, the disease presents with extraintestinal symptoms, although gastrointestinal disease is usually present if sought.[17] A long interval (6-36 months) may exist between onset of symptoms and diagnosis in children.[17,18]

Gastrointestinal Manifestation

Initial mild inflammation may be heralded by vague symptoms such as early satiety, anorexia and behavioral change. More severe disease presents with anemia, weight loss, abdominal pain or diarrhea, but symptoms manifest according to the affected site. Malabsorption secondary to mucosal inflammation or bacterial overgrowth results in diarrhea. Children with small bowel disease may have altered enterohepatic bile salt circulation exacerbating their diarrhea, and an increased incidence of mineral and vitamin deficiencies.[19] Colonic involvement presents with diarrhea, abdominal cramping and tenesmus. Rectal bleeding occurs in 20-30% of cases and may be indistinguishable from UC. Perianal disease is often associated with Crohn's colitis and may help to distinguish between CD and UC.[20-22]

Alternatively, patients may present with complications of the disease such as bowel obstruction, fistulas, abscesses or perforation.

Extraintestinal Manifestation

Pathology of every system in the body has been described in association with CD.[17] The majority of CD children (50-80%) have systemic manifestations such as fever, fatigue and weight loss.[18] Bone and joints involvement occurs in 13-22% of patients. Skin disease occurs in 10-14%, and the oral mucosa is often affected by aphthous stomatitis that follows the course of iptestinal disease.[23,24] Ocular disease is found in 30% of children. Long-term ophthalmic surveillance is recommended in all children with inflammatory bowel disease.[25] Liver disease is less common in children than adults. but 15% of children will have abnormal serum transaminases during the course of the disease.[17,26] Kidney and gallstones may occur secondary to malabsorption. Hypercoagulable states with thrombocytosis are commonly associated with active disease and hematological parameters may be used to monitor disease activity.[23,27]

Growth Abnormalities and Nutritional Deficiencies

Extraintestinal manifestations with growth retardation result in more subtle presentation. These patients may have poor growth and delayed puberty with nonspecific signs of intestinal inflammation such as anorexia and general malaise. The pubertal growth spurt accounts for about 16% of normal adult height with a doubling of body weight.[28] Such accelerated growth requires increased nutritional intake that cannot be met by children with active disease, often resulting in permanent deficits in adult height and maturation. Delayed sexual maturation is also a common feature.

Inadequate caloric intake is the single most important factor in the pathogenesis of growth failure.[29] Fever and sepsis increase energy requirements, but most patients have normal basal energy requirements.[30] Vitamin and trace element deficiencies are seen in 20-40% of children with CD.[29] Endocrine hormone levels are generally normal and are not the cause of growth failure.[31] Therapeutic interventions, such as extensive small bowel resection and prolonged corticosteroid and immunosuppressive drug administration, contribute significantly to malnutrition and growth failure.[32] Growth failure needs to be aggressively treated and should influence acute and long-term medical and surgical management decisions.

DIAGNOSIS

Early diagnosis of CD in a child requires a high index of suspicion. The most frequent presenting symptoms include diarrhea with discharge of blood or mucus, abdominal pain, nausea, vomiting, weight loss, fever and general malaise. Signs of malabsorption are found in 60% of children and 10% are growth retarded at diagnosis.

History and Physical Examination

A detailed history including gastrointestinal and extraintestinal manifestations, growth, sexual development, family history, recent infections and antibiotic use should be obtained. Physical examination should include a careful abdominal examination including inspection of the mouth and perineum. Signs of extraintestinal manifestations such as uveitis, clubbing, skin rashes and arthritis should be elicited. A detailed assessment of growth, development and nutritional status, often neglected in surgical practice, should routinely be performed in the diagnosis and follow-up of all inflammatory bowel patients. Height, weight, percent height for age, growth velocity and standard anthropometric measurements should be recorded at each visit.[33,34]

Laboratory Assessment

Laboratory tests are not diagnostic in inflammatory bowel disease and cannot differentiate between Crohn's colitis and UC.[20] However, they are useful in monitoring disease activity, nutritional state and effect of therapy, and may exclude other causes of mucosal inflammation such as infectious agents. Anemia (70% of cases), leukocytosis (60%), thrombocytosis (60%), elevated erythrocyte sedimentation rate (80%) and hypoalbuminemia (60%) are most commonly seen in active CD.[17,35] More specialized tests of disease activity are indicated in clinical studies but not routinely used in patient management.[31,35,36]

Nutritional status is monitored by measuring serum proteins with rapid turnover (albumin, prealbumin, retinol binding protein, transferrin), vitamin (B_{12} and A,D,E,K) and trace element levels (folate, iron parameters, calcium, phosphate, magnesium and zinc) as well as liver function tests.[20,31,35,37]

Infectious diseases may mimic inflammatory bowel disease. The presence of infectious pathogens mandates treatment, but does not exclude the diagnosis of inflammatory bowel disease.

Endoscopy

Endoscopy with biopsy is more sensitive than radiographic studies for initial diagnosis, and detection and monitoring of mild mucosal disease.[38] In the diagnosis of CD, endoscopy should include visualization of the entire colon and terminal ileum.[39,40] Esophagogastroduodenoscopy should also be performed because of the high incidence of upper gastrointestinal disease in children.[16,41,42] Biopsies from multiple sites should be obtained to characterize the extent of the disease and to differentiate between CD and UC. Although the histopathologic features of the two are characteristic, none are pathognomonic.

Radiology

Contrast radiographic imaging remains the cornerstone in the detection of fistulas, strictures, perforations and the depth of ulceration.[43] In most tertiary care centres, double contrast barium enema is reserved for complicated colonic disease or where colonoscopy has been suboptimal.

Small bowel contrast radiographic imaging is important in the initial evaluation and subsequent monitoring of the child with CD. This may be done by upper gastrointestinal series with small bowel follow-through using orally ingested contrast material and insufflation of air per rectum to improve visualization of the terminal ileum, with a sensitivity of 42%.[44] Alternatively, enteroclysis, a small bowel enema with tube placement in the third part of the duodenum, may be used with a sensitivity of 100% and specificity of 98.3%.[45] The former approach is considerably more comfortable for the patient, but the latter allows more detailed imaging of the bowel, especially if combined with esophagogastroduodenoscopy.

Computed tomography, transabdominal and transrectal ultrasonography are useful in identifying extraluminal and pelvic complications such as abscesses, phlegmons and fistulas.[46,47] With improvements in interventional radiology, both of these modalities may be used therapeutically as well as diagnostically.

MEDICAL AND NUTRITIONAL MANAGEMENT

The goal of medical and surgical therapy is to control symptoms and prevent complications while minimizing toxicity, affording the patient a reasonable quality of life. Because the disease cannot be eradicated, the patient's clinical condition rather than laboratory data or evidence of placebo.[48,49] Although pediatric data is lacking, following the adult experience, high dose disease should guide management. Growth disturbance is an important consideration both as a symptom of disease activity and as an effect of therapy. Maintenance of normal growth is of paramount importance in the management of the child with CD. The intent of medication is to treat active inflammation, induce remission or suppress chronically active disease. In CD, the role and use of effective therapy to maintain remission is debatable.

Pharmacologic Therapy

The pharmacologic management of CD often realise on the use of multidrug therapy with synergistic effects. A variety of 5-aminosalicylate (5-ASA) agents are currently used to induce remission and to prevent recurrence after surgery in CD (17). The action of 5-ASA is topical. Various carrier agents have been compounded to the 5-ASA moiety, which are split off by gut or bacterial action to allow delivery of the active drug at a particular site in the intestine, preventing more proximal metabolism. After inducing medical or surgical remission of CD, a two-year follow-up study showed that these drugs reduced disease recurrence by 50% compared with placebo (48, 49). Although pediatric data is lacking, following the adult experience, high dose maintenance therapy is required (50-60 mg/kg/d). This may be tapered slowly at about a year until a critical dose is reached where patient symptoms recur.

A variety of immunosuppressive agents are used in treating CD. Corticosteroids are able to induce remission in most patients with small or large bowel disease. Steroids should be used when disease is refractory to other agents, in extensive small bowel disease, in acute severe or fulminant disease, in extraintestinal complications and for postoperative recurrence.[50] High dose steroid therapy is associated with significant side-effects and is usually not effective in maintaining remission of CD. Prolonged use of steroids is not recommended. The only long-term indication is to control chronically active disease resistant to other drugs. In this instance, alternate day low dose steroid therapy after induction of remission with daily steroids, is recommended.[51,52] Steroid effect on growth is variable. Some patients grow only after steroids induce disease remission. while others only grow once disease is in remission and steroids are tapered.[53]

Side-effects often limit the use of systemic corticosteroids. Budesonide, a new corticosteroid with high topical anti-inflammatory activity and low systemic levels because of rapid hepatic metabolism, is efficacious against active CD in adults.[54,55] Side-effects are less than with prednisone, but pediatric effects have not yet been determined.

Other immunosuppressive agents include 6-mercaptopurine, azathioprine, methotrexate and cyclosporine. These drugs are used in cases of steroid dependency, steroid toxicity and for medical intractability (particularly when surgery is not feasible). With the exception of cyclosporine, early reports of the efficacy of these drugs in children are promising, but more detailed studies are required.[56-60]

Antibiotics such as sulfasalazine, metronidazole and ciprofloxacin are effective against acute inflammatory flare-ups especially in the colon and perianally, but are less effective in small bowel disease.[61] Broad-spectrum antibiotics are used to treat acute infections and their complications such as abscesses. An empiric course of antibiotics in patients with fever and localizing symptoms suspicious for microperforation is useful. Addition of ciprofloxacin to metronidazole synergistically enhances its efficacy in the treatment of terminal ileal and perianal disease.[62] Ciprofloxacin is not recommended in children younger than 10-12 years. Metronidazole therapy should be restricted to 6 months as it may cause peripheral neuropathy.[63]

Developments in immunotherapy appear to be a promising new step in the goal-directed medical therapy of chronic active CD. Proinflammatory cytokines play a significant role in CD. Neutralization of cytokines secreted by cells in the immune system, such as tumor necrosis factor-alpha (TNFα.) may prove useful in decreasing bowel inflammation and aid in the closure of fistulas. Alternatively, upregulating or administering immunosuppressive cytokines such as IL-l0, has shown great potential in treating CD.[64-66]

Prospective multicenter randomized trials of the anti-TNFα drug, infliximab (Remicade), a chimeric monoclonal antibody form of anti-TNFα), given over short courses, have demonstrated a high degree of benefit lasting 8-12 weeks after termination of drug administration. Infliximab has been effective in the short-term reduction of chronic active inflammation as well as rapid closure of fistulae in children.[64,65] Similar trials using IL-l0 have demonstrated significant clinical benefit over placebo. However, return of disease activity suggests that combination drug strategies may be required for long-term effect.[66]

Nutritional Therapy

Enteral nutrition is no longer recommended as primary treatment for active CD.[67] But, nutrition as an adjunctive therapy to prevent or reverse malnutrition and micronutrient deficiencies and to maintain remission, is integral to the management of the child with CD to regain and maintain metabolic homeostasis, replace ongoing losses, promote catch-up growth to premorbid percentiles, and promote progression through puberty.[20,53] Particular attention to complete nutritional supplementation should be paid when children are placed on bowel rest or elemental diets, or when they have unusual losses secondary to their disease or therapy.

In children undergoing elective surgery for CD, the risk of developing postoperative complications is directly related to their nutritional status.[68] Preoperative parenteral and enteral nutritional support in malnourished patients significantly reduces the risk of developing postoperative complications.[69]

SURGICAL MANAGEMENT

Indications for Operation

Indications for operation vary with the site of disease: In small bowel disease, 80% of operations are for obstruction and internal fistulas. In colonic disease, persistent acute or subacute bleeding, fulminant colitis with or without toxic megacolon, obstruction, perforation, abscess, internal and external fistulas and perianal disease are indications for surgery. However, with improved medical, endoscopic and radiologic interventional skills and equipment, many of these complications are treated without the need for operative intervention.[70] Obstructive hydronephrosis due to chronic phlegmonous inflammation may require surgical release. Surgery is also required for refractory symptoms, including growth failure, despite maximal medical and nutritional therapy. Steroid dependency and toxicity are also an indication for surgery, although the use of immunosuppressive agents may offer an alternative in such patients.

CD patients are often tolerant of complications of their disease. Symptomatic discomfort from a complication is more often an indication for surgery than simply the presence of the complication. Surgeons should consider disease in the context of symptoms rather appearance and should also be perceptive to quality of life issues. Ongoing active CD may lead to social invalidism, especially during adolescence, which may be an indication for operative intervention.

Protein-energy malnutrition due to insufficient caloric intake has been identified as the primary reason for growth failure. In active CD, children are often food intolerant because of early satiety, abdominal pain, partial bowel obstruction, diarrhea related to malabsorption and a central anorexia mechanism. Nutritional supplementation may reverse growth failure, but does not address the reason for insufficient caloric consumption. Surgical resection should induce remission from disease and symptoms, allowing children to increase caloric intake, regain metabolic homeostasis and achieve premorbid growth percentiles.

Patients with CD for more than 10 years are at increased risk of developing both small bowel and colorectal cancer. A strict regime of endoscopic and radiological surveillance should be maintained, and any evidence of dysplasia or carcinoma is an indication for surgical resection.[71-73]

Surgical Approaches

Prior to elective surgery, the extent and nature of the disease should be determined by endoscopy and contrast radiography. The patient's preoperative nutritional status should be optimized. If inflammatory masses or local peritoneal signs are present, preoperative bowel rest and intravenous antibiotics may reduce the extent of surgery and postoperative complications.

Minimally invasive surgery is becoming increasingly useful as a diagnostic tool with therapeutic advantages and greater acceptance among physicians and patients. As technical expertise is gained, minimally invasive procedures will dominate surgery in these patients, especially those undergoing their first operation.

Bowel Resection

Two broad categories of diseased bowel are found at surgery. Firstly, when the surgery is performed for acute complications, the bowel is inflamed and edematous, often with abscess formation or fistulization. Anatomy is difficult to identify, with poor tissue plane separation. It is imperative to adopt a minimalist approach in this scenario. Extensive dissection and adhesiolysis often results in iatrogenic injury and sacrifice of bowel that would have had the potential to 'cool off and recover function. Disease recurrence is inevitable, but multiple anastomoses or short bowel syndrome is a disaster. In this situation, a period of preoperative bowel rest is of great benefit to the surgeon and patient. In the second instance, surgery is performed for chronic symptoms such as growth failure, recurrent obstruction due to stricture or chronic fistulas. The serosa and mesentery are not acutely inflamed and tissue planes are identifiable. Resection or repair of an isolated segment is feasible without compromising uninvolved bowel.

Midline laparotomy is the best approach in children as it allows for dealing with unexpected findings, access to the pelvis. better stoma placement and easier access in the event of recurrent surgery.

Resection margins should be just sufficient to provide grossly normal bowel for anastomosis or stoma. There is no role for microscopic evaluation of resection margins as microscopic involvement does not affect the rate of anastomotic disease recurrence. Resection back to microscopically normal bowel results in unnecessarily radical resection.[74,75]

A proximal diverting ileostomy should only be used if the tissues are so edematous and inflamed that distal anastomoses warrant such protection or if the remnants of an abscess wall would come to lie adjacent to a suture line. However, ileostomy is associated with a significantly lower early recurrence rate than following anastomosis. Therefore, it should be considered in patients with aggressive disease or after multiple operations for recurrence.[76]

Crohn's toxic megacolon should be treated with partial colon resection without anastomosis.[70] In the presence of generalized peritonitis (free perforation or abscess rupture), limited resection is preferred with exteriorization or anastomosis depending on the degree of contamination. Surgical drains are best avoided but may be used for discrete, mature abscesses when, after debridement, residual contamination is suspected. However, uncomplicated abscesses are nearly always amenable to guided percutaneous drainage. Postoperative abscesses may occur in up to 10% of cases, and these too, may be drained percutaneously.

Duodenal CD is seen more frequently in children than adults. Differentiation from peptic ulcer disease is difficult, even in those patients with known CD. Full medical management for both peptic ulcer and CD should be attempted before elective operative repair is considered. Chronic obstruction, hemorrhage, perforation or recurrent pancreatitis are indications for surgery. Gastrojejunostomy with or without selective vagotomy to prevent marginal ulcer while preventing postvagotomy diarrhea, is the procedure of choice, although stricturoplasty has been used.[77]

It is difficult to predict the postoperative frequency and consistency of bowel movements. Patients should be monitored closely until fluid and nutritional homeostasis can be maintained. If growth failure was an indication for surgery, placement of a gastrostomy at the time of surgery may be of great benefit in the postoperative period.

Stricturoplasty

The concept of minimal surgery for extensive CD is relatively new. Stricturoplasty epitomizes this concept and is the new approach to the surgical management of CD. Short strictures (5-8 cm long) are widened using a Heineke-Mikulicz pyloroplasty-type procedure, while longer narrowed segments (up to 30 cm), including the ileocecal valve and previous anastomotic sites, may be widened using the Finney technique.[78,79] Guidelines indicating the tightness of strictures requiring stricturoplasty are well documented in the adult literature, but clearly do not apply to children.[80] In view of the safety of stricturoplasty, 'prophylactic' stricturoplasty may be performed on all recognizable strictures except for those sites where the luminal caliber is not compromised. Several groups have adopted this practice despite a lack of documented evidence.[80]

In addition to surgical stricturoplasty, two endoscopic techniques, divulsion and ablation, been developed for treating strictures. Divulsion techniques dilate the stricture by tearing tissue at the weakest section, thus providing a larger lumen. Dilatation of esophageal, gastroduodenal, ileocecal, colonic, anorectal and anastomotic strictures is accepted practice among therapeutic endoscopists. More recently, ablation techniques using electrocautery or laser have employed with success in treating chronic fibrous strictures. Multiple therapies combining dilatation and ablation may reduce the risk of injury and improve the chances of successful endoscopic stricturoplasty.[81] Long-term results of these endoscopic techniques in pediatric CD have not been reported.

Management of Granulomatous Colitis

The initial management of acute Crohn's colitis is identical to that of acute UC. Marked colonic dilatation with mucosal islands or a perforation mandates immediate surgery. If the radiologic picture is less severe, further investigation and medical management with daily abdominal views is instituted. Surgery is performed if the clinical or radiological picture deteriorates. In Crohn's colitis, perforation may occur without preceding dilatation. At surgery, the rectum should be preserved leaving a distal mucus fistula or tacking a Hartmann pouch subcutaneously. Perforation or leakage from an intra-abdominal Hartmann pouch stump may cause significant morbidity. Only if there is no other option because of disintegrative rectal disease or massive bleeding from an undefined site, should primary proctectomy be performed. However, despite rectal conservation, the likelihood of subsequent anastomosis is low and secondary proctectomy high. Initial operative conservatism also allows an opportunity to confirm the diagnosis of CD which is not known in more than half the cases. If it turns out to be UC, ileoanal restoration may be performed.[82]

The unpredictability of findings despite pre-operative investigations and the possibility of a stoma, either temporary or permanent should be discussed with the patient and family before any abdominal operation for CD. The results of surgery for CD of the colon are less than satisfactory and surgical intervention should be limited to those patients who have complications severe enough to justify an operation.

Management of Intestinal Fistulas

The presence of an internal fistula is not an indication for surgery. However, in 'high-low' fistulas that produce torrential diarrhea, and fistulas that connect to the urinary tract, surgery is recommended. En bloc resection of the diseased intestine and fistula with primary anastomosis is the preferred treatment, but temporary exteriorization of the intestinal ends should be undertaken in those patients compromised by extensive sepsis or profound malnutrition.[83]

Duodenal fistulas are the exception, where failure to heal following primary closure occurs more frequently with disastrous results. Duodenal fistulas should be closed primarily, then protected by a jejunal serosal patch. This buttresses the defect increasing the healing potential, but should breakdown occur, preferential duodenojejunal fistulization occurs rather than retroperitoneal leakage.[83]

Proximal temporary loop colostomy should be used to protect repairs of fistulas in diseased colon or rectum, but primary repair is feasible when these structures are not grossly diseased.

Although medical management of external fistulas has good early results, recurrence is common and local management unpleasant and painful. Therefore, early operative treatment is recommended. Bowel resection is required and the chronic granulation tissue of enterocutaneous fistula tracts should be cored out and the adjacent peritoneum closed from within the abdomen. The external opening is left open to heal by secondary intention.

Diagnosis of rectovaginal fistulas in premenarchal girls is difficult and a high index of suspicion is required, often requiring evaluation under anesthesia to demonstrate the communication. All fistulas secondary to CD are considered complex. Up to 50% of rectovaginal fistulas will close with aggressive medical management of rectal disease, including the use of nocturnal rectal budesonide infusion, metronidazole and immunosuppressive agents. Surgical repair is elective and should not be done in the presence of active local disease. Failure of medical control of rectal disease may require a diverting colostomy prior to repair of the fistula.

Management of Abscesses

Percutaneous ultrasound or CT - guided drainage of abscesses is a useful option as primary therapy or as a temporizing measure to allow acute inflammation to settle prior to surgery. Drainage without subsequent resection has a high recurrence rate.[84] Local antibiotics within the abscess cavity have not shown to be of any benefit, but long-term administration of broad-spectrum systemic antibiotics has been effective in eradicating abscesses and decreasing recurrence rates. Patients and their families should be made aware that abscess recurrence and fistula development following abscess drainage should always be expected in CD.

Management of Perianal Disease

In the initial management of perianal and perineal disease the presence, extent and location of bowel involvement should be established by performing endoscopy. The incidence of perianal disease increases in association with colonic involvement and is highest in patients with active rectal disease.[21]

Local CD should be aggressively treated, including the use of topical steroid preparations. Surgery is indicated for failure to heal, anal stenosis and fissures associated with abscesses. The presence of an underlying fistula should be excluded. Anal sphincterotomy is the operation of choice. The fissure, sentinel pile and enlarged anal papilla should not be excised. Dilatation is not recommended in CD patients because it is generally more traumatic and less effective.[85]

CD is a common cause of anorectal strictures resulting in a stiff, non-compliant anorectum and anal incontinence: Surgical management ranges from four quadrant incisions through scar tissue followed by internal sphincterotomy and dilatation to anoplasty with a Y-V advancement flap. The most important criterion for success is the absence of active anorectal disease at the time of surgery.

Recurrent perianal abscesses are often a presenting feature of CD and are managed the same way as in patients without CD. Rectal CD should be treated along with abscess drainage. Oral metro-nidazole and ciprofloxacin (in older children) may be used until the abscess is healed, irrespective of the presence of rectal disease. Up to 30% of patients will be left with a fistulous tract after abscess drainage. Surgical treatment of fistula-in-ano is based on the patient's symptoms.[85] Many children have minimal symptoms from their fistulas, and as long as the tract is kept clean without recurrent abscess formation, no fistulotomy is required. The disease rarely progresses and spontaneous healing may occur. In patients with significant symptoms or recurrent abscesses, those with active CD require systemic treatment before perianal surgery (abscesses should be drained). Postoperative oral antibiotic therapy appears to decrease recurrence.[86] A 63-68% primary healing rate after fistulotomy may be achieved in this way.[85,87]

In complex fistula-in-ano or in patients with chronic rectal disease despite full medical therapy, temporary fecal diversion via colostomy followed by definitive fistulotomy may improve the chances of healing.[88] Setons are useful in complex or high fistulas to facilitate staged surgical fistulotomy or prolonged drainage while minimizing impairment of continence by avoiding external anal sphincter disruption. Alternative management of high fistulas including the use of endorectal advancement flaps and wide external drainage, or posterior approaches such as those described by York-Mason and Kraske have high morbidity and low success rates and should only be undertaken with the knowledge that the next step is proctectomy.

While failure to heal the fistula is the commonest complication, the gravest one is to injure the sphincter mechanism resulting in fecal incontinence. In CD, as in non-inflammatory perianal disease, incontinence is likely to be the result of aggressive surgery, not of aggressive disease, creating social invalids out of these children.[89] Of all patients with any type of perianal fistula coming to surgery, 8-12% will end up having a proctectomy and end-colostomy.[85,87]

Management of Extraintestinal Manifestations

A myriad of nonspecific inflammatory conditions involving almost every organ and system in the body has been described as part of the extraintestinal manifestations of inflammatory bowel disease. Treatment involves a combination of close monitoring, organ- or system-specific therapy. Management of the underlying intestinal inflammation and generalized supportive measures.

Joint involvement is the most common extraintestinal manifestation of CD, with an incidence of up to 25%.[90] Treatment is aimed at the underlying intestinal disease. Acetaminophen is the drug of choice for pain relief. Aspirin and nonsteroidal anti-inflammatory agents which may exacerbate the CD should be avoided Ankylosing spondylitis and sacroileitis occur less frequently in CD than UC. There is usually no improvement with treatment of the underlying bowel disease, so that therapy is primarily supportive.

Up to 4% of CD patients may develop primary sclerosing cholangitis.[91] Ursodeoxycholic acid may slow progression, but there is no proven cure for the disease. Many of these patients ultimately come to liver transplantation. Granulomatous hepatitis is seen in 1% of patients and is part of the spectrum of somatic granulomatous disease associated with CD. Treatment is that of the underlying bowel disease. The incidence of cholelithiasis is increased in CD, and gallstones develop at a younger age, especially in adolescents with terminal ileitis or after ileal resection and disturbance of enterohepatic bile circulation. Laparoscopic cholecystectomy is the operation of choice.

Mucocutaneous lesions seen in children with inflammatory bowel disease should be biopsied. Treatment includes that of the underlying intestinal disease as well as topical and intralesional corticosteroids.[92]

Uveitis and iritis occur in 2-4% of children with predominantly colonic CD and if left untreated may progress to scarring and blindness. Episcleritis is seen more commonly, but does not lead to permanent injury. Regular surveillance and prompt treatment of eye involvement is recommended for all children with CD.

PROGNOSIS

No reliable criteria are available to identify patients likely to have early symptomatic recurrence (within 36 months of surgery) once their disease is in remission due to medical or surgical intervention. Nearly 75% of patients have peri-anastomotic recurrence within 1 year of resection of macroscopically diseased bowel.[93] Patients requiring an ileostomy have significantly lower early recurrence rates than those having single or multiple anastomoses. The number of anastomoses and the presence of microscopic disease at the resection margin in patients having multiple anastomoses also results in a significantly increased incidence of early recurrence. Multiple site disease has a three-fold increased recurrence rate over single-site disease.[76]

Restoration of the fecal stream seems to have a significant effect on the development of early recurrence. In children with a temporary diverting ileostomy, recurrent distal disease usually develops after closure of the stoma.

In a long-term study of children and adolescents with CD, 69% of patients had at least one surgical intervention within 7.7 years of diagnosis.[94] In a similar study, 95% of patients with ileocolonic, 83% with colonic and 56% with small bowel disease underwent surgery over a 15 year follow-up period. The mean interval between diagnosis and surgery was 1.7 years for ileocolonic and 4 years for colonic disease.[95-97] The time between the onset of symptoms and the first operation is shorter in children compared with adults.[70] While surgeons have become more aggressive in terms of earlier operative intervention in children, maximal bowel conservation should be practiced.

The long-term risk of recurrence increases with disease duration before surgery, and relapse occurs earlier in patients undergoing surgery for failed medical therapy as opposed to specific complications.[97] Rates of reoperation are high depending on the site of disease, varying from 50% at 10 years for disease limited to the small bowel to 65% when the colon is involved.[76,98]

SMALL AND LARGE BOWEL RECURRENCE AND COMPLICATIONS

Anatomic location of disease, indication for surgery and preoperative duration of symptomatic disease are the most important factors influencing the rate of postoperative symptomatic recurrence of CD in childhood.[99] Children with diffuse ileocolonic disease (50% at 1 year) have the quickest recurrence, while isolated small bowel disease (50% at 5 years) is slowest to recur. Failure of medical therapy as the indication for surgery results in significantly earlier recurrence than when surgery is done for specific intestinal complications. If patients require surgery within one year of diagnosis, the majority have a long disease-free interval with only 30% recurrence by 8 years, compared with 50% recurrence in 3 years if duration of disease is more than 4 years. When these results are combined with the knowledge that significant postoperative catch-up growth in prepubertal children will occur if they remain in remission, a strong argument can be made for early operative intervention in newly diagnosed patients with limited disease.

CD of the terminal ileum recurs in a predictable sequence proximal to the ileocolic anastomosis after resection. Pre-anastomotic endoscopic recurrence is seen within 3 months of resection in up to 74% of CD patients. At 3 months, aphthous ulcers are seen in the neoterminal ileum with progression to larger ulcers and stricture in most patients. This pattern occurs irrespective of whether anastomosis occurred at the time of resection, or if there was an intervening ileostomy period. This signifies new inflammation rather than persistent disease or incomplete anastomotic healing. Recurrent disease causes anastomotic stricture; disease recurrence is not due to a stricture or tight anastomosis. However, only one third of patients with endoscopic disease recurrence are symptomatic.[100]

The length of bowel resected is statistically correlated with disease recurrence. Technically adequate resections of 25-50 cm of small bowel or combined small and large bowel are associated with a decreased probability of disease recurrence or reoperation. Longer resection (50-100 cm) does not correlate with lower recurrence rates. This statistic reflects the improved outcome of surgery in patients with limited small bowel disease as opposed to those with diffuse or colonic disease and does not mean that by limiting the length of resection, a given patient will have a better outcome.[101]

Several studies have demonstrated that the reoperation rate for pediatric CD is related to the site of the initial disease, because the site of disease is directly related to disease recurrence.[70,99] Diffuse or panenteric disease usually recurs after surgery, and in 95% of cases requires l or more re-operations. In children with colitis, recurrence and reoperation depends on the type of initial operative procedure. Staged colonic resections with primary anastomoses or ileostomy with fecal diversion have disease recurrence or persistence in more than 90% of cases with reoperation rates between 62-88%. In contrast, subtotal colectomy with ileostomy as the primary procedure remain well 89% of the time, and require surgery in less than 1% of cases.[94] Patients with limited small bowel or ileocolic disease have sustained remission in 85 and 80% respectively, with reoperation rates even lower.[95-97] In a small series of children with limited terminal ileal and right colonic disease, early resection resulted in 91% (10 of 11 children) long-term remission with no postoperative morbidity or mortality. Other subgroups of disease location have not met with similar success after early surgery. These excellent results with early resection in this subgroup emphasize the importance of accurate preoperative disease identification and location. The study also substantiates the need for differential management strategies based on the predicted nature of the disease in each subgroup.[99]

In a cohort study comparing CD parameters in a group of adults with a similar group of children, it has been noted that the incidence of toxic megacolon is significantly higher in children than in adults (9.5% versus 0.4%), which the authors explained by a more aggressive pattern to CD occurring at a younger age. In the adult group, 50% of patients had their first bowel resection within 6-8 years of the onset of symptoms. In the pediatric group, with approximately the same frequencies of localization, 50% of children had their first resection within 3 years of initial symptoms, again arguing for a more aggressive disease pattern.

Acute CD of the colon requiring emergency surgery is uncommon but may be increasing in frequency. In a large adult study, of 215 patients requiring surgery for acute inflammatory bowel disease, only 18 had CD (8%), with similar results reported in the pediatric population. Only 2 of these 18 patients do not have a stoma, and 10 of 16 patients with a stoma have required proctectomy. Thus, despite a policy of rectal conservation, it is very unlikely that acute colonic CD will be amenable to restorative surgery.[82]

In colonic CD, prolonged (greater than 15 years) spontaneous or drug-induced remission occurs at all sites: Right-sided disease (11%), extensive colonic disease (21%) and left-sided disease (38%). Prolonged remission may also occur after resection for CD, however, the overall reoperation rate is 76%.[102]

In a 7-year follow-up period of juvenile onset CD in Scotland, 79% of patients underwent a total of 135 operative procedures (71 major, i.e. intra-abdominal, 64 minor). In several similar series, major operative rates ranged from 62-80%. In the Scottish study, 50% of patients had one major operation within 5 years of diagnosis, and 94% by 15 years, with 59% of these patients requiring a second major procedure within 5 years of the first. Within 7 years of diagnosis, 20% of juveniles have a permanent stoma. Overall mortality is between 0 and 3% at 5 years and 10-20% at 20 years from diagnosis. The common causes of death include overwhelming sepsis following acute perforation and postoperative complications such as perforation, obstruction, hemorrhage and sepsis.[94]

In comparing this juvenile onset group with an adult onset group, the younger group had significantly more diagnostic laparotomy (17% versus 2% of all major operations), fewer total small bowel resections and fewer abdominoperineal resections as the first procedure. In the juvenile group, 88% of patients having a diagnostic laparotomy required a second major operation with resection. No patient having only small bowel resection has required colonic surgery, despite several requiring repeat small bowel resection. Of 7 patients whose first operation was colectomy with ileostomy, none have had disease recurrence. However, recurrence of disease after total proctocolectomy depends on whether the terminal ileum was involved at the time of surgery. Nearly 70% of patients with ileal disease have relapse within 10 years of surgery compared with less than 10% with disease limited to the colon.[103]

The long-term success (mean follow-up 8 years) of ileorectal anastomosis is directly dependent on the presence or recurrence of proctitis. When mild or no proctitis is present distal to the anastomosis, all patients retained a functioning anastomosis, however, when moderate to severe proctitis recurred, 81% had either a proctectomy or defunctioning stoma. Although the indication for rectal excision or exclusion was disease distal to the anastomosis, 63% of these patients also had small bowel disease compared with 11% in the group that had a functional astomosis. In this series, 88% of patients with intestinal, perforation required permanent ileostomy, whereas only 23% of patients with non-perforating colorectal disease required permanent ileostomy.[103]

Symptomatic recurrence rates as high as 60% at five years and 94% at 15 years, with re-operation rates of 10-40% at 10 years are not unusual in the literature.[104]

Within 20 years of the diagnosis of CD, the cumulative risk of having any stoma is 41%, and 14% of all patients will have a permanent stoma (40% of patients with colonic disease). Revision surgery for stomal complications is more common after colostomy than ileostomy. Increased risk of having any stoma is associated with rectal inflammation, perianal fistula or abscess and absence of small intestinal disease. Interestingly, despite a higher rate of disease recurrence, long-standing symptomatic disease before the first operation reduces the risk of having a stoma. The likelihood of stoma reversal is 75% when used for anastomotic protection or avoidance, 79% after postoperative complications and 40% for perianal disease or rectal inflammation.[105]

Patients with diffuse or pan-enteric disease, representing about 20% of children with CD, pose major problems in medical and surgical management with high morbidity and mortality (up to 15% in this subgroup). Surgery is more often for complications such as chronic obstruction due to stricture within diseased segments of bowel rather than resection of diseased bowel to attain remission. Therefore, disease recurrence and reoperation is very common and this group is at the highest risk for developing short bowel syndrome, Everything possible should be done to avoid this complication, including stricturoplasty, endoscopic divulsion or ablation of strictures instead of resection for obstruction, and tolerance of mild to moderate symptoms to avoid repeated surgeries. Nevertheless, over 60% of these children are permanently growth and height retarded.[97]

Short bowel syndrome is characterized by steatorrhea, mineral and vitamin losses and undernutrition. Parenteral hyperalimentation is required initially to achieve nutritional homeostasis, and then is used chronically to supplement inadequate gastrointestinal absorption. Parenteral hyperalimentation is fraught with problems and complications that add to those of the underlying CD. Effective management depends on accurate determination of nutritional deficiencies and a carefully supervised, highly specialized oral feeding program. Long-term uninterrupted control permits physiologic adaptation of the residual bowel and may decrease the need for medication and dietary limitations. The degree of morphologic and physiologic intestinal adaptation after small bowel resection or colectomy is dependent on the length of residual bowel and the age of the child. Younger children have a large adaptive capacity which is another reason for earlier surgical intervention in preadolescent children with CD, which may result in restoration of complex bowel functions not possible in older patients. If the residual bowel is too short to allow effective adaptation, small bowel transplantation, although still experimental, has become a viable option. Immunosuppressive drugs required for the transplanted bowel may have the added effect of suppressing CD in these children. Until the etiology of CD is elicited and specific therapy can be developed, bone marrow transplantation may be the last resort in salvaging those few patients with unrelenting resistant disease. Having stressed the benefits of surgery, it is important to recognize the potential for postoperative complications, most commonly sepsis, fistula formation, obstruction, short bowel syndrome and recurrence.

Crohn's ileitis or ileocolitis may first be diagnosed at laparotomy or laparoscopy often performed for suspected appendicitis. After incidental appendectomy the, fistula rate is about 50% in CD patients as opposed to 0.3% in normal patients, but most of these fistulas are from the terminal ileum rather than the appendiceal stump. Indeed, laparotomy alone is associated with a 10-39% risk of fistula formation, whereas the fistula rate after bowel resection for CD is 2-5%. The debate on the role of incidental appendectomy in CD continues, but if the cecum is soft, pliable and uninvolved, most surgeons would perform an appendectomy.[105,106] Unexpected chronic CD (fat wrapping, fibrosis, woody thickening and fibrosis with a short thickened mesentery and possibly a mass or fistula) should be dealt with—according to the patient's symptoms and gross evidence of complicated disease or stricture. A conservative approach to the unexpected finding of CD at laparotomy is best.[106]

Crohn's colitis must be differentiated from UC because of the implications of management. However, diagnostic error occurs in 6-10% of patients.[107,108] Evidence of non-colonic CD, endoscopy and histology are used to differentiate between the two diseases. The rectum is always involved in UC, whereas 40% of Crohn's colitis children have rectal sparing, irrespective of anal involvement. Toxic megacolon and perforation is rare in CD, usually occurring early on and may be mistaken for UC.

Proctocolectomy with end-ileostomy is the conventional operative approach for the treatment of granulomatous colitis involving the rectum or anus. Another approach in patients with mild to moderate rectal involvement, is to create a temporary diverting ileostomy and rectal mucus fistula or Hartmann, pouch with delayed ileorectal anastomosis if the anorectal disease heals. If the anorectal disease does not heal, an abdominoperineal or perineal proctectomy may be performed later. In patients in whom Crohn's colitis was initially mistaken for UC, and who underwent ileoanal anastomosis, complication rates are very high.[107,108] Based on results of these studies, the creation of ileal pouches and ileoanal anastomosis is contraindicated in patients known to have CD. The creation of a continent ileostomy such as a Kock's pouch is also controversial because of the high complication and failure rates.[109] Recurrence of CD following proctocolectomy when the disease was confined to the colon, is between 10 and 20%.

For patients with colonic CD and rectal sparing, colectomy and primary or delayed ileorectal anastomosis is the optimal procedure. For children and adolescents, avoidance of an ileostomy during the years of their physical and emotional development is desirable even though one third of these children will subsequently develop severe enough disease to warrant proctectomy or divertion.

Perianal Disease

Treatment failure of perianal and genital fistulous disease is the commonest indication for primary stoma creation (64% of all patients with stomas). Considerable controversy exists on the rate of success of temporary fecal diversion in the management of complicated perianal or refractory rectal disease. Once patients require fecal diversion, 20-66% will have some improvement, although new fistulas may arise despite diversion. The best criterion of success is restoration of intestinal continuity. This is successful in only 10-31% of patients.[110] Even after proctectomy, fistulas or genital problems may persist and continue to impair quality of life.[111] Nevertheless, it is often psychologically better not to perfom non-reversible procedures such as proctectomy as long as there is hope of life without a permanent stoma. A Hartmann procedure followed later by perineal proctectomy (if required) once the patient has come to terms with the inevitability of a permanent stoma may be of significant psychological benefit for patients living with this chronic illness. However, in a study of three groups of children with CD, a stoma group, an ileorectal anastomosis group and a non-surgical group, no difference was found in psychosocial adjustment, self-esteem and quality of life. Children seem far better able to cope with the sequelae of early onset CD than when the disease presents in late adolescence or later.[112]

Growth Failure and Sexual Maturation

Linear growth following surgery is directly related to pubertal status. Following surgery, Tanner Stage I and II patients achieve normal or near normal height velocity and regain their pre-illness height percentiles within 1-5 years. Tanner Stage III patients have a growth spurt after surgery, but usually not to full pre-illness percentiles, whereas Tanner Stage IV and V patients had no increase in height velocity.[113] Patients with limited, surgically resectable disease in whom surgical remission with symptomatic relief is possible, will benefit most in terms of growth failure. Persistence or early recurrence of active disease negates the benefit of surgery for growth failure.[113] Nutritional supplementation should continue following surgery, providing 120-30% of the age-recommended daily nutritional requirements.[114] Placement of a gastrostomy for postoperative nutritional supplementation should be considered at the time of surgery. Postoperatively, steroids should be tapered and discontinued, but maintenance 5-aminosalicylate therapy has been shown to prolong remission. When patients with CD and growth failure are prepubertal and surgery is performed primarily because of failure of medical therapy or other complications, a postoperative growth spurt may be expected within one year.[113] Despite the almost inevitable postoperative recurrence of disease, the potential for a period of remission makes early surgical intervention justifiable for carefully selected patients with localized disease.[115]

Chronic disease refractory to medical and nutritional therapy is the main indication for surgery in most pediatric series. Patients with localized disease have the best outcomes. In children with preoperative evidence of linear growth retardation, surgical resection of localized CD, followed by adequate nutritional support results in catch-up growth and a prolonged symptom- and drug-free period in most patients, although this may be limited by their age or stage of puberty.

Fertility of either sex is unaffected by CD unless malnutrition or inflammatory damage to reproductive organs occurs. Disease activity is usually not affected by pregnancy, but occasionally may improve. Exacerbation may occur following delivery. There appears to be no risk of maternal disease affecting the fetus, although medications should be reviewed and may need to be altered.

Although morbidity is high, mortality is low and most children with CD can expect to grow and mature relatively normally, leading productive lives with good general health. Sexual function may be affected on psychological grounds of altered body image, especially in patients with a stoma. However, patients in whom CD developed in childhood are far better adapted in terms of body image than when the onset of disease occurs in adulthood.[112]

Carcinoma

The risk of developing adenocarcinoma of the small or large bowel is increased in patients with longstanding CD. Carcinoma usually develops within a site of chronic disease including along fistulas tracts. The risk for colon cancer is between 4 and 20 times greater than the general population. In patients whose CD was diagnosed before 21 years of age, the risk of developing colorectal cancer is 20 times the general population.[116] The risk of developing small bowel carcinoma is estimated at 114 times the general population, but these data are skewed because of the low incidence of the disease in the general population. Historically, 40% of small bowel carcinoma occurred in excluded loops of small bowel, and since this practice is now almost obsolete, the overall incidence of cancer of the small bowel should be much lowet.[104] Patients with CD are also at greater risk of developing extraintestinal carcinoma. Unlike UC, the association of colonic mucosal dysplasia with carcinoma is not sufficiently established to warrant prophylactic colectomy.

A subgroup of CD patients has been identified for being at greatest risk for the development of colorectal carcinoma. These patients are typically diagnosed before the age of 40, have long- standing proctocolitis of more than 10 years duration and frequently have co-existing strictures, fistulas and bypassed segments. Because of their background disease symptomatology, the development of colorectal cancer often goes unnoticed until well advanced and is consequently associated with poor survival. Surveillance colonoscopy with biopsy is recommended in these patients and appears to impart a significant survival benefit since mortality rates from cancer are decreasing with current surveillance strategies.[73]

CONCLUSION

In a 15-year long-term follow-up study of children with CD presenting before the age of 16 years, two of three had no evidence of residual disease, one in four were clinically well, although evidence of macroscopic disease was present, and one in ten were symptomatic.[97]

The management of CD in children is complex. A positive attitude and the patient's willingness to become actively involved in disease management, as well as a trusting relationship between physician and patient, especially through the demands of adolescent development, is essential to the long-term care and outcome of this disease.

REFERENCES

1. Crohn B, Ginsberg L, Oppenheimer G. Regional ieitis: Pathologic and clinical entity. JAMA 1932;99:1323.
2. Calkins BM, et al. Trends in incidence rates of ulcerative colitis and Crohn's disease. Dig Dis Sci 1984;29:913.
3. Barton JR, Gillon S, Ferguson A. Incidence of inflammatory bowel disease in Scottish children between 1968 and 1983; marginal fall in ulcerative colitis, threefold rise in Crohn's disease. Gut 1989;30:618-22.
4. Cosgrove M, Al-Atria RF, Jenkins HR. The epidemiology of paediatric inflammatory bowel disease. Arch Dis Child 1996;74:460-61.
5. Chong SKF, et al. Prospective study of colitis in infancy and early childhood. J Pediatr Gastroenterol Nutr 1986;5:352-58.
6. Whelen G. Epidemiology of inflammatory bowel disease. Med Clin North Am 1990;74.
7. Bennett RA, Rubin PH, Present DH. Frequency of inflammatory bowel disease in offspring of couples both presenting with inflammatory bowel disease. Gastroenterology 1991;94:603.
8. Sofaer J. Crohn's disease: The genetic contribution. Gut 1993;34:869.
9. McDonald GB, Lopez-Curbero SO, Sullivan KM. Prolonged remission of Crohn's disease following allogeneic marrow transplantation. Gastroenterology A798;1997.
10. Katz JA, Fiocchi C. Causes and mechanisms of Crohn's disease. In Prantera C, Korelitz HI (Eds): Crohn's disease. New York, Marcel Dekker, Inc 1996;9-56.
11. Snook J. Are the inflammatory bowel diseases autoimmune disorders? Gut 1990;31:961-63.
12. Abreu MT, Targan SR. The future of Crohn's disease: New developments in etiopathogenesis and therapeutics. In Prantera C, Korelitz BI (Eds): Crohn's disease. New York, Marcel Dekker, Inc 1996;561-86.
13. Fanner RG, Hawk WA, Tumbu11 RB. Clinical patterns in Crohn's disease: A statistical study of 615 cases. Gastroenterology 1975;68:627.
14. Wolff BG, et al. Anorectal Crohn's disease: A long tenI1 perspective. Dis Colon Rectum 1985;28:709.
15. Rotterdam H, Korelitz B, Sommers SC. Microgranulomas in grossly normal rectal mucosa in Crohn's disease. Am J Clin Pathol 1977;67:550.
16. Mashako MNL, et al. Crohn's disease lesions in the upper gastrointestinal tract: Correlation between clinical, radiological, endoscopic and histological features in adolescents and children. J Pediatr Gastroenterol Nutr 1989;8:442-46.
17. Hyams JS. Crohn's disease in children. Pediatr Clin North Am 1996;43:255-77.

18. Burbidge PJ, Huang S, Bayless TM. Clinical manifestations of Crohn's disease in children and adolescents. Pediatrics 1915;55:866-11.
19. Sandbom WJ, Phillips SF. Pathophysiology of symptoms and clinical features of inflammatory disease. In Kirsner JB, Shorter RG (Eds): Inflammatory bowel disease. Baltimore, Williams and Wilkins 1995;407-28.
20. Hofley PM, Piccoli DA. Inflammatory bowel disease in children. Med Clin North Am 1994;78:1281-302.
21. Palder SB, Shandling B, Bilik R. Perianal complications of pediatric Crohn's disease. J Pediatr Surg 1991;26:513-15.
22. Markowitz J, et al. Perianal disease in children and adolescents with Crohn's disease. Gastroenterology 1984;86:829-33.
23. Hyams JS. Extraintestinal manifestations of inflammatory bowel disease in children. Pediatr Gastroenterol Nutr 1994;19:7.
24. Plauth M, Jenss H, Meyle J. Oral manifestations of Crohn's disease: An analysis of 79 cases. J Clin Gastroenterol 1991;13:29-37.
25. Salmon JF, Wright JP, Murray ADN. Ocular inflammation in Crohn's disease. Ophthalmology 1991;98:480-84.
26. Kane W, Miller K, Sharp HL. Inflammatory bowel disease presenting as liver disease during childhood. J Pediatr 1980;97:775-78.
27. Lloyd-Still JD, Tomasi L. Neurovascular and thromboembolic complications of inflammatory bowel disease in childhood. J Pediatr Gastroenterol Nutr 1989;9:461-66.
28. Booth IW. The nutritional consequences of gastrointestinal disease in adolescence. Acta Pediatr Scand 1991;375 (suppl):91.
29. Seidman EG, et al. Nutritional issues in pediatric inflammatory bowel disease. J Pediatr Gastroenterol Nutr 1991;12:424.
30. Kuschner RF, Schoeller DA. Resting and total energy expenditure in patients with inflammatory bowel disease. Am J Clin Nutr 1991;53:161-65.
31. Barth JA, Grand RJ. Crohn's disease in childhood and adolescence. In Prantera C, Korelitz BI (Eds): Crohn's disease. New York, Marcel Dekker, Inc 1996;561-86.
32. Hyams JS, Carey DE. Corticosteroids and growth. J Pediatr 1988;113:249.
33. Hildebrand H, Karlberg J, Kristiansson B. Longitudinal growth in children and adolescents with inflammatory bowel disease. J Pediatr Gastroenterol Nutr 1994;18:165-73.
34. Griffiths AM, et al. Growth and clinical course of children with Crohn's disease. Gut 1993;34:939-43.
35. Beck IT. Laboratory assessment of inflammatory bowel disease. Dig Dis Sci 1987;32:265.
36. Jewell PM, et al. Technitium-99m-HMP AO labeled leucocytes in the detection and monitoring of inflammatory bowel disease in children. Br J Radio 1996;169:508-14.
37. Thomas DW, Sinatra FR. Screening laboratory tests for Crohn's disease. West J Med 1989;150:63.
38. Stringer DA. Imaging inflammatory bowel disease in the pediatric patient. Radiol Clin North Am 1987;25:93-113.
39. Hassall E, Barclay GN, Ament ME. Colonoscopy in childhood. Pediatrics 1984;73:594-99.
40. Habet GB. Role of endoscopy 32: 16S(suppl); 1987 In inflammatory bowel Disease. Dig Dis Sci 1987;32 :16 (S).
41. Schmidt Sornmerfeld E, Kirschner BS, Stephens JK. Endoscopic and histologic findings in the upper gastrointestinal tract of children with Crohn's disease. J Pediatr Gastroenterol 1990;11:448.
42. Lenaerts C, et al. High incidence of upper gastrointestinal tract involvement in children with Crohn's disease. Pediatrics 1989;83:777-81.
43. Dijkstra J, Reeders JW AJ, Tytgat GNJ. Idiopathic inflammatory bowel disease: Endoscopic- radiologic correlation. Radiology 1995;197:369-75.
44. Jobling JC, et al. Investigating inflammatory bowel disease -white cell scanning, radiology and colonoscopy. Arch Dis Child 1996;74:22-26.
45. Maglinte DDT, et al. Crohn's disease of the small intestine: Accuracy and relevance of enteroclysis. Radiology 1992;184:541-45.
46. Jabra AA, Fishman EK, Taylor GA. Crohn's disease in the pediatric patient: CT evaluation. Radiology 1991;179:495-98.
47. Faure C, et al. Ultrasonographic assessment of inflammatory bowel disease in children: Comparison with ileocolonoscopy. J Pediatr 1997;130:147-51.
48. Gendre JP, et al. Oral mesalamine (Pentasa) as maintenance treatment in Crohn's disease: A multicenter placebo-controlled study. Gastroenterology 1993;104:435.
49. Prantera C, et al. Oral 5-aminosalicylic acid (Asacol) in the maintenance treatment of Crohn's disease. Gastroenterology 1992;103:363.
50. Malchow H, et al. European co-operative Crohn's disease study: Results of drug treatment. Gastroenterology 1984;86:249.
51. Kirschner BS. Ulcerative colitis and Crohn's disease in children. Gastroenterol Clin North Am 1995;24:99-117.
52. Bello C, Goldstein F, Thomton 11. Alternate-day prednisone treatment and treatment maintenance in Crohn's disease. Am J Gastroenterol 1991;86:460.
53. Statter, MB, Hirschl RB, Coran AG. Inflammatory bowel disease. Pediatr Clin North Am 1993;40:1213-31.
54. Greenberg OR, et al. Oral budesonide for active Crohn's disease. N Engl J Med 1994;331:836.
55. Rutgeerts P, et al. A comparison of budesonide with prednisolone for active Crohn's disease. N Engl J Med 1994;331:842.
56. Nicholls $, et al. Cyclosporin as initial treatment for Crohn's disease. Arch Dis Child 1994;71:243-47.
57. Mahdi G, Israel DM, Hassall E. Cyclosporine and 6-mercaptopurine for active, refractory Crohn's colitis in children. Am J Gastroenterol 1996;91:1355-59.
58. Markowitz J, et al. Long-term 6-mercaptopurine treatment in adolescents with Crohn's disease. Gastroenterology 1990;99:1347-51.

59. Verhave M, Winter HS, Grand RJ. Azathioprine in the treatment of children with inflammatory bowel disease. J Pediatr 1990;117:809-14.
60. Gohkale R, Kirschner B. Methotrexate (MTX) therapy in children with severe Crohn's disease (CD): Preliminary results. Gastroenterology 1997;IIO:A916.
61. Hildenbrand H, et al. Treatment of Crohn's disease with metronidazole in childhood and adolescence. Gastroenterol Clin Bio 1980;121:19-25.
62. Peppercorn MA. Is there a role for antibiotics as primary therapy in Crohn's ileitis? J Clin Gastroenterol 1993;17:235-37.
63. Duffy LF, et al. Peripheral neuropathy in Crohn's disease patients treated with metronidazole. Gastroenterology 1985;88:681-84.
64. Hyams JS, Markowitz J, Wylie R. Use of infliximab in the treatment of Crohn's disease in children and adolescence. J Pediatr 2000;137(2):192-96.
65. Present DH. Review article: the efficacy of infliximab in Crohn's disease -healing of fistulae. Aliment Phamlacol Ther Suppl 1999;4:23-28.
66. Papadakis KA, Targan SR. Role of cytokines in the pathogenesis of inflammatory bowel disease. Ann Rev Med 2000;51:289-98.
67. Griffiths AM, et al. Meta-analysis of enteral feeding as a primary treatment of active Crohn's disease. Gastroenterology 1995;108:1056-67.
68. Polk DB, Hattner JAT, Kemer JA. Improved growth and disease activity after intermittent administration of a defined formula diet in children with Crohn's disease. J Parenter Enter Nutr 1992;16:499-504.
69. Blair GK, Yaman M, Wesson DE. Preoperative home enteral nutrition in complicated Crohn's disease. J Pediatr Surg 1986;21:769.
70. Aronson DC, et al. Surgical treatment of Crohn's disease in children and adolescents; How conservative can the paediatrician be? Bur J Pediatr 1993;152:727-29.
71. Kirchmann HMA, Bender SW. Intestinal obstruction in Crohn's disease in childhood. J Pediatr Gastroenterol Nutr 1987;6:79-84.
72. Munkholm P, et al. Intestinal cancer risk and mortality in patients with Crohn's disease. Gastroenterology 1993;105:1716-23.
73. Persson P-G, et al. Crohn's disease and cancer: Gastroenterology. A population-based cohort study. 1994;107:1675-79.
74. Heuman R, et al. The influence of disease at the margin of resection on the outcome of Crohn's disease. Br J Surg 1983;70:519-21.
75. Kotanagi H, et al. Do microscopic abnormalities at resection margins correlate with increased anastomotic recurrence in Crohn's disease? Dis Colon Rectum 1991;34:909-16.
76. Heiman TM, et al. Prediction of early symptomatic recurrence after intestinal resection in Crohn's disease. Ann Surg 1993;218:294-99.
77. Handelsman JC. Crohn's disease of the small bowel. In: Cameron JL. Ed. Current surgical therapy. St Louis, Mosby Yearbook, Inc 1995.
78. Alexander-Williams J, Haynes IG. Conservative operations for Crohn's disease of the small bowel. World J Surg 1985;9:945-51.
79. Oliva L, et al. The results of stricturoplasty in pediatric patients with multifocal Crohn's disease. J Pediatr Gastroenterol Nutr 1994;18:300-10.
80. Fazio VW, et al. Stricturoplasty in Crohn's disease. Ann Surg 1989;210:621-25.
81. Haber G, Oz MC, Forde KA. Endoscopic alternatives in the management of colonic strictures. Surgery 1990;108:513-19.
82. Mortensen NJ, et al. Surgery for acute Crohn's colitis: Results and long term follow-up. Br J Surg 1984;71:783-84.
83. Pettit SH, Irving MH. The operative management of fistulous Crohn's disease. Surg Gynecol Obstet 1988;167:223-28.
84. Katz S, Shulman N, Levin L. Free perforation in Crohn's disease. A report of 33 cases and review of the literature. Am Gastroenterol 1987;81:31-43.
85. Weaver RM, et al. Manual dilatation of the anus versus lateral subcutaneous sphincterotomy in the treatment of chronic fissure-in-ano: Results of a prospective, randomized clinical trial. Dis Colon Rectum 1987;30:420-23.
86. Levien DH, Surrell J, Mazier WP. Surgical treatment of anorectal fistula in patients with Crohn's disease. Surg Gynecol Obstet 1989;169:133-36.
87. Brandt LJ, et al. Metronidazole therapy for perineal Crohn's disease: A follow-up study. Gastroenterology 1982;83:383-87.
88. Bernard D, Morgan S, Tasse D. Selective surgical management of Crohn's disease of the anus. Can J Surg 1986;29:318-21.
89. Orking BA, Telander RL. The effect of intra abdominal resection or fecal diversion on perianal disease in pediatric Crohn's disease. J Pediatr Surg 1985;20:343-47.
90. Alexander-Williams J, et al. Perianal Crohn's disease. Gut 1974;15:822.
91. Gravallese EM, Kantrowitz FG. Arthritic manifestations of inflammatory bowel disease. Am J Gastroenterol 1988;83:703-09.
92. Schrumpf E, et al. Hepatobiliary complications of inflammatory bowel disease, Semin Liver Dis 1988;8:201-09.
93. Warner AS, MacDermott RP. Extraintestinal manifestations. In Prantera C, Korelitz BI (Eds): Crohn's disease. New York. Marcel Dekker, Inc 1996;9-56.
94. Olafson Q, Smedh K, Sjodahl R. Natural course of Crohn's disease after ileocolic resection: Endoscopically visualized ulcers preceding symptoms. Gut 1992;33:331-35.
95. Sedgewick DM, et al. Population-based study of surgery in juvenile onset Crohn's disease. Br J Surg 1991;78:171-75.

96. Davies G, et al. Surgery for Crohn's disease in childhood: Influence of site of disease and operative procedure on outcome. Br J Surg 1990;77:891-94.
97. Farmer RG, Michener WM. Prognosis of Crohn's disease with onset in childhood or adolescence. Dig Dis Sci 1979;24:752-57.
98. Puntis J, McNeish AS, Allan RN. Long term prognosis of Crohn's disease with onset in childhood and adolescence. Gut 1984;25:329-36.
99. Castille RG, et al. Crohn's disease in children: Assessment of the progression of disease, growth, and prognosis. J Pediatr Surg 1980;15:462-69.
100. Coran AG, Klein MD, Sarahan TM. The surgical management of terminal ileal and right colon Crohn's disease in children. J Pediatr Surg 1983;18:592-94.
101. Kahn E, et al. The morphologic relationship of sinus and fistula formation to intestinal stenoses in children with Crohn's disease. Am J Gastroenterol 1993;88:1395-98.
102. Ellis L, et al. Postoperative recurrence in Crohn's disease. Ann Surg 1984;199:340-47.
103. Andrews HA, Lewis P, Allan RN. Prognosis after surgery for colonic Crohn's disease. Br J Surg 1989;70:1184-90.
104. Chevalier JM, et al. Colectomy and ileorectal anastomosis in patients with Crohn's disease. Br J Surg 1994;81:1379-81.
105. Greenstein AJ, Sachar DB, Smith H. A comparison of cancer risk in Crohn's disease and ulcerative colitis. Cancer 1981;48:2742-45.
106. Siminowitz DA, Rusch VW, Stevenson JK. Natural history of incidental appendectomy in patients. Am J Surg 1982;143:171-73.
107. Handelsman JC. Crohn's disease of the small bowel. In: Cameron JL, Ed. Current surgical therapy. St Louis, Mosby Yearbook, Inc 1995.
108. Fazio VW, et al. Ilealpouch-anal anastomoses complications and function in 1005 patients. Ann Surg 1995;22:120-27.
109. Coran AG. A personal experience with 100 consecutive total colectomies and straight ileoanal endorectal pull-through for benign disease of the colon and rectum in children and adults. Ann Surg 1990;212:242-48.
110. Kelly KA. Anal Sphincter-saving operations for chronic ulcerative colitis. Am J Surg 1992;163:5-11.
111. Post S, et al. Experience with ileostomy and colostomy in Crohn's disease. Br J Surg 1995;82:1629-33.
112. Scammell BE, Keighley MRB. Delayed perineal wound healing after proctectomy for Crohn's colitis. Int J Colorectal Dis 1990;5:49-52.
113. Lask B, et al. Psychosocial sequelae of stoma surgery for inflammatory bowel disease in children. Gut 1987;28:1257-60.
114. Alperstein G, et al. Linear growth following surgery in children and adolescents with Crohn's disease: Relationship to pubertal status. J Ped Surg 1985;20:129-33.
115. McLain BI, et al. Growth after gut resection for Crohn's disease. Arch Dis Child 1990;65:760-62.
116. Weedon DD, et al. Crohn's disease and cancer. N Engl J Med 1973;283:1099-102.

Ulcerative Colitis

Robert Cywes, Arnold G Coran

HISTORICAL OVERVIEW

Ulcerative colitis (UC) was first described as an inflammatory bowel disease distinct from infectious colitis by Wilks and Moxon in 1875, but it was not until 1960 that criteria were established to differentiate UC from Crohn's colitis.[1,2] Today, there remains a significant overlap between the two diseases, with up to 15% of colitis cases being assigned an indeterminate diagnosis, suggesting a similar etiology and pathogenesis.[3] UC is an idiopathic chronic relapsing inflammatory disease limited to the colonic and rectal mucosa, and is associated with significant extra-intestinal manifestations.

Early management strategies for severe UC included intestinal diversion which provided good initial results, but was a poor long-term solution. This was followed by appendicostomy and antegrade lavage, which also had marginal success. In 1913, Browne revisited the concept of bowel rest by total fecal diversion using an ileostomy and this became the standard of care.[4] In 1944, Strauss described proctocolectomy with ileostomy for management of severe UC.[5] Technical and staged improvements in this approach were described by Cattell in (three-stage procedure) and Gardner in 1951 (two-stage procedure).[6,7] In 1952 and 1954, Ripstein and Goligher respectively, described a one-stage ileostomy with proctocolectomy approach, which together with the Brooke ileostomy described in 1952 has become the current elective standard curative operation for UC patients.[8-10]

Together with advances in the surgical treatment of UC came advances in stomal care that have been instrumental in improving the quality of life of UC patients and has led to greater acceptance of the surgical cure for this disease. Major advances have included the Brooke eversion ileostomy creation, improvements in nursing care and stomal appliances. In 1969, Kock described a technique for creating a continent ileostomy using an internal reservoir and nipple valve that requires interval tube irrigation without the use of stomal appliances.[11] Although associated with a high complication rate, the Kock's pouch has benefited a significant number of patients requiring permanent stomas.

While it is recognized that total proctocolectomy is curative for UC, anal sphincter-saving alternatives to permanent ileostomy have been sought for over 50 years. Early efforts included ileosigmoidostomy and ileoproctostomy. In a 1985 meta-analysis of 17 studies on patients with ileoanal anastomoses for UC. Parc reported excellent functional results in terms of number of bowel movements per day (4.5) and continence (>99%).[12] However, 5% of patients required proctectomy for recurrent disease and up to 20% of patients developed carcinoma of the retained large bowel. This operation is now reserved for special circumstances only.

Complete proctocolectomy with sphincter-saving ileoanal anastomosis was initially unsuccessful because of unacceptable frequency and urgency. Even when Ravitch and Sabiston modified the ileoanal anastomosis by including a rectal mucosectomy functional results were mostly unacceptable in terms of quality of life.[13] However, in 1973, Safaie reported successful results in familial polyposis patients using a straight ileo-endorectal pull-through procedure

(ERPT) that included a distal rectal mucosectomy that was based upon the success of the Soave endorectal pull-through developed for Hirschsprung's disease.[14,15] This procedure was further improved by Martin in 1977 and most recently by Coran.[16,17]

Concerns remained in terms of frequency, urgency and soiling because of the lack of a neorectal reservoir. In 1955, Valiente developed an ileal pouch proximal to the ileoanal anastomosis.[18] Various modifications of this concept have developed over the years, including S, W and J shaped pouches. Such pouches were combined with rectal mucosectomy by Parks in 1978 to create the current standard ileoanal pouch anastomosis.[19,20] The physiology and relative merits of the various pouch configurations have been extensively reviewed.[21] Most large series report a high degree of patient satisfaction regardless of the type of ERPT.

The final improvement to this restorative proctocolectomy has come with the advent of minimally invasive surgical techniques where the proctocolectomy is performed laparoscopically with the rectal mucosectomy and ileoanal anastomosis performed via a perineal approach. Ileal pouch construction may be performed through a small Pfannenstiel incision.

EPIDEMIOLOGY

Pediatric epidemiological studies have confirmed a recent rise in the incidence of Crohn's disease (CD), while the incidence of UC, despite annual fluctuations, has remained stable to the point where the incidence of CD is now greater than that of UC.[4] The most consistent risk factor for inflammatory bowel disease (10 times greater risk) is a positive family history which is seen in 15-40% of children with UC. Within families, the two forms of disease appear to run true. No other postulated risk factors are statistically significant. While the prevalence remains high in certain groups such as Ashkenazi Jews, the prevalence has increased in certain groups who have migrated from low to high incidence areas, suggesting an environmental influence on the disease. Males and females are equally likely to get the disease. Age distribution is bimodal with peaks occurring in the second and third, and fifth and sixth decades. In 15-40% of all patients with UC, the diagnosis is made before 20 years of age.

ETIOLOGY

UC is an idiopathic inflammatory bowel disease. The most plausible current etiology is an inappropriate response to environmental factors resulting from direct or indirect dysregulation of the immune system at a genetic level. Genetic predisposition is supported by HLA-W27 testing in patients with UC, ankylosing spondylitis and uveitis. An altered cytokine response to an environmental trigger may result in an inflammatory cascade causing the disease. An autoimmune etiology is given weight by the finding of autoantibodies in over 70% of UC patients.[5] A genetic/autoimmune etiology would explain the extraintestinal manifestations of the disease as well. Confounding factors such as psychosocial and psychosomatic effects, while not causing the disease, may have a significant exacerbating influence.

PATHOLOGY

UC is defined by inflammation limited to the rectal and colonic mucosa. The rectum is involved in all cases with proximal extension into the colon in 90%. The colon may be involved for varying distances towards the ileocecal junction, but inflammation is continuous from the rectum proximally. Pancolitis is more common in children than adults, while 15% have isolated rectal involvement and 20% have limited left-sided disease only. Perianal involvement is so rare that should it occur, a diagnosis of CD must be entertained. Although, by definition, the small bowel is not involved, a phenomenon of 'backwash ileitis' has been described to explain the finding of macroscopic inflammation in the terminal ileum in up to 15% of patients with pancolitis. 'Backwash ileitis is a clinical finding described as nonspecific chronic inflammation microscopically, and is therefore not a pathological entity. However, if polymorphonuclear leukocytes are seen in the lamina propria of the terminal ileum, the diagnosis of CD must be considered. Pathological examination of biopsies from clinically inflamed terminal ileum should distinguish 'backwash ileitis' from true ileal inflammatory bowel disease.

In active colitis, crypt abscesses lead to mucosal ulceration on a background of diffuse continuous inflammation with hemorrhage and edema. Islands of regenerating epithelium developing into pseudopolyps may be present. Because inflammation is limited to the mucosa, disease activity is usually underestimated when viewed from the serosal surface at operation. However, the bowel becomes distended with little peristalsis. The disease may acutely progress to toxic megacolon. In chronic UC, the repeated inflammatory episodes result in fibrosis of the muscularis with thickening, shortening and loss of haustral folds. The mucosa becomes atrophic and may develop dysplasia or neoplastic changes. Diagnosis and disease activity is confirmed by mucosal biopsy.

CLINICAL MANIFESTATIONS

Gastrointestinal Manifestation

Over 95% of patients with UC present with gastrointestinal manifestations of varying intensity resulting in early diagnosis of inflammatory bowel disease. The majority present with insidious onset diarrhea, mild rectal bleeding, and vague abdominal pain without systemic signs or symptoms. Such disease tends to be localized to the left colon and rectum and the course usually remains mild. About 30% of patients have moderate disease with pus and bloody diarrhea, *cramps, abdominal tenderness, urgency and tenesmus. Systemic symptoms include anorexia,* weight loss, low-grade fever and mild anemia. Severe colitis requiring hospitalization and *occasionally emergency surgery occurs in about* 10% of patients. *This disease is usually* a fulminant pancolitis characterized by five or more bloody stools per day, diffuse abdominal tenderness and distension. fever. tachycardia, anemia. leukocytosis and hypoalbuminemia with weight loss and malnutrition. In less than 5% of patients, extraintestinal features dominate the clinical picture as is commonly seen in CD. These patients may present with growth failure, arthropathy, erythema nodosum or liver disease such as sclerosing cholangitis and mayor may not have active colitis at the time of presentation.[22]

Limited disease usually maintains its course but occasionally may extend beyond its initial involvement. In most cases, the course and severity of disease activity are similar in intensity to' that of its onset. The course of UC in most patients is one of remission with periodic relapses often related to emotional stress or intercurrent infection. Fewer than 8% of all UC patients will require surgical intervention before 20 years of age. However, up to 50% children with pancolitis *will require surgery. A single attack with complete remission never requiring surgical* intervention is seen in less than 10% of all children.

The incidence of carcinoma is 3% *in the first decade of disease, with* a 10-15% *increment in* each subsequent decade. While carcinoma rarely presents in children, it is most common in patients where the diagnosis of UC is made early in life, in those with pancolitis or in those with frequent acute recurrences.[23] Surveillance colonoscopy with biopsy is recommended for all patients.

Extraintestinal Manifestation

Extraintestinal manifestations of inflammatory bowel disease may involve any system or organ in the body, lending credence to the autoimmune etiology theory. Bone and joint involvement occurs in 20-25% of patients, more commonly than with CD. Osteoporosis and osteomalacia occurs secondary to poor calcium and fat soluble vitamin absorption, while nephrolithiasis occurs due to chronic dehydration secondary to diarrhea.

Dermatologic lesions such as pyoderma gangrenosum and erythema nodosum often present during an exacerbation of gastrointestinal disease activity. *Pyoderma gangrenosum is* a progressive deep ulceration that may complicate healing of surgical incisions and stoma sites. It may be refractory to medical therapy, occasionally requiring excision and skin grafting. Aphthous stomatitis is common during flare-ups.

Sclerosing cholangitis is the most severe extraintestinal manifestation of UC. Its course is generally progressive and independent of the activity of the bowel disease. Ursodeoxycholic acid may slow the progression, but ultimately patients will require liver transplantation for long-term survival.[24]

Routine ophthalmic surveillance is recommended in the management of all children with inflammatory bowel disease because of the frequent occurrence of uveitis, episcleritis, conjunctivitis and steroid-associated eye problems.[25]

Growth abnormalities and nutritional deficiencies seen in UC children are thought to be due to a combination of anorexia, rapid intestinal transit, malabsorption and psychosomatic disturbance. Delayed sexual maturity may be as a result of low levels of gonadotrophins.[26] These conditions are seen far less frequently than in CD because of the lack of small bowel involvement.

DIAGNOSIS

Clinical Examination

A detailed history and physical examination directs the physician to the lower gastrointestinal tract in over 95% of cases. Growth and maturation, irrespective of disease activity, should carefully be monitored Radiologic and endoscopic findings confirm the presence of inflammatory bowel disease, but the diagnosis of UC can only be made by recognizing the pattern of disease manifestation and excluding other causes of inflammation such as infections. Occasionally, the presence of infectious agents such as *Clostridium difficile* may mask underlying UC. About 15% of cases are labeled indeterminate colitis because the distinction between CD and UC cannot definitively be made, and in 2-5% of patients the wrong diagnosis is made which may lead to inappropriate management decisions. An important pitfall to avoid is to underestimate the severity of the colitis. The presence of fever, orthostatic hypotension, dehydration, focal abdominal tenderness or masses indicates severe disease requiring hospitalization.

Laboratory Assessment

There are no laboratory tests for inflammatory bowel disease. Anemia occurs in two thirds of patients and an elevated erythrocyte sedimentation or prolonged prothrombin time is common. Nutritional status may be monitored by following levels of serum proteins such as albumin. Iron and magnesium stores may be low because of chronic blood loss.

Gastrointestinal bacteria, viruses, fungae, ova and parasites should be excluded as a cause for the bowel inflammation. In particular, *Clostridium difficile* enterocolitis is more prevalent in UC patients than the general population, and should be screened for whenever disease activity changes. The identification of a pathogen requires specific treatment but does not exclude the diagnosis of UC. Indeed, infectious agents may often trigger acute flare-ups of disease in patients known to have inflammatory bowel disease.

Endoscopy

Flexible colonoscopy into the terminal ileum with mucosal biopsies at varying sites along the bowel including the ileum, provides the most sensitive and specific evaluation of intestinal inflammation and may make barium contrast studies unnecessary.[27] Full colonoscopy of pediatric patients of all age groups, including infants, is now possible.[28,29] In long-standing disease, surveillance for dysplasia should include full colonoscopy in all patients regardless of the extent of disease, because of the high incidence of dysplasia in the 'normal' proximal colon. For the same reason, any child with UC undergoing colonic surgery should have a total colectomy irrespective of the extent of proximal extension of the disease. Colonoscopy is contraindicated in acute severe colitis and toxic megacolon because of the risk of perforation and hemorrhage. Bowel inspection should be limited to proctosigmoidoscopy with minimal air insufflation.

The mucosa of active UC is diffusely edematous. erythematous and friable. The distal colon is usually most severely affected, but this is not always the case. Rectal sparing is suggestive of CD, but may be seen following topical treatment of proctitis. Histology of endoscopically normal areas may reveal acute cryptitis or chronic changes such as architectural distortion of crypts or granulomas. Such detail is especially important in evaluating patients who have been medically treated on the basis of a clinical diagnosis of UC in whom surgery is being contemplated. Where doubt exists, upper endoscopy and biopsy may be performed. Children with atypical features of UC or CD are categorized as having indeterminate colitis (10-15%). Patients in this group should be restudied at intervals. If no specific diagnosis can be assigned, they should be treated as a separate group.

Radiology

With the emergence of flexible endoscopy, radiology has assumed a confirmatory and back-up role in the diagnosis and management of inflammatory bowel disease. Abdominal radiographs are useful in establishing a baseline for later comparisons. In acute severe UC and toxic megacolon, daily abdominal series are useful to monitor progress of the disease and diagnose complications such as perforation. Contrast studies should be avoided in acute severe disease because contrast medium may exacerbate edema and inflammation. Barium enema is useful as an adjunct to colonoscopy when the latter is poorly tolerated or technical difficulty precludes passage of the endoscope to the terminal ileum. Barium enema in chronic UC may show a narrow shortened rigid colon with loss of haustral folds and pseudopolyp formation.

An upper gastrointestinal series and small bowel follow-through with fluoroscopic study of the terminal ileum or enteroclysis is useful to diagnose small bowel involvement and exclude a diagnosis of UC. Barium is the contrast of choice, and the study is only deemed complete once contrast is seen in the right colon.[30]

In complicated inflammatory bowel disease, ultrasound or computed tomography is useful diagnostically and therapeutically for identifying phlegmons and draining abscesses, although such complications are more commonly associated with CD.

Before surgery, the diagnosis of inflammatory bowel disease should always be revisited. A specific diagnosis should only be assigned when complete histological, clinical and radiological evaluation of the entire intestinal tract is in agreement. Although the histopathologic features of the two forms of inflammatory bowel disease are characteristic, none are pathognomonic. When doubt exists, inappropriate surgery may have severe consequences.

MEDICAL AND NUTRITIONAL MANAGEMENT

The goal of medical therapy in children is to control disease, prevent relapse and allow for normal growth and maturation. Steroids, 5-aminosalicylate compounds and antibiotics remain the primary pharmacological agents for treatment of UC.

Several 5-ASA products that deliver the active 5-ASA to the colon are available with differing properties, side effects and tolerance levels. Budesonide, a rapidly metabolized steroid with decreased systemic toxicity is being used more frequently, although it has not yet been adequately evaluated in children. Corticosteroid preparations are useful in disease exacerbations but should be weaned as soon as possible. Steroid use should be accompanied by gastric acid inhibitors. Immunosuppressive agents may be administered as adjuncts to steroid therapy, Methotrexate, azathioprine and its active metabolite, 6-mercaptopurine, may be useful in refractory colitis or to decrease steroid dependency. While most children do respond, median response time is 3 months. and the drugs are not indicated for acute flare-ups. Cyclosporine is effective in treating severe UC with a mean response time of seven days, but efficacious use in children requires such high doses as to preclude its use in this population group.[31] The antibiotic metronidazole significantly increases remission rates following exacerbation of colitis and is useful in combination with 5-ASA products and steroids.[32] Ciprofloxacin may also have a synergistic effect when used with metronidazole in age-appropriate children.

Antidiarrheal medications such as diphenoxylate hydrochloride with atropine sulphate (Lomotil) or loperamide hydrochloride (Imodium), or opiates such as codeine are useful to reduce cramping and frequency, but may induce toxic megacolon.[33]

Dietary manipulation and supplemental (elementary) nutrient formulas have an important role in managing UC. In addition, patients may occasionally require blood and albumin infusions. Psychotherapy and support groups also play an important role in the overall well being of UC patients to reduce emotional stress that may trigger a flare-up.

Medical management of colitis depends upon the severity and extent of colonic involvement proximal to the rectum. Mild colitis is managed at home with a low residue diet and 5-ASA products in incremental doses. Response time is approximately two weeks, with reduction in cramps, bleeding and stool frequency.

Moderate colitis with systemic signs is managed in hospital. Bed rest, with initial bowel rest and total parenteral nutrition or a low residue elemental diet and oral steroids are the mainstay. As an adjunct, 5-ASA products may have an additional benefit and once disease is controlled and steroids are tapered, these agents may be useful in maintaining remission. Patients should be monitored for anemia and malnutrition.

Severe disease with copious bloody diarrhea, malnutrition and weight loss, fever, abdominal distension and tenderness. anemia and leukocytosis should be treated as a medical emergency. Patients require intense fluid, electrolyte and blood product management, parenteral nutrition, high dose intravenous steroids, and broad spectrum antibiotic coverage. Frequent radiographic monitoring is required. Colectomy should be performed for failed initial response to treatment, life-threatening complications such as toxic megacolon, severe hemorrhage or perforation. Patients with persistent severe disease refractory to treatment after 2-3 weeks should also be considered for colectomy. Our experience has shown that an emergency colectomy and ileo-anal pull-through can be done without mortality or increased morbidity.[34] If the operation needs staging, a subtotal colectomy and ileostomy with a Hartmann turn-in or mucus fistula should be done initially. One of the disadvantages of this approach for severe rectal disease or hemorrhage is postoperative continuation of symptoms. Acute severe exacerbation of UC is a relative indication for surgery, and most patients should be considered for early colectomy and ileodistal anastomosis following resolution of such a flare-up.

Localized rectal and left-sided disease may be managed topically with 5-ASA suppositories or enemas or non-absorbable steroid enemas or foam. Budesonide may also be given topically via a fine-bore rectal catheter as a rectal infusion.

While nutritional support is less likely to induce remission in UC than CD. Correction of nutrient deficiencies and maintenance of adequate nutritional status to ensure appropriate growth and development is essential. During exacerbation of disease, nutritional balance may only be achieved at 140-150°/n of recommended daily allowance, usually requiring enteral supplementation with elemental diets or total parenteral nutrition. Following surgery, enteral intake is usually resumed within one to two days when an ileostomy is created.

SURGICAL MANAGEMENT

Indications for Operation

All patients with UC will eventually come to colectomy. Total proctocolectomy is curative for gastrointestinal disease. Medical management is used initially, while surgery is reserved for failure to respond to full medical therapy, complications of medical therapy or prolonged steroid requirement, nutritional and growth failure, dysplasia or carcinoma, or long-standing disease (usually greater than 15-20 years). Such elective surgery should be performed when epiphyses are still open to allow for adequate catch-up growth 'and maturation. In 20% of children, surgery is performed emergently for acute complications such as acute fulminant colitis or toxic megacolon, perforation, severe hemorrhage or bowel obstruction secondary to stricture.

Preparation for surgery includes optimization of nutritional and electrolyte abnormalities. Children should be fully prepared mentally for postoperative changes including dealing with a stoma. Formal bowel cathartic bowel preparation should be avoided as it may cause a flare in disease. Children should be placed on clear fluid restriction 48 hours prior to surgery. Oral antibiotics such as erythromycin, neomycin and metronidazole should be used in the 24 hours before surgery, while intravenous broad spectrum antibiotics should be administered 2 hours preoperatively. Most children are on steroids at the time of their surgery. While one-stage proctocolectomy and ileoanal anastomosis without temporary ileostomy may be used in stable children off steroids, we recommend temporary diverting ileostomy for children who are malnourished or those on steroids at the time of surgery. This is to avoid higher incidence of complications, specifically abscess formation and poor wound healing.

Surgical Approaches

Colectomy with Ileoanal Pull-through

Straight pull-through: A large experience with ERPT for the definitive management of Hirschsprung's disease has been reported.[15,17,35] The first significant experience with straight ERPT for the management of UC in 17 adolescents was published by Martin in 1977.[16] We have pursued this approach using ERPT and straight ileoanal anastomosis as the primary alternative to abdominal wall ileostomy in children requiring total colectomy for UC (Figs 69.1A to H).

In children, the operation is usually performed as a two-stage procedure with initial total colectomy, rectal mucosectomy and ileoanal anastomosis with a protective diversionary loop ileostomy which is closed at 8-12 weeks. Under less optimal conditions, a subtotal colectomy, ileostomy and sigmoid mucus fistula or Hartmann's turn-in may be performed acutely, followed weeks to months later by rectal mucosectomy and ileoanal anastomosis.[36,37]

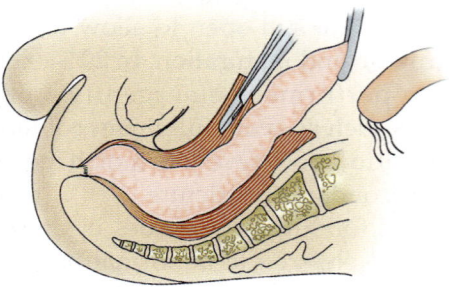

Fig. 69.1A: The endorectal dissection is carried out between the submucosa and muscularis of the rectum

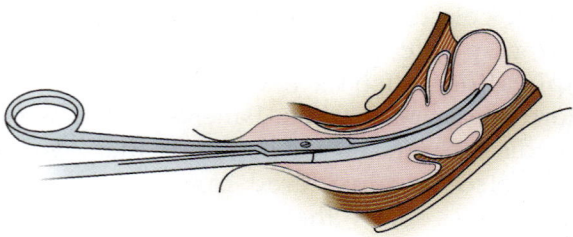

Fig. 69.1B: The rectal mucosal-submucosal tube is everted outside the anal opening

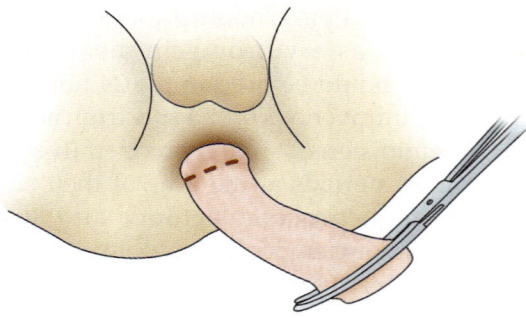

Fig. 69.1C: The everted mucosal-submucosal tube is incised anteriorly at the pectinate line

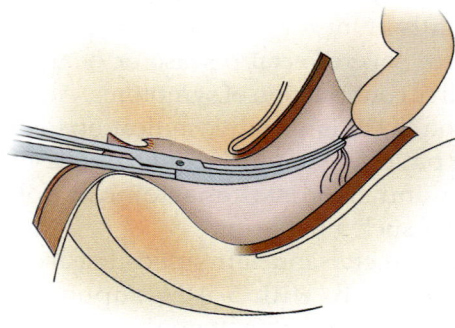

Fig. 69.1D: A clamp is passed through the opening in the inverted tube in order to grasp the terminal ileum

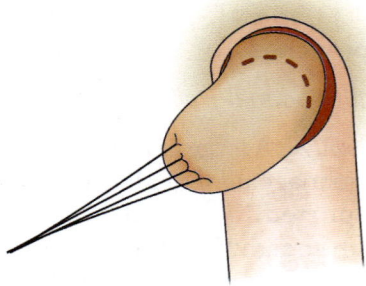

Fig. 69.1E: The anterior wall of the terminal ileum is incised

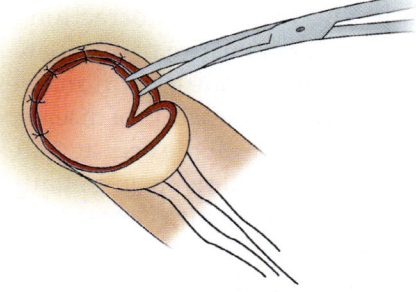

Fig. 69.1F: An anterior anastomosis is created between the terminal ileum and the anorectal mucosa

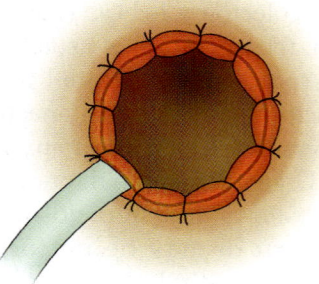

Fig. 69.1G: The anastomosis is completed and a drain may be left between the rectal cuff and the ileum

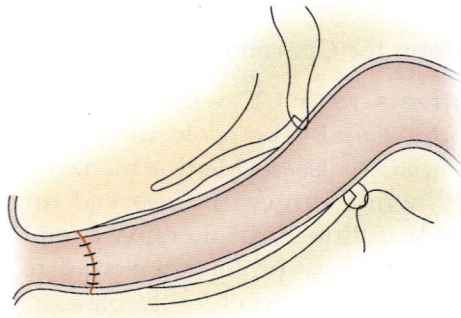

Fig. 69.1H: The top of the rectal cuff is tacked to the ileum

The endorectal dissection may be performed via an abdominal approach or transanally, although it is more difficult to remove an intact mucosal-submucosal tube using the latter approach. A 4-5 cm rectal muscular cuff is left and the terminal ileum is brought down through the rectal muscular cuff and anastomosed to the rectal mucosa at the dentate line. This technique affords optimal protection to the nervi erigenti, seminal vesicles in boys and vagina in girls, since the endorectal dissection is started proximally just below the peritoneal reflection and the entire distal dissection occurs within the wall of the rectum.

Anal continence is defined by the ability to defer defecation voluntarily, maintain control nocturnally " and have the ability to discriminate between flatus and stool in the neorectal vault.

The anatomic and physiologic requirements for normal anal continence include preservation of the anorectal angle by the levator muscle complex and puborectalis sling, maintenance of the anal sphincter function, anorectal sensation and the presence of reservoir capacity compliance within the rectal ampulla. These requirements are all preserved or recreated after ERPT (Fig. 69.2).

Pouches

A major factor in early continence is the size and compliance of the neorectal reservoir. Anorectal continence may also be affected by stool frequency, i.e. the regularity and rapidity with which stool collects in the neorectal ampulla, as well as by the consistency of that stool. reservoirs have been adapted to increase rectal capacity and alter prograde peristaltic waves reaching the anus, thereby reducing stool frequency.[36] Four types of reservoir configuration are used clinically: the J-shaped double loop reservoir (most widely used), the S-shaped triple loop reservoir (useful to reduce mesenteric tension in reaching the anus in long thin patients), the W-shaped quadruple reservoir and the lateral side-to-side or isoperistaltic reservoir. Irrespective of the type of pouch used, care must be taken to construct short pouches <12 cm long) and to avoid leaving a spout that results in stasis and prevents complete evacuation resulting in pouchitis.

Usually, when pouch procedures are employed, unlike the straight ERPT procedure the rectal dissection continues on the outside of the rectum all the way down to the dentate line. This dissection increases the likelihood of injury to the parasympathetic nerves as well as to the posterior wall of the vagina or seminal vesicles. As the pouch is placed in the pelvis, the pouch suture line may lie against the dissected posterior wall of the vagina, increasing the likelihood of pouch-vaginal fistulae. In addition, full-thickness ileal pouch is anastomosed to full thickness distal rectum, and this is often a stapled anastomosis, increasing the likelihood of pelvic fistulae and abscesses as well as low fistulae to the vagina, since the protection afforded by the rectal cuff is not present.[37] If an endorectal dissection is employed, care should be taken to avoid constriction by the muscular cuff or leaving a spout that may result in pouch obstruction and inflammation.

Irrespective of the type of ileoanal anastomosis, care should be taken to avoid tension on the mesenteric vessels as ischemia may result in leaks, poor healing or anastomotic structuring. Careful dissection of the superior mesenteric vessels and opening distal arcades will reduce anastomotic tension.

If a temporary ileostomy is constructed, this should be of the loop type, with the proximal end Brooked, and the distal end sutured level with the skin. This will allow some stool to spillover into the distal limb over time and allow the patient to maintain anal sensation and continence. It will also maintain mucosal integrity, preventing atrophy.

Steroids are tapered postoperatively and once the patient is off all medication, the ileostomy is closed. Following closure of the ileostomy, patients may be maintained on metronidazole and combinations of anti-diarrheal and anti-peristaltic medications as

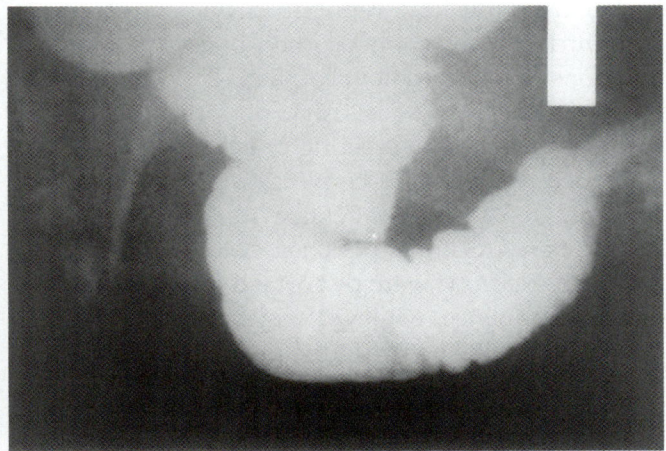

Fig. 69.2: Barium enema demonstrating a neorectum 1 year following straight endorectal pull-through and ileoanal anastomosis

needed. Commonly used drugs include diphenoxylate hydrochloride, loperamide hydrochloride, codeine and kaopectate. Perineal barrier creams are also vital to prevent excoriation of the perianal skin. Dilatation of the anastomosis may be necessary.

Other Procedures

The authors do not recommend subtotal colectomy with ileorectal anastomosis, end-ileostomy or Kock continent ileal reservoir as a primary procedure in UC patients. Subtotal colectomy with ileoproctostomy may be appropriate in older patients, but it is not a procedure that should be considered in the pediatric population because of its attendant risks of ongoing inflammation, medication and the risk of cancer. Permanent Brooke end-ileostomy is associated with a 30% complication rate. Complications of end-ileostomy include adhesive bowel obstruction, dehydration and malnutrition, and local stoma problems including retraction, herniation, prolapse and obstruction. Kock's continence ileostomy procedures involve the creation of an S-shaped pouch with the exit site on the abdominal wall. The incidence of complications with Kock's pouches is 64% with a high morbidity rate often resulting in the loss of the Kock's continent ileostomy with concomitant loss of the small bowel required to create the pouch.[38,39] These procedures should be used in cases of failed ileoanal anastomoses or when such an anastomosis cannot be performed.

SURGICAL OUTCOME

In a recent report by Telander, the primary indications for colectomy in a group of 100 children with UC included intractable disease (64%), refractory growth failure (14%), toxic megacolon (6%), massive hemorrhage (4%), perforation (3%) and cancer prophylaxis (2%).[40]

While there are several large series reporting results with ileal pouch-anal anastomosis in adults, the University of Michigan Medical Center (UMMC) straight ERPT series and the UCLA Medical Center ileal pouch-anal anastomosis series are the only ones large enough to permit statistical comparison in children.[41-46] In the UMMC review of 164 patients, 116 patients underwent straight ERPT for UC, while UCLA reported 116 children younger than 19 years of age of which 94 had UC.

Both procedures are safe. The operative mortality rate was 1% in both series. Of all the deaths, only one patient died as a direct result of the operative procedure, namely postoperative sepsis in the UCLA series.

In the UCLA series, 52% of patients developed complications, including ileoanal stenosis with reservoir outlet obstruction (16%), elongated ileal spout (2.3%), elongated ileal reservoir greater than 15 cm (4.6%), where a combination of outflow obstruction and reservoir enlargement caused stasis, and adhesive intestinal obstruction (8.6%). Further complications included pelvic abscesses and fistulas, wound infection, incisional hernias anal stricture, rectovaginal fistulas and pouch hemorrhage. The reoperation rate was 32%. Sixty per cent of complications occurred in the first 30 patients. Only three of the last 40 patients had reoperation. Four children (two with Crohn's disease) returned to a permanent ileostomy (4.9%); 10 had a temporary ileostomy. Five straight pull-throughs were converted to a reservoir because of stool frequency; 22% underwent reservoir reconstruction because of stasis. However, 91% of children are well following their surgery and resolution of complications.

In combined adult and pediatric series from the Mayo and Cleveland Clinics, pelvic sepsis following pouch creation occurred in 5-8.2% of patients with 2.5-6% of patients requiring operative drainage of abscesses. This resulted in pouch loss in 2% of patients. Overall, septic complications were noted in 18.3% of all patients in the Cleveland study. This is significantly higher than the 1.8% reported pelvic sepsis rate in straight ERPT in whom 1% had operative drainage and none required removal of the ERPT. This is one of the key factors in our decision to perform straight pull-throughs rather than creating pouch reservoirs.

Pouch excision and conversion to end-ileostomy occurred in 3.4-5% of patients, with an additional 1% having non-functional pouches. Between 0.7 and 1% of pouch excisions were performed for incapacitating fecal incontinence, while 0:1% of patients had pouch infarction. By the nature of the procedure, no patients required pouch excision in the straight ERPT group, but 3.5% were converted to end-ileostomy, 2% because of increased stool frequency. However, resection of a pouch results in significantly greater small bowel loss than does conversion of a straight ERPT.

All pouches in the Mayo study had handsewn ileal pouch-anal anastomoses, while two thirds of the Cleveland series pouch-anal anastomoses were stapled with preservation of the anal transition zone 1-2 cm above the dentate line. This group has reported fewer complications and better postoperative sphincter pressures using the stapled technique because it involves less anal sphincter manipulation. However, because of the residual mucosal cuff, these patients require annual biopsies of the transitional zone to exclude dysplastic and malignant changes. All of the straight ERPT anastomoses performed at the University of Michigan have been handsewn with resection of the mucosa to the dentate line. A 2.9% anastomotic leak or separation rate was noted in the Cleveland group, while the straight ERPT group only had a single iatrogenic anastomotic separation caused by postoperative passage of a rigid sigmoidoscope.

From the patient's perspective, the most significant determinants of a successful operation are stool frequency and continence. Frequency, as assessed by the number of bowel movements in 24 hours, ranged between 4-8 stools per day for patients with pouches, while stool frequency 3 years after straight ERPT was 7.4 stools per day. Two percent of straight ERPT patients were converted to end-ileostomy because of dissatisfaction with high stool frequency (10-15 per day). All of these patients were continent during the day and night. Stool frequency for patients having straight ERPT for total colonic Hirschsprung's disease was 3.5 per 24 hours. These patients were operated on at a significantly younger age (20.6 years for UC patients versus 17 months for Hirschsprung's patients). This decreased stool frequency is a good representation of increased bowel adaptability when the operation is performed at a younger age.

Perfect fecal continence without inadvertent seepage of liquid or solid stool was present in 75% of patients during the day and 45% of patients at night in the handsewn pouch Mayo series. Nocturnal continence improved over time with 25% having occasional incontinence 4 years after closure of their ileostomy. Similarly, in the Cleveland series which had two-thirds stapled pouch anastomoses, 71% of patients had perfect continence with 82% daytime and 71% night time continence. In the University of Michigan series of straight ERPT, daytime continence was 98% 3 months after ileostomy closure, with 100% continence at 1 year. Nocturnal continence was 96% at 1 year with 100% continence by 2 years.

The volume of fecal output can be decreased by one-third by the use of loperamide hydrochloride, while bulking agents such as kaopectate thicken stools but do not decrease output. Up to 44% of patients are on some form of dietary restriction to help limit frequency and incontinence.

The most significant complication of pouch creation was a 23-28% incidence of symptomatic pouchitis, which was completely avoided by straight ERPT. Symptomatic pouchitis is diagnosed by a history of "rectal" cramping, diarrhea and occasionally hematochezia. Malaise, fever, anorexia and extraintestinal manifestations of UC such as arthritis, uveitis or erythema nodosum may be found.[47] Nicholls and others have reported that 90% of pouch reservoirs showed evidence of chronic and acute inflammation on biopsy.[42,48] This inflammation is thought to be due to stasis and bacterial overgrowth. Thus, frequent, complete pouch emptying minimizes pouchitis and therapy includes the use of drugs such as metronidazole, ciprofloxacin, pouch washouts and even topical steroids. Rectal dilatation is also helpful.

All of the straight ERPT patients have undergone annual or semiannual biopsy of their pull-through ileum. No patient has had evidence of significant inflammation. Further complications related to pouch creation included a 3.8% incidence of bleeding from the pouch suture line and a 4.2% incidence of pouch-vaginal fistulas, complications avoided by not creating a pouch. However, the straight ERPT series did have a 1.4% rectovaginal fistula rate.

Because of the endorectal pelvic dissection, straight ERPT patients did not develop postoperative major sexual or urinary dysfunction. However, following pouch creation, 3-6% of patients had transient sexual dysfunction, including 1-4% of patients with retrograde ejaculation and 0.1% with impotence. Dyspareunia was noted in 1-7% of female patients. Urinary dysfunction occurred in less than 1% of pouch patients.

The incidence of postoperative small bowel obstruction ranged from 15 to 25.3% for pouch patients with about a third in each series requiring operative intervention. In the straight ERPT group, 8% developed bowel obstruction with 4% requiring surgical intervention.

Anal anastomotic strictures were found in 14% of pouch patients and 6% of straight ERPT patients. All of these patients responded well to periodic anal dilatation, but 0.3% of pouch patients eventually required reoperation for stricture.

A recent trend to avoid a diverting ileostomy in selected patients undergoing restorative proctocolectomy has reduced the expense and hospital time associated with the surgery, but may have slightly higher complication rates.[49,50] About 10% of the most favorable patients in the Cleveland study had one-stage procedures with a similar complication rate to those having multiple stage procedure. However, this cohort of optimal patients should intuitively have a lower complication rate with multiple stage procedures, therefore it is difficult to assess the true benefits of the single-stage procedure until similar cohorts of patients are compared" We have performed such one-stage ERPT procedures successfully on patients with familial polyposis and total colonic Hirschsprung's disease without an increased incidence of complications.

A relatively new development in this field of surgery is laparoscopic or laparoscopically-assisted colectomy and endorectal pull-through. We and others have recently begun to use this technique in selected patients, but while preliminary results are promising, it is still too early to make long-term comparisons.

In all studies, the cohort of patients having the highest complication rates from their ileoanal procedures with or without pouch creation, were the 4-8% who subsequently proved to have CD. While the focus of this chapter is inflammatory bowel disease, none of the large series on ileal pouch-anal anastomoses and straight ERPT differentiate between diagnostic subgroups. However, more than 75% of patients in all three series had a diagnosis of UC. and as a group, UC patients did have more complications than patients having either procedure for familial polyposis or Hirschsprung's disease.

Overall, functional results and quality of life improved with time and stabilized approximately year after closure of the ileostomy. Quality of life as assessed by growth and development, dietary limitations, return to school or work, sport and recreational activity, sexual activity, fertility and reproduction was considered excellent in 93-95% of patients irrespective of the type of procedure performed.

In patients with pancolitis, the observed risk of cancer at 35 years after diagnosis is 30% for all patients, but 40% for those diagnosed before 15 years of age.[51] In a group of Danish patients who underwent surveillance management, the cumulative cancer incidence was 3.1% over 25 years of follow-up, with 32% of patients having a colectomy during that period. The cancer rate in this carefully followed group was not different from that in the general population.[52] Based on this and other reports, surveillance colonoscopy is recommended beginning 8 years after diagnosis in children with pancolitis.[53]

CONCLUSION

Almost all children with UC should be managed medically until surgery is indicated by worsening disease, medical complications or growth and developmental retardation. Prior to definitive surgery, the diagnosis of CD should be excluded. Surgery (i.e. total proctocolectomy) should be curative for gastrointestinal UC in children.

The major surgical decision is whether to create a reservoir or not. The sole purpose of a reservoir is to increase rectal capacity and thereby decrease stool frequency. We have shown that the neorectum created by the straight ERPT progressively dilates during the first 2 years after operation and develops a normal rectal appearance on barium enema (suggesting normal rectal capacity). This is consistent with the clinical observation that initially the stool frequencies on average are higher with the straight ERPT than pouch procedures, but these differences equilibrate 1-2 years after the procedure.

REFERENCES

1. Wilks S, Moxon W. Lectures on pathological anatomy, Edn 2. J and A Churchill, London 1875.
2. Lockhart-Mummery H, Morson B. Crohn's disease (regional enteritis) a pathological entity. Gut 1960;1:87.
3. Kirsner JB. Problems in the differentiation of ulcerative colitis from Crohn's disease of the colon: The need for repeated diagnostic evaluation. Gastroenterology 1975;68:187-91.
4. Browne JY. Value of complete physiological rest of large bowel in ulcerative and obstructive lesions. Surg Gynecol Obstet 1913;16:610-14.
5. Strauss AA, Strauss SF. Surgical treatment of ulcerative colitis. Surg Clin North Am 1994;24;211-22.
6. Cattell RE. The surgical treatment of ulcerative colitis. Gastroenterology 1948;10:63-66.

7. Gardner C, Miller CG. Total colectomy for ulcerative colitis. Arch Surg 1951;63:370-77.
8. Ripstein CB. Results of the surgical treatment of ulcerative colitis. Ann Surg 1952;135:14-18.
9. Goligher JC. Primary excisional surgery in the treatment of ulcerative colitis. Ann Roy Coll Surg Engl 1954;15:316-19.
10. Brooke BN. The management of an ileostomy including its complications. Lancet 1952;2:102-04.
11. Kock NO. Intra-abdominal reservoir in patients with permanent ileostomy: preliminary observations on a procedure resulting in fecal continence in five ileostomy patients. Arch Surg 1969;99:223-28.
12. Parc R, et al. Current results: ileorectal anastomosis after total abdominal colectomy for ulcerative colitis. In: Dozois RR, Editor: Alternatives to conventional ileostomy. Chicago, 1985, Year Book Medical Publishers.
13. Pavitch MM, Sabiston DC. Anal ileostomy with preservation of the sphincter. A proposed operation in patients requiring total colectomy for benign lesions. Surg Gynecol Obstet 1947;84:1095-99.
14. Safaie S, Soper RT. Endorectal pullthrough procedure in the surgical treatment of familial polyposis coli. J Pediatr Surg 1973;8:711-14.
15. Soave R. A new surgical technique for treatment of Hirschsprung's disease. J Ped Surg 1964;56:1007-11.
16. Martin L W, LeCoultre C, Schubert WK. Total colectomy and mucosal proctectomy with preservation of continence in ulcerative colitis. Ann Surg 1977;186:477-80.
17. Coran AG, Weintraub WH. Modification of the endorectal procedure for Hirschsprung's disease. Surg Gynecol Obstet 1976;143:277-82.
18. Valiente MA, Bacon HE. Construction of pouch using "pantaloon technique for pull-through following total colectomy. Am J Surg 1955;90:6621-25.
19. Parks AG, Nichols RJ. Proctocolectomy without ileostomy for ulcerative colitis. Br Med J 1978;2:85-89.
20. Orkin BA, et al. The surgical management of children with ulcerative colitis: the old vs. the new. Dis Colon Rectum 1990;33:947-51.
21. Wong WD, Rothenberger DA, Goldberg SM. Ileoanal pouch procedures. Curr Prob Surg 1985;22:1-78.
22. Motil K, Grand R. ulcerative colitis and Crohn's disease in children. Pediatr Rev 1987;9:109-20.
23. Ekbom A, et al. Ulcerative colitis and colorectal cancer, a population based study. N Engl J Med 1990;323:1228-30.
24. Beuers U, Spengler U, Kruis W, et al. Ursodeoxycholic acid for treatment of primary sclerosing cholangitis: A placebo-controlled trial. Hepatology 1992;16:707-14.
25. Hyams JS. Extraintestinal manifestations of inflammatory bowel disease in children. Pediatr Gastroenterol Nutr 1994;19:7-21.
26. McCaffery TD, et al. Severe growth retardation in children with inflammatory bowel disease. Pediatrics 1970;45:386-440.
27. Leichner AM, Jackson WD, Grand RJ. Ulcerative colitis. In: Walker A W. Drurie PR. Hamilton JR, et al, Eds. Pediatric Gastrointestinal Disease. Mosby- Year Book, Inc 1996.
28. Williams CB, Laage NJ, Campbell CA, et al. Total colonoscopy in childhood. Arch Dis Child 1982;57:49-53.
29. Hassall E, Barclay GN, Ament ME. Colonoscopy in childhood. Pediatrics 1984;73:594-99.
30. Winthrop ill, Balfe DM, Shackelford GD, et al. Ulcerative and granulomatous colitis in children. Radiology 1985;154:657-60.
31. Ramakrishna J, Langhans N, Calenda K, Grand RJ, Verhave M. Combined use of cyclosporine and azathioprine or 6-mercaptopurine in pediatric inflammatory bowel disease. J Pediatr Gastroenterol Nutr 1996;22:296-302.
32. Sachar DB. Maintenance therapy in ulcerative colitis and Crohn's disease. Gastroenterol 1995;20:117-22.
33. Garrett JM, Sauer WG, Moertel CG. Colonic motility in ulcerative colitis after opiate administration. Gastroenterology 1967;53:93-97.
34. Coran AG. New surgical approaches to ulcerative colitis in children and adults. World J Surg 1985;9:203-13.
35. Boley SI. An endorectal pull-through operation with primary anastomosis for Hirschsprung's disease. Surg Gynecol Obstet 1968;127:353-57.
36. Coran AG. Surgical management of ulcerative colitis. Can J Surg 1982;25:498-500.
37. Reissman P, Piccirillo M, Ulrich A, et al. Functional results of the double-stapled ileoanal reservoir. J Am Coll Surg 1995;181:444-50.
38. Beahrs OH. Use of ileal reservoir following proctocolectomy. Surg Gynecol Obstet 1975;141:363-67.
39. Sagar PM, Pemberton JH. Update on the surgical management of ulcerative colitis and ulcerative proctitis: Current controversies and problems. Inflam Bowel Dis 1995;1:299-312.
40. Telander RL, et al. Long-term follow-up of the ileoanal anastomosis in children and young adults. Surgery 1990;108-11.
41. Coran AG. A personal experience with 100 consecutive total colectomies and straight ileoanal endorectal pull-throughs for benign disease of the colon and rectum in children and adults. Ann Surg 1990;212:242-48.
42. Becker JM, Raymond JL. Ileal pouch-anal anastomosis. A single surgeon's experience with 100 consecutive cases. Ann Surg 1986;204:375-83.
43. Fazio VW, Ziv Y, Church JM, et al. Ileal pouch-anal anastomoses complications and function in 1005 patients. Ann Surg 1995;22:120-27.
44. Kelly KA. Anal Sphincter-saving operations for chronic ulcerative colitis. Am J Surg 1992;163:5-11.
45. Coran AG. The surgical management of ulcerative colitis, familial polyposis and total colonic agangliosis in infants and children (in Press).

46. Fonkalsrud EW, Loar N. Long-term results after colectomy and endorectal ileal pull-through procedure in children. Ann Surg 1992;215(1):57-62.
47. Mignon M, Stettler S, Phillips SF. Pouchitis a poorly understood entity. Dis Colon Rectum 1995;38:100-03.
48. Nicholls RJ. Restorative proctocolectomy with various types of reservoir. World J Surg 1987;1:751-62.
49. Winslet MC, Barsoum G, Pringle W, et al. Loop ileostomy after IF AA –is it necessary? Dis Colon Rectum 1991;34:267-70.
50. Binderow SR, Wexner SD. Current surgical therapy for mucosal ulcerative colitis. Dis Colon Rectum 1994;37:610-24.
51. Ekbom A, Helmick CG, Zack M, et al. Survival and causes of death in patients with inflammatory bowel disease: A population-based study. Gastroenterology 1992;103:954-60.
52. Langholz E, Munkholm P, Davidsen M, et al. Colorectal cancer risk and mortality in patients with ulcerative colitis. Gastroenterology 1992;103:1444-51.
53. Grundfest SF, Fazio YW, Weiss RA, et al. The risk of cancer following colectomy and ileorectal anastomosis for extensive mucosal ulcerative colitis. Ann Surg 1981;193:9-14.

CHAPTER 70

Polyposis Syndromes

AF Scharli

This chapter mainly deals with hereditary neoplastic polyposes, but some other syndromes involving the colon and rectum are also described.

NEOPLASTIC POLYPOSES

Familial adenomatous polyposis (FAP) is the disease associated with the highest risk of development of cancer. Affected individuals are virtually certain to develop a colorectal carcinoma if preventive colectomy is not performed. Furthermore, FAP is the best model to support the hypothesis of the adenoma-carcinoma sequence. Because of its autosomal dominant inheritable characteristics, it has stimulated investigators to look into genetic and molecular biology approaches to elucidate the etiology of the disease (Fig. 70.1).

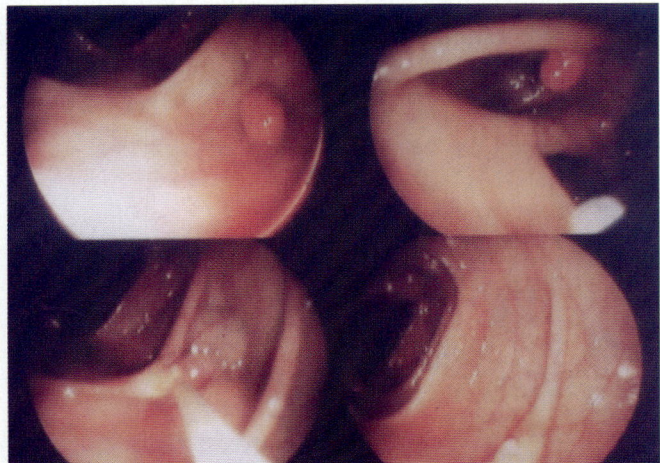

Fig. 70.1: Endoscopic view of multiple polyposis of the colon and rectum in a 4 year old boy

Numerous adenomas are present primarily in the colon, but polyps may also occur elsewhere in the digestive tract. The most important feature is that one or more of the adenomas in the large bowel will develop into cancer, usually before the age of 40 years. In fact, thousands of polyps are usually present in patients with FAP. Bodmer et al[1] found that FAP is caused by a mutation in the APC gene on the long arm of chromosome.[2]

Despite the inherited nature of the condition, in approximately 20% of patients there is no clear family history.

The size of the polyps varies from case to case, but rarely exceeds 1 cm in diameter. Very occasionally, there is a lack of polyps in the cecum and right colon.

Histologically, the adenomatous polyps seen in FAP are similar to those seen in nonpolyposis patients. They are predominantly tubular adenomas. The coexistence of stomach and duodenal polyps is more frequent than previously realized.

Jagelman et al found that the incidence of malignancy of the Upper 61 tract was 4.5% in 1255 FAP patients.[3] In addition to extracolonic polyps, many other lesions have been described in FAP. The most frequent include the following.[2]

Eye Lesions

A total of 75-80% of individuals with FAP have congenital hypertrophy of the retinal pigmented epithelium.[4] These Patchy lesions are due to 1 freckle-like increased content of melanin granules. Hence, ophthalmological examination to detect epithelial lesions may be useful screening technique for FAP.

Skin Lesions

First described by Gardner and Richards.[5] They consist of epidermal cysts, usually multiple and on the face.

Endocrine Gland Lesion

The best-documented association of FAP is with papillary carcinoma of the thyroid.[6]

Desmoid Tumors

Desmoid tumors are rare, and since there is a well-documented association with polyposis. All patients who present with such lesions should be investigated for FAP.

Bone Tumors

The so-called osteomas occurring in FAP are exostoses and endostoses and tend to arise on long bones.[5]

Liver and Biliary Tree Tumors

There is an increased incidence of hepatoblastoma in children of families affected by FAP.

Dental Lesions

Teeth abnormalities, distinct from osteomas of the jaw, have been described in 11-80% of individuals with FAP. As they often appear at an early age, dental anomalies are helpful in the diagnosis of FAP.

DIAGNOSIS

The natural history of FAP is variable. Adenomas usually appear during puberty, with subsequent development of cancer in early childhood. Many subjects with polyposis are asymptomatic and the diagnosis is only made when screening the family of a known patient.

Since the rectum is rarely spared, digital examination, sigmoidoscopy, and biopsy are usually all that is required to confirm the diagnosis of FAP. Sigmoidoscopy and barium enema will usually distinguish between these two conditions. It may as well provide evidence for the diagnosis of FAP. Colonoscopy with histological examination should follow in order to evaluate the extension of the disease. For investigation of manifestations of variants of the disease outside the GI tract, it is worth performing skull and jaw radiography to determine whether osteomata are present and computed tomography (CT) scan to rule out other lesions.

MANAGEMENT

Treatment of FAP is influenced by the natural history of the disease. If patients are left long enough without a colectomy, they will develop carcinoma. The average age at which symptoms develop is about 20 years.[7]

The procedure of choice for FAP is still the subject of much debate. The options are proctocolectomy or colectomy and rectal mucosectomy without restoration of GI continuity, colectomy and ileorectal anastomosis, or restorative proctocolectomy.

Although an ileostomy patient can have a full and active life, it is difficult for a young and active family member, usually asymptomatic, to accept such a procedure.

The advantages of colectomy with ileorectal anastomosis are that GI continuity is restored and bowel function is reasonable.

Furthermore, there is evidence suggesting that carcinoma can develop de novo even in rectal mucosa not occupied by polyps.

The ileum should be divided at approximately 10 cm from the ileocecal junction and its lumen inspected for the presence of polyps (Fig. 70.2).

In patients who develop numerous polyps following ileorectal anastomosis which fulguration fails to control, restorative proctocolectomy should be considered. If this operation is contraindicated because

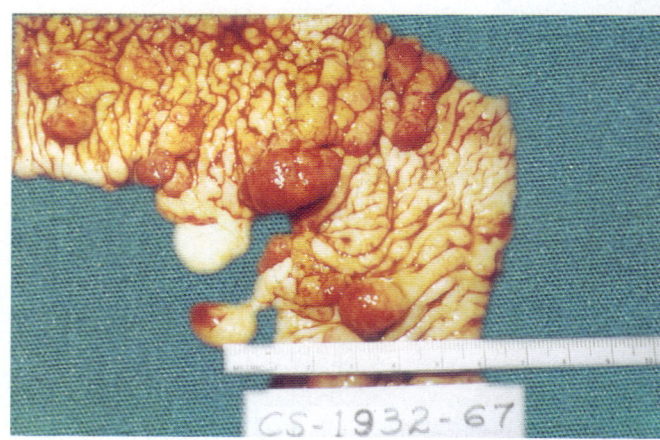

Fig. 70.2: Multiple polyposis of the colon in a 10 year old boy. Histology was suggestive of adenomatoid disease

of poor anal function or ileal polyposis, the entire rectum should be removed and a permanent ileostomy constructed.

Restorative proctocolectomy is the operation of choice for patients with numerous polyps in the rectum. This procedure is performed in the same manner as for ulcerative colitis. All anal mucosa above the dentate line should be excised.

The approach taken in many units still involves performing colectomy and ileorectal anastomosis in the first instance. Patients with 20-100 polyps are treated by colectomy and ileorectal anastomosis. All others are advised to have an ileoanal pouch.

Desmoid tumors in the abdominal wall should be removed if there is progressive enlargement or if they produce symptoms.

GARDNER'S SYNDROME

Gardner's syndrome was originally described as consisting of cutaneous cysts, osteomata, and fibromata associated with the polyposis. Later, other extracolonic lesions were described. Today, Gardner's syndrome is no longer regarded as a separate entity, but merely as one group of patients in the whole spectrum of FAP.

TURCOT'S SYNDROME

Turcot's syndrome is an eponym given to familial polyposis in association with malignant tumors of the central nervous system. The neurological condition may become apparent before the polyposis.[8] Turcot's syndrome is thought to be a distinct entity from FAP, unlike Gardner's syndrome.[9]

HAMARTOMATOUS POLYPOSIS

Juvenile Polyposis

Originally described in 1964, this rare condition is characterized by multiple polyps, predominantly in the large bowel.[10] Nonfamilial cases may have other associated congenital abnormalities. Although it was initially believed that there was no danger of cancer development, further studies demonstrated that some of the polyps show adenomatous features with malignant potential.[11] Several authors found frank malignancy within polyps from these patients. True juvenile polyposis is now considered to be a premalignant condition akin to adenomatous polyposis, and the current trend is to treat it in the same radical way as FAP, with colectomy and ileorectal anastomosis or restorative proctocolectomy.[12]

Diagnosis

The first office evaluation must include a careful and gentle digital rectal examination, with concomitant stool examinations to rule out the presence of enteric pathogens and the presence of blood. The finding of a firm polypoid mass or an irregular firmness in the rectal mucosa suggests the need for proctosigmoidoscopy.

Juvenile Retention (Inflammatory) Polyps

These lesions are often silent, but they may cause blood-streaking on the stools. Sharp rectal bleeding from the stalk occurs after spontaneous avulsion of the polyp, but exsanguinating hemorrhage and anemia do not occur. Occasionally the polyp appears as a purple colored protruding mass in the anal canal. A prolapsed polyp can descend to the anal canal from the rectosigmoid junction or even higher, and it may not be palpable to digital examination.

Rigid or flexible proctosigmoidoscopy will permit the diagnosis of rectal polyps in over 85 percent of the cases. Because any polyp can contain adenomatous or other malignant elements, it is essential to secure one or more of the lesions for histologic examination (Fig. 70.3).

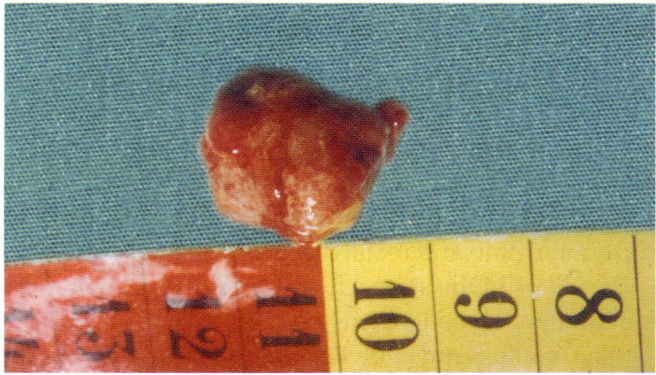

Fig. 70.3: Rectal hamartoma (Juvenile polyp) in a 4 year old boy

Gross and Microscopic

Appearance of the Juvenile Polyp

These common polyps have a smooth, round, oval or slightly lobulated surface and a reddish or reddish-brown appearance. On cut section, large numbers of mucus-filled irregular cysts are seen to be lined by mucin-containing columnar cells.

Treatment

Unless multiple large polyps are present, anemia is rarely a problem. The 15 cm pediatric rigid procto-sigmoidoscope is adequate for identifying and removing at least 75 percent of juvenile polyps. The stalk can be sectioned by an electrocautery snare or by cutting through it with simple biopsy forceps. There may be brisk bleeding from the vessels in the stalk. All visible polyps should be removed.

Juvenile polyps can be intermixed with true adenomatous polyps. Patients should therefore be followed more carefully than has suggested in the past.

PEUTZ-JEGHERS SYNDROME

Peutz-Jeghers syndrome is a very rare, usually familial, syndrome of pigmentation of the mouth and other parts of the body together with GI polyps and was first described by Peutz in 1921.[13,14] Jeghers later reported several patients with the disease. Although it is almost invariable a familial disease with an autosomal dominant inheritance, sporadic cases do occur.

The most frequent site for polyps is the upper small bowel, but they may also occur in the stomach and large bowel.

Peutz-Jeghers syndrome occurs equally in both sexes. The age of onset of manifestations is commonly in childhood or adolescence. Cutaneous pigmentation often precedes polyp formation and may disappear after puberty. The most common symptoms are abdominal pain and rectal bleeding. The risk is greater with polyps in the stomach and small bowel, whereas for colonic polyps it seems negligible (Fig. 70.4).

The management of Peutz-Jeghers syndrome is usually conservative. Surgery is sometimes performed for complications such as intussusception or massive hemorrhage.[15]

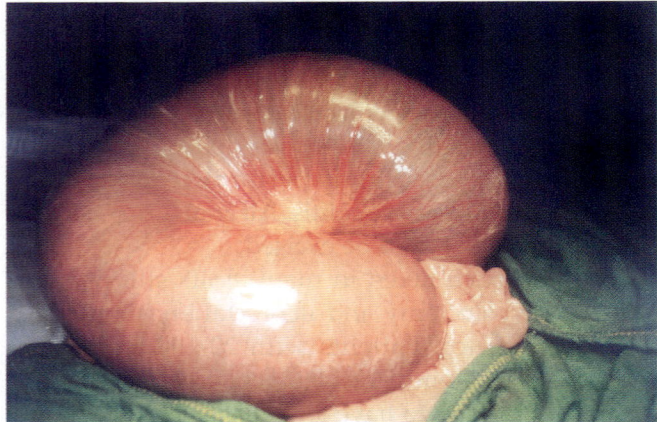

Fig. 70.4: Operative photograph of Peutz-Jeghers syndrome of the ileum with intussusception

CANADA-CRONKHITE SYNDROME

Canada-Cronkhite syndrome[16] is one of the rare generalized GI polypoid syndromes of which the components have only recently been classified. There are five cardinal features:
1. Presence of multiple hamartomatous polyps of the juvenile variety
2. Ectodermal changes, consisting of alopecia, onychodystrophy, and hyperpigmentation
3. Absence of a family history
4. Adult onset
5. Eventual development of diarrhea and weight loss.

Anemia, edema, and tetany result from malabsorption, and hypokalemia is common. The hyperpigmentation takes the form of brown macular lesions which occur most frequently on the upper and lower extremities and on the face. The nails are dystrophic, fragile, discolored, and sometimes absent. The appearance of multiple, rounded filling defects on barium examination is characteristic.

An aggressive treatment may result in long periods of remission. Patients need fluid and electrolyte correction, nutritional support, treatment of anemia and coagulation defects, and prophylaxis for peptic ulcer.

The risk of developing carcinoma is insufficient to justify prophylactic colectomy.

CONCLUSION

Intestinal polyposis encompasses a spectrum of abnormal growths. These syndromes vary from discrete polyps and cancer to Gardner's syndrome with its dramatic extracolonic manifestations. FAP and Turcot's syndrome are both part of a systemic overgrowth pattern, and the associated soft tissue, bony, glandular, and brain tumors illustrate the wide spectrum of this disorder.

Our understanding of the contribution of a genetic susceptibility to the development of GI polyps and cancer is increasing rapidly.

Treatment has also made great strides. Recognition of the familial tendency allows the detection of asymptomatic patients before cancer develops. Prophylactic operations are now well accepted. The choice between colectomy/ileorectal anastomosis, with the remaining risk of rectal cancer, and proctocolectomy/permanent ileostomy has been altered by the appearance of the ileoanal pouch procedure. We should therefore be able to treat every patient with neoplastic polyposis so as to avoid the development of colon cancer.

REFERENCES

1. Bodmer WF, Bailey CJ, Bodmer J, et al. Localisation of the gene for familial adenomatous polyposis on chromosome 5. Nature 1987;328:614-16.
2. Dick JA, owen WJ, McColl I. Rectal sparing in familial polyposis coli. Br J Surg 1984;71:664.
3. Jagelman DG, De Cosse JJ, Bussey HJR. Upper gastrointestinal cancer in familial adenomatous polyposis. Lancet 1988;i:1149-50.
4. Chapman PD, Church W, Burn J, Gunn A. The detection of congenital hypertrophy of retinal pigment epithelium (CHRPE) by indirect ophtalmoscopy: a reliable clinical feature of familial adenomatous polyposis. Br Med J. 1989;298:353-54.
5. Gardner EJ, Richards RC. Multiple cutaneous lesions occurring simultaneously with hereditary polyposis and osteomatosis. Am J Hum Genet 1953;5:139-48.
6. Plail RO, Bussey HJR, Glazer G, Thomson JPS. Adenomatous polyposis: an association with carcinoma of the thyroid. Br J Surg 1987;74:377-80.
7. Bussey, HJR. Familial polyposis coli. The John Hopkins University Press, Baltimore 1975.
8. Turcot J, Depres JP, St. Pierre F. Malignant tumours of the central nervous system associated with familial polyposis of the colon. Dis Colon Rectum 1959;2:465-66.
9. Rothman D, Su CP, Kendall AB. Dilemma in a case of Turcot's (glioma polyposis) syndrome. Report of a case. Dis Colon Rectum 1975;18:514-15.
10. McColl I, Bussey HJR, Veale AMC, Morson BC. Juvenile polyposis coli. Proc R Soc Med 1964;57:896.
11. Jarvinen H, Franssila KO. Familial juvenile polyposis coli: increased risk of colorectal cancer. Gut 1984;25:792-800.
12. Grigioni WF, Alampi G, Martinelli G, Piccaluga A. Atypical juvenile polyposis. Histopathology 1981;5: 361-76.
13. Jeghers H. Pigmentation of skin. New Engl J Med, 1944;231:88-100.
14. Peutz JLA. Very remarkable case of familial polyposis of mucous membrane of intestinal tract and nasopharynx accompanied by peculiar pigmentations of skin and mucous membrane. Nederl Maandschr V. Geneesk 1921;10:134-46.
15. Williams CB, Goldblatt M, Delaney P. Top and tail endoscopy and follow-up in Peutz-Jeghers syndrome. Endoscopy 1982;14: 82-84.
16. Daniel ES, Ludwin SL, Lewis KJ, et al. The Cronkhite Canada syndrome. An analysis of clinical and pathological features and therapy. Medicine (Balt) 1982;61:293-309.

Anorectal Malformations: Anatomy and Physiology

Pradip Mukherjee, MK Bhattacharyya

A mother, in true sense of the term, can never say 'No' to her child however, serious congenital malformation the child might have. But when the child has fecal (and or urinary) incontinence a day does come when the mother turns her face. Thousands of suns cannot put light to the life of the child. Thus, normal continence has rightly been called "God's greatest gift for mankind". So the surgeon operating upon a child with ARM must have the highest degree of knowledge of anatomy so that the sphincter muscles and nerves are not damaged during operation and thus the prospect of continence is not jeopardized for ever.

Willis Pots wrote in 1959, "In general, the atresia of the rectum is more poorly handled than any other congenital anomaly of the newborn.[1] A properly functioning rectum is an unappreciated gift of greatest price. The child who is so unfortunate as to be born with an imperforate anus may be saved from a lifetime misery and social seclusion by the surgeon, who with skill, diligence and judgement performs the first operation on the malformed rectum."

HISTORY

From Webster's article we get a beautiful description of the way to deal with this common anomaly.[2] Initially the procedure was done by the Byzantine Physician Paul of Aegina. The bowel was opened by plunging a bistoury through the perineum and then dilating the passage with bougies. This method of treatment was followed throughout the next thousand years. In 1787, Benjamin Bell performed perineal dissection and could locate the blind rectal ampulla.[2] Amussat recognized the severe complications of these methods.[3] He opened the rectum and sutured it to the skin margins. Perhaps this was the first definitive anorectoplasty in the history of management of ARM. In 1833, Roux had stressed on the importance of keeping the perineal dissection strictly in the midline.[2] Splitting, dislocating or excising the coccyx were practiced by many surgeons and a few deliberately opened the pelvis to gain extra length of the bowel.

For the low anomalies most of the surgeons used to perform a perineal anoplasty without a colostomy during the first sixty years of the 20th century. For high anomalies a colostomy used to be done in the newborn period and it was later followed by an abdominoperineal pull-through operation. The decision to create the colostomy was based mainly on the radiological information obtained from the invertogram. While doing abdominoperineal pull-through operation surgeons used to keep close to the sacrum in order to avoid trauma to the genitourinary tract. In 1880 Neil Mcleod performed a combined and perineal exploration. It was accepted and modified by many surgeons.[2] As early as 1948 Rhoades et al successfully ventured one stage abdominoperineal procedure in the newborn.[4]

First objective anatomic studies on human specimens were done by Stephens.[5,6] In 1953, he proposed an initial sacral approach, followed by an abdominoperineal operation when necessary. His main idea was to avoid injury to the puborectal sling which was considered to be the most important factor in maintaining fecal continence. Since then various modifications have been done by many surgeons.

Submucosal resection was done independently by Rehbein and Kiesewetter.[7-10] Advantage of this procedure is that it can avoid damage to the pararectal nerves and muscles. Mollard's anterior dissection to define the puborectalis muscles just adjacent to the urethra has proved another milestone in the operation of ARM.[11-14] It is considered to be a good approach when the standard approaches have failed and the surgeon wants to go through a virgin field.

Posterior Sagittal Anorectoplasty (PSARP) for the treatment of ARM was first performed by de Vries and Pena in September, 1980.[15,16] They published it in 1982. This approach allowed good exposure of this complex anatomic area. Since the advent of this approach pull-through operation for ARM is no more a blind procedure, and the clinical results have become more predictable. So with due reasons PSARP is now the standard operation done throughout the world.

EMBRYOLOGY

The exact mechanism of development of anorectum is still mysterious and controversial. Two main events are thought to be important for the differentiation of the cloaca. The conventional view is that downgrowth of the urorectal septum divides cloaca into urogenital (anterior) and anorectal (posterior) parts (Fig. 71.1). Controversy does still persist whether the division takes place by downward frontal septum (Tourneux fold), median fusion of lateral folds of Rathke or a combination of both. The cloacal membrane is divided into anal and urogenital membranes.

Three theories are there:
1. Conventional
2. Chatterjee and Roy (1978)
3. Van der Putte (1986).

Conventional Theory

The foregut has a ventral diverticulum which develops into a completely different system, i.e. respiratory system. Similarly the hindgut has a ventral diverticulum that too develops into a separate system. This diverticulum is called 'Allantois'. In stage 10 of the developmental process there is reorganization of the caudal region of the embryo. As a result a part of the allantois is drawn into the body cavity.

Now the hindgut has a dorsal part extending from the caudal intestinal portal to the cloacal membrane, and a ventral part, i.e. the allantois.

The dilated cavity receiving the hindgut proper and allantois is lined by endoderm and is called endodermal cloaca. Ventrally endodermal cloaca is closed by cloacal membrane. Endodermal cloaca with hindgut proper and allantois are together surrounded by mesenchyme. At the junction of the hindgut and allantois there is proliferation of the mesenchyme and endoderm, and as a result a septum develops called the urorectal septum. Classically the urorectal septum is formed by the downgrowth of the Tourneux's fold

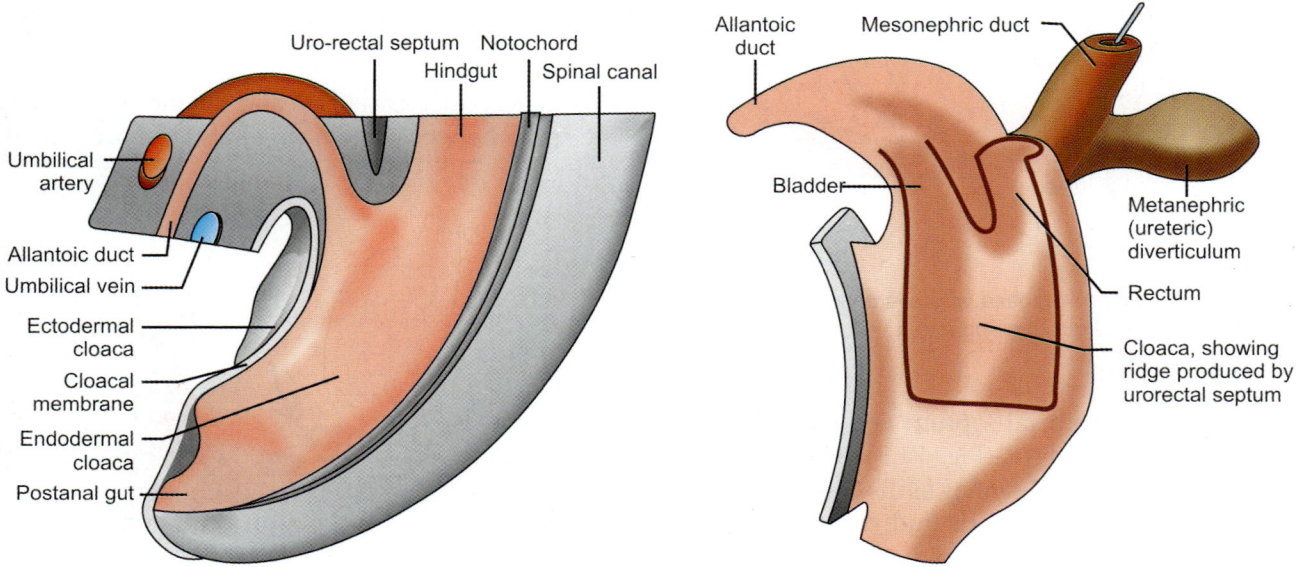

Fig. 71.1: Division of endodermal cloaca by the urorectal septum

and ingrowth of the lateral folds of Rathke that fuse in the midline. This septum grows further to divide the endodermal cloaca into a dorsal part and a ventral part. The dorsal part develops into rectum and anal canal. The ventral part develops into vesicourethral part and urogenital sinus. The vesicourethral part gives rise to the bladder and the proximal part of prostatic urethra in male, and bladder and the whole of the urethra in female. The urogenital sinus develops into the rest of the urethra in male, and caudal five-sixths of vagina in female.

The urorectal septum also divides the cloacal membrane. The posterior part is called the anal membrane and the anterior part is called the urogenital membrane. Perineal body develops at the junction of these two membranes.

Theory of Chatterjee and Roy[17]

As the conventional theory fails to explain all the anomalies Chatterjee and Roy put forward a different hypothesis.

a. Internal cloaca with allantois and hindgut opening into it: It is separated from external cloaca by cloacal membrane. Arrow is in the mesodermal urorectal septum (Fig. 71.2).

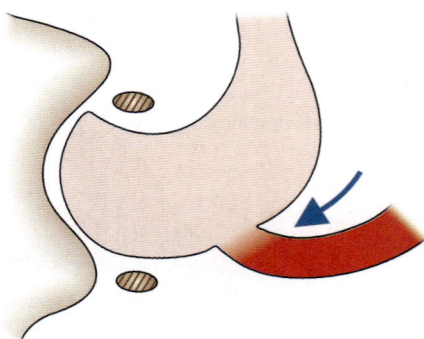

Fig. 71.2: Internal cloaca with allantois and hind gut opening into it

b. Descent of the urorectal septum and cloacal duct and growth of hindgut (Fig. 71.3): The internal cloaca is now the urogenital sinus and Wolffian duct opens into it. A ureteric bud grows from the terminal end of each Wolffian duct.

Wolffian duct opens into it. A ureteric bud grows from the terminal end of each Wolffian duct.

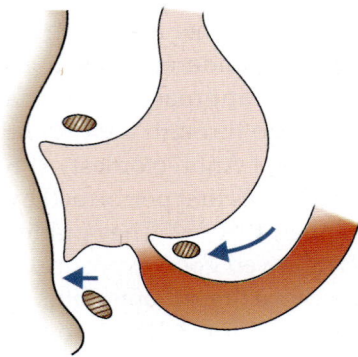

Fig. 71.3: Descent of cloacal duct and urorectal septum and growth of hind gut

c. The growing tip of the hindgut reaches the posterior margin of the cloacal membrane and thus opens into the external cloaca (Fig. 71.4).

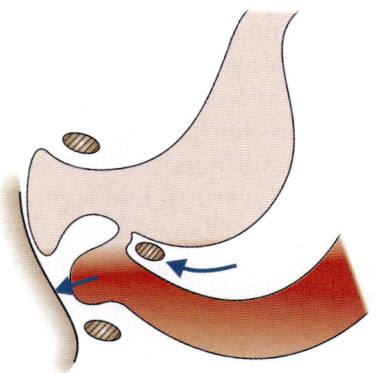

Fig. 71.4: The growing tip of hindgut reaches the posterior margin of the cloacal membrane

d. The cloacal duct has closed and the mesoderm fills the space between the hindgut and the urogenital sinus (Fig. 71.5).

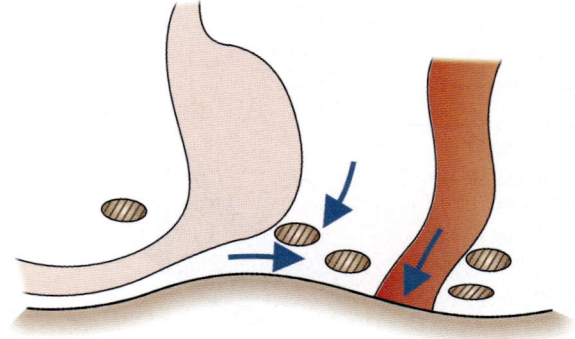

Fig. 71.5: Mesoderm fills space between the hind gut and urogenital sinus

e. The surface ectoderm around the opening of the hindgut is drawn in to form the lining of the lower half of the anal canal (Fig. 71.6).

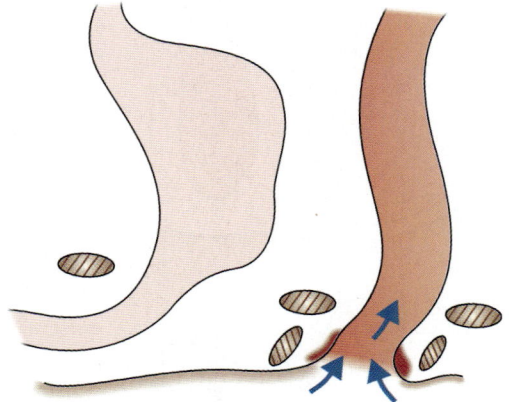

Fig. 71.6: The lower lining of the anal canal is formed by the surface ectoderm

f. The anal opening migrates backwards to reach the posterior perineum (Fig. 71.7).

They agreed that hindgut developed by growth and caudal migration. The growing tip was not at the cloacal opening, but distal to the opening. When it reaches the normal anal site the cloacal opening closed. This closure was brought about by the frontal and lateral septa described earlier.

The majority of the malformations are due to the growth failure of the hindgut or agenesis. Arrest of growth takes place at varying distances from the cloacal membrane giving rise to high, intermediate or low malformations. In these anomalies, the whole of the cloacal membrane is taken up by urogenital sinus. Surface ectoderm at the normal anal site forms the normal skin without any dimple. Mesoderm intervenes between the endoderm and surface ectoderm. It differentiates normally to form the pelvic diaphragm, the levator sling around the urogenital tubes and striated muscle complex at the normal anal site.

Abnormal Development due to Anorectal Agenesis (Figs 71.8A to D)

a. The connection between the hindgut and the urogenital sinus may remain patent as a fistulous opening into the urinary bladder, prostatic or bulbar urethra in male or unsplit rectovaginal passage, the vagina or the vestibule in the female.
b. Cloacal duct closes and leaves a blind terminal bowel.
c. Original connection may close and a new connection can develop.
d. New connection may persist with non-obliteration of the cloacal duct leading to formation of two openings.

Abnormal Development without Anorectal Agenesis (Figs 71.9A to D)

a. Persistence of the cloacal duct leading to a fistula with normal anorectum.
b. Anterior perineal anus—failure of posterior migration
c. Covered anus—anus covered by genital folds.
d. Normal anus with atresia.

Theory of Van der Putte

After working on pig embryos he has shown that previous theories are not acceptable. He showed that future urinary passage, future anorectum and tail gut open into the cloaca. Cloacal plate, made of multilayered solid epithelium, separates cloaca from the amniotic cavity. The cloacal plate extends dorsally to the tail groove and ventrally to the tip of the genital tubercle. The urorectal septum is not a true septum, but a large mesenchymal mass with two tubular structures which are the future urinary and anorectal

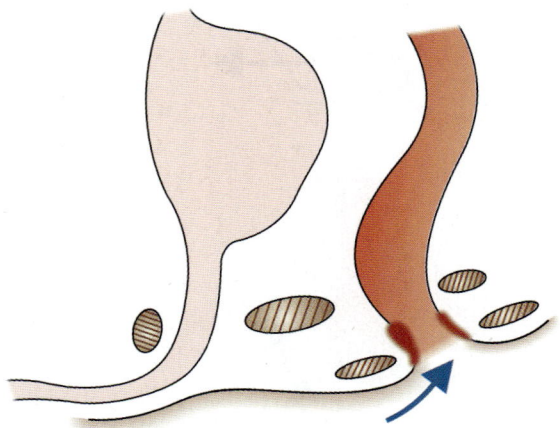

Fig. 71.7: The anal opening migrates backwards

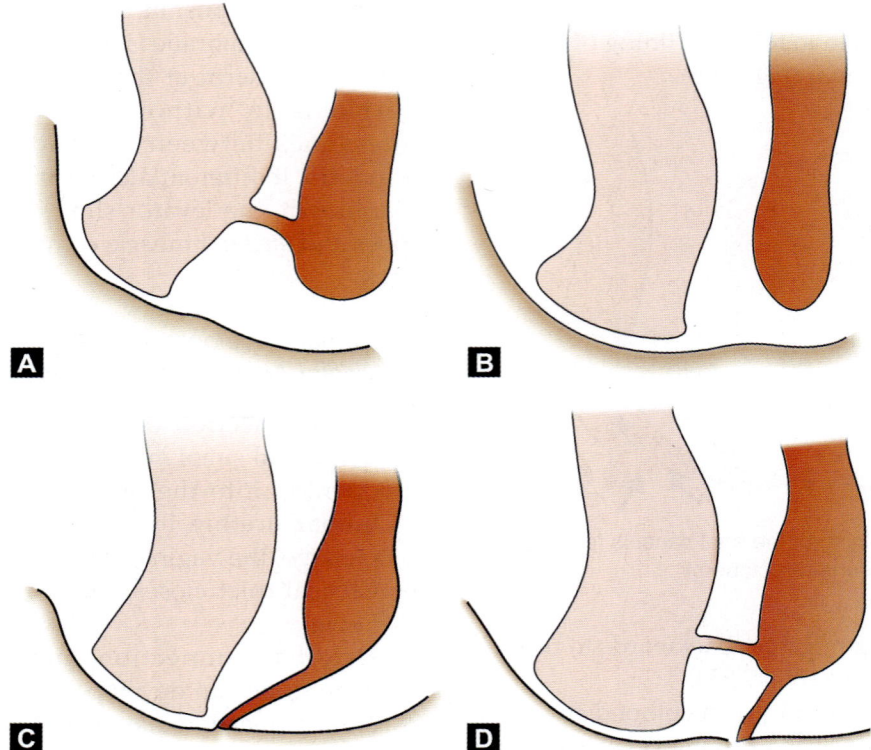

Figs 71.8A to D: A. Connection between hindgut and urogenital sinus **B.** Blind terminal bowel **C.** New connection between terminal bowel and exterior **D.** New connection with non-obliteration of cloacal duct

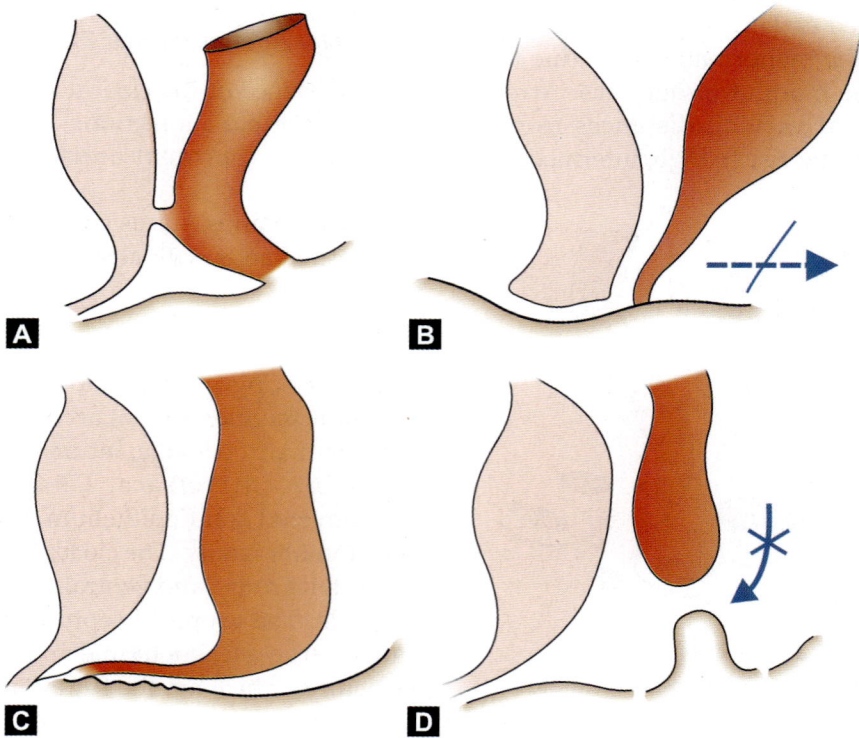

Figs 71.9A to D: A. Persistence of cloacal duct **B.** Anterior perineal anus **C.** Covered anus **D.** Rectal atresia

passages. He suggested 'uroenteric region' to be a more appropriate term for the urorectal septum. In the older embryo (15 -18 mm.) the urorectal septum was never to fuse with the cloacal plate. The classically described downgrowth of the urorectal septum was brought about by the changes that occur in the dorsal part of the cloacal membrane. When the dorsal part of the cloacal membrane breaks, the future urinary tract and the anorectum are simultaneously exposed. The urorectal septum broadens and the distance between the urogenital sinus and the anorectum increases.

He postulated the followings:
a. Agenesis of the whole cloacal membrane gave rise to absence of both urethral and anorectal orifices.
b. Agenesis of the dorsal part of the cloacal membrane gave rise to the anorectal agenesis, stenosis and ectopia. Superficial defects were thought to give rise to low malformations like simple stenotic anus, complete and incomplete covered anus and anterior perineal anus in male and female, and vestibular anus or rectovaginal fistula in the female. Defects extending deeper were responsible for anal or anorectal agenesis with rectobulbar, rectoprostatic, rectovesical fistulae in the male, and rectovaginal and rectovestibular fistulae in the female. In the same way anorectal agenesis without communication and regressive changes in the epithelium of these communications were found in a number of embryos he studied.
c. Agenesis of the ventral part of the cloacal membrane gave rise to stenosis and ectopia of the urethral orifice, hypospadias or urethral agenesis with communications to the anorectum.
d. Interruption of the dorsal part by an isolated defect produced a double anus or a combination of an ectopic anus and a fistula with the urogenital system.
e. Interruption of the ventral part by an isolated defect produced a double urethral orifice.
f. Excessive formation of the cloacal membrane with extension too far ventralwards gave rise to epispadias and exstrophies.

ANATOMY

Structures responsible for anorectal continence are gut, muscles, nerves and higher centers.

Gut

Sensory elements:
a. Rectal wall nerve endings and stretch receptors
b. Puborectalis
c. Striated muscle complex
d. Anal mucosa

Motor elements:
a. Rectal wall
b. Levator ani
c. Puborectalis
d. Striated muscle complex
e. Internal sphincter
f. External sphincter: Superficial, deep and subcutaneous.

Muscles

Important muscles for anorectal continence are internal sphincter, external sphincter, puborectalis and striated muscle complex. Levator ani, except its puborectalis part, has a less important role.

i. *Internal anal sphincter:* Classically it is described as a condensation of circular smooth muscle around the upper three-fourths of the anal canal. It starts at the anorectal junction and ends at white line. Normally it remains tonically contracted. When feces enters the rectum the internal sphincter gets dilated reflexly. About 80% of the resting anal pressure is due to the internal anal sphincter.

Sympathetic nerve supply comes from plexuses around superior rectal artery and hypogastric plexus. Parasympathetic nerve supply comes from pelvic splanchnic nerves (S_2, 3, 4).

ii. *External anal sphincter:* Classically it has three parts—deep, superficial and subcutaneous (Fig. 71.10).
   a. *Deep part:* It is a thick band of muscle encircling the upper part of the internal sphincter. It has no bony attachments. Its proximal and deeper fibers blend with puborectalis, a part of levator ani. Anteriorly after encircling the anal canal some fibers decussate into superficial transverse perineal muscles (Fig. 71.11).
   b. *Superficial part:* Only this part of the external sphincter has bony attachment. It is attached

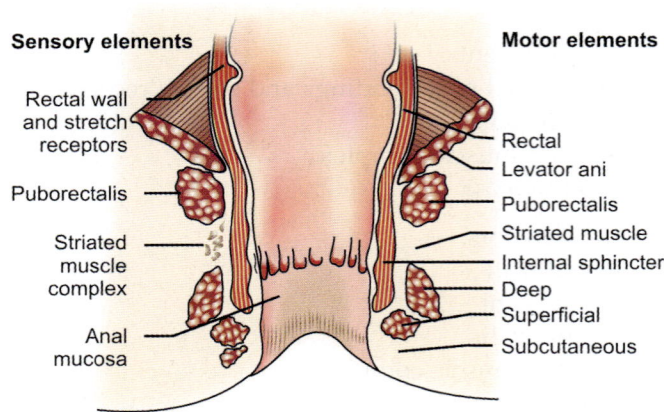

Fig. 71.10: The external and sphincter has three parts: deep, superficial, subcutaneous

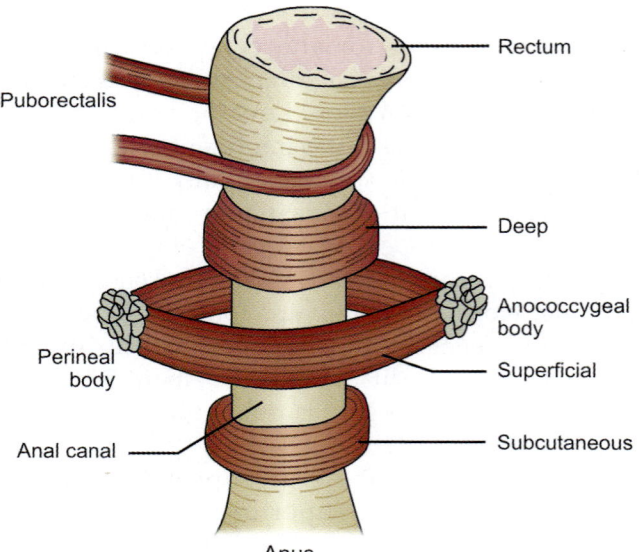

Fig. 71.11: The fibers of the deep part of the external and sphincter merge with the puborectalis

multiple parts and functions are concerned it is the most complex muscle of the body. It has the following parts.

a. *Pubococcygeus:* Anteriorly it is attached to the posterior surface of the body of the pubic bone of the same side. Posteriorly it is attached to the anterior surface of the coccyx. Medial part of pubococcygeus has the following subdivisions:
   – Fibers related to sphincter urethrae in both sexes and levator prostatae in male.
   – Some fibers are attached to vaginal wall, called pubovaginalis.
   – Some fibers are attached to the perineal body and anal canal, called puboanalis.
   – Puborectalis: It forms a sling around the anorectal junction (Described below in details).

b. *Iliococcygeus:* It is thinner than pubococcygeus. Anterolaterally it arises from obturator fascia and ischial spine. Posteriorly it forms the anococcygeal ligament and is attached to the sides of the last two pieces of coccyx.

Medial fibers of levator ani have important role in fecal continence. During PSARP operation the surgeon deals with these fibers. The puborectalis part of levator ani increases the strength of external sphincter.

iv. Puborectalis: Histologically it is a skeletal muscle. It is the medial most part of levator ani. Puborectalis of both sides form a muscular sling around the posterior aspect of the anorectal junction. Anteriorly each puborectalis is attached as a band to the pubic bone of the same side. Anterior to the anorectal junction only a few fibers of each side unite with each other—thus forming some sort of a complete ring. Puborectal sling causes an acute angle at the anorectal junction.

Arrangement of the muscle fibers of the puborectalis and the different parts of the external sphincter is complex. Muscle tone of both external and internal sphincters keeps the anal canal and anus closed except during defecation. Their contractions increase when the intra-abdominal pressure rises during forced expiration, straining, coughing, etc. The purpose is to prevent soiling. The external sphincter, being a striated muscle, can also be voluntarily contracted to occlude the anus more firmly. The external sphincter is more effective than the internal sphincter. The latter is unable to close the anal canal

posteriorly to the last piece of coccyx through the anococcygeal raphe. Anteriorly it is attached to the perineal body. This part encircles the lower part of the internal sphincter.

c. *Subcutaneous part:* It encircles the lower end of anal canal. Motor supply of external sphincter comes from the inferior rectal branch of the pudendal nerve ($S_{2,3}$) and from the perineal branch of the 4th sacral nerve.

iii. *Levator Ani:* Levator ani of both sides form the major part of the pelvic floor. So far as the

completely. Puborectalis forming a sling round the posterior aspect anorectal junction pulls the upper part of the canal forwards to form an acute angle at the anorectal junction, thus assisting its closure.

In resting conditions the anal sphincters undergo periodic increased contractions at the rate of about 15/min with some reversal of peristaltic action, presumably helping to prevent leakage and returning the fecal debris to rectum and upwards.

vi. *Striated Muscle Complex:* Puborectalis and the deep part of the external anal sphincter fuse together to form striated muscle complex.

Nerves (Figs 71.12A and B)

i. *Parasympathetic:* Sacral$_{3,4}$ are motor to the bowel and inhibitor to the sphincters and carries sensation for rectal distension.

ii. *Sympathetic:* Arises from the lumbar$_{2,3,4}$ ganglia, and they form preaortic plexus. These are inhibitor to the bowel and motor to the internal sphincter.

iii. *Somatic:* Anterior roots of S$_{2,3,4}$ via pudendal nerve, then through the perineal branch of the 4th sacral nerve. These fibers supply puborectalis and external sphincter.

iv. *Sensory:*
1. Pain is carried by free nerve endings.
2. Touch sensation is carried by Meissner's corpuscles.
3. Cold sensation is carried by end bulb of Krause.
4. Sensation of Tension is carried by Pacinian corpuscles and Golgi Mazzini.
5. Sensation of friction is carried by genital corpuscles.

Muscular coordination required for the complex activities depends on reflex control involving the smooth muscles of the internal sphincter, enteric plexuses and associated autonomic and visceral sensory nerves. For the skeletal muscle of the external sphincter, puborectalis and associated perineal muscles, regulation is partly reflex and partly voluntary through the visceral and somatic afferent nerves.

Rich sensory innervation of the rectal and anal canal linings and proprioceptive fibers in the muscles and surrounding tissues is essential for normal anorectal continence. Neural integration of these sensory inputs and appropriate motor control are performed at many levels in the nervous system including the spinal cord, brain stem, thalamus and the cortex. Process of defecation is regulated by these operations. Moreover, the integrity of the sensory nerves and the higher center enables the child to differentiate between flatus and feces, and between solid and liquid stool. This differentiation is essential for normal anorectal continence.

CONCEPT OF DE VRIES AND PENA

The knowledge of anatomy of the pelvic floor muscles and anorectal sphincters, and their role in the maintenance of continence was standing more or less in the same place for a long time. Two decades ago Alberto Pena the Mexican Pediatric surgeon introduced the revolutionary operation, i.e. Posterior Sagittal Anorectoplasty (PSARP) for the management of ARM.[18,19]

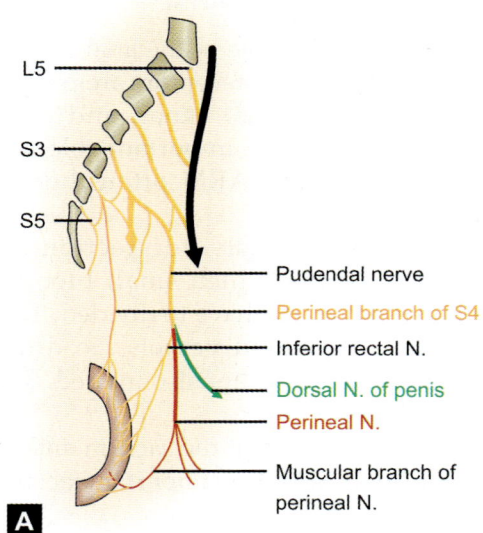
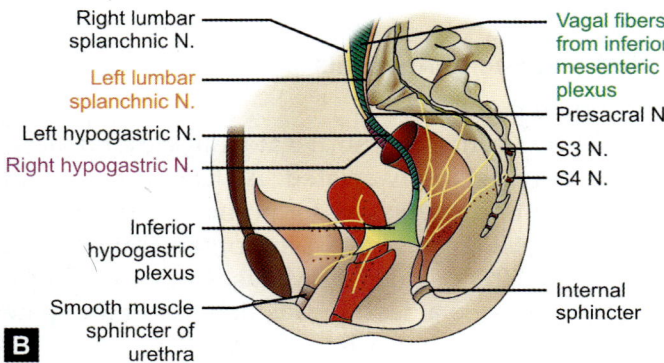

Figs 71.12A and B: Nerve supply of the anorectal region **A.** Sympathetic and parasympathetic, **B.** Somatic supply (N = Nerve)

Several authors studied levator ani muscles for the presence of puborectal sling and formation of the rectal sphincters. Their views were accepted without modification. Pena performed anatomical dissection and electrical dissection of the pelvic muscles and CT scan for the pelvic musculature. He found that the levator ani of both sides constituted a funnel shaped structure around the rectum and anal canal. On each side of the rectum and anal canal there is a sheet of parasagittal fibers. He also stated that these muscle fibers run parallel to each other on either side of the mid sagittal plane. His concept not only challenged the various components (e.g. subcutaneous, superficial and deep) of external sphincter, but also questioned the very existence of the puborectal sling, which was once considered as the key factor in maintaining anorectal continence.

So it can be concluded that:
1. External anal sphincter is represented by two sets of fibers :
   a. Parasagittal fibers running from the tip of the coccyx to the anal skin parallel to the midline in the sagittal plane.
   b. Vertical fibers running medial and perpendicular to the parasagittal fibers.
2. The levator ani fibers are continuous below with the upper part of the vertical part of the external sphincter and they are inseparable from each other.
3. Separate existence of the puborectal sling cannot be ascertained.

Pena says that the most of the muscle fibers run in a cephalocaudal direction. The muscles have their nerve supply from the respective sides. So if the muscles are divided exactly in the midline, no damage is done because the parallel muscle fibers are actually separated, not divided.

Pena and his associates showed that their views were proposed by Amussat[3](1835) long ago. But no detail descriptions were given.

Pena's views have been challenged by Prof Durham Smith (1987), the father figure of Pediatric Surgery with a mammoth contribution in the field of ARM.[20] He criticized the deliberate division of the muscle complex and considered that the deep portions (deep external sphincter and puborectalis) were essential muscles for continence and the patient would never gain continence since the puborectalis has been considered a key structure for fecal continence (Konar H).[21] Direct exposure of the anatomy allows one to recognize that the divided muscle do not retract, as expected. Although there are some horizontal fibers, most of the muscle fibers run in a cephalocaudal direction, so one is separating parallel muscle fibers. In addition, there is a very thin midline fascia and raphe hat requires a meticulous technique to be identified and posterior sagittal approach is based on the fact that the nerves do not cross the midline. So keeping exactly in the midline ensures preservation of nerves of all important pelvic structures. Moreover, suturing all the muscles behind the pulled-through rectum will restore the functional efficacy of these muscles.

Good results of PSARP operation done by most of the surgeons all over the world support the golden concept of Pena.

ANATOMIC CONSIDERATIONS

Poor Continence in High ARM

a. In high ARM the whole of the anal canal may be absent. As the sensory receptors are present in the distal half of the anal canal, and as sensory receptors have a very important role in normal continence, in high ARM often there is poor continence.
b. In high ARM extensive dissection becomes necessary, during which small blood vessels supplying the rectum have to divided. The nerves accompany the blood vessels. So during this procedure fine nerves are also injured. So there is poor continence.
c. Associated anomalies of the sacrum and vertebral column in high ARM is an important factor for poor continence.
d. Sphincter muscles are often poorly developed in high ARM.

ARM and Sacral Agenesis

Important points are:
1. Development of sacrum, levator muscles and sacral nerves are closely related. At least three sacral segments are necessary for normal continence.
2. 30% of ARM cases have spinal or sacral anomalies. About 50% of high ARM cases have vertebral anomalies. So at least a straight X-ray of the spine must be done in all cases of ARM.
3. In caudal regression syndrome vertebral anomalies are associated with urinary and gastrointestinal anomalies.

4. Sacral anomalies may be symmetric or asymmetric. Types of sacral deformities are butterfly, dysplastic and hemivertebra.
5. 1% of the diabetic mothers have offspring with sacral agenesis. 16% of children with sacral agenesis have insulin-dependent diabetes mellitus.
6. Clinical diagnosis can be made by the absence of bony prominence just behind the normal anal site. Gluteal cleft is usually absent and the buttocks are flat.
7. Degree of neurologic deficit cannot be predicted from the number of absent sacral segments. Motor involvement is more common than sensory involvement. In 75% cases of sacral agenesis perianal sensation does persist.

Problems of Common Wall in ARM

The problems are:
1. In rectourethral fistula in male invariably there is a common wall. The lower the level of rectourethral fistula, the more is the length of the common wall. Common wall between the rectum and the urethra makes the dissection difficult, and there is risk of injury to the urethra. Persistence of cloacal duct explains blind ending rectum, rectourinary fistula and a common wall.
2. In anovestibular or rectovestibular fistula in female there is a common wall between the rectum and the vagina.

Anatomic Abnormalities and Urinary Tract Injuries in ARM

Problems are :
1. As there is failure of complete separation between the anorectum and the urinary tract, they are in more close proximity than in normal children. So during dissection of the blind anorectum there is risk of injury to the bladder and urethra. Placing a urethral dilator in the urethra helps identification of the urethra better than placing a Foley's catheter. Before opening up the bowel it is a good practice to aspirate with a syringe-needle. Of course a catheter introduced through the distal colostomy opening helps identification of the blind rectal end.
2. Rarely an ectopic ureter may get injured during dissection of the rectum.
3. Sometimes the most distal structure is the bladder (or urethra) and not the rectum. So it is better to open the bowel 1 cm proximal to the end of the blind rectum.

PHYSIOLOGY

Anorectal continence depends on :
A. *Propulsive force:* It depends on the volume of feces, voluntary contraction of the striated muscles (abdominal and diaphragm) and contraction of the smooth muscles of the colon and rectum.
B. *Resistance at the outlet:* Resistance at rest is offered by anorectal angulation, tonicity of the internal sphincter, contraction of striated muscle complex and congested veins of the pelvic floor.
C. *Sensation:* Exquisite sensation in the normal individual resides in the anal canal. Except for the patients for rectal atresia most patients with ARM are born without an anal canal, therefore the sensation does not exist or is rudimentary. Still the distension of the rectum is felt in many of these patients, provided the rectum has been placed properly within the muscles. This sensation appears to be due to stretching of the voluntary muscle (proprioceptive). The most important clinical problem is that liquid stool or soft fecal material may not be perceived by the patients with anorectal malformations as the rectum is not distended. Thus, to achieve some degree of sensation and bowel control, the patient must have the capacity to form solid stool.
D. *Bowel motility:* Perhaps the most important factor in fecal continence is bowel motility. However, motility has been largely underestimated. In a normal individual the rectosigmoid remains quiet for periods of 12 hours to several days. So if there is motility disorder that has to be corrected.

CONCLUSION

If anorectal reconstruction is done early in ARM it is perhaps true that new nerves do develop in the pulled-down bowel. As in other cases perhaps locally acting growth factor is responsible for this neural advancement.

After all these detailed discussions it boils down like this:
1. Pena has not shown any new anatomical concept of the muscles of the anorectal region. If it would have been so, his concept would have been included in all the current text books of Anatomy. A thorough search was made in all the recent text

books of Anatomy as also on the internet, but there is no reference of Pena's article.
2. Discussions with the anatomists about the concept of Pena revealed that if we go down from above—levator ani, puborectal sling, deep part of the external sphincter, superficial part of the external sphincter—it will look like a funnel. Parasagittal fibers are nothing but superficial part of the external sphincter.

What Pena has impressed us all?
Previously we were afraid of cutting the puborectal sling and the vertical component of the muscle in the pre-Pena era with a mental block that if we cut the puborectal sling and vertical component it will lead to incontinence. In order to avoid cutting the puborectal sling people had to operate on an area where there was so little space to work in sacroperineal or sacroabdominoperineal approach. In this approach there was unnecessary overstretching of the puborectal sling and in some of the cases one could not place the bowel within this sling and thereby compromising with the continence.

What Pena has shown to all of us?
If we stay exactly in the midline and cut all the muscles from the sacrum down to the anus :
1. There is no chance of damaging the nerves.
2. Excellent operative visualization.
3. If we suture all the components in the midline after bringing the bowel down to the anus—there is no compromise with the continence. Pena has demonstrated this by his operation and postoperative results.

Many ill-treated cases of ARM are leading a miserable life with fecal incontinence. As ARM is a common anomaly, and as fecal incontinence is a serious hindrance for a child to live meaningfully in a society, and as failure cases are very difficult to manage, it is perhaps well justified to build up a separate discipline to deal with ARM only.

REFERENCES

1. Potts WJ. The Surgeon and the Child. WB Sounders, Philadelphia 1959.
2. Lister J, Irving IM. Neonatal Surgery (3rd ed). Butterworth and co (Publishers Ltd.) 1990.
3. Amussat J. Observation Su rune Operation d' anus artificiel practiquee avee success par un nouveaunprocede. Gaz Med Paris 1836;28:28.
4. Rhoades JE, Piper RL, Randall JP. A simultaneous abdominal and perineal approach in operations for imperforate anus with atresia of rectum and rectosigmoid. Ann Surg 1948;127:552-56.
5. Stephens FD, Durham Smith E. Classification, identification and assessment of surgical treatment of anorectal anomalies. Ped Surg Int 1986;1:200-05.
6. Stephens FD. Imperforate rectum: A new surgical technique. Med J Aust 1953;1:202-06.
7. Rehbein F. Operations for anal and rectal atresia with rectourethral fistula. Chirurgie 1959;30:417-19.
8. Rehbein F. Imperforate anus: Experiences with abdominoperineal and abdominosacroperineal pull-through procedures. J Pediatr Surg 1967;2:99-105.
9. Kiesewetter WB, Chang JHT. Imperforate anus. A 5 to 30 yr. follow up prospective. Prog Ped Surg 1977;10:111-21.
10. Kiesewetter WB, Sukarochana K, Sieber WK. The frequency of aganglionosis associated with imperforate anus surgery 1977;58:877-80.
11. Mollard P, Marechal JM, de Beaujeu MJ. Surgical Treatment of High Imperforate anus with definition of puborectal sling by an anterior perineal approach. J Pediatr Surg 1978;13:499-504.
12. Mollard P, Marechal JM, de Beaujeu, M. J Le reperage de la Sangle du releveur an cours du traitement des imperforations ano-rectales hautes. Ann chir Inf 1975;16:461-68.
13. Mollard P, Soucy P, Louis D, et al. Preservation of infralevator structures in Imperforate Anus repair. J Pediatr Surg 1989;24:1023-26.
14. Mollard P. Surgery for Anorectal Anomalies: Anterior Perineal approach. Rob and Smith's Operative Surgery (Pediatric Surgery) edited by Lewis Spitz and Arnold G Coran. 5 th edition (Chapman and Hall Medical).
15. de Vries PA, Pena A. Posterior Sagittal Anorectoplasty: Important technical considerations and new applications. J Pediatr Surgery 1982:17:796-881.
16. de Vries PA, Pena A. Posterior Sagittal Anorectoplasty. J Pediatr Surg 1982:17:638-43.
17. Chatterjee Subir K. Anorectal Malformations: A Surgeon's Experience. Oxford University Press 1991.
18. Pena A. Posterior Sagittal Anorectoplasty : results in the management of 332 cases of anorectal malformations. Pediatr Surg Int 1988;3:94-104.
19. Pena A. The surgical management of persistent cloaca: Results in 54 patients treated with Posterior Sagittal approach. J Pediatr Surg 1989:24:590-98.
20. Stephens FD, Durham Smith E. Classification, identification and assessment of surgical treatment of anorectal anomalies. Ped Surg Int 1991;1:200-05.
21. Konar H. A study for the Muscle arrangements for Anorectal Continence. A Thesis submitted for Master of Surgery (Anatomy) 1992;94.

Anorectal Malformations: Diagnosis and Management

SN Kureel, RK Tandon

Whenever a baby is born with absence of anal opening in perineum, the condition has been traditionally named as "imperforate anus". It is actually an overt clinical presentation of a wide spectrum of malformations involving the agenesis of anal canal and/or rectum with variable development of sphincteric muscles of continence. It is more often associated with fistula and possibilities of associated visceral and skeletal anomalies. These anomalies of imperforate anus are more accurately termed as anorectal malformations (ARM). Wide spectrum of defects ranges from non-complex low malformations to very complex high malformations of anorectum. Low anorectal malformations are associated with well developed rectum, anal canal, sphincters and sensory receptors with prospects of good prognosis whereas high malformations are complicated due to poor development of sphincters and its innervation with associated genitourinary anomalies which are difficult to treat and associated with prospects of poor prognosis.

Precise diagnosis of pathological anatomy, effective and efficient therapeutic approach and meticulous technique of repair in planned manner by an expert, is the only hope to save these babies from life time misery and offer the control of defecation. In 1959, Potts, then Surgeon in Chief at Children's Memorial Hospital in Chicago wrote "In general, atresia of the rectum is more poorly handled than any other congenital anomaly of the newborn.[1] A properly functioning rectum is an unappreciated gift of greatest price. The child who is so unfortunate as to be born with an imperforate anus can be saved a life time of misery and social seclusion by the surgeon who with skill, diligence and judgement performs the first operation on the malformed rectum.

More than forty years later despite enormous advancement in understanding of abnormal anatomy, advances in imaging and plethora of technical breakthrough above statement stands true even today. Approximately 50% of babies with high ARM fail to achieve normal continence despite being treated with perfection in best hands and the figure will swiftly go up with inappropriate decision and wrong technique forcing more children towards life long misery and permanent colostomy.[2] Therefore, surgeons carry great responsibility in management of this problem and cannot afford a casual approach. This chapter will review the diagnosis and current management of ARM.

MAGNITUDE OF THE PROBLEM

Average worldwide incidence of ARM is reported to be 1 in 5000 live births.[3] However, in India Chatterjee reported incidence of 1 in 1862 births in Calcutta and approximately 13,223 babies with anorectal malformations are born every year in India.[4] Even this may be an underestimate. Firstly because some cases may never reach the hospital and low anomalies with fistula may not attend the hospital in neonatal period.

CLASSIFICATION

Importance of determination of exact type of malformation and level of patent rectum cannot be overemphasized (Figs 72.1 to 72.5). It will not only guide the management strategy but also help in comparing the clinical results of one technique with those of another.

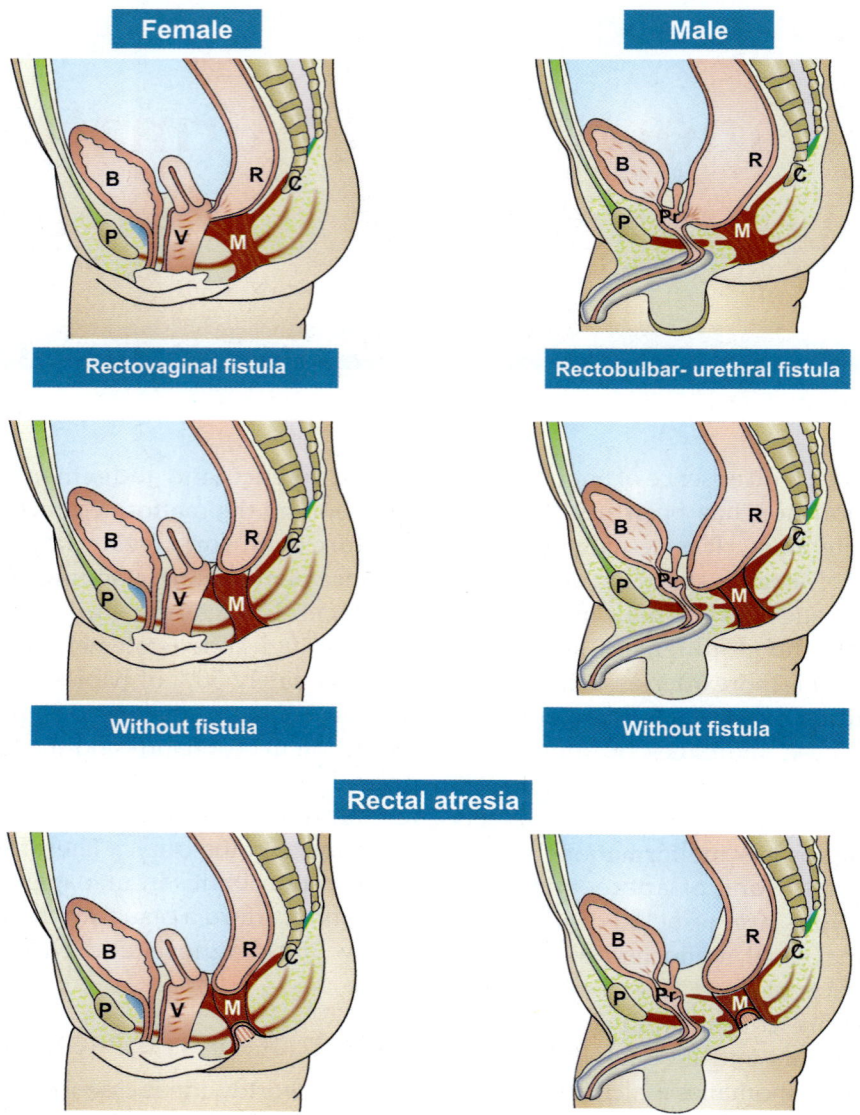

Fig. 72.1: Anatomy of high ARM showing level of rectum, site of fistula and relation to sphincter muscle

In addition to records of earlier classification first modern classification of ARM was described by Ladd and Gross in 1934.[5] Denis Browne first conceived the necessity of classifying the Ladd-3 type of anorectal malformations into "High" and "low" depending upon whether the gut terminated above or below the pelvic floor.[6] Douglas Stephens recognized the importance of puborectalis sling in defecation and fecal continence and divided these lesions into high or supralevator where bowel terminates on cranial side of the levator muscle and low or infralevator anomalies in whom the bowel extends through most of the levator and sphincter muscles.[3,7]

The International Classification of 1970 was proposed in an attempt to ensure that surgeons were describing the same condition and Intermediate or translevator group of anomalies were added with other diverse anomalies.[8] In practice, it proved unwieldy and complex. The Wingspread classification of 1984 is a simpler version that combines anatomic details with what is known of the embryology (Table 72.1).[7]

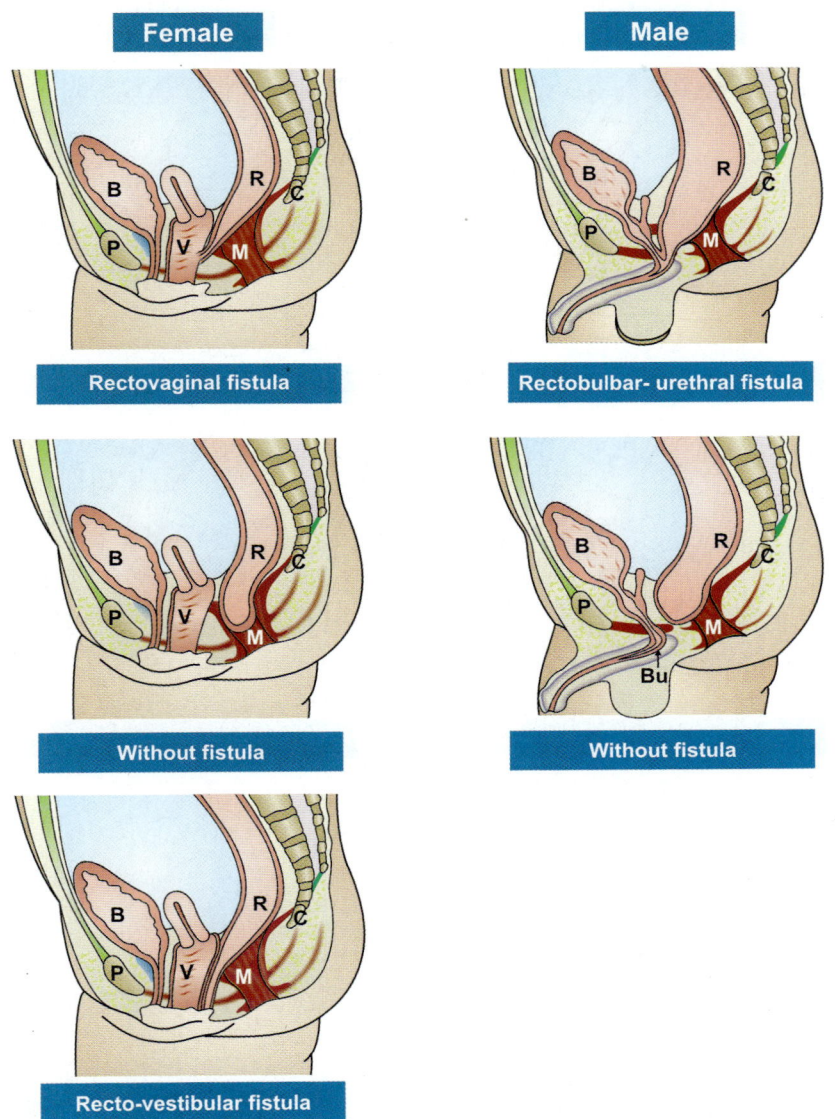

Fig. 72.2: Anatomy of Intermediate ARM showing level of rectum, site of fistula and relation to sphincter muscle

A descriptive classification based on initial management decision more related to surgical imperatives was proposed by Alberto Pena to decide whether a colostomy is required or not (Table 72.2) which was subsequently modified by Rintala.[9,10]

Irrespective of the method used for classification basic essential features remain unchanged which are:
1. Most female babies with ARM are intermediate and low anomalies while majority of malformation in male are high or intermediate anomalies.
2. In female baby with ARM rectum or anal canal almost always opens as fistula either in vagina, vestibule or perineum, wide enough to permit passage of gas and stool, therefore, these patients may not present as intestinal obstruction.
3. In male baby with ARM rectum may open in bladder neck, prostatic urethra or bulbar urethra with narrow fistula insufficient to decompress the colon or a fistula may not be present at all and these patients present with intestinal obstruction.

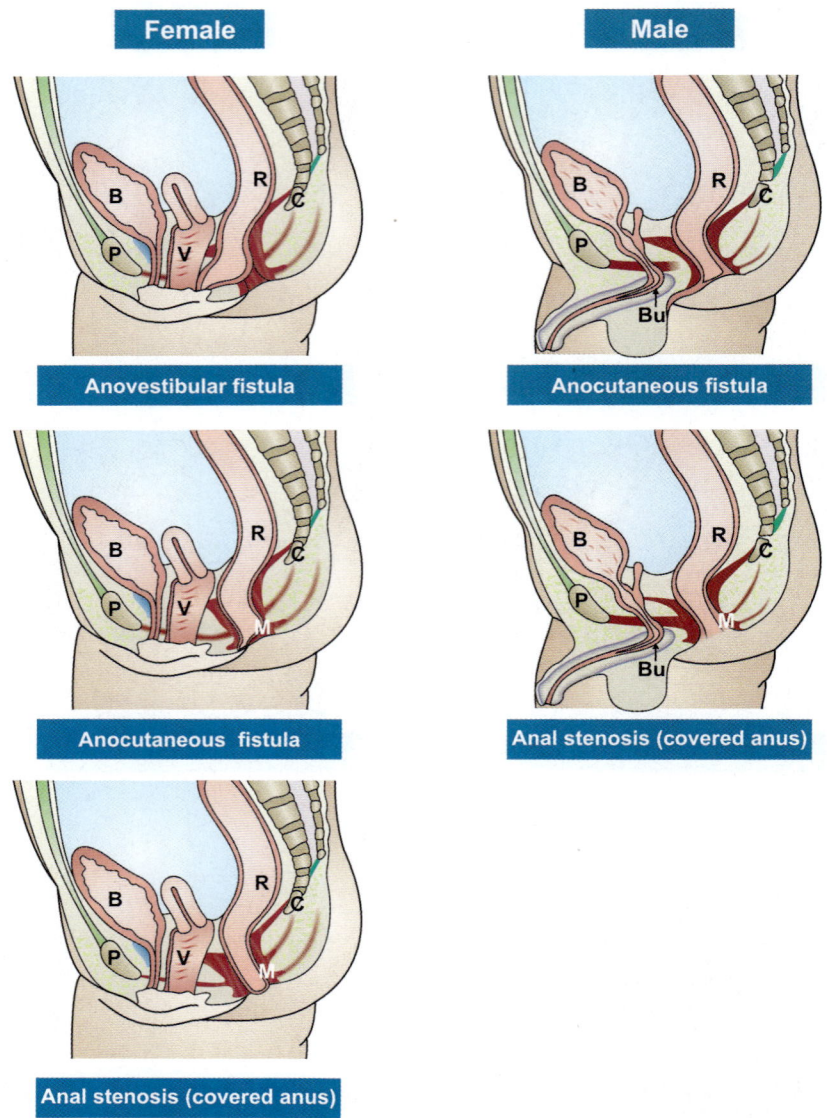

Fig. 72.3: Anatomy of Low ARM showing level of rectum, site of fistula and relation to sphincter muscle

DIAGNOSIS AND INVESTIGATIONS

Antenatal Diagnosis

The normal anal canal in the fetus can be appreciated on ultrasound as circular rim of hypoechogenic tissue in the perineum with central linear echogenic stripe (Guzman et al).[11] The sonographic evidence of ARM is non specific in the form of dilated fetal bowel and abnormal appearance which is suggestive but not diagnostic of ARM. Associated anomalies like esophageal atresia, caudal regression syndrome, hydrometrocolpos and renal anomalies are readily identified by antenatal sonography.

Neonatal Assessment

Diagnosis of absence of anal opening is usually straight forward, it is surprising but not uncommon that such obvious anomaly is often missed and discovered at second look when abdominal distension begins or baby does not pass stool for 24 hours.[4]

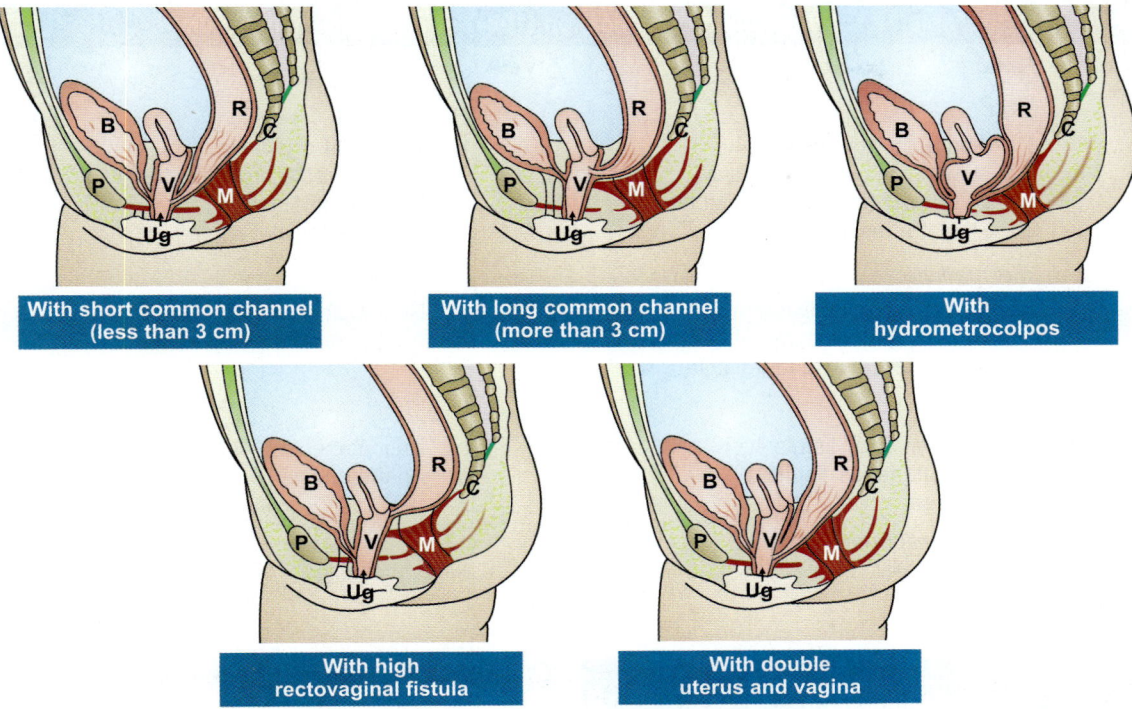

Fig. 72.4: Anatomy of cloacal malformations showing level of fistula and relation to sphincter muscle

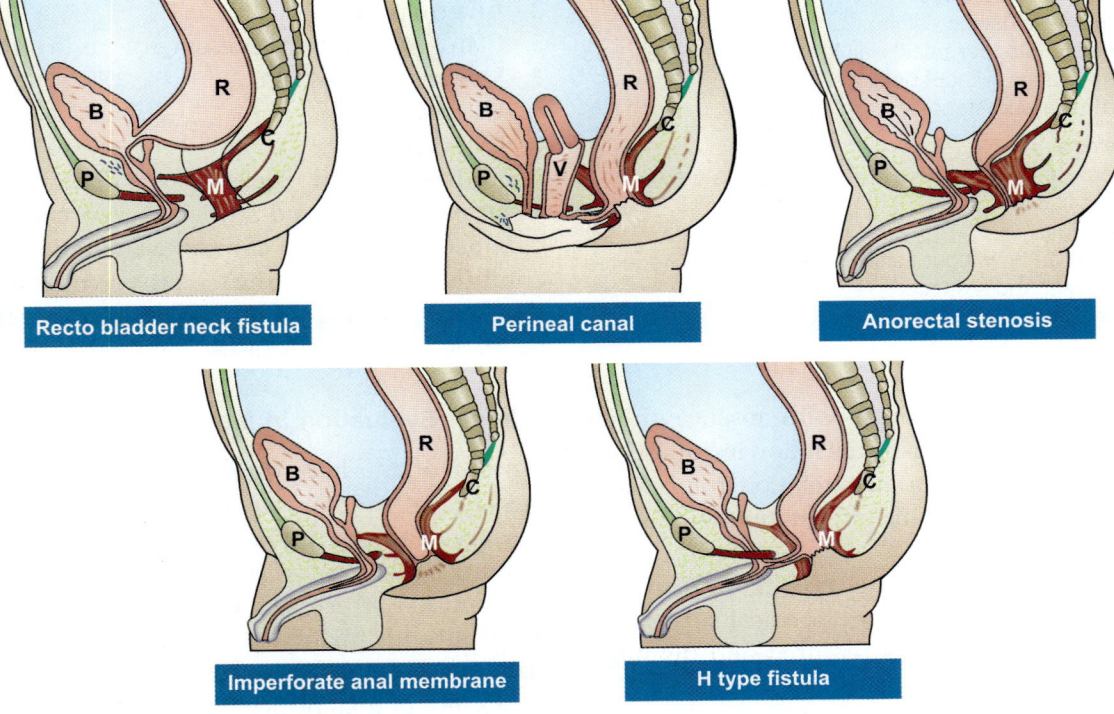

Fig. 72.5: Rare ARM showing level of fistula and relation to sphincter muscle

Table 72.1: Wingspread classification (1984) of anorectal malformations

Female	Male
High	*High*

1. Anorectal agenesis
   a. with rectovaginal fistula
   b. without rectovaginal fistula
2. Rectal atresia
	1. Anorectal agenesis
	   a. with recto-prostatic urethral fistula
	   b. without fistula
	2. Rectal atresia

Intermediate	*Intermediate*
1. Rectovestibular fistula 2. Rectovaginal fistula 3. Anal agenesis without fistula	1. Rectobulbar urethral fistula 2. Anal agenesis without fistula
Low	*Low*
1. Anovestibular fistula 2. Anocutaneous fistula 3. Anal stenosis	1. Anocutaneous fistula 2. Anal stenosis
Cloacal malformations *Rare anomalies*	*Rare anomalies*

Table 72.2: Pena's classification of anorectal malformations

Male defects

1. Cutaneous fistula and stenosis, anal membrane	No colostomy
2. Rectourethral bulbar fistula 3. Rectourethral prostatic fistula 4. Rectovesical (bladder neck) fistula 5. Imperforate anus without fistula 6. Rectal atresia and stenosis	Colostomy is required

Female defects

1. Cutaneous (perineal fistula)	No colostomy
2. Vestibular fistula 3. Vaginal fistula 4. Imperforate anus without fistula 5. Rectal atresia and stenosis 6. Persistent cloaca	Colostomy is required

Initial assessment of a neonate with absence of anal opening is aimed at answering the following questions:

A. What is the level of rectum, in relation to sphincters and where is fistula. This information will help in deciding.
 1. Can the anomaly be corrected without colostomy by single stage perineal surgery?
 2. Whether colostomy is required and definitive surgery is to be done later on?
B. Is there any other associated anomaly which needs immediate or subsequent correction?
C. What is the integrity of neuromuscular component?

Assessment of level of malformation, and fistula in relation to sphincters can be done by:[12]
1. Clinical examination of baby and examination of urine in males
2. Invertogram
3. Plan X-ray showing presence of gas in other viscera
4. Dye study of fistula
5. Ultrasound
6. CT scan
7. Endoscopy and Electromyography.

In neonatal period sufficient information can be obtained with careful clinical examination alone and combined with findings of invertogram, correct decision regarding initial operative management can be made in almost all cases.

Clinical Evaluation in Male

Mother of the baby may give information about passage of meconeum per urethra (meconuria), passage of air per urethra (pneumaturia) or history of staining of clothing with meconeum coming out from unidentified orifice. Occasionally, baby is brought to hospital with history of abdominal distension and absolute constipation since birth absolutely unaware of absence of anal orifice. In India, it is not rare to see patients with ARM reaching hospital with perforation-peritonitis, severe respiratory distress and septicemia.

History of regurgitation of feeds with drooling of saliva may be present if the patient of ARM has associated esophageal atresia.

In addition to general examination and assessment of associated anomalies local inspection of perineum may reveal valuable information regarding the type of anomaly and level of rectum. Perineal inspection should always be done under good shadowless light with baby held in lithotomy position and if needed magnifying glass may be used for inspection of median raphe.

Inspection starts at the point where normal anal opening should have been present and proceeds anteriorly along the medium raphe. Appearance of perineum, natal cleft, and presence of skin fold or pigmentation at anal dimple, configuration of genitalia and presence of an orifice on medium raphe from frenulum to anal dimple are noted. Careful inspection of perineum will reveal either of the three possibilities

1. Absent anal orifice with clinical evidence of perineal or urethral fistula.
2. Normal looking anal orifice with anorectal malformation.
3. Absent anal orifice with no external evidence to indicate the level of rectum and fistula. In this group presence of meconeum or squamous epithelial cells in voided urine sample may provide the clue. If urine examination is also normal, invertogram is must for decision making.

Description of physical sign and diagnosis by inspection of perineum with management decision in male ARM is given in Table 72.3.

Pena has described a decision making algorithm for ARM in male.[13] It essentially gives three options.
  i. A perineal fistula indicates low malformation and baby can be managed with anoplasty without colostomy.
  ii. Meconeum in urine indicates recto-urethral fistula and initial colostomy is needed followed by definitive surgery.

In case no perineal fistula and no meconeum in urine is discovered further decision making is based on Invertogram/prone cross table X-ray findings.

Clinical Evaluation in Female

In female patients with ARM, almost always mother will complain that baby passes stool through genital orifice with absence of anal opening.

Rare anomaly like anorectal agenesis without fistula and rectal atresia will present with abdominal distension. Patients with perineal canal will present with history of passage of stool through normal anal orifice and genital orifice as well.

Decision-making involving opening of colostomy in female is an easier process and rarely radiological investigations are needed. By and large female ARM will have a fistulous communication through which they pass meconeum and diagnosis can nearly always be predicted by examination of genitalia and perineum.

For perineal inspection, importance of good shadowless light, adequate prior cleaning of genitalia and vestibule which may be full of stool or meconeum and identification of abnormal orifice in vestibule by probing with lubricated red rubber catheter or hegar's dilator cannot be overemphasized.

In cases of closed vulva repeat examination under general anesthesia and midline division of fused labial folds may be needed.[12] Description of findings of perineal inspection, diagnosis and decision-making is given in Table 72.4.

In malformations without fistula which is very rare, help of invertogram or prone cross table X-ray is sought for decision-making process.

Invertogram

Invertogram is the single most important investigation that helps in deciding the level of rectum in relation to sphincters. The use of plain radiograph for determination of level of rectal pouch was first described by Wangensteen and Rice in 1930 and subsequently modified by Stephen in 1953, Kelly in 1969.[14-16]

Basic Principle

Soon after birth, with each breath, baby starts swallowing air which traverses through the gastrointestinal tract to reach the rectum in 4 to 12 hours and by 18 hours rectum is well distended. X-ray, true lateral view of the pelvis at birth shows following relevant bony landmarks.
  1. Anterior most boomerang shaped shadow is casted by superior pubic ramii and ospubis. The angle of junction of the boomerang corresponds to upper border of pubic symphysis which forms the p point (The ossification of the pubis

Table 72.3: Decision making in male ARM

Absent anal orifice with evidence of fistula

Findings	Diagnosis	Decision
Pinpoint orifice on median raphe (Fig. 72.6A)	Anocutaneous fistula (rarely recto cutaneous fistula) (Perineal fistula according to Pena's classification)	Anoplasty No colostomy
Fly speck of meconeum and passage of gas bubble through minute orifice on median raphe (Fig. 72.6B)	-do-	-do-
Fine bluish line on median raphe (Meconeum trapped along the track of median raphe) (Fig. 72.6C)	-do-	-do-
White epithelial pearls on median raphe (Fig. 72.7A)	-do-	-do-
Stenotic anal orifice hidden in folds at normal anal site (Fig. 72.7B)	Covered anus (anal stenosis)	-do-
Bucket handle band deformity (Fig. 72.7C) with meconeum/staining/without meconeum stain	Covered anus (anal stenosis) inpredictable	-do-
Meconeum shining through thin skin (Fig. 72.8A)	Covered anus	-do-
Massage of bulbar urethra revealing meconeum at external meatus (Black eye urethra) (Fig. 72.8B)	Rectobulbar urethral fistula	Colostomy
Atypical hypospadias with cleft scrotum (Fig. 72.8C)	Rectobulbar uretheral fistula (Confirmation with invertogram needed)	Colostomy
Meconeum jelly or squamous epithelial cells in voided urine	High ARM	Colostomy

ARM with normal looking anus

Normal looking anal orifice but anteriorly placed and patent (tested by passing lubricated red rubber catheter) (Fig. 72.8D)	Anterior ectopic anus	Anoplasty
Normal looking anus but red rubber catheter could not be passed beyond 2 cm (Figs 72.9A and B)	Rectal atresia	Rectal atresia colostomy
Normal looking anus but red rubber catheter could not be passed beyond dentate line Presence of bulging anal membrane at dentate line	Imperforate anal membrane (rare)	Anoplasty
Passage of ribbon stools with narrowing at dentate line	Anal membrane stenosis (rare) Anorectal stenosis (rare)	Anoplasty Colostomy

ARM with no external evidence of level of rectum

No meconeum in urine	Diagnosis not predicted	Invertogram
No external clinical evidence		

begins at second fetal month under the acetabulum and extends along the superior ramus to body.

2. Posterior most bony shadows are five ossified segments of sacrum, fifth sacral segment at birth appears as small ossific ring (ossification begins at 4th mouth of gestation) coccyx is not ossified at birth hence not visible, but a point just caudal (5 mm) to fifth ossific center of sacrum corresponds to coccyx and is marked as C point. Line drawn between P and C point is called pubococcygeal line (PC line).

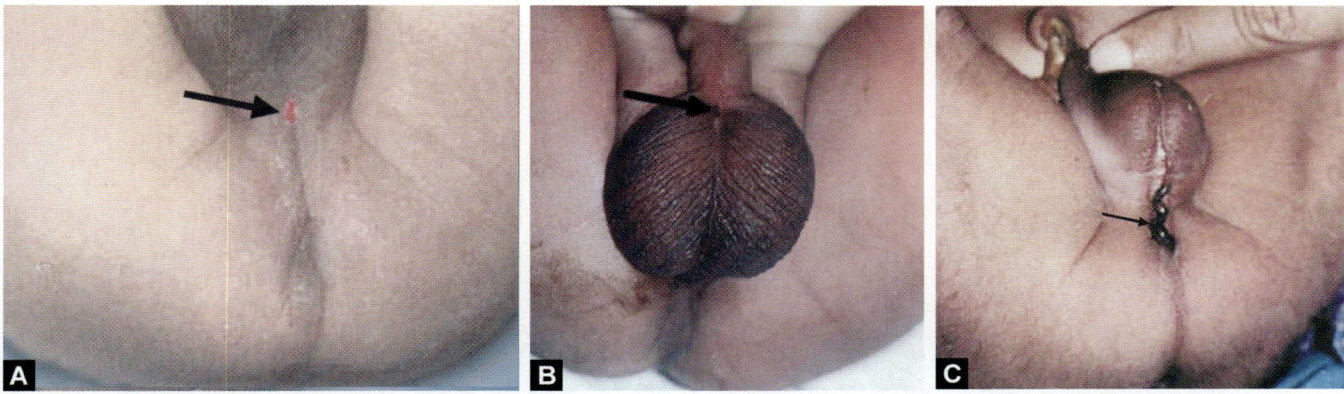

Figs 72.6A to C: A. Pin point orifice on median raphe in a case of low ARM with anocutaneous fistula **B.** Fly speck of meconeum seen through minute orifice on median raphe at penoscrotal junction in a case of low ARM with anocutaneous fistula **C.** Fine bluish line on median raphe seen (meconeum trapped along the track) in a case of anocutaneous fistula

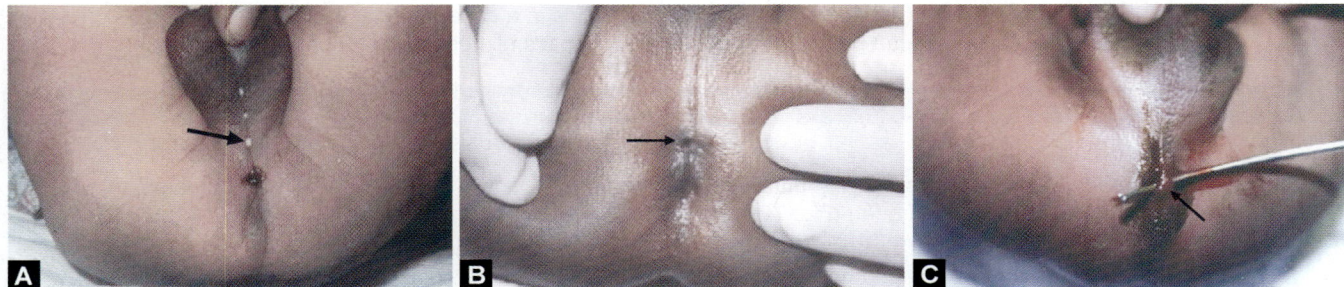

Figs 72.7A to C: A. White epithelial pearls seen on median raphe with fly-speck of meconeum in a case of anocutaneous fistula **B.** Covered anus with anal stenosis; stenotic anal orifice seen hidden in folds at anal dimple **C.** Covered anus with bucket handle deformity. Bucket handle skin fold is lifted up on Hegar's dilator

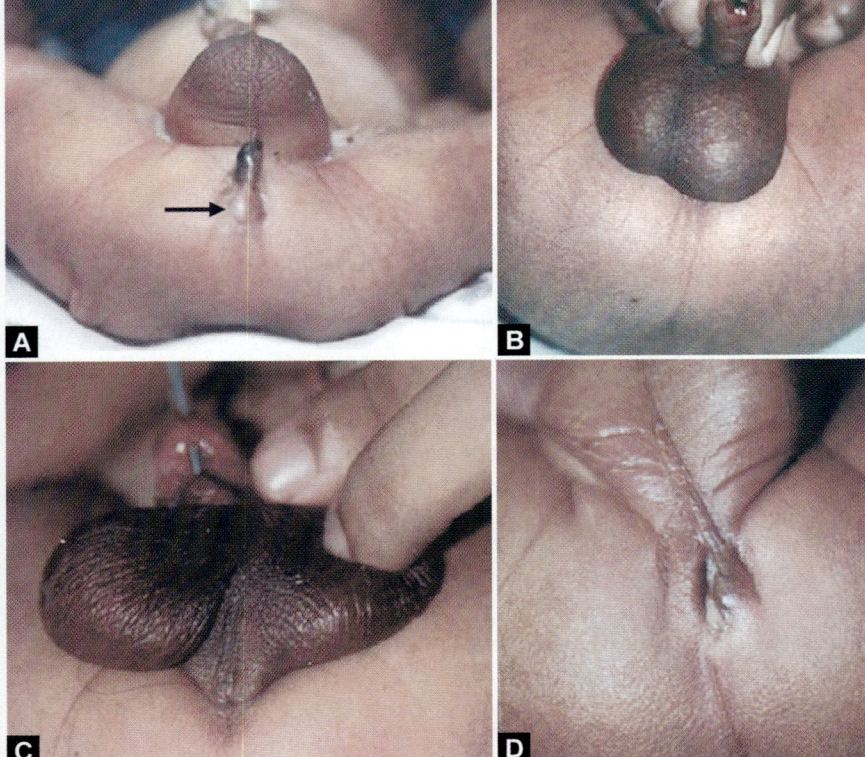

Figs 72.8A to D: A. Meconeum shining through thin skin at anal dimple and median raphe in a case of low ARM **B.** Black eye urethra in a case of intermediate ARM with rectobulbar urethral fistula **C.** A case of atypical hypospadias with cleft scrotum; the patient had rectobulbar urethral fistula **D.** Anterior ectopic anus; normal looking anal orifice but anteriorly placed. Patient presented with constipation

796 Pediatric Surgery—Diagnosis and Management

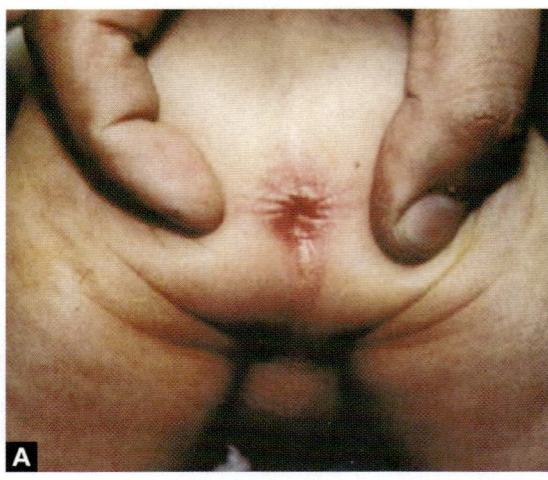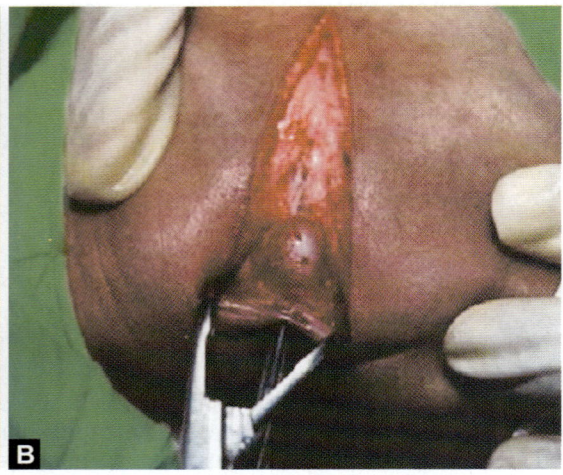

Figs 72.9A and B: A. Normal looking anal orifice in a case of rectal atresia **B.** Blind anal canal can be seen during PSARP. Hegar's dilator stops at 2 cm depth

Table 72.4: Decision making in female ARM

Findings	Diagnosis	Decision
A. Only one orifice seen in vestibule discharging urine and meconeum. Separate vaginal and anal orifice not seen (Fig. 72.10A)	Cloaca	Colostomy
B. Two orifices seen (Fig. 72.10B): (1) Urethral orifice; (2) Vaginal orifice Stool coming out of vagina, third opening not present in vestibule	Rectovaginal fistula (rarely rectovestibular fistula with vaginal atresia) (Fig. 72.10C)	Colostomy
C. Three orifices seen separately: • Urethral orifice; • Vaginal orifice Third orifice seen either as fistula or as normal anus	Diagnosis and decision is given below	
I. Third orifice present as vestibular fistula		
i. Hegar's dilator put in vestibular orifice goes upwards and its tip cannot be palpated at anal dimple (Figs 72.11A and B)	Rectovestibular fistula	ASARP / Colostomy
ii. Three orifices seen • Urethral • Vaginal • Vestibular Hegar's dilator in vestibular orifice goes posteriorly and its tip palpable at anal dimple (Figs 72.12A and B).	Anovestibular fistula (Vulvar anus - Anovulvar fistula)	ASARP - no colostomy
iii. Four orifices seen (Fig. 72.13A) • Urethral orifice • Two vaginal orifice • Vestibular orifice	Rectovestibular fistula with septate vagina	Colostomy / ASARP
II- Third Orifice seen outside vestibule (Perineal fistula)		
i. Normal caliber third orifice sited forward in perineum near the vulva (Fig. 72.13B)	Anterior perineal anus	Anoplasty No colostomy
ii. Stenotic anal orifice present anteriorly	Anocutaneous fistula (Fig. 72.13C)	Anoplasty No colostomy

Contd...

Contd...

	IIIa. Third orifice seen as normal anal orifice (No intestinal obstruction)		
i.	Stool coming out from anal orifice as well as vestibular fistula	Perineal canal (Fig. 72.14) No colostomy	ASARP
ii.	Normal anal orifice with red moist groove between anus and fourchette	Perineal groove	Anoplasty No colostomy
	IIIb- Third orifice seen as normal anal orifice (with intestinal obstruction)		
i.	Anal orifice present but with intestinal obstruction. Red rubber catheter can not be passed beyond 2 cm	Rectal atresia	Colostomy
ii.	Anal orifice present but with intestinal obstruction. Red rubber catheter can not be passed beyond 1 cm	Imperforate anal membrane	Anoplasty
iii.	Anal orifice present but with intestinal obstruction. Red rubber catheter can not be passed beyond 1 cm with ribbon stool.	Anal membrane stenosis (rarely anorectal stenosis)	Anoplasty
iv.	Third orifice seen as stenotic anal orifice	Covered anal stenosis	Anoplasty
	IV- No external orifice or fistula seen (rare)		
i.	No orifice discovered with absence of anus (rare) (Fig. 72.15)	Diagnosis can not be predicted	Investogram

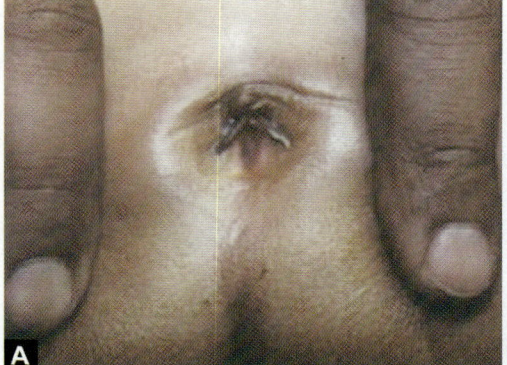 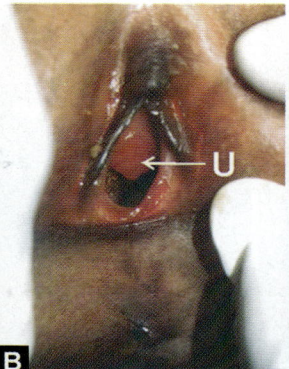 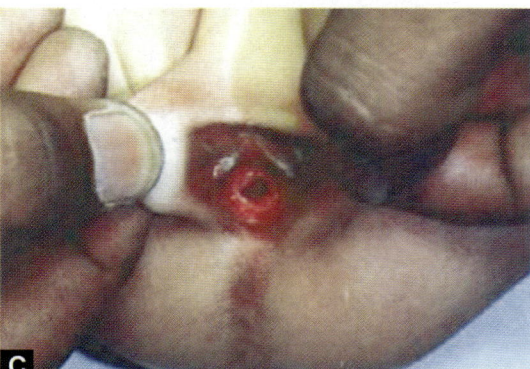

Figs 72.10A to C: A. Appearance of perineum in a case of cloaca; only one orifice is seen **B.** Perineal appearance in rectovaginal fistula. Urethral meatus (U) is seen separate from vaginal orifice. Stool is coming out from vaginal orifice **C.** Perineal appearance in a case of rectovestibular fistula with vaginal atresia; urethral and vestibular orifices are seen

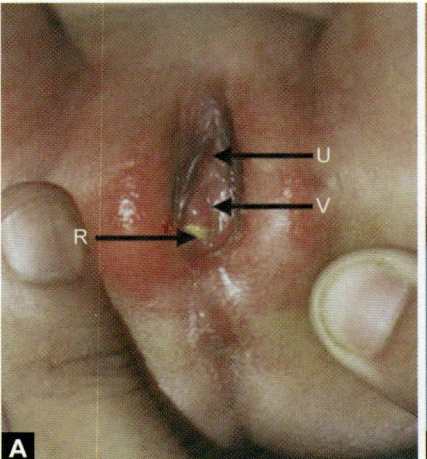 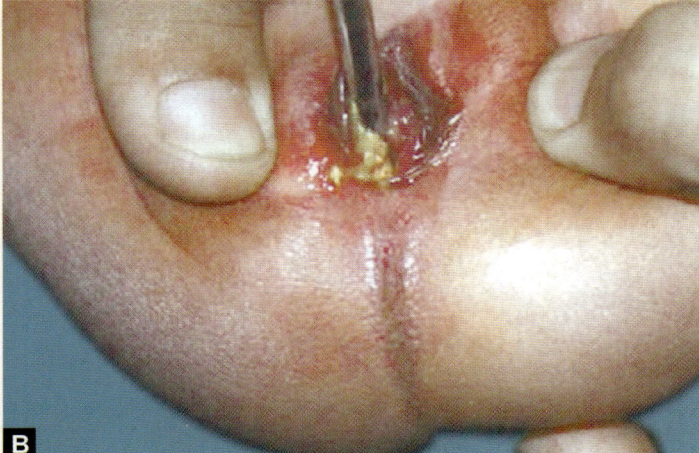

Figs 72.11A and B: A. Rectovestibular fistula. Examination reveals urethral meatus (U), vaginal orifice (V) and third vestibular orifice (R) from which stool is coming out **B.** Hegar's dilator passed through vestibular fistula goes cranially parallel to vagina and its tip is not palpable at anal dimple

798 Pediatric Surgery—Diagnosis and Management

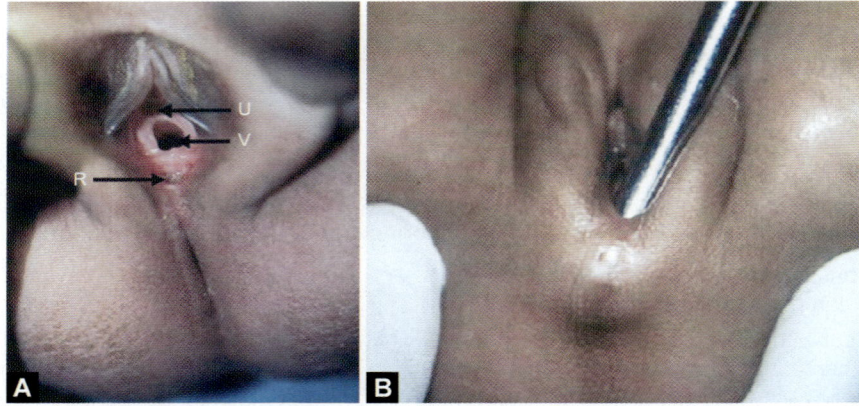

Figs 72.12A and B: A. Anovestibular fistula, urthral orifice (U), vaginal orifice (V) and third vestibular (R) orifice seen, **B.** Hegar's dilator in vestibular fistula goes posteriorly and its tip can be palpated at anal dimple

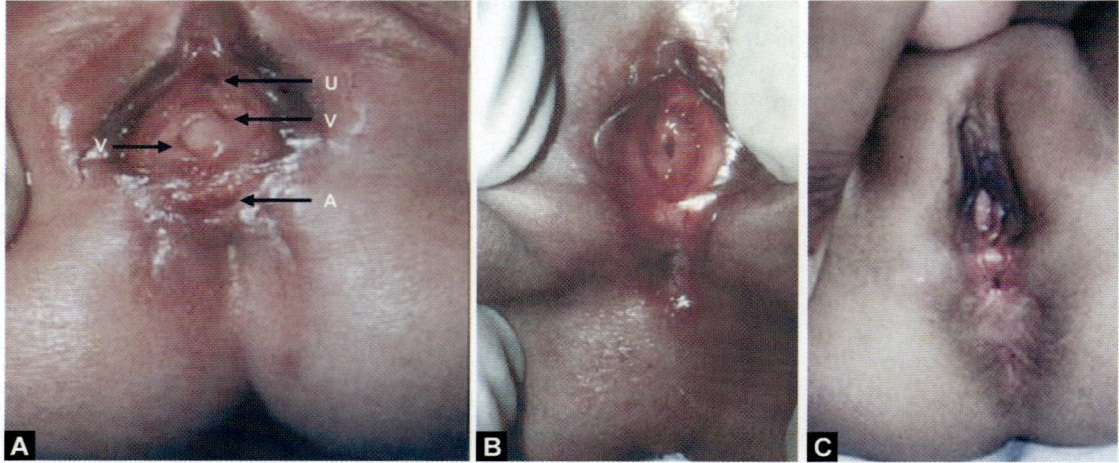

Figs 72.13A to C: A. Perineal appearance in case of anovestibular fistula with septate vagina. Urethral orifice (U), two vaginal orifices (V) and fourth vestibular orifice (A) is seen, **B.** Anterior perineal anus; normal calibre anus sited forward in perineum near the vulva, **C.** Anocutaneous fistula; stenotic and anteriorly placed anal orifice

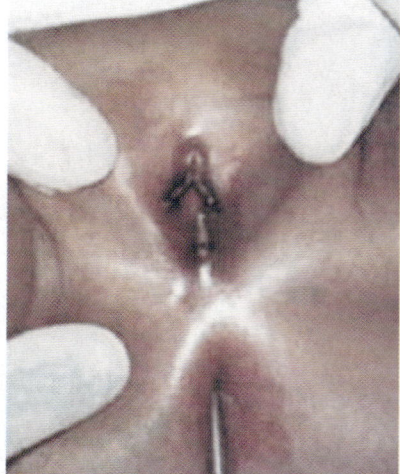

Fig. 72.14: Perineal canal; Hegar's dilator can be passed through fistula between vestibule and anal canal

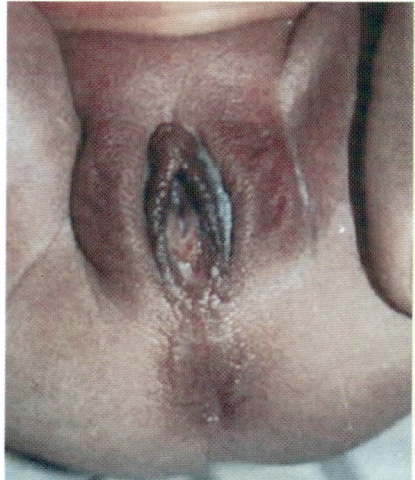

Fig. 72.15: A case of female ARM with no fistula, invertogram revealed intermediate malformation

3. In between P point and C point comma shaped shadow of ossified ischium is seen and PC line crosses it through the junction of caudal 3/4 and cranial 1/4 of ischial shadow. Anterior and inferior end of ischial comma is marked as I point. In cases of sacral agenesis PC line can be drawn between P point and the points at the junction of caudal 3/4 and cranial 1/4 of ischial comma (Fig. 72.16).

Stephens has demonstrated that *PC line* crosses through bladder neck, verumontanum, peritoneal reflection from prostate to rectum in male (Fig. 72.17). In female PC line crosses through bladder neck, external os of cervix and peritoneal reflection from vagina to rectum. Puborectalis and diaphragm part of levator lie caudal to PC line (Fig. 72.18).

Technique

For correct interpretation, invertogram should not be done before 18 hours of birth and relevant points in technique should be adhered to.

A true lateral view with accurate centering on greater trochanter is essential to ensure that two shadows of faintly ossified centers of pubes are superimposed with superimposition of shadows of two ischial bones.

The baby should be held upside-down for 3 minutes to allow displacement of meconeum and accumulation of gas in terminal rectal pouch. A marker or thin barium smear accurately applied at natal cleft on anal dimple helps in measurement of skin bowel distance in invertogram film.

Repeat films may be taken if gas shadow remains proximal to ischial line and abdominal distension is minimal.

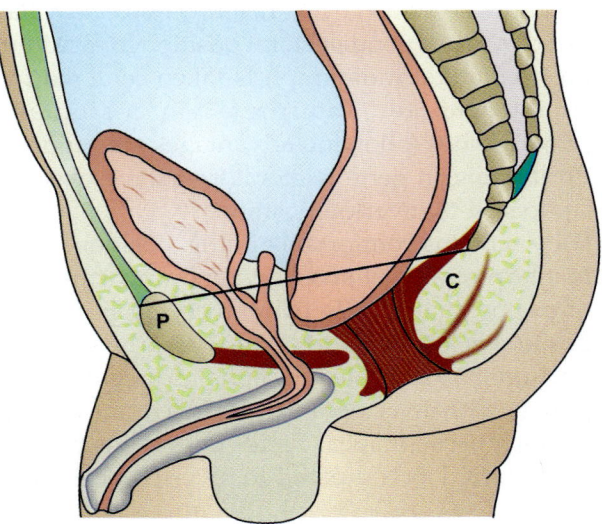

Fig. 72.17: Diagram shows PC line crosses bladder neck and peritoneal reflection from prostate to rectum in male

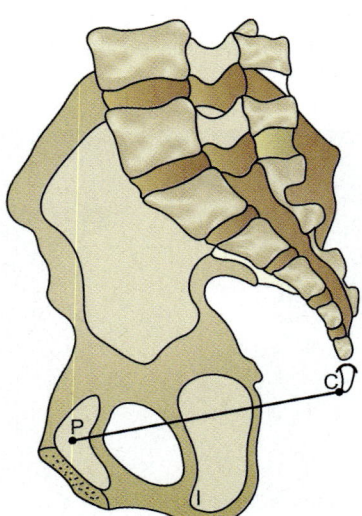

Fig. 72.16: Illustration shows medial surface of right innominate bone and sacrum. Ossified area at birth are marked as yellow color. P point, I point, and C point are marked. Pubococcygeal line crosses the junction of upper ¼ and lower ¾ of ossified ischial tuberosity

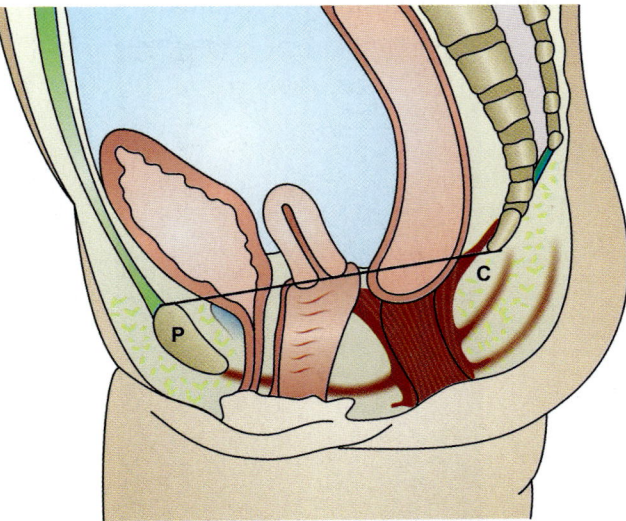

Fig. 72.18: Diagram to illustrate PC line crossing bladder neck, external os of cervix and peritoneal reflection from vagina to rectum in female

If X-ray is taken earlier than 18 hours, time allowed after inversion is less than 3 minutes, meconeum remains stuck to terminal rectum, active contraction of pulsorectalis occurs or gas escapes through fistula an intermediate or low ARM may be wrongly interpreted as high anomaly.

Prone Cross-table Lateral X-ray

An alternative to invertogram is prone cross table lateral X-ray described by Narasimha Rao et al.[17] Baby is placed in prone genu pectoral position for 3 minutes and a true lateral radiograph is taken centered over greater trochanter. Interpretation is similar to invertogram but following advantages are reported:
1. Positioning in genu pectoral position is easier as compared to inverted position.
2. Baby remains comfortable in this position, fallacy in interpretation of invertogram due to contraction of puborectalis while baby is crying in inverted position is less likely to occur with prone position.
3. Rectum may be pulled in cephalic direction due to gravity with invertogram but not in prone position.
4. In tracheo-esophageal fistula prone position will be preferred as compared to inverted position.

Interpretation

I. Gas shadow ends proximal to PC line → High anomaly → Colostomy is required (Fig. 72.19).
II. Gas shadow ends in between two lines → intermediate anomaly → Colostomy is required (Fig. 72.20).
III. Gas shadow crossing the I point → Low anomaly → Perineal proctoplasty is required - no colostomy (Fig. 72.21).

In place of anatomical landmarks, Pena prefers to measure skin bowel distance which if shorter than 1 cm, anomaly is treated as low and if skin bowel

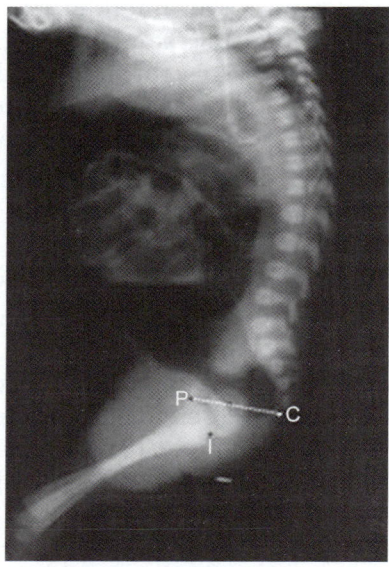

Fig. 72.20: Invertogram of a case of intermediate malformation. Gas shadow in rectum has crossed the PC line but remains proximal to I point

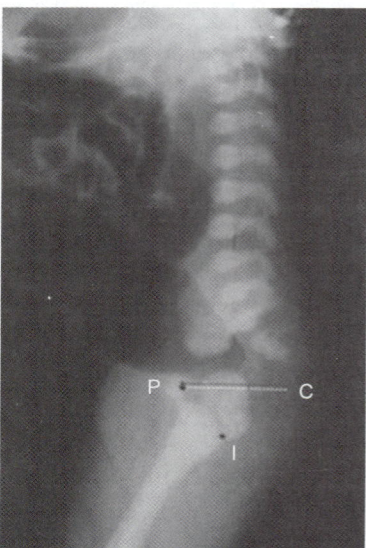

Fig. 72.19: Invertogram of a patient of high ARM with partial sacral agenesis. PC line is drawn through P point transacting the shadow of ischial tuberosity at the junction of cranial ¼ and caudal ¾. Rectal gas shadow is above the PC line

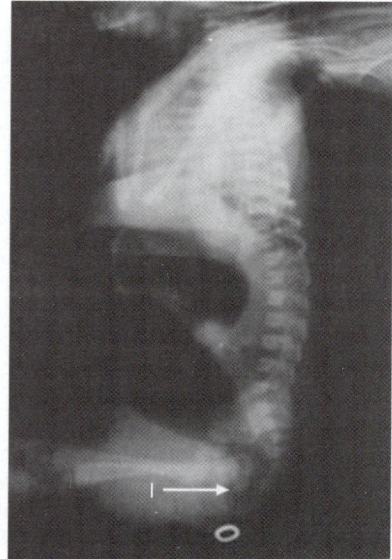

Fig. 72.21: Invertogram of case of low ARM, rectal gas shadow has crossed well beyond the I point

distance is more than 1 cm, colostomy is recommended, however, author finds use of anatomical landmarks a more reliable method in decision making (Fig. 72.22). It may not be possible to accurately identify the 'P' point if the centering of patient is inaccurate. If identification of 'P' point becomes difficult, even in repeated films either because of inaccurate centering or due to superimposition of shadow of femur specially in prone cross table lateral films, decision regarding creation of colostomy versus anoplasty can be made by observing the rectal gas shadow in relation to 'I' point.

Apart from rectal gas shadow, study of distribution of gas in other viscera in anteroposterior and lateral films may provide valuable information. Presence of congenital short colon is diagnosed if single large gas shadow occupies half of the abdominal width in anteroposterior film (Fig. 72.23). Presence of gas in bladder may indicate rectovesical fistula (Fig. 72.24).

Ultrasound Examination

Abdominal ultrasound will help in assessing genitourinary anomalies while perineal ultrasound can help to decide the distance between skin and rectal pouch as an alternative or supplement to information provided by invertogram.[18,19]

Dye Study of Fistula (Figs 72.25A and B)

It is not an essential investigation because site of external visible orifice mostly indicates the pattern of internal anatomy. However, in female ARM it may be helpful in distinguishing rectovestibular from anovestibular fistula and the investigation can be used for assessment of length of fistula specially in cases of anorectal stenosis.

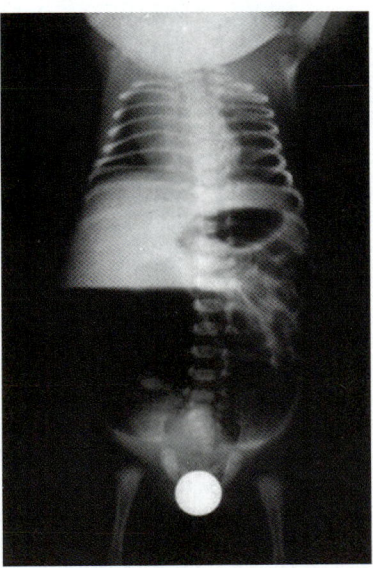

Fig. 72.23: Congenital short colon; inverted X-ray AP view shows single large gas shadow occupying half of the width of abdomen

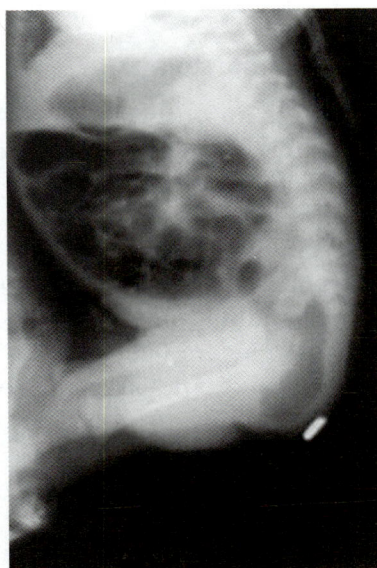

Fig. 72.22: Invertogram of a case of low ARM; skin bowel distance is less than 1 cm

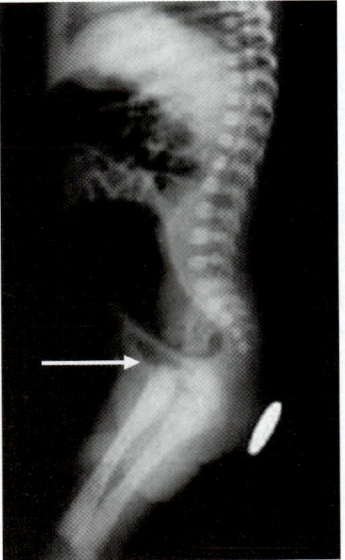

Fig. 72.24: Invertogram showing presence of air in urinary bladder. Patient had rectovesical fistula

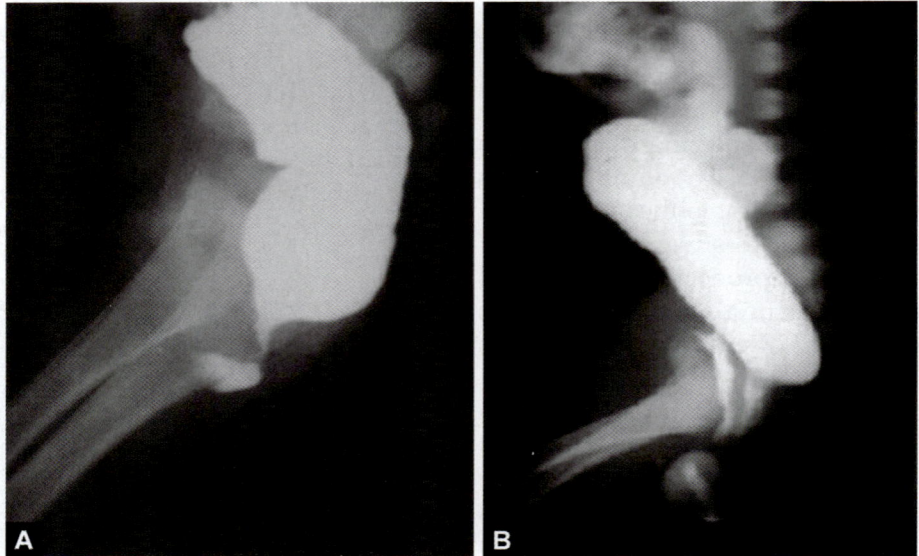

Figs 72.25A and B: Dye study in a case of vestibular fistula - **A.** Anovestibular fistula. **B.** Rectovestibular fistula - long narrow fistula runs parallel to vagina

Direct percutaneous needle aspiration and injection of contrast in the rectal pouch have been described but in practice we do not prefer it because of invasiveness of the procedure while other non-invasive methods are quite satisfactory.

Finally, it cannot be overemphasized that in case level of rectum is not certain and doubt persists after investigations, a colostomy is done to leave the sphincters intact for subsequent planning and appropriate surgery. Currently, it is inexcusable to explore the perineum blindly and cause irreversible damage to continence mechanism.

Preliminary Assessment of Associated Anomalies in Neonatal Period

In addition to examination of a neonate, as a whole; recording gestational age, weight, temperature, color, cry, respiration, jaundice, abdominal distension, signs of respiratory distress, septicemia and dehydration, one should look for any other associated occult congenital malformation in general, and VACTERL syndrome in particular [V = Vertebral; A = Anorectal; C = Cardiac; TE = Tracheo-esophageal fistula with esophageal atresia; R = Radial and Renal, and L = Limb or skeletal anomalies]. Some of these anomalies are life threatening and need immediate correction. Esophageal atresia should be ruled out by passage of no. 8 red rubber catheter down to stomach. Plain X-ray of baby on a large plate will quickly reveal condition of chest, abdomen, short colon, presence of gas in other viscera and an overview of spine and skeletal anomaly. If general condition of baby permits and facility is available, emergency ultrasound and echocardiography may be included in part of neonatal assessment.

Assessment after Colostomy

Patients with high or intermediate ARM with colostomy are subjected to further investigations before planning definitive reconstruction. Purpose of the investigations are following :

Once acute emergency is over and intestinal obstruction is relieved detailed assessment of baby with colostomy is aimed at obtaining maximum possible information regarding:
1. Configuration, size and level of rectum and information regarding presence or absence of fistula.
2. Integrity of neuromuscular component and development of sphincters.
3. Detailed evaluation of urogenital system, spine, heart and other associated anomalies :

The most important investigation after colostomy is distal cologram which provides excellent information about the level of rectum and presence or absence of fistula.

Distal cologram: Keiller was first to use barium suspension into the distal limb of colostomy to demonstrate the site of fistula but in current practice a water soluble contrast medium is used in place of barium.[20]

Before performing this valuable investigation distal loop of colostomy should be thoroughly washed with saline ensuring complete evacuation of any residual fecal matter in the rectum. Cologram performed with residual meconeum or feces in the rectum will give inaccurate information regarding level of rectum and fistula will not be demonstrated even if it is present.

A Foley catheter is passed in distal stoma of colostomy and balloon is sufficiently inflated to block the distal lumen, purpose is to prevent reflux of contrast outside the distal stoma while injecting the contrast medium under pressure.

Patient is positioned to obtain true lateral view of the pelvis.

Organic iodine solution (we prefer urograffin 76% diluted with equal volume of saline) is pushed in distal lumen under pressure through Foley's catheter.

Volume of contrast instilled in distal lumen should be sufficient enough to distend the rectum under pressure for demonstration of exact level of rectum and fistula is opened up under pressure even if it is narrow.

Inadequate volume of contrast not injected under pressure will give false information regarding the level of rectum and presence of fistula.

Cologram, performed with precision, provides excellent information regarding shape, size and level of rectum with delineation of size and site of fistula, which is of immense value while performing the definitive repair (Figs 72.26A to 72.27B).

Micturating cystourethrography and retrograde urethrogram (MCU and RGU): Combined with cologram (MCU and RGU), can provide better information regarding the site of fistula. It will also provide information regarding vesicoureteric reflux and other associated anomaly in bladder and urethra.

Assessment of Sphincters and its Nerve Supply

Radiograph of the sacrum and lumbar spine are obtained for assessment of levator muscle. Smith has described a closed relationship between development of sacrum and extent of formation of levator muscle.[12]

i. Normal spine and well developed all segments of sacrum are the indicators of normal levator function and innervation.
ii. Deficiency of fourth and fifth sacral vertebrae usually allow normal innervation of bladder and levator.
iii. Deficiency of third, fourth and fifth sacral vertebrae is associated with variable innervation

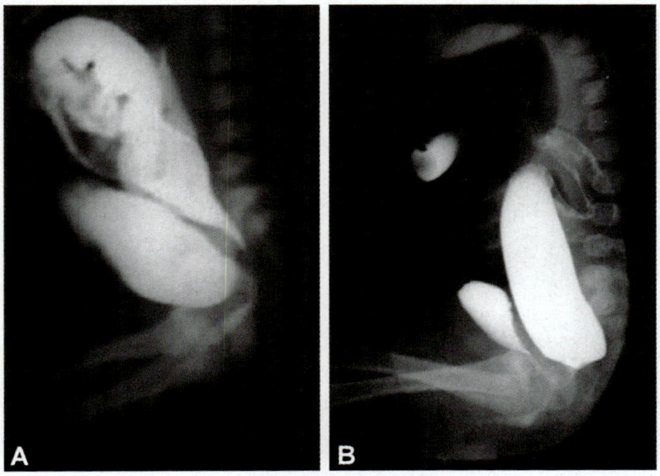

Figs 72.26A and B: A. Distal cologram; rectovesical fistula **B.** Distal cologram; rectoprostatic urethral fistula is present, contrast has gone into bladder and urethra

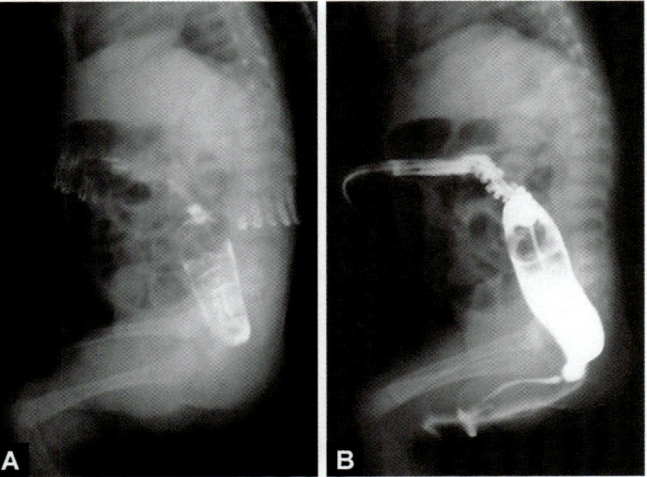

Figs 72.27A and B: A. Distal cologram performed with insufficient volume and pressure fails to demonstrate the fistula **B.** Repeat film with adequate volume of contrast and pressure has demonstrated recto bulbar-urethral fistula

and muscle development, most patients are incontinent.

iv. Deficiency of first and second sacral segment is always associated with incontinence.
v. Presence of lumbosacral myelomeningocele is almost always associated with serious defect in innervation.
vi. Presence of hemisacral defects is associated variable innervation and muscle development.

In order to improve the prognostic accuracy Pena has devised a sacral ratio based on sacral abnormalities.[10] One ratio calculated from anteroposterior and lateral radiograph of sacrum in children with good prognosis is about 0.7-0.8 but those with a ratio of less than 0.4 tend to have high malformation with poor functional prognosis (Fig. 72.28).

Assessment of Sphincters with Magnetic Resonance Imaging (MRI)/Computerized Tomography (CT) Scan

With use of MRI and CT scans, components of sphincter can be visualized and their quality can be assessed before surgery. Level of rectum in relation to sphincter can be visualized in sagittal cut MRI (Figs 72.29A and B). The value of CT scan for patients

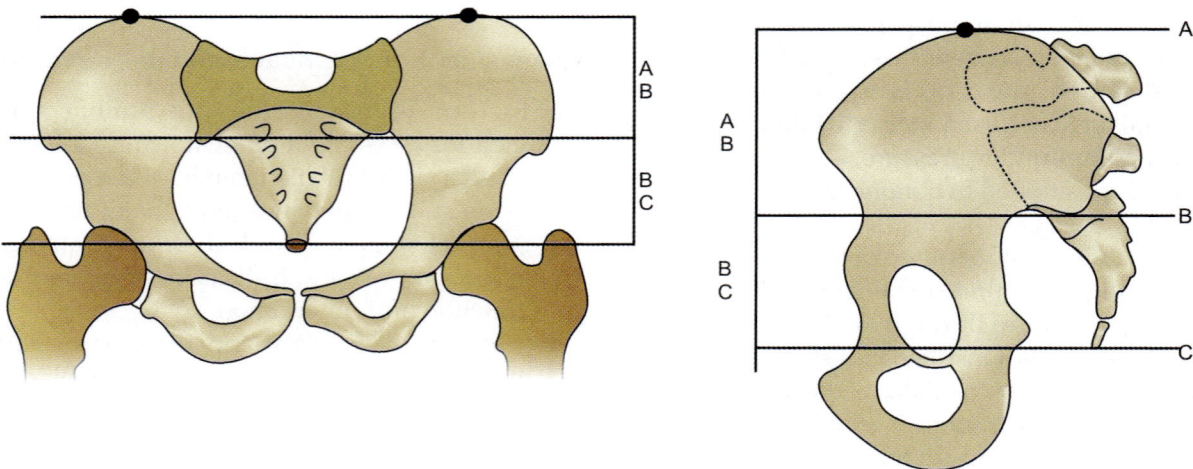

Fig. 72.28: Diagram to show calculation of sacral ratio. Line A drawn through highest point of iliac crest, line B through lower most point of sacroiliac joint and line C passes through coccyx. Ratio of AB/BC should be 0.7 to 0.8. Ratio of less than 0.4 indicates poor prognosis (from Pena)

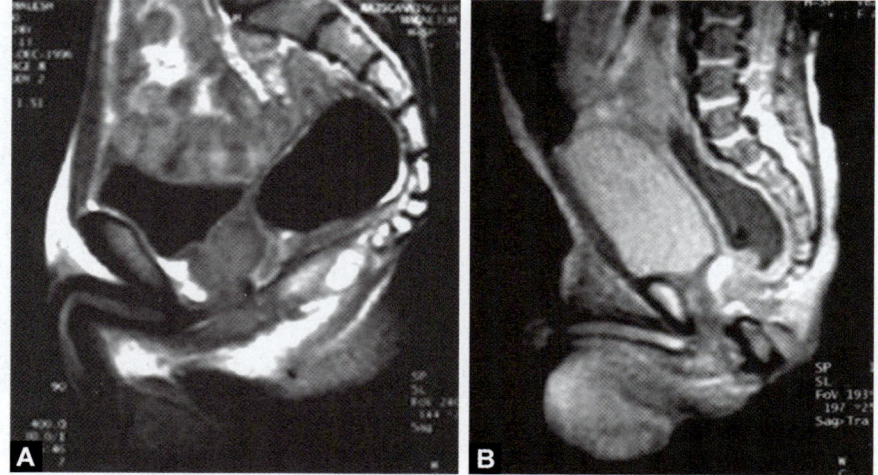

Figs 72.29A and B: A. MRI: Sagittal cut study in case of recto prostatic urethral fistula patient presented at the age of 20 year for definitive repair **B.** MRI: Sagittal cut study in a case of rectal atresia. Distance between proximal rectum, distal and canal is well demonstrated

with anorectal malformation was first reported by Ikawa in 1985.[21,22] Pringle in 1987 reported use of MRI in delineating the anatomy of sphincters before and after corrective surgery.[23] Since then numerous reports on role of CT/MRI scan have come up describing the morphology of sphincters. Before performing the definite surgery, CT/MRI imaging of sphincters helps in better planning of definitive surgery.[24-27] After surgery objective demonstration of deviation or placement of the rectum in the muscle complex is best possible with CT and MRI.

Sacral Outflow Tests for Sphincter Innervations

Second, third and fourth sacral segments innervate levator ani, sphincters, bladder parasympathetics and perineal dermatomes. Therefore, analysis of bladder and perineal sensation may provide important information about hidden pelvic floor innervation. History of voiding pattern may reveal almost continuous dribbling or overflow leakage. Bladder expressibility is most constant sign of paretic bladder. Presence of expressible bladder with or without bladder lamp heralds poor innervation of pelvic musculature.

Perineal sensations: Absence of response to pin prick sensation indicates defective innervation, however, normal perineal sensation does not mean normal sphincters.

Detailed Assessment of Genitourinary System, Spine and Heart

Children with ARM have a high incidence of genitourinary and lumbosacral spine anomalies. Some genitourinary anomalies are associated in approximately 66-71% in high ARM and 25% in low ARM.[28] Vesicoureteric reflux, voiding dysfunction and sacral agenesis being more common. Therefore, ultrasound examination or IVP, micturating cystourethrogram and urodynamic studies are desirable.[28] Cardiac anomalies most commonly encountered are ventricular septal defect, patent ductus arteriosus, atrial septal defect and tetralogy of Fallot's should be identified and will effect the survival.[29]

Associated Defects

These have been dealt with in a chapter 74.

OPERATIVE MANAGEMENT OF LOW ANORECTAL MALFORMATIONS AND SINGLE STAGE PERINEAL REPAIR

Low anorectal malformations are easier to correct because rectum and anal canal are well developed with its sensory receptors and is embraced by the striated muscle complex for control of defecation. The muscles are mostly well developed without loss of innervation or sacral vertebral segments. The surgical procedure is basically aimed at re-establishing a satisfactory anal orifice at normal site by simple perineal anoplasty. If low malformation presents with anterior ectopic fistula the orifice is transferred back to normal site. Results with all the techniques are good provided there is no stenosis of stoma, residual persistent posterior ledge or there is no infection and scarring. In emergency anal stenosis can be relieved by dilatation only and anoplasty be planned subsequently. The common surgical procedures in practice are:

Anal Cutback

This procedure was first described by Denis Browne in 1951. It was initially favoured because of simple technique and low complications. Cutback was described as a life saving procedure for a surgeon with limited experience and facility.

One blade of a pair of straight scissors is placed along the horizontal fistula and perineal tissue is cut back exactly in midline to the site of neoanal orifice. Mucosa is sutured to the skin. Alternatively, Hegar's dilator is passed in the fistula and midline division of all structures from fistula to anal site can be completed with a knife followed by mucocutaneous anastomosis (Figs 72.30A and B). It has been used as first aid procedure in patient with anovestibular fistula with severe stenosis having low birth weight and poor general condition to relieve the obstruction. Anocutaneous fistula, covered anus, anterior ectopic anus and anal stenosis have been managed with this technique with quite satisfactory results.[30,31]

Presently, it has gone into disrepute due to nonscientific basis and resulting severe incontinence.

YV Anoplasty[31]

An alternative procedure for low ARM with or without perineal fistula in YV anoplasty also known as

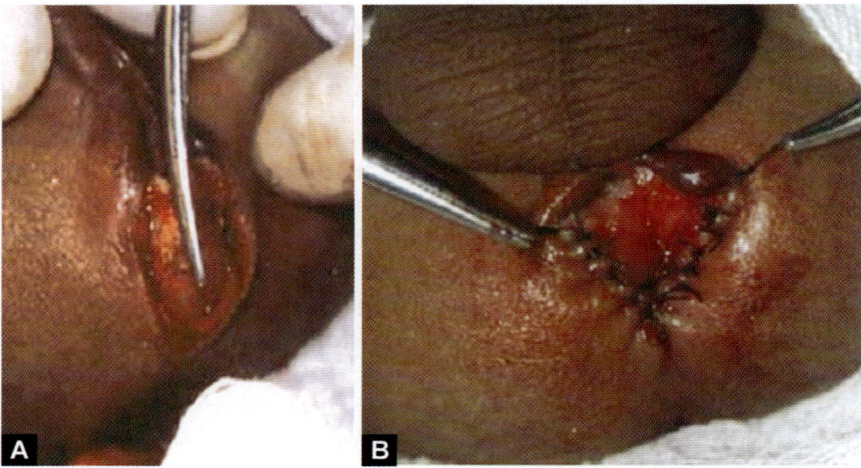

Figs 72.30A and B: Cut back anoplasty for low ARM in male

Barrow's flap anoplasty. A V-shaped skin flap is raised posteriorly with apex at posterior margin of fistula. Vertical incision through full thickness of bowel is made on posterior wall of anal canal which opens the bowel and creates a defect for advancement of skin flap into anal canal.

Anal Transposition

The anovestibular fistula is dissected all around and brought out through a separate incision given only above the proposed anal site.

Limited Posterior Sagittal Anoplasty (PSAP)

Pena has described minimal posterior mobilisation of fistula within the limits of external sphincter and anoplasty in prone position but author prefers to use the technique of anterior sagittal anorectoplasty for reconstruction of low malformations.

Anterior Sagittal Anorectoplasty (ASARP)

Anovestibular fistula and rectovestibular fistula in girls and anocutaneous or rectocutaneous fistula in boys are best managed with this technique as single stage perineal surgery. This procedure demands greater surgical skill and meticulous dissection because from anterior fistula to the proposed site of normal anal opening skin, and muscles are divided exactly in midline. The anus and rectum are dissected free from vagina or urethra and mobilized to be transposed posteriorly. Perineal body is reconstructed anterior to rectum and anoplasty is performed at proposed normal site well embraced by sphincter. The procedure reported by Okada and Wakhlu et al offers excellent results in anovestibular fistula and rectovestibular fistula in female.[32,33] It can also be used for anocutaneous fistula in males. Author prefers single stage correction of all cases of anovestibular and rectovestibular fistula without colostomy.

Anatomical Basis

In anovestibular fistula and rectovestibular fistula levator muscle and adjacent part of muscle complex embraces the bowel at the cranial end, but downwards muscle complex runs posteriorly to terminate at anal dimple while anorectum courses anteriorly out of muscle complex to terminate in vestibule. Mid line incision from fistula to anal dimple will divide the caudal end of muscle complex and anterior segment of parasagittal fibers in two half without damaging its nerve supply exposing the posterior wall of rectum. Wide anatomic exposure allows separation of bowel from vagina under vision. Bowel is placed in the centre of bisected muscle complex with midline reconstruction of perineal body, muscles, vestibule and neoanal orifice.

Indications

The procedures can be used for single stage correction of anovestibular fistula, vulvar anus, anterior ectopic

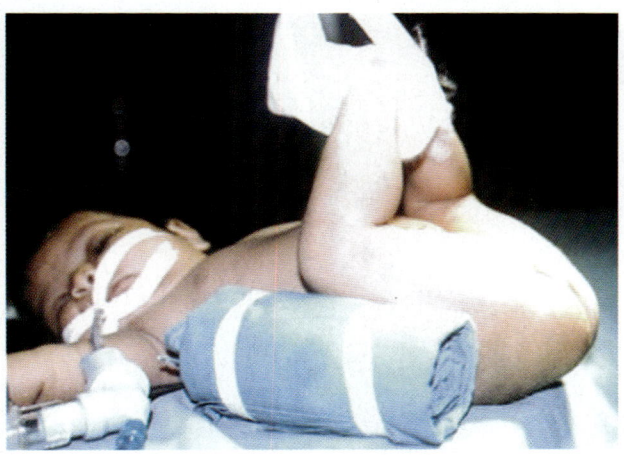

Fig. 72.31: Position of the patient for ASARP. Feet joined together suspended in mid line with flexion at hip and knee joint. A roll of towel placed adjacent to thigh stabilizes the position

anus and perineal canal. Uncomplicated cases of rectovestibular fistula can also be corrected with this technique without colostomy by a surgeon well versed with the technique.

Technique

In general anesthesia, patient is placed in lithotomy position with feet joined together, suspended in mid line, with forward eversion of perineum. Soft bolsters are placed on both sides adjacent to lateral aspect of thigh. This position provides adequate exposure for the procedure (Fig. 72.31). Proposed site of neo anal orifice is identified by inspection of pigmented anal dimple or skin fold and confirmed with electro-stimulation. Its posterior limit is marked.

Incision is made exactly in mid line starting from fourchette proceeding posteriorly just beyond the posterior limit of neoanal orifice. Skin, subcutaneous tissue and fibers of muscle complex are divided exactly in mid line exposing the posterior wall of anal canal and rectum (Fig. 72.32A). Divided structures are held retracted laterally either with stay sutures or retractors. Lateral wall of the rectum and vestibular fistula is easily separated from parasagittal fibers, transverse perineal muscles and fibro fatty tissue by blunt sharp dissection in relatively avascular plane bleeding points are coagulated (Fig. 72.32B).

Vestibular fistula is now to be separated from posterior wall of vagina which is technically the most important and difficult part of dissection but usually completed without complications, provided meticulous technical details are adhered to. It is elaborated herewith. For uniform traction, 3-5 stay sutures are placed on posterior edge of vestibular orifice which is retracted downward and posteriorly, inspecting vaginal orifice hymen and posterior vaginal wall (Fig. 72.32C).

Separation of initial 1-1.5 cm of posterior wall of vagina adherent to anterior wall of rectum and vestibular fistula is started with sharp dissection. Infiltration of 1:150000 adrenaline in posterior wall of vagina makes dissection easier. Initial sharp dissection proceeds from lateral to midline in a plane just outside the longitudinal muscle coat of the bowel taking great care not to open the bowel. The plane of dissection is kept very close to vaginal wall even if accidental hole is made in vagina. It is acceptable at the cost of separating the intact bowel. Commonest site of vaginal wall injury is at a recess present at the junction of posterior vaginal wall and hymen at 8'o clock and 4'o clock position. This injury can be prevented if dissection proceeds just outside the longitudinal muscle coat of bowel but at the same time very thin vaginal wall remains all the time identified by placing the tip of a forceps, through vaginal orifice. Its tip can be seen through intact but thin vaginal wall. Once initial 1-1.5 cm of vagina is separated in correct plane remaining part can be easily and quickly separated with by sweeping it off the rectum with help of a pledget and sharp dissection.

Higher up, two constant vessels (branches of middle rectal artery) running on lateral wall of rectum are to be coagulated for hemostasis. If the bowel is sufficiently mobilised, vestibular fistula should lie at neoanal orifice site without tension, and without tendency for upward retraction.

If it is not so, bowel is further mobilised and lengthened by dividing fascial bands. Once dissection is complete rectum is placed in between bisected muscle complex, muscle complex is reapproximated posterior and anterior to rectum. Anoplasty is completed by suturing the vestibular fistula to neoanal orifice. Anterioir midline cut in bowel may be made if orifice is narrow.

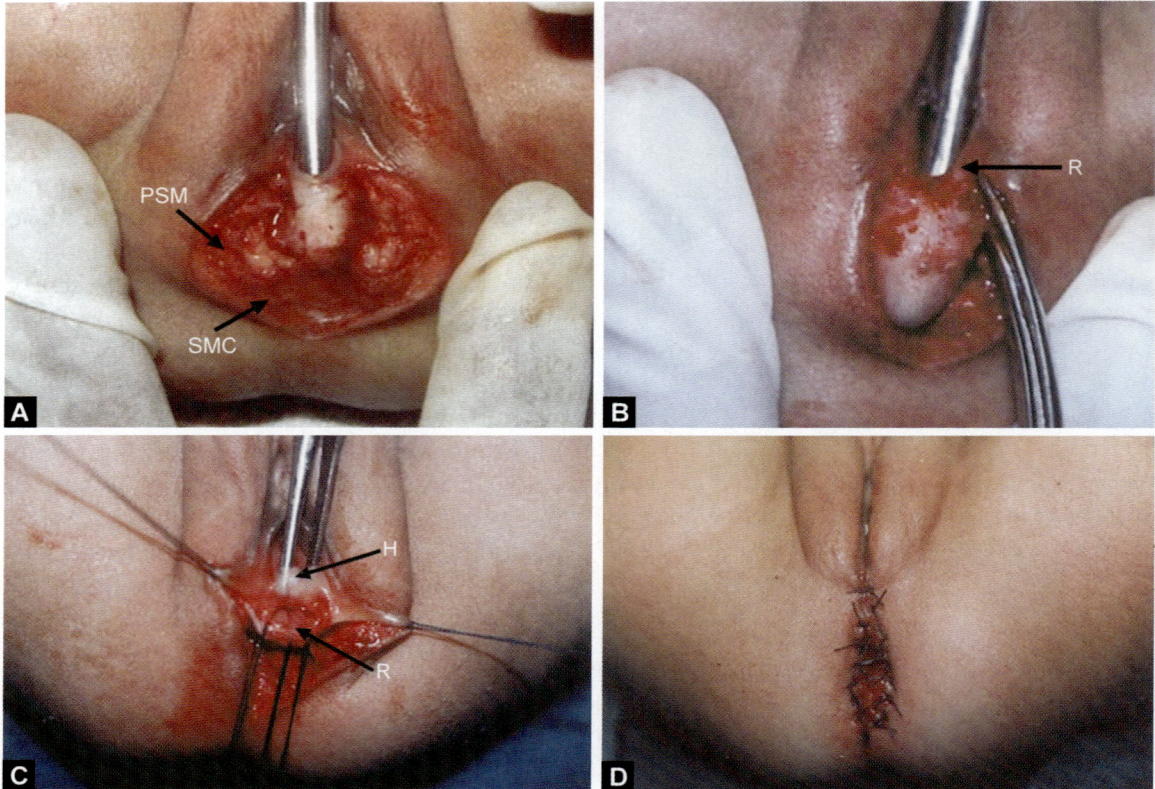

Figs 72.32A to D: A. Skin incision from fourchette to the point just posterior to anal dimple. Parasagittal muscle (PSM) running parallel to skin incision. Vertically oriented fibers of sphincter muscle complex (SMC) split in mid line at anal dimple, Hegar's dilator in vestibular fistula. Posterior wall of anorectum is exposed **B.** Lateral wall of rectum and vestibular fistula(R) are being separated with sharp dissection **C.** Stay sutures are placed on posterior edge of vestibular orifice (R). Tip of the forcep placed in vagina can be seen through very thin hymen (H) **D.** Repair is completed with anoplasty, reconstruction of vestibule, fourchette and median raphe

Between vagina and rectum, perineal muscles are reapproximated in midline, perineal body is reconstructed with interrupted vicryl sutures. After anoplasty, the procedure is completed by reconstruction of vestibule, fourchette and midline raphe (Fig. 72.32D).

Postoperative Care

Patient may be orally allowed as soon as recovery from general anesthesia occurs. Perineal dressing applied in OT can be removed when patient passes urine and wound is best managed with open care without dressing. Sitz bath or local warm saline compresses without rubbing at stitches after each bowel movement will keep the perineum clean. Three weeks after surgery assessment is made regarding the need for dilatation. Most patients are not constipated and anal orifice admits no. 16 Hegars. In case orifice is narrow, dilatation may be continued for three months.

Complications

Two major complications associated with this technique are related to technical difficulty which are entirely preventable.

i. **Complete wound dehiscence and anterior migration of anus** is almost always secondary to inadequate mobilisation of bowel and anoplasty performed under tension. Intact bowel mobilised adequately to lie at neoanal orifice even without suturing is the only and surest way to prevent this complication.

ii. *Recurrent fistula:* Occurs if during separation of bowel from vagina, a hole in anterior wall of rectum is made. This complication will never occur if bowel is mobilised off the vagina without injuring its anterior wall. Adherence to meticulous technique will prevent this complication. **If you have opened the anterior rectal wall during mobilisation the best option is to repair it and perform a protective colostomy.**

iii. *Persistent posterior ledge:* If incision is not extended little beyond the posterior limit of anal dimple, residual posterior ledge can be troublesome and persistent constipation may necessitate secondary procedure like cutback, anoplasty.

Other complications recorded with the technique include postoperative retention of urine, bleeding, wound infection, edema and perianal excoriation.

Advantages

Though the basic principle and approach is eventually the same as described in procedure of limited PSARP for vestibular fistula by Pena but anterior sagittal anorectoplasty allows far better exposure. Direct vision of vaginal orifice as well as vestibular fistula is of great help in mobilisation of intact full thickness bowel from vagina. Mobilized full thickness bowel placed in sphincter muscle obviates the need for colostomy.

There is no need to perform colostomy because bowel is mobilised full thickness and placed in muscle complex which is split from anterior to posterior in lower part only leaving intact levator muscle and upper segment of muscle complex.

Superficial muscles of perineum and reconstruction of perineal body prevents anterior migration of anus. Overall appearance of the perineum becomes identical to normal.

Results

Till date we have successfully treated more than 528 cases of vestibular fistula, 58 perineal canal, and 31 cases of perineal ectopic anus with this technique without significant complications. Follow-up analysis of 326 patients revealed normal looking perineum and normal defecation in 291. Constipation was present in 35 patients. Persistent posterior ledge was found responsible in 25 and treated with cut back anoplasty. Anal stenosis was present in 6 (Barrow flap anoplasty done in 4) while 4 patients had functional constipation.

OPERATIVE MANAGEMENT OF HIGH ANORECTAL MALFORMATIONS

Colostomy

A divided and separated proximal sigmoid colostomy is recommended by Pena to achieve complete defunctioning of the distal loop. We have found that simple loop colostomy done at the junction of descending and sigmoid colon with adequate spur works very well to relieve the obstruction in emergency and defunctioning of distal loop is also obtained provided that loop is adequately exteriorized with no tendency of recession.

Transverse colostomy is not preferred because of the disadvantages which are:

1. Colostomy diarrhea is poorly tolerated with transverse colostomy as compared to sigmoid colostomy.
2. Stagnation of urine and severe metabolic acidosis may occur with transverse colostomy if wide recto-urinary fistula is present and there is reflux of urine in colon through fistula.
3. Distal loop wash outs are difficult and it is difficult to obtain good quality of cologram with transverse colostomy.

However, in cases of type IV congenital short colon, bladder neck fistula and complex malformations of cloaca, sigmoid colostomy may not be preferred because it is necessary to preserve the blood supply of rectum during colostomy and its subsequent closure. With sigmoid colostomy in these conditions, firstly, it may be difficult to mobilise rectum to gain sufficient length during abdominal exploration for a definitive repair. Secondly during colostomy closure blood supply of the pulled through rectum may be damaged leading to ischemia of the rectum. In these cases transverse colostomy may be preferred alternative to obviate these problems.

Overview of Operative Procedure

The ultimate cherished goal to be attained is provision of anal opening with perfect fecal continence. With endeavour to utilize the functional contribution of available sphincter muscle and avoid damage to innervation of already existing sphincters yet providing anal orifice has led to innovation of numerous techniques and advancement concomitant with advancement in understanding of pathological anatomy and physiology.

Norris in 1943 and Rhoads in 1944, reported one stage abdominoperineal rectoplasty in neonate describing abdominal exploration, disconnection of fistula and pull through anterior to sacrum with perineal anoplasty.[34,35] At that time concept of the puborectalis sling was non-existent.

Stephens by the early 1960s described the importance of puborectalis sling, a principal muscle of continence which hugs the urethra in male and vagina in female.[3,15] He emphasized that by sacroperineal route, a narrow plane anterior to but within the sling of muscle can be defined and rectum must be routed through it for continence.

Based on this information, Swenson and Donnellan modified the abdominoperineal approach.[36] After disconnection of fistula through abdominal route; puborectalis sling was identified, space was created between the sling and posterior urethra and the rectum was pulled through the space and sutured in perineum creating a neoanus. No importance was given to striated muscles of external sphincter.

Retbein who earlier proposed submucosal resection of rectum and abdominoperineal rectoplasty to minimize injury to the nerves and blood vessels; modified the procedure to palpate the levator with a finger above and below to define a plane anterior to puborectalis and passed rectum through it.[37,38]

It was Stephens contention that the entrance to the tunnel can never be seen by an abdominal approach nor can it be palpated; only gentle blunt probing with a right angle clamp can actually open the plane in front of sphincter muscle against urethra or vagina and for this reason he favored sacroperineal approach.[3,15] However, when fistula was higher up, in addition laparotomy was performed (Sacro-abdominoperineal pull-through).

Kieswester's sacro-abdomino perineal pull through was essentially a combination of Stephen's sacro-perineal approach and Rehbein's submucosal dissection.[39]

Mollard's operation reported in 1975 is essentially a Rehbein's technique with identification of puborectalis sling via anterior sagittal perineal approach in anterior sagittal plane just behind the urethra.[40]

Congenital Pouch Colon and ARM

This is described in detail in chapter 76.

Posterior Sagittal Anorectoplasty

Posterior sagittal approach (PSARP) since its introduction by Pena and de Vries has practically replaced all earlier techniques because of obvious advantages.[41] In this technique via midline perineal approach all striated sphincter muscles are divided exactly in midline aided by electrostimulation (Fig. 72.33). After splitting the coccyx in midline and levator ani muscle posterior aspect of rectum is exposed (Figs 72.34A to F). Its distal most segment is opened in midline and through lumen of the rectum fistula is directly visualized. Fistula, is disconnected and closed under vision and mobilised rectum is placed exactly in the center of sphincter muscles which are meticulously, reapproximated around rectum.

In this overview of operative procedures it is intriguing to see history moving in a full circle from perineal exposure of the nineteenth century through numerous modifications away from perineum and now back to the perineum again. Smith ED in 1987 has excellently described an overview of surgery of anorectal anomalies.[42]

The PSARP procedure has been discussed in chapter 73.

Postoperative Management

Posterior sagittal incision is relatively painless and the course is usually smooth. If repair is not combined with laparotomy patient is orally allowed after recovery from anesthesia.

We remove urethral catheter after 5 days in repair of rectourethral fistula but if catheter was accidentally dislodged earlier, all patients passed urine and no recurrent fistula was noted.

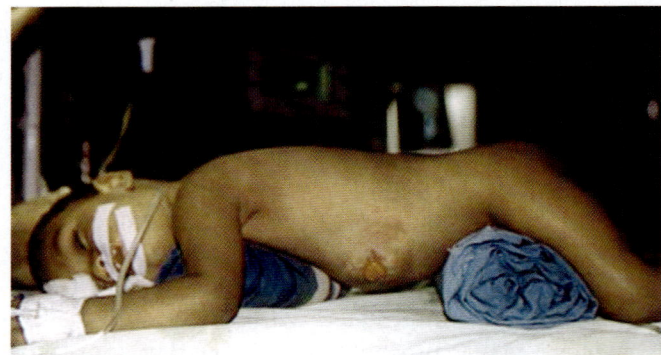

Fig. 72.33: Position of the patient for PSARP. Lateral view showing placement of paddings and free abdomen wall

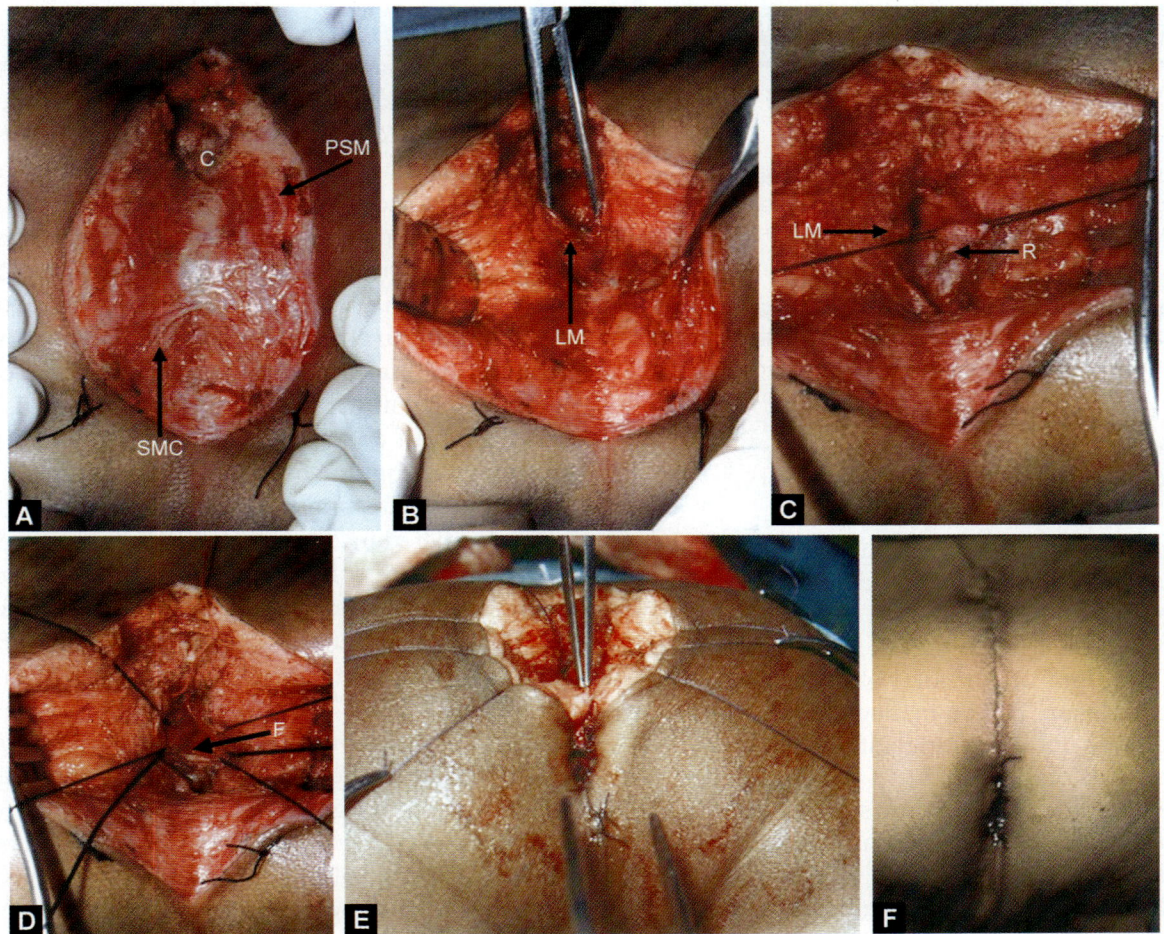

Figs 72.34A to F: A. Showing mid line division of parasagittal muscle (PSM) and vertically running sphincter muscle complex (SMC). Tip of coccyx is seen (C) and mid line plane is avascular with thin white fascia **B.** Right angle hemostat is passed through split coccyx and held up to lift the levator ani muscle (LM) which is divided in mid line **C.** Through split open Levator ani muscle (LM). Posterior wall of rectum (R) is held up in stay sutures and will be opened in mid line **D.** Edges of the opened posterior rectal wall are held with stay sutures and fistula is seen (F) **E.** After completion of anoplasty rectum is repositioned to create some recession of neoanus and reapproximating sutures to muscle complex are tied **F.** Closure is completed with reapproximation of all the layers

Dressing is removed after 48 hours, open care of the wound with application of antibiotic ointment is preferred.

Intravenous antibiotics are administered for 48 hours followed by oral antibiotics for 7 days. Patient can be discharged as soon as urethral catheter is removed and patient had spontaneous voiding.

Hospital stay is longer in patients of bladder neck fistula, congenital short colon and cloaca with abdominal exploration.

Pena recommends anal dilatation 2 weeks after surgery but we find if dilatation is started at 3 weeks after surgery, chances of minor bleeding are minimized occurring at the time of first dilatation by parents.

Parents are trained to dilate the orifice twice a day with size of dilator which goes in neoanus without resistance and without causing undue stretching.

Every week parents are called and given progressively increasing size of dilator until the desired size of anal orifice is achieved (Table 72.5).

Table 72.5: Desired size of dilators and protocol for tapering anal dilatations for different ages

Age	Hegar size	Protocol
1-4 months old	#12 Hegar	Once a day for 1 month
4-8 months old	#13 Hegar	Every other day for 1 month
8-12 months old	#14 Hegar	Twice a week for 1 month
1-4 years old	#15 Hegar	Once a week for 1 month
Older than 4 years	#16 Hegar	Once a month for 3 months

Table 72.6: Protocol for tapering anal dilatations

Age	Hegar size
1-4 months old	#12 Hegar
4-8 months old	#13 Hegar
8-12 months old	#14 Hegar
1-4 years old	#15 Hegar
Older than 4 years	#16 Hegar

Colostomy is now closed but programme of anal dilatation is not abruptly stopped but tapered. Protocol for tapering the anal dilatation is described by Pena and given in Table 72.6.

The problem of perianal skin excoriation after colostomy closure can be managed with reassurance, barrier creams, local cleaning without rubbing the skin and treatment of diarrhea.

After six months patients develops an individualized bowel movement pattern and prospect of prognosis is assessed. Patients will be toilet trained by 2.5 to 3 years of age but patients with indicators of poor prognosis and bad prognostic signs are put on bowel management program. The bowel management program has been discussed in chapter 81.

COMPLICATIONS

In series of 1102 patients reported by Pena following complications were noted:
1. Wound infection
2. Anal strictures
3. Devascularization of rectum during mobilisation
4. Constipation
5. Urethrovaginal fistula
6. Acquired atresia of vagina
7. Transient femoral nerve palsy
8. Recurrent rectourethral fistula
9. Ureteric injury
10. Neurogenic bladder
11. Injury to Vas

The complications are discussed in detail in chapter 75.

RESULTS

In the Department of Pediatric Surgery, K.G. Medical College, Lucknow, 1088 patients (749 male, 339 females) of ARM were admitted from 1990 to 2001. Out of 741 patients of high or intermediate malformations, colostomy was done in 700 patients (601 male, 99 male). Type of anomalies in male patients were: congenital short colon 60, rectal atresia 7, rectovesical fistula 25 and 501 patients of rectoprostatic, rectobulbar urethral fistula and without fistula. Among 99 females type of malformations were: cloaca 41, pouch colon with cloaca 8, rectovaginal fistula 30, rectal atresia 1 and in 19 patients type of anomaly was not clear as per records. PSARP was done in 291 patients (243 males and 48 females). Colostomy closure was completed in 204 patients. Follow-up assessment was completed in 106 patients (78 males 28 females). Using Wing Spread criteria good results were noted in 50 (47%), fair in 30 (28%) and poor in 26 (25%) patients. Complications noted during PSARP are given in Tables 72.7 and 72.8.

Stephens and Smith concluded that "discussion is not required in the translevator deformities as most authors agree on good results or 70-95%.[30,43] Recent long-term studies suggest that good bowel control is usually achieved after correction of anomalies in 90% of patients.[44,45] However, long-term bowel dysfunction especially in the form of constipations has often been troublesome.

The rate of continence after correction of high anomalies by older techniques has been reported as disappointing. Older procedure such as abdominoperineal, sacroperineal or sacroabdominoperineal procedures are not associated with good results but improvement in continence is reported because most patients organize their lives to minimize the occurrence and effects of soiling. Improved continence has also been reported with procedures where terminal bowel was preserved and used for anorectoplasty.

Experience with posterior sagittal anorectoplasty is clearly encouraging than previous procedures but more time is needed to permit evaluation of long-term result and quality of life in adulthood.

Some careful follow-up studies on results of PSARP indicate that achievement of continence is possible in 50% cases of high ARM.[2,46-48]

Table 72.7: Intraoperative complications of PSARP encountered with 261 patients operated in KGMC, Lucknow

S.No.	Complications	No.
1.	Difficulty in identification of rectum	1
	a. Septate vagina and rectum was in the septum	3
	b. Deviation from midline (cause—rectum very high and long narrow fistula entering the prostate)	
2.	Incision of prostate misidentified as rectum	2
3.	Injury to prostate while mobilising the rectum	2
4.	Injury to bulbous urethra while mobilising the rectum	1
5.	Injury to vas (partial)	3
6.	Complete detachment of vas and seminal vesicles	1
7.	Opening up of bladder in cases of sacral agenesis	1
8.	Gross deviation from midline	1
9.	Wound dehiscence because of	
	a. Poor bowel preparation and fecal contamination	
	b. Receded colostomy and continued passage of stools through neorectum	3
10.	Very high rectum—excessive mobilization causing rectal stenosis	2

Data by Bliss et al and Templeton indicate that continence results of PSARP are no different form those obtained with other operations currently in use while Rintala showed that 35% of these patients had apparently normal continence with PSARP.[2,43,49]

Rintala et al has reported improvement in continence at adolescence in patients having undergone PSARP procedure for high ARM because severity of constipation diminishes with passage of time.[50]

Follow-up study with comparison of results of PSARP and conventional methods has been reported by Tsuji et al using Kelly's clinical scoring system.[51] Overall results were found to be better in PSARP but long-term bowel management was needed in all patients of high and intermediate malformations.

Longterm follow-up result in 48 patient, with modified technique of PSARP was reported by Lien NT et al revealing very good function in 4%, good function in 54%, fair in 38% and poor results in 4%.[52]

Obviously it is apparent that more careful long-term follow-up studies are needed to determine the place of this technique and identify patients who are likely to achieve total continence and those going to remain incontinent.

PRIMARY NEONATAL PULL-THROUGH

There has been a recent interest again in primary neonatal PSARP or neonatal laparoscopic pull-through without colostomy. Moore has recommended operative repair within the first 7 days without a prior colostomy because activity driven anocortical neurocircuitry develops in perinatal period and within few days after birth.[53] If act of defecation is not initiated soon after birth by primary repair, the advantage is lost. One stage PSARP has been reported by Goo, Albanse and S Chooramani Gopal.[54-56] Laparoscopic primary neonatal pull-through is also reported.[57]

Table 72.8: Delayed complications of PSARP encountered in 261 patients, operated in KGMC, Lucknow (encountered in the study group)

Complications	No.
Infection	10
Dehiscence and scarring	3
Mucosal prolapse	5
Anal stenosis	3

SUMMARY

Reconstruction of normal anatomical anal opening and provision of normal continence remains the cherished goal to be achieved in cases of ARM. Correction of associated anomalies is also mandatory. In cases of low ARM with good available sphincters not associated with loss of sacral segment and loss of innervation, it is possible to achieve good results in 95% of cases. Procedure of choice is single stage perineal proctoplasty by various techniques but anterior sagittal anorectoplasty is currently the procedure of choice. High ARM is best managed with staged procedure, i.e. colostomy, definitive reconstruction and colostomy closure. PSARP is the technique of choice today for definitive reconstruction of high ARM after colostomy. It has to be combined with abdominal exploration in cases of rectovesical fistula, congenital short colon and some cases of cloaca. Results are dependent firstly on meticulous repair with perfect technique, placing the bowel with its preserved sensory receptors and internal sphincter in the centre of muscle complex and secondly on quality of available sphincter muscle complex which can be judged with CT and MRI. Early neonatal surgery may help to establish the normal activity driven anocortical neurocircuitry. Patients of ARM with poorly developed sphincters are helped by medical bowel management program, biofeedback therapy, Malon's antigrade continent enema or permanent colostomy.

ACKNOWLEDGEMENTS

Author is grateful to Mr Varun for secretarial assistance and Dr Ravi Kanojia for organizing the figures.

REFERENCES

1. Potts WJ. The surgeon and the child. Philadelphia, WB Saunders 1959;203.
2. Bliss Jr DP, Tapper D, Anderson JM, et al. Does posterior sagittal anorectoplasty in patients with imperforate anus provide superior fecal continence? J Pediatr Surg 1996;31:26-32.
3. Stephens FD. Congenital imperforate rectum, rectourethral and rectovaginal fistula. Aust NZJ Surg 1953;22:161-67.
4. Chatterjee SK. A surgeon's experience. In: Anorectal malformations. New York, Oxford University Press, 1993.
5. Ladd WE, Gross RE. Congenital malformations of the anus and rectum. Report of 162 cases. Am J Surg 1934;23:176-83.
6. Browne D. Congenital deformities of the anus and rectum. Arch Dis Child 1955;30:42-47.
7. Stephens FD, Smith ED. Classification, identification and assessment of surgical treatment of anorectal anomalies. Pediatr Surg Int 1986;1:200-21.
8. Santulli TV, Kieswetter WB, Bill AH. Anorectal malformations: A suggested international classification. J Pediatr Surg 1970;5:281-87.
9. Pena A. Surgical management of anorectal malformations: A unified concept. Pediatr Surg Int 1988;3:82-93.
10. Pena A. Anorectal malformations. Semin Pediatr Surg 1995;4:35-37.
11. Guzman E, Ranzini A, Day-Salvatore D. The prenatal ultrasonographic visualization of imperforate anus in monoamniotic twins. J Ultrasound Med 1995;14:547.
12. Smith ED, Cywes S. Diagnosis and investigations. In: Stephens FD, Smith ED (Eds.). Anorectal malformations in children. Update 1988. Birth defects: Original article series. New York: Alan R, Liss 1988;24:247-99.
13. Pena A. Current management of anorectal anomalies. Surg Clin North Am 1992;72:1393-416.
14. Wangensteen OH, Rice CO. Imperforate anus: A method of determining the surgical approach. Arch Surg 1930;92:77-81.
15. Stephens FD. Malformations of the anus. Aust NZ Surg 1953;23:9-18.
16. Kelly JH. The radiographic anatomy of the normal and abnormal neonatal pubis. J Pediatr Surg 1969;4:432-35.
17. 17 Narasimharo KL, Prasad GR, Katariya S, et al. Prone cross table lateral view: An alternative to invertogram in imperforate anus. Am J Roentgenol 1983;140:227-29.
18. Sultan AH, Nicholls RJ, Kamm MA, et al. Anal endosonography and correlation with in vitro anatomy. Br J Surg 1993;80:508-11.
19. Law PJ, Bartman CL. Anal endosonography: Technique and normal anatomy. Gastrointest Radiol 1989;14:349-53.
20. Keiller VH. Imperforate anus with report of 3 cases. Texas J Med 1924;20:278-49.
21. Ikawa H. The use of computerised tomography to evaluate ano-rectal anomalies. J Pediatr Surg 1985;20:640-44.
22. Khoda E, Fujioka M, Ikawa H, Yakoyama J. Congenital ano-rectal anomaly: CT evaluation. Radiology 1985;57:349-52.
23. Pringle KC, Sato Y, Soper RT. Magnetic resonance imaging as an adjunct to planning an ano-rectal pullthrough. J Pediatr Surg 1987;22:571-74.
24. Edward J, Daolin C, Thomas Black, et al. Rectal manometry. Computed tomography and functional results of anal atresia surgery. Journal of Paediatric Surgery 1993;28(2):195-98.
25. Fondelli P, Taccone A, Martuciello G, et al. CT and ARM. their Post operative evaluation. Radiol Med. Torino 1989;77(4):361-64.
26. Shigeru Uno, Seishichi, Yokoyama, et al. Three dimensional display of the pelvic structure of anorectal malformations based on CT and MRI. Journal of Pediatric Surgery 1995;30(5):682-86.
27. Teaccone A, Marzoli A, Martuciello G, Saloman G, et al. CT Vs. MRI in the diagnosis of anorectal anomalies. Radiol Med Torino 1991;82(5):638-43.
28. Nakayama DK. Imperforate anus. In: Nakayama DK, Bose CL, Chescheir NC, Valley RD (Ed.). Critical care of the surgical newborn. New York: Futura 1997;449-73.
29. Noonan JA. Syndromes: In: Long WA (Ed.). Fetal and neonatal cardiology. Philadelphia, WB Saunders 1990:662.
30. Nixon HH. Operative management of low anomalies in girls. In: Stephens FD, Smith ED (Eds.). Anorectal malformations in children. Update 1988, Birth Defects, Original article series. New York, Alan R Liss 1988;24:309-16.

31. Smith ED. Operative management of low anomalies in males. Translevator type. In: Stephens FD, Smith ED (Eds.). Anorectal malformations in children. Update 1988. Birth defects: Original article series. New York: Alan R Liss, 1988;24:301-07.
32. Okada A, Kamata S, Imura K, et al. Anterior saggital anorectoplasty for rectovestibular and anovestibular fistula. J Pediatr Surg 1992;27:85-89.
33. Wakhlu A, Prasad A, Pandey A, et al. Anterior sagittal anorectoplasty for ARM and perineal trauma in the female child. J Pediatr Surg 1996;31(9):1236-40.
34. Norris WJ, Brophy TW III, Brayton D. Imperforate anus: A case series and preliminary report of the one-stage abdomino-perineal operation. Surg Gynecol Obstet 1949;88:623-32.
35. Rhoads JE, Piper RL, Randall JP. A simultaneous abdominal and perineal approach in operation for imperforate anus with atresia of the rectum and rectosigmoid. Ann Surg 1948;127:552-56.
36. Swenson O, Donnellan WL. Preservation of the puborectalis sling in imperforate anus. Surg Clin J Am 1967;47:172-93.
37. Rehbein F. Operation for anal and rectal atresia with recto-urethral fistula. Chirugie 1959;30:417-22.
38. Rehbein F. Imperforate anus: Experiences with abdominoperineal and abdomino-sacro-perineal pull through procedures. J Pediatr Surg 1967;2:99-101.
39. Kieswetter WB. Imperforate anus II. The rationale and technique of the sacro-abdomino-perineal operation. J Pediatr Surg 1967;2:106.
40. Mollard P, Marechal JM, Jaubert de Beaujeu M. Surgical treatment of high imperforate anus with a definition of puborectalis sling by an anterior perineal approach. J Pediatr Surg 1978;13:499-504.
41. Pena A, deVries PA. Posterior sagittal anorectoplasty: Important technical considerations and new applications. J Pediatr Surg 1982;17:796-811.
42. Smith ED. The bath water needs changing, but don't throw out the baby: an overview of anorectal anomalies. J Pediatr Surg 1987;22:335-36.
43. Rintala RJ, Lindahl H. Is normal bowel function possible after repair of intermediate and high anorectal malformations? J Pediatr Surg 1995;30:491.
44. Rintala RJ, Mildh L, Lindahl HG. Fecal continence and quality of life in adult patients with operated low anorectal malformations. J Pediatr Surg 1992;27:902-05.
45. Yeung CK, Kiely EM. Low anorectal anomalies. A critical appraisal. Pediatr Surg Int 1991;6:33-35.
46. Pena A. Posterior sagittal anorectoplasty: Results in the management of 332 cases of anorectal malformation. Pediatr Surg Int. 1988;3:94-104.
47. Kureel SN, Tandon RK, Wakhlu AK, et al. Place of posterior sagittal anorectalplasty in management of high and intermediate anorectal malformations in 64 cases. J Surg 1994;23:176-83.
48. Rintala RJ, Lindahl H and Louhimo. Anorectal malformations: results of treatment and long-term follow up in 208 patients. Pediatr Int Surg 1991;6:36-41.
49. Temleton Jr JM, Ditesheim JA. High imperforate anus. Quantitative results of long term fecal continence. J Pediatr Surg 1985;20:645-52.
50. Rintala RJ, Lindale HG. Fecal continence in patients having undergone PSARP procedure for high ARM improves at adolescence as constipation disappears. J Pediatr Surg 2001;36(8):1218-21.
51. Tsuji H, Okada A, Nakai H, et al. Follow-up studies of anorectal malformations after posterior sagittal anorectoplasty. J Pediatr Surg 2002;37(11):1529-33.
52. Lien NT, Hau BD. Long term follow up results of the treatment of high and intermediate ARM using a modified technique of PSARP. Eur J Pediatr Surg 2001;11(4): 242-45.
53. Moore TC. Advantages of performing the sagittal anoplasty operation for imperforate anus at birth. J Pediatr Surg 1990;25:276-77.
54. Goo HK. Repair of anorectal anomalies in the neonatal period. Pediatr Surg Int 1990;5:246-49.
55. Albanese CT, Jennings RW, Lopoo JB, et al. One-stage correction of high imperforate anus in the male neonate. J Pediatr Surg 1999;34:834-36.
56. Gopal S Chooramani. Single stage PSARP in neonates. In:Textbook of neonatal surgery. Edited by: DK Gupta. Modern Publishers 2000:249-53.
57. Sydorak RM, Albanese CT. Laparoscopic repair of high imperforate anus. Semin Pediatr Surg 2002;11(4):217-25.

CHAPTER 73
Anorectal Malformations: Pena's Perspectives

Shilpa Sharma, Alberto Pena

The management of anorectal malformation (ARM) has seen a major change in the surgical approach with the introduction of the Posterior Sagittal Anorectoplasty (PSARP) by Alberto Pena, popularly known as the PSARP approach.[1-9] Anorectal malformations represent a spectrum of defects. Of the many available techniques, the best is the one that could be performed easily and with least postoperative complications. The surgeon should use the technique with dedication, perseverance and inclination to adopt changes as and when required. This includes evolving toward less aggressive approaches, less number of operations and minimal invasive procedures. The crux of treatment lies in proper identification of the anomaly, so that the child is benefited with a well planned surgery to get the best possible outcome.

If a particular operation is done for a particular anomaly over a long time, sufficient expertise is acquired to handle complicated cases and even those treated earlier by other surgeons.[3,10] The results of re-operations in good hands are thus far superior to primary operations in inexperienced hands.[11]

Management of anorectal malformations requires an accurate clinical diagnosis, proper newborn treatment, meticulous anatomic reconstruction, and comprehensive postoperative care with the goal of having a child who is clean and dry, with an excellent quality of life, because they either have the capacity for continence or can be kept artificially clean with a comprehensive bowel management program.[12] The surgical treatment has evolved to proper reconstruction, avoid complications and understand mechanisms of incontinence, ultimately leading to improved quality of life for patients. Figures 73.1 and 73.2 outline the algorithm suggested for management.

COLOSTOMY

Colostomy is still a widely accepted procedure for high and complex malformations. The circumstances vary from one institution to another and from one country to another. Experienced pediatric surgeons are now managing some of the newborns even without a protective colostomy. A colostomy is mandatory in premature and very sick babies, when they suffer from severe associated defects, or in case of complex malformations, e.g. cloacal anomalies.

A descending colostomy is recommended as all colostomies performed in a mobile portion of colon have a tendency to prolapse. Fixation of the distal mucus fistula to the anterior abdominal wall or making the mucus fistula small (around 5 mm in diameter) is recommended as the purpose of creation of such a mucus fistula is to use the same for chronic irrigation or high pressure distal colostogram. A divided

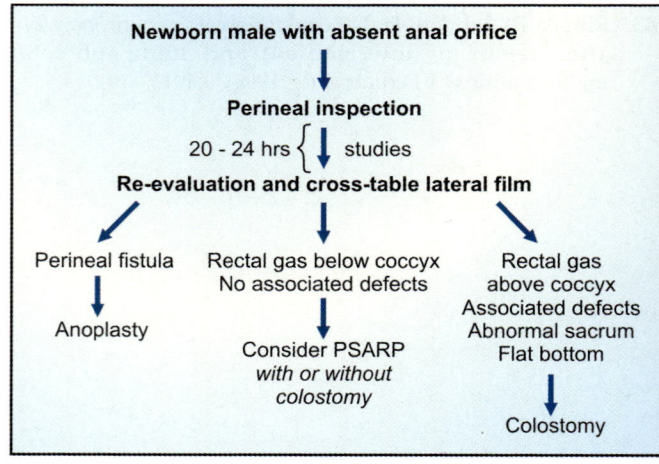

Fig. 73.1: Pena's decision-making algorithm for male ARM

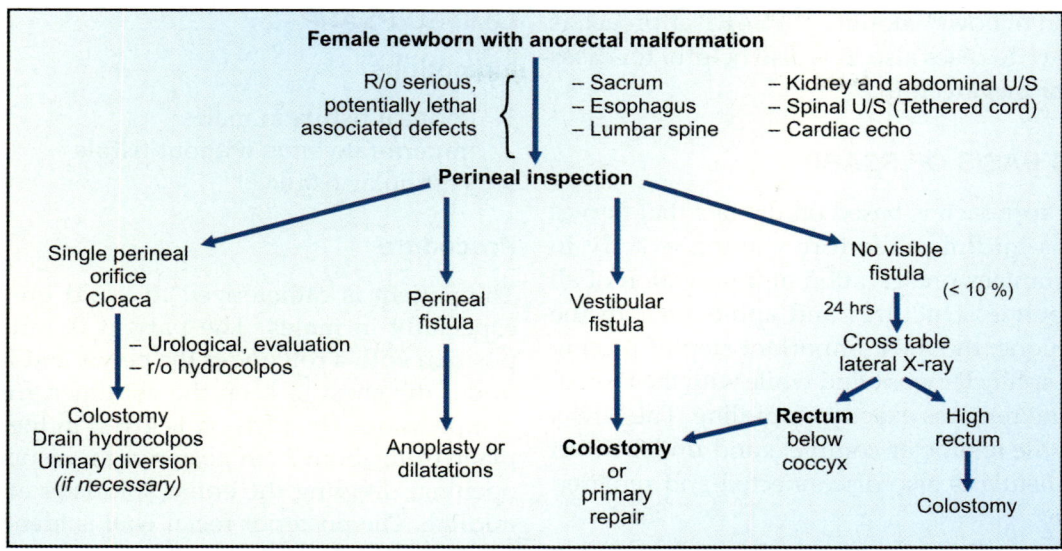

Fig. 73.2: Pena's decision-making algorithm for female ARM

colostomy is preferred. The loop colostomy has a tendency to prolapse and it does not provide complete diversion of stool. Also fecal impaction in the distal rectum may also contaminate the urinary tract with feces.

The incision is placed in the left lower quadrant long enough to place both stomas sufficiently separated with a skin bridge so as to accommodate the stoma bag only over the proximal stoma. On abdominal exploration the surgeon should select the first portion of the mobile sigmoid just distal to the descending colon. One can place a purse string suture over the distended colon and make an orifice in the center, pass a catheter to irrigate the colon until all the meconium has been removed. This helps to create a better colostomy, without contaminating the field.

Many surgeons still continue performing a loop colostomy. This is only justified provided the colostomy is completely diverting with the help of spur formation between both the loops.

TIMING OF THE DEFINITIVE REPAIR

The timing of the definitive surgery depends upon the expertise of the surgeon. Primary repair is feasible for perineal fistula and vestibular fistula. PSARP can be performed by 3-6 weeks when baby is investigated and thriving well. In cases of cloaca, the surgery may be delayed upto 3-6 months after birth.

UTILITY OF PSARP

The posterior sagittal approach was also used for the treatment of acquired conditions including tumors, post-trauma and post-radiation fistulae and other postoperative complications. A historic review of the posterior approach disclosed that Cripps, a British surgeon, published his experience with a posterior trans-sphincteric approach to the rectum nine years before Kraske, a German surgeon, whose name has been traditionally associated with the leadership in this approach. Kraske actually approached the rectum through a paramedian incision and never performed a real trans-sphincteric incision. An experimental study done in dogs by the senior author demonstrated that it is not harmful to divide the sphincteric mechanism.[13]

The posterior sagittal approach represents a useful alternative to treat many pelvic conditions and, therefore, it must be a part of the armamentarium of the colorectal surgeons. Co-ordinated rectosigmoid motility is the most important single factor in fecal continence and, thus, our efforts to help patients suffering from fecal incontinence must be aimed at the manipulation of bowel motility.[14] PSARP approach is beneficial in redo cases also. It is also helpful for cases of excision of megarectum.

SCIENTIFIC BASIS OF PSARP

The PSARP approach is based on the fact that nerves do not cross midline therefore staying exactly in midline guarantees preservation of innervation of all important pelvic structures and sphincters. In the earlier technique, the most important step of placing the bowel in sphincter was blind while with the PSARP approach, one remains exactly in midline. The bowel is placed in the sphincter complex, and under direct vision. The fistula is also disconnected and repaired under vision.

Posterior sagittal anorectoplasty is based upon complete exposure of the anorectal region by means of a median sagittal incision that runs from the sacrum to the anal dimple, cutting through all muscle structures behind the rectum. It was learned through this procedure that the external sphincter is a functionally useful prominent structure. No puborectalis sling, as such, could be identified.

However, it was possible to recognize a muscle continuity from the skin to the sacral insertion of the levator ani.[1] In the PSARP approach, as the skin incision extends from the sacrum to the perineum (ventral aspect of the anal dimple), it provides an excellent exposure for evaluation and mobilization of the terminal bowel. It also enables one to construct an anal canal, suture the bowel wall to the striated musculature and the mucosa to the skin, thereby reducing or avoiding the complications of prolapse and stenosis.[2]

In males, with a rectourethral fistula, a transrectal closure of the mucosa at the fistula site, leaving the rectal longitudinal smooth muscle insertions on the prostatic capsule, avoids the possibility of any damage to the nerves and genital structures.[2]

Through PSARP approach, the full understanding of the anatomic damage is obtained and consequently a rational reconstructive plan can be designed in each case.[3] Tapering that was done in the past was possible only by this approach.[3] It is now required only in cases of megarectum.[3]

LIMITED PSARP

Indications

1. Perineal fistula in males
2. Imperforate anus without fistula
3. Vestibular fistula.

Procedure

The patient is catheterized to avoid urethral injury, especially in males. The patient is put in a prone position with a roll under the pelvis and folded towel under the chest to keep the abdomen free from any compression. The incision is given in the midsagittal plane from about 2 cm posterior to the proposed anal opening, dividing the entire sphincter exactly in the midline. The posterior rectal wall is identified with a characteristic whitish appearance. Stay sutures may be applied on the either side of the incision to provide uniform traction to facilitate dissection. The dissection is preceded towards both the lateral walls turn by turn to maintain symmetry and eventually towards the anterior rectal wall. Special care should be taken during anterior dissection to remain very close to the rectal wall to avoid urethral injury in males, as there is no plane of separation between the rectum and the urethra. Moreover, it should be taken into consideration that the anomaly is a spectrum with possibility of the rectum lying very close to the urethra. The dissection should be based on clinical experience to identify the correct plane and proceeded slowly especially during anterior dissection. The rectum is mobilized sufficient enough to be placed within the limits of the sphincter complex without any tension and at the same time avoiding any prolapse. The sphincter at the proposed anal site is identified with the help of an electrical stimulator. This usually coincides well with the visual pigmentation of the sphincter at the proposed anal site. The perineal body is reconstructed with long-term absorbable sutures. In case the rectal pouch is a little higher and the dissection has proceeded above the upper limits of the sphincter, it is beneficial to place a stitch high up anteriorly also to approximate both the sides of the incised sphincter, so as to construct a funnel of the sphincter mechanism all around the rectum.

In cases of imperforate anus without fistula, the rectum is usually located at approximately 1-2 cms above the perineal skin, at the level of the bulbar urethra. This is seen in 5% of all cases of ARM and half of these have Down's syndrome. This defect has a good prognosis, the rectum is located about 2 cm above the perineal skin, the sacrum is normal, and the sphincter mechanism is good.[15] Almost 95% of patients who have associated Down's syndrome have this type of anomaly. Care should be taken in these cases as the rectum is intimately attached to the posterior urethra. The surgeon must open the posterior wall and create a place of dissection between the anterior rectal wall and the urethra. All these patients have urinary continence.[15]

The anoplasty is performed within the limits of the sphincter with 16, 6/0 circumferential long-term absorbable sutures.

The baby is kept nil orally for 24-48 hrs with intravenous antibiotics. The duration of the total parental nutrition, if given, depends upon the type of anomaly, the degree of mobilization and the presence or absence of diverting colostomy.

There is a controversy whether or not to operate cases of perineal fistula. The repair of a perineal fistula in females is not only for esthetic reasons but it also potentiates the protection against rectal injury during the vaginal delivery and improves the sexual function. These patients have a good prognosis, good sacrum and good sphincters. About 90% of these without Down's syndrome have a good bowel control, while 80% of those with Down's syndrome have a good bowel control.

POSTERIOR SAGITTAL ANORECTOPLASTY (PSARP)

The patient is catheterized to avoid urethral injury, especially in males.

Position

Patient is placed in prone jack knife position with foam bolsters or soft cotton rolls placed under the chest and groin ensuring that the abdomen is not compressed and there is adequate space for abdominal wall movement with respiration. The level of pelvis is little higher than thorax. The lower limbs are positioned on frog-leg fashion symmetrically to avoid any distortion of natal cleft.

Incision and Midline Division of Sphincteric Muscles

The site of the neoanus is identified with electro-stimulation which usually corresponds, to midline pigmented skin fold or anal dimple and the limits are marked with back of knife or the silk sutures. The incision is given in the midsagittal plane, from the middle of the sacrum to the anterior limit of the anal dimple that is identified with electrical stimulation. A fine needle tip cutting diathermy with current of 700-800 mA is used.

The incision is given exactly in the midline dividing the entire sphincter mechanism. The incision goes through the skin, subcutaneous tissue, parasagittal fibers, muscle complex and levator muscle. Stay sutures may be applied on the either side of the incision to provide uniform traction to facilitate dissection. In the region of anal dimple mass of vertically oriented sphincter muscle complex, the fibers are present running from levator mechanism to the skin at anal dimple crossing the parasagittal fibers. In this region, the incision is deepened taking utmost care to stay in midline. As the lateral limits of the vertically running sphincter muscle are very narrow as compared to the antero-posterior limits, the surgeon can easily deviate leading to unequal division of muscle complex. Deviation from the midline may also be avoided by dividing the posterior edge of vertically running muscle complex first where it is perpendicular to and decussates with parasagittal fibers and tested with stimulator for equal contraction or both sides. If the deviation from the midline is identified by appreciating unequal contraction of muscle, the mistake is corrected at this stage before further splitting the muscle complex. At the upper end of incision, the tip of the coccyx corresponds to midline which is split in two halves. In the midline a fine midline fascia divides the anatomy in two half. In this region, staying in the midline is identified by stimulation of deep parasagittal muscle fibers. Deviation from midline is also identified by herniation of fat through the midline fascia. The midline plane is also avascular. The posterior rectal wall is identified with a characteristic whitish appearance. A mastoid retractor may be used for application of uniform traction in depth.

In cases with rectobulbar urethral fistula, the bulging rectum is seen as soon as the levator muscle is divided. In case of rectoprostatic urethral fistula the rectum is much smaller and may not bulge through the incision. In such cases, the rectum may be identified immediately below the coccyx. Searching for a rectum in the lower part of the incision in case of rectoprosthetic urethral fistula is the main source of complications in this operation.[16] The surgeon must keep in mind that there is a white fascia that covers the rectum posteriorly and laterally that MUST be incised. The rectal dissection is continued staying as close as possible to the rectal wall without injuring the wall itself. The dissection is done in both the lateral directions turn by turn to maintain symmetry. Stay sutures are applied over the midline of the posterior rectal wall at the lower limit and an incision is given exactly in the midline. The incision is continued distally, staying in the midline while applying stitches in the edges of the rectum. Uniform traction is helpful. At the distal end of incision, a rectourethral fistula is identified as a 1-2 mm opening. Multiple 6/0 sutures are placed in a semi-circumferential manner around the fistula, above and lateral to it to give uniform traction.

An incision is given just distal to these sutures and the dissection is now done in the submucosal plane for 5-10 mm. This is then continued to a full thickness dissection till the rectum is completely separated from the urinary tract. The separation of the urethra from the rectum requires meticulous dissection and is the most important step of the operation. The fistula is closed with 3-4, 6/0 long-term absorbable sutures. The dissection is proceeded till the rectum is mobilized enough to be placed within the limits of the sphincter without any tension and at the same time avoiding any prolapse.

The rectum is then examined to judge the need for tapering. This is usually not required now due to early referral of cases, decreased incidence of megarectum and the good diverting colostomies.[16]

The limits of the sphincter are determined electrically and marked with temporary silk sutures. The anterior limits of the sphincter must be reconstructed. The posterior edge of the levator, muscle is electrically determined and rectum is placed anterior to it. The levator is repaired with interrupted 5/0 absorbable sutures taking a bite of the posterior rectal wall to fix it in a proper position to avoid retraction and rectal prolapse. The perineal body is reconstructed. The wound is closed in the midline in layers. The anoplasty is performed within the limits of the sphincter with 16, 6/0 circumferential long-term absorbable sutures. The damaged or the ischemic part of the rectum is trimmed off. The distal rectal smooth muscle, resected during correction of anorectal malformations, shows similarities to the function reported previously on normal anal smooth muscle evaluated *in vitro* and thus has the functional properties of a sphincter and should be preserved as far as possible.[17]

Patients with rectourethral bulbar fistulae, have an 80% chance of having a bowel control by the age of three. Patients with rectoprostatic have a higher incidence of associated defects (60%) as compared to those with the rectourethral bulbar fistulae (30%). The patients with rectoprostatic fistula require a more demanding perirectal dissection to mobilize the rectum that is located higher in the pelvis.

RECTOVESTIBULAR FISTULA

Cases of rectovestibular fistula with a narrow and long fistulous tract who develop constipation soon after birth should be differentiated from the patients with vestibular anus who have a good and muscular anus. The later do not require any management in the newborn period if not constipated. The baby may be kept on dilatation and a single stage PSARP at 3-6 months of age is justified in these without any colostomy. However, cases of vestibular fistula that have constipation do merit a colostomy.

The important feature here is that the rectum and the vagina share a long common wall that must be separated by creating a plane of dissection between the two. This enables the complete mobilization of the rectum so that it can be put in the proper place. The patient is placed in the prone position with pelvis elevated with a roll. The incision is given from the coccyx to the fistula site. Multiple sutures are placed in a circumferential manner around the fistula opening to provide uniform traction. Most of the dissection is the same as that for PSARP in the lateral directions. The difference is that the rectum is not opened in the midline. After lateral mobilization the dissection proceeds from caudal to cranial direction anterior to the rectum. During the dissection, two walls are made out of one, taking care to avoid perforations either in the rectal wall or the vaginal wall. If it is to happen at all, it should be avoided in the rectum. Once the separation is complete, the limits of the sphincter are determined electrically. The perineal body is reconstructed bringing together the anterior limits of sphincter. The rest of the procedure is the same as PSARP.

Patient with vestibular fistula have an excellent prognosis, with 93% of patients having bowel control.[16] About 70% have constipation that is incurable but manageable.

CLOACA

Cloaca is defined as a defect in which the urinary tract, the vagina and the rectum are all fused, creating a single common channel, and opening into an orifice at the site of the normal urethra.[18]

This represents a spectrum of malformations. The treatment differs on whether the common channel is less than or more than 3 cm in length on the cystoscopy measured from the proximal end of the common channel up to the perineum.[19,20] About 2/3rd of patients have a short common channel.

The patient is placed in lithotomy position and cystoscopy is done to assess the length of the common channel.

Plan of Surgery according to Length of Common Channel

Length of common channel	Plan of surgery
Less than 1 cm	No urogenital mobilization
1 - 2.5 cm	Urogenital mobilization
2.5 -3 cm	Rectum mobilization + urogenital mobilization
3 - 5 cm	Extended transabdominal urogenital mobilization
More than 5 cm	Transabdominal urogenital mobilization

For short common channel the patient is placed in the prone position with the pelvis elevated with a roll. The incision is given from the middle portion of the sacrum to the single perineal orifice. The entire sphincter mechanism is divided in the midline and the rectum is exposed. During the last decade, a total urogenital moblization has been found to be beneficial for these patients.[21] The rectum is separated from the vaginal wall by creating two walls out of one. Multiple 6/0 silk sutures are placed taking the edges of the common channel, along with the edges of the vaginal walls, to exert uniform traction. The urethra and the vagina are mobilized together. Another set of sutures are placed transversally 5 mm proximal to the clitoris and the entire common channel is mobilized as one. The dissection is proceeded till a vascular fibrous structure is identified and divided. This step allows a gain of 2-4 cm length of the urogenital structures. The purpose is to place the urethral meatus at its normal location just below the clitoris. The edges of the vagina are sutured to skin of the perineum forming the new labia. The initial common channel is divided in the midline to make two flaps that are sutured on either side. About 80% of these patients with a good sacrum have bowel control and most of them can empty their bladder voluntarily. However, remaining 20% of patients with a short common channel would require CIC.[18]

Patients with long common channel more than 5 cm are approached through the abdomen with an incision in the midline. If the channel is between 3-5 cm the posterior sagittal approach may be tried and a total urogenital mobilization may be attempted.[16] The separation requires delicate surgery and the decision should be made by an experienced surgeon. Seventy percent of all patients with a common channel longer than 3 cm require intermittent catheterization to empty their bladder.[18]

Further operation depends upon the anatomy of each case. If the vagina is large as in cases of hydrometrocolpos, then it may easily reach the perineum. In cases with a short vagina, a switch procedure may be feasible in cases with two joined hydrocolpos with separate hemiuteri. In such cases, the septum may be divided and one entire Mullerian structure may be resected. The blood supply to one side should be preserved to provide the blood supply to the side that is being switched down.

If the vagina is very short, small and high, a replacement is needed. The first choice for vaginal replacement is to use a part of the rectum in babies with a megarectum. The rectum is divided longitudinally to form both, the new vagina and the neorectum. If the patient has internal genitalia, the segment of neovagina is sutured to it. If not, the upper part of the neovagina is closed. The second choice for the vaginal replacement is the use of sigmoid colon, followed by segment of small bowel. Patients with long common channel have a high frequency of complex associated anomalies. Approximately 50% of the patients with cloaca have hydrocolpos that may lead to bilateral megaureters and hydronephrosis.

During the first 24 hrs of life, emphasis is placed on the recognition and treatment of potentially lethal associated defects, mainly urologic, esophageal or cardiac. The baby should not be taken to the operating room without ruling out these associated defects.[18] The most common associated anomalies involved are those of the urinary tract with renal agenesis, renal dysplasia, vesicoureteral reflux and megaureter. These children may exhibit some form of masculinization of the external genitalia with the accessory urethra or cloacal channel assuming a phallic position in an enlarged clitoris.[22]

All babies with cloacal anomaly should undergo an ultrasound of the kidneys and pelvis before surgery. If a hydrocolpos is present, it should be drained at the same time the colostomy is performed. The colostomy should be completely diverting so as to prevent contamination of the urinary tract.

In cases of extremely long common channel that lies usually near the trigone, the bladder neck is closed and a vesicostomy is done. About 30% of these patients have duplicated Mullerian structures. The prognosis should be explained to the patients well in advance and the complications that may arise, especially during pregnancy, may be explained.

UROGENITAL SINUS WITH NORMAL RECTUM

A perineal approach with or without a skin flap seems to be effective for those patients with a low implantation of the vagina. However, in patients with a high vaginal implantation, this treatment frequently fails to provide a good, functional vagina due to a narrow and strictured vaginal opening. For patients with a high urogenital sinus with normal rectum a posterior sagittal transanorectal approach with a protective colostomy provides excellent exposure to the urogenital sinus.[23]

The pelvis is approached through a midsagittal posterior incision; the coccyx is split and the entire anorectal sphincteric mechanism is divided in the midline. The rectum is bivalved in the midline including both the posterior and anterior rectal walls. The vagina is then fully separated from the urogenital sinus, mobilized and sutured to the perineum. The rectum and the sphincteric mechanism are meticulously reconstructed. A midline incision assures the preservation of anorectal innervation, and provides excellent exposure to the pelvis. Anal dilatations are not necessary to maintain a patent and supple anorectal opening because the rectum has two suture lines, one in front of the other.[23] After the colostomy is closed, most patients have appropriate bowel control for their age.

GYNECOLOGICAL OPERATIONS FOR CASES WITH ANORECTAL MALFORMATIONS

It is best to do a vaginoscopy at the time of PSARP to identify a vaginal septum. The presence of vaginal agenesis is noted. The Mullerian structures are identified with delineation of the uterine anatomy. The benefits of the early repair of Mullerian anomalies include adequate repair, decreased chances of injury and good sexual functional outcome. For hydrocolpos, a vaginostomy may be done. A vesicostomy is an alternative option.

In cases with vestibular fistula or perineal fistula, a normal delivery may be planed. Cloacal anomalies would require a cesarean section for delivery. Vaginal replacement is done early for cases with cloaca. It may be done later for cases with Mayer-Rokitansky syndrome. Introitoplasty should be done after puberty but before the onset of menstruation. Vaginal dilatation may also be helpful for cases with a pliable vaginal wall.

Short-term vaginal dilatation may be done from Hegar-dilator number 14-17, if menstrual function is not adequate. Asymmetry of the duplicated uterus indicates increased chances of atresia of the less developed side. The incidence of vaginal atresia is 25% of all cases of anorectal malformations. The incidence of vaginal agenesis is 5% of all cases.

Gynecologic anomalies are common in patients with persistent cloaca, but, except for hydrocolpos, these patients remain asymptomatic in the neonatal period.[24] To prevent future problems, the management of the neonatal cloaca must include the early clarification of the gynecologic anatomy, specifically the patency of Mullerian structures. Unilateral atretic structures and tubes connected to atretic uteri should be resected.[24] One must be suspicious of menstrual problems in teenagers operated on early in life for persistent cloaca.

POSTERIOR CLOACA

This rare entity is identified with a separated pubic bone, with the clitoris placed posteriorly, a single orifice is located posteriorly through which both the urine and stool come out. It is defined as a defect in which urethra and vagina are fused together forming a urogenital sinus that deviates posteriorly and opens in the anterior rectal wall at the anus or immediately anterior to it.[25] The rectum is essentially normal or may be minimally anteriorly mislocated. The diagnosis requires a suspicious observer and a meticulous examination of the female genitalia. A complete urologic evaluation is mandatory because 88% of these patients have important associated urologic defects. A posterior sagittal transanorectal approach allows a full dissection and mobilization of urethra and vagina together to be placed in a normal location. Rectal dissection and mobilization is avoided to preserve the bowel control. Most patients enjoy bowel and urinary control.

ASSOCIATED TETHERED CORD

Tethered cord has been found to be associated in 24% of all patients with anorectal malformations.[26] The prevalence varies from 43% in the complex group to 11% in patients with rectovestibular fistula.[26] Patients with tethered cord have a lateral sacral ratio lower than that of patients without tethered cord (0.410 versus 0.702). Tethered cord is reported to be present in 90% of patients with myelodysplasia, 60% in patients with a presacral mass, 57% of patients with sacral hemivertebrae and 56% of patients with a single kidney. The risk of having tethered cord is also reported to increase with the number of associated anomalies present. Patients with tethered cord have worse functional prognosis than those without tethered cord.[26] A study also showed that the tethered cord occurred more frequently in patients with severe anorectal defects, sacral hypodevelopment, myelodysplasia, presacral mass, sacral hemivertebrae, or a single kidney, or in those with an anorectal defect with poor functional prognosis. Presently, there is no evidence to support the concept that tethered cord by itself affects the functional prognosis of patients with anorectal malformations. Also, there is no good evidence demonstrating that surgical untethering improves the prognosis.[26]

FOLLOW-UP

Globally, 75% of all patients with ARM following PSARP have voluntary bowel movements.[27] Though, half of the patients in this group still soil their underwear occasionally.[27] Therefore, about 37.5% of all cases are considered totally continent. Constipation has been reported as the most common sequelae. Urinary incontinence was relatively common after the repair of cloacas. Male patients rarely suffer from urinary incontinence. Twenty-five percent of all cases have been found to suffered from fecal incontinence but they significantly improved their quality of life when subjected to a bowel management program.[27] All patients born with anorectal malformations can be kept clean of stool and dry of urine, either because they achieve bowel control or because they are subjected to a bowel management program.[27]

Bowel management consisting of enemas, laxatives, and medications is successful when administered in an organized manner.[28] It is vital to determine the type of fecal incontinence from which the patients suffer and to target their treatment accordingly.[28]

Bowel management was found to be successful in 93% of patients in the constipation group and 88% in the diarrhea group.[28] About 97% patients in a group of patients who had no potential for bowel control became continent for stools. Continent appendicostomy may be used to change the route of enema administration, but in only those patients for whom bowel management with rectal enemas has proved successful.[29] This operation further improves their quality of life. The appendix must thus be preserved whenever possible in patients at risk for fecal incontinence. Segmental dilatation of the sigmoid colon may be a source of fecal pseudoincontinence and, therefore, should be ruled out when the surgeon is evaluating patients with fecal incontinence.[30]

SUMMARY

Anorectal malformations comprise a spectrum of defects. Some of these defects are minor, with an excellent functional prognosis. Others are complex and may be associated with other defects in the urinary tract that may risk the patient's life. The decision-making process for the management of a newborn with anorectal malformations is crucial; the timing and establishment of priorities are the key to success.[31]

A simplified well planned approach helps to avoid the most common errors in the management of anorectal malformation.[8] Yet, there are still many children born with severe anatomic deficiencies who cannot expect normal bowel function. For this group, a bowel management program is available to help improve their quality of life. This is discussed in detail in chapter 81.

REFERENCES

1. Peña A, Devries PA. Posterior sagittal anorectoplasty: important technical considerations and new applications. J Pediatr Surg 1982;17(6):796-811.
2. deVries PA, Peña A. Posterior sagittal anorectoplasty. J Pediatr Surg 1982;17(5):638-43.
3. Peña A. Posterior sagittal anorectoplasty as a secondary operation for the treatment of fecal incontinence. J Pediatr Surg 1983;18(6):762-73.
4. Peña A. Posterior sagittal approach for the correction of anorectal malformations. Adv Surg 1986;19:69-100.
5. Peña A. Potential anatomic sphincters of anorectal malformations in females. Birth Defects Orig Artic Ser 1988;24(4):163-75.
6. Peña A. Surgical treatment of female anorectal malformations. Birth Defects Orig Artic Ser 1988;24(4):403-23.
7. Peña A. Advances in the management of fecal incontinence secondary to anorectal malformations. Surg Annu 1990;22:143-67.
8. Peña A. Current management of anorectal anomalies. Surg Clin North Am 1992;72(6):1393-416.
9. Peña A. Anorectal malformations. Semin Pediatr Surg 1995;4(1):35-47.
10. Peña A, Hong AR, Midulla P, Levitt M. Reoperative surgery for anorectal anomalies. Semin Pediatr Surg 2003;12(2):118-23.
11. Peña A, Grasshoff S, Levitt M. Re-operations in anorectal malformations. J Pediatr Surg 2007;42(2):318-25.
12. Levitt MA, Peña A. Outcomes from the correction of anorectal malformations. Curr Opin Pediatr 2005;17(3):394-401.
13. Peña A, Amroch D, Baeza C, Csury L, Rodriguez G. The effects of the posterior sagittal approach on rectal function (experimental study). J Pediatr Surg. 1993;28(6):773-78.
14. Peña A. The posterior sagittal approach: implications in adult colorectal surgery. Harry E. Bacon Lectureship Dis Colon Rectum 1994;37(1):1-11.
15. Torres R, Levitt MA, Tovilla JM, Rodriguez G, Peña A. Anorectal malformations and Down's syndrome. J Pediatr Surg 1998;33(2):194-97.
16. Pena A. Anorectal anomalies. In Atlas of Children's Surgery, 1st edition, Ed. GHWillital, EKielly, Amin Gohary, Devendra K Gupta, Minju Li, Y.Tsuchida, PABST Publishers, Germany 2005;196-209.
17. Hedlund H, Peña A. Does the distal rectal muscle in anorectal malformations have the functional properties of a sphincter? J Pediatr Surg 1990;25(9):985-89.
18. Peña A, Levitt M. Surgical management of cloacal malformations. Semin Neonatol 2003;8(3):249-57.
19. Peña A. The surgical management of persistent cloaca: results in 54 patients treated with a posterior sagittal approach. J Pediatr Surg 1989;24(6):590-98.
20. Peña A, Levitt MA, Hong A, Midulla P. Surgical management of cloacal malformations: a review of 339 patients. J Pediatr Surg 2004 Mar;39(3):470-79; discussion 470-79.
21. Peña A. Total urogenital mobilization--an easier way to repair cloacas. J Pediatr Surg 1997;32(2):263-67; discussion 267-68.
22. Karlin G, Brock W, Rich M, Peña A. Persistent cloaca and phallic urethra. J Urol 1989;142(4):1056-59.
23. Pena A, Filmer B, Bonilla E, Mendez M, Stolar C. Trans-anorectal approach for the treatment of urogenital sinus: preliminary report. J Pediatr Surg 1992;27(6):681-85.
24. Levitt MA, Stein DM, Peña A. Gynecologic concerns in the treatment of teenagers with cloaca. J Pediatr Surg 1998;33(2):188-93.
25. Peña A, Kessler O. Posterior cloaca: a unique defect. J Pediatr Surg 1998;33(3):407-12.
26. Levitt MA, Patel M, Rodriguez G, Gaylin DS, Pena A. The tethered spinal cord in patients with anorectal malformations. J Pediatr Surg 1997;32(3):462-68.
27. Peña A, Hong A. Advances in the management of anorectal malformations. Am J Surg 2000;180(5):370-76.
28. Peña A, Guardino K, Tovilla JM, Levitt MA, Rodriguez G, Torres R. Bowel management for fecal incontinence in patients with anorectal malformations. J Pediatr Surg 1998;33(1):133-37.
29. Levitt MA, Soffer SZ, Peña A. Continent appendicostomy in the bowel management of fecally incontinent children J Pediatr Surg 1997;32(11):1630-33.
30. Peña A, el Behery M. Megasigmoid: a source of pseudo-incontinence in children with repaired anorectal malformations. J Pediatr Surg 1993;28(2):199-203.
31. Peña A. Management of anorectal malformations during the newborn period. World J Surg 1993;17(3):385-92.

Anomalies Associated with Anorectal Malformations

D K Gupta, Shilpa Sharma

Anorectal malformations (ARM) are often associated with other significant anomalies, which can be a cause of morbidity and even mortality. The overall incidence of associated malformations in ARM varies between 30-60%.[1-2]

This wide variation reflects the difference in the screening protocol adopted by each center. The incidence of associated anomalies also varies according to size and sample of study population, facilities of diagnostic investigations and zeal with which associated anomalies are looked for. Because anorectal malformations occur at the critical age of embryonic differentiation (2-8 weeks), associated multisystem anomalies are not uncommon and may be seen in 40-70% of patients. Patients with high malformations are more likely to have more associated defects. It is now increasingly being recognized that associated malformations (especially urological anomalies) are the prime cause of morbidity associated with ARM. It is therefore the responsibility of the treating surgeon to observe a rigid protocol for screening these patients for the associated anomalies and instituting an early treatment. Table 74.1 enlists these associated malformations.

VACTERAL association:[3] Vertebral defects, anorectal, cardiac, tracheo-esophageal fistula, esophageal atresia, renal anomalies and radial dysplasia and limb defects.

Curarino syndrome:[4] Partial sacral agenesis, presacral mass (sacrococcygeal teratoma or anterior meningocele) and anal stenosis. Typically there is hemisacrum with preserved first sacral segment.

Table 74.1: Associated malformations with ARM

1. Genitourinary malformations (20-54%)
   Renal–Agenesis, dysplasia, ectopia, hydronephrosis, duplex
   Ureter– VUR, ectopia, megaureter, ureterocele
   Bladder– Hutch diverticulum, megacystis, exstrophy, neurogenic bladder
   Urethra– Atresia, congenital urethral fistula, PUV, hypospadias, megalourethra (Figs 74.1A and B)
   Genital– Urogenital sinus anomaly, Vaginal atresia, double vagina, hemiuterus, bifid scrotum., cryptorchidism
2. Sacrospinal anomalies (~ 13%)
   Sacral agenesis (caudal regression syndrome) ~25%
   Vertebral segmentation anomalies, limb anomalies
3. Spinal cord anomalies
   - Myelodysplasia
   - Occult spinal dysraphism (Tethered cord syndrome)
   - Syringohydromyelia
4. Cardiac anomalies (10-15%) –Tetralogy of Fallot, VSD, ASD
5. Gastrointestinal malformations (20%)
   - Esophageal atresia—6-10%
   - Duodenal obstructions—1-2%
   - Abdominal wall defects
   - Hirschsprung's disease—3-5%
6. Chromosomal anomalies—Down's syndrome, trisomy 18
7. Associated syndrome

Townes-Brocks syndrome:[5] ARM with hand and ear anomaly. There may be cardiovascular, genitourinary malformations and mental retardation.

FG syndrome:[6] ARM, mental retardation, neurological defects (marked constipation), facial dysmorphism, hand abnormality (broad thumbs) and genital abnormality.

Cat-eye syndrome:[7] ARM with coloboma of iris, choroid, micro-ophthalmia and ear anomalies.

Klein-Waardenberg syndrome:[8] Facial dysmorphism, pigmentary defects and ARM.

Caudal regression syndrome:[7,9] ARM, spinal cord anomaly, genitourinary and lumbosacral defects.

GENITOURINARY MALFORMATIONS

Vesicoureteric reflux (VUR) is most common associated urologic anomaly. Rectovesical fistula and cloaca may have 90% chance of an associated genitourinary anomaly while in low defects like perineal fistula, the incidence of associated anomalies is quite low (< 10%).[10] Some series have reported higher incidence of genitourinary anomaly in low defects also. With lumbosacral spinal defects, the incidence of urological involvement is 50%.[11] Genital anomalies in girls most commonly involve vaginal and uterine septation defects and vaginal agenesis.[12]

The initial approach in ARM management involves decision making regarding the need for a colostomy and screening for associated malformations. The genitourinary tract is the most frequent and serious site of associated defects in anorectal malformations. The 1969 report of the surgical section of the American Academy of Pediatrics (AAP) reported a 26% incidence of associated significant urologic malformations.[2] Parrott noted that around 40% of patients with high anomalies, 21% of intermediate anomalies and 14% of low anomalies have associated urologic malformations.[13] Rich et al showed a 52% incidence of urologic anomalies in males with a bladder neck fistula, whereas almost 30% of females with a cloaca had associated urologic anomalies.[14] The higher the level of the lesion, higher is the incidence of genitourinary anomalies.[13-15] Overall, urinary tract anomalies occur in more than 40% of all patients with ARM (~20% in low, 50% in high).

Screening: An ultrasound of the genitourinary tract performed 72 hours after birth is used as the primary method of screening for urinary tract anomalies. The kidneys, ureters, bladder and urethra should all be assessed (Figs 74.1 to 74.4). The role of the voiding cystourethrogram (VCUG) is clear when there is upper tract dilatation on ultrasonography. However, most centers now recommend a VCUG in all newborns with imperforate anus. The points in favor for performing a VCUG are:

i. High incidence of VUR noted with high lesions and even in low anomalies.[16]
ii. The morbidity associated with missed VUR and reflux nephropathy is significant but can be easily prevented by chemoprophylaxis.
iii. Urethral anomalies can be missed in males if VCUG not done.
iv. Voiding film may give additional information about the site of fistula.

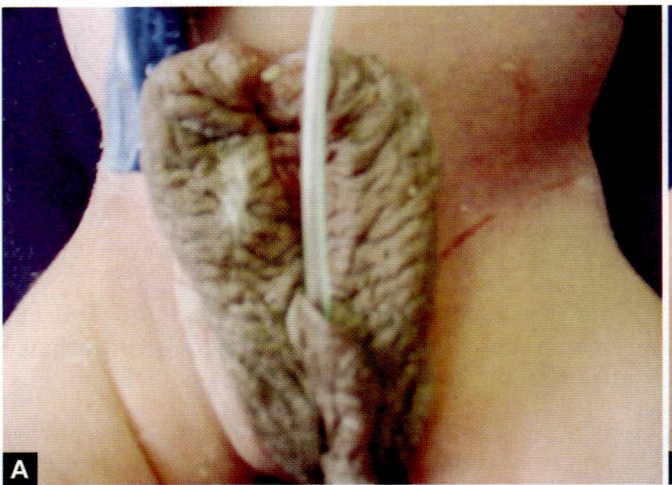 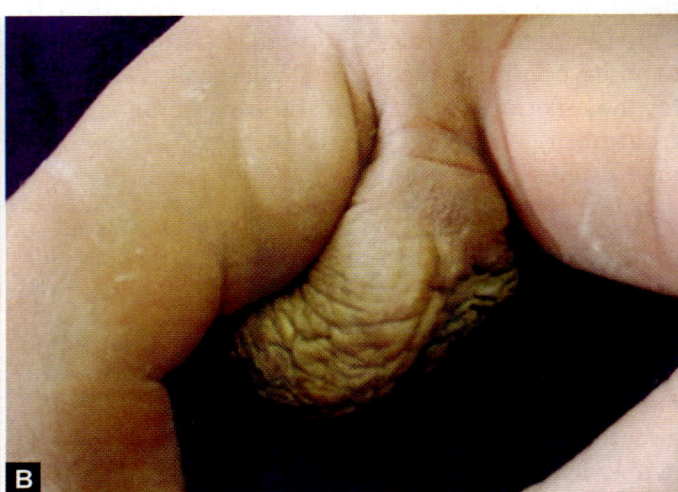

Figs 74.1A and B: Megalourethra with hypospadias

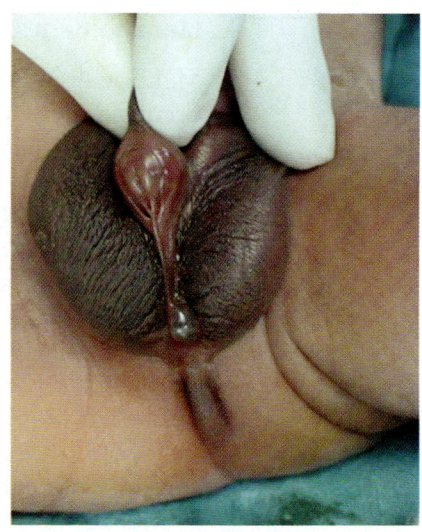

Fig. 74.2: Anorectal malformation with scrotal hypospadias

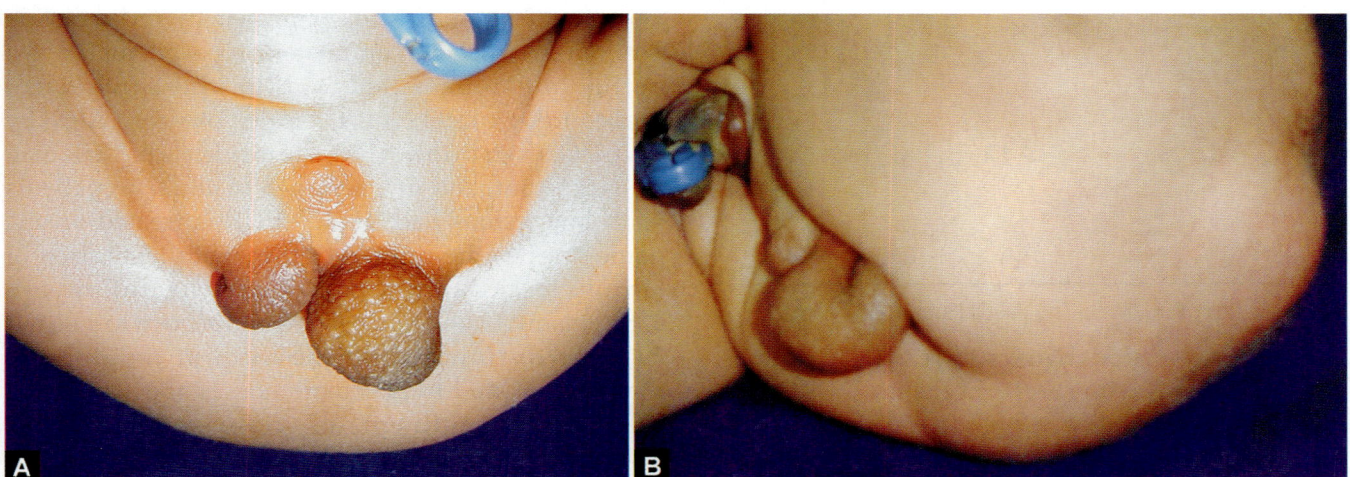

Figs 74.3A and B: Anorectal malformation with
A. Bifid scrotum and flat bottom **B.** Same patient with lumbosacral spina bifida also

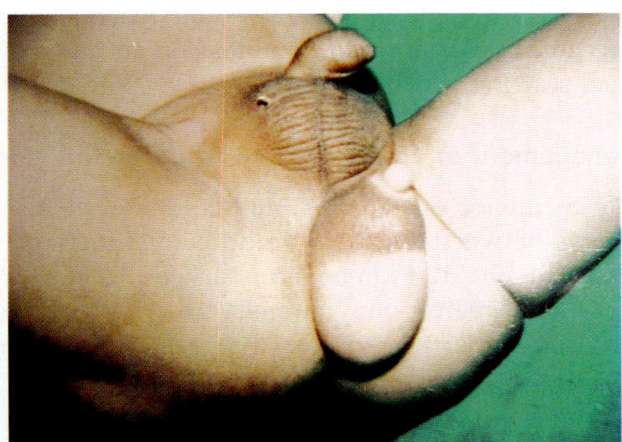

Fig. 74.4: Ectopic lipomatous scrotum

v. Reflux into seminal vesicles and vas may be detected thus identifying boys who may be in risk for recurrent epididymitis and future infertility.

vi. VCUG can also identify signs, which suggest a neurogenic bladder like VUR, trabeculated bladder and high post void residue. Early management of these patients ensures preservation of upper tracts.

The ARGUS protocol devised by Boemer's et al is ideal in evaluating newborns with ARM.[17] This protocol shown below ensures that associated anomalies are not missed without performing unnecessary investigations (Fig. 74.5). This protocol states that ultrasound KUB, a VCUG and a plain X-ray of the spine and sacrum is mandatory in all

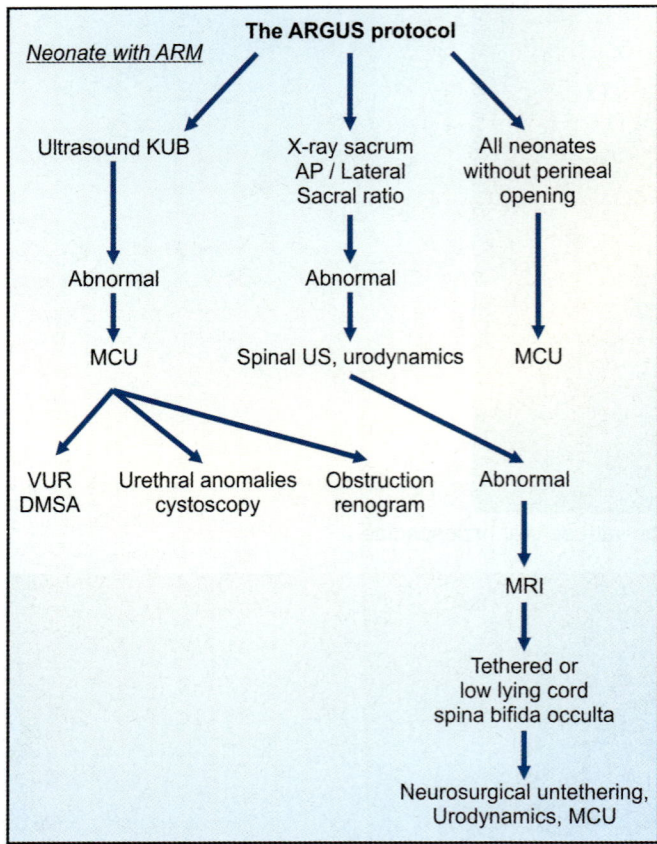

Fig. 74.5: The ARGUS protocol

Indications for urodynamics in ARM
I. All patients with sacral anomalies
II. Cloacal anomalies
III. All patients with transabdominal dissection of distal bowel
IV. All patients with tethered or low lying cord

patients. Radionuclide studies and IVP or preferably a magnetic resonance urogram are indicated only in the presence of abnormal findings noted on US or VCUG examination, e.g. horse shoe kidney, ectopic ureter/s, ureterocele. In addition, all children with ARM and associated sacral abnormalities must have an early urodynamic evaluation. Postoperative urodynamics is also recommended in boys with rectourethral fistula who have associated sacral agenesis, in girls with cloacal anomaly and in all patients who have had transabdominal mobilization of the distal bowel. Cystometry is also recommended in all patients with voiding dysfunction following PSARP and those who have undergone detethering of the cord.

Management of Urologic Anomalies

McLorie et al found that mortality from renal failure occurred in up to 6.4% of patients with high anomalies and even in 1.1% patients who had low anomalies.[18] The morbidity and mortality of the genitourinary anomalies in ARM clearly exceeds those related to the ARM itself. Before undertaking the definitive repair for ARM, it is essential to avoid urinary tract infections which may be caused by a rectourogenital fistula or reflux. This is best accomplished by ensuring a completely diverting proximal sigmoid colostomy and washes of the distal pouch. Hyperchloremic acidosis may occur due to intestinal absorption of urine in the presence of a large fistula.

Renal agenesis and dysplasia including the common multicystic kidney disease, can be diagnosed on ultrasonography and confirmed by radionuclide scanning. Associated contralateral renal anomalies and reflux must be ruled out in these children. Vesicoureteric reflux must be ruled out in all ARM by a VCUG. Even in low ARM, the incidence of VUR may be significant, and in a series 18 of 48 (37%) patients with low lesions had VUR.[16] VUR is treated on the same lines as the primary reflux, with institution of prophylactic antibiotics and close follow-up. Urodynamic evaluation becomes important to rule out bladder dysfunction in the form of uninhibited contractions and hypocompliance. In these patients, additional treatment of co-existent bladder dysfunction is also needed. Early institution of anticholinergics increases the chances of resolution of VUR. Surgical intervention is indicated for the breakthrough infections, Grade IV-V reflux, in the presence of a single kidney, deterioration of the upper tract function or onset of hypertension and the new renal scarring.

Management of Lower Urinary Tract Dysfunction

The incidence of neuropathic bladder with ARM ranges between 7-18%.[19] Voiding dysfunction in patients with ARM can be secondary to:
  i. Caudal regression syndrome with sacral agenesis.
 ii. Associated tethered cord syndrome or overt spinal dysraphism.
iii. Secondary to operative trauma during PSARP.

The reported incidence of urinary incontinence in low anomalies varies between 0-10%. However, up to

33% of patients with high anomalies have urinary incontinence.[20-22] The PSARP procedure by itself does not lead to a higher incidence of neurogenic bladder as compared to other traditional procedures. Pena reported a 10% incidence of incontinence in 233 children who underwent PSARP for a high or intermediate anomaly.[20] The incidence of urinary incontinence was 69% inpatients with a high confluence cloaca. The incontinence inpatients with a high cloacal malformation is usually due to inability to empty the bladder and not from bladder neck incompetence.

Early urodynamic evaluation helps in instituting clean intermittent catheterization (CIC) early. It is well documented that early institution of CIC (preferably before 3 months) leads to better compliance by the parents and the child. Clean intermittent catheterization allows complete bladder emptying at low pressures and prevents upper tract deterioration. The CIC is indicated in:[23]

1. High pressure bladders (> 30 cm H_2O filling pressure).
2. Presence of functional outlet obstruction in the form of detrusor sphincter dys-synergia.
3. Poor detrusor contraction leading to high residual urine.

Chronic constipation and fecal impaction following PSARP can itself lead to bladder outflow obstruction and induce detrusor instability. Proper management of constipation alone in such cases will lead to resolution of UTI and enuresis. It has also been documented that treatment of constipation can sometimes lead to urinary incontinence by reducing the leak point pressures. Prophylactic antibiotics are indicated in patients with VUR, neurogenic bladder and upper tract dilatation and also in boys with urethro-ejaculatory reflux. Anticholinergics, usually with CIC, are used inpatients with detrusor hyper-reflexia or detrusor hypocompliance. It must be kept in mind that anticholinergics decrease bowel motility, which may adversely affect postoperative bowel function.

SKELETAL ANOMALIES

Skeletal anomalies described in relation to ARM include radial aplasia, major lower limb defects, rib and vertebral anomalies. Expertise help from pediatric orthopedic surgeon would be required to repair or reconstruct the defects as much as found feasible, including the use of prosthesis and physiotherapy, to improve cosmesis and function.

Spinal Anomalies

Vertebral defects of lumbosacral region are most common and the overall incidence of lumbosacral anomalies noted on plain radiographs in patients with ARM ranges from 30-45% (Fig. 74.6).[24-29] The sacral ratio devised by Pena is helpful in assessing sacral hypodevelopment.[21] In the AP view, a line is traced from the most superior aspect of the iliac crest on both sides. A second line is drawn between the two posterior inferior iliac spines. A third line is drawn parallel to the other two, joins at the lowest radiologically visible part of the sacrum. The sacral ratio is obtained by dividing the distance between the two lower lines by the distance between the two upper lines. The average ratio in 100 normal children was 0.74 and lower ratio represented sacral hypodevelopment. The same ratio obtained on a lateral view of the spine X-ray, was 0.77 and considered more reliable.

All patients with ARM and a sacral defect should undergo a screening spinal ultrasound examination in the newborn period (before 3 months of age when the ossification of the posterior lamina begins). MRI of the spine should be obtained in older patients and inpatients with an abnormal finding on spinal ultrasonography.[17] A normal plain film of the spine

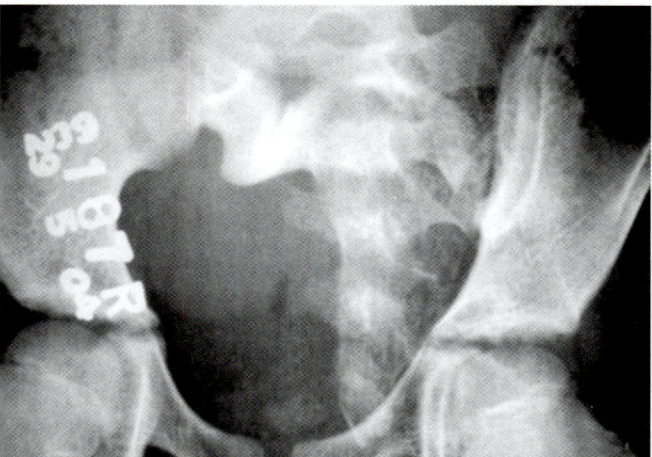

Fig. 74.6: Skiagram Lumbosacral region AP view depictive of a hemisacrum

does not always rule out a tethered cord. Tethered cord syndrome can lead to neurogenic bladder, back pain and gait disturbances. It is not clear whether the tethered cord directly affects fecal continence. Though, untethering may prevent subsequent neurogenic bladder or other complications, at present, it is unknown whether it will be beneficial for improving the anorectal function.[24-26] These patients require close follow-up and urodynamic evaluation at 1 and 6 months after surgery as recurrent tethering may occur. Vertebral anomalies may signify an underlying occult lesion and the hemivertebral anomalies can result in scoliosis and therefore may require bracing or operative spinal fusion to prevent further deterioration in posture.

SPINAL CORD ANOMALIES

With advent of magnetic resonance imaging, spectrum of spinal anomalies has been well documented and appreciated but all of them may not be significant.

Tethered cord has been found in 20-50% of patients with ARM but in absence of functional sequelae, detethering may not be indicated. Table 74.2 outlines the indications for MRI screening for telthered cord syndrome. In presence of other unequivocal neurological symptoms with bowel dysfunction, untethering may be beneficial.[30] Following spinal cord abnormalities have been reported:

- Tethered cord
- Spinal canal stenosis
- Myelomeningocele
- Spinal cord syrinx
- Diastematomyelia
- Diplomyelia
- Dermoid cyst
- Neurogenic bladder
- Sacrococcygeal teratoma.

Table 74.2: Indications for MRI screening for tethered cord syndrome in ARM

Absolute	Recommended
• Myelodysplasia	• Bladder neck fistulas
• Sacral ratio of < 0.6 on lateral view	• Cloaca with common channel > 3 cm
• Complex defects	• Presacral mass
• Cloacal exstrophy	• Hemivertebrae
• Neurogenic bladder	• Poor result despite good surgery and good prognosis defect

Caudal Regression Syndrome

Rectal, genitourinary and lumbosacral spine anomalies associated with an anorectal malformation may represent a syndrome of 'caudal regression.[9,31]

Sacral agenesis is defined as the absence of all or part of two or more vertebral bodies at the lower end of the spinal column. This is associated with defective development of the S2-S4 sacral nerves. Isolated sacral agenesis occurs more frequently in babies born to diabetic mothers. Overall, up to 25% of patients with ARM have associated sacral agenesis and 75% of these patients have lower urinary tract dysfunction.[24,26] Classically, these patients have a flat buttock and a low or absent gluteal cleft. The urodynamic pattern in children with sacral agenesis is varied. Boemers et al studied 13 patients with partial sacral agenesis and ARM.[32] Three patients had normal urodynamic findings, 5 showed a hyper-reflexic pattern and 5 others had a hyporeflexic study. In 1999, these abnormalities were grouped together using the term ARGUS (Anorectal, genitourinary, sacral). Guzman et al demonstrated an upper motor lesion in 35% patients (detrusor hyper-reflexia, detrusor sphincter dys-synergia) whereas 40% had a lower motor neuron lesion with absent sacral reflexes and detrusor areflexia.[33] The remaining 25% of patients had a normal study. There is no correlation between the number of affected vertebrae and the type of motor neuron lesion present. A VCUG and MRI of the spine are also recommended in these children. Treatment usually involves with CIC and prophylactic antibiotic therapy.

GENITAL ANOMALIES

Females with high ARM frequently have vaginal and uterine septation defects and vaginal agenesis. Pena recommends evaluating the patency of the fallopian tubes and uterus in babies with common cloaca. An intraoperative hysterosalpingogram is performed during the colostomy closure to rule out atresias of the uterus and vagina. Vaginal scarring secondary to the pull through procedure often leads to coital problem (dyspareunia) and the difficulty in vaginal delivery. Vaginal delivery in patients with a history of a vestibular fistula may also worsen fecal continence. Adult males may have ejaculatory duct obstruction, weak or absent erections and retrograde ejaculation. It has also been noted that a significant number of adults operated for high anorectal anomalies avoid sexual contact because of fecal incontinence. Careful follow-up and examination is required to assess these anomalies.[34] Psychological support and even surgical correction of these defects are required.

GASTROINTESTINAL ANOMALIES

Either as a part of VACTERAL association or in isolation, following gastrointestinal anomalies may be seen with ARM.[35]

- Esophageal atresia with tracheo-esophageal fistula
- Duodenal atresia
- Malrotation
- Hirschsprung's disease
- Duplication cyst
- Intestinal atresia

The treatment of most congenital gastrointestinal anomalies found in association with ARM, is usually done at the time of colostomy formation. Associated Hirschsprung's disease and other intestinal dysganglionosis, though uncommon (4%) and existence controversial, do not manifest early and are usually diagnosed after definitive repair of the ARM. The congenital pouch colon, classified under the group of rare lesions in the Krickenbeck classification, is not uncommon in certain areas, including in northern India, Pakistan and Bangladesh.[36] The incidence has been found as high as 20% of all high ARM cases from the authors center, and 63.6% of these having other associated anomalies.[37,38] Sometimes, very rare anomalies are encountered as a pouch colon opening into the bladder and also exteriorly as a patent intestinal fistula (Figs 74.3A and B). The management of this anomaly quite complex and deserves a separate chapter.[39-44]

CARDIOVASCULAR ANOMALIES

Incidence ranges from 8-20%. In patients with VACTERAL, the associated cardiac anomalies may be present in 50-80% cases. Most common anomalies are ventricular septal defect, patent ductus arteriosus, atrial septal defect and tetralogy of Fallot . Reconstruction of major malformations even in an association with serious cardiac anomalies, are though, feasible in most tertiary care level centers, yet it is expensive and requires repeated hospital visits for many surgeries and follow-ups. In absence of the support from insurance or the national health delivery system, an ethical based decision may have to be taken, if the local circumstances and economic status of the parents do not permit so.[45]

REFERENCES

1. Lerone M, Bolino A, Martucciello G. The genetics of associated malformations. A complex matter. Sem Paediatr Surg 1997;6:170-79.
2. Santulli TV, Schullinger IN, Kiesewetter WB, et al. Imperforate anus. A survey from the members of the surgical section of the American Academy of Pediatrics. J Pediatr Surg 1971;6:484-87.
3. Quan L and Smith DW. The VATER association. J Pediatr Surg 1973;82:104-07.
4. Currarino G, Coln D and Votteler T. Triad of anorectal, sacral and presacral and presacral anomalies. Am J Roentgenol 1981;137:395-98.
5. Townes PL and Brocks ER. Hereditary syndromes of imperforate anus with hand, foot and ear anomalies. J Pediatrics 1972;81:321-25.
6. Opitz JM, Richieri-da Costa A, Aase JM, et al. FG syndrome update 1988: note of 5 new patients and bibliography. Am J Med Genet 1988;30:309-28.
7. Lerone M, Bolino A and Martucciello G. The genetics of anorectal malformations: a complex matter. Semin Pediatr Surg 1997;6:170-79.
8. Nutman J, Nussenkorn I, Varsano I, Mimouni M and Goodman RM. Anal atresia and the Klein-Waardenberg syndrome. J Med Genet 1981;18:239-41.
9. Duhamel B. From the mermaid to anal imperforation: the syndrome of caudal regression. Arch Dis Child 1961;36:152-57.
10. Rich MA, Brock WA and Pena A. Spectrum of genitourinary malformations in patients with imperforate anus. Pediatr Surg Int 1988;3:110-13.
11. Parrott TS. urological implications of anorectal malformations. Urol clin North Am 1985;12:13-21.
12. Hall R, Fleming S, Gysler M and McLorie G. The genital tract in female children with imperforate anus. Am J Obstet Gynecol 1985;151:169-71.
13. Parrott TS. Urologic implications of anorectal malformations. Urol Clin North Am 1985;12:13-21.
14. Rich MA, Brock W A, Pena A. Spectrum of genitourinary malformations in patients with imperforate anus. Pediatr Surg Int 1988,3: 110-13.
15. Sheldon CA, Gilbert A, Levis AG, et al. Surgical implications of genitourinary tract anomalies in patients with imperforate anus. J Urol1992, 152: 196-99.
16. Misra D, Mushtaq I, Drake P, et al. Associated urologic anomalies in low imperforate anus are capable of causing significant morbidity: A 15-year experience. Urology 1996;48:281-83.

17. Boemers TML, Beek JF A, Bax NMA. Guidelines for the urological screening and initial management of lower urinary tract dysfunction in children with anorectal malfonnations – The ARGUS protocol. Br. J Urol. 1999;8:662-71.
18. McLorie GA, Sheldon CA, Fleischer M, et al. The genito-urinary system in patients with imperforate anus. J Pediatr Surg 1987;22:1100-04.
19. Brock W, Pena A. Urologic implications of imperforate anus. AUA update series 1991;10:202-07.
20. Pena A. Anorectal malformations. Semin Pediatr Surg. 1995;4: 35-47.
21. Rintala R, Mildh L, Lindahl H. Fecal continence and quality of life in adult patients with an operated low anorectal malformation. J Pediatr Surg 1992;27:902-05.
22. Rintala R, Lindahl H. Internal sphincter saving PSARP for high and intermediate anorectal malformations: technical considerations. Pediatr Surg. Int 1995;10:345-49.
23. Ralph Dl, Woodhouse CRJ, Ransley PG. The management of the neuropathic bladder in adolescents with imperforate anus. J Urol 1992;148:366-68.
24. Rivosecchi M, Lucchetti MC, Zaccara A, et al. Spinal dysraphism detected by magnetic resonance imaging in patients with anorectal anomalies. Incidence and clinical significance. J Pediatr Surg 1995;30:488-90.
25. Long FL, Hunter N, Mahboubi S, et al. Tethered cord and associated vertebral anomalies in children and infants with imperforate anus. Evaluation with MR imaging and plain radiography. Radiology 1996;2000:377-82.
26. Carson JA, Barnes PD, Tunell WP, et al. Imperforate anus: The neurologic implications of sacral abnormalities. J Pediatr Surg 1984;19:838-42.
27. Tsakayannis DE, Schamberger RC. Association of imperforate anus with occult spinal dysraphism. J Pediatr Surg 1995;30:1010-12.
28. Levitt MA, Patel M, Rodriguez G, et al. The tethered spinal cord in patients with anorectal malformations. J Pediatr Surg 1997;32:462-68.
29. Greenfield SP and Fera M. Urodynamic evaluation of the patient with an imperforate anus: a prospective study. J Urol 1991;146:539-41.
30. Levitt MA, Patel M, Rodriguez G, et al. The tethered spinal cord in patients with anorectal malformations. J Pediatr Surg 1997;32:462-68.
31. Loewy JA, Richards DG and Toi A. In-utero diagnosis of the caudal regression syndrome: report of three cases. J Clin Ultrasound 1987;15:469-71.
32. Boemers TM, Van Gool JD, De Jong TPVM, et al. Urodynamic evaluation of children with the caudal regression syndrome. J Urol 1994;151:1038-40.
33. Guzman L, Bauer SB, Hallet M, et al. The evaluation and management of children with sacral agenesis. Urology 1983;23:506-08.
34. Gupta DK, Sharma Shilpa. Current trends in Anorectal Malformations In "Current trends in Pediatrics" Vol 3 Ed Mathur GP, Mathur S. Nepal publ. Academa. 2006; 16: 161-73.
35. Paidas CN and Pena A. Rectum and anus. In Oldham KT, Colombani PM and Foglia RP (Eds) Surgery of infants and children: Scientific principles and practice, Philadelphia: Lippincott-Raven 1997;1323-61.
36. Holschneider A, Hutson J, Pena A, Beket E, Chatterjee S, Coran A, Davies M, Georgeson K, Grosfeld J, Gupta D, et al. Preliminary report on the International Conference for the Development of Standards for the Treatment of Anorectal Malformations. J Pediatr Surg. 2005;40:1521-26.
37. Gupta DK. Ethical Issues in Pediatric Surgery – Guest Lecture delivered during the Round Table Meet, 1st World Congress of Association of Pediatric Surgeons, Zagreb, Croatia, 2004.
38. Kumar A, Agarwala S, Srinivas M, Bajpai M, Bhatnagar V, Gupta DK, Gupta AK, Mitra DK. Anorectal malformations and their impact on survival. Indian J Pediatr 2005;72:1039-42.
39. Gupta DK. Management of Associated anomalies with anorectal malformation. Guest lecture delivered during the International Workshop on Anorectal Malformations, Varanasi, India 2001.
40. Gupta DK, Sharma Shilpa. Congenital Pouch Colon, in Anorectal Malformations, 1st edition, Ed. John Hutson and Alex Holschneider, Springer Heidelberg. 2006;11:211-22.
41. Gupta DK, Sharma Shilpa. Congenital pouch colon – Then and now. J Indian Assoc Pediatr Surg 2007;12:5-12.
42. Gupta DK. Congenital pouch colon: Present lacunae. J Indian Assoc Pediatr Surg 2007;12:1-2.
43. Sharma Shilpa, Gupta D K, Bhatnagar V, Bajpai M, Agarwala S. Management of Congenital Pouch Colon in Association with ARM 2005;10 (Suppl 1: S22).
44. Gupta DK. Editorial: Anorectal malformations- Wingspread to Krickenbeck. Journal of Ind Assoc. Ped Surg. 2005;10:79.
45. Greenwood RD, Rosenthal A and Nadas AS. Cardio-vascular malformations associated with imperforate anus. J Pediatr 1975; 86: 576-79.

Complications Following PSARP

Alex Holschneider, DK Gupta

The posterior sagittal anorectoplasty (PSARP) performed for infants and children with anorectal malformations (ARM) is a technically demanding operation and requires strict adherence to the finer operative details to achieve good results. The postoperative care of the wound, catheterization of the urinary bladder postoperatively for 7-10 days for appropriate healing of the rectourethral fistula and than a careful anal dilatation program for 10-12 weeks until the elasticity of the sphincter fibers is secured and the anus is growing itself, are vital to avoid severe complications.

These complications encountered following PSARP are listed in Table 75.1.[1-5] This list does not include the complications that may be encountered with the opening and closure of colostomy. The associated malformations in ARM also have an important bearing on postoperative results and morbidity. This article discusses the management of complications following PSARP. It also stresses the technical points which are important to avoid most of the complications as listed in Table 75.1. PSARP procedure in anorectal malformations is not usually associated with mortality, however mortality if any (10-20%) is related to associated cardiac defects, associated cerebral malformations, neonatal septicemia and very low birth weight.[4] Severe early complications following PSARP are rare. In a series of 792 patients reported by Alberto Pena, only 2% had complications requiring major re-operative surgery.[2] It is important to note, however, that lack of experience and non-adherence to the finer details of PSARP procedure can lead to significant and serious complication, many of them may continue even life-long.

The most important long-time complications after PSARP procedure is chronic constipation. It is astonishing that in the period from 1953 when Douglas Stephens presented first his sacral approach, being very similar to Pena's technique, up to 1982 (when Pena and de Vries introduced PSARP) fecal incontinence represented the main postoperative problem.[6,7] After the introduction of PSARP, primary fecal incontinence disappeared almost completely but secondary chronic constipation with overflow incontinence became the most important postoperative problem. The reconstruction of the anal sphincters was now improved but bowel rectal motility became disturbed.[5]

EARLY AND LATE COMPLICATIONS FOLLOWING PSARP

These are outlined in Table 75.1.

1. Wound infection or dehiscence is one of the most common complications following PSARP. It is recommended that a divided diverting colostomy should be constructed initially which decreases the incidence of infection following PSARP. A thorough cleaning of the bowel should also be done preoperatively.
2. Meticulous hemostasis and proper closure of the wound without leaving any dead space also decreases the incidence of wound infection. A deep infection of the wound may suggest dehiscence of the rectal tapering and needs aggressive management.
3. Inadequate dilatation, perianal sepsis, ischemia of the pulled down rectal pouch due to either an excessive or an inadequate mobilization leading to

Table 75.1: Early and late complications following PSARP

Early	Delayed
1. Wound infection, bleeding	1. Anocutaneous stenosis
2. Mis-located anus	2. Anorectal stricture
3. Wound dehiscence	3. Anal stenosis
4. Bowel retraction	4. Rectal mucosal prolapse
5. Recurrent fistula	5. Functional problems chronic constipation with overflow incontinence, primary fecal incontinence
6. Transient femoral nerve palsy	6 Urethral stricture
7. Injury to urethra, bladder, vas deferens, ureters	7. Urethral diverticulum
8. Peritonitis	8. Neurogenic bladder
9. Perineal skin excoriation	9. Fibrosis of vagina in cloacas
10. Bladder dysfunction	

tension on the neoanus can all lead to anocutaneous or anorectal stricture.

4. Tension on the anocutaneous anastomosis and infection can also lead to retraction of the bowel. Injury to the bladder neck, vas deferens and ectopic ureter can also occur if proper care is not taken during mobilization of the rectal pouch.
5. Transient femoral nerve palsy has been reported in adolescent patients' secondary to direct nerve compression in the prone position. Deviating from the strict midline approach of PSARP and improper (deep) placement of the self-retaining retractors can cause pudendal nerve damage and lead to postoperative neurogenic bladder.

Urethral stricture, diverticulum or recurrent fistula can all result due to improper closure of the fistula during surgery. Adequate postoperative catheterization for 12 days is also important to allow healing of the urethral suture line. Rectal mucosal prolapse can be prevented by proper fixation of the neoanus under adequate tension.

The management of primary fecal incontinence and constipation with secondary overflow incontinence would be dealt with in some detail.

DEFECATION PROBLEMS

Long-term results of surgery for high ARM has shown that at least 25-30% of children will suffer from fecal incontinence.[2,8-10] An additional 30 % will have varying degree of constipation, occasional soiling and fecal incontinence during periods of diarrhea. Though in some cases, fecal incontinence is a complication of surgery (a mislocated rectum), in most children, fecal incontinence is secondary to the defect. Fecal incontinence, therefore depends on the type of lesion and the original reconstructive procedure. Children with sacral agenesis, and males with a rectobladder neck fistula have the highest rates of fecal incontinence followed by the females with a high confluence cloaca.

It is also now well recognized that fecal continence does not improve with time and the future continence can be predicted within weeks of stoma closure. The earlier belief that fecal continence improves with time is a manifestation of the adaptation and adjustments made by the patient himself to achieve a socially acceptable status. Regular bowel movement with evidence of straining and observation by the mother of signs suggestive of imminent defecation without staining of the napkins suggests a good outcome.

Therefore, the etiology of defecation problems after PSARP is multi-factorial and includes
 I. Sacral malformations
 II. Sphincteric insufficiency
 III. Altered rectosigmoid motility
 IV. Secondary psychological problems.

Clinical Evaluation of a Child with Fecal Incontinence following PSARP

All children with fecal incontinence should be evaluated systematically to identify the causative factors. In this connection it is most important to distinguish between problems arising from insufficiency of the sphincter/levator muscle complex leading to true or primary incontinence (use score A) and disturbed rectal motility resulting in chronic constipation with secondary overflow incontinence

Table 75.2: Clinical score for incontinence (A)

Symptoms	Findings	Score
Frequency of stools	Normal: 1-2/day	2
	Frequent: 3-5/day	1
	Very frequent >/day	0
Consistency of stools	Normal/formed	2
	Mushy	1
	Liquid	0
Soiling	Never	2
	Under stress/diarrhea	1
	Always	0
Feeling of fullness	Normal	2
	Uncertain	1
	Absent	0
Discrimination	Normal	2
	Uncertain	1
	Absent	0
Need of care (e.g. napkins)	Not necessary	2
	Sometimes	1
	Always	0

Evaluation: 10-12 Points: Good continence, 6-9 points: fair (sufficient for social life = partial continence), 0-5 points: poor (incontinent)

Table 75.3: Clinical score for chronic constipation and overflow incontinence (B)

Symptoms	Findings	Score
Frequency of stools	Normal: 1-2/day	2
	Frequent: 3-5/day	1
	Less than every 3rd day	0
Consistency of stools	Normal/formed	2
	Hard	1
	Fecalomas (with enterocolitis)	0
Overflow soiling	Never	2
	Sometimes	1
	Always	0
Laxatives necessary	Never	2
	Sometimes	1
	Always	0
Washout necessary	Never	2
	Sometimes	1
	Always	0
Evacuation on defecography (3 hr post-examination)	Almost complete	2
	Rectum not emptied	1
	Higher parts not emptied	0

Evaluation: 10-12 points: No/almost no constipation (equal to good continence); 6-9 points: fair, sufficient for social life with aids; 0-5 points: bad (severe constipation)

(use score B). The situation is similar to the problem of vesicourethral reflux where we have to distinguish between refluxing and obstructive ureters.

Table 75.2: Lists the individual factors, which should be assessed for the different kinds of complaints.

In the very few patients achieving only 0-2 points, continent improving operations may be considered.

Score A should be used for true or primary incontinence based on hypoplasia of sphincter muscles. It is like others scores published by Kelly, Holschneider, Rintala and others not useful for overflow incontinence secondary to chronic constipation.[5,8,11] Rintala modified Holschneiders score from 1983 by the addition of 4 more criteria.[12] But only 2 dealt with chronic constipation which is the most frequent sequel after PSARP. Therefore, this score too can not be representative for all post PSARP problems. It seems, therefore to be justified to use two different scores for the two different post PSARP diseases: Dysmotility of the rectum and the sphincter incompetence.

For patients with rectal motility disorders resulting in chronic constipation and secondary overflow incontinence score B should be taken (Table 75.3).

Table 75.4: Classification of postoperative treatment according to scoring A and B (Tables 75.2 and 75.3)

Nor or almost no treatment necessary (Type I, Type II a)
10-12 points score A/B

Motility problems, chronic constipation (Type II b) (score B)
6-9 points: Diet, laxative drugs, defecation training
3-5 points: Washouts
0-2 points: Anterior resection/Soave

Sphincter insufficiency (Type II c) (Score A)
6-9 points: Biofeed back training, anal plugging
3-5 points: Motility reducing drugs (with washouts)
0-2 points: Continence improving operations

In patients getting only 0-2 points, resection of the non motile rectum might be necessary. Concerning the treatment necessary, the scores A and B can be summarized in Table 75.4. Besides, according to the treatment, a classification of the type of post-PSARP sequelae, can be introduced which seems to be more practical and more objective than the usual grading of the severity of postoperative incontinence (Table 75.5).

Table 75.5: Types of anorectal continence according to the postoperative treatment if necessary

Total continence: No soiling, no constipation, voluntary bowel movements

Partial continence
- Type A: Continent with dietary management and/or laxatives
- Type B: Constipation with overflow soiling, clean with enemas
- Type C: Partially insufficient muscle complex, occasional soiling, no constipation

Incontinence
- Type D: Complete insufficient muscle complex, encopresis
- Type E: Severe motility problems, constipation not manageable

According to Table 75.5, three main and five subgroups of continence problems can be distinguished.[5] One should consider any more of "degrees" of continence. The maingroups are:
1. Patients who are continent
2. Patients who are partial continent (either due to chronic constipation or incontinence)
3. Patients who are incontinent.

There are no aspects of clinical examination considered in these two scores because there is unfortunately only a very poor correlation between the morphology and the function. However, rectal palpation of the sphincter tone and its elasticity are the first and most important examination in children with PSARP.

CLASSIFICATION

Patients who are continent do not soil, are not constipated and have regular voluntary bowel movements. Patients with partial continence can by classified in three subgroups depending on the therapy necessary to get regular bowel movements.

The patients of the first subgroup, Type A, are continent with a few adjuvants like occasional diet and laxatives. The second subgroup, Type B, is the constipation group and the largest group of sequels after PSARP. These patients can be helped with enemas and a regular laxative diet. They are constipated due to more sever motility problems in the rectum, but can be treated successfully conservatively. The primary defect in this group of patients is dysmotility of the bowel, which progressively can lead to megarectum.

The treatment of constipation in this dysmotility group is a challenging problem and requires a patience and methodical approach based on sound clinical judgment. Patient have care giver confidence and motivation is absolutely essential. The treatment of constipation is based on the following principles:
1. Explaining the problem fully
2. Supporting the child and family
3. Using minimal therapeutic input
4. Ensuring complete evacuation of retained stools,
5. Establishing effective toilet routines
6. Maintaining regular bowel movements.

Prior to initiating the bowel management program, the bowel must be completely cleared by using enemas or manual evacuation. Regular use of stool softeners (such as docusate sodium), a high fiber diet and adequate fluid intake follow this. Regular bowel emptying is established using laxatives like senna, dulcolax and sodium picosulfate. This program should start early to avoid the development of a megarectum. Older children can be taught to push against a closed glottis to evacuate. Enemas are ideally given soon after a meal to act concomitantly with the gastrocolic reflex. The aim is to establish one to two bowel movements per day by adjusting the regimen. The dietary adjustments are vital for any bowel management program. Excessive milk or cheese intake should be avoided. Vegetables, fruits and other traditional high fiber foods are initiated. Cisapride has also been used successfully to treat constipation as it improves colonic motility. It is important to remember that treatment has to be continued for at least 6 months to 1 year following normalcy as recurrence or relapse rates are high. Success is dependent on perseverance and initiating treatment early.

In more severe constipated children the use of smaller or larger volume enemas or colonic irrigation are necessary to keep the colon clean. It is believed that in the presence of a clean colon, the underlying bowel hypomotility will prevent soiling. In the presence of accidents or radiological evidence of retained stools, a larger volume of enema is used. In 44 patients in Pena's study, 41 (93%) achieved success and it took an average of 4.4 days to reach continence.[13]

The third subgroup, Type C, focuses on fecal incontinence. These patients suffer from hypoplasia of the muscle complex, sensory deficit and lack of smooth muscle fibers. For these children laxative measures are not suitable. Their diet must rather be constipating. The more solid consistency of the stools increases the feeling of rectal fullness, better discrimination and allows therefore better evacuation. The use of soft anal tampons may help after sufficient bowel cleaning. These patients are not constipated do not show overflow incontinence but soil occasionally due to their partial sphincter insufficiency. However, this symptom can be treated by conservative means. With these aids the patients are sufficient continent for social life. One reason for primary fecal incontinence sometimes combined with a tendency for diarrhea is a resection of the rectum or at least a part of their sigmoid colon during the pull-through procedure. The barium enema will show absence of the sigmoid with a straight non-dilated colon running straight down from the splenic flexure to the anus. The management involves daily use of small enemas to keep the colon clean. A strict constipating diet is used along with loperamide (1-2 mg orally 3 times daily) or diphenoxylate hydrochloride with atropine (0.05-0.1 mg/kg, orally, four times daily). Sometimes probiotics are helpful too. Accidents in this group are usually secondary to failure to reduce motility of the colon. Of the 128 patients in this subgroup in Pena's study, 112 (88%) were successfully managed by this protocol.[13]

However, the treatment plan has sometimes to be individualized episodes of soiling or large unexpected bowel movements are termed as accidents. In the constipation subgroup, an accident represents failure to completely clean the colon whereas in the diarrhea subgroup it meant that the colonic motility was not adequately decreased. A larger volume of enema or increasing the concentration of NaCl or adding Bisacodyl can be tried in the constipation subgroup. In the presence of a clean colon on plain radiograph, a more constipating diet or increase in drug dosage can be tried in the diarrhea subgroup. The bowel management program is considered successful if the patients remain clean for at least 3 days consecutively. Such patients can be offered the MACE (Malone Antegrade Continent Enema) procedure as an alternative to rectal enemas. Failure after 10 days of continuous trial means that a permanent colostomy may be the only alternative in these patients.

Biofeedback is useful in patients with ARM with preserved rectal sensation. The intra-anal plug electrode can be used for supervised training and can increase the sphincter tone. However, surface electrode is more comfortable in most of the cases. Biofeedback can be successful in patients with minor problems and children who are able to cooperate. Severe defects usually do not respond and the technique is suitable only between 8-10 years of age.[14] Soft anal plugs are very successful additional help for patients who are able to empty their bowel almost completely. The plugging can not avoid involuntary bowel movements, bowel accidents and stool staining.[15]

The last main group, the incontinent group represents children who are completely incontinent. This, on one hand (Type D), may be caused by a completely insufficient muscle complex, sacral agenesis or poor prognostic defects (high rectobladder neck fistula, high confluence cloaca) or, on the other hand (Type E), rectal motility can be disturbed so seriously that it leads to an overflow incontinence with most severe constipation that can hardly be remedied even by washouts. This problem is also called pseudoincontinence.

Pseudoincontinent patients include children with good sphincters, normal sacrum, children with good prognosis defect, a preserved and well placed rectum and a technically good operation. However, they all have had a history of most severe constipation, followed by history of fecal soiling. Pseudo-incontinence should be suspected if there is a delayed onset of soiling after a period of fecal continence and a history of constipation.

A contrast enema typically shows a megasigmoid. It is important to differentiate this defect from the subgroup (Type B) which has constipation with fecal incontinence. It is recommended that such children should initially be disimpacted and then put on laxatives to provoke bowel movements. The laxatives are increased over the next few days till a spontaneous bowel movement can be induced without enemas or suppositories. If the patient remains continent then he is assigned as true overflow incontinence and will benefit from sigmoid resection. If the patient remains incontinent then he is treated as the subgroup of fecal incontinence with constipation. As mentioned above, in group E a resection of the hypoperistaltic rectum might be required or a MACE stoma considered if some motility for the transport of the cleaning liquids were preserved. Only the rare first subgroup of children with primary total incontinence due to sphincter insufficiency (type D) may benefit from continence improving sphincter operations like gracilis transposition. This procedure is successful in one-third of the patients, improves their situation in an other third of the children but fails in the others. The stimulation of the gracilis muscle by pacemakers can not be recommended in children at present.[16]

Physical Examination (Table 75.6)

Beside clinical evaluations, the investigation of patients with anorectal malformations involves a complete review of the history including the type of defect, the pre-PSARP findings on distal cologram, the initial assessment of the spine and the gluteal cleft, and the quality of sphincter muscles noted during surgery. It is very important to review details of the PSARP technique especially the extent of the preparation on the rectal muscle wall because this part of the mobilization cuts the neurovascular fibers of the nervi erigentes resulting in disturbed rectal motility. A plain radiograph of the spine and the sacral ratio according to Pena might be calculated. A detailed history of the bowel pattern, soiling pattern and constipation is noted. Physical examination should assess the location and caliber of the neoanus, the anal tone and the configuration of the perineum and the buttocks. A barium enema and defecography can delineate the length and elasticity of the anal canal, the caliber of the bowel, the anorectal angle and the descent of the pelvic diaphragm.

Manometry

Electromanometric investigations are very useful to distinguish between fecal incontinence due to an insufficiency of the anorectal sphincter structures and overflow incontinence. With special regard to incontinence, the most important parameters are the anorectal resting pressure profile and the squeezing pressure profile where as in chronic constipation the adaptive reaction/compliance of the rectum and the course of propulsive waves are important.[12] Manometry is the ideal objective means to assess anorectal function, however, it does not always correlate well with the clinical status because not only the force of the anorectal sphincters are measured but also that of gluteal and adductor muscles as well.[17]

Table 75.6: Physical examination

History
I. Type of defect
II. Operative details

Examination
III. Status of neoanus, sacrum and spine
IV. Cutaneous markers of occult spinal dysraphism Sacral pieces as seen on skiagram
V. Gluteal folds, perineal sensation, anocutaneous reflex
VI. Per rectal examination for anal tone, posterior shelf, pouch, fecalomas

Investigations
VII. Plain films of spine and sacrum (AP and lateral view) for spina bifida, sacral pieces. Ganglion cells on histology
VIII. Barium enema—assess for stenosis, dilatation (mega-sigmoid), postevacuation residue
IX. MRI/CECT pelvis—to assess the relationship of bowel to sphincters, evaluate spinal cord (ruleout tethered cord syndrome)
X. US, KUB and VCUG, manometry
XI. Anal sphincter myography.

Two other reliable findings on manometry are: Presence of an inhibitory rectoanal, which is a good prognostic factor and the decreased rectal sensitivity to distension, which is a poor prognostic sign.

Anal sphincter myography has also been used to objectively assess the sphincter function.[18] Dynamic defecography has been replaced by CT scan and MRI to assess-the location of the pulled through bowel in relation to the sphincters and the anorectal angle.[19,20] These studies also assess the quality of the sphincter complex and help in ruling out any occult spinal lesions.

OTHER COMPLICATIONS AFTER PSARP TREATMENT

1. Urethral diverticulum results from improper division of the fistula during the primary procedure. The diverticulum can lead to recurrent UTI, post-micturition dribbling or calculi formation. Treatment is by surgical excision preferably through the posterior sagittal route or through an anterior perineal approach.
2. A recurrent fistula usually manifests in the first 6 weeks. If a colostomy is not present, a redo colostomy is the initial step in treatment. A redo posterior sagittal approach and transrectal excision

of the fistula by the Kraske approach is advisable.[21] The rectal suture line is rotated so as not to overlap the site of fistula closure.

3. Anal stenosis may respond to dilatations. In refractory cases an anoplasty or even excision of the scar tissue may be required.
4. Colostomy closure is often followed by development of redness and edema of the perineum. The redness may also be seen following primary PSARP (Fig. 75.1). Perineal excoriation may be real nuisance and is caused by fecal urease, which converts urea to ammonia (Fig. 75.2). Aggressive treatment with zinc oxide paste, warm compresses and perineal hygiene is required. Sucralfate and Karaya gum powder has also been used recently to heal the excoriated skin.

TREATMENT OF POSTOPERATIVE COMPLICATIONS

Most of the postoperative complications are preventable (Fig. 75.3). It is pertinent to stress the important technical hints-of the PSARP procedure. These are:
1. Following a strictly midline approach
2. Preservation of rectosigmoid
3. Careful not too extensive preparation of the blind pouch close to the rectal wall
4. Proper relocation of the pulled through bowel in relation to the vertical and parasagittal fibers
5. Skin lined anal canal
6. Postoperative good toilet training and dilatation program, early treatment of constipation and avoiding liquid stools.

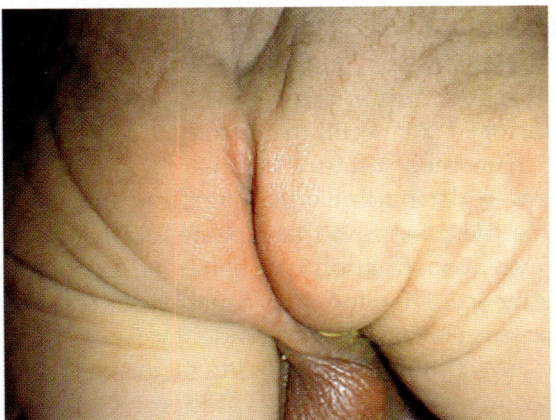

Fig. 75.1: Redness over the suture line may be seen following primary PSARP

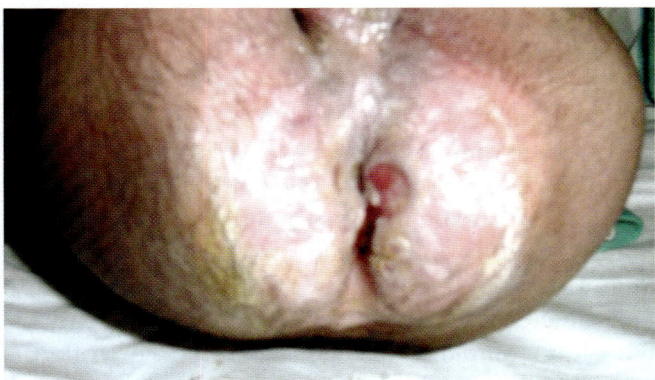

Fig. 75.2: Perineal excoriation in a child with fecal incontinence, considered for permanent stoma

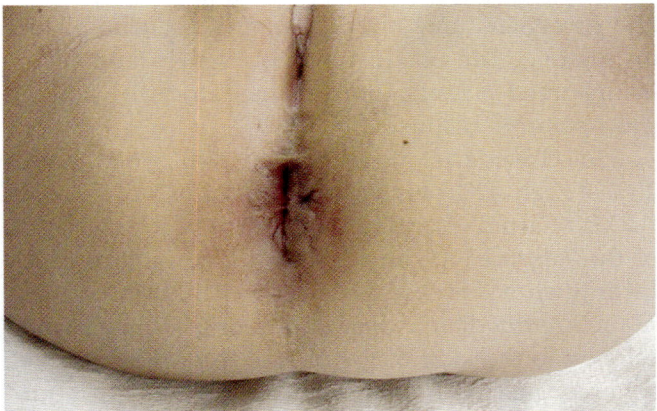

Fig. 75.3: Normal looking anus following PSARP in a child with good continence

The cutting of the neurovascular fibers penetrating Waldeyer's fascia destroys the nerve erigentes and reduces bowel motility which leads to chronic constipation. That is the reason why patients with little mobilization of the blind pouch like low and high type anorectal malformations suffer less frequently from chronic constipation than intermediate or higher types mobilized extensively from behind.

Dilatation should not exceed more then 1-3 month. The anal orifice should have been calibrated intraoperatively upto Hegar's 12. During the following month it should grow elastically to Hegar's 13 until the end of the first year of life.

Results of the Treatment of Chronic Constipation following PSARP

The incidence of constipation following PSARP varies between 10-73%.[2,19,20] The incidence of constipation is higher in intermediate anomalies as compared to high anomalies. Yeung et al, evaluated 35 children with low anomalies followed up for 1-7 years.[19] In this study 17 (53%) patients had constipation and 9% had soiling. Rintala et al also showed that 42% children (n = 40) with low anomalies had constipation and 10% had soiling.[16] Low anomalies, especially rectovestibular fistulas, are frequently associated with constipation following repair. In the same report, Rintala et al using a quantitative scoring method modified from Holschneiders score, showed that only 60% of patients with low anomalies had good continence while the completely normal bowel function was observed in only 15%.[8,12,16] This study shows that objective evaluation of bowel function is important as patients and caregivers may not always give the true picture on history. The use of objective scores and of the Wingspread classification is mandatory to compare postoperative results.[6]

Holschneider et al reported in 2001 continence in 20% of high, 42% of intermediate and 79% of low type ARM.[22] Partially continent were 56% of the high, 47% of the intermediate and 21% of the low deformities. Incontinence was observed in 24% of the high and 11% of the intermediate types. Comparing constipation in relation to the kind of the operative procedure used, severe constipation occurred much less in abdominoperineal pull-through procedures (n = 0) and perineo-proctoplasties (3.6%) than after the PSARP (52.1% and abdomino PSARP (52.4%).

Using the new above mentioned classification according to the kind of postoperative treatment necessary, Holschneider observed in 2002[5] total or near total continence (Type A) 35.3% of the high. 40.9% of the intermediate and 2 children in the low type of ARM in the constipation group.[5] Partial sphincter insufficiency (Type C) occurred in 26.5% of the high and 13.6% of the intermediate types of deformities. Fecal incontinence needing further surgical treatment (Type D and E) were reported in 10 patients most of them having high type abnormalities.

Secondary Operations following PSARP

Redo Pull-through

A redo pull-through operation is indicated in good prognosis defects with a normal sacrum where the pulled through bowel has not been placed correctly in the muscle complex. This is suggested by findings of disparity in the muscle sling thickness on either side of the pulled through bowel on a CT scan. The presence of fat around the bowel also suggests an eccentrically placed bowel. The recommended treatment for this group of patients involves a redo PSARP under colostomy-cover. The reported outcome in terms of fecal continence have been variable following redo-pull through. Pena reported a significant improvement in 52%, mild improvement in 18% and no improvement in 12%.[2] Mulder et al reported that 25% of their 20 patients became continent over a follow up of 3.5 years.[23] Rintala et al followed-up 16 patients with redo pull-through.[24] The clinical continence status and manometric findings initially improved in 13 patients (81%). However, on longer follow-up till adulthood, only 4 (25%) were clinically continent. Therefore, the results of secondary surgery are variable and on long-term follow-up may not be very encouraging. This further stresses the fact that there lies a considerable responsibility on the surgeon performing the primary reconstructive procedure.

Severe Chronic Constipation, Rectal Resection

As mentioned above only the very small group of patients with severe motility disturbance of the rectum may benefit from a resection of parts of the rectum/mobilized not propulsive blind pouch (Type E, score B). The mean reason for this most severe problem are (a) aplastic and hypoplastic desmosis of the rectal wall and (b) injury to the nervi erigentes responsible for rectal motility.[23,25,26]

In the period before the introduction of PSARP the main postoperative problem was stool incontinence because the blind pouch was at least partially resected by Rehbein-Romualdi-Kiesewetter's procedure.[27-29] In contrast, after Stephens abdomino-sacro-perineal pull-through technique, the results were much more satisfactory.[5,6,30,31] With the introduction of PSARP in 1982, true incontinence almost disappeared and chronic constipation with overflow incontinence became the most important postoperative problem. However, constipation can better be handled than incontinence. Therefore, it is a matter of the feasibility of the surgeon to use the tendency to constipation factor as a continence improving factor in addition to the reconstruction of the sphincter complex but without achieving severe chronic constipation.

For eventual rectal resection deep anterior resection according to Rehbein's technique should be used keeping 4-5 cm of the blind pouch *in situ* and with special care of the variability of the sigmoid vessels.[32]

Continence Improving Operations

a. Gracilloplasty has been a common method for secondary sphincter reconstruction.[32-35] Early results shown increase in the resting and squeeze pressure. However, long-term results are far from encouraging as the muscle wrap tends to weaken over time.[36] Continuous electrical stimulation of the gracilis muscle wrap induces a transition in muscle composition, from fatigable type II fibers to fatigue resistant type I fibers.[33] This so-called dynamic gracilloplasty used an implanted muscle stimulator to maintain a constant anal tone. Baeten et al showed promising results using dynamic gracilloplasty; more than half of the patients became continent and the anal pressures were maintained high but most of them were adults.[33]
b. Gluteus maximus transfer operation involves dissecting the medial parts of the muscle bilaterally, splitting the ends and suturing them to each other both anterior and posterior to the rectum.[37]
c. Levatorplasty involves detaching the lateral and posterior attachments of the levator muscle and plicating it over the pulled through bowel. The short-term results are encouraging.[38] The improvement following levatorplasty is probably related to creation of an acute anorectal angle rather than by increasing the actual resting or squeeze pressures. Long-term outcomes in adults has not been encouraging.[38,39]
d. Smooth muscle free or flapped transpositions have also been successfully used by Holschneider and others.[40]
e. Other secondary procedures for attaining fecal continence include free transplantation of palmaris longus muscle, secondary reconstruction of a used gracilis sling and the artificial anal sphincter.[41]
f. Mucosal ectopy and sensitivity improvement (Figs 75.4A and B): To improve anorectal sensitivity and correct rectal prolapse, a three flap anoplasty or Nixon's flap plasty are very useful (Figs 75.5A to D).[7,42,43] Various other types of anoplasty have also been tried (Figs 75.6A to C). Mucosal rectal prolapse may be trimmed and a redo anoplasty has good results (Figs 75.7A and B).

Antegrade Continence Enema (ACE)

The Malone ACE procedure was initially reported in 1990 and was based on the fact that complete colonic emptying could produce fecal continence.[44] The success of the Mitrofanoff principle was applied to provide a continent, intermittent, catheterizable access to the proximal colon. The operation is simple, but attention to detail is very important to avoid complications.

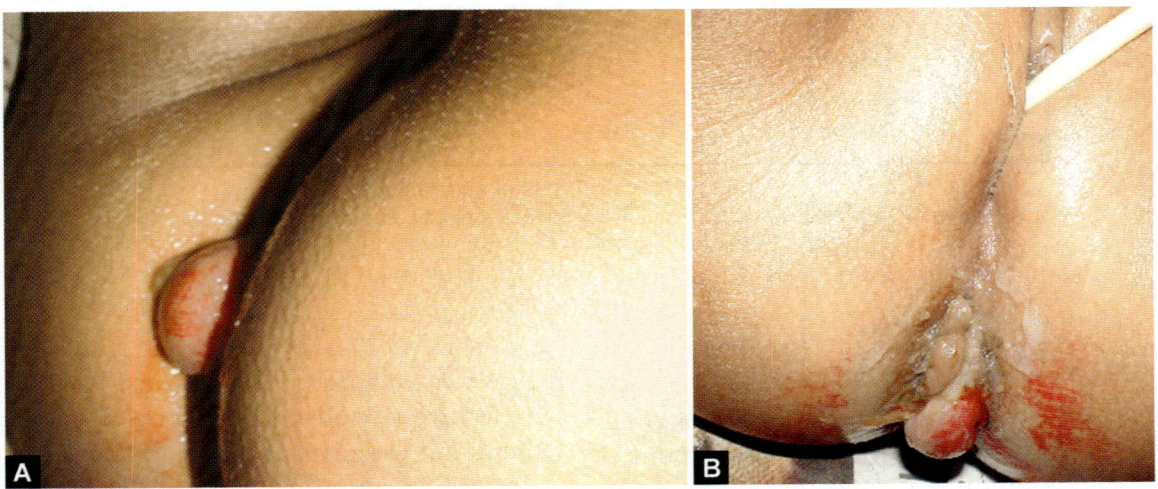

Figs 75.4A and B: Mucosal prolapse following PSARP

842 Pediatric Surgery—Diagnosis and Management

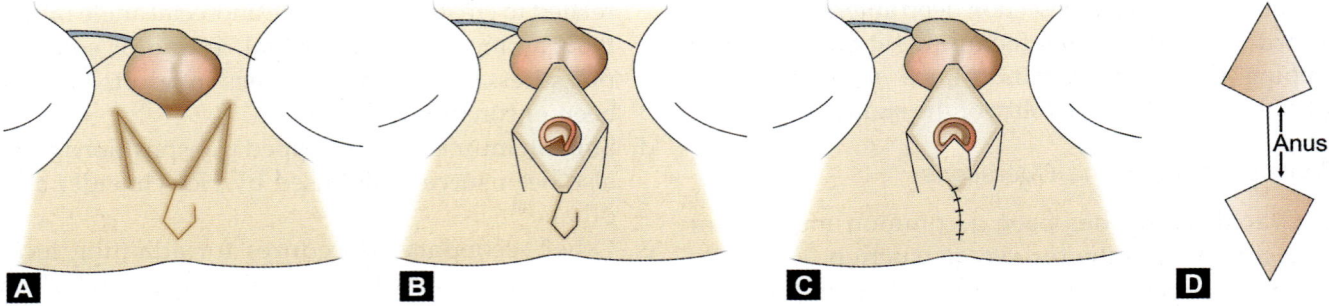

Figs 75.5A to D: **A to C.** Steps of Mollard's (Caouette-Laberge) three– flap anoplasty, **D.** Nixon's flap anoplasty

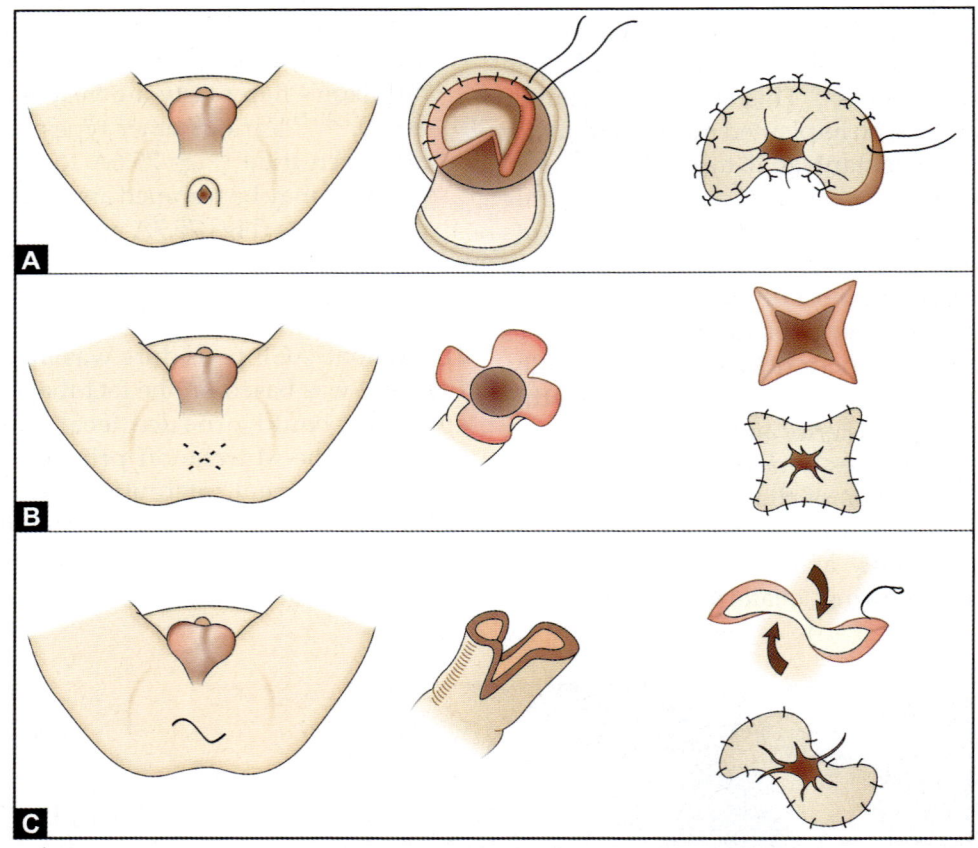

Figs 75.6A to C: Types of anoplasty
A. Posterior flap anoplasty, **B.** Cruciate incision anoplasty, **C.** Lateral flap anoplasty

Patient Selection for MACE Procedure

Pena believes that the MACE procedure should only be used when traditional bowel management is successful and is simply a more acceptable route for giving enemas.[45] In one of every twenty patients in their series, the procedure was unsuccessful, if there was failure of conservative bowel management. Patient and caregiver motivation and counseling is absolutely mandatory. Continued postoperative support and motivation is also important. Curry et al

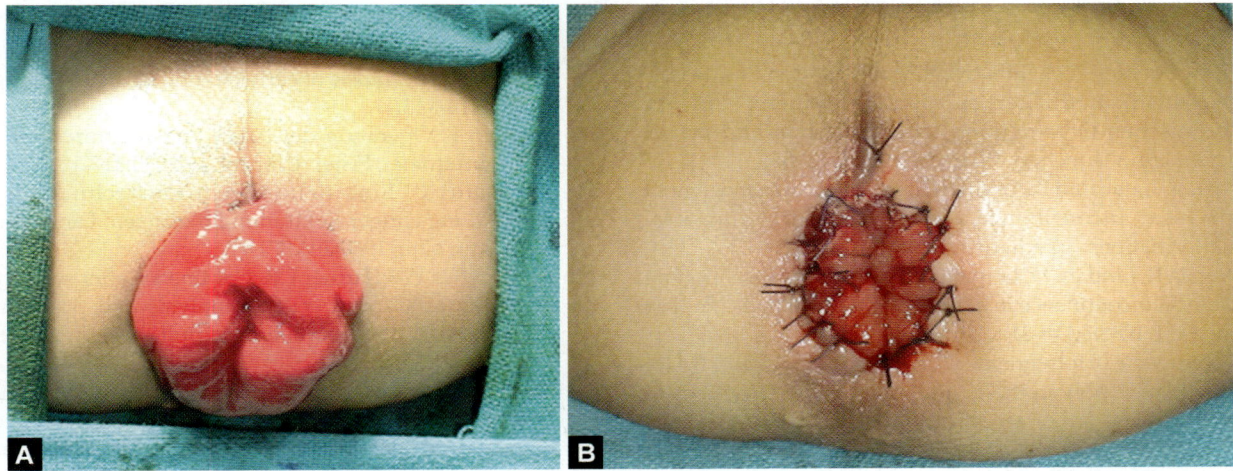

Figs 75.7A and B: A. Rectal mucosal prolapse following PSARP, **B.** Postoperative photograph of the same case

have also noted that age at operation is a significant factor in determining success; there was a 70% failure rate for patients less than 5 years as compared with 24% for those older than 5 years.[46] The MACE procedure is not free from complications and therefore should be used as only a means for providing a more convenient and acceptable channel for enemas.[46-48]

The initial procedure devised by Malone involved dividing the appendix at its base and reimplanting it submucosally in a reverse manner into the cecum. A thorough bowel preparation and preoperative broad-spectrum antibiotics are used. The modified MACE procedure involves *in situ* plication of the cecum around the appendix. The tip of the appendix is divided and after each plicating suture a catheter is passed to check patency. The cecum and right colon are mobilized toward the midline and the appendix is exteriorized using interposition skin flaps through the deepest part of the umbilicus. The neoappendix can also be created from the medial portion of the ascending colon or the Monti principle can be used.[48] Recently, laparoscopic appendicostomy without cecal plication has been used with success indicating that in some cases the native valve mechanism of the appendix may be sufficient.[49]

Results of Malone ACE Procedure

Levitt et al reported a 95% complete continence in 19 of 20 patients.[45] Stomal stricture occurred in 2, and 3 patients developed leakage at the appendicostomy site. In 1999, Curry et al reported a 72% complete and 17% partial success in ARM patients with the MACE procedure.[46]

REFERENCES

1. Pena A. Postop care, complications and results In: Atlas of surgical management of anorectal malformations. Ed: A Pena, Springer Verlag, N York 1990;91-95.
2. Pena A. Anorectal malformations. Semin Pediatr Surg 1995;4:35-47.
3. Rintala R, Lindahl H, Louhimo I. Anorectal malformations: results of treatment and long-term follow-up of 208 patients. Pediatr Surg Int 1991;6:36-41.
4. Hecker WC, Holschneider AM, Kraeft H, et al. Complications, lethality and long-term results after surgery of anorectal atresia. Z Kinderchir 1980;29:238-44.
5. Holschneider AM, Jesch NK, Stragholz E, Pfrommer W. Surgical methods for anorectal malformations from Rehbein to Pena - Critical assessment of score systems and proposal for a new classification. Eur J Pediatr Surg 2002:12:73-82.
6. Stephens FD, Smith ED. Paul NW. Anorectal malformations in children: Update 1988. Alan R. Liss, New York , March of Dimes Birth Defect Foundation, Birth Defect Original Series 1988;124:4.
7. Stephens FD, Smith ED. Anorectal malformations in children. Year book Medical Publishers, Chicago 1971.
8. Rintala RJ, Lindahl HO. Is normal bowel function possible after repair of intermediate and high anorectal malformations. J Pediatr Surg 1995;30:491-99.
9. Rintala R, Mildh L, Lindahl H. Fecal continence and quality of life in adult patients with an operated low anorectal malformation. J Pediatr Surg 1992;27:902-05.
10. Rintala R, Lindahl H. Internal sphincter saving PSARP for high and intermediate anorectal malformations: technical considerations. Pediatr Surg Int 1995;10:345-49.

11. Kelly JH. Cineradiography in anorectal malformations J Pediatr Surg 1969;6:538-46.
12. Holschneider AM. Elektromanometrie des Enddarms. Diagnostik und Therapie der Inkontinenz und der chronischen Obstipation. Auflage, Urban and Schwarzenberg, Munchen, Wien, Baltimore, 1983.
13. Pena A, Guardino K, Tovilla JM, et al. Bowel management for fecal incontinence in patients with anorectal malformations. J Pediatr Surg 1998;33:133-37.
14. Rintala R, Lindahl H, Louhino I. Biofeedback conditioning for fecal incontinence in anorectal malformations. Pediatr Surg Int 1988;3:418-21.
15. Pfrommer W, Holschneider AM, LOffler N, Schauff B, Ure BM. A new polyurethane anal plag in the treatment of incontinence after atresia repair. Eur J Pediatr Surg 2000;10:187-91.
16. Rintala RJ, Lindahl HG, Rasanen M. Do children with repaired low anorectal malformations have normal bowel function. J Pediatr Surg 1997;32:823-26.
17. Hedlund H, Pena A, Rodriguez G, et al. Long-term anorectal function in imperforate anus treated by posterior sagittal anorectoplasty: manometric investigation. J Pediatr Surg 1992;27:906-09.
18. Iwai N, Kaneda H, Tamiguchi T, et al. Postoperative continence assessed by electromyography of the external sphincter in anorectal malformations. Z Kinderchir 1985;40:87-90.
19. Young CK, Kiely EM. Low anorectal anomalies: A critical appraisal. Pediatr Surg Int 1991;6:333-35.
20. Ong NT, de Campo M, Fowler R. Computerised tomography in the management of inperforate anus patients following rectoplasty. Pediatr Surg Int 1990;5:241-45.
21. Huber A, Hochstetter ARC, Allgower M. Transsphinktere Rektumchirurgie. Topographische Anatomie und Operationstechnik. Berlin, Heidelberg. New York, Tokyo Springer 1983.
22. Holschneider AM, Koebke I, Meier-Ruge, Land N, Iesch NK: Pathophysiology of chronic constipation on anorectal malformations. Longterm results and preliminary anatomical investigations. Eur I Pediatr Surg 2001;11:305-10.
23. Mulder W, de long E, Wauters I, et al. Posterior sagittal anorectoplasty: functional results of primary and secondary operations in comparison to the pull-through method in anorectal malformations. Eur I Pediatr Surg 1995;5:170-73.
24. Rintala R, Lindahl H. Secondary PSARP for anorectal malformations: A long-term follow- up extending beyond childhood. Pediatr Surg Int 1995;10:414-17.
25. Holschneider AM, Ure BM, Pfrommer W, Meier-Ruge WM. Innervation patterns of the rectal pouch and fistula in anorectal malformations: A preliminary report. I Pediatr Surg 1996;31:357-62.
26. Meier-Ruge WA, Holschneider AM, Scharli AF. New pathogenetic aspects of gut dysmotility in aplastic and hypoplastic desmosis of early childhood. Pediatr Surg Int 2001;17:140-43.
27. Rehbein F. Operation der Anal- und Rektumatresie mit Rekto-urethraler Fistel. Chirurg 1959;30:417-18.
28. Romualdi P. Eine neue Opemtionstechnik fur die Behandlung elmger Rektummi Bbidungen. Langenbeck's Arch Klin Chir 1960;296:371-77.
29. Kiesewetter WB, Turner CR. Continence after surgery for imperforate anus. A critical analysis and preliminary experience with the sacroperineal pull-through. Ann Surg 1963;158:498-512.
30. Holschneider AM, Pfrommer W, Gerresheim B. Results in the treatment of anorectal malformations with special regard to the histology of the rectal pouch. Eur I Pediatr Surg 1994:4:303-09.
31. Rehbein F. Kinderchirurgische Operationen. Hippokrates Verlag Stuttgart 1976.
32. Raffensperger I. The gmcilis sling for faecal incontinence. I Pediatr Surg 1979;14:794-97.
33. Baeten CGM1, Konsteri I, Heineman E, et al. Dynamic gracioplasty for anal atresia. J Pediatr Surg 1994;29:922-25.
34. Holschneider AM., Lahoda F. Electromyographic and electromanometric studies after gracilis -transplantations following Pickrell's procedure. Z. Kinderchirurgie 1974;14:288-303.
35. Holschneider AM, Poschl, Kraeft H. Hecher WCh. Pickrell's Gracilis muscle transplantation and its effect on anorectal continence. A five year prospective study. Z Kinderchir 1979;27:135-44.
36. Holschneider AM. Flapped and free muscle transplantation in the treatment of anal incontinence. Z Kinderchir. 1981;32:244-58.
37. Hentz VR. Construction of a rectal sphincter using the origin of the glutieus maximus muscle. Plast Reconstr Surg 1982;70:82-85.
38. Kottmeier PK, Velcek FT, Klotz DH, et al. Results of levatorplasty for anal incontinence. J Pediatr Surg 1986;21:647-50.
39. Ninan GK, Puri P. Levatorplasty using a posterior sagittal approach in secondary fecal incontinence. Pediatr Surg Int 1999;9:17-20.
40. Holschneider AM, Hecker WCh. Reverse smooth muscle plasty: A new method of treating anorectal incontinence in infants with high anal and rectal atresia. J Pediatr Surg 1981;16:917-20.
41. Holschneider AM. Secondary sagittal posterior anorectoplasty. Progress in Pediatric Surgery, Springer Berlin -Heidelberg 1990;25:103-17.
42. Caouette-Calrrge L, Yazbeck S, Laberge JM. Multiple- flap anoplasty in the treatment of rectal prolapse after pull-through operations for imperforate anus. J Pediatr Surg 1987;22:65-67.

43. Nixon HH. In: Stephens FD, Smith ED. Anorectal malformations in children: Update 1988. AlanR. Liss, Inc. New York 1988;381.
44. Malone PS. Ransley PG, Kiely EM. Preliminary report: The antegrade continence enema. Lancet 1990;336:1217-18.
45. Levitt MA, SofTer SZ, Pena A. Continent appendicostomy in the bowel management of incontinent children. J Pediatr Surg 1997;11:1630-33.
46. Curry JL, Osbome A, Malone PS. The MACE procedure. Experience in the United Kindgon. I Pediatr Surg 1999;34:338-40.
47. Osbome II, Malone PSI. How to achieve a successful malone ante grade continence enema. J Pediatr Surg 1998;33:138-41.
48. Sugaman ID, Malone PS, Terry TR, et al. Transversely tulularized ileal regiments for the MitrofanofT or Malone ante grade continence enema procedures: The Monti Principle. Br I Urol 1998;81:253-56.
49. Webb-HW, Barraza MA, Crump JM. Laparoscopic appendicostmy in the treatment of fecal incontinence. I Pediatr Surg 1997;32:457-58.

Congenital Pouch Colon

Shilpa Sharma, DK Gupta

Congenital pouch colon (CPC), an entity found in association with anorectal malformation, particularly from south Asian subcontinent has recently gained momentum.[1-4] Initially the disease entity was not very well recognized and was thus various names were coined for describing the same condition. The anomaly, mostly reported from a few major centers in North India has now been well recognized at the international forum, with its inclusion under rare anomalies in the Krickenbeck classification of anorectal malformations.[5,6]

With the proper description elucidated, more and more cases are being reported from various parts of the world.[7-9] A changing trend has been seen in the most common type of CPC seen over the years from complete congenital pouch colon that accounted for more than 70% of cases earlier to incomplete pouch colon that is more commonly seen now.[2]

NOMENCLATURE AND RELEVANT HISTORY

The entity was first described in 1912 by Spriggs in a London Hospital Museum specimen.[1,10] Table 76.1 outlines the important historical landmarks for this anomaly.[1,2,5,6,10-22]

The terms commonly used to describe this anomaly are the "congenital short colon" and the "congenital pouch colon". Pouch colon needs to be differentiated from the entity short colon and the congenital segmental dilatation of the colon, both these without

	Table 76.1: Important historical landmarks for congenital pouch colon[1,2,5,6,10-22]	
1912	Spriggs	Absence of the left-half of colon and rectum
1959	Truslerin	Pouch like dilatation of shortened colon associated with high ARM
1965	Spencer	Typical/ atypical extrophia splanchnica
1967	Blunt	An absence of colon and rectum
1971	Shafie	Cystic dilatation of colon
1972	Singh S and Pathak	Short colon
1976	Chiba et al.	Described coloplasty
1977	Singh A et al	First described anatomy
1978	Gopal	Colonic reservoir
1981	Li	Congenital atresia of anus with short colon malformation
1984	Narsimha Rao et al	Pouch colon syndromeclassification into types I-IV
1990	Wu YJ	Association of Imperforate anus with short colon (AIASC) and Association of imperforate anus with extrophia splanchnica (AIAES).
1996	Wakhlu AK et al.	Classification into partial and complete based on presence of 8 cm or less of normal colon.
2005	Gupta and Sharma[1,2]	Paradigm shift in classification of congenital pouch colon in two main types - complete and incomplete
2005	Gupta et al.[5,6]	Inclusion of pouch colon as rare anomalies in Krickenbeck Classification of ARM

any anorectal anomaly. The term "short colon" refers to a shortened length of the left colon without the anorectal anomaly, that is also narrow in caliber and the babies are usually born to the diabetic mothers.

DEFINITION OF CONGENITAL POUCH COLON

In this anomaly, whole or part of the colon is replaced by a pouch like dilatation that communicates distally with the urogenital tract by a large fistula. The supralevator anomaly is associated with a colonic pouch of variable length and diameter (5-15 cm). The mesentery is very short and poorly developed, the taenia coli are absent or ill defined, the haustrations and the appendices epiploicae are also absent.

The following anatomical criteria for description of congenital pouch colon have been described by the authors[1,2]

1. There is anorectal agenesis.
2. Total length of the colon is short
3. Colon has a pouch formation for a varying length in the form of a saccular or a diverticular pouch with the collection of meconium or the fecal matter in it.
4. The blood supply to the pouch is abnormal. The main pouch is supplied by the branches arising from the superior mesenteric artery, that forms a leash of vessels around the pouch.
5. The colon wall is uniformly thick and muscular, with mucosal hypertrophy.
6. The fistula with the genitourinary tract is wide, muscular and closely adherent with the bladder wall.
7. Fistulous communication is with the bladder in the males and either in the vaginal wall, the vaginal septum between the hemivaginae or in the perineum in the females.
8. There is no transitional zone between the pouch colon and the normal bowel. The bowel pattern changes suddenly and sharply.
9. The associated major anomalies, specially the genitourinary anomalies are quite frequent.

INCIDENCE AND EPIDEMIOLOGY

The incidence varies in different parts of the world with an increased incidence in the northern part of the Indian subcontinent and only sporadic cases reported from the other parts of the world. The cause of this unique geographical distribution has not yet been ascertained.

The incidence of pouch colon has been reported to be between 5-15% of all cases of anorectal malformation in Northern India, 8-10% in Pakistan and 1.7% in Bangladesh.[2] The incidence is much higher (23%) with the high anomaly and as low as 5% with the low type of anomaly. Also, pouch colon is commonly seen in tertiary care centers catering to more serious and redo cases of anorectal malformation. There is a male preponderance that varies from 3:1 to 7:1.[2]

EMBRYOGENESIS

The exact embryogenesis is unknown. The following hypotheses have been proposed:

1. *Dickinson:* Aborted hindgut development following obliteration of the inferior mesenteric artery early in fetal life.[23]
2. *Chatterjee:* Improper development of the postaxial midgut or presplenic gut due to a primary disorder of the proximal end of the hindgut or postsplenic gut.[24]
3. *Wu:* Faulty rotation and fixation of the colon leads consequently to a disturbed longitudinal growth.[21]
4. *Chadha:* Varying extents of vascular insult at the time of the partitioning of the cloaca by the urorectal septum could explain the different types of the malformation.[25]
5. *Wakhlu:* The anomaly is a stage in the development of cloacal exstrophy and is the combined effect of defective development of the splanchic layer of the caudal fold and failure of rotation of the gut causing defective longitudinal growth of the colon.[22]
6. *Gupta and Sharma:* Role of pesticides, micronutrients or the vitamin deficiency in a largely vegetarian community with poor socioeconomic status, affecting the vascular supply in the growing hindgut of the fetus at a critical window period of gestation.[2] Any genetic link, though suggestive of a strong geographical distribution of the anomaly still needs to be confirmed.

Thus, the following factors may have a role to play[2]

1. *Early vascular insult:* This cannot be ruled out as the blood supply is always abnormal to the pouch. It is only the superior mesenteric artery that is prominent and supplies the whole distal bowel. The

inferior mesenteric artery is present only in 50% cases of the distal pouch colon.
2. *Environmental factors:* The high density of cases in the northern Indian subcontinent strongly suggests environmental factors with deficiency of iodine or vitamin B as the possible factors contributing to this anomaly. In this region, the land is very fertile and farming is the main occupation. Pesticides and fungicides are used liberally and the population is mainly vegetarian. Also, most cases of anorectal anomalies belong to the low socioeconomic status. These factors may be responsible for precipitating the anomaly at a window time after the conception when the hindgut is developing and differentiating into urinary and intestinal tracts.
3. Genetic predisposition needs to be ruled out in view of the typical geographical distribution.

CLASSIFICATION

Various classifications have been described to identify the type of anomaly. A widely accepted classification was based on the length of normal colon present proximal to the dilated pouch as given by Narsimha Rao et al. (Table 76.2).[20]

Wakhlu et al. simplified the classification, depending on the length of normal colon and the management planning in relation to the need for coloplasty (Table 76.3).[22] However, this classification was not found practical as the length of 8 cm was not sufficient for performing a pull through.

The Krickenbeck classification of anorectal malformation laid stress on the classification of anomalies that best decide the management options to keep the descriptions universal and to compare the results globally. Thus the authors had classified the anomaly into "Incomplete" and "Complete" pouch colon based on the feasibility to use the remaining colon that would be more important while performing the pull through (Table 76.4).[1,2]

Initially, in India, complete congenital pouch colon was more commonly seen and accounted for more than 70% of cases till 1985. Interestingly, during the past two decades, it is the incomplete pouch colon that has become much more common now (75-80%). Associated genitourinary malformations (cloacal anomalies, double vagina, exstrophy) are also more common in girls.

In complete congenital pouch colon, a large dilated thick walled pouch occupies most of the left side of abdomen. Cecum, if present almost always opens into the sac from right side. It may be associated with an absent, rudimentary or double appendix. There is associated malrotation. The pouch with poorly developed mesentery is supplied by the superior mesenteric artery on the superior and right side and an arcuate extension of superior mesenteric artery on the left side.[26] Inferior mesenteric artery is present only in incomplete pouch colon and supplies the lower half of left lateral side of pouch. The genitourinary fistula of the pouch opens into the posterior wall of the bladder in males. Fistula is usually quite broad and thick walled. In females, colocloacal fistula is the most common followed by colovaginal and colovestibular fistulas. There may be double or septate vagina and the fistulous communication may open in one of the hemivaginae or between the two into the cloaca.

HISTOPATHOLOGY OF THE POUCH

Grossly, the wall of the pouch is thick, the taenia coli are absent or ill defined, haustration and the appendices epiploicae are absent. The main pouch is supplied by a leash of vessels around it. The authors have found the following histological features in patients with pouch colon.

The most salient feature is the disorganization of the muscle coat in an arborhizing manner.[1] This is possibly responsible for the absence of normal

Table 76.2: Types of pouch colon-based on length (1984)

Type I	Normal colon is absent and the ileum opens directly into the colonic pouch.
Type II	The ileum opens into a short segment of cecum which then opens into the pouch.
Type III	Presence of a significant length of normal colon between the ileum and the colonic pouch.
Type IV	Presence of near normal colon with only the terminal portion of colon (sigmoid and rectum) converted into a pouch.

Table 76.3: Types of pouch-colon based on need for coloplasty (1996)

Type A.	Partial short colon length of normal colon proximal to the pouch > 8 cm.
Type B.	Complete short colon absent normal colon or the length of colon proximal to pouch < 8 cm.

Table 76.4: Classification of congenital pouch colon based on presentation at Krickenbeck (2005)[1,2] (Figs 76.1 A and B)		
Type	Description	Management
Incomplete congenital pouch colon	Length of the normal colon is adequate enough for performing the pull through, without the need for doing a coloplasty	Excision of pouch with an end colostomy at birth and a definitive pull through later. Or a single stage pull through in the newborn stage if the condition of the baby permits
Complete congenital pouch colon	There is either no or little normal colon left that is not enough for performing the pull through	A coloplasty procedure would be required to retain only 10-15 cm length of pouch colon in the form of a tube, to be brought out as an end colostomy. A pull through procedure at the time of performing coloplasty should not be preferred in the newborn stage as it is associated with high morbidity and mortality

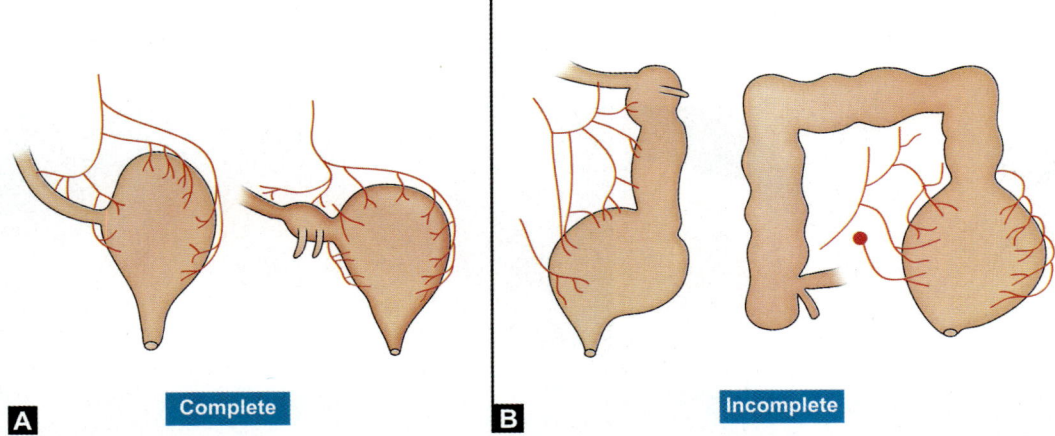

Figs 76.1A and B: Classification of congenital pouch colon (2005) *Reproduced from Gupta DK, Sharma Shilpa. Congenital Pouch Colon, in Anorectal Malformations, 1st edition, Ed. John Hutson and Alex Holschneider, Springer Heidelberg. 2006 Chapter 11:211-22 with kind permission in children of Springer Science and Business Media)*

peristaltic activity in these cases, requiring the removal of dilated pouch and retaining only the normal bowel.

1. The muscle coat is not clearly differentiated into inner circular and outer longitudinal muscles, and is arranged in a decussating pattern. The circular muscle may be incomplete in 50% cases (Fig. 76.2A).
2. The ganglion cells are mature and present in all cases with the presence of normal or occasionally hypertrophic nerve bundles. The pouch wall consists of normal ganglion cells though these may be reduced in number and smaller in size.[2] However, giant ganglia are also seen in 10% cases (Fig. 76.2 B). Nerve bundle hypertrophy has also been reported but is not the regular feature.[26]
3. Congestion of the mucosa and focal hemorrhages are seen commonly.
4. Ectopic heteroplastic tissue has also been reported.[27]

CLINICAL PRESENTATION

The presentation is usually in the early neonatal period with an absent anal opening and distension of the abdomen with or without meconurea (Figs 76.3A and B). There may be associated bilious vomiting with early gross distension of abdomen. In the female child, the anomaly is often associated with a cloacal anomaly and the baby passes meconium from the abnormal opening. Colonic perforation may occur early in cases of grossly distended pouch colon presenting with

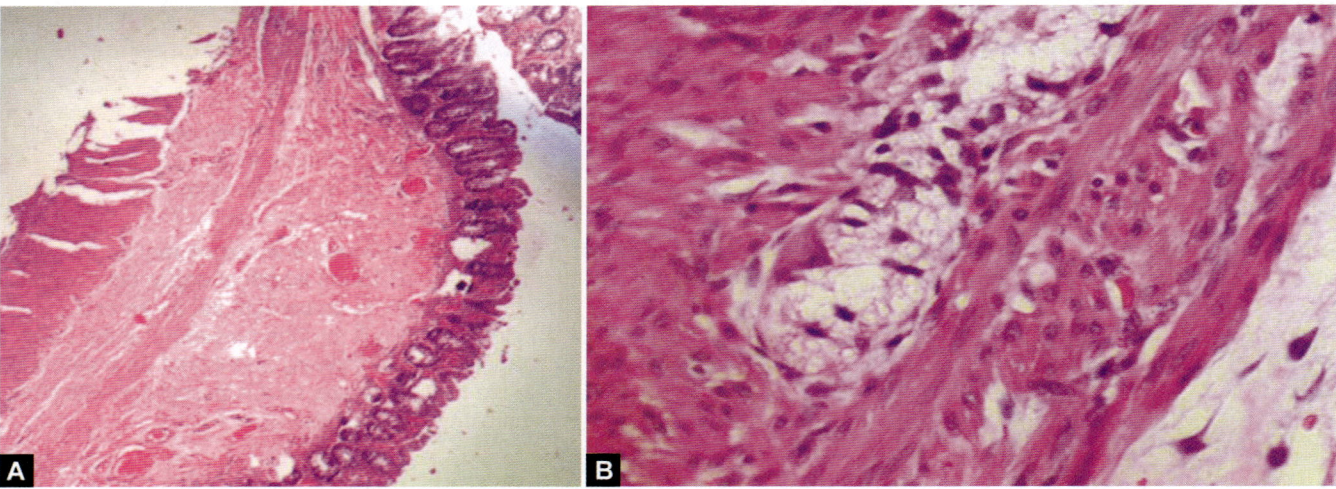

Figs 76.2A and B: A. Photomicrograph showing flattened mucosa, widened submucosa, discontinuation of circular muscle coat (10X), **B.** Photomicrograph showing giant ganglion cell in between the muscle coat (40X)

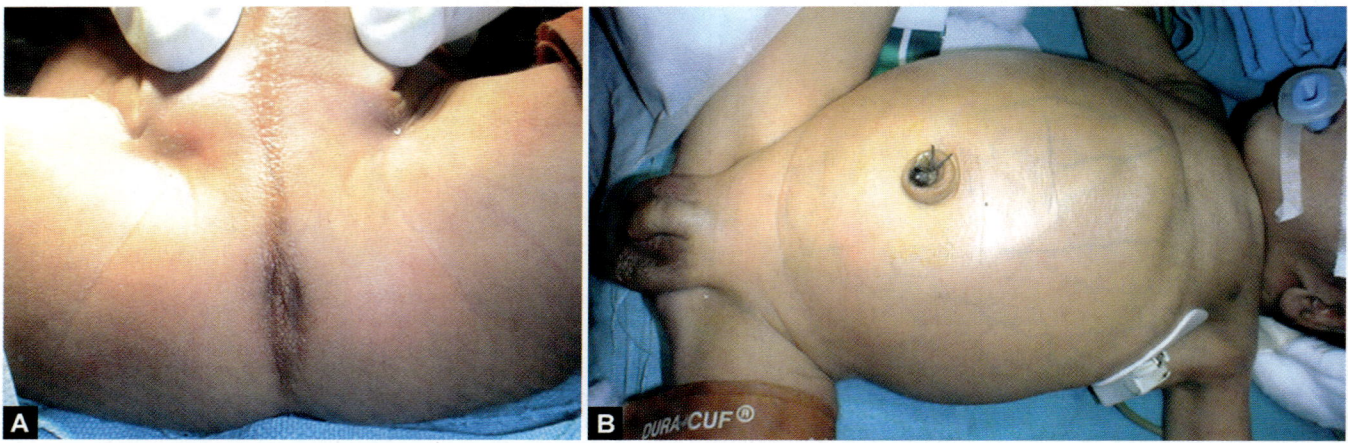

Figs 76.3A and B: A newborn with absent anal opening. **B.** The shiny grossly distended abdomen with redness and visible veins in a particular geographical area is suggestive of pouch colon

septicemia, gross abdominal distension and features of peritonitis.

Late presentation may be seen in a female child with a large colocloacal fistula as the child remains decompressed. The child may also present with a colostomy done by a person not aware of this condition, as an undiagnosed case.

INVESTIGATIONS

In cases with suspected pouch colon with gross abdominal distension in geographical areas where it has high incidence, the diagnosis may be made with an erect skiagram in addition to the conventional invertogram done for anorectal malformations (Figs 76.4A and B). A large loop of bowel with single air fluid level occupying more than half of the total width of abdomen and displacing the small bowel to one side (usually right) is the classical picture seen. The pouch is proximal to the pubococcygeal line in the invertogram. An early perforation is also suggestive of pouch colon especially if the baby comes from an area where pouch colon is commonly seen.

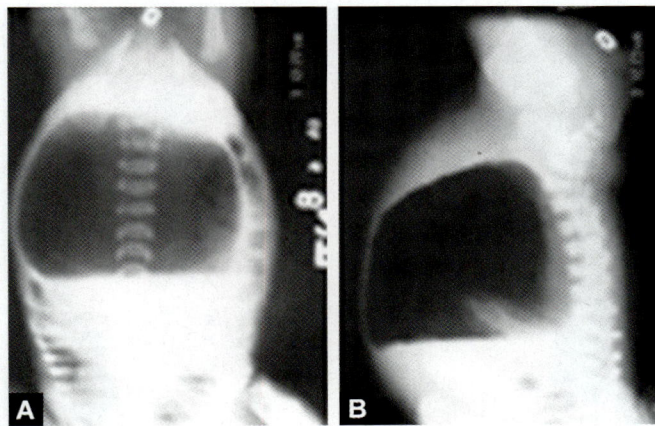

Figs 76.4A and B: Invertogram (AP and lateral) showing large Air—Fluid level occupying more than half of the total width of abdomen, pushing the small bowel loops on one side, suggestive of pouch colon

A detailed work up of the baby at the time of definitive surgery includes ultrasound of abdomen, intravenous urogram and voiding cystourethrography and echocardiography to evaluate for associated anomalies. Spiral CT with 3-D reconstruction of pelvic musculature or MRI of pelvis are optional to study pelvic musculature.

Fallacies in Diagnosis

The following causes may lead to fallacies in diagnosis:
- Massive dilatation of sigmoid in anorectal malformation.
- Hydrometrocolpos (with fistula).
- Pneumoperitoneum.
- Localized pneumoperitoneum following perforation in patients with anorectal malformation presenting late.
- In female babies with rectouterine fistula where the massive dilatation of uterus with meconium and gas may mimic pouch colon.[26]
- If colon is fully decompressed by a large fistula, with the genitourinary tract.

ASSOCIATED ANOMALIES

Genitourinary system is most commonly involved with associated anomalies followed by gastrointestinal, vertebral, limb and cardiac anomalies. Table 76.5 summarizes associated anomalies found with congenital pouch colon.[2] The most common associated anomalies are veisoureteric reflux, kidney anomalies, absent appendix, double appendix and bicornate uterus.

Table 76.5: Common associated anomalies reported in literature[2]

Anomalies

I. Genitourinary system
- Vesicoureteric reflux
- Hydronephrosis
- Renal dysplasia/Agenesis/Ectopia
- Pseudoexstrophy bladder
- Cryptorchidism
- Hypospadias
- Urethral anomalies — diverticulum, duplication, megalourethra, stricture
- Prune belly syndrome
- Bicornuate uterus
- Double uterus/vagina
- Septate vagina

II. GI system
- Absent appendix
- Double appendix
- Malrotation
- Meckel's diverticulum
- Duplication of colon
- Oesophageal atresia

III. Vertebral and limb anomalies
- Sacral agenesis, other vertebral anomalies
- Hemivertebrae
- Meningomyelocele
- Congenital talipes equinovarus

IV. Congenital heart disease

MANAGEMENT

Timely diagnosis and planned management is essential to get the best outcome for any case. Preoperative resuscitation is mandatory as in all cases with anorectal malformation presenting in the newborn age with nasogastric decompression and catheterization of the bladder.

The aim of surgery is to utilize the available length of colon for absorption and storage capacity as well as capability for propelling fecal matter onward with a continent anal opening.

Figure 76.5 outlines the algorithm for the surgical management of pouch colon that depends upon the choice of the surgeon, condition of baby at presentation, technical skill of the surgeon and the available facilities.

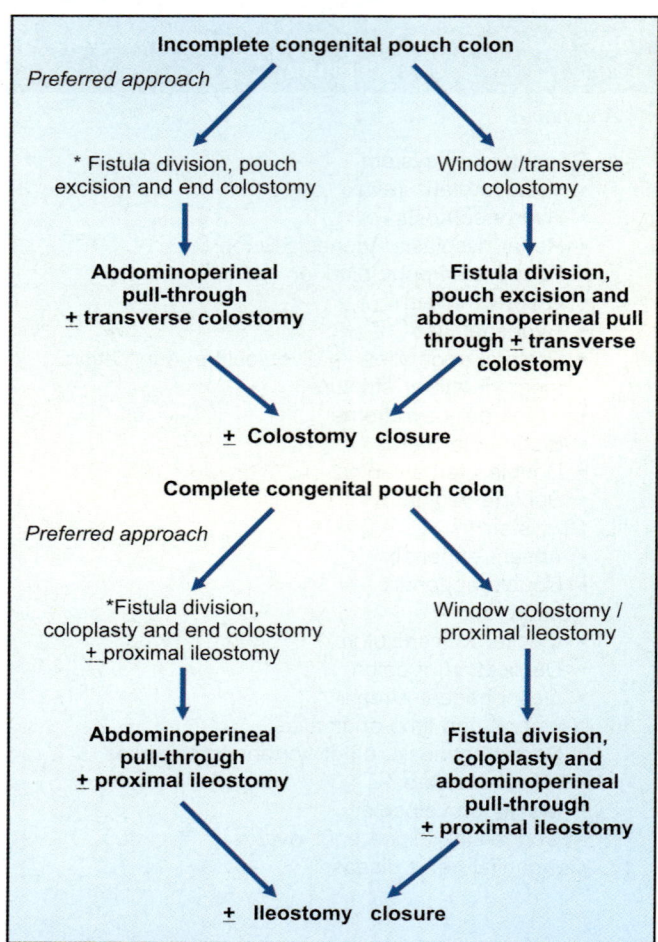

Fig. 76.5: Algorithm for management of congenital pouch colon

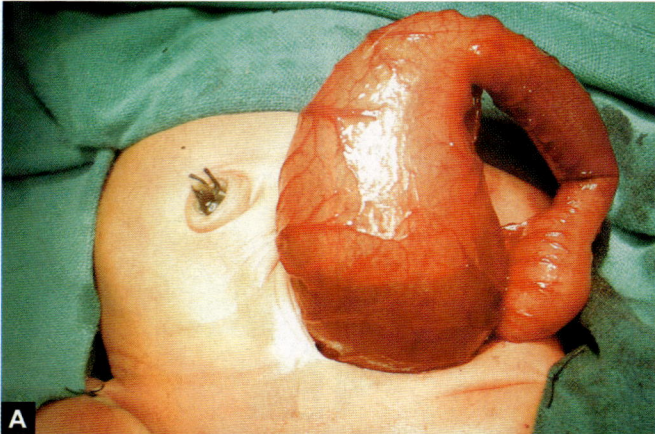
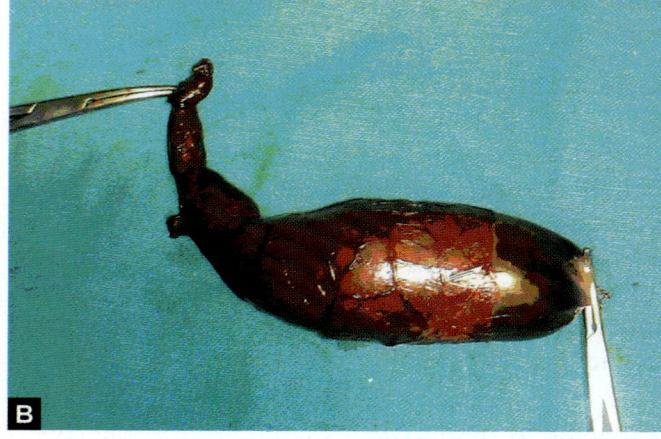

Figs 76.6A and B : A. Operative photograph of an incomplete congenital pouch colon. **B.** An operative specimen of an incomplete pouch colon that was excised

In incomplete congenital pouch colon, the pouch can be excised (Figs 76.6A and B). In complete congenital pouch tubularisation of the pouch in the form of coloplasty is needed (Fig. 76.7). A tube length of about 15 cm is just enough to serve the purpose of colon for adequate propulsion of fecal matter as well as to utilize the colonic surface for water absorption and form formed stools and to avoid the complications of a long and non-functional bowel (Figs 76.8A and B). At present single stage surgery for congenital pouch colon is not routinely advocated as there is unacceptably high mortality associated with it.

With the most common type of CPC now being incomplete congenital pouch colon (than the complete congenital pouch colon that was more commonly seen earlier), better results are expected after surgery as it is preferred to excise and do away with the abnormal colon and its related complications.

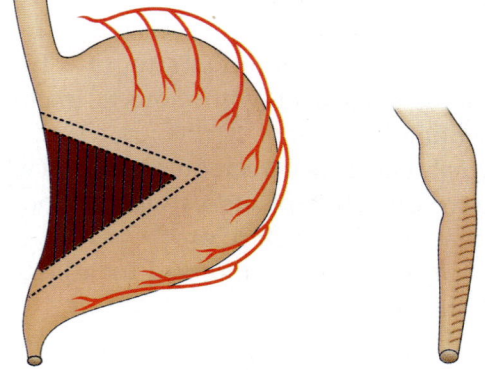

Fig. 76.7: To perform coloplasty, a tube is formed along the antimesenteric border to lengthen the colon preserving the vascular arcade. (Reproduced from Gupta DK, Sharma Shilpa. Congenital pouch colon, in Anorectal Malformations, 1st edition, Ed. John Hutson and Alex Holschneider, Springer Heidelberg. 2006;11:211-22 with kind permission of springer science and business media)

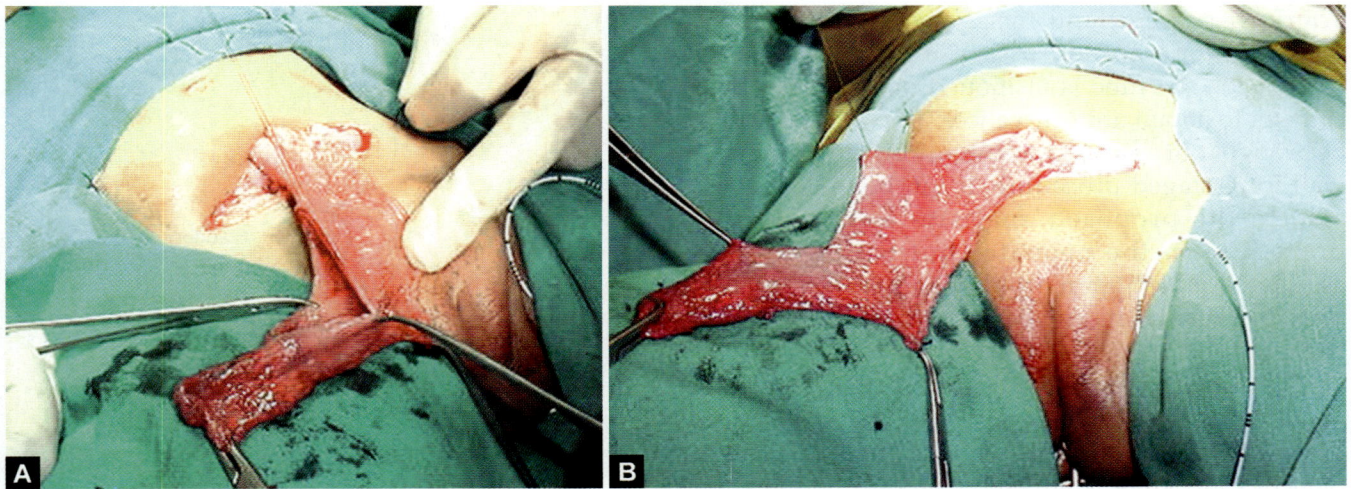

Figs 76.8A and B: Operative photograph of a coloplasty procedure

Table 76.6: Complications associated with congenital pouch colon
1. Related to window colostomy—Recurrent urinary tract infection, incomplete decompression, massive prolapse, bleeding from the prolapsed bowel, recession and stenosis, pouchitis, enterocolitis, adhesive obstruction, septicemia failure to thrive
2. Related to colostomy—Anemia, skin excoriation, diarrhea, poor weight gain, prolapse, stenosis
3. Related to coloplasty—Suture line leak, wound dehiscence, constipation, dilatation, high mortality
4. Related to pull-through—Mucosal prolapse, Anal stenosis, Colonic dilatation, incontinence, mucus discharge; skin excoriation
5. Related to short-length of colon—Recurrent watery diarrhea, poor weight gain

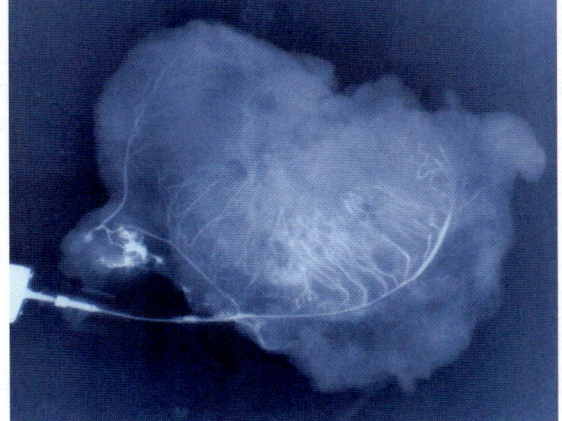

Fig. 76.9: Angiogram of a specimen of pouch colon showing the peculiar blood supply of congenital pouch colon

The preferred approach is proximal diversion in the form of "End colostomy" after division of fistula and (i) excision of the pouch in incomplete pouch colon and (ii) coloplasty in complete pouch colon. The other forms of proximal diversion are: (i) Proximal ileostomy in complete pouch colon and (ii) Transverse Colostomy in incomplete pouch colon.

A window colostomy is a simple surgery in which an opening is made on the anterior surface of the colonic pouch without attempting to ligate the fistulous connection. It can be done with minimum anesthesia especially in a sick neonate, may provide adequate decompression and a time period to allow for weight gain and be fit for second stage. However, it is associated with the well known complications and a mortality as high as 15-20% and is thus not favored by most including the authors (Table 76.6). The mortality rate following the coloplasty procedure performed with an end colostomy in the newborn period, is also reported to be high, hence it is wiser to perform an ileostomy at birth and defer the coloplasty for a later date.

Excision of the pouch in toto with an end colostomy (using normal colon) is the preferred procedure, wherever feasible. An attempt should be made to close the fistulous communication with the urinary tract and excise the pouch even in cases presenting with colonic perforation.

The coloplasty is done after mobilising the pouch completely by division of the inferior mesenteric artery (if present) and incising the pouch on the antimesenteric border, preserving the vascularity (Fig. 76.9). The tube is fashioned over a red rubber catheter to obtain uniform calicer. The coloplasty may be brought out as an end colostomy on the abdominal wall for a staged procedure. It can be pulled down also to the proposed anal site as a definitive procedure in the neonates but it is risky and associated with high morbidity and even mortality. Variable results have been reported by different authors.[1,2,28,29]

The pouch has been used to reconstruct the vagina and the anorectum both at the same time. In this case, the pouch was split longitudinally in analogy with Bianchi's intestinal lengthening procedure and used to create the vagina and reconstruct the anorectum with the preserved blood supply.[30]

COMPLICATIONS

Most of the complications associated with congenital pouch colon are related to the window colostomy (Table 76.6). Recurrent urinary tract infection occurs due to persistent colourinary fistula and associated vesicoureteric reflux. Incomplete decompression of pouch through the window colostomy requires regular washouts.

Suture line leak following the coloplasty has become negligible ever since proximal ileostomy has been used. Minor wound dehiscence occurs in 4-5% of patients. Mortality following coloplasty has been reduced to less than 5% since it is being performed as a staged procedure.

Colonic dilatation has been a problem following pull through procedure utilizing the coloplasty segment in long-term follow-up of patients. This may be due to the fact that the colonic pouch is abnormal histologically and due to the disorganized muscle coat and the abnormal peristalsis, has a tendency to dilate. The utilization of a shorter segment of the pouch for coloplasty is thus recommended.

RARE VARIANTS

There are few cases that are unique and different from the usually seen cases of pouch colon.

A case with imperforate anus associated with duplication of descending colon, double pouch colon type IV, duplication of the urinary bladder, and a bifid penis has been described.[31]

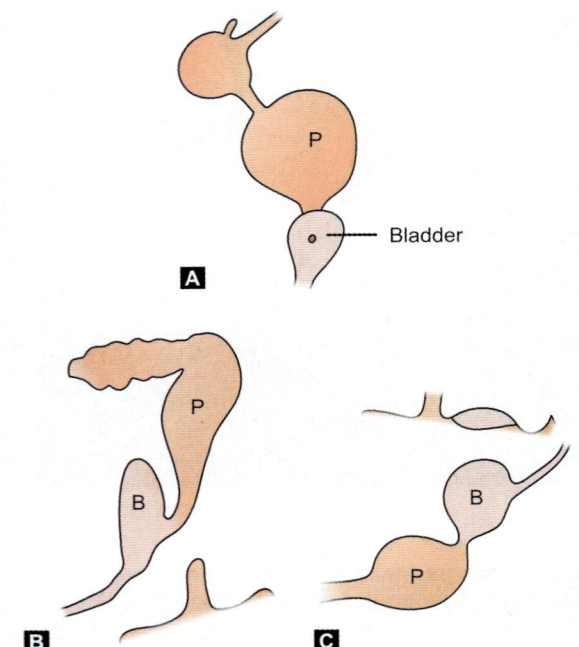

Figs 76.10A to C: Variants of congenital pouch colon **A.** Two segments of pouch colon (P) with an intervening segment of normal colon opening with a fistula into the bladder, **B.** Incomplete pouch colon opening into the bladder associated with rectal atresia. **C.** Pouch colon associated with duplicated exstrophy bladder

Other unusual variants include the presence of two pouches with an intervening segment of normal colon, presence of associated rectal atresia, pseudoexstrophy bladder and associated duplicated exstrophy bladder (Figs 76.10A to C).[32-34] The lower urinary tract and part of the hindgut develop from the allantoic diverticulum. The embryologic basis of the association of pouch colon with duplicate bladder exstrophy has been proposed as malposition of allantoic diverticulum with the yolk sac resulting in anorectal malformation or sequestration of a part of allantois, infraumbilically and improper mesodermal progression giving rise to duplicate bladder exstrophy.[34]

The authors have encountered a case in which there was a lumen opening through the umbilicus giving the appearance of a patent vitellointestinal duct through which stool was coming out (Figs 76.11A to C). On exploration, the opening led to a structure that was composed-half of bladder wall and mucosa and the other half of colonic wall and mucosa. This was an abnormal pouch colon opening with a fistula into the bladder. There was no segment of normal colon. The ileum opened into the structure made of

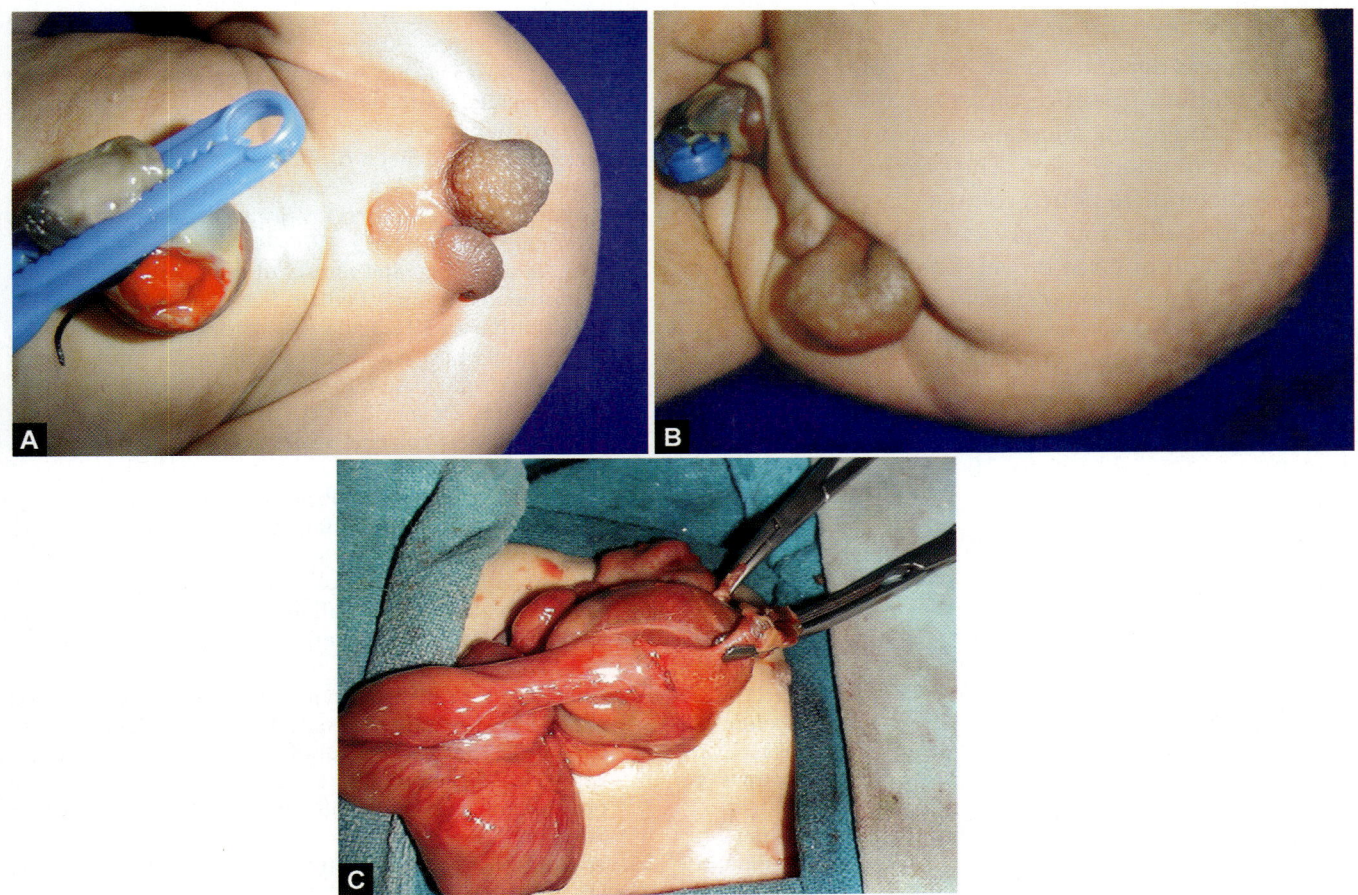

Figs 76.11A to C: A. Newborn presenting with a patent pouch colon opening at the umbilicus, **B.** The baby had associated bifid scrotum and meningomyelocele **C.** Operative photograph demonstrating the pouch made up of colonic and bladder wall

bladder and colonic tissue directly. Ileostomy was done. The pouch colon variant composed of bladder and colonic wall was excised and the bladder fistula was closed.

RESULTS

The results depend on the condition of the perineum, muscle complex and associated anomalies. The presence of a good perineum is essential to attain good continence results and prevent mucosal prolapse. A bad perineum with sacral agenesis in a complete congenital pouch colon may suffer from poor continence status postoperatively.

During the initial follow-up, the baby passes frequent loose stools but subsequently the frequency of defecation decreases and the consistency becomes semisolid to solid. The colon on follow-up examination shows normal caliber in most of the cases; however, dilatation of the tube coloplasty is a serious problem, though rare.

In author's experience, as the anatomy and the histology of the pouch colon is abnormal, even the tube made from the dilated pouch does not work well and does not contribute effectively to the colonic motility.

The continence results vary in different series due to many factors including the available infrastructure, the NICU care and the surgical expertise. Babies with incomplete pouch colon fair comparatively well with normal continence and physical, motor and behavioral development. Cases of complete pouch suffer from increased frequency of stools, rectal prolapse and skin excoriation, especially during the initial years though the frequency decreases with the growth of the child and the dietary modifications. Many children operated for pouch colon and who had been totally incontinent, have attained continence at puberty.

PROGNOSIS

The prognosis depends on the weight of the child, age at presentation, presence of sepsis and perforation, associated congenital anomalies and most importantly on the type of pouch colon. The prognosis is better in cases of incomplete pouch colon as cases of complete pouch colon suffer from recurrent watery diarrhea due to short length of large bowel. The presence of other serious associated anomalies also affects the prognosis. Excision of the pouch and end enterostomy has been associated with maximal survival.

Overall mortality of congenital pouch colon in the newborn age was previously as high as 30-40% but has now come down to 10-20% with growing awareness of this condition and improvement in the surgical management and neonatal care.[4]

REFERENCES

1. Gupta DK, Sharma Shilpa. Congenital Pouch Colon, in Anorectal Malformations, 1st edition, Ed. John Hutson and Alex Holschneider, Springer Heidelberg. 2006;11:211-22.
2. Gupta DK, Sharma Shilpa. Congenital pouch colon — Then and now. J Indian Assoc Pediatr Surg 2007;12:5-12.
3. Gupta DK. Congenital pouch colon: Present lacunae. J Indian Assoc Pediatr Surg 2007;12:1-2.
4. Sharma Shilpa, Gupta D K, Bhatnagar V, Bajpai M, Agarwala S. Management of Congenital Pouch Colon in Association with ARM. 2005;10 (Suppl 1: S22).
5. Gupta DK. Editorial: Anorectal malformations-Wingspread to Krickenbeck. Journal of Ind Assoc. Ped Surg. 2005;10:79.
6. Holschneider A, Hutson J, Pena A, Beket E, Chatterjee S, Coran A, Davies M, Georgeson K, Grosfeld J, Gupta D, et al. Preliminary report on the International Conference for the Development of Standards for the Treatment of Anorectal Malformations. J Pediatr Surg. 2005;40:1521-26.
7. Donkol RH, Jetley NK, Al Mazkary MH. Congenital pouch colon syndrome in a Saudi Arabian neonate: J Pediatr Surg. 2008;43(1):e9-11.
8. Demirogullari B, Ozen IO, Afsarlar C, et al. Congenital pouch colon associated with anorectal malformation: report of 2 cases: J Pediatr Surg. 2007;42(10):E13-16.
9. Bhat NA. Congenital pouch colon syndrome: a report of 17 cases. Ann Saudi Med. 2007;27(2):79-83.
10. Spriggs NJ. Congenital occlusion of the gastrointestinal tract. Guys Hosp. Rep. 1912;766:143.
11. Trusler GA, Mestel AL, Stephens CA: Colon malformation with imperforate anus. Surgery 1959;45:328.
12. Spencer R: Exstrophia splanchnica. Surgery 1965; 57: 751.
13. Blunt A, Rich GF. Congenital absence of the colon and rectum, Am. J. Dis. Child. 1967;114:405.
14. El Shafie M: Congenital short intestine and cystic dilatation of the colon associated with ectopic anus. J. Pediatr. Surg 1971;6:76.
15. Singh S, Pathak IC: Short colon associated with imperforate anus. Surgery 1972;71:781-86.
16. Chiba J, Kasai M, and Askura Y: Two cases of coloplasty for congenital short colon. Arch. Jpn. Chir. (Nippon Geva Hokan) 1976;45:40.
17. Singh A, Singh R, Singh A. Short colon malformation with imperforate anus. Acta Pediatr. Scand. 1977;66:589.
18. Gopal G. Congenital rectovaginal fistula with colonic reservoir. Indian J. Surg. 1978;40:446.
19. Li Z, et al. Congenital atresia of anus with short colon malformation. Chin J. Pediatr. Surg 1981;2:30-32.
20. Narasimharao KL, Yadav K., Mitra SK, Pathak IC1 Congenital short colon with imperforate anus (pouch colon syndrome). Ann. Pediatr. Surg 1984;1:59.
21. Wu YJ, Du R, Zhang GE, Bi ZG. Association of imperforate anus with short colon: a report of eight cases. J. Pediatr. Surg. 1990;25:282-84.
22. Wakhlu AK, Wakhlu A, Pandey A, Agarwal R, Tandon RK, Kureel SN. Congenital short colon. World J Surg 1996;20:107-14.
23. Dickinson SJ. Agenesis of the descending colon with imperforate anus. Correlation with modern concepts of the origin of intestinal atresia. Am J Surg 1987;113:279-81.
24. Chatterjee S K. In Anorectal malformations, A surgeons experience. Oxford University Press, 1991;170-75.
25. Chadha R, Bagga D, Malhotra CJ, Mohta A, Dhar A, Kumar A. The embryology and management of congenital pouch colon associated with anorectal agenesis. J Pediatr Surg 1994;29:439-46.
26. Wakhlu AK, Pandey A. Congenital pouch colon. In : Gupta DK. Textbook of Neonatal Surgery 2000;38:240-48.
27. Agarwal K, Chadha R, Ahluwalia C, Debnath PR, Sharma A, Roy Choudhury S. The histopathology of congenital pouch colon associated with anorectal agenesis. Eur J Pediatr Surg 2005;15:102-06.
28. Upadhyaya P. Pouch colon syndrome: A high anorectal anomaly. Ann. Pediatr. Surg 1984;1:155-57.
29. Gangopadhyay AN, Shilpa S, Mohan TV, Gopal SC. Single-stage management of all pouch colon (anorectal malformation) in newborns. J Pediatr Surg 2005;40:1151-55.
30. Wester T, Lackgren G, Christofferson R, Rintala RJ. The congenital pouch colon can be used for vaginal reconstruction by longitudinal splitting. J Pediatr Surg 2006;41:e25-28.
31. Pimpalwar A, Chowdhary SK , Rao KLN. Duplication of pouch colon associated with duplication of the lower genitourinary tract. Journal of Pediatric Surgery 2003;38: E1.
32. Mathur P, Prabhu K, Jindal D. Unusual presentations of pouch colon Journal of Pediatric Surgery 2002;37:1351-53.
33. Chadha R, Sharma A, Bagga D, et al. Pseudoexstrophy associated with congenital pouch colon. J Pediatr Surg 1998;33:1831-33.
34. Mathur P, Rana YPS, Simlot A, Soni V. Congenital pouch colon with duplicate bladder exstrophy. Journal of ped surg. 2008 [In press].

Persistent Cloaca

DK Gupta, Shilpa Sharma, Alex Holschneider

The presence of a cloaca is physiological in some reptiles, birds and a few mammalians. However, in humans it represents a malformation occurring at a very early stage of development. A cow with a malformation resulting from the confluence of the genital, urinary, and intestinal tracts was first described by Aristotle.[1] Johann Friedrich Meckel introduced the term "cloaca congenita" in the early 1800s.[1] However, cloacal malformations were only rarely reported until 50 years ago.[2]

Persistent cloaca is considered as the most challenging of all types of anorectal malformations. The surgery of the most complex of these anomalies should only be performed by one specially trained in these anomalies to achieve the desired goal of bowel and bladder control. Hendren has published the most comprehensive reports on cloacal malformation repair.[3-9] The posterior sagittal anorectovaginourethroplasty (PSARVUP) allowed direct exposure to the complex anatomy and the voluntary muscles of urinary and fecal continence. Pena has contributed greatly to the treatment of this malformation with the introduction of the total urogenital mobilization after the use of PSARP worldwide.[10-16] The treatment differs on whether the common channel is less than or more than 3 cm in length on the cystoscopy measured from the proximal end of the common channel up to the perineum.[11-17] About 65% of the patients have a short common channel.

This anomaly had a poor prognosis until a few decades ago, with a mortality rate greater than 50%.[18] The prognosis has improved considerably in recent years, and surgical repair with good functional outcome is now possible.

DEFINITION

A persistent cloaca is defined as a confluence of the rectum, vagina, and urethra into a single common channel at the site of the normal urethra.[17] The incidence of these malformations reported previously varied between 1 per 40,000 and 1 per 250,000 live births.[19] However, with growing awareness, the incidence is now considered around 1 in 50,000 live births, comprising around upto 10% of all cases of anorectal malformations. The incidence of cloacal exstrophy still remained much rare with an expected incidence of 1 in 2,50,000 live births.

EMBRYOLOGY

The aetiology of persistent cloaca is unknown but an embryological basis does exist. Cloacal malformations result from the failure of the urorectal septum to join the cloacal membrane during the fourth to sixth weeks of embryonic development. This failure could result in a persistent communication between the rectum and the urogenital sinus.[20]

The tail gut immediately distal to hindgut starts to regress by apoptosis on day 12th of gestation in a craniocaudal direction and has regressed completely by day 13.5.[21,22] The tail gut regression and the urorectal septum play an important role in the process of cloacal separation by cellular proliferation and differentiation. Rupture of the anal membrane plays an additional role. However, Kluth et al reported that the embryonic cloaca never passes through a stage that is similar to any form of anorectal malformations in neonates including the cloaca.[23] They feel that the development of the septum is more passive than active. Based on studies in appropriate animal models, the process of maldevelopment starts early in the embryo.[23] The cloacal membrane is always too short in its dorsal part in abnormal embryos and the region of the future anal opening is missing in contrast to normal mice embryos.[24] The hindgut remains attached to the sinus urogenitalis, thus forming the recto-urethral fistula.[23]

Several experimental models of anorectal malformations including persistent cloaca exists. They are based on the teratogenic effect of ethylenethiourea in the rat, adriamycin exposition of rat fetuses or etretinate a long-acting Vitamin A analog in mice.[25-27] A molecular basis for anorectal malformations was first shown by Kimmel et al.[28] In the murine model of ARM, Gli3-/-mutants had anal stenosis and ectopic anus, Gli2-/-mutants showed imperforate anus and rectourethral fistula. Gli2-/-Gli3+/- mutants developed a cloacal abnormality. Possible etiologic role for homeobox genes, such as HLXB9 with mutations resulting in anorectal- and spine abnormalities have also been suggested.[29]

The cloacal plate, a vertically orientated midline plate of epithelial cells in the caudal half of the genital tubercle, is the key structure to understanding early anorectal and urogenital development that varied between the different animal models.[30] In rats the plate maintained a vertical height along its length, while in humans and pigs it reverted to a two-layer membrane dorsally, shortly before it degenerated, to expose both the anorectal and urogenital tracts. In sheep the plate was taller ventrally than in the other species but also reverted to a short membrane dorsally that exposed the hindgut when it degenerated. The anterior part of the cloacal plate persisted in all embryos as the urethral plate, which then participated in the formation of the urethra in the male and the vestibule in the female. Given the similarities between porcine and human development, the pig may be the most legitimate animal model for the study of anorectal and urogenital anomalies in humans.[30] Persistent Cloaca may occur either in an isolated fashion or as part of a spectrum of anomalies involving multiple organs.

CLASSIFICATION

Classification of Persistent Cloaca

A detailed description of the varying anatomy of cloacal malformations has been published by Hendren and Pena in many publications.[3-7] Hendren distinguishes between anomalies of the perineum, sinus urogenitalis, vagina and rectum.

Hendren's Description of Various Cloacal Anomalies

Perineum

According to Hendren there is a wide range of deformities of each pelvic structure. At the mild end of the spectrum of perineal malformations there is an almost normal looking vaginal opening with an anal orifice which is situated very close but not incorporated in the urogenital sinus. In the next degree the vaginal introitus might be incompletely formed and the anus displaced forward with a dysplastic perineum between both openings. There might be a large sinus urogenitalis opening and the anal opening just behind it, or a single perineal opening covered by the clitoris which could be hyper- or hypoplastic. In a very few cases an accessory hypoplastic urethra can be observed at the tip of the phallus in addition to the proximal urethra fusing with the urogenital sinus. The accessory urethra may have a large diverticulum also. The perineal skin can be covered by an hemangioma and abnormal pigmentation.

Sinus Urogenitalis Variations

The urogenital sinus (UGS) may show an ending on the tip of the clitoris, a subclitoral meatus, a wide opening to a short common channel or a long sinus with the junction of urethra, Vagina(s) and rectum above the PC line. By using this anatomical projection of the upper border of the prostate and the I-point representing the plane of the upper border of the internal anal sphincter, high, intermediate and low types of cloaca can be distinguished according to the Wingspread classification of anorectal malformations.[31] However, there are so many variations of anomalies of the vagina, urethra and rectum in cloacas, that this classification was not very helpful to classify cloacas.

Nevertheless it is important to distinguish between high and low cloacal deformities because a urogenital sinus less than 3 cm of length can be treated by total sinus urogenitalis advancement whereas in longer channels an abdominal approach is necessary.[11]

Vaginal Variations

The two most common variations are a single vaginal opening in the upper urethra with the rectal opening below this orifice and a double side by side vagina with the rectum ending on the septum between both vaginas. In cases of hemivaginas and an incomplete septum the rectal fistula can be situated high on the septum, in cases with two separated vaginas it can usually be found between both vaginal openings.

There might be variations, e.g. two vaginas but atresia or even absence of one, double diverging vaginas, two separate vaginas or one or two vaginas entering the bladder.

Rectal Variations

The rectum can enter the UGS separate and below the vagina, may enter the posterior wall the vagina or even in the bladder coursing between the two halves of the uterus. It can be positioned between and anterior of two vaginal openings or it may run as a long fistula all along the posterior wall of the vagina down to the urogenital sinus. The fistulous tract may open in the septum between two hemivaginae. The rectal pouch at the upper end of the fistula is very high up in these cases, sometimes even above the peritoneal reflection.

Pena's Description

Pena has now the largest world experience in the management of cloacal malformations.[11-16] As cloaca has a spectrum of anomalies, it can not be classified in separate groups. However, Pena has classified these anomalies into two main groups: (a) those with a common channel length of less than 3 cm and (b) those with a common channel length of more than 3 cm. The length of the channel may be as long as 10 cm.

Holschneider Classification of Persistent Cloacas, 2006[32]

Type I: Forme fruste anteposition of anus with ultra short UGS and normal female genitalia

Type II: Low cloacal malformation short UGS < 3 cm (confluence below PC line)

Type III: High cloacal malformation long UGS > 3 cm (confluence at or above PC line)

Type IV: Vagina and/or rectum into bladder cavity.

Posterior cloaca and cloacal exstrophy have been grouped as rare cloacal malformations.

In the Authors' Opinion, the Following Considerations Need to be Kept in Mind while Managing a Case of Common Cloaca

1. Firstly, the true common cloaca needs to be differentiated from a urogenital sinus with a normal or anteposed anal opening. The exact anatomy may be delineated by good clinical examination, dye study, imaging or panendoscopy
2. The presence of a pouch colon (not uncommon in Indian Subcontinent) needs to be ruled out as it affects the management plan in a child born with common cloaca.
3. It is also very important to establish whether the bowel is opening in the cloaca as a fistula or as a normal sized muscular bowel. Patients having a fistulous anomaly require urgent fecal diversion.
4. Presence of associated hydrometrocolpos. The presence of a valvular opening between the urethra and the vagina may lead to one way flow of urine to the vaginal cavity leading to dilatation of vagina, infection and foul smell.
5. Presence or absence of associated other anomalies, which are not uncommon in babies born with persistent cloaca, e.g. unilateral renal agenesis.
6. Whether the urogenital sinus is stenosed or not. A narrow UGS may be just enough to be utilized for the purpose of reconstruction of a new urethra. However, if a girl presents at a higher age with a wide urogenital sinus, the anomaly may possibly be managed with a perineal approach to reconstruct the urethra and the vagina and perform an anal transposition.
7. The presence of urinary incontinence suggests a higher malformation and thus the need to consider surgical options including urinary diversion procedures well in advance.
8. Whether the cloacal opening is a true opening or a covered anomaly giving the appearance of a cloaca.

Babies born with vesico-intestinal fissures require urinary and bowel diversions and despite all advancements can not be ensured a continent and normal quality of life. Parents need to be counselled properly so that they can have the treatment options.

Types of Persistent Cloacal Anomalies

The exact anatomy of the anomaly needs to be defined for proper management. For all practical purposes, a 3 cm length may be described as the borderline between low and high anomalies as advocated by Pena.

Figure 77.1 describes various types of persistent cloaca from a practical point of view. These have been described in Table 77.1. A number of rare variants have also been reported in literature.

Cloacal exstrophy is much rare. The clinical presentation includes the presence of an exomphalos, exstrophied caecum flanked by two hemibladders containing ureteric orifices. A proximal opening leads to the ileum that may prolapse. Two appendiceal appendages may be seen. The distal opening leads to a blind large bowel segment that may be of variable length. The diagnosis of the other rare variants of cloaca requires a high index of suspicion.[33]

Anterior and Posterior Cloacal Malformations

A new entity called posterior cloaca has also been described by Pena and Kessler.[34] It is an extremely rare variant (< 1% as only a few cases are reported till date). In these patients, the rectum is placed at the normal site or minimally mislocated anteriorly. The vagina and urethra fuse together to form the UGS but the UGS instead of opening in the perineum, opens in the anterior rectal wall. As most cloacal anomalies are anterior, thus in reference interms of location, most cloacas would mean an anterior cloacal anomaly in almost 99% cases.

Association with Congenital Pouch Colon

An association with congenital pouch colon is not uncommon. In such cases, the rectum is quite high, very much dilated and opens in the bladder or the vagina with a wide fistula. The wall is thick and the blood supply is also abnormal.[35-37] The rectum may open as a fistula or with a normal sized opening. The fistula may be long and run parallel to the posterior wall of the bladder and the urethra. The opening of the fistula may be located in the vaginal septum or in one of the hemivaginae or in the bladder.

Table 77.1: Types of Persistent cloacal anomalies

Type	Anomaly
I	Low confluence cloaca
II	Low UGS with high rectovaginal fistula (RVF)
III	High UGS with low rectal anomaly
IV	High confluence cloaca
Rare variants	Cloacal exstrophy
	Low confluence with vaginal agenesis
	High confluence with vaginal agenesis
	low/high UGS + Rectovestibular fistula
	Posterior Cloaca
	Low/High UGS with double vagina with rectum opening in vaginal septum/hemi vagina
	Low/High UGS with double vagina with rectum opening in bladder
	UGS with Pouch Colon opening in bladder
	UGS with double vagina with Pouch Colon opening in vaginal septum
	Low UGS with normal rectum
	High UGS with normal rectum

CLINICAL PRESENTATION

The most striking clinical feature that brings the patient to the doctor is the absence of anal opening and the presence of a single perineal orifice (Figs 77.2A and B). The external genitalia appear smaller and are under developed. The newborn may present with an abdominal mass, due to a distended vagina (hydrocolpos) and is present in 50% of patients with persistent cloaca. The sacrums should be examined. The presence of associated anomalies should be looked for.

There have been instances when the diagnosis could not be made in the newborn period and the children have presented as late as at the age of 10-13 years.[38] Girls with a single opening on their perineum should always be suspected to suffer from a cloacal malformation. Rarely cloacas have been reported in boys in whom the urethra and rectum are coalescing into a common channel that connected to the external surface in the perineal or anal area.[39] In girls, an abdominal mass and severe abdominal distension can be observed resulting from hydrometrocolpos and/or rectal obstruction. Additional malformations of the lower limbs, genitalia, the skin (hemangioma), the urogenital tract, vertebras and cardiac, gastrointestinal and other deformities may occur.

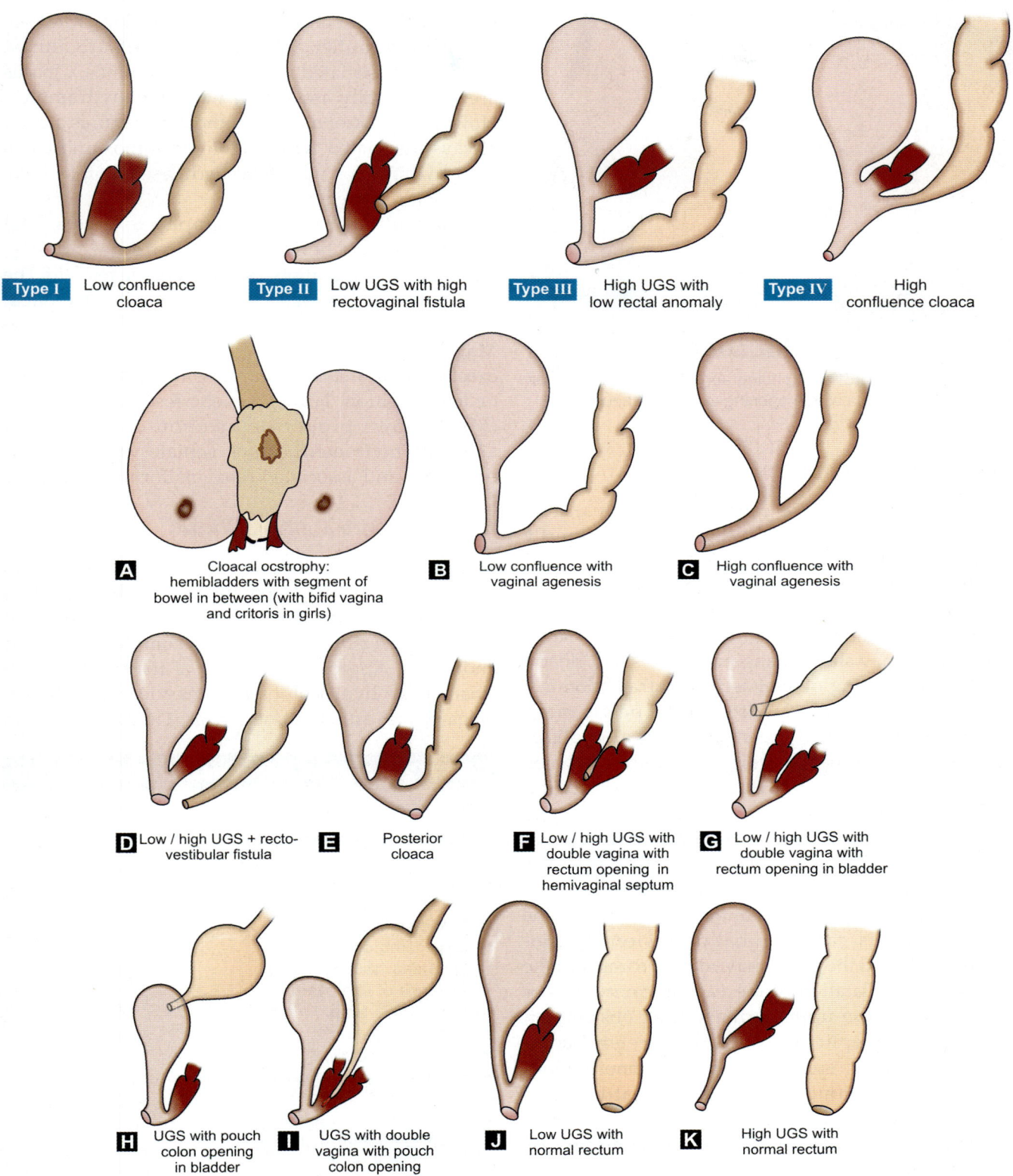

Fig. 77.1: Types of persistent cloacas. The main types are type I to IV. The rare variants include A-K. UGS: Urogenital sinus

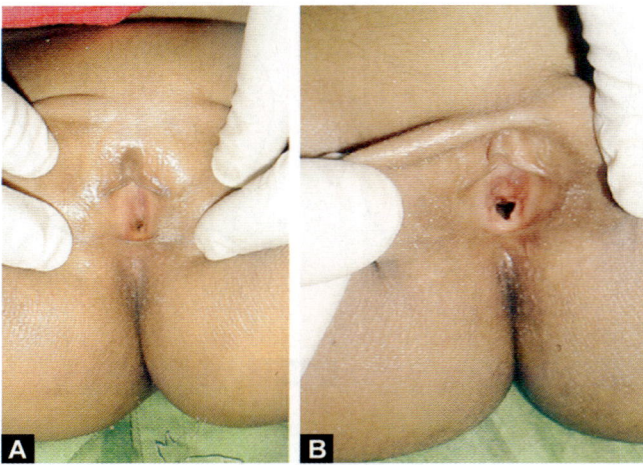

Figs 77.2A and B: Clinical photograph of a case of common cloaca with a single opening in the perineum

ANTENATAL DETECTION

Cloacal anomalies are rare and have variable presentations, these are difficult to diagnose correctly by ultrasonography antenatally.[40-43]

The anatomy of cloacal malformations is variable, thus ultrasonography findings could vary according to the type of anomaly in different cases.[44-49] Serial ultrasounds may show changing features of a cloacal anomaly, consisting of fetal ascites, intra-abdominal cystic structures with debris, a cystic pelvic mass, hydrometrocolpos, hydronephrosis, and oligohydramnios.[40,43] Linear calcifications in the abdomen along the peritoneal surface indicate calcified meconium from meconium peritonitis.[52] This may occur, apart from intestinal perforation, in cloacal malformations, when meconium spills into the peritoneal cavity through the fallopian tubes.[53] As the condition progresses, an inflammatory reaction in the fallopian tubes causes tubal occlusion, hydrometrocolpos, and the progressive disappearance of the ascites.[52] The dilatation of the vaginal cavity further contributes to the upper urinary tract obstruction (hydroureteronephrosis) by direct ureteral compression. Urologic, spinal, and cardiac abnormalities are the most commonly associated features and account for 50-68% of all cases.[41]

Maintenance of amniotic fluid is a dynamic process involving fetal urine production, fetal swallowing, secretion of the oral and respiratory tracts, and intramembranous flow (fluid transfer across the placenta, the umbilical cord, and fetal skin). The lack of a urinary outlet and renal agenesis are almost invariably associated with oligohydramnios. Cloacas are thus usually associated with oligohydramnios. However, occasionally the pathologic features are not always associated with oligohydramnios and cases with hydramnios with fetal hydrometrocolpos have also been reported.[43]

The ability of ultrasonography to detect fetal anomalies may be limited by maternal obesity, amniotic fluid alteration, and inadequate fetal lie. The prenatal ultrasonographic diagnosis of cloacal anomalies may be confirmed by the use of a Fetal Magnetic resonance imaging (MRI) that reveals excellent fetal images regardless of maternal obesity or fetal position. Fetal Magnetic resonance imaging (MRI) allows proper delineation of the cloacal anomaly, hydrometrocolpos, septate vagina, uterus didelphys and associated renal malformations.

ASSOCIATED MALFORMATIONS

More than 80% of all patients with a cloaca have an associated urogenital anomaly. Sacrum and vertebral anomalies are common. Patients with long common channel have a high frequency of complex associated anomalies. Approximately 50% of the patients with cloaca have hydrocolpos that may lead to bilateral mega ureters and hydronephrosis. The most common

Table 77.2: Anomalies associated with persistent cloaca

Vesicoureteral reflux
- Malformations of the kidneys
- Tethered cord
- Neurogenic bladder
- Diastematomyelia
- Myelomeningocele
- Lower limb deformities
- Occluded fallopian tubes
- Absence of one ovary
- Hypoplastic labia
- Absence of uterus
- Bladder exstrophy
- Gastrointestinal duplications
- Pouch colon
- Cardiac malformations
- Vertebral deformities
- Esophageal atresia
- Cerebral anomalies
- Abnormalities of the central nervous system

associated urinary tract anomalies involved are renal agenesis, renal dysplasia, vesicoureteral reflux and megaureter.

During the immediate assessment of the newborn, emphasis is placed on the recognition and treatment of potentially lethal associated defects, mainly urologic, esophageal or cardiac anomalies (Table 77.2). Some of the children exhibited masculinization of the external genitalia with the accessory urethra or cloacal channel assuming a phallic position in an enlarged clitoris.

All babies with cloacal anomaly should undergo an ultrasound of the kidneys and pelvis before surgery. If a hydrocolpos is present, it should be drained at the same time the colostomy is performed. The colostomy should be completely diverting so as to prevent contamination of the urinary tract. In cases of extremely long common channel that lies usually near the trigone, the bladder neck is closed and a vesicostomy is done. About 30% of these patients have duplicated Mullerian structures. The prognosis should be explained to the patients well in advance and the complications that may arise, especially during pregnancy, may be explained.

Tethered Cord

A tethered spinal cord, intravertebral fixation of the filum terminale has a known association with anorectal malformations and is particularly common in patients with persistent cloaca (in approximately 40% of patients). Preoperative ultrasound can give suspicion of tethered cord syndrome sometimes associated with lipoma of the spinal cord or diastematomyelia. Anomalies of the sacrum are commonly associated with the tethered cord. Patients with anorectal malformations and tethered cord have a worse functional prognosis regarding bowel and urinary function. Motor and sensory disturbances of the lower extremities may result. Controversy still exists on whether or not an asymptomatic child with an incidentally diagnosed tethered cord should be operated or not. Many patients who had been untethered have been reported to have a retethering postoperatively due to postoperative scarring. If the child suffers from incontinence and there is neither sacral agenesis nor deficient muscle complex, surgical de-tethering is recommended.

INVESTIGATIONS

A skiagram lumbosacral spine is useful to look for associated vertebral defects. Plain radiography of the sacrum in the anterior-posterior and lateral projections can reveal sacral anomalies, such as a hemisacrum and sacral hemivertebrae. The skiagram should be performed in a strict sagittal position with the legs elevated and the anal dimple marked. The complete lumbosacral spine should be visible. There is a clear correlation between the degree of vertebral and sacral malformations and the occurrence of neurogenic voiding and defecation disorders. A complete destruction of S2- S4 is called Lower Motor Neuron Lesion (LMNL) and shows clinically as an always dribbling bladder. A severe deformity of higher lumbar neurons with intact sacral reflex activity, resulting in an autonomic or reflex bladder, is called Upper Motor Neuron Lesion.[54] However, the majority of the patients suffer from a Mixed Motor Neuron Lesion (MMNL) with a varying amount of residual urine and uninhibited detrusor contractions.[54]

The sacral ratio measured by the distance from the coccyx to the sacroiliac joint divided by the distance from the sacroiliac joint to the top of the pelvis in a lateral radiograph gives an idea about the functional prognosis. Normal sacrum has a ratio of 0.77. Bowel control has never been observed in patients with ratios less than 0.3 by Pena's team. Abdominal and pelvic ultrasonography may be done to look for associated anomalies before the baby is discharged. Spinal ultrasonography in the first 3 months of life is useful to look for tethered cord. At a later age, MRI may be used.

After birth, once the colostomy has been created, a high pressure hydro soluble contrast distal colostogram may help to delineate the detailed anatomy. A properly performed genitogram through the single perineal opening may further elucidate the anatomy (Figs 77.3A and B).

Cystoscopy and vaginoscopy are essential components for evaluation of the patient with persistent cloaca. The combination of imaging, dye study and panendoscopy, provides reasonable information whether a laparotomy will be required in addition to the perineal approach, and the assessment of the internal organs, the vagina(s), rectal fistula, bladder neck and urethral orifices besides measuring the length of the common channel .Without endoscopic

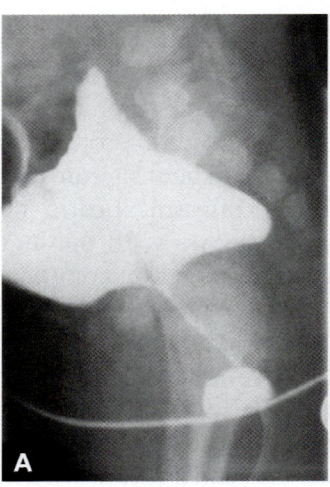 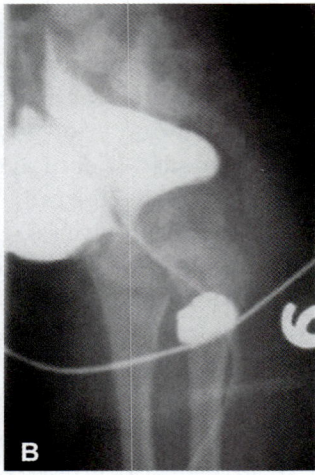

Figs 77.3A and B: Contrast study of a patient with common cloaca delineating the double vaginae separated by a long septum. There was associated bilateral hydrocolpos

aid it is usually not possible to catheterize the bladder because the fusion of the proximal urethra with the UGS is almost sharply angulated in the direction of the pubic bone. This may be helpful to teach the parents to allow later intermittent catheterization by the mother until the final reconstruction is performed. In many cases however, the urine is first passed in the vagina before being evacuated through the common channel. In these patients it is sufficient to perform intermittent catheterization in the vagina. Only very few children with cloaca need a vesicostomy or vaginostomy.

The investigations should also be directed to identify the associated urologic anomalies and presence of hydrocolpos that need to be managed within the newborn period to avoid serious complications. An obstructive uropathy may be overlooked and later present with life threatening sepsis and acidosis.

TREATMENT

The goals of management in cases of persistent cloaca in the newborn period are:
1. Achieve satisfactory diversion of the gastrointestinal tract
2. To detect associated anomalies
3. Identify and manage a distended vagina, if present
4. Divert the urinary tract, when indicated.

Colostomy

The preliminary intervention should consist of a colostomy either in the transverse colon (or rarely even the high sigmoid colon) keeping in mind that the left colic- and the sigmoidal arteries are essential for later reconstructive pull-through procedures. Diversion of the fecal stream using the transverse colostomy, is most commonly employed. Transverse colostomy placed in the ascending colon and a distal mucous fistula are recommended. The defunctionalized colon so obtained, is used for the future rectal pull-through; thus, adequate length must be ensured when the colostomy location is chosen. Also, an access to this distal colon is vital for radiological evaluation. Complete diversion of the fecal matter is necessary to prevent urinary infections.

Drainage of the Hydrometrocolpos

A catheter drainage or open drainage should be introduced in the bladder and/or vagina in case of hydrometrocolpos. The distended vagina is a common cause of an obstructed urinary tract with pressure on the trigone; therefore, once the vagina is decompressed, the urinary tract may no longer be obstructed. If the hydrocolpos is not drained during the newborn period, it can become infected and can lead to vaginal scarring. Many patients require antimicrobial prophylaxis for urinary tract infections for associated vesicoureteral reflux. After the recovery of the baby, further detailed studies especially by endoscopy are necessary with introduction of stents in all visible urethral, vaginal and rectal openings. These probes are important for a detailed X-ray study immediately after the endoscopy.

Definitive Repair of Cloacal Malformations

The final goals of management in cases of persistent cloaca during definitive repair are:
1. To place all the three orifices at their normal locations, with good cosmesis.
2. To achieve bowel control
3. To attain urinary control
4. To attain ability for normal sexual function.

It may be difficult to attain all these goals in complicated cases. The prognosis depends on the length of the common channel, sacral development and the presence of associated anomalies.

Principles of Surgery

The length of the common channel determines the extent of surgical repair.[17] The length of the common channel can vary from 1cm to sometimes more than 5 cm at the time of definitive repair. If the common channel is quite short about a cm, a perineal approach may be sufficient if the surgical access is allowed. For a common channel of 1-3 cm, the posterior sagittal approach should be used to repair the defect without an abdominal approach. For patients with a common channel longer than 3 cm, a laparotomy is usually required. The plan of surgery depends on the length of common channel and the anomaly. Figures 77.4 and 77.5 describes the algorithm for options of management for these cases.

The surgical procedure combines the advantages of the Posterior Sagittal Anorectoplasty (PSARP) introduced by De Vries and Pena in 1982 with the classical abdomino perineal approach.[10] However, the appropriate technique depends on the individual case and malformation. The repair can usually be performed using only the posterior sagittal approach. For more complex anomalies, an abdominal approach is added to mobilize a very high vagina or the rectum.

The principle previously followed was to separate the rectum from the vagina, the vagina from the sinus urogenitalis to pull both structures down to the perineum and to reconstruct the urethra from the UGS. Often, the vagina and urinary tract were separated to gain length. With the introduction of the total urogenital mobilization, the rectum is mobilized first. Then, the vagina and urinary tract are mobilized together (total urogenital mobilization), with the goal that these structures reach the perineum. If total urogenital mobilization does not adequately lengthen the vagina, the vagina and urethra must be separated, which is a technically challenging maneuver. Care must be taken not to cause any ischemic injury to the urethra or the vagina. Vaginourethral fistulae are more likely after this. The rectum is placed within the limits of the sphincter mechanism, determined with an electrical stimulator.

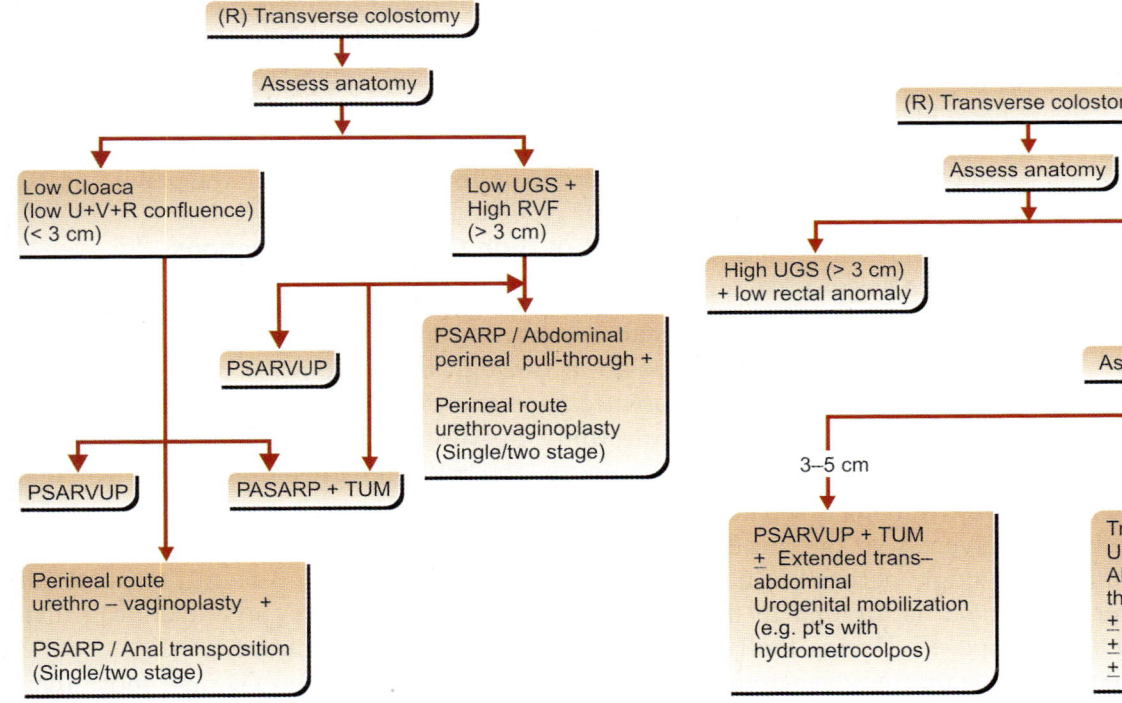

Fig. 77.4: Flow chart for management of cloaca with low confluence

Fig. 77.5: Flow chart for management of cloaca with high confluence

U = Urinary bladder, V = Vagina, R = Rectum
UGS = Urogenital sinus, RVF = Rectovaginal fistula, TUM = Total urogenital sinus mobilization

The main challenge involves the repair of the vagina, the urethra, and the associated urologic defects. The surgeon must be prepared to open the bladder and to reimplant the ureters, if necessary. Complex vaginal mobilizations are often required, and vaginal replacement with small intestine or colon is frequently necessary.

A large vagina can be mobilized more easily and has more alternatives for vaginal repair. A vaginostomy performed in the newborn period must be taken down at the time of the definitive repair as it may be tethered to the abdominal wall and prevent mobilization of the vagina. Approximately half of the patients have various degrees of vaginal or uterine septation that can be totally or partially repaired during the main operation or deferred for definitive repair until puberty.

Operative Procedure

The patient is placed in lithotomy position and pan-endoscopy is done to assess the length of the common channel, the bladder, the vagina and the rectum/fistula.

Perineal Urethrovaginoplasty

For low anomalies or anomalies with a low urogenital sinus, the perineal route can be used for the urethrovaginoplasty. A low urogenital sinus with a vaginal septum can be handled at the same time (Figs 77.6A to M). This approach is particularly useful for the cases that have had a PSARP in the past, leaving the UGS as such or a misdiagnosed UGS.

Total Urogenital Sinus Mobilization (TUM)

For short common channel the patient is placed in the prone position with the pelvis elevated with a roll. A posterior sagittal approach is used initially to separate the rectum. The incision is given from the middle portion of the sacrum to the single perineal orifice. The entire sphincter mechanism is divided in the midline and the rectum is exposed. During the last decade, a total urogenital moblization has been found to be beneficial for these patients.[17] The rectum is separated from the vaginal wall by creating two walls out of one. Multiple 6/0 silk sutures are placed taking the edges of the common channel, along with the edges of the vaginal walls, to exert uniform traction. The urethra and the vagina are mobilized together. Another set of sutures are placed transversally 5 mm dorsal to the clitoris and the entire common channel is mobilized as one. Gentle uniform traction on all these sutures distributes tension and avoids damage to the very thin structure of the UGS. The wall of the urogenital sinus is then divided completely ventral to the sutures and dorsal to the clitoris. The dissection proceeds lateral and ventral to the UGS and includes step by step the vagina and urethra together. The dissection is proceeded with till a vascular fibrous structure is identified and divided. These vascular fibrous ligaments attached to the pelvic rim must now be divided to free the vagina, urethra and bladder without dividing the blood supply to these structures. The dissection goes on until enough length has been gained to connect the vaginal edges to the perineum. This step allows a gain of 2 to 4 cm length of the urogenital structures. The purpose is to place the urethral meatus at its normal location around 5-8 mm below the clitoris. The edges of the vagina are sutured to skin of the perineum forming the new labia. The initial common channel is divided in the midline to make two flaps that are sutured on either side. By this procedure the urethra and the vagina are shortened but without any loss of function. The uterus and the bladder are pulled down deeper in the pelvis.

Repair of High Cloacal Malformations

The baby is prepared and draped circumferentially so that the surgeon can work with the patient in supine position through the abdominal route, jack-knife position for the posterior sagittal access and in lithotomy position for the perineal stage of the procedure. The baby should be draped in a way that it can easily be turned to each position inside sterile drapes.

If the channel is between 3-5 cm the posterior sagittal approach may be tried and a total urogenital mobilization may still be attempted.[17]

Patients with long common channel more than 5 cm are approached through the abdomen with an incision in the midline. The separation requires delicate surgery and the decision should be made by an experienced surgeon.

Persistent Cloaca 867

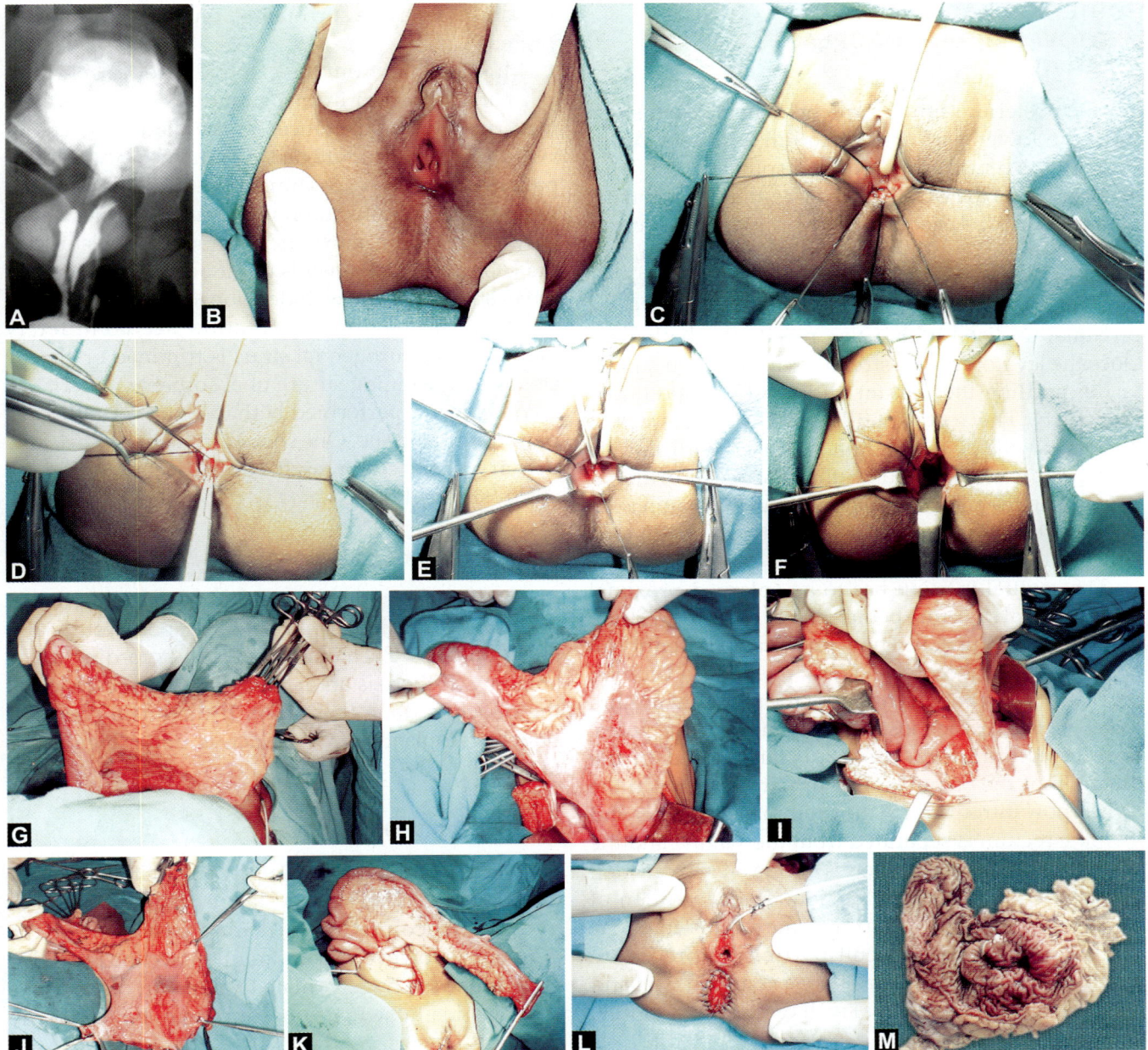

Figs 77.6A to M: Operative steps in the management of a case of common cloaca (Type II- Low UGS and High rectovaginal fistula). The girl was 3 yrs old with pouch colon and was on colostomy from 3 months of age **A.** Contrast study of a patient with common cloaca delineating the double vaginae and the fistulous tract of a pouch colon opening in the vaginal septum, **B.** Clinical photograph of the same baby, **C.** The urethra catheterized, **D.** The exposed vaginal septum, **E.** The division of the vaginal septum in process, **F.** The divided vaginal septum, **G.** Abdominal exploration and colostomy mobilized, **H.** An incomplete pouch colon was identified with adequate length of the bowel, **I.** The fistulous tract of the pouch colon into the vaginal septum, **J.** The fistula divided and the incomplete pouch colon ready for excision **K.** Adequate mobilization of bowel assessed, **L.** Completed urethrovaginoplasty and abdominperineal pull-through, **M.** Excised specimen of pouch colon

POSTERIOR SAGITTAL ANO RECTOVAGINOURETHROPLASTY (PSARVUP)

For the posterior sagittal approach, the incision starts from the lower part of the sacrum and goes down through the centre of the external sphincter ani fibers to the orifice of the UGS. The parasagittal and sphincter fibers are divided exactly in the midline. The coccyx is divided and split in the midline for about 1 cm. It is easier to find the levator structures close to the coccyx than in the anal region and to open them from proximal to distal with a fine needle tip diathermy. Once the levator muscle structures are divided strictly in the midline the rectum and the UGS should be identified. The rectal fistula usually enters at the posterior wall of the vagina. In cases with double vaginas it is not infrequent that the rectal orifice is situated on the septum separating the two vaginas. In a few cases it can only be reached by an abdominal approach.

The sagittal incision has to be enlarged proximal to the visceral structure being in most cases the rectum, in others the vagina. It is now important to identify all openings which become evident: one or two vaginas, the rectal fistula and the orifice of the proximal urethra which is usually the most distal opening in the cloaca. Besides, the urethra is sharply angulated in the direction of the os pubis. The urinary catheter in the UGS is now introduced in the urethra and bladder and then the rectum is separated from the Vagina and the vagina from the urethra. Series of fine 6-0 silk traction sutures may be used for traction. The separation of the rectum from the vagina and the vagina from the urethra is the most difficult part of the procedure because rectum and vagina share a common wall and the vagina covers the dorsal wall of the bladder neck. The urethra may be surrounded on its lateral sides by vagina.

Muscle fibers from the external bladder sphincter can hardly be seen in this situation and the ureters may run to ectopic orifices in the bladder neck. To avoid urinary incontinence, as much as possible the paraurethral tissue should be preserved. The separation of the rectum and vagina becomes easier only up to 1-2 cm above the entrance of the fistulae in the UGS because the walls of the rectum, vagina and the urethra are now well developed.

Once the vagina and rectum are completely mobilized, the urogenital sinus is trimmed or simply closed by a running suture of absorbable material. A second layer is performed with interrupted sutures of para-urethral tissue. One should try to reconstruct the urinary sphincter which could be identified by electrostimulation.

Associated Pouch Colon

The pouch colon associated with persistent cloacas require prior diagnosis to achieve good results and avoid mishaps. Each case is handled according to the anatomy. If there is an incomplete pouch, excision of the pouch is done (Fig. 77.6). If there is a complete pouch, coloplasty of the pouch is done (Figs 77.7A to C).[35]

Vaginal Reconstruction

Further operation depends upon the anatomy of each case. If the vagina is large as in cases of hydrometrocolpos, then it may easily reach the perineum. However, lot of careful dissection is needed to mobilize the hugely dilated vagina. In cases with a short vagina, a switch procedure may be feasible in

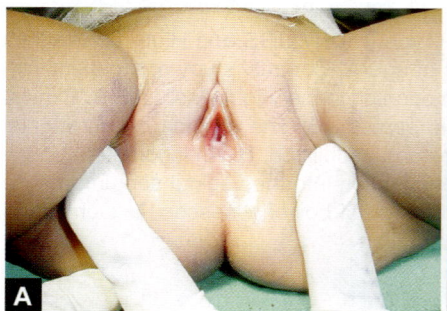
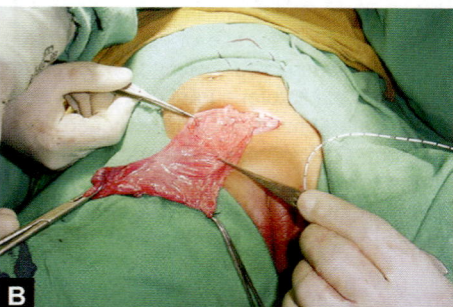
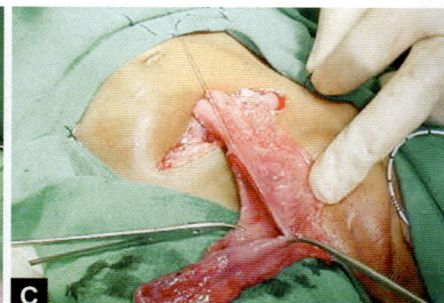

Figs 77.7A to C: A. Clinical photograph of a case of commom cloaca
B. On abdominal exploration there was complete pouch colon, **C.** Coloplasty in process

cases with two joined hydrocolpos with separate hemiuteri. In such cases, the septum may be divided and one entire Mullerian structure may be resected. The blood supply to one side should be preserved to provide the blood supply to the side that is being switched down.

If the vagina is very short, small and high, a replacement is needed. The first choice for vaginal replacement is to use the part of the rectum in babies with a mega rectum. The rectum is divided longitudinally to form both, the new vagina and the neo rectum. These structures are based on the sigmoid vessels for the vagina and of the descending colon based on the left colic artery for the rectum. If the patient has internal genitalia, the segment of neovagina is sutured to it after the free passage of the fallopian tubes has been secured. In absence of these, the upper part of the neovagina is closed. The second choice for the vaginal replacement is the use of sigmoid colon, followed by the segment of the small bowel.

The lower rectum can also be used according the technique of Harrison in form of a J-loop with one single long arcade.[50-51] The distal part of the J-loop forms the vagina, while the proximal segment, the new rectum. The deepest point of the J is implanted in the perineum to create the separate vaginal and rectal orifices. However, the procedure requires meticulous care to preserve the blood supply (Fig. 77.8).

In case of a vaginal perforation during this procedure, the vagina is rotated by 90 degree so that the urethral suture line and the vaginal sutures are separated and rectovaginal fistula are avoided. The vagina should be implanted next to the urethral orifice and inside the labia. A perineum of 1.5 cm of length is then constructed and the rectum fixed inside the external anal sphincter fibers. Nixon's cutaneous flap anoplasty has also been used to increase anorectal sensibility.[52]

POSTOPERATIVE CARE

The urinary catheter remains in place for approximately 10-14 days. In complicated cases, one may have to resort to a suprapubic cystostomy tube. Anal calibration is performed 2 weeks after the operation, followed by a program of anal dilatations. The anus must be dilated twice daily, and the size of the dilator is increased every week. The final size to be reached depends on the age of the patient. Once the desired size is reached, the colostomy can be closed.

COMPLICATIONS

To avoid complications, in most cases of cloaca, the rectal pull-through should not be performed first as an isolated procedure. In the majority of cases, all three systems, i.e. rectum, vagina, and urinary tract can be repaired simultaneously.[7] Most complications can be preventable or reduced by adhering to specific principles.[53]

1. *Urethrovaginal fistulae:* This is the main operative complication. It requires a reoperation. Cystoscopy and vaginoscopy may be performed before colostomy closure to ensure that there is no urethrovaginal fistula
2. Vaginal stricture or atresia
3. Urethral strictures
4. Inadequate drainage of hydrocolpos may lead to urinary tract infections, pyocolpos, and/or vaginal perforation.
5. Colostomy complications, including a colostomy sited too distally
6. Persistent urogenital sinus after rectal reconstruction.
7. *Fecal incontinence:* Continence is more likely in patients with a low cloaca and in those with a normal sacrum. About 80% of patients with a low cloaca and good sacrum have bowel control. Approximately, 70% of patients can achieve voluntary movements. For patients with

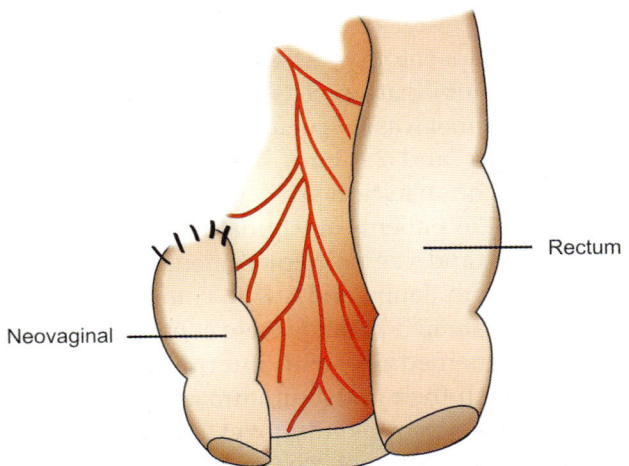

Fig. 77.8: The lower rectum can be used as a J-loop to form neovagina and rectum

incontinence, a bowel management program is successful in keeping the patient clean and dry. In those in whom bowel management is unsuccessful (< 3%), a colostomy may be the best option to ensure good quality of life.

8. *Urinary incontinence*: Urinary control varies based on the length of the common channel. Intermittent catheterization is required in 70% of patients with persistent cloaca who have a common channel longer than 3 cm, compared with 20% in the group with a common channel shorter than 3 cm. In patients with urinary incontinence, urinary diversions, such as the Mitrofanoff procedure and the use of intermittent catheterization, are usually successful in keeping the patient dry of urine. In most patients, the bladder neck is competent and the patients who require catheterization remain dry between micturitions. If catheterization is not performed, overflow incontinence occurs. Occasionally, the bladder neck is not competent in these patients, a urinary diversion, such as a Mitrofanoff procedure may be helpful. Seventy percent of all patients with a common channel longer than 3 cm require intermittent catheterization to empty their bladder.[17]

9. *Gynaecological problems*: The precise gynecologic anatomy must be ascertained during the main repair or at the time of the colostomy closure. Approximately one third of the patients may have obstructed Müllerian structures that can lead to severe problems due to retrograde menstruation.[17]

OUTCOME

Most patients of common cloaca can be repaired with a satisfactory functional and anatomic result with the posterior sagittal midline approach, often together with an abdominoperineal approach.[7] Hendren in 1998 reported on 195 cases of cloacal repair.[3] Out of a follow up of 141 cloacal patients, 82 had spontaneous bowel movements and satisfactory control, 38 used enemas to evacuate, 9 had a colostomy and 7 suffered from fecal soiling. Regarding urinary control, 83 voided spontaneously, 40 patients catheterized to empty, 4 had urinary diversion, 1 had a continent diversion and 5 patients were wet. Also, 24 of these were the adult patients when followed up. Seventeen had experienced coitus and 7 had babies, all except one by caesarian section.

Patients with cloacal malformation have a high incidence of bladder dysfunction with recurrent urinary infections and incontinence.[54] Urodynamic assessment has been reported to be necessary to detect bladder dysfunction in these patients. Some authors have reported that surgical reconstruction by total urogenital mobilization can cause further deterioration of bladder function, particularly in the group with a long common channel.[54]

Gynecologic results in 22 teenagers were reported by Levitt et al.[55] Seven girls are menstruating, six had primary amenorrhea because of absent or atretic uteri. Nine patients suffered from obstruction of one or more Mullerian structures that did not allow menstruation. Renal outcome is less favorable. Warne et al identified 64 patients with cloacal malformations aged 0.5-19 years at the time of the study.[56] Also, 83% were born with a structural abnormality of the urinary tract, including renal dysplasia (27%), ectopic kidney (14%), solitary kidney (13%), duplex kidneys (9%), and uretropelvic junction obstruction (5%).[52] VUR was observed in 53%, sacral abnormalities in 57% of the patients. Chronic renal failure developed in 32 (50%) patients with a glomerular filtration rate of less than 80 ml per minute per 1.73 m². Moreover, 17% progressed to end stage renal failure, 6% required renal transplantation and 4 died of chronic renal failure. Therefore careful postoperative follow up is obligatory in these patients.

Pena has recently reported a review of 339 cases of cloaca.[17] A total of 265 patients underwent primary operations and 74 were secondary. All patients were approached posterior sagittally; 111 of them also required a laparotomy. Also, 122 underwent total urogenital mobilization. The average length of the common channel was 4.7 cm for patients that required a laparotomy and 2.3 cm for those who did not. Vaginal reconstruction involved a vaginal pull-through in 196 patients, a vaginal flap in 38, vaginal switch in 30, and vaginal replacement in 75 (36 with rectum, 31 with ileum, and 8 with colon).[17] A total of 54% of all evaluated patients were continent for urine and 24% remained dry with intermittent catheterization through their native urethra and 22% through a Mitrofanoff-type of conduit. Seventy-eight percent patients with a common channel longer than 3 cm required intermittent catheterization compared with 28% when their common channel was shorter than 3 cm. Sixty percent of all cases have voluntary bowel movements (28% of them never soiled, and 72% soiled occasionally). Forty percent were incontinent for stools but remained clean when subjected to a bowel management program.[17]

CLOACAL EXSTROPHY

In cloacal exstrophy, the results are worse and the mortality and morbidity is high.[57] However, Lund and Hendren achieved an overall survival rate of 98% in 50 cases observed over a period of 25 years.[58] Of the 40 reconstructed cases, 31 were dry. Acceptable bowel continence was achieved with wash out enemas in 19 of 25 pull-throughs.

Patients with cloacal exstrophy have complex anomalies of the genitourinary and gastrointestinal tract with a spectrum of colonic length. Often, colon is lost during the initial management by use of ileostomies and for urologic and genital reconstruction.[59]

In a series of 53 patients of cloacal exstrophy treated over a 26-year period, including typical cloacal exstrophy,[27] or a covered variant (16), and complex anorectal malformations with short colon (10), the patients' ability to form solid stool was assessed via bowel management involving a constipating diet, antidiarrheals, bulking agents, and a daily enema through the stoma.[59] Patients who underwent successful bowel management through the stoma were offered a pull-through. Of 20 available for follow-up after pull-through, 17 are clean with bowel management (85%), 2 (10%) have voluntary bowel movements with occasional soiling, and 1 is incontinent but noncompliant.[59]

Indication for pull-through depends on successful bowel management through the stoma, which depends on the ability to form solid stool. To maximize this potential, it is crucial to use all available hindgut for the initial colostomy and avoid use of colon for urologic or genital reconstruction. Most patients have poor prognosis for bowel control but can remain clean with bowel management.[59]

OTHER UNUSUAL FORMS OF CLOACA

These have been described in Fig. 77.1. Their management requires a high suspicion for accurate diagnosis.

The rare forms of cloaca like urogenital sinus with anteriorly placed rectum can be managed with PSARVUP with or without TUM. Vaginal reconstruction will be needed for cases with vaginal agenesis. If the Mullerian structures are present and are patent, the upper part of the neo vagina can be anastomosed to the Cervix. Cases of posterior cloaca need to be tackled with a different approach altogether. Fortunately these are extremely rare.[33,34] Pena has also operated upon a few cases with a transpubic approach.

SUMMARY

In conclusion, the surgical management of a persistent cloaca represents the most serious technical challenge in pelvic pediatric surgery. It should be performed in specialized pediatric surgical centers by a team of pediatric surgeons/urologists who are well trained in the management of cloacal anomalies. A careful lifelong follow-up of the patients into adulthood is necessary.

REFERENCES

1. Bodenhamer W. A Practical Treatise on the Aetiology, Pathology and Treatment of the Congenital Malformation of the Rectum and Anus. New York, NY: Wood 1860:225-77.
2. Gough MH. Anorectal agenesis with persistence of cloaca: Proc R Soc Med 1959;52:886-89.
3. Hendren WH. Cloaca, The most severe degree of imperforate anus. Experience with 195 cases. Annals of Surgery 1998;228:331-46.
4. Hendren WH. Cloacal malformations. In Walsh PC, Retik AB, Stamey TA, et al. (Eds) Campbell's urology 6th ed. Philadelphia, WB Saunders, 1992;1822-48.
5. Hendren WH, Donahoe P. Correction of congenital abnormalities of the vagina and perineum. J Pediatr Surg 1980;15:751-63.
6. Hendren WH. Further experience in reconstructive surgery for cloacal anomalies. J Pediatr Surg 1982;17:695-717.
7. Hendren WH. Repair of cloacal anomalies: current techniques. J Pediatr Surg 1986;21:1159-76.
8. Hendren WH. Urological aspects of cloacal malformations. J Urol 1988;140:1207-13.
9. Hendren WH. Cloacal malformations. Experience with 105 cases. J Pediatr Surg 1992;27:890-901.
10. Pena A, de Vries P. Posterior sagittal anorectoplasty. J Pediatr Surg 1982;17:796-881.
11. Pena A. Total Urogenital Mobilisation-An easier way to repair cloacas. J Pediatr Surg 1997;32:263-68.
12. Pena A. Atlas of surgical management of anorectal malformations. New York, Berlin Heidelberg, Springer 1990.

13. Pena A. Anorectal malformations. Semin Pediatr Surg 1995;4:35-47.
14. Pena A. The surgical management of persistent cloaca: Results in 54 patients treated with a posterior sagittal approach. J Pediatr Surg 1989;24:590-98.
15. Pena A, Hong A. Advances in the management of anorectal malformations. Am J Surg 2000;180:370-76.
16. Pena A. Imperforate anus and cloacal malformations. In: Ashcraft KW, Murphy JP, Sharp RJ, Sigalet DL, Snyder CHS (Eds): Pediatric Surgery Third edition, Philadelphia, London, New York, WB Saunders Company 2000.
17. Peña A, Levitt MA, Hong A, Midulla P. Surgical management of cloacal malformations: a review of 339 patients. J Pediatr Surg 2004 Mar;39(3):470-79.
18. Chen CP, Liu FF, Jan SW, Chang PY, Lin YN, Lan CC. Ultrasound-guided fluid aspiration and prenatal diagnosis of duplicated hydrometrocolpos with uterus didelphys and septate vagina. Prenat Diagn 1996;16:572-76.
19. Cilento BG, Benacerraf BR, Mandell J. Prenatal diagnosis of cloacal malformation. Urology 1994;43:386-88.
20. Jirasek JE. Morphogenesis of the genital system in the human. Birth Defects 1977;13:13-39.
21. Qi, Bao Quan Beasley Sp. W, Williams AK, Frizelle F. Apoptosis during regression of the tailgut and septation of the cloaca. J Pediatr Surg 2000;35:1556-61.
22. Nievenstein RA, van der Werff JF, Verbeek FJ, Valk J, Vermeij. Keers C: Normal and abnormal embryonic development of the anorectum in human embryos. Teratology (United States) 1998;57:70-78.
23. Kluth D, Lambrecht W. Curent concepts in the embryology of anorectal malformations. Semin Pediatr Surg 1997;6:180-86.
24. Kluth D, Hillen M, Lambrecht W. The principles of normal and abnormal hindgut development. J Pediatr Surg 1995;30:1143-47.
25. Arana J, Villanueva A, Guarch R, Aldazabal P, Barriola M. Anorectal atresia. An experimental model in the rat. Bur J Pediatr Surg 2001;11:192-95.
26. Liu MI, Hutson JM. Cloacal and urogenital malformations in adriamycin-exposed rat fetuses. Bill Int 2000;86:107-12.
27. Kubota Y, Shimotake T, Yanaghira J, Iwai N. Development of anorectal malformations using etretinate. J Pediatr Surg 1998;33:127-29.
28. Kimmel SO, Mo R, Hui CC, Kim PC. New mouse models of congenital anorectal malformations. J Pediatr Surg 2000;35:227-30.
29. Keppler-Noreuil KM: OBIS complex (omphalocele, extrophy, imperforate anus, spinal defects) a review of 14 cases. Am J Med Genet 2001;99:271-79.
30. Penington EC, Hutson JM. The cloacal plate: the missing link in anorectal and urogenital development. BJU Int. 2002;89(7):726-32.
31. Stephens FD, Smith ED. Anorectal malformations in children: Up date 1988. New York, Alan R. Liss inc. 1988.
32. Holschneider AM, Scharbatke H. Persistent cloaca – clinical aspects. In Anorectal Malformations in children Holschneider and Hutson (Ed). Springer 2006;10:201-09.
33. Chatterjee SK. Rare/regional Variants. In Anorectal Malformations in children Ed Holschneider and Hutson. Springer 2006;15:251-62.
34. Pena A, Kessler O. Posterior cloaca: A unique defect. J Pediatr. Surgery 1998;33:407-12.
35. Gupta DK, Sharma S. Congenital Pouch Colon. In Anorectal Malformations in children Ed Holschneider and Hutson. Springer 2006;11:211-22.
36. Gupta DK, Sharma S. Congenital Pouch Colon– Then and now. J Indian Assoc Pediatr Surg 2007;12:5-12.
37. Sharma S, Gupta DK, Bhatnagar V, et al. Management of Congenital Pouch Colon in Association with ARM. Journal of Indian Association of pediatric surgeons 2005;10: S22.
38. Pintér A, Farkas A, Vajda P, Juhász Z, Oberritter Z. Late reconstructive surgery for cloaca malformations Magy Seb. 2002 Dec;55(6):379-83.
39. Wheeler PG, Weaver DD. Partial urorectal septum malformation sequence: a report of 25 cases. Am J Med Genet 2001;103:99-105 Male cloacas
40. Ohno Y, Koyama N, Tsuda M, Arii Y. Antenatal ultrasonographic appearance of a cloacal anomaly Obstetrics and Gynecology 2000;95:1013-15.
41. Odibo AO, Turner GW, Borgida AF, Rodis JF, Campbell WA. Late prenatal ultrasound features of hydrometrocolpos secondary to cloacal anomaly: case reports and review of the literature. Ultrasound Obstet Gynecol 1997;9:419-21.
42. Zaccara A, Gatti C, Silveri M, et al. Persistent cloaca: Are we ready for correct prenatal diagnosis? Urology 1999;54:367.
43. Cianciosi F, Mancini P, Busacchi A, Carletti D, de Aloysio, and C Battaglia. Increased amniotic fluid volume associated with cloacal and renal anomalies. J Ultrasound Med 2006;25:1085-90.
44. Sahinoglu Z, Mulayim B, Ozden S, et al. The prenatal diagnosis of cloacal dysgenesis sequence in six cases: can the termination of pregnancy always be the first choice? Prenat Diagn 2004; 24:10–16.
45. Warne S, Chitty LS, Wicox DT. Prenatal diagnosis of cloacal anomalies. BJU Int 2002; 89:78-81.
46. Hayashi S, Sago H, Kashima K, et al. Prenatal diagnosis of fetal hydrometrocolpos secondary to a cloacal anomaly by magnetic resonance imaging. Ultrasound Obstet Gynecol 2005;26:577-79.
47. Wheeler PG, Weaver DD, Obeime MO, Vance GH, Bull M, Escobar LF. Urorectal septum malformation sequence: report of thirteen additional cases and review of the literature. Am J Med Genet 1997;73:456-62.
48. Qureshi F, Jacques SM, Yaron Y, Kramer RL, Evans MI, Johnson MP. Prenatal diagnosis of cloacal dysgenesis sequence: differential diagnosis from other forms of fetal obstructive uropathy. Fetal Diagn Ther 1998;13:69-74.

49. Bear JW, Gilsanz V. Calcified meconium and persistent cloaca. AJR Am J Roentgenol 1981;137:867-68.
50. Holschneider AM, Iesch NK, Stragholz E, Pfrommer W. Surgical methods for anorectal malformations from Rehbein to Pena -Critical assessment of score systems and proposal for a new classification. Europ J Pediatr Surg 2002;12:73-82.
51. Harrison MR, Glick PL, Nakayama DK, de Lorimier AA.: Loop colon rectovaginoplasty for high cloacal anomaly. J Pediatr Surg 1983;18:885-86.
52. Nixon HH. A modification of the proctoplasty for rectal agenesis. In: Stephens FD, Smith (Eds): Anorectal malformations in children: Update 1988 (Eds). 1988;18:380.
53. Peña A, Grasshoff S, Levitt M. Reoperations in anorectal malformations J Pediatr Surg 2007;42(2):318-25.
54. Warne SA, Godley ML, Wilcox DT. Surgical reconstruction of cloacal malformation can alter bladder function: a comparative study with anorectal anomalies. J Urol 2004;172(6 Pt 1):2377-81; discussion 2381.
55. Levitt MA, Stein DM, Pena A. Gynecologic concerns in the treatment of teenagers with cloaca. J Pediatr Surg 1998;33:188-93.
56. Warne SA, Wilcox DT, Ledermann SE, Ransley PG. Renal outcome in patients with cloaca. J Urol 2002;167:2548-51.
57. Wagner G, Holschneider AM, Gharib M. A complex high cloacal malformation: case report. Europ J Pediatr Surg 1998:8:182-85.
58. Lund DP, Hendren WH, Cloacal exstrophy: A 25-Year experience with 50 cases. J Pediatr Surg 2001;36:68-75.
59. Levitt MA, Mak GZ, Falcone RA Jr, Peña A. Cloacal exstrophy—pull-through or permanent stoma? A review of 53 patients. J Pediatr Surg 2008;43:164-8; discussion 168-70.

Anorectal Malformations: Current Perspectives

DK Gupta, Shilpa Sharma

Albeit, there has not been much development in the understanding of the embryological and clinical aspects of patients with anorectal malformations (ARM), yet, the surgical management of these children has seen a major paradigm shift with the development of posterior sagittal anorectoplasty (PSARP) as proposed by Alberto Pena in 1982.[1] Another recent development has been the review of the subject by the world experts and proposing the new classification in 2005 at Krickenbeck (Germany), with an attempt to include all types of anorectal malformations, both major and minor, and the rare anomalies and evaluating the postoperative outcome based on various operative techniques practiced world wide.[2,3]

Recent Advances in the Field of ARM Include[4]

1. Attempt on the antenatal detection- Introduction of Fetal MRI.
2. Utilizing the new Krickenbeck Classification for ARM — 2005.
3. Referral of cases with ARM to trained pediatric surgeons at tertiary care level.
4. Avoiding the colostomy at primary center in favor of single stage repair.
5. Investigations in relation to muscle complex and associated anomalies.
6. Appropriate diagnosis of ARM before performing colostomy.
7. Increasing recognition of associated tethered cord.
8. Early single stage definitive surgery – even in the newborn period.
9. Laparoscopic assisted pull through.
10. Robotic pull through, if the facility and the expertise is available.
11. Regular follow-up for assessment of continence.
12. Bowel management program to make the patient socially acceptable.

The aim of management of ARM is now shifted from saving life to ensuring a near normal quality of life.[4] Though antenatal detection has been attempted yet the features to detect this anomaly before birth are often missed on prenatal ultrasonography. Thus, the incidence of prenatal detection of babies with ARM is almost negligible at present.

Management is now based on the accurate scientific information about the muscle complex and the associated malformations. The investigations like echocardiogram, ultrasonography for various abdominal organs and the magnetic resonance imaging have helped to delineate the associated anomalies in detail.[5] A high pressure distal colostogram and a 3D spiral MRI have helped to delineate the anatomy of the defect, level of the lower end of the pouch, the presence and also the size of the fistulous communication thus offering the information for adopting the most appropriate surgical procedure for the correction of the defect in a particular baby.[6] The definitive surgery is now done at an earlier age with the increasing popularity of the single stage procedures not only in females but in males also, not only in infancy but in the newborn period also, not only for the full-term but for the premature babies as well.[4,7,8]

A regular follow-up for the assessment of continence is quite essential for successful management.[9] Finally, a dedicated bowel management program can provide the patients with a happy and acceptable quality of life, free from routine hassles due to incontinence.[10]

ETIOLOGY

Despite much generated interest to elucidate the exact etiology, it still remains poorly understood. These malformations however are believed to result from arrests or abnormalities in the embryological development of the anus, rectum and urogenital tract.

Genetic predisposition has been seen in only a few families. Sex linked and autosomal dominant inheritances have been suggested.

If anorectal malformation is the only abnormality in the family, an autosomal dominant mode of inheritance may be likely.[11] However, the presence of multiple associated malformations may indicate recessive inheritance and subsequent pregnancies should be regarded as high risk requiring full antenatal investigative workup.[11]

Trisomy 13 is associated with anorectal malformations.[12] It is also seen in association with trisomy 21,18 and Townes Brocks syndrome.[6] Currarino syndrome is associated with mutations of the homeobox gene HLXB9.[13] Apparently there is no racial predilection. Pena has noticed a positive family history in cases of rectoperineal fistula.[6]

The etiology of ARM may be multifactorial. The anomaly has usually been found in families from developing countries with lower socioeconomic status, thus suggesting possibly the role of nutritional and environmental factors like liberal use of pesticides in the fields, leading to the embryological defects.[4]

A significantly higher incidence has recently been reported from Italy, in children born after assisted reproductive techniques (odds ratio 13.31, 95% confidence limits 4.0-39.6).[13] This is in agreement with the result of a recent epidemiological study in Sweden. Though, further studies are necessary to define the risks involved and identify the causes, the couples undergoing assisted reproductive techniques, should be informed of the general risks of the congenital anomalies, especially ARM.[14]

An increased incidence of ARM has also been seen in fetuses whose mothers have had diabetes or thalidomide toxicity.[15]

INCIDENCE

The global incidence of ARM anomaly is taken as 1:5000 live births, However, few geographical areas have reported a higher incidence of this anomaly, e.g. 1:1832 from Calcutta.[16] A recent study on the incidence of anorectal malformations in the province of Alberta, Canada has reported the incidence as high as 1: 2162 with a marked rise in male predominance (1.7:1).[15]

ANTENATAL DETECTION

There have been recent attempts to diagnose anorectal malformations antenatally with the development of sophisticated equipment.[17-22] The initial reports held that anorectal atresia can be diagnosed only from 22 week gestation onwards.[17] However, recent reports have picked up the anomaly as early as 12 weeks of gestation by transvaginal ultrasonography as a cystic echogenic structure, with a distal tapered appearance low down within the abdomen and pelvis.[18] Also, a dilated colon may be picked up on ultrasound examination in a fetus at 12 weeks of gestation. Dilatation of the colon has been reported to be clearly seen in the first and the third trimester of pregnancy, but it is difficult to detect it in the second trimester.[20]

Meconium, as a semisolid mixture of enteric secretions and sloughed cells, usually appears in the fetal colon from approximately 15 week onwards as a normal physiologic process. Apart from the small size of fetal structures early in pregnancy, the difficulty of diagnosis results from the changing physiologic characteristics of the fetal gastrointestinal tract.[14] The presence of isoechoic meconium within the dilated bowel may cause the loss of the cystic appearance. Decompression of the fluid-filled bowel into the urinary tract, via the fistula, may cause disappearance of the dilated bowel.

Fetal meconium is usually hypoechoic or isoechoic to adjacent abdominal structures on antenatal sonography. Hyperechoic meconium is associated with pathologic conditions, such as meconium ileus, meconium peritonitis, and anorectal malformations, though hyperechoic meconium has been reported as a normal variant, particularly in the third trimester.[21] The sonographic detection of a meconium concretion in the fetal bladder strongly suggests the presence of an enterovesical fistula.[22]

Enterolithiasis with anorectal malformation has been described in which the intra-luminal calcification was identified using an ultrasound. Ultrasonography can thus differentiate between enterolithiasis and meconium peritonitis and the prenatal diagnosis of rectourinary communication may be made when enterolithiasis is present.[23]

In one of the series, fetal MRI has been found useful to pick up four cases of anorectal malformations including one with cloacal malformation.[24] A prenatal diagnosis of fatal VACTERL association, may allow the medical termination of pregnancy.[25]

WINGSPREAD, USA (1984)

The ARM conference organized by D Stephens and Durham Smith from May 25-27, 1984 in Wingspread, Winconsin, USA, formed a platform for the international authorities on the subject to share their experiences and suggest a universal classification.[3] The emphasis then was laid on the relation of the rectal pouch to the levator muscle complex which was like a hammock. This allowed the classification of the anorectal anomalies into high, intermediate and low, depending upon if the terminal rectal pouch had crossed the levator sling or not (Fig. 78.1). Also, the surgical procedures were aimed at passing the rectal pouch through the puborectalis muscle sling, so as to reach the proposed anal site, using a perineal or a sacroperineal approach, with or without combining the same with the additional abdominal route.

PSARP ERA: NEED FOR A NEW CLASSIFICATION

Things changed substantially with the popularity of Posterior Sagittal Anorectoplasty (PSARP) approach

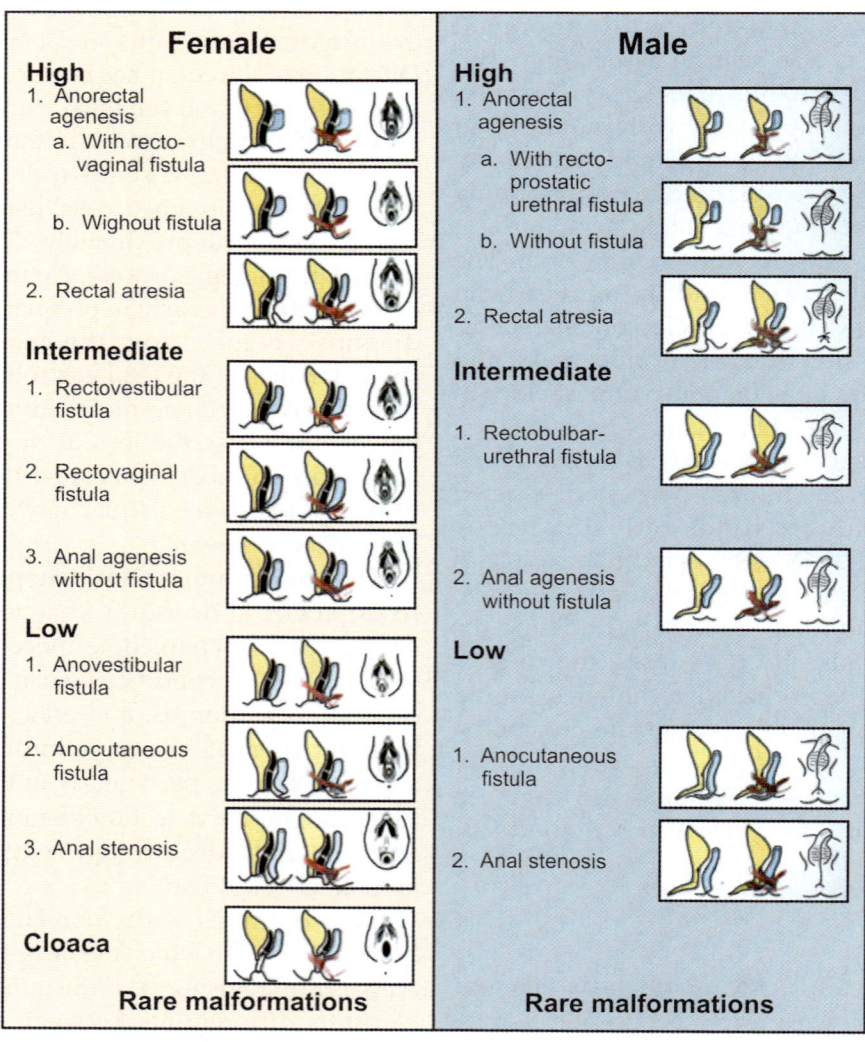

Fig. 78.1: Classification of anorectal malformations 1984 (Wingspread Classification)

described by Alberto Pena in early 1980s, for the surgical correction of all types of the anomalies (high, intermediate and low). This approach is now practiced worldwide for its simplicity and accuracy in defining the structures by remaining strictly in the midline posteriorly.

A number of rare anomalies, not previously recognized but included in the Wingspread classification, were also reported, e.g. perineal groove, H-type of anorectal anomalies, rectal ectasia, rectal atresia and most importantly the pouch colon, mostly reported from the Indian subcontinent.

Additional associated anomalies were also reported, like the tethered cord (25% of all ARM anomalies). Consequently, there was lot of confusion regarding the nomenclature and the uniformity in the clinical diagnosis and the investigative and surgical approach for these malformations. The postoperative results were also difficult to be assessed and compared in the presence of many operative techniques being followed, despite the fact that a number of complicated scoring systems were described in the literature. A need was thus felt for new international classification and development of international standards for assessing the postoperative outcome.

KRICKENBECK CLASSIFICATION (GERMANY, 2005)

The Krickenbeck classification was formed during the expert group conference held in Krickenbeck, Germany from 17-20 May, 2005 (Fig. 78.2).[2]

The goals of the Krickenbeck Conference on ARM was to develop standards for an International Classification of ARM based on a modification of the type of fistula and adding the rare and regional variants, and design a system for the comparable follow up studies incorporating all known major surgical techniques being practiced world wide.[2]

Table 78.1 outlines the Krickenbeck classification.[2] The lesions were classified into major clinical groups based on the fistula location (perineal, rectourethral, rectovesical, or the vestibular), cloacal lesions, those with anal stenosis and no fistula. Rare and regional variants of ARM included pouch colon, rectal atresia or stenosis, rectovaginal fistula, H-fistula and others.[3]

The Krickenbeck classification also enabled various operative procedures used for the treatment of various types of malformations, to be more comparable to each

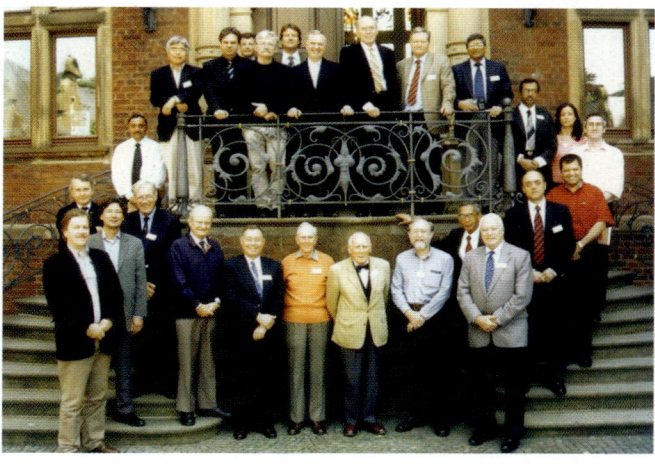

Fig. 78.2: Krickenbeck, a scenic and beautiful place was a perfect venue for holding a serious meeting like this. The conference hotel Krickenbeck castle is close to Düsseldorf, but miles away from all the hustle and bustle of the city. It is situated in a nature reserve, tucked away amongst the 7 Krickenbeck lakes and surrounded by ancient oaks and beeches. The castle dating back to the 13th century, is located 75 miles away from Cologne, amidst lakes, library and forests. It was a home away from all active business centers, major cities, airports, train stations and any habitation. An 1100 hectare property belonging to the West LB with 693 Billion DM as assets in early 1998, was very popular amongst the academicians and researchers

Table 78.1: Standards for diagnosis international classification (Krickenbeck)

Major clinical groups	Rare/regional variants
Perineal (cutaneous) fistula	Pouch colon
Rectourethral fistula	Rectal atresia/stenosis
– Prostatic	Rectovaginal fistula
– Bulbar	H-fistula
Rectovesical fistula	Others
Vestibular fistula	
Cloaca	
No fistula	
Anal stenosis	

other than with the Wingspread classification.[2] Also it was decided that for the follow-up studies, not only the site of the fistula should be documented but also an additional grouping according to the operative procedure should be done, e.g. perineal operation, anterior sagittal approach, sacroperineal procedure, posterior sagittal anorectal plasty (PSARP), abdominosacroperineal pull-through, abdominoperineal pull-through and laparoscopically assisted pull-through (Table 78.2).

Table 78.2: International grouping (Krickenbeck) of surgical procedures for follow up

Operative procedures
1. Perineal operation
2. Anterior sagittal approach
3. Sacroperineal procedure
4. Posterior sagittal anorectal plasty (PSARP)
5. Abdominosacroperineal pull-through
6. Abdominoperineal pull-through
7. Laparoscopically assisted pull-through

Associated conditions
1. Sacral anomalies
2. Tethered cord

Table 78.3: Method for assessment of outcome established in Krickenbeck 2005 (patient age > 3 years, no therapy)

1. Voluntary bowel movements — Yes/No
   (Feeling of urge, capacity to verbalize, hold the bowel movement)
2. Soiling — Yes/No
   - Grade 1 Occasionally (once or twice per week)
   - Grade 2 Every day, no social problem
   - Grade 3 Constant, social problem
3. Constipation — Yes/No
   - Grade 1 Manageable by changes in diet
   - Grade 2 Requires laxatives
   - Grade 3 Resistant to laxatives and diet

It was emphasized that the groups should be analyzed on the basis of the associated conditions such as sacral anomalies and tethered cord. A standard method for postoperative assessment of continence was also determined as outlined in Table 78.3.

The new International diagnostic classification system, operative groupings and a method of postoperative assessment of continence was developed by consensus of a large group of experts representing all the continents and involved in the management of patients with ARM. This allowed for a common standardization of diagnosis, management and comparing the postoperative results.

The need for the change in classification was felt, as the earlier classifications did not pertain to the management options adopted. Also, the rare anomalies seen in some parts of the world especially pouch colon from South East Asia were included.[2,3]

CONGENITAL POUCH COLON (CPC)

Congenital pouch colon is a condition associated with anorectal malformation defined as an anomaly in which all or part of the colon is replaced by a pouch-like dilatation, which communicates distally with the urogenital tract via a large fistula.[26-29] The mesentery of the colonic pouch of variable size (5-15 cm in diameter) is short and poorly developed, the wall is very thick, the *Taenia coli* are absent or ill defined, and haustration and the appendices epiploicae are absent. The main pouch is supplied by the branches arising from the superior mesenteric artery, which form a leash of vessels around it. This condition is more common in the northern India, although sporadic cases have also been reported from other parts of India, Nepal, Pakistan, Bangladesh as well as from the rest of the world.[30,31]

Due to the paradigm shift seen with this anomaly in the recent past in its clinical presentation, the authors had proposed a simple and practical new classification.[26]

1. *Incomplete CPC:* Where the length of the normal colon is adequate for performing the pull-through, without the need for doing a coloplasty. The procedure would involve excision of the pouch with an end colostomy at birth and a definitive pull-through later. A single-stage pull-through in the newborn stage can also be undertaken in experienced hands, if the condition of the baby also permits.
2. *Complete CPC:* Where there is either no or insufficient length of the normal colon left to permit a pull-through procedure. In this situation, a coloplasty procedure would be required to retain only about 15 cm length of CPC in the form of a tube, to be brought out as an end colostomy. A pull-through procedure should be attempted later and not at the time of performing coloplasty in the newborn stage, otherwise it may result in high morbidity and even mortality.

In this anomaly, all babies present with an absent anal opening. The distal communication of the pouch is in most instances with the genitourinary system. Most patients would present within the first 2-3 days of life.

The male baby presents early with anorectal agenesis and gross abdominal distension. As the fistulous communication is usually large and with the urinary baldder, the passage of gas or frank meconium per urethra is a good indicator pointing the presence of pouch colon. The association of bilious vomiting with gross abdominal distension in a case of ARM, is also strongly suggestive of CPC in endemic areas.

The female baby presents with perineal fistula in the vestibule or a common cloacal malformation. In patients with CPC and colonic perforation, the baby may present with septicemia, gross abdominal distension (pneumoperitoneum) with prominent veins, fluid and electrolyte imbalance and peritonitis.

The aim of surgery is to utilize the available length of colon for the absorptive function and storage capacity as well as for propelling the fecal matter onward with a continent anal opening. However, as the pouch musculature is abnormal, the authors prefer to excise the pouch if it is found feasible, as in cases with incomplete CPC where there is an adequate length of normal colon present.[26] However, in babies with the complete CPC, an attempt is always made to do coloplasty and retain a limited length of colon (15 cm or less) and preserve its functions as much as possible. It is important that the length of the coloplasty segment should not be more than 15 cm, lest, it starts dilating and causes re-pouching, fecoloma formation and constipation in the postoperative period.

RECTAL ATRESIA

This entity has also been included under rare variants in the Krickenbeck classification.[2] Rectal atresia is characterized by the presence of the proximal rectum, which ends at or above the pubococcygeal (PC) line, and a well-formed distal anus that is in its normal location and has a normal appearance, which is about 1-3 cm in depth. The two pouches may be connected to each other by a fibrous strand surrounded by the puborectalis sling. The anal canal and lower rectum are well surrounded by the sphincter complexes and hence the outcome after surgery is generally good.[32]

Classification of Rectal Atresia (Fig. 78.3)[32]

Type I: Rectal stenosis (rare)
Type II: Rectal atresia with a septal defect
Type III: Rectal atresia with a fibrous cord between the two atretic ends (common)
Type IV: Rectal atresia with a gap
Type V: Multiple rectal atresia with stenosis (A), and multiple atresia (B)

INVESTIGATIONS FOR ARM

There has been an improvement in the sophistication of the investigative modalities. The associated anomalies can be scanned in a reasonably short time by a careful clinical examination, abdominal ultrasonography including echocardiography, an invertogram and babygram including the chest, abdomen and spine. The cross table prone lateral invertogram is an alternative technique that can be utilized to replace the invertogram for the same purpose.

The level of the terminal bowel can also be determined by ultrasonography.[33] In a recent series, the authors have used infracoccygeal transperineal USG using a 7-10-MHz linear-array transducer to determine the type of imperforate anus correctly in all cases.[33]

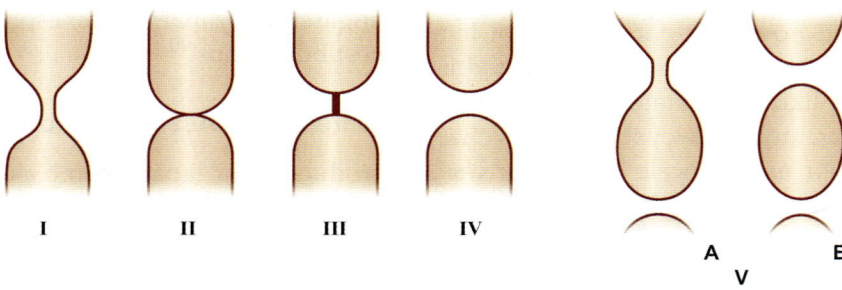

Fig. 78.3: Classification of rectal atresia (Reproduced with kind permission from Springer science and Business Media)[32]

A pouch to perineal distance of less than 1 cm is suggestive of a low anomaly. The relationship of the terminal bowel to the sacrum, the urogenital organs and the surface can thus be visualized. Sensitivity of invertography performed in 22 patients was only 27% with a mean error of measurement of 0.84 cm, and the difference between measurements and real distance was statistically significant.[34] While the sensitivity of perineal USG (22 children) was 86 % (mean error 0.12 cm) and with no significant difference between measurements and the intraoperative findings (p > 0.001). This study reported that perineal US was extremely useful in the newborn period and provided reliable information on which the decision can be based for either preliminary colostomy or a definitive operation.[34]

The high distal colostogram is very useful tool to delineate the anatomy prior to definitive surgery.[6] It has recently been recognized that there is a close relationship between spinal cord tethering (SCT) and congenital anorectal malformation (ARM).[6,35,36] Pena has advocated the use of spinal ultrasound in babies less than 3 months age to detect a tethered cord. The incidence may be as high as 25% in children with ARM. Spiral computed tomography with three-dimensional reconstruction of the pelvic musculature, or magnetic resonance imaging of the pelvis are optional for studying the pelvic musculature.[6]

Whether any surgical treatment in the form of prophylactic detethering is needed, remained a controversial issue. Some authors recommend routine MRI of patients with ARM and early untethering surgery in children with the spinal cord tethering.[36] However, most surgeons including the authors are of the opinion that such children should be kept under observation and treated surgically only if the symptoms appear due to tethered cord, e.g. Weakness of legs, recurrent urinary tract infection, loss of control over the bladder and bowel, in-cordination of leg movements. Surgery would however, be indicated if associated anomalies like diastematomyelia with or without a bony spur, dermoid cyst, diplomyelia, syringomyelia, anterior meningocele co-exist or else if the parents insist for the surgery. The surgery should be performed by the specialists in the field and the risks, if any should be explained to the parents beforehand.

MANAGEMENT OF ARM

The surgical approach using PSARP allowed surgeons to view the anatomy of these defects clearly, repair them under direct vision, and learn about the complex anatomic arrangement of the junction of rectum and genitourinary tract.[37]

The main concerns in correcting these anomalies for the surgeon today remain the bowel control, urinary control and the sexual function.[37] Adherence to specific principles in technique can prevent a large number of the postoperative complications.[38]

Repair in the Neonatal Age

Moore has recommended operative repair within the first 7 days without a prior colostomy because the anocortical neurocircuitry pathways develop in the perinatal period or within first few days after birth.[8] If act of defaecation is not initiated soon after birth by doing a primary repair, the advantage is lost.[7]

There is now a declining trend for performing a colostomy in cases with ARM.[39] It is being avoided wherever feasible to reduce the number of surgical procedures and also the nuisance to the patient and the parents. However, the risks involved must be weighed with the benefits expected.[4] The neonatal single stage posterior sagital anorectoplasty (PSARP) is a significant change in the management of anorectal malformations in the recent past. This can be done safely both in males and females with or without a fistula.[39] It is possible to perform a pull through operation even in the premature babies in the neonatal age, but should be done only by the experienced surgeons and under good anesthesia cover in the neonatal ICU setup.[39] It is expected that these babies are likely to have better continence due to development of efficient nerve pathways from birth itself. Many surgeons today are routinely performing a single stage primary repair especially in females with a vestibular anus.[40]

Laparoscopic Assisted Anorectal Pull-through

Introduction of laparoscopic assisted anorectal pull through (LAARP) for high imperforate anus by Georgeson et al in 2000 has opened a new alternative for repair of high imperforate anus, with the possible advantage that the rectum can be placed in the center of sphincters without any midline surgical division. In LAARP performed in 11 patients of high ARM, seven patients (1 girl and 6 boys) underwent divided sigmoid colostomy at birth and 4 boys underwent primary LAARP without colostomy.[41]

Laparoscopic Technique

With a sharp and diathermy dissection, the rectal pouch is exposed laparoscopically, down to the urethral or vaginal fistula. The fistula is then clipped at two places and divided in between. The pelvic floor musculature is then assessed and the levator sling identified. Externally, an electrostimulation is used to define the center of the anal dimple. An 8 mm skin incision is made, centered at the strongest cephalad contraction. Using a minimal blunt dissection on the perineum, a hemostat is guided by transillumination from the laparoscopic light source. A trocar, consisting of a radially expandable sheath over a Varess needle, is passed through this defined plane in the external sphincter muscle complex and advanced into the pelvis between the 2 bellies of the pubococcygeus muscle guided by the laparoscopic visualization. This perineal trocar therefore formed a passage through the center of the striated muscle complex and the levators. The rectal pouch, which had been dissected out laparoscopically, is now grasped using the perineal trocar and exteriorized to the perineum. Anorectal anastomosis is performed with absorbable interrupted suture. In this series, all the patients had a brisk and symmetrical anal contraction with perineal electrostimulation.

Yamataka et al used the laparoscopic muscle stimulator to identify the center of contraction of the levator ani muscle from above and the center of contraction of the external sphincter muscle was identified transcutaneously from below.[42] An intravenous canula was then passed from center of contraction of external sphincter muscle to the center of contraction of levator ani muscle under laparoscopic vision and laparoscopic muscle stimulator in place. Subsequently, a guide wire was passed through intravenous canula and a series of dilators were passed to create a tunnel exactly in the center of sphincter muscle through which laparoscopically mobilized rectum was pulled down for completing the anorectoplasty.

Yamataka et al also reported the use of endosonographic probe to enhance the accuracy of positioning of rectum in the muscle complex during the laparoscopic pull through.[43] Endosonographic probe was inserted into the proposed route of dissection in the muscle complex, and utilized to measure the thickness of surrounding muscle. With this, it is possible to make an immediate assessment of the symmetrical distribution of muscle complex just before the completion of the actual pull-through.

Thus, laparoscopic pull-through offers the advantages of minimal invasion, dissection of fistula, under vision deep in the pelvis, with laparoscopic magnification, placement of rectum in the center of the muscle complex without actually dividing the muscle complex. However, follow-up studies regarding the quality of continence achieved following this technique are awaited.

Kubota et al, reported the initial experience with the use of a combination of laparoscopic dissection, pinpointing the center of anal sphincter by electrostimulation and identification of the urethra by using ultrasonographic images from the perineum, to facilitate the creation of an appropriate pull through canal in the muscle complex.[44] However, only a limited expertise is available with this technique at present.

CONTINENCE

Using the PSARP approach, the reported results of continence have improved markedly worldwide, as has been outlined in Table 78.3. The fecal and urinary incontinence can occur even with an excellent anatomic repair, due mainly to associated problems such as a poorly developed muscle complex, deficient sacrum (specially if more than 3 pieces are missing), deficient nerve supply, and spinal cord anomalies. For these patients, an effective bowel management program, including enema and dietary restrictions has been devised to improve the quality of life.[37] The bowel management program has been discussed in a separate chapter.

Artificial bowel sphincter is not popular in children and has however, been used successfully in 2 patients with anorectal malformation with fecal incontinence.[45]

RESEARCH IN ANORECTAL MALFORMATIONS

An experimental model for anorectal anomalies has been induced by ethylene thiourea (ETU),[46] in fetuses from rats that received ETU on the 11th day of gestation at the dose of 125 mg/kg, diluted in distilled water to 1% concentration (12.5 ml/kg). On the 21st day of gestation, when the animals were sacrificed by causing hypoxia in a carbon dioxide chamber. The laparotomy was done to remove the fetuses and assess them for anomalies like the vertebral column malformation and urological structural alterations. In the experimental group, 71% presented with anorectal anomaly, 80% presented vertebral column alterations and 35% presented with urological alterations.[46]

REFERENCES

1. Peña A, De Vries P. Posterior sagittal anorectoplasty: Important technical considerations and new applications. J Pediatr Surg 1982;17:796-811.
2. Holschneider A, Hutson J, Pena A, Beket E, Chatterjee S, Coran A, Davies M, Georgeson K, Grosfeld J, Gupta D, Iwai N, Kluth D, Martucciello G, Moore S, Rintala R, Smith ED, Sripathi DV, Stephens D, Sen S, Ure B, Grasshoff S, Boemers T, Murphy F, Soylet Y, Dubbers M, Kunst M. Preliminary report on the International Conference for the Development of Standards for the Treatment of Anorectal Malformations. J Pediatr Surg 2005;40:1521-26.
3. Gupta Devendra K. Anorectal malformations- Wingspread to Krickenbeck. JIAPS 2005;10:75-77.
4. Gupta DK, Sharma S. Current trends in Anorectal Malformations In "Current trends in Pediatrics" Mathur GP, Mathur S (Ed). Nepal publ. Academa. Chap 2006;(3)16:161-73.
5. Gupta DK Anorectal Malformation – A pictorial depiction. In Textbook of Neonatal Surgery. Ed. Gupta DK (1st ed.) Modern Publishers. New Delhi 2000;37:233-39.
6. Pena A. Lecture delivered in 43rd workshop on Pediatric Anorectal and Colorectal Surgical problems, Cincinnati, 2007;6-8.
7. Gopal Chooramani S. Single stage PSARP in Neonates. In Textbook of Neonatal Surgery. Ed. Gupta DK 1st Ed. Modern Publishers. New Delhi 2000;39:249-53.
8. Moore TC. Advantages of performing the sagittal anoplasty operation for imperforate anus at birth. J Pediatr Surg 1990;25:276-77.
9. Sharma S, Gupta DK. Long-term Outcome of Anorectal malformations using the Krickenbeck Criteria. Journal of Indian Association of pediatric surgeons 2006;11:161.
10. Pena A, Guardino K, Tovilla JM, et al. Bowel management for fecal incontinence in patients with anorectal malformations. J Pediatr Surg 1998;33:133-37.
11. Boocock GR, Donnai D. Anorectal malformation: familial aspects and associated anomalies. Arch Dis Child 1987;62(6):576-79.
12. Lewis NA, Lander AD. Trisomy 13 is associated with anorectal malformations Arch Dis Child. 2007 Feb;92(2):185. Erratum in: Arch Dis Child. 2007 Apr;92(4):375.
13. Riebel T, Köchling J, Scheer I, Oellinger J, Reis A. Currarino syndrome: variability of imaging findings in 22 molecular-genetically identified (HLXB9 mutation) patients from five families. Rofo. 2004 Apr;176(4):564-69.
14. Midrio P, Nogare CD, Di Gianantonio E, Clementi M. Are congenital anorectal malformations more frequent in newborns conceived with assisted reproductive techniques? Reprod Toxicol. 2006 Nov;22(4):576-77. Epub 2006 May 16.
15. Lowry RB, Sibbald B, Bedard T. Stability of prevalence rates of anorectal malformations in the alberta congenital Anomalies surveillance system 1990-2004 J Pediatr Surg 2007;42(8):1417-21.
16. Chatterjee SK. Anorectal Malformations, Oxford University Press, Oxford 1993.
17. Harris RD, Nyberg DA, Mack LA, Weinberger E. Anorectal atresia: prenatal sonographic diagnosis. Am J Radiol 1987;149:395-400.
18. Lam YH, Shek T, Tang MHY. Sonographic features of anal atresia at 12 weeks. Ultrasound Obstet Gynecol 2002;19:523-24.
19. Gilbert C E, Hamill J, Metcalfe R F, Smith P, Teele RL. Changing Antenatal Sonographic Appearance of Anorectal Atresia From First to Third Trimesters. J Ultrasound Med 2006;25:781-84.
20. Taipale P, Rovamo L, Hiilesmaa V. First-trimester diagnosis of imperforate anus. Ultrasound Obstet Gynecol 2005;25(2):187-88.
21. Hill LM, Rivello D, Martin JG. Intraluminal bladder calcifications: an antenatal sign of an enterovesical fistula. Obstet Gynecol 1990 Sep;76(3 Pt 2):500-02.
22. Paulson EK, Hertzberg BS. Hyperechoic meconium in the third trimester fetus: an uncommon normal variant. J Ultrasound Med. 1991;10(12):677-80.
23. Anderson S, Savader B, Barnes J, Savader S. Enterolithiasis with imperforate anus. Report of two cases with sonographic demonstration and occurrence in a female. Pediatr Radiol 1988;18(2):130-33.
24. Veyrac C, Couture A, Saguintaah M, Baud C. MRI of fetal GI tract abnormalities Abdom Imaging. 2004;29(4):411-20. Epub 2004 May 12.
25. Tongsong T, Chanprapaph P, Khunamornpong S. Prenatal diagnosis of VACTERL association: A case report. J Med Assoc Thai. 2001;84(1):143-48.
26. Gupta D K, Sharma Shilpa. Congenital Pouch Colon. In Anorectal Malformations in children Ed Holschneider and Hutson Springer 2006;11:211-22.
27. Gupta DK. Congenital pouch colon: Present lacunae. Journal of Indian Association of pediatric surgeons 2007;12:1-22.
28. Gupta DK, Sharma S. Congenital Pouch Colon – Then and now. J Indian Assoc Pediatr Surg 2007;12:5-12.
29. Sharma S, Gupta DK, Bhatnagar V, et al. Management of Congenital Pouch Colon in Association with ARM. Journal of Indian Association of pediatric surgeons 2005;10:S22.

30. Bhat NA. Congenital pouch colon syndrome: a report of 17 cases Ann Saudi Med 2007 Mar-Apr;27(2):79-83.
31. Demirogullari B, Ozen IO, Afsarlar C, et al. Congenital pouch colon associated with anorectal malformation: report of 2 cases. J Pediatr Surg 2007 Oct;42(10):E13-6.
32. Gupta DK, Sharma Shilpa. Rectal Atresia and Rectal Ectasia. In Anorectal Malformations in children (Ed). Holschneider and Hutson Springer 2006 Chap 12;223-30.
33. Han TI, Kim IO, Kim WS. Imperforate anus: US determination of the type with infracoccygeal approach. Radiology. 2003;228(1):226-29.
34. Niedzielski JK. Invertography versus ultrasonography and distal colostography for the determination of bowel-skin distance in children with anorectal malformations. Eur J Pediatr Surg. 2005 ;15(4):262-67.
35. Robinson AJ, Russell S, Rimmer S. The value of ultrasonic examination of the lumbar spine in infants with specific reference to cutaneous markers of occult spinal dysraphism. Clin Radiol. 2005 Jan;60(1):72-77. Comment in: Clin Radiol. 2005;60(8):935.
36. Uchida K, Inoue M, Matsubara T, et al. Evaluation and treatment for spinal cord tethering in patients with anorectal malformations. Eur J Pediatr Surg 2007;17(6):408-11.
37. Levitt MA, Peña A. Anorectal malformations. Orphanet J Rare Dis. 2007;26;2:33.
38. Peña A, Grasshoff S, Levitt M. Reoperations in anorectal malformations. J Pediatr Surg 2007;42(2):318-25.
39. Gupta DK, Sharma Shilpa. Changing trends in neonatal surgery. In Surgery of the Newborn – diagnosis and management Gupta DK (Ed), Jaypee Brothers, Delhi. 2008 (In press).
40. Gangopadhyay AN, Gopal SC, Sharma S, Gupta DK, Sharma SP, Mohan TV. Management of anorectal malformations in Varanasi, India: a long-term review of single and three stage procedures. Pediatr Surg Int. 2006;22(2):169-72. Epub 2005 Nov 29.
41. Georgeson KE, Inge TH, Albanese CT. Laparoscopically assisted anorectal pull-through for high imperforate anus – A new technique. J Pediatr Surg 2000;35:927-31.
42. Yamataka A, Segawa O, Yoshida R, et al. Laparoscopic muscle electrostimulation during laparoscopy-assisted anorectal pull-through for high imperforate anus. J Pediatr Surg 2001; 36(11): 1659-61.
43. Yamataka A, Yoshida R, Kobayashi H, et al. Intraoperative endosonography enhances laparoscopy-assisted colon pull-through for high imperforate anus. J Pediatr Surg 2002;37(12):1657-60.
44. Kubota A, Kawahara H, Okuyama H, Oue T, Tazuke Y, Tanaka N, Okada A. Laparoscopically assisted anorectoplasty using perineal ultrasonographic guide: a preliminary report. J Pediatr Surg 2005;40:1535-38.
45. Hoch J, Skába R, Jech Z. Artificial sphincter in patients with congenital anorectal malformations Rozhl Chir 2007;86(4):170-73.
46. Macedo M, Martins JL, Meyer KF. Evaluation of an experimental model for anorectal anomalies induced by ethylenethiourea. Acta Cir Bras 2007;22(2):130-36.

Rectal Ectasia

Shilpa Sharma, DK Gupta

Rectal Ectasia is defined as a state of massive focal dilation of the rectum and sigmoid colon due to primary muscle defect or a secondary response to obstructive anorectal condition.[1,2] Rectal ectasia may thus be occasionally encountered either as a separate entity or associated with anorectal anomalies.[3] Ectasia should thus be suspected not only in all patients with chronic constipation but also in association with anorectal malformation.

Various terminologies that have been used in the past to describe this entity include; balloon like rectum, colonic inertia, megarectum, terminal fecal reservoir syndrome, congenital funnel anus, pseudo-Hirschsprung's disease and rectal inertia.[4-6]

CLASSIFICATION

Rectal Ectasia can be broadly classified into two types based on the etiology:[1]

A. *Primary rectal ectasia:* This is congenital in origin with no known cause for the ectasia. It may occasionally be due to midanal sphincter defect or the deficiency of the rectal musculature. However, 2-5% cases of anorectal malformations may present with congenital rectal ectasia.

B. *Secondary rectal ectasia:* This develops after birth, usually as a result of distal obstruction, secondary to fecal impaction or surgery at the anorectum. Postoperative anal stricture after an otherwise good surgical repair of anorectal malformation may also result in rectal ectasia. The dilatation of the ectatic rectum will depend on the degree and duration of the obstruction. The presence of fecoloma in the rectum initiates a vicious cycle and worsen the dilatation further.

EMBRYOLOGY AND PATHOPHYSIOLOGY

Various theories have been proposed to explain the development of primary rectal ectasia.

1. The cloaca that is divided by the urorectal septum into urinary and rectal passages may be initially more voluminous than normal before partition in cases of anorectal malformation with consequent oversized passage or passages after partition.[2]
2. The rectum is normally modelled into two ampullae, one in midrectum that becomes the mature rectum and one in the region of the future anal canal. Primary rectal ectasia occurring in association with anorectal anomalies may be an example of developmental overgrowth of the upper or lower primitive ampullae or both.[2]
3. The temporary tail gut, an extension of the undivided cloaca is initially quite voluminous, but becomes atrophic and disappears before partition of the cloaca is complete. Incorporation and persistence of part of the tail gut into the rectum may result in anorectal ectasia.[2]
4. It may be a variant of segmental dilatation of the intestine that is a well-known cause of obstruction.[2]
5. Primary hypomotility of distal rectum has been proposed.[7]
6. Weakness of the posterior rectal wall or defect in the external anal sphincter. The authors have found a primary deficiency of the musculature of the posterior rectal wall and the external anal sphincter, resulting in rectal inertia followed by rectal ectasia. This explains the clinically and radiologically evident posterior rectal shelf in few cases of primary rectal ectasia. A mid-sphincteric defect as the possible cause of constipation in anterior perineal anus has also been suggested.[8]

The primary pathology in the causation of primary rectal ectasia is deficiency in the smooth muscle wall causing weakening and dilatation of rectal wall.[3] Secondary rectal ectasia develops as a result of outflow obstruction. Elasticity of the rectal wall permits the normal rectum to expand to approximately double the caliber but it returns to its normal size. In the newborns, ectasia beyond this diameter is predictive of a primary developmental ectasia.[1] If the rectal ampulla is developmentally ectatic, the dilation may persist and lead postoperatively to fecal accumulations, further enlargement, troublesome constipation, and soiling. Hypertrophy and dilation may occur as a result of propulsive activity against an obstruction or upon a retained meconium bolus in the terminus of the bowel after a defunctioning colostomy.[9] On histological background primary and secondary rectal ectasia can be differentiated by examining rectal specimens–hypertrophy and hyperplasia of smooth muscle cells in acquired cases, normal or smaller size in newborns indicating primary or developmental anomaly.[1] Dysplastic nitrergic neurons in the rectum of a patient with rectal ectasia have also been demonstrated.[10]

The ectatic bowel has been reported to show a proliferation of nerve fibers in keeping with the degree of circular smooth muscle hypertrophy, thus representing a reactive phenomenon secondary to the functional obstruction.[10] Rectal ectasia may also present in adults as a result of a neuropathic process as an underlying mechanism.[11]

CLINICAL PRESENTATION

Rectal ectasia usually presents with refractory constipation either primarily or persistent constipation after a reconstructive surgery for a known cause of obstruction usually anorectal malformation. The patients usually present after 6 months of age, the most common period being around 1-3 years.[1] However, secondary rectal ectasia may present in adults also Rectal ectasia may or may not be associated with megasigmoid colon.[11,12]

Paradoxical diarrhea may occur due to peristalsis pushing the feces against the puborectalis sling and levator diaphragm. These muscles fatigue, relax, and temporarily lose the important sphincter functions that control the entrance to the rectoanal canal. Soft feces are then propelled by peristalsis over the fecal masses to escape constantly from the anus called "hold back-dyschesia cycle or pseudo-incontinence" inspite of good surgery.[7,9]

Paradoxical diarrhea and incontinence resulting from anatomically defective sphincters must be differentiated by rectal examination. Digital palpation of strongly contracting sphincters of the anal canal or satisfactory pressure profiles in the anal canal indicates that the leakage is more likely to be paradoxical. The proximal ectatic bowel remains large and dilated even after a defunctioning colostomy.

Adults diagnosed as rectal ectasia are usually symptomatic since childhood with the most common symptom being soiling and impaction.[13]

A per rectal examination is essential in all cases. This may be repeated after cleaning the rectum with repeated enemas for better defining the anatomy and feeling the sphincter complex.

Posterior Rectal Shelf

This entity can be well appreciated if looked for with suspicion in any case of unexplained constipation. It may be picked up on a barium enema or on per rectal examination (Fig. 79.1). The posterior rectal shelf is ballooning of the rectum only posteriorly in which the finger in the rectum can be brought very close to the

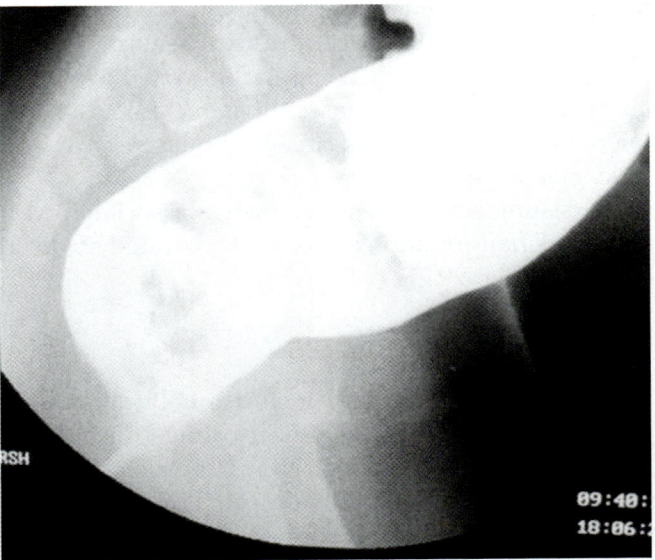

Fig. 79.1: Contrast study delineating the posterior rectal shelf

perineum with very less intervening tissue. Typically, the child presents with chronic constipation, straining at stool and ability to pass small amount of hard fecal matter by rubbing the bottom against the floor/ toilet seat.[1] A posterior shelf on barium study requires careful evaluation for the mid-sphincteric and rectal wall defects.

INVESTIGATIONS

The most useful investigation is barium enema. However, it is difficult to distinguish between primary and secondary rectal ectasia unless there is a history of previous surgery or anal stenosis or a anal stricture. Contrast study may delineate the dilated rectum with or without a posterior rectal shelf (Fig. 79.1).

Manometry will usually show a normal rectoanal inhibitory reflex unlike in patients with Hirschsprung's disease.

On rectometrographic studies, the elasticity coefficient of the rectal wall has been reported as decreased in patients of rectal ectasia as compared to controls (P less than 0.01).[14] The colonic transit time may show rectosigmoid stagnation. Rectal pressure was similar at the level of conscious sensation of filling, regardless of rectal capacity, suggesting a motor, rather than a sensory, abnormality. The amplitude of the rectoanal inhibitory reflex has been reported as decreased (P less than 0.001) as compared to controls in a series, thus sometimes mimicking the findings of Hirschsprung's disease, but increasing rectal distension always induced a relaxation of the internal anal sphincter.[14] The megarectum in rectal ectasia thus tolerates large amounts of fluid without sensation and lacks elasticity.[14]

Persisting ectasia in infancy when associated with anorectal malformation can be demonstrated by distal cologram (Fig. 79.2).

DIFFERENTIAL DIAGNOSIS

The differential diagnosis includes habitual constipation, ultrashort segment Hirschsprung's disease and Pouch colon syndrome. Rectal punch or suction biopsy should be performed to rule out Hirschsprung's disease in suspected cases.[15] Segmental dilatation of the colon that also causes chronic constipation in children is also an important differential diagnosis.[13,16] Sigmoid volvulus is a reported complication of segmental dilatation of the colon.[13]

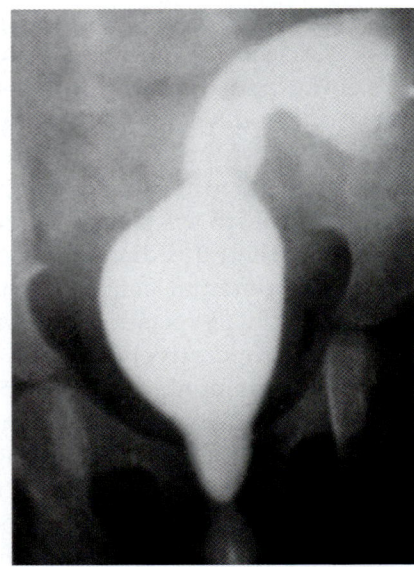

Fig. 79.2: Distal cologram suggestive of rectal ectasia

TREATMENT

An effective medical therapy would be helpful in the majority; however, surgery may be needed if the ectasia is too much and for too long in which the symptoms are not likely to improve with the conservative medical management.[1] The initial treatment depends on the consistency of the stool as judged by digital examination.

Medical Management

Medical management is indicated only in those cases where no inciting factor can be identified. The principles of medical management are to keep the bowel clean till the ectatic segment reduces to its original size. This is done with dietary modifications, laxatives and if the need arises then suppositories, enemas and manual evacuation. Bulk forming agents are given. Constipating agents are to be avoided. Fecoliths may need digital disintegration and saline washouts. Toilet training is an essential component of the medical management. The child is trained to attend to the toilet everyday at a fixed time and spend enough time till he is successful in evacuating the bowel by using his abdominal muscles additionally. Medication in adequate amounts is needed to maintain a suitable stool consistency. While the rectal ectasia persists, relapses are prone to occur, necessitating vigilance and even repeating the local bowel toilet regimen. A minimum trial with medical management of 6 months duration should be given under continuous supervision before resorting to surgical options. Patient with associated huge megacolon, with consequent constipation are usually refractory to conservative treatment.[6]

Surgical Treatment

The surgical management depends on the primary pathology and is considered only if the medical management fails. The main principle is to excise or plicate the redundant bowel to prevent postoperative incontinence or constipation. Resection or tailoring of the ectatic segment should be done during primary reconstructive procedure if rectal ectasia is recognized peroperatively in association with anomalies like anorectal malformation or anal stenosis. The large bulk of the walls of the intact wide rectum may impair the reconstruction of the sphincter muscles at the time of the anorectoplasty, thus lessening the ultimate degree of continence.[1]

Figure 79.3 shows the operative photograph of a case of rectal ectasia.

If a prominent posterior shelf is identified, a rectal wall plication may be done with effective results.[1] A mid-sphincteric defect, if detected on surgical dissection can be repaired in layers.

Various techniques have been used for treating rectal ectasia:

1. Posterior sagittal route tailoring. Tapering of the dilated segment of rectum through posterior sagittal route has also been a preferred method with desirable results.[17]
2. Endorectal pull-through. Resection of the abnormal bowel by an endorectal pull-through has been reported to give good to excellent results.[7,18]
3. Swenson's pull-through.[18]
4. Duhamel's pull-through has also been tried in few cases with good postoperative results.[18]
5. Plication of the dilated segment through posterior sagittal route. The authors prefer this method as it has less morbidity, preserves the sphincter complex, pelvic nerve plexus is not disturbed, strengthens the deficient rectal muscle and has been found to produce good postoperative results.
6. Anterior resection.[19] This is indicated for patients with hugely dilated rectum, not amenable to evacuation and medical management. Excision of the dilated bowel is done and the normal sized bowel is anastomosed to the distal rectum at the peritoneal reflection.
7. Resection of an ectatic sigmoid segment with colorectal anastomosis has been done with good postoperative outcome (Fig. 79.4). Resection of the terminal bowel may be done up to the dentate line when associated with low anorectal malformation.[5] If rectal ectasia is not recognized at the time of surgical reconstruction it may lead to megarectosigmoid, resulting in severe constipation and overflow incontinence postoperatively.[15,18]
8. Sphincteromyectomy and-plasty.[20] An incision is placed on the dentate line at 6 o'clock and the internal sphincter muscle is identified. The

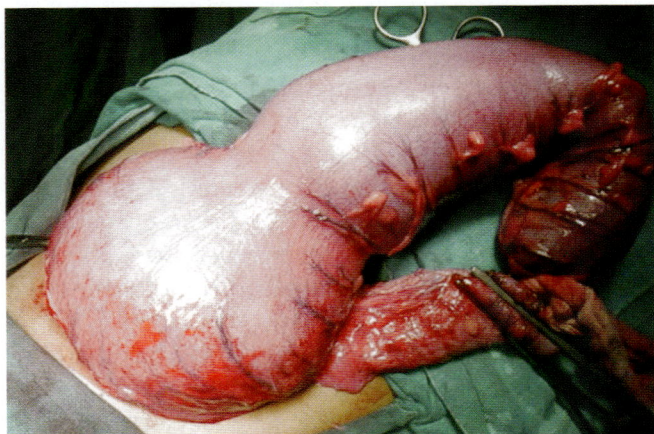

Fig. 79.3: Peroperative photograph showing the ectatic rectosigmoid segment with prominent but ineffective peristalsis (Reproduced from with permission of Springer science and business media)[1]

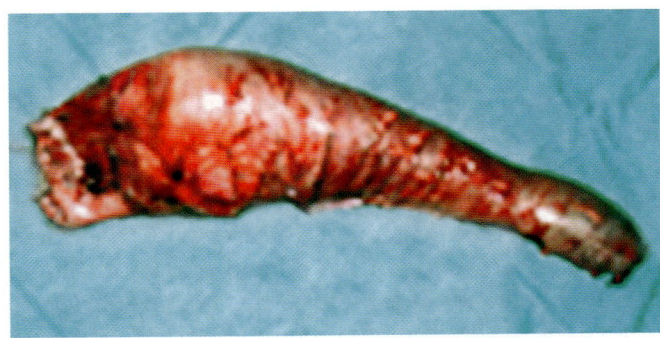

Fig. 79.4: Resected ectatic segment followed by colorectal anastomosis

incision is extended to this muscle and blunt dissection is done between the internal and external sphincter muscles advanced cranially 5 cm from the dentate line. All layers of anus and lower part of rectum upto 5 cm are clamped 1 cm apart. The mucosal and muscular layers are then divided for the 1 cm strip. The rectum at the proximal end of the strip is pulled through to the dentate line and anastomosed thus forming the posterior part of the anus.

9. Vertical reduction rectoplasty (VRR) has also been found to be beneficial in correcting rectal diameter, compliance and sensory function in most patients with rectal ectasia.[21] It has been reported to have low morbidity.[21]
10. Formation of a J pouch has also been described to treat patients with rectal ectasia associated with megasigmoid.[22]

PROGNOSIS

The prognosis of primary rectal ectasia is usually good if diagnosed appropriately and well in time. The prognosis of cases with secondary rectal ectasia depends upon the etiological factor responsible for the ectasia and its management. In cases with associated megacolon, resection of the dilated part of the colon and low coloanal anastomosis has been reported to relieve the severe constipation in all cases.[6]

REFERENCES

1. Gupta DK, Sharma Shilpa. Rectal Atresia and Rectal Ectasia in Anorectal Malformations, 1st edition, Ed. John Hutson and Alex Holschneider, Springer Heidelberg 2006;12:223-30.
2. Stephens FD. Rectal Ectasia: primary and secondary associated with anorectal anomalies. Birth Defects Orig Artic Ser 1988;24(4):99-104.
3. Brent L, Stephens FD. Primary rectal ectasia. A quantitative study of smooth muscle cells in normal and hypertrophied human bowel. In Rickham PP, Hecker W, and Prevot J: "Progress in Pediatric Surgery." Berlin: Urban and Schwarzenberg 1976;41-62.
4. Cloutier R, Archambault H, D'Amours C, Levasseur L, Ouellet D. Focal ectasia of the terminal bowel accompanying low anal deformities. J Pediatr Surg 1987;22(8):758-60.
5. Powell RW, Sherman JO, Raffensperger JG. Megarectum: a rare complication of imperforate anus repair and its surgical correction by endorectal pull-through. J Pediatr Surg 1982;17(6):786-95.
6. Rintala RJ, Jarvinen HJ. Congenital funnel anus. J Pediatr Surg 1996;31:1308-10.
7. Pena A, El Behery M. Megasigmoid: A source of pseudo-incontinence in children with repaired anorectal malformations. J Pediatr Surg 1993;28:199-203.
8. Upadhyaya P. Midanal sphincteric malformation, cause of constipation in anterior perineal anus. J Pediatr Surg 1984;19(2):183-86.
9. Stephens FD. Anorectal continence and idiopathic constipation. In Holter TM and Ashcraft KW: "Pediatric Surgery" Philadelphia: WB Saunders 1980;418-28.
10. Cuffari C, Bass J, Rubin S, Krantis A. Dysplastic nitrergic neurons in the rectum of a patient with rectal ectasia. J Pediatr Surg 1997;32(8):1237-40.
11. Chiarioni G, Bassotti G, Germani U, et al. Idiopathic megarectum in adults. An assessment of manometric and radiologic variables. Dig Dis Sci 1995;40(10):2286-92.
12. Stabile G, Kamm MA, Phillips RK, et al. Partial colectomy and coloanal anastomosis for idiopathic megarectum and megacolon. Dis Colon Rectum 1992;35(2):158-62.
13. Gattuso JM, Kamm MA. Clinical features of idiopathic megarectum and idiopathic megacolon. Gut 1997;41(1):93-99.
14. Verduron A, Devroede G, Bouchoucha M, et al. Megarectum. Dig Dis Sci 1988;33(9):1164-74.
15. Nguyen L, Shandling B. Segmental dilation of the colon: a rare cause of chronic constipation. J Pediatr Surg 1984;19(5):539-40.
16. Martinez MA, Conde J, Bardaji C, et al. Congenital segmental dilatation of the colon. Cir Pediatr 1989;2(1):43-44.
17. De Vries PA, Pena A. Posterior sagiltal anorectoplasty. J Pediatr Surg 1982;17:638.
18. Zia-ul-Miraj, Brereton RJ. Rectal ectasia associated with anorectal anomalies. Journal of Pediatric Surgery 1997;32:621-23.
19. Hallows MR, Lander AD, Corkery JJ. Anterior resection for megarectosigmoid in congenital anorectal malformations. J Pediatr Surg 2002;37:1464-66.
20. Hata Y, Shinada Y, Sasaki F, et al. Surgical treatment of chronic constipation with megarectum in children. Nippon Geka Gakkai Zasshi 1986;87:531-35.
21. Gladman MA, Williams NS, Scott SM, et al. Medium-term results of vertical reduction rectoplasty and sigmoid colectomy for idiopathic megarectum. Br J Surg 2005;92(5):624-30.
22. Stewart J, Kumar D, Keighley MR. Results of anal or low rectal anastomosis and pouch construction for megarectum and megacolon. Br J Surg 1994;81(7):1051-53.

Fecal Incontinence and Constipation

Anju Goyal, Paul D Losty

Fecal incontinence and constipation are common chronic problems affecting the pediatric surgical population. Constipation accounts for 3% of all pediatric outpatients visits.[1] It may be a manifestation of an underlying medical or surgical disorder although can be acquired as a functional problem in infancy, childhood and adolescence. Almost 95% of all cases of childhood constipation are idiopathic in etiology.[2] Fecal incontinence is a socially embarrassing condition. The child and parents often deny the problem and therefore the true incidence is underestimated. Disturbed defecation patterns often have a disruptive influence on family life. Most conditions leading to fecal incontinence in children are congenital in origin and present during the early crucial years of life interfering with the child's social and educational development. Even in Western societies with improved support structures, incontinent patients attain significantly lower educational levels than the normal population.[3] Many patients experience double incontinence (fecal and urinary incontinence) so there is a need to develop comprehensive support services in pediatric surgical centers to cater for children with this severe disability. Greater understanding of the long-term outcome of congenital colorectal malformations may also lead to improved care pathways for successful management.

NORMAL ANATOMY AND PHYSIOLOGY

Fecal continence is an individual's ability to perceive rectal distension, distinguish between solid, liquid and gas content and achieve evacuation in a socially acceptable environment. This is achieved through the presence of normal anorectal anatomy and physiology. Knowledge of normal mechanisms promoting continence is crucial to understand and manage fecal incontinence and constipation effectively.

ANATOMY

The rectum is normally empty and acts as a reservoir. It joins the anal canal at the level of the levator ani muscle. The puborectalis muscle slings around the anorectal junction and forms an angle of approximately 90 degrees at rest and helps maintain continence during periods of raised intra-abdominal pressure as encountered during coughing and sneezing episodes. The circular smooth muscle layer continues as the internal anal sphincter and is in a tonically contracted state. The external anal sphincter is a striated muscle, which along with the puborectalis forms an important voluntary continence mechanism (Fig. 80.1).

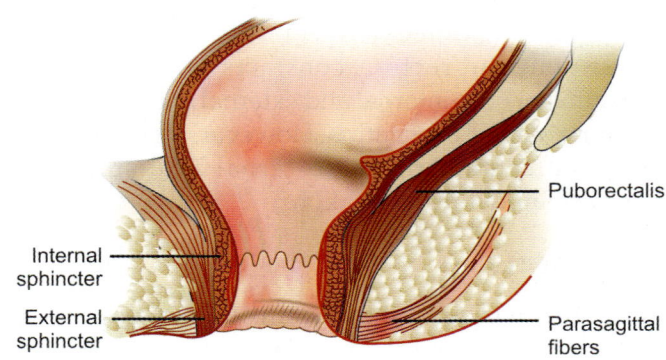

Fig. 80.1: Normal anatomy of anorectal region

PHYSIOLOGY

Physiology of fecal continence depends on:
1. Normal rectal sensation which perceives stretching on rectal distension. It triggers the rectoanal inhibitory reflex which promotes the reflex relaxation of the internal anal sphincter.
2. Normal anal sensation which differentiates between solid, liquid and gas contents.
3. Voluntary contraction of the puborectalis and external anal sphincter (innervated by the pudendal nerves) which inhibits defecation under socially inappropriate circumstances.
4. Intact internal sphincter tone (controlled by sympathetic and parasympathetic fibers), which prevents soiling. Its rhythmic relaxation allows sampling which helps differentiate between solid and fluid matter.

NORMAL DEFECATION

Normal defecation depends on the ability of the colon to deliver feces to the rectum. The colon has 2 types of physiological contractions: (a) the segmental non-propagated contractions that allow mixing and (b) high amplitude propagated contractions (HAPC) that empty the colon contents into the rectum. There are 2 main stimulants of HAPC: (i) awakening from sleep and (ii) ingestion of meals (gastrocolic reflex). These contractions by distending the rectum with feces initiate the rectoanal inhibitory reflex leading to relaxation of the internal anal sphincter. This allows sampling by the sensitive anal mucosa that differentiates between fluid and feces. This is perceived at cortical level leading to the desire to defecate and depending upon whether the circumstances are socially convenient, defecation is either facilitated or the desire to defecate over-ridden. If socially convenient the rectum contracts with complete relaxation of both internal and external anal sphincters resulting in stool evacuation. However, if over-ridden, the puborectalis and the external anal sphincter contracts inhibiting defecation.

DEFINITIONS

Incontinence is defined as the involuntary passage of stools in a socially inappropriate environment. It is usually due to deficient neural or muscular control of the anorectal sphincter mechanism.

Constipation is more difficult to define and definition varies according to person, age, and culture. Since defecation patterns vary widely among children, it is almost impossible to give a single definition that is acceptable and applicable to all. The infrequent and difficult evacuation of hard stools less than 3 times per week is a useful criteria.[4]

Though fecal incontinence is easier to define, grading is more difficult. Soiling, smearing and accidents are various terms used to define degrees of incontinence but there is no universally agreed definition for these terms. This makes comparison and evaluation of various treatments for fecal incontinence and constipation difficult. Constipation and incontinence can occur alone or they can coexist in same individual. Broad management strategies for treating these entities are similar therefore they may be classified together based on etiology (Table 80.1).

Table 80.1: Classification of constipation and fecal incontinence based on etiology

Idiopathic functional constipation

Idiopathic fecal incontinence[5]
Motility disorders
- Functional gastrointestinal dysmotility of prematurity
- Slow transit constipation

Medical disorders
- Cow's milk protein allergy
- Endocrine disorders such as hypothyroidism, hyperparathyroidism
- Drugs, e.g. opiates, vinca alkaloids
- Cystic fibrosis
- Generalised hypotonic disorders, e.g. Down's syndrome

Surgical disorders congenital
- Anorectal malformations (ARM)
- Hirschsprung's disease and allied neuropathies such as neuronal intestinal dysplasia(NID), hypoganglionosis
- Myelodysplasia
- Mechanical obstruction due to duplication cyst or pelvic masses, e.g. sacrococcygeal tumor type IV

Acquired
- Anal fissure
- Operative trauma following anorectal surgery, e.g. for Hirschsprung's disease, sacrococcygeal tumor
- Colorectal strictures, e.g. secondary to necrotising enterocolitis (NEC) or inflammatory bowel disease (IBD)
- Spinal trauma and direct trauma to the anorectal region

HISTORY AND CLINICAL EXAMINATION

Thorough history regarding time of onset, severity, progression and response to treatment is very helpful in suggesting a diagnosis. Time of passage of meconium is essential as 94% of full-term neonates and 76% of preterm babies pass meconium within 24 hrs of life and failure to do so is highly suggestive but not diagnostic of HD.[6] Gestational age at birth is important as premature babies are slow to open their bowels. A history of onset of constipation after the first month of life makes a diagnosis of Hirschsprung's disease unlikely. Associated urinary symptoms should be recorded and may suggest deficient neurological control. The onset of constipation may coincide with weaning or change in diet. Dietary history and medications should be reviewed. Clinical examination of the abdomen, spine and perineum is important. The abdominal findings give information on the degree of fecal loading. Examination of the spine may detect spina bifida occulta. Inspection of the perineum provides useful knowledge about the development of the anorectal muscle complex in ARM patients, as a flat perineum is associated with poor sphincters. Subtle anorectal malformations such as anal stenosis, anterior perineal anus may be detected which are important causes of constipation.[7-10] A digital rectal examination is not mandatory.[11] However, when performed may provide information regarding sphincter tone. An explosive bowel action after withdrawal of the finger may suggest Hirschsprung's disease.

INVESTIGATIONS

The investigative protocol is shown in Table 80.2.

Table 80.2: Protocol for investigations

Investigations
Biochemical investigations
Radiological investigations
- Abdominal X-ray
- Contrast enema
- Colon transit studies

Rectal biopsy
Anorectal manometry
MRI spine
MRI anorectal region

Biochemical Examination

Hypocalcemia and hypothyroidism may lead to constipation. Thyroid function tests and serum calcium are part of the investigative protocol for constipation in newborns. In babies with delayed passage of meconium, gene probe analysis should be performed to rule out cystic fibrosis, which is especially common in Caucasian populations.

Radiology

Abdominal X-ray: It may demonstrate the degree of fecal loading (Fig. 80.2). In those patients with severe fecal impaction it may guide the first line of management, e.g. manual evacuation. Spinal anomalies may also be readily apparent.

Colon transit studies: Transit time is closely related to defecation frequency. In 1-3 month old babies transit time from mouth to anus is approximately 8 hours, by 2 years it is 16 hours and in school age children ranges from 26-36 hours.[12-14] The study involves ingestion of ten radio-opaque beads daily for 6 consecutive days and an abdominal X-ray is performed on day seven (Fig. 80.3).[15] This investigation helps to differentiate pancolonic dysmotility (colonic inertia) and evacuation obstruction by the pattern of bead distribution. In colonic inertia, e.g. pancolonic dysmotility "scattered beads" are apparent on the X-ray study whereas in evacuation disorders where there is delayed transit principally in the descending and rectosigmoid regions "beads" are confined to the left colon/rectum.[16]

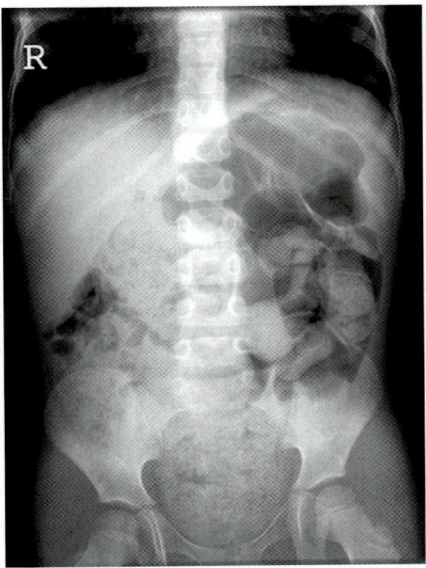

Fig. 80.2: X-ray showing gross fecal loading

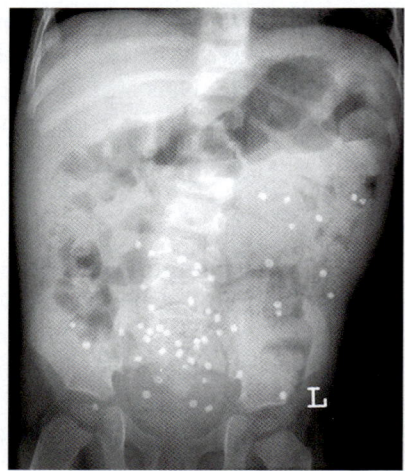

Fig. 80.3: Colon transit study showing concentration of beads at rectosigmoid level suggesting evacuation obstruction

Contrast enema: Contrast studies can prove diagnostic in conditions such as Hirschsprung's disease. It provides information about the degree of fecal impaction and recto sigmoid dilatation in patients with constipation, which can aid in planning treatment, e.g. bowel resection, ACE procedure.

Rectal biopsy: A suction rectal biopsy is carried out in infants with suspicion of HD, whereas in older children a formal full thickness rectal biopsy is indicated. Though full thickness biopsy is the gold standard, the advantage of suction biopsy is that it does not require general anesthesia. The specimen must be deep enough to contain submucosal tissue and should be taken from an area at least 2-3 cm above the dentate line to avoid the normal hypoganglionic region. The absence of ganglion cells along with the presence of numerous thickened acetylcholinesterase positive nerve fibers is diagnostic of HD. Other features that may be seen on rectal biopsy are hypoganglionosis, giant ganglia, etc. Laparoscopy may also be utilised to obtain serial biopsies from the colon, rectum and small bowel.[17]

Anorectal Manometry

Manometry is a useful adjunct in the investigative protocol for constipation and incontinence. It can suggest the diagnosis of HD by the absence of the rectoanal inhibitory reflex in older children (Fig. 80.4).

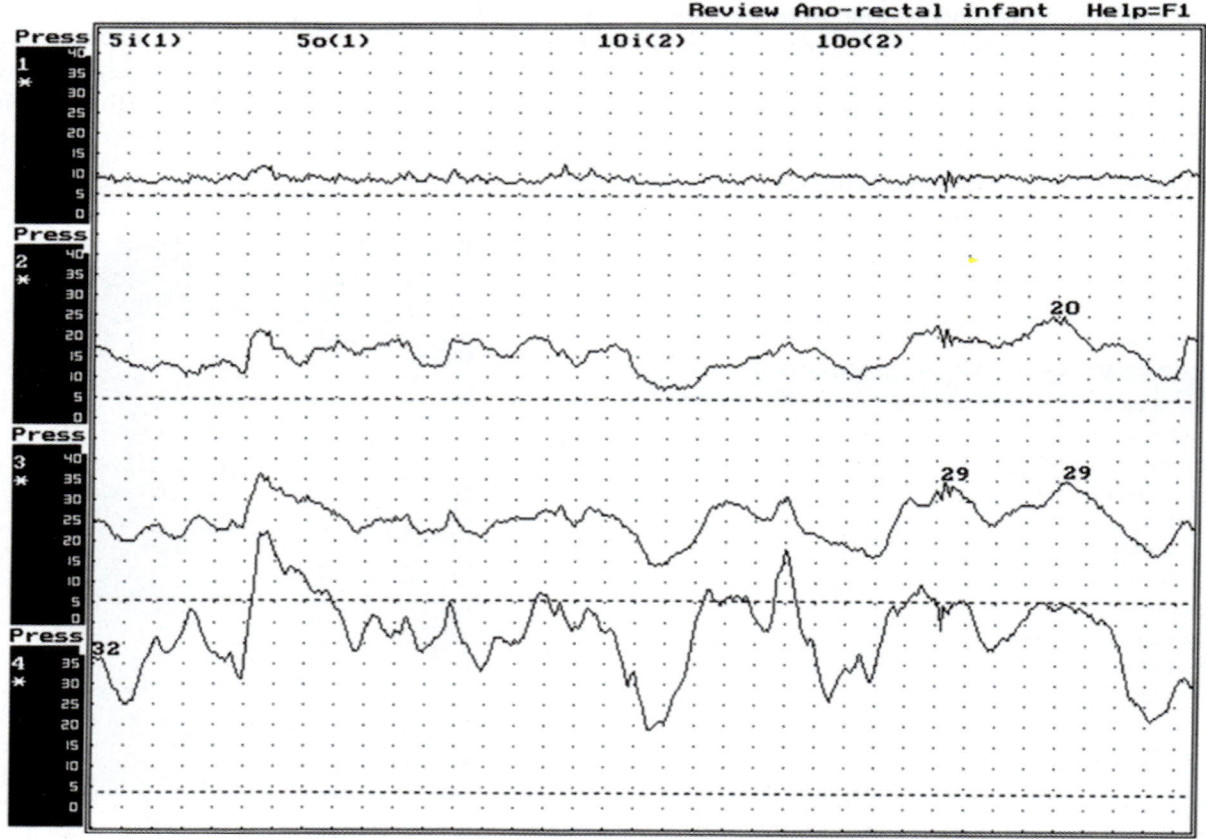

Fig. 80.4: Abnormal manometry trace showing absence of rectoanal inhibitory reflex

It is not reliable in newborns. It can be performed at the outpatient department and involves placement of a transducer probe in the anal canal and an inflatable balloon in the rectum. The balloon is inflated to distend the rectum and initiate the rectoanal inhibitory reflex. Normally, distension of the rectum by balloon inflation causes relaxation of the internal anal sphincter. The transducer probe detects the basal tone of the internal sphincter and records the decrease in tone when the rectoanal reflex causes the sphincter to relax (Fig. 80.5). It may also note paradoxical contractions during defecation, which are found in a group of children with delayed transit due to rectosigmoid colonic dysmotility (evacuation obstruction).[16]

MRI Anorectal Region

MRI of the anorectal region is a good modality to evaluate the development of the sphincter muscle complex. In patients who have had previous anorectal reconstruction it can provide information about the anatomy of the "pull through bowel" in relation to the muscle complex.[18]

MRI of the spinal cord MRI demonstrates the extent of cord involvement in patients with spina bifida and also in patients with spinal tumor and spinal injury. In individuals with anorectal malformation (both high and low) it can detect associated tethered cord, which may be a further cause of constipation/incontinence. Golonka et al report an incidence of tethered cord in 26.8% of high ARM anomalies and 50% of low malformations.[19]

TREATMENT

Treatment of the underlying medical cause where identifiable such as hypothyroidism or hyperparathyroidism should be undertaken.

The therapeutic options available are given in Table 80.3.

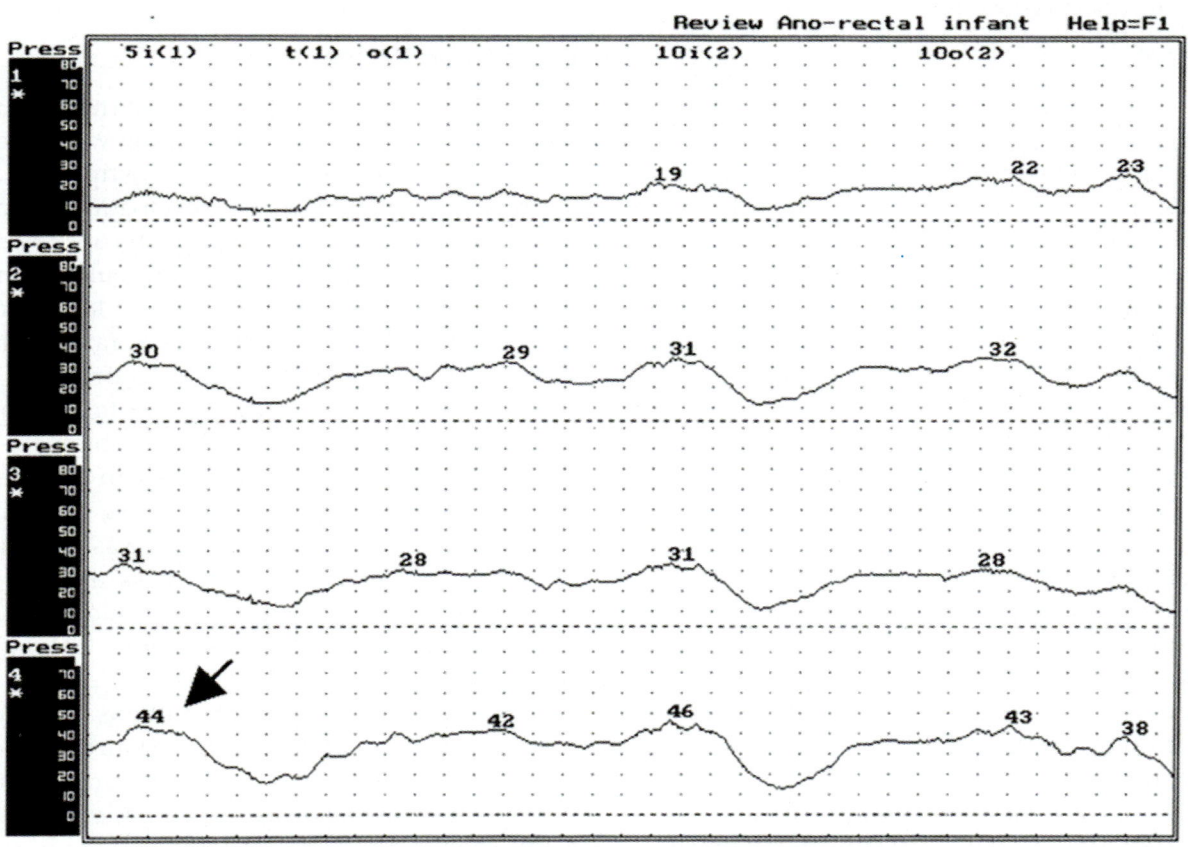

Fig. 80.5: Normal manometry trace demonstrating lowering of internal sphincter tone (arrow indicates fall in pressure in anal canal) on rectal distention

> **Table 80.3: Therapeutic strategies in the management of chronic constipation and fecal incontinence**
>
> **Medical treatment**
> - Dietary manipulation
> - Laxatives suppositories
> - Enemas
> - Prokinetic agents (e.g. Cisapride)
> - Bowel training program
> - Biofeedback
> - Anal plug
> - Botulinum toxin injection (internal sphincter achalasia)[23]
>
> **Surgery**
> - Manual evacuation
> - Antegrade continence enema (ACE)
> - Colon resection (partial or total)
> - Diverting stomas (permanent or temporary)
> - Anorectal myectomy (Hirschsprung's disease, internal sphincter achalasia)[24]
> - Artificial sphincter
> - Gracilus neosphincter

MEDICAL MANAGEMENT

Constipation

Aggressive medical management is the mainstay of treatment for constipation and fecal incontinence. The main aim is to ensure regular bowel emptying to evacuate the rectum and prevent fecolith formation. Though first line treatments may entail dietary manipulation, it is unclear if this is as effective in children as in adult practice.[20] Measures adopted include increased fiber intake and regular fluid intake. Recently cow's milk protein allergy has been shown to be an important cause of constipation.[21] An aggressive laxative regime provides the next option and a combination of various osmotic, stimulant and bulk laxatives are commenced depending on the obstinacy of constipation. Doses can be modified according to response. The type of laxative(s) utilised are varied and include bulk-forming agents (e.g. ispaghulla husk), stimulant laxatives (e.g. bisacodyl, docusate, senna or sodium picosulphate). Fecal softeners (e.g. liquid paraffin, olive oil) or osmotic laxatives (e.g. lactulose, polyethylene glycol) are useful. The key to the success of medical management is adequate parental counseling. This enables the carers to understand the mechanisms involved, the goals of treatment and the importance of active participation as well as expectations of the time scale involved to achieve satisfactory outcomes. The aims are to ensure regular bowel emptying to reduce fecaloma formation. In refractory cases of constipation (fecalomas and soiling), manual evacuation of the bowel is generally recommended prior to commencing laxative therapy. Manual evacuation not only disimpacts the megarectum, it also achieves temporary dilatation of the anal sphincter. Thus by breaking the vicious cycle of painful defecation and sphincter spasm may permit anal fissure(s), if present, to heal. These measures may cure up to 50% of children.[1] Other children will need further evaluation and investigations. Some patients require regular enemas or suppositories on a long-term basis to aid regular evacuation. Cisapride, a prokinetic agent has been shown also to benefit selected cases.[22] Botulinum toxin is an option in the treatment of chronic constipation due to internal sphincter achalasia as an alternative to internal sphincterotomy that was used for postoperative cases of Hirschspring's disease having constipation.[23,24]

Fecal Incontinence

Fecal incontinence is due to inadequate neuromuscular control or may be seen in association with 'overflow' states in children with severe constipation. While appropriate management of constipation can control fecal incontinence due to constipation and 'overflow', problems due to deficient neuromuscular control are more difficult to manage and require long-term care and support. Normal continence is rarely achieved with treatment and the aim is to promote social continence. If the bowel can be emptied adequately and regularly at socially convenient intervals then a reasonable degree of continence can be achieved. Various methods used to attain these goals include regular suppositories, daily bowel washouts and/or enemas. In patients with gross incontinence constipating agents such as loperamide (imodium) may be of use. Biofeedback is another option before contemplating surgery.

Biofeedback training is a technique, which can be used as an adjunct to other measures to control incontinence.[25] It is based on the principle of learning through reinforcement using the patient's ability to control bodily functions. An air filled manometric anal probe is attached to a color monitor and the amplitude and duration of voluntary anal sphincter contractions are assessed and demonstrated to the patient. Visual feedback cues are provided to demonstrate how the muscles work and the children are then taught to identify sphincter contractions from gluteal and abdominal effort (e.g. valsalva maneuver) and to perform sphincter exercises during the sessions and while at home. The overall aim is to enhance the child's understanding of their condition and to promote the individual's sense of control and self-esteem.

SURGICAL MANAGEMENT

Antegrade Continence Enema (ACE)

The formation of a continent stoma to perform antegrade colonic enemas (ACE) has been an important development in the management of children/adolescents with troublesome constipation and fecal incontinence. The procedure was first reported in 1990 by Malone et al.[26] The ACE is based on the principle of administration of a large volume enema via an appendicostomy stoma.[27] It works on the basis of the Mitrofanoff principle. Though originally described for patients with incontinence, its use has been extended to children with intractable functional constipation/soiling where it may be of some benefit. Stoma reversal can be performed in some patients when normal bowel motility has been restored.

Procedure: Though originally described as an appendico-cecostomy by reversing and reimplanting the appendix in a submucosal cecal tunnel thereby creating a continent stoma; pediatric surgeons now perform a simple orthotopic appendicostomy by imbricating the cecum with a series of sutures around the base of the appendix (optional) creating a similar continent channel. We employ a mini-abdominal incision below the "bikini line" and prefer to site the stoma in the right iliac fossa. Other surgeons prefer to site the stoma at the umbilicus. The stoma is fashioned by means of a broad based lateral skin flap that is tubularized and sutured to the mouth of the appendix hence burying the appendix and reducing skin discharge.

Various modifications have been reported to prevent stomal complications.[28] The procedure has also been performed laparoscopically.[29] If appendix is not available (e.g. previous appendicetomy or utilized for a Mitrofanoff) tubularized cecum, ileum, or ureter can be employed.[28] Recently a button device has been described.[30] Based on the principle of percutaneous endoscopic gastrostomy (PEG), a cecostomy catheter can be inserted percutaneously with the aid of a colonoscope.[31] If large volumes of enema are needed to achieve effective "washouts" particularly in patients with a large redundant sigmoid colon a modified left continent colonic ACE (sigmoid ACE) can be created to permit effective evacuation of the distal colon.[32]

An indwelling catheter is left *in situ* for 2-3 weeks to permit the stoma to mature and washouts can be started on the fourth postoperative day. Washout regimes include use of normal saline or tap water with one teaspoon of salt per 0.5 liters (volume varying from 100 to 1000 ml), given using an IV administration set while the child sits on the toilet. Each patient develops his or her own individual regimen by a process of trial and error. Most regimes employ a phosphate enema followed by a saline washout at 24, 48 or 72 hourly intervals. The technique of catheterization is easy and more acceptable to the child than retrograde enemas. On average it takes about 30 minutes every other day to ensure regular bowel emptying. Children can opt for an indwelling catheter or a button device in preference to regular intermittent self-catheterization. Crucial to good outcomes is appropriate patient selection and involvement of a nurse specialist who provides counseling and support for the child and family. Caution should be exercised when contemplating the ACE in young children. We rarely offer the procedure in those less than 5 years, as cooperation is required to achieve regular catheterization. The younger child may also fail to comprehend the intended benefits of the operation. Inadequate colonic washouts, stomal complications including stenosis, fecal and flatus problems are reported with this procedure.[33] Hyperphosphatemia has been described with use of phosphate enemas in young children.[34] Good functional outcomes are best achieved in those patients with adequate bowel motility and a degree of sphincter function.[35]

Colonic Resection

Partial or total colonic resection is performed in intractable cases of constipation who do not respond to maximal medical therapy or the ACE operation. The extent of resection may be guided by contrast studies and colonic transit time. In patients with anorectal malformations there is a tendency to develop megarectum and sigmoid colon inertia, which can lead toward stubborn constipation/soiling. Anterior resection of the megarectum in selected cases is associated with good results.[36]

Stomas

Stomas are further options in children with intractable constipation or gross fecal incontinence. They may be employed temporarily to allow the megacolon or rectum to regain normal caliber. Whilst patients with fecal incontinence may benefit from colostomy, ileostomy is an alternative in patients with pancolonic dysmotility.[37] Wherever possible a stoma should be considered a temporary solution. Other continence promoting strategies offer a better quality of life and patient independence.

Artificial Sphincter

The artificial sphincter is a fully implantable prosthetic device (Fig. 80.6). Initially introduced in 1996 which consist of an inflatable cuff tunnelled around the anal canal with an "activating" pump located in the labia in the female or scrotum in males.[38] Pediatric experience is limited although success rates varying from 33-75% have been reported in adult series.[39]

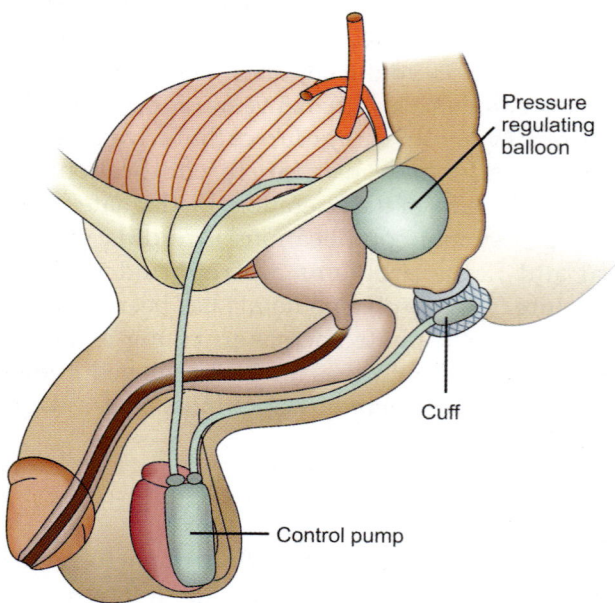

Fig. 80.6: Artificial anal sphincter

Dynamic Graciloplasty

The gracilis sphincter was originally described by Pickrell in 1952 and later modified by Williams et al.[40,41] The procedure involves mobilizing the gracilis muscle and wrapping it around the anal canal. Continuous electrical stimulation via an implantable electrode provides a continent mechanism. Results are good in almost two thirds of adults undergoing graciloplasty, however, pediatric experience is limited.

Specific pediatric surgical problems presenting with constipation and fecal incontinence are discussed here to provide a better perspective on individualized management.

ANORECTAL MALFORMATIONS

The principles of management of anorectal malformations are to surgically correct the anomaly keeping in mind that continence is influenced by neural (absent sacrum, deficient sacrum) and muscular development at birth. Surgery is integral to good outcomes and special expertise is mandatory to achieve such results. Most patients with imperforate anus do not have normal anal sensation and also have impaired rectal sensation as well as altered colonic motility.[42] They are not able to recognize liquid stool content and rectal distension adequately. Continence is never normal in these patients. Control is dependent on the extent of sphincter muscle development present at birth. Rectosigmoid motility is altered in patients with anorectal malformations and constipation is common. Pena considers abnormal rectosigmoid motility the most important single factor influencing bowel control and continence. Ensuring daily regular bowel emptying should ensure many patients remain "clean" even if they have inadequate sphincters. Patients with low anomalies have a tendency to constipation and soiling. Those with high or intermediate anomalies experience incontinence, soiling and/or constipation. Management begins at the time of colostomy formation where the two stomas should be sited with an adequate gap to prevent spillage of bowel content into the distal rectum thus ensuring it is kept empty and narrow in caliber. Washouts should also be given periodically to empty the defunctioned rectum. An anal dilatation program to prevent stenosis of the neoanus should follow the "pull through". Following colostomy closure, vigilant follow-up is required to assess the adequacy of bowel emptying. If emptying is not adequate or the child has developed incontinence a bowel management program should be initiated with the aim of emptying the rectum and distal colon daily so that soiling is minimized. A good laxative program should be commenced where constipation is a major problem. Regular emptying is achieved by use of suppositories, enemas or high colonic washouts. If colonic transit is fast, a combination of the above regimes with constipating agents like loperamide may be useful. The bowel management program needs to be individualized for each patient. If retrograde enemas are not having good results then formation of an ACE stoma should be considered. Those patients with severe constipation where a contrast enema study shows severe segmental dilatation of the rectosigmoid, should be considered candidates for megasigmoid resection. A "redo" pull through may be considered if the MRI suggests that the rectum has not been positioned adequately in relation to the sphincter complex. However, outcomes following "redo" PSARP are not good.[43]

A further important group of patients are those with "pouch" colon where there is usually no rectosigmoid and thus reservoir function is lost. The colon is like a cesspool. These children have increased frequency of stools due to lack of colonic absorption capacity. They are difficult to manage. The response to bowel management programs is not good. A permanent stoma may be an option in these patients. Gracioplasty may be considered in grossly incontinent patients although pediatric experience is limited. Aids like the anal plug (based on tampon principle) are also useful in achieving improved quality of life.[44] These are easy to use and offer useful control for short periods of time.

MYELODYSPLASIA

Spina bifida patients are characterized by inadequate voluntary sphincter function and poor anorectal sensation. Colonic motility is also disturbed.[45] Urinary incontinence is also variable. Bowel function depends upon the level of the spinal lesion. Patients with high lesions (thoracic or thoracolumbar) have slow colonic motility and absent anorectal sensation with loss of voluntary sphincters and internal sphincter dysfunction. These patients are prone to fecal loading and very difficult to manage. Those with lumbosacral lesions have slow left colonic transit time however, they can usually achieve bowel emptying by using the gastrocolic reflex to prevent fecal loading.[45] Intact anal resting tone implies that fecal leakage is unusual in these children. The main problem is the "automatic" nature of bowel emptying. A regimen of rectal stimulation at appropriate time intervals will help to achieve an acceptable level of continence. Patients with sacral spinal lesions usually have some voluntary sphincter activity and some anorectal sensation so they are continent but deficient rectal sensibility predisposes them to constipation.[45] Management consists of dietary modifications, regular rectal stimulation, enemas and washouts. The ACE procedure has been used in difficult cases but careful patient selection is required to achieve optimum results.

SUMMARY

Patients with fecal incontinence and constipation constitute a significant proportion of the pediatric surgical workload in many units. While constipation is often self-limiting, incontinence is usually incurable and this disability requires long-term comprehensive management to provide an acceptable quality of life. Problems should be anticipated and support should be provided at an early stage to pre-empt deterioration of anorectal function. A multidisciplinary approach (radiologists, gastroenterology technicians and surgeons) including family liaison with a clinical nurse specialist remains pivotal to a successful bowel management program.

REFERENCES

1. Loenig-Baucke V. Constipation in early childhood: Patient characteristics, treatment and long-term follow up. Gut 1993; 34:1400-04.
2. Loenig-Baucke V. Encopresis and soiling. Pediatr Clin North Am 1996;43:279-98.
3. Hassink EA, Rieu PN, Brugman AT, et al. Quality of life after operatively corrected high anorectal malformation. A long-term follow-up study in patients 18 years of age and older. J Pediatr Surg 1994;29:773-76.
4. Clayden G, Agnarsson U. Constipation in Childhood. Oxford. England, OUP 1991.
5. Griffiths DM. The Physiology of Continence: Idiopathic Fecal Constipation and Soiling. Semin Pediatr Surg 2002;11(2):67-74.
6. Clark DA. Times of first void and first stool in 500 newborns. Pediatrics 1977;60:457-59.
7. Leape LL, Ramanofsky ML. Anterior ectopic anus: A common cause of constipation in children. J Pediatr Surg 1978;13:627-30.

8. Upadhyaya P. Midanal sphincteric malformation, cause of constipation in anterior perineal anus. J Pediatr Surg 1984;19(2):183-86.
9. Hendren WH. Constipation caused by anterior location of the anus and its surgical correction. J Pediatr Surg 1978;13:627-30.
10. Reisner SH, Sivan Y, Nitzan M, et al. Determination of anterior displacement of the anus in newborn infants and children. Pediatrics 1984;73:216-17.
11. Jesudason EC, Walker J. Rectal examination in pediatric surgical practice. Br J Surg 1999;86:376-78.
12. Foman SJ. Infant Nutrition, Philadelphia, PA, Saunders 1984.
13. Triboulet H. Duree de la Traversee chez l' enfant malade epreuve du carmin. Bull Soc Pediatr Paris 1909;11:512-29.
14. Dimson SB. Carmine as an index of transit time in children with simple constipation. Arch Dis Child 1970;45:225-32.
15. Bouchoucha M, Devroede G, Arhan P, et al. What is the meaning of colorectal transit time measurement? Dis Colon Rectum 1992;35:773-82.
16. Gutierrez C, Marco A, Nogales A, et al. Total and segmental colonic transit time and anorectal manometry in children with chronic idiopathic constipation. J Pediatr Gastroenterol Nutr 2002;35:31-38.
17. Carvalho JL, Campos M, Soares-Oliveira M, et al. Laparoscopic colonic mapping of dysganglionosis. Pediatr Surg Int 2001;17(5-6):493-95.
18. Sachs TM, Applebaum H, Touran T, et al. Use of MRI in evaluation of anorectal anomalies. J Pediatr Surg 1990;25(7):817-21.
19. Golonka NR, Haga LJ, Keating RP, et al. Routine MRI evaluation of low imperforate anus reveals unexpected high incidence of tethered spinal cord. J Pediatr Surg 2002;37:966-69.
20. Roma E, Adamidis D, Nikolara R, et al. Diet and chronic constipation in children: The role of fiber. J Pediatr Gastroenterol Nutr 1999;28:169-74.
21. Iacono G, Cavataio F, Montalto G, et al. Intolerance of cow's milk and chronic constipation in children. N Engl J Med 1998;339:1100-04.
22. Nurko S, Garcia-Aranda JA, Worana LB, et al. Cisapride for the treatment of constipation in children: A double blind study. J Pediatr 2000;136:35-40.
23. Messineo A, Codrich D, Monai M, et al. The treatment of internal anal sphincter achalasia with botulinum toxin. Pediatr Surg Int 2001;17:521-23.
24. Blair GK, Murphy JJ, Fraser GC. Internal sphincterotomy in post-pull-through Hirschsprung's disease. J Pediatr Surg 1996;31:843-45.
25. Olness K, mcParland FA, Piper J. Biofeedback: A new modality in the management of children with fecal soiling. J Pediatr 1980;96:505-09.
26. Malone PS, Ransley PG, Kiely EM. Preliminary report: The antegrade continence enema. Lancet 1990;336:1217-18.
27. Shandling B, Gilmour RF. The enema continence catheter in spina bifida: successful bowel management. J Pediatr Surg 1987;22:271-73.
28. Griffiths DM, Malone PS. The Malone antegrade continence enema. J Pediatr Surg 1995; 30(1):68-71.
29. Robertson RW, Lynch AC, Beasley SW, et al. Early experience with the laparoscopic ACE procedure. Aust N Z J Surg 1999;69(4):308-10.
30. Duel BP, Gonzalez R. The button caecostomy for the management of fecal incontinence. Pediatr Surg Int 1999;15(8):559-61.
31. De Peppo F, Iacobelli BD, De Gennaro M, et al. Percutaneous endoscopic cecostomy for antegrade colonic irrigation in fecally incontinent children. Endoscopy 1999;31(6):501-03.
32. Gauderer MW, Decon JM, Boyle JT. Sigmoid irrigation tube for the management of chronic evacuation disorders. J Pediatr Surg 2002;37(3):348-51.
33. Dey R, Ferguson C, Kenny SE, et al. After the honeymoon-medium term outcome of antegrade enema procedure. J Pediatr Surg 2003;38(1):65-68.
34. Hunter MF, Ashton MR, Griffiths DM, et al. Hyperphosphatemia after enemas in childhood: prevention and treatment. Arch Dis Child 1993;68(2):233-34.
35. Shankar KR, Losty PD, Kenny SE, et al. Functional results following the antegrade continence enema procedure. Br J Surg 1998;85(7):980-82.
36. Hallows MR, Lander AD, Corkery JJ. Anterior resection for megarectosigmoid in congenital anorectal malformations. J Pediatr Surg 2002;37(10):1464-66.
37. Villarreal J, Sood M, Zangen T, et al. Colonic diversion for intractable constipation in children: colonic manometry helps guide clinical decisions. J Pediatr Gastroenterol Nutr 2001;33(5):588-91.
38. Wong WD, Jensen LL, Bartolo DC, et al. Artificial anal sphincter. Dis Colon Rectum 1996;39:1345-51.
39. Wong WD, Congliosi SM, Spencer MP, et al. The safety and efficacy of the artificial bowel sphincter for fecal incontinence: results from a multicentre cohort study. Dis Colon Rectum 2002;45(9):1139-53.
40. Pickrell K, Broadbent R, Masters F, et al. Construction of a rectal sphincter and restoration of anal continence by transplanting the gracilis muscle. Ann Surg 1952;135:853-62.
41. Williams NS, Hallan RI, Koeze TH, et al. Construction of a neoanal sphincter by transposition of the gracilis muscle and prolonged neuromuscular stimulation for the treatment of fecal incontinence. Ann R Coll Surg Engl 1990;72:108-13.
42. Pena A. Anorectal Malformations. Semin Pediatr Surg 1995; 4:35-47.
43. Rintala R, Mildh L, Lindahl H. Faecal continence and quality of life in adult patients with an operated high or intermediate anorectal malformation. J Pediatr Surg 1994; 29: 777-80.
44. Pfrommer W, Holscneider AM, Loffler N, et al. A new polyurethane anal plug in the treatment of incontinence after anal atresia repair. Eur J Paed Surg 2002;10(3):186-90.
45. Rintala RJ. Fecal incontinence in anorectal malformations, neuropathy and miscellaneous conditions. Semin Pediatr Surg 2002;11(2):75-82.

CHAPTER 81

Bowel Management

Shilpa Sharma, DK Gupta, Alberto Pena

The main goal of a bowel management program is to improve the quality of life in children with fecal incontinence.[1] A well established bowel management program needs dedication, determination and consistency with an aim to keep the child clean for 24 hours.[1] At the Krickenbeck Conference, besides a new International diagnostic classification system, a method of postoperative assessment of continence was developed by the expert group to manage patients with ARM.[2] These methods should allow for a common standardization of comparing postoperative results. The initial management options already adopted by the patient include; alterations in diet, suppositories, laxatives and enemas. Some authors advocate perineal exercises but the results are equivocal and depend a lot on patient's compliance and anatomy.

PRELIMINARY ASSESSMENT

As a surgeon, it is imperative that the child is examined thoroughly to assess the need of a second operation that may treat the incontinence. This is relevant especially in cases of anorectal malformation if

a. The child was born with a good sacrum, good sphincter mechanism and a malformation with good functional prognosis.
b. The rectum is mislocated.[3]
c. The length of the colon is intact with a demonstrable rectosigmoid region.

The redo PSARP (posterior sagittal anorectoplasty) can be performed and the rectum can be relocated within the limits of the sphincter mechanism. Approximately 50% of the children re-operated by experienced surgeons under these circumstances have a significant improvement in bowel control and do not require bowel management to remain clean.[1] In a large series of 303 who had undergone re-operation for anorectal malformations, a mislocated rectum was present in 76 cases.[3] Surgery may be beneficial in the management of children with chronic intractable constipation and documented abnormalities in motility.[4]

If constipation is a persisting problem with overflow and rectal ectasia is documented, the surgical treatment may be warranted. Anterior resection is considered if the rectum is hugely dilated. Surgical results in patients with gross megarectum are good.

Indications of Bowel Management

1. Anorectal malformations[-9]
2. Spina bifida[10]
3. Chronic idiopathic constipation[11]
4. Hirschprung's disease[12]
5. Inflammatory bowel disease[13]
6. Trauma causing fecal incontinence[14]
7. Operated case of rectal carcinoma
8. Colonic dysmotility
9. Other colorectal disorders.

Fecal continence is an important achievement in a child's development and is an important assessment for evaluating the results in the diseases mentioned as above.

Functional soiling is a self-limiting problem and usually disappears at puberty. The high incidence and importance of chronic idiopathic constipation as an entity in itself and a contributing factor to fecal incontinence has been recognized.[11] Organic fecal incontinence is a consequence of congenital malformations affecting the anorectum, anal sphincters or the spinal cord. Inability to control bowel function may be permanent, as in patients with myelodysplasia; self-limiting, as in patients who have fecal soiling after a pull-through operation for Hirschsprung's disease; or partial, as in many patients who have undergone repair of an anorectal malformation.[12]

Management of anorectal malformations requires an accurate clinical diagnosis, proper planning of treatment in the newborn, meticulous anatomic reconstruction, and comprehensive postoperative care with the goal of having a child who is clean and dry, with an excellent quality of life, because they either have the capacity for continence or can be kept artificially clean with a comprehensive bowel management program.[6] Globally, 75% of all patients of anorectal malformations have voluntary bowel movements. Half of this group still soils their underwear occasionally. Therefore, only about 37.5% of all cases are considered totally continent.[5]

Objectives of a Bowel Management Program

The goal of a well established bowel management program is to teach patients and their parents or guardians how to administer a daily enema in order to clean the colon and prevent incontinence.

The bowel management program includes:
1. Use of daily enemas tailored to each patient.
2. Observation with supervision for a week.
3. Parents are taught how to give the enema everyday in a controlled environment.
4. Daily abdominal skiagram to assess the result of the enema.
5. Psychological support.

Through trial and error, the correct amount and type of enema suitable for each patient is determined. The medical staff also considers what, if any, dietary restrictions or medications are needed to help the child control his/her bowels.

Fecal Incontinence

Fecal incontinence is defined as the incapacity to voluntarily hold feces in the rectum.

A child with fecal incontinence must be evaluated so that the medical team can distinguish between actual fecal incontinence and pseudoincontinence (overflow fecal incontinence).

Real Fecal Incontinence

The presence, the passage of stool and the perception to differentiate between solid and liquid stool and gas, is damaged. The etiology for fecal incontinence in anorectal malformation and some cases of Hirschsprung's disease is a defect in the sphincter mechanism and the striated muscle complex that surrounds the normal rectum, apart from neurologic deficiency associated with sacral agenesis. In cases of spina bifida, the contraction and relaxation of the muscles, as well as sensation, are both deficient.

Pseudoincontinence

In over flow fecal incontinence, the child suffers from severe constipation and fecal impaction. When the impaction is treated and the patient receives enough laxatives to pass stool, he or she becomes continent.

Overflow fecal incontinence results due to dilatation of the rectum and the sigmoid, a condition defined as megarectosigmoid. These children also suffer from a hypomotility disorder that interferes with the complete emptying of the rectosigmoid.[1] Fecal impaction and pseudo overflow fecal incontinence can occur in a child with a good prognosis type of defect who though underwent a technically correct operation yet did not receive an appropriate treatment for constipation.

Physical Causes of Fecal Incontinence

About 70-80% of all children with anorectal malformations who have undergone a correct and successful operation will have voluntary bowel movements after the age of 3. About half of these patients soil their underwear on occasion usually related to constipation.[1] If the constipation is treated properly, the soiling frequently disappears. Thus, approximately 40% of all children have voluntary bowel movements and no soiling.

Children with good bowel control still may suffer from temporary episodes of fecal incontinence, particularly severe diarrhea. About 25% of all children with anorectal malformations despite a good operation suffer from real fecal incontinence and they must undergo bowel management to stay clean.[5]

Physical Elements of Fecal Incontinence in Anorectal Malformations

Children born with anorectal malformation often do not experience the following:

1. Sensation within the Rectum
2. Motility of the Rectosigmoid

Normally, the rectosigmoid acts as a reservoir and remains quiet for periods of 24-48 hours, then a peristaltic wave allows the complete emptying of the rectosigmoid after which it remains quiet. If the rectosigmoid is slow, the stool stays stagnant and constipation occurs. As a result, the child may suffer from overflow incontinence and will soil. In the absence of a rectosigmoid, the child passes stool constantly, which may result in colonic hypermotility.

3. Muscles

Children with anorectal malformations lack some degree of development of the muscle complex or voluntary sphincters that normally surround the rectum and anus and therefore are incapable of holding in stool. The more complex the defect, the less developed is the muscle complex.

Prognosis for Bowel Control (Table 81.1)

It is possible for a surgeon with wide experience to predict in advance the functional prognosis of a child with anorectal malformation after definitive repair.[1]

A normal sacrum and a prominent midline groove with good gluteal muscles are indicators of good bowel control vis-a-vis an abnormal sacrum with a flat perineum and poorly developed muscles.

Children with anomalies with good prognosis like vestibular fistula, perineal fistula, rectal atresia, rectourethral bulbar fistula, imperforate anus with no fistula and a common cloaca with common channel less than 3 cm have a strong likelihood to have voluntary bowel movements by age 3.[1] However, the child will still need supervision to avoid fecal impaction, constipation and soiling.

Children with anomalies with poor prognosis for bowel control include a very high cloaca with a common channel longer than 3 cm, recto-bladder-neck fistula and complex malformations.[1] These children will most likely need a bowel management program to remain clean and be socially acceptable at 3-4 years age.

For children with rectoprostatic urethra fistula, there is a 50% chance that they will have voluntary bowel movements.[1] Toilet training is recommended for these children by the age of 3. If this is unsuccessful, bowel management should be implemented at the time of potty training so that the child can remain clean and avoid social discomfort.

Table 81.1: Prognostic signs for bowel control

Good	Poor
No soiling	Constant soiling and passage of stools
Good bowel movements 1-2/day	
Sensation of passing stool or gas present (pushing, making faces)	No sensation (no pushing)
Urinary control present	Urinary incontinence, dribbling of urine

MANAGEMENT

Pseudoincontinence

Enemas and/or colonic washouts are used to clean the mega-rectosigmoid and remove the impaction. Then the constipation is prevented through administration of large doses of laxatives.[1] The laxative dosage is adjusted daily until the proper amount of laxative is reached in order to completely empty the colon every day.

The diagnosis of overflow pseudoincontinence is made if the child becomes continent after the constipation is treated adequately. In case medical treatment fails due to a severe megasigmoid, surgical resection of the dilated sigmoid colon may be considered. After the sigmoid resection, the amount of laxatives required to treat these children can be significantly reduced or possibly even abolished.

However, before this is done, real fecal incontinence with constipation should be ruled out. A fecally incontinent constipated child subjected to this management would be changed to the one with diarrhea, which becomes much more difficult to manage.

Constipation (Colonic Hypomotility)

Constipation is the most common sequelae of anorectal malformations.[5] The aim is to teach the parents to clean their child's colon once a day with an enema or a colonic irrigation. No special diet or medications are necessary for children with colonic hypomotility or constipation.[1] Their condition guarantees that they will remain clean in between enemas. The real challenge is to find an enema capable of cleaning the colon completely. Soiling episodes or severe "accidents" occur when there is an incomplete cleaning of the bowel.

Loose Stools and Diarrhea (Colonic Hypermotility)

This group is more difficult to manage. Most of these patients have been treated before the invention of PSARP with operations that included resection of the rectosigmoid (reservoir). Rapid transit of stool results in frequent episodes of diarrhea as even when an enema cleans the colon rather easily, stool keeps on passing fairly quickly from the cecum to the descending colon. Diarrhea is the most common aggravating factor for fecal incontinence, and antidiarrheal medications such as loperamide and diphenoxylate or bile acid binders may help.[15] Thus a constipating diet and/or medications are needed to slow down the colon.

The treatment starts with enemas, a very strict diet, and under medical supervision, Imodium may be prescribed.

Once clean, the child can choose one new food every two to three days observing the effect on his or her colonic activity.[1] If the child soils after eating a newly introduced food, parents are advised to eliminate that food from the diet on a permanent basis. The most liberal diet possible should be sought for the child. If he or she remains clean with a liberal diet then the dose of the medication can gradually be reduced to the lowest dose effective. Often the strict diet does not need to last forever. After two months of successful bowel management a child may have one of the "no eat" foods that he or she has been craving for. If the child soils after eating that food, then it stays on the no-eat list. The parents may introduce just one new food a week and observe the effect on the bowel movement pattern.

Teamwork

The bowel management program is most successful when the parents and skilled health professionals work together. Each member of the team should understand the sensitivity of the issue with a good communication and rapport between the members to achieve a successful outcome.

The bowel management program is tailored to individual patients and differs from child to child. A routine is usually achieved within a week while the family, patient, physician, and nurse undergo a process of trial and error designing the program to the specific patient. This requires a lot of dedication and the results are gratifying.

Enema

The type and amount of daily enema required to control the bowels varies from patient to patient.

There are different types of solutions to use for enemas. There are available as the prepared solutions or solutions that can be prepared at home based on water and salt. One and a half teaspoon of table salt added to a liter of tap water is the right combination to use as a home made enema solution. Children should never receive more than one phosphate enema a day because of the risk of phosphate intoxication. Children with impaired renal function should also use phosphate enemas with caution. The "right" enema is the one that can empty the child's colon and allow him to stay clean for the following 24 hours. This can be achieved only by trial and error. A larger volume of saline solution is necessary in those children who have hypomotility as compared to those who have hypermotility who tend to empty their colon more rapidly. The solution of the enema should be at body temperature to decrease cramping. The consistency and the amount of stool evacuated after the enema should be examined to determine if it was effective. Administered on a regular basis, the enema should result in a bowel movement followed by a period of 24 hours of complete cleanliness. If one enema is not enough to clean the colon, (as demonstrated by an X-ray, or if the child keeps soiling), then the child requires a more aggressive treatment. If the saline enema produces inadequate results, then other additives can be added to increase the potency of the enema. The additives that can be added to the saline enema include phosphate, mild soap, glycerine and castile soap. The use of phosphate enemas is convenient and can be added to saline enemas.

A Foley catheter (22/24 Fr) is used as an alternative to the normal catheter when the enema solution administered leaks. The goal of this procedure is to use a balloon to act as a plug to avoid leaking during the enema process.

Best Time of the Day to Administer an Enema

The timing of the enema plays a role in how efficiently it cleans the bowel. The recommendation is to give an enema after the main meal of the day in order to take advantage of the gastrocolic reflex (this reflex happens after each meal), but more importantly, the enema should be given when it is the best time for the parents and the child to have time to do the enema efficiently and have one hour to devote to the administration.

It is advisable to give the enema at the same time every day in order to create a routine. It is also important to consider that if the enema is given every other day, the child should expel the amount of stool due for two days. No more than 48 hours should elapse between enemas.

Steps for Administering the Enema[1]

1. The child should be in a position that facilitates delivery of the fluid as high up into the colon as possible. A small child can be placed on the parent's lap with the head down and buttocks on the lap. The older child may lie prone on a bed with a pillow under their abdomen or in a knee-chest position (Figs 81.1A to C). Adolescents may try self-administration of these enemas with the knee-chest position while lying on their side. Lying on right or left side to administer enema may be just as effective if comfortable.
2. A lubricated 22-24 F Foley catheter should be gently introduced through the anus for approximately 4-6 inches.
3. Using a 30 cc syringe filled with air or warm water, 15 cc is in stilled and then the catheter is pulled back. If the balloon comes out, the catheter is pushed back and the remaining 5 cc of water is instilled then pulled back again. This may be continued till the full 30 cc. The balloon should never be inflated right at the anus.
4. As soon as the balloon is inflated, the syringe from the catheter is removed to prevent the balloon from deflating. While keeping tension on the catheter to avoid leaking, the flow of enema fluid is started.
5. When the enema is complete, the solution should not be released for 5-10 minutes for optimal effect. The enema fluid should be retained as long as possible and this depends on the child and the quantity of fluid introduced.
6. When retention time is up, the child is placed on the toilet and at this point is deflated the balloon allowing the catheter to slip out.
7. The child should sit on the toilet for 45 minutes to allow enough time for the enema to be most effective for complete emptying of the colon. It is very important to be sure that the child empties

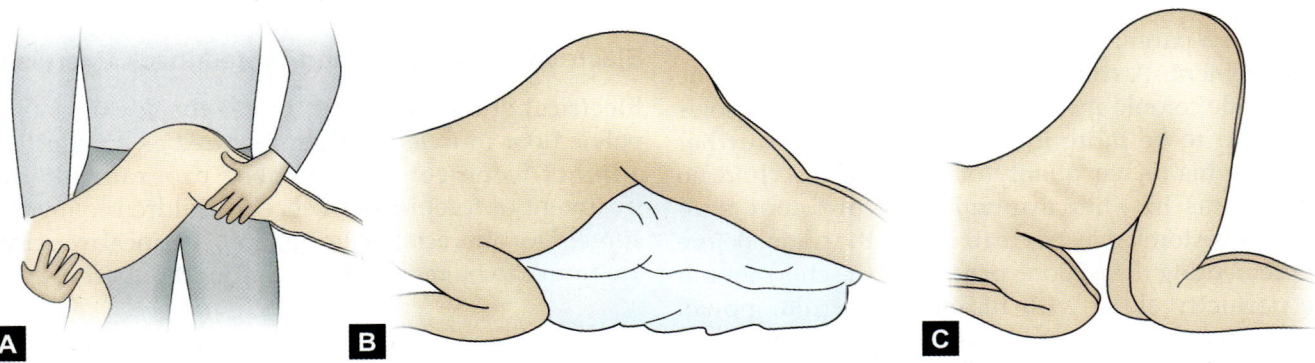

Figs 81.1A to C: A. Small baby on the lap **B.** Older child raised on a pillow in prone position **C.** Knee-elbow position for easy access taking the advantage of gravity to push the enema solution

his or her colon, otherwise a more aggressive enema is necessary which can cause additional discomfort.

Toilet Training

Toilet training for stool is a long-term goal for children with anorectal malformations. Parents of children born with a good prognosis type of defect should be encouraged to use the same strategies for toilet training as those followed by families with typical children.

Between ages 2-3 years old, parents are advised to sit their child on the toilet after every meal. Allowing him or her to play with toys is encouraged while on the toilet. Just as in training any child, parents are encouraged to toilet train as a game and not as a punishment.

Parents should sit with their child and not argue or force the child to remain seated. If the child gets up, the parents should put the toys away.

The child should be rewarded for a bowel movement or voiding while on the toilet.

If the child is not successfully toilet trained by school age, a family has two alternatives: Not to send the child to school for another year and continue attempts at toilet training or begin the Bowel Management program.

It is recommended to begin the bowel management program by the time their child is 3-4 years old. The family may decide when and how to start bowel management with the goal to have the child in school wearing a normal underwear without being ridiculed by his or her classmates who are already toilet trained.

Continent Catheterizable Channel

Adolescents often feel their privacy is being infringed on when a parent continues to help them with bowel management. A continent appendicostomy (Malone antegrade colonic enema or MACE procedure) allows the child to be more independent and can further improve his or her quality of life.[1,16] If the child no longer has his/her appendix, a continent neo-appendicostomy may be created from the colon. Before implementing the Malone procedure the child should be perfectly clean with his or her regular bowel management and should be absolutely motivated, both in terms of the surgery and the administration of the enemas as well as in his or her ability to evaluate the effects.

To manage overflow incontinence of children with anorectal malformations and Hirschsprung's disease, laparoscopic technique to allow antegrade enema treatment has been described as a technically straightforward, effective, and reversible method for the placement of a cecostomy button.[17]

Duration of the Program

Patients with a poor prognosis type of anorectal defect will require the bowel management program life long. However, as anorectal malformations is a spectrum of defects, it is conceivable that later in life, some children may stop using enemas and remain clean, following a specific regimen of a disciplined diet with regular meals (three meals per day and no snacks) to provoke bowel movements at a predictable time. Discontinuing the daily enemas may be attempted if the child is completely clean with bowel management, cooperative and understands that there's a risk it won't work and one might have to return to the bowel management program by daily enemas. For children with constipation, a daily laxative given at the same time each day is recommended. The dose of the laxative can be adjusted by trial and error. It is best to first try the less aggressive and natural types of laxative, and then, depending on the child's response, use medications with more active ingredients. The first choice is a laxative type of diet; the next choice is a bulk forming agent. If this medication does not work, a laxative with senna is indicated. After a few weeks, the family and child can decide whether they want to continue with the new regimen or go back to the bowel management program. This decision is up to the family and the child, and is based on the quality of life experienced with each method.

Electrical Stimulation and Biofeedback Exercise

Electrical stimulation and biofeedback exercise of pelvic floor muscle has been reported as an effective adjunct to bowel management program for the treatment of fecal incontinence in children following surgery for anorectal malformation.[7] Perineal exercises are found to be more effective around puberty.

RESULTS

More than 90% of the children who follow bowel management remain artificially clean and dry for the entire day and can have a completely normal life. The bowel management program has been in practice for over 20 years.[1] There are no known negative effects that can be attributed to the use of enemas or colonic irrigations. If the specific recommendations of the manufacturer are followed for a phosphate enema, problems of phosphorus intoxication or hypocalcemia have not been seen.[1] Too much salt in the saline solution can lead to sweating, feelings of nausea, and hypernatremia.

Sometimes after a period of successful bowel management, the child becomes incontinent again. This is an indication that something has changed in the child's habits and a thorough evaluation becomes necessary. If the abdominal skiagram shows a large amount of stool in the colon after the enema, the enema solution needs to be adjusted. It can take a week of enemas and skiagrams to make this determination. If the skiagram shows a clean colon then the "accidents" are due to increased motility and it may be necessary to introduce some medications to slow down the colon and to observe a more strict diet.

There are centers where at longer follow-up, there is a significant percentage of subjects who still soil while following a bowel management program. This is explained by the small number of nurses and bowel management specialists who are involved in the rehabilitation process and by the lack of appropriate information about functional prognosis that are conveyed to the parents. Thus psychologic support in bridging the gap between cure and care is critical.[18]

Twenty-five percent of all cases of anorectal malformations that suffered from fecal incontinence significantly improved their quality of life when subjected to a bowel management program.[5]

At good centers, almost all patients born with anorectal malformations can be kept clean of stool and dry of urine, either because they achieve bowel control or because they are subjected to a bowel management program.[5,19-23]

ACKNOWLEDGEMENTS

The authors acknowledge the team of Bowel Management program at Children's Hospital, Cincinnati for carrying out a successful bowel management program. The active members of the team are Alberto Peña, Mark Levitt, Cathy Bauer, Tracy Ashworth and Lindsey Foley. This chapter is based on the 42nd and 43rd workshop on Pediatric Anorectal and Colorectal Surgical workshop, June, 2006 and 2007 at Cincinnati, USA led by Alberto Peña and Mark Levitt.

REFERENCES

1. Peña A, Levitt M. Brocheur of the Bowel Management Program. Colorectal Center for Children Cincinnati Children's Hospital Medical Center. USA 2006.
2. Holschneider A, Hutson J, Peña A, et al. Preliminary report on the International Conference for the Development of Standards for the Treatment of Anorectal Malformations. J Pediatr Surg 2005;40:1521-26.
3. Peña A, Grasshoff S, Levitt M. Reoperations in anorectal malformations. J Pediatr Surg 2007;42:318-25.
4. Youssef NN, Pensabene L, Barksdale E Jr, et al. Is there a role for surgery beyond colonic aganglionosis and anorectal malformations in children with intractable constipation? J Pediatr Surg 2004;39:73-77.
5. Peña A, Hong A. Advances in the management of anorectal malformations. Am J Surg 2000;180:370-76.
6. Levitt MA, Peña A. Outcomes from the correction of anorectal malformations. Curr Opin Pediatr 2005;17: 394-401.
7. Leung MW, Wong BP, Leung AK, et al. Electrical stimulation and biofeedback exercise of pelvic floor muscle for children with fecal incontinence after surgery for anorectal malformation. Pediatr Surg Int 2006;22:975-78.
8. Hamid CH, Holland AJ, Martin HC. Long-term outcome of anorectal malformations: the patient perspective Pediatr Surg Int. 2007 Feb;23(2):97-102. Epub 2006 Dec 14.
9. Uba AF, Chirdan LB, Ardill W, et al. Anorectal anomaly: a review of 82 cases seen at JUTH, Nigeria. Niger Postgrad Med J 2006;13:61-65.
10. Krogh K, Lie HR, Bilenberg N, Laurberg S. Bowel function in Danish children with myelomeningocele. APMIS Suppl 2003;(109):81-85.
11. Griffiths DM. The physiology of continence: idiopathic fecal constipation and soiling. Semin Pediatr Surg 2002;11(2):67-74.
12. Rintala RJ. Fecal incontinence in anorectal malformations, neuropathy, and miscellaneous conditions. Semin Pediatr Surg 2002;11:75-82.
13. Gerasimidis K, McGrogan P, Hassan K, et al. Dietary modifications, nutritional supplements and alternative medicine in paediatric patients with inflammatory bowel disease. Aliment Pharmacol Ther. 2007 Oct 17 [Epub ahead of print].
14. Oztürk H, Onen A, Dokucu AI, et al. Management of anorectal injuries in children: an eighteen-year experience. Eur J Pediatr Surg 2003 Aug;13(4):249-55.
15. Whitehead WE, Wald A, Norton NJ. Treatment options for fecal incontinence. Dis Colon Rectum 2001;44(1): 131-42; discussion 142-44.
16. Krogsgaard SM, Milling MD, Qvist N. Appendicostomy in the treatment of severe defecation disorders in children Ugeskr Laeger 2006 Feb 13;168(7):692-94.

17. Yagmurlu A, Harmon CM, Georgeson KE. Laparoscopic cecostomy button placement for the management of fecal incontinence in children with Hirschsprung's disease and anorectal anomalies. Surg Endosc 2006;20:624-27.
18. Aminoff D, La Sala E, Zaccara A. AIMAR (Italian Parent's Association of Children Born with ARM). Follow-up of anorectal anomalies: the Italian parents' and patients' perspective. J Pediatr Surg 2006;41:837-41.
19. Levitt M, Pena A. Treatment of fecal Incontinence. In Anorectal malformations in children, 1st edition, Ed. John Hutson and Alex Holschneider, Springer Heidelberg 2006; 29:377-83.
20. Peña Alberto. Bowel Management. Lecture delivered during the 20th Congress of Asian Association of Pediatric surgeons. New Delhi 2006.
21. Gupta DK. Anorectal malformations-Wingspread to Krickenbeck. Lecture delivered at Beijing Children hospital, Beijing, China, October 2005.
22. Gupta DK, Sharma Shilpa. Current trends in Anorectal Malformations in Current trends in Pediatrics Vol 3 Ed GP Mathur and Sarla Mathur. Nepal publ. Academa 2006;16:161-73.
23. Sharma Shilpa, Gupta DK. Long-Term outcome of Anorectal Malformations Using the Krickenbeck Criteria. Journal of Indian Association of pediatric surgeons 2006; 11:161.

Pediatric Surgery
Diagnosis and Management
Volume 2

Editor

Devendra K Gupta MS, MCh, FAMS, FAAP, FRCSG (Hon.), DSc (Hon. Causa)
Professor and Head
Department of Pediatric Surgery
All India Institute of Medical Sciences
New Delhi, India

Associate Editor

Shilpa Sharma MS, MCh
Diplomate National Board
Assistant Professor of Pediatric Surgery
Postgraduate Institute of Medical Education and Research
(Dr RML Hospital, New Delhi)
PhD Scholar, Department of Pediatric Surgery
All India Institute of Medical Sciences
New Delhi, India

Guest Editor

Richard G Azizkhan MD, PhD (Hon.), FACS, FAAP
Surgeon-in-Chief
Lester W Martin MD Chair of Pediatric Surgery
Cincinnati Children's Hospital Medical Center
Professor of Surgery and Pediatrics
University of Cincinnati College of Medicine
Cincinnati, Ohio, USA

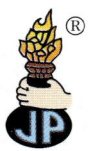

JAYPEE BROTHERS MEDICAL PUBLISHERS (P) LTD
New Delhi • Ahmedabad • Bengaluru • Chennai • Hyderabad • Kochi • Kolkata • Lucknow • Mumbai • Nagpur

Published by
Jitendar P Vij
Jaypee Brothers Medical Publishers (P) Ltd

Corporate Office
4838/24, Ansari Road, Daryaganj, **New Delhi** 110 002, India
Phone: +91-11-43574357

Registered Office
B-3, EMCA House, 23/23B Ansari Road, Daryaganj, **New Delhi** 110 002, India
Phones: +91-11-23272143, +91-11-23272703, +91-11-23282021, +91-11-23245672
Rel: +91-11-32558559 Fax: +91-11-23276490, +91-11-23245683
e-mail: jaypee@jaypeebrothers.com, Website: www.jaypeebrothers.com

Branches

- 2/B, Akruti Society, Jodhpur Gam Road Satellite
  Ahmedabad 380 015   Phones: +91-79-26926233,   Rel: +91-79-32988717
  Fax: +91-79-26927094,   e-mail: ahmedabad@jaypeebrothers.com

- 202 Batavia Chambers, 8 Kumara Krupa Road, Kumara Park East
  Bengaluru 560 001   Phones: +91-80-22285971, +91-80-22382956, +91-80-22372664
  Rel: +91-80-32714073, Fax: +91-80-22281761   e-mail: bangalore@jaypeebrothers.com

- 282 IIIrd Floor, Khaleel Shirazi Estate, Fountain Plaza, Pantheon Road
  Chennai 600 008   Phones: +91-44-28193265, +91-44-28194897,   Rel: +91-44-32972089
  Fax: +91-44-28193231,   e-mail: chennai@jaypeebrothers.com

- 4-2-1067/1-3, 1st Floor, Balaji Building, Ramkote Cross Road
  Hyderabad 500 095   Phones: +91-40-66610020, +91-40-24758498   Rel:+91-40-32940929
  Fax:+91-40-24758499, e-mail: hyderabad@jaypeebrothers.com

- No. 41/3098, B & B1, Kuruvi Building, St. Vincent Road
  Kochi 682 018, Kerala   Phones: +91-484-4036109, +91-484-2395739, +91-484-2395740
  Fax: +91-844-2395740,   e-mail: kochi@jaypeebrothers.com

- 1-A Indian Mirror Street, Wellington Square
  Kolkata 700 013   Phones: +91-33-22651926, +91-33-22276404, +91-33-22276415
  Rel: +91-33-32901926 Fax: +91-33-22656075,   e-mail: kolkata@jaypeebrothers.com

- Lekhraj Market III, B-2, Sector-4, Faizabad Road, Indira Nagar
  Lucknow 226 016   Phones: +91-522-3040553, +91-522-3040554
  Fax: +91-522-3040553 e-mail: lucknow@jaypeebrothers.com

- 106 Amit Industrial Estate, 61 Dr SS Rao Road, Near MGM Hospital, Parel
  Mumbai 400012   Phones: +91-22-24124863, +91-22-24104532,   Rel: +91-22-32926896
  Fax: +91-22-24160828,   e-mail: mumbai@jaypeebrothers.com

- "KAMALPUSHPA" 38, Reshimbag, Opp. Mohota Science College, Umred Road
  Nagpur 440 009 (MS)   Phone: Rel: +91-712-3245220, Fax: +91-712-2704275
  e-mail: nagpur@jaypeebrothers.com

USA Office
1745, Pheasant Run Drive, Maryland Heights (Missouri), MO 63043, USA
Ph: 001-636-6279734   e-mail: jaypee@jaypeebrothers.com, anjulav@jaypeebrothers.com

Pediatric Surgery—Diagnosis and Management
© 2009, Editors

All rights reserved. No part of this publication and DVD ROM should be reproduced, stored in a retrieval system, or transmitted in any form or by any means: electronic, mechanical, photocopying, recording, or otherwise, without the prior written permission of the editor and the publisher.

> This book has been published in good faith that the material provided by contributors is original. Every effort is made to ensure accuracy of material, but the publisher, printer and editor will not be held responsible for any inadvertent error(s). In case of any dispute, all legal matters are to be settled under Delhi jurisdiction only.

First edition: **2009**
ISBN 978-81-8448-439-7
Typeset at JPBMP typesetting unit
Printed at: Ajanta Offset & Packagings Ltd., New Delhi.

Pediatric Surgery
Diagnosis and Management

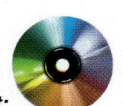

System requirement:
- **Windows XP or above**
- **Power DVD player (Software)**
- **Windows Media Player version 10.0 or above**
- **Quick time player version 6.5 or above**

Accompanying DVD ROM is playable only in Computer and not in DVD player.

Kindly wait for few seconds for DVD to autorun. If it does not autorun then please follow the steps:
- Click on my computer
- Click the **drive labelled JAYPEE** and after opening the drive, kindly double click the file **Jaypee**

DVD CONTENTS

DVD – 1

- **Gastric Transposition** — *DK Gupta*
- **Colonic Interposition** — *A Hamza, DK Gupta*
- **Thal Fundoplication** — *KW Ashcraft*
- **Kasai's Portoenterostomy** — *R Ohi, M Nio*

DVD – 2

- **PSARP in a Male** — *A Pena*
- **PSARP in a Female** — *A Pena*
- **Common Cloaca** — *A Pena*

Contributors

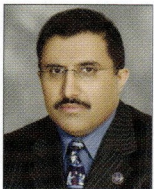

Aayed Al-Qahtani MD, FRCSC, FACS, FAAP
Associate Prof and consultant of
Pediatric surgery,
College of Medicine
King Saud University
PO Box-84147
Riyadh-11671, Saudi Arabia

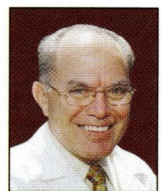

Alberto Pena MD
Director, Colorectal Division
Cincinnati Children's Hospital
Medical Center, University of
Cincinnati College of Medicine, 3333
Burnet Avenue, Cincinnati
Ohio/USA 45229-3039

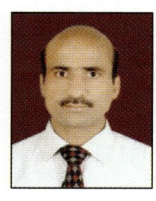

Abhinit Kumar MD
334, South Point Clinic
Vardman City Plus Mall
Dwarka
Sector 22
New Delhi-75

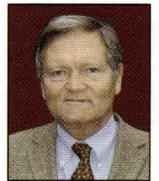

Alex Holshneider MD
Former Professor of Pediatric Surgery
Immenzaun, 6 A
51429 BERG
Gladbach, Koln
Germany

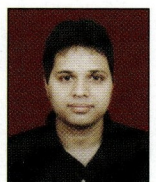

Ajay Kumar MD, PhD, DNB, MNAMS
Post-Doctoral Fellow, Pediatrics and
Neurology, Children Hospital of
Michigan School of Medicine,
Wayne State University, 3901 Beaubien
Street, Detroit MI, 48201, USA

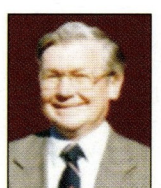

Alois F Scharli MD
Formerly, Professor and Head
Department of Pediatric Surgery
Pilatusstrasse 1 CH6003
Lucerne
Switzerland

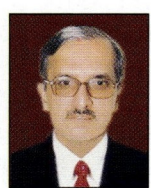

AK Mahapatra MS, MCh
Director
Professor and Head
Department of Neurosurgery
Sanjay Gandhi Postgraduate Institute
Lucknow, India

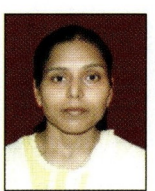

Alpana Prasad MS, MCh
Senior Consultant
Pediatric Surgeon
Fortis Hospital
Noida

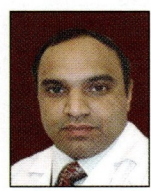

Akshay Chauhan MBBS, MCh
Fellow, Pediatric Urology
Surgical Services
Cincinnati Children Hospital and
Medical Center, Cincinnati
Ohio-45209

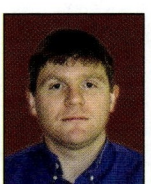

Alun R Williams FRCS
Consultant Pediatric Surgeon
Department of Pediatric Surgery
University Hospital
Queen's Medical Center Nottingham
NG7 2UH (UK)

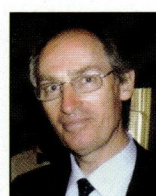

Alastair JW Millar MBBS
FRCS (Eng), (Ed) FRACS, DCH
Charles F M Saint Professor of
Pediatric Surgery, University of Cape
Town and Red Cross Children's
Hospital, University of Cape Town
Cape Town, South Africa

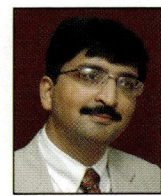

Amar Shah MS MCh, FRCS (Ped. Surgery)
Amardeep Multispeciality Children
Hospital, 65
Pritamnagar Society, Ellisbridge
Ahmedabad-06
India

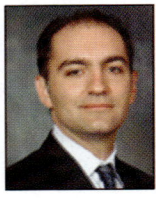

Amir Kaviani MD
Staff Surgeon
Vascular lab
Association of South Bay Surgeons
Torrance, CA

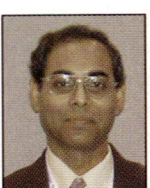

Amit K Dinda MD, PhD
Additional Professor
Department of Pathology and
Sub-Dean (examination)
All India Institute of Medical
Sciences, New Delhi-29

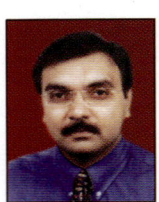

Amulya K Saxena MD, PhD
Associate Professor
Department of Pediatric and
Adolescent Surgery, Medical
University of Graz
Auenbruggerplatz-34
A-8036, Graz, Austria

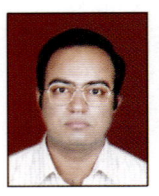

Anand Sharma MBBS, MD, FRCA
Specialist registrar, Anesthesia and
Intensive care, Addenbrookes
University Hospital, Hills Road
Cambridge, Cambridgeshire
CB22QQ, United Kingdom

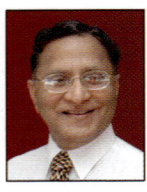

Anirudh Shah MS, FRCS(Eng), FRCS (Edin)
Director
Amardeep Multispeciality Children
Hospital, 65, Pritamnagar Society
Ellisbridge, Ahmedabad-380006
India

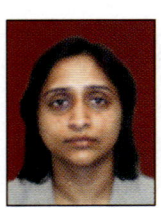

Anju Goyal MBBS, MS, MCh(Paed Surg),
MRCS, FRCS(Paed)
Specialist Registrar in Pediatric
Surgery and Urology, Royal
Manchester Children's Hospital
Hospital Road
Manchester, M27 4HA, UK

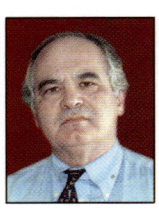

Antonio Dessanti MD, PhD
Professor of Pediatric Surgery
Head of Unit of Pediatric Surgery
University of Sassari, Azienda
Ospedaliero Universitaria. Viale S
Pietro, 43. 07100, Sassari, Italy

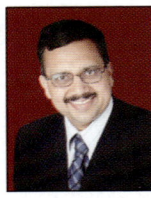

Anurag Bajpai MBBS, MD, FRACP
Consultant Pediatric Endocrinologist
Department of Endocrinology and
Diabetes, Royal Children's Hospital
Flemington Road, Parkville
Victoria, Melbourne-3052

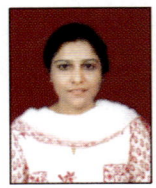

Archana Puri MS, MCh
Assistant Professor of Pediatric
Surgery, Lady Hardinge Medical
College and Associated Kalawati
Saran Children's Hospital
New Delhi-1

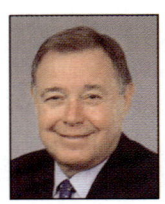

Arnold Coran AB, MD
Professor of Pediatric Surgery
University of Michigan Medical
School, C.S. Mott Children's Hospital,
F3970 Pediatric Surgery 1500 E
Medical Center Drive
Ann Arbor, MI, USA 48109-5245

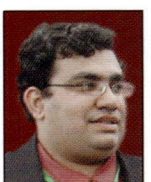

Arun Choudhary MD
Research Fellow in Medicine
(Gastroenterology), Center for
Swallowing and Motility Disorders
VA Boston Healthcare System
Harvard Medical School and Beth
Israel Deaconess Medical Center
Boston, USA.

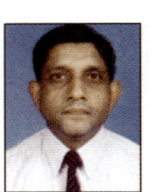

Arun Kumar Gupta MD
Professor and Head
Department of Radiology
All India Institute of Medical Sciences
New Delhi-29
India

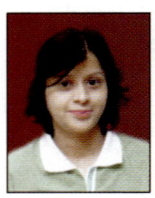

Arundhati Panigrahi MSc, PhD
Scientist, Department of
Transplantation and Immunogenetics
All India Institute of Medical Sciences
New Delhi-29
India

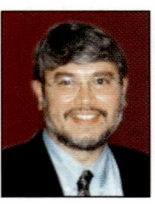

Ashley D'cruz MS, MCh
Former Professor and Head
Department of Pediatric Surgery
St John's Medical College Hospital
Bangalore-560034

Contributors vii

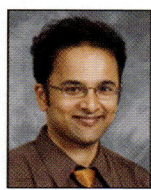
Ashok Srinivasan MD
Clinical Assistant Professor
Division of Neuroradiology
Department of Radiology
University of Michigan
USA

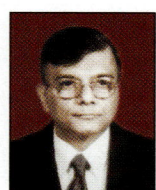
Ashoke K Basu MS, MCh
Consultant
Pediatric Surgeon
90, Ballygunge Place
Kolkata
West Bengal

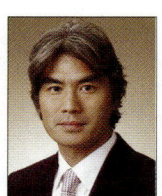
Atsuyuki Yamataka MD, PhD
Professor and Head
Pediatric General and Urogenital
Surgery, Juntendo University School
of Medicine, 2-1-1
Hongo, Bunkyo
Tokyo, 113-8421, Japan

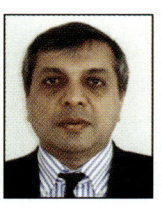
Azad B Mathur MS, MCh,
FRCS (Eng), FRCS (G)
Consultant Pediatric Surgeon
Jenny Lind Department of Pediatric
Surgery, Norfolk and Norwich
University, Hospital, Norwich Colney
Lane, NR4 7UY, United Kingdom

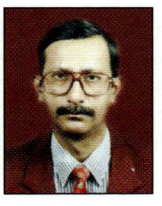
B Mukhopadhyay MS, MCh, FRCS
Professor and Head
NRS Medical College
Kolkata
West Bengal

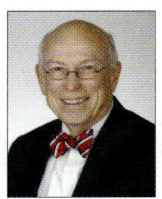
B Othersen Jr MD
Professor of Surgery and Pediatrics
Emeritus chief Pediatric Surgery
Medical University of South Carolina
Charleston, SC, USA

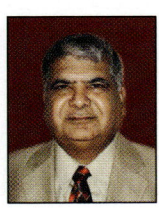
Bikramjit S Sangha MD
Attending Neonatologist
Kaiser Permanente–
Los Angeles Medical Center
USA

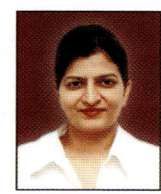
Bobby Batra MD
Director of Pediatrics
Detroit Medical Group
8125 Chatham Drive
Canton, MI
48187, USA

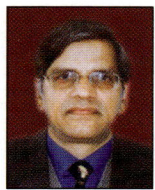
BS Sharma MS, MCh
Professor and Head
Department of Neurosurgery
All India Institute of Medical Science
Ansari Nagar
New Delhi

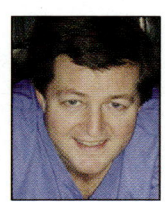
Carl F Davis MBMCh, FRCS(I)
FRCS (Glas), FRCS (Paed)
Consultant Pediatric Surgeon and
Neonatal Surgeon
Royal Hospital for Sick Children
Yorkhill, Glasgow G3 8 SJ
Scotland

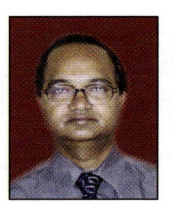
Chandersen K Sinha
MS, FRCS, MChMS, FRCS, MCh (Paed Surg)
Senior Specialist Registrar
Department of Pediatric Surgery
Denmark Hill
London SE5 9RS, UK

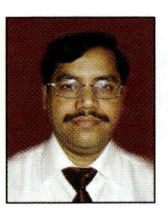
CS Bal MD
Professor
Department of Nuclear Medicine
All India Institute of Medical Sciences
New Delhi, India

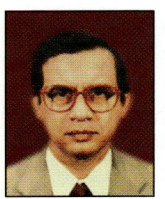
D Basak MS, MCh
Consultant Pediatric Surgeon
Pediatric Surgery
Peerless Hospital
223, C. R. Avenue
Kolkata

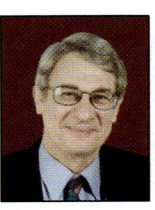
David A Lloyd MChir (Cantab)
FCS(SA), FRCS(Eng), FRCS(C), FACS
Professor of Pediatric Surgery
Department of Child Health
Alder Hey Children's Hospital
Eaton Road, Liverpool, L12 2AP

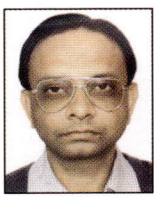
Deep N Srivastava MD
Professor, Department of Radiology
All India Institute of Medical Scinces
New Delhi-29, India

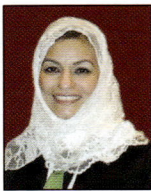
Enaam Raboei MD, PhD
Consultant Pediatric Surgeon
Chief of Pediatric Surgery
King Fahd Armed Forces Hospital
Jeddah 21159, PO Box-9862
Kingdom of Saudi Arabia

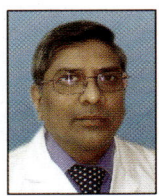
Devendra K Gupta MS, MCh
FAAP, FRCSG (Hon.), FAMS, DSc (Hon. Causa)
Professor and Head
Department of Pediatric Surgery
All India Institute of Medical Sciences
New Delhi-29, India

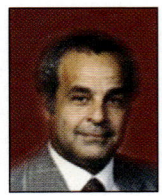
Essam El-Sahwi MD
5 Ahmed Abdel-Salam Street
El Sultan Hussein
El Attarin, Alexandria
Egypt

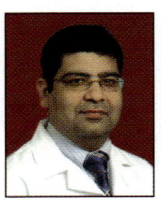
Dheeraj Gandhi MBBS, MD
Director
Interventional Neuroradiology
Assistant Professor of Radiology and
Neurosurgery, 1500 E Medical
Center Drive, Ann Arbor, MI 48109

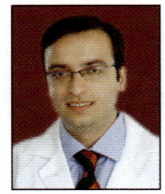
Faiz-ud-din Ahmad MBBS, MCh
Fellow, Pediatric Neurosurgery
Jackson Memorial Hospital
Miller school of Medicine, University
of Miami, Lious Pope Life Centre
1400 NW, 10th Avenue 2nd Floor
(Neurosurgery) Florida USA, 33136

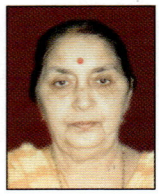
DK Agarwal MD
Ex-Prof and Head Pediatrics
Institute of Medical Sciences Varanasi
D-115, Sector 36
Noida- 201301

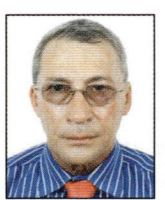
Gabriel O Ionescu MD, PhD
Professor, Iasi, Romania
Pretoria, RSA
Tawam Hospital
UAE

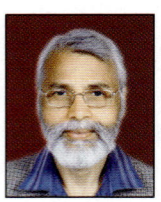
DK Pawar MD
Professor
Department of Anesthesiology
All India Institute of Medical Scinces
New Delhi-29, India

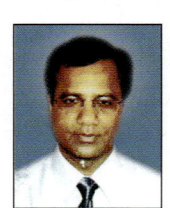
Ganga Prasad MD
Additional Professor
Department of Anesthesiology
All India Institute of Medical Sciences
New Delhi-29, India

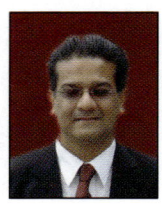
DN Jha MS
Consultant ENT Surgeon
Apollo Hospital
Colombo
Srilanka

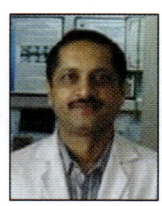
GD Satyarathee MS, MCh
Assistant Profeesor
Department of Neurosurgery
All India Institute of Medical Sciences
New Delhi-29, India

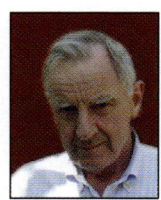
Edward Kiely FRCS
Consultant Pediatric Surgeon
The Hospital for Sick Children
Great Ormond Street
London
WC1N 3JH, UK

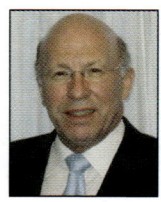
GH Willital MD, PhD
Chief of the International Institute for
Children's Surgery,
Münster Research Institute
Hansaring 94, Greven Münster 48268
Germany

Contributors ix

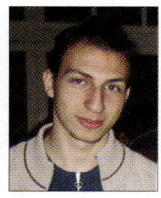
Giacomo Parigi BS
Department of Computer Sciences
Faculty of Engineering
University of Pavia
Italy

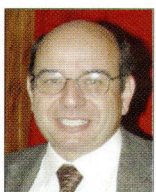
Gian Battista Parigi MD, FEBPS
Director, Specialization School in
Pediatric Surgery
Associate Professor of Pediatric
Surgery, University of Pavia
Pavia, Italy

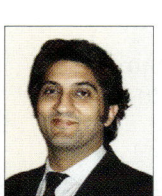
Gunninder Soin FRCS
Brownlow Group Practice
70 Pembroke Place
Liverpool
L69 3GF
UK

GVS Murthi
Department of Surgical Pediatrics
Royal Hospital For Sick Children
Yorkhill, Glasgow G3 8 55
Scotland

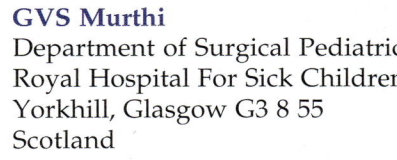
Htut Saing MD, PhD
Emeritus Professor
University of Hong Kong
2512 Aspen Valley Lane
Sacramento, CA 95835
USA

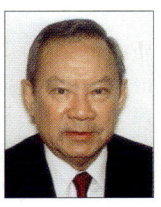
Hussam S Hassan MS, FRCS
Lecturer of Pediatric Surgery
Tanta University
Egypt

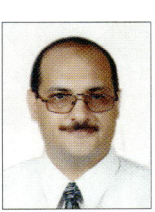
IC Pathak MS, FRCS
Professor Emeritus
Department of Pediatric Surgery
Post Graduate Institute of Medical
Education and Research
Chandigarh, India

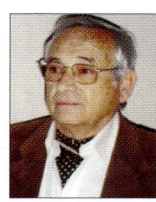
J Boix-Ochoa MD, PhD
Emeritus Professor
Can Tio
PO Box-308490
Tordera-BCN
SPAIN

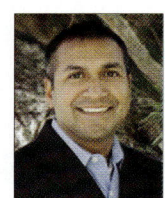
Jayant Agarwal MS
Assistant professor
Department of Surgery, Division of
Plastic Surgery, University of Utah
School of Medicine, Huntsman
Cancer Institute, 2000 Circle of Hope
Salt Lake City, UT 84112, USA

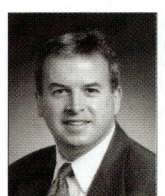
John J Aiken MD
Associate Professor
Division of Pediatric SurgeryMedical
College of Wisconsin Children's
Hospital of Wisconsin, 999 N
92nd Street, Ste. 320 Milwaukee
WI 53226

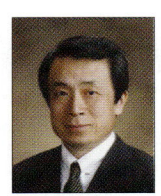
K Hashizume MD, PhD
Formerly, Professor and Head
Department of Pediatric Surgery
Graduate School of Medicine
The University of Tokyo
Tokyo, Japan

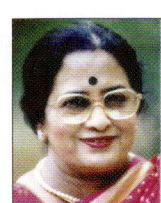
K Mathingi Ramakrishnan FRCS (Eng)
FRCS (Edin), MCh, DSc, DSc (Hon CAusa, BHU), FAMS
Director, CHILDS Trust Medical
Research Foundation, Chief of
Pediatric Burns Intensive Care Unit
and Department of Plastic Surgery
KK CHILDS Trust Hospital
Chennai-600034

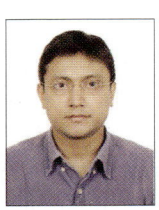
Kamalesh Pal MS, MCh
PO Box- 40129 Assistant Professor
Pediatric Surgery Division
King Fahad Hospital of the
University, Al Khobar 31952
Kingdom of Saudi Arabia

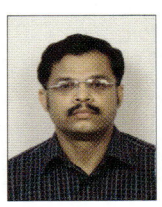
Kanishka Das MS, MCh
Professor and Head
Department of Pediatric Surgery
St John's Medical College Hospital
Bangalore-56003

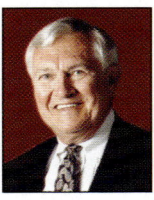
Keith Ashcraft MD
Emeritus Professor of Surgery
University of Missouri at Kansas City
School of Medicine, Former Surgeon-
in-Chief, Children's Mercy Hospital
Kansas City, Missouri

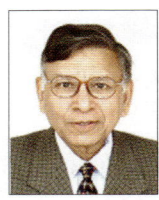
KN Agarwal MD
Hon. Scientist, Indian National
Science Academy and President
health Care and Res Ass for
Adolescents, D-115, Sector 36
Noida-201301

Kurush Paya MD
Associate Professor of Pediatric
Surgery, Dept of Surgery,
Div. of Pediatric Surgery
Medical University of Vienna
Waehringerguertel 18-20
Vienna, Austria

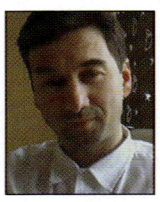
Lalit Parida MBBS, MCh
Pediatric Surgeon
King Fahad Specialist Hospital
PO Box-15215
Dammam 31444
Saudi Arabia

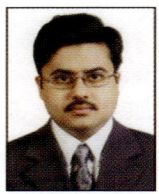
Leela Kapila FRCS, OBE
Formerly, Consultant Pediatric
Surgeon
University Hospital Queen's
Medical Centre, Nottingham
NG7 2 UH UK

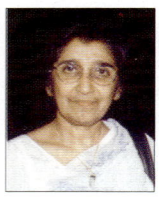
Li Long MD, PhD
Department of Pediatric Surgery
The Capital Institution of Pediatrics
Yabao Rd. 2, Beijing-100020
China

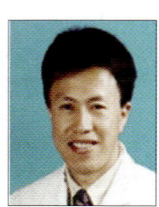
LW Martin MD
Chair of Pediatric Surgery, Cincinnati
Children's Hospital Medical Center
Professor of Surgery and Pediatrics
University of Cincinnati School of
Medicine, 3333 Burnet Avenue
Cincinnati, Ohio 45229

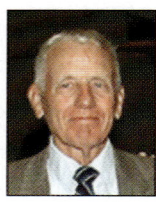

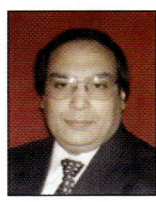
M Bajpai MS, MCh,
Diplomate National Board, PhD
Professor
Department of Pediatric Surgery
All India Institute of Medical Sciences
New Delhi-29, India

M Charles Washington MSc, MPhil
Professor, Child Health Nursing
Department, St John's College of
Nursing, SJNAHS, Sarjar Road
Bangalore, India

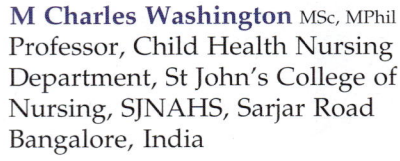

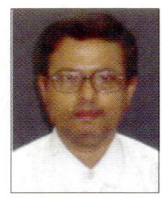
M K Bhattacharya MS, MCh
Asstt Professor
Department of Pediatric Surgery
Dr. B. C. Roy Memorial Hospital for
Children, Kolkata

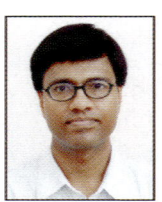
M Srinivas MS, MCh
Associate Professor
Department of Pediatric Surgery
All India Institute of Medical Sciences
New Delhi, India

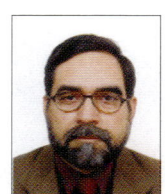
Mahesh K Arora MD
Professor
Department of Anesthesiology
All India Institute of Medical Sciences
New Delhi-29, India

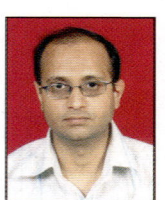
Manish Pathak MBBS, MCh
51, Shanti Niketan Colony
Barkat Nagar
Jaipur, Rajasthan-302015
India

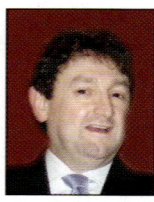
Mark Davenport ChM, FRCS (Paed Surg)
FRCS (Eng), FRCPS (Glas)
Consultant Pediatric Surgeon
Department of Pediatric Surgery
Kings College Hospital
Denmark Hill, London, SE5 9RS

Contributors xi

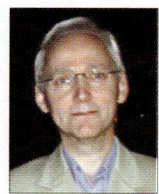

Mark Stringer BSc, MS, FRCS, FRCS (Paed.), FRCP, FRCPCH
Consultant Pediatric Surgeon Clinical Anatomist (Former Professor of Pediatric Surgery), Anatomy and Structural Biology, Otago School of Medical Sciences, University of Otago, Great King Street, Dunedin
New Zealand-9054

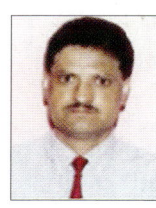

Nissar Ahmed Bhat MS, MCh
Assistant Professor
Department of Pediatric Surgery
Shere Kashmere Institute of Medical Sciences, Srinagar
Jammu and Kashmir, India

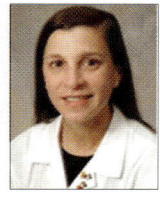

Mindy Statter FRCS
Associate Professor of Surgery and Pediatric Surgery
Section of Pediatric Surgery
University of Chicago
Chicago, IL, USA 60637

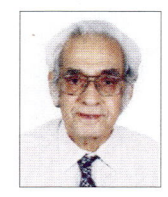

P Madhok MS, FRCS
Ashwani Nursing Home
15th Road
Khar
Mumbai-400052

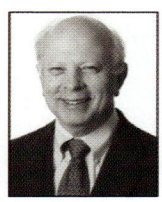

Moritz M Ziegler MD
Surgeon-in-Chief and the Ponzio Family Chair, The Children's Hospital, 13123 East 16th Avenue B323 Aurora, Colorado
USA 80045

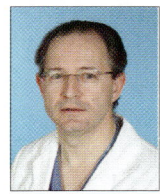

Paul D Losty MD, FRCSI, FRCS(Eng) FRCS(Ed), FRCS(Paed)
Professor, Department of Pediatric Surgery Institute of Child Health
Royal Liverpool Children's Hospital (Alder Hey) & The University of Liverpool, UK

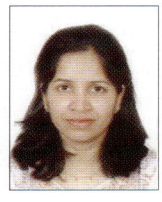

Mrunalini Chavarkar MD, MCh
Department Of Pediatrics
Louisiana State University
New Orleans
LA-70118, USA

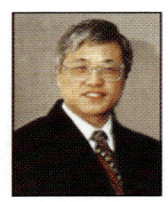

Paul KH Tam
Pro Vice Chancellor
Division of Pediatric Surgery
Department of Surgery
Queen Mary Hospital, K 15
Pokfulam, Hong Kong SAR
University of HongKong, China

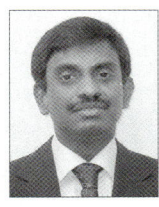

N Kumaran MS, MCh, FRCS
Formerly, Specialist Registrar in Pediatric Surgery, Mailpoint 44
Southampton General Hospital
Southampton SO16 6YD
United Kingdom

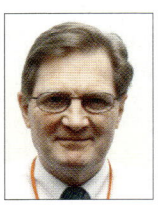

Peter AM Raine FRCS
Formerly, Professor
Royal Hospital for Sick Children
Yorkhill Glasgow
G3 8 SJ, Scotland

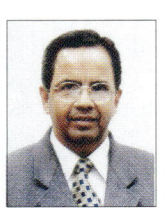

Narinder K Mehra MD, DSc
Professor and Head
Department of Transplantation and Immunogenetics
All India Institute of Medical Sciences
New Delhi-29, India

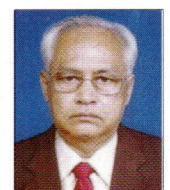

Pradip Mukherjee MS, MCh
Formerly, Professor and Head
Department of Pediatric Surgery
N. R. S. Medical College
Kolkata

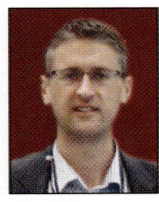

NC Featherstone FRCS
Specialist Registrar Pediatric Surgery
Norfolk and Norwich University
Foundation Trust Hospital
Colney lane, Norwich, UK

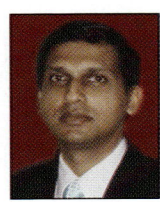

Prakash Agarwal MS, MCh
Associate Professor
Department of Pediatric Surgery
Sri Ramachandra University
Porur, Chennai-600116

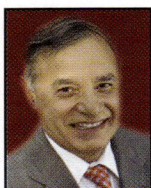

Prem Puri MS, FRCS
Consultant Pediatric Surgeon and
Director of Surgical Research
Children's Research Centre
Our Lady's Children's Hospital
Crumlin, Dublin 12, Ireland

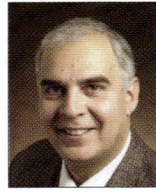

Richard Azizkhan MD, PhD, FACS, FAAP
Surgeon-in-Chief, Lester Martin Chair
in Pediatric Surgery, Cincinnati
Children's Hospital Medical Center
University of Cincinnati College of
Medicine, 3333 Burnet Avenue
Cincinnati, Ohio/USA 45229-3039

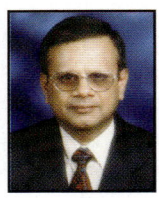

PSN Menon MD, MNAMS(Ped)
Consultant and Head
Department of Pediatrics
Jaber Al-Ahmed Armed Forces
Hospital, Kuwait

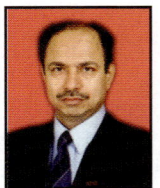

RK Batra MD
Professor
Department of Anesthesiology
All India Institute of Medical Sciences
New Delhi-29, India

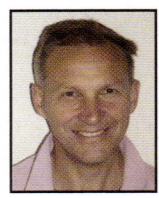

RA Wheeler MS, LLB, FRCS
Consultant Pediatric Surgeon
Lecturer in Medical Law Wessex
Regional Centre for Pediatric Surgery
Southampton General Hospital
Southampton
SO16 6YD, UK

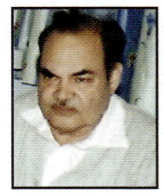

RK Tandon MS, MCh
Professor and Head
Department of pediatric Surgery
C.S.M. Medical University
Lucknow-226003

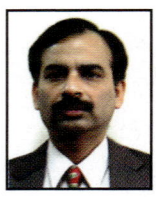

Rajesh Malhotra MS
Professor
Department of Orthopedics
All India Institute of Medical Sciences
New Delhi-29, India

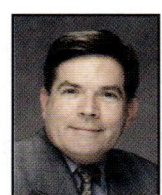

Robert Arensman MD, PhD
Emeritus Professor of Surgery and
Pediatrics, Northwestern University
and University of Chicago, Former
Surgeon-in-Chief, Children's
Memorial Hospital and the Wyler
Children's Hospital, Chicago, USA

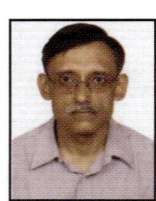

Rajiv Chadha DA, MS, MCh
Professor, Department of Pediatric
Surgery, Lady Hardinge Medical
College and Associated Kalawati
Saran Children's Hospital
New Delhi-01, India

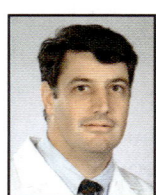

Robert Cywes MD, PhD, FRCS
Director Jacksonville Surgical
Associates, PA Wolfson
Children's Hospital
USA

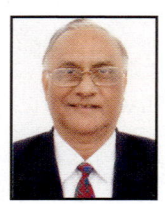

RC Deka MS, FAMS
Dean,
Professor and Head
Department of Otorhinolaryngology
All India Institute of Medical Sciences
New Delhi-29, India

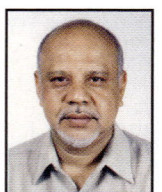

Supriyo Ghose MS
Professor and Head
Chief of Centre for Ophthalmic
Sciences
All India Institute of Medical Sciences
New Delhi-29, India

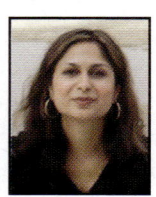

Reena Bhargava MD, FRCSC
Bariatric Health Centres
200 Fairview Road West
Toronto, Ontario
L5B 1K8, Canada

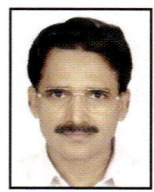

S N Kureel MS, MCh
Professor
Department of Pediatric Surgery
CS M Medical University
Lucknow-226003

Contributors xiii

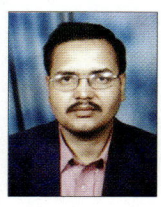

S Nainiwal MD, DNB, MNAMS
Asstt Professor, Ophthalmology
JLN Medical College
Ajmer, Rajasthan

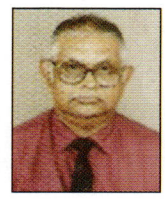

SK Mitra MS, MCh, FRCS
Formerly, Professor and Head
Department of Pediatric Surgery
Postgraduate Institute of Medical
Sciences, Chandigarh

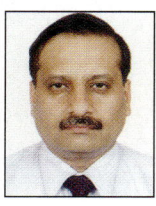

Sandeep Agarwala MBBS, MCh
Associate Professor
Department of Pediatric Surgery
All India Institute of Medical Sciences
New Delhi-29, India

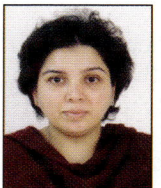

Sonika Aggarwal MD
Senior Resident
Department of Gynecology/
Obstetrics, All India Institute of
Medical Sciences, New Delhi-29
India

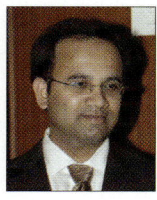

Sangamalai Manoharan FRCS
Specialist Registrar, Pediatric
Urology/Surgery, Nottingham
University Hospitals NHS Trust
Queens Medical Centre
Derby Road, Nottingham NG7 2UH
United Kingdom

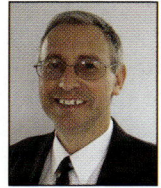

Spencer Beasley MBChB (Otago)
MS (Melb), FRACS
Consultant Pediatric Surgeon
Department of Pediatric Surgery
Christchurch Hospital
Christchurch, New Zealand

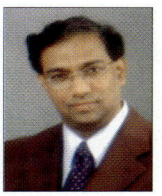

Sanjay Oak MS, MCh
Dean, Professor and Head
Dept of Pediatric Surgery
B Y L Nair Hospital
Mumbai

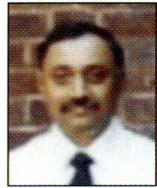

Sudipta Sen MS, MCh
Professor and Head
Department of Pediatric Surgery
Christian Medical College
Vellore

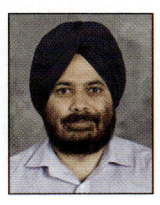

Shailinder Jit Singh MS, DNB, MCh, FRCSI
FRCS (Eng), FRCS (Paed. Surgery)
Consultant Pediatric Surgeon and
Programme Director, University
Hospital, Queen's Medical Centre
Nottingham (UK)
NG7 2UH

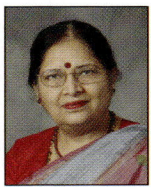

Suneeta Mittal MD, FAMA, FRCOG
FICOG, FICMCH, FIMSA
Professor and Head, Department of
Gynecology
All India Institute of Medical Sciences
New Delhi-29, India

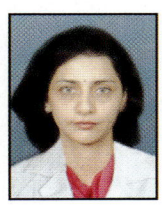

Shilpa Sharma MS, MCh, DNB
Assistant Professor
Postgraduate Institute of Medical
Education and Research
Dr RML Hospital, PhD Scholar
Department of Pediatric Surgery
All India Institute of Medical Sciences
New Delhi-29, India

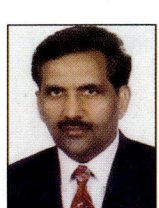

Suresh Chandra Sharma MS
Professor
Department of Otorhinolaryngology
All India Institute of Medical Sciences
New Delhi-29, India

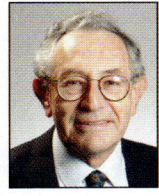

Sid Cywes MD, FACS (Ped), FRCS(Eng)
FRCS(Edin), FRCPS(Glas), FAAP (Hon.), FCS (SA)
(Hon), DSc (UCT) (Hon.)
Emeritus Professor, Department of
Pediatric Surgery, School of Child
and Adolescent Health, Red Cross
War Memorial Children's Hospital
University of Cape Town

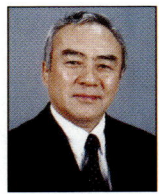

Takeshi Miyano MD, PhD
Emeritus Professor
Department of Pediatric Surgery
Juntendo University School of
Medicine, 2-1-1 Hongo, Bunkyo-ku
Tokyo-113-8421, Japan

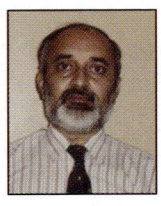
V Bhatnagar MS, MCh, FNASc, FIMSA, FAMS
Professor
Department of Paediatric Surgery
All India Institute of Medical Sciences
New Delhi 29, India

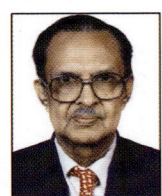
V Ravi Kumar MS, MCh
Consultant Peditatric Surgeon
GKNM hospital
Pappanayakkan palayam
Coimbatore-38

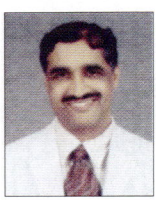
V Jayaraman MS, MCh
Consultant Plastic Surgeon, CHILDS Trust Hospital, Pediatric Burns Intensive Care Unit and Department of Plastic Surgery, K.K. CHILDS Trust Hospital, Chennai-600 034

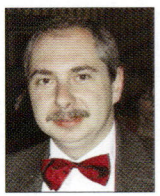
Vadim Kapuller MD, FRCS
Surgery Alef Department
Kaplan Medical Center
PO Box 1, Rehovot, Israel

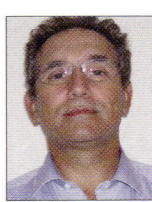
V Martinez Ibañez MD, PhD
Chairman, Department of Pediatric Surgery Hospital, Vall d'Hebron
Autonomous University of Barcelona
Spain

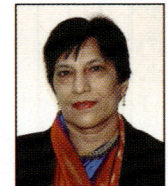
Veena Kalra MD, FAMS
Former Professor and Head
Department of Pediatrics
All India Institute of Medical Sciences
New Delhi-29, India

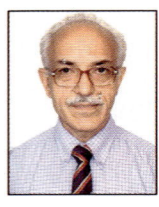
V P Choudhary
MD, FIAP, FIMSA, FIACM, FISHTM
Former Professor and Head
Department of Hematology
All India Institute of Medical Science
New Delhi-29, India

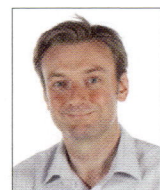
Walker Gregor M BSc(Hons), MBChB, MD FRCS(Ed), FRCS(Paed)
Consultant Pediatric Surgeon and Neonatal surgeon
Royal Hospital for Sick Children
Yorkhill, Glasgow, G3 8 SJ, Scotland

Foreword

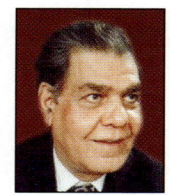

This book marks an important milestone in the growth of pediatric surgery in India. Its significance is indicated by the fact that it has been officially sponsored by IAPS, the Indian Association of Pediatric Surgeons.

The IAPS has grown, from a modest beginning in 1965, into a vibrant organization with more than 900 members. Thirty to thirty-five new members join each year after completing their training in 23 centers in the country. It is, therefore, time for it to have its own standard compendium of information relevant to the needs of its members. Trainees too need an authoritative textbook written by experts who are familiar with the needs of a developing country like India. Unfortunately, books written and published in the West are too exhaustive, often prohibitively expensive and largely unrealistic for our needs. I have no doubt that pediatric surgical trainees in neighboring countries of Asia will also appreciate the significance of this book.

There are more than 400 million children below the age of 12 years in India and the volume of surgical work is simply astounding. The kind of experience that a pediatric surgeon gets in India is the envy of many a surgeons in the developed world. Yet it is not very often that Indian authors find a place in the list of contributors to books published in the west and one gets the impression that children's surgery hardly exists in this vast subcontinent. Our authors need to be recognized for their rich and authentic experience. At the same time, our trainees need to be acquainted with the wide range of expertise from abroad. They need to have a broad vision, yet focused to the needs of a country like India. This is another valid reason for bringing out this book.

It is commendable that Professor Devendra K Gupta, Chief of pediatric surgery at the All India Institute of Medical Sciences has been chosen as the Editor. Professor Gupta is a highly regarded leader in pediatric surgery, recognized nationally and internationally for his writings. He has a wide base of valuable experience, which is admirably reflected in his editorship of this book. He has, very wisely, taken a younger colleague Dr Shilpa Sharma as Associate Editor to bring in, open-minded dynamism of the youth in the editing process. Significantly, he has also succeeded in getting the able guidance of Prof Richard Azizkhan, of Cincinnati, USA, as Guest Editor.

Professor Gupta has chosen contributors who are either working in India or who have been associated with Indian departments of pediatric surgery for some time. In fact, nearly one third of the contributors are working in countries abroad. It is noteworthy that authors have been selected not so much for their prominence in the profession as for proficiency in their fields of interest. In the fast changing world of medicine, dynamic young surgeons have acquired new expertise and amassed enormous experience that would be unimaginable in the West. I heartily welcome this move to include younger authors. They may not be well known today, but they certainly need to be taken note of, for they will be the leaders of tomorrow.

It usually takes several years to produce a multi-authored book – it is hard work collecting manuscripts and making the matter suitable for publication. Often, the information is outdated, if not obsolete, by the time the book is published. I would like to compliment the editors for bringing out this book as quickly as they have. The information provided is current, and presented with clarity of expression. Surgical techniques are described in a way that facilitates understanding. Wherever necessary, the subject has been discussed by more than one author so that varying points of view are accommodated.

I feel assured that this book will become an invaluable aid to pediatric surgeons not only in India but also in other parts of the world. With this book the editors have given an international identity to Indian pediatric surgery. This in itself is a commendable achievement.

Purushottam Upadhyaya MS, FRCS, FAMS
Emeritus Professor and Advisor
Himalayan Institute of Medical Sciences
Dehra Dun, India

Foreword

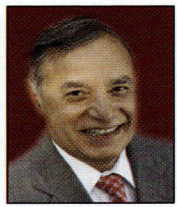

Professor Devendra Gupta deserves to be congratulated for his enormous effort in producing this valuable textbook in pediatric surgery. This book which comprises 130 chapters and 132 contributors from all five continents of the world provides an authoritative, comprehensive and complete account of various surgical conditions in children. This detailed reference text is suitable for both specialist pediatric surgeons as well as trainees in pediatric surgery as it covers both common and uncommon paediatric surgical conditions. The book has the added attraction because it covers recent developments in the care of children with congenital malformations and acquired surgical conditions. There are full chapters devoted to ethics in pediatric surgery, robotics, stem cell therapy, tissue engineering, laser applications in pediatric surgery, nanotechnology and computers.

Professor Gupta was successful in persuading well known pediatric surgeons to provide an authoritative and complete account of their respective topics. Pediatric surgical community should find this book a useful reference in the management of childhood surgical disorders.

We applaud the efforts of Professor Gupta and contributors for this comprehensive textbook in pediatric surgery.

Prem Puri MS, FRCS, FRCS (Ed), FACS
President, World Federation of Associations of Pediatric Surgeons

Preface

*" It is not enough to begin. Continuance is necessary.
The reason of failure in most cases is lack of perseverance."*

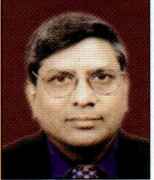

Though there are number of high quality books available in pediatric surgery, yet most of them are not accessible to the majority of pediatric surgeons in the world due to their high cost. The proposal from the Indian Association of Pediatric Surgeons (IAPS) to publish a multi-authored pediatric surgery book that was complete in all respects and still affordable, was quite a challenge. The Editor accepted this responsibility to bring out a book that would be of international quality, high in scientific value and still low in cost. To accomplish this task, the help and support received from Dr Shilpa Sharma as the Associate Editor and Prof Richard Azizkhan as the Guest Editor were simply outstanding and are greatly acknowledged.

The initial concept for the book was to include many pediatric surgical sub-specialties, e.g. General Pediatric Surgery, Neonatal Surgery, Pediatric Oncology, Pediatric Urology, Cardiothoracic Surgery and others, all in a single book. However, since the contents became too voluminous, this book was restricted to "Pediatric Surgery—Diagnosis and Management", primarily to cover general pediatric surgery; yet still these required two volumes to keep the book handy.

The scope of the book remains very broad and covers the spectrum of General Pediatric Surgery. It includes some relevant basic science, embryology and pathophysiology, diagnosis and management, as well as complications and includes long-term results. The descriptions and pictures of operative procedures have also been added wherever indicated. Many subjects have been covered by more than one expert still without duplicating the text.

The book with about 1200 figures (Clinical photographs, flow charts, X-rays and the ones drawn by the artist) makes it unique. The book also includes chapters on Nanotechnology, Minimal invasive procedures, Endoscopic procedures, Lasers, Robotic surgery, Stem cell regeneration, Tissue engineering, Computers and Molecular genetics to offer state-of-the-art information to the pediatric surgical community. The book also extends to adolescent surgery as it includes the chapters on Empyema, Intestinal obstruction, Bariatric surgery, Tuberculosis, Hydatid disease and Bezoars.

The authors in this book have been outstanding. Their contributions have been excellent. I was rather bestowed with faith to edit their work (Chapters, photographs, charts, tables, references, etc.), so as to maintain uniformity and regular flow of thoughts.

A foreword for this book has been written by Prof P Upadhyaya who had not only been my teacher and the Founder Professor and the Chief of the Department of Pediatric Surgery at the All India Institute of Medical Sciences, New Delhi, but also a perfectionist, and an academician with utmost human values. Prof Prem Puri, President of WOFAPS who is known internationally for his deep interest in research and surgical care has not only applauded our efforts but written a Foreword as well.

The support received from the colleagues and the staff from the department at All India Institute of Medical Sciences, New Delhi (AIIMS), especially from Mr Ved Grover, is greatly appreciated. I also thank my wife, Dr Rani and the daughters Dr Malvika and Deepika, for being the force behind to complete this book.

The book has been published by M/s Jaypee Brothers, the reputed exclusive Medical Publishers from New Delhi. Shri JP Vij, Chairman and Managing Director; Mr Tarun Duneja, the Director (Publishing), had shown special interest while publishing this book.

It is hoped that the book would serve its purpose if it reaches the pediatric surgical community in the developed and the developing world alike, for its scientific contents, quality of production, affordability and balanced approach.

When you light a lantern for another, it brightens up your path as well —Nichiren Daishonin.

Devendra K Gupta

Message

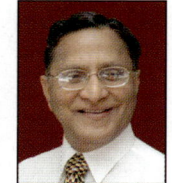

On behalf of the Indian Association of Pediatric Surgeons (IAPS), I take great honour and privilege to write a brief message for the long awaited book *"Pediatric Surgery—Diagnosis and Management"*, edited by Prof DK Gupta. The book published by Jaypee Brothers, New Delhi has been creditably supported by the rich experience of Prof Richard Azizkhan from Cincinnati Children Hospital, USA and Dr Shilpa Sharma from New Delhi.

It was the year 2000 that after the success of *"Textbook of Neonatal surgery"* published by Dr DK Gupta, the IAPS wanted more such books in the specialty and thus requested Dr Gupta to bring out the much needed book in Pediatric Surgery that would be complete, informative, affordable and at the same time matched with the best international standards in its presentation and scientific contents. It is commendable that the editors have accomplished this daunting task so well that would be beneficial for the pediatric surgical community.

This book, Pediatric Surgery—Diagnosis and Management, is first of its kind from the developing part of the world. It is well divided in sections, and covers the complete spectrum of diseases including recent advances. Despite being a multi-authored book, it has been dominated by the Indian contributors, reflecting the maturity of pediatric surgery specialty in India. Many chapters have been covered by more than one expert known for their professional standing in the field, so as to incorporate the differing views of various experts. Chapters have been supplemented generously with operative techniques, line diagrams, charts and clinical photographs to make the book educative and informative.

I am sure this book would be an asset and reach a large number of pediatric surgeons. It should serve as a reference book in general pediatric surgery not only to the postgraduates and the pediatric surgeons but also the institutional libraries across the world.

Anirudh Shah
President, Indian Association of Pediatric Surgeons
Ahmedabad

Acknowledgements

The Editors would like to thank the Indian Association of Pediatric Surgeons (IAPS), for giving us the singular honour and the major responsibility to write this book for the benefit of the pediatric surgical fraternity especially from the developing world.

The editors admire the support that has been received from the authors from around the world. The willingness, with which all of them gave us their valuable time, leaves us personally indebted.

The Editors acknowledge the blanket permission granted by MBD publishers to reproduce the published material free of charge (text, photographs, diagrams, charts, tables, etc.) from the Textbook of Neonatal Surgery, edited by DK Gupta, New Delhi 2000, in various chapters of this book. Though, every effort has been taken by the contributors to acknowledge the published text, color photographs, charts and diagrams reproduced/quoted from the books and the journals, an inadvertent error, if any, in any chapter of this book, would only be due to an oversight.

We also appreciate the support and the encouragement received from the World Federation of Association of Pediatric Surgeons (WOFAPS), Asian Association of Pediatric Surgeons (AAPS), the Federation of Association of Pediatric Surgeons from SAARC Nations (FAPSS) and the International Foundation for Pediatric Surgery and Research for producing the book aimed at improving the surgical care of children around the globe.

Finally, our appreciation to Shri JP Vij, Chairman and Managing Director of Jaypee Brothers, Mr Tarun Duneja, and members of the publishing team, including the artists, for their hard work and special interest taken to produce a book of this quality.

*To
The students of Pediatric Surgery,
"at all levels",
in their quest for knowledge*

Contents

VOLUME-I

SECTION 1: BASIC PEDIATRIC SURGERY

1. Pediatric Surgery—Overview of the Specialty 03
   DK Gupta
2. Evolution of Pediatric Surgery 10
   IC Pathak
3. Molecular Biology and the Pediatric Surgeon 21
   Arun Chaudhury, M Srinivas
4. Growth and Development in Pediatric Surgical Practice 34
   KN Agarwal, DK Agarwal
5. Fluid and Electrolytes in Pediatric Surgery 48
   V Ravikumar, M Srinivas
6. Shock in Children—Surgeon's Perspective 65
   DK Gupta, Archana Puri
7. Blood Component Therapy 82
   VP Choudhry
8. Ventilatory Support in Children 90
   DK Pawar
9. Pediatric Anesthesia—General Considerations 103
   Ravinder K Batra, Anand Sharma
10. Relief of Postoperative Pain in Children 123
    MK Arora, G Prasad
11. Common Radiological Procedures in Pediatric Surgery 131
    AK Gupta, Ashok Srinivasan
12. Nuclear Imaging in Pediatric Surgery 140
    CS Bal, Ajay Kumar
13. Pediatric Interventional Radiology 168
    Deep N Srivastava, Bobby Batra, Dheeraj Gandhi
14. Postoperative Care 180
    Bikramjit Singh Sangha
15. Antimicrobials and Antimicrobial Prophylaxis in Pediatric Surgery 199
    V Ravikumar, M Srinivas
16. Fungal Infections in Pediatric Surgical Patients 210
    Nissar A Bhat, DK Gupta
17. Ethics in Pediatric Surgery 215
    P Madhok
18. Esophagoscopy 222
    B Othersen Jr, HS Hassan
19. Pediatric Bronchoscopy 229
    DK Gupta, Shilpa Sharma
20. Management of Terminal Illnesses 238
    Kanishka Das, M Charles, Ashley L J D'Cruz

SECTION 2: TRAUMA

21. **Pediatric Trauma** 253
    Azad B Mathur, NC Featherstone
22. **Head Injuries in Children** 264
    BS Sharma, Feiz Uddin Ahmad
23. **Pediatric Abdominal Trauma** 272
    David A Lloyd, Gunninder Soin
24. **Soft Tissue Trauma** 286
    DK Gupta, Lalit Parida
25. **Vascular Injuries in Children** 298
    Nagarajan Kumaran, Rob A Wheeler
26. **Pediatric Burns** 307
    K Mathingi Ramakrishnan, V Jayaraman
27. **Traumatic Hemobilia in Children** 321
    Shilpa Sharma, DK Gupta

SECTION 3: THORACIC SURGERY

28. **Gastroesophageal Reflux in Children** 329
    J Boix-Ochoa
29. **Thal Fundoplication** 357
    Keith W Ashcraft
30. **Achalasia Cardia** 363
    Shilpa Sharma, DK Gupta
31. **Esophageal Strictures** 369
    Shailinder J Singh, Leela Kapila
32. **Esophageal Replacement with Colon** 382
    D K Gupta, Shilpa Sharma
33. **Gastric Tube Esophageal Replacement** 391
    Gabriel O Ionescu
34. **Gastric Transposition** 409
    D K Gupta, Shilpa Sharma
35. **Jejunal Interposition as a Substitute of Esophagus** 422
    Kohei Hashizume, Antonio Dessanti
36. **Colon Patch Esophagoplasty** 426
    Enaam Raboei
37. **Esophageal Perforation** 432
    HS Hassan, B Othersen
38. **Principles of Lung Resection** 437
    DK Gupta, Shilpa Sharma
39. **Lung Anomalies** 448
    John Aiken
40. **Bronchiectasis and Lung Abscess** 471
    Shilpa Sharma, DK Gupta
41. **Pulmonary Tuberculosis in Children** 478
    Shilpa Sharma, DK Gupta
42. **Chylothorax** 491
    Spencer W Beasley

43. **Empyema Thoracis** 495
    Shilpa Sharma, DK Gupta
44. **Chest Wall Deformities** 510
    Amulya K Saxena, Günter H Willital

SECTION 4: GASTROINTESTINAL SURGERY

45. **Disorders of the Umbilicus** 523
    Sudipta Sen
46. **Inguinal Hernia and Hydrocele** 527
    AR Williams, SJ Singh, L Kapila
47. **Rare Pediatric Hernias** 534
    DK Gupta, Shilpa Sharma, Kamlesh Pal
48. **Peritonitis in Childhood** 544
    Rajiv Chadha
49. **Infantile Hypertrophic Pyloric Stenosis** 564
    Sengamalai Manoharan, Azad B Mathur
50. **Gastric Volvulus** 570
    Shilpa Sharma, DK Gupta
51. **Gastrointestinal Bleeding** 575
    AK Basu, D Basak
52. **Idiopathic Primary Intussusception** 581
    Essam El-Sahwi
53. **Meckel's Diverticulum** 587
    M Gregor Walker, F Carl Davis
54. **Appendicitis** 596
    Kurosh Paya
55. **Short Bowel Syndrome** 618
    DK Gupta, Shilpa Sharma
56. **Intestinal Obstruction** 633
    Alpana Prasad, Rajiv Chadha
57. **Abdominal Tuberculosis** 646
    Shilpa Sharma, DK Gupta
58. **Alimentary Tract Duplications** 659
    Richard G Azizkhan
59. **Bezoars in Children** 671
    Shilpa Sharma, DK Gupta
60. **Ascariasis Lumbricoides** 678
    Essam-El-Sawhi
61. **Hirschsprung's Disease** 681
    Edward Kiely
62. **Total Colonic Aganglionosis** 696
    Lester W Martin
63. **Variant Hirschsprung's Disease** 701
    Prem Puri
64. **Swenson's Pull-through** 709
    DK Gupta, Shilpa Sharma

65. **Duhamel's Pull-through** 717
    Sandeep Agarwala
66. **Soave's (Boley Scot) Endorectal Pull-through** 723
    DK Gupta, Manish Pathak, Shilpa Sharma
67. **Transanal Endorectal Pull-through** 733
    DK Gupta, Shilpa Sharma
68. **Crohn's Disease** 741
    Robert Cywes, Arnold G Coran
69. **Ulcerative Colitis** 758
    Robert Cywes, Arnold G Coran
70. **Polyposis Syndromes** 771
    AF Scharli
71. **Anorectal Malformations: Anatomy and Physiology** 776
    Pradip Mukherjee, MK Bhattacharyya
72. **Anorectal Malformations: Diagnosis and Management** 787
    SN Kureel, RK Tandon
73. **Anorectal Malformations: Pena's Perspectives** 816
    Shilpa Sharma, Alberto Pena
74. **Anomalies Associated with Anorectal Malformations** 825
    DK Gupta, Shilpa Sharma
75. **Complications Following PSARP** 833
    Alex Holschneider, DK Gupta
76. **Congenital Pouch Colon** 846
    Shilpa Sharma, DK Gupta
77. **Persistent Cloaca** 857
    DK Gupta, Shilpa Sharma, Alex Holschneider
78. **Anorectal Malformations: Current Perspectives** 874
    DK Gupta, Shilpa Sharma
79. **Rectal Ectasia** 884
    Shilpa Sharma, DK Gupta
80. **Fecal Incontinence and Constipation** 889
    Anju Goyal, Paul D Losty
81. **Bowel Management** 899
    Shilpa Sharma, DK Gupta, Alberto Pena

VOLUME-II

SECTION 5: HEPATOBILIARY SYSTEM

82. **Diseases of the Gallbladder in Children** 909
    Mark Devenport
83. **Hepatic Hemangiomas** 918
    Mark Devenport
84. **Liver Abscess in Children** 925
    Mark D Stringer
85. **Hydatid Disease** 936
    SN Oak, Prakash Agarwal, M Chavarkar
86. **Liver Resections and Allograft Preparation** 949
    Mark D Stringer

87. **Transplant Immunogenetics** 969
   Narinder K Mehra, Arundhati Panigrahi
88. **Liver Transplantation** 988
   AJW Millar, S Cywes
89. **Biliary Atresia** 1002
   CK Sinha, DK Gupta, Mark Davenport
90. **Choledochal Cyst** 1013
   Takeshi Miyano, Long Li, Atsuyuki Yamataka
91. **Pancreatic Pseudocyst** 1026
   Shilpa Sharma, DK Gupta
92. **Pancreatitis** 1033
   GVS Murthi, PAM Raine
93. **Management of Portal Hypertension** 1044
   M Bajpai
94. **Persistent Hyperinsulinemic Hypoglycemia of Infancy** 1051
   Shilpa Sharma, DK Gupta
95. **Pancreas and Intestinal Transplantation** 1058
   V Martinez Ibanez
96. **Spleen** 1066
   Amir Kaviani, Moritz M Ziegler

SECTION 6: VASCULAR DISORDERS

97. **Hemangiomas** 1079
   Richard G Azizkhan
98. **Vascular and Lymphatic Anomalies** 1099
   Robert Arensman, Jayant Agarwal, M Statter
99. **Picibanil (OK-432) in Lymphangiomas** 1108
   DK Gupta, Shilpa Sharma

SECTION 7: PEDIATRIC NEUROSURGERY

100. **Hydrocephalus** 1117
    DK Gupta, Shilpa Sharma
101. **Encephaloceles** 1148
    AK Mahapatra, GD Satyarthee
102. **Microcephaly** 1163
    Shilpa Sharma, Veena Kalra
103. **Spina Bifida** 1168
    DK Gupta, Shilpa Sharma

SECTION 8: HEAD AND NECK SURGERY

104. **Craniosynostosis** 1193
    M Bajpai
105. **Cleft Lip and Palate** 1201
    Peter AM Raine
106. **Neck Anomalies** 1222
    B Mukhopadhyay, SK Mitra
107. **Torticollis** 1230
    DK Gupta, Manish Pathak, Shilpa Sharma

SECTION 9: PEDIATRIC SURGICAL SPECIALITIES

108. **Common Eye Problems in Children** 1239
 Supriyo Ghose, Sanjeev Nainiwal
109. **Pediatric Otolaryngology** 1257
 RC Deka, DN Jha
110. **Pediatric Larynx and Trachea** 1265
 Abhinit Kumar, Suresh C Sharma
111. **Orthopedic Problems in Children** 1299
 Rajesh Malhotra
112. **Conjoined Twins** 1349
 Htut Saing, DK Gupta
113. **Heteropagus Twinning** 1364
 DK Gupta, Shilpa Sharma
114. **Gynecological Problems in Children** 1370
 Suneeta Mittal, Sonika Agarwal
115. **Ovarian Cysts** 1381
 Shilpa Sharma, DK Gupta
116. **Vaginal Anomalies and Reconstruction** 1387
 Akshay Chauhan, Shilpa Sharma, DK Gupta
117. **Adrenal Disorders** 1404
 Anurag Bajpai, PSN Menon
118. **Childhood Obesity** 1415
 Anurag Bajpai, PSN Menon
119. **Surgery for Pediatric Morbid Obesity** 1421
 Reena Bhargava, Shilpa Sharma, Azad B Mathur

SECTION 10: RECENT ADVANCES

120. **Molecular Genetics of Hirschsprung's Disease** 1433
 Paul KH Tam, Mercè Garcia-Barcelo
121. **Duhamel's Pull-through Using Staplers** 1450
 SN Oak, Prakash Agarwal
122. **Pediatric Laparoscopy** 1455
 Anirudh Shah, Amar Shah
123. **One Port Laparoscopically Assisted Appendectomy** 1463
 Vadim Kapuller
124. **Robotic Pediatric Surgery** 1468
 Aayed R Al-Qahtani
125. **Tissue Engineering: Present Concepts and Strategies** 1482
 Amulya K Saxena
126. **Stem Cell Therapy** 1491
 DK Gupta, Shilpa Sharma
127. **Nanotechnology: Technology to Revolutionize the Future of Medicine** 1503
 Amit K Dinda
128. **Laser Applications in Pediatric Surgery** 1512
 V Bhatnagar
129. **Pediatric Surgeon and the Computer** 1518
 Gian Battista Parigi, Giacomo Parigi
130. **Pediatric Surgery in Europe: Problems and Perspectives** 1552
 Gian Battista Parigi

 Index 1565

SECTION 5

Hepatobiliary System

Diseases of the Gallbladder in Children

Mark Davenport

ANATOMY AND EMBRYOLOGY

Normally the gallbladder lies on the undersurface of the liver in a slight depression of the anatomical right lobe (Fig. 82.1). It is composed of a fundus that protrudes from the margin of liver substance, a larger body and becomes somewhat narrower at the neck before connecting to the common bile duct by an occasionally tortuous cystic duct. The lining mucosa assumes a valve like spiral configuration (of Heister) toward the neck and there is often a pouch-like arrangement (of Hartmann) where gallstones may lodge. The junction of cystic and common bile duct is normally "T" shaped although occasionally the cystic duct runs alongside the CBD or shares a common wall before entering it distally. Calot's triangle is bordered by the cystic duct, common hepatic duct and the liver and contains the cystic artery and a fairly constant lymph node (of Lund). The venous drainage is via multiple veins running directly into liver substance across the gallbladder bed.

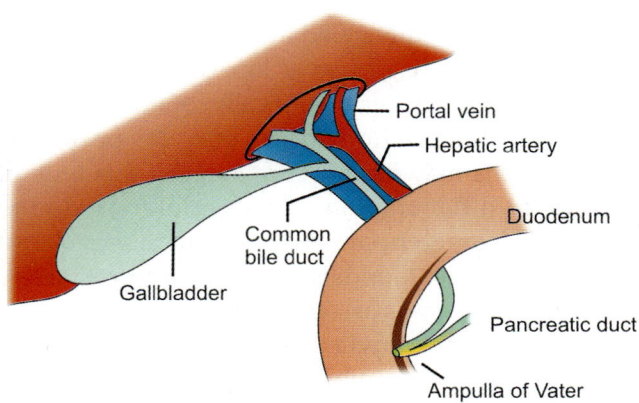

Fig. 82.1: Normal anatomy of gallbladder

Embryologically, bile ducts are derived from two distinct elements. Intrahepatic bile ducts appear from about 7 weeks while the extrahepatic bile ducts are derived from the budding foregut endoderm. Each branch of portal vein is surrounded by a layer of mesenchyme and a cylindrical double cell layer of darkly staining cells derived from hepatoblasts termed the ductal or limiting plate. Remodeling of this layer occurs to form a network of interconnected bile ducts enveloped into the mesenchyme but retaining the connections with the intrahepatic bile canaliculi. This process begins at the porta hepatis and extends back into the more peripheral areas of liver tissue. Bile is first observed in cholangioles and then the fetal gut from 12-14 weeks gestation implying completion of biliary continuity.

CONGENITAL ANOMALIES OF THE GALLBLADDER

The majority of configuration anomalies of the gallbladder are asymptomatic and therefore usually incidental findings. Thus, bilobed gallbladders, duplications and diverticula have all been described either as findings at cholecystectomy or in anatomical postmortem reviews. Similarly, the position of the gallbladder may vary and it has been found on the left side of liver or buried within the liver substance as an intrahepatic gallbladder. The classic paper documenting these type of anomalies is that of Robert Gross who recorded several anatomical variants in an extensive literature review in 1934.[1]

Gallbladder agenesis, can occur as an isolated anomaly but is usually found in association with biliary atresia or with duodenal atresia. In cases where biliary atresia is the predominant defect, the anomaly is simply a reflection of a generalised development defect of the biliary tree with the affected infant presenting with conjugated jaundice. Coughlin et al reported two infants with duodenal atresia (one also with an imperforate anus and hypospadias) where at operation an otherwise normal common bile duct was found but no evidence of a gallbladder.[2] There were no sequelae.

A septate or multiseptate gallbladder arises from incomplete vacuolation of the lumen during development and has been reported.[3-5] The septum may include muscle fibers within its structure, which supports it as a congenital anomaly. Occasionally in adults, an acquired septum may form due to recurrent inflammation. Such septation appears to predispose to stone formation secondary to bile stasis.[4] However, even in the absence of complications these anomalies can be symptomatic.[4,5] St-Vil et al described a three-year-old boy found to have an "hour-glass" deformity due to a gallbladder diaphragm with a pin-hole separating both elements.[3] The fundal part appeared inflamed and long-standing abdominal discomfort and failure to thrive was cured by cholecystectomy. Tan et al have described a case of multiseptate gallbladder in association with a fusiform choledochal cyst malformation.[5]

Sometimes, although structurally normal, the histological architecture of the gallbladder may vary. For instance, Santonja et al described a case of histological replacement with tissue resembling gastric wall architecture.[6]

INFLAMMATORY CONDITIONS OF THE GALLBLADDER

Acute Hydrops

Hydrops of the gallbladder is the term used for an acute, symptomatic, distension of the gallbladder, which can occur in the absence of inflammatory change, calculi or any congenital anomaly. The etiology is not clear although the condition frequently follows upper respiratory tract infections and non-specific viral illness.[7] Mesenteric adenitis and Kawasaki disease (mucocutaneous lymph node syndrome) have been reported as associated conditions.[8] The largest series in children is that of Chamberlain and Hight who reviewed 29 cases with a mean age at presentation of 5 years and a preponderance of boys.[9] The presenting symptoms included abdominal pain, vomiting, tenderness in the right hypochondrium and, in about half of all cases, a palpable gallbladder. Hydrops is commonly misdiagnosed as appendicitis in the older child or intussusception in infants although a correct diagnosis can be made without difficulty with ultrasonography. It can be differentiated from a mucocele of the gallbladder by the demonstrable absence of gallstones and by the absence of pyrexia or leucocytosis.

Hydrops may be treated conservatively with intravenous fluids, gastrointestinal rest and usually antibiotics. This is largely successful with the function of the gallbladder returning eventually. If, however, the case is diagnosed at laparotomy then either cholecystectomy or cholecystostomy is appropriate.

Acute Acalculous Cholecystitis

Acalculous cholecystitis (AC) may occur without a history of any preceding illness but certainly in developed countries it is more usually a complication of trauma or sepsis. Associated illnesses have included leptospirosis, cholera, AIDS, scarlet fever, burn wound infection with *pseudomonas* and *Salmonella typhimurium* and typhoid fever.[10] Some authors have speculated that, unlike gallstone-associated cholecystitis, there is an underlying ischemic component in some cases. There appears to be an increased prevalence of AC in some sub-saharan African countries such as Nigeria, although the cause is unknown. Rarely, infection of the biliary tree with the nematode worm, Ascaris lumbricoides, may cause cholecystitis by blockage of the cystic duct. AC can occur in the neonatal period, although it is usually misdiagnosed as necrotizing enterocolitis and diagnosed at laparotomy.[11]

Septicemia and fever are typically found and a mass in the right hypochondrium may be palpable. Complications may be more frequent in this type of gallbladder inflammation. Thus perforation due to necrosis and gangrene are not uncommon sequelae of untreated disease. Jaundice occurs in approximately one-third of the cases associated with another illness although it is not clear whether this is due to the effects of the sepsis or a mechanical obstruction to the adjacent common hepatic or bile duct.

A laparotomy may be indicated either because of difficulty in diagnosis, failure of resolution with antibiotic therapy or complications such as necrosis and abscess formation. A tube cholecystostomy is all that is needed for the majority of cases although on occasion cholecystectomy may be indicated, particularly for complicated disease. Interventional radiologists have described percutaneous techniques for drainage in adults.

A rare variant of gallbladder inflammation in children, xanthogranulomatous cholecystitis, has been described in a 10-year-old child who presented with a five month history of abdominal pain complicated by jaundice.[12] The jaundice was secondary to involvement of the common bile duct in the inflammatory process. Cholecystectomy was performed and histological examination showed the typical features of a destructive inflammatory process, fibrosis and nodules of lipid-laden macrophages.

Acquired stenosis of the cystic duct may occur even in the absence of gallstones. We have recently treated a 14-year-old boy with sclerosing cholangitis who developed right upper quadrant pain with a palpable gallbladder (Fig. 82.2). At surgery he had a tense mucocele of the gallbladder with complete stenosis of the cystic duct, presumed to be due to the sclerosing process.

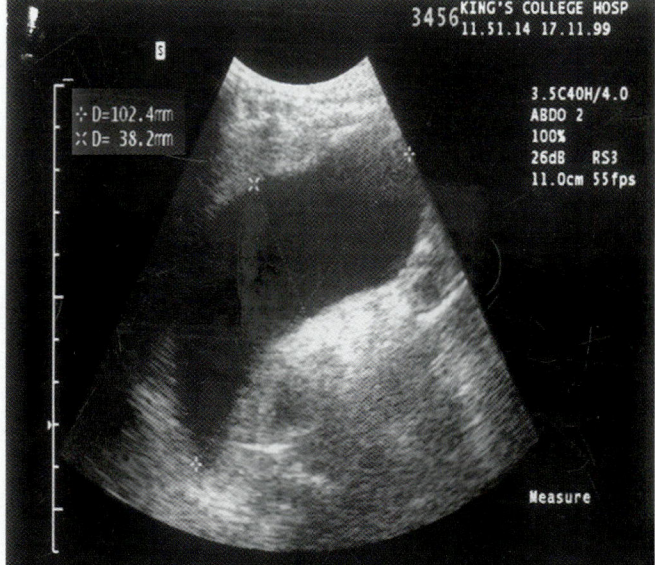

Fig. 82.2: Ultrasonographic appearance of chronic mucocele and grossly distended gallbladder (10 x 5 cm) associated with cystic duct stenosis and sclerosing cholangitis

Cholelithiasis and Acute Cholecystitis

There are three types of gallstones, depending on their composition, which are generally termed cholesterol, pigment or mixed. Normally, cholesterol exists in a supersaturated form in bile and is kept in solution by lecithin, primary and secondary bile salts. Physiochemical alteration of this balance can render the bile lithogenic and cholesterol may precipitate as a consequence. Similarly, bilirubin is excreted in a water-soluble conjugated complex molecule by the biliary canalicular apparatus. The increased excretion of bilirubin which, for instance, occurs in chronic hemolysis increases the concentration of bilirubin and potential precipitation as calcium bilirubinate. Cholesterol stones tend to be large, smooth and solitary while pigment stones are multiple, black and spiky. The contribution of infection to the formation of stones in children is not known but in adults some bacteria present in bile may produce β-glucuronidase an enzyme known to hydrolyse bilirubin glucuronide to insoluble bilirubin and glucuronic acid.

INCIDENCE AND ETIOLOGY

Although compared with adults, cholelithiasis is unusual in children it is certainly not rare.[13] One ultrasound screening program performed in children between 6 and 15 years of age showed a prevalence of 0.13 %.[14] For comparison, the prevalence among screened adults would be about 10%.

Table 82.1 lists a number of associated causes or predisposing factors in the development of gallstones in the pediatric population while Table 82.2 selectively illustrates some of the more recent large pediatric series of gallstones from around the world.[15-20]

Pigment stones are certainly more prevalent in this age group than in comparable adult series and in these children, the sex ratio is the same. Common hemolytic disorders include congenital disorders of the red cell membrane such as spherocytosis, eliptocytosis and stomatocytosis and the more prevalent, thalassemia (α and β), hemoglobin C and sickle cell disease (SCD). Within each predisposing group, the prevalence of stones varies. Thus almost 60 % of children and adolescents with congenital spherocytosis will have gallstones compared to a somewhat lower prevalence in homozygous sickle cell disease, ranging from 13- 37% of cases.[17,21] In one cohort study from Jamaica,

Table 82.1: Associated factors and underlying causes of gallstones in children

Predisposing factors in gallstone formation	Mechanism	Reference
Sickle cell disease	Hemolysis	16, 20
Congenital spherocytosis, eliptocytosis, etc.	Hemolysis	17
Thalassemia	Hemolysis	38
Ileal resection/ileostomy	Impaired bile salt recirculation, dehydration	17
Parenteral nutrition	Gallbladder stasis	31
Prematurity	Hemolysis, impaired enteral nutrition, sepsis	35
Choledochal malformation	Stasis, infection	32
Childhood malignancy	? Blood transfusions	33
Bone marrow transplant	Blood transfusions	33
Immunoglobulin A deficiency		54
Adolescent pregnancy	Metabolic, estrogen	17, 18

Table 82.2: Illustrative series of gallstones in children reported during 1990's

Series (ref.)	N	%pigmented	Mean age (years)	Comments
Grosfeld Indianapolis, USA[17]	169 (67% female)	?	35% < 10 years	39% idiopathic
Reif Buffalo, USA[18]	50	36	12	20% idiopathic
Bruch Ontario, Canada[19]	74 (55% female)	0	11	81% idiopathic
Walker Jamaica[20]	114	100	n/a	24% of cohort with SCD

n/a - not applicable

gallstones developed in 96 (57%) of 167 patients. Actual symptoms were however uncommon as only 7 children required a cholecystectomy.[20] Biliary sludge has also been recognised as a predisposing feature to actual stones in children with SCD. In one study from Saudi Arabia, some 16% of a SCD population had sludge present, compared with 20% who had actual stones.[22]

Cholelithiasis in the neonatal period has been noted with increasing frequency and has been attributed to the increased use of total parenteral nutrition (TPN) and perhaps to an increased availability of ultrasonography. The genesis of TPN-related gallstones is unclear but may include physiochemical alterations in bile due to amino acid infusion or to a lack of enteral stimulation.[23] Biliary sludge also appears to predate true stones and has been identified in approximately 40% of neonates receiving TPN.[24]

Heaton et al described 9 infants with an obstructed biliary tree caused by bile and sludge in seven infants aged 2-12 weeks and by gallstones in two infants aged four and six months.[25] Underlying factors such as prematurity or hemolysis were not present in most of these infants but there was a high incidence of congenital anomalies of the biliary tree. Spontaneous resolution of "cholelithiasis" in infants has been reported particularly if the stones are not calcified and a conservative policy is probably justified although later complications can occur.[26-28]

Disease of the ileum or surgical resection of the ileum may be associated with the formation of predominantly pigment gallstones. This is caused by a disturbance of the enterohepatic recycling of bile salts and an increased lithogenicity of bile.[29-31]

Congenital structural anomalies of the bile duct such as choledochal cysts and less commonly the gallbladder such as duplication or septation, may predispose to stone formation.[4,32] This is presumably because of biliary stasis, which allows precipitation of insoluble complexes.

Recently an increased prevalence of gallstones in children with cancer has been observed, specifically following bone marrow transplant. Safford et al reported 20 (8.5%) cases of cholelithiasis in 235 cases of bone marrow transplant that had also undergone abdominal ultrasonography.[33] Among the reasons

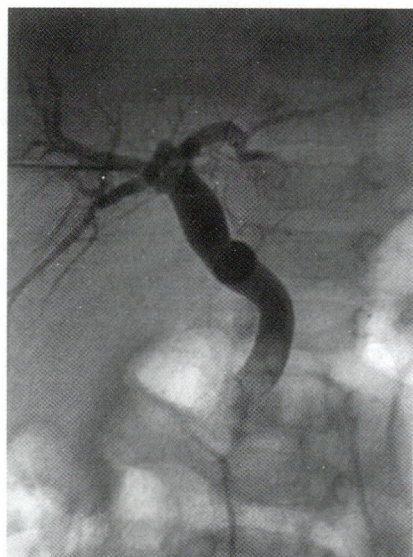

Fig. 82.3: Percutaneous transhepatic cholangiogram showing radiolucent filling defect impacted in distal common bile duct (choledocholithiasis)

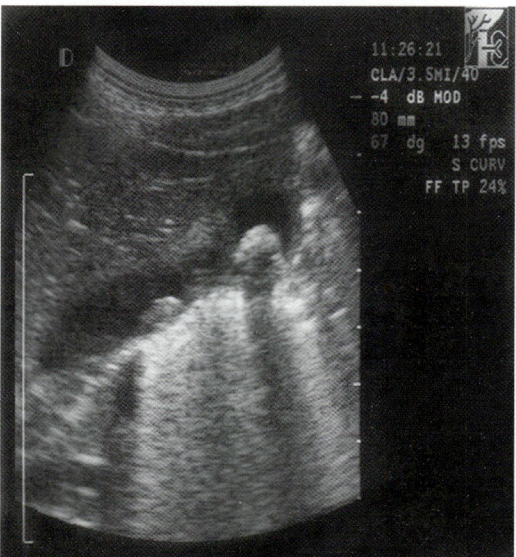

Fig. 82.4: Ultrasonographic imaging of 8-year-old boy with homozygous sickle cell disease and intermittent right upper quadrant pain showing multiple gallstones and prominent acoustic shadowing

suggested for this include, repeated blood transfusions, parenteral nutrition, and irradiation therapy.

CLINICAL FEATURES

Gallstones may cause abdominal pain, and the diagnosis should certainly be considered in cases of recurrent abdominal pain, even in children. The typical relationship to meals may be established in older children and adolescents. Most can be localised to the right hypochondrium with a degree of tenderness even between attacks. Palpation of a mass in an otherwise well child implies the formation of a mucocele of the gallbladder due to complete obstruction of the cystic duct (Fig. 82.2).

Stones in the common bile duct (choledocholithiasis) (Fig. 82.3) will present as a conjugated jaundice with pale stools and dark urine and has been estimated to occur in from 2 - 6% of cases.[13] Secondary infection and ascending cholangitis are uncommon complications in children but must be considered if there are features of jaundice, pyrexia and marked right-upper quadrant tenderness.[18] Occasionally Mirizzi's syndrome can occur where a gallstone impacts in Hartman's pouch causing inflammation and obstructive jaundice due to narrowing of the adjacent common hepatic duct.[34] Small gallstones particularly

Table 82.3: Suggested preoperative regimen in children with sickle cell disease	
Rehydration	IV fluids—6 hours prior to start time.
Avoidance of Peripheral Cooling	Wrap limbs in cotton wool, heating blanket, core temperature monitoring
Transfusion	Packed cell transfusion in previous week. Aim for Hb > 10 g/dl

may pass through the sphincter of Oddi temporarily obstructing the main pancreatic duct to cause acute pancreatitis. This occurred in up to 8% of an unselected series of children with gallstones in one American series.[18] Such children may well present with pancreatitis and hyperamylasemia, having otherwise asymptomatic gallstones. If the symptoms do not subside quickly on conservative management then an ERCP is indicated in the acute phase with stone removal and sphincterotomy.

The diagnosis of gallstones is easily established by ultrasonography (Fig. 82.4) although in children with sickle cell disease for instance, it can be difficult to determine their relationship to symptoms. Recurrent jaundice, fever and leucocytosis and abdominal pain occurs in sickling crises and the concomitant changes in liver function are often similar to those seen with biliary tract obstruction. The combination of ultrasonography and biliary tract scintigraphy can be useful for differentiating sickling crises from gallstone induced abdominal pain although Serafini et al found a low predictive value for either test when used alone.[35]

The management of gallstones in children is straightforward if they are symptomatic-elective cholecystectomy. However, where they are asymptomatic or indeed if symptoms are atypical then a more conservative approach may be indicated. This is true whether the stones are pigmented or not. For instance, Bruch et al prospectively studied 74 children with gallstones where 33 (45%) required cholecystectomy and 41 were followed without intervention.[19] In the follow-up only group, 34 (83%) remained symptom-free or had responded to dietary manipulation.

CHOLECYSTECTOMY

Cholecystectomy through a right subcostal muscle-cutting incision was the standard procedure until relatively recently. In many centers however, this has been replaced by the technique of laparoscopic cholecystectomy with excellent results reported. This minimally invasive procedure has proved beneficial particularly to the children with sickle cell disease because of a reduced morbidity from respiratory complications.[36,37]

Sometimes the question of an incidental cholecystectomy is raised. Thus a preoperative ultrasound scan of the gallbladder should be performed if splenectomy is being considered for hemolytic disorders to detect gallstones in these children and concomitant cholecystectomy has been recommended even for asymptomatic stones.[38]

LAPAROSCOPIC CHOLECYSTECTOMY IN CHILDREN

Laparoscopic cholecystectomy (LC) was initially performed by French surgeons at the end of the 1980's.[39] Since then it has become the procedure of choice for cholecystectomy in adults with low morbidity and mortality in several large series.[40] Nevertheless it may be prone to occasional complications which can be life-threatening such as common bile duct damage and biliary leaks. Many authors have emphasised that there is a "learning curve" in the acquisition of the necessary manual skills and techniques. It is a debatable point whether the general pediatric surgeon will acquire enough expertise to be able to remove the occasional gallbladder laparoscopically in the same way that they had once removed gallbladders at open operation.

Pediatric-specific series have been reported.[41,42] Although there is no technical reason why even infants cannot undergo LC, for instance Sanada et al.[43] have described its use in an eight-month-old girl with gallstones, a common-sense approach should be adopted as the actual benefits of such a challenging procedure in an infant are marginal.

Typically four ports will be used: Umbilical, epigastric and two lateral ports placed in the right lower quadrant in smaller children or in the flank in the older child or adolescent (Figs 82.5 and 82.6). Although all these ports can be 5 mm in diameter, if a 10 mm port is used through the umbilicus it facilitates final removal of the gallbladder. Most surgeons would now place the initial port by open dissection at the umbilicus (Hassan approach) although the alternative using a Veress-type needle is still widely performed. A CO_2 pneuoperitoneum is then induced with a maximum pressure of about 10-12 mm Hg. At this point the anesthetist may well have to increase the inspired minute volume to reduce the tendency to hypercarbia. Some authors describe gasless laparoscopic procedures using devices designed to "tent" the abdominal wall and this may be particularly useful in very small children and infants.[43]

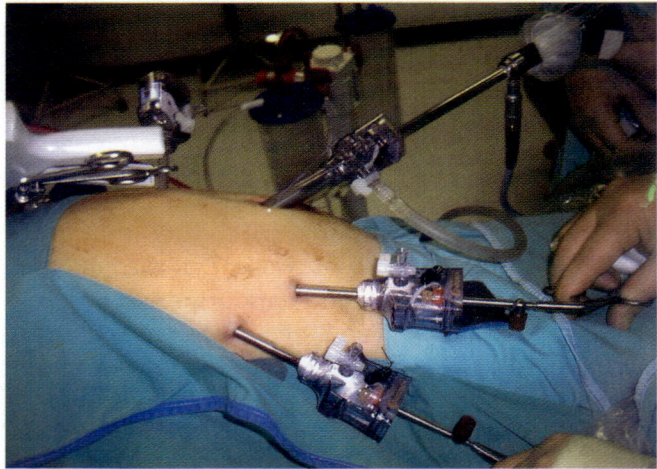

Fig. 82.5: Typical appearance of laparoscopic ports (x4) required for cholecystectomy. The uppermost is a 10 mm disposable port sited at the umbilicus with camera in place. The two in the foreground are 5 mm disposable ports used for grasping the gallbladder. The epigastric port (left and unfocused in picture) is used for dissection and diathermy

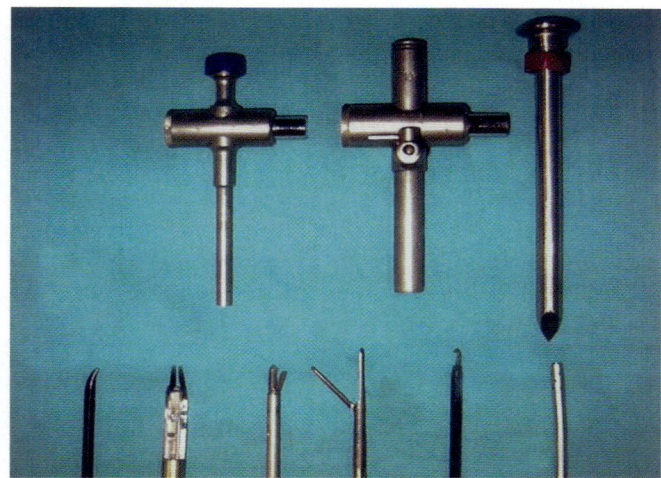

Fig. 82.6: Array of pediatric laparoscopic instruments. Top from left to right: 5 mm reusable port, 10 mm reusable port and trocar for insertion. Bottom from left to right: curved Petelin dissection forceps, 10 mm Ligaclip applicator, 5 mm Ligaclip applicator, grasping forceps, diathermy hook and suction/ lavage catheter

Dissection of the cystic artery and duct is exactly the same as the open procedure and once identified these may be clipped or ligated. The gallbladder is taken off its bed by diathermy (bipolar or monopolar) and removed through the largest available point using heavy grasping forceps.

Perioperative Medical Preparation

The commonest single group requiring cholecystectomy in many centers will be children with homozygous sickle cell disease. Careful preoperative preparation of these children is important to minimise medical and hematological complications and must include hydration, antibiotic administration, avoidance of anemia and pre- and perioperative oxygen saturation monitoring.

Formerly an aggressive preoperative transfusion regimen was advocated in order to reduce the sickle percentage (to < 30%) and increase the hemoglobin levels (to > 10 g/dl).[44] Recently this approach has changed and currently in many centers a more conservative approach is taken with blood transfusion being undertaken only to the level required to raise the hemoglobin to > 10 g/dl.[45] This has been associated without change in perioperative morbidity and with much less transfusion-related problems.

There are specific medical complications peculiar to sickle cell disease which may be precipitated by surgery. For instance, the acute chest syndrome (ACS) is a post-operative phenomenon where there is sickling and sequestration of red cells in the pulmonary vasculature. In children this presents as fever, cough and respiratory distress with hypoxia. The mortality ranges from 10 - 25% and laparoscopic procedures do not appear to offer much protection. In one recent series, ACS occurred in 6 (10%) of 59 children with SCD undergoing a surgical procedure.[46] Although in the surgical population, risk factors have been hard to define, in other studies ACS appears more commonly in children aged 2-4 years of age and in those with the SS genotype

MISCELLANEOUS CONDITIONS OF THE GALLBLADDER

Biliary Dyskinesia

This is a poorly defined condition that has been described in detail in only a single pediatric series.[47] The key features are chronic right-upper quadrant pain without gallstones, an absence of other causes of pain and objective delayed gallbladder emptying. The later feature may be difficult to satisfy outside of a specialised center but involves a cholecystokinin (CCK)-stimulated gallbladder ejection fraction as assessed using a radionuclide hepatobiliary isotope (e.g. Technetium labelled -imino-diacetic acid). Normally 90-100% emptying should be achieved following CCK administration; in biliary dyskinesia, < 40% is all that should be achieved. Gollin et al described 29 children with a median age of 13 years who fulfilled these criteria and who were subjected to cholecystectomy.[47] Symptoms were relieved in 23 (79%) suggesting the validity of this entity.

Gallbladder Torsion

Daux reported the first case of torsion of the gallbladder identified at postmortem in 1925.[48] Although the condition is typically found in elderly women, a few cases have been reported in children.[49,50] About 50 cases have been documented in the literature with about 14 of those being in children. Invariably it is related to a mobile gallbladder with its own mesentery and pedicle consisting of cystic artery and duct.

In children it presents as an acute-onset right-sided pain with features of right upper quadrant peritonism.

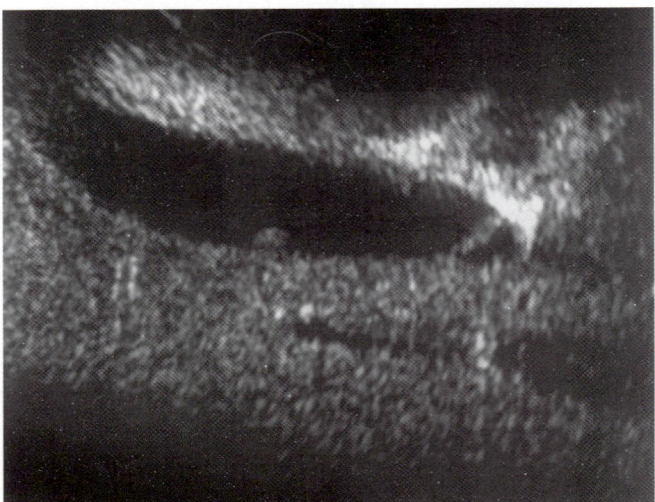

Fig. 82.7: Ultrasound imaging of gallbladder in 12-year-old girl with history of right upper quadrant pain, showing a small (5 mm) polyp arising from anterior wall. Removed at laparoscopic cholecystectomy with subsequent resolution of pain

A single case of torsion following blunt abdominal trauma has also been reported.[51] A palpable mass may be found in about 10% of cases. It is possible to diagnose the condition on ultrasound or CT scan although this is uncommon. Kitagawa et al have suggested the following ultrasonographic signs (1) a collection of fluid between gallbladder and fossa, (2) horizontal rather than vertical appearance of gallbladder, (3) edema and wall-thickening.[50] In addition there is often marked enhancement of the cystic duct, lying to the right of the gallbladder which can be apparent on CT or ultrasonography.

Cholecystectomy is usually required as the gallbladder is typically gangrenous at laparotomy. Percutaneous cholecystostomy has also been suggested by Quinn et al although perhaps only as a temporising measure.[52]

Polypoid Lesions and Adenomyomatosis of the Gallbladder

Hyperplastic mucosal polyps occur either singly (Fig. 82.7) or multiple. Adenomyomatosis is a benign neoplastic condition which occasionally occurs in children. It may be defined as localised or diffuse hyperplastic extensions of the mucosa into the muscular layer and beyond. In adults it has been reported to be premalignant. The youngest such case in the pediatric literature appears to be a five-year-old child reported by Alberti et al.[53]

ACKNOWLEDGEMENTS

Figures 82.2, 82.4 and 82.7 were kindly supplied by Mrs Pat Farrant and Figure 82.3 by Dr J Karani, both of the Department of Radiology at Kings College Hospital.

REFERENCES

1. Gross RE. Congenital anomalies of the gallbladder: a review of 148 cases, with report of a double gallbladder. Arch Surg 1936;32:131-62.
2. Coughlin JP. Rector FE and Klein MD. Agenesis of the gallbladder in duodenal atresia: Two case reports. J Pediatr Surg 1992;27:1304.
3. St-Vil D, Luks FJ, Hancock BJ et al. Diaphragm of the gallbladder: a case report. J Pediatr Surg 1992;27:1301-03.
4. Esper E, Kaufman DB, Crary GS, et al. Septate gallbladder with cholelithiasis: a cause of chronic abdominal pain in a 6-year-old child. J Pediatr Surg 1992;27:1560-62.
5. Tan CEL, Howard ER, Driver M, Murray-Lyon IM. Noncommunicating multiseptate gallbladder and choledochal cyst: a case report and review of the literature. Gut 1993;34:853-56.
6. Santonja C, Rollan V. Gallbladder malformation with gastric wall-like architecture. J Pediatr Surg 1996;31:1292-93.
7. Rumley TO, Rodgers BM. Hydrops of the gallbladder in children. J Pediatr Surg 1983;18:138-40.
8. Maglavy DB, Speert P, Siver TM. Mucocutaneous lymph node syndrome, report of 2 cases complicated by acute hydrops and diagnosed by ultrasound. Pediatrics 1978;61:699-702.
9. Chamberlain JW, Hight DW. Acute hydrops of the gallbladder in childhood. Surgery 1970;68:899-905.
10. Roca M, Sellier N, Maensire A, et al. Acute acalculous cholecystitis in Salmonella infection. Pediatr Radiol 1988;18:421-23.
11. Fernandes ET, Hollabaugh RS, Boulden TF, Angel C. Gangrenous acalculous cholecystitis in a premature infant. J Pediatr Surg 1989;24:608-09.
12. Ayling RM, Heaton ND, Davenport M, et al. Xanthogranulomatous cholecystitis in a 10-year-old boy. Pediatr Surg Inter 1993;8:170-72.
13. Rescorla FJ. Cholelithiasis, cholecystitis and common bile duct stones. Curr Opin Pediatr 1997;9:276-82.
14. Palasciano G, Portincasa P, Vinciguerra V, et al. Gallstone prevalence and gallbladder volume in children and adolescents: an epidemiological ultrasonographic survey and relationship to body mass index. Am J Gastrol 1989;84:1374-82.

15. Bailey PV, Connors RH, Tracy TF Jr, et al. Changing spectrum of cholelithiasis and cholecystitis in infants and children. Am J Surg 1989;158:585-86.
16. Webb DK, Darby JS, Dunn DT, et al. Gallstones in Jamaican children with homozygous sickle cell disease. Arch Dis Child 1989;89:693-96.
17. Grosfeld JL, Rescorla FJ, Skinner MA, et al. The spectrum of biliary tract disorders in infants and children: experience with 300 cases. Arch Surg 1994;129:513-20.
18. Reif S, Sloven DG, Lebenthal E. Gallstones in children. Characterisation by age, etiology and outcome. Am J Gastroenterol Nutr 1991;145:105-08.
19. Bruch SW, Ein SH, Rocchi C, Kim PCW. The management of non-pigmented gallstones in children. J Pediatr Surg 2000;35:729-32.
20. Walker TM, Hambleton IR, Serjeant GR. Gallstones in sickle cell disease: observations from the Jamaican cohort. J Pediatr 2000;136:80-85.
21. Flye MW, Silver D. Biliary tract disorders and sickle cell disease. Surgery 1972;72:361-67.
22. Al-Salem AH, Qaisruddin S. The significance of biliary sludge in children with sickle cell disease. Pediatr Surg Inter 1998;13:14-16.
23. Presig R, Rennert O. Biliary transport and cholestatic effects of amino acids. Gastroenterology 1977;73:1240.
24. Matos C, Avni EF, Van Gausbeke D, et al. Total parenteral nutrition and gallbladder disease in neonates. Journal of Ultrasound Medicine 1987;6:243-48.
25. Heaton ND, Davenport M, Howard ER. Intraluminal biliary obstruction. Arch Dis Childh 1991;66:1395-98.
26. Keller MS, Markle BM, Laffey PA, et al. Spontaneous resolution of cholelithiasis in infants. Radiology 1985;157:345-48.
27. Holgerson LO, Stolar C, Berdon WE, Hilfer C, Levy JS. Therapeutic implications of acquired choledochal obstruction in infancy: spontaneous resolution in three infants. J Pediatr Surg 1990;25:1027-29.
28. St-Vil D, Yazbeck S, Luks FI, et al. Cholelithiasis in newborns and infants. J Pediatr Surg 1992;27:1305-07.
29. Pellerin D, Bertin P, Nihoul-Fekete CL, Racour CL. Cholelithiasis and ileal pathology in childhood. J Pediatr Surg 1975;10:35-41.
30. Heubi JE, Soloway RD, Balisteri WF. Biliary lipid composition in healthy and diseased infants, children and young adults. Gastroenterology 1982;82:1295-99.
31. Roslyn JJ, Berquist WE, Pitt HA, et al. Increased risk of gallstones in children receiving total parenteral nutrition. Pediatrics 1983;71:784-89.
32. Stringer M, Dhawan A, Davenport M, et al. Choledochal cysts: lessons from a 20 year experience. Arch Dis Child 1995;73:528-31.
33. Safford SD, Safford KM, Martin P, Rice H, Kurtzberg J, Skinner MA. Management of cholelithiasis in pediatric patients who undergo bone marrow transplantation. J Pediatr Surg 2001;36:86-90.
34. Mirizzi PL. Sindrome del conducto hepatico. J Int Chir 1948;8:731-32.
35. Serafini AN, Spoliansky G, Sfakianskis GN, et al. Diagnostic studies in patients with sickle cell anemia and acute abdominal pain. Arch Int Med 1987;147:1061-62.
36. Newman KD, Marmon LM, Attorri R, Evans S. Laparoscopic cholecystectomy in pediatric patients. J Pediatr Surg 1991;26:1184-85.
37. Holcombe GW, Olsen DO, Sharp KW. Laparoscopic cholecystectomy in the pediatric patient. J Pediatr Surg 1991;26:1186-90.
38. Pappis CH, Galanski S, Moussatos G, et al. Experience of splenectomy and cholecystectomy in children with chronic hemolytic anaemia. J Pediatr Surg 1989;24:543-46.
39. Perissat J, Collet DR, Belliard R. Gallstones: laparoscopic treatment, intracorporeal lithotripsy followed by cholecystostomy or cholecystectomy - a personal technique. Endoscopy 1989;21:373-74.
40. Fiore NF, Ledniczky G, Wiebke EA, et al. An analysis of perioperative cholangiography in one thousand laparoscopic cholecystectomies. Surgery 1997;122:817-23.
41. Sigman HH, Laberge JM, Croitoru D, et al. Laparoscopic cholecystectomy: a treatment option for gallbladder disease in children. J Pediatr Surg 1991;26:1181-83.
42. Moir CR, Donohue JH, van Heerden JA. Laparoscopic cholecystectomy in children: initial experience and recommendations. J Pediatr Surg 1992;27:1066-70.
43. Sanada Y, Yamaguchi M, Chiba M, et al. Endoscopic sphincterotomy and laparoscopic cholecystectomy in an infant with cholecysto-choledocholithiasis. J Pediatr Surg 1998;33:1312-14.
44. Banerjee AK, Layton DM, Rennie JA, Bellingham AJ. Safe surgery in sickle cell disease. Br J Surg 1991;78:516-17.
45. Vichinsky E, Haberkern CM, Neumayr L, et al. A comparison of conservative and aggressive transfusion regimens in the perioperative management of sickle cell disease. N Eng J Med 1995;333:206-13.
46. Delatte SJ, Hebra A, Tagge EP, et al. Acute chest syndrome in the postoperative sickle cell patient. J Pediatr Surg 1999;34:188-92.
47. Gollin G, Raschbaum GR, Moorthy C, Santos. Cholecystectomy for suspected biliary dyskinesia in children with chronic abdominal pain. J Pediatr Surg 1999;34;854-57.
48. Daux F. Volvulus de al vesicule biliaire. J Chir 1925;25: 356-58.
49. Levard G, Weil D, Barret D, Barbier J. Torsion of the gallbladder in children. J Pediatr Surg 1994;29:569-70.
50. Kitagawa H, Nakada K, Enami T, et al. Two cases of torsion of the gallbladder diagnosed preoperatively. J Pediatr Surg 1997;32:1567-69.
51. Salman AB, Yildirgan MI, Celebi F. Post-traumatic gallbladder torsion in a child. J Pediatr Surg 1996;31:1586.
52. Quinn SF, Fazzio F, Jones E. Torsion of the gallbladder: findings on CT and sonography and role of percutaneous cholecystostomy. Am J Roentgen 1987;148:881-82.
53. Alberti D, Callea F, Camoni G, et al. Adenomyomatosis of the gallbladder in childhood. J Pediatr Surg 1998; 33:1411-12.

CHAPTER 83
Hepatic Hemangiomas

Mark Davenport

Although the precise figure can never be known with certainty perhaps 10% of all liver masses are of vascular origin. These are mostly benign vascular tumors termed hemangioma or hemangioendothelioma (HAE). Such lesions can present in many ways; from being entirely asymptomatic, incidental lesions to multiple tumors almost entirely replacing liver tissue and causing life-threatening cardiac failure. As with hemangiomas in other parts of the body, the natural history of most lesions in the liver is to undergo initial rapid proliferation within the first 6-12 month of life and then spontaneous involution over the next 5 -10 years. Hepatic angiosarcoma, not covered in this chapter, is the malignant counterpart of a hemangioma, which in adults is associated with environmental exposure to vinyl chloride monomer and rarely presents in childhood.

HISTORICAL ASPECTS

Isolated reports of hemangiomatous lesions of the liver appearing in infancy exist in the 19th century literature although they were often referred to as angiosarcoma or hemangio-endotheliosarcoma. Kundstadler in a classic review of hepatic hemangiomatous lesions during childhood reported a case and reviewed the literature up to 1933, identifying 14 other cases.[1] All of the cases reported died within a month of presentation.

Anemia was frequently mentioned by early authors as one manifestation, although it was not directly related to red cell destruction within the liver lesions. The association of thrombocytopenic purpura and a giant capillary hemangioma of the skin was first reported by Haig Kasabach and Katharine Merritt in 1940 of New York and applied by later authors to a similar phenomenon in extensive liver hemangiomas.[2]

EPIDEMIOLOGY AND PREVALENCE

Cavernous hemangiomas of the liver are considered the second most common hepatic tumor, in the general population, exceeded only by hepatic metastases. Most, however, are clearly incidental lesions usually presenting in later life. In these, there is a female predominance although this seems to be less marked in children.

HISTOLOGICAL AND IMMUNOHISTOCHEMICAL FEATURES

Although there is a broad histological division between the predominantly solitary cavernous hemangioma and the often multifocal and bilobar hemangioendotheliomas, this may mean little in clinical practice. There can be histological overlap and commonly, no actual tissue is ever obtained for histological analysis. In most reports, there is no particularly precision to either of the two terms.

Hemangiomas and hemangioendotheliomas (HAE's) are histologically benign tumors arising from the hepatic mesenchyme. Their cut surface varies from grey to reddish brown with a spongy consistency. There may be areas of fibrosis, calcification, cystic degeneration and overt hemorrhage.

Hemangioendotheliomas may be isolated or multiple and tend to have smaller vascular spaces than hemangiomas. Dehner and Ishak subdivided them into two histological types with the most common, Type

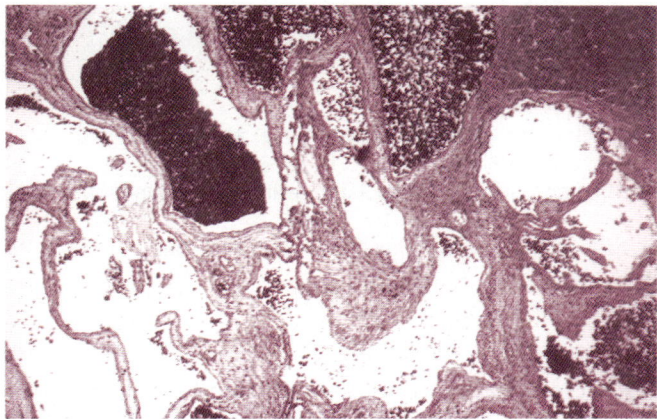

Fig. 83.1: Low power photomicrograph of resected hemangio-endothelioma from a four-year-old girl showing large irregular vascular spaces, lined by normal sinusoidal endothelium. Relative reduction in liver parenchyma

1, being composed of multiple small vascular channels lined by immature endothelial cells and separated by a fibrous stroma that may contain biliary ductules (Fig. 83.1).[3] Type 2 HAE's are less common lesions where the vascular spaces are lined by more pleomorphic and even frankly malignant-looking endothelial cells. These tend to form papillary-like structures budding into the vascular spaces and are without stromal bile ductules. Type 2 HAE's tend to present outside of the neonatal period and there is a definite tendency for malignant transformation into overt angiosarcoma.

The immunohistochemical characteristics of HAE's have been reported by Selby et al in a large series of 91 cases.[4] In this series, about 20% were Type 2. Immunohistochemical staining for factor VIII was usually present. Bile ducts demonstrable by cytokeratin staining, were present in all cases, although largely confined to the periphery of the tumor. Other vascular cell receptors may be expressed such as vimentin, intercellular adhesion molecule (ICAM-l) and PECAM/CD3l but interestingly not vascular cell adhesion molecule (VCAM) or e-selectin. The underlying stromal cells can express α-smooth muscle actin (α-SMA) and vimentin had no aortic disparity, whereas this was almost invariably observed in those who had percutaneous angiograms some weeks later. Nevertheless, the reports from the obstetric literature detailed above do show definite prenatal examples of cardiac failure.

Rupture of a liver hemangioma and hemoperitoneum has been reported rarely, both in children and adults, and usually with fatal consequences.[5,6]

Jaundice may occur in up to 50% of cases and is multifactorial in origin. Commonly it is caused by increased hemolysis and a reduced erythrocyte life, span consequent upon "sumping" in the dilated tortuous vascular channels of the hemangioma. Occasionally, hemangiomas at the hilum appear to be a direct cause of obstructive jaundice. For instance, Hase et al described a four-month-old boy who presented with conjugated jaundice who had a 4 cm.[7] tumor arising in the hepatoduodenal ligament extending to the hepatic hilum, which had caused biliary obstruction. This was unresectable and treated by internal biliary stenting. Spontaneous resolution of the tumor occurred by 20 months, allowing stent removal and an excellent outcome.

Occasionally, gastrointestinal symptoms such as diarrhea and even malabsorption may be apparent although the mechanism of this in the absence of arterioportal hypertension is obscure.[5]

Liver hemangiomas may be part of a multiple hemangioma syndrome. The commonest sites aside from the skin, are the lungs and the central nervous system.[8] Other rarer sites have been the small bowel, larynx and trachea, vertebral column and spleen.[5] Table 83.1 illustrates the occurrence of liver hemangiomas that have been reported as part of a recognised malformation syndrome. Isolated cases have been reported of liver hemangiomas in association with congenital heart defects.[9]

It has been recently recognized that hemangiomatous tissue may also secrete protein, hormones or hormone-like substances. Clinical manifestations of this phenomenon are however rare. The commonest example of this is the secretion of α-fetoprotein and abnormally high serum levels may cause diagnostic confusion between hepatoblastomas and solitary hemangiomas. A definite association with thyroid hormone abnormalities has recently been identified.[10,11] A recent analysis at our institution identified seven infants with multifocal liver HAE who had abnormal biochemical thyroid function. In seven, this was characterised by a raised TSH with otherwise variable plasma thyroxine levels. Autopsy liver material from one child showed positive immuno-

Table 83.1: Known associations of liver hemangioma and hemangioendotheliomas	
Association	Features
Beckwith - Wiedemann syndrome	Overgrowth syndrome, with macroglossia, hypoglycemia, exomphalos and hepatomegaly. Association with Wilm's tumor
Hemihypertrophy syndrome	Disparity in size between sides of body. Association with hepatoblastoma and Wilm's tumor
Cornelia de Lange syndrome	Characteristic facies, gastroesophageal reflux, developmental delay. Association with Wilm's tumor
Multiple cavernous angioma syndrome	Cerebral and retinal angiomas

histochemical staining for TSH thought to be evidence for secretion of a TSH-like substance by the hemangiomatous tissue capable of causing inappropriate stimulation of the thyroid gland.

CLINICAL FEATURES

Antenatal

The antenatal liver hemangiomas have been reported although with markedly different clinical outcomes. For instance, Dreyfus et al identified a large markedly vascular, septated liver mass in a fetus.[15] No intervention was necessary and indeed postnatal investigations showed spontaneous regression of the tumor. In contrast, Morris et al reported a fetus initially diagnosed at 17 weeks gestation to have a liver hemangioma with later antenatal ultrasound evidence of heart failure.[13] This was treated with maternal and later postnatal corticosteroids with ultimate resolution.

Fetal liver hemangiomas may have effects upon the mother. Certainly, associated vascular anomalies of the placenta such as chorioangiomas have been reported.[14]

Postnatal

Hemangiomas may well be entirely asymptomatic, particularly if small. Increasing size and vascularity make symptoms more likely and typically these can include a palpable abdominal mass hepatomegaly, failure to thrive, respiratory distress, cardiac failure, jaundice, anemia, thrombocytopenia and disseminated intravascular coagulation. Often the specific diagnostic clue is the presence of cutaneous hemangiomas, which have been described in up to 60% of cases.[9]

Cardiac failure is high-output in nature and due to the huge, yet futile, hepatic artery to hepatic vein shunt through the liver. This can account for up to 50% of cardiac output in some cases and will be manifest as cardiomegaly, systolic cardiac murmurs, an abdominal bruit and marked aortic disparity above and below the origin of the relevant hepatic artery. It is not uncommon for the cardiac features to be so prominent that the actual cause of the failure is sometimes disregarded leading to a delay in diagnosis.

The hemodynamic changes, which accompany the rapid enlargement of the lesions, are usually considered as a postnatal phenomenon. Thus Stanley et al showed that all those infants who had angiography via the umbilical artery within one week of life has usually been ineffective.[9] Holcomb et al described liver irradiation in five children who received from 350-2000 rads, apparently with reasonable tumor control in three.[15] They also noted that an early case died later at the age of 12 years of leukemia.

DIAGNOSIS

Although the diagnosis of hemangiomatous lesions may not be straightforward. For most symptomatic lesions presenting in infancy a combination of ultrasonography, Doppler flow studies and dynamic contrast CT scanning should be adequate. Occasionally, plain radiographs may show hepatomegaly and intratumoral calcification with features such as cardiac enlargement and pulmonary plethora due to cardiac failure.[8]

Ultrasonography and Doppler flow studies are not in themselves characteristic and may show hypoechoic, complex or even hyperechoic lesions.[8] Dilatation of the draining hepatic veins may be seen and is consistent evidence of increased vascularity and a high flow shunt.

The characteristic CT appearance of hemangiomas is of a mass of lower attenuation than surrounding liver with an immediate intense peripheral enhancement and centripetal frond-like extensions following intravenous contrast administration (Fig. 83.2). More delayed scans will show contrast retained within periphery although there may be sequential central enhancement. Magnetic resonance imaging (MRI) shows decreased signal on T1-weighted images and increased signal on T2-weighted Most are usually discrete and best seen on T2-weighted images as high intensity lesions (Figs 83.3A and B). Functionally they exhibit fast flow, which are seen as flow voids on spin-echo images and high signal intensity on gradient recalled echo images. Hepatic angiography has been used extensively to study the vascular nature of these tumors. The blood supply may be very variable although typically it is predominantly from the hepatic arteries and may be manifest as hypertrophy of the right and left hepatic arteries. The development of both collaterals and accessory arteries (e.g. phrenic arteries) is also common. Most lesions exhibit a rapid homogenous capillary blush, while others show peripheral egg shell opacification. Some hemangiomas may have predominantly a portal venous rather than arterial blood supply—which is angiographically apparent as late re-opacification of hepatic lesions. Occasionally direct portal vein to hepatic vein communications can be demonstrated with a minimal systemic arterial collateral circulation. Clearly, attempts at therapeutic embolization or arterial ligation will be completely ineffective for this latter type.

MANAGEMENT

The management of both symptomatic hemangiomas and HAE's is controversial and there is widespread disagreement between authors as to the most appropriate choice of therapy. Figure 83.4 illustrates a suitable management algorithm developed at our institution for hepatic hemangiomas/HAE's. Most asymptomatic lesions can simply be managed expectantly perhaps using serial ultrasonography to

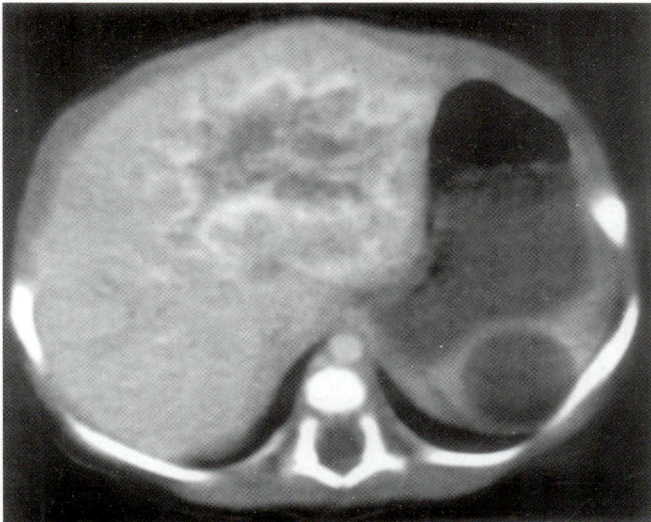

Fig. 83.2: Contrast enhanced CT scan of mass in left lobe of liver in one month old asymptomatic boy. The mass involves segment IV and shows peripheral and central enhancement

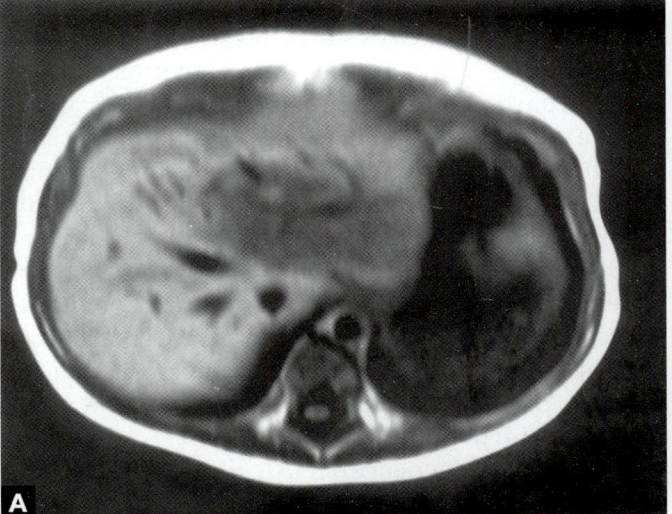
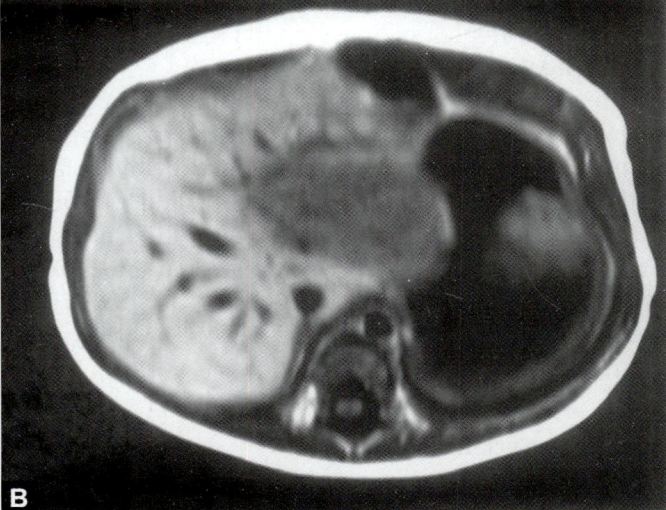

Figs 83.3A and B: MRI imaging of same case as Fig. 83.2, at **B.** six months of age, with overall reduction in size

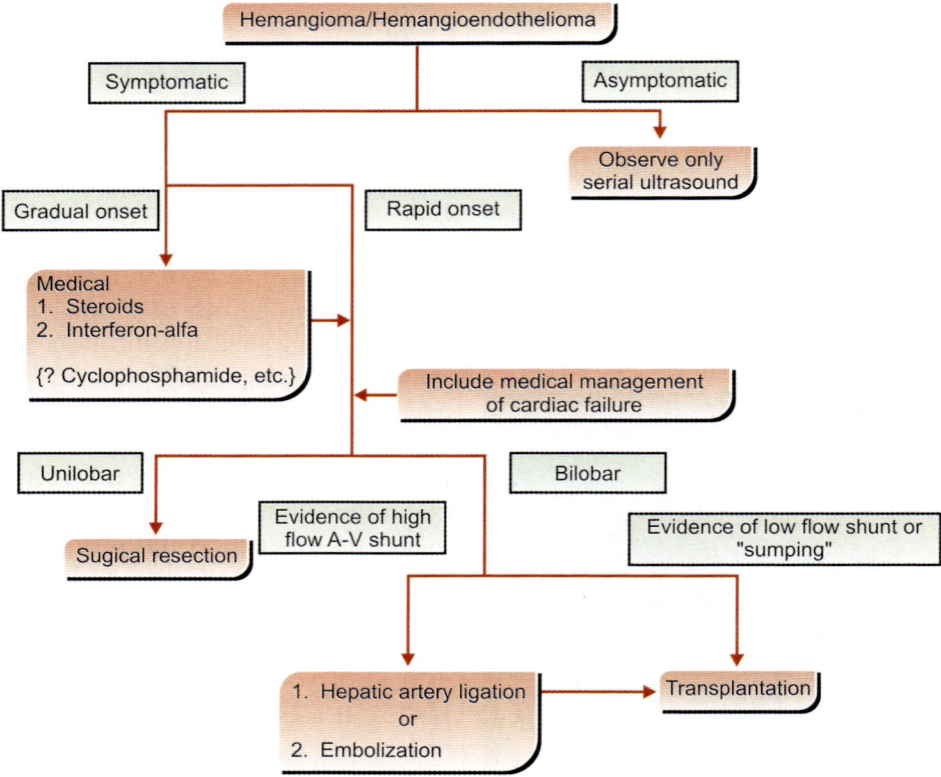

Fig. 83.4: Management algorithm of hemangioma/hemangioendothelioma of childhood

document the expected pattern of resolution. However, at the other end of the symptom scale, those infants who present with catastrophic cardiac and respiratory failure will need emergency therapy effective immediately. This usually implies interventional strategies such as hepatic resection, hepatic arterial ligation or embolization.

The medical treatment for liver HAE and hemangiomas has not been standardized but in addition to the specific agents detailed below infants with clinical signs of cardiac failure will also require fluid restriction, digitalization and diuretics as supportive therapy. Occasionally epsilonaminocaproic acid (EACA) has also been suggested as supportive therapy to counter the intravascular coagulation seen in multiple HAE's.

Hepatic Arterial Ligation

Early reports of successful hepatic arterial ligation (HAL) by De Lorimier et al.[16] in 1967 in infants with cardiac failure and multiple liver hemangiomas showed the value of selective arterial devascularization. At that time there was 80-90% mortality in infants who were conservatively treated and this was the first effective treatment for the high-output cardiac failure due to shunting through typically unresectable, bilobar lesions. Further reports have confirmed its value in the management of multiple lesions particularly when associated with cardiac failure.

The effectiveness of HAL arises from the biological observation that liver hemangiomas and HAE are preferentially supplied by hepatic arterial rather than portal venous sources. Consequently, dearterialization causes selective ischemia in abnormal hemangiomatous tissue sparing normal hepatic parenchyma. In humans, and unlike dogs, hepatic necrosis is not a consequence of HAL provided that sepsis and shock can be avoided.

The largest experience of HAL in symptomatic RAE is from our institution, which described eight infants who had presented at a median age of four weeks with symptomatic cardiac failure.[9] HAL was extremely successful in controlling the high flow shunt and cardiac failure in six.

At operation it is important to look for all possible arterial sources in order to dearterialise the liver effectively including accessory arteries in the lesser omentum from the right gastric artery and an aberrant right hepatic artery from the superior mesenteric artery. A cholecystectomy should also be performed, as the cystic artery will be ligated. Bile duct ischemia due to devascularization is a possible sequel and we have had one child who developed a spontaneous duodeno-biliary fistula manifest some years after HAL as recurrent cholangitis.

Hepatic Artery Embolization

Transcatheter arterial embolization of the feeding vessels was introduced in the 1980's to control the high-output cardiac failure in infants with RAE.[17] Numerous materials have since been used to achieve thrombosis including gelatin sponge particles (Gelfoam), polyvinyl alcohol particles (Ivalon), silicone balloons, cyanoacrylate and coils.

The procedure requires a high degree of skill and experience in pediatric angiography is essential. A variety of technique-related complications have been reported including hepatic necrosis, renal infarction and pulmonary embolism. Femoral artery damage is common although fortunately this does not usually lead to clinical sequelae due to collateral formation. Nevertheless, a possible late manifestation of femoral artery damage is inequality of lower limb growth.

The effectiveness of dearterialization (either HAL or embolization) procedures will depend upon the scale of the arterial input, the type of arteriovenous shunt and its contribution to symptoms. If the blood supply to the hemangiomatous tissue is predominantly from the portal vein then arterial embolization will not be helpful and is contraindicated.[15] Dearterialization is also unlikely to be of benefit in infants where the clinical manifestations are more characteristic of low-flow "sumping" (e.g. consumption coagulopathy and anemia) rather than a high-flow arteriovenous shunt (e.g. cardiac failure).

Hepatic Resection

Unilobar tumors may be effectively treated by partial hepatectomy (right, left or non-anatomical). Nevertheless, resection of a large hemangioma can be formidable as the liver is soft and friable in the early weeks of life coupled with the difficult dissection necessary to control the invariably dilated hepatic veins. Resection is usually the most suitable treatment for the late-presenting solitary tumor, particularly if there is doubt about its histological nature. In some centers, liver resection has been the only alternative to medical treatment. For instance, Luks et al.[18] in Montreal described 7 of 16 cases where resection was carried out without morbidity or mortality, the other cases being managed entirely medically.

Some novel techniques have been used to aid safe resection surgery. For instance, Ranne et al.[19] reported the use of hypothermic circulatory arrest and liver resection in two infants with cardiac failure and liver hemangiomas. The first, a four-day-old infant, underwent closure of an atrial septal defect and a left partial hepatectomy for hemangioma and the second, a 12 day-old infant, an extended right hepatectomy for HAE.

Transplantation

The option of complete liver excision and transplantation arrived with the advent of successful liver transplant programs in the early 1990's. However, real evidence of its value is still lacking and there are still considerable logistical problems related to lack of suitable size-matched donor organs and the urgency in which therapy is often needed.

The first successful liver excision and orthotopic liver transplantation (OLT) was reported in a child with RAE in 1994 by Egawa et al.[20] At the time of transplant she was six months old and had required ventilation due to the massive size of her tumor. Daller et al from the Thomas Starzl Transplant Institute in Pittsburgh, USA have recently reported their experience with infantile HAE.[21] Thirteen infants and children were referred for treatment for symptomatic HAE and giant hemangiomas at a median age of 14 days. Aside from the range of medical therapies, a variety of interventional techniques were used including resection (n = 5), embolization (n = 6), HAL (n = 2) and OLT (n = 3). However, the overall results were not good and only six (46%) children survived. Of the three infants who underwent OLT, one was for bilobar disease and the other two for Budd-Chiari syndrome following attempted resections. Only one remains alive, the others have died from transplant-related complications.

CAVERNOUS HEMANGIOMAS IN ADOLESCENTS AND ADULTS

Although the majority of cavernous hemangiomas will be incidental findings, some of the larger examples may become symptomatic, usually causing a dull ache or feelings of dragging. Cardiac failure is not seen and consumption coagulopathy is exceptional. A relationship with estrogens use has been suggested although with the female predominance this may well be incidental. Most surgical series concentrate on those > 4 cm in diameter and anything smaller tends to be ignored as trivial. For instance, Trastek et al.[22] reported the Mayo Clinic experience of 118 adult patients with cavernous hemangiomas. Of these 49 (41%) were > 4 cms in diameter and 12 (10%) were resected. No complications occurred in 35 who were followed expectantly for an average of five years. Reading et al reported the Kings College Hospital experience of 24 adults (mean age 43 years) with cavernous hemangiomas of which 15 were symptomatic.[23] Resection and/or gelfoam embolization were performed in cases. The later treatment was usually associated with reduction in symptoms but seldom with a reduction in size and furthermore in two of the larger examples multiple liver abscesses occurred.

REFERENCES

1. Kundstadler RH. Hemangioendothelioma of the liver in infancy. Am J Dis Child 1933;46:803-10.
2. Kasabach HA, Merritt KK. Capillary hemangioma with extensive purpura: report of a case. Am J Dis Child 1940;59:1063-70.
3. Dehner LP, Ishak KG. Vascular tumours of the liver in infants and children: a study of 30 cases and review of the literature. Arch Pathol 1971;92:101-11.
4. Selby DM, Stocker JT, Waclawiw MA, Hitchcock CL, Ishak KG. Infantile hemangioendothelioma of the liver. Hepatology 1994;20:39-45.
5. Samuel M, Spitz L. Infantile hepatic haemangioendothelioma: the role of surgery. J Pediatr Surg 1995;30:1425-29.
6. Ehren H, Mahour GH, Issacs H. Benign liver tumors in infancy and childhood: report of 48 cases. Am J Surg 1983;145:325-29.
7. Hase T, Kodama M, Kishada A, et al. Successful management of infantile hepatic hilar hemangioendothelioma with obstructive jaundice and consumption coagulopathy. J Pediatr Surg 1995;30:1485-87.
8. Stanley P, Geer GD, Miller JH, et al. Infantile hepatic hemangiomas: clinical features, radiologic investigations and treatment of 20 patients. Cancer 1989;64:936-49.
9. Davenport M, Hansen L, Heaton ND, Howard ER. Hemangioendothelioma of the liver in infants. J Pediatr Surg 1995;30:44-48.
10. Huang SA, Tu HM, Harney JW, et al. Severe hypothyroidism caused by Type 3 iodothyronine deiodinase in infantile hemangiomas. N Eng J Med 2000;343:185-89.
11. Ayling RM, Davenport M, Hadzic N, et al. Hepatic hemangioendothelioma associated with production of humoral thyrotropin-like factor. J Pediatr 2001;138:932-35.
12. Dreyfus M, Baldauf JJ, Dadoun K, Becmeur F, Berrut F, Ritter J. Prenatal diagnosis of hepatic hemangioma. Fetal Diagnosis and Therapy 1996;11:57-60.
13. Morris J, Abbott J, Burrows P, Levine D. Antenatal diagnosis of fetal hepatic hemangioma treated with maternal corticosteroids. Obstet Gynecol 1999;94:813-15.
14. Drut R, Drut RM, Toulouse JC. Hepatic hemangioendothelioma, placental chorioangiomas and dysmorphic kidneys in Beckwith- Wiedemann syndrome. Pediatr Pathol 1992;12:197-203.
15. Holcomb OW, O'Neil JA, Mahboubi S, Bishop HC. Experience with hepatic hemangioendothelioma in infancy and childhood. J Pediatr Surg 1988;23:661-66.
16. de Lorimier AA, Simpson EB, Baum RS, et al. Hepatic artery ligation for hepatic hemangiomatosis. N Eng J Med 1967;277:333-37.
17. Burrows PE, Rosenberg HC, Chuang HS. Diffuse hepatic hemangiomas: percutaneous transcatheter embolization with detachable silicone balloons. Radiology 1985;156:85-88.
18. Luks PI, Yazbeck S, Brandt ML, et al. Benign liver tumors in children: a 25 year experience. J Pediatr Surg 1991;26:1326-30.
19. Ranne RD, Ashcraft KW, Holder TM, et al. Hepatic hemangioma: resection using hypothermic circulatory arrest in the newborn. J Pediatr Surg 1988;23:924-26.
20. Egawa H, Berquist W, Garcia-Kennedy R, et al. Respiratory distress from benign liver tumors: a report of two unusual cases treated with hepatic transplantation. J Pediatr Gastro Nutr 1994;19:114-17.
21. Daller JA, Bueno J, Gutierrez J et al. Hepatic hemangioendothelioma: clinical experience and management strategy. J Pediatr Surg 1999;34:98-106.
22. Trastek VF, van Heerden JA, Sheedy PF, Adson MA. Cavernous hemangiomas of the liver: resect or observe? Am J Surg 1983;145:49-53.
23. Reading NO, Forbes A, Nunnerley HB, Williams R. Hepatic haemangioma: a critical review of diagnosis and management. Q J Med 1988;67:431-45.

CHAPTER 84

Liver Abscess in Children

Mark D Stringer

Liver abscess is a relatively rare but life-threatening condition in childhood. Failure to diagnose and treat the abscess(es) promptly and appropriately may cause serious morbidity or death. Accounts of the condition date back to Hippocrates (460-375 BC) who included abscesses in his accounts of liver disease and stated that they were least dangerous when opened externally. In modern times, it was not until 1938 that the first detailed study was published.[1] Most liver abscesses are either pyogenic or amebic.

PYOGENIC LIVER ABSCESS

EPIDEMIOLOGY

The variable incidence of pyogenic liver abscess in different communities probably reflects the distribution of predisposing factors. In adults in industrialised countries, the incidence is as low as 1.1 per 100,000 person years.[2] In children incidence figures of 3-25 per 100,000 hospital admissions have been recorded.[3-6] In some parts of the world, such as Southern India and Brazil, this figure is much higher but the true population incidence is difficult to determine because of local referral patterns.[7,8]

Pyogenic liver abscesses may affect any age group, including neonates. In a series of 98 patients with pyogenic liver abscess from Cape Town, South Africa, the mean age was 4.5 years whilst in Brazil the mean age of 65 affected children was 7.5 years.[8,9] Boys out number girls by approximately 2:1.[5,8] In children with underlying chronic granulomatous disease, there is a much greater male preponderance.

ETIOLOGY

Pyogenic liver abscess may develop in apparently healthy children, particularly in developing communities where protein calorie malnutrition and worm infestation are probable predisposing factors.[6,7,9] In developed communities, liver abscess is more often seen in immunocompromized children, especially those with chronic granulomatous disease (see below).[3,5]

Several pathways of infection may result in a liver abscess:
- *Biliary tract:* Ascending bacterial infection via the biliary tract or directly from the gallbladder
- *Portal vein:* From acute appendicitis or intra-abdominal sepsis
- *Hepatic artery:* From septicemia originating from a distant source, or bacteremia resulting in infection of a pre-existing hepatic lesion such as a hematoma or focal infarction
- *Direct:* From penetrating trauma or spread from contiguous intra-abdominal sepsis.

In the immunocompetent child, biliary tract disease is the commonest overall source. There still remains a substantial group of patients with cryptogenic abscess. Potential predisposing factors to pyogenic liver abscess are shown in Table 84.1.

Biliary Tract Diseases

This includes a wide variety of pathologies which can cause ascending bacterial cholangitis and intrahepatic abscess formation. Choledocholithiasis, cholecystitis

Table 84.1: Potential predisposing factors to pyogenic liver abscess

- Biliary tract diseases, e.g. calculi, choledochal cyst, Caroli's, cholecystitis, biliary atresia, etc.
- Intra-abdominal sepsis, e.g. appendicitis, NEC, Crohn's disease, foreign body perforation, etc.
- Distant sepsis/septicemia, e.g. osteomyelitis, pneumonia, bacterial endocarditis
- Structural liver lesions, e.g. cysts (parasitic or simple)
- Blunt or penetrating liver trauma
- Hepatic artery thrombosis, e.g. after liver transplantation
- Sickle cell anemia
- Chronic granulomatous disease
- Immunosuppression
- Recent measles infection
- Protein energy malnutrition
- Ascariasis
- Toxocariasis
- Papillon-Lefévre syndrome
- Ventriculo-peritoneal shunts
- Cirrhosis (adults)
- Underlying hepatic malignancy (adults)

(calculous or acalculous), sclerosing cholangitis, and choledochal cyst may all be complicated by pyogenic liver abscess. After Kasai portoenterostomy, children with biliary atresia may develop an intrahepatic bilioma which may be complicated by ascending infection and abscess formation.[10]

Oriental cholangiohepatitis or recurrent pyogenic cholangitis is especially prevalent in South-East Asia and the Far East with 3% of all cases occurring in children.[11] It is characterized by recurrent attacks of ascending cholangitis and associated hepatolithiasis, biliary stricturing and dilatation.[12] Pathologically, the intra- and extrahepatic ducts are dilated and contain soft, pigment stones and pus. The cause of the disease is not known, but associations with clonorchiasis, ascariasis, and nutritional deficiency have been suggested. Sonographic and CT findings include intra- or extrahepatic duct stones, ductal dilatation, segmental hepatic atrophy, and pyogenic liver abscesses. The latter are typically small and multiple and may contain biliary sludge and stones.

The finding of intact ascaridae within some liver abscesses suggests that migration through the ampulla of Vater and invasion of intrahepatic biliary radicles by Ascaris lumbricoides may result in abscess formation in endemic areas.[13] Ascariasis may also cause liver abscess by obstruction of the biliary tree and ascending bacterial cholangitis. In addition, several authors have suggested that helminthic infestations such as ascariasis and toxocariasis, in which larvae migrate through the liver, may indirectly predispose to pyogenic liver abscess.[8,9,14,15] Helminths can reduce the microbicidal activity of phagocytes and promote a granulomatous reaction encouraging trapping of bacteria in the liver.

Intra-abdominal Sepsis

Acute appendicitis may be complicated by portal pyemia and liver abscess. In a literature review, Sorensen et al (1983) identified acute appendicitis as the cause of pyogenic liver abscess in only 8% of reported cases.[16] This complication may present with nonspecific symptoms and signs either before or after a diagnosis of acute appendicitis but should be suspected in a persistently unwell child with signs of sepsis and hypoalbuminemia. In such children, an abdominal ultrasound scan may reveal a focal liver mass of low-to-mixed echogenicity and/or evidence of portal vein inflammation (Fig. 84.1).[17] Portal vein thrombosis is a potential complication of portal pyemia.[18]

Bacteria can be isolated from portal venous blood samples in up to one-third of patients undergoing surgery but the hepatic reticuloendothelial system normally prevents these pathogens from causing disease.[19] In acute appendicitis, portal bacteremia occurs more frequently. In one study, bacteria were isolated from superior mesenteric venous blood samples in at least 40% of patients with appendicitis.[20] Bacteroides spp. and *Escherichia coli* were most frequently identified. When the liver is compromised as a result of poor perfusion or disease or when the hepatic defence systems become overwhelmed by excessive numbers of bacteria, as in some cases of intra-abdominal sepsis, suppurative infection may supervene. In addition to appendicitis, other sources of intra-abdominal sepsis may be complicated by a pyogenic liver abscess. These include inflammatory bowel disease, necrotizing enterocolitis, and foreign body perforation of the gut.[12,21-23]

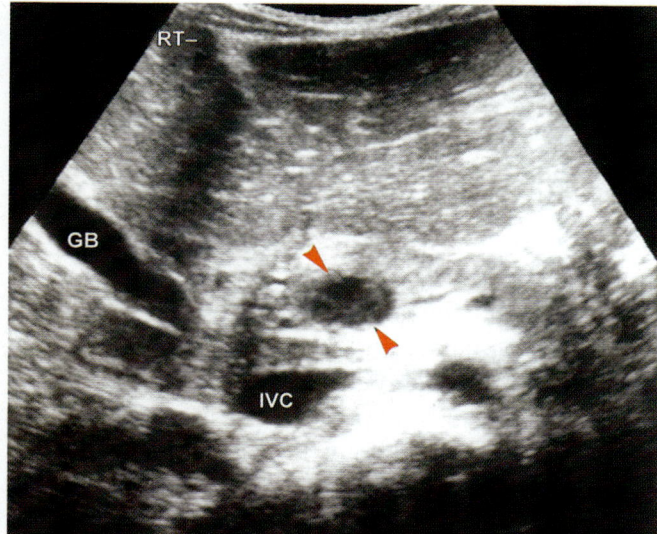

Fig. 84.1: A transverse abdominal ultrasound scan demonstrating non-occluding thrombus within the portal vein (arrowed) in a boy with portal pyemia complicating suppurative appendicitis. GB = gallbladder, IVC = inferior vena cava, RT

Distant Sepsis

Septicemia from a distant site of infection may cause the development of a pyogenic liver abscess. For example, bacterial endocarditis, osteomyelitis and pneumonia may be complicated in this way; multiple small hepatic abscesses are more common than solitary lesions.

Trauma

An intrahepatic abscess may form after blunt or penetrating liver trauma. Penetrating wounds may lead to direct contamination of injured liver and after blunt trauma, hematogenous infection of a hematoma may result in abscess formation.[24]

Structural Liver Lesions

A variety of structural abnormalities in the liver, both congenital, and acquired, may be complicated by infection and hepatic abscess formation. Caroli's disease is a congenital segmental saccular dilatation of the intrahepatic bile ducts with intervening ducts of near normal caliber. It may affect the liver diffusely or be localized to one lobe, more often the left. The condition typically causes recurrent cholangitis which may present with fever, jaundice or abdominal pain. Hepatosplenomegaly is common and intrahepatic abscess and/or stone formation may complicate the disease. Most cases present as young adults but pediatric examples have been reported.[25] Simple liver cysts rarely become infected unless there have been attempts to drain them. In endemic regions, hydatid cysts may be complicated by pyogenic infection. Mesenchymal hamartoma may rarely become infected but, unlike adults, liver abscess in children is almost never the presenting feature of an underlying hepatic malignancy. In adults, cirrhosis of the liver is associated with a higher incidence of pyogenic liver abscess because of impaired immunity and macrophage function, and the potential for abdominal infection but this association has not been documented in children.[2,26]

Other Causes of Pyogenic Liver Abscess

Children with chronic granulomatous disease, an inherited disorder of neutrophil function, are particularly susceptible to infection with catalase-positive organisms such as *Staphylococcus aureus*, gram negative bacteria such as *Escherichia coli* and *Serratia marascens*, and fungi such as *aspergillus* and *candida species*. These children typically present in early childhood with recurrent pyogenic abscesses which may involve the liver.[27]

Hepatic allografts which are retained after hepatic artery thrombosis following liver transplantation are often complicated by focal infarction and/or biliary complications, both of which predispose to hepatic abscess formation.[28] Liver abscess may also complicate sickle cell disease either as a consequence of biliary tract pathology (including choledocholithiasis) or after a vaso-occlusive crisis with segmental hepatic infarction.[29,30]

Rarely, pyogenic liver abscess has been reported as a complication of ventriculoperitoneal shunting for hydrocephalus.[31] The shunt partially erodes into the liver resulting in the formation of an intrahepatic cyst which becomes secondarily infected. Along with treatment of the abscess, the peritoneal part of the shunt must be externalized.

Papillon-Lefevre syndrome is an autosomal recessive condition characterized by palmoplantar keratosis and severe periodontopathy. The disease is related to defects in cell-mediated immunity and neutrophil function which, together with possible bacteremia from dental disease, are responsible for infections at other sites, including liver abscesses.[32]

PATHOLOGY

Abscesses may be single or multiple, unilocular or multilocular. Multiple abscesses are more often associated with biliary tract diseases. The right lobe is the site of abscess formation in more than two-thirds of patients.

Staph. aureus and *E.coli* account for most cases of pyogenic liver abscess (Table 84.2).[5,7,33] In the Western Cape Province of South Africa, *Staph. aureus* was identified in 85% of children with a pyogenic liver abscess.[6] The *Streptococcus milleri* group of bacteria (which includes *Str. intermedius* and *Str. anginosus*) are important pathogens in adults with a liver abscess and may be the causative organism in some children. An occult hepatic abscess should be suspected if blood cultures are positive for *Streptococcus milleri*.[34] These bacteria may be mistaken for anaerobes but are resistant to metronidazole and usually sensitive to penicillin. However, anaerobic organisms should always be suspected if the abscess contains gas. Hemophilus influenzae and other haemophilus species may rarely cause pyogenic liver abscess in unvaccinated children.[35] Cat-scratch disease is an infection caused by a gram-negative bacillus, Bartonella henselae, and is another rare cause of liver and spleen abscesses in children.[36]

CLINICAL FEATURES

Pyogenic liver abscess usually presents with fever and general malaise. Most school age children complain of upper abdominal pain. The duration of symptoms is variable but usually less than 3 weeks. Other symptoms may include anorexia, nausea and vomiting, weight loss, cough, and abdominal distension. Clinical signs include fever, tender hepatomegaly, and jaundice especially in those with biliary tract diseases and/or multiple liver abscesses. A right-sided pleural effusion may be present.

Routine laboratory investigations typically show anemia and leucocytosis with elevated inflammatory indices (C-reactive protein, plasma viscosity, and erythrocyte sedimentation rate) and hypoalbuminemia. Abnormalities of biochemical liver function are found in half the patients and include raised serum alkaline phosphatase and, to a lesser extent, bilirubin and transaminase levels. Blood cultures may be positive in up to 50% of patients.[7] Suspicion of chronic granulomatous disease may be confirmed by nitroblue tetrazolium test.

DIAGNOSIS

A pyogenic liver abscess should be suspected in any child with fever, abdominal pain and hepatomegaly. A plain chest radiograph may show an elevated right hemidiaphragm or pleural effusion or, rarely, gas or a fluid level within the abscess. Ultrasonography has proved to be sensitive method of detecting liver abscesses but may miss smaller lesions and those in the dome of the liver.[37-39,41] Lesions are typically hypoechoic and round to oval with illdefined margins and variable internal echoes (Figs 84.2A and 84.3A). A ring of hypoechogenic liver edema often surrounds the lesion. Computed tomography (CT) is the most sensitive imaging modality for liver abscess.[40,41] (Figs 84.2B and 84.3B). Appearances are variable and include low-density areas, cavities and more complex images. US and CT also provide other useful information about the cause of the pyogenic liver abscess. It has been suggested that, unlike fungal or mycobacterial microabscesses, small pyogenic abscesses tend to cluster, or aggregate, in a pattern that suggests the beginning of coalescence into a single, larger abscess cavity.[42]

Conventional radionuclide scans are of limited diagnostic value but gallium scanning and labelled white cell scans may have a role in selected cases.[41,43,44] With any imaging technique, pyogenic liver abscesses must be distinguished from liver cysts, tumors, pseudotumor, vascular malformations, and hematomas.

Table 84.2: Common pathogens in pyogenic liver abscess		
	Gram-negative	*Gram-positive*
Aerobes	Escherichia coli Klebsiella pneumonia	Staphylococcus aureus Streptococcus pyogenes Streptococcus milleri group
Anaerobes	Bacteroides spp. Fusobacterium spp.	Peptostreptococcus spp. Clostridium spp.

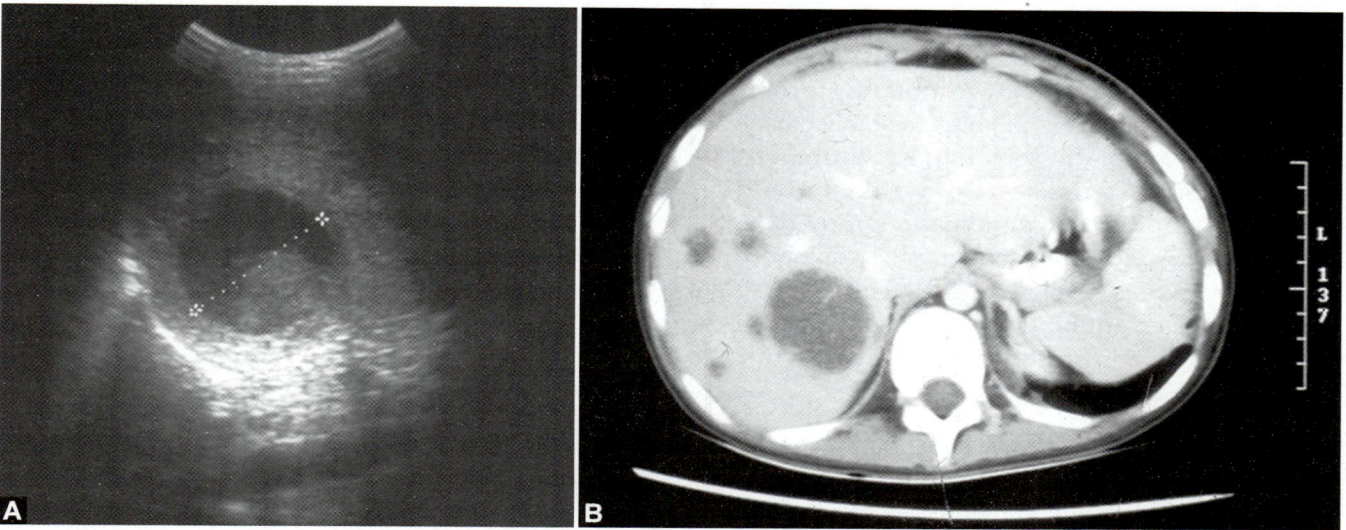

Figs 84.2A and B: A-13 year-old girl with a large predominantly solitary pyogenic abscess cavity in the right lobe of the liver. **A.** Ultrasonography shows a hypoechoic cavity with internal echoes and a surrounding rim of liver edema. **B.** CT scan shows the abscess with adjacent smaller abscesses

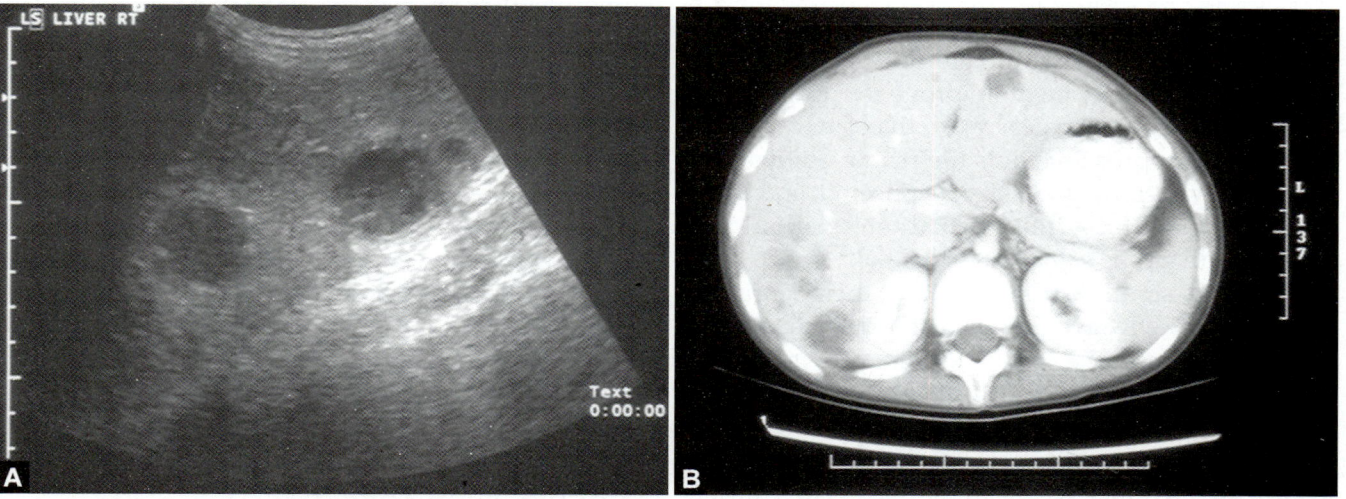

Figs 84.3A and B: Multiple liver abscesses demonstrated by **A.** ultrasound and **B.** CT scan in a girl with acute appendicitis soon after repair of coarctation of the aorta. She was treated successfully with intravenous broad spectrum antibiotics and subsequently underwent an uneventful interval appendicectomy

TREATMENT

This is guided by three basic principles:
- Confirm the diagnosis and determine the anatomy of the abscess(es).
- Treat with broad-spectrum intravenous antibiotics
- Drain the abscess if there is no prompt clinical response to therapy.

The success of an initial non-operative approach has been verified by many authors in recent years.[7,45]

In addition to the above measures, the patient will require correction of severe anemia and any fluid and electrolyte imbalance. Any underlying condition and associated diseases will require specific treatment.

Antibiotic Therapy

These must be an appropriate antibiotic given for an adequate duration. A penicillinase-resistant penicillin with an aminoglycoside and metronidazole is a suitable initial antibiotic regimen but a third generation cephalosporin and aminoglycoside is a reasonable alternative. In patients not responding promptly, percutaneous drainage will help to establish bacterial profiles and antibiotic sensitivities. Antibiotics are usually administered for 6-8 weeks but this is somewhat empirical. Symptomatic improvement is usually swift but complete sonographic resolution may take up to 8 weeks. In children with chronic granulomatous disease, antibiotic therapy may need to be supplemented with interferon gamma therapy to achieve abscess resolution.[27]

Percutaneous Drainage

Ultrasound-guided percutaneous needle aspiration/drainage should be considered in patients not responding to conservative therapy within 48 hours, i.e. those with persistent toxemia, tenderness and/or peritonism, and also in patients where the abscess is deemed to be at risk of imminent rupture.[29] Some have recommended earlier drainage for left-sided liver abscesses which may be more prone to rupture.[45] An anterior subcostal approach rather than a mid-axillary transpleural approach avoids the risk of empyema.[29] Lavage may increase the risk of septicemia and is not routinely used but drainage catheters should be flushed with sterile saline 4-6 times daily.[46]

Although simple aspiration can be therapeutic it is generally less effective than catheter drainage. Rajak et al (1998), compared the efficacy of repeated sonographically guided percutaneous needle aspiration and percutaneous catheter drainage (both with appropriate antimicrobial therapy) in the treatment of liver abscesses larger than 3 cm in adults and found the latter to be superior.[47] With catheter drainage, 8-12 French pigtail or sump catheters are introduced into the abscess cavity under ultrasound or CT guidance using a Seldinger's technique. Percutaneous catheter drainage is now the procedure of choice in the drainage of pyogenic abscesses.[29,48,49] Drainage is continued until abscess resolution is evidenced by defervescence, cessation of catheter drainage and ultrasound scan.[50]

Open Surgical Drainage

This is applicable in children with larger abscesses not responding to more conservative measures and in those undergoing *laparotomy to treat a primary* source of infection. A *large perforated tube drain* (18-24 Fr) is inserted into the abscess cavity, the wall of which should be biopsied to exclude amebic infection.

Rarely, hepatic resection is required. Indications include a chronically infected fibrotic cavity and focal hepatic involvement in Caroli's disease. For oriental cholangiohepatitis and biliary ascariasis, interventional endoscopic procedures may also be necessary.

RESULTS AND COMPLICATIONS

The most serious complications of a pyogenic liver abscess are septicemia and rupture, both of which may be fatal. Rupture may lead to a subphrenic abscess, empyema or peritonitis.[44,45] Liver abscess may rarely cause hemobilia manifesting as gastrointestinal bleeding this should be managed by angiography and selective arterial embolization. Metastatic septic endopthalmitis has also been reported in patients with Klebsiella liver abscess.[51-53]

Mortality from pyogenic liver abscess is now less than 10%.[6,45] In a series of 98 pyogenic and 26 amebic abscesses in children from South Africa, Moore et al (1994) reported no fatalities in those treated by an initial nonoperative approach. Kumar et al (1998) recorded an 11% mortality in 18 children with pyogenic liver abscess from Southern India, but one of the two deaths in this series presented with septic shock.[7,15] At greater risk of mortality and morbidity are immunodeficient children and those with other underlying diseases, patients with multiple abscesses, and those experiencing treatment complications.[54]

AMOEBIC LIVER ABSCESS

Amoebic liver abscess is the commonest extraintestinal manifestation of amebiasis and affects up to 10% of infected adults. The disease is less common in children but is associated with significant morbidity and mortality.[55,56]

EPIDEMIOLOGY

Amoebiasis is endemic in much of Asia, Africa, Central and South America and is frequently associated with poor sanitation, malnutrition, and concomitant infectious diseases. Amoebic liver abscess is most common in India, Pakistan and the Far East.[56,57] There is a slight male preponderance in children with amoebic liver abscess.[45,57] The mean age of affected children was 2 years in the Cape Town series and three-quarters of patients were less than 10 years in a report from Karachi, Pakistan.[45,56]

PATHOLOGY

Hepatic amoebiasis originates from intestinal infection by the protozoan parasite, entamoeba histolytica. Amoebic liver abscesses develop after the trophozoites enter the portal venous system via the gut. Thrombosis of small portal venous radicles results in foci of liquefactive necrosis and the formation of characteristic "anchovy sauce" pus. Small abscesses coalesce to form large abscesses which expand and may rupture. Multiple abscesses occur more often in children than adults but in some series solitary lesions predominate.[56] As with pyogenic abscesses, right lobe lesions are more common. A solitary left lobe abscess is present in approximately 10% of patients.

CLINICAL FEATURES

The typical presentation is a young debilitated child with a fever, right upper quadrant abdominal pain, and tender hepatomegaly. A previous history of bloody diarrhea is common but evidence of active amoebic colitis is unusual.[58] Jaundice is uncommon. Some patients present with a pyrexia of unknown origin or with the consequences of abscess rupture. In some cases, acute abdominal signs may cause confusion by suggesting perforated appendicitis.[56,59]

DIAGNOSIS

The key elements to diagnosis are imaging and serology. Investigations frequently show anemia and hypoalbuminemia and there may be a leucocytosis. Biochemical liver function tests are often normal or only minimally deranged. Cysts or trophozoites in the stool can only be isolated in one-third of patients.[11] There exists a wide variety of serologic tests for invasive amoebiasis but they cannot differentiate between previous and current infection. They depend on the detection of anti-amoebic antibodies. In children with amoebic liver abscess serology is almost invariably positive but these tests are less reliable in affected infants.[60]

A chest radiograph may show an elevated right hemidiaphragm, right pleural effusion, or right lower lobe changes. As with pyogenic liver abscess, ultrasound scanning and CT are sensitive imaging techniques. Ultrasound provides excellent anatomical information and demonstrates a characteristic peripheral halo with central liquefication.[45,61,62] However, it does not reliably distinguish between amoebic and pyogenic liver abscess. Both ultrasound and CT are useful in detecting transdiaphragmatic pleural involvement. Magnetic resonance imaging shows no specific image or intensity pattern and is comparable to ultrasound and CT in the detection of amoebic abscess.[63]

Diagnostic percutaneous aspiration of the abscess may be used in diagnosis; the aspirate is odorless and bacteriologically sterile (unless complicated by secondary bacterial infection) and may contain trophozoites. The characteristic "anchovy sauce" appearance is a variable finding. Recently, polymerase chain reaction technology has been successfully used to identify E. histolytica DNA in liver abscess pus.[64]

TREATMENT

This consists of antimicrobial therapy with or without abscess drainage.

Antimicrobial Therapy

Small uncomplicated amebic liver abscesses can be successfully managed by antimicrobial therapy alone.[55,56,58] Metronidazole is effective against both liver and intestinal parasites and is the drug of choice for amoebic liver abscess. The recommended doses are age related, ranging from 100 mg orally tds for children aged 1-3 years to 200 mg orally qds for 7-10 year old. The duration of treatment is 10-14 day. Most patients will respond clinically within 48-72 hours. Some authors recommend initial treatment with intravenous metronidazole and broad-spectrum antibiotics, discontinuing the later once the diagnosis of amoebic liver abscess is confirmed.[56] This has the merit of treating co-existent secondary bacterial infection of the abscess.[65]

Clinical response is the major determinant of successful treatment. Clinical and hematologic parameters return to normal within days and weeks, respectively but sonographic resolution takes months.[65] This delay in sonographic resolution does not warrant additional or prolonged therapy.

Abscess Drainage

Ultrasound guided percutaneous aspiration or catheter drainage of amoebic liver abscess may be indicated for the following reasons:

1. To distinguish pyogenic from amoebic abscess in nonendemic areas.
2. In cases failing to respond to metronidazole (lack of clinical and sonographic improvement within 48 hours).
3. For abscesses with signs of impending rupture (e.g. lesions >7cm diameter).
4. For large left lobe abscesses.

Percutaneous needle aspiration has yielded excellent results.[58,67] In a series of 48 consecutive children with amoebic liver abscesses from Pakistan, 28 required aspiration, and 9 required repeat aspiration.[56] No patient required open surgical drainage and all recovered without relapse.

Open surgical drainage is now reserved for the treatment of complications.

RESULTS AND COMPLICATIONS

The commonest complication is rupture into the pleural cavity and lung which results in pleural effusion, empyema and bronchopleural fistula. Chest tube drainage is required in addition to treatment of the liver abscess. The most serious complication is pericardial erosion from a left lobe abscess; this may lead to cardiac tamponade which requires urgent drainage of the liver abscess with or without pericardiocentesis. Intraperitoneal rupture causes peritonitis and intra-abdominal abscess formation, erosion of adjacent viscera such as the stomach can cause hematemesis,[68] and, rarely, hemobilia may develop. Many of these complications require laparotomy but localized intraperitoneal rupture can be treated by percutaneous drainage of the abscess and intravenous metronidazole.[56] In recent years, patients with ruptured amebic liver abscesses have been increasingly managed successfully by percutaneous catheter drainage irrespective of the extent of extrahepatic contamination.[69]

Morbidity and mortality from amoebic liver abscess have declined as a result of improved public health, earlier and more accurate diagnosis, and effective antimicrobial therapy. Overall mortality is significantly increased if the abscess ruptures or if it occurs in infancy.[60,70,71]

Although hepatic amoebiasis can be treated effectively, it remains an important cause of morbidity and mortality in endemic regions. The future lies in prevention which demands socioeconomic interventions to improve public health and, hopefully, the development of a vaccine.[72]

NEONATAL LIVER ABSCESS

Liver abscess is rarely encountered in neonates. Moss and Pysher (1981) identified only 24 cases in the literature prior to their report of 13 autopsy cases seen over a 20 year period.[73] Infection may occur through several routes: following umbilical vein cannulation[74] via the portal vein after intra-abdominal infection or surgery for necrotizing enterocolitis[12] via the hepatic artery as part of a generalized septicemia, when abscesses are more often multiple; and as a complication of catheter migration and infusion of parenteral nutrition into the hepatic vein.[12,74,75] Infusion of hypertonic solutions (such as 8.4% sodium bicarbonate or parenteral nutrition) and direct bacterial contamination may be significant factors with umblical venous catheter sepsis. Given the frequency of portal vein gas in necrotizing enterocolitis, it is perhaps surprising that liver abscess does not occur more often in this setting. In endemic areas, amebic liver abscess may also occur in the neonatal period.[56]

Clinical presentation and laboratory findings are frequently non-specific but indicative of sepsis. Hepatomegaly, abdominal tenderness and distension, with or without respiratory symptoms and signs may suggest the diagnosis.[76] Leucocytosis, thrombocytopenia and abnormal liver enzymes are common. Sonography may show a solitary abscess but multiple, small abscesses are more commonly found. The causative organism is usually *Staph. aureus*, gram negative bacteria such as *Klebsiella, Pseudomonas* and *E. coli*, or *Candida sp*. Most cases can be managed medically with appropriate intravenous antibiotic therapy. Solitary abscesses may require percutaneous catheter drainage.[76]

OTHER CAUSES OF LIVER ABSCESSES

Other rare causes of liver abscess include candidiasis (particularly immunocompromised children and neonates), actinomycosis, tuberculosis, listeriosis, brucellosis, and echinococcal disease.[77,78]

REFERENCES

1. Oschner A, Debakey M, Murray S. Pyogenic liver abscess. II. An analysis of 47 cases with review of the literature. Am J Surg 1938:40;292-319.
2. Molle I, Thulstrup AM, Vilstrup H, Sorensen HT. Increased risk and case fatality rate of pyogenic liver abscess in patients with liver cirrhosis: a nationwide study in Denmark. Gut 2001;48:260-63.
3. Chusid MJ. Pyogenic hepatic abscess in infancy and childhood. Pediatrics 1978;62:554-59.
4. Arya LS, Ghani R, Abdali S, Singh M. Pyogenic liver abscess in children. Clinical Pediatrics 1982;21:89-93.
5. Pineiro-Carrero VM, Andres JM. Morbidity and mortality in children with pyogenic liver abscess. Am J Dis Child 1989;143:1424-27.
6. Hendricks MK, Moore SW, Millar AJ. Epidemiological aspects of liver abscesses in children in the Western Cape Province of South Africa. J Trop Pediatr 1997;43:103-05.
7. Kumar A, Srinivasan S, Sharma AK. Pyogenic liver abscess in children – South Indian experiences. J Pediatr Surg 1998;33:417-21.
8. Ferreira MA, Pereira FE, Musso C, Dettogni RV. Pyogenic liver abscess in children: some observations in the Espirito Santo State, Brazil. Arq Gastroenterol 1997;34:49-54.
10. Tam PKH, Saing H, Lau JTK. Three successfully treated cases of nonamoebic liver abscess. Arch Dis Child 1983;58: 828-29.
11. Joseph VT. Hepatic abscesses. In: Howard ER, ed. Surgery of Liver Disease in Children. Oxford: Butterworth-Heinemann, 1991;193-210.
12. Lim JH. Oriental cholangiohepatitis: pathologic, clinical, and radiologic features. Am J Roentgenol 1991;157:1-8.
13. Javid G, Wani NA, Gulzar GM, et al. Ascaris-induced liver abscess. World J Surg 1999;23:1191-94.
14. Pereira FE, Musso C, Castelo JS. Pathology of pyogenic liver abscess in children. Pediatr Dev Pathol 1999;2:537-43.
15. Moreira-Silva SF, Pereira FE. Intestinal nematodes, Toxocara infection, and pyogenic liver abscess in children: a possible association. J Trop Pediatr 2000;46:167-72.
16. Sorensen MR, Baekgaard N, Kirkegaard P. Pyogenic liver abscess. A case report with a short review of current concepts of diagnosis and management. Acta Chir Scand 1983;149:437-39.
17. Slovis TL, Haller JO, Cohen HL, Berdon WE, Watts FB Jr. Complicated appendiceal inflammatory disease in children: pylephlebitis and liver abscess. Radiology 1989;171:823-25.
18. Chan SC, Chan FL, Chau EM, Mok FP. Portal thrombosis complicating appendicitis: ultrasound detection and hepatic computed tomography lobar attenuation alteration. J Comput Tomogr 1988;12:208-10.
19. Schatten WE, Desprez JD, Holden WD. A bacteriologic study of portal-vein blood in man. Arch Surg 1955;71:404-09.
20. Juric I, Primorac D, Zagar Z, et al. Frequency of portal and systemic bacteremia in acute appendicitis. Pediatr Int 2001;43:152-56.
21. Weinberg RJ, Klish WJ, Brown MR, Smalley JR, Emmens RW. Hepatic abscess as a complication of Crohn's disease. J Pediatr Gastroenterol Nutr 1983;2:171-74.
22. Lowry P, Rollins NK. Pyogenic liver abscess complicating ingestion of sharp objects. Pediatr Inf Dis J 1993;12:348-50.
23. Lim CT, Koh MT. Neonatal liver abscess following abdominal surgery for necrotizing enterocolitis. Pediatr Surg Int 1994;9:30-31.
24. Eng RH, Tecson-Tumang F, Corrado ML. Blunt trauma and liver abscess. Am J Gastroenterol 1981;76:252-55.
25. Pinto RB, Lima JP, da Silveira TR, et al. Caroli's disease: report of 10 cases in children and adolescents in Southern Brazil. J Pediatr Surg 1998;33:1531-35.
26. Pitt HA, Juidema GD. Factors influencing mortality in the treatment of pyogenic hepatic abscess. Surgery, Gynecology and Obstetrics 1975;140:228-34.
27. Hague RA, Eastham EJ, Lee REJ, Cant AJ. Resolution of hepatic abscess after interferon gamma in chronic granulomatous disease. Arch Dis Child 1993;69:443-45.
28. Stringer MD, Marshall MM, Muiesan P, et al. Survival and outcome after hepatic artery thrombosis complicating pediatric liver transplantation. J Pediatr Surg 2001;36:888-91.
29. Vachon L, Diament MJ, Stanley P. Percutaneous drainage of hepatic abscesses in children. J Pediatr Surg 1986;21:366-68.
30. Lama M. Hepatic abscess in sickle cell anaemia: a rare manifestation. Arch Dis Child 1993;69:242-43.
31. Huang LT, Chen CC, Shih TT, Ko SF, Liu C. Pyogenic liver abscess complicating a ventriculoperitoneal shunt. Pediatr Surg Int 1998;13:6-7.
32. Oguzkurt P, Tanyel FC, Buyukpamukcu N, Hicsonmez A. Increased risk of pyogenic liver abscess in children with Papillon-Lefevre syndrome. J Pediatr Surg 1996;31:955-56.
33. Frey CF, Zhu Y, Suzuki M, Isaji S. Liver abscesses. Surg Clin North America 1989;69:259-71.
34. Corredoira J, Casariego E, Moreno C, et al. Prospective study of Streptococcus milleri hepatic abscess. Eur j Clin Microbiol Infect Dis 1998;17:556-60.
35. Hartwig NG, Sinaasappel M, Robben SG, de Groot R. Liver abscess caused by Haemophilus influenzae b in an infant. Pediatr Infect Dis J 1995;14:245-46.
36. Dunn MW, Berkowitz FE, Miller JJ, Snitzer JA. Hepatosplenic cat-scratch disease and abdominal pain. Pediatr Infect Dis J 1997;16:269-72.

37. Glen PM, Noseworthy J, Babcock DS. Use of intraoperative ultrasonography to localise a hepatic abscess. Arch Surg 1984;119:347-48.
38. Laurin S, Kaude JV. Diagnosis of liver-spleen abscesses in children – with emphasis on ultrasound for the initial and follow-up examinations. Pediatr Radiol 1984;14:198-204.
39. Salama HM, Abdel-Wahab MF, Farid Z. Hepatobiliary disorders presenting as fever of unknown origin in Cairo, Egypt: the role of diagnostic ultrasonography. J Trop Med Hyg 1988;91:147-49.
40. Halvorsen RA Jr, Foster WL Jr, Wilkinson RH Jr, Silverman PM, Thompson WM. Hepatic abscess: sensitivity of imaging tests and clinical findings. Gastrointest Radiol 1988;13:135-41.
41. Halvorsen RA, Korobkin M, Foster WL, Silverman PM, Thompson WM. The variable CT appearance of hepatic abscesses. Am J Roentgenol 1984;141:941-46.
42. Jeffrey RB Jr, Tolentino CS, Chang FC, Federle MP. CT of small pyogenic hepatic abscesses: the cluster sign. Am J Roentgenol 1988;151:487-89.
43. Sty JR, Starshak RJ. Comparative imaging in the evaluation of hepatic abscesses in immunocompromised children. J Clin Ultrasound 1983;11:11-15.
44. Denison H, Wallerstedt S. Diagnosis of pyogenic liver abscess via liver scanning with indium-111 labelled granulocytes. Scand J Infect Dis 1989;21:345-48.
45. Moore SW, Millar AJW, Cywes S. Conservative initial treatment for liver abscesses in children. Br J Surg 1994;81:872-74.
46. Taguchi T, Ikeda K, Yakabe S, Kimura S. Percutaneous drainage for post-traumatic hepatic abscess in children under ultrasound imaging. Pediatric Radiology, 1988;18:85-87.
47. Rajak CL, Gupta S, Jain S, Chawla Y, Gulati M, Suri S. Percutaneous treatment of liver abscesses: needle aspiration versus catheter drainage. Am J Roentgenol 1998;170:1035-39.
48. Greenwood LH, Collins TL, Yrizarry JM. Percutaneous management of multiple liver abscesses. American Journal of Roentgenology 1982;139:390-92.
49. Skibber JM, Lotze MT, Garra B, Fauci A. Successful management of hepatic abscesses by percutaneous catheter drainage in chronic granulomatous disease. Surgery 1986;99:626-29.
50. Liu KW, Fitzgerald RJ, Blake NS. An alternative approach to pyogenic hepatic abscess in childhood. J Pediatr Child Health 1990;26:92-94.
51. Larsen LR, Raffensperger J. Liver abscess. J Pediatr Surg 1979;14:329-31.
52. Khalil A, Chadha V, Mandapati R, et al. Hemobilia in a child with liver abscess. J Pediatr Gastroenterol Nutr 1991;12:136-38.
53. Chiu CT, Lin DY, Liaw YF. Metastatic septic endophthalmitis in pyogenic liver abscess. J Clin Gastroenterol 1988;10:524-27.
54. Northover JMA, Jones BJM, Dawson JL, Williams R. Difficulties in the diagnosis and management of pyogenic liver abscess. British Journal of Surgery 1982;69:48-51.
55. Porras-Ramirez G, Harnandez-Herrera MH, Porras-Harnandez JD. Amebic hepatic abscess in children. J Pediatr Surg 1995;30:660-64.
56. Moazam F, Nazir Z. Amebic liver abscess: spare the knife but save the child. J Pediatr Surg 1998;33:119-22.
57. Das BN, Mitra SK, Walia BNS, Mahajan RC, Pathak IC. Amoebic liver abscess in children: a report of five cases. Indian Pediatrics 1976;13:113-17.
58. Wiersma R, Hadley GP, Luvuno FM. Amoebiasis in children: pathology, diagnosis, and treatment. Pediatr Surg Int 1990;5:406-10.
59. Harrison Hr, Crowe CP, Fulginiti VA. Amebic liver abscess in children: clinical and epidemiologic features. Pediatrics 1979;64:923-28.
60. Johnson JL, Baird JS, Hulbert TV, Opas LM. Amebic liver abscess in infancy: case report and review. Clin Infect Dis 1994;19:765-67.
61. Ralls PW, Colletti PM, Quinn MF, Halls J. Sonographic findings in hepatic amebic abscess. Radiology 1982;145:123-26.
62. Hayden CK jr, Toups M, Swischuk LE, Amparo EG. Sonographic features of hepatic amebiasis in childhood. Journal of Canadian Association of Radiology 1984;35:279-82.
63. Ralls PW, Henley DS, Colletti PM, et al. Amebic liver abscess: MR imaging. Radiology 1987;165:801-04.
64. Zaman S, Khoo J, Ng SW, Ahmed R, Khan MA, Hussain R, Zaman V. Direct amplification of Entamoeba histolytica DNA from amoebic liver abscess pus using polymerase chain reaction. Parasitol Res 2000;86:724-28.
65. Gathiram V, Simjee AE, Bhamjee A, et al. Concomitant and secondary bacterial infection of the pus in hepatic amoebiasis. S Afr Med J 1984;65:951-53.
66. Sharma MP, Dasarathy S, Sushma S, Verma N. Long-term follow-up of amebic liver abscess: clinical and ultrasound patterns of resolution. Trop Gastroenterol 1995;16:24-28.
67. Singh JP, Kashyap A. A comparative evaluationof percutaneous catheter drainage of resistant amebic liver abscesses. American Journal of Surgery 1989;158:58-62.
68. Angel C, Chand N, Sankar A, Rowen J, Murillo C. Gastric wall erosion by an amebic liver abscess in a 3-year-old girl. Pediatr Surg Int 2000;16:429-43.
69. Baijal SS, Agarwal DK, Roy S, Choudhuri G. Complex ruptured amebic liver abscesses: the role of percutaneous catheter drainage. Eur J Radiol 1995;20:65-67.
70. Jessee W F, Ryan J M, Fitzgerald JF, Grosfeld J L. Amebic liver abscess in childhood. Clinical Pediatrics 1985;14:134-45.
71. Meng XY, Wu JX. Perforated amebic liver abscess: clinical analysis of 110 cases. South Med J 1994;87:985-90.
72. Huston CD, Petri WA Jr. Host-pathogen interaction in amebiasis and progress in vaccine development. Eur J Clin Microbiol Infect Dis 1998;17:601-14.

73. Moss TJ, Pysher TJ. Hepatic abscess in neonates. American Journal of Diseases of Children 1981;135:726-28.
74. Brans YW, Ceballos R, Cassady G. Umbilical catheters and hepatic abscesses. Pediatrics 1974;53:264-66.
75. Raffensperger JG, Ramenofsky MI. A fatal complication of hyperalimentation. A case report. Surgery 1970;68:393-94.
76. Vade A, Sajous C, Anderson B, Challapalli M. Neonatal hepatic abscess. Comput Med Imaging Graph 1998;22:357-59.
77. Jain R, Sawhney S, Gupta RG, Acharya SK. Sonographic appearances and percutaneous management of primary tuberculous liver abscess. J Clin Ultrasound 1999;27:159-63.
78. Vallejo JG, Stevens AM, Dutton RV, Kaplan SL. Hepatosplenic abscesses due to Brucella melitensis: report of a case involving a child and review of the literature. Clin Infect Dis 1996;22:485-89.

Hydatid Disease

SN Oak, P Agarwal, M Chavarkar

HISTORY

The word "Echinococcosis" is of Greek origin and means "hedgehog berry". It was first used by "Rudolphi" in the period between 1801 and 1808.

It is clear that human cystic hydatid disease was already known to Hippocrates and Galen and that the parasitic nature of this disease was strongly suspected in the 17th century. It was first noted in Talmud and was known to Hippocrates as "livers full of water".[1] "Hydatid" is also of Greek origin and means "drop of water" or a "water vesicle". Siebolt in 1853 and Haubner in 1855 experimentally confirmed the cycle of the parasite. Hydatid cysts was demonstrated to be a zoonosis in 1862. It was only during the present century, however, that significant advances were made in accurate diagnosis and effective treatment of hydatid disease in the human. After World War II, enormous advances were achieved in surgical techniques and organ imaging techniques, as well as in immunologic diagnosis, so that the stage has been reached when both the diagnosis and treatment of human hydatid disease is at a most effective and sophisticated level. During the past 50 years an increasing understanding of the surgical pathology of human-hydatid disease and innovative developments in surgical technique have resulted in a very marked decrease in the mortality of human hydatid disease and, even more importantly, a very significant decrease in the morbidity that, in the past, often followed surgery for hydatid disease.

EPIDEMIOLOGY

E. granulosus thrives in environments as diverse as Arctic tundra and the deserts of North Africa. Cysts have been detected in up to 10% of the population in Northern Kenya and Western China. Among developed countries, the disease is well known in Italy, Greece and Australia. In the United States there is transmission in Alsaka, as well as foci in sheep herding areas of the Western States and Isle Royale on Lake Superior, where there is a wolf/moose cycle.

The disease is common in several Mediterranean countries and in a continuous belt eastwards up to the Indian subcontinent.[2] In India, it is mainly reported amongst the south Indians and Indian Tamils.[3] It is most frequently reported in the states of Tamilnadu, Andhra Pradesh, Gujarat.[4-6] It is also common in Maharashtra, Madhya Pradesh, West Bengal, Himachal Pradesh and Punjab.[7]

LIFE CYCLE (FIG. 85.1)

E. granulosus has a well established life cycle, which is shown in the following cycle:

Host Range

Definitive Hosts

Dog, wolf, dingo, and other canidae.

Intermediate Host

Herbivore (sheep, bovines, swine, goats, equine, camelids) and man.

Infectious Dose

Not known.

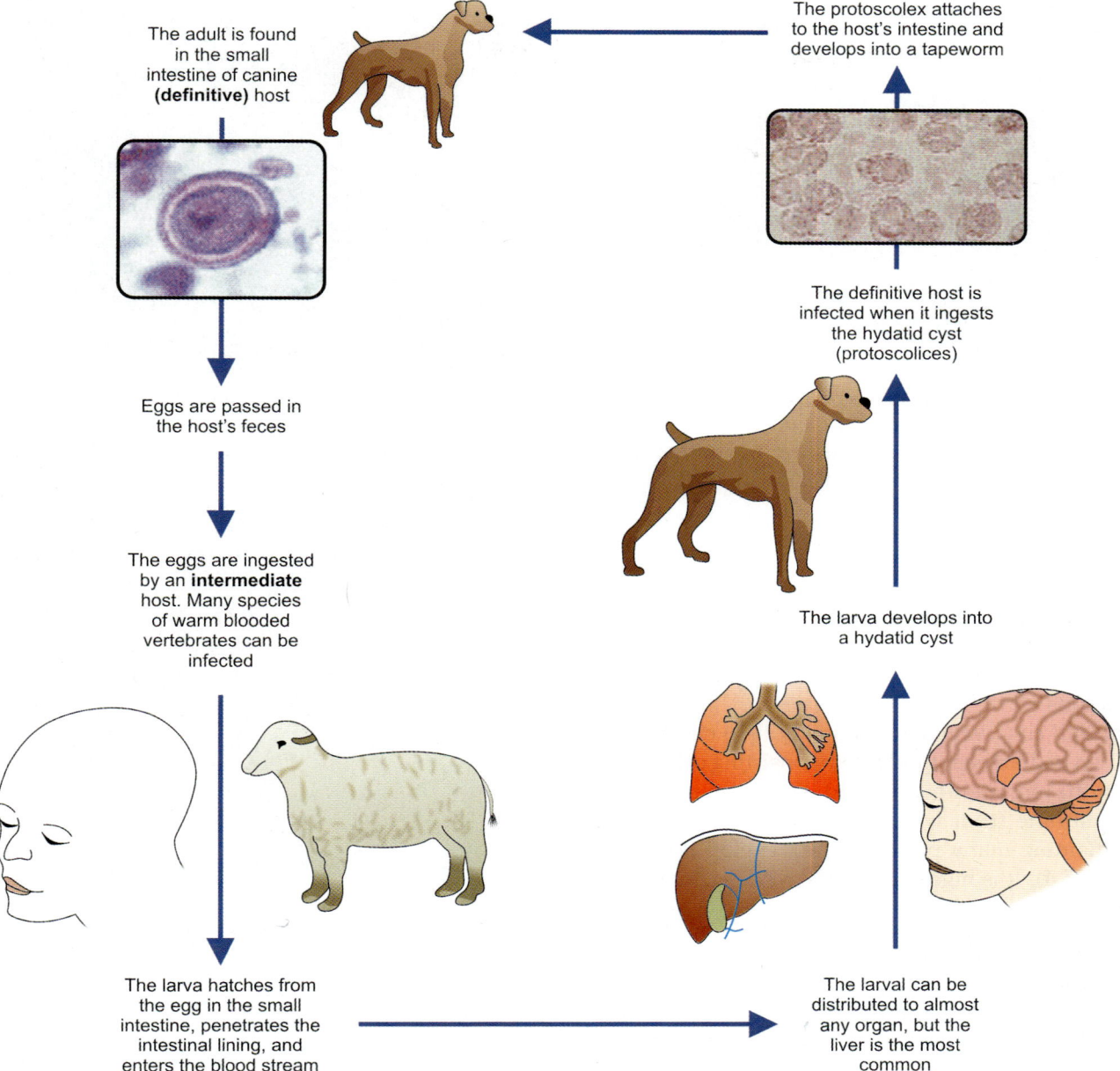

Fig. 85.1: Life cycle of Echinococcus granulosus

Mode of Transmission

Hand to mouth transfer of eggs from dog Feces; fecally contaminated food and water; in Northwest Cananda disease is maintained by wolf- Moose cycle, from which the dog bring the parasite to people.

Incubation Period

It is variable, from 12 months to years, depending on the site and number of cysts.

Communicability

It is not directly transmitted from person to person, Dogs begin to pass eggs 7 weeks after infection.

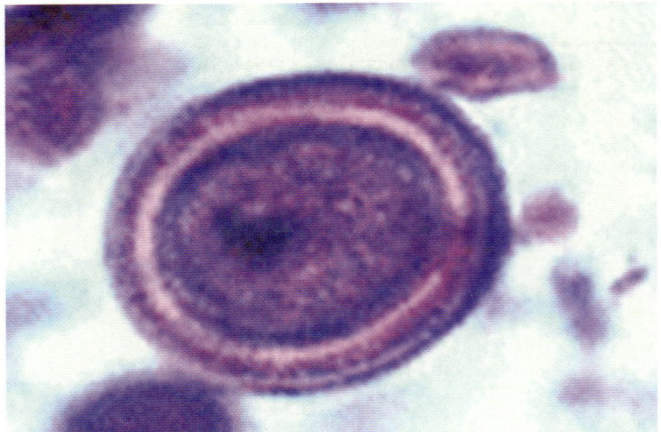

Fig. 85.2: Egg of Echinococcus granulosus

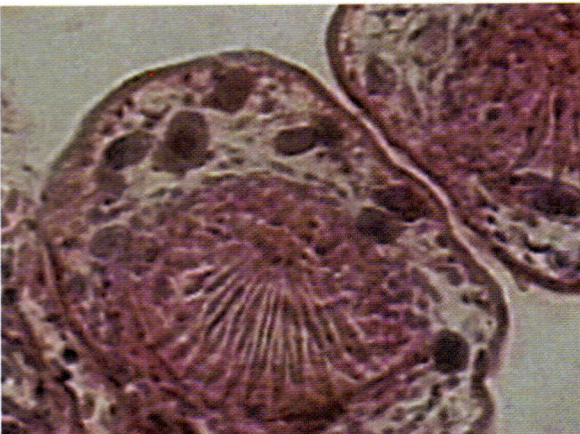

Fig. 85.3: Proctoscolises enlarged view

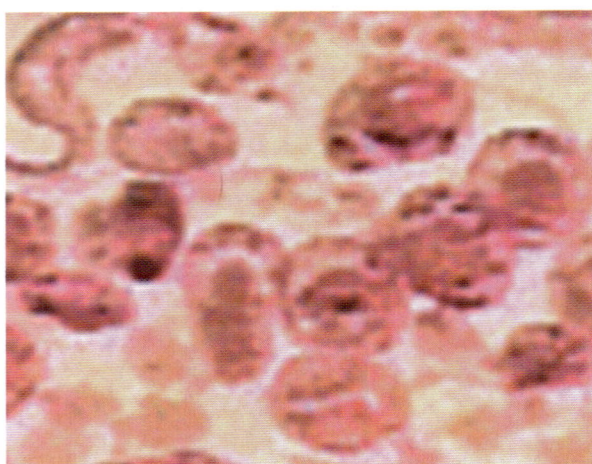

Fig. 85.4: Proctoscolises miniature view

Though most infections subside after 6 months; adult worms may survive for 2-3 years.

Morphology

- *Adults:* 2-7 mm long; usually has only 3-4 segments; Scolex has 4 suckers and the rostellum has 2 rows of hooks.
- *Eggs:* (Fig. 85.2) Typical of taeniids, 32-36 × 25-30 microns.
- *Hydatid cyst (unilocular):* Usually 5-10 cm, but up 50 cm in diameter, fluid filled; consisting of an outer laminated membrane and an inner germinal membrane from which multiple brood capsules containing many protoscolices develop (Figs 85.3 and 85.4). It is highly infective.

The ova, which are ingested by the human from the feces of the tapeworm-infected dog, reach the stomach, where they hatch, then penetrate the wall of the intestine and pass to the liver through a portal vein radicle. Some are destroyed in the liver, some develop there into a hydatid cyst, and others pass through the hepatic veins into the systemic circulation to develop as hydatid cysts anywhere else in the body. In any of these sites, the development of cysts in the human is very slow but appears to be variable in its rate, possibly related to the immunologic interplay between the human and the hydatid parasite. It is emphasized that in the human, within the abdominal cavity, extra-hepatic hydatids can also develop following either extrusion from the liver of a hydatid cyst or rupture of a hydatid cyst through the liver capsule and dissemination within the abdominal cavity, either spontaneously or, more commonly, during hepatic hydatid cyst surgery.

PATHOLOGY

The most common unilocular hydatid cyst is caused by *Echinococcus granulosus*, while the alveolar type is caused by *E. multilocularis*. Approximately 70 % of hydatid cysts are located in the liver, and in one-quarter to one-third of these cases there are multiple cysts. The right lobe is affected in 85 % of patients. Cysts are usually superficial and are composed of three layers.

1. *The adventitia (pseudocyst)*, consisting of fibrous tissue, is the result of reaction of the liver to the parasite, is grey in color and blended intimately with the liver, from which it is inseparable.

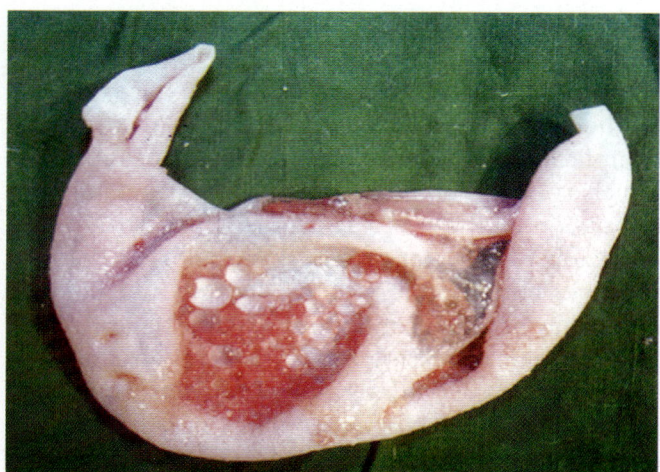

Fig. 85.5: Laminated membrane of hydatid cyst showing daughter cysts

2. *The laminated membrane (ectocyst)* (Fig. 85.5) formed of the parasite itself is whitish and elastic, and contains the hydatid fluid. Indeed, this membrane closely resembles a child's uncolored balloon filled with water, and unless bacterial infection has occurred it peels readily from the adventitia.
Hydatid fluid is crystal-clear; it registers a specific gravity of 1.005-1.009, has a high pressure of approximately 300 mm of water. It is slightly alkaline, contains no albumin, and when not too old, also has hooklets and scolices. The cyst grows very slowly.

3. *The only living part of a hydatid cyst is a single layer of cells (germinal epithelium) lining the cyst (endocyst):* This secretes: (a) internally: the hydatid fluid; (b) externally: the laminated membrane. Brood capsules within the cyst develop from the germinal epithelium and are attached by pedicles to its innermost wall. Within the brood capsules, scolices (heads of future worms develop. Should the laminated membrane become damaged, it disintegrate, and the brood capsules, becoming free, grow into daughter cysts. In this event the mother cyst ceases to exist as such, the hydatid fluid and its content being confined by the adventitia only.

Extension is commonly into the peritoneal cavity, but progressive intrahepatic expansion may result in the replacement of liver parenchyma. In contrast to the unilocular hydatid cysts, the alveolar hydatid is a growth without a capsule and with a tendency toward multiple metastases. As growth progresses, the center becomes necrotic, and the periphery invades the blood vessels and lymphatic channels.

CLINICAL FEATURES

The clinical features of hydatid disease depends on the site, size, stage of development, whether the cyst is alive or dead and whether the cyst is infected or not.

Clinically hydatid cyst may present as an asymptomatic cyst or symptomatic cyst due to infection, pressure effects, rupture and bile duct communication.

Asymptomatic Presentation

The outstanding feature of a simple, uncomplicated, liver hydatid cyst is its clinical latency. The hydatid produces few symptoms until complications occur.

Symptomless unsuspected, cysts can be detected during routine examinations, or at operations or autopsy. In the absence of complications and with an annual growth rate of 1-2 cm, the cyst may be as old as the patient. the only complaint may be a dull ache in the right upper quadrant, and a feeling of abdominal distention associated with hepatomegaly. An exception is 'hydatid cachexia', when an infected child, harboring a large cyst, becomes cachectic.

Symptomatic Presentation

Infection

An asymptomatic hydatid cyst may become infected. Leakage of the cyst is an essential preliminary to infection, as entry of serum into the cyst makes it an excellent medium for rapid bacterial growth.[8] Secondary invasion by pyogenic organisms follows rupture into the biliary passage. The clinical presentation is as a pyogenic abscess and the parasite dies. The most frequently isolated organism is *Escherichia coli*.

Pressure

A viable liver hydatid cyst is a space-occupying lesion with a tendency to grow. In confined areas, such as the central nervous system, small cysts cause serious symptoms. In less restricted areas the symptoms depend on the site and size of the cyst. Symptoms may result from direct pressure or distortion of neighboring structures or viscera. An enlarging liver cyst causes compression atrophy of surrounding hepatocytes and fibrosis. This can lead to compensatory hypertrophy of the remaining liver tissue. Frequently an entire liver lobe can be replaced by an enormous cyst. The cyst grows in the direction of the least resistance.

Rupture

It may be of various forms,
- Obscure – as a result of rupture of the endocyst only, content is retained by the pericyst.
- Communicant – where the content enters the biliary or bronchial tree.
- Free – the hydatid contents disseminate throughout the peritoneal pleural and pericardial cavity.

Live hydatid cysts can rupture into:
- Physiologic channels—e.g. biliary or bronchial tree.
- Free body cavities—peritoneal, pleural or pericardial cavities.
- Adjacent organs—digestive tract.

Intraperitoneal rupture can present in several forms.[9]
- As acute abdominal symptoms due to peritoneal irritation by the cyst.
- As anaphylactic shock with severe circulatory collapse which may be fatal, tends to mask the abdominal manifestations.
- It may be totally silent with the patient presenting years later with disseminated abdominal hydatidosis.
- Rarely as herniation of the laminated membrane through the adventitial pericyst presenting as a 'dumb-bell hepato-peritoneal cyst'. This condition mimics ascites and aspiration can lead to allergic manifestations.

The cyst can rupture into adjacent organs, e.g. into the stomach, duodenum or small intestine.

These patients develop hydatidemesis (hydatid cysts and membranes in the vomitus) and hydatidenteria (passage of hydatid membranes in the stools) with diminishing of clinical symptoms Hydatiduria has been described.[10,11] Rupture into the aorta, the inferior vena cava into pericystic blood vessels, the gallbladder, and into the heart with subsequent embolism has been described.[12-16]

Hydatid cysts located in the dome of the liver close to the diaphragm tend to generate intrathoracic complications. A sympathetic pleural effusion occurs which is sterile on culture. Infection and continued expansion of the cyst causes pressure erosion and adhesion to the diaphragm. Expansion of the cyst stretches and ruptures the diaphragm and the cyst eventually becomes contiguous with the pleural space. In time, with increasing intracystic pressure, the cyst ruptures into the pleural cavity. Empyema forms and the pus (hydatopiothorax) contains necrotic hydatid debris and innumerable daughter cysts.

Upward extension of a subdiaphragmatic cyst can cause dry cough, dyspnea, chest pain and toxemia. Rupture into the lumen of a bronchiole may lead to the appearance of daughter cysts in the sputum. Expectoration of bile tinged sputum is a sign of bronchobiliary fistula.

Compression and displacement of biliary ducts is frequent. A triad of symptoms characterizes rupture into the bile ducts:
  a. Biliary colic
  b. Partial intermittent or complete ductal obstruction with cholangitis and jaundice
  c. Germinative membranes in the feces.

A cyst developing close to the porta hepatis can cause obstruction by compressing the common bile duct or the hepatic ducts, thus not all patients with biliary tract obstruction have intrabiliary rupture.

Dominant symptoms of liver hydatidosis
- Asymptomatic
- Abdominal pain
- Dyspepsia
- Vomiting
- Fever
- Weight loss
- History of jaundice

DIAGNOSIS

Imaging Techniques

Plain Radiograph

a. *Abdomen:* A calcified ring may be seen in the liver zone which may indicate that a hydatid cyst is present in the liver. It does not necessarily mean that the hydatid cyst is dead.

b. *Chest:* It may reveal an elevated right hemidiaphragm or
Concurrent hydatid cyst or lung pleurisy.

Radionuclide Scanning

A dynamic radionuclide scan, using agents such as technetium, show a hydatid cyst as filling defect, distinguishing it from solid vascular masses such as malignant tumors of the liver. Small cysts situated peripherally in the liver can be missed.

Ultrasonography (Figs 85.6 and 85.7)

Ultrasonography can demonstrate the cystic nature of the lesion and will sometimes show the presence of unmistakable daughter cysts within the main cyst cavity thus providing a definitive diagnosis.

CT Scan

CT probably yields the most information regarding the position and the extent of intrabdominal hydatid disease. CT, however is the method of choice to accurately diagnose extrahepatic intra-abdominal or extra-abdominal (Brain and thorax) hydatid cyst.

MRI

The real value of MRI in hydatid disease is in monitoring skeletal and vertebral disease and in cardiac hydatidosis.

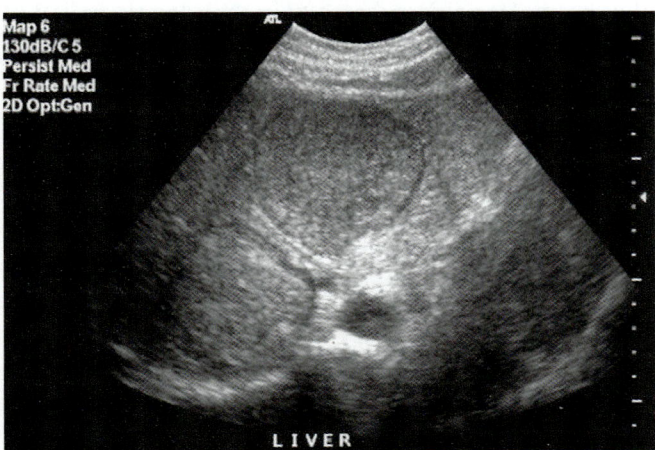

Fig. 85.6: USG of liver showing hydatid cyst (Courtesy: Dr. Nitin Chaubal, Thane Diagnostic USG Centre)

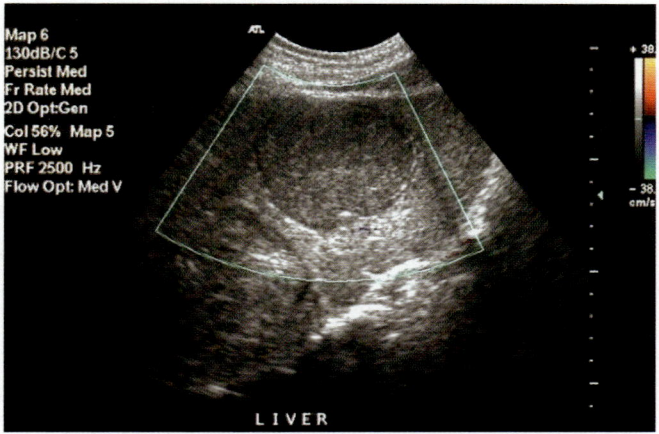

Fig. 85.7: Doppler USG showing no blood flow in the cyst to rule out a tumor (Courtesy: Dr. Nitin Chaubal, Thane Diagnostic USG Centre)

ERCP

It is of particular value when obstructive jaundice is caused by hydatid membrane.

Immunologic Techniques

Immunologic diagnosis using hydatid serology has become extremely sophisticated in the last few years and has assumed an increasing role, not only in primary diagnosis of hydatid disease but also in the screening of susceptible populations as well as in the post-surgical follow-up of hydatid cases for recurrent hydatid disease.

It is emphasised that the Casoni or intradermal test, though time honored, now has no place in diagnosis and because of its high rate of false-positives, its persistence after successful treatment and the occasional problem of anaphylaxis.

A number of laboratory tests have been used in recent years, these are described below.

Immunoelectrophoresis

This investigation depends on its positivity, upon the formation of a specific arc of precipitation (called "Arc 5") produced by the interaction of the serum from the hydatid patient with the antigen, compared to a control. It is highly specific.

Indirect Hemagglutination Test

This is a simple and sensitive test. It gives a positive reaction for *E.granulosus* and also for other parasitic infestation. This limits its usefulness in primary diagnosis in those countries in which these infestations are common.

Latex Agglutination Test

This is a reasonably specific, sensitive, and simple test and has no cross-reactions with other parasitic infestations, so that its very useful for large-scale screening of susceptible populations. Positive titers often persists for long periods after treatment and therefore it is not useful for post-surgical follow up: However, it is more sensitive than the immuno-electrophoresis test and does produce a number of false positives.

Complement Fixation Test

This was the first hydatid immunologic investigation and has been used since-the beginning of this century. The test is extremely sensitive and therefore has a limited value in the primary diagnosis of human hydatid disease because of an unacceptably high positive reaction in other diseases. However, it returns to negative and is therefore useful in postoperative follow-up of hydatid patients.

Enzyme-linked Immunosorbent Assay (ELISA)

This investigation is automated, giving it a great advantage in large scale screening or in epidemiologic studies of hydatid disease. Only small amounts of hydatid antigen are required, which again makes it most useful for screening of susceptible populations. ELISA is a most valuable investigation in primary diagnosis. As the titer do not revert to normal for some years, ELISA is not useful in follow-up.

TREATMENT

Primary prevention is the most important step in the control this disease. The control measures are as follows,
- Decontamination of all wastes before disposal; steam sterilization, clinical disinfection, incineration
- Avoid feeding offal to dogs
- Periodically treat dogs with cestocides
- Humans must use good sanitary habits
- Laboratory staff must wear coat with gloves when skin contact with infectious material is unavoidable. Working with this parasite should be conducted in a biosafety cabinet or its equivalent
- Allow aerosols to settle; wearing protective clothing gently cover the spill with absorbent paper towel and apply 1% sodium hypochlorite starting at the perimeter and working toward the center; allow sufficient contact time (30 min) before clean up.

Secondary prevention includes the drug treatment or the surgical treatment depending upon the indication.

DRUG THERAPY

Indications

- Unusual site,
- multiple cysts (e.g. disseminated peritoneal disease),
- or other diseases in the patient, making operation and anesthesia hazardous.

Contraindications

- Pregnant and lactating mothers,
- Large hepatic cysts with cyst/biliary communications as chemotherapy will not prevent the discharge of cyst debris into the biliary system,
- Debris causing biliary obstruction or cholangitis.

Antimony, arsenic, thymol derivatives, iodides and mercury have been tried without concrete evidence of success. Variable success of mebendazole was first demonstrated in 1977.[17] Mebendazole kills the larval stage by limiting their cellular glucose uptake and lowering the glycogen levels. The drug causes death of the germinal membrane cells and the cyst looses its ability to maintain homeostasis and integrity. Parasites undergo senile degeneration and death. However, the drug has to be given in high doses for longer periods. 20-50 mg/kg body weight divided into three equal doses per day for 21-30 days cycles for 3-12 months. Brandimarte et al (1980) and Morris and Gould (1982) showed limited absorption of mebendazole leading to low blood concentration and even lower cyst fluid concentrations.[18,19]

Albendazole is the only drug that is ovicidal, larvicidal, and vermicidal. Albendazole studies have been encouraging. It is the preferred drug for the treatment of cystic hydatidosis. It is given in the dosage of 15 mg/kg/day in three divided doses for 28 days and taken with a fatty meal to improve the absorption. The absorption of albendazole is far better than mebendazole. The course is usually repeated three to four times with 15 days drug free intervals. Careful monitoring of the white blood cells and the liver function tests during therapy are mandatory. A positive response is seen in 40-60% patients. Side effects of Albendazole includes, elevation in transaminase, jaundice, pyrexia, alopecia and leucopenia.

Praziquantel has much less dramatic effect on the germinal layer than on the protoscolices and it appears to be less effective than albendazole. It is probably the best prophylactic agent for prevention of implantation of spilled protoscolices, and a dose of 50 mg/kg day would certainly achieve active concentrations.

Medical therapy slows the progression of alveolar hydatid. It can be effective in approximately 30% of patients with E. granulosus infestation. It is most effective for pulmonary hydatid, less so for liver infections. Success is progressive shrinkage and solidification of the cyst.

Ultrasound indications for successful therapy are change in shape from spherical to elliptical or flat, progressive increase in echogenicity, and detachment of membranes from the capsule (Water lily sign); another CT criteria are reduction in diameter and augmented density of cyst fluid up to that of other tissues.

SURGICAL MANAGEMENT

Indications for Operation

The decision to operate for hepatic hydatidosis depends on the condition of the patient and the cyst characteristics. Surgery offers the only consistently effective treatment for living abdominal hydatid cysts of the E.granulosus; and it is recommended for both symptomatic as well as asymptomatic cases. Some cysts are reported to die without ever being symptomatic; however the natural history of the disease is of growth; complications of rupture into adjacent organs with serious, life threatening complications. The consensus dictates that uncomplicated, large peripherally located, viable hydatid cysts require operation, as do all complicated cysts.[20,21]

A small, deep parenchymal cysts measuring no more than 4 cms can be managed conservatively for several reasons. Hydatid cysts grow peripherally and will eventually reach the liver capsule if they survive. Small deep located cysts are difficult to manage and radical operation can cause unnecessary damage to the liver parenchyma. Such cysts should be monitored by repeated ultrasound. Once the cyst reaches subcapsular position, the risk of complication increases and the justification for operation is obvious.

Asymptomatic calcified cysts at a younger age require special consideration. The chances of major complications from the presence of a calcified dead, hydatid cyst are minimal and are less than the risks of surgery. Once the semisolid contents of the cyst are drained and the redundant portion of the roof resected; the rigid; calcified cyst wall does not collapse and biliary leaks may become persistent. Subphrenic abscesses, secondary infection in the cyst and sloughing of calcified adventitia are morbid complications, which may occur after the surgery of a calcified hydatid cyst. Segmental resection may become necessary in the case of a large calcified hydatid cyst.

Surgical treatment over the years has become progressively safer with a minimal mortality.[22] The points in the evolution of surgical technique are over-simplification of operation, near complete elimination of postoperative biliary fistulae in liver hydatids, minimization of postsurgical major sepsis, decrease in recurrent cystic hydatid disease and reducing the disabling complications.

This should be achieved by:
1. Preventing spillage of living hydatid material
2. Removing all cyst elements
3. Sterilization of the residual hydatid cavity
4. Using an appropriate non-toxic scolicidal agent.
5. Intraoperative and postoperative complications can be avoided by the use of hydatid cones. Saidi and Nazarian (1971) first described the use of a cryogenic cone, which they adhered to the cyst surface by freezing.[23] They were also the first to advocate the use of freshly prepared 0.5% silver nitrate solution as a good scolicidal agent.

In 1983 subsequently Aarons of Kune described a suction cone that adheres to the cyst wall.[24] This instrument is simpler, safer and more effective that the cryogenic cone. In the recent past laparoscopy has offered minimally invasive option to treat hepatic hydatidosis.

Preparation for Operation

Antibiotic prophylaxis (single dose of cephalosporin) is administered to all patients with uncomplicated hydatid cysts. Septic patients are started on broad-spectrum antibiotic regimen. One may even add an antihistaminic and a steroid in premedication. A preoperative course of mebendazole (50 mg/kg/day) for a period of 1-8 wk is recommended.[25]

The anesthetist should have adrenaline and steroid on the trolley and operating room personnel should adhere to strict regulations for contaminated procedures. Bronchospasm needs to be treated with conventional intravenous bronchodilators. In the event of a hypotension due to anaphylaxis, blood transfusion, plasma expanders and IV drug therapy is of significance. Protective goggles are recommended.

Operative Procedures

- Marsupialization
- Closed total cystectomy
- Partial pericystectomy
- Partial pericystectomy with capitonnage
- Partial pericystectomy with omentoplasty
- Liver resection -Typical, atypical, anatomic
- Laparoscopic methods.

Inscision and Exploration

The usual preference is for a long subcostal incision. An upward extension in the midline is sometimes necessary. On exploring the peritoneal cavity, spleen, pancreas, retroperitoneal areas, pelvis, inguinal canals must be looked carefully. Adhesions must be separated with great care since they might be overlying an unidentified abdominal cyst. The liver should be completely mobilized and bimanual palpation and inspection of both lobes is necessary.

The diaphragm should be dissected away from the superficially located cyst and full mobility restored. A large posterior cyst in the liver is dangerous and the liver must be mobilized adequately before handling such a cyst. If available, intraoperative ultrasound should be employed at this stage to note the intrahepatic extent, associated cysts and the relationship cyst to the inferior vena cava and the hepatic veins, and the complete patency of the CBD.

Right lobe is more commonly affected. In a series described by Al-Bassam et al of 21 patients over a period of 11 yrs, 11 children had a single cyst, 8 of which were in the right lobe.[25] Ten children had multiple cysts occupying both liver lobes. Khoury et al report a series of 108 hydatid cysts of liver and spleen in 83 patients treated laparoscopically.[26] In 42 patients (53%) the liver cysts were located in the right lobe; 21 patients (26%) in the left lobe and in both lobes in 16 patients (21%). The most frequently involved segment is; segments V, segment VI and segment VII.

Conservative Operation

Aim: Safe Decompression of the Cyst

Salient Features
a. Protect the skin around the entire space around the mobilized liver with packs and drapes soaked in 10% saline(green or blue drapes).
b. Put a pack behind the right lobe.
c. Treat all cysts as if they are viable and infectious.
d A cyst will have contents under high pressure, therefore determine the point of entry and make actual working area as small as possible with additional packing.
e. 2 drains with a powerful suction must be available. Use a sump type cannula. The suction reservoirs should have a large capacity avoiding frequent changing.
f Penetrate the cyst with a large gauge needle connected by a transparent plastic tubing to one of the drain. Observe the color of the hydatid fluid.
g. Aspirate at least 50 ml; then the cyst pressures lower and then take three stay sutures close to the inserted needle. Remove the needle. Hold the stay with upward traction. Incise the cyst with electrocautery and insert large gauge sump drain inside.
h. Incise the cyst further to about 3 cm; to allow direct vision inside and sump suck freely within the cavity. Inject warm saline solution intermittently

to keep the suction working and to evacuate the hydatid sand.

i. Evaluation of the cyst contents is important. The typical contents of a viable cyst are clear, containing sand and debris of brood capsules. Sometimes the contents may be stained with bile. Bile duct communications should always be looked for. Cyst may contain viable daughter cysts and the fluid may be infective.

j. The appearance of toothpaste like material blocking the suction cannula is a sign that the cyst is dead. Once all the liquid has been drained the laminated membrane collapses into the cavity and the cyst contents can be evacuated. The laminated membrane can be best managed with a Babcock's forceps and progressive screwing type of movements with gentle traction. Daughter cysts should be sucked with wide bore suction. It is sometimes necessary to use a spoon to evacuate daughter cysts. When all the visible daughter cysts have been evacuated, the cavity is rinsed with 3-5% warm saline.

k. The redundant portion of the cyst roof is excised (Fig. 85.8). The adventitia and thinned out liver are cut with electrocautery or ultrasonic shears. The cut edges are oversewn using a reabsorbable suture material.

A careful search for daughter cysts is essential. Exogenic cyst can be incised and evacuated. The interior of the cyst should be carefully scrapped with sponges soaked in 5% sodium chloride. Curettage with sharp instruments is dangerous as it may injure adjacent hepatic veins. 3-5% of saline is left in the cystic cavity for 10 mins. To sterilize the cyst. Use a sponge immersed in formalin to gently scrub the interiors of the cyst cavity.

Scolicidal Agents

Scolicidal agents	Strength	Reported negative effects
Sodium chloride	3-20 %	Caustic sclerosing cholangitis
Ethanol	75-95	Caustic sclerosing cholangitis
Cetrimide	0.1-0.5	Cholangitis, metabolic acidosis
Povidone	1	Colors cystic cavity-difficult to identify bile duct communications
Formalin	4-10	Anaphylaxis, toxicity
Hydrogen peroxide	1.5-3	Bursting, spillage, air-embolism
Chlorhexidine	10	Metabolic acidosis
Silver nitrate	0.5	Sclerosing cholangitis

Protoscolicidal agents are no substitute for meticulous surgical technique. Even the most effective agents may not kill all the protoscolices or the germinal layer. Inadequate sterilization usually results from lack of contact with all the daughter cysts or low concentration of the protoscolicidal agent in large volume cysts.[27] Protoscolicides cannot penetrate the wall of the cysts. During operation, a protoscolicidal agent should not be injected into an unopened hydatid cyst.

Complications of Protoscolicidal Agents[28, 29]

1. Acute toxic reactions
2. Anaphylactic shock
3. Hypernatremia
4. Gas embolism
5. Immediate postoperative death
6. Sclerosing cholangitis
7. Abscess formation.

Management of Bile Duct Communications

Diagnosis of bile duct communications
1. Large cysts > 10 cm
2. Cysts occupying several liver segments
3. Episodes of cholangitis
4. Intraoperative cholangiography
5. Intraoperative ultrasound
6. Endoscopic retrograde cholangiopancreaticography

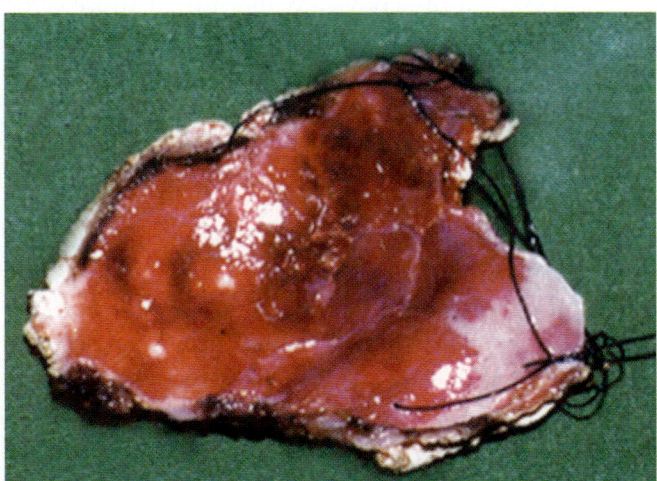

Fig. 85.8: Calcified wall of a hepatic hydatid cyst

7. Fill the cyst with saline, inject air and watch for bubbles at the site of leak
8. Appearance of bile stains in a cavity packed with hypertonic saline packs.

Type of procedures on bile ducts in patients with cyst bile duct communications.
1. Suture
2. Suture + tube
3. Roux-en-Y jejunostomy
4. Intracavitary reconstruction(Roux-en-Y intracystic hepaticojejunostomy)
5. Liver resection
6. Choledochoduodenostomy.

Gahukamble DB (2000) has analyzed 30 children with hydatid cysts of the liver who were treated by partial pericystectomy and external tube drainage.[30] In 21% of cases in which clear hydatid fluid was observed during surgery developed biliary leakage in spite of appropriate precautions taken during surgery. Histological examination of the pericyst wall confirmed the presence of openings of small bile ducts in the cyst, which probably caused the biliary leak. The series also emphasizes on the fact that in children; the leak is likely to cease spontaneously, providing distal biliary duct obstruction is ruled out and external tube drainage is used to prevent accumulation of bile in the pericyst cavity.

Management of Residual Cavity

Methods of obliterating the residual cyst cavity:
1. Simple cyst closure
2. Leave the cyst open
3. Marsupialization
4. External drainage
5. Introflexion
6. Capitonage
7. Omentoplasty
8. Roux-en-Y cystojejunostomy
9. Hepatic resection.

Omentoplasty as described by Papadmitiou and Mandrakas (1970), involves suturing of omentum into place, and if the cavity has a large volume, a drain is also placed.[31] If the omentum is not available the cyst cavity can frequently be obliterated by capitonnage. This technique involves infolding the redundant cyst wall into the depths of the cyst with successive layers of sutures. Capitonnage is not possible when the volume the cyst is large and when the walls are calcified and rigid. Care should be taken not to place sutures deep into the cyst wall since hepatic veins can be injured. Marsupialization consists of suturing the adventitia to the parietes thereby allowing free and direct drainage of the cavity into the exterior.

An infected cyst should be treated like a liver abscess.

Radical Operation

Radical operation includes the procedure of closed cystpericystectomy, anatomic liver resection, typical liver resection and liver transplantation. Resection is reserved for peripherally placed cysts, usually in the left lateral segment, for pedunculated lesions extrahepatic intra-abdominal cysts. It is to be avoided for cysts impinging upon the major hepatic veins; IVC and close to the liver hilum. It is an ideal procedure for multivescicular cysts and for calcified cyst. In atypical liver resection the cyst is dissected en-bloc with a thin layer of hepatic tissue disregarding the anatomy of the liver. Hepatic resection should be done only if there is no other surgical alternative.

Laparoscopic Treatment of Hepatic Hydatidosis

The technical development in laparoscopic instruments and increasing skill of surgeons has encouraged them to attempt a laparoscopic approach. 4-6 ports may be required. Cyst puncture and initial decompression is important and can be done by a special 10/12 mm cannula with aspirator.[32,33]

The trocar cannula have a wider lumen, more force of suction and 2 side channels one for gas insufflation and one for suction. The special cannula is introduced perpendicularly into the cyst under supraumbilically inserted laparoscopic guidance. Cetrimide soaked pad is used to protect the trocar wound externally. Constant suction on the side suction cannula prevents spillage while introducing the trocar. Continuous irrigation and simultaneous suction removes fragments. Confirmation of extraction of entire cyst is checked by introducing operating laparoscope onto the cyst through the trocar. The wall of the cyst is carefully inspected for biliary leak and biliary communication can be sutured using vicryl. More than one hydatid cyst can be managed by multiple introduction of trocars.

Management of Extrahepatic Intraperitoneal Hydatid Cysts

These cysts may be either in a solid organ such as the spleen, pancreas or the kidney, or ovary.[34] The other forms of extrahepatic peritoneal hydatidosis is usually the result of spillage of living hydatid material during surgery on a liver hydatid. Peritoneal hydatids need to be each individually removed with its host capsule intact. When part of the host capsule forms from the bladder, bowel or some viscus the cyst should then be treated in a fashion similar to primary liver cysts. When they are in the spleen the usual surgical treatment is splenectomy. Bhatnagar et al have reported successful enucleation of a deep seated splenic hydatid cyst and preservation of the spleen.[35] Cysts located in the pancreas should be evacuated using a hydatid cone. Ismail K in his series of pancreatic hydatids has performed distal pancreatectomies, cystectomy and marsupialization in others.[36] Hydatid cyst of the kidney has also been reported. It is possible to excise a small cyst.[6] Partial or total nephrectomy is generally advisable.

Apart from the kidney, hydatid cyst may develop in retroperitoneal tissues. They arise in psoas sheath and progressively enlarge. It is difficult to excise the retroperitoneal cysts. They are densely adherent to adjacent structures and cannot be enucleated. Incision into the cyst after injecting 10% of formalin; evacuation of all the contents of the cyst and the laminated membrane and marsupialization are only possible.

Pulmonary Hydatidosis

Symptoms produced by hydatid cyst may not be severe, surgical treatment is always necessary to prevent a complication of rupture. Cyst may rupture into a bronchus or into the pleura. This may lead to anaphylactic reactions. The patient may develop aspiration pneumonia, disseminated disease, abscess or an empyema.

Thoracotomy is indicated in all cases of hydatid disease in lungs

1. *Barrets maneuver* – For a closed cyst which is not infected and which is situated near the surface of the lungs, it is possible to incise the thin adventitia and allow the cyst to separate itself from the

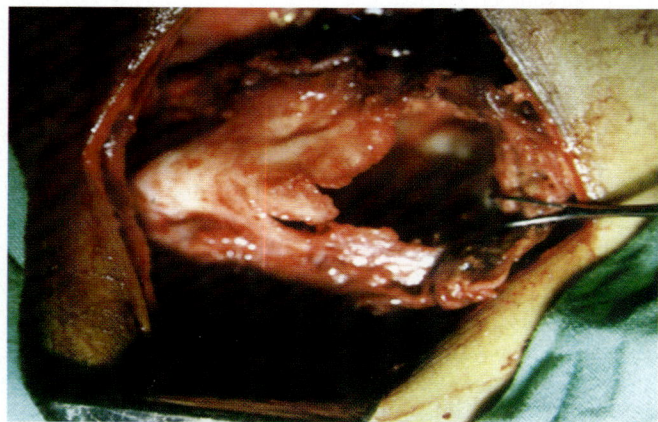

Fig. 85.9: Pulmonary hydatid cyst being excised

   adventitia while the anesthetist blows the lungs intermittently.
2. *Removal of cyst* (Fig. 85.9) – After preliminary aspiration of the cyst the laminated membrane is dissected away from the pericyst. Any openings of the minor bronchi are carefully closed and purse string sutures are taken to carefully obliterate the cavity.
3. *Pulmonary resection* – Pulmonary resection is indicated when the cyst is infected; when it is too large or when it arises from the middle lobe.

   The anatomical site of the lesion determines whether the resection be lobectomy, segmental resection or only a wedge resection. Results of pulmonary resection and other conservative measures are generally good and rewarding.
4. *Pneumonostomy* – After excision of the cyst a separate catheter is fixed within the residual lung cavity and brought through the adjacent chest wall; effectively marsupializing the residual cavity to the atmosphere.[37]

Other Sites

Hydatids at the hip bone, lower third of tibia/femur calf, psoas, sternomastoid, in the diploic layer of skull bones, intracranial, temperoparietal, and periorbital region may need excision. Spinal hydatids may be intra or extra dural, vertebral or paravertebral, and may lead to progressive weakening of the lower limbs. Laminectomy is required to relieve the compression of the cord. The cavities have to be freely opened and curetted. Early decompression has good results.

REFERENCES

1. Blumgart LH, Y Fong. Surgery of the liver and biliary tract, Hydatid disease, Vol II, 3rd edn, edited by M N Milicevic. WB Saunders Company limited 2000;1167-204.
2. Joshi Manohar. Surgical disease in the tropics, Hydatid disease,1st edn, Macmillan India limited 1982;151-69.
3. Dissanalike AS, Paramanathan DC. 'On the occurrence and significance of hydatids cysts in the Ceylone Sambhur'. Ceylon J Med Sci, 1962;11:1.
4. Devadasan C. 'Hydatid disease in India'. Acta Trop., 1974;31:4, 378, Trop Dis Bull, 1975;72, 6. Abstr. 1531.
5. Shah HS, Kanvinde MS, Shukla BK, Meheta KN. 'Hydatid disease: A comparative review of its incidence with that in other parts of India'. Indian J Med Sci 1969;23:38.
6. Upadhyaya GH, Prahlad Rai, Shah PK. Clinical study of hydatid disease in Jamnagar. J Ind Med Assoc 1974;63:213.
7. Bhandarkar LD, Talwalkar GV, 'Hydatoid disease': A report of 35 cases. Indian J. Med Sci 1973;27:11,849.
8. Loewenthal J, Way LW. Echinococcosis. In: Surgery of the gallbladder and bile ducts. Way L, Pellegrini CAP(Eds) WB Saunders company, Philadelphia 1987;557-68.
9. el-mufti M. Surgical management of hydatid disease. Butterworths, London 1989;1-55.
10. Thomas S, Mishra MC, Kriplani AK, Kapur BM. Hydatidemesis: a bizarre presentation of abdominal hydatidosis. Australian and New Zealand Journal of Surgery 1993;63:496-98.
11. Chopra JS, Kakar R, Madan TR. Hydatiduria resulting from rupture of hydatid cyst of the kidney (a case report). Journal of the Association of Physicians of India 1970;18:523-24.
12. Hadijat N, Graba A, Mansouri H. Rupture of retroperitoneal hydatid cyst into the abdominal aorta. Annals of vascular surgery 1987;1:483-85.
13. Blasco NavaJpotro MA, Corraks Rodriguez dc Tembleque M, Poza Jimenez A, Sanchez Gomez Navarro J: Anaphylactic shock caused by spontaneous rupture of hepatic hydatid cyst into inferior vena cava (letter). Shock anafilactico por rotura espontanea de unquiste hidatidico hepatico en la vena cava inferior. Revista Clinjca Espanola 1993;192:49-50.
14. Eyal I, Zveibil F, Stamler B. Anaphylactic shock due to rupture of a hepatic hydatid cyst into a pericystic blood vessel following blunt abdominal trauma. Journal of Paediatric Surgery 1991;26:217-18.
15. Singh R, Sinha SN, Sinha RS. Rupture of infected hydatid cyst of liver into the gallbladder causing Empyema with obstructive jaundice, Journal of the Indian Association 1984;82:375-76.
16. Atias A, Pizzaro D, Levia A, Gomez G, Naquira N. Intracardiac rupture of a hydatid cyst of the left ventricle with arterial hydatidic emboli and gangrene of leg. Rupture de un quiste hidatidico del ventriculo izquierdo con embolia hidatidica arterial y gangrene de un meimbro inferior. Boletin Chileno de Parasitologia 1966;21:124-26.
17. Bekhti A, Schaaps JP, et al. Treatment with hepatic hydatid disease with Mebendazole: Preliminary results in four cases. Br Med J 1977;2:1047.
18. Brandimarte C, Attili AF, et al. Serum and hydatid cystic fluid levels of mebendazole in patients with liver hydatidosis. Ital J Gastrenterol 1980;12:212.
19. Morris DL, Gould SE. Serum and cyst concentrations of mebendazole and flubendazole in hydatid disease. Br Med J 1982;285:175.
20. Morl M. Echinoccocosis. Rational diagnosis and therapy. Fortschritte der medezin 1982 ;100:1131-36.
21. Langer JE, Rose DB, Keystone JS, Taylor BR, Langer B. Diagnoses and management of hydatid disease of the liver. A 15 year North American experience. Annals of surgery 1984;199:412-17.
22. Bornes SA, Lillemoe KD. Hydatid disease in maingots abdominal operations. (Ed) Zinner MJ. Appleton and Lange 1997(10):1534-45.
23. Saidi F, Nazarian T. Surgical treatment of hydatid cysts by freezing of cyst wall and instillation of 0.5% silver nitrate solution. N Eng J Med 1971;284:1346.
24. Arons B J, Kune GA. A suction cone to prevent spillage during hydatid surgery. Aust NZ J Surg 1983;53:471.
25. Al- Bassam A, Hassab H, Al-Olayat y, Shadi M, Al-Shami G, Al-Rabeeah A, Jawad A. Hydatid disease of the liver in children. Ann Trop Paediatr 1999;19(2):191-96.
26. Khoury G, Abiad F, Geagea T, Nabout G, et al. Laparoscopic treatment of hydatid cysts of the liver and spleen. Surg Endosc 2000; 14(3):243-45.
27. Pawlowski ZS, Which Protoscolicidal agent if any? Echinomed 1992;3-4:4-5.
28. Belghiti J, Perniceni T, Kabbej M, Fekere F. Complications of preoperative sterilization of hydatid cysts of the liver. Apropos of 6 cases Chirurgie 1991;117:343-46.
29. Warren KW, Athanassiades S, Monge JI. Primary sclerosing cholangitis. A study of 42 cases. American J of Surgery 1966;111:23-38.
30. Gahukambale DB, Kjamage AS, Gahukambale LD. Outcome of minimal surgery for hydatid cysts of the liver in children with reference to post operative biliary leakage. Ann Of Trop Paed 2000;20(2):147-51.
31. Papadimitiou J, Mandrekas A. The surgical treatment of hydatid disease of liver. BJS 1970;57:431-33.
32. Alper A, Emre A, Hazar H, Ozden I, Bilge O, Acarli K, Arioglu O. Laparoscopic surgery of hepatic hydatid disease:initial results and early follow up of 16 patients. World Journal of surgery 1995;19:725-28.
33. Palanivelu C. Textbook of surgical laparoscopy published by Gem Digestive Foundation, Coimbatore; 2002.
34. Brown RA, Millar AJ, Steiner Z, Krige JE, Burkemisher D, Cywes S. Hydatid cyst of the pancreas - a case report in a child. Eur J Paed Surg 1995;5(2):121-23.
35. Bhatnagar V, Agarwal S, Mitra D K. Conservative surgery for splenic hydatid cyst. J Paed Surg 1994;29(12): 1570-71.
36. Ismail K, Haluk GI, Necati O. Surgical treatment of hydatid cysts of the pancreas. Int Surg 1991;76(3):185-88.
37. Anand V, Sen S, Jacob R, Chacko J, Zacharia N, Thomas E, Mammen KE. Pneumonostomy in the surgical treatment of bilateral hydatid cysts of the lung. Paed. Surg. Int 2001;7(1):29-31.

CHAPTER 86

Liver Resections and Allograft Preparation

Mark D Stringer

Liver resection in childhood is required for a variety of reasons but the commonest indication is for the treatment of liver tumors. All pediatric surgeons should be familiar with the principles and practice of the more basic techniques. Anatomically or pathologically complex lesions are best dealt with in an experienced center by a multidisciplinary team consisting of a specialist hepatobiliary surgeon and radiologist, supported by pediatric anesthesia, hepatology, oncology, intensive care, and nursing. This approach should minimize the risk of mortality and morbidity and yield the optimum long-term results from what is a potentially major undertaking.

HISTORICAL ASPECTS

The regenerative powers of the liver have been recognized since ancient times. They were hinted at in the legend of Prometheus who was bound to a rock in the Caucasus mountains because he stole fire to give to man. Every day, eagles came to devour his liver which then regrew each night. The study of liver anatomy began in earnest with Leonardo da Vinci's observations gleaned from anatomical dissections. However, it was Francis Glisson's *Anatomia Hepatis* published in 1654 that marked the beginnings of modern liver anatomy and surgery. In the late 1880s, after the introduction of anesthesia and antisepsis, adult liver resections were first performed by pioneers such as Langenbuch, Loreta, and others. Further advances in anatomy were made by Rex in Germany and Cantlie in England and in the early 1900s Pringle developed his maneuver for controlling hemorrhage.

The subsequent revolution in liver resectional surgery began in the 1950s and was inspired by Couinaud's studies of segmental liver anatomy. The first right hepatectomy was undertaken by Lortat-jacob in Paris in 1952. It was not until the 1980's that advanced techniques of liver resection became available, pioneered by surgeons such as Bengmark, Bismuth, and Blumgart. In particular, the different types of anatomical liver resection were refined[1] and the problem of hemorrhage was successfully addressed.[1] Liver transplantation ushered in the next wave of advances in resectional liver surgery and most recent progress has largely come from centers specializing in both fields.

In recent times, the three major advances in liver resectional surgery have been the definition of hepatic anatomy, the application of accurate imaging techniques, and the development of liver transplantation. It is against this background that pediatric hepatobiliary surgery has emerged as a specialist discipline.

INDICATIONS FOR LIVER RESECTION

Although liver tumors are the commonest reason for liver resection in childhood, there are a variety of other indications (Table 86.1).

Table 86.1: Indications for liver resection in childhood

- Tumors – benign and malignant neoplasms
  – cysts, abscesses, pseudotumors, etc.
- Vascular or biliary malformations or complications (e.g. Caroli's disease, localized hemangioendothelioma)
- Trauma
- Transplantation
- Miscellaneous, e.g. open fetal surgery for congenital diaphragmatic hernia

Table 86.2: Classification of liver tumors (Stringer 2000)

Liver tumors	
Benign	Hemangioma/Hemangioendothelioma
	Focal nodular hyperplasia
	Adenoma (and adenomatosis)
	Mesenchymal hamartoma
	Other hamartomas
	Lymphangioma (and lymphangiomatosis)
	Nodular regenerative hyperplasia
	Cystadenoma
	Teratoma
	Myxoma
Malignant	Hepatoblastoma
	Hepatocellular carcinoma (and fibrolamellar variant)
	Undifferentiated embryonal sarcoma
	Rhabdoid tumor
	Rhabdomyosarcoma
	Epithelioid hemangioendothelioma
	Angiosarcoma
	Liposarcoma
	Fibrosarcoma
	Malignant germ cell tumor Non-Hodgkin's lymphoma
	Metastases: neuroblastoma, Wilms' tumor, rhabdomyosarcoma, germ cell tumor, lymphoma, leukemia, Langerhans' cell histiocytosis, choriocarcinoma, pancreatoblastoma, carcinoid
Bile duct tumors	
Benign	Granular cell tumor
	Inflammatory pseudotumor
Malignant	Rhabdomyosarcoma
	Adenocarcinoma
	Cholangiocarcinoma
Cysts	Parasitic
	Non-parasitic (Peliosis hepatis)
Other liver 'tumors'	Inflammatory pseudotumor
	Liver abscesses
	Fetus-in-fetu
	Hematoma/Biloma

Tumors

There is a wide spectrum of pediatric liver tumors (Table 86.2) but only the more common lesions requiring hepatic resection are described in this section. The rarity and complexity of these tumors indicates that they should be managed in centers with appropriate oncological and surgical expertise.

Malignant Liver Tumors

In Western societies, primary malignant liver tumors have an incidence of approximately 1-1.6 per million children per year and account for just over 1% of all childhood cancers.[2,3] Hepatoblastoma (HB) and hepatocellular carcinoma (HCC) comprise more than two-thirds of childhood primary liver malignancies.

Hepatoblastoma

HB is the commonest primary malignant liver tumor in infants and children, with a peak incidence in the first 3 years of life. Presentation is usually with a combination of abdominal distension, pain or a mass. Rarely, the tumor ruptures and causes intraperitoneal bleeding. Most cases of HB are sporadic but familial cases associated with Beckwith-Wiedemann syndrome or familial adenomatous polyposis are described. Serum alpha-fetoprotein is elevated in more than 90% of cases and is a valuable diagnostic and prognostic marker. Biopsy is advisable for histological confirmation. Ultrasound scan (US) and computerized tomography (CT) are useful in assessing the primary tumor but chest radiography and CT are required to exclude metastases.

In the USA and Germany, the staging system for HB and HCC is based on operative findings and histological features, i.e. *postsurgical*. In Europe, the staging system adopted by the Societe Internationale d'Oncologie Pediatrique (SIOP) is a *pretreatment* grouping based on the results of imaging studies.[4] In the latter, the liver is divided into four sections comprising the left lateral section (segments 2 and 3), a left medial section (segment 4 and part of 1), a right medial section (segments 5 and 8 and part of 1) and a right posterior section (segments 6 and 7). The number of liver sections involved by the tumor, and the presence of tumor involving the portal vein, vena cava, or extrahepatic sites are recorded.

Effective chemotherapy and complete surgical resection of the tumor are the mainstays of therapy. Various chemotherapy regimens have been advocated.[5] In the USA, the traditional focus has been on initial laparotomy, surgical resection where possible, and postoperative chemotherapy (e.g. cisplatin, vincristine and 5-fluorouracil). Neoadjuvant chemotherapy is given for initially unresectable tumors.[6,7] The SIOP studies have concentrated on preoperative chemotherapy. In SIOPEL-1, all patients except those with small peripheral tumors were treated by preoperative chemotherapy with cisplatin and doxorubicin (PLADO) which induced tumor necrosis and shrinkage.[8]

The presence of multifocal tumor, involvement of more than three liver sectors, evidence of caval or main portal vein invasion, or distant metastases are the usual reasons for unresectable disease. However, HB resectability has progressively improved since the introduction of chemotherapy for unresectable disease.[9-12] After PLADO cytotoxic therapy, 70-85% of unresectable tumors become operable. Preoperative chemotherapy renders most tumors smaller, better demarcated from the surrounding liver, and more likely to be completely resected.[13]

Patients who respond to chemotherapy but have unresectable tumors with no evidence of persistent metastases should be considered for orthotopic liver transplantation (OLT). A careful search for extrahepatic disease prior to OLT is important and chemotherapy should be continued until the time of transplant. Published experience is limited but the indications are that this approach offers a greater than 50% chance of disease-free survival if patients are carefully selected, despite the need for long-term immunosuppression.[14-16]

During the last 30 years, there has been a progressive improvement in survival after treatment of HB. In SIOPEL-1 overall 5 year survival was 75% and in the German Cooperative Liver Tumor Study 82% at 3 years.[8,17] Results from SIOPEL-1 indicate that tumor extent at presentation (pretreatment grouping) and presence of distant metastases are possibly the most important prognostic variables.[18]

Hepatocellular Carcinoma

HCC (hepatoma) accounts for less than a quarter of all pediatric malignant liver tumors in Western societies but is much more frequent in parts of Asia, South America and Africa where hepatitis B infection is endemic.[19] HCC typically occurs in older children (10-14 years) and more commonly affects boys. Presenting features include an abdominal mass, weight loss and fever.

Fewer than 10% of tumors in Western children are associated with cirrhosis or underlying liver disease.[5] This is not the case in the Far East, where vertical transmission of Hepatitis B is an important cause of HCC and almost all affected children are infected with the virus and have chronic liver disease.[20] A national hepatitis B vaccination program in Taiwan has significantly reduced the incidence of HCC in recent years.[21]

HCC spreads by lymphatic and vascular invasion. Bilobar, multifocal disease is common and at least half the patients have metastases or extrahepatic spread at presentation.[22] Serum AFP is elevated in two-thirds or more of cases but not in the fibrolamellar variant of HCC which occurs in adolescents and young adults in the absence of underlying cirrhosis and is associated with elevated serum levels of the vitamin B12 binding protein, transcobalamin (Fig. 86.1).

The tumor is much more resistant to chemotherapy than HB. If possible, complete excision of HCC should be attempted but the presence of multifocal tumor or underlying cirrhosis may preclude resection. Children with unresectable tumors and no evidence of extrahepatic spread should be assessed for transplant.[16]

Children with HCC had a 41% 2 year survival in SIOPEL-1 but disease-free survival was only 27% in the German studies with longer follow-up.[23,24] Currently, the role of chemoembolization, intra-arterial chemotherapy, ultrasound guided percutaneous intralesional injection of ethanol, intraoperative cryotherapy and radiofrequency ablation, all of which have their advocates in adult practice, remains uncertain in children and, where possible, liver resection offers the best chance of survival.

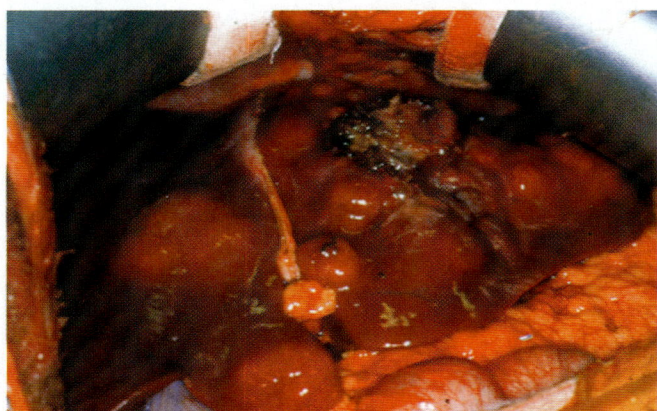

Fig. 86.1: Operative appearance of a fibrolamellar hepatocellular carcinoma in a 15-year-old boy just prior to left hemihepatectomy. Adherent omentum (previous biopsy site) was excised with the liver tumor

Other Malignant Liver Tumors

Undifferentiated (embryonal) sarcoma usually occurs in school age children (Fig. 86.2). Treatment is by chemotherapy and liver resection but local recurrence is common and the prognosis generally poor.[25]

Rhabdomyosarcomas are mostly found in the extrahepatic biliary tree of pre-school children and presentation is with obstructive jaundice and abdominal pain. Histologically they are locally invasive embryonal or botryoid rhabdomyosarcomas. Approximately 20% of children have metastases at presentation. Surgical excision (assisted by intraoperative cholangiography and frozen section histology), multiagent chemotherapy, and in some cases radiotherapy have resulted in a significantly improved survival. The Intergroup Rhabdomyosarcoma Study Group reported their experience of 25 children with biliary rhabdomyosarcoma treated by chemotherapy and surgery.[26] They concluded that (i) surgical exploration is required to accurately identify regional non-nodal metastases, and (ii) surgery should be used principally to determine histological diagnosis and extent of disease; if possible, endoscopic stent placement should be used to achieve biliary drainage. Estimated 5 year overall survival was 66% but was better in children without distant metastases at diagnosis.

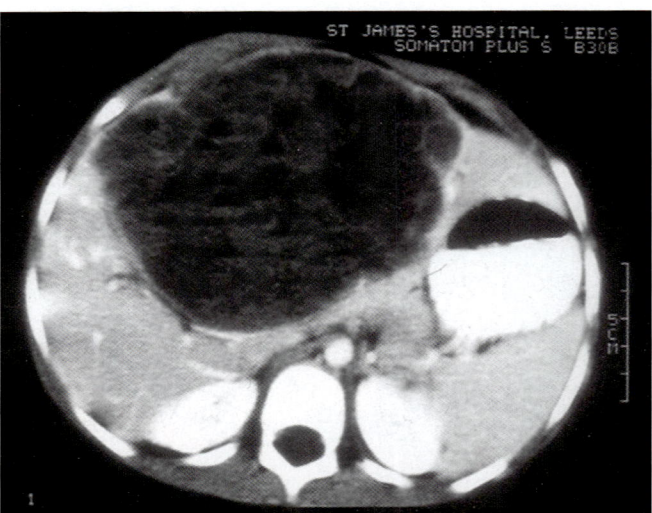

Fig. 86.2: A large undifferentiated sarcoma in a 7-year-old girl. The tumor showed a partial response to chemotherapy and was successfully excised by left trisectionectomy. She remains well 4 years later

A variety of other rare malignant liver tumors may be encountered in children (Table 86.2) and with the exception of lymphoma, may require resection. Surgical excision may also be indicated for isolated liver metastases from Wilms' tumor.

Benign Liver Tumors

Several benign liver tumors are best treated by complete excision.

Mesenchymal Hamartoma

These are large, multicystic liver tumors usually found in infants and pre-school children but occasionally presenting in older persons.[27,28] After hemangiomas, mesenchymal hamartomas are the second commonest benign hepatic tumor in childhood. They typically present with an abdominal mass or distension from progressive accumulation of serous or mucoid fluid within the cysts. Tumors may be very large, sometimes exceeding a diameter of 20 cm and weighing up to 3 kg.

Mesenchymal hamartomas are best treated by complete excision, either by conventional hepatic resection or non-anatomical excision with a rim of normal liver. An excellent prognosis can be anticipated after complete excision.[27] Incomplete resection should be avoided because of the long-term risk of malignant change, namely the development of an undifferentiated (embryonal) sarcoma, and the possibility of late symptomatic recurrence.[28,29] Marsupialization may lead to intractable local complications.

Focal Nodular Hyperplasia

This benign liver tumor is most often seen in young women; children account for only 7% of reported cases.[30] It most commonly presents as an asymptomatic solitary liver mass but may cause discomfort. The lesion is not premalignant, and asymptomatic patients with a confirmed diagnosis can be managed conservatively. In children, the lesion often remains static in size and asymptomatic for many years.[31] Symptomatic cases have been treated by resection, embolization or hepatic artery ligation.

Hemangiomas

These are the commonest liver tumors in children ranging from small asymptomatic lesions to large life-threatening tumors. Most hemangiomas and many hemangioendotheliomas regress spontaneously but treatment is indicated for cardiac failure, respiratory symptoms, or abdominal pain and distension. Specific measures to control the hemangioma may be required. Corticosteroids or alpha-interferon can induce gradual regression in some but not all cases. For bilobar disease complicated by cardiac failure, hepatic artery ligation or embolization may be effective.[32,33] Large symptomatic hemangiomas localized to one or other half of the liver can be resected.[32] Buttressed compression sutures may be a useful adjunctive surgical treatment in unresectable cases.[34] Rarely, liver transplantation is the only therapeutic option.

Adenoma

Although rare, hepatic adenomas may affect children of any age and either sex. They are usually single and well circumscribed with a thin fibrous capsule. In young women, there is a well established association between hepatic adenomas and the combined oral contraceptive pill. In children, hepatic adenomas may be idiopathic, associated with exogenous sex steroid therapy, or linked to various rare disorders.[5,35] Symptomatic or large hepatic adenomas generally require resection to control pain or avert potential complications such as hemorrhage, rupture, and the small risk of malignant transformation.

Other pediatric liver 'tumors' which may occasionally require liver resection include large or symptomatic non-parasitic cysts, inflammatory pseudotumors (usually only if symptomatic or if there is diagnostic uncertainty), and rarely, chronic abscesses and parasitic cysts.[36]

Trauma

Most pediatric liver trauma is successfully managed non-operatively. Nevertheless, a child with a liver injury who is hemodynamically unstable after basic resuscitation (at least 40 ml/kg of intravenous fluid) requires an urgent laparotomy and control of intra-abdominal bleeding. Direct suture ligation and perihepatic packing are frequently sufficient to control ongoing hemorrhage. Anatomical resection following acute liver trauma has a high mortality rate when performed in the presence of coagulopathy, acidosis, and associated injuries which often complicate major liver injury. In contrast, non-anatomical resectional debridement, i.e. the removal of devitalized liver parenchyma along lines of injury rather than anatomical planes (after inflow occlusion) is valuable.[37] However, formal hepatic resection can be useful for more delayed complications of liver trauma such as in the child with localized hepatic necrosis or in those with biliary complications not amenable to biliary reconstruction.

SURGICAL ANATOMY AND IMAGING

Any surgeon operating on the liver must be thoroughly familiar with normal hepatic anatomy and common variants. Unfortunately, the nomenclature for describing normal hepatic anatomy and the common types of hepatic resection is often confusing. In recent years, Strasberg has attempted to introduce a more consistent terminology.[38]

The right and left liver lobes are the classic lobes of *surface anatomy* separated by the attachment of the falciform ligament superiorly and the umbilical fissure and ligamentum venosum inferiorly. The internal anatomy of the whole organ can be subdivided on three levels:

1. The right and left *hemilivers* are divided by the midplane that lies between the medial margin of the gallbladder fossa and the left side of inferior vena cava (previously known as Cantlie's line).
2. Each hemiliver is divided into two *sections* based on the internal anatomy of the hepatic artery and bile duct. Thus the right hemiliver has anterior (segments 5 and 8) and posterior (segments 6 and 7) sections and the left hemiliver has medial (segment 4) and lateral (segments 2 and 3) sections.
3. Segmental anatomy is based on Couinaud's 8 *segments* which relate to the intrahepatic divisions of the portal vein but each segment is also subserved by branches of the hepatic artery and bile duct. The caudate lobe is segment 1 and is based on surface anatomy (Fig. 86.3).

There are three main hepatic veins—right, middle and left. The venous drainage of segment 2 is always solitary. Segment 3 has a single vein in 30%, two veins in 50%, and three veins in 20%. Segment 4 drains to the middle hepatic vein in 50% of cases, to the left hepatic vein in 10%, and to both in 40%. Almost 20% of adults have a sizeable right inferior hepatic vein (> 5 mm) which usually drains segment 4 but has good

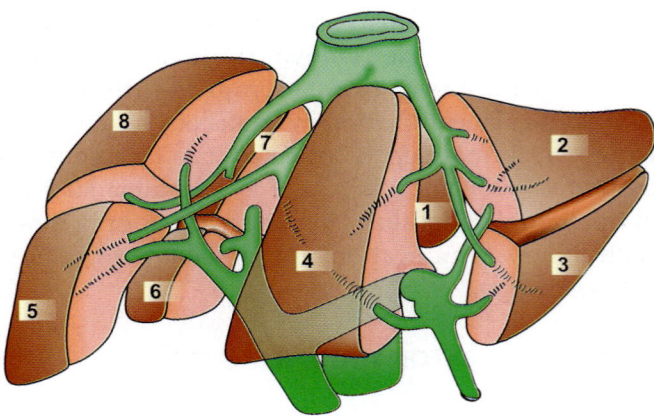

Fig. 86.3: Segmental anatomy of the liver

confluence are shown in (Fig. 86.5).[40,41,42] It is also important to note that the right posterior sectional duct (draining segments 6 and 7) typically loops around the medial sectional branch of the portal structures ('Hjortsjo's crook') (Fig. 86.6) where it is vulnerable to injury during a left trisectionectomy.

Anatomical variations in the origin and course of the hepatic artery/arteries are common and the more frequent variations are shown in (Fig. 86.7).[43,44] The arterial supply of the common bile duct has been studied in detail by Northover and Terblanche (1979) and is of relevance to liver resection and transplantation because of the need to avoid bile duct

collateral flow to other segments. The left and middle veins usually unite to form a short common trunk before entering the inferior vena cava.[39] Consequently, the left hepatic vein is potentially vulnerable during a right trisectionectomy and the middle hepatic vein during left hemihepatectomy. The middle hepatic vein occupies the midplane of the liver and the right vein lies in the right intersectional plane. Only the terminal portion of the left hepatic vein occupies the left intersectional plane. During liver resection, the hepatic veins can be approached and ligated prior to parenchymal dissection or they may be controlled from within the liver substance.

The left branch of the portal vein and the left hepatic duct have a longer, more horizontal extrahepatic course (Fig. 86.4). The anatomy of the left portal vein is more constant than the right; the right portal vein trifurcates in about 15% of individuals. Common variations in the anatomy of the hepatic duct

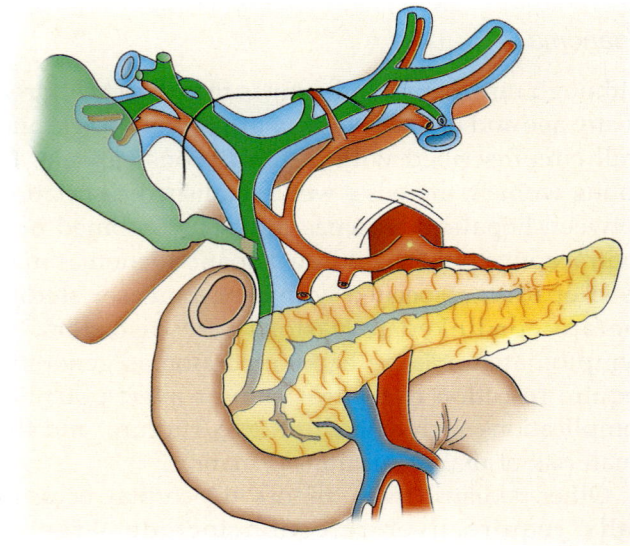

Fig. 86.4: The bifurcation of the portal triad. Note the longer and relatively horizontal course of the left portal vein and left hepatic duct

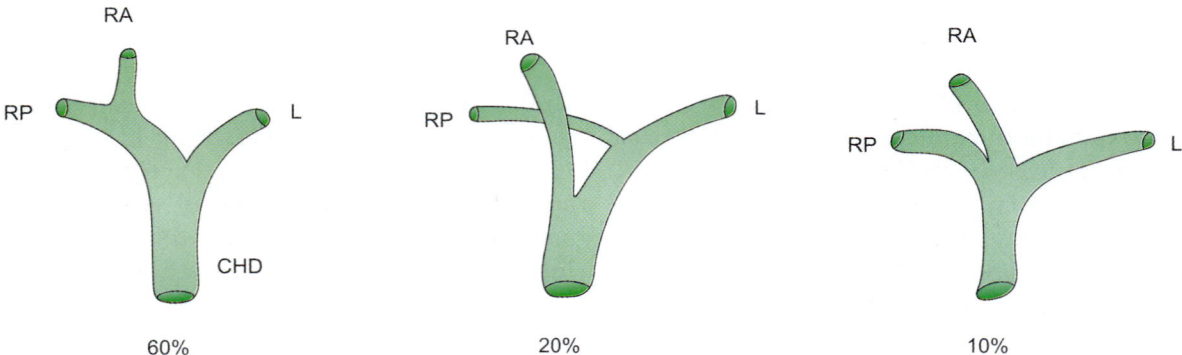

Fig. 86.5: Common variations in the anatomy of the hepatic duct confluence (Couinaud 1981)

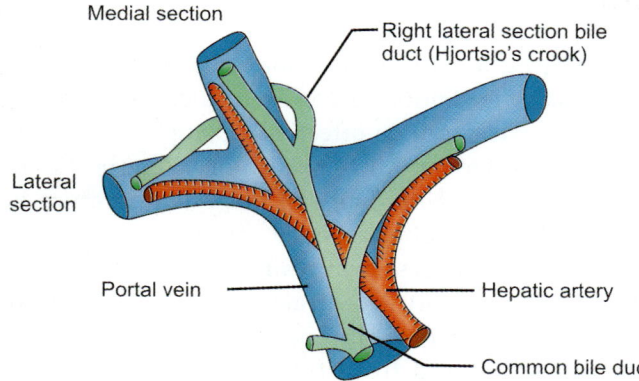

Fig. 86.6: Relationship of the right lateral sectional bile duct to the intrahepatic bifurcation of the right portal structures

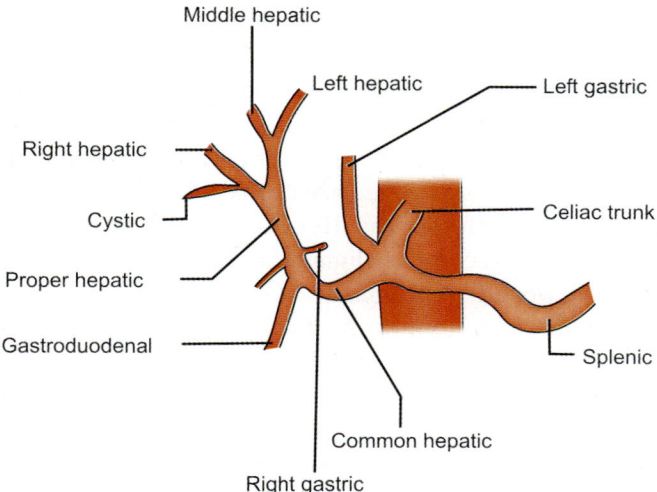

Fig. 86.7: Patterns of hepatic arterial anatomy. The diagram shows the usual arterial arrangement found in ~60-70% of cases. Common variations include:
- The right hepatic artery (RHA) arises partially (accessory) or completely (replaced) from the superior mesenteric artery (SMA) in ~15%
- The left hepatic artery (LHA) arises partially (accessory) or completely (replaced) from the left gastric artery (LGA) in ~10%
- The liver is supplied by a common hepatic artery and a replaced or accessory RHA from the SMA and a replaced or accessory LHA from the LGA in ~7%
- The RHA and LHA originate independently from the celiac trunk or close to the origin of the common hepatic artery. Rarely, the common hepatic artery arises directly from the SMA or aorta

ischemia.[45] The supraduodenal duct receives arterial blood from the right hepatic artery above and the retroduodenal and gastroduodenal arteries below; the small arterial branches on the duct run in an axial direction and are mainly located at 3 and 9 o'clock.

Most liver tumors present with abdominal distension and/or a mass. Initial investigation using ultrasonography (US) will confirm whether the mass is hepatic, cystic or solid, and single or multiple. Doppler ultrasound studies provide information about its vascularity. Computerized tomography (CT) with intravenous contrast enhancement defines the anatomy of the lesion as a guide to surgical resection. Definition can be improved further by using faster scanners, CT arterioportography, or spiral CT.

Additional investigations prior to surgery may include hepatic angiography but in our experience this has been largely supplanted by a combination of imaging using duplex ultrasonography and gadolinium-enhanced magnetic resonance angiography (MRA).[46] The latter is particularly good at demonstrating vascular anatomy, including the vena cava and hepatic veins (Fig. 86.8). Hepatic masses are well characterized by magnetic resonance imaging after obtaining both T1 and T2 weighted images.[47] MR cholangiography offers the ability to non-invasively assess the biliary tree and is particularly useful prior to a planned trisectionectomy.

RESECTABILITY OF LIVER TUMORS

CT, MR and sonography are all capable of providing images in the transaxial, sagittal and coronal planes which affords the surgeon considerable confidence when assessing hepatic vascular anatomy and tumor

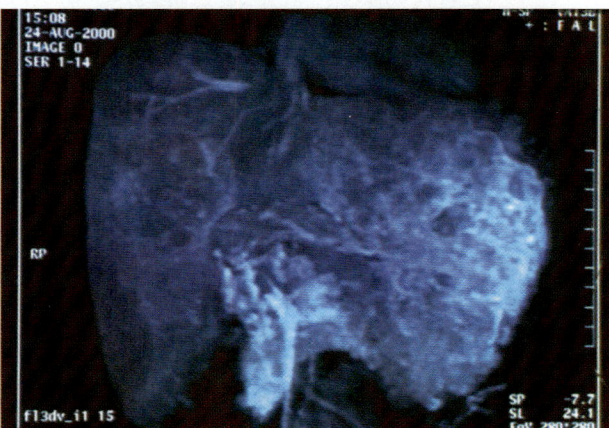

Fig. 86.8: Magnetic resonance angiogram in a girl with multifocal hepatocellular carcinoma. Note the presence of tumor in the portal vein

resectability.[48] Prior to surgical resection of any liver tumor it is essential to determine the presence and extent of extrahepatic disease. The resectability of a liver tumor can generally determined by accurate preoperative imaging but it is only finally possible to be sure at laparotomy. The greatest dificulty arises with tumors adjacent to the hilar structures or to the hepatic vein confluence or inferior vena cava. The size of the tumor *per se* is not a contraindication to resection. Intraoperative US can be extremely useful in defining the extent of a tumor adjacent to the cava or major hepatic veins; application of a high frequency transducer directly to the surface of the liver increases the sensitivity of conventional transabdominal ultrasound examination (Fig. 86.9).[49]

Laparoscopy may also have a role in assessing the resectability of some liver tumors but there is little experience of using the technique for this purpose in children. Caval/hepatic vein assessment is best performed using other methods. In adults, laparoscopic liver resection with 'hand port' assistance has been described.

TECHNIQUES OF LIVER RESECTION

With tumors, the aim of surgery is complete excision of the mass leaving the remaining liver with an adequate arterial and portal supply, intact biliary drainage and satisfactory venous outflow.

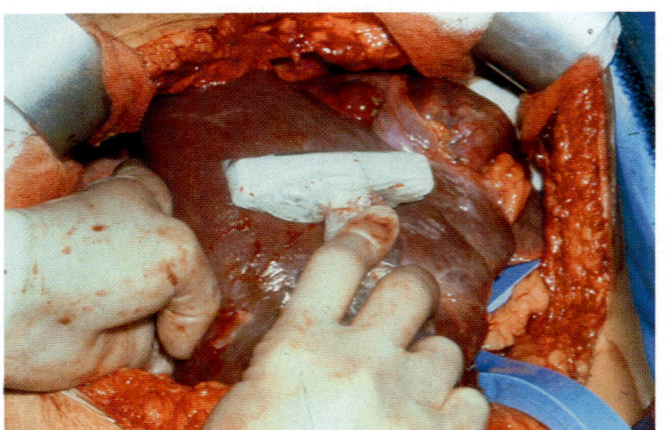

Fig. 86.9: Intraoperative ultrasound is useful in assessing the extent of a liver tumor and its relationship to major hepatic vessels. The liver has been mobilized prior to scanning

Preparation

Preoperative coagulopathy should be corrected and prophylactic antibiotics given on induction. Epidural analgesia can produce effective postoperative pain relief and help to minimize respiratory complications. Intraoperative maintenance of body temperature is important and can be achieved in a variety of ways (e.g. warming mattress, warm air devices and ambient temperature control). A central venous line is inserted for pressure monitoring and rapid transfusion. Cross-matched blood and fresh frozen plasma should be available.

Exposure

Good surgical access is achieved via a curved bilateral subcostal incision with or without a midline xiphoid extension. Rarely, a thoracoabdominal approach may be indicated for paracaval tumors.[50] A roll or gel pad may be placed under the thoracolumbar spine to facilitate exposure. After preliminary laparotomy, the liver is mobilized by division of the falciform, triangular and coronary ligaments and the retrohepatic cava exposed. A versatile self-retaining retractor attached to the operating table such as the Omni-Tract® (Minnesota Scientific, Inc., USA) enables the costal margins to be retracted in a superior, lateral and anterior direction (Fig. 86.10). Intraoperative US imaging is useful at this stage in selected cases.[51]

Inflow Occlusion

The portal triad is slung to allow subsequent inflow occlusion (Pringle maneuver) which reduces blood loss during subsequent parenchymal transection.[52] A warm ischemic period of up to one hour is well tolerated by the normal adult liver and intermittent portal triad clamping is safe up to two hours.[53] Prolonged periods of ischemia may be better tolerated after a brief period of ischemia followed by temporary reperfusion and then sustained inflow occlusion, so called ischemic preconditioning.[54] The underlying mechanism may be related to downregulation of apoptotic pathways in hepatocytes. Venous congestion of the gut can be a problem with temporary portal vein occlusion, especially in those patients with no pre-existing portal hypertension.

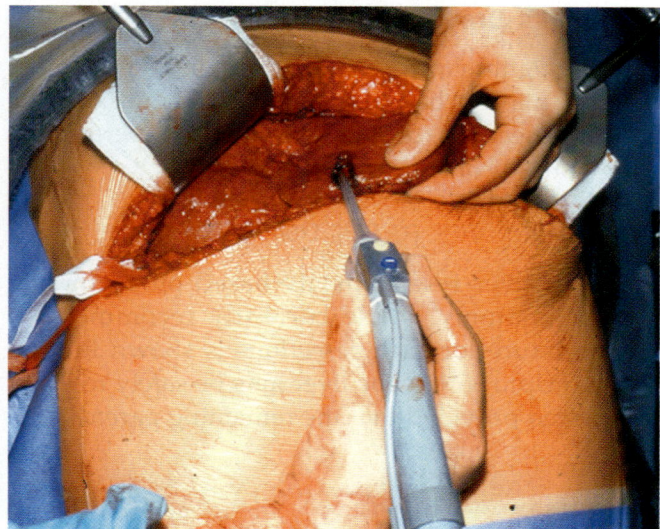

Fig. 86.10: The Omni-Tract® enables the costal margins to be retracted to provide good operative exposure and the ultrasonic surgical aspirator (CUSA) can be used to divide the hepatic parenchyma and expose larger vessels for ligation/suturing

Parenchymal Transection

A variety of techniques can be used to transect the liver parenchyma and control vascular and biliary radicles (Table 86.3).[55-58]

The author uses a combination of bipolar diathermy, ultrasonic aspiration, suture ligation, argon beam and fibrin glue but any technique which safely minimizes blood loss and prevents bile leakage is acceptable. The Cavitron ultrasonic surgical aspirator contains a transducer that oscillates longitudinally at high frequency and to which a hollow conical titanium tip is attached (Fig. 86.10). Irrigation and suction channels are incorporated. The hepatic parenchyma, with its high water content, is cavitated and fragmented but blood vessels and bile ducts are relatively spare.[59,60] Hepatic veins, however, are more vulnerable. The harmonic scalpel operates at a higher frequency than the ultrasonic surgical aspirator and tissue dissection is achieved more by compression and sawing than cavitation.

Once surgical bleeding points have been controlled, the raw surface of the liver should be carefully inspected for bleeding and bile leaks. Oozing from small vessels on the cut-surface of the liver can be controlled in various ways. The argon beam coagulator is particularly good; the non-combustible argon gas provides a safe medium for the transmission of electrosurgical current leading to less smoke, non contact coagulation, and reduced tissue adhesion. Suture sites should be avoided since the argon beam may damage these. Fibrin sealant is also valuable; fibrinogen and thrombin are sprayed on to the raw surface of the liver using compressed air interacting rapidly to produce a stable fibrin clot. There is a theoretical risk of viral transmission with current products. Other topical hemostatic agents include oxidized regenerated cellulose, gelatin sponge, and collagen fleece.

A vascular stapler (Endo GIA®) can be used to control large hepatic veins in older children.

Central Venous Pressure

Maintenance of a low central venous pressure (0-4cms H_2O) helps to minimize blood loss during the phase of parenchymal transection and this is facilitated by a slight head down tilt.[61] The CVP should be above 0 cm H_2O to avoid the risk of air embolism when hepatic veins are opened.

Total Vascular Exclusion

Normothermic total vascular exclusion (TVE) is occasionally necessary for lesions adjacent to the hepatic veins or inferior vena cava; the non-cirrhotic liver will tolerate up to one hour of warm ischemia.[62,63,64] This technique requires complete mobilization of the liver with vascular inflow occlusion (Pringle manouver), supra and infrahepatic caval clamping and control of the right adrenal vein and

---

Table 86.3: Technical aids to liver resection and cut-surface hemostasis

- Crushing forceps, e.g. Kelly clamp
- Diathermy (monopolar and bipolar)
- Suture/ligation
- Metal clips, e.g. titanium ligaclips
- Ultrasonic surgical dissector
  - Cavitron ultrasonic surgical aspirator (CUSA®)
  - Harmonic scalpel
- Water jet dissector
- Neodymium YAG laser
- Argon beam coagulator
- Topical hemostatic agents—fibrin glue, oxidized cellulose, gelatin sponge, collagen fleece
- Vascular stapler

any accessory hepatic arteries. Hemodynamic disturbances, particularly a fall in cardiac output, must be anticipated by appropriate expansion of the intravascular volume. Hemodynamic changes may be minimized by synchronous portosystemic veno-venous bypass.[65] The addition of supraceliac aortic clamping has been largely abandoned. *In situ* perfusion of the isolated liver with cold preservative solution has been used in adults to extend the period of total vascular exclusion.

Cardiopulmonary bypass with hypothermic circulatory arrest has been advocated in special circumstances but is not without hazard.[66,67]

Abdominal Drainage

After straightforward hemihepatectomy, abdominal drainage may not be required but after more extensive hepatic resections, drainage with a soft, perforated, wide-bore silicone drain is advisable.

TYPES OF LIVER RESECTION

Standard liver resections are based on segmental hepatic anatomy.[40,1] The currently recommended nomenclature for such resections is shown in (Fig. 86.11).[38] Upto 85% of the liver may be safely resected in children provided that the remaining parenchyma

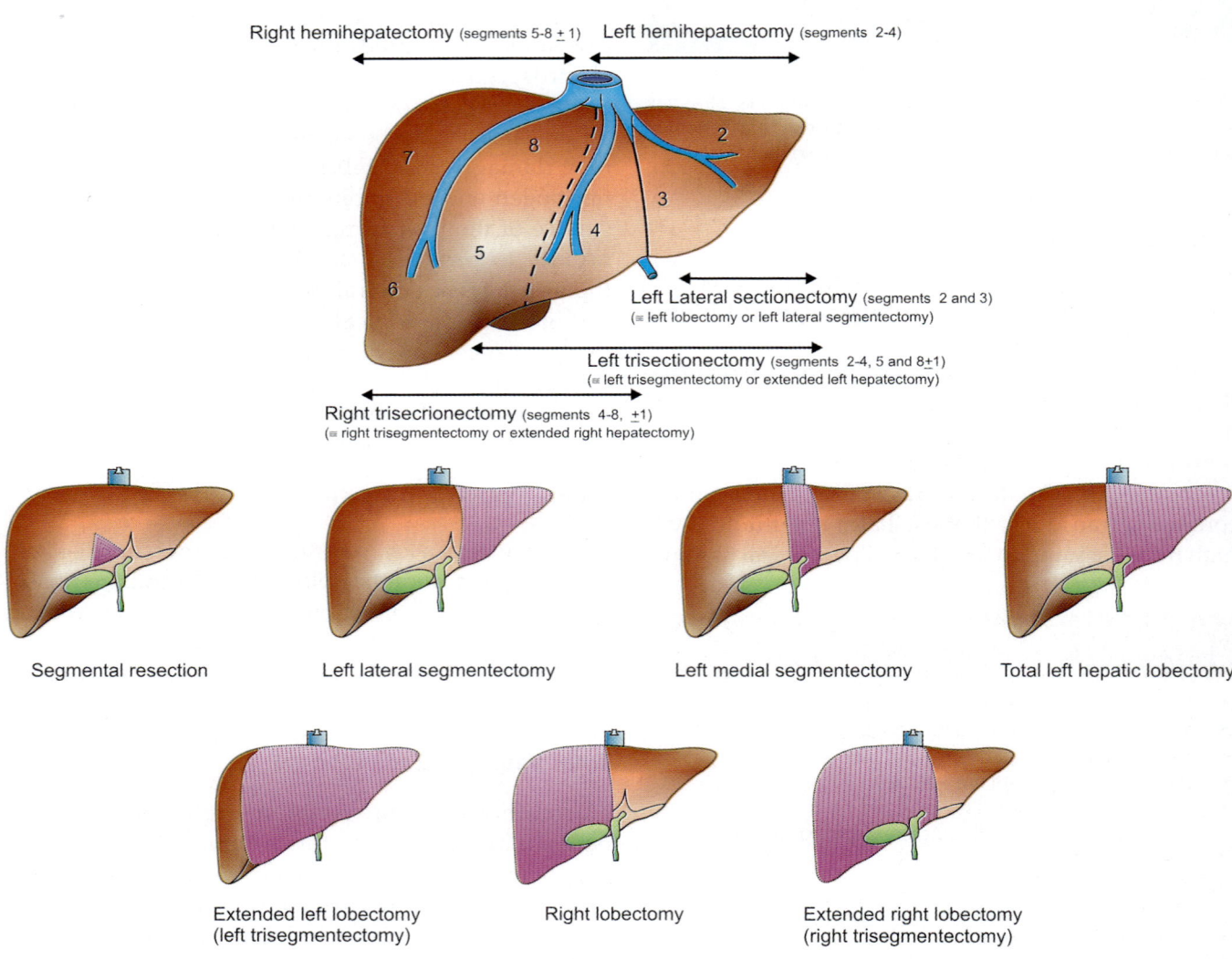

Fig. 86.11: Standard liver resections based on segmental hepatic anatomy

is healthy and the arterial and portal inflow and hepatic venous outflow are safeguarded.[57,68] Major resections are better tolerated if there has been compensatory hypertrophy of remaining healthy liver as a result of the disease process. A right trisectionectomy leaves a remnant volume of between 15 and 35% (median 20%).

The approach to liver resection is illustrated by consideration of two "standard" resections.

Right Hemihepatectomy

The liver is mobilized by division of its ligamentous attachments and the portal triad is slung. The retrohepatic cava is exposed by dividing the venous branches from the caudate lobe. Superiorly, the hepatocaval ligament is divided to expose the right hepatic vein. This vein can be divided between vascular clamps and oversewn with a non-absorbable suture at this stage or from within the liver parenchyma at a later stage of the operation, depending on ease and preference.

After cholecystectomy, the right hepatic artery is dissected and divided close to the hilum of the liver, usually to the right of the common hepatic duct. Left hepatic arterial pulsation should be confirmed prior to ligation. The right portal vein is mobilized by dividing any posterior caudate branches; it is then divided and oversewn. The hilar plate is lowered by incising Glisson's capsule anteriorly at the base of segment 4 to expose the common hepatic duct bifurcation. The right hepatic duct is usually divided well away from the bifurcation at a later stage, after hepatic transection. The plane of hepatic transection lies just to the right of the midplane, proceeding along the right margin of the middle hepatic vein (Fig. 86.12). This is initially outlined by diathermy on the liver surface. If the caudate lobe is retained, the portal structures must be divided distal to their caudate branches. Positioning packs behind the right lobe brings it anteriorly and medially and renders the transection plane close to the sagittal.

Left Trisectionectomy

Previously known as extended left hepatectomy or left trisegmentectomy, this resection involves the excision of segments 2, 3, 4, 5 and 8. Occasionally, the caudate lobe (segment 1) is also removed. This resection was

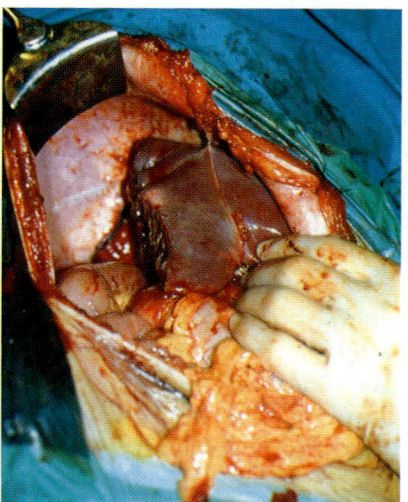

Fig. 86.12: The liver remnant after right hemihepatectomy just prior to spraying with fibrin sealant

first described in detail by Starzl et al (1982) and Blumgart et al (1993) and has been utilized in the treatment of extensive pediatric liver tumors by others.[11,69,70] More recently, a specific description of the technique applied to children has been reported.[58]

Vascular structures are controlled outside the liver before dividing the hepatic parenchyma. The left hepatic artery and left branch of the portal vein are dissected by incising Glisson's capsule and lowering the hilar plate; both vessels are then ligated. The obliterated ductus venosus is identified by retracting segments 2 and 3 anteriorly and division of this fibrous band exposes a recess at its upper limit which runs under the confluence of the middle and left hepatic veins. The suprahepatic cava is exposed by incising the falciform ligament posteriorly and careful dissection now enables the confluence of the middle and left hepatic veins to be isolated and slung. The confluence is then divided between vascular clamps and oversewn with a non-absorbable monofilament suture. A vascular stapler can be used in teenagers.

Control of the vascular inflow to segments 5 and 8 is achieved by dissecting the hepatic parenchyma surrounding the right portal vein and right hepatic artery as far as the right anterior sectional pedicle. This is initially clamped to demarcate segments 5 and 8 after which it is ligated. If segment 1 is to be retained, the left portal vein and left hepatic artery should be ligated distal to their caudate branches. The hepatic parenchyma is then transected in a coronal plane with or without temporary inflow occlusion.

Thus, in hemihepatectomy and trisectionectomy procedures, preliminary hilar dissection is necessary prior to hemihepatic vascular occlusion. If the relevant hepatic vein can be safely clamped extrahepatically, this allows a form of localized total vascular exclusion which helps to reduce the need for blood transfusion.

Liver tumors should be excised en bloc with any localized area of tumor adherence, such as the diaphragm or omentum, to ensure complete tumor excision. Caudate lobe hepatoblastomas are uncommon but typically adherent to the cava and/or porta hepatis, show signs of early vascular invasion and dissemination and are technically difficult to resect.[71,72] An understanding of segmental hepatic anatomy also renders atypical liver resections possible such as central or transverse hepatectomies.[73] For more detailed accounts of hepatic resections and a description of individual segmentectomy procedures, the reader is advised to consult Blumgart (2000).[41]

Non-anatomic Hepatic Resection

Despite the advantage of anatomical resections there are indications for non-anatomical procedures such as removal of small benign tumours, excision of a small hepatocellular carcinoma in liver cirrhosis, re-resection following a previous major hepatectomy, and liver trauma.

Pledgetted sutures can be useful for dealing with cut surface bleeding after resection or after reduced-size transplantation; it is important that such sutures are placed *superficially* on the cut surface and tied to produce compression. Strangulation and necrosis of deeper areas of parenchyma must be avoided. This technique has been extended by Sandler et al (2001) to non-anatomical liver resection in small children by prior placement of Teflon felt pledgetted sutures. It may be particularly advantageous in small children who have a relatively soft liver parenchyma and in whom a non-anatomical resection is planned.

Most hepatic resections are relatively straightforward but tumors which are complex, either because of size or location, should be managed in centers with hepatobiliary surgical expertise. These include large central tumors and those involving the hepatic vein confluence or IVC. Innovative techniques have been used to treat tumors of borderline resectability, thus avoiding the need for liver transplantation.

Extending the Limits of Hepatic Resection

i. **Neoadjuvant chemotherapy** or transarterial chemoembolization have effectively extended the limits of resection for hepatoblastoma. Between one and two-thirds of patients present with unresectable primary tumors or distant metastases and after PLADO cytotoxic therapy, 70-85% of unresectable tumors become operable.[6,9,11,74]

ii. **Preoperative portal vein embolization.** This may encourage growth of an anticipated liver remnant consequently permitting a more extensive hepatic resection to be performed. Kaneko et al 2001 reported preoperative portal embolization of the right hemiliver and caudate lobe one month before right trisectionectomy for an inflammatory pseudotumor involving the hepatic hilum in a 6 year old boy.[36] The volume of the left lateral segment assessed by CT increased from 217 cm^3 to 250 cm^3 prior to resection. A similar although spontaneous process enabled Shuto et al (1993) to perform a massive liver resection for a giant mesenchymal hamartoma, leaving only the hypertrophied caudate lobe behind.[75]

iii. **Caval repair/reconstruction.** Minimal tumour involvement of the inferior vena cava is best dealt with by local resection and repair, with or without an autologous vein patch. More extensive involvement has been treated in adults by prosthetic replacement which requires hypothermic hepatic perfusion with preservative solution and *ex-vivo* bench surgery.[65,76] Takayama et al 1991 reported excision of the retrohepatic cava en bloc with a left trisectionectomy for a hepatoblastoma in the caudate lobe which had invaded the cava.[71,72] The retrohepatic cava was not reconstructed because it had been chronically occluded by tumor and fibrosis and the patient already had well established collateral venous pathways.

iv. **Liver transplantation.** This is the ultimate hepatic resection for an otherwise unresectable liver tumor where there is no evidence of persistent extrahepatic disease. The results are critically dependent on the type of tumor and case selection

(Table 86.4).[5] Extended hepatic resection with transplant back-up has been proposed for tumors of borderline resectability by the Cape Town group.[77] This innovative strategy may encourage a more aggressive attempt at tumor resection in the knowledge that transplantation is an option but the logistics are potentially problematic.

v. **Resection of the hepatic vein confluence.** Liver tumors that surround the three major hepatic veins are generally considered unresectable. Superina et al (2000) have described a new technique: the left hepatic artery, left branch of the portal vein, and the three hepatic veins are occluded with vascular clamps.[67] Perfusion of the remaining liver is through the right hepatic artery and portal vein. An extensive resection of segments 2, 3, 4, 7 and 8 is possible if there is adequate venous drainage of the right hemiliver via the retro-hepatic veins (most likely if there is a sizeable accessory right inferior hepatic vein). If the liver remains soft and does not become tense or mottled, the three major hepatic veins can be divided and the tumor resected. If venous drainage is inadequate, the procedure must be abandoned and the patient considered for liver transplantation.

vi. **Staged resection** of multiple tumors has been recommended as a means of allowing intervening parenchymal regeneration in cases where residual hepatic sufficiency is in doubt but this would probably only be applicable to benign tumors in children.[84]

vii. **Ex-vivo dissection and auto-transplantation** involves total hepatectomy, placing the patient on caval and portal veno-venous bypass, and, after extracorporeal bench surgery, transplanting the healthy liver remnant back into the patient.[85,65] Such an approach has not yet been used in children.

Before any liver tumor resection, close liason with the pathologist is important so that resection margins can be adequately assessed and the tumor appropriately characterized. This will often mean submitting the liver resection specimen in the intact, fresh, and unfixed state.[86]

POSTOPERATIVE MANAGEMENT

The patient is supported with dextrose saline and albumin infusions for two or three days after a major hepatic resection; vitamin K and fresh frozen plasma may be necessary to correct coagulopathy.[80] After major resection, gastric hyperacidity and temporary portal hypertension predispose to bleeding from gastric erosions and gastric protection with H2 blockers or Sucralfate is advisable until enteral feeding is re-established. A fever above 38°C is commonly seen for a few days after an uncomplicated major hepatic resection. Prophylactic antibiotics are usually given for 24 hours.

Table 86.4: Results of liver transplantation for hepatoblastoma and hepatocellular carcinoma

Author	Year	No	Survival
Hepatoblastoma			
Koneru et al[14]	1991	12	6 (50%) @ mean 44 m
Tagge et al[78]	1992	6	5 (83%) @ mean 16 m
Bilik and Superina[79]	1997	5	4 (80%) @ 1-5y
Al-Qabandi et al[80]	1999	8	5 (63%) @ median 22 m
Perilongo and Shafford[15]	1999	11	9 (82%) @ median 46 m
Reyes et al[16]	2000	12	92% actuarial survival @ 1y, 83% @ 5y
Hepatocellular carcinoma			
Tagge et al[78]	1992	9	4 (44%) @ mean 27 m
Broughan et al[81]	1994	4	3 (75%) @ mean 63 m
Otte et al[82]	1996	5	3 (60%) @ median 49 m
Superina and Bilik[83]	1996	3	3 (100%) @ 1-5y
Reyes et al*[16]	2000	19	79% actuarial survival @ 1y, 63% @ 5y

*Includes 7 patients with "incidental" HCC discovered within the explanted liver

Standard biochemical liver function tests are initially abnormal after hepatic resection because of loss of functioning hepatocytes and relative portal hypertension secondary to reduced hepatic mass and venous outflow. Typically, the prothrombin time returns to normal by the fourth postoperative day and liver enzymes and bilirubin within 10-14 days, but albumin levels may take 6 weeks to normalize.[57,87] Hepatic regeneration is particularly rapid in children and, despite perioperative chemotherapy, liver volume is restored within 90 days in most cases and remains almost normal for age with continued growth.[88,89] Cisplatin interferes little with hepatic regeneration but chemotherapy is best avoided 10 days either side of surgery.[90]

An injured or fatty liver shows slower and/or incomplete regeneration and liver regeneration is slowed by extrahepatic complications such as sepsis. Cirrhotic livers have a significantly impaired capacity to regenerate and postoperative liver function is disturbed more and for longer. Biliary obstruction also impedes hepatic repair.[88] In the vast majority of cases, liver function is restored and continues to be normal years later.[88]

COMPLICATIONS

Major intraoperative risks are hemorrhage, air embolism, tumor embolus, hyperkalemia from tumor lysis and primary or secondary (ischemic) bile duct injury.[9,11,91-95] Excessive blood loss during surgery correlates with increased postoperative morbidity. Median intraoperative blood loss is very variable but is generally less for hemihepatectomy compared to trisectionectomy.[11,58] With modern techniques, hepatic resection is associated with a substantially reduced blood loss. Indeed, blood transfusion may be unneccessary in some standard hemihepatectomies.

Postoperative complications include hemorrhage, bile leak, subphrenic abscess, pulmonary complications, hepatic insufficiency, adhesive bowel obstruction, catheter-related blood stream infection, and wound problems. A bile leak is usually from the parenchymal cut-surface and tends to resolve spontaneously with drainage but major duct injury or ischemia are possible causes. Persistent or large volume bile leaks require investigation by radionuclide scan and/or endoscopic retrograde cholangiography. Temporary stenting of the common bile duct encourages transduodenal bile flow which may accelerate resolution. Persistent or infected fluid collections can be successfully treated by percutaneous catheter drainage. Hepatic insufficiency and ascites is rare except in patients with cirrhosis.

The mortality from elective liver resection in children has progressively fallen and is now below 5%. Most patients recover rapidly and can be discharged home within 7-10 days.

LIVER RESECTION IN PEDIATRIC LIVER TRANSPLANTATION

Liver transplantation is the treatment of choice for end-stage liver disease in children. The commonest indication for pediatric liver transplantation is biliary atresia and the majority of these patients are infants. A shortage of size-matched pediatric donors stimulated the development of innovative surgical techniques to produce smaller allografts from adult donors. Many of these techniques and associated aspects of liver function are relevant to liver resection.

The theoretical liver volume of an individual is related to body weight and in children corresponds to 2.5 ml per 100 g (i.e. 2.5% of body weight). When procuring liver grafts from living donors, the aim is to obtain a minimum graft to recipient body weight ratio of 1%.[96] Clearly, the function of the graft depends not only on this critical liver mass but also on a wide variety of other graft and host factors. Small-for-size grafts (< 0.8% graft to recipient body weight ratio) are associated with lower graft survival, and reduced metabolic and synthetic capacity.

The adult liver mass is somewhere between 1300 and 1700 g and is reached at 15-20 years of age. The weight of the adult organ depends not only on age and sex (M > F) but also on body mass, alcohol consumption and steatosis. The left lateral segment (segments 2 and 3) comprises approximately 20-25% of the liver weight and the left lobe 40%. Implantation of a large for size graft is also associated with an increased morbidity and a greater risk of graft failure. Table 86.5 provides a guide to the maximum donor:recipient weight mismatch which is usually tolerated in liver transplantation in children.

Table 86.5: Guide to donor:recipient weight mismatch in pediatric liver transplantation
• Whole graft—up to 1.5:1 (depending on recipient size, hepatomegaly, ascites etc) • Right lobe—up to 1.5:1 • Left lobe—up to 3:1 • Left lateral segment—up to 10:1 • Monosegment—up to 15:1

TYPES OF LIVER GRAFT

- Full-size or whole liver graft
- Reduced-size graft (=cut-down or partial graft)

In a reduced-size graft, a single smaller liver graft is prepared from a larger donor by excision of part of the liver. Reduced or split livers now account for more than 50% of all pediatric grafts.[97,98]

The first successful reduced-size graft was reported by Bismuth and Houssin in 1984 but these allografts only gained wide acceptance when methods of graft preservation improved to allow an adequate cold ischemic time for the necessary graft dissection.[99] Further technical refinements led to the development of both right (segments 5-8 ± 4) and left (2-4) lobe grafts and the left lateral segment (2 and 3) graft. For a reduced right or left lobe graft the retrohepatic cava is usually retained with the lobe but for the left lateral segment graft (Fig. 86.13) the left hepatic vein of the donor graft is anastomosed to the recipient's retrohepatic inferior vena cava.[100,101]

Split-liver Graft

In a split-liver graft, the donor liver is divided for implantation into two recipents, either as a left lateral segment and a right lobe graft (Fig. 86.14) or as right and left lobe grafts. In 1988, Pichlmayr in Germany and Bismuth in France simultaneously performed the first split-liver transplant.[102,63,64] For optimum results in split-liver transplantation, a graft must be prepared from a hemodynamically stable donor aged between 10 and 50 years with normal biochemical liver function and a macroscopically healthy liver with minimal steatosis.

Most liver splits are performed on the back table after cadaveric organ retrieval (*ex-situ* splitting) but, where logistic and organizational aspects permit, *in situ* splitting in the donor has some advantages.[103] These include better cut-surface hemostasis and a potentially shorter cold ischemic time.

Living Donor Liver Graft

The liver graft is procured from a living donor, usually a close relative. The left lateral segment graft for children was popularized at first but adult to adult right lobe transplantation has since become increasingly common.[104] Donors require an intensive physical and psychological work up to assess their suitability. The first successful pediatric living donor liver transplant was performed by Strong et al (1990) who implanted a left lobe graft from the pediatric

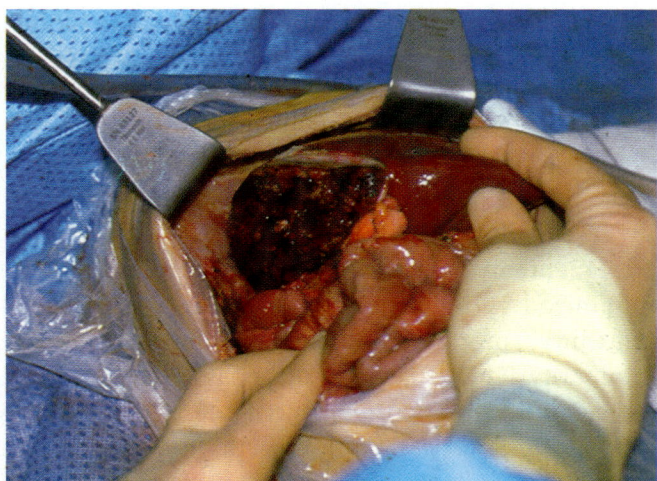

Fig. 86.13: A cadaveric left lateral segment orthotopic liver graft transplanted into an infant with biliary atresia

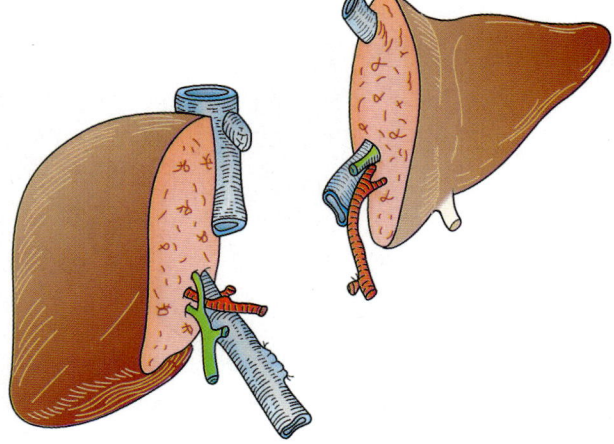

Fig. 86.14: Split-liver preparation. The donor liver has been divided to produce two transplantable grafts: a left lateral segment graft and a right lobe graft

recipient's mother.[105] Broelsch et al subsequently reported the first successful series.[106]

Monosegmental Grafts

The left lateral segment graft (segments 2 and 3) can be used to overcome a size discrepancy from donor to recipient of up to 10:1. Monosegmental grafts (segment 2 or 3) from pediatric donors have been used successfully to transplant small infants weighing as little as 2.9kg (Fig. 86.15).[107,108] Long, thin left lateral segments are more suitable than short, thick grafts.

GRAFT PREPARATION

Most split-liver grafts are prepared on the bench and this process may take 2-3 hours. Close communication with the recipient hepatectomy team is important to make adjustments according to liver size and vessel allocation in split procedures. The donor liver must be kept immersed in preservative solution (e.g. University of Wisconsin solution) at a temperature of 4°C throughout the dissection. After conventional preparation of the liver and major vessels, an early assessment of vascular and biliary anatomy is important to ensure that there is no anatomical contraindication to splitting, such as an absent portal vein bifurcation, a segment 3 vein draining directly into the middle hepatic vein, atrophy of the left lobe, or an accessory right hepatic artery arising from the left hepatic artery.[109-111] Many of the commoner arterial anomalies are not a bar to splitting.[112]

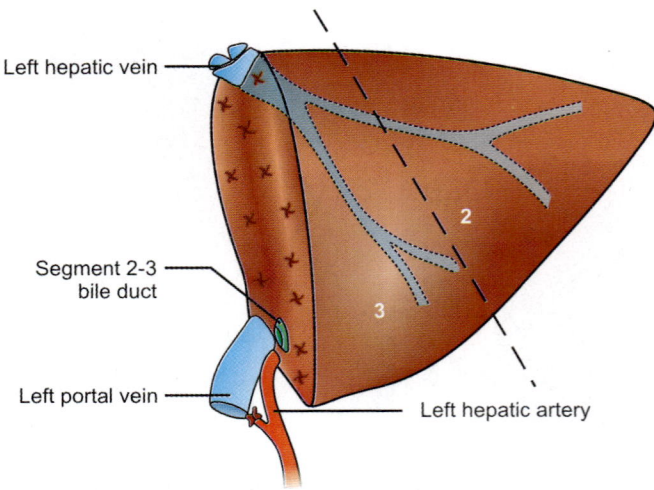

Fig. 86.15: A left lateral segment graft (segments 2 and 3) can be reduced further to produce a monosegmental graft

The plane of parenchymal transection is dictated by the type of graft being prepared—this is close to the midplane with right and left lobe grafts and about 1 cm to the right of the falciform ligament in left lateral segment grafts. The middle hepatic vein is retained with left lobe grafts. The liver parenchyma may be divided with forceps, an ultrasonic dissector, and/or diathermy. Individual vessels and bile ducts are ligated and divided within the parenchyma. On the cut surface, superficial circular monofilament purse string sutures from the liver capsule are useful in securing hemostasis. The integrity of the cut surface can be tested by gentle injection of preservative solution into the hepatic artery, portal vein and bile duct. After implantation of the graft, argon beam coagulation and fibrin sealant are helpful.

In right/left lobe splits, preliminary back-table cholangiography is valuable. The vessels and bile ducts are divided from within the parenchyma, leaving the division of porta hepatis structures until later. In contrast, the extrahepatic vessels are divided early in the preparation of the left lateral segment graft (usually the portal vein trunk remains with the right lobe but the common hepatic artery may be allocated to either graft depending on recipient vessels); the left hepatic duct is divided well away from the porta hepatis adjacent to the cut surface of the graft. After preparation of the left lateral segment graft, there is some controversy as to whether segment 4 should be preserved with the right lobe or removed.[111] This is partly because the arterial supply to segment 4 is often divided when dissecting free the left lateral segment graft.

CONCLUSIONS

Liver resection is an uncommon procedure in children but potentially hazardous. The risks of surgery can be minimized by a thorough understanding of surgical anatomy, meticulous surgical technique, and familiarity with all aspects of hepatobiliary surgery. Occasionally, the surgeon must be prepared to be innovative. Many hepatic resections are relatively straightforward but lesions which are complex because of their size or location are best managed in centers with hepatobiliary surgical expertise.

REFERENCES

1. Bismuth H, Houssin D, Dastaing D. Major and minor segmentectomies "reglees" in liver surgery. World J Surg 1982;6:10-24.
2. Mann JR, Kasthuri N, Raafat F, et al. Malignant hepatic tumours in children: incidence, clinical features and aetiology. Paediatr Perinat Epidemiol 1990;4:276-89.
3. Miller RW, Young JL, Novakovic B. Childhood cancer. Cancer 1994;75:395-405.
4. MacKinlay GA, Pritchard J. A common language for childhood liver tumors. Pediatr Surg Int 1992;7:325-26.
5. Stringer MD. Liver tumors. Seminars in Pediatric Surgery 2000;9:196-208.
6. Ortega JA, Krailo MD, Haas JE, et al. Effective treatment of unresectable or metastatic hepatoblastoma with cisplatin and continuous infusion doxorubicin chemotherapy: a report from the Childrens Cancer Study Group. J Clin Oncol 1991;9:2167-76.
7. Douglass EC, Reynolds M, Finegold M, et al. Cisplatin, vincristine, and fluorouracil therapy for hepatoblastoma: a Pediatric Oncology Group study. J Clin Oncol 1993;11:96-99.
8. Pritchard J, Brown J, Shafford E, et al. Cisplatin, doxorubicin, and delayed surgery for childhood hepatoblastoma: a successful approach - results of the first prospective study of the International Society of Pediatric Oncology. J Clin Oncol 2000;18:3819-28.
9. Filler RM, Ehrlich PF, Greenberg ML, et al. Preoperative chemotherapy in hepatoblastoma. Surgery 1991;110:591-97.
10. Reynolds M. Conversion of unresectable to resectable hepatoblastoma and long-term follow-up study. World J Surg 1995;19:814-16.
11. Stringer MD, Hennayake S, Howard ER, et al. Improved outcome for children with hepatoblastoma. Br J Surg 1995;82:386-91.
12. Fuchs J, Bode U, von Schweinitz D, et al. Analysis of treatment efficiency of carboplatin and etoposide in combination with radical surgery in advanced and recurrent childhood hepatoblastoma: a report of the German Cooperative Pediatric Liver Tumor Study HB 89 and HB 94. Klin Padiatr 1999;211:305-09.
13. Seo T, Ando H, Watanabe Y, et al. Treatment of hepatoblastoma: less extensive hepatectomy after effective preoperative chemotherapy with cisplatin and Adriamycin. Surgery 1998;123:407-14.
14. Koneru B, Flye MW, Busuttil R, et al. Liver transplantation for hepatoblastoma. The American experience. Ann Surg 1991;213:118-21.
15. Perilongo G, Shafford EA. Liver tumours. Eur J Cancer 1999;35:953-59.
16. Reyes JD, Carr B, Dvorchik I, et al. Liver transplantation and chemotherapy for hepatoblastoma and hepatocellular cancer in childhood and adolescence. J Pediatr 2000;136:795-804.
17. von Schweinitz D, Byrd DJ, Hecker H, et al. Efficiency and toxicity of ifosfamide, cisplatin and doxorubicin in the treatment of childhood hepatoblastoma. Study Committee of the Cooperative Paediatric Liver Tumour Study HB89 of the German Society for Paediatric Oncology and Haematology. Eur J Cancer 1997;33:1243-49.
18. Brown J, Perilongo G, Shafford E, et al. Pretreatment prognostic factors for children with hepatoblastoma - results from the International Society of Paediatric Oncology (SIOP) study SIOPEL 1. Eur J Cancer 2000;36:1418-25.
19. Moore SW, Hesseling PB, Wessels G, Schneider JW. Hepatocellular carcinoma in children. Pediatr Surg Int 1997;12:266-70.
20. Chen WJ, Lee JC, Hung WT. Primary malignant tumor of liver in infants and children in Taiwan. J Pediatr Surg 1988;23:457-61.
21. Chang MH, Chen CJ, Lai MS, et al. Universal hepatitis B vaccination in Taiwan and the incidence of hepatocellular carcinoma in children. Taiwan Childhood Hepatoma Study Group. N Engl J Med 1997;336:1855-59.
22. Chen JC, Chen CC, Chen WJ, et al. Hepatocellular carcinoma in children: clinical review and comparison with adult cases. J Pediatr Surg 1998;33:1350-54.
23. Plaschkes J, Perilongo G, Shafford E, et al. Preoperative chemotherapy—Cisplatin (PLA) and Doxorubicin (DO) PLADO for the treatment of hepatoblastoma (HB) and hepatocellular carcinoma (HCC)—results after 2 years follow-up. Med Pediatr Oncol 1996;27:256 (abstract O-182).
24. von Schweinitz D. Treatment of liver tumors in children. In Malignant Liver Tumors. Current and emerging therapies. Ed Clavien PA, Blackwell Science, Inc., Massachusetts, 1999;323-40.
25. Babin-Boilletot A, Flamant F, Terrier-Lacombe MJ, et al. Primitive malignant nonepithelial hepatic tumors in children. Med Pediatr Oncol 1993;21:634-39.
26. Spunt SL, Lobe TE, Pappo AS, et al. Aggressive surgery is unwarranted for biliary tract rhabdomyosarcoma. J Pediatr Surg 2000;35:309-16.
27. DeMaioribus CA, Lally KP, Sim K, Isaacs H, Mahour GH. Mesenchymal hamartoma of the liver. A 35 year review. Arch Surg 1990;125:598-600.
28. Murray JD, Ricketts RR. Mesenchymal hamartoma of the liver. Am Surg 1998;64:1097-103.
29. Ramanujam TM, Ramesh JC, Goh DW, et al. Malignant transformation of mesenchymal hamartoma of the liver: case report and review of the literature. J Pediatr Surg 1999;34:1684-86.
30. Stocker JT, Ishak KG. Focal nodular hyperplasia of the liver: a study of 21 pediatric cases. Cancer 1981;48:336-45.
31. Lack EE, Ornvold K. Focal nodular hyperplasia and hepatic adenoma: a review of eight cases in the pediatric age group. J Surg Oncol 1986;33:129-33.

32. Davenport M, Hansen L, Heaton ND, Howard ER. Hemangioendothelioma of the liver in infants. J Pediatr Surg 1995;30:44-48.
33. Daller JA, Bueno J, Gutierrez J, et al. Hepatic hemangioendothelioma: clinical experience and management strategy. J Pediatr Surg 1999;34:98-106.
34. Rokitansky AM, Jakl RJ, Gopfrich H, et al. Special compression sutures: a new surgical technique to achieve a quick decrease in shunt volume caused by diffuse hemangiomatosis of the liver. Pediatr Surg Int 1998;14:119-21.
35. Resnick MB, Kozakewich HP, Perez-Atayde AR. Hepatic adenoma in the pediatric age group. Clinicopathological observations and assessment of cell proliferative activity. Am J Surg Pathol 1995;19:1181-90.
36. Kaneko K, Ando H, Watanabe Y, et al. Aggressive preoperative management and extended surgery for inflammatory pseudotumor involving the hepatic hilum in a child. Surgery 2001;129:757-60.
37. Feliciano DV, Pachter HL. Hepatic trauma revisited. Curr Probl Surg 1989;26:453-524.
38. Strasberg SM. Terminology of liver anatomy and liver resections: coming to grips with hepatic babel. J Am Coll Surg 1997;184:413-34.
39. Nakamura S, Tsuzuki T. Surgical anatomy of the hepatic veins and the inferior vena cava. Surgery 1981;152:43-50.
40. Couinaud C. Controlled hepatectomies and exposure of the intrahepatic bile ducts. Anatomical and technical study. C. Couinaud, Paris 1981.
41. Blumgart LH, Hann LE. Surgical and radiologic anatomy of the liver and biliary tract. In Surgery of the Liver and Biliary Tract. (3rd edn). Eds LH Blumgart and Y Fong. WB Saunders Co Ltd., London 2000;3-33.
42. Blumgart LH. Liver resection for benign disease and for liver and biliary tumors. In Surgery of the Liver and Biliary Tract. (3rd edn). Eds LH Blumgart and Y Fong. WB Saunders Co Ltd, London 2000;1639-713.
43. Hiatt JR, Gabbay J, Busuttil RW. Surgical anatomy of the hepatic arteries in 1000 cases. Ann Surg 1994;220:50-52.
44. Gruttadauria S, Foglieni CS, Doria C, et al. The hepatic artery in liver transplantation and surgery: vascular anomalies in 701 cases. Clin Transplant 2001;15:359-63.
45. Northover JMA, Terblanche J. A new look at the arterial supply of the bile duct in man and its surgical implications. Br J Surg 1979;66:379-84.
46. Tonkin ILD, Wrenn EL, Hollabaugh RS. The continued value of angiography in planning surgical resection of benign and malignant hepatic tumors in children. Pediatr Radiol 1988;18:35-44.
47. Laub G. Principles of contrast-enhanced MR angiography. Basic and clinical applications. Magn Reson Imaging Clin N Am 1999;7:783-95.
48. Mukai J, Stack CM, Turner DA, et al. Imaging of surgically relevant hepatic vascular and segmental anatomy. Part 1. Normal anatomy. AJR 1987;149:287-92.
49. Castaing D, Emond J, Bismuth H, Kunstlinger F. Utility of operative ultrasound in the surgical management of liver tumours. Ann Surg 1986;204:600-05.
50. Torzilli G, Makuuchi M, Midorikawa Y, et al. Liver resection without total vascular exclusion: hazardous or beneficial? An analysis of our experience. Ann Surg 2001;233:167-75.
51. Bismuth H, Castaing D, Garden OJ. The use of operative ultrasound in surgery of primary liver tumours. World J Surg 1987;11:610-14.
52. Man K, Fan ST, Ng IOL, et al. Prospective evaluation of Pringle maneuver in hepatectomy for liver tumors by a randomized study. Ann Surg 1997;226:704-13.
53. Belghiti J, Noun R, Malafosse R, et al. Continuous versus intermittent portal triad clamping for liver resection. A controlled study. Ann Surg 1999;229:369-75.
54. Clavien PA, Yadav S, Sindram D, Bentley RC. Protective effects of ischemic preconditioning for liver resection performed under inflow occlusion in humans. Ann Surg 2000;232:155-62.
55. Price JB, Schullinger JN, Santulli TV. Major hepatic resections for neoplasia in children. Arch Surg 1982;117:1139-41.
56. Schmittenbecher PP. The neodymium YAG laser in surgery of parenchymatous organs in childhood. Prog Pediatr Surg 1990;25:23-31.
57. Filler RM. Liver resections. In Pediatric Surgery, Eds Spitz L and Coran AG. Chapman and Hall Medical, London, 1995;579-89.
58. Glick RD, Nadler EP, Blumgart LH, LaQuaglia MP. Extended left hepatectomy (left hepatic trisegmentectomy) in childhood. J Pediatr Surg 2000;35:303-08.
59. Fasulo F, Giori A, Fissi S, et al. Cavitron ultrasonic surgical aspirator (CUSA) in liver resection. Int Surg 1992;77:64-66.
60. Hodgson WJB, Morgan J, Byrne D, et al. Hepatic resections for primary and metastatic tumors using the ultrasonic surgical dissector. Am J Surg 1992;163:246-50.
61. Rees M, Plant G, Wells J, Bygrave S. One hundred and fifty hepatic resections: evolution of technique towards bloodless surgery. Br J Surg 1996;83:1526-29.
62. Huguet CL, Nordlinger B, Bloch P, et al. Tolerance of the human liver to prolonged normothermic ischaemia. Arch Surg 1978;113:1448-51.
63. Bismuth H, Castaing D, Garden OJ. Major hepatic resection under total vascular exclusion. Ann Surg 1989;210:13-19.
64. Bismuth H, Morino M, Castaing D, et al. Emergency orthotopic liver transplantation in two patients using one donor liver. Br J Surg 1989;76:722-24.
65. Lodge JPA, Ammori BJ, Prasad KR, Bellamy MC. Ex vivo and in situ resection of inferior vena cava with hepatectomy for colorectal metastases. Ann Surg 2000;231:471-79.
66. Ein SH, Shandling B, Williams WG, et al. Major hepatic tumor resection using profound hypothermia and circulation arrest. J Pediatr Surg 1981;16:339-42.

67. Superina RA, Bambini D, Filler RM, Almond PS, Geissler G. A new technique for resecting 'unresectable' liver tumors. J Pediatr Surg 2000;35:1294-99.
68. Starzl TE, Putnam CW, Groth CG, et al. Alopecia, ascites, and incomplete regeneration after 85 to 90 per cent liver resection. Am J Surg 1975;129:587-90.
69. Starzl TE, Iwatsuki S, Shaw BW, et al. Left hepatic trisegmentectomy. Surg Gynecol Obstet 1982;155:21-27.
70. Blumgart LH, Baer HU, Czerniak A, et al. Extended left hepatectomy: technical aspects of an evolving procedure. Br J Surg 1993;80:903-06.
71. Takayama T, Makuuchi M, Kosuge T, et al. A hepato-blastoma originating in the caudate lobe radically resected with the inferior vena cava. Surgery 1991;109:208-13.
72. Takayama T, Makuuchi M, Takayasu K, et al. Resection after intra-arterial chemotherapy of a hepatoblastoma originating in the caudate lobe. Surgery 1990;107:231-35.
73. Scheele J. Anatomical and atypical liver resections. Chirurg 2001;72:113-24.
74. Ninane J, Perilongo G, Stalens JP, et al. Effectiveness and toxicity of cisplatin and doxorubicin (PLADO) in childhood hepatoblastoma and hepatocellular carcinoma: a SIOP pilot study. Med Pediatr Oncol 1991;19:199-203.
75. Shuto T, Kinoshita H, Yamada C, et al. Bilateral lobectomy excluding the caudate lobe for giant mesenchymal hamartoma of the liver. Surgery 1993;113:215-22.
76. Miller CM, Schwartz ME, Nishizaki T. Combined hepatic and vena caval resection with autogenous caval graft replacement. Arch Surg 1991;126:106-08.
77. Millar AJW, Hartley P, Khan D, Spearman W, Andronikou S, Rode H. Extended hepatic resection with trans-plantation back-up for an "unresectable" tumour. Ped Surg Int 2001; 17:378-81.
78. Tagge EP, Tagge DU, Reyes J, et al. Resection, including transplantation, for hepatoblastoma and hepatocellular carcinoma: impact on survival. J Pediatr Surg 1992;27:292-97.
79. Bilik R, Superina R. Transplantation for unresectable liver tumors in children. Transplant Proc 1997;29:2834-35.
80. Al-Qabandi W, Jenkinson HC, Buckels JA, et al. Orthotopic liver transplantation for unresectable hepatoblastoma: a single center's experience. J Pediatr Surg 1999;34:1261-64.
81. Broughan TA, Esquivel CO, Vogt DP, et al. Pretransplant chemotherapy in pediatric hepatocellular carcinoma. J Pediatr Surg 1994;29:1319-22.
82. Otte JB, Aronson D, Vraux H, et al. Preoperative chemotherapy, major liver resection, and transplantation for primary malignancies in children. Transplant Proc 1996;28:2393-94.
83. Superina R, Bilik R. Results of liver transplantation in children with unresectable liver tumors. J Pediatr Surg 1996;31:835-39.
84. Adam R, Laurent A, Azoulay D, et al. Two-stage hepatectomy: a planned strategy to treat irresectable liver tumors. Ann Surg 2000;232:777-85.
85. Pichlmayr R, Grosse H, Hauss J, et al. Technique and preliminary results of extracorporeal liver surgery (bench procedure) and of surgery on the in situ perfused liver. Br J Surg 1990;77:21-26.
86. Stocker JT. An approach to handling pediatric liver tumors. Am J Clin Pathol 1998;109 (Suppl 1):S67-S72.
87. Stone HH. Major hepatic resections in children. J Pediatr Surg 1975;10:127-34.
88. Shamberger RC, Leichtner AM, Jonas MM, LaQuaglia MP. Long-term hepatic regeneration and function in infants and children following liver resection. J Am Coll Surg 1996;182:515-19.
89. Wheatley JM, Rosenfield NS, Berger L, LaQuaglia MP. Liver regeneration in children after major hepatectomy for malignancy—evaluation using a computer-aided technique of volume measurement. J Surg Res 1996;61:183-89.
90. Engum SA, Sidner RA, Miller GA, Galliani C, Grosfeld JL. Early use of cisplatin is safe after partial hepatectomy. J Pediatr Surg 1993;28:411-19.
91. Mahour GH, Wogu GU, Siegel SE, et al. Improved survival in infants and children with primary malignant liver tumors. Am J Surg 1983;146:236-40.
92. Dorman F, Sumner E, Spitz L. Fatal intraoperative tumor embolism in a child with hepatoblastoma. Anesthesiology 1985;63:692-93.
93. Gauthier F, Valayer J, Thai BL, et al. Hepatoblastoma and hepatocarcinoma in children: analysis of a series of 29 cases. J Pediatr Surg 1986;21:424-29.
94. Brown TCK, Davidson PD, Auldist AW. Anaesthetic considerations in liver tumor resection in children. Pediatr Surg Int 1988;4:11-15.
95. Lobe TE, Karkera MS, Custer MD, et al. Fatal refractory hyperkalaemia due to tumor lysis during primary resection for hepatoblastoma. J Pediatr Surg 1990;25:249-50.
96. Kiuchi T, Kasahara M, Uryuhara K, et al. Impact of graft size mismatching on graft prognosis in liver transplantation from living donors. Transplantation 1999;67:321-27.
97. Sindhi R, Rosendale J, Mundy D, et al. Impact of segmental grafts on pediatric liver transplantation—a review of the United Network for Organ Sharing Scientific Registry data (1990-1996). J Pediatr Surg 1999;34:107-10.
98. European Liver Transplant Registry web site http://www.eltr.org.
99. Bismuth H, Houssin D. Reduced-sized orthotopic liver graft in hepatic transplantation in children. Surgery 1984;95:367-70.
100. Strong R, Ong TH, Pillay P, Wall D, Balderson G, Lynch S. A new method of segmental orthotopic liver trans-plantation in children. Surgery 1988;104:104-07.

101. Ringe B, Pichlmayr R, Burdelski M. A new technique of hepatic vein reconstruction in partial liver transplantation. Transpl International 1988;1:30-35.
102. Pichlmayr R, Ringe B, Gubernatis G, Hauss J, Bunzendahl H. Transplantation of a donor liver to 2 recipients (splitting transplantation)—a new method in the further development of segmental liver transplantation. Langenbecks Arch Chir 1988;373:127-30.
103. Rogiers X, Malago M, Gawad K, et al. In situ splitting of cadaveric livers. The ultimate expansion of a limited donor pool. Ann Surg 1996;224:331-41.
104. Pomfret EA, Pomposelli JJ, Jenkins RL. Live donor liver transplantation. J Hepatol 2001;34:613-24.
105. Strong RW, Lynch SV, Ong TH, et al. Successful liver transplantation from a living donor to her son. N Engl J Med 1990;322:1505-07.
106. Broelsch CE, Whitington PF, Emond JC, et al. Liver transplantation in children from living related donors. Surgical techniques and results. Ann Surg 1991;214:428-37.
107. Srinivasan P, Vilca-Melendez H, Muiesan P, et al. Liver transplantation with monosegments. Surgery 1999;126:10-12.
108. DeSantibanes E, McCormack L, Mattera J, et al. Partial left lateral segment transplant from a living donor. Liver Transplantation 2000;6:108-12.
109. Rat P, Paris P, Friedman S, Favre JP. Split-liver orthotopic liver transplantation: How to divide the portal pedicle. Surgery 1992;112:522-26.
110. Rela M, McCall JL, Karani J, Heaton ND. Accessory right hepatic artery arising from the left. Transplantation 1998;66:792-814.
111. Rela M, Vougas V, Muiesan P, et al. Split liver trans-plantation. King's College Hospital Experience. Ann Surg 1998;227:282-88.
112. Shaw BW Jr, Wood RP, Stratta RJ, et al. Management of arterial anomalies encountered in split-liver trans-plantation. Transpl Proc 1990;22:420-22.

CHAPTER 87

Transplant Immunogenetics

Narinder K Mehra, Arundhati Panigrahi

The modern era of '*Omics*' has heralded a new beginning in our understanding of the molecular aspects of Clinical Immunology with considerable impact on developing new perspectives in the field of organ transplantation. While proteomics and functional genomics have significantly enhanced our understanding of how genes, transcripts and proteins interact, the science of '*immunomics*' has helped in identifying a variety of genes, involved in immune regulation. Of the 20-25,000 genes estimated to comprise the human genome, > 4000 are broadly associated with the immune system. Immune tolerance holds the key to controlling unwanted immunological attacks on self and transplanted tissues/organs. The major determinant of acceptance or rejection of a technically perfect graft is the magnitude of immunologically mediated response against graft, based on the ability to differentiate 'self from nonself'. It has long been recognized that the specificity of antigens involved in graft rejection is under genetic control. Thus while grafts can be freely exchanged among genetically identical individuals, the same is not true in the highly outbreed human species.

The genetic difference between recipient and the donor is predominantly determined by a set of immune response genes clustered together as human leukocyte antigen (HLA) system, which is an analogue of the major histocompatibility complex (MHC) that exists in almost all species. These antigens play an important role in immune discrimination between self and non-self (foreign) and effectively promote detection and elimination of foreign macromolecules. Accordingly, immune mechanisms are associated with the recognition of alloantigens in allogeneic transplantation.[1,2] This article attempts to provide a simplified review of basic features of the HLA system and its role in long and short-term survival of a renal allograft. Also discussed are other immunological factors that influence the graft outcome. Critical among these are the influence of *de novo* development of anti donor and lymphocytotoxic antibodies on the overall graft survival and protocols for their removal.

MAJOR HISTOCOMPATIBILITY COMPLEX (MHC)

Developments in the field of histocompatibility have largely been related to the progress in technology, computer aided programs of data storage and analysis. In the MHC region, a total of 224 genes have been identified, of which 128 are assumed to be functional genes and 96 are pseudogenes. More than 40% of the genes have one or more assigned immune functions.[3] Four inherent features of the MHC, namely i) extraordinary polymorphism, ii) tight linkage among its various loci, iii) nonrandom association of alleles and iv) its multi-peptide binding ability make the system of particular interest in biology and medicine. The MHC molecules are the peptide-display molecules of the immune system that bind peptide fragments derived from protein antigens (e.g. viruses, bacterial peptides and mismatched transplant antigens) and display them on the surface of APCs, evoking effector responses upon recognition by the T-cell receptor (TCR). As the number of peptides that can be generated is very large, there is a biological need for an extensive MHC gene pool. Apart from being an invaluable tool in organ and bonemarrow transplantation, MHC is specifically relevant with respect to its causative role as an important immunogenetic marker of 'risk prediction' for several diseases. In recent years, there has been an upsurge of information on MHC ligands, peptide motifs and structural requirements of their optimal binding. Knowledge on these lines has been utilized effectively for designing immune intervention therapies in autoimmune and infectious diseases.[4,5]

In the area of transplantation, experience of several centers suggests that a critical factor that determines the success of a renal allograft is through better understanding of the immunobiology of the human MHC and more precise and comprehensive immunogenetic matching between the donor and recipient. This is based on the notion that 'better' the matching, better the transplant outcome". In addition to this, other immunological factors also influence graft survival to a large extent. These include the presence of antibodies and sensitization status of the recipient, HLA versus non-HLA humoral immunity, involvement of the MHC class I A (MICA) antigen system and genetic constitution of the host.[6-9] Although acute rejection episodes are important risk factors for the success of a renal allograft, the major challenge today remains in the area of chronic rejection.

GENETICS OF HLA

The human MHC gene cluster (HLA molecule) spans a region of approximately 4000 kb (4×10^6 nucleotides) on chromosome 6 (position 6p21.1 to 21.3) and contains several genes, only some of which are related to histocompatibility. These genes are grouped into three distinct sets of molecules, each comprising of a cluster of immune response (Ir) genes (Fig. 87.1). The most centromeric segment is the class II region that spans around 1100 kb, and contains the HLA-DP, DQ and DR loci: The class I region, on the other hand lies at the telomeric end and contains the classical HLA-A,B,C and related loci spread over a region of approximately 2 MB. Both class I and II gene products show important differences in structure, function and tissue distribution. They represent the major transplantation antigen system. Matching donors and recipients for class I and class II antigens during organ and bone marrow transplantation is therefore critical to the survival of a graft.[10,11] In contrast, the central 'non-HLA' or class III region contains genes whose products are involved in the complement cascade and various non-immunological functions.

HLA Class I Genes

HLA class I molecules are expressed on all nucleated cells. Upto 35 genes have been defined in this region

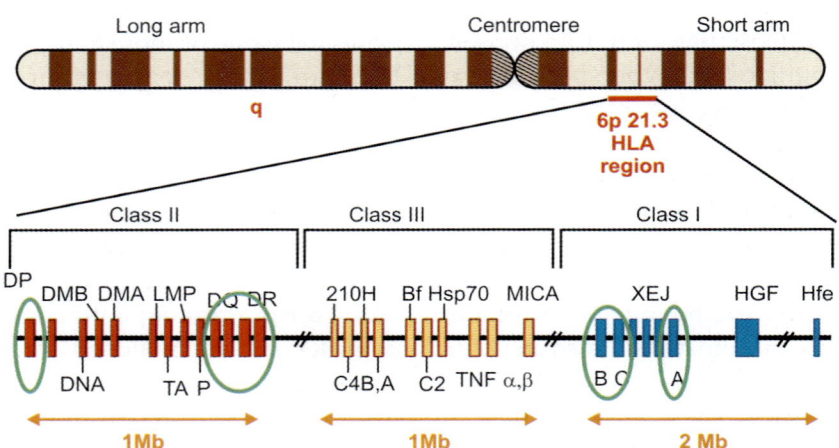

Fig. 87.1: Human major histocompatibility complex (MHC) with chromosomal location and gene map showing multiple genes on the short-arm of chromosome 6 (6p21.3). The two way array shows the genetic distance covered by the respective regions on the chromosome. The circled loci are highly polymorphic. Note that MICA (MHC class I related chain A) is situated in close proximity to the HLA-B locus

so far although HLA –A, –B and –C are most important since their products have been well defined as 'classical transplantation antigens'. Several other human class I genes with less defined gene products have been identified and include HLA –E, –F, –G, –H and –J. All these genes are polymorphic. Using tools of molecular biology and DNA typing methods, 238 alleles have been identified in locus A, 451 in locus B, and 238 in locus Cw. Conventional serology, on the other hand, can define much less number of alleles in each of these loci (23 in locus A, 47 in B, and 8 in C locus).

Biochemically, HLA class I molecules are heterodimeric glycoproteins consisting of an MHC-encoded alpha or heavy chain of about 44,000 daltons molecular weight and non MHC encoded light chain (beta-2 microglobulin) of 12,000 dalton molecular weight. The alpha chain is about 350 amino acid residues long and can be divided into three functional regions: external, transmembrane and intracytoplasmic (Fig. 87.2). The extracellular portion of the heavy chain is folded into three globular domains, α_1, α_2 and α_3, each of which contains stretches of about 90 amino acids long, and encoded on separate exons. The transmembrane region spans the lipid bilayer of the plasma membrane while the cytoplasmic region has elements of the cytoskeleton.

The β_2 microglobulin (β_2m) is a soluble protein encoded by a gene located on chromosome 15 in man and associates noncovalently with the heavy alpha chain. Cells lacking β_2m are deficient in the expression of MHC class I molecules. The X-ray crystallography of class I molecule has provided an understanding of the three-dimensional structure of the MHC:[12,13]

a. The membrane proximal structures (α_3 and β_2m) are essentially conserved and folded to form immunoglobulin (Ig) like domains. The α_3 and β_2m are responsible for imparting general shape to the class I molecule by providing a platform to the top lying polymorphic domains.

b. The region distal from the membrane is formed by α_1 and α_2 domains which take part in antigen binding. Structurally, therefore, the peptide-binding groove of the MHC class I molecule is made up of only one polypeptide chain, while two chains contribute to the peptide-binding groove of the MHC class II molecule. The two alpha helixes form the sides of a cleft whose floor is formed by a plane of eight anti parallel beta pleated sheets. The dimensions of this cleft (25Å×10Å×11Å) are sufficiently large as to accommodate foreign peptides which are about 9 amino acids long.

c. Most of the polymorphic residues of the MHC class I molecules are clustered in the cleft and those critical for recognition of class I molecules by T lymphocytes are located around it, accounting for the differential ability of different allelic forms of class I molecules to bind to a variety of peptides.

d. Functionally, MHC class I molecules bind to CD8 co-receptor molecules on the T-cells and therefore present antigen to CD8 T-cells. MHC class II molecules bind to CD4 co-receptors molecules on T-cells and hence they present antigen to CD4 helper T-cells.

HLA Class II Genes

The HLA-class II region of the human MHC extends over 1000-1200 kb with at least six subregions termed DR, DQ, DO, DN, DM and DP (Fig. 87.1). They are expressed as heterodimers on the cell surface and are composed of two genes that traverse the plasma membrane: an α (alpha) gene and a β (beta) gene (Fig. 87.2). The alpha genes encode glycoproteins of 34000 dalton molecular weight which are much less polymorphic compared to beta genes (mol. wt. 29000 daltons) which are highly polymorphic. The tissue distribution of class II molecules is relatively restricted. They are expressed on specific cells of the immune system involved in antigen presentation (APCs). These include B lymphocytes, macrophages, monocytes, epithelial cells, dendritic cells, Langerhan's cells and Kuppfer cells. In addition, some other cell types such as keratinocytes, thyrocytes and human T lymphocytes are known to express class II molecules under certain situations, e.g. following viral infection and induction due to gamma interferon-like factors.

X-ray crystallographic studies have revealed overall similarity in the structure of class II HLA molecules with that of class I molecules.[14] The alpha and beta chains consist of two extracellular domains of 90 amino acids each. The α_2, β_2 domains are close to the plasma membrane, whereas the α_1, β_1 domains are on the top of the molecule. Long peptides of at least

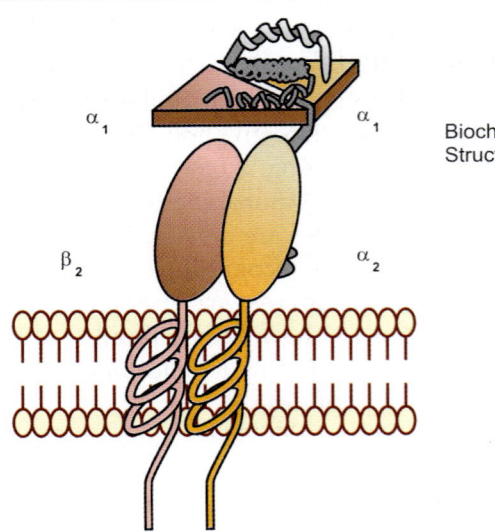 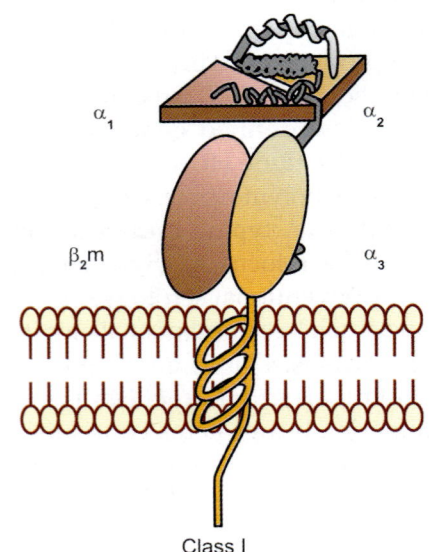

Fig. 87.2: Schematic view of HLA class II and class I molecular structures showing the peptide binding cleft formed between α_1 and β_1 domains in case of class II and α_1 and α_2 domains in case of class I molecules. The membrane proximal domains (α_2, β_2 of class II and $\beta_2 m$ and α_3 of class I) are non-polymorphic

15 residues are seen to be bound on the class II molecule.

Currently, 438 DRB1, 71 DQB1 and 59 DPB1 alleles can be recognized using DNA typing methods of PCR and oligonucleotide probes. Of course, the number of alleles defined by serology remains very small (14 DR, 9 DQ and 6 DP).

Non-MHC Genes in Human Class II Region

In addition to the classical HLA class II genes, two groups of non-HLA genes have recently been identified in the MHC class II regions. There are two genes in the first group named as TAP-1 and TAP-2 genes for 'transporter associated with antigen processing'. These belong to a large family of transporters called ABC (ATP-binding cassette) transporters. The second group is proteasome-related low-molecular-mass polypeptide (LMP) complex that includes LMP2 and LMP7 genes. Both the LMP as well as TAP genes are polymorphic.

Class III Genes (Central Genes)

At least 39 genes have now been located in a 1000 kb stretch of DNA within the class III region interposed between class I and class II regions. This includes the complement genes C2, C4 and Bf (factor β), the TNF-α and TNF-β genes and the Hsp 70 (heat shock protein) genes. In addition, genes with no obvious association with the immune system have also been identified in this region. This includes G7α (valyl-tRNA synthetase) and CYP21B (steroid 21-hydroxylase).

HLA Class I and Class II Molecules Differ in Antigen Presentation

The determination of the crystal structure of the human MHC class I and class II molecules and the identification of the putative peptide binding cleft established that MHC molecules are the principal antigen binding and presenting molecules to the T-cells. Thus peptide antigens alter the HLA molecule by occupying the cleft to be scrutinized by the T-cell. This concept was first put forward by Zinkernagel and Doherty whose studies of anti-viral T-cell recognition led to their award of the Nobel Prize for Medicine in 1996.[15]

The fundamental difference in the above process is that whereas class I MHC molecules bind 'endogenous' peptides and eliminate them through the process of cytotoxic T-cell killing (inside out mechanisms), the class II molecules, on the other hand, bind peptides derived from 'external' sources (exogenous) and present them to $CD4^+$ helper T-cells (outside in mechanism). The processing pathway in both situations utilizes highly specialized cell machinery that works most effectively. The endogenous proteins in the cytoplasm of the cells are digested into 9-10 amino acid peptides by the LMP complex, a distinct subset of the cellular pool of proteasome. Peptides in the cytoplasm may gain access to the TAP transporter on the membrane of the endoplasmic reticulum (ER) via a specific transporter. Peptides transported into the ER lumen bind to class I molecules, inducing a conformational change that may facilitate their export to the cell surface. The $CD8^+$ cytotoxic T lymphocytes see this MHC-peptide complex through the T-cell receptor and other co-receptors, subsequently causing killing of the targe T-cell.

In the class II pathway, antigens taken from outside the cell by endocytosis are digested by the proteolytic enzymes in the endosomal compartment into small peptide fragments. The MHC class II molecule with its α and β chains assembles in the ER with the invariant chain to form a stable trimolecular complex which inhibits the binding of endogenous or self-peptides in the ER. The trimolecular complex is efficiently transported out of the ER and is targeted to a post-Golgi compartment in the peripheral cytoplasm. The invariant chain is subsequently cleaved in endosomes, opening up the cleft for peptide occupancy.

The development of accurate and reproducible high-resolution DNA-based HLA typing methods have significantly improved our capabilities to define HLA alleles at a single nucleotide difference. Further advanced technologies based on sequencing, mass spectroscopy and DNA chips have now opened up a whole new dimension of studying SNPs, i.e. polymorphism at a single nucleotide level. Using these procedures, an appreciable number of 'novel alleles' and unique HLA haplotypes have been discovered in the Indian population.[16,17]

LEVEL OF HLA MATCHING IN TRANSPLANTATION

Owing to its inherent extreme polymorphic diversity, the MHC has proven to be a major barrier in selection of HLA matched donors for patients requiring organ transplantation. Theoretically, the likelihood of finding a match among any two unrelated individuals sharing the same genotype is less than 1 in 10 billion. Although the HLA system comprises multiple Class I and class II genes, most matching strategies for renal transplantation consider only HLA-A, HLA-B and HLA-DR loci. Because of the co-dominant expression of HLA genes, the degree of compatibility ranges from 0 to 6 matches (two for each locus).

The degree of HLA matching required for successful organ grafting depends upon the donor category and nature of the graft. In renal and other solid organ transplantation, a large body of data indicates a direct relationship between graft survival and the level of matching.[18-20] As outlined in Table 87.1, four types of donors are generally available for renal transplantation. Family donors include parents, siblings and offspring and their match status is determined by the parental haplotype inheritance and whether they share one, both or no HLA haplotypes.

An haplotype refers to a set of HLA alleles on one chromosome inherited together from one parent and defined through family studies (Fig. 87.3). Accordingly biological parents and offspring always share atleast one haplotype and such donors are referred to as 'haploidentical. On the other hand, as per the Mandelian segregation analysis, atleast 25% of the siblings have an opportunity to share both haplotypes with each other and kidneys exchanged amongst them are called '*HLA-identical*' sibling transplants. In bone marrow or hematopoitic stem cell transplantation (HSCT), the level of HLA matching is much more critical than solid organ transplants because of the risk of graft versus host diseases (GVHD) where T-cells in the stem cell graft react against allogeneic host HLA molecules expressed in all tissues. Thus while HSCT is limited to *HLA-identical* sibling donors, renal transplants with live related donors involves mostly haploidentical parental/sibling or offspring donors and very few are HLA-Id donors.

Most grafts from unrelated donors that include cadaver (or deceased), spousal or other unrelated donors are mismatched at one or more HLA loci. Thus it is not unusual to see patients transplanted with a graft bearing a 6/6 (HLA-A, B and DR loci) mismatch, even though, statistically, graft survival in these patients is significantly reduced compared with the survival in better matched (0/6 mismatch, or 1, 2/6 mismatch or family donors) patients.

Table 87.1: Donor categories for renal transplantation and probability of HLA match

Donor category	Match probability	Match designation
A. Family donors		
Parents	50% match or one haplotype match	Haploidentical
Siblings	25% chance of full match	HLA identical
	50% chance of one haplotype match	Haploidentical
	25% chance of no haplotype match	HLA -unidentical
Offsprings	50% match or one haplotype match	Haploidentical
B. Cadaver donor	Generally poor	Expressed as mismatch (mm) for the number of HLA antigens shared in HLA– A, B, and DR loci : for example 'full house' match (0/6 mm) or grades of 1 to 6 antigen mm
C. Spousal donor	Generally poor	
D. Unrelated donor	Generally poor	

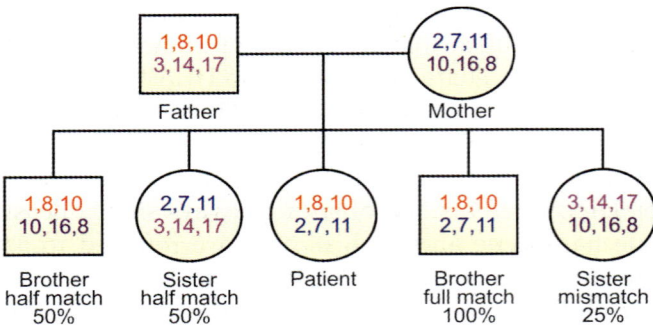

Fig. 87.3: Segregation of HLA haplotypes in a family. The sibs inherit one haplotype from each parent and accordingly four different haplotypic combinations are possible. In this case, the patient is HLA-identical with his younger brother, HLA-unidentical with his younger sister and shares only one haplotype (haploidentical) with his elder brother and sister

Fig. 87.4 summarizes the results of long-term renal graft survival compiled by the University of California los Angeles (UCLA) registry involving a large number of transplants.[20] The ten year graft survival of 70% seen in the HLA identical sibling grafts is significantly reduced to 50% for the HLA haploidentical parental donor grafts and < 40% for those involving poorly matched cadaver donors. Further, the data is expressed as 'half-life' that indicates the period at which atleast half the grafts are still functioning. While it is 25 years for well matched HLA-Id sibling grafts, it is 11.5 years for parental donors and only 7.8 years for cadaver donor grafts which are generally mismatched. Again, there is no significant difference in the half life of the latter grafts in the period between 1996-2006 despite introduction of highly effective immunosuppressive agents including Tacrolimus and Sirolimus.

It may be mentioned here that optimal HLA matching of renal grafts using cadaveric donors is greatly improved by organ sharing schemes such as within Europe, UK, North America, Japan and other developed countries. Systematic organ sharing involving HLA matching practiced by the Large Organ Transplant Organizations such as Eurotransplant Foundation (Netherlands), United Network of Organ Sharing (UNOS) USA, ScandiaTransplant, etc. have proven extremely useful in making available 6/6 or 5/6 matched donors for renal transplantation. HLA matching is logisticaly less achievable for heart/lung and liver transplantation which almost invariably results in some mismatching between the host and graft.

Since the passage of the Transplantation Act of Human organs by the Indian Parliament in 1994 (TAHO 1994), a large number of spousal transplants have been conducted in India. As expectedly, most of these are poorly matched and are from wives to the husband. The Act also has a provision of permitting unrelated voluntary donors provided they are motivated through altruistic reasons and are approved by the Hospital Authorization Committee. Again such donors are poorly matched and long-term graft survival with these is not very encouraging.

DIRECT AND INDIRECT ALLORECOGNITION

The term allorecognition refers to T-cell recognition of genetically encoded polymorphism between members of the same species. The immunological

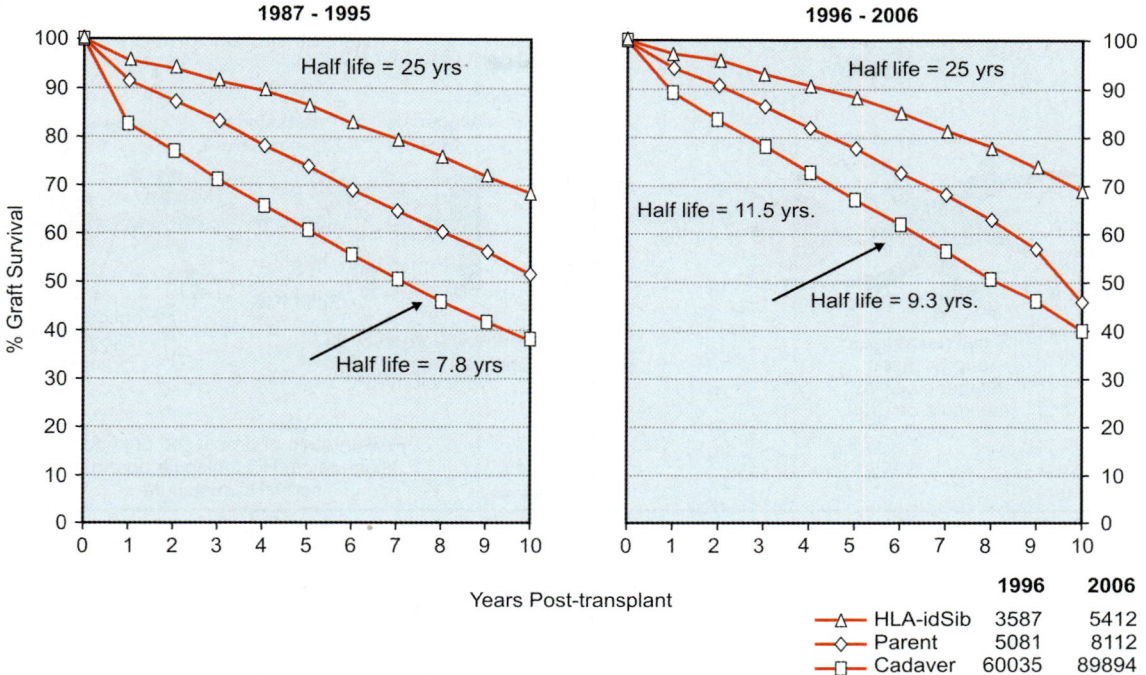

Fig. 87.4: UCLA data involving large series of kidney transplants showing the HLA matching effect followed for at least 10 year period. The HLA-identical sibling donor transplants have 70% graft survival compared to 50% for haploidentical parental grafts and < 40% for mismatched cadaver donor grafts. The half life of the HLA-Id grafts is 25yrs which drops significantly to 7.8 yrs (1987-95 block) and 9.3 yrs (1996-2006 block) for the cadaver donors. Source: Kaneku et al 2006

event(s) that initiate graft rejection involves interaction between the donor derived peptides and major histocompatibility complex (MHC) molecules on antigen presenting cells (APCs) and the T-cell receptor on $CD4^+$ recipient T-cells.[21-23] The latter can recognize donor alloantigens through either of the two pathways of allorecognition. In the *direct pathway*, the host T lymphocytes recognize native MHC molecules expressed on graft-associated APCs. In the *indirect pathway*, on the other hand, the same cell recognizes donor alloantigen-derived peptides in the context of self MHC molecules expressed on recipient APCs (Figs 87.5A and B). Historically evidence favors a predominant role of the direct pathway especially during acute rejection. Host T cells primed through the direct pathway have the ability to engage the allograft directly and thus to efficiently mediate effector functions. Further, the proportion of host T-cells that can respond to native alloantigens is substantially greater than the proportion of host T-cells that can respond through the indirect pathway to donor-derived peptides presented in the context of self MHC. It is likely that the direct pathway predominates early post-transplant and is a major factor in acute rejection since donor derived APCs expressing donor alloantigens rapidly migrate from the graft and enter the secondary lymphoid tissues, where they can encounter and prime the allospecific T-cells.

On the other hand, indirect pathway of alloantigen recognition involves recipient T-cells that recognize allogenic peptides presented by MHC molecules on self-APCs.[22] Donor MHC molecules are presumed to be shed off from the allograft into the recipients circulation, phagocytosed by the recipient APCs, processed into peptides and presented on the cell surface by self MHC Class II molecules. The recipient $CD4^+$ T-cells recognize this foreign peptide-self MHC complex and get activated, proliferate, differentiate and secrete various cytokines from the effector cells which in turn destroy the graft. A variety of cell types, that include cytotoxic T lymphocytes, B cells, macrophages and natural killer cells are recruited in a graft undergoing rejection. The three main

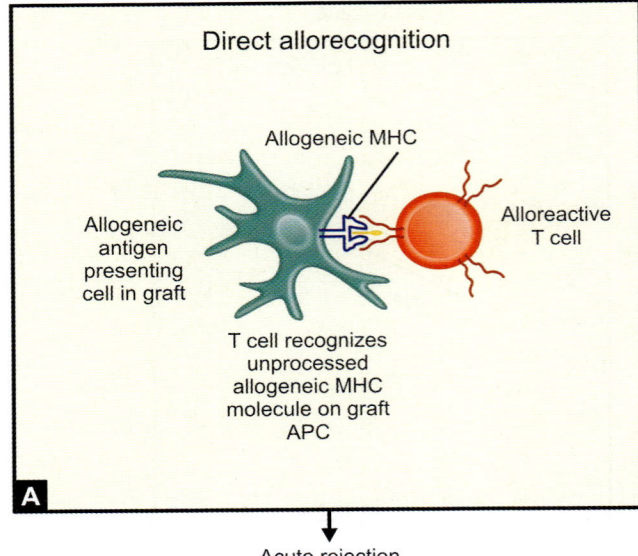
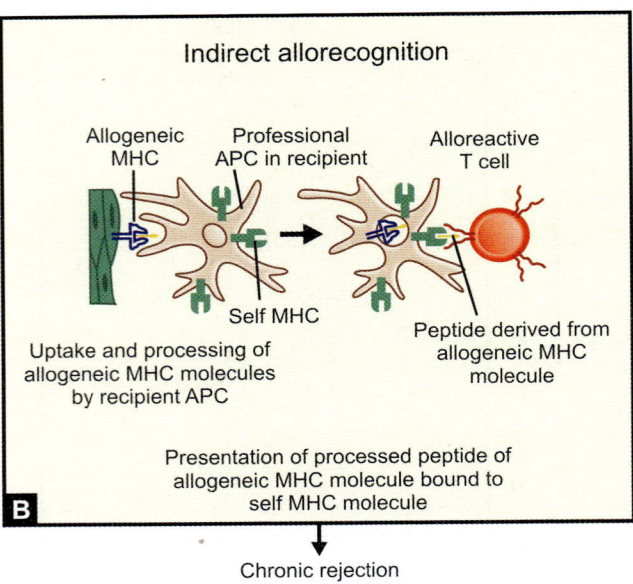

Figs 87.5A and B: The pathways of allorecognition that cause problems in organ transplantation as a result of HLA mismatching. **A.** Direct pathway. The alloreactive responses of recipient T-cells to donor APC expressing incompatible antigens. **B.** Indirect Pathway. Allogeneic HLA antigens are taken up and processed by the recipient APCs and presented in the context of autologous (self) HLA molecules to recipient T-cells. Antigen-presenting cell trigger CD4 and CD8 cells, and as a result local and systemic immune response develops. Cytokine recruitment and activation of specific T cells, NK cells and macrophage-mediated mechanisms lead to cytotoxicity and finally the allograft destruction

mechanisms implicated for graft destruction are cell-mediated cytotoxicity, delayed type hypersensitivity and antibody-dependent-cellular cytotoxicity. Of these, direct antibody mediated damage and development of donor-specific alloantibodies that can cause rejection has been found to be the most critical and lends support to the importance of antibodies in graft rejection. It is now amply clear that the pre and post-transplant development of IgG antibodies against donor epithelium and/or endothelium may predict the risk of allograft rejection.[24,25] Thus, humoral mechanisms appear to play the most critical role both in chronic as well as acute rejection.

PRE-TRANSPLANT EVALUATION OF ANTIBODIES

Anti-donor Antibodies

The most important factor in organ transplantation is the meticulous evaluation of the possible occurrence of antidonor antibodies before transplantation. This is referred to as the 'cross-match test' and is usually carried out by the complement dependent lymphocytotoxicity (CDC) assay. In this test, the donor lymphocytes are first incubated with the patient serum, followed by the rabbit complement and finally the lysis of lymphocytes is assessed by the uptake of an extravital dye like trypan blue or eosin red. A positive CDC crossmatch is generally a contraindication for organ transplantation because of the presence of IgG antibodies in the recipient leading to antibody-mediated (hyperacute) rejection. This applies particularly for kidney transplants whereas the liver allograft shows a relative resistance to antibody-mediated injury. In kidney transplantation, several cross match assays have been developed with the purpose of increasing the sensitivity and specificity of the test and depending upon the type specificity of the antibody to be detected. These include the anti human globulin (AHG), flow cytometry and ELISA based test systems. Serum treatment with dithiothreitol (DTT) is used to distinguish clinically less relevant IgM type antibodies.

Crossmatch assays detect different types of antibodies, some of which are deleterious while others may be harmless or even beneficial for the graft. Generally, the auto reactive T and B cells detect IgM, cold reactive auto antibodies that are not harmful. Many investigators have reported that successful transplantation can be performed with a positive donor specific cross match due to IgM antibodies after their reduction using dithiothreitol.[26,27] Also most centers agree that neither the short nor the long-term graft survival of deceased donor kidneys is influenced by a positive flow B-cell IgG cross match.[28] Further transplantation can be performed in the presence of a negative cross match with a current serum sample and a historical positive serum sample particularly in the case of first grafts.[29]

The greatest drawback of the CDC test is that in addition to the HLA specific antibodies, it detects non-HLA auto antibodies. This can be circumvented by incubating the test at 37°C (and not at room temperature) to avoid reaction of cold auto antibodies and by the addition of dithiothreitol to the serum to inactivate IgM antibodies. It may be noted, however that some strong auto antibodies, present particularly in patients with systemic lupus erythematosus (SLE), are of IgG type and therefore DTT treatment in such situations does not completely solve the problem of excluding extraneous reactions. Ultimately a better technique with increased specificity and sensitivity is required to detect donor specific antibodies for meticulous evaluation of anti-donor antibodies.

Panel Reactive Antibodies

Transplant candidates often become sensitized due either to a prior transplant, pre-transplant blood transfusions or previous pregnancies/abortions. Serum screening for generalized lymphocytotoxic antibodies (not necessarily anti-donor) against a random cell panel derived from healthy volunteers (covering diverse HLA antigen specificities) provides an assessment of the degree of sensitization expressed as the percentage panel reactive antibody (PRA). Generally, a panel of upto 50 volunteers is sufficient to cover the known broad HLA specificities. The PRA test result is expressed as 0-10% (non-sensitized), 1-50% (moderately sensitized) and 51-100% indicating a high degree of sensitization. Patients with high PRA values are more likely to have anti-donor antibodies in addition and are therefore prone to graft rejection.

These patients generally require longer time before a transplant can be planned on them since their antibody levels must come down to the threshold level. Meticulous evaluation of the recipient sensitization status both during pre- and post-transplant periods provides highly useful information on the state of allo-sensitization. Graft survival analyzed with respect to the post-transplant PRA at a 2 year follow up time indicates that the overall survival is significantly compromised in the highly sensitized group as compared to the non-sensitized patients, alongwith high incidence of acute and chronic rejection episodes.[30] The PRA test is equally important both in live related as well as cadaver donor transplant situations. Most highly sensitized patients show persistence of the same pattern of antibody specificity against one or a few shared epitopes. A better understanding of the antibody specificity improves the selection of renal transplant donors with acceptable HLA mismatches, and significantly improved graft outcome.

Flow Cytometric Crossmatch (FCXM)

Flow cytometry is a more sensitive technology for the detection of anti-donor antibodies during renal transplantation. The assay detects the anti-donor antibodies with a 10 to 250 fold greater sensitivity than the CDC test and characterizes their isotype(s) using fluorescent labelled secondary anti-human antibodies. Further, it is possible to determine if these antibodies are directed against class I and/or class II HLA determinants. T and B lymphocytes are generally used as targets to distinguish anti-HLA class I from class II reactivity. By using fluorescent labeled anti-human globulin isotype-specific antibodies like, anti-human IgG or anti-human IgM, isotype of the antibody can be easily determined. Finally, the intensity of the reaction, which is related to the ratio of antibody molecules per target antigen, can be determined quantitatively by median channel shift or relative change in fluorescence ratio (Figs 87.6A to F). However, determining the HLA specificity of the anti-donor antibodies is generally difficult, mainly due to the requirement of lymphocytes derived from a diverse pool of donors.

Detection of anti-donor antibodies by flow-cytometry is of immense value for the clinicians in the field of transplant immunology. Mismatched HLA antigens in the transplant may induce the formation of specific antibodies against the donor antigens. The conventional serological cytotoxic cross match (CTXM) is sometimes unable to detect sub threshold levels of donor specific antibodies (DS-Abs), which can be otherwise detected by flow cytometry. In the post-transplant scenario, FCXM is helpful in differentiating acute rejection episodes from other causes of declining graft function like cyclosporin-A (CsA) nephrotoxicity and acute tubular necrosis (ATN). Our data on the live related donor transplants carried out at the AIIMS center has shown that a comprehensive assessment of anti-donor antibody repertoire using both CDC as well as flow cytometry assays provides a more sensitive system of assessing sensitization status of the recipient and can prove to be of immense prognostic value in renal transplantation.[31]

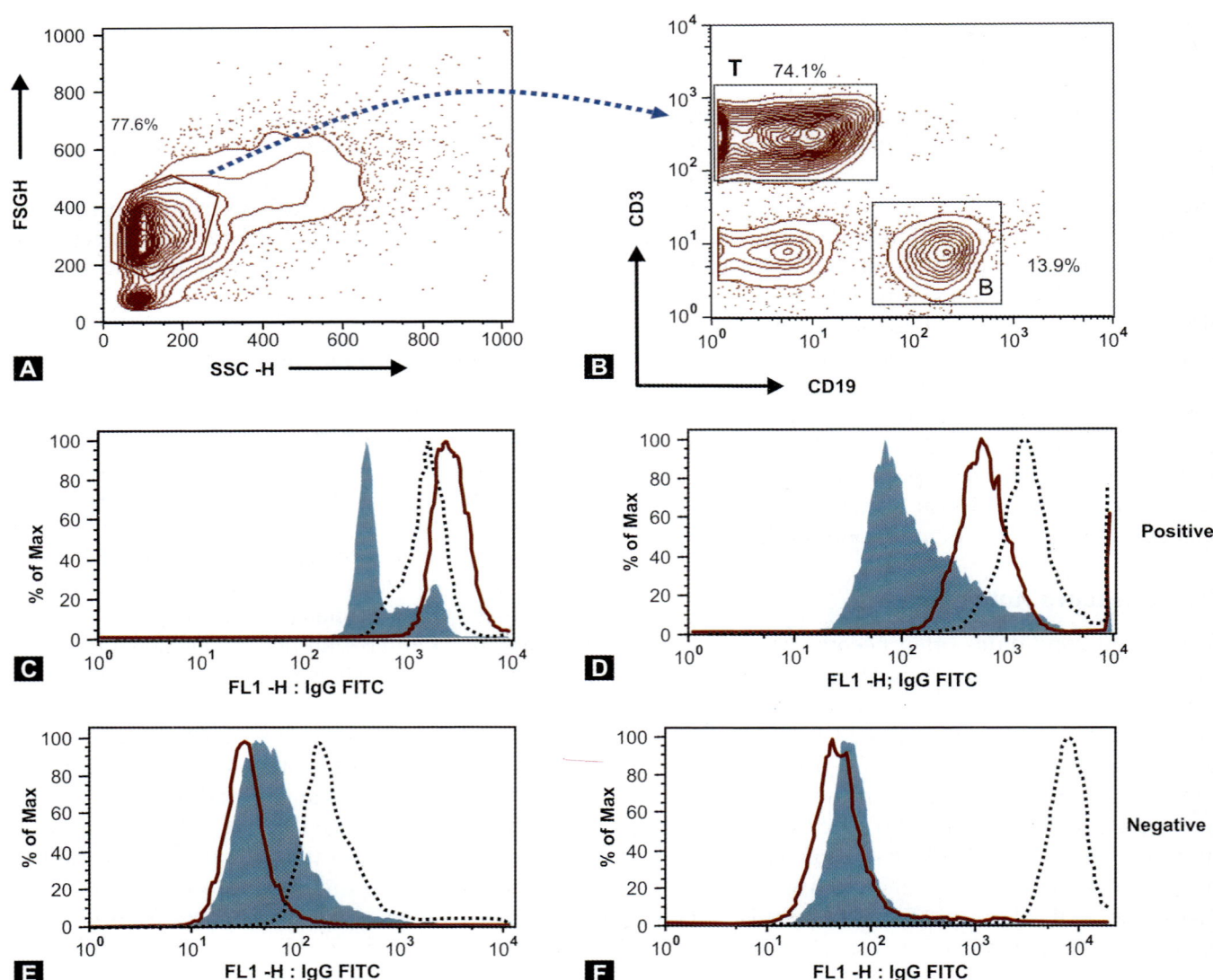

Figs 87.6A to F: Representative samples of the flow cytometric cross match (FCXM) showing negative (shaded line) and positive (dotted line) control peaks as compared to patient (thick line) sample. A mean peak shift to the right of > 40 is taken as the positive result (A)

Enzyme Linked Immunosorbant Assay (ELISA)

Use of the ELISA based method for the determination of HLA antibodies was introduced in 1993 to detect IgG and IgA antibodies to HLA antigens.[32] Purified HLA antigens are adhered to a microplate, and antibody reactivity is measured using a sandwich assay. Experience of several centers suggests that ELISA detects HLA antibodies with greater sensitivity than the CDC test. Although the conventional colorimetric substrates of ELISA are probably less sensitive than flow cytometry, fluorescent substrates may be as sensitive. The main advantage of the test is that ELISA readers are readily available and are far less expensive than flowcytometers. Moreover, many reactions can be examined in a 96-well plate, thus permitting determination of the specificity of HLA antibodies. As with flow cytometry, complement fixation is not required and the antibody isotype can be readily resolved. Nevertheless a major disadvantage of the ELISA test is that it does not provide information on the presence of anti-donor antibodies. Indeed in most centers, the donor cells are often not available for the determination of donor-specific activity following transplantation. Therefore, most ELISA assays detect anti-HLA antibodies reactive against a panel of antigens. We have recently made a comparison of the CDC versus FCXM and ELISA based tests for determination of alloantibody development following renal transplantation. Our data indicate that while FCXM is a sensitive test for the detection of donor specific antibodies, ELISA offers the additional advantage of detecting anti-HLA antibodies, which are detrimental for the graft survival.[33]

CLINICAL RELEVANCE OF POST-TRANSPLANT ANTI-HLA AND NON-HLA ANTIBODIES

In the previous section, we have observed that occurrence of pretransplant anti-HLA antibodies plays a central role in graft survival, particularly in kidney transplantation. The presence of such preformed donor specific anti-HLA antibodies is always excluded before transplantation by performing crossmatches using current and historic recipient serum samples. However, in recent years, it has become clear that several HLA antibodies that develop denovo post transplant and are not necessarily donor specific, are also associated with poor graft survival. It is therefore advisable to monitor routinely the post-transplant development of such antibodies, which could be a predictive marker for allograft function.[34-36] Indeed the presence of circulating anti-HLA antibodies along with positive C4d staining on allograft biopsies has been reported to have strong correlation with the development of chronic rejection in kidney transplant recipients.[37] Long-term follow-up of these patients is necessary to establish whether patients who subsequently reject their grafts come from the antibody-positive group. Our results are also consistent with those of others that renal transplant patients with anti-HLA antibodies, even though they are not donor specific (cross-match negative) have significantly poor graft survival as compared to the negative group.[38]

Despite the availability of potent immuno-regulatory drugs and other biologic agents, allograft rejection still remains a formidable challenge in renal transplantation. The presence of donor lymphocyte-reactive HLA-specific antibodies before and after transplantation is associated with rejection episodes and renal allograft loss.[39] Nevertheless, rejections may still occur in the absence of detectable lymphocytotoxic antibodies, suggesting that non-HLA antigenic systems may also play a role in hyperacute and acute renal allograft rejections.[8,39] Amongst these, the MHC class I related chain (MICA) is a locus situated on chromosome 6 linked to HLA and determines a polymorphic series of antigens similar to HLA. The MICA and MICB genes are located in close proximity to the HLA-B locus and encode for 62 kDa cell-surface glycoproteins. MICA is expressed on the cell surface of endothelial cells that makes this polymorphic molecule a target for both cellular and humoral immune responses. Indeed MICA has been reported to be an important polymorphic alloantigen capable of inducing synthesis of specific allo-antibodies in transplant patients and as a target for humoral immunity associated with irreversible rejection of kidney allograft.[8,40] Recently, it has been reported that antibodies to MICA are produced in the course of immunization by pregnancy and kidney transplantation, and they occur more frequently in patients experiencing rejection episodes compared to those with well functioning grafts.[8] Presensitization of kidney-transplant recipients against MICA antigens is associated with an increased frequency of graft loss and this might contribute to allograft loss among recipients who are well matched for HLA and have otherwise no evidence of the presence of anti HLA antibodies.

Studies carried out by us on LRD renal transplants have revealed that MICA is an important antibody target towards graft destruction. Patients who develop both anti HLA and MICA antibodies reject their grafts more frequently than those having either of these antibodies.[8,41] Thus, post-transplant monitoring of both these antibodies could not only be predictive of renal allograft failure, but also as an important prognostic marker in renal transplant subjects.

GRAFT REJECTION

Since transplant immunity leads to rejection primarily due to genetic disparity between donor and the recipient, it is plausible that the patient and donor are matched for HLA gene loci as completely as possible. Although full HLA compatibility is possible only among genetically identical twins (syngeneic grafts) and to a lesser extent between HLA-identical siblings, the vast majority of transplants come from HLA incompatible unrelated donors. These include parental and/or sibling donors, a majority of whom are HLA haploidentical (50% match grade). Deceased and spousal donors are likewise poorly matched. Accordingly, immunosuppressive drugs are given to control the host immunity steaming out of the HLA disparity so that rejection can be prevented or controlled and the recipient develops long-term acceptance (or tolerance) of the graft. Rejection can be mediated by antibodies, lymphocytes or both and can manifest itself in different ways: hyperacute rejection (during the early post-transplant period, within hours), acute rejection (may occur at any time) and chronic rejection (a slowly developing process causing a progressive decline in graft function).

Hyper-acute Rejection

Hyperacute rejection is mainly due to the presence of preformed donor specific alloantibodies in the presensitized recipients. Vascularized organs (especially kidney and heart) are at risk for hyperacute rejection if the patient has preformed donor-specific alloantibodies. This humoral presensitization (or alloimmunization) may be caused by a previous transplant, blood transfusions and pregnancy. The primary target of the donor-specific antibodies is the vascular endothelium of the grafted organ. The most common target antigens are HLA class I, and ABO, although other less-well defined antigens are also involved. HLA class II antigens seem less relevant in hyperacute rejection because they are not strongly expressed on the vascular endothelium. Antibodies mediating hyperacute rejection are almost always complement-fixing and could be of IgG or IgM type or both. Alloreactive T lymphocytes are rarely involved in hyperacute rejection. A critical step in alloantibody-mediated rejection is the initiation of the Complement cascade that involves binding and activation of C1q, which requires at least two Complement-fixing sites on the antigen/antibody complex. This requires close proximity between antigens and complement such that activation will not occur if the antigen density is too low on the cell surface. Activation of the Complement cascade leads to the release of various inflammatory mediators and the initiation of the coagulation and fibrinolytic systems. Hyperacute rejection is manifested by rapid vascular constriction, edema and thrombotic occlusion.[42] Endothelium stimulation and exposure to sub-endothelial basement membrane proteins activate platelets which then adhere and aggregate in the vasculature. Soon afterwards, polymorphonuclear leukocytes (PMN) adhere to the vascular endothelium, leading to its damage.

Acute Rejection

Acute cellular rejection is mediated by lymphocytes which have become alloactivated against donor transplantation antigens. *In vivo* stimulation of alloreactive T-cells takes places primarily in the peripheral lymphoid tissues of the recipient although intragraft sensitization may also occur. The strongest stimulus is provided by donor dendritic cells in the allograft which enter the circulation and end up on the lymphoid tissues of the recipient. These dendritic cells function as antigen-presenting cells and provide a strong stimulus of HLA class II reactive CD4 cells, which can stimulate the growth and differentiation of HLA class I reactive $CD8^+$ cytotoxic lymphocytes. Alloreactive lymphocytes enter the circulation and react with allograft vascular endothelium, which is the primary target of the initial stage of cellular rejection.

The lymphocyte-endothelial interactions depend on the expression of appropriate target antigens on the endothelium. HLA class I antigens are constitutively expressed at the cell surface whereas HLA class II antigen expression (with the exception of the APCs) must be induced by various cytokines, especially gamma interferon (IFN-γ). Furthermore, adhesion molecules like intercellular adhesion molecules (ICAMs), vascular cellular adhesion molecules (VCAMs), integrins, selectins, play an important role in the cell surface interaction between lymphocytes and endothelium, their activation and release of inflammatory mediators including cytokines and, chemokines.[43] These processes lead to migration of lymphocytes through the vascular wall to the grafted tissues.

Graft-infiltrating lymphocytes can mediate various effector mechanisms of allograft immunity. Besides a direct cytotoxic effect on graft parenchymal cells, lymphocytes can mediate a delayed type hypersensitivity leading to graft rejection. The latter involves the recruitment of macrophages and release of various cytokines. Other inflammatory cells may also be seen during rejection, including neutrophils, eosinophils, B lymphocytes and NK cells. Varying proportions of CD4 and CD8 lymphocytes are found in cellular infiltrates of rejecting allografts. Many of them express T-cell activation markers, like IL-2 receptors and these activated T-cells, probably through release of IFN-γ and other cytokines, increase expression of HLA antigens (especially class II) on the vascular endothelium and other target cells in the graft parenchyma. Consideration must be given to additional immunological mechanisms of graft injury secondary to infection, especially by viruses. This means that other types of lymphocytes may infiltrate the graft and these could mediate effector immune responses against virus infected cells in the graft. Another possibility is that graft infiltrating lymphocytes mediate recurrent autoimmune disease processes.

Chronic Rejection

This major complication, affecting most long-term transplant survivors, is not completely understood. Chronic rejection is characterized by vasculopathy, fibrosis and a progressive loss of the organ function. Its pathogenesis probably involves both humoral as well as cellular immune mechanisms.[44] Chronic rejection may be mediated by low-grade, persistent delayed type hypersensitivity response in which activated macrophages secrete mesenchymal cell growth factors leading to fibrosis. Of potential importance are persistent viral infections which induce cellular immune responses simultaneously along with the donor-specific alloreactive T-cells. Chronic rejection may also reflect chronic ischemia secondary to injury of the blood vessels by antibody or cell-mediated mechanisms. Vascular occlusion may occur as a result of smooth muscle cell proliferation in the intima of the arterial walls.

IMMUNE PROFILING: PREDICTIVE VALUE OF HLA ANTIBODIES

The humoral theory of transplantation states that antibodies cause allograft rejection, lead to C4d deposits associated with early kidney graft failure, are a good indicator of presensitization leading to early acute rejection, are present in a large majority of patients who reject a kidney graft, are associated with chronic rejection and appear in circulation well before rejection.[45] One of the challenges for organ transplantation today is development of diagnostic criteria for humoral rejection, assess the relevance of immune profiling, develop potential immunologic paradigms and develop effective treatment protocols for removal of alloantibodies. A positive CDC or AHG cross match result poses a high risk of humoral rejection or early graft loss. A positive CDC cross match is a contraindication to transplantation particularly when antibody in the recipient cannot be reduced with desensitization protocols. A positive flow or historic CDC cross match result poses intermediate risk for early acute rejection that may require intensive immunosuppression. Recipients with a negative flow or AHG crossmatch have low risk of acute humoral rejection with conventional immunosuppresion. Hence it is essential that antibody specificity and cross match should always be assessed prior to transplantation. Table 87.2 summarizes strategies for cross matching depending on the 'risk' status of the patients.

Diagnosis of acute and chronic humoral rejection is based on clinical, pathologic and serological criteria. When recipients have deteriorating function and other

Table 87.2: Strategies of crossmatching

A. For low risk patients (i.e. first transplant, patients with PRA < 10%, non-transfused, nulliparous female patients)
- CDC cross match alongwith HLA matching
- Pre-transplant cross match by CDC. If positive, repeat by CDC, DTT and flowcytometry
- CDC PRA screening alongwith HLA matching

B. For high risk patients (i.e. retransplants, Patients with PRA >10% multitransfused individuals, parous female patients)
- CDC cross match alongwith good HLA matching
- Pretransplant Crossmatch by CDC, DTT, FCXM
- CDC PRA screening alongwith HLA matching
- If PRA >10%, ELISA PRA/ Flow PRA to be done

potential causes such as cellular rejection or drug toxicity are ruled out, clinicians normally resort to allograft biopsy to make a definitive diagnosis. However, it is often difficult to distinguish humoral rejection form other forms of graft dysfunction, so current experience depends mainly on the results of the existence of circulating antibody for diagnosis.

Strategies to diagnose and treat acute humoral rejection involves four parameters: allograft dysfunction, circulating HLA or DSA antibody, C4d deposition in peritubular capillaries and other rejection morphology on allograft biopsy. These parameters help in defining four levels of rejection. Types 1-3 represent subclinical grades where there is evidence of humoral rejection but no measurable graft dysfunction Type 1 classification for patients with detectable antibody (DSA) indicates a biopsy would be informative to determine the severity of rejection. Type 2 indicates C4d staining is observed in the absence of other histologic parameters, while type 3 indicates both C4d and histologic evidence of humoral rejection is present. If type 4 dysfunction is observed with the other three parameters, treatment for antibody removal is recommended.

TREATMENT OF HUMORAL REJECTION

Two treatment protocols are currently being used to remove donor specific antibodies for patients awaiting renal transplant: i) one protocol uses high dose intravenous immunoglobulin (IVIG) to reduce or eliminate antibody reactivity. Desensitization is more durable with this protocol in comparison to the second protocol, although not all patients respond to treatment. ii) The second protocol uses plasmapheresis, and a lower dose of IVIG. Most patients respond to this treatment, but the procedure is expensive and rebound of antibody can occur if the patient does not undergo kidney transplantation immediately after completion of the protocol.

Terasaki and Ozawa through a large collaborative study of 2231 transplanted patients have concluded that regular screening of HLA antibodies post-translantation is predictive of subsequent graft failure and this predictive value can be enhanced among patients with higher serum creatinine values.[46] Thus if HLA antibody testing is to be used for monitoring, then the value of testing will depend on serum creatinine value at any given time. If the creatinine is low, one can expect that the graft will function well for some years, and the antibody results will give a warning far in advance of failure. If Kidney damage develops, as shown by higher serum creatinine levels, then the results of the antibody screening will require rapid action, if graft failure is to be stopped.

CYTOKINES AND CYTOKINE GENE POLYMORPHISMS IN RENAL GRAFT OUTCOME

Cytokines are known to play a central role in directing both the magnitude and type of the immune response directed against the grafted tissue. Since immunologic processes like antigen recognition and proliferation of lymphoid cells, mark the beginning of graft dysfunction, their products (cytokines and antibodies) appear quite early in the circulation following transplantation.

Current immunologic protocols fail to detect acute rejection at an early stage before the onset of clinically observable rejection episode, a time point by which already certain level of irreversible damage to the graft tissue has take place. Since the cytokines produced by the alloactivated T-cells play an important role in the initiation and maintenance of alloimmune response, an assessment of their profile could provide an important predictive marker of post-transplant immune activation and may provide useful clues for tailoring immunosuppressive regimen leading to improved clinical care.[47-49] Our own data indicates that monitoring intracellular cytokine expression profile of primed peripheral T-cells is important and that estimation of circulating sIL-2 levels post transplantation provides not only a useful prognostic tool but also a better alternative for functional assessment of immune-suppression for follow up of transplant subjects.[50]

Quantitative estimation of cytokines at the site of the allograft is a useful indicator of graft function and helps to determine accelerating or suppressing rejection. The level of cytokine production has been associated with polymorphisms in cytokine gene promoters.[51-53] It is now accepted that promoter region polymorphisms can directly or indirectly affect the binding of transcription factors and consequently increase or decrease the production of mRNA, thus regulating cytokine production. Cytokines can be categorized into two broad groups : i) the so-called Th1-type cytokines, including interleukin-2 (IL-2), tumor necrosis factor-α(TNF-α), TNF-β and interferon-γ (IFN-γ), that mediate cellular immune responses and are proinflammatory ii) cytokines described as the Th2 type, which include IL-4, IL-5, and IL-10, that have been shown to inhibit the development and function of Th1 cells, suppress inflammation, and enhance humoral pathways of the immune response. These are designated as the anti-inflammatory cytokines.

The proinflammatory cytokine TNF-α, which stimulates macrophage function and increases MHC class II antigen expression, has been implicated both in acute as well as chronic rejection. It has been shown that a G to A polymorphism at position –308 on the TNF-α gene promoter, giving alleles TNF1 and TNF2, respectively, is associated with a six to seven fold increase in transcription of the TNF-α gene *in vitro*.[54] Similarly, the activation of endothelial cells and the subsequent expression of intercellular adhesion molecule-1 (ICAM-1) induced by TNF-α can enhance vascular permeability and therefore augment the infiltration of proinflammatory granulocytes into the graft. The expression of ICAM-1 on the vascular endothelium has been associated with acute rejection in kidney transplants. Conversely, IL-10 has the ability to inhibit APC function, TNF-α production, and ICAM-1 expression *in vitro*. Evidence from animal transplant models has suggested a role for the immunoregulatory cytokine IL-10 in promoting graft survival. However, others have provided evidence supporting the role of IL-10 in rejection.[55]

The exact relationship between transforming growth factor beta-1 (TGFβ-1) and the development of chronic graft nephropathy remains uncertain. However, it appears that TGFβ-1 is up-regulated at the protein and mRNA levels during the first year following cadaveric renal transplantation and the effect of 'high producer' gene polymorphism is important. This up-regulation of TGFβ-1 in plasma may provide a novel noninvasive means of identifying early fibrotic damage before it becomes clinically apparent thus allowing an opportunity for intervention for grafts that may otherwise fail.

Infection remains a significant cause of morbidity and mortality after solid organ transplantation. Genetic background has an influence on the incidence of infection. Kidney transplant recipients with -511 IL-1β CC genotypes or with -1188 IL-12 CA and CC genotypes have been reported to be at higher risk of developing infections in the first year after transplantation. Such patients with genetic susceptibility to infection may therefore benefit from less potent immunosuppressive therapy and more intense preventive measures.[56]

Quantitation of soluble interleukin receptor-2 (sIL-2R) has also been found to be useful in the detection of rejection in recipients of heart and liver allo-grafts. It has been suggested that sIL-2R assays offer a rapid, reliable and noninvasive indicator of allo-reactivity, response to therapy and prognosis in conditions associated with T and B cell activation. It may also reflect immune activation in other tissues or fluid compartments as the IL-2R generated in these sites may enter the circulation. Impaired renal function has been reported to show elevated serum sIL-2R as this molecule is likely to be actively transported into the urine. The preoperative and serial postoperative measurement of sIL-2R level has been used to distinguish rejection from cyclosporin A (CsA) nephrotoxicity in renal transplant recipients but not rejection from infection. Data generated from our group showed that sIL-2R levels are generally higher in patients undergoing acute rejection, chronic rejection cases and even those with infective episodes.[33] However, there was no difference in patients with CsA nephrotoxicity and those with ATN despite elevation of their serum creatinine levels.

Similarly, soluble CD30 (sCD30), a marker for T-helper 2-type cytokine-producing cells reflects on the immune state of the graft and could be used as a predictor for kidney graft survival. Elevated pre transplant serum sCD30 levels have been found to be detrimental for graft survival, hence could be a better predictor of allograft rejection.[57-59] The permissible and immunogenic HLA mismatches reflected in cytotoxic T-lymphocyte precursor frequencies could be used in clinical settings, whereby significantly lower CTLp frequency is correlated with permissible HLA mismatches and better graft survival compared to immunogenic HLA mismatches. Therefore, use of multiple parameters for assessing recipient's immune profile can predict graft outcome more accurately and help in subsequent individualization and optimization of immuno-suppression.

TRANSPLANT TOLERANCE AND MOLECULAR THERAPEUTICS

Although the goal of transplantation is to achieve long-term acceptance of the allograft, little is known about the mechanisms responsible for this successful outcome. Induction of immunological tolerance has long been thought to be the ultimate goal of research in the field. As graft rejection is the major cause and primarily mediated by immunological reactivity against the donor antigens, attempts to induce a state of tolerance as observed in case of self antigens seems most rational. Self tolerance is brought about mainly by central and peripheral mechanisms. Central mechanism relies on the deletion and/or functional incapacitation of self reactive T-cells during the ontogeny of the immune system and manipulating these mechanisms may not be directly relevant to the clinical induction of graft tolerance. However, studying the underlying mechanisms has greatly facilitated our knowledge on the immunological basis of tolerance. On the other hand, peripheral tolerance is mediated by mechanisms actively suppressing the auto and/or alloreactive T-cells and understanding of the cellular and molecular mechanism may contribute in the translational research leading to the development of effective protocols for tolerance induction following allografting.

Recent advances in the field of peripheral tolerance have paved the way for the induction of transplant tolerance. This is best exemplified by the standard immuno-suppressive regimen used in clinical management of organ transplant. Currently used immuno-suppressive drugs like cyclosporine, Tacrolimus, Sirolimus, etc. are all known to mediate their therapeutic action by inhibiting the clacineurin pathway of T-cells activation. However, they suffer from the major limitation of non-specifically suppressing T-cell function indiscriminately, thus compromising the function of T-cells involved in controlling the infections and immune surveillance. Therefore, alternate routes of specifically inhibiting the T-cells responsible for alloreactivity need to be developed. Recent findings suggest that donor specific hypo responsiveness induced by Foxp3+ T regulatory (Treg) cells or by manipulating the co-stimulatory pathway may be a potential approach to achieve a state of immune tolerance among transplant patients.[60] Blocking the co-stimulatory pathways of T-cell activation namely CD28-CD80/86 and CD40-CD40L has met with considerable degree of success in various transplant models. However, their inclusion in the clinical protocols for use in humans still remains controversial. Similarly genetically engineered CTLA4-Ig fusion protein has been tried for effective blockage of the co-stimulatory pathway leading to induction of T-cell anergy with encouraging success.[61] Many of these molecular approaches alone may offer an effective state of tolerance, but their use as adjunct molecular therapy seems quite promising and may offer more specific and effective immunosuppressive or tolerogenic regimen for therapeutic management of patients following renal transplantation.

CONCLUSION

Newer insights into the cellular and molecular basis of the allograft rejection have delineated novel targets for immunosuppressive therapy. Recent advances in the immunological techniques also promise improved management of transplant patients by developing newer assays to predict the pending rejection episodes before irreversible and terminal damage of the grafted tissue. HLA matching effect has been proven both for short as well as long-term survival of the renal allograft and involving live related or cadaver donors. Further, antibody development following transplantation has been directly correlated with the HLA match status of the donor and recipient—the poor match status frequently associated with more vigorous antibody response. Molecular approaches for clinical monitoring of the post-transplant immune status and identifying the best functionally matched donor before the transplant procedures are among the key area of futuristic research in the area of clinical transplantation. Appreciation of the mechanisms underlying T-cell recognition of alloantigen has generated scopes for the use of synthetic peptides in prevention of graft rejection. Furthermore, a better understanding of the importance of adhesion molecules in transplant rejection has encouraged the introduction of clinical trials with anti-ICAM-1 monoclonal antibodies for the prevention of acute graft rejection. Hopefully, continuing progress in unraveling the molecular mechanisms of graft rejection will facilitate further refinements in immunosuppressive protocols and soon achieve the ultimate goal of long-term acceptance of organ allograft through tolerance induction.

ACKNOWLEDGMENTS

The authors wish to thank the Department of Biotechnology (DBT), Ministry of Science and Technology, Govt of India and the Indian Council of Medical Research (ICMR) for financial assistance of our studies on organ transplantation.

REFERENCES

1. Thorsby E. Transplantation Immunology : A brief update. Transplant Proceed 1997;29:3129-34.
2. Jin Y, Hernandez A, Fuller L, Rosen A, Cirocco R, Esquenazi V, Ciancio G, Burke GW, Miller J. A novel approach to detect donor/recipent immune responses between HLA- Identical pairs. Hum Immunol 2006; 68(5):350-61.
3. Shiina T, Tamiya G, Oka A, Takishima N, Yamagata T, Kikkawa E, et al. Molecular dynamics of MHC genesis unraveled by sequence analysis of the 1,796,938bp HLA class I region. Proc. Natl Acad Sci USA 1999;96:13282-87.
4. Mehra NK, Kaur G. MHC-based vaccination approaches: progress and perspectives. Expert Rev Mol Med 2003; 5: 1-17.
5. Mehra NK, Kaur G. HLA genetics and disease with particular reference to Type 1 diabetes and HIV infection in Asian Indians. Expert Rev of Clini. Immunol 2006;2: 901-13.
6. Sumitran-Holgersson S. HLA-specific alloantibodies and renal graft outcome. Nephrol Dial Transplant 2001;16: 897-904.
7. Sumitran-Holgersson S, Wilczek HE, Holgersson J, Soderstrom K. Identification of the nonclassical HLA molecules, mica, as targets for humoral immunity associated with irreversible rejection of kidney allografts. Transplantation 2002;74:268.
8. Mizutani K, Shibata L, Ozawa M, Esquenazi V, Rosen A, Miller J, Terasaki PI. Detection of HLA and MICA antibodies before kidney graft failure. Clin Transpl 2006;255-64.
9. Zou Y, Stastny P, Süsal C, Döhler B, Opelz G. Antibodies against MICA antigens and kidney-transplant rejection. N Engl J Med 2007; 357:1293-300.
10. Sheldon S, Poulton K. HLA typing and its influence on organ transplantation. Methods Mol Biol 2006;333: 157-74.
11. Little AM. An overview of HLA typing for hematopoietic stem cell transplantation. Methods Mol Med 2007;134: 35-49.
12. Bjorkman PJ, Saper MA, Samraoui B, Bennett WS, Stromonger JL, Wiley DC. Structure of the human class I histocompatibility antigen, HLA-A2. Nature 1987a; 329:506-12.
13. Bjorkman PJ, Saper MA, Samraoui B, Bennett WS, Stromonger JL, Wiley DC. The foreign antigen binding site and T-cell recognition regions of class I histocompatibility antigens. Nature 1987b;329:512-18.
14. Stern LJ, Brown JH, Jardetzky TS, Gorga JC, Urban RG, Stromonger JL, Wiley DC. Crystal structure of the human class II MHC protein HLA-DR1 complexed with an influenza virus peptide. Nature 1994;368:215-21.
15. Zinkernagel RM, Doherty PC. MHC-restricted cytotoxic T-cells: studies on the biological role of polymorphic major transplantation antigens determining T-cell restriction-specificity, function, and responsiveness. Adv Immunol 1979;27:51-177.
16. Mehra NK, Jaini R, Rajalingam R, Balamurugan A, Kaur G. Molecular diversity of HLA-A*02 in Asian Indians: predominance of A*0211. Tissue Antigens. 2001;57: 502-07.
17. Jaini R, Kaur G, Mehra NK. Heterogeneity of HLA-DRB1*04 and its associated haplotypes in the north Indian population. Hum Immunol 2002;63:24-29.
18. Opelz G, Wujciak T, Döhler B, Scherer S, Mytilineos J. HLA compatibility and organ transplant survival. Collaborative Transplant Study. Rev Immunogenet 1999;1:334-42.
19. Claas FH, Dankers MK, Oudshoorn M, van Rood JJ, Mulder A, Roelen DL, Duquesnoy RJ, Doxiadis. Differential immunogenicity of HLA mismatches in clinical transplantation. Transpl Immunol 2005;14:187-91.
20. Kaneku HK, Terasaki PI. Thirty year trend in kidney transplants: UCLA and UNOS Renal Transplant Registry. Eds Terasaki PI, Clin Transpl 2006;1-27.

21. Côté I, Rogers NJ, Lechler RI. Allorecognition: Transfus Clin Biol 2001;8:318-23.
22. Hornick P. Direct and indirect allorecognition. Methods Mol Biol 2006;333:145-56.
23. Bharat A, Mohanakumar T. Allopeptides and the alloimmune response. Cell Immunol 2007;248:31-43.
24. Scornik JC, Salomon DR, Lim PB, Howard RJ, Pfaff WW. Posttransplant antidonor antibodies and graft rejection. Evaluation by two-color flow cytometry. Transplantation 1989;47:287-90.
25. Yard B, Spruyt-Gerritse M, Claas F, Thorogood J, Bruijn JA, Paape ME, Stein SY, van Es LA, van Bockel JH, Kooymans-Coutinho M, et al. The clinical significance of allospecific antibodies against endothelial cells detected with an antibody-dependent cellular cytotoxicity assay for vascular rejection and graft loss after renal transplantation. Transplantation 1993;55:1287-93.
26. Tellis VA, Matas AJ, Senitzer D, Louis P, Glicklich D, Soberman R, Veith FJ. Successful transplantation after conversion of a positive crossmatch to negative by dissociation of IgM antibody. Transplantation 1989;47:127-29.
27. Khodadadi L, Adib M, Pourazar A. Immunoglobulin class (IgG, IgM) determination by dithiothreitol in sensitized kidney transplant candidates. Transplant Proc 2006;38:2813-15.
28. Bryan CF, Wakefield M, Reese JC, Shield CF 3rd, Warady BA, Winklhofer FT, Murillo D. Renal graft survival is not influenced by a positive flow B-cell crossmatch. Clin Transplant 2007;21:72-79.
29. Thielke J, DeChristopher PJ, Sankary H, Oberholzer J, Testa G, Benedetti E. Highly successful living donor kidney transplantation after conversion to negative of a previously positive flow-cytometry cross-match by pretransplant plasmapheresis. Transplant Proc 2005;37:643-44.
30. Deka R, Panigrahi A, Aggarwal SK, Guleria S, Dash SC, Mehta SN, Pandey RM, Mehra NK. Influence of pretransplant panel reactive antibodies on the posttransplant sensitization status. Transplant Proc. 2002;34:3082-83.
31. Panigrahi A, Deka R, Bhowmik D, Tiwari SC, Mehra NK. Immunological monitoring of posttransplant allograft sensitization following living related donor renal transplantation. Transplant Proc 2004;36:1336-39.
32. Monien S, Salama A, Schönemann C. ELISA methods detect HLA antibodies with variable sensitivity. Int J Immunogenet 2006;33:163-66.
33. Panigrahi A, Deka R, Bhowmik D, Dash SC, Tiwari SC, Guleria S, Mehta SN, Mehra NK. Functional assessment of immune markers of graft rejection: a comprehensive study in live-related donor renal transplantation. Clin Transplant 2006;20:85-90.
34. Cardarelli F, Pascual M, Tolkoff-Rubin N, Delmonico FL, Wong W, Schoenfeld DA, Zhang H, Cosimi AB, Saidman SL. Prevalence and significance of anti-HLA and donor-specific antibodies long-term after renal transplantation. Transpl Int 2005;18:532-40.
35. Terasaki P, Lachmann N, Cai J. Summary of the effect of de novo HLA antibodies on chronic kidney graft failure. Clin Transpl 2006;4:455-62.
36. Girnita AL, Webber SA, Zeevi A. Anti-HLA alloantibodies in pediatric solid organ transplantation. Pediatr Transplant 2006;10:146-53.
37. David-Neto E, Prado E, Beutel A, Ventura CG, Siqueira SA, Hung J, Lemos FB, de Souza NA, Nahas WC, Ianhez LE, David DR. C4d-positive chronic rejection: a frequent entity with a poor outcome. Transplantation 2007;84:1391-98.
38. Panigrahi A, Deka R, Mehra NK. Clinical relevance of donor specific and non-donor anti HLA class-I antibodies in live related donor renal transplantation. In: Immunobiology of the human MHC, Proceeding of the 13th International Histocompatibility workshop and conference. Vol II. Eds. John A Hansen, IHWG Press, Seattle USA P 2006;591-96.
39. Terasaki PI, Ozawa M, Castro R. Four-year follow-up of a prospective trial of HLA and MICA antibodies on kidney graft survival. Am J Transplant 2007;7:408-15.
40. Zafar MN, Terasaki PI, Naqvi SA, Rizvi SA. Non-HLA antibodies after rejection of HLA identical kidney transplants. In Clinical Transplants 2006, eds Michael Cekka, Terasaki PI, Published by UCLA Immunogenetics centre, USA P 2006;421-26.
41. Panigrahi A, Gupta N, Siddiqui JA, Margoob A, Bhowmik D, Guleria S, Mehra NK. Monitoring of anti-HLA and anti-Major histocompatibility complex class I related chain. A antibodies in living related renal donor transplantation. Transplant Proc 2007;39(3):759-60.
42. Racusen LC, Haas M. Antibody-mediated rejection in renal allografts: lessons from pathology. Clin J Am Soc Nephrol 2006;1:415-20.
43. Wecker H, Auchincloss H Jr. Cellular mechanisms of rejection. Curr Opin Immunol 1992;4:561-66.
44. Hayry P. Molecular pathology of acute and chronic rejection. Transplant Proc 1994;26:3280-84.
45. Treasaki PI. Humoral theory of transplantation. Am J Transplant 2003;3:66S-73.
46. Terasaki PI, Ozawa M. Predictive value of HLA antibodies and serum creatinine in chronic rejection: Results of a 2 year prospective trial. Transplantation 2005;80:1194-97.
47. van den Boogaardt DE, van Miert PP, de Vaal YJ, de Fijter JW, Claas FH, Roelen DL.The ratio of interferon-gamma and interleukin-10 producing donor-specific cells as an in vitro monitoring tool for renal transplant patients. Transplantation 2006;82:844-48.
48. Bellisola G, Tridente G, Nacchia F, Fior F, Boschiero L. Monitoring of cellular immunity by interferon-gamma enzyme-linked immunosorbent spot assay in kidney allograft recipients: preliminary results of a longitudinal study. Transplant Proc 2006;38:1014-17.
49. Israeli M, Yussim A, Mor E, Sredni B, Klein T. Proceeding the rejection: in search for a comprehensive post-transplant immune monitoring platform. Transpl Immunol 2007;18(1):7-12.

50. Basak U, Mitra DK, Panigrahi A, Guleria S, Agarwal S, Mehta SN, Dash SC, Mehra NK. Clinical relevance of monitoring cytokine production following living donor renal transplantation. Transplant Proc 2003; 35: 404-06.
51. Awad M, Pravica V, Perrey C, El Gamel A, Yonan N, Sinnott PJ, Hutchinson IV. CA repeat allele polymorphism in the first intron of the human interferon-gamma gene is associated with lung allograft fibrosis. Hum Immunol 1999;60:343-46.
52. Pravica V, Asderakis A, Perrey C, Hajeer A, Sinnott PJ, Hutchinson IV. In vitro production of IFN-gamma correlates with CA repeat polymorphism in the human IFN-gamma gene. Eur J Immunogenet 1999;26:1-3.
53. Hoffmann SC, Stanley EM, Cox ED, DiMercurio BS, Koziol DE, Harlan DM, Kirk AD, Blair PJ. Ethnicity greatly influences cytokine gene polymorphism distribution. Am J Transplant 2002;2:560-67.
54. Pawlik A, Domanski L, Rozanski J, Florczak M, Dabrowska-Zamojcin E, Dutkiewicz G, Gawronska-Szklarz B IL-2 and TNF-alpha promoter polymorphisms in patients with acute kidney graft rejection. Transplant Proc 2005;37:2041-43.
55. Amirzargar M, Yavangi M, Basiri A, Moghadam SH, Khosravi F, Solgi G, Gholiaf M, Khoshkho F, Dadaras F, Mahmmodi M, Ansaripour B, Amirzargar A, Nikbin B. Genetic association of interleukin-4, interleukin-10, and transforming growth factor-beta gene polymorphism with allograft function in renal transplant patients. Transplant Proc. 2007;39:954-57.
56. Rodrigo E, Sánchez-Velasco P, Ruiz JC, Fernández-Fresnedo G, López-Hoyos M, Piñera C, Palomar R, Gómez-Alamillo C, González-Cotorruelo J, Leyba-Cobián F, Arias M. Cytokine polymorphisms and risk of infection after kidney transplantation. Transplant Proc 2007;39: 2219-21.
57. Slavcev A, Honsova E, Lodererova A, Pavlova Y, Sajdlova H, Vitko S, Skibova J, Striz I, Viklicky O. Soluble CD30 in patients with antibody-mediated rejection of the kidney allograft. Transpl Immunol 2007;18:22-27.
58. Truong DQ, Darwish AA, Gras J, Wieërs G, Cornet A, Robert A, Mourad M, Malaise J, de Ville de Goyet J, Reding R, Latinne D. Immunological monitoring after organ transplantation: potential role of soluble CD30 blood level measurement. Transpl Immunol 2007;17:283-87.
59. Wang D, Wu GJ, Wu WZ, Yang SL, Chen JH, Wang H, Lin WH, Wang QH, Zeng ZX, Tan JM. Pre- and post-transplant monitoring of soluble CD30 levels as predictor of acute renal allograft rejection. Transpl Immunol 2007;17:278-82.
60. Bestard O, Cruzado JM, Mestre M, Caldés A, Bas J, Carrera M, Torras J, Rama I, Moreso F, Serón D, Grinyó JM. Achieving donor-specific hyporesponsiveness is associated with FOXP3+ regulatory T-cell recruitment in human renal allograft infiltrates. J Immunol 2007;179: 4901-09.
61. Benigni A, Tomasoni S, Turka LA, Longaretti L, Zentilin L, Mister M, Pezzotta A, Azzollini N, Noris M, Conti S, Abbate M, Giacca M, Remuzzi G. Adeno-associated virus-mediated CTLA4Ig gene transfer protects MHC-mismatched renal allografts from chronic rejection. J Am Soc Nephrol 2006;17:1665-72.

CHAPTER 88

Liver Transplantation

AJW Millar, S Cywes

INTRODUCTION

Until recently, treatment options for the debilitating effects of liver disease in children were limited to supportive therapy and immunosuppressive agents. With surgical conditions such as biliary atresia, some success has been achieved with timely diagnosis and early surgical intervention. However, in many cases even with expert management there is inevitable progression of liver disease. Liver transplantation offers the only chance of a cure for these unfortunate children. Early experimental studies were conducted in the 1950's and early 60's in Boston and Denver. Although the first attempted human transplant was performed in 1963, it was not until five years later that long-term success was achieved.[1] In 1983, the National Institutes of Health Consensus Development Conference in the USA accepted liver transplantation in children and adults as deserving a wider clinical application. Advances in surgical technique, anesthetic management, pre- and postoperative care and refinements in immunosuppression over the last three decades have resulted in a much improved outcome and wide acceptance of liver transplantation among pediatricians with an ever-increasing list of indications being identified (Table 88.1).

The full story of liver transplantation for children has yet to be told but the current expected five-year survival is now greater than 85% in some centres.[2,3] Excellent quality of life is the rule rather than the exception.[4] The longest survivor is well nearly 40 years after transplantation. Current anxieties over organ donor scarcity, long-term side effects of the immunosuppressive therapy, financial implications and some ethical issues remain. The focus of attention has now

Table 88.1: Indications for which liver transplantation has been performed in children

I. Metabolic (inborn errors of metabolism)
   a. Alpha-1 antitrypsin
   b. Tyrosinemia
   c. Glycogen storage disease type III and IV.
   d. Wilson's disease
   e. Perinatal hemochromtosis
   f. Hypercholesterolemia
   g. Cystic fibrosis
   h. Hyperoxaluria (+ renal transplant)
   i. Hemophilia A + B
   j. Protein C deficiency
   k. Crigler-Najjar syndrome

II. Acute and chronic hepatitis
   a. Fulminant hepatic failure (viral, toxin or drug induced).
   b. Chronic hepatitis (B, C, etc. toxin, autoimmune, idiopathic)

III. Intrahepatic cholestasis:
   a. Neonatal hepatitis
   b. Alagille syndrome
   c. Biliary hypoplasia
   d. Familial cholestasis

IV. Obstructive biliary tract disease
   a. Biliary atresia
   b. Choledochal cyst with cirrhosis

V. Neoplasia
   a. Hepatoblastoma
   b. Hepatocellular carcinoma
   c. Sarcoma
   d. Hemangioendothelioma

VI. Miscellaneous
   a. Cryptogenic cirrhosis
   b. Congenital hepatic fibrosis
   c. Caroli's disease
   d. Budd-Chiari syndrome
   e. Cirrhosis from prolonged parenteral nutrition

shifted from an initial target of early post-transplant survival to quality of life in the long-term. The transformation of a miserable jaundiced invalid into an active healthy child remains a powerful stimulant for pediatricians and transplant surgeons alike.

Shortage of donor organs has been tackled in an imaginative way with increasing use being made of size reduction of the donor liver for transplantation, splitting the liver into two functioning units for two recipients, as well as the use of segments of liver from living related donors. Transplantation in developing countries initially lagged behind, due mainly to inadequate resources and the unavailability of cadaver donors. However, many of these countries are now forging ahead with living donor transplantation.

INDICATIONS

Liver disease has been generally underestimated as a cause of death in children.[3] This is probably because many liver conditions in children have led to rapid deterioration and death in the past. Almost all forms of liver disease in children can be complicated by hepatocellular failure.[5,6] These would include acute and subacute liver failure from metabolic, toxic or viral insults and chronic parenchymal disease of varying causes of which biliary atresia, biliary hypoplasia, chronic active hepatitis, post-viral hepatitis and some metabolic diseases are the most common.[6-11] In some metabolic diseases, the manifestation is as in hepatocellular disease and in others there may be more widespread effects such as tyrosinemia, Wilson's disease, hyperglycoproteinemia, some glyco-storage diseases and hyperoxaluriatable.[1]

Assessment

In general, liver transplantation should be considered as a therapeutic option in all cases of chronic liver disease before the condition of end stage liver disease is realised.[12,13] This allows for a thorough assessment of the child and the family and gives time for full and frank discussions of treatment options which can prepare all concerned as much as possible for the transplant procedure and afterwards. The family's capacity to sustain long-term compliance after transplantation, so crucial to the success of this endeavour, must also be assessed. Transplant candidacy inevitably results in enormous emotional stress for parents while waiting for the appropriate donor as their child's condition often deteriorates with bleeding from gastrooesophageal varices and episodes of systemic infection. Family life may become disrupted. Those that live afar may feel constrained to relocate, which in itself could cause major domestic distressed families. The value of a sympathetic social worker to provide support cannot be overstated.

There are indeed few reasons for refusal for transplantation (Table 88.2).[12,13] These include uncontrolled systemic bacterial, viral or fungal infections, malignancy outside the liver, cyanotic pulmonary arteriovenous shunting with pulmonary hypertension, active chronic hepatitis B, HIV/AIDS as well as other major cardiorespiratory, neurological or renal disease which would be incompatible with quality long-term survival.[14] To a certain extent these are all relative contraindications. Psychosocial factors may be a reason for refusal. Parental substance abuse, severe psychiatric problems and poor preoperative compliance with therapy need to be factors carefully examined.

Compliance is more difficult to predict in children with acute hepatic failure, as time from presentation to decision to transplant is much shorter. As the outcome of the operation is so much better in recent years, indications for early transplant would be evidence of impaired synthetic function, including prolonged prothrombin time, reduced serum cholesterol levels and low serum albumin. Clinical indicators include presence of ascites, bleeding from esophageal varices not controlled by sclerotherapy and poor response to nutritional resuscitation. Those with acute hepatic failure who develop encephalopathy, hypoglycemia, a prothrombin time of greater than 50 seconds and a Factor V level of less than 20% should be considered for transplant, as almost all of these children die without transplantation.

Table 88.2: Contraindications

- Inadequate vascular supply
- Uncontrolled systemic infection
- Malignancy outside the liver
- Cyanotic pulmonary arteriovenous shunting
- Hepatitis B, HBeAg positive, HIV/AIDS
- Disease in other organs incompatible with quality survival
- Psychosocial factors

All patients require initial confirmation of the diagnosis, intensive medical investigation and nutritional resuscitation to treat the complications of the liver disease, portal hypertension and nutritional deprivation (Tables 88.3, 88.4,). Immunization status must be reviewed and supplemented with hepatitis A and B immunization, Hemophilus influenzae, pneumoccocal and meningococcal vaccine in most cases. Blood group identical or compatible donors are much preferred as the long-term survival with blood group incompatible donors is significantly less. Patients are generally listed according to urgency on a score from 1 to 4 with 1 being the most urgent.

SURGICAL TECHNIQUE

Donor organ suitability and function is difficult to predict. Increasingly marginal donors are being used with a surprisingly low incidence of primary poor or non-function. Age limits are being extended.[15] However, stable donors from patients with a short intensive care unit stay (less than 3 days), little requirement for inotropic support and normal or near normal liver function are preferred, with an expected <5% incidence of impaired function after transplant. Liver biopsy is useful if steatosis is suspected. Greater than 50% fatty infiltration would preclude the use of the liver in most centers. Viral screening of the donors is essential. This would include Hepatitis A, B and C, CMV, EBV and HIV screening. Core HBV antibody and HCV positive donors would only be considered in selected viral infected recipients.

Surgical techniques used for donor retrieval and recipient liver removal and engraftment have evolved over the last 30 years.[16,17] The majority of donor livers are removed as part of a multiorgan procurement procedure, which would include various combinations of kidneys, liver, heart or heart and lungs, small bowel and pancreas. University of Wisconsin solution is widely used as the preservation solution of choice.

The principle two techniques are a careful dissection and excision technique or the so-called rapid technique described by Starzl.[17,18] A mid-line incision is made from the suprasternal notch to the pubis. The sternum is opened and spread with a sternal retractor. The subcostal diaphragm is incised on each side to obtain better exposure. The abdominal part of the operation includes control of the aorta above the celiac axis by incision of the right crus of the diaphragm, being careful to avoid entering esophagus. The aorta is encircled with tape to enable cross clamping prior to infusion of preservation solution. The inferior vena cava and aorta are identified, dissected and encircled with tapes below the renal vessels. The inferior mesenteric artery may be ligated in continuity to prevent loss of preservation fluid into the bowel. After a careful search for any vascular abnormalities, which would include most frequently, a left hepatic branch from the left gastric artery and an accessory or replaced

	Table 88.3: Investigation of the liver transplant candidate	
A.	Full symptom history and physical examination.	
B.	Hematology	Complete blood count, clotting profile Blood group and tissue typing Serum biochemistry and liver function tests.
C.	Radiology	Chest and abdominal X-ray X-ray wrists and long bones.
D.	Imaging	Ultrasound with Doppler for size and flow in the portal vein and unusual anatomy. CT with contrast or magnetic resonance angiogram if vascular anomaly is suspected.
E.	Renal function	Urine analysis, biochemistry and creatinine clearance.
F.	Cardiopulmonary	Full evaluation particularly if hepatopulmonary syndrome is evident.
G.	Serology	Hepatitis A, B, C, CMV, EBV, HSV, HIV, measles and varicellla.
H.	Infection screen	Cultures of urine, sputum, blood, stool, ascites fluid and swabs from nose and throat.
I.	Nutritional evaluation	Micronutrients iron, zinc, selenium, manganese and vitamin levels A and E.
J.	Developmental assessment	
K.	Psychosocial assessment	

Table 88.4: Vitamin and nutrient intake/supplement of patients being prepared for transplantation

Formula	Suitable Age Group	Formula Characteristics
Breastmilk	Birth - 2 yrs	Contains lipase which makes fat and fat soluble vitamins availability high, also high biological protein availability
PreNan (Nestle)	Birth - 1 yr	Polymeric, contains 40% MCT's
Pediasure (Abbott)	1-10 yrs	Polymeric, contains 40% MCT's
Nutren Jnr. (Nestle)	1-10 yrs	Polymeric, contains 30% MCT's
Pregestimil (Mead Johnson)	Birth - 1 yr	Semielemental, contains 43% MCT's and hydrolyzed casein protein. This formula should only be used during periods of diarrhea, as patient compliance is limited due to taste. Relatively costly.
Alfaré (Nestlé)	Birth - 1 yr	Semielemental, contains 42% MCT's + hydrolyzed whey protein. This formula should only be used during periods of diarrhea, as patient compliance is limited due to taste. Relatively costly.
Pepti Jnr (Nutricia)	Birth to 10 yrs	Semielemental, contains 42% MCT's, hydrolyzed whey and casein protein. This formula should only be used during periods of diarrhea, as patient compliance is limited due to taste. Relatively costly.
Peptamen Jnr (Nestle) or Peptamen	1-4 yrs 21+yrs	Semielemental, contains 42% MCT's, hydrolyzed whey and casein protein. This formula should only be used during periods of diarrhea, as patient compliance is limited due to taste. Relatively costly.

Supplements

Supplements need to be added to the formula, enteral feed or the food of the patient. They require 160 kcal/kg/d and 12-15% protein, or (± 4 g/kg/d if < 1yr.), and an ordinary daily intake would not allow them to reach such high caloric and protein intake. Failing to reach these requirements will result in failure to thrive. The supplements need to be added with detailed calculations, as the ratios and total percentages of the final product will determine tolerance and continual growth.

Type	Characteristics
Polycose (Abbott)	Carbohydrate supplement
Promod (Abbott)	Protein supplement
Protifar (Nutricia)	Protein supplement
MCT oil (Nutricia)	Fat supplement

Vitamins (Daily)

Fat soluble: A (15,000 units), 1 alpha vitamin D (1 μgm), E (300-1,000 units, K (2.5-5 mg)

Water Soluble: B_1, B_6, C and folate as multivitamin syrup.

Micronutrients and minerals: Zinc, Selenium, Manganese, Iron.

Calcium and phosphate : Monitor serum Ca^{++} and PO_4 and urinary Ca^{++} excretion.

---

right hepatic from the superior mesenteric artery, which may run through the head of the pancreas and behind the common bile duct, the liver is mobilized by division of the left coronary ligament. An appropriate sized cannula is placed in the inferior mesenteric or superior mesenteric vein so that the tip lies at the junction with the splenic vein. A large bore cannula is placed in the aorta with the tip approximately opposite the renal arteries, the distal common iliac vessels are tied off and the donor is given a heparin (3 gm/kg). A large bore cannula may be placed in the inferior vena cava, which is connected to an away suction. The gallbladder and biliary tree are thoroughly irrigated with saline.

Procurement commences with infusion of preservation solution through both the portal vein and aorta after cross clamping the aorta at the level of the diaphragm and incising the suprahepatic vena cava within the pericardium. Normally one to two liters of preservation solution is infused through each cannula according to the size of the donor. If the superior mesenteric artery is not ligated the bowel will blanche and this will allow portal perfusion as well as arterial perfusion particularly if the inferior mesenteric vein is used for access. The porta hepatis is divided distal to the gastroduodenal artery, which is ligated and the portal vein is divided at the junction with the splenic vein. The proximal part of the superior mesenteric artery is defined and is dissected down to the aorta on its left side preserving 2 to 3 cm if accessory or replaced right hepatic arteries are present.

The liver is now removed with a patch of aorta including the base of the superior mesenteric and the celiac axis particularly if abnormal arterial supply has been identified. The liver is then removed from above downwards. The resected liver includes a cuff of diaphragm around the bare area along with the retrohepatic cava and part of the right adrenal gland, which is cut through. The infrahepatic inferior vena cava is divided above the renal veins. Once the organs have been removed, they are placed in a plastic bag and the liver is further perfused with 500 ml of preservation solution via the portal vein, hepatic artery and through the bile ducts. The liver then is placed in a further two plastic bags and packed in ice for transportation. Once the kidneys are removed, the iliac arteries and veins are retrieved in case of subsequent vascular reconstructions.

The **recipient operation** is commenced so that the estimated hepatic graft ischemic time is less than 12 hours. Much longer preservation times have been recorded, but this leads to an increased incidence of cholestasis and graft dysfunction. The recipient operation commences with a laparotomy incision, which may be subcostal or extended in the midline to the xiphoid process for extra exposure. Self-retaining subcostal retractors are an essential aid in obtaining the necessary exposure. Careful suture ligation of large thin walled veins in the abdominal wall, adhesions and omentum are required to keep blood loss to a minimum. Once the infrahepatic and subcostal areas are freed from the surrounding structures and liver, the flaps of abdominal wall are sewn back over the costal margins and the subcostal self-retaining retractor such as is inserted. The porta hepatis is dissected first and in children with biliary atresia, this requires the portoenterostomy to be taken down with preservation of the Roux-en-Y loop for later anastomosis.

It is useful at this stage to dissect out the hepatic artery at least as far back as the gastroduodenal in preparation for revascularization; this avoids unnecessary delay at the engraftment stage of the procedure. The portal vein is dissected and isolated. The rest of the liver is carefully mobilized. This includes the gastrohepatic ligament, the falciform and triangular ligaments together with the right retroperitoneal reflection. Mobilization of the liver off the inferior vena cava which is frequently preserved to facilitate reduced size transplantation or piggy-back engraftment should be done and is assisted by carefully dividing the vena cava ligament and right adrenal vein. The suprahepatic and infrahepatic vena cava are dissected and encircled with tape.

Backtable preparation of the donor liver would depend on whether a reduced size liver graft is to be used (Fig. 88.1). The liver is placed with the inferior surface uppermost within the inner plastic bag and is surrounded by packed sterile ice. Upper and lower cava are defined and redundant diaphragmatic muscle is excised, phrenic veins are ligated and sutured closed and the arterial and venous anatomy clearly dissected. The plane of transection when size reduction is planned is usually just to the right of the falciform ligament in left lateral segment transplants and in the median plane for left liver transplants (Fig. 88.2).

Even more careful dissection is required where split liver transplantation is being used; that is the liver is divided into two functional units for two recipients;

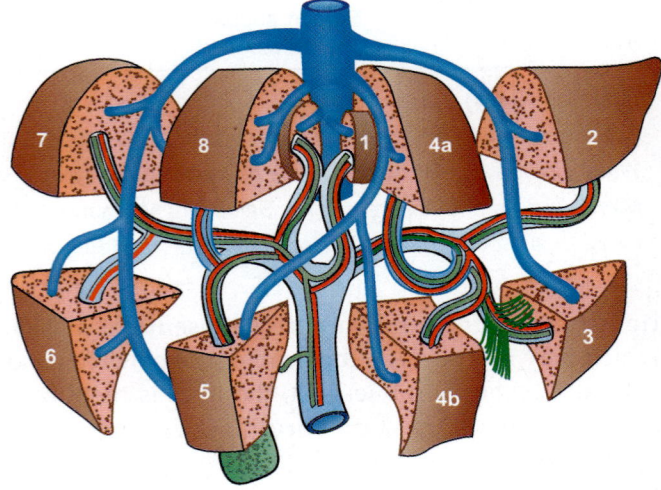

Fig. 88.1: Based on the segmental anatomy of the liver as depicted here diagrammatically, large livers can be reduced in size by ratios of up to 10:1 by bench work dissection. Usually segments 2 + 3 or segments 2, 3 and 4 are transplanted, or the liver is "split" into two functional units, i.e. segments 5-8 and 2 + 3

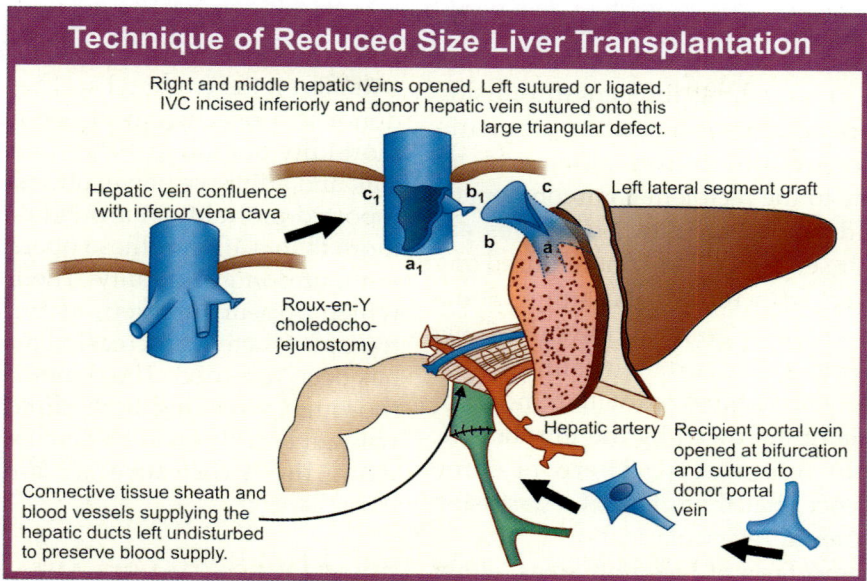

Fig. 88.2: This shows a reduced size liver (segments 2 and 3) at transplantation with its vascular and biliary anastomoses. In this case the recipient vena cava has been preserved and the hepatic vein of the donor is sutured onto the IVC

and decisions must be made as to which porta hepatis structures will go with which graft. To a certain extent, this depends on local preference but many centers opt to export the right-sided graft with the full compliment of structures of bile duct, portal vein and hepatic artery keeping the left lateral segment for the local graft in much the same way as a living donor transplant. Where a reduced size liver is used, the caudate lobe is always excised. The division of liver tissue may be performed using the standard forceps clamp or bipolar diathermy technique with suture and ligation of vascular and biliary structures. The ultrasonic dissector or harmonic scalpel may also be used. The cut edge of the liver is then sprayed with two layers of tissue glue. Once the recipient liver has been removed meticulously, hemostasis of the retroperitoneum must be ensured with a combination of suture ligation and cautery. If the recipient inferior vena cava is to be preserved, this is simplest done by carefully incising the diseased liver clear of the cava and when the liver has been removed individually suturing all small areas of leakage from divided direct caudate lobe hepatic veins. The IVC is prepared for the donor liver by dividing the bridges between the separate hepatic veins. This creates a wide orifice for the hepatic vein to cava anastomosis. The inferior vena cava should be incised distally for approximately 1-2 cm to make a triangular orifice for the 'piggy-back' graft.

Engraftment should begin with the upper caval anastomosis, which is usually performed with continuous posterior sutures of polypropylene and interrupted anterior sutures if a conventional transplant is being done. Prior to completion of the anastomosis, the liver is flushed of preservation solution via the portal vein with normal saline or a colloid solution. The lower cava anastomosis is then performed if required being sure not to cause any stricture or kinking, a growth factor of about a third of the diameter of the vessel is usually sufficient to prevent this occurring. The recipient portal vein is usually used for the anastomosis and in reduced size transplants where the donor liver is of large diameter, the bifurcation of the recipient portal vein is opened to create a trumpeted end for anastomosis. If the portal vein is hypoplastic, then the anastomosis is done at the level of the confluence the splenic vein after careful dissection under the head of the pancreas.

Another technique is to place a graft from the donor iliac vein onto this area first during the anhepatic phase. The portal vein anastomosis is carefully performed using continuous posterior and interrupted anterior sutures or the use of a generous growth factor.

In reduced size grafts, plenty of portal vein length should be left to avoid having any tension on the vein, which may result in stretching thus compromising flow. The donor hepatic artery is flushed with heparin saline to remove air and blood clots and an anastomosis is done to the recipient common hepatic artery. End to end microvascular techniques are preferred and in our series, we have not required any vascular grafts even with retransplantation. Some centers have used vascular grafts to the infra-renal aorta or from the supra-celiac aorta with success. The donor liver is usually revascularized with removal of the suprahepatic clamp followed by the infrahepatic clamp portal vein and artery. There is some experimental evidence that there is less reperfusion injury with early arterial revascularization.

After careful hemostasis of bleeding areas, either from the free edge of a reduced size liver or from any of the other major bleeding points, the operation is completed, by performing the biliary reconstruction. The bile duct is trimmed back such that good bleeding from the edges is obtained. In biliary atresia patients and those with a reduced size graft, a Roux-en-Y choledochojejunostomy is performed with fine absorbable sutures.[19-23]

Occasionally in pediatric cases, a duct-to-duct anastomosis may be performed with a whole liver graft in a recipient with a normal extrahepatic biliary system. Stents or T tubes are optional with some evidence of increased biliary complications associated with their use. The only real advantage is access to the biliary system during the postoperative period. Finally hemostasis is obtained and the wound closed with drainage to the suprahepatic and infrahepatic spaces.

LIVING RELATED DONORS

Living related donation of the left lateral segment, first successfully performed by Strong, has become widely accepted as a method of acquiring a liver graft in the face of severe donor shortages, particularly in countries with cultural or religious reticence to accept brain death in a ventilated heart-beating donor.[24] There are clear advantages in the planned nature of the procedure preferably before end stage liver disease in the recipient, the excellent quality of the graft and short ischemic time.

The use of a living donor also increases the availability of donor organs in general for other patients on the waiting list. The only advantage to the donor is a psychological one and there is a current morbidity of around 10% (wound sepsis, hernia, bile leak and adhesive bowel obstruction). There is also a reported mortality of around 0.2% although in Japan more than a 1000 of these operations have been done without donor mortality. There are ethical concerns, which appear justified, as with more widespread transplant activity increasing mortality and morbidity has been recorded. The donor should first undergo a thorough screening both clinical and psychological without coercion and be given an option to withdraw from the procedure at any time before the transplant.[25,26]

SPLIT LIVER TRANSPLANTATION

The liver of the donor is divided into two functional units thus making maximum use of this very scarce resource (Figs 88.3A and B). The procedure may be performed *in situ*, which has been associated with less post-reperfusion bleeding from the cut surfaces and improved graft function. However, this technique is time-consuming and may not be feasible in many cases. Early results with *ex-situ* dissection on the back table were poor and this was in part due to a technical learning curve, prolonged preservation times and the use of grafts, for only those recipients in the worst condition. Recent results are much improved. Clearly, the infrastructure must be in place to either perform two transplants simultaneously or alternatively one hemi-liver graft is exported to another center.

The *in situ* technique is similar to a living related transplant. Cholangiography is essential as there is considerable variety in the intrahepatic biliary anatomy.[27] Angiography is desirable but not essential. Some centers leave the hepatic artery with the right lobe making it more acceptable as an 'export'. The left lateral segment graft remaining is then used locally. Segment 4 should be used with the left graft if size is compatible, otherwise it is better to resect it prior to transplant as the segment 4 duct usually drains into the left hepatic duct. Likewise arterial anatomy is carefully examined and apportioned to each hemi-liver. There is usually a sufficient periductular vascular network to ensure adequate blood supply to the relevant ductal systems so long as the main hepatic artery branch to each hemi-liver is preserved. Accessory arteries can be ligated.

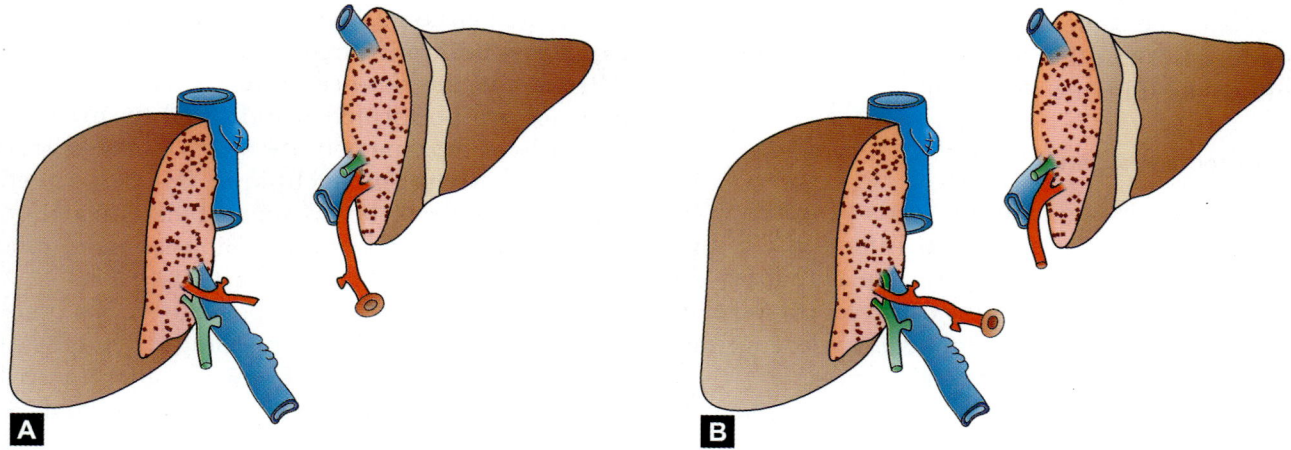

Figs 88.3A and B: Two arrangements of liver split are depicted. Segments 2 and 3 with and without the main arterial trunk. Segment 4 is discarded and the right lobe graft., segments 5,6,7 and 8, retains the inferior vena cava. Segment 1 is resected in all forms of reduced size liver

MEDICAL MANAGEMENT

Immunosuppression

Most protocols employ triple therapy with cyclosporin, azathioprine and methylprednisolone. Increasingly, particularly for small children, tacrolimus is used as primary immunosuppression. In addition, there are a number of other strategies in place to reduce the amount of nephrotoxicity, which is a toxic side effect to both calcineurin II inhibitors. Thus, mycophenolate mofetil, an inosine monophosphate dehydrogenase inhibitor may be used instead of azathioprine and a monoclonal interleukin-2 antibody may also be used with some steroid-sparing.[28,29] Rapamycin, a drug structurally similar to tacrolimus, which prevents proliferation of T cells but acts at a different stage of T cell activation than either cyclosporin or tacrolimus, has the advantage that it is not nephrotoxic and does not interfere with transcription and production of interleukin II, rather it antagonises the action of interlerukin II on its receptor. It has no adverse effects on liver function and may be synergistic with cyclosporin.

With cyclosporin in the microemulsion formulation (Neoral) 5 mg/kg is given immediately before the operation and is continued in the postoperative period as an oral dose. In infants and small children, there is some advantage to giving it as a three times a day dose initially, aiming at a trough level of around 350 ng/ml initially or a C2 (2 hour post dose) peak level of greater than 800-1200 ng/ml. The C2 appears to be a more effective measure of dosing as it reflects the area under the pharmacodynamic curve more accurately than the trough level. The dose must be frequently adjusted in the postoperative period, as particularly in small children absorption is erratic. Azathioprine (1-2 mg/kg) and methylprednisolone (10 mg/kg) are given at the time of reperfusion of the graft. The methylprednisolone dosage is reduced over the first week to about 1 mg/kg/day for the first month and then reduced to a level of 0.3 mg/kg/day to 0.2 mg/kg as maintenance. This can be later reduced in some patients to alternate day therapy or even withdrawn completely.

The azathioprine dose of 1 to 0.5 mg/kg/day is monitored keeping the leucocyte count above 4000 per mm^2 and is continued for 3 to 6 months. Tacrolimus can be used as rescue therapy for an acute rejection that does not respond to three or four daily pulses of intravenous methylprednisolone (10 mg/kg per dose) or it can be used as primary immunotherapy with steroids. Both mycophenolate mofetil and rapamycin can be used as renal sparing should nephrotoxicity become evident. Use of humanised anti-CD25 monoclonal antibodies given before and during the first week of the transplant have reduced the incidence of acute rejection in the first three months by around 30% but long-term graft survival is essentially the same as when these agents have not been used. The other polyclonal anti-lymphocyte immunoglobulins are rarely used.

Anti-infection Agents

Immunosuppression naturally leads to susceptibility to bacterial, fungal and viral infections. Fungal prophylaxis is given before the transplant as mycostatin orally to reduce *Candida* colonization of the gut and after transplant as amphotericin lozenges and continued for a period of several months.

From two to three weeks after the transplant, for at least the first year, trimethoprin-sulphamethoxazole is given at a dose of 6 mg/kg/day in two divided doses three days a week for prevention of *pneumocystis carinii* infection. Intravenous ganciclovir 5 mg/kg/dose, 12 hourly is used as prophylaxis against cytomegalovirus (CMV) and Epstein-Barr virus (EBV) infection, initially for two weeks and this may be extended for up to three months in high-risk patients who have not previously been exposed to CMV or EBV but have received a donor graft with previous exposure. This considerably reduces the incidence of both cytomegalovirus disease and post-transplantation lymphoproliferative disorder. Either hyper-immune cytomegalovirus globulin or immunoglobulin is also given to assist viral prophylaxis. Leucocyte filtered blood products are used throughout to reduce CMV load.

Prophylactic antibiotics are given with induction of anesthesia and continued for three to five days. These are changed according to cultures taken of blood, secretions, sputum and urine. Anti-tuberculosis prophylaxis is given only if the reason for transplant is a reaction to anti-tuberculosis drugs with fulminant hepatic failure, where evidence of tuberculosis is found before surgery and if a close family contact has tuberculosis.

Ofloxacin, rifampicin and ethambutol or ethionamide may be used in addition to isoniazid but very careful monitoring of liver function tests is required because all of these drugs may be hepatotoxic and particularly rifampicin may result in a decrease in the levels of cyclosporin or tacrolimus levels due to enzyme P450 induction with increased drug metabolism.

Postoperative care: Patients are monitored intensively postoperatively and usually require ventilation for a period of 24-48 hours. Liver ultrasound with color flow Doppler is performed frequently to confirm vascular patency and the absence of biliary dilatation. Liver biopsies are performed if indicated by increasing serum liver enzyme activity or by bilirubin levels, using the Menghini technique (Hypafix needle (Braun), diameter 1.4 mm), unless biliary dilatation is observed on ultrasonography. Biopsies are routinely assayed for viral and bacterial activity.

Diagnosis of rejection can be made on the basis of clinical, biochemical and histologic changes and usually presents in the first few weeks after transplant with fever malaise, a tender graft and loose stools. The grade of rejection is assessed according to established histological criteria on a scale of 0 to 4.

Acute rejection is treated with four doses of methyl predisnolone 10 mg/kg for the first three doses on successive days and the fourth on the fifth day after commencing treatment. Monoclonal antibodies and antilymphocyte globulin are very rarely used for steroid resistant rejection. If rejection persists, immunosuppressive protocols can be changed or the dosage increased. The tacrolimus starting dosage of 0.3 mg/kg/day in two divided doses is usually given to obtain a trough level of between 10 and 15 ng/ml initially. Once rejection is under control and liver function tests have returned to normal, the dosage can be reduced to a maintenance dose, obtaining trough levels of around 5 ng/ml. Hypertension is almost universal in pediatric transplantation and can be initially managed with nifedipine sublingually in conjunction with diuretic agents. Subsequently calcium channel blockers may be given in appropriate dosage. Aspirin 3 mg/kg given on alternate days is used as prophylaxis against arterial thrombosis and a proton pump inhibitor is given for gastric mucosal protection.

Nutritional and vitamin supplementation should be commenced within 72 hours of surgery and may be supplemented by nasogastric feeding or parenteral nutrition in the early phase if there is a delay in restoration of bowel function. Phosphate and magnesium deficiency is common and requires replacement therapy in nearly all patients.

SURGICAL COMPLICATIONS (TABLE 88.5)

Surgical complications may be reduced to an absolute minimum with meticulous technique.[30-32] These may

Table 88.5: Summary of common postoperative problems

1. Biliary tract
   a. Stenosis or stricture
   b. Anastomotic leak - often associated with hepatic artery thrombosis.
   c. Infection.
2. Rejection
   a. Acute
   b. Chronic (vanishing bile duct syndrome)
3. Infection
   Bacterial, viral, (CMV, EBV, Herpes Zoster, hepatitis B), fungal (*Candida, Aspergillus*), parasitic (pneumocystis)
   a. Abdominal (peri- or intrahepatic abscess)
   b. Biliary tree
   c. Pulmonary
   d. Reactivated virus
   e. Gastrointestinal tract
   f. Catheter associated (intravenous, urinary tract)
4. Graft vascular injury (thrombosis, stenosis)
   a. Hepatic artery
   b. Portal vein
   c. Inferior vena cava (supra- and infrahepatic)
   d. Hepatic vein (left lateral segment grafts), Budd-Chiari recurrence
5. Renal dysfunction
   a. Cyclosporin or other drug induced injury
   b. Tubular necrosis due to hypoperfusion
   c. Pre-existing disease (hepatorenal syndrome)
   d. Hypertension
6. Miscellaneous
   a. Encephalopathy (cyclosporin, tacrolimus, hypertensive, metabolic)
   b. Bowel perforation (steroid, diathermy)
   c. Diaphragm paresis/paralysis
   d. Gastrointestinal hemorrhage (peptic ulceration, variceal)
   e. Obesity (steroids)
   f. Other drug side effects.

present early and late. Biliary complications continue to be a significant problem with an overall incidence of between 10 and 20%, particularly in living related left lateral segment grafts.[33] These complications include bile leak, anastomotic strictures, and non-anastomotic strictures of the donor bile duct with sludge formation.

It is imperative with all suspected biliary complications to ensure that the hepatic artery is patent using Doppler ultrasound or angiography, as hepatic artery thrombosis will cause ischemia and necrosis of the biliary tree.

Simple bile leaks are diagnosed in the early postoperative period by the presence of bile in drainage fluid or in percutaneous aspirate of fluid collections around the liver. Early biliary complications are best treated by immediate surgery and re-anastomosis if required. Late stricture formation may be satisfactorily dealt with by endoscopic or percutaneous balloon dilatation or stenting. Graft ischemia either from hepatic artery thrombosis or portal vein thrombosis can be a devastating complication.[34] The incidence is much less frequent with the use of reduced size liver transplants and microsurgical techniques for living donor transplants. Nevertheless, when it occurs it may lead to graft necrosis, intrahepatic abscess, biliary necrosis and bile leakage. A massive rise in enzyme activity, particularly in the first few days after transplant, may be the first signs. Immediate intervention with thrombectomy and re-anastomosis is only occasionally successful. Bowel perforation is also a well recognized complication with predisposing factors, which include previous surgery (Kasai porto-enterostomy), steroid therapy and hypoxemia due to porto-pulmonary syndrome.[35] Rarely, diaphragmatic hernia has also been reported.[36]

Late presentations may be less acute and typically present with gram-negative sepsis, liver abscess or biliary complications.[37-39] An early hepatic artery thrombosis usually means that the patient will require an urgent liver retransplant. Late thrombosis may be asymptomatic and if so can be ignored. Although technical factors usually account for most cases, it is advisable to maintain the hematocrit at around 30% to improve microvascular flow. Portal vein thrombosis usually presents with a degree of liver dysfunction with prolonged clotting and portal hypertension, which may be heralded by an esophageal variceal bleed. Immediate thrombectomy may be successful.

Where portal vein thrombosis is established, a meso-portal (Rex) shunt, with a vein graft taken from the internal jugular vein and interposed between the superior mesenteric vein and the left branch of the portal vein, may be curative.[39] Inferior vena cava thrombosis or venous outflow obstructions are now rare, particularly since the triangular technique of caval anastomosis has been practiced. Thrombosis in the IVC may develop either in the immediate postoperative period presenting with ascites and lower body edema or later on due to regeneration of the graft and twisting of the caval anastomosis. Thrombolytic therapy may be successful in late thromboses but should be avoided in early thromboses as uncontrollable bleeding may occur from raw surfaces particularly if a reduced size liver was transplanted. Hepatic venous outflow obstruction is suspected if there is persistence of ascites and is confirmed by liver biopsy findings of congestion, and ultrasound and red cell extravasation around central veins.

MEDICAL FOLLOW-UP AND LATE COMPLICATIONS[40-54]

Most patients can be discharged from the intensive care unit within the first week after transplantation. The majority of infections can be prevented. However, should the patient require excessive immunosuppression for persistent rejection, almost inevitably they will develop some opportunistic infections.

In this situation, not only must specific therapy be directed at the pathogen but also immunosuppression must be reduced. Cytomegalovirus is best monitored with PP65 antigen and polymerase chain reaction (PCR) measurement of the virus.

Post-transplantation lymphoproliferative disorder (PTLPD) presents from the first few weeks after transplant to several years later with a mean time of onset around nine months. A typical presentation is initially with acute membranous tonsillitis and associated cervical lymphadenopathy, which is resistant to antibiotic therapy. However, the disease may be widespread and gastrointestinal and central nervous system involvement is common.

Management strategies include reduction of immunosuppression, which may require complete withdrawal along with standard anti-lymphoma chemotherapy, particularly with the monoclonal type. Mortality varies from 20 to 70% or more. Prophylactic intravenous ganciclovir given for a prolonged period may be effective in preventing EBV activation, which is the promoter of PTLD in most cases. Hepatitis B infection has been a problem particularly if hepatitis B core antibody positive donors are used where HBV in the graft occurs in up to 80% of cases. There is frequently progression to active hepatitis although antiviral therapy using famciclovir or lamivudine along with hepatitis B immunoglobulin may be effective in controlling the virus, which is monitored with regular DNA levels.

Most children are hypertensive and require some anti-hypertensive agent for a period of time post-transplant. A degree of renal impairment is almost inevitable in those patients suffering from chronic liver disease and with the additional burden of the use of nephrotoxic immunosuppressive drugs such as cyclosporin and tacrolimus many have significant renal impairment of function in the long-term. The importance of renal sparing strategies in immunosuppression is becoming increasingly evident as long-term survivors present with drug induced renal failure.

Chronic rejection is an irreversible phenomenon, which is chiefly intrahepatic and ductular rather than a vascular phenomenon in contrast to other organ transplants. This is usually manifested by disruption of bile duct radicals with development of the vanishing bile duct syndrome. The incidence seems less frequent with tacrolimus based immunosuppressive regimens as opposed to cyclosporin where an incidence of up to 10% has been recorded. Late chronic rejection may also be associated with a vasculopathy affecting larger arteries.

RETRANSPLANTATION

Ten to 20% of patients may suffer graft failure at some time and need retransplantation. Early indications may be primary non-function, early hepatic arterial thrombosis, severe drug resistant acute rejection and established chronic rejection. Early retransplantation is technically a much less traumatic procedure than the original transplant although the patient may be in a poorer condition. Outcome largely depends on the indication for retransplantation and is quite good for technical causes but less satisfactory for rejection and infection. An increasingly poorer outcome can be expected after third and fourth retransplants and the efficacy and ethics of these interventions are in question.

LONG-TERM SURVIVAL AND QUALITY OF LIFE

One year survival of > 95% is being achieved in the best centers with predicted 10-year survivals of around 70-75%. Patients grafted for acute liver failure have done less well with a higher early death rate usually associated with cerebral complications and multi-organ failure. Excellent quality of life can be achieved and most children are fully rehabilitated.

It is however increasingly evident that prolonged cholestatic jaundice and malnutrition in infancy may have late effects and despite good physical rehabilitation evidence of significant cognitive deficits, which present during early schooling as learning difficulties and attention deficit disorder, are common. As with any immunosuppressed patient, the incidence of neoplasia in a lifetime is greatly increased.

RESULTS

Liver transplantation for infants and children has been available in South Africa for more than a decade. Concerns have shifted from an initial target of short-term survival to quality of life in the long-term. Since 1985, more than 300 patients have been assessed with 124 being accepted for transplantation. Ninety-two have undergone liver transplantation, 90 at the Red Cross Children's Hospital and 2 abroad. Biliary atresia (52%) was the most frequent diagnosis followed by acute liver failure (ALF) (16%). Waiting list mortality has remained high (15%), particularly for the ALF group (50%).

Sixty-three patients survive (72%), 2 months to 22 years post-transplant. Survival since 1996, when HBV core antibody positive donors were excluded and an active anti-viral prophylaxis program was instituted has been > 80%. Early post-transplant mortality was low (7%) but late morbidity and mortality (23%) was mainly due to viral infections: de novo hepatitis B (5 patients and 2 deaths), EBV-related PTLPD (6 patients and 4 deaths), and CMV disease (10 patients and 5 deaths), were most frequently implicated. Tuberculosis prophylaxis, required in 6 cases, resulted in major morbidity in 1. Hypertension requiring medication along with some compromise of renal function has been present in all but 2 patients. However, all those of school going age attend school normally and remain in good health. Only 3 of the survivors have abnormal liver function tests.

Successful liver transplantation is possible in a developing country with limited resources. Scarcity of virus free donors (HIV and HBV) has led to waiting list mortality and infrequent retransplantation. The consequences of prolonged immunosuppression, infections, lymphoma and renal toxicity remain challenges. Compliance problems with medication particularly amongst teenagers, has required constant vigilance and supervision.

CONCLUSION

Careful planning, extensive preparation of personnel and a broad base of skills along with good teamwork between health professionals are required for the development of a successful pediatric transplant program. Surgical technique, anesthetic skills, and medical care of the highest order are essential.

A patient with a liver transplant is a patient for life and requires complete commitment from the transplant medical and surgical team, which cannot be abrogated after discharge from hospital. Endemic viral and bacterial infections particularly HBV, CMV, EBV and tuberculosis, impact negatively on any program in the setting of a developing country.

Extended hospital stay may be required and this, along with long-term therapy may be expensive. Hepatitis B acquired with the liver graft is a tragic occurrence and is not a benign disease. Pretransplant immunization and avoiding the use of hepatitis B core antibody positive donors will reduce the incidence to almost nil but is likely to greatly reduce the numbers of cadaver donor livers presenting particularly if hepatitis B is endemic in the local population. Unfortunately, prophylactic therapeutic measures are costly.

The need for pediatric liver transplants has been assessed at approximately 1 to 2 children per million per year. Thus, transplant activity should be concentrated in specific centers preferably doing more that 12 transplants a year. The shortage of donor organs will continue and future efforts must be focused on maximum use of cadaver donors and increasing living related donation. Transplant activity is rapidly increasing throughout the developing world. This endeavour should be strongly supported as poor socio-economic status is not a contraindication to transplantation and we have frequently been impressed by how parents with relatively few material resources have been able to diligently care for their children. No child with end stage liver disease should be denied the opportunity of receiving appropriate treatment. As with any new development, knowledge and experience improves, costs decline and success is ensured.

These challenges must be met to offer any infant or child requiring liver replacement a chance of a life. The ultimate aim is to restore the child to normal health such that he/she can grow up into a productive healthy adult who can make his/her contribution to society and develop all of his/her human potential.

REFERENCES

1. Eiseman B. The puzzle people: memoirs of a transplant surgeon. Arch Surg, 1992;127(9):1009-11.
2. Vilca-Melendez H, Heaton ND, Paediatric liver transplantation: the surgical view. Postgrad Med J, 2004; 80(948):571-76.
3. Otte JB. Paediatric liver transplantation—a review based on 20 years of personal experience. Transpl Int, 2004;17(10):562-73.
4. Otte JB. History of pediatric liver transplantation. Where are we coming from? Where do we stand? Pediatr Transplant, 2002;6(5):378-87.
5. Shepherd RW. The treatment of end-stage liver disease in childhood. Aust Paediatr J, 1988;24(4):213-16.
6. Baker A, Dhawan A, Heaton N, Who needs a liver transplant? (new disease specific indications). Arch Dis Child, 1998;79(5):460-64.
7. McDiarmid SV, et al. Indications for pediatric liver transplantation. Pediatr Transplant, 1998;2(2):106-16.
8. Le Coultre, C, et al. Biliary atresia and orthotopic liver transplantation 11 years of experience in Geneva. Swiss Surg, 2001;7(5):199-204.
9. Francavilla, R, et al. Prognosis of alpha-1-antitrypsin deficiency-related liver disease in the era of paediatric liver transplantation J Hepatol, 2000;32(6):986-92.
10. Burdelski M, et al. Treatment of inherited metabolic disorders by liver transplantation. J Inherit Metab Dis, 1991;14(4):604-18.
11. Sokal, EM, et al. Liver transplantation in mitochondrial respiratory chain disorders. Eur J Pediatr, 1999;158 Suppl 2:S81-84.
12. Cox, KL, WE Berquist, RO Castillo. Paediatric liver transplantation: indications, timing and medical complications. J Gastroenterol Hepatol, 1999;14 Suppl:S61-66.
13. Shneider, BL. Pediatric liver transplantation in metabolic disease: clinical decision making. Pediatr Transplant, 2002;6(1):25-29.
14. Van Obbergh LJ, et al. Hepatopulmonary syndrome and liver transplantation: a review of the peroperative management of seven paediatric cases. Paediatr Anaesth, 1998;8(1):59-64.
15. Otte JB, et al. Organ procurement in children—surgical, anaesthetic and logistic aspects. Intensive Care Med, 1989;15 Suppl 1:S67-70.
16. Christophi C, B Morgan, I McInnes. A comparison of standard and rapid infusion methods of liver preservation during multi-organ procurement. Aust N Z J Surg, 1991; 61(9):692-94.
17. de Ville de Goyet J, et al. Standardized quick en bloc technique for procurement of cadaveric liver grafts for pediatric liver transplantation. Transpl Int, 1995;8(4): 280-85.
18. Miller C MV. Makowka L, Gorgon RD, Todo S, Bowman J, Morris M, Ligush J, Starzl TE. Rapid flush technique for donor hepatectomt: safety and efficacy of an improved method of liver recovery for transplantation. Transplant Proc, 1988; 20 (Suppl 1):948-50.
19. Tan KC, et al. Surgical anatomy of donor extended right trisegmentectomy before orthotopic liver transplantation in children. Br J Surg, 1991;78(7):805-08.
20. Badger IL, et al. Hepatic transplantation in children using reduced size allografts. Br J Surg, 1992;79(1):47-49.
21. Neuhaus P, KP Platz. Liver transplantation: newer surgical approaches. Baillieres Clin Gastroenterol, 1994;8(3):481-93.
22. Spearman CW, et al. Liver transplantation at Red Cross War Memorial Children's Hospital. S Afr Med J, 2006;96(9 Pt 2): 960-63.
23. Millar, AJ, et al. Liver transplantation for children—the Red Cross Children's Hospital Experience. Pediatr Transplant, 2004;8(2):136-44.
24. Settmacher U, et al. Living-donor liver transplantation— European Experiences. Nephrol Dial Transplant, 2004;19 Suppl 4:iv16-21.
25. Krenn CG, P Faybik, H Hetz. Living-related liver transplantation: implication for the anaesthetist. Curr Opin Anaesthesiol, 2004;17(3):285-90.
26. Baker A, et al. Assessment of potential donors for living related liver transplantation. Br J Surg, 1999;86(2):200-05.
27. Muiesan P, Vergani D, Mieli-Vergani G, Liver transplantation in children. J Hepatol, 2007;46(2):340-48.
28. Reding R, et al. The paediatric liver transplantation program at the Universite catholique de Louvain. Acta Gastroenterol Belg, 2004;67(2):176-78.
29. Reding R, et al. Steroid-free liver transplantation in children. Lancet, 2003;362(9401):2068-70.
30. Lloret J, et al. Biliary complications in hepatic transplantation in children. Cir Pediatr, 1993;6(2):63-65.
31. Chardot C, et al. Biliary complications after paediatric liver transplantation: Birmingham's experience. Transpl Int, 1995; 8(2):133-40.
32. Lopez-Santamaria M, et al. Late biliary complications in pediatric liver transplantation. J Pediatr Surg, 1999;34(2): 316-20.
33. Griffith JF, John PR, Imaging of biliary complications following paediatric liver transplantation. Pediatr Radiol, 1996;26(6):388-94.
34. Stringer MD, et al. Survival and outcome after hepatic artery thrombosis complicating pediatric liver transplantation. J Pediatr Surg, 2001;36(6):888-91.
35. Vilca Melendez, H, et al. Bowel perforation after paediatric orthotopic liver transplantation. Transpl Int, 1998;11(4): 301-04.

36. McCabe AJ, et al. Right-sided diaphragmatic hernia in infants after liver transplantation. J Pediatr Surg, 2005;40(7):1181-84.
37. Duncan KA, King SE, Ratcliffe JF. Intraperitoneal fluid collections following liver transplantation in a paediatric population. Clin Radiol, 1995;50(1):40-43.
38. Lo CM, Liu CL, Fan ST, Correction of left hepatic vein redundancy in paediatric liver transplantation. Asian J Surg, 2005;28(1):55-57.
39. Chardot C, et al. Portal vein complications after liver transplantation for biliary atresia. Liver Transpl Surg, 1997; 3(4):351-58.
40. Sokal EM, Quality of life after orthotopic liver transplantation in children. An overview of physical, psychological and social outcome. Eur J Pediatr, 1995;154(3):171-75.
41. Bouchut, JC, et al. Postoperative infectious complications in paediatric liver transplantation: a study of 48 transplants. Paediatr Anaesth, 2001;11(1):93-98.
42. Debray D, et al. Therapy for acute rejection in pediatric organ transplant recipients. Paediatr Drugs, 2003;5(2):81-93.
43. Britton, PD, et al. The role of hepatic vein Doppler in diagnosing acute rejection following paediatric liver transplantation. Clin Radiol, 1992;45(4):228-32.
44. Lang T, et al. Elevated biliary interleukin 5 as an indicator of liver allograft rejection. Transpl Immunol, 1995;3(4):291-98.
45. D'Antiga L, et al. Late cellular rejection in paediatric liver transplantation: aetiology and outcome. Transplantation, 2002;73(1):80-84.
46. Davison SM, et al. Chronic hepatitis in children after liver transplantation: role of hepatitis C virus and hepatitis G virus infections. J Hepatol, 1998;28(5):764-70.
47. Mellon, A, et al. Cytomegalovirus infection after liver transplantation in children. J Gastroenterol Hepatol, 1993; 8(6):540-44.
48. McGavin JK, Goa KL. Ganciclovir: an update of its use in the prevention of cytomegalovirus infection and disease in transplant recipients. Drugs, 2001;61(8):1153-83.
49. Couchoud C. Cytomegalovirus prophylaxis with antiviral agents for solid organ transplantation. Cochrane Database Syst Rev, 2000(2):CD001320.
50. Hardikar W, et al. Successful treatment of cytomegalovirus-associated haemophagocytic syndrome following paediatric orthotopic liver transplantation. J Paediatr Child Health, 2006;42(6):389-91.
51. Rombaux. P, et al. Post-transplant lymphoproliferative disorder with supraglottic involvement. B-Ent, 2005;1(1):53-56.
52. Meru, N, et al. Epstein-Barr virus infection in paediatric liver transplant recipients: detection of the virus in post-transplant tonsillectomy specimens. Mol Pathol, 2001;54(4):264-69.
53. Lee TC, et al. Use of cytokine polymorphisms and Epstein-Barr virus viral load to predict development of post-transplant lymphoproliferative disorder in paediatric liver transplant recipients. Clin Transplant, 2006;20(3):389-93.
54. Adetiloye VA, John PR. Intervention for pleural effusions and ascites following liver transplantation. Pediatr Radiol, 1998;28(7):539-43.
55. Avitzur Y, et al. Health status ten years after pediatric liver transplantation—looking beyond the graft. Transplantation, 2004;78(4):566-73.
56. Burdelski M, et al. Liver transplantation in children: long-term outcome and quality of life. Eur J Pediatr, 1999;158 Suppl 2:S34-42.
57. Noujaim HM, et al. Techniques for and outcome of liver transplantation in neonates and infants weighing up to 5 kilograms. J Pediatr Surg, 2002;37(2):159-64.
58. Le Coultre C, Mentha G, Belli DC. Liver transplantation in children: past, present and future. Eur J Pediatr Surg, 1997; 7(4):221-26.

Biliary Atresia

CK Sinha, DK Gupta, Mark Davenport

Jaundice is the clinical description for the yellowish tinge to the skin, mucous membranes and sclera caused by raised levels of bilirubin in the blood. The word itself derives from Old French (Jaundice = yellow). Interestingly the alternative medical term, icteric, derives from the Greek word (Ikteros) for a variety of yellow bird. It was believed that a sufferer from jaundice would be cured by gazing at such a bird!

The normal range of total and conjugated bilirubin are < 1 mg/dL (< 17 µmol/L) and < 0.25 mg/dL (< 5 µmol/L) respectively, although jaundice can only be appreciated when total bilirubin is greater than 4 mg/dL (~50 µmol/L).

BILIRUBIN METABOLISM

Bilirubin is an open chain tetrapyrrole with eight side chains (Mol. wt. = 585) and a metabolic by-product of red cell breakdown (largely in the spleen). Hem is converted (enzyme: hem oxygenase via biliverdin) to bilirubin which is transported (on albumin) to the liver in an unconjugated fat-soluble form. Hepatocyte uptake occurs with (enzyme: UDPGT) conversion to the water soluble form by conjugation with glucuronic acid. This is then excreted into the biliary canaliculus.

Further metabolism occurs in the ileum (to urobilinogen which is absorbed and re-excreted in urine) and colon (stercobilinogen - excreted in stools) although the process is poorly developed in infancy.

PHYSIOLOGICAL JAUNDICE

Physiological jaundice (always unconjugated) occurs from 2nd to 10th days of life and is due to a number of factors including immaturity of neonatal liver enzymes and shortened postnatal red cell survival. Prematurity, growth retardation, breast feeding and cephalohematoma tend to exacerbate the intensity and duration of physiological jaundice. Usually, serum bilirubin levels do not rise above 8 mg/dl in a full-term and 12 mg/dl in a premature infant. At high levels, unconjugated bilirubin can cross the blood-brain barrier and cause brain injury (kernicterus). The usual therapy for unconjugated jaundice is phototherapy and occasionally exchange transfusion.

MEDICAL CAUSES OF CONJUGATED JAUNDICE

There are important medical causes of conjugated jaundice which include Alpha-1- antrypsin deficiency, giant cell hepatitis, cytomegalovirus hepatitis, Alagille's syndrome (biliary hypoplasia, abnormal vertebrae, pulmonary stenosis, odd facies), cystic fibrosis and galactosemia (due to defect in enzyme galactose-1-phosphate uridyl transferase).

From 2-15% of neonates will remain clinically jaundiced beyond 2 weeks. Although only in 0.2-0.4% neonates, will this be a conjugated jaundice due to hepatobiliary disease of either medical or surgical origin. All infants with persistence of jaundice beyond 2 weeks and in the absence of an apparent medical cause should be investigated for a potential surgical cause. Figure 89.1 illustrates a suitable investigation algorithm used to discriminate between the various causes of surgical jaundice.

The most common surgical causes included biliary atresia, choledochal malformation, inspissated bile syndrome, spontaneous perforation of bile duct and rarely the tumors.

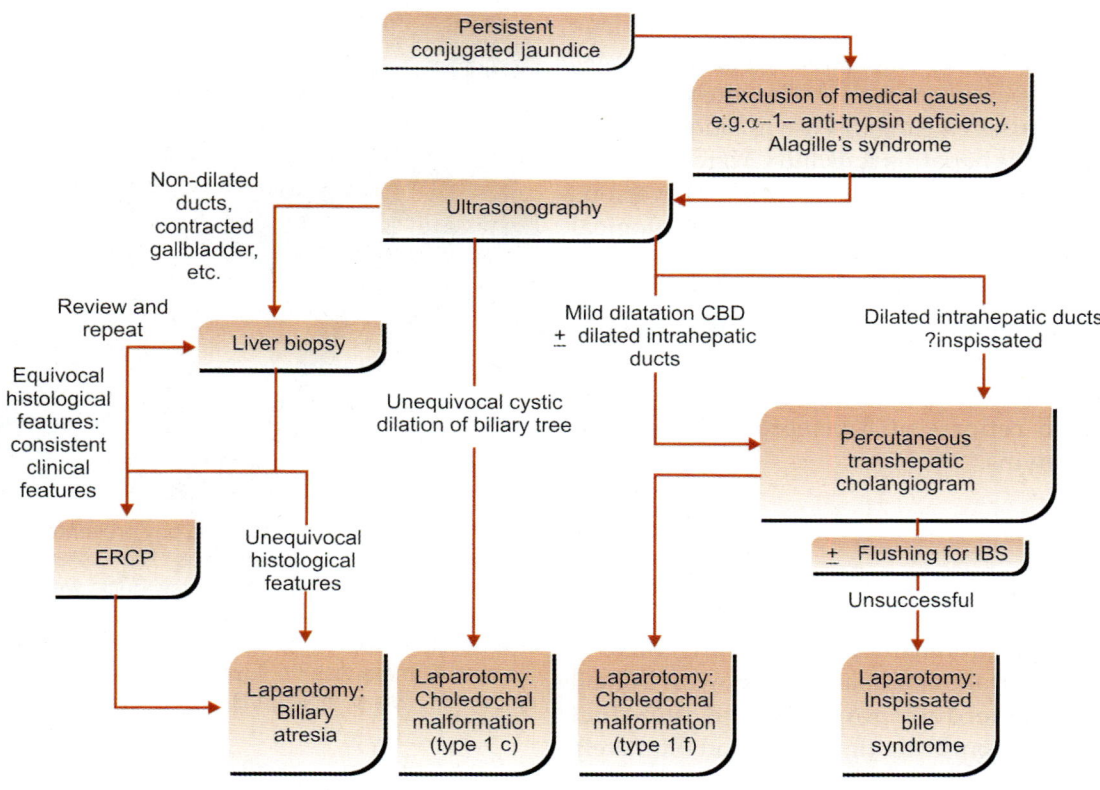

Fig. 89.1: Algorithm for investigating case of surgical jaundice

BILIARY ATRESIA

Biliary atresia (BA) is a cholangio-destructive disease affecting both the intra- and extra-hepatic biliary tract ultimately leading to obliteration of the ducts, cirrhosis and liver failure. The incidence is higher in Japan and China (1 in 9,000) than in Europe and the UK (1 in 16,000).[1,2]

ETIOLOGY AND PATHOGENESIS

The exact etiology of BA remains obscure, and hypotheses abound. Whatever the cause, the process leads to complete obliteration of the lumen of extrahepatic bile ducts and progressive cellular inflammation of the intra-hepatic ducts.[3,4]

1. In some infants there is evidence to suggest that the process begins early in gestation. Thus antenatal ultrasonography allows detection of that subgroup of BA that show cystic changes within the extrahepatic ducts.[5] Furthermore, about 10% cases of all cases have other congenital anomalies.[6,7] These anomalies are unusual but characteristic such as polysplenia, asplenia, situs inversus, absence of inferior vena cava and pre-duodenal portal vein, for which the term Biliary Atresia Splenic Malformation (BASM) syndrome has been coined.[6] In these infants there is a high incidence of first trimester maternal problems such as diabetes and it is a reasonable supposition that all of the constituent anomalies occur during the critical period of organogenesis within that period.

There are similarities between the appearance of developing bile ducts at the porta hepatis at 12-14 weeks gestation and the appearance of the residual biliary ductules at the porta hepatis in BA patients, suggesting that even some cases of isolated BA may be due to alteration in bile duct development and remodeling.[8]

Alternatively, BA may arise due to damage of a fully-developed biliary tract at some point in postor at least perinatal life. Thus, some studies report an association of a host of various gastrointestinal viral infections with BA including reovirus type 3, cytomegalovirus respiratory syncitial virus, Epstein-

Barr virus, human papillomavirus and rotavirus type A.[9-18] Other similar studies on the same viruses, however have been negative.[19-21] The most common hepatotropic viruses causing disease in older children and adults (such as hepatitis A, B and C) have not been related to BA in infants.[22-23] There are also various animal models which can mimic the pathological features of BA and rely upon exposure of the newborn animal to viruses such as rotavirus.[24-26]

Genetics may play a role in the pathogenesis of BA, although this is probably a fairly minor role in most. Familial cases of BA have been rarely reported, but there are also reports of BA seen in discordant monozygotic twins.[27-34]

PATHOLOGY

The gross appearance of the extrahepatic biliary tract varies from an inflamed, hypertrophic occluded biliary tract to an atrophic remnant. Histologically, the liver has features of portal tract inflammation, with a small cell infiltrate, bile duct plugging and bile duct proliferation. Later on, bridging fibrosis and ultimately biliary cirrhosis occurs.

The lumen of the extrahepatic duct is obliterated at a variable level and this forms the basis for the commonest classification in clinical use as suggested by the Japanese Society of Pediatric Surgeons (JSPS) (Table 89.1). In the Type I BA, the atresia involves the common bile duct only. In type II, the atresia involves the common hepatic duct only. Type III BA, is the commonest (~ 90% cases) type and involves the whole of the extrahepatic biliary tree, including the porta hepatic. In this type, there are no visible ducts present.

An important variation is that of cystic change, seen in about 5% of cases, within some part of the extrahepatic biliary tract. Some cysts contain mucus, while others contain bile. The cyst is usually small, about a cm in diameter (Figs 89.2A and B) while rarely it could attain a large size and is very thin walled and transparent, filled with bile stained fluid (Figs 89.3A and B). If it is bile, there may be diagnostic confusion with that of a true choledochal cyst. In cystic biliary atresia, the wall is invariably thickened, lacks an epithelial lining and communicates poorly with abnormal non-dilated intrahepatic ducts. This should be evident at operative or percutaneous cholangiography.[35,36]

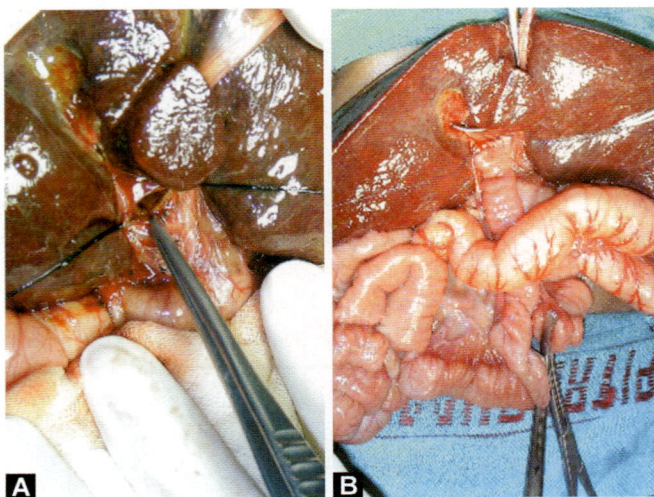

Figs 89.2A and B: A 3-month-old boy presented as EHBA with a cyst (1x1cm) at the portahepatis. The liver was cirrhotic and the LFT were deranged. Intrahepatic ducts were absent. HIDA showed no excretion even after 24 hrs. USG failed to pick up a small cyst, about 1x1 cm, at the porta hepatic. After opening the cyst **A.** there was no flow of bile. Cystojejunostomy with a Roux-en-Y was completed **B.**

PRESENTATION

All patients with BA present with varying degree of jaundice, clay-colored stools and dark yellow urine. The severity of jaundice increases steadily and it is not unusual to find bilirubin levels around 20 mg% at the time of first presentation in developing countries. Failure to thrive, coagulopathy and anemia are not uncommon. Some will present with signs of advanced disease and cirrhosis such as ascites, umbilical hernia, prominent abdominal veins and respiratory discomfort. In comparison to European or North American experience, most cases in developing countries present late. In a review of BA, only 5% cases were seen below 60 days of age, 40% between 2 and 3 months, 30% between 3 and 4 months and 25% presented beyond 4 months of age. Hepatomegaly was seen in all and 60% patients had a palpable spleen.[37]

Table 89.1: Types of biliary atresia	
Type I	Atresia of the common bile duct
Type II	Atresia of the common hepatic duct
Type III	Atresia of the whole extrahepatic biliary tree up to the portahepatis

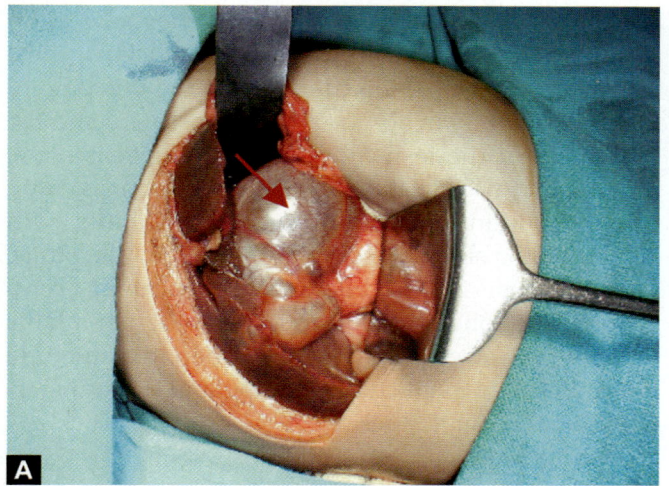 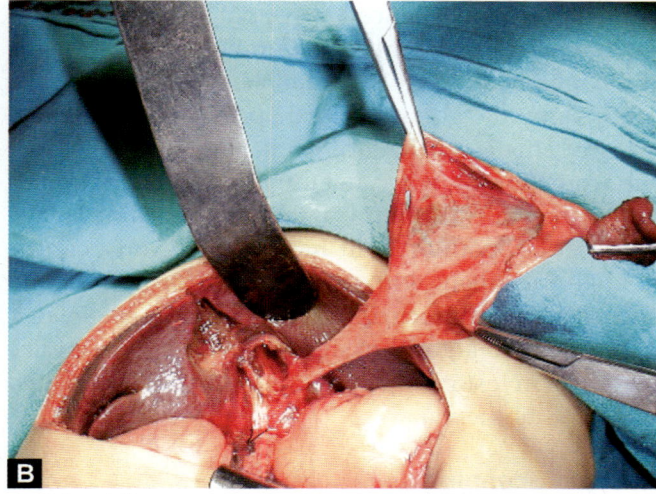

Figs 89.3A and B: A 5-month-old girl presenting with features resembling biliary atresia was found to have a large cyst (arrow) **A.** The wall of the cyst was transparent and thin **B.** Preoperatively, MRCP was suggestive of the diagnosis of a large choledochal cyst. However, intrahepatic biliary ducts were not dilated. Liver was cirrhotic. The fluid was bile stained but the cyst did not have any communication above or below. Such large cysts in association with biliary atresia are very uncommon. Hepaticoportoenterostomy was performed. Prognosis is guarded

A fair idea can be made in over 80% cases using the bedside clinical scoring system whether it is a case of biliary atresia or neonatal hepatitis.[38]

DIAGNOSIS

The clinical diagnosis of BA is usually quite obvious in late-presenting cases. However, in infants of < 60 days, the diagnosis can be difficult. Key investigations include ultrasonography, biochemical liver function tests, nuclear imaging, viral serology, and a percutaneous liver biopsy. In some centers, duodenal intubation and measurement of intralumenal bile is practiced as the routine test for BA. Newer modalities such as ERCP and MRCP have been used at times, although the former is clearly highly operator-dependent and the latter not sufficiently precise in its delineation of infantile biliary anatomy to offer real advantage.[39] Possibly in most surgical centers, operative cholangiography remains the principal investigation in demonstrating biliary patency. This can also be performed laparoscopically with apparently good results.[40]

Liver Function Tests (LFTs)

LFTs are abnormal in all patients of BA and neonatal hepatitis. There is a rise in total serum bilirubin (mainly conjugated) and fall in serum proteins (especially albumin) and a reversal of the albumin/globulin ratio in advanced cases. Alkaline phosphatase and transaminase (e.g. SGOT, SGPT) levels all rise. Deranged LFTs correspond to the degree of parenchymal damage rather than the duration of disease. Serum γ-Glutamyl transpeptidase (GGTP) levels more than 250 units are suggestive of obstruction due to biliary atresia while the GGTP levels less than 150 units are indicative of neonatal hepatitis.[41]

Imaging

Hepatobiliary ultrasound after 12 hours of fasting (with intravenous fluid support) is perhaps the initial investigation of choice. Certainly BA is highly unlikely if a dilated intrahepatic biliary duct is found (being more indicative of an obstructed choledochal cyst, or inspissated bile syndrome). Percutaneous liver biopsy after exclusion of medical causes of cholestatic jaundice (e.g. Alpha 1-antitrypsin deficiency, Alagille's syndrome, and neonatal hepatitis) is a helpful investigation in diagnosis, but relies upon expert pathological interpretation. Negative ultrasonography and positive histology results should be able to establish the correct preoperative diagnosis in about 85% cases of BA.[42] In our series, an incorrect (typically giant-cell hepatitis) or nonspecific biopsy diagnosis was reported in about 15% of those eventually shown to have BA.[42] ERCP may be considered in infants with equivocal biopsy results, although it should be noted that this diagnosis depends crucially on failure to show a biliary tree, and hence appropriate experience and judgment are essential.[42] Percutaneous transhepatic cholangiography (PTC) is valuable in those diagnostic groups in which dilated intrahepatic bile ducts are a feature. This is particularly so in the inspissated bile syndrome group, when not only can the diagnosis be established but an attempt at therapeutic saline lavage also can be made. About half of this group can be treated effectively without the need for laparotomy and without any recurrence or long-term sequelae.[42] The simplified algorithm shown in Fig. 89.1 should be helpful in investigating these children with conjugated hyperbilirubinemia.

Nuclear Scanning

Excretion of Technetium labeled isotopes into the gut within 24 hours, establishes the patency of the biliary tract. However, a negative scan even after 24 hours may still be consistent with both BA and advanced stage of neonatal hepatitis. Negative HIDA scans may be repeated after one week of phenobarbitone therapy, if clinically indicated. Phenobarbitone is known to stimulate the hepatic enzymes and increase the flow of bile. One study showed that 40% patients with neonatal hepatitis excreted the isotope into the gut within 24 hours in postluminal HIDA scan while that of BA again failed to do so.[43] Alternatively, further improvements have been suggested with the addition of betamethasone to phenobarbitone prior to HIDA scanning.[43] To improve the efficacy and also importantly without loosing any time, it is recommended that the infants with suspected biliary atresia undergoing nuclear imaging, should be primed by both, the phenobarbitone and the betamethasone for a week instead of phenobarbitone alone. Though the exact mechanism is not known, yet the steroids serve not only as choleretics but also as anti-inflammatory and antifibrotic agents. These are also known to stabilize the cell membrane of the red blood cells to prevent their early breakdown thus reducing the bilirubin load to the liver.

Percutaneous Needle Biopsy

Sometimes the interpretation of biopsy can be difficult and need experienced pathologist as there is a lot of overlapping in the histologic finding of BA and neonatal hepatitis. There is also an inherent risk of bleeding in performing needle biopsy. While this forms a regular armamentarium of the diagnostic workup of the patient under care of the pediatricians, most pediatric surgeon do not depend on the outcome of this investigation in absence of the sensitivity and the specificity of the test. Infants with choletasis show inflammatory infiltrate, hepatocellular necrosis, mild portal proliferation and fibrosis. The infants with biliary atresia show bile duct proliferation, bile plugs, portal fibrosis with well preserved normal architecture. The common features on histology in infants with biliary atresia and neonatal hepatitis include multinucleated giant cells, pseudoglandular transformation and hematopoesis.

Duodenal Drainage Test

A 4 hourly duodenal aspiration is done to confirm the presence of bile in it. Again, the test may be false-negative in patients of neonatal hepatitis with severe cholestasis. A presence of bile in the aspirate confirms patency of the biliary tree. Before resorting to surgery, neonatal hepatitis can still be suspected if the liver is soft, the jaundice is fluctuating, the color of the urine is not dark, the GGTP values are less than 150 units. HIDA may or may not show excretion depending on the degree of cholestasis.

Peroperative Cholangiogram

In most centers, having excluded medical causes of jaundice and failed to show isotope excretion in a HIDA scan, then progression to peroperative cholangiogram is a reasonable option. The key observation at laparotomy is presence or absence of bile in the gallbladder. Clearly in the presence of bile, apart from the rare type 1 cases, then BA can be excluded. Cholangiogram through the gallbladder should demonstrate the entire biliary tree, but in those cases, where only the distal common bile duct (CBD) opacifies an attempt should be made to delineate the proximal intrahepatic tree by application of a distal vascular clamp in the common bile duct.

SURGICAL MANAGEMENT

Currently BA is being Managed in Two Phases

First Phase

An attempt to preserve the infant's own liver. This usually involves the Kasai operation which essentially excises all extrahepatic biliary remnants leaving a transected portal plate, followed by biliary reconstruction using a Roux loop onto that plate as a portoenterostomy.

Second Phase

If bile flow is not restored at exploration or life-threatening complications of cirrhosis ensue, then consideration should be given to liver transplantation. Sometimes this is done as a primary procedure, in those who present late with features of advanced cirrhosis.

Preoperative Preparation

Preoperative preparation includes broad-spectrum antibiotics, vitamin K, correction of anemia, hypoproteinemia, chest infection and ascites.

Surgical Technique

The major breakthrough in the surgery for biliary atresia was seen in 1959 when Morio Kasai reported the operative relief of biliary obstruction in infants traditionally considered to have non-correctable biliary atresia.[44] As described by Kasai and modified subsequently by others, the surgical steps of portoenterostomy starts with opening of the abdomen through a right upper transverse incision, a peroperative cholangiogram (if required) and a wedge liver biopsy. Once the diagnosis of BA is established the liver should be mobilized fully, outside of the abdominal cavity (by division of its suspensory ligaments), to ensure maximal exposure of the porta hepatis and facilitate a detailed dissection (Figs 89.4A to C). The atretic gallbladder, cystic duct and the entire remnant extrahepatic biliary tree are excised up to the level of the porta hepatis. The portal dissection itself must be wide extending from exposure of the origin of the umbilical vein from the left portal vein (in the Rex fossa) to the bifurcation of the right portal vein pedicle. Small veins from the portal vein to the portal remnant should also be divided to expose the caudate lobe posteriorly. The correct level of transaction is flush with the liver capsule, where the plane is usually self-evident. Transgression into actual liver parenchyma, however, adds nothing to the success of surgery. Most transected ductules are found in the marginal areas,

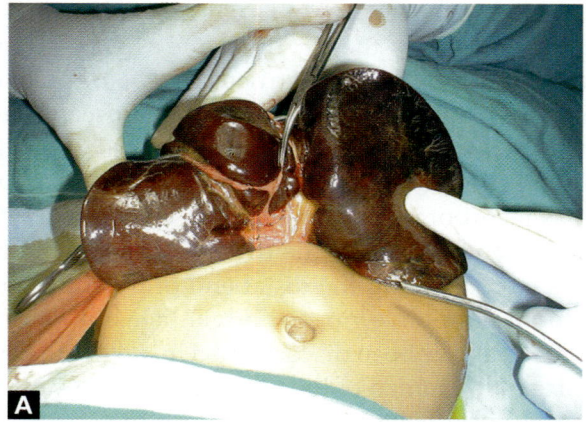
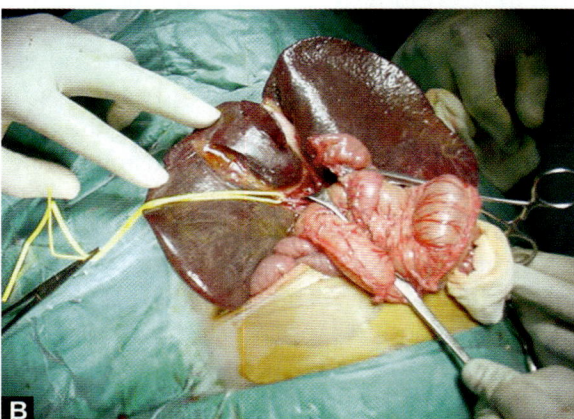
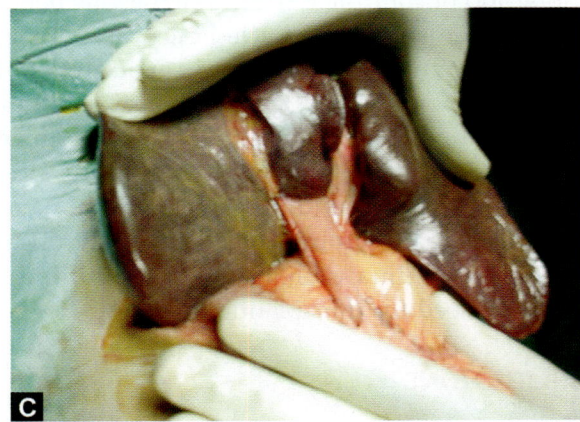

Figs 89.4A to C: Operative procedure for Kasai's hepatico-portoenterostomy (HPE). **A.** The liver has been exteriorized. The gall bladder and the extrahepatic atretic biliary tree has been dissected. The fibrous tissue as the solid cord at the porta hepatic is identified and ready to be transected. **B.** The fibrotic tissue at the porta hepatic has been transected. The portal vein has been retracted downwards gently with a retractor. The right branch of the hepatic artery has been placed in the vessel loop. **C.** The Roux-en-Y loop (about 40 cm long) has been anastomosed to the porta hepatic, to drain the bile into the gut

recapitulating the normal biliary arrangement, and it is important to allow these to drain into a long (~40 cm) Roux loop of jejunum (retrocolic). A single layer anastomosis is performed between the transected end at the porta hepatic and the jejunal loop, using absorbable interrupted sutures (Fig. 89.4C). Modifications such as incorporation of an intussus-ception valve in the ascending limb near the distal end, creation of a stomas or implanting the distal end of the Roux into the duodenum have no real advantages in clinical practice and have been discontinued in most centers.[35] The size of the lumen of the ducts found on histology from the porta hepatic have been grouped as > 150 micron, 50-150 micron and < 50 micron in size. Smaller the size, poorer is the bile flow and the prognosis.

Various technical variants have been proposed according to the anatomical pattern of the biliary remnant. In Type 1 BA, hepaticojejunostomy may be an option. Sometimes the gallbladder may be used as the conduit to the transected portal plate (portocholecystostomy) with a consequent reduction in postoperative cholangititis.[45] The appendix has also been described as a conduit (appendico-duodenostomy).[46]

A number of drugs have been suggested to try and improve postoperative results. For instance, there are anecdotal and uncontrolled studies suggesting benefit from corticosteroids ursodeoxycholic acid and Chinese herbs.[47-51] However, none have been universally accepted and subjected to extensive clinical acceptable scientific scrutiny. The initial results of a randomized double-blind, placebo controlled trial using postoperative prednisolone (2 mg/kg/day) showed a reduction in initial bilirubin levels but no significant difference in ultimate clearance of jaundice or reduction in need for transplantion.[52]

COMPLICATIONS

Early postoperative complications include: cholangitis, bleeding, leak from anastomosis, prolonged ileus, and intestinal obstruction. Late complications include: cessation of bile flow, recurrent cholangitis, portal hypertension, ascites, hepatopulmonary syndrome/pulmonary hypertension, formation of bile-filled cavities in liver and cirrhosis.

Cholangitis

Cholangitis occurs in 30-60% of cases of biliary atreisa after HPE. The attacks are more frequent during the first two years following the Kasai procedure.[52,53] The severity can vary from mild to fulminant sepsis. Clinically, the patient will develop fever or hypothermia, vomiting, jaundice, hepatosplenomegaly, abdominal pain/distension and acholic stools. The diagnosis can be confirmed by blood culture (and conduit cultures if present) and/or liver biopsy.[52] However, although gram-negative organisms or a mixed flora can be seen, mostly cultures are negative. The cause of cholangitis is not clear but there must be an intestinal-biliary communication and therefore the most favored hypothesis is that of an ascending infection from the gut.

Treatment includes resuscitation, intravenous fluid, broad spectrum antibiotics, (and in some centers high doses of steroids) for 7-10 days. In recurrent or late-onset cholangitis, obstruction to the drainage of the Roux loop should be considered.[54] In those where a mechanical cause can not be found, a prolonged course of antibiotics should be considered.[45]

Historically various measures have been tried with to reduce cholangitis although none have stood the test of time. These include creation of external stomas or placing catheters in the proximal limb of the Roux loop, use of an omental wrap applied to the porta hepatis, jejunal loop "valves", creation of an intussuscepted ileocecal conduit and use of an appendiceal conduit based on its vascular pedicle.[46,55-59] Biliary stomas may cause problems such as prolapse, retraction, fluid and electrolyte loss, bleeding and malabsorption due to bile losses. As a routine practice, a valve is incorporated in patients with biliary atresia in the ascending limb of the Roux-en-Y loop with the presumption that the intestinal contents would not be allowed to go up and cause cholangitis.

Portal Hypertension

The incidence of portal hypertension is about 75% after Kasai operation and has a clear relationship with liver fibrosis. In a recent study, it was found that increased portal pressure (measured at the time of Kasai operation) is a bad prognostic sign.[60,61] These patients will have higher chances of developing portal hypertension, even if bilirubin level normalizes after operation. This study reported that portal pressure index (height of the saline level column above the liver surface level) was safe, simple and better predictor of postoperative outcome than the hepatic fibrosis score.[62] Portal hypertension may cause clinically significant variceal formation at the esophagus, stomach, Roux loop and/or rectum. In patients with good liver function, varices are treated with endoscopic sclerotherapy or banding, but in those with persisting jaundice, poor synthetic liver function, then this will only be temporizing and liver transplantation is the only really successful option.[63] Interventional radiological techniques such as transjugular intra-hepatic portosystemic shunts (TIPS) are possible for some cases, as a bridge to transplantation, but requires skill and perseverance if good results are to be obtained. Portal vein hypoplasia may preclude this option. In those unusual cases of life-threatening bleeding, but non-progressive liver disease and good liver function, a conventional portosystemic shunts should be considered, particularly if transplantation is not an option.

Hepatopulmonary syndrome: Hepatopulmonary (HP) syndrome is characterized by hypoxia, cyanosis, dyspnea and clubbing and is due to development of pulmonary arteriovenous shunts. This seems to be due to gut derived vasoactive substances that are not cleared by the cirrhotic liver. The diagnosis is made by pulmonary scintigraphy. HP syndrome can be reversed after liver transplantation.[64,65]

Biliary Lakes

Bile containing cysts can develop in liver post-operatively even in patients with complete clearance of jaundice. These bile lakes could be drained either externally or by cystoenterostomy if infection supervene or they cause pressure on portal veins. Ultimately, liver transplantation may be required in these cases.

Malignancies

In cirrhotic liver patients of biliary atresia, a number of malignancies have been reported including hepatocellular carcinoma, hepatoblastoma and cholangiocarcinoma.[66,67]

OUTCOME

The outcome following Kasai operation can be assessed in two ways:
  i. Clearance of jaundice
 ii. Proportions of native liver survival.

Clearance of jaundice (< 2 mg/dL or < 34 μmol/L) after Kasai has been reported to be around 60%, whereas five year survival with native liver ranges from 35-64%.[68-72] Long-term (10 years or greater) survival have been reported in the range of 27 - 53%.[1,70-72] Only about 15% will have a true long term survival with no jaundice, normal liver biochemistry and no signs of liver disease or portal hypertension.[73] However, even in this apparently "cured" group, liver histology still remains abnormal.[73]

In the children with a failed Kasai operation, liver transplantation is the only hope. The main problems associated with this major operation are lack of a suitable donor, small size of the recipient abdomen, immunosuppression and a significant postoperative morbidity and even mortality. At present, 3-year survival after liver transplantation in good centers is 85-90%.[74,75]

PROGNOSTIC FACTORS

Biliary atresia is a rare disease and surgical outcome following biliary atresia depends upon adequate dissection and restoration of bile flow, together with effective treatment of the two major complications (cholangitis and portal hypertension). A number of factors contribute to good outcome and may be listed as:
  i. Operator experience and size and experience of referral center.
 ii. Extent of the pre-existing liver damage
iii. Frequency of cholangitis
 iv. Syndromic (e.g. BASM) patients have poorer prognosis than non-syndromic group. This may be due to severe cardiac disease and hepatopulmonary syndrome.[6,76]
  v. Age at operation—The age at Kasai operation has an effect on outcome, but it is not as clear-cut as was once thought. There is no real cut-off (e.g. six or eight weeks or 60 days). These were simply the arbitrary values from earlier small studies. There is no doubt that the fibrotic element of the hepatopathology is progressive but beyond what

age an attempt at a Kasai portoenterostomy is pointless, is not known. Some infants will come to surgery early with very soft, non-fibrotic livers, at 20 days for instance, but because they have few residual ductules at the porta hepatis, that their Kasai's will fail. In contrast, some infants will be operated late (beyond 100 days) and 10 year survival in these infants could be 40%.[77]

It is unfortunate that despite ongoing research in the field, biliary atresia remained a dreadful disease, especially in the underdeveloped nations.[78] About 25% infants still present beyond 4 months of age not only with the features of biliary atresia, portal hypertension and ascites but also with severe anemia, chest infections and malnutrition. HPE is a major undertaking and if performed in such advanced cases of biliary atresia (with bilirubin > 10 mg%, age more than 120 days, liver fibrotic), it carries a high morbidity and mortality. In such cases, a modified approach is safer and better in the interest of the patient. This includes the benefit of the surgical exploration, dissection at porta hepatic to assess for the flow of bile and HPE only if there is a bile flow. In absence of bile flow, the porta hepatis is drained with a sump drain for 5-7 days. In the postoperative period, choleresis is induced and even if there is no flow of bile noted in the contents of the drain, it is simply pulled out and the prognosis is explained.[79, 80]

The results of HPE are not satisfactory in the long run and most patients would require liver transplantation, the facilities for which however, remain limited to major centers in the developed world. The availability of live related donors is a serious issue and the waiting list for liver transplant is quite long. Majority infants die during the waiting period alone. Also the surgical expertise, the cost for transplant, the maintenance cost for immunosuppression are also important considerations while considering this option. Thus attempt for finding an alternate procedure remains alive amongst the researchers in the field. Efforts are on to use the modern technology of tissue engineering to produce liver in the laboratory however, the success is still far away due to the complex nature of tissues (biliary system, blood vessels and the hepatocytes) involved in liver regeneration. Artificial liver on the pattern of renal dialysis, is another option but not yet fully successful and easily available. Recently, a significant interest has been generated to use stem cells to treat the damaged liver cells, with the hope that once transplanted the stem cells would repair or replace the diseased hepatocytes to prolong or obviate the need for liver transplantation.[81] With the use of stem cells, the hepatic fibrosis has been shown to have regressed over months and years. However, lot of work is needed to prove this further.[82]

REFERENCES

1. Nio M, Ohi R, Miyanot, et al. Five and 10 year survival rates after surgery for biliary atresia: a report from the Japanese Biliary Atresia Registry. J Pediatr Surg 2003;38:997-1000.
2. McKiernan PJ, Baker AJ, Kelly DA. The frequency and outcome of biliary atresia in the UK and Ireland. Lancet 2000;355:25-29.
3. Balistreri WF, Grand R, Hoofnagle JH, Suchy FJ, Ryckman FC, Perlmutter DH, et al. Biliary atresia: current concepts and research directions. Hepatology 1996;23:1682-92.
4. Fischler B, Haglund B, Hjern A. A population based study on the incidence and possible pre- and perinatal etiological risk factors of biliary atresia. J Pediatr 2002;141:217-22.
5. Hasegawa T, Sasaki T, Kimura T, Sawai T, Nose K, Kamata S, et al. Prenatal ultrasonographic appearance of type IIId (uncorrectable type with cystic dilatation) biliary atresia. Pediatr Surg Int 2002;18:425-28.
6. Davenport M, Savage M, Mowat AP, Howard ER. The Biliary Atresia Splenic Malformation syndrome. Surgery 1993;113:662-68.
7. Kataria R, Kataria A, Gupta DK. Spectrum of Congenital Anomalies Associated with Biliary Atresia. Ind J Pediatr 1996;63 (5):651-54.
8. Tan CE, Driver M, Howard ER, Moscoso GJ. Extrahepatic biliary atresia: A first-trimester event? Clues from light microscopy and immunohistochemistry. J Pediatr Surg 1994;29:808-14.
9. Glaser JH, Balistreri WF, Morecki R. Role of reovirus type 3 in persistent infantile cholestasis. J Pediatr 1984;105:912-15.
10. Morecki R, Glaser JH, Cho S, Balistreri WF, Horwitz MS. Biliary atresia and reovirus type 3 infection. N Engl J Med 1982;307:481-84.
11. Morecki R, Glaser JH, Johnson AB, Kress Y. Detection of reovirus type 3 in the porta hepatis of an infant with extrahepatic biliary atresia: ultrastructural and immunocytochemical study. Hepatology 1984;4:1137-42.
12. Tyler KL, Sokol RJ, Oberhaus SM, Le M, Karrer FM, Narkewicz MR, Tyson RW, Murphy JR, Low R, Brown WR. Detection of reovirus RNA in hepatobiliary tissues from patients with extrahepatic biliary atresia and choledochal cysts. Hepatology 1998;27:1475-82.
13. Fischler B, Ehrnst A, Forsgren M, Orvell C, Nemeth A. The viral association of neonatal cholestasis in Sweden: a possible link between cytomegalovirus infection and extrahepatic biliary atresia. J Pediatr Gastroenterol Nutr 1998;27:57-64.

14. Hart MH, Kaufman SS, Vanderhoof JA, Erdman S, Linder J, Markin RS, Kruger R, Antonson DL. Neonatal hepatitis and extrahepatic biliary atresia associated with cytomegalovirus infection in twins. Am J Dis Child 1991;145:302-05.
15. Nadal D, Wunderli W, Meurmann O, Briner J, Hirsig J. Isolation of respiratory syncytial virus from liver tissue and extrahepatic biliary atresia material. Scand J Infect Dis 1990;22:91-93.
16. Weaver LT, Nelson R, Bell TM. The association of extrahepatic bile duct atresia and neonatal Epstein-Barr virus infection. Acta Paediatr Scand 1984;73: 155-57.
17. Drut R, Drut RM, Gomez MA, Cueto Rua E, Lojo MM. Presence of human papillomavirus in extrahepatic biliary atresia. J Pediatr Gastroenterol Nutr 1998;27: 530-35.
18. Petersen C, Biermanns D, Kuske M, Schakel J, Meyer-Junghanel L, Mildenberger H. New aspects in a murine model for extrahepatic biliary atresia. J Pediatr Surg 1997;32:1190-95.
19. Brown WR, Sokol RJ, Levin MJ, Silverman A, Tamaru T, Lilly JR, Hall RJ, Cheney M. Lack of correlation between infection with reovirus 3 and extrahepatic biliary atresia or neonatal hepatitis. J Pediatr 1988;113:670-76.
20. Dussaix E, Hadchouel M, Tardieu M, Alagille D. Biliary atresia and reovirus type 3 infection. N Engl J Med 1984;310:658.
21. Steele MI, Marshall CM, Lloyd RE, Randolph VE. Reovirus 3 not detected by reverse transcriptase-mediated polymerase chain reaction analysis of preserved tissue from infants with cholestatic liver disease. Hepatology 1995;21:697-702.
22. A-Kader HH, Nowicki MJ, Kuramoto KI, Baroudy B, Zeldis JB, Balistreri WF. Evaluation of the role of hepatitis C virus in biliary atresia. Pediatr Infect Dis J 1994;13: 657-59.
23. Balistreri WF, Tabor E, Gerety RJ. Negative serology for hepatitis A and B viruses in 18 cases of neonatal cholestasis. Pediatrics 1980;66:269-71.
24. Bangaru B, Morecki R, Glaser JH, Gartner LM, Horwitz MS. Comparative studies of biliary atresia in the human newborn and reovirus-induced cholangitis in weanling mice. Lab Invest 1980;43:456-62.
25. Rosenberg DP, Morecki R, Lollini LO, Glaser J, Cornelius CE. Extrahepatic biliary atresia in a rhesus monkey (Macaca mulatta). Hepatology 1983;3:577-80.
26. Petersen C, Biermanns D, Kuske M, Schakel K, Meyer-Junghanel L, Mildenberger H. New aspects in a murine model for extrahepatic biliary atresia. J Pediatr Surg 1997, 32:1190-95.
27. Cunningham ML, Sybert VP. Idiopathic extrahepatic biliary atresia: recurrence in sibs in two families. Am J Med Genet 1988;31:421-26.
28. Gunasekaran TS, Hassall EG, Steinbrecher UP, Yong SL. Recurrence of extrahepatic biliary atresia in two half sibs. Am J Med Genet 1992;43:592-94.
29. Lachaux A, Descos B, Plauchu H, Wright C, Louis D, Raveau J, Hermier M. Familial extrahepatic biliary atresia. J Pediatr Gastroenterol Nutr 1988;7:280-83.
30. Silveira TR, Salzano FM, Howard ER, Mowat AP. Extrahepatic biliary atresia and twinning. Braz J Med Biol Res 1991;24:67-71.
31. Smith BM, Laberge JM, Schreiber R, Weber AM, Blanchard H. Familial biliary atresia in three siblings including twins. J Pediatr Surg 1991;26:1331-33.
32. Hyams JS, Glaser JH, Leichtner AM, Morecki R. Discordance for biliary atresia in two sets of monozygotic twins. J Pediatr 1985;107:420-22.
33. Poovorawan Y, Chongsrisawat V, Tanunytthawongse C, Norapaksunthorn T, Mutirangura A, Chandrakamol B. Extrahepatic biliary atresia in twins: zygosity determination by short tandem repeat loci. J Med Assoc Thai 1996;79 (Suppl 1):S119-S124.
34. Strickland AD, Shannon K, Coln CD. Biliary atresia in two sets of twins. J Pediatr 1985;107:418-20.
35. Davenport M. Biliary atresia. Outcome and management. Ind J Pediatr 2006;73:825-28.
36. Hinds R, Davenport M, Mieli-Vergani G, Hadzic N. Antenatal presentation of biliary atresia. J Pediatr 2004;144: 43-46.
37. Gupta DK. Experience with Biliary Atresia Disease at AIIMS during the Past Decade. Jour. IAPS, 1999;4(2): 84-89.
38. Gupta DK, Srinivas M, Bajpai M. AIIMS Clinical Score: A reliable rate to distinguish neonatal hepatitis from extra hepatic biliary atresia Ind. J Pediatr 2001;68:605-08.
39. Ohnuma N, Takahashi H, Tanabe M, Yoshida H, Iwai J. The role of ERCP in biliary atresia. Gastrointest Endosc 1997;45:365-70.
40. Okasaki T, Miyano G, Yamataka A, et al. Diagnostic laparoscopy-assisted cholangiography in infants with prolonged jaundice. Pediatr Surg Int 2006;22:140-43.
41. Arora NK, Kohli RK, Gupta DK, Bal CS, Gupta AK. Hepatic Technetium-99m mebroferrin iminodiacetate scans and Serum y-Glutamy1 transpeptidase (GGTP) levels interpreted in series to differentiate exthepatic biliary atresia and neontal hepatitis. Acta pediatr 2001;90:1-7.
42. Davenport M, Betalli P, D'Antinga L, et al. The spectrum of surgical jaundice in infancy. J Pediatr Surg 2003;38: 1471-79.
43. Gupta DK. Use of Phenobarbital and Betamethasone before ^{99m}Tc-HIDA scintigraphy in the evaluation of neonatal Jaundice. Jour Ind Assoc Pediatr Surg 1999;4: 97-100.
44. Kasai M, Suzuki S. A new operation for non-correctable biliary atresia-hepatic portoenterostomy. Shujitsu 1959;13:733-39.
45. Lilly JR. Hepatic portocholecystostomy for biliary atresia. J Pediatr Surg 179;14:301-04.
46. Gupta DK, Rohatgi M. Use of appendix in biliary atresia. Indian J Pediatr 1989;56:479.
47. Dillon PW, Owings E, Cilley R, et al. Immunosupression as adjuvant therapy for biliary atresia. J Pediatr Surg 2001;36:80-85.
48. Meyers R, Book LS, O'Gorman M, et al. High dose steroids, ursodeoxycholic acid and chronic intravenous antibiotics improve bile flow after Kasai procedure in infants with biliary atresia. J Pediatr Surg 2004;38:406-11.

49. Rattan J, Rohatgi S, Gupta DK, Rattan S. A controlled trial of choleretic and hepatoprotective actions of livzon and dehydrocholic acid in a rat model of obstructive Jaundice. Tohoku J Exp Med 1997;181(1):161-66.
50. Linuma Y, Kubota M, Yag M, et al. Effects of the herbal medicine Inchinko-to on liver function in postoperative patients with biliary atresia—a pilot study. J Pediatr Surg 2003;38:1607-11.
51. Davenport M, Stringer MD, Tizzard S, et al. Randomized double-blind placebo-controlled trial of corticosteroids after Kasai portoenterostomy for biliary atresia. Hepatology (in press).
52. Burnweit CA, Coln D. Influence of diversion on the development of cholangitis after hepatoportoenterostomy for biliary atresia. J Pediatr Surg 1986;21:1143-46.
53. Ecoffey C, Rothman E, Bernard O, Hadchouel M, Valayer J, Alagille D. Bacterial cholangitis after surgery for biliary atresia. J Pediatr 1987;111:824-49.
54. Houben C, Phelan S, Davenport M. Late-presenting cholangitis and Roux loop obstruction after Kasai portoenterostomy for biliary atresia. Pediatr Surg Int 2006;41:1159-64.
55. Stellin GP, Uceda JE, Lilly LR. Conduit decompression of biliary atresia. J Pediatr Surg 1983;18:782-83.
56. Kasai M. Long-term results in 189 patients of biliary atresia. In: Long-term Results in Congenital Anomalies, Kiesewetter WB (Ed), Tokyo: Ishuke 1980;1-9.
57. Altman RP. The portoenterostomy procedure for biliary atresia: a five year experience. Ann Surg 1978;188: 351-62.
58. Shim WKT, Zhang JZ. Antirefluxing Roux-en-Y biliary drainage valve for hepaticoportoenterostomy: animal experiments and clinical experience. J Pediatr Surg 1985;20: 689-92.
59. Endo M, Katsumata K, Yokoyama J, Morikawa Y, Ikwawa M, et al. Extended dissection of the porta hepatis and creation of an intussuscepted ileocolic onduit for biliary atresia. J Pediatr Surg 1983;18:784-93.
60. Kasai M, Okamoto A, Ohi R, Yabe K, Matsumura Y. Changes of portal vein pressure and intrahepatic blood vessels after surgery for biliary atresia. J Pediatr Surg 1981;16:152-59.
61. Ohi R, Mochizuki I, Komatsu K, Kasai M. Portal hypertension after successful hepatic portoenterostomy in biliary atresia. J Pediatr Surg 1986;21:271-74.
62. Duche M, Fabre M, Kretzschmar B, Serinet M, Gauthier F, Chardot C. Prognostic value of portal pressure at the time of Kasai operation in patients with biliary atresia. J Pediatric Gastroenterology and Nutrition 2006;43:640-45.
63. Sasaki T, Hasagawa T, Nakajima K, et al. Endoscopic variceal ligation in the management of gastroesophageal varices in postoperative biliary atresia. J Pediatr Surg 1998;33:1628-32.
64. Yonemura T, Yoshibayashi M, Uemoto S, Inomata Y, Tanaka K, Furusho K. Intrapulmonary shunting in biliary atresia before and after living-related liver transplantation. Br J Surg 1999;86:1139-43.
65. Losay J, Piot D, Bougaran J, Ozier Y, Devictor D, Houssin D, Bernard O. Early liver transplantation is crucial in children with liver disease and pulmonary artery hypertension. J Hepatol 1998;28:337-42.
66. Tatekawa Y, Asonuma K, Uemoto S, Inomata Y, Tanaka K. Liver transplantation for biliary atresia associated with malignant hepatic tumors. J Pediatr Surg 2001;36:436-39.
67. Kulkarni PB, Beatty E Jr. Cholangiocarcinoma associated with biliary cirrhosis due to congenital biliary atresia. Am J Dis Child 1977;131:442-44.
68. Hung PY, Chen CC, Chen WJ, et al. Long-term prognosis of patient with biliary atresia: a 25 year summary. J Pediatr Gastrol Nutr 2006;42:190-95.
69. Davenport M, Ville de Goyet J, Stringer MD, et al. Seamless management of biliary atresia. England and Wales 1999-2002. Lancet 2004;363:1354-57.
70. Davenport M, Kerkar N, Mieli-Vergani G, et al. Biliary atresia - The King's College Hospital experience (1974 - 1995). J Pediatr Surg 1997;32:479-85.
71. Chardot C, Carton M, Spire-Bendelac N, et al. Prognosis of biliary atresia in the era of liver transplantation: French national study from 1986 to 1996. Hepatology 1999;30: 606-11.
72. Altman RP, Lily JR, Greenfield J, et al. A multivariable risk factor analysis of the portoenterostomy (Kasai) procedure for biliary atresia: twenty-five years of experience from two centers. Ann Surg 1997;226:348-53.
73. Hadzic N, Tizzard S, Davenport M, Mieli-Vergani G. Long-term survival following Kasai portoenterostomy: is chronic liver disease inevitable? J Pediatr Gastro Nutr 2003;37:403-33.
74. Barshes NR, Lee TC, Balkrishnan R, et al. Orthotopic liver transplantation for biliary atresia: the US experience. Liver Transpl 2005;11:1193-1200.
75. Utterson EC, Shepherd RW, Sokol RJ, et al. Biliary atresia: clinical profiles, risk factors, and outcomes of 755 patients listed for liver transplantation. J Pediatr 2005;147:180-85.
76. Davenport M, Tizzard S, Underhill J, et al. The biliary atresia splenic malformation: a 28 year single center retrospective review. J Pediatr 2006;149:393-400.
77. Davenport M, Puricelli V, Farrant P, et al. The outcome of the older (> 100 days) infant with biliary atresia. J Pediatr Surg 2004;39:575-81.
78. Gupta DK. Editorial: Biliary Atresia; Still a Dreadful Disease for the poor nations Jour IAPS 1999;4(2):52-57.
79. Gupta DK, Srinivas M, Bajpai M. Advanced Biliary Atresia : Is Portoenterostomy Justified in all infants. Ind Jour Pediatr 2001;68(5):405-57.
80. Gupta DK, Agarwala S. A simple alternative to Hepatoportoenterostomy (HPE) in Advanced Biliary atresia. ? Asian Jour Surg 2005;28:13.
81. Gupta DK, Sharma Shilpa. Stem cell therapy—Hope and scope in pediatric surgery. Journal of Indian Association of Pediatric Surgeons. July - September 2005:10;138-41.
82. Gupta DK, Sharma S, Venugopal P, Kumar L, Mohanty S, Dattagupta S. Stem cells as a therapeutic modality in pediatric malformations. Transplant Proc 2007;39:700-02.

CHAPTER 90

Choledochal Cyst

Takeshi Miyano, Long Li, Atsuyuki Yamataka

Choledochal cyst is an uncommon anomaly of the biliary tract. First reported by Douglas in 1852, it was not until early this century that precise clinical recognition and surgical treatment were developed.[1] There is little doubt that choledochal cyst is a congenital lesion with a strong hereditary component, which may explain the higher incidence seen in Asia, and its familial occurrence in siblings and twins.[2-4] Incidence in the newborn has been increasing in recent years due to advances in diagnostic imaging techniques and in our series about 20% of patients were detected either neonatally or antenatally.[5-15]

Choledochal cyst is commonly associated with pancreaticobiliary malunion (PBMU) through which the pancreatic fluid can reflux into the biliary system and bile can flow into the pancreatic duct, and in recent years, combined anomalies of the common channel, pancreatic duct and intrahepatic duct are being recognized with increasing frequency, underlying the importance of cholangiography for visualizing the pancreaticobiliary system in its entirety.

EMBRYOLOGY

The extrahepatic biliary duct system and the ventral pancreas arise from the hepatic diverticulum during the fourth to sixth weeks of life. On day 22 of gestation, a small endodermal thickening, the hepatic plate, appears on the ventral side of the duodenum.[15] The cells in the plate proliferate and form a hepatic diverticulum, which rapidly enlarges and divides into three parts: the large cranial part (the liver bud), the cystic diverticulum, and the small caudal part (the ventral pancreatic bud). On day 26 of gestation, another duodenal bud (the dorsal pancreatic bud) appears opposite the hepatic diverticulum. The cells at the junction of the liver, cystic, and ventral pancreatic buds proliferate and form the common bile duct.[16]

Initially, the main duct of the ventral pancreatic bud develops near the entry of the common bile duct develop into the duodenum. As the duodenum rotates to the right (clockwise) and becomes C-shaped, the ventral pancreatic bud is carried dorsally with the bile duct and fuses with the dorsal pancreas. Later it comes to lie posterior to the dorsal pancreatic bud and fuses with it. The ventral pancreatic bud forms the uncinate process and part of the head of the pancreas.[16,17]

The ventral pancreas fuses with a pair of ventral buds in the fifth week of fetal life and is connected by two ducts to the primitive hepatic duct. The left ventral duct regresses with development.[18,19] The duct of the right ventral pancreas divides into superior and inferior branches. As the pancreatic buds fuse, the superior ventral branch joins the dorsal pancreatic duct to form the main pancreatic duct, which merges with the common bile duct, inserting into the duodenum via the papilla of Vater.[20]

ETIOLOGY

The etiology of choledochal cyst has not been fully clarified. Choledochal cyst is believed to be caused by two factors, i.e. weakness of the wall and an obstruction distal to it. Spitz stressed on the role of an obstructive factor in the early developmental stage, based on his experimental study on sheep, in which cystic dilatation of the common bile duct was produced by ligation of the distal end of the choledochus in a neonatal lamb, but not at later stages of development.[21]

Our research in different animals confirmed this hypothesis.[22-27] Similarly, our radiological and histological studies on patients with Choledochal cyst clearly demonstrate that distal segmental stenosis is closely associated with the cystic dilatation of the common bile duct and the site of stenosis is related to the abnormal choledochopancreatic ductal junction.[23-27] In recent years, improved accuracy of cholangiography has drawn attention to a close association between choledochal cyst and anomalous arrangement of the pancreaticobiliary ductal system. In 1969, Babbit first proposed this long common channel theory.[28] Since then, pancreaticobiliary malunion (PBMU) has been reported in choledochal cyst from endoscopic retrograde cholangio-pancreaticography (ERCP) and intraoperative cholangiography. High amylase levels in the aspirated cyst fluid from cases of choledochal cyst would appear to support this association. Between 1969 and 1997, we treated 210 patients with choledochal cyst. All had PBMU proven by cholangiography, and most had high amylase levels in the cyst fluid. Both a dilated common channel and anomalous pancreatic duct are also frequently observed, and may be related to the formation of protein plugs or pancreatic stones, which may cause pancreatitis.

In spite of these findings, controversy surrounds the cause of the stenosis that lies distal to the dilated common bile duct. Babbit stressed that the pancreatic fluid is the most basic causative factor for edema and subsequent fibrosis in the distal common bile duct as well as weakness of the choledochal wall.[28] However, the chemical reaction of the refluxed pancreatic fluid in the bile duct appears to be extremely mild, according to our animal experiments in which choledo-chopancreaticostomy was performed in puppies to allow pancreatic fluid to regurgitate into the bile duct.[29] In this animal model, fusiform dilatation rather than cystic dilatation of the common bile duct was induced. Also, a number of patients with PBMU and high amylase level in the gallbladder do not have dilatation of the choledochus, although some had gallbladder carcinoma.[30] The chemical effect of pancreatic fluid on the bile duct has not been clarified in the antenatal period. However, choledochal cyst can now be diagnosed as early as the 15th-20th weeks of gestation, a period when pancreatic acini are only just beginning to appear, and zymogen granules are immature, and there is no evidence of secretion seen on electron microscopy.[8,11-13,31] Even in the newborn, the pancreas has not matured enough to produce functional enzymes, so the role of pancreatic fluid in choledochal cyst formation may be overemphasized.[32]

Jona suggested that choledochal cyst is related to faulty budding of the primitive ventral pancreas.[33] Tanaka proposed that canalization of the ventral pancreatic duct and regression of the terminal choledochus is responsible for PBMU formation.[34,35] Based on human fetus observation, Wong demonstrated that choledopancreatic junction lies outside the duodenal wall before eighth week of gestation then moves inward and towards the duodenal lumen as age advanced, suggesting that an anomalous junction can be caused by arrest of this migration.[36]

Therefore, based on these radiological and experimental studies, we believe that an anomalous choledochopancreatic ductal junction combined with congenital stenosis are the basic causative factor of choledochal cyst rather than weakness caused by the reflux of pancreatic fluid, at least in perinatal and young infants. The anomalous choledochopancreatic junction and stenosis may cause abnormal development of the ventral pancreatic duct and biliary ductal system by unknown genetic associations.

CLASSIFICATION

Choledochal cyst can be roughly classified into two types according to the shape of the common bile duct: cystic dilatation and fusiform dilatation.[37] It could be intra or extrahepatic or both. Both Todani and Komi have described classifications for choledochal cyst based on cholangiographic studies of the pancreaticobiliary ductal system (Figs 90.1A to E).[38,39]

However, the authors prefer to classify Choledochal cyst into groups according to the presence or absence of PBMU (Figs 90.2A to F).
  i. *With PBMU:* (A) cystic dilatation of the extrahepatic bile duct*. (B) Fusiform dilatation of the extrahepatic bile duct*. (C) Forme fruste choledochal cyst+.
  ii. *Without PBMU:* (D) Cystic diverticulum of the common bile duct. (E) Choledochocele (a diverticulum of the distal common bile duct). (F) Intrahepatic bile duct dilatation alone (Caroli's disease).

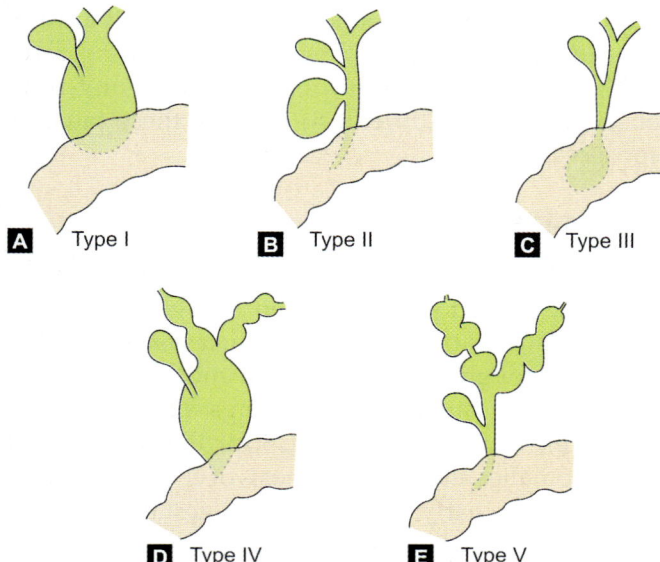

Figs 90.1A to E: Classification of choledochal cysts: **A.** Cystic or fusiform dilatation of the extrahepatic bile duct. **B.** Cystic diverticulum of the common bile duct. **C.** Choledochocele (a diverticulum of the distal common bile duct). **D.** Intrahepatic and extrahepatic bile duct dilatation **E.** Intrahepatic bile duct dilatation alone (Caroli's disease)

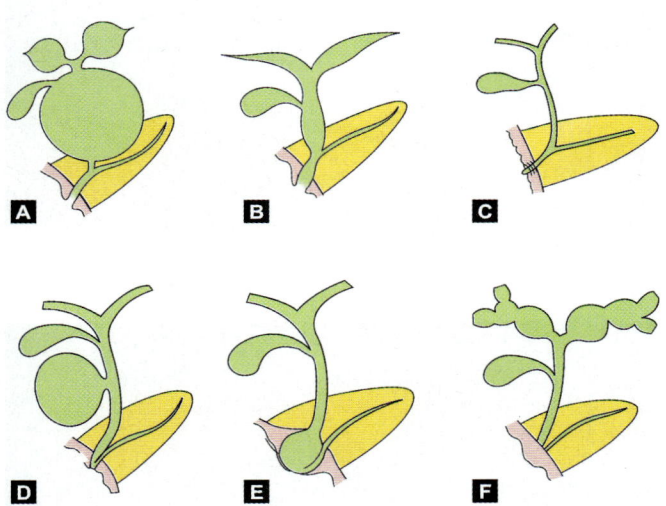

Figs 90.2A to F: Classification of choledochal cysts with PBMU: **A.** Cystic dilatation of the extrahepatic bile duct* **B.** Fusiform dilatation of the extrahepatic bile duct* **C.** Forme fruste choledochal cyst+ without PBMU **D.** Cystic diverticulum of the common bile duct. **E.** Choledochocele (adiverticulum of the distal common bile duct). **F.** Intrahepatic bile duct dilatation alone (Caroli's disease). * With or without intrahepatic bile duct dilatation. +Minimal or negligible extra and intrahepatic bile duct dilatation. PBMU- pancreaticobiliary malunion

CLINICAL PRESENTATION

The clinical manifestations of choledochal cyst differ according to the age of onset. Neonates and young infants usually present with an abdominal mass, jaundice, and acholic stools. Some present with a huge upper abdominal mass with or without jaundice. Since the advent of routine antenatal ultrasound (US) for the detection of fetal anomalies, the number of neonates being detected with incidental choledochal cyst has increased.[5-14] According to our investigations, the ratio of cystic to fusiform type antenatally or neonatally is 20:1, in contrast to an overall ratio of 5:3.[14] In older children, the classical triad of pain, mass and jaundice may be present. Fever and vomiting may also occur. The pattern of pain has been described as being similar to that of recurrent pancreatitis in which a high serum amylase level is often present. However, in our series, there was little clinical evidence of pancreatitis in the newborn, because amylase levels were not found to be elevated.

Asymptomatic Neonatal Choledochal Cyst

There are very few reports on the management of asymptomatic choledochal cyst detected in the antenatal or neonatal period. Some pediatric surgeons recommend primary cyst excision soon after diagnosis, but our experience had been that cyst excision need not be performed hastily in these young infants; rather, they should be thoroughly assessed and surgery should be planned.[7,10,12,14,40-43]

PBMU with Nondilatation or Minimal Dilatation of the Common Bile Duct

In children who present with recurrent pancreatitis, PBMU must be suspected even if the common bile duct appears to be normal. Treatment of choledochal cyst today is primary excision of the cyst followed by hepaticoenterostomy. However, PBMU without dilatation of the biliary tract is often encountered and its treatment is controversial.[44] In adults, simple cholecystectomy without biliary reconstruction is usually performed, because PBMU presents with gallbladder related symptoms.

Over 30 years, we have treated eight patients with nondilatation or minimal dilatation of the common bile duct at our institution, approximately 4.4% of the whole choledochal cyst population (Fig. 90.3).[45,46]

These patients presented with signs and symptoms of pancreatitis, i.e. abdominal pain associated with elevation of serum amylase levels. Five of those had jaundice or a history of pale colored stools.

At presentation, ERCP showed that five (62.5%) of these eight patients had dilatation of the common channel, a finding that is usually seen in about 30% of the choledochal cyst cases. Three cases (37%) also had protein plugs or debris at the level of the common channel, a finding that is usually only observed in 16% of choledochal cyst cases. Histopathologically, there was mild to moderate inflammation and mucosal hyperplasia manifested in the gallbladder and epithelial denudation and fibrosis also observed in the common bile duct.

The extrahepatic bile duct was excised with the gallbladder followed by a Roux-en-Y hepaticojejunostomy in six cases and a hepaticoduodenostomy in two cases for biliary reconstruction. No postoperative complications were encountered. All patients had resolution of their symptoms after operative repair on follow-up (average duration 4.3 years).

Since clinical symptoms in patients with PBMU arise from stasis or protein plugs at the level of the common channel, caused by reflux of the pancreatic secretions and chronic inflammation, we believe that radical treatment by pancreaticobiliary separation should be selected to prevent serious long-term complications. Based on our close and long-term observation, it is difficult to manage these patients conservatively.

INVESTIGATIONS

Currently, abdominal US is the best method for detecting choledochal cyst even though it does not permit visualization of the entire duct system and it is not clear enough to demonstrate an undilated common channel and pancreatic duct (Figs 92.4 and 90.5). However, routine antenatal US for the detection of fetal anomalies allow the diagnosis of choledochal cyst to be made as early as 15th week of gestation.[11] For a complete diagnosis of choledochal cyst, it is also

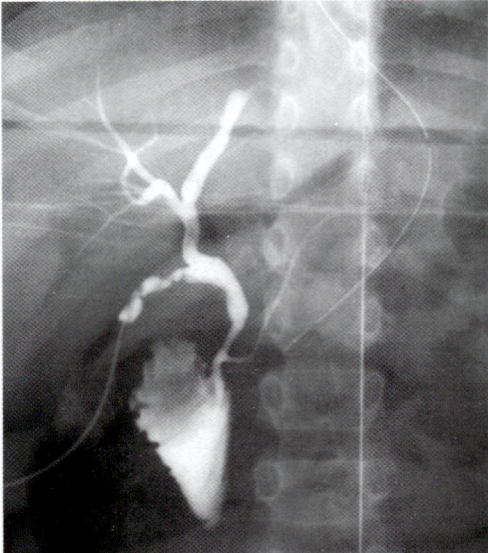

Fig. 90.3: Intraoperative cholangiopancreatography. An anomalous junction between the pancreatic and common bile ducts followed by a long common channel is demonstrated. Normal proportion of the biliary tree is maintained

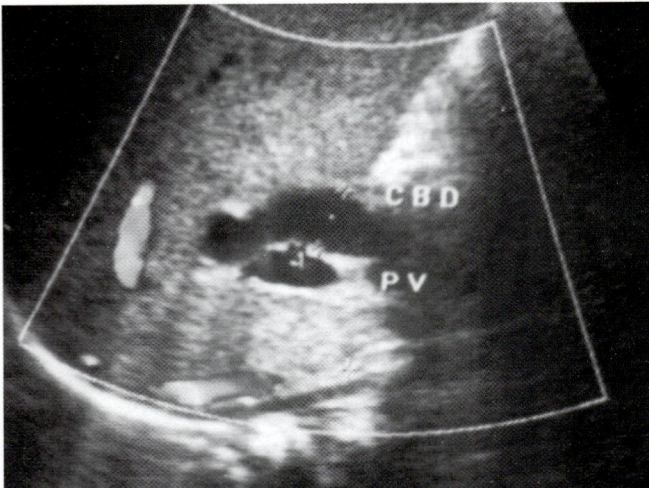

Fig. 90.4: Ultrasonography depicting a fusiform choledochal cyst (Courtesy: Prof DK Gupta, New Delhi)

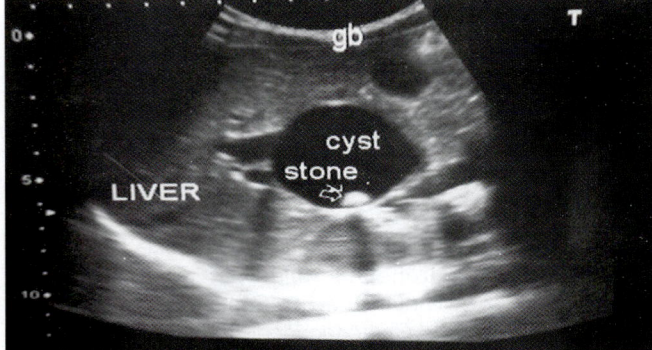

Fig. 90.5: Ultrasonography showing a cystic type of choledochal cyst with a stone (a rare association) (Courtesy: Prof DK Gupta, New Delhi)

important to investigate for coexisting PBMU, abnormalities of the pancreatic duct, intrahepatic ducts and extrahepatic duct. ERCP can accurately visualize the configuration of the pancreaticobiliary ductal system in detail, and is unlikely to be replaced by other investigations, especially in cases where fine detail is required preoperatively. ERCP is routinely performed in the diagnosis of biliary malformations in infants and the newborn in many centers in Japan, with a reasonable success rate.[47] However, it is invasive and therefore unsuitable for repeated use, and is contraindicated during acute pancreatitis.

We have shown that magnetic resonance cholangiopancreatography (MRCP) can provide excellent visualization of the pancreaticobiliary system in patients with choledochal cyst allowing narrowing, dilatation and filling defects to be detected with medium to high degrees of accuracy (Figs 90.6 and 90.7).[48,49] Because MRCP is noninvasive, it can partially replace ERCP as a diagnostic tool for the evaluation of anatomical anomalies of the pancreaticobiliary tract. Another advantage of MRCP over ERCP is that the pancreatic duct can be visualized upstream to an obstruction or area of stenosis. So far, there are limitations of patient's size, weight and age for using MRCP. Once the quality of MRCP improves, ERCP may become optional.

If preoperative imaging can clearly visualize the entire pancreaticobiliary ductal system, including the intra- and extrahepatic bile ducts, and pancreatic duct in detail, intraoperative cholangiography is unnecessary; however, if sufficient information is not

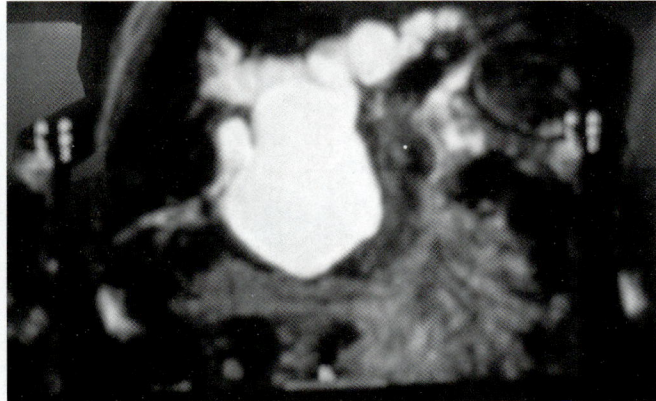

Fig. 90.6: MRCP delineating a large cystic choledochal cyst with intrahepatic biliary dilatation

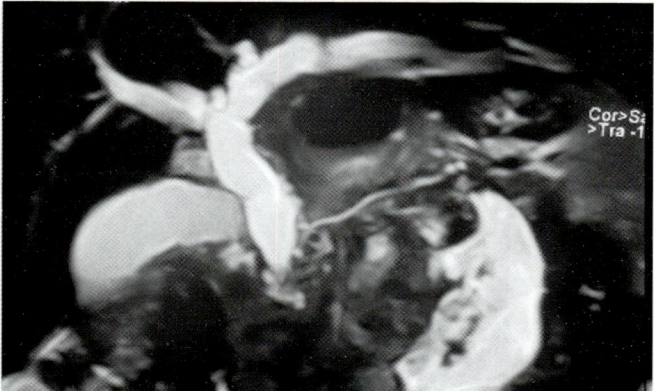

Fig. 90.7: MRCP delineating a fusiform choledochal cyst (intra and extrahepatic, both) with a distended gallbladder. Pancreatic duct is also shown in the section

obtained, it must be performed (Figs 90.8A and B). Also, if the cyst is too large, intraoperative cholangiography via the gallbladder or directly via the common bile duct is useless. In such cases, intraoperative cholangiography should be performed separately for the intrahepatic bile duct and distal common bile duct by a selective technique during excision of the cyst. Rarely, intraoperative cholangiogram may help to diagnose unsuspected anomalies if MRCP was not done earlier (Figs 90.9A to D).

DIFFERENTIAL DIAGNOSIS

Choledochal cyst can be diagnosed without difficulty using abdominal US and ERCP. Caroli's disease, congenital stricture of the common bile duct, correctable biliary atresia, congenital hepatic fibrosis and pancreatic disorders with bile duct obstruction, need to be considered in the differential diagnosis. In such cases, there is usually a normal pattern of pancreaticobiliary union. The typical feature of Caroli's disease is cystic dilatation of the intrahepatic ducts, which resemble a string of beads. There is usually a normal extrahepatic bile duct without PBMU. In fully developed biliary atresia, the bile duct may be obstructed distally with dilated extrahepatic bile ducts. On such occasions, Choledochal cyst can be differentiated from biliary atresia because there is a patent communication with the duodenum and a well-developed intrahepatic bile duct tree (Figs 90.10A and B).

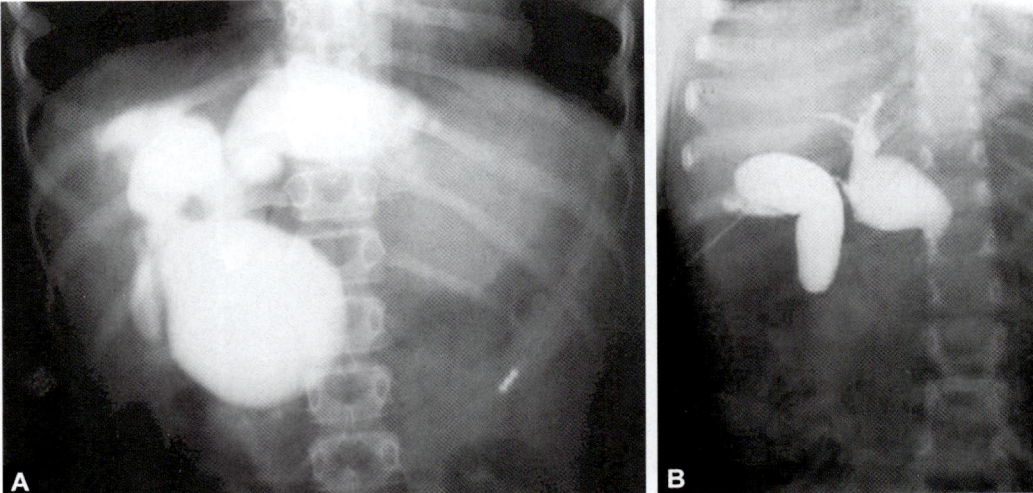

Figs 90.8A and B: A. Preoperative cholangiogram showing type IV large choledochal cyst with intra and extrahepatic dilatations **B.** Peroperative cholangiogram showing a dilated gallbladder communicating with the choledochal cyst (courtesy: Prof DK Gupta, New Delhi)

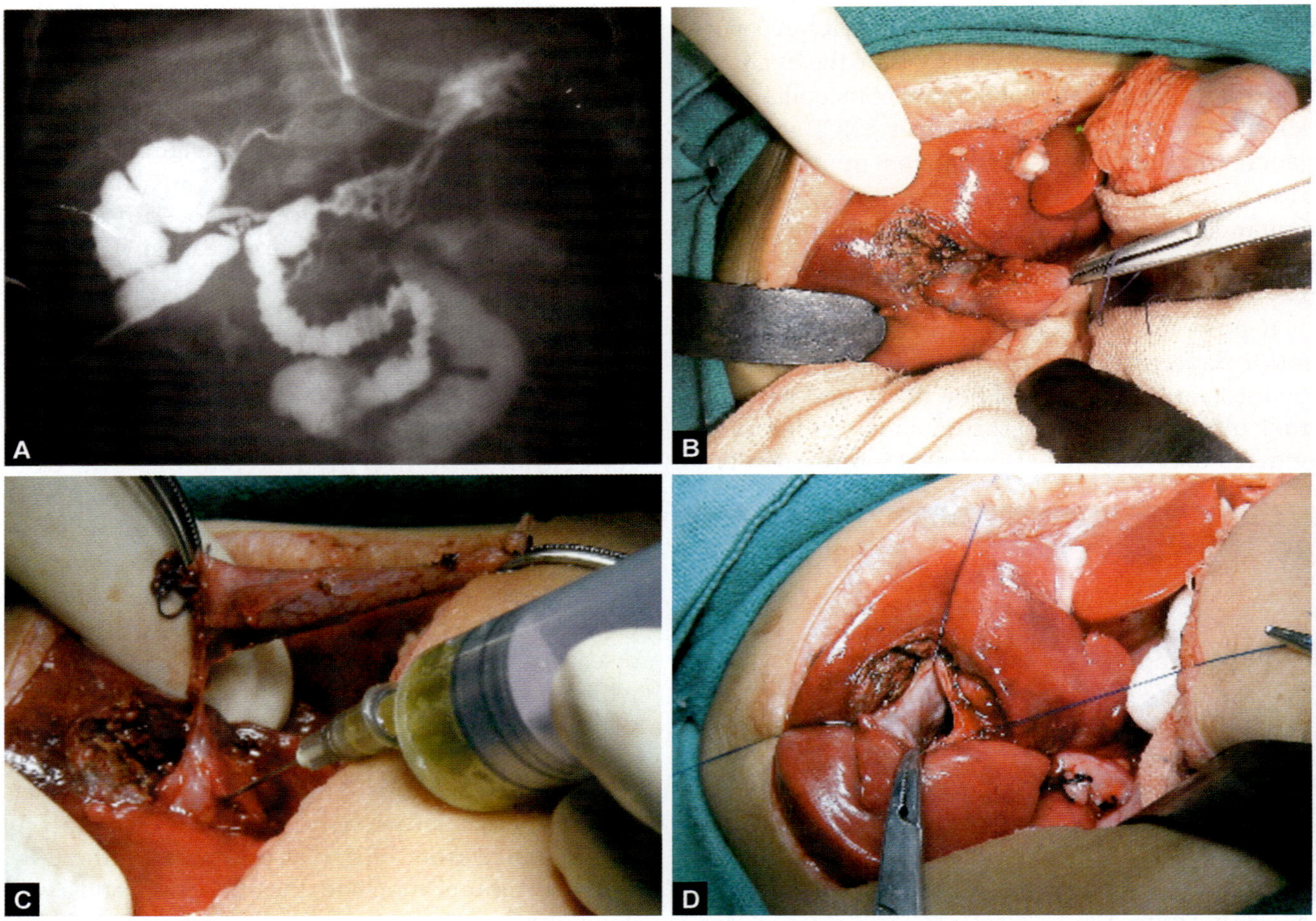

Figs 90.9A to D: A seven-year-old girl with intrahepatic choledochal cyst. **A.** Operative cholangiogram demonstrating an intrahepatic cyst in the right lobe of liver communicating with the gallbladder bed **B.** The gallbladder being dissected off the choledochal cyst **C.** The cyst being aspirated while still connected with the gallbladder near its fundus. **D.** The cyst was deroofed and a Roux-en Y cystojejunostomy made (Courtesy: Prof DK Gupta, New Delhi)

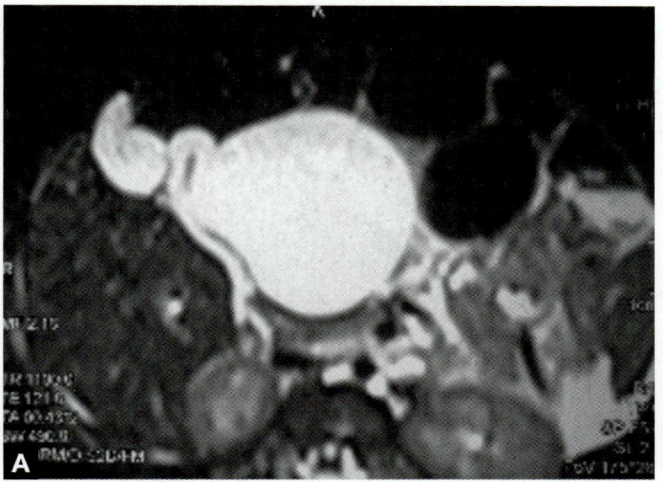
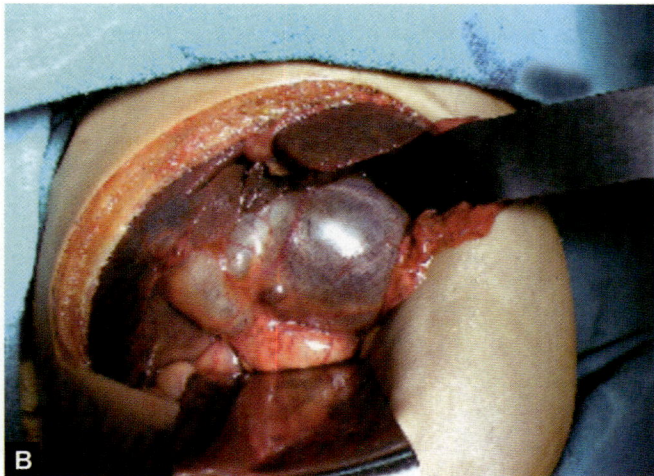

Figs 90.10: **A.** MRCP demonstrating a large choledochal cyst and gallbladder. **B.** operative photograph of the tense and thin walled cyst. The proximal end showed only minute openings at the porta as pits but there was neither a lumen nor the bile flow. There was also no distal communication with the duodenum (Courtesy: Prof DK Gupta, New Delhi)

SURGERY

Choice of Operative Procedure

Cyst excision with Roux-en-Y hepatoenterostomy is the definitive treatment of choice in all patients with Choledochal cyst, regardless of age or symptomatology (Fig. 90.11). In patients who have already had internal drainage without cyst excision, revision with cyst excision is strongly recommended if there is any symptom of postoperative biliopancreatic dysfunction. By doing so, a good prognosis can be expected. However, there is high morbidity and high risk of carcinoma after internal drainage without cyst excision, a commonly used treatment in the past.

Complete Excision

In newborn and young infants, choledochal cyst is usually cystic type. Complete cyst excision (full thickness of the cyst) is much easier in young infants, because the wall of the dilated common bile duct is generally thin and there are fewer adhesions to the surrounding vital structure, such as portal vein.[50,51] Aspiration of the cyst prior to dissection makes surgery easier, if the cyst is large and tense. Care is also taken if the cyst is infected and the gallbladder is turgid (Fig. 90.12). The cyst should be opened at the midportion close to the duodenum, because there is often an anomalous opening of the hepatic duct, i.e. a separate opening or opening to the distal part of the

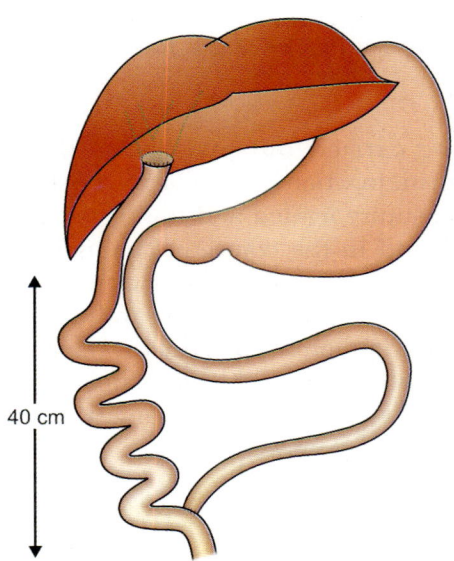

Fig. 90.11: Line diagram showing Roux-en-Y hepaticodocho jejunostomy, the most commonly preferred operative procedure for choledochal cyst after the complete excision of the cyst

cyst. The cyst is then transected midportion after careful circumferential dissection from the hepatic artery and portal vein. Calculus, if any, in the cyst is carefully removed (Fig. 90.13). Subsequently, dissection of the distal portion is carried out. It is important that the cyst be completely excised at the level of caliber change, in order to avoid malignant changes in the remaining cyst epithelium. If there is no distinct caliber change (i.e. fusiform type), excision

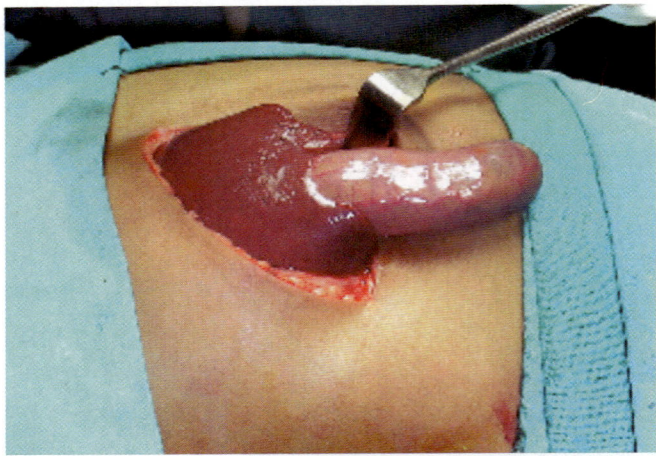

Fig. 90.12: A girl with infected choledochal cyst presenting with features of cholangitis. The cyst and the gallbladder were tense cystic with full of pus. The liver was enlarged and edematous. A two stage procedure may be preferred in these cases, to allow the inflammation to subside before resorting to cyst excision and definitive operative procedure with internal drainage (*courtesy:* Prof DK Gupta, New Delhi)

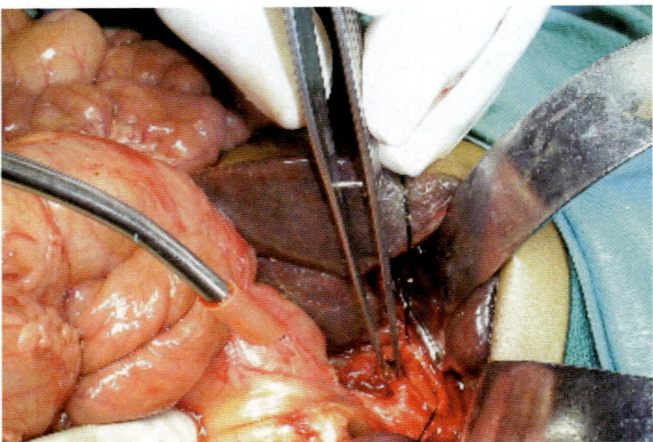

Fig. 90.13: A small calculus being removed from the lower end of the choledochal cyst (Courtesy: Prof DK Gupta, New Delhi)

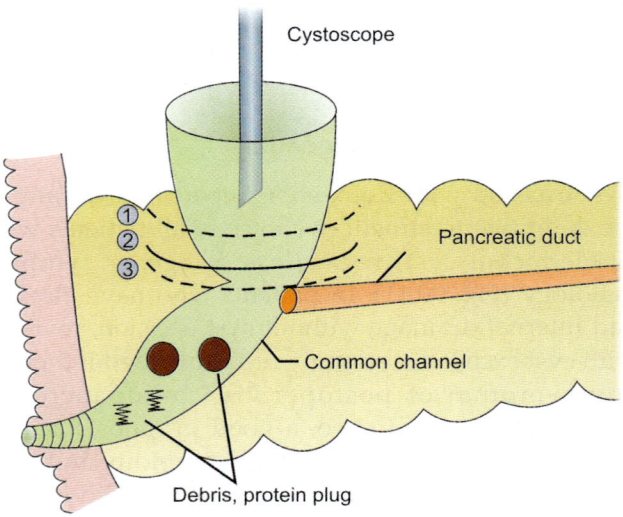

Fig. 90.14: Diagram of intraoperative endoscopy showing the bile duct distal to the cyst with debris and protein plug. After identification of the orifice of the pancreatic duct, the cyst is excised at level 2. (1) likelihood of leaving the residual cyst, (2) adequate excision level of the cyst, (3) likelihood of injuring the pancreatic duct

should be carried out just above the choledochopancreatic junction (Fig. 90.14).[52] The stump should be double-suture ligated and transected. If a protein plug is found in the common channel, it must be washed out toward the duodenum to avoid postoperative stone formation and pancreatitis.[42] Finally, the common hepatic duct is transected at the level of distinct caliber change. Since proximal cyst mucosa is prone to malignant changes, it must not be left for large anastomosis.[43]

Mucosectomy

In a patient in whom complete excision of the distal portion of the cyst is difficult, mucosectomy of the distal portion of the cyst is recommended in order to avoid not only damage to the pancreatic duct, hepatic artery and portal vein, but also to avoid cancer arising from the remaining epithelium of the distal portion of the cyst.

Staged Procedure

If primary excision is considered to be difficult, for example, in the case of perforated bile peritonitis, severe cholangitis or severe general condition, or in neonates, external biliary drainage is recommended by open drainage, precutaneous transhepatic cholangiodrainage or direct precutaneous cyst drainage. Subsequently, delayed primary excision may be carried out one or two months later.[14,42,43]

Biliary Reconstruction

Most surgeons use a Roux-en-Y hepaticojejunostomy, however some surgeons recommend a wide anastomosis at the level of the hepatic hilum to allow free drainage of bile to prevent postoperative anastomotic stricture and stone formation.[52,53] Based on a wealth of experience from a large number of series, we recommend conventional hepaticoenterostomy as the treatment of choice.[54] Hepaticoenterostomy at the hepatic hilum is indicated in specific cases only, such as in patient's with dilated intrahepatic bile duct with stenosis in the common hepatic duct or adolescent patient with severe inflammation of the common hepatic duct. Although we initially used end-to-side anastomosis, we now prefer end-to-end, because drainage is smoother and more direct, with less possibility of stasis (Figs 90.15A to C). With end-to-side anastomoses, we have experienced overgrowth of the blind end, which caused bowel obstruction in one case, and bile stasis in the blind pouch, which caused bowel obstruction in one case.[54] Bile stasis in the blind pouch can also cause stone formation in the pouch or dilatation of intrahepatic bile ducts.

However, our results do not compel us to resort to other procedures such as hepaticoenterostomy at the hilum and valved jejunal interposition hepaticoduodenostomy to prevent reflux of digested food into the intrahepatic bile duct, which are appealing theoretically, but offer no significant improvement in morbidity.[53] Hepaticoenterostomy at the hepatic hilum also appears to be more difficult than conventional hepaticoenterostomy, particularly in small children without the dilatation of intrahepatic bile duct.

A hepaticoduodenostomy has a limited indication and is found useful if the lumen of the duct is less than one cm in diameter after the cyst has been excised. Duodenum should be mobilized so as to reach the portahepatis comfortably. A single layer anastomosis is made with the duct and the superoposterior aspect of the first part of the duodenum. The area should always be drained as 10% leak is reported. The valved jejunal interposition hepaticoduodenostomy though practiced by a few surgeons, is a rather complicated procedure and is not preferred for routine use.

Role of Intraoperative Endoscopy

Since 1986, we have routinely performed intraoperative endoscopy of the common channel, pancreatic duct and intrahepatic ducts to examine the duct system directly for stone debris and ductal stenosis and remove any stone debris by irrigation with normal saline.[54] Intraoperative endoscopy with a pediatric cystoscope or fine fiberscope with a flush channel is also recommended as a valuable adjunct to determine the transection level of the common hepatic duct, irrigating the common channel and to determine the level of excision of the distal end of the cyst to avoid injuring to the pancreatic duct, leaving only a minimal intrapancreatic terminal choledochus.[55]

Laparoscopic Cyst Excision

Recent advances in laparoscopy have enabled pediatric surgeons to perform minimally invasive surgery for Choledochal cyst.[56,57] Although technically demanding and long-term follow-up results remain unknown, experienced laparoscopic surgeons can obtain results as good as those for open surgery. The disadvantages are mainly the longer operating time and the higher costs, which, however, may be offset by a shorter hospital stay.

ASSOCIATED CONDITIONS

Intrahepatic Bile Duct Dilatation

Recently, more attention has been paid to the treatment of intrahepatic ductal disease such as intrahepatic bile

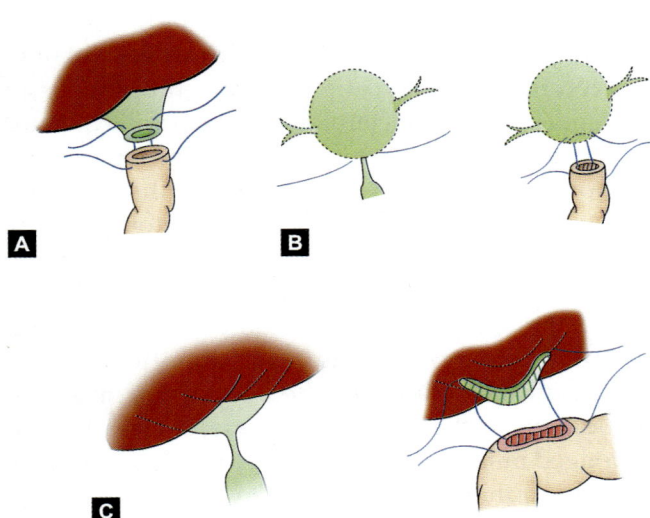

Figs 90.15A to C: A. Conventional hepaticoenterostomy. **B.** Intrahepatic cystoenterostomy after excision of the stenosed portion of the common hepatic duct **C.** Hepaticoenterostomy at the hepatic hilum, with a wide stoma created by an incision along the lateral wall of the hepatic ducts

duct dilatation with downstream stenosis, which is closely associated with late postoperative complications.[54,58-63] Intrahepatic bile duct dilatation can be managed by segmentectomy of the liver, intrahepatic cystoenterostomy or balloon dilatation of the stenosis at the time of cyst excision.[38,60,61] In three cases in our series, we performed an intrahepatic ductoplasty and cystojejunostomy or hepaticojejunostomy at the hepatic hilum for stricture of he intrahepatic bile duct at the hepatic hilum to create a wide stoma by incising along the lateral walls of the hepatic ducts following excision of the narrowed segment of the common hepatic duct.[54,62] By using intraoperative endoscopy, the ideal level of resection of the common hepatic duct can be safely determined without injuring the orifices of the hepatic duct or leaving any duct remnant.[62]

Disorders of Pancreatic Duct and Common Channel

With the advent use of endoscopy, more anomalies of the pancreatic duct and common channel have been identified. These include protein plugs or stones in the common channel, stenosis of papilla of Vater, stricture of the pancreatic ducts, or even septate common channel.[63-65] Stone debris in the common channel and intrahepatic duct are responsible for abdominal pain, pancreatitis and jaundice. If nor removed at the time of radical surgery, they can be the cause of recurrent pancreatitis or calculi formation in pancreatic and biliary system postoperatively. We use a pediatric cystoscope for intraoperative pancreatoscopy of the common channel and intrahepatic duct.[62,63] A neonatal cystoscope with a flush channel can also be used and is finer and more flexible (1.9-2.0 mm). We have performed intraoperative pancreatoscopy in 67 patients with Choledochal cyst. Stone debris in pancreatic duct distal to the common channel was detected in eight cases (11.9%). All eight patients had a dilated long common channel with PBMU and presented with acute pancreatitis. They are all well after a mean follow-up period of 7.3 years.

COMPLICATIONS AND OUTCOME

Cyst excision combined with hepaticoenterostomy (CEHE) is the treatment of choice for choledochal cyst A satisfactory surgical outcome with early low morbidity is expected after this standard surgical procedure.

We have reviewed 200 children and 40 adults who underwent CEHE and found 9.0% (18/200) of children, and 42.5% (17/40) of adults had post-CEHE complications.[45,54] The complication rate in children was significantly lower than in adults. No stone formation was seen in the children who had CEHE before the age of five years.

The post-CEHE complications recorded were cholangitis, intrahepatic bile duct stone formation, stone formation in the intrapancreatic terminal choledochus or pancreatic duct, and bowel obstruction. No complications were found in the 70 children who had intraoperative endoscopy in our series. Stone formation was seen in seven of the 55 children (12.7%) aged over five years at the time of CEHE. There was no stone formation in the 145 children who had CEHE before the age of five years. Stones developed in seven (17.5%) adults. One patient presented with relapsing pancreatitis owing to a stone within the residual segment of an intrapancreatic cyst, six years after excision of a fusiform-type dilatation of the common bile duct with hepaticojejunostomy. One patient was found to have stones in the blind pouch of an end-to-side anastomosis.

Reoperation was required in 15 children-revision of hepaticoenterostomy in four, percutaneous transhepatic cholangioscopic lithotomy in one, excision of intrapancreatic terminal choledochus in tow, endoscopic sphincterotomy of the papilla of Vater in one, pancreaticojejunostomy in one, and laparotomy for bowel obstruction in six. Ten adults required reoperations-revision of hepaticoenterostomy in two, percutaneous transhepatic cholangioscopic lithotomy in two, exploratory laparotomy in two, adhesiolysis in one, endoscopic sphincterotomy in two, and left lobectomy of liver in one. Anastomotic stricture appears to be related to the severity of mucosal denudation in the common hepatic duct and/or to prolonged inflammation secondary to bile stasis in the dilated intrahepatic bile duct. On such occasions, a hepaticojejunostomy should be performed at the hepatic hilum to create a wide stoma by incising along the lateral walls of the hepatic ducts following excision of the narrowed segment of the common hepatic duct, because the inflammation of the walls of the extrahepatic cyst is more chronic and fibrotic and the

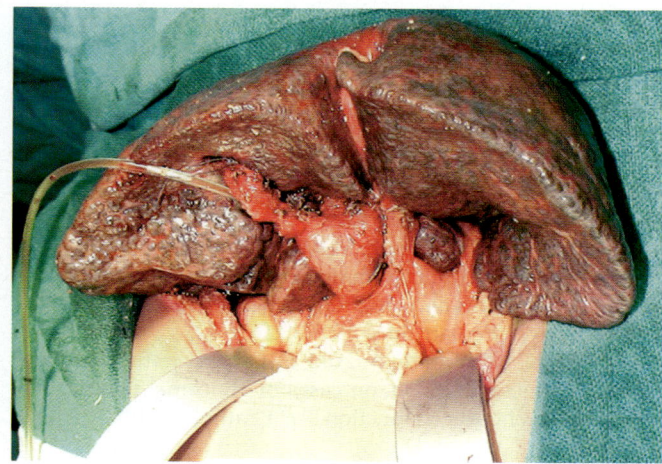

Fig. 90.16: A case of choledochal cyst in 2-year-old girl with cirrhotic liver, portal hypertension and neovascularisation (Courtesy: Prof DK Gupta, New Delhi)

wall of the intrahepatic bile ducts also may be severely and irreversibly damaged, resulting in poor resolution of the intrahepatic bile duct dilatation. Patients who present late during infancy or childhood with liver cirrhosis, portal hypertension, associated pancreatitis and superadded infection have poor prognosis (Fig. 90.16).

Careful long-term follow-up is required, particularly in patients who have had intrahepatic bile duct dilatation and also dilatation of the remaining distal bile duct, pancreatic duct and common channel, because of chronic inflammation, calculus formation as well as the possibility of carcinoma arising at a later stage.

REFERENCES

1. Douglas AH. Case of dilatation of the common bile duct. Monthly J Med Sci (London) 1852;14:97.
2. Iwafuchi M, Ohsawa Y, Naito S. Familial occurrence of congenital bile duct dilatation. J Pediatr Surg 1990;25:353-55.
3. Ando K, Miyano T, Fujimoto T, Ohya T, Lane G, Tawa T, Tokita A, Yabuta K. Sibling occurrence of biliary atresia and biliary dilatation. J Pediatr Surg 1996;31:1302-04.
4. Lane GJ, Yamataka A, Kobayashi H, Segawa O, Miyano T. Different types of congenital biliary dilatation in dizygotic twins. Pediatr Surg Int 1999;15:403-4.
5. Dewbury KC, Aluwihare APR, Birch SJ, et al. Prenatal ultrasound demonstration of a choledochal cyst. Br J Radiol 1980;53:906-7.
6. Frank JL, Chirathivat S, Sfakianakis GN, et al. Antenatal observation of a choledochal cyst by sonography. Am J Roentgenol 1981;137:166-68.
7. Howell CG, Templeton JM, Weiner S, et al. Antenatal diagnosis and early surgery for choledochal cyst. J Pediatr Surg 1983;18:387-93.
8. Marchildon MB. Antenatal diagnosis of choledochal cyst: the first four cases. Pediatr Surg Int 1988;3:431-36.
9. Wiedman MA, Tan AA, Martinez CJ. F, et al. sonography and neonatal scintigraphy of a choledochal cyst. J Nucl Med 1985;26:893-96.
10. Elrad H, Mayden KL, Ahart S. Prenatal ultrasound diagnosis of choledochal cyst. J Ultrasound Med 1985;4:893-96.
11. Schroeder D, Smith L, Prain HC. Antenatal diagnosis of choledochal cyst at 15 weeks gestation: Etiologic implications and management. J Pediatr Surg 1989;24:936-38.
12. Bancroft JD, Buncuvalas JC, Ryckman FC. Antenatal diagnosis of choledochal cyst. J Pediatr Gastroenterol Nutr 1994;18:142-45.
13. Galliran EK, Crombleholme TM, D'Alton ME. Early prenatal diagnosis of choledochal cyst. Prenat Diagn 1996;16:934-37.
14. Lane GJ, Yamataka A, Kohno S, Fujiwara T, Fujimoto T, Sunagawa M. Choledochal cyst in the newborn. Asian J Surg 1999;22:310-12.
15. Hayes MA, Bishop CC. The developmental basis for bile duct anomalies. Surg Gyn Obst 1958;107:447-56.
16. Schwegler RA, Boyden EA. The development of the pars intestinalis of the common bile duct in the human fetus, with special reference to the origin of the ampulla of Vater and the sphincter of Oddi. I. The involution of the ampulla. Anat Rec 1937;67:441-67.
17. Kanagasuntheram R. Some observations on the development of the human duodenum. J Anat 1960;94:231-40.
18. Odergers PNB. Some observations on the development of the ventral pancreas in man. J Anat 1930;65:1-7.
19. Lewis FT. The bi-lobed form of the ventral pancreas in mammals. Am J Anat 1912;12:389-400.
20. Dawson W, Langman J. An anatomical-radiological study on the pancreatic duct pattern in man. Anat Rec 1961;139:58-68.
21. Spitz L. Experimental production of cystic dilatation of the common bile duct in neonatal lambs. J Pediatr Surg 1977;12:39-42.
22. Miyano T, Suruga K, Kimura K, Suda K. A histopathologic study of the region of the ampulla of Vater in congenital biliary atresia. Jpn J Surg 1980;10:34-8.
23. Suda K, Matsumoto Y, Miyano T, et al. A narrow duct segment distal to choledochal cyst. Am J Gastroenterol 1991;86:1259-63.
24. Miyano T, Suruga K, Chen SC. A clinicopathological study of choledochal cyst. Word J Surg 1980;4:231-38.

25. Miyano T, Suruga K, and Suda K. Abnormal choledocho-pancreatico ductal junction related to the etiology of infantile obstructive jaundice. J Pediatr Surg 1979;14:16-25.
26. Suda K, Miyano T. An abnormal pancreatico-choledochal-ductal junction in cases of biliary tract carcinoma. Cancer 1983;52:2086-88.
27. Miyano T, Takahashi A, Suruga K. Congenital stenosis associated with abnormal choledocho-pancreatico joining concerning the pathogenesis of congenital dilatation of biliary tract. Jpn J Pediatr Surg 1978;10:539-54.
28. Babbit DP. Congenital choledochal cyst: new etiological concept based on anomalous relationships of common bile duct and pancreatic bulb. Ann Radiol 1969;12:231-41.
29. Miyano T, Suruga K, Kuda K. "The choledocho-pancreatic common channel disorders" in relation to the etiology of congenital biliary dilatation and other biliary tract disease. Ann Acad Med 1981;10:419-26.
30. Tanaka K, Nishimura A, Yamada K, Ishibe R, Ishizaki N, Yoshimine M, Hamada N and Taira A. Cancer of the gallbladder associated with anomalous junction of the pancreatobiliary duct system without bile duct dilation. Br J Surg 1993;80:622-24.
31. Laitio M, Lev R, Orlic D. The developing human fetal pancreas: An ultrastructural and histochemical study with special reference to exocrine cells. J Anat 1974;117:619-34.
32. Lebenthal E, Lee PC. Development of functional response in the human exocrine pancreas. Pediatrics 1980;66:556-60.
33. Jona JZ, Babbit DP, Starshak RJ, et al. Anatomic observations and etiologic and surgical considerations in choledochal cyst. J Pediatr Surg 1979;14:315-20.
34. Tanaka T. Embryological development of the duodenal papilla and related diseases: primitive ampulla theory. Am J Gastroenterol 1993;88:1980-81.
35. Tanaka T. Pathogenesis of choledochal cyst. Am J Gastroenterol 1995;90:685.
36. Wong KC, Lister J. Human fetal development of the hepatopancreatic duct junction; a possible explanation of congenital dilatation of the biliary tract. J Pediatr Surg 1981;16:139-45.
37. Alonso-Lej F, Rever WB, Pessagno GJ, et al. Congenital choledochal cyst, with a report of 2, and an analysis of 94 cases. Internat Abstr Surg 1959;108:1-30.
38. Todani T, Narusue M, Tabuchi K, Okajima K. Management of congenital choledochal cyst with intrahepatic involvement. Ann Surg 1977;187:272-80.
39. Kom N, Takehara Hi, Kunitomo K, Miyoshi Y, Yagi T. Does the type of anomalous arrangement of pancreatico-biliary ducts influence the surgery and prognosis of choledochal cyst? J Pediatr Surg 1992;27:728-31.
40. Burnweit CA, Birken GA, Heiss K. The management of choledochal cysts in the newborn. Pediatr Surg Int 1996;11:130-33.
41. Suita S, Shono K, Kinugasa Y, Kubota M, Matsuo S. Influence of age on the presentation and outcome of choledochal cyst. J Pediatr Surg 1999;34:1765-68.
42. Miyano T. Congenital biliary dilatation. In Newborn Surgery. Edited by Puri P. Oxford: Butterworth-Heinemann: 1996;433-39,46.
43. Miyano T, Yamataka A. Choledochal cysts. Curr Opin Pediatr 1997;9:283-88.
44. Ando H, Ito T, Nagaya M, Watanabed Y, Seo T, Kaneko K. Pancreaticobiliary maljunction without choledochal cysts in infants and children: clinical features and surgical therapy. J Pediatr Surg 1995;30:1658-62.
45. Suda K, Miyano T, Suzuki F. Clinico-pathologic and experimental studies on cases of abnormal pancreatico-choledocho-ductal junction. Acta Pathol Jpn 1987;37:1549-62.
46. Miyano T, Ando K, Yamataka A. Lane G, Segawa O, Kohno S, Fujiwara T. Pancreaticobiliary maljunction associated with nondilatation or minimal dilatation of the common bile duct in children: Diagnosis and treatment. Eur J Pediatr Surg 1996;6:334-37.
47. Iinuma Y, Narisawa R, Iwafuchi M, et al. The role of endoscopic retrograde cholangiopancreatography in infants with cholestasis. J Pediatr Surg 2000;35:545-49.
48. Yamataka A, Kuwatsuru R, Shima H, Kobayashi H, Lane GJ, Segawa O, Katayama H, Miyano T. Initial experience with non-breath-hold magnetic resonance cholangi-opancreatography: A new noninvasive technique for the diagnosis of choledochal cyst in children. J Pediatr Surg 1997;32:1560-62.
49. Shimizu T, Suzuki R, Yamashiro Y, Segawa O, Yamataka A, Miyano T. Progressive dilatation of the main pancreatic duct using magnetic resonance cholangiopancreatogrphy in a boy with chronic pancreatitis. J Pediatr Gastroenterol Nutr 2000;30:102-4.
50. Filler RM, Stringel G. Treatment of choledochal cyst by excision. J Pediatr Surg 1980;15:437-42.
51. Somasundaram K, Wong TJ, Tan KC. Choledochal cyst: a review of 25 cases. Austral NZ J Surg 1985;55:443-46.
52. Todani T, Watanabe Y, Toki A, et al. Reoperation for congenital choledochal cyst. Ann Surg 1988;207:142-47.
53. Todani T, Watanabe Y, Mzuguchi T, et al. Hepatico-duodenostomy at the hepatic hilum after excision of choledochal cyst. Am J Surg 1981;142:584-87.
54. Miyano T, Yamataka A, Kato Y, Segawa S, Lane G, Takamizawa S, Kohno S and Fujiwara T. Hepatico-enterostomy after excision of choledochal cyst in children: A 30-year experience with 180 cases. J Pediatr Surg 1996;31:1417-21.
55. Yamataka A, Ohshiro K, Okada Y. Complications after cyst excision with hepaticoenterostomy for choledochal cysts and their surgical management in children versus adults. J Pediatr Surg 1997;32:1097-1102.
56. Shimura H, Tanaka M, Shimizu S, Mizumoto K: Laparoscopic treatment of congenital choledochal cyst. Endosc 1998;12:1268-71.

57. Farello GA, Cerofolini A, Rebonato M, Bergamaschi G, Ferrari C, Chiappetta A: Congenital choledochal cyst: video-guided laparoscopic treatment. Surg Laparosc Endosc 1995;5:354-58.
58. Ohi R, Yaoita S, Kamiyama T, et al. Surgical treatment of congenital dilatation of the bile duct with special reference to late complications after total excision operation. J Pediatr Surg 25:13-17.
59. Ando H, Ito T, Kaneko K, Seo T, Ito F. Intrahepatic bile duct stenosis causing intrahepatic calculi formation following excision of a choledochal cyst. J Am Coll Surg 1996;183:56-60.
60. Engle J, Salmon PA. Multiple choledochal cysts. Arch Surg 1964;88:345-49.
61. Tsuchida Y, Taniguch F, Nakahara S, Uno K, Kawarasaki H, Inoue Y, Nishikawa J. Excision of a choledochal cyst and simultaneous hepatic lateral segmentectomy. Pediatr Surg Int 1996;11:496-97.
62. Miyano T, Yamataka A, Kato S, Kohno S and Fujiwara T. Choledochal cyst: special emphasis on the usefulness of intraoperative endoscopy. J Pediatr Surg 1996;30:482-84.
63. Yamataka A, Segawa O, Kobayashi H, Kato Y and Miyanot. Intraoperative pancreatoscopy for pancreatic duct stone debris distal to the common channel in choledochal cyst. J Pediatr Surg 2000;35:1-4.
64. Miyano T, Suruga K, Shimonura H. Choledochopancreatic elongated common channel disorders. J Pediatr Surg 1984;19:165-70.
65. Kaneko K, Ando H, Ito T. Protein plugs cause symptoms in patients with choledochal cysts. Am J Gastroenterol 1997;92:1018-21.

Pancreatic Pseudocyst

Shilpa Sharma, DK Gupta

Pancreatic pseudocysts are the most common cystic lesions of the pancreas; accounting for 75-80% of such masses. Pancreatic pseudocysts in children are usually a sequelae of pancreatic blunt trauma though it may rarely be associated with chronic pancreatitis and parenchymal disease. Imaging studies, such as ultrasound, computed tomography scan and endoscopic retrograde cholangiopancreatography are helpful in establishing diagnosis. Most of the diagnoses are usually made by an ultrasonogram or a CT scan abdomen.

DEFINITION

A pancreatic pseudocyst is a collection of fluid around the pancreas as a result of acute or chronic pancreatitis bound to the pancreas by inflammatory tissue.[1] The true incidence of pancreatitis in children is unknown. Pseudocysts complicate acute pancreatitis in approximately 10-30% cases.[2] The incidence of pancreatic pseudocysts is greater than 50% when associated with traumatic injury to the abdomen.

ETIOLOGY

Pancreatic ductal disruption in children leading to pseudocyst formation may occur secondary to:
1. Trauma.
2. Ductal obstruction.
3. Acute pancreatitis.
4. Chronic pancreatitis from strictures or ductal calculi.[3]
5. Pancreaticobiliary malformations, most commonly pancreatic divisum, bifid duct.[4]
6. Chronic pancreatitis resulting from systemic diseases like Systemic Lupus Erythematosus.[5]
7. Chronic relapsing pancreatitis resulting from hereditary pancreatitis.[4]
8. Drug induced acute pancreatitis—Valproic acid for epilepsy, L-asparaginase in pediatric malignancies.[6-8]
9. Cholelithiasis.[4]
10. Pancreatic neoplasms
11. Idiopathic.[4]

The most common etiology of the pancreatic pseudocyst identified in children is post-traumatic, being upto 80-100% of the cases in different series.[9,10] Idiopathic causes comprised up to 25% of the cases in a series of pediatric pseudocysts.[4]

PATHOPHYSIOLOGY

The formation of a pseudocyst usually requires four or more weeks from the onset of pancreatitis-acute or chronic. Pseudocysts have a higher incidence in chronic pancreatitis as compared to acute pancreatitis. Acute pancreatitis can cause necrosis. Chronic pancreatitis can cause elevated pancreatic duct pressures. Crushing or blunt abdominal trauma can injure the pancreas by compression against the vertebra.

A pancreatic pseudocyst is a fluid collection contained within a well-defined thick capsule of fibrous or granulation tissue or a combination of both.

Typically, the wall of a pancreatic pseudocyst lacks an epithelial lining, and the cyst contains pancreatic juice or amylase-rich fluid. The location of the pseudocyst is in the lesser peritoneal sac in proximity to the pancreas. It may involve any part of the pancreas, head, body and tail.[11] Large pseudocysts can extend into the paracolic gutters, pelvis, mediastinum, neck or scrotum.

More than 90% of the cysts are single though they can be multiple.[12] The cyst may be loculated. The fluid in the pseudocyst has similar electrolyte concentrations to plasma and a high concentration of amylase, lipase and enterokinases such as trypsin.

Pancreatitis originates with blockage or disruption of the collecting ducts and damage to the acinar cell, that leads to activation and release of digestive enzymes that autodigest the pancreatic parenchyma. The localized collections of pancreatic secretions become walled off by granulation tissue and form a pseudocyst either within the pancreatic tissue or immediately adjacent to it.

CLINICAL PRESENTATION

Though the most common etiology is post-traumatic in children, yet a negative history of trauma is not uncommon. This is so as the trauma is often subtle and long forgotten and the history from children may not be reliable. The cysts have been detected from 3-57 days after injury.[13] It is more common in boys.[13]

The most common presenting symptom is epigastric pain.[14] Other symptoms include mass, nausea, vomiting, feeling of bloating or a deep ache in the abdomen (Figs 91.1A to C). Additional symptoms include jaundice, chest pain, anorexia, weight loss, ascites and rarely gastrointestinal hemorrhage. If infection has set in, the child may present with fever, worsening abdominal pain and systemic signs of sepsis. The child may also present with failure to thrive.[4]

On examination, a tender epigastric mass may be palpaple. It is usually tense cystic.

COMPLICATIONS

These include:
1. Infection of the pseudocyst with a pancreatic abscess. About 10% pseudocysts become infected.[15]
2. Bleeding into the pseudocyst.
3. Intestinal obstruction.
4. Rupture.[16]
5. Pleural effusion.[17]
6. Thrombosis—Splenic vein is the most common site.
7. Pseudoaneurysm formation—Splenic artery is the most common site; other sites include gastroduodenal artery and pancreato duodenal artery.[16]
8. Spread into the mediastinum. Mediastinal pancreatic pseudocyst is a rare occurrence in children and may be difficult to diagnose.[18]

INVESTIGATIONS

Blood Investigations

Blood investigations may reveal leukocytosis, and persistent elevation of serum amylase. The initial serum amylase level has been found to correlate with neither the time of resolution nor the appearance of cyst after the trauma.[13] Genetic testing may detect established risk factors for chronic pancreatitis like homozygous SPINK1-N34S mutation.[3]

Plain Skiagram

Plain skiagram may demonstrate nonspecific findings ranging from a distended loop of small intestine (sentinel loop), calcifications, dilation of the transverse colon (cutoff sign), peripancreatic extraluminal gas bubbles, ileus, left-sided basal pleural effusion and

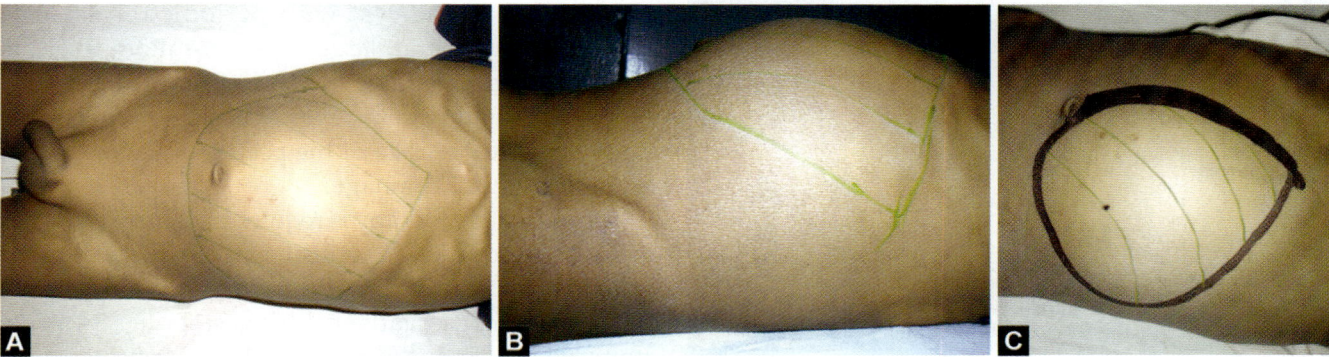

Figs 91.1A to C: A. Post-traumatic pseudocyst in a boy presenting as acute intestinal obstruction due to mass effect. The boy had bilious vomitings. He was managed conservatively with total parenteral nutrition and octreotide started on day 5. **B.** Lateral view of the same in which the mass can be seen extending up to below the umbilicus. **C.** The mass reduced in size gradually after 3 weeks and the boy could be discharged

blurring of the left psoas margin to pancreatic calcifications from chronic or recurrent pancreatitis. A soft tissue shadow of the pseudocyst may be identified. Concretions in the main pancreatic duct may be picked up.[3]

Ultrasonography

This is the primary screening tool for evaluation of the pediatric pancreas. Ultrasonography findings may identify a pseudocyst as a well-defined, hypoechoic mass that may be multilocular. Pancreatitis may be identified with a focally or diffusely enlarged, hypoechoic, sonolucent, or edematous pancreas; dilated pancreatic ducts; a fluid collection or peripancreatic fluid or an abscess. Ascites is easily picked up on ultrasonography. Endoscopic Ultrasonography (EUS) can also be added to the armamentarium. Serial sonogram examinations play an important role in monitoring the progress of pancreatic pseudocysts.[13]

Computed Tomography Scan

CT scan is a better modality to detect chronic pancreatitis and its complications, pancreatic trauma and neoplastic conditions. A pseudocyst with a well-defined wall or capsule and central area of low attenuation is well appreciated (Fig. 91.2). CT scanning is also a better modality for evaluating the presence and the extent of pancreatic necrosis and inflammation of peripancreatic fat.

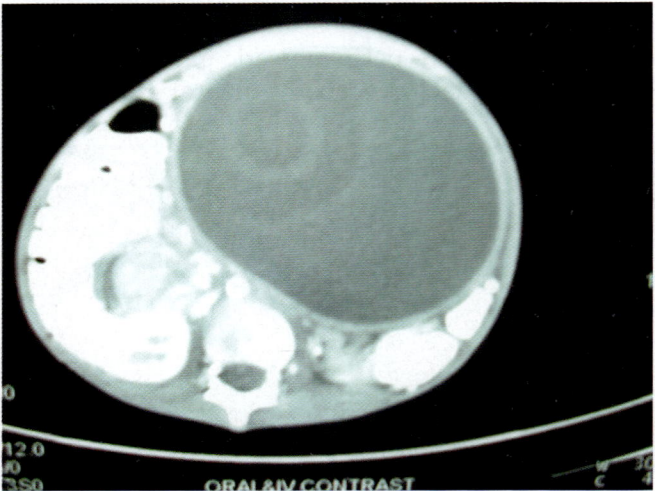

Fig. 91.2: CT scan of the pseudocyst of the boy in Figure 91.1 showing a well demarcated thin wall lined pseudopancreatic cyst as a hypodense lesion occupying the central abdomen

Endoscopic Retrograde Cholangiopancreatography (ERCP)

ERCP is essential for evaluation of pancreatic and biliary anomalies and has been found useful in establishing pancreas divisum as the etiology.[18] It can identify various ductal abnormalities or obstructions. It is also an important tool as a therapeutic intervention. ERCP is also essential to assess pseudocyst communication with the pancreatic duct to determine definitive operative therapy.

Magnetic Resonance Imaging (MRI) and Magnetic Resonance Cholangiopancreatography (MRCP)

Magnetic resonance imagining (MRI) is another modality to diagnose pancreatitis and is used for the same indications as CT scan. Magnetic resonance cholangiopancreatography (MRCP) is a noninvasive alternative to ERCP but lacks therapeutic capabilities.

MANAGEMENT

The aim of treatment for pseudocyst is the avoidance of complications. It has been reported that pseudocysts from nontraumatic etiologies are more likely to benefit from surgical interventions, whereas pseudocysts from traumatic etiology are more amenable to conservative management.[4]

Observation

All cysts do not require treatment. In many cases the pseudocysts resolve without interference and require only supportive care.[19] In a child with a cyst less than 6 cm that is not causing any symptoms, careful observation of the cyst with periodic CT scans is indicated. In general, larger cysts are more likely to become symptomatic or cause complications. However, some patients even with larger collections do well; therefore, size of the pseudocyst alone is not an indication for drainage.

Conservative therapy is required for approximately 4-6 weeks to allow the cyst wall to mature drug induced pancreatitis complicated by a pseudocyst may be managed conservatively by just stopping the drug. Valproic acid induced pancreatitis complicated by a pseudocyst has been reported to resolve spontaneously in four weeks.[7]

Conservative Medical Treatment

Medical therapy reduces the pancreatic stimulation and favors the resolution or the maturation of the pseudocyst.[9] Many patients with pancreatic pseudocysts can be managed conservatively if the presenting symptoms can be controlled.[20]

If the child is symptomatic with pain abdomen, an intial supportive management may be given till there is relief in symptoms. This consists of adequate rehydration, keeping the child nil orally and on nasogastric decompression. Total parenteral nutrition may be added if there is no relief within five days (Fig. 91.1). Octreotide can be useful to decrease the amount of pancreatic secretions.[21] Antacids or H_2-histamine blockers are useful to prevent gastritis and reduce duodenal acid exposure. Antibiotics may be added if the cyst is infected. Acute pancreatitis should resolve in 2-7 days with adequate resuscitation. In chronic relapsing pancreatitis, pancreatic enzyme supplementation, insulin and elemental or low-fat diets are useful adjuncts to maximize nutritional status. About 1/3-1/2 of the pseudocysts resolve spontaneously.

INTERVENTION

The management of pseudocysts in children should be individualized as suggested for management of pancreatic injuries in children.[22]

Certain indications for operative interventions have been identified. If a pseudocyst is persistent over 6 weeks or causing symptoms, then surgical treatment of the cyst is required. Indications for drainage include enlargement of the cyst to more than 6 cm, setting in of complications, symptoms and concerns about possible malignancy.[23]

Surgical intervention is also indicated for the management of congenital anatomic defects like pancreatic divisum.

The methods of intervention include percutaneous drainage, endoscopic drainage and surgical drainage.

Percutaneous Drainage

Percutaneous catheter drainage is the procedure of choice for treating infected pseudocysts. Octreotide can be useful as adjunct to catheter drainage.[24] Percutaneous continuous drainage may be done until the output is < 50 ml/day or the serum amylase is normal. The failure rate is about 15% and recurrence rate is 7%. The complications include conversion into an infected pseudocyst (10%), catheter-site cellulitis, gastrointestinal hemorrhage, pancreatico-cutaneous fistula and damage to the adjacent organs.

L-asparaginase (used for acute lymphocytic leukemia) induced pancreatitis, complicated with pseudocyst formation has been treated by percutaneous external drainage, total parenteral nutrition (TPN), administration of octreotide and antibiotic therapy for one month.[8] Percutaneous external drainage proved to be an effective, noninvasive method in this special case with a systemic disorder and the high risk of mortality should a surgical intervention have been performed.[8]

Endoscopic Drainage

Recently, there has been an increasing trend towards the use of endoscopic treatment for the management of pancreatic pseudocysts in children with success rates as high as 85%.[25,26] Some authors suggest that endoscopic treatment should be the first choice and surgical treatment can be reserved for cases that fail to the endoscopic treatment.

Endoscopic drainage may be either transpapillary (via ERCP) or transmural (transenteric).[27,28] The procedure adopted requires careful patient selection to ensure success and safety.

The indications for endoscopic drainage include; mature cyst wall < 1 cm thick, cyst adherent to the duodenum or posterior gastric wall and a history of previous abdominal surgery or significant co-morbidities. The contraindications for endoscopic drainage include bleeding dyscrasias, gastric varices, acute inflammatory changes that may prevent cyst from adhering to the enteric wall, evidence of intrapancreatic ductal obstruction, presence of thick debris and multiloculated cyst.

Transpapillary drainage is feasible as 40-70% of pseudocysts communicate with pancreatic duct. The usual procedures adopted are ERCP with sphincterotomy, balloon dilatation of pancreatic duct strictures, and stent placement beyond strictures. Endoscopic transpapillary nasopancreatic drainage placement is a safe and effective modality for the treatment of multiple and large pseudocysts, especially when there is partial ductal disruption, and the disruption can be bridged.[29]

Large pseudocysts of the pancreas have been successfully treated in the short-term by minimally-invasive stent placement to create an internal cyst-gastric communication.[30]

Endoscopic placement of stents has been found successful in the treatment of pancreatic pseudocysts in children, in even a baby as young as 17-month-old.[2,31,32]

Transmural drainage may be cystogastrostomy or cystoduodenostomy. Endoscopic transmural drainage is a minimally invasive, effective and safe approach in the management of pancreatic pseudocysts and abscesses.[33,34]

Cystogastrostomy and cystoduodenostomy have been created with an interventional linear echoendoscope under endosonographic and fluoroscopic control by the endoscopic insertion of straight or double pigtail stents.[34]

Complications have been seen more frequently in patients with a recent episode of acute pancreatitis.[34]

The majority of major complications in endoscopic drainage may be prevented by using pigtail stents instead of straight stents and by taking a more aggressive approach to the prevention and treatment of secondary cyst infection.[35] The technical success rate of the drainage procedure has been reported as 97 %. Complications include hemorrhage caused by erosion of a straight endoprosthesis through the cyst wall, secondary infection and perforation.[35]

Surgical Treatment

Pancreatic pseudocysts with associated major ductal disruption or a transected pancreas require operative therapy with cyst enterostomy.

Surgical internal drainage is the procedure of choice and has a success rate of 85-90%.[36] Surgical drainage is the standard criteria against which all therapies are measured.

Patients who failed non-operative measures should have a period of stabilization prior to operation. This is important to reverse sepsis and to improve nutritional status prior to intervention.

The type of surgical procedure depends on the location of the cyst. For cysts that occur in the body and tail of the pancreas either a cysto-jejunostomy or cystogastrostomy is performed depending on the location of the cyst in the abdomen. For pseudocysts that occur in the head of the pancreas a cysto-duodenostomy is usually performed. A cysto-duodenostomy may be complicated by duodenal fistula and bleeding at anastomotic site.

Successful enucleation of the pseudocyst has also been reported.[11] However, since the anterior wall of the pancreas forms a wall of the cyst, it is not at all advisable to attempt this procedure in most cases. Larger cysts and those located in the head and neck, tend to be drained, while smaller and distal cysts have more often been resected.[37]

Some surgeons have performed an intraoperative pancreatic ductography in adults with chronic pancreatitis to determine the site of ductal disruption and adopt the most appropriate operative procedure. Ductal anatomy on ERCP has been used as a guide to the choice of modality. Cases with a normal duct with a noncommunicating or a communicating pseudocyst have been managed non-operatively. Cases with an isolated ductal segment and chronic pancreatitis have been managed operatively.

Definitive management with subtotal or total pancreatectomy is associated with considerable morbidity and mortality due to loss of both endocrine and exocrine functions of the pancreas. Generally, pancreatectomy is not indicated in children; however, it may be considered in cases of intractable pain and diffuse parenchymal damage without ductal dilation. Distal pancreatectomy may also be considered when the pseudocyst is in the tail of the gland.

Surgical options for chronic pancreatitis include distal pancreatectomy with Roux-en-Y pancreaticojejunostomy (i.e. Duval procedure), lateral pancreaticojejunostomy (Puestow procedure), or ERCP sphincteroplasty. In presence of a dilated pancreatic duct with multiple calculi, a transverse pancreaticojejunostomy is justified after removal of the calculi.[11]

Pancreatic pseudocyst has been reported to account for 6% of the 253 cases undergoing distal pancreatectomy.[38] Cyst wall biopsy obtained confirmed the diagnosis of pseudocyst in 8 of 10 cases while a true cyst with epithelial lining was found in only 2 cases in a series.[39]

A mediastinal pseudocyst has been approached thoracoscopically.[18]

Laparoscopic cystojejunostomy and cystogastrostomy have been successfully performed in children with pancreatic pseudocysts.[40,41] A technique combining upper endoscopy with percutaneous transgastric minilaparoscopic instrumentation for the formation of pancreatic cystgastrostomy has been performed safely and effectively for the internal drainage of pancreatic pseudocysts.[42] Ports have been placed through the anterior abdominal and gastric walls, and into the lumen of the stomach for access to the posterior gastric wall. Using electrocautery diathermy, an incision was made through the posterior gastric wall and into the adjacent pseudocyst to obtain complete and unobstructed drainage.

MORBIDITY AND MORTALITY

Management of pancreatic pseudocysts has been associated with considerable morbidity (15-25%).[21] These morbidities include pancreatic leak, wound infection, failure to thrive and insulin-dependent diabetes.[4] The mortality is however 0-1%.

AIIMS EXPERIENCE

At AIIMS, most pseudocysts were seen following trauma. Post-pancreatitis pseudocysts were uncommon in our setup. Most of these were large and unilocular. Only a few were multiloculated. While ultrasonography offers the diagnosis, CT scan was mandatory to evaluate the pancreas properly. Children without any symptoms or the cysts less than 5 cm in size were observed with serial monthly ultrasonography. Larger cysts, if found feasible were drained with a pigtail catheter under ultrasonographic control. The amount of the daily output of the pancreatic fluid and the amylase content was monitored. Cystogastrostomy was performed for the infected cysts or the cysts that fail to resolve even with after 3 months. The cyst fluid drained into the stomach and the cyst disappeared completely in a few months. Authors' have no experience with the endoscopic management of the pseudocyst of the pancreas.

REFERENCES

1. Gupta DK, Sharma Shilpa. Abdominal Cysts in Adolescence in Textbook of Adolescent Medicine. Ed Swati Bhave. Jaypee Brothers, Delhi 2006; 20.6: 670-74.
2. Bridoux-Henno L, Dabadie A, Rambeau M, et al. Successful endoscopic drainage of a pancreatic pseudocyst in a 17-month-old boy. Eur J Pediatr 2004;163:482-84.
3. Kahn AC, Teich N, Caca K, et al. Chronic pancreatitis with pancreaticolithiasis and pseudocyst in a 5-year-old boy with homozygous SPINK1 mutation. Pediatr Radiol 2005;35:902-05.
4. Teh SH, Pham TH, Lee A, et al. Pancreatic pseudocyst in children: the impact of management strategies on outcome J Pediatr Surg 2006;41:1889-93.
5. Al-Mayouf SM, Majeed M, Al-Mehaidib A, et al. Pancreatic pseudocyst in paediatric systemic lupus erythematosus Clin Rheumatol 2002;21:264-66.
6. Queizán A, Hernández F, Rivas S. Pancreatic pseudocyst caused by valproic acid: case report and review of the literature. Eur J Pediatr Surg 2003;13:60-62.
7. Houben ML, Wilting I, Stroink H, et al. Pancreatitis, complicated by a pancreatic pseudocyst associated with the use of valproic acid Eur J Paediatr Neurol 2005;9: 77-80.
8. Karabulut R, Sanmez K, Afayarlar C, et al. Pancreas pseudocyst associated with L-asparaginase treatment: a case report. Acta Chir Belg 2005;105:667-67.
9. Kisra M, Ettayebi F, Benhammou M. Pseudocysts of the pancreas in children in Morocco. J Pediatr Surg 1999;34:1327-29.
10. Rosenthal R, Vogelbach P. Post-traumatic pancreatic pseudocyst in a child Swiss Surg 2001;7(5):225-28.
11. Rehman S, Jawaid M. Enucleation of Pancreatic Pseudocyst in a patient suffering from chronic pancreatitis. Pak J Med Sci 2005;21:380-84.
12. Pitchumoni CS, Agarwal N. Pancreatic pseudocysts. When and how should drainage be performed? Gastroenterol Clin North Am 1999;28:615-39.
13. Tiao MM, Chuang JH, Ko SF, et al. Pancreatic pseudocysts in children. Chang Gung Med J 2000;23:761-67.
14. van Leeuwaarde R, Kneepkens CM, Ekkelkamp S, et al. Three children with pancreatic (pseudo) cysts as the cause of undefined abdominal pain. Ned Tijdschr Geneeskd 2006;150:500-04.
15. Hamel A, Parc R, Adda G. Bleeding pseudocysts and pseudoaneurysms in chronic pancreatitis. Br J Surg 1991;78:1059-63.
16. Afzal M, Ghous SG, Siddiq K. Spontaneous rupture of pancreatic pseudocyst J Coll Physicians Surg Pak 2004;14:370-71.
17. Poddar B, Singh K, Kochar S, et al. Pancreatopleural fistula presenting as hemorrhagic pleural effusion. Indian Pediatr 1999;36:310-13.
18. Bonnard A, Lagausie P, Malbezin S, et al. Mediastinal pancreatic pseudocyst in a child. A thoracoscopic approach. Surg Endosc 2001;15:760.
19. Yeo CJ, Bastidas JA, Lynch-Nyhan A. The natural history of pancreatic pseudocysts documented by computed tomography. Surg Gynecol Obstet 1990;170:411-17.
20. Cheruvu CV, Clarke MG, Prentice M, et al. Conservative treatment as an option in the management of pancreatic pseudocyst. Ann R Coll Surg Engl 2003;85:313-16.
21. Tissières P, Bugmann P, Rimensberger PC, et al. Somatostatin in the treatment of pancreatic pseudocyst

complicating acute pancreatitis in a child with liver transplantation. J Pediatr Gastroenterol Nutr 2000;31: 445-47.
22. Stringer MD. Pancreatic trauma in children. Br J Surg 2005;92:467-70.
23. Warshaw AL, Rutledge PL. Cystic tumors mistaken for pancreatic pseudocysts. Ann Surg 1987;205:393-98.
24. D'Agostino HB, van Sonnenberg E, Sanchez RB. Treatment of pancreatic pseudocysts with percutaneous drainage and octreotide. Work in progress. Radiology 1993;187:685-88.
25. Mas E, Barange K, Breton A, et al. Endoscopic cystostomy for post-traumatic pseudocyst in children J Pediatr Gastroenterol Nutr 2007;45:121-24.
26. Haluszka O, Campbell A, Horvath K. Endoscopic management of pancreatic pseudocyst in children. Gastrointest Endosc 2002;55:128-31.
27. Beckingham IJ, Krige JE, Bornman PC. Long-term outcome of endoscopic drainage of pancreatic pseudocysts. Am J Gastroenterol 1999;94:71-74.
28. Binmoeller KF, Seifert H, Walter A. Transpapillary and transmural drainage of pancreatic pseudocysts. Gastrointest Endosc 1995;42:219-24.
29. Bhasin DK, Rana SS, Udawat HP, et al. Management of multiple and large pancreatic pseudocysts by endoscopic transpapillary nasopancreatic drainage alone. Am J Gastroenterol 2006;101:1780-86.
30. Breckon V, Thomson SR, Hadley GP. Internal drainage of pancreatic pseudocysts in children using an endoscopically-placed stent. Pediatr Surg Int 2001;17: 621-23.
31. Kimble RM, Cohen R, Williams S. Successful endoscopic drainage of a post-traumatic pancreatic pseudocyst in a child. J Pediatr Surg 1999;34:1518-20.
32. Al-Shanafey S, Shun A, Williams S. Endoscopic drainage of pancreatic pseudocysts in children. J Pediatr Surg 2004;39:1062-65.
33. Patty I, Kalaoui M, Al-Shamali M, et al. Endoscopic drainage for pancreatic pseudocyst in children. J Pediatr Surg 2001;36:503-55.
34. Lopes CV, Pesenti C, Bories E, et al. Endoscopic-ultrasound-guided endoscopic transmural drainage of pancreatic pseudocysts and abscesses. Scand J Gastroenterol 2007;42:524-29.
35. Cahen D, Rauws E, Fockens P, et al. Endoscopic drainage of pancreatic pseudocysts: long-term outcome and procedural factors associated with safe and successful treatment. Endoscopy 2005; 37:977-83.
36. Heider R, Meyer AA, Galanko JA. Percutaneous drainage of pancreatic pseudocysts is associated with a higher failure rate than surgical treatment in unselected patients. Ann Surg 1999;229:781-89.
37. Usatoff V, Brancatisano R, Williamson RC. Operative treatment of pseudocysts in patients with chronic pancreatitis. Br J Surg 2000; 87:1494-99.
38. Lillemoe KD, Kaushal S, Cameron JL, et al. Distal pancreatectomy: indications and outcomes in 235 patients. Ann Surg 1999 May;229(5):693-98; discussion 698-700.
39. Ezzedien Rabie M, Ghaleb AH, Al-Ghamdi MA, et al. Drainage of pancreatic pseudocysts. The importance of cyst wall biopsy in the recent era. Saudi Med J 2005;26: 289-93.
40. Saad DF, Gow KW, Cabbabe S, et al. Laparoscopic cystogastrostomy for the treatment of pancreatic pseudocysts in children. J Pediatr Surg 2005;40:e13-17.
41. Seitz G, Warmann SW, Kirschner HJ, et al. Laparoscopic cystojejunostomy as a treatment option for pancreatic pseudocysts in children-a case report. J Pediatr Surg 2006;41:e33-35.
42. Heniford BT, Iannitti DA, Paton BL, et al. Minilaparoscopic transgastric cystgastrostomy. Am J Surg 2006; 192:248-51.

CHAPTER 92

Pancreatitis

GVS Murthi, PAM Raine

Pancreatitis is encountered far less commonly in children when compared to its frequent presentation in adult clinical practice. A major reason is that some of the principal causative or predisposing factors—alcohol, gallstone disease, drug abuse, multisystem disorders—are fortunately less prevalent in childhood; idiopathic, traumatic, hereditary and congenital causes are more common. Pancreatitis in childhood usually runs an acute self-limiting course and is often less severe than in adults, but it can be associated with a considerable long-term morbidity and a significant mortality. A high index of suspicion and a special interest is necessary to make the diagnosis in a child with unexplained or recurrent abdominal pain.[1]

INCIDENCE

The incidence of pancreatitis in childhood is difficult to establish with accuracy. Reports vary partly due to different policies regarding the inclusion of adolescent and young adult patients in series. An estimate of 1:50,000 for the incidence of pancreatitis has been made but variations occur between different populations, particularly in relation to the prevalence of sickle cell disease and gallstones.[2,3] Major pediatric centers often see only a handful of cases each year. The sex ratio is equal. A carefully analysed study of all ages in the Netherlands suggests a gradually increasing incidence but a reducing mortality over the decade 1985-1995.[4]

ETIOPATHOGENESIS

Clinically, pancreatitis can be classified as acute, chronic or relapsing.

Acute pancreatitis presents a spectrum from a relatively mild inflammatory disorder to severe hemorrhagic destruction of the gland itself.[5-7] The precise mechanisms of initiation of pancreatitis are poorly understood though factors such as obstruction, toxins and ischemia are implicated. Injury to acinar cells disturbs the formation and transport of zymogen granules and leads to the activation of precursor digestive enzymes (e.g. trypsinogen to trypsin).[8] In turn, this activates other enzymes such as kallikrein, elastase and phospholipase 2. This precipitates a cascade of events progressing to autodigestion and necrosis of pancreatic tissue. Macroscopically, mild disease consists of interstitial edema whilst severe disease produces extensive peripancreatic fat necrosis and outpouring of hemorrhagic fluid into the peritoneal cavity. A massive coagulation necrosis of both pancreatic and peripancreatic tissue may result—necrotising pancreatitis.

Recent work has centered on the possibility of pancreatitis being related to ischemia–reperfusion injury and the role of inflammatory mediators such as arachidonic acid, interleukin 6, tumor necrosis factor alpha and platelet activating factor is being explored.[8,9] Cytokine activation and the generation of toxic oxygen free radicals during reperfusion is considered a potent source of damage to cell membranes and tissues.[8] Secondary gram-negative bacterial infection of the necrotic pancreas is relatively common (40-60%) and an abscess may form.[10]

The systemic effects of acute pancreatitis include vasodilatation, capillary permeability, coagulopathy, respiratory distress, renal insufficiency, CNS effects, hypocalcemia and shock. In turn, multi-system organ failure may supervene.

Chronic pancreatitis may follow a recurrent or relapsing course and is often based on an identifiable underlying cause (systemic infection, hereditary pancreatitis, cystic fibrosis, hyperlipoproteinemia, inborn errors of metabolism, inflammatory bowel disease) or is secondary to a definable anatomical abnormality (pancreas divisum, annular pancreas).[11] Similar mechanisms to those in play in the pathogenesis of acute pancreatitis (viz. cytokine release and free radical generation) are responsible for cellular damage in chronic pancreatitis.[8] The process may be focal, segmental or diffuse and can progress to lobular fibrosis of acini, duct dilatation and lesions of the duct epithelium.[7,12] Precipitation of protein in pancreatic ducts is related to lithostathine (pancreatic-stone protein) secretion and leads to plugging.[13] Subsequently, calcification and stone formation occur. Eventually some degree of irreversible exocrine and endocrine pancreatic dysfunction develops.[14]

The causes of pancreatitis can be classified under broad categories as: idiopathic, hereditary, traumatic, drug-related, secondary to bilio-pancreatic tract anomaly, infection, multisystem disorder or metabolic disorder. Whether an acute or chronic illness develops depends to some extent on the eradication or persistence of the underlying cause.

Idiopathic: Between 10 and 30% of cases of pancreatitis are of unknown cause.[10,13,15] Some of these patients will subsequently develop recurrent pancreatitis and have an underlying anatomic abnormality identified by endoscopic retrograde cholangiopancreatography or by magnetic resonance cholangiopancreatography.[16,17]

Hereditary pancreatitis has an autosomal dominant pattern with variable expressivity and incomplete penetrance (up to 80%).[18-22] It is described only in Caucasians and diagnosis is usually based on the finding of a positive family history in one or more first-degree relatives. Recently, a mutation in the cationic trypsinogen gene has been identified as the cause of hereditary pancreatitis.[23] It is a relatively severe form of chronic relapsing pancreatitis that leads more often to surgical treatment usually in the form of a longitudinal pancreatico-jejunostomy.[24]

Drugs may predispose to pancreatitis by interfering with the normal responses to infection and inflammation or by impairing metabolic pathways and cellular mechanisms and causing secondary toxic effects. A hypersensitivity/allergic mechanism has also been postulated and a single overdose may lead to pancreatitis.[5,10] Organ transplantation is associated with pancreatitis probably in relation to immunosuppressive therapy. Over 100 drugs have been reported to be associated with pancreatitis and some are listed in Table 92.1.

Trauma is probably the commonest cause of acute pancreatitis (about 20%) and is usually blunt (accidental or non-accidental) though both open and endoscopic surgical injury may occur.[10] A trivial injury in a child such as a fall on a handle-bar is sufficient to cause pancreatitis. The fixed retroperitoneal position of the pancreas astride the arch of the vertebral bodies renders it particularly susceptible to direct compression and to shearing and tearing forces. Postoperative pancreatitis may be related to hypotension in complex abdominal and thoracic surgery.[10] Ischemic and hypothermic injuries also cause pancreatitis.

Biliopancreatic tract anomalies have been diagnosed with increasing frequency as anatomical definition has become readily possible using endoscopic retrograde pancreatography (ERCP) and magnetic resonance cholangiopancreatography (MRCP).[17,25-28] Variations on the "standard" anatomy of the common bile duct and the ducts of Wirsung and Santorini (accessory pancreatic ducts) are not unusual. A long common channel, ectopic sphincter of Oddi, annular pancreas, pancreas divisum and duplications of pancreas and stomach may be found. These may be associated with duct stenosis, stricture, dilatation and both intrinsic and extrinsic obstruction. Whether these are the cause or the result of pancreatitis is not always clear.

Table 92.1: Drugs associated with Pancreatitis

Azathioprine	Trimethoprim
6 – mercaptopurine	Sulfamethoxazole
Cyclosporine	Tetracycline
Pentamidine	Metronidaole
Didanosine	Sulphasalazzine
Steroids	Erythromycin
Thiazides	L–asparaginase
Valproate	Acetaminophen
Diazoxide	Oral contraceptives
Cimetidine	Narcotic dependency
Ranitidine	Alcohol abuse

Infective causes of pancreatitis include a wide variety of viruses; mumps, Coxsackie, Epstein-Barr, influenza A, hepatitis A and B, measles, Guillain-Barre, enterovirus and rubella. Pancreatitis has a complex relationship with HIV infection involving immunocompromise, opportunistic infection and the drug treatment itself and may follow a severe and prolonged course.[29] Syphilis and toxoplasmosis have also been implicated. Secondary bacterial infection is recognised as a potentially lethal complication of acute necrotising enterocolitis.[30] Venoms from bites by snakes, scorpions and spiders and parasitic infections (e.g. ascariasis) are risks in many parts of the world.

Metabolic problems arise in hyperlipidemia, hyperparathyroidism, alpha-1-antitrypsin deficiency, cystic fibrosis, glucose-6-phosphate dehydrogenase deficiency, diabetes, aminoaciduria (lysine, cystine, arginine), malnutrition and spherocytosis. Such problems usually give rise to a chronic relapsing pattern of pancreatitis that may lead eventually to fibrosis and calcification and, in the long-term, to pancreatic insufficiency. Gallstone disease, giving rise to pancreatic duct obstruction, may complicate the metabolic abnormality.[11] Malnutrition, associated with alcohol or narcotic drug abuse, leads to severe pancreatic damage.[14] Malnutrition has been associated with but not proven as the cause of tropical pancreatitis – a form of chronic pancreatitis in young non-alcoholic adults found in South India, Africa and other tropical areas.[31]

Multisystem disorders such as hemolytic uremic syndrome, systemic lupus erythematosus, polyarteritis nodosa and Reye's syndrome may be complicated by severe acute pancreatitis. Although in general there is no clear correlation between the cause of pancreatitis and the pathological findings, mortality is higher in the context of multisystem disorders.[7,15]

PRESENTATION

Pain is the pre-eminent presenting feature in up to 95% of cases, though the characteristics vary.[2] It is most often a continuous epigastric pain (30%), but it may be focused in the right upper quadrant or umbilical areas, or may be diffuse; radiation to the back is a feature.[15] The intense boring nature of the pain may be severe enough to induce anxiety and psychological disturbance. Severity of pain also causes the child to lie still with knees flexed.[6] The pain may be exacerbated by eating. The pain needs to be differentiated from other causes of abdominal pain (Table 92.2).

Nausea and anorexia are common and vomiting occurs in approximately 60%; when bilious, it may be related to paralytic ileus.[7,15] Fever is low grade (37.5-38.5 °C) initially. Jaundice occurs particularly in chronic relapsing cases in which a fibrosing pancreatitis progresses to common bile duct obstruction.[21,32] In recurrent chronic pancreatitis, weight loss and diarrhea develop.[12,19,33] Additional pointers to the diagnosis of pancreatitis are a previous history of similar pain, a family history of pancreatitis, associated biliary disease or parotid or testicular enlargement suggesting mumps.

The initial clinical finding is localised epigastric tenderness with rebound tenderness progressing to guarding and rigidity in more severe cases. Abdominal distension may be related to ileus or ascites in 10-20%.[7,15] Pleural effusions, usually left sided, occur in up to 40%.[7] These add to the respiratory problems caused by the tendency to hypoventilation.

In the most severe hemorrhagic pancreatitis, in which massive outpouring of fluid occurs, hemoconcentration and hypotension may supervene.[5] Metabolic disturbances follow rapidly due to fluid and electrolyte imbalance, hypocalcemia and hyperglycemia. Tetany occasionally occurs. Retroperitoneal hemorrhage may become manifest as bruising in the flanks (Grey-Turner's sign) or around the umbilicus (Cullen's sign).[6] Severity of pancreatitis can be assessed using a variety of clinical scoring systems and criteria.[34-36]

Table 92.2: Conditions presenting with abdominal pain and raised amylase

- Acute appendicitis
- Perforated duodenal ulcer
- Bowel infarction
- Salivary gland inflammation
- Biliary tract disorders
- Hepatitis
- Renal failure
- Tumors
- Intestinal obstruction
- Peritonitis
- Diabetic ketoacidosis
- Basal pneumonia

INVESTIGATION AND DIAGNOSIS

The diagnosis of pancreatitis is usually based on a suggestive or typical clinical picture supported by biochemical and radiological investigations. The presence of an inflammatory disorder is suspected by the raised white cell count, raised C-reactive protein, raised erythrocyte sedimentation rate and fall in hematocrit. Hypocalcemia, hyperglycemia and raised bilirubin and liver enzymes are all suggestive of pancreatitis and biliary tract obstruction/inflammation.

Biochemical Investigations

Raised amylase though often a mainstay of diagnosis of pancreatitis, is not pathognomonic: However, the test is rapid. It is elevated in a variety of other disorders presenting with abdominal pain that may potentially cause diagnostic confusion (Table 92.3). Only approximately 40% of serum-amylase (P-isoamylase) is derived from the pancreas and 60% (S-isoamylase) is salivary.[2] Normal serum levels in childhood are in the range 48+/− 29 mg/dl (Somogyi units) with elevation to three times normal in most cases of pancreatitis and occasionally up to 1000 mg/dl.[5] However, serum amylase may be normal in up to 10% of cases.[6,37] Sensitivity is therefore about 95% but specificity is only 86%.[2,6] The level of serum amylase is not a predictor of severity of disease.[3,10]

Amylase is a small molecule and is rapidly cleared in pancreatitis due to decreased renal tubular absorption. Urinary amylase is therefore a more specific indicator of pancreatitis. Renal clearance of amylase is related to renal clearance of creatinine to give a ratio with an upper limit of normal of 4%, and a ratio greater than 5% is strongly suggestive of pancreatitis.[21,38]

Other pancreatic enzymes, such as lipase, elastase and immunoreactive cationic trypsin, also show elevated serum levels.[15] Lipase is more specific (up to 99%) for pancreatitis and, although measurement takes longer, it also clears more slowly from the blood stream. The diagnosis of chronic pancreatitis may be made in the quiescent phase using a morphine-prostigmine stimulation test to evoke symptoms of pancreatitis and measure elevation of serum enzymes.[1] More detailed tests of pancreatic function involve collection and analysis of duodenal juice after stimulation, measurement of chymotrypsin in stool and measurement of products of pancreatic digestion which are absorbed and excreted in urine.[13] Such tests are, of necessity, complex and time consuming and of limited application in pediatrics.

C-reactive protein rises rapidly and in proportion to the severity of disease.

Radiological Investigations

Th relative roles and value of different radiological modalities in the diagnosis of pancreatitis have been assessed in detail.[39] Available techniques include plain radiography, upper small bowel contrast, ultrasound (US), contrast-enhanced computed tomography (CT), magnetic resonance imaging (MRI), endoscopic retrograde cholangiopancreatography (ERCP), transhepatic cholangiography and angiography. Which is most appropriate depends on local circumstances and expertise but, overall, contrast-enhanced CT scanning, ERCP and magnetic resonance cholangiopancreatography (MRCP) probably have most to offer.

Plain radiographs may show ileus, sentinel loop (Fig. 92.1), mass, colon cut-off, calcification and abscess (air-fluid level).[3,6,15,40] Up to 55% of plain radiographs may be abnormal, and therefore suggest a significant intraperitoneal problem, though many signs are nonspecific. Chest radiograph may show a left-sided pleural effusion or elevation of the left hemidiaphragm due to fluid collection.

Upper small bowel contrast may show displacement, expansion (Fig. 92.2), distortion or obstruction of the duodenal loop.

Table 92.3 : Criteria used in prediction of outcome from acute pancreatitis[34,35]

- Age of patient
- White cell count
- Blood urea nitrogen
- Lactic dehydrogenase
- Serum albumen
- Serum calcium
- Serum glucose
- Partial pressure of oxygen (PaO_2)
- Base deficit (after 48 hours)
- Fluid deficit (after 48 hours)

Ultrasound has the great advantage of being rapid, non-invasive, readily repeated and available at the bedside. However, interpretation can be difficult due to the concealed retroperitoneal position of the gland and distension of overlying bowel and a high level of expertise is needed. The size and shape of the pancreas can be defined (Fig. 92.3) and features such as edema, calcification, duct dilatation and pseudocyst formation (Fig. 92.4) can be recognised.[3,6,15] Doppler ultrasound gives additional information by delineating vascular flow (Fig. 92.5). Endoscopic ultrasound gives greater definition and may detect pathology (e.g. stones) not seen with transabdominal ultrasound.[41] Peroperative ultrasound may assist in definition and location of cysts in both closed and open drainage procedures. Fine needle aspiration of the pancreas under ultrasound control is helpful in determining the presence of infection and indicating the need for surgical drainage.[42]

CT scanning (contrast-enhanced) (Fig. 92.6) is the method of choice in diagnosis of acute or chronic pancreatic changes, viz. pancreatic necrosis, infected necrosis, acute fluid collection, pseudocyst formation (Fig. 92.7), abscess and hemorrhage.[10,39,43] The clear anatomical detail shown on CT scan is especially helpful in identification of the safest and most effective route for percutaneous drainage of fluid collections.[39,44]

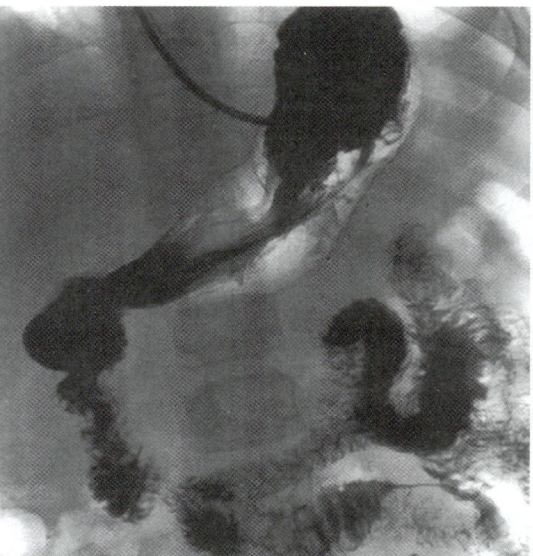

Fig. 92.2: Barium meal showing expanded duodenal loop due to enlarged head of pancreas

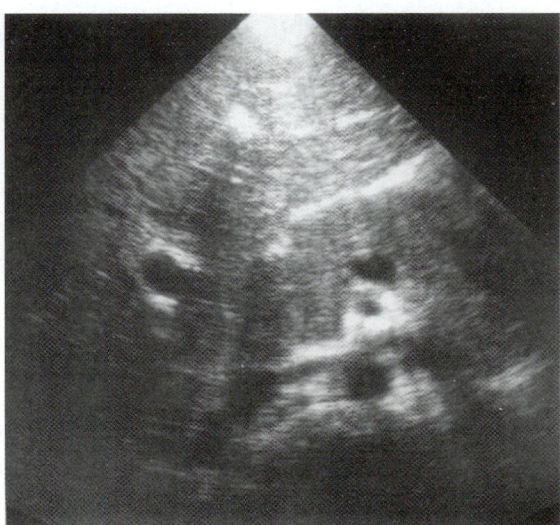

Fig. 92.3: Ultrasound scan showing enlarged body of pancreas overlying portal vein, superior mesenteric artery aorta and inferior vena cava with liver and gallbladder to the right

ERCP offers fine detail of duct and gland anatomy that is important if operative resection or drainage procedures are planned.[3,33] Larger series in childhood report over 90% technical success.[25,27,28,45-48] Morbidity related to flare-up of pancreatitis is commoner than in adults though it usually resolves rapidly: Bleeding occasionally occurs. The indications for ERCP are acute non-resolving recurrent or chronic pancreatitis and abnormal findings are noted in about 50% of all examinations.[2,12,21,25,40] The abnormalities include:

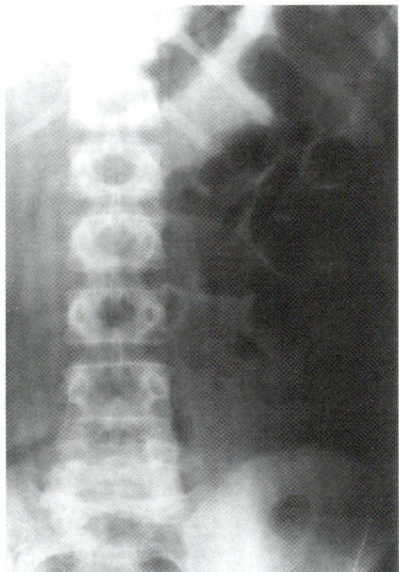

Fig. 92.1: Plain abdominal radiograph showing sentinel loop of bowel caused by inflamed pancreas

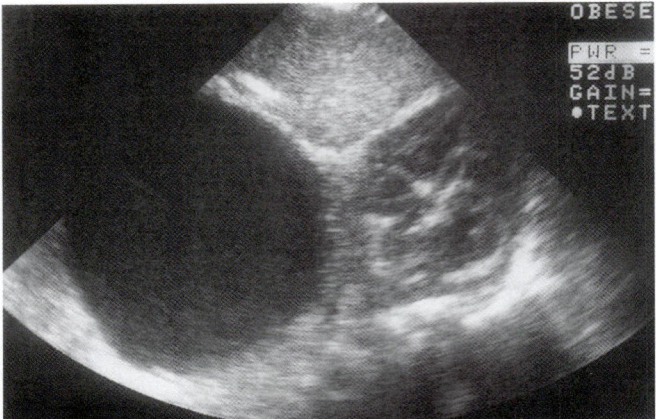

Fig. 92.4: Ultrasound scan showing pancreatic pseudocyst

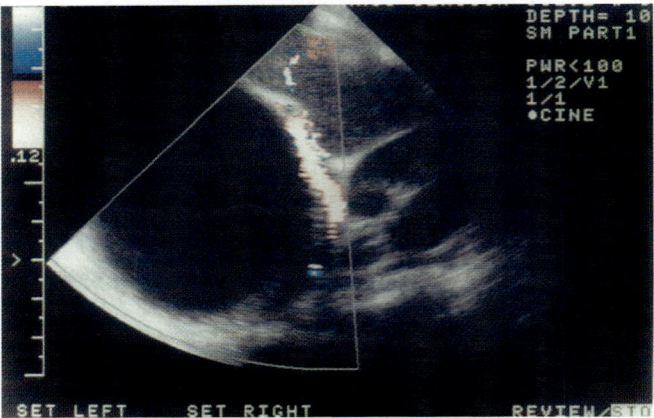

Fig. 92.5: Doppler ultrasound scan showing pancreatic pseudocyst with splenic vessels coursing around

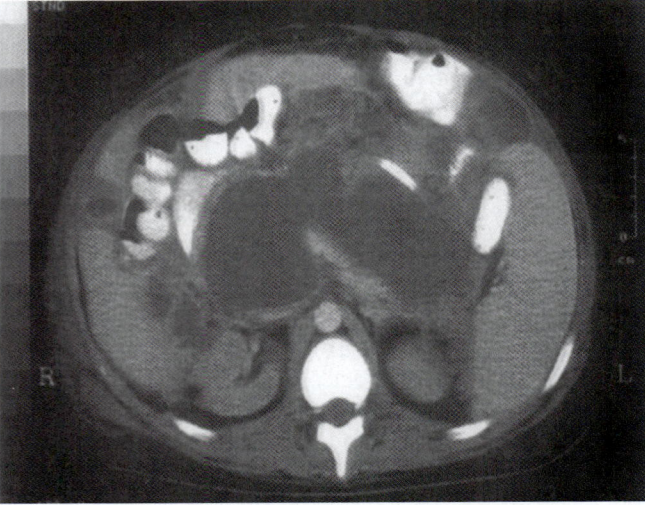

Fig. 92.6: Computed tomography scan showing enlarged necrotic pancreas

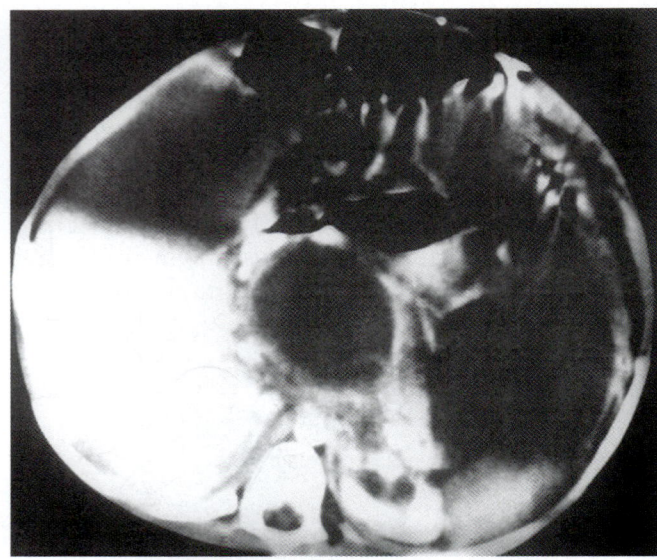

Fig. 92.7: Computed tomography scan showing pancreatic pseudocyst

Anomalous union of the pancreas and biliary ducts, pancreas divisum, stone in the duct, stricture, sclerosis and deformity of the duct, duct dilatation and choledochal cyst.[26,49,50] At ERCP, the resting pressure at the sphincter of Oddi can be measured and procedures such as dilatation of narrowed ducts, removal of stone, insertion of stents and sphincterotomy can be performed safely.[46,51] However, the expertise to perform ERCP in children is not readily available in all centers and may lead to consideration of earlier surgical intervention.

Magnetic resonance cholangiopancreatography (MRCP) (Fig. 92.8) has the advantages of being fast, non-invasive and reproducible.[17] It allows visualization of biliary and pancreatic ductal anatomy and will detect stones, strictures, intraductal tumors and duct compression.[52] Secretin may improve visualization and false negative results are rare.

MEDICAL MANAGEMENT

The medical management of acute or chronic pancreatitis has three main elements:
- Resuscitation and supportive treatment
- Elimination of the underlying cause of the pancreatitis

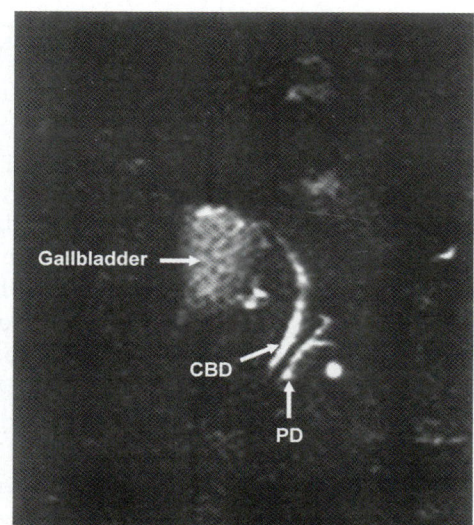

Fig. 92.8: Magnetic resonance cholangiopancreatogram showing gallbladder (PD), common bile duct (CBD) and pancreatic duct

- Specific therapy directed against the pancreatitis process.

The principal objectives of treatment in clinical terms are to relieve pain, minimise shock, limit electrolyte disturbance and reduce pancreatic exocrine excretion.[2,36] The speed of onset of symptoms and signs of pancreatitis and the potential for rapid clinical deterioration call for sure judgement and decisive action. The use of guidelines and treatment protocols may facilitate this.

RESUSCITATION AND SUPPORTIVE TREATMENT

The immediate assessment of the requirement for resuscitation is based on measurements of full blood count and hematocrit, arterial partial pressure of oxygen, urea and electrolytes (including calcium and glucose) and monitoring of pulse, blood pressure, respiratory rate and temperature. Intravascular monitoring of arterial pressure, central venous pressure and pulmonary artery wedge pressure may be needed to keep track of fluid replacement when massive losses are occurring into the third space (retroperitoneal tissues and peritoneal cavity). Adequate and timely intravenous rehydration is essential to avoid prerenal failure. Crystalloid or colloid solutions can be used; blood transfusion may be needed particularly in the case of hemorrhagic necrosis of the pancreas. Calcium gluconate should be given in the presence of hypocalcemia or tetany and soluble insulin is administered on a sliding scale to control hyperglycemia. Pain relief requires narcotic analgesia. Pethidine, which can be potentiated by the addition of promethazine, is less likely than morphine to cause spasm of the sphincter of Oddi.[2,38]

Elimination of the Underlying Cause

When pancreatitis is drug-related any further administration should obviously be stopped whenever possible. Alcohol is occasionally a factor in pancreatitis in childhood and should be strictly avoided. Relief of pancreatic duct obstruction, (e.g. by removal of impacted gallstone), is important in reversing the inflammatory process.

Specific Therapy Directed Against the Pancreatitis Process

The aim of therapy against the process of pancreatitis is to reduce stimulation of the gland to a minimum and to neutralise or inactivate the various exocrine gland secretions and inflammatory agents.

Insertion of a nasogastric tube and aspiration of gastric contents serves both to prevent risks of vomiting and inhalation in the presence of ileus and also to remove the stimulus of food and gastric secretions. Insertion of a long feeding tube beyond the ligament of Treitz allows continued enteral nutrition. Complete fasting and total parenteral nutrition are sometimes necessary in an acute episode but low fat dietary intake may be helpful in reducing pain and risk of relapse in chronic pancreatitis. Medium chain triglycerides (MCT) are absorbed in the absence of pancreatic enzymes or bile salts.

Pancreatic "rest" and the consequent possibility of reduction of pain and complications of pancreatitis, may also theoretically be promoted by anticholinergics, H_2-receptor antagonists, exogenous enzyme administration, enzyme inhibitors, cholecystokinin-receptor antagonists, glucagon, somatostatin analogues and the protease inhibitor gabexate.[13,53,54] However, evidence of consistent clinical effectiveness is at present sparse.

Similarly, the role of prophylactic antibiotics remains inconclusive except in severe necrotising pancreatitis when they are of proven benefit in reducing bacterial translocation to necrotic tissue.[55] In the presence of bacterial superinfection or acute septic necrosis, antibiotics such as imipenem or cefuroxime with good penetration into pancreatic tissue produce therapeutic benefit.[10] Recognition of the role of free radicals in the inflammatory process has led to trials of the use of antioxidants such as N-acetylcysteine, vitamin C and sodium selenite but proof of effectiveness is awaited.[8] Antagonists of platelet activating factor (lexipafant) may also have a role.

SURGICAL MANAGEMENT

Surgery in pancreatitis is usually reserved for the problems caused by the complicated, relapsing and chronic cases. Inevitably however, pancreatitis will be first diagnosed in some cases at laparotomy when acute abdominal signs have led to emergency surgery. In this circumstance debridement and drainage of necrotic pancreatic tissue is the best option.[38] If possible, the biliary tree should also be examined to exclude gallstones. Subsequent surgery to deal with abscess formation or encysted fluid collections and definitive surgery for pancreatic or biliary duct abnormalities may be needed. Biliary tract disorders associated with pancreatitis may require cholecystectomy or bile duct drainage using a Roux-en-Y loop of jejunum (bilio-enteric bypass).

The indications for surgery in relapsing and chronic pancreatitis include; failure to respond to medical treatment, frequent relapse, disabling pain, the need to limit further pancreatic damage, pseudocyst formation, duct dilatation, strictures and stones.[12] When severe acute pancreatitis progresses to necrosis and infection, necrosectomy is necessary but carries a high mortality.[56] If infection can be excluded, a conservative non-surgical approach is advocated.[42] Fine-needle aspiration guided by US or CT is a valuable and accurate technique in resolving the question of an infected necrosis.[57] Up to 60% of patients may benefit from surgical intervention at some stage in the course of pancreatic disease–particularly when trauma, biliary tract disease or congenital abnormalities are the cause.[3] Relief of pain and reduced hospitalization are the principal benefits whilst improvement in exocrine and endocrine function is minimal. Pseudocysts can be drained percutaneously by catheter insertion under CT or US guidance but there is a risk of pancreatic fistula formation.[58] If the cyst is managed conservatively until a surrounding capsule has formed, internal drainage by cyst-jejunostomy or cyst-gastrostomy should be curative.

Information from ERCP and MRCP, from transduodenal retrograde cholangiopancreatography or from operative cholangiography allows the choice of the most appropriate procedure in view of the duct anatomy and the presence of stone, stenosis, obstruction or dilatation.[10,21] ERCP therapeutic procedures give direct benefit in terms of pain relief and well-being but long-term follow-up studies are needed to assess the full impact.[46-51]

Operative options consist of sphincteroplasty (endoscopic or open), stent placement to improve drainage and direct pancreatic drainage via an enteric fistula. Distal pancreatectomy and Roux-en-Y pancreaticojejunostomy (Duval procedure) has been shown to be more effective than longitudinal pancreaticojejunostomy (Puestow procedure) in most childhood pancreatitis and is more effective than sphincteroplasty in severe disease.[54,59] In hereditary pancreatitis, however, both longitudinal pancreaticojejunostomy and stenting have proved effective.[60,61] Pancreatic resection, either partial or sub-total, may be necessary in the most severe cases to achieve relief of symptoms. Total pancreatectomy and pancreaticoduodenectomy (Whipple procedure) are not normally considered in childhood. Major pancreatic surgery now carries minimal mortality and complication rates of about 20%.[38,62] The most significant complications are pancreatic fistula, intra-abdominal and wound infection and pneumonia.

COMPLICATIONS

Complications following pancreatitis arise both from the inflammatory process itself and also from damage to the function of the pancreas. Problems can occur acutely or in the long-term.

Complications due to the Inflammatory Process

Systemic effects of acute pancreatitis may be shock, sepsis, respiratory distress syndrome, acute renal failure due to tubular necrosis and coagulopathy.[6] Hypocalcemia and hyperglycemia, complicate electrolyte and fluid imbalance. The multisystem organ failure that may supervene can be fatal.

Outpouring of pancreatic secretions and fluid from the inflamed gland causes ascites and loculation of the fluid leads to pseudocyst or abscess formation. Portal vein thrombosis may result from the intense inflammatory reaction and cavernous transformation of the vein and portal hypertension may be long-term sequelae.[18] Pancreatic fistulae can be internal or external and may form spontaneously or follow external drainage procedures. Upper gastrointestinal bleeding occurs from diffuse ulceration, duodenal stress ulceration, portal vein obstruction or erosion of the neovascular tissue of the inflammatory mass.[10,40] Subphrenic inflammation may cause pleural effusion, usually on the left side.

Complications due to Pancreatic Damage

Both exocrine and endocrine functions of the pancreas are affected by pancreatitis. Insufficiency of exocrine secretion leads to malabsorption and steatorrhea in 5–19% of chronic pancreatitis and after extensive resection in which more than 90% of the gland is removed.[13,24] Pancreatic endocrine failure leads to diabetes mellitus in 3–12% of cases.[20,24,40]

Although there is a potential risk of carcinoma developing in chronic pancreatitis, which is assessed in about 4% after 20 years disease,[13] there are no reported cases of carcinoma in larger pediatric series of chronic pancreatitis.[13,18,20,24] However in hereditary pancreatitis, carcinoma has been reported in older family members.[18] Patients with tropical pancreatitis are at increased risk of carcinoma and this occurs at a younger age.[63]

PROGNOSIS

The prediction of outcome from acute pancreatitis has been assessed in detail using various criteria related to the acute episode.[34-35] The criteria are shown in Table 92.3. Measurement of various markers of oxidative stress have also been correlated with the criteria in an attempt to improve predictive value of severity but do not offer any added value.[64]

The application of such methods to children have some value, as does assessment using the Acute Physiology and Chronic Health Evaluation (APACHE) II system.[3,36,37] However, accurate prediction of outcome in childhood acute pancreatitis is certainly not possible. Mortality in the acute episode has been reported to be as high as 15–25% with up to 86% in severe hemorrhagic pancreatitis.[2,5,10,38] Necrosis and infection are bad prognostic indicators.[56] Recurrence of acute pancreatitis is more likely when the initial episode is of unknown etiology or when the problem is structural or metabolic.[15] The underlying cause persists in these situations.

Chronic pancreatitis may be a less severe disease when onset is in early life rather than later and mortality is low.[14,65] In some cases, disease progression is self-limiting with eventual burn-out.[12]

REFERENCES

1. Buntain WL. Chronic relapsing pancreatitis in childhood. The American Surgeon 1985;51:180-88.
2. Mader TJ, McHuqh TP. Acute pancreatitis in children. Pediatric Emerqengy Care 1992; 8.157-61.
3. Ziegler DW, Long JA, Philippart AI, Klein MD Pancreatitis in childhood Ann Surg 1988;207:257-61.
4. Eland IA, Sturkenboom MJ, Wilson JH, et al. Incidence and mortality of acute pancreatitis between 1985 and 1995. Scand. J Gastroenterol 2000;35:1110-16.
5. Jordon SC, Ament ME. Pancreatitis in children and adolescents. J Pediatr 1977;91:211-16.
6. Kornberg AE. Pancreatitis in Reisdorff EJ, Roberts MR, Weigenstein JG (Eds) Pediatric Emergency Care WB Saunders, Philadelphia 1993;359-65.
7. Nguyen T, Abramowsky C, Ashenburg C, Rothstein F. Clinicopathologicat studies in childhood pancreatitis. Human Pathology 1988;19:343-49.
8. Johnson CD. Pathogenesis of pancreatitis: in Taylor I, Johnson CD (Eds) Recent Advances in Surgery (18) Churchill Livingstone, Edinburgh 1995;1-16.
9. Formela LJ, Galloway SW, Kingsnorth AN. Inflammatory mediators in acute pancreatitis. B J Surg 1995;82:6-13.
10. Steinberg W, Tenner S. Acute pancreatitis. New Eng. J Med 1995;330:1198-210.
11. Trapnell JE. Management of chronic relapsing pancreatitis in adolescents. World J Surg 1990;14:48-52.
12. Mathew P, Wyllie R, Caulfield M, Steffen R, Kay M. Chronic pancreatitis in late childhood and adolescence, Clinical Pediatrics 1994; 88-94.
13. Steer ML, Waxman I, Freedman S. Chronic pancreatitis New Eng. J Med 1995;332:1482-90.
14. Little JM, TaitN, Richardson A, Dubois R. Chronic pancreatitis beginning in childhood and adolescence. Arch Surg 1992; 127:90-92.
15. Weizman Z, Durie PA. Acute pancreatitis in childhood. J Pediatr 1988;113:24-29.
16. Guelrud M, Mujica C, Jaen D, Pial J, Arias J. The role of ERCP in the diagnosis and treatment of idiopathic recurrent pancreatitis in children and adolescents. Gastrointest Endosc 1994;40:428-36.

17. Arcement CM, Meza MP, Arumanla S, et al. MRCP jn the evaluation of pancreaticobiliary disease in children. Pediatr Radiol 2001:31;92-97.
18. Konzen KM, Perrault J, Moir C, Zinsmeister AR. Long-term follow-up of young patients with chronic hereditary or idiopathic pancreatitis. Maya Clin Proc 1993;68:449-53.
19. Elitsur V, Hunt JA, Chertow BS. Hereditary pancreatitis in the children of West Virginia. Pediatrics 1994;93:528-31.
20. Sibert JR. Hereditary pancreatitis in Enqland and Wales J Med Genet 1978;15:189-201.
21. Ghishan FK, Greene HL, Avant G, a'Neill J, Neblett WN Chronic relapsing pancreatitis in childhood. J Pediatr 1983:102:514-18.
22. Rothstein FC, Wyllie R, Gauderer MWL. Hereditary pancreatitis and recurrent abdominal pain of childhood. J Pediatr Surg 1985;20:535-37.
23. Whitcomb OC, Gorry MC, Preston RA, Furey W, Sossenheimer MJ, Ulrich CD, Martin SP, Gates LK Jr, Amann ST, Toskes PP, Liddle R, McGrath K, Uomo G, Post JC, Ehrlich GD. Hereditary pancreatitis is caused by a mutation in the cationic trypsinogen gene (see comments) Nat Genet 1996;14:141-45.
24. Moir CR, Konzen KM, Perrault J. Surgical therapy and long-term follow-up of childhood hereditary pancreatitis J Pediatr Surg 1992;27:282-87.
25. Brown CW, Werlin SL, Geenen JE, Schmalz M. The diagnostic and therapeutic role of endoscopic retrograde cholangiopancreatography in children. J Pediatr Gasroenterol Nutr 1993;17:19-23.
26. Mori K, Nagakawa T, Ohta T, Nakano T, Kayahara M, Akiyama T, Kanno M, Ueno K, Konishi I, Izumi R, Konishi K, Miyazaki I. Pancreatitis and anomalous union of the pancreaticobiliary ductal system in childhood. J Pediatr Surg 1993; 28:67-71.
27. Allendorph M, Werlin SL, Geenen JE, Hagan WJ, Venu RP, Stewart ET, Blank EL. Endoscopic retrograde cholangiopancreatography in children. J Pediatr 1987;110:206-11.
28. Buckley A, Connon JJ. The role of EACPin children and adolescents. Gastrointestinal Endoscopy 1990;36:369-37.
29. Koranyi KI, Brady MT, Stock K, et al. Pancreatitis in children infected with human immunodeficiency virus. Pediatr AIDS HIV infect 1996;7:261-65.
30. Isenmann R, Buchler MW. Infection and pancreatitis B J Surg 1994;81:1707-08.
31. Balakrishnan V, Sauniere JF, Hariharan M, Sarles H Diet. Pancreatic function and chronic pancreatitis in South India and France. Pancreas 1988:3:30-35.
32. Sylvester FA, Shuckett B, Cutz, et al. Management of fibrosing pancreatitis in children presenting with obstructive jaundice Gut 1998: 43:715-20.
33. O'Neill JA, Greene H, Ghishan FK. Surgical implications of chronic pancreatitis. J Pediatr Surg 1982;17:920-26.
34. Ranson JHC, Pasternak BS. Statistical methods for quantifying the severity of clinical acute pancreatitis. J Surg Res 1977; 22:79-91.
35. Imrie CW, Benjamin IS, Ferguson JC. A single centre double blind trial of trasylol therapy in primary acute pancreatitis. Br J Surg 1978;65:337-41.
36. Tran DO, Cuesta MA. Evaluation of severity in patients with acute pancreatitis. Am J Gastroenterol 1992;87:604-08.
37. Haddock G, Coupar G, Youngson GG, MacKinlay G, Raine PAM. Acute pancreatitis in children; a 15-year review. J Pediatr Surg 1994;29:719-22.
38. Synn AV, Mulvihill SJ, Fonkalsrud EW. Surgical management of pancreatitis in childhood. J Pediatr Surg 1987;22:628-32.
39. Balthazar EJ, Freeny PC, van Sonnenberg E Imaging and intervention in acute pancreatitis Radiology 1994;193; 297-310R.
40. Festen C, Severijnen R, VD Staak F, Rieu P. Chronic relapsing pancreatitis in childhood. J Pediatr Surg 1991;26:182-83.
41. Norton SA, Alderson D. Endoscopic ultrasonography in the evaluation of idiopathic acute pancreatitis. Br J Sura 2000: 87: 1650-55.
42. Buchler MW, Gloor B, Muller CA, et al. Acute necrotising pancreatitis treatment strategy according to the status of infection Ann Surg 2000;232:627-29.
43. King LR, Siegel MJ, Balfe DM. Acute pancreatitis in children– CT findings of intra- and extrapancreatic fluid collections. Radiology 1995;195:196-200.
44. London NJM, Lavelle JM. Acute pancreatitis: CT scanning in diagnosis and management. Hospital Update 1994; 369-76.
45. Caulfield M, Wyllie R, Sivak MV, Michener W, Steffen R. Upper gastrointestinal tract endoscopy in the pediatric patient. J Pediatr 1989:115:339-45.
46. Poddar U, Thapa BR, Bhasin DK, et al. Endoscopic retrograde cholangiopancreatography in the management of pancreaticobiliary disorders in children. J Gastroenterol Heoatol 2001:16:927-31.
47. Prasil P, Laberge JM, Barkun A, et al. Endoscopic retrograde cholangiopancreatography in children: A surgeon's perspective. J Pediatr Surg 2001; 36:733-35.
48. Keil R, Snajdauf J, Stuj J, et at. Endoscopic retrograde cholangiopancreatography in infants and children. Indian J Gastroenterol 2000;19:175-77.
49. Yedin ST, Dubois AS, Philippart AI. Pancreas divisum: a cause of pancreatitis in childhood. J Pediatr Surg 1984;19:793-94.
50. Okada A, Higaki J, Nakamura T, Fukui V, Kamata S. Pancreatitis associated with choledochal cyst and other anomalies in childhood BJ Surg 1995;82:829-32.
51. Hsu RK, Draganov P, Leung JW, et al. Therapeutic ERCP in the management of pancreatitis in children. Gastrointest Endosc 2000;51:396-400.
52. Hirohashi S, Hirohashi R, Uchida H, Akira M, Itoh T, Haku E, Ohishi H. Pancreatitis; evaluation with MR cholangiopancreatography in children. Radiology 1997;203:411-15.
53. Buchler MW, Binder M, Friess H. Role of somatostatin and its analogues in the treatment of acute and chronic pancreatitis Gut 1994;35(suool):815-19.

54. Neblet WW, O'Neill JA. Surgical management of recurrent pancreatitis in children with pancreas divisum. Ann Surg 2000; 231:899-908.
55. Kramer KM, Levy H. Prophylactic antibiotics for severe acute pancreatitis: the beginning of an era. Pharmacoltherapy 1999; 19:592-602.
56. Poves I, Fabregat J, Biondo S, et al. Results of treatment in severe acute pancreatitis. Rev Esp Enferm Dig 2000;92: 586-94.
57. Rau B, Pralle U, Mayer JM, et al. Role of ultrasonographically guided fine-needle aspiration cytology in the diagnosis of infected pancreatic necrosis Br J Sura 1998; 85:179-84.
58. Huizinga WKJ , Baker LW. Treatment of persistent and complicated pancreatic pseudocysts. J R Coll Surg Edinb 1992;37: 373-76.
59. Weber TR, Keller MS. Operative management of chronic pancreatitis in childen. Arch Surg 2001;136:550-54.
60. Dubay D, Sandier A, Kimura K, et al. The modifed Puestow procedure for complicated hereditary pancreatitis in children. J Pediatr Surg 2000;35:343-48.
61. Vaughan D, Imrie G, Kelleher J, et al. Pancreatic duct stenting as a treatment for hereditary pancreatitis Pediatrics 1999:104:1129-33.
62. Fernandez-del Castillo C, Rattner DW, Warshaw AL. Standards for pancreatic resection in the 1990S Arch Surg 1995;130:295-300.
63. Thomas PG, Augustine P, Ramesh H, Rangabashyam N. Observations and surgical management of tropical pancreatitis in Kerala and southern India World J Surq 1990;14:32-42.
64. Abu-Zidan FM, Bonham MJ, Windsor JA. Severity of acute pancreatitis; a multivariate analysis of oxidative stress markers and modified Glasgow criteria. Br J Surg 2000;87:1019-23.
65. Forbes A, Leung JWC, Cotton P8. Relapsing acute and chronic pancreatitis. Arch Dis Child 1984;59:927-34.

CHAPTER 93
Management of Portal Hypertension

M Bajpai

Portal hypertension may be defined as a portal pressure gradient of 12 mm Hg or greater. Portal hypertension is less common in children as compared to adults. The significant clinical manifestations are esophageal variceal hemorrhage, ascites and hypersplenism. Portal hypertension in children is commonly due to extrahepatic obstruction from portal vein thrombosis.

PATHOPHYSIOLOGY

Portal hypertension is characterized by a pathologic increase in portal venous pressure that leads to the formation of an extensive network of portosystemic collaterals that divert a large fraction of portal blood to the systemic circulation, bypassing the liver. An increased vascular resistance to portal blood flow[1] is the initial factor responsible for the increase in portal pressure. This resistance is exerted along the hepatic and portal-collateral circulation. At a later stage, an increased portal venous blood inflow, promoted by splanchnic vasodilation, contributes to maintenance and aggravation of portal hypertension. Humoral vasodilatory agents play an important role in the splanchnic vasodilation. Several vasodilators are likely to be involved, including glucagon, prostacyclin, endotoxins, and nitric oxide. The splanchnic vasodilation is associated with a hyperkinetic systemic circulation, with reduced arterial pressure and peripheral resistance and increased cardiac output. The splanchnic circulation is probably the vascular territory in which the vasodilation is more pronounced. Therefore, splanchnic and systemic vasodilation probably share some pathophysiologic events. An expanded plasma volume is observed in all forms of portal hypertension. Expansion of plasma volume is due to renal sodium retention, which has been shown to precede the increase in cardiac output and can be prevented or reversed by sodium restriction and spironolactone. The expanded blood volume represents another mechanism that contributes to further increases in portal pressure.

Management of a child with portal hypertension is largely determined by the cause of obstruction to portal venous flow. The cause may be prehepatic, hepatic presinusoidal or hepatic postsinusoidal. Less common is suprahepatic obstruction, i.e. Budd-Chiari syndrome. Management is related to the underlying cause of the portal hypertension. In children with intrahepatic disease, management is usually temporary, stabilizing measures until liver transplantation can be performed. Over the years sclerotherapy has increasingly replaced shunt procedures. Extrahepatic obstruction in children has been treated successfully by both endoscopic techniques and shunts. Although used sparingly, sometimes, approaches directed at interruption of the varices, such as esophageal transection or Suguira's procedure are the only choice.

INVESTIGATIONS

Patients undergoing portosystemic shunt procedures should be stable and not actively bleeding. The source of hemorrhage can be documented endoscopically. In addition to a complete blood count, liver function tests and coagulation studies, the patient should undergo radiological studies. Barium swallow and endoscopy, both can be used to grade the varcies. CT portovenography and MRI are being increasingly used nowadays.

Laboratory Studies

Lab studies are carried out when portal hypertension is due to cirrhosis. The general aim being investigating the etiologies of cirrhosis. These studies consist of: Liver function tests, prothrombin time, albumin, viral hepatitis serologies, platelet count, antinuclear antibody, antimitochondrial antibody, antismooth muscle antibody, Iron indices, Alpha1-antitrypsin deficiency, Ceruloplasmin, 24-hour urinary copper - in children who have unexplained hepatic, neurologic, or psychiatric disease.

Imaging Studies

Duplex-Doppler Ultrasonography

Ultrasound (US) is a safe, economical and effective method for screening for portal hypertension. It also can demonstrate portal flow and helps in diagnosing cavernous transformation of the portal vein, portal vein thrombosis, or splenic vein thrombosis.

Features suggestive of hepatic cirrhosis with portal hypertension include, nodular liver surface. However, this finding is not specific for cirrhosis and can be observed with congenital hepatic fibrosis and nodular regenerative hyperplasia. Splenomegaly is a suggestive finding. Patients may demonstrate the presence of collateral circulation.

Limitations of US include—Reproducibility of data as well as variables, such as circadian rhythm, meals, medications, and the sympathetic nervous system which affect portal hemodynamics.

CT Scan

CT scan is a useful qualitative study in cases where sonographic evaluations are inconclusive. It is not affected by patients' body habitus or the presence of bowel gas.

With improvement of spiral CT scan and 3-dimensional angiographic reconstructive techniques, portal vasculature may be visualized more accurately. Findings suggestive of portal hypertension include: Collaterals arising from the portal system and dilatation of the IVC are also suggestive of portal hypertension.

Limitations of CT scan are inability to demonstrate the venous and arterial flow profile. Also, intravenous contrast agents cannot be used in patients with renal failure or contrast allergy.

Magnetic Resonance Imaging (MRI)

MRI provides qualitative information similar to CT scan when Doppler findings are inconclusive. It detects the presence of portosystemic collaterals and obstruction of portal vasculature. MRI also provides quantitative data on portal venous and azygos blood flow.

MANAGEMENT OF ACUTE VARICEAL BLEEDING[2]

A rapid and detailed assessment is done for the extent of blood loss already taken place and the rate of current loss. Patient's vitals are recorded, venous access is gained and blood samples are taken for hematocrit, platelet count and prothrombin time, liver function tests and electrolytes. A sample is send for cross matching. Urinary bladder is catheterized.

Blood volume is restored by blood, crystalloid and colloid transfusion.

A nasogastric tube is inserted to assess the severity of bleeding and gastric lavage.

Pharmacologic Treatment

The aim of the pharmacotherapeutic approach is to decrease the portal venous pressure gradient below 12 or even 10 mm Hg. Reduction of this gradient will significantly reduce the risk of re-bleeding. Pharmacological approach following acute bleeding include vasopressin, somatostatin or octreotide. Vasopressin is no more used in view of its marked peripheral vasoconstrictive effect, and is now replaced by somatostatin or octreotide. Acute variceal bleeding originating from gastric varices can be effectively controlled by endoscopic injection of tissue adhesive agent (n-butyl 2 cyanoacrylate).

Endoscopic therapy has largely replaced balloon temponade.

Endoscopic Sclerotherapy

Endoscopic sclerotherapy is successful in controlling acute esophageal variceal bleeding in majority of patients. Control should be obtained with 1-2 sessions. Patients continuing to bleed after 2 sessions should be considered for alternative methods to control their bleeding. Sodium tetradecyl sulphate and ethanolamine are commonly used as a sclerosants.

Serious complications related to sclerotherapy have been reported in 15-20% of patients, with an associated mortality rate of 2%. Complications of sclerotherapy may include mucosal ulceration, bleeding, esophageal perforation, mediastinitis, and pulmonary complications. Long-term complications, such as esophageal stricture formation, also may occur.

Endoscopic Variceal Ligation (Banding)

Endoscopic variceal ligation is based on the widely used technique of rubber-band ligation of hemorrhoids. The esophageal mucosa and the submucosa containing varices are ensnared, causing subsequent strangulation, sloughing, and eventual fibrosis, resulting in obliteration of the varices. Rebleeding occurs less frequently with endoscopic variceal ligation than with endoscopic sclerotherapy (26% vs 45%). Recent trials have demonstrated that ligation and sclerotherapy achieved similar rates of initial hemostasis in patients whose varices were actively bleeding at the time of treatment. Local complications are less common with ligation compared to sclerotherapy.

Transjugular intrahepatic portosystemic shunting (TIPS) is a viable option and is less invasive for those whose bleeding is not controlled. However, if TIPS is not available, then staple transection of the esophagus is an option when endoscopic treatment and pharmacological therapy have failed. TIPS is a useful procedure for continued bleeding despite medical and endoscopic treatment. It is effective only in portal hypertension of hepatic origin.

For prevention of rebleeding when pharmacological therapy and/or endoscopic therapy have failed, surgery is considered.

SHUNT AND NON-SHUNT OPTIONS

Decisions regarding the advisability of porto-systemic shunts as opposed to nonshunt options are often difficult. Important factors include the clinical status of the patient, the cause of portal hypertension and the expertise of the treating unit. It is often difficult to predict at the outset regarding outcome of the therapeutic procedures: re-bleeding, hepatic decompensation or encephalopathy.

Shunt Therapy for Extrahepatic Portal Obstruction[3]

The goal of any portosystemic shunt is effective decompression of the gastroesophageal veins. There are two distinct types of protosystemic shutns: those that are associated with total diversion of portal blood away from the liver (total shunts) and those that maintain portal blood supply to the liver (selective shunts). Examples of total shunts include portacaval, mesocaval and central splenorenal shunts.

Portosystemic shunts provide a means of decompressing the high-pressure portal system and thus esophageal varices. Although these procedures provide effective decompression and reduce the incidence of variceal bleeding there is a risk of long-term complications. These are: hepatic encephalopathy, accelerated hepatic deterioration and may make future hepatic transplant difficult.

Presently excellent results with portal decompression by shunt procedures in infants and children have been achieved in many centres and age and size are no more the limiting factors.

Non-shunt Therapy

Non-shunt therapies have limited application in children. Transthoracic ligation of varices or direct ligation by an abdominal approach are temporizing procedures.

Devascularization Procedures[4]

Sugiura and Futagawa advocated extensive esophagogastric devascularization combined with esophageal transection and re-anastomosis.

Siguira's Procedure[4]

This procedure consists of lower esophageal transection and anastomosis, devascularization of the lower esophagus and stomach and splenectomy. It was devised to avoid many of the complications of portosystemic shunts. However, experience in children is limited. This procedure remains an option for controlling esophageal varices due to intrahepatic or extrahepatic portal hypertension when endoscopic methods fail and portosystemic shunts are not possible (Fig. 93.1).

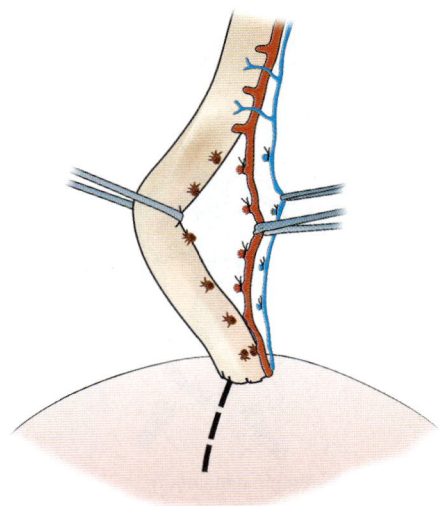

Fig. 93.1: Siguira's procedure

DISTAL SPLENORENAL SHUNT (DSRS)[5]
Selective Shunting

The concept of selective shunting was first introduced by Warren and his associates in 1967. These authors emphasized the increased morbidity and mortality associated with liver failure and hepatic encephalopathy following total shunting procedures. They attributed these problems to loss of liver portal perfusion. Their goal for the ideal operation for the treatment of patients with variceal bleeding was to achieve effective variceal decompression while preserving portal blood flow to the liver. Since the splenorenal anastomosis is not in direct communication with the superior mesenteric or portal veins, the pressure in these vessels remains elevated. Such pressure elevation is crucial in maintaing portal blood flow to the liver. For its success a complete spleno-pancreatic disconnection is essential which includes interruption of the coronary gastroepiploic and inferior mesenteric veins. The operation they devised to achieve these objective was the DSRS.

DSRS is created by anastomosing the medial end of the divided splenic vein to the side of left renal vein. The portal end of the splenic vein is oversewn. A functioning DSRS achieves variceal decompression by establishing a route for gastric venous drainage that offers less vascular resistance than the anastomotic channels between the gastric and esophageal veins. This route finally leads to the left renal vein (Figs 93.2A and B). Reversal of hypersplenism has been demonstrated by DSRS.

Central Splenorenal Shunt[6]

In a central splenorenal shunt, the principal direction of portal flow is to the systemic circulation. Reversal of blood flow from the portal to systemic circulation

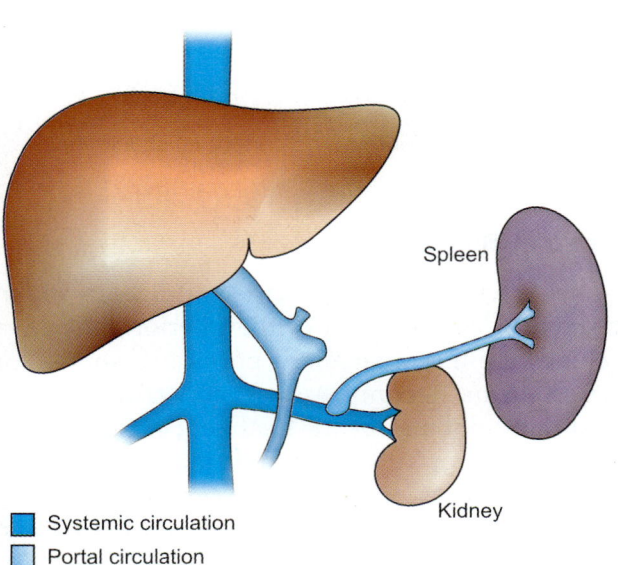

Fig. 93.2A: Distal splenorenal shunt (Warren)

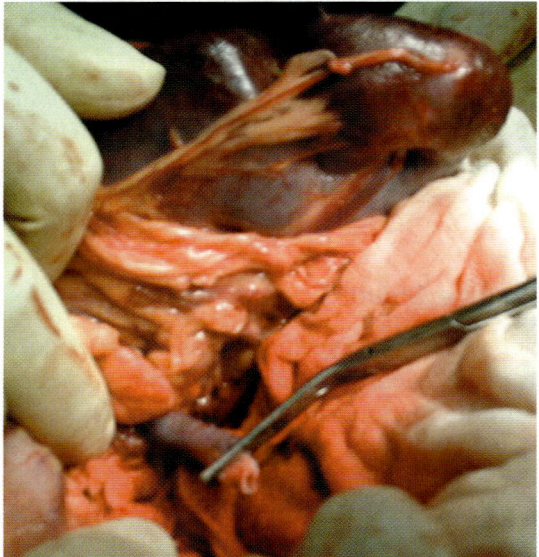

Fig. 93.2B: Operative photograph of distal splenorenal shunt: End of the splenic vein to be anastomosed to the left renal vein

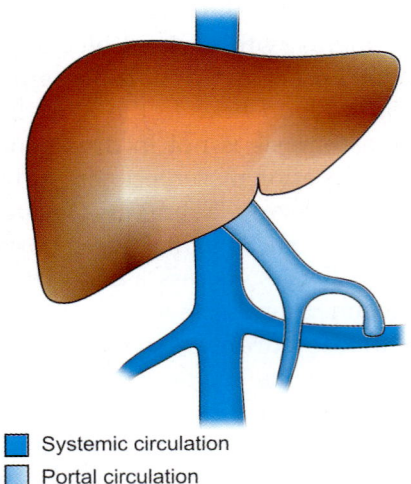

Fig. 93.3: Central (Proximal) splenorenal shunt

with hepatic deprivation is a hazard most serious with this option. In this procedure the spleen is removed and the central end of the splenic vein is anastomosed to the side of the left renal vein (Fig. 93.3).

Mesocaval Shunt[7]

In this shunt anastomosis or graft anastomosis of the side of the superior mesenteric vein to the proximal end of the divided inferior vena cava is performed as a means of controlling portal hypertension. The inferior vena cava is exposed by mobilizing the right mesocolon. The duodenum is reflected by a Kocher maneuver. After exposure the inferior vena cava is mobilized from the renal veins to below the caval bifurcation. Individual ligation of several lumbar veins is often required. A tunnel is made in the retroperitonium and posterior mesentery, often thick and edematous, to reach the superior mesenteric vein (Fig. 93.4).

Side-to-side Shunt[8,9]

Mitra et al have reported an extensive experience with side-to-side splenorenal shunt without splenectomy in children with noncirrhotic portal hypertension with 87% patency.[9] The technique involves extensive mobilization of spenic vein while maintaining its medial (portal) and lateral (splenic) attachments. Reversal of blood flow from the portal to systemic circulation, which allows the vein to act as an outflow tract, remains a potential consequence (Fig. 93.5).

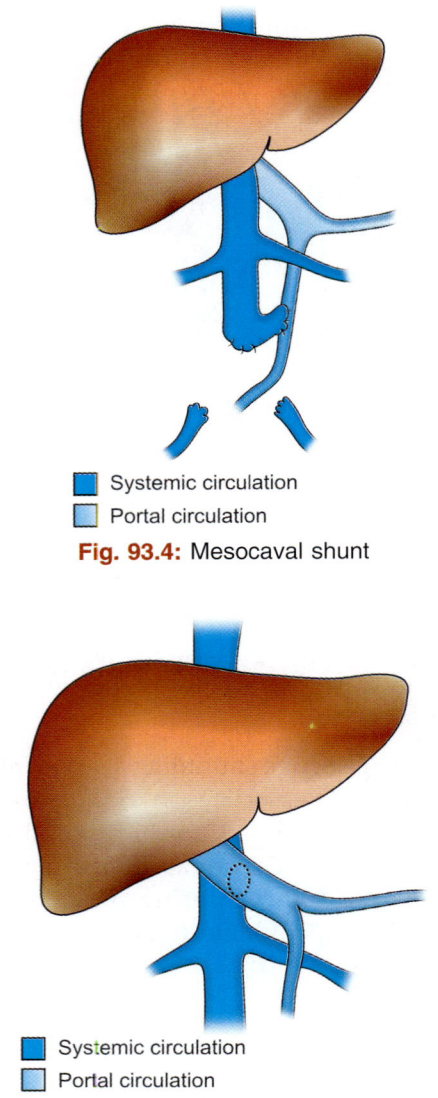

Fig. 93.4: Mesocaval shunt

Fig. 93.5: Side-to-side portocaval shunt

Mesoatrial Shunt[10]

In patients with the Budd-Chiari syndrome in whom occlusion or compression of the inferior vena cava precludes the use of standard portacaval shunts for portal venous decompression, construction of a mesoatrial shunt may be the treatment of choice. This shunt is a Dacron or Gortex graft that is interposed between the superior mesenteric vein and the right atrium. The occlusion rate of these shunts is high because of their long length and slow flow rates (Fig. 93.6).

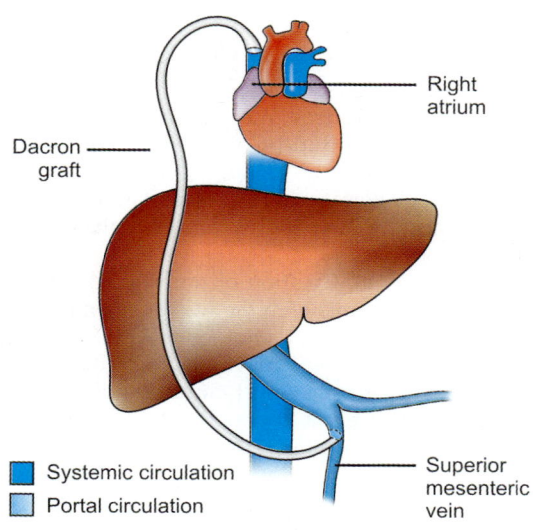

Fig. 93.6: Mesoatrial shunt

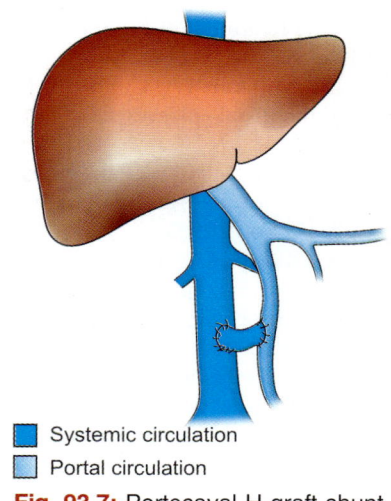

Fig. 93.7: Portocaval H-graft shunt

Portocaval H-Graft Shunt[11]

Small diameter H graft portacaval shunts (HGPCSs) effectively treat bleeding varices due to cirrhosis, although the effects of such shunts on hepatic blood flow are not well established. Proponents of HGPCS believe that portal flow diverted through the shunt is regained through increased hepatic arterial inflow while others argue that this flow is never recovered; resulting in compromised nutrient flow (Fig. 93.7).

Transjugular Intrahepatic Portosystemic Shunting (TIPS)[12]

This procedure provides the same shunting benefits as the major shunt procedures. It is carried out by an interventional radiologist. TIPS eliminates the disadvantage of altering the extrahepatic venous anatomy. By this technique, an intrahepatic communication is established between the hepatic venous outflow and the portal venous inflow. The portosystemic communication is accomplished under fluoroscopic guidance. It is dilated and the intrahepatic tract secured by insertion of an expandable stent. These procedures are routinely successful in decreasing the portal pressure and eliminating the dangerous gradient between the portal and systemic venous systems. Ascites is regularly resolved with TIPS.

The TIPS procedure has been proven effective for controlling bleeding esophageal and gastric varices even when other measures have failed. Accepted indications for TIPS include acute variceal bleeding or recurrent bleeding refractory to pharmacological measures for which sclerotherapy has failed. Contraindications to TIPS include right-sided heart failure (elevated central venous pressure) and severe hepatic failure.

Meso-Rex Bypass

The recent introduction of the meso-Rex bypass raises a possible paradigm shift in the therapeutic approach to extrahepatic portal vein obstruction (EHPVO). Long-term follow-up of patients with EHPVO has revealed a variety of complications including variceal hemorrhage, hypersplenism, biliopathy, growth/development retardation and neuropsychiatric disease. The meso-Rex bypass restores physiologic blood flow to the liver. Thus, when feasible, the meso Rex bypass should be considered in patients with clinically significant manifestations of EHPVO.[13]

REFERENCES

1. Karrer FM. Portal hypertension. Seminar Pedatr Surg 1: 134;192.
2. Williams SG, Westaby D. Management of variceal haemorrhage. BMJ 1994;308(6938):1213-17.
3. Maksoud JG, Mies S. Distal splenorenal shunt in children. Ann Surg 1982;195:401.

4. Siguiura M, Futagawa S. Further evaluation of the Sugiura procedure in the treatment of oesophageal varices. Arch Surg 1977;112:1317.
5. Henderson JM, Millikan WJ, Galloway JR. The Emory perspective of the distal splenorenal shunt in 1990. Am J Surg 1990;160:54.
6. Zhang H, Zhang N, Li M, Jin W, Pan S. Surgical treatment of portal vein cavernous transformation. World J Surg 2004;28(7):708-11. Epub 2004.
7. Mercado MA, Orozco H, Guillén-Navarro E, Acosta E, López-Martínez LM, Hinojosa C, Hernández J, Tielve M. Small-diameter mesocaval shunts: a 10-year evaluation.: J Gastrointest Surg 2000;4(5):453-57.
8. Kraft RO, Fry WJ. The demonstration of hepatofugal flow following side-to-side portacaval anastomosis. Surg Gynecol Obstet 1964;118:124.
9. Mitra SK, Rao KL, Narasimhan KL, Dilawari JB, Batra YK, Chawla Y, Thapa BR, Nagi B, Walia BN. Side-to-side lieno-renal shunt without splenectomy in noncirrhotic portal hypertension in children. J Pediatr Surg 1993;28(3): 398-401; discussion 401-02.
10. Cameron JL, Maddrey WC. Mesoatrial shunt: a new treatment for the Budd-Chiary syndrome. Ann Surg 1978;187:401.
11. Sarfeh IJ, et al. Portacaval H-grafts: relationships of shunt diametr, portal flow patterns, and encephalopathy. Ann Surg 1983;197:422.
12. LeBerge JM, et al. Creation of transjugular intrahepatic portosystemic shunts with the wall stent endoprosthesis: results in 100 patients. Radiology 1993;187:413.
13. Riccardo Superina, Benjamin Shneider, Sukru Emre, Shiv Sarin, Jean de Ville de Goyet. Surgical guidelines for the management of extra-hepatic portal vein obstruction. Pediatric Transplantation 2006;10 (8):908-13.

CHAPTER 94

Persistent Hyperinsulinemic Hypoglycemia of Infancy

Shilpa Sharma, DK Gupta

Persistent hyperinsulinemic hypoglycemia of infancy (PHHI) is a challenging disease both to establish the diagnosis well in time and also to treat as PHHI can lead to brain damage or death secondary to severe hypoglycemia.

TERMINOLOGY

The term persistent hyperinsulinemic hypoglycemia of infancy (PHHI) is synonymous with nesidioblastosis, congenital hyperinsulinism, nesidiodysplasia and isletcell dysmaturation syndrome.

The term 'nesidioblastosis', derived from the Greek words nesidion, for islet, and blastos, for germ, was originally conceived by Laidlaw in 1938.[1] Severe infantile hypoglycemia was first associated with nesidioblastosis in 1970.[2]

This term has now been replaced by persistent hyperinsulinemic hypoglycemia of infancy (PHHI), to describe the neoformation or neodifferentiation of islets of Langerhan's from pancreatic ductal epithelium.[3,4] Hyperinsulinism is the most common cause of persistent neonatal hypoglycemia.

EMBRYOLOGY

The endocrine and exocrine pancreas arise from endodermal buds from which primitive pancreatic ducts and acini develop by repeated branchings.[5] At birth, increased numbers of islet cells are found throughout the lobule as single cells and as clusters of cells, in addendum to the islets of Langerhans.

In PHHI, the pancreas resembles the third-trimester fetal and neonatal pancreas. This finding has also been found in teratomas.[6] It has been suggested that nesidioblastosis may be the result of improper development of the endocrine pancreas progressing beyond birth and neonatal life.[7]

The diffuse pattern of development in the fetal and newborn endocrine pancreas makes the diagnosis of nesidioblastosis therefore rather challenging.[8]

ETIOPATHOGENESIS

1. Unknown etiology. Most cases of PHHI are sporadic. In more than 50% cases, no known genetic abnormality is found.
2. High rates of consanguinity have been noted in some series.[9]
3. Familial forms of PHHI have been reported.[10] These involve autosomal recessive or dominant defects in Beta-cell high-affinity sulfonylurea receptor gene (SUR1). Inwardly rectifying potassium channel gene (Kir 6.2), glucokinase gene (GK) and glutamate dehydrogenase gene (GUD1).
4. The advances in molecular genetics have contributed enormously to our understanding of nesidioblastosis.[11,12] The underlying genetic defects of β-cell regulation include a severe recessive disorder of the sulphonylurea receptor, a milder dominant form of hyperinsulinism, and a syndrome of hyperinsulinism plus hyperammonemia.
5. In the focal form, maternal loss of heterozygosity in chromosome region 11p15 in the cells of the hyperplastic area have been observed without loss in the normal pancreatic cells.[13] This has not been observed in the diffuse form of PHHI.
6. Lately, the pathogenesis is now divided into K-channel disease [hyperinsulinemic hypoglycemia, familial (HHF) 1 and 2], which can mandate surgery, and other metabolic causes, HHF 3-6, which are treated medically in most patients.[13]

7. The diffuse form is inherited as a recessive gene on chromosome 11, whereas most cases of the focal form are caused by a sulfonylurea receptor 1 defect inherited from the father, which is associated with a maternal loss of heterozygosity on chromosome 11.[13]

PATHOPHYSIOLOGY

PHHI may be focal or a diffuse abnormality of the islets. Abnormalities in the insulin secretory or glucose-sensing mechanism result in a failure to reduce pancreatic insulin secretion in presence of hypoglycemia. High insulin levels in turn promote hepatic and skeletal muscle glycogenesis, resulting in a decrease in the amount of free blood glucose available and suppression of the formation of free fatty acid (FFA), an alternative energy substrate for the brain. Thus a vicious cycle is established resulting in life-threatening hypoglycemia.

EPIDEMIOLOGY

The incidence varies from 1 in 40000 live births in northern Europe and USA to 1/2675 live births in areas where consanguineous marriages are common.[9,14] The male-to-female ratio is 1.2:1 in diffuse forms and 1.8:1 in focal lesions. The overall incidence is slightly higher in males with a male-to-female ratio of 1.3:1.

AGE AT PRESENTATION

PHHI usually present from birth to 18 months of age, with most cases diagnosed at about one month after birth. PHHI represents the most common cause of hyperinsulinism in neonates.[15-17] PHHI is usually found during the first two years of life and is unusual to find after that. Although PHHI was initially thought to affect only infants and children, various cases have been reported in adults.[18,19]

CLINICAL PRESENTATION

The babies may present soon after birth with symptoms of hypoglycemia that include jitteriness, lethargy, apnea, seizures and hunger.[20] Hypoglycemia should be documented during the symptoms. Hypoglycemia is persistent, requiring frequent or continuous glucose infusions or feedings to maintain adequate blood glucose levels.

Older children may also show diaphoresis, confusion, behavior changes or peripheral neurological symptoms like altered gait and motor weakness.

Presenting symptoms of PHHI reported in adults include confusion, headaches, dizziness, syncope, and loss of consciousness. These symptoms may be exacerbated by fasting and may improve after eating. The characteristic Wipples triad is seen in adults for diagnosing an insulinoma. This comprises of symptoms of hypoglycemia, documented hypoglycemia and subsiding of symptoms on giving glucose.

The physical examination findings are usually normal during euglycemia.

DIFFERENTIAL DIAGNOSIS

The presence of hepatomegaly suggests a metabolic disorder, such as glycogen storage disease, galactosemia, or fructosemia. The presence of syndromic or dysmorphic features suggests a different diagnosis. PHHI is not usually associated with a genetic syndrome or characteristic physical features. The babies may be large for their gestational age because of the influence of chronic hyperinsulinism in utero. The differential diagnosis include hypopituitarism, transient hypoglycemia of the newborn, erythroblastosis fetalis, effects of drugs like tocolytics and quinine, infant of diabetic mother, Patau syndrome, insulinoma, ketotic hypoglycemia and Beckwith-Weidemann syndrome. Hyperinsulinism can be caused by pancreatic islet cell tumors such as insulinoma and associations with multiple endocrine neoplasia syndromes.[21]

INVESTIGATIONS

Blood Investigations

1. PHHI is characterized by severe recurrent hypoglycemia associated with an inappropriate elevation of serum insulin, C-peptide, and proinsulin.
2. Serum glucose, ketone, and insulin levels should be obtained while the patient is hypoglycemic (serum glucose level < 60 mg/dL). The definition of hypoglycemia in neonates is dependent upon gestational age, and the threshold may be lower.

3. Nonketotic hypoglycemia with elevated insulin levels (>10 mU/mL) and normal levels of FFA supports the diagnosis of hyperinsulinism.
4. The insulin-to-glucose ratio may range from 0.4-2.7 (normal < 0.3).
5. Other tests for differential diagnosis include cortisol and growth hormone levels, serum metabolic screens, pH, lactate, ammonia studies, urinary ketones, amino acids, and reducing-substances. Hyperinsulinism with hyper-ammonemia and elevated levels of FFA suggests a fatty acid oxidation disorder. Hyperinsulinism with hyperammonemia and normal levels of FFA suggest the diagnosis of hyperinsulinism with hyperammonemia.
6. Requirement of sustained glucose to remain symptom free in excess of 10 mg/kg/min are consistent with exaggerated insulin activity.
7. Catheterization of the portal and pancreatic veins with venous sampling may help distinguish between focal and diffuse PHHI. Selective pancreatic venous sampling may help to identify focal lesions. Pancreatic venous sampling has been studied widely now, even in neonates.
8. Selective intra-arterial calcium stimulation has been described to a lesser extent in children. An excessive insulin response from calcium stimulation in a single artery suggests a focal lesion.[22,23]

Imaging Studies

Ultrasonography, CT scanning, or MRI are helpful to locate a focal mass in the pancreas. The focal lesion is commonly too small to be identified on imaging studies. No form of imaging currently available reveals the diffuse form of PHHI.

A preoperative PET scan with fluorodihydroxy-phenylalanine has been found useful to pick up focal lesions.[13]

Histopathology

The morphologic characteristic features are ductoendocrine proliferation, numerous small endocrine cell groups and large endocrine areas.[24] PHHI may be focal or diffuse.[25] The diffuse form is more common (60-70% cases). The focal lesion contains islet like cell clusters with ductoinsular complexes, hypertrophic insulin cells with giant nuclei. Nuclear abnormalities include greatly increased size or crescent or ovoid shapes of beta-cells.

Immunohistochemical staining shows an increased proportion of insulin-containing cells (Fig. 94.1). The focal lesion may occur in any part of the pancreas, although the tail and body are the most common locations. The rest of the pancreas appears normal. Most patients with the focal form have a solitary lesion, though the lesions may be multifocal in 25% cases. Malignant potential based on clinical findings should be ruled out in solitary lesions.[26]

In the diffuse form, findings are similar throughout the pancreas with irregularly sized islets. Grossly, the pancreas appears normal (Fig. 94.2).

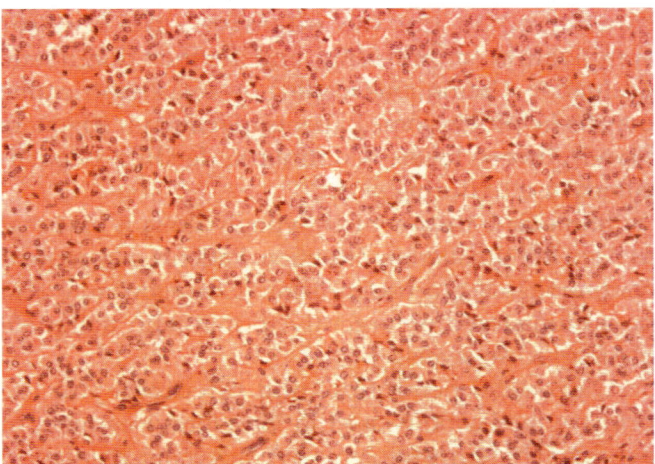

Fig. 94.1: Histopathology of the pancreas in a case of persistent hyperinsulinemic hypoglycemia of infancy

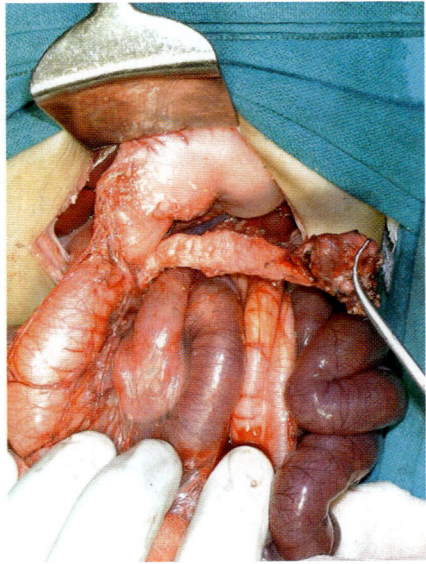

Fig. 94.2: The pancreas grossly appears normal

De novo formation of intermediate cells (acinar-islet cells) is a phenomenon which is clearly associated with nesidioblastosis.[27] Nesidiodysplasia has been proposed to describe apparently increased and possibly maldistributed and/or malregulated endocrine cells associated with hyperinsulinemic hypoglycemia.[28] Future classifications related to the underlying genetic defects may result in appropriate modification of the existing nomenclature.[29]

MEDICAL TREATMENT

Newborns with persistent hypoglycemia should be transferred to the the intensive care unit for stabilization, monitoring, and further diagnostic evaluation. Continuous feeding by a nasogastric tube may be helpful in some patients to maintain adequate blood glucose levels. Continuous feeding is particularly useful during sleep.

Immediate treatment of hypoglycemia is essential as it is a life-threatening situation. Patients may require continuous IV glucose infusion. Glucagon may also be administered emergently to maintain adequate blood glucose levels.

Diazoxide, octreotide, and nifedipine are the primary medications used in long-term treatment of persistent hyperinsulinemic hypoglycemia of infancy. Some also recommend using chlorothiazide in conjunction with diazoxide for a synergistic effect.

Oral diazoxide is used usually for the treatment of hypoglycemia. Diazoxide promotes opening of the potassium adenosine triphosphate channel, which inhibits pancreatic secretion of insulin, stimulates glucose release from the liver, and stimulates catecholamine release. Intravenous use may cause hypotension. Diazoxide is given in a dose of 8-10 mg/kg/d in three divided doses in neonates and infants and 3 mg/kg/d in older children, titrated to effect.

Octreotide, a long-acting somatostatin analogue inhibits insulin release but tolerance may develop over time. The dose is 1-10 mcg/kg/d SC divided 6-8 hourly.

Nifedipine has also been used successfully for ionic control of beta cell function.[30-32]

The doses and selection of drugs, must be highly individualized on the basis of therapeutic response and adverse-effect tolerance. Many children require years of drug therapy, and regular reassessment and dose adjustments are required besides ensuring compliance.[33]

SURGICAL TREATMENT

PHHI is often poorly responsive or unresponsive to medical management, necessitating 95% or near-total pancreatectomy (Figs 94.3A and B). However, a more conservative approach is now possible after the recognition of a nonrecurring focal form, which is cured by partial surgery, and a diffuse form, which necessitates total pancreas removal only in cases of medical treatment failure.[13] In infants, surgery is usually performed within the first 2 months of life. Laparoscopic procedures can be done in all age groups.

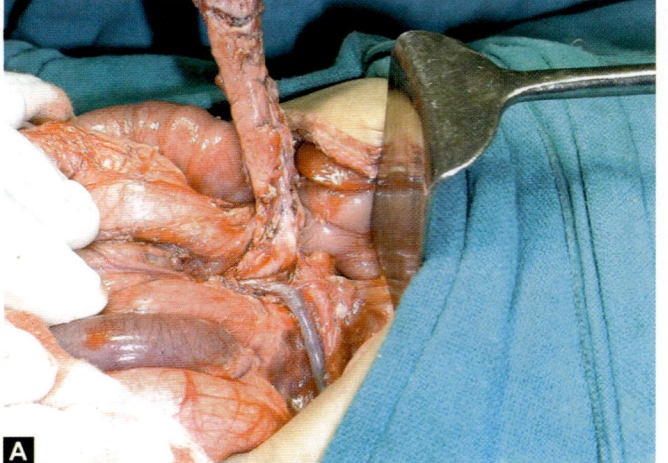 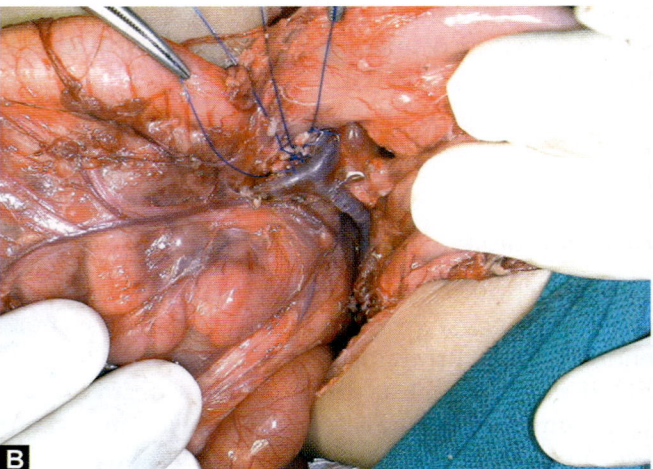

Figs 94.3A and B: A. Near total pancreatectomy in process with the pancreas lifted off its bed. **B.** The pancreatic bed showing the denuded splenic vein and superior mesenteric vein after near total pancreatectomy

Indications of Surgical Intervention

1. Medical therapy fails to maintain normoglycemia.
2. A focal lesion.
3. Noncompliance to medical therapy.
4. Recurrent symptoms following partial pancreatectomy.

Identification of a Focal Lesion

The distinction between focal and diffuse lesions is critical in planning surgical intervention. Every effort should be made, pre and perioperatively to identify or rule out a focal lesion. Limited pancreatic resection prevents future development of diabetes mellitus. Most focal lesions are too small to identify by CT scanning, MRI, ultrasonography, or even intraoperative palpation. Pancreatic venous sampling or intra-arterial calcium stimulation may help identify a focal lesion.[34] Preoperative localization of focal insulin hypersecretion by percutaneous pancreatic venous sampling has allowed to limit the amount of pancreatic resection.[34]

A routine intra-arterial calcium stimulation test with venous sampling (IACS test) may help to identify an occult insulinomas.[35]

An intraoperative ultrasound may supplement in detecting an occult lesion as it is able to identify nonpalpable lesions.[36] This in turn may be guided by the calcium stimulation test.[35] Occult lesions identified by intraoperative ultrasound have been treated by 40% or 60-70% distal pancreatectomies when insulin gradients were demonstrated on calcium stimulation to the splenic or to the superior mesenteric artery, respectively.[35]

A rapid intraoperative insulin assay has been recently developed that yields results within several minutes and confirms complete resection of insulinoma.[37] It is a valuable adjunct to determination of complete excision in complicated cases of recurrent or questionable insulinoma.[37] Children may especially benefit from this novel assay to confirm complete resection and to differentiate multiple etiologies of hyperinsulinism in the pediatric population.[37]

Care should to taken so as not to miss multiple focal lesions. Intraoperative glucose monitoring during a trial of glucose-free IV fluids may guide the surgeon in determining the need to search for additional lesions. If there is normoglycemia without IV glucose, after removal of a focal lesion, it is unlikely that there is another lesion.

The surgical approach involves taking multiple biopsy samples from different parts of the pancreas (head, body, isthmus, and tail). Intraoperatively frozen-section evaluation helps to determine whether the pathology is diffuse or focal.[13,38]

Abnormal beta-cell nuclei in all specimens suggests a diffuse lesion necessitating extensive pancreatectomy. In contrast, if only one specimen contains abnormal beta-cell nuclei, a focal lesion may be present.

If no focal lesion is found a near total pancreatectomy may be performed. Varying degrees of pancreatic resection from 85-95% in infants and children have been reported.[36] Albeit being a controversial issue, subtotal pancreatectomy or 95% or is the most widely accepted procedure for infants and children. The tail, body, uncinate process, and most of the head of the pancreas are removed, leaving a portion of pancreas to the right of the common bile duct and a thin rim along the second portion of the duodenum and the pancreaticoduodenal arteries. Resection of less than 95% of the pancreas is associated with a higher rate of treatment failure and need for reoperation. The more aggressive, 98% pancreatectomy removes all but a few small islands of pancreatic tissue along the pancreaticoduodenal arteries. This procedure is associated with a higher rate of postoperative diabetes mellitus. However, patients with even lesser degrees of pancreatic resection are at risk for development of diabetes mellitus. To remain on the safer side, some authors advocate a more conservative initial procedure, with reoperation later if hypoglycemia persists.

COMPLICATIONS

Preoperative

1. Permanent neurologic dysfunction (e.g., seizures, developmental delay, focal neurologic deficits).
2. Death secondary to severe, prolonged hypoglycemia may occur if PHHI goes untreated or is inadequately treated.
3. Adverse effects of medications.

Postoperative

Early Complications

1. Bleeding
2. Wound infection
3. Pancreatic fistula[36]
4. Persistent hypoglycemia.

Late Complications

1. Pancreatic exocrine insufficiency and glucose intolerance.
2. Diabetes mellitus following total pancreatectomy. The risk of diabetes mellitus appears to increase with the extent of pancreatic resection; however, the risk is significant even with conservative surgical procedures. Upto 15% of children with diffuse lesions may develop diabetes mellitus, regardless of the surgical procedure performed. The mean time from surgery to development of diabetes mellitus was 9.6 years. Diabetes mellitus is extremely rare following resection of focal lesions.
3. *Persistent hypoglycemia:* Hypoglycemia often persists even after a 95-98% pancreatectomy. Hypoglycemia may be easier to control after partial pancreatectomy and may resolve months or years later or persist throughout life.
4. *Neurological developmental delay:* A high incidence of mental retardation, developmental delay, and nonhypoglycemic seizures has been reported by some, attributed to minimal brain damage from early hypoglycemic events. It has been thus suggested that patients with early, severe disease treated with early, aggressive surgery may have a better neurodevelopmental outcome.

FOLLOW-UP

Long-term follow-up is essential to prevent delay in the diagnosis of disease recurrence, glucose intolerance, or diabetes mellitus.

Regardless of the surgical procedure used, hypoglycemia may recur, and the patient may require continued medical therapy.[39] Additional pancreatic resection may be indicated if optimal medical management cannot provide adequate glycemic control. In refractory cases, which are rare, total resection of the pancreas has been performed.

In a series evaluating the residual pancreas in children diagnosed with nesidioblastosis and who had undergone 90-95% pancreatectomy, it was reported that most patients showed complete or incomplete pancreatic regeneration during follow-up.[40] These patients were asymptomatic and showed normal laboratory tests.[40]

Ultrasound measurements indicated normal age-dependent growth after near-total resection in 54% of patients. The function and echogenicity of the regenerated pancreas indicated that the increase in organ size was due to normal pancreatic tissue.[40]

PROGNOSIS

If a solitary focal lesion can be identified and excised, the patient usually remains euglycemic without medication or continuous feedings. The results following surgery for diffuse disease have not been encouraging in most series. Rates of initial failure to control hypoglycemia are high, followed by, paradoxically, high rates of subsequent development of diabetes mellitus. About half of the patients undergoing 95% or greater pancreatectomy have been cured at a mean follow up of 5 years. 40-60% of patients managed with medical therapy alone have had late remission of hypoglycemia. Later onset of disease has been correlated with a higher likelihood of being able to discontinue medical therapy. Future advances in medical therapy may provide better glycemic control with fewer side effects, permitting less radical pancreatic resection.

REFERENCES

1. Laidlaw GF. Nesidioblastoma, the islet tumor of the pancreas. Am J Path 1938;14:125-34.
2. Brown RE, Young RB. A possible role for the exocrine pancreas in the pathogenesis of neonatal leucine-sensitive hypoglycemia. American Journal of Digestive Diseases 1970;15: 65-72.
3. al-Rabeeah A, al-Ashwal A, al-Herbish A. Persistent hyperinsulinemic hypoglycemia of infancy: experience with 28 cases. J Pediatr Surg 1995;30:1119-21.
4. Kaczirek K, Niederle B. Nesidioblastosis: an old term and a new understanding. World J Surg 2004;28:1227-30.
5. Moore KL. The Developing Human - Clinically Oriented Embryology, (5th ed) KL Moore (Ed). Philadelphia. 1993:264-65.
6. Resnick JM, Manivel JC. Immunohistochemical characterization of teratomatous and fetal neuroendocrine pancreas. Archives of Pathology and Laboratory Medicine 1994;118:155-59.
7. Heitz PU, Klöppel G, Hacki WH, Polak JM, Pearse AG Nesidioblastosis. The pathologic basis of persistent hyperinsulinemic hypoglycemia in infants. Morphologic and quantitative analysis of seven cases based on specific immunostaining and electron microscopy. Diabetes 1977;26 632-42.
8. Dahms BB, Landing BH, Blaskovics M, et al. Nesidioblastosis and other islet cell abnormalities in hyperinsulinemic hypoglycemia of childhood. Human Pathology 1980;11:641-49.
9. Mathew PM, Young JM, Abu-Osba YK, et al. Persistent neonatal hyperinsulinism. Clinical Pediatrics 1988;27: 148-51.

10. Bianchi C, Corbella E, Beccaria L. A case of familial nesidioblastosis: Prenatal diagnosis of foetal hyperinsulinism. Acta Paediatr 1992;81(10):853-55.
11. Glaser B, Thornton P, Otonkoski T. Genetics of neonatal hyperinsulinism. Arch Dis Child Fetal Neonatal Ed 2000;82:F79-86.
12. Milner RDG. Nesidioblastosis unravelled. Archives of Diseases in Childhood 1996;74:369-72.
13. Delonlay P, Simon A, Galmiche-Rolland L, et al. Neonatal hyperinsulinism: Clinicopathologic correlation Hum Pathol 2007;38:387-99.
14. Bruining GJ. Recent advances in hyperinsulinism and the pathogenesis of diabetes mellitus. Current Opinion in Pediatrics 1990;2:758-65.
15. Shepherd RM, Cosgrove KE, O'Brien RE. Hyperinsulinism of infancy: Towards an understanding of unregulated insulin release. European Network for Research into Hyperinsulinism in Infancy. Arch Dis Child Fetal Neonatal Ed 2000;82:F87-97.
16. Lovvorn HN 3rd, Nance ML, Ferry RJ Jr. Congenital hyperinsulinism and the surgeon: Lessons learned over 35 years. J Pediatr Surg 1999;34:786-92.
17. Tyrrell VJ, Ambler GR, Yeow WH. Ten years' experience of persistent hyperinsulinaemic hypoglycaemia of infancy. J Paediatr Child Health 2001;37:483-88.
18. Babinska A, Jaskiewicz K, Karaszewski B. Nesidioblastosis— A rare cause of hypoglycaemia in adults. Exp Clin Endocrinol Diabetes 2005;113(6):350-53.
19. Kim HK, Shong YK, Han DJ. Nesidioblastosis in an adult with hyperinsulinemic hypoglycemia. Endocr J 1996;43:163-67.
20. de Lonlay-Debeney P, Poggi-Travert F, Fournet JC. Clinical features of 52 neonates with hyperinsulinism. N Engl J Med 1999;340:1169-75.
21. Sempoux C, Guiot Y, Jaubert F. Focal and diffuse forms of congenital hyperinsulinism: The keys for differential diagnosis. Endocr Pathol 2004;15:241-46.
22. Abernethy LJ, Davidson DC, Lamont GL. Intra-arterial calcium stimulation test in the investigation of hyperinsulinaemic hypoglycaemia. Arch Dis Child 1998;78:359-63.
23. Cucchiaro G, Markowitz SD, Kaye R. Blood glucose control during selective arterial stimulation and venous sampling for localization of focal hyperinsulinism lesions in anesthetized children. Anesth Analg 2004;99:1044-48.
24. Goudswaard WB, Houthoff HJ, Koudstaal J, et al. Nesidioblastosis and endocrine hyperplasia of the pancreas: A secondary phenomenon. Human Pathology 1986;17:46-54.
25. Taguchi T, Suita S, Hirose R. Histological classification of nesidioblastosis: efficacy of immunohistochemical study of neuron-specific enolase. Journal of Pediatric Surgery 1991;26:770-74.
26. Gupta DK, Sharma S. Pancreatic Tumors in Childhood in Pediatric Oncology-Surgical and Medical Aspects. Gupta DK and Carachi Robert (Ed). Jaypee Brothers, New Delhi 2007;42: 427-36.
27. Bani D, Bani Sacchi T, Biliotti G. Nesidioblastosis and intermediate cells in the pancreas of patients with hyperinsulinemic hypoglycemia. Virchows Archives B (Cell Pathology Including Molecular Pathology) 1985;48:19-32.
28. Gould VE, Memoli VA, Dardi LE, et al. Nesidiodysplasia and nesidioblastosis of infancy: Ultrastructural and immunohistochemical analysis of islet cell alterations with and without associated hyperinsulinaemic hypoglycaemia. Scandinavian Journal of Gastroenterology 1981;70 (Suppl):129-42.
29. Zumkeller W. Nesidioblastosis Endocrine–Related Cancer 1999;6:421-28.
30. Shanbag P, Pathak A, Vaidya M. Persistent hyperinsulinemic hypoglycemia of infancy-successful therapy with nifedipine. Indian J Pediatr 2002;69:271-72.
31. Lindley KJ, Dunne MJ, Kane C. Ionic control of beta–cell function in nesidioblastosis. A possible therapeutic role for calcium channel blockade. Arch Dis Child 1996;74:373-78.
32. Bas F, Darendeliler F, Demirkol D. Successful therapy with calcium channel blocker (nifedipine) in persistent neonatal hyperinsulinemic hypoglycemia of infancy. J Pediatr Endocrinol Metab 1999;12:873-78.
33. Thornton PS, Alter CA, Katz LE. Short- and long-term use of octreotide in the treatment of congenital hyperinsulinism. J Pediatr 1993;123:637-43.
34. Maniati-Christidis M, Psychou F, Nihoul-Fekete C. Persistent hyperinsulinemic neonatal hypoglycemia caused by focal nesidioblastosis. Preoperative diagnosis by pancreatic venous sampling. Hormones (Athens) 2003;2:67-71.
35. Tseng LM, Chen JY, Won JG, et al. The role of intra-arterial calcium stimulation test with hepatic venous sampling (IACS) in the management of occult insulinomas. Ann Surg Oncol 2007;14:2121-27.
36. Casanova D, Polavieja MG, Naranjo A, et al. Surgical treatment of persistent hyperinsulinemic hypoglycemia (PHH) (insulinoma and nesidioblastosis). Langenbecks Arch Surg 2007;392:663-70.
37. Strong VE, Shifrin AL, Inabnet WB. Rapid intraoperative insulin assay: A novel method to differentiate insulinoma from nesidioblastosis in the pediatric patient. Ann Surg Innov Res 2007;24;1:6.
38. Suchi M, Thornton PS, Adzick NS. Congenital hyperinsulinism: Intraoperative biopsy interpretation can direct the extent of pancreatectomy. Am J Surg Pathol 2004;28:1326-35.
39. Cade A, Walters M, Puntis JW. Pancreatic exocrine and endocrine function after pancreatectomy for persistent hyperinsulinaemic hypoglycaemia of infancy. Arch Dis Child 1998;79:435-39.
40. Berrocal T, Luque AA, Pinilla I, Lassaletta L. Pancreatic regeneration after near-total pancreatectomy in children with nesidioblastosis. Pediatr Radiol 2005;35:1066-70.

Pancreas and Intestinal Transplantation

V Martinez Ibanez

In spite of the considerable improvements in conventional diabetes therapy during the past years, insulin-dependent diabetes mellitus ranks as one of the major disease entities in the world. The life expectancy of the diabetic patient is approximately one-third less than that of the general population. Since the metabolic abnormalities that prevail in diabetes mellitus are due to non-functioning B-cells in the islets of Langerhans, it would be logical to treat this disease by the transplantation of a normally functioning pancreas. This procedure should correct the metabolic abnormalities and presumably prevent or delay the onset of severe secondary complications. Clinical application has been limited because of immunologic and technical problems, but these problems are gradually being overcome. From the 1980s the number of diabetic patients treated with pancreatic transplantation has increased rapidly and the results improved markedly.[1]

PATIENT SELECTION

In spite of the mortality and morbidity associated with insulin-dependent diabetes mellitus, the disease is not immediately life-threatening, and pancreatic transplantation unlike heart and liver transplantation, cannot be considered a life-saving procedure. Instead the potential benefits of pancreatic transplantation on the quality of life and on the secondary complications of diabetes must be weighed against the risks of the surgical procedure and by the immunosuppression required after transplantation. Until recently the difficult question of whether it was justifiable to try to cure diabetes by a major surgical procedure which was to be followed by long-term immunosuppressive therapy has largely been circumvented by accepting diabetic patients with end-stage renal disease for pancreatic and renal transplantation. In the diabetic patients with end-stage renal disease, pancreatic transplantation has been performed either concomitantly with a renal transplantation, with both the organs coming from the same donor, or alternatively, with a diabetic patient already having a renal graft has been given a subsequent pancreatic graft. Since end-stage renal disease usually develops after 20-30 years of insulin-dependent diabetes, these patients have been in the 25-45 years age range. Most patients have had various diabetic stigmata in addition to renal damage such as retinopathy and neuropathy.

The diabetic patients accepted for combined transplantation have been the patients who would otherwise have been accepted for renal transplantation only. When pancreatic transplantation has been carried out in diabetic patients already having a renal graft, the patient selected are those who have had few or no rejection episodes.

Uncorrectable malignancy and psychosis constitute contraindications for organ transplantation. Any acute disease, whether related to the patient's diabetes or not, should be treated and preferably corrected before transplantation. Infections are especially important in this regard. Some severe disabilities caused by the diabetes constitute contraindications to pancreatic transplantation, for instance ongoing peripheral gangrene, severe coronary insufficiency with angina or intractable cardiac in compensation and severely incapacitating peripheral neuropathy such as in the case of bedridden patients. An upper age limit in the 50-60 years range is usually applied.

PREOPERATIVE PATIENT EVALUATION

Because of the high incidence of coronary artery disease in the diabetic patient population, an exercise ECG should always be performed. If there is any indication of coronary artery disease, coronary angiography should be carried out. If a significant stenosis is found the patient should be evaluated for bypass surgery before pancreatic transplantation. Angiography of the iliac arteries, one of which is used for the anastomosis of the graft artery, is indicated if the femoral pulses are weak or absent or if the patient has significant claudication. If there is a history of gastroparesis or gastric candidiasis, an upper GI series or gastroscopy should be performed. If there is a history of urinary bladder dysfunction, cystoscopy should be performed. In patients with pre-uremic nephropathy, glomerular filtration rate should be determined repeatedly to establish the extent of deterioration.

To establish the effects of the pancreatic transplantation on the secondary complications of the disease a careful preoperative evaluation of the patient's neurologic and ophthalmologic status should be carried out. In patients with pre-uremic nephropathy a baseline biopsy from the native kidneys should be obtained.

THE PANCREATIC DONOR GRAFT

All cadaveric donors considered for kidney donation should be considered also for pancreas graft donation, providing there is no history of diabetes mellitus, chronic pancreatitis or pancreatic damage by trauma. Blood glucose and serum amylase should be examined in the donor. If a high blood glucose level exists, our practice is to give the donor a non-glucose-containing infusion solution for a few hours. If the blood glucose remains more than a twice normal, we are hesitant to use the pancreas. Valuable further information concerning the state of the endocrine pancreas can be obtains by determination of glycosylated hemoglobin (HbA1) with a rapid screening method. Hyperamylasemia may exist and some evidence has been presented that this can be a consequence of the cerebral infarction.

The final decision concerning the suitability of the pancreas for transplantation is made during its actual removal. The normal pancreas is yellowish, soft and has a homogeneous consistency. If sclerotic, calcified or markedly discolored, the pancreas should not be used.

In some instances relatives have served as donors for segmental pancreatic grafts. The rationale for using living related donors for pancreas grafts is that provides for a better immunological match, presumably reducing the risk for graft rejection.

THE CADAVERIC DONOR OPERATION

Most pancreases are obtained from multiorgan donors. The heart and liver are usually harvested prior to the removal of the pancreas and kidneys. Previously most pancreatic transplantations were performed using a segmental-body and tail-graft. Today more and more groups use a pancreatico-duodenal graft consisting of the entire pancreas and a segment of the duodenum.

The following is a brief description of the steps required for removal of pancreatico-duodenal graft. A long midline or a cruciate incision is used. The lesser sac is opened by ligating and dividing the gastrocolic ligaments from the pylorus to the short gastrosplenic vessels. The stomach is retracted cranially and the body and the tail of the pancreas are inspected and palpated. The spleen is mobilized or alternatively, the splenic vessels are ligated in the splenic hilum. The pancreatic tail is then reflected medially and the dissection is carried out towards the portal vein following the lower margin until the superior mesenteric vein (SMV) is reached. The inferior mesenteric vein is identified and ligated. At the upper margin the dissection is carried out until the trifurcation of the celiac axis is reached. The left gastric artery is ligated. The diaphragm is incised to provide access to the aorta and the roots of the celiac axis and the superior mesenteric artery (SMA).

The duodenum and the pancreatic head are mobilized by a Kocher maneuver. The common bile duct is divided and ligated, and the hepatic artery is ligated and divided distally to the gastroduodenal artery. The right gastric and gastroepiploic arteries are divided. The portal vein is then dissected free. The SMV and the SMA are ligated where they ride over the duodenum. The duodenum is divided just distal to the pylorus and the lower bend. The cut ends are usually closed with staples. Finally dissection is carried out towards the aorta behind the SMA.

The aorta is crossclamped above the celiac axis, and organ cooling and flushing are accomplished by intra-aortic infusion of a cold electrolyte solution by a tube inserted in the lower aorta. Thus, the pancreas and also the two kidneys are perfused. The pancreatic graft is then removed with an aortic patch containing the two arteries. The portal vein is divided to provided a length of 2-3 cm. If the whole pancreas and the liver are to be harvested from the same donor, the common hepatic artery is usually required for the vascular pedicle of the liver. In this case the gastroduodenal artery is ligated at its origin from the common hepatic artery, and the pancreatic head and the duodenum will then derive their arterial supply from the inferior pancreatico-duodenal artery arising from the SMA. If the celiac axis is also taken with the liver, the severed splenic artery can be anastomosed end-to-side to the SMA or a Y-extension graft (from the donor iliac artery bifurcation) can be used to join the splenic artery and the SMA.

If a segmental pancreatic graft is to be obtained from a cadaveric or living related donor, the dissection is carried from the tail to the level of the portal vein as describe above. A finger is passed between the pancreatic neck and the portal vein, and the pancreatic neck is cut with scissors. In the cadaveric donor this maneuver can be facilitated by first dividing the common bile duct and the gastroduodenal artery.

PANCREATIC GRAFT PRESERVATION

The techniques used for flushing, cooling and storage of the pancreatic graft have been similar to those used for kidney grafts. Thus, until recently most groups flushed the graft with electrolyte solution with intracellular electrolyte content as suggested by Collins. With these, cold storage time has usually been kept under eight hours. In 1987 the University of Wisconsin (UW) group introduced a solution containing lactobionate and raffinose as impermeable osmotic agents. This solution is also devoid of glucose and, therefore, avoids lactic acid production in the organ. It has proved to be an excellent solution for flushing the pancreas and allows storage for 24 hours and perhaps even longer.[2]

THE RECIPIENT OPERATION

In the very first series of pancreatic transplantation's performed in man, pancreatic-duodenal grafts were used. The graft duodenum was anastomosed end-to-end to a recipient Roux-loop thereby accomplishing enteric exocrine diversion. However, following the occurrence of necrosis and fistulas in the duodenum in some patients, this type of graft fell into disrepute and segmental body and tail grafts became standard from the early 1970s onwards. However, the pancreatic-duodenal graft was reintroduced by Starzl in 1990s.[1] By now, most groups are using such grafts (Fig. 95.1). The duodenal complications previously encountered are now hardly seen, probably due to better techniques for tissue preservation and better protocols for avoiding graft rejection.

Intestinal transplant alone may also be done as a separate procedure (Fig. 95.2).

Management of the Exocrine Pancreas

As for the handling of the exocrine secretion of the pancreatic graft, there are three options.

1. *Pancreatic ducto-occlusion:* One technique introduced by Dubernard of France is ductal filling with a polymer.[3] By such filling the exocrine secretion is prevented from escaping or indeed even from being formed. The procedure is appealing in that it reduces the intervention in the patient to the vascular anastomosis. However, it has recently become clear that monitoring of amylase in the exocrine secretion is crucial for the diagnosis of graft rejection. Since ductal filling makes this impossible, the interest in this technique has diminished.

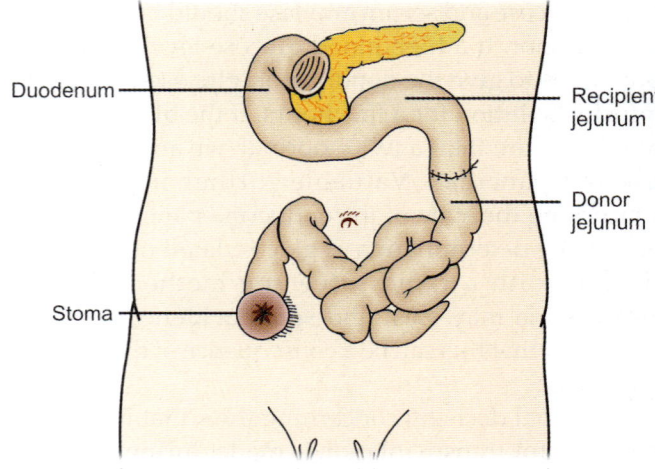

Fig. 95.1: Pancreatico duodenal graft

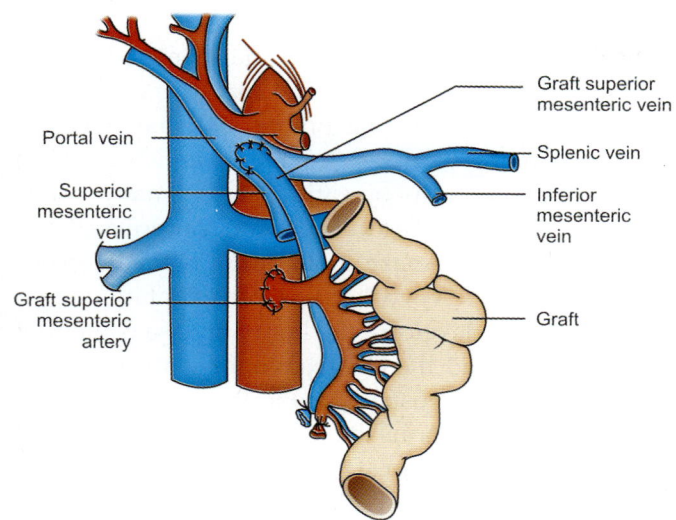

Fig. 95.2: Intestinal transplant

2. *Diversion to the urinary bladder:* In the early 1970s Gliedman suggested that exocrine diversion should be accomplished via the patient's ureter.[4] In so doing the bowel did not have to be entered and the risk for infection was thereby reduced. The concept was reintroduced in the 1980s by Sollinger, who suggested that a duodenal patch of the graft should be anastomosed to the patient's bladder instead.[5] Today most groups favour pancreatic-duodenal grafts with bladder drainage.

The graft is placed intraperitoneally with the head of the pancreas pointing downwards. Vascular anastomoses are made to the iliac vessels on the right side. The antimesenteric side of the duodenal segment is anastomosed to the top of the bladder with a two layer anastomosis or with help of a stapler. A segmental pancreatic graft can also be anastomosed to the bladder.

A disadvantage of urinary tract diversion is that it causes a significant bicarbonate loss sometimes leading to metabolic acidosis requiring replacement therapy.

3. *Exocrine diversion to the bowel:* Diversion to the bowel offers the most physiological way of handling the exocrine secretion. The graft is placed intraperitoneally. Previously, when segmental grafts were used, a pancreatic-enterostomy was created by telescoping the cut end of the pancreas into the end of a jejunal Roux-loop.

When pancreatic-duodenal grafts are used, the anastomosis consists of an entero-entero anastomosis performed either to a Roux-loop or directly end-to-side to the recipient's jejunum. The arterial anastomosis is to the iliac vessels. Since the head of the graft should point upward, the portal vein is usually anastomosed to the lower caval vein. The Stockholm group uses a pancreatic duct catheter to divert the exocrine secretion to the exterior for the first few weeks after transplantation. Pure pancreatic juice is then made available for monitoring graft function.

POSTOPERATIVE MANAGEMENT AND MONITORING

Infection and Thrombosis Prophylaxis

Most groups use prophylaxis with antibiotics during surgery and for the first 2-5 postoperative days. Also various drug protocols aimed at reducing the risk of graft vascular thrombosis are used by most groups. The treatment may consist of dextraninfusion given intravenously for one or several days followed by either aspirin or warfarin sodium given for weeks or months.

Immunosuppression

Immunosuppression is usually similar to that used in renal transplantation although quadruple drug therapy may be somewhat more common with pancreatic transplantation.

Monitoring the Graft

For monitoring the pancreatic graft, blood glucose, glycosylated hemoglobin and serum amylase levels are routinely assayed. In addition, many groups assay the serum C-peptide as a measure of graft insulin production. If the graft has been anastomosed to the patient's bladder, the amylase excretion is measured by amylase assay in the urine. If, alternatively, the pancreatic secretion has been exteriorized by means of a ductal catheter, amylase and inflammatory cells are assayed directly in the juice. If an abdominal drain is used, the amylase activity in the discharge should be measured daily. An elevated level may disclose an anastomotic leakage.

GRAFT-RELATED COMPLICATIONS

Most of the graft-related complications seen after pancreatic transplantation reflect well-known pancreatic pathophysiological conditions. Examples of such conditions are pancreatis, peripancreatic fluid collections, anastomotic leaks, fistulas and peri- and intrapancreatic abscesses. With all these conditions, wound infections are common. Another characteristic graft-related complication has been graft thrombosis.

Pancreatitis

In almost all patients some symptoms and signs typical of pancreatitis (pain and tenderness related to the pancreatic graft in combination with hyperamylasemia) appear during the first few days after transplantation. This early postoperative pancreatitis is believed to be a consequence of injury to the pancreas which occurs during the actual transplant procedure, i.e. specifically ischemic damage. In some patients hyperamylasemia appears without any specific symptoms but in others severe pain and tenderness at the graft site appear. The longer the cold ischemia, the greater the risk of pancreatitis. Still, severe pancreatitis may appear even with relatively short ischemia time.

The treatment of graft pancreatitis is similar to that of common pancreatitis, the patient is kept fasting and IV replacement is given. In case of severe local symptoms, laparotomy should be performed with evacuation of peripancreatic fluid collections. Sometimes resection of necrotic areas on the pancreatic surface might also be necessary followed by peritoneal lavage for a few days. Usually endocrine function is unaffected even during severe attacks of graft pancreatitis. Nonetheless if the pancreatitis is very severe, graft-removal offers the safest remedy.

Pancreatic Exocrine Sweating

With pancreatitis or any pancreatic injury, a fluid high in amylase and other enzymes seeps out from the pancreatic graft and accumulates around the gland, a phenomenon often referred to as pancreatic sweating. The pancreatic sweating usually abates a few days after transplantation but may continue for 1-2 weeks. By tube drainage of the operative site, the risk for fluid accumulation will be much reduced.

Anastomotic Leaks and Fistulas

When the pancreatic graft is anastomosed to the patient's bowel or urinary tract for diversion of the exocrine secretion, an anastomotic leak may develop. This leak may give rise to a pancreatic fistula to the exterior. Also, a peripancreatic abscess usually forms. The symptoms include local pain and tenderness, fever and leucocytosis. Anastomotic leaks typically occur during the first few weeks after transplantation. If an exterior fistula develops, the high amylase content of the discharge and the skin reddening caused by the digestive enzymes usually make the diagnosis easy. If only an abscess forms the diagnosis may be difficult since pancreatitis, graft rejection and intestinal obstruction may give similar symptoms.

Early re-exploration should be considered as soon as the patient experiences unexplained abdominal pain and fever. The chances of repairing an anastomotic leak and of successfully draining fluid collections are much enhanced if the operation is performed promptly.

Intrapancreatic Abscesses

In some patients intrapancreatic abscesses have developed several weeks after transplantation. The symptoms are persistent fever, pain at the graft site and a gradual deterioration of blood glucose control. Serum amylase is unaffected. Such intrapancreatic abscesses are probably due to subacute or chronic rejection with ensuing destruction of the exocrine part of the graft. They may also be due to primary cytomegalovirus infection of the pancreas. If an intrapancreatic abscess develops, the pancreatic graft must be removed.

Graft Thrombosis

Vascular thrombosis has been observed to be responsible for 10-20% of all graft losses. One possible reason for the propensity of graft thrombosis lies in the abnormal hemodynamic situation that exists in the pancreatic graft. Arterial revascularization is achieved by anastomosing large arterial trunks, such as the celiac axis or splenic artery and the SMA, with their distal ends ligated. These large trunks are then left to drain via the small pancreatic branches thus creating a low outflow situation. Pancreatitis with ensuing swelling of the exocrine pancreas may also be a predisposing factor. Thrombosis may be arterial or venous. It usually occurs during the first week after transplantation, and many thromboses occur within the first 24 hours.

With arterial graft thrombosis the characteristic findings are a sudden increase in blood glucose level and a fall in serum amylase levels. If a pancreatic duct catheter is used, the typical finding is a gradual decline in output and bloodstaining of the pancreatic juice. Pain and tenderness over the graft is common.

Grafts that thrombose early should be removed while grafts undergoing late arterial thrombosis can be left *in situ* unless local symptoms occur. To prevent graft thrombosis most groups use anticoagulation therapy as primarily mentioned. With such therapy a reduction in the incidence of thrombosis has occurred, but a price has been paid since an increased incidence of bleeding has resulted. The risk of bleeding is lowest when only dextran and aspirin only are used.

DIAGNOSIS OF REJECTION

When rejection occurs in recipients of combined renal and pancreatic graft, signs of impaired renal function, such as increasing creatinine and BUN, usually precede signs of impaired pancreatic function by a few days. Often signs of pancreatic graft rejection may be absent. This finding may be explained by the pancreas being less prone to rejection than the kidney, or alternatively, the parameters used for diagnosing pancreatic graft rejection might be less sensitive. In patients subjected to single pancreatic transplantation and in those given a pancreatic transplantation after a renal transplantation–with the grafts coming from different donors–the diagnosis of acute rejection must been found that elevation of blood glucose is a very late sign of rejection, the rise occurring only when about 90% of the pancreatic graft has been destroyed. C-peptide assays seem to be a somewhat more sensitive marker of endocrine function, but the test is time-consuming and usually not performed on a daily basis. As a result of the above, interest has focused on measurements of exocrine function as possible rejection markers. So far, there are no reliable serum assays reflecting pancreatic graft rejection. Serum amylase levels sometimes show a transient rise during the first few days of an acute rejection episode, but the level may be unchanged or even decrease. At the present time the most widely used marker of acute pancreatic graft rejection is the amylase level in the pancreatic juice. If the exocrine graft has been anastomosed to the patient's urinary tract, urinary amylase level reflects the amylase content in the juice. Some investigators prefer to use the 12-hour amylase output as the parameter thereby avoiding the influence of variations in urinary output. The diversion of the pure pancreatic juice to the exterior by means of a catheter also makes possible daily determinations of amylase output. In addition this technique makes possible studies of pancreatic juice cytology. During the first days after transplantation the pancreatic juice contains large amounts of granulocytes probably as a reflection of ischemic graft pancreatitis. During rejection, inflammatory cells appear in the juice. Monocytes usually appear first to be followed one or two days later by lymphocytes and lymphoblasts. Following antirejection treatment the lymphoblasts disappear and the pancreatic juice again becomes devoid of cells. The appearance of inflammatory cells has been found to precede the decline in amylase by one or two days. Thus pancreatic juice cytology is probably a more sensitive and more specific marker for rejection than the amylase content.

Various radiological examinations such as angiography, scintigraphy, ultrasonography and MRI may also aid in the diagnosis of acute rejection. On angiography acute rejection is reflected in poor staining of the parenchyma. If the rejection is severe, there are also irregularities in the small arteries. In scintigraphy a reduced perfusion index and a reduction in the staining of the graft is indicative of rejection. In ultrasonography with Doppler measurement of blood flow, an increase in the resistance index as well as swelling of the graft and peripancreatic fluid collections are taken as signs of rejection. With MRI the normal pancreas allograft has a signal intensity similar to that of normal renal cortex on T:1 weighted images and less than that of urine or kidney on T:2 weighted images. During acute rejection, the pancreatic parenchyma has an abnormal focal or diffuse signal intensity less than that of normal renal cortex and similar to that of muscle on T:1 weighted images and brighter or equal to that of urine or kidney on T:2 weighted images.

Chronic graft rejection may occur months or years after transplantation, and a slowly rising blood glucose level, indicative of a progressive destruction of the endocrine capacity, is a characteristic laboratory finding. Usually the rise is seen first in the postprandial blood glucose. At the same time there is a progressive decline in the C-peptide level.

Ultimate confirmation of rejection requires microscopic evaluation of a biopsy specimen from the graft. Characteristic findings are diffuse mononuclear cell infiltrates in the pancreatic parenchyma and acute or chronic vasculitis. Since the pancreatic graft is placed intraperitoneally among the intestines, a laparotomy is necessary for a safe biopsy. Fine needle aspiration biopsies can be carried out with little or no risk of enteric damage.

OUTPATIENT FOLLOW-UP

Patients are seen in the outpatient clinic, initially twice weekly then over longer and longer intervals. At each visit, pancreatic graft function is assessed by measuring fasting and postprandial blood glucose levels, glycosylated hemoglobin and serum amylase. In patients with graft with urinary tract diversion, urinary amylase is measured. Between visits the patients may perform home monitoring of blood glucose levels. The patients with urinary diversion are also recommended to monitor urinary pH since a reduction of the exocrine secretion from the graft is reflected in an increased pH.

Every three or six months the endocrine capacity of the pancreatic graft is examined by intravenous and oral glucose tolerance test. Retinopathy and neuropathy is reassessed every six months after transplantation. In pre-uremic patients the course of the nephropathy is followed by regular assays of serum-creatinine, BUN and EDTA clearance. The immunosuppressive treatment is tapered.

EFFECT OF TRANSPLANTATION ON METABOLIC CONTROL

Usually normoglycemia occurs within a few hours after pancreas transplantation, and exogenous insulin therapy can be discontinued. However, hyperglycemia requiring treatment with exogenous insulin may exist for days or even weeks in some patients. Such post-transplantation hyperglycemia may be due to ischemic damage to the graft, and it may be aggravated by the intravenous glucose infusions given in the early postoperative phase. When conditions have stabilized, fasting and postprandial blood glucose should be normal or almost normal. When glycosylated hemoglobin is measured, it is found normal in approximately two-third of the patients and slightly elevated in the remaining one-third. The oral glucose tolerance is normal in most of the patients while the intravenous glucose tolerance is normal only in some 50% of the patients. These abnormalities in glucose metabolism are probably mainly due to immunosuppression. Graft injury, due to sustained ischemic damage or rejection, might be a contributing factor in some patients. In spite of the difference in islet mass provided there seems to be no significant difference in blood glucose control whether pancreaticoduodenal or segmental grafts are used. It is clear that the long-term metabolic control seen after successful pancreatic transplantation is superior to that which can be achieved with any other method today.

EFFECT OF TRANSPLANTATION ON QUALITY OF LIFE AND ON THE SECONDARY COMPLICATIONS OF DIABETES

After successful pancreatic transplantation there is a distinct improvement in the quality of life of the recipient. Insulin injections can be dispensed with and all dietary restrictions abandoned. These changes have considerable social and psychological implications for most patients. Also general wellbeing is often improved and can be objectively measured in factors such as social, physical and psychological functions.

As for the effects on the secondary complications of the disease, such as retinopathy, neuropathy and nephropathy, there are some unfavourable and some more favourable findings. Thus combined renal and pancreatic transplantation in uremic recipients seems to have little or only moderate effect on established diabetic retinopathy or neuropathy. However these findings may be explained by the fact that most recipients transplanted so far, have had very advanced secondary complications, complications that could hardly be expected to be reversed or even halted. An important conclusion to be drawn from these findings is that pancreatic transplantation needs to be performed earlier in the course of the disease. So far, only limited clinical data are available concerning the effect on the secondary complications in this situation. It has been reported however, that in recipients of combined pancreatic and renal grafts diabetic lesions in the transplanted kidney are avoided while such lesions develop after two years in diabetic patients who have received a kidney only. In addition there is some preliminary data showing that early diabetic lesions in a previously transplanted renal graft or the patient's native kidneys can be halted or perhaps even reversed following pancreatic transplantation. Also following single pancreatic transplantation in non-uremic recipients the progression of diabetic polyneuropathy may be halted. These findings confirm several animal studies where pancreatic transplantation has been shown to prevent or reverse secondary lesions if performed early on in the course of the disease.[6-8]

FUTURE

Pancreas transplantation has become increasingly effective for the treatment of human diabetes. Islet cell transplants have thus far been successful only in the laboratory. Unless islet cell yield can be improved and methods to reduce immunogenicity can be made practical, pancreas transplantation is the only practical method of total endocrine replacement therapy in diabetes that can succeed. Potentially, pancreas transplantation could be applied on as large scale as renal transplantation is. Eventually, pancreas transplantation may be routinely performed at a sufficiently early stage to prevent the development of diabetic nephropathy and other complications and may supersede kidney transplants and other procedures in the management of complication-prone diabetic patients.

REFERENCES

1. Starzl TE, Iwatsuki S, Shaw P, et al. Pancreatico-duodenal transplantation in humans. Surg Gynec Obstet 1984;159: 265-72.
2. Wahlberg JA, Love R, Landegaard L, et al. 72-hour preservation of the canine pancreas. Transplantation 1987;43:5-8.
3. Dubernard JM, Sanseverino R, Martinenghi S, et al. Duct obstruction of segmental grafts in pancreas transplantation. Transplant Proc 1989;21:2799-800.
4. Gliedman ML, Gold M, Whittaker J, et al. Clinical segmental pancreatic transplantation with ureter pancreatic duct anastomosis for exocrine drainage. Surgery 1973;74:171-80.
5. Sollinger HW, D'Alessandro AM, Startta RJ, et al. Combined kidney/pancreas transplantation with pancreaticocystostomy. Transplant Proc 1989;21: 2837-38.
6. Bohman SO, Tyden G, Wilczek H. Prevention of kidney graft diabetic nephropathy by pancreas transplantation in man. Diabetes 1985;34:306-08.
7. Bilous RW, Mauer SM, Sutherland DER, et al. The effects of pancreas transplantation on the glomerular structure of renal allografts in patients with insulin dependent diabetes mellitus. N Engl J Med 1989;321: 80-85.
8. Kennedy WR, Navarro X, Goetz F, et al. Effects of pancreatic transplantation on diabetic neuropathy. N Engl J Med 1990;322:1031-37.

CHAPTER 96

Spleen

Amir Kaviani, Moritz M Ziegler

Modern-day understanding of the role of the spleen both in health and disease can be traced back to Virchow's detailed anatomic and histologic descriptions in the 19th century.[1] In the hundred years that followed, little knowledge was gained about the exact function of the spleen, and as recently as fifty years ago, it was believed that the spleen could be removed with impunity. In the early 1950's, it was recognized that removal of the spleen may have life-threatening consequences, particularly in young children.[2] In the past 20 years, much has been learned about the important role of the spleen in the immune processes of the body. This knowledge has led to a more conservative approach in the surgical management of splenic disease. Important new aspects of splenic surgery in children include splenic preservation, laparoscopic approaches, and autotransplantation. Furthermore, more evidence has accumulated supporting a nonoperative approach in the management of splenic trauma in a majority of cases.

EMBRYOLOGY AND ANATOMY

Normal

The spleen is unique in that it is the only unilateral and completely mesenchymal organ in humans.[3] It arises at about the fifth week of gestation from the mesenchyme of the dorsal pancreatic bud. With the normal longitudinal rotation of the stomach, the spleen is carried into the left upper quadrant where it occupies a position superior and dorsal to the stomach and anterior to the left adrenal and kidney. By the twelfth week of gestation, the spleen assumes a triangular shape, with a parietal convex surface abutting the diaphragm and a concave visceral surface directly adjacent to the stomach, kidney, and colon. The dorsal mesentery surrounding this structure gives rise to the peritoneal layer that envelops the spleen, as well as an inner capsule containing a network of connective tissue fibers. An extensive network of sinusoids develops in this capsule in the fifth to seventh weeks of gestation. During the second trimester, the spleen supplements the liver in its hematopoietic function.[4] The weight of the spleen increases more quickly during this time than the body weight until the fetus reaches 200 grams. The rapidity of this rise corresponds with the increasing hematopoietic function of the fetal spleen. At the splenic hilum, the leaves of the dorsal mesentery coalesce to form the gastrosplenic and splenorenal ligaments, providing fixation and enveloping the splenic pedicle. Other lesser attachments develop between the spleen and the colon, diaphragm, and pancreas.

At birth, the normal spleen weighs between 10 to 15 grams and measures approximately 5 cm at its greatest dimension. Its main arterial blood supply, the splenic artery, arises from the celiac trunk.[5] Additional arterial blood supply is obtained from the short gastric arteries, branches of the left gastroepiploic artery. The splenic artery divides into several smaller trabecular arteries at the hilum. These trabecular arteries branch into smaller central arteries that supply the splenic parenchyma, named as a result of their central position in the white pulp. The central arteries send numerous radial branches into the white pulp, terminating as the penicillate arteries and arterioles in the capillaries of the red pulp. It is this radial orientation of vessels from a central hilum that facilitates the technical performance of a partial splenectomy. These capillaries are sheathed with phagocytic cells, and communicate with the venous system either directly or indirectly in the splenic substance.[6] The circulation of blood through the red pulp, which is lined entirely by endothelium is termed "closed circulation," whereas circulation into the phagocyte lined sinuses (Billroth's cords) is referred to as the "open circulation".

Venous drainage of the splenic parenchyma begins in the sinuses located in the red pulp. These structures empty directly into venules and veins coursing the trabecular arteries which eventually join to form the splenic vein near the hilum. Near the tail of the pancreas, the splenic vein coalesces with the inferior mesenteric vein which more medially is joined by the superior mesenteric vein giving rise to the portal vein.

The red and white pulp within the splenic parenchyma have specialized functions.[7] The red pulp, so named because of the slow flow of blood through the sinusoids, forms the majority of splenic substance. It is composed of cords of loose trabecular tissue containing capillaries and reticuloendothelial cells interspersed among venous sinuses. The white pulp is composed of lymphoid tissue and reticular substance and surrounds the central artery and arterioles. Within the white pulp, B-cells are arranged as follicles surrounding a germinal center. T-cells are arranged densely around the central artery, and more dispersed peripherally. This precise microarchitecture is critical to the normal physiologic and immunologic function of the spleen.

Abnormal

Asplenia and Polysplenia

Asplenia and polysplenia are unusual defects arising from a failure of normal symmetric organogenesis, and are associated with other major congenital anomalies.[8] The incidence of asplenia in man is between 1:632 and 1:3214 in series reporting on this syndrome, with a slight male predominance. Congenital asplenia (Ivemark syndrome) occurs as a result of bilateral right-sidedness.[9] Other structures derived from the dorsal mesogastrium are also affected, including the stomach and omentum. Associated cardiac anomalies often include transposition of the great arteries, septal defects, truncus arteriosus, pulmonary artery stenosis or atresia, anomalous venous return, and atrioventricular canal defects. In most cases, both lungs are trilobed, and the stomach is located on the right with a centrally located liver. Splenic absence is suggested by examination of a peripheral blood smear in the newborn revealing Howell-Jolly bodies and siderocytes. Patients should be placed on asplenia prophylaxis (as discussed later) as soon as the diagnosis is made. Acquired asplenia is encountered after removal or sequestration of the spleen in sickle cell anemia.

In contrast, polysplenia results from bilateral left-sidedness. The multiple spleens are usually located along the greater curvature of the stomach. Cardiac defects are often present, however, not as severe as those accompanying asplenia. The lungs are usually bilobed, and the liver may be bilateral. Other associated lesions of surgical significance include a higher incidence of biliary atresia, and a preduodenal portal vein. Splenic function is usually normal.

Accessory Spleen

Accessory spleen refers to small (1 to 10 cm), functioning splenic nodules, in addition to a normal, functioning spleen.[10] It represents by far the most common anomaly of the spleen, and one of the most common anomalies of the body overall, reportedly occurring in between 10-30% of the general population. In most cases, a single accessory spleen is present, but multiple accessory spleens have also been reported. Accessory spleens are usually found in the splenic hilum, along the curvature of the stomach, in the omentum, and adjacent to the pancreas. The nodules often resemble small lymph nodes, but may proliferate quickly if overlooked during splenectomy performed for hematologic disease, thereby allowing for recurrence of the original disorder.

Splenogonadal Fusion

Splenogonadal fusion refers to a rare developmental anomaly that results in the presence of splenic tissue in the left scrotum or adnexa. The aberrant tissue is often connected to the normal spleen by a band of fibrous tissue with or without additional splenic tissue along its course. The most-likely etiology is the adherence of the splenic anlage with the mesonephric ridge in the developing embryo.[11] Splenogonadal fusion is often found in association with limb or anorectal anomalies. In males, these lesions typically present as left undescended testicle, presumed hernia or even an "acute scrotum", the latter secondary to acute congestion of the ectopic splenic tissue. In most cases, the splenic tissue can be safely removed from the underlying testicle, however, this may be complicated in cases in which there is direct fusion with the testicular tissue underlying the tunica.

Splenic Ectopia (Wandering Spleen)

Splenic ectopia describes a condition where the laxity of the splenic ligaments allows the spleen to be located anywhere in the peritoneal cavity other than its normal position in the left upper quadrant.[12] The exact etiology is unknown, however, the abnormality most likely results from the failure of the dorsal mesogastrium to give rise to the major supporting ligaments of the spleen. The long splenic pedicle predisposes the spleen to torsion which can result in infarction, an acute surgical condition. A child with a wandering spleen may present with chronic abdominal pain or a painless abdominal mass, although the most common presentation is acute abdominal pain secondary to torsion and infarction. The classic physical exam findings of a notched, elliptical, freely mobile abdominal mass are highly suggestive of a wandering spleen. Diagnosis may be confirmed by ultrasound or computed tomography which demonstrates a mass with morphologic characteristics of a spleen in the absence of a spleen in its normal expected position in the left upper quadrant.[13] Once detected, therapy is based on the indications for operation. Splenectomy is required in cases of infarction, however, if spleen viability is found at operation or if an incidentally discovered wandering spleen is discovered, it may be treated by splenopexy in which the spleen is placed into an extraperitoneal pouch. The use of polyglactin mesh as a buttress to secure the splenic capsule to the diaphragm and retroperitoneum may be a useful adjunct.[14]

PHYSIOLOGY

Normal

Hematologic Function

In many mammalian species, the spleen serves as a major reservoir of erythrocytes; however there is little evidence of this role in humans. In contrast, the human spleen serves as a reservoir for platelets, with up to 50% of the platelet pool sequestered in the spleen at any given time.[15] In hypersplenic states, this proportion is increased. As a result, splenectomy leads to loss of this platelet reservoir, and a rapid increase in the number of circulating platelets which may lead to thrombotic complications. These complications often involve the mesenteric circulation, and are exceedingly rare in children.

The spleen plays an important role in the normal homeostasis of erythrocytes. Immature erythrocytes (reticuloendothelial cells) are retained by the spleen and released into the circulation after achieving maturation.[16] This process involves remodeling of the cell membrane, loss of reticulum, and shrinkage of cell volume. The spleen is responsible for removing intraerythrocytic inclusions such as (Howell-Jolly bodies) and Heinz bodies. This process is commonly referred to as "pitting" and is a direct result of the microarchitecture of the splenic sinusoids. Erythrocytes which have traversed the splenic cords re-enter the circulation through the fine interendothelial gap junctions of the splenic sinus. Normal erythrocytes are distensible, and traverse the small spaces with ease. Cells containing inclusion bodies become less distensible, and are unable to complete this journey intact. A small portion of the cell membrane is pinched off with the cell wall at the splenic sinus aperture, effectively removing the inclusion bodies from the circulation. Other abnormal erythrocytes (spherocytes, poikilocytes) cannot deform sufficiently to enter the splenic sinus, and are trapped in the splenic cords where they are phagocytosed by cells of the reticuloendothelial system. This includes aged red cells in which the membrane is less deformable in part as a result of diminished adenosine triphosphate activity. In addition to decreased deformability, aged erythrocytes acquire immunoglobulin G (IgG) antibody on the cell surface which is recognized by monocytes and phagocytes of the spleen. Immunoglobulin-mediated destruction of these aged erythrocytes takes place after subsequent slow passage through the splenic reticuloendothelial system.

Immunologic Function

Normally, the spleen serves as a major storage center for lymphoid cells, accounting for up to 30% of the

T-cell pool, and 15 to 20% of the B-cell population at any given time.[17] There is constant flux of the circulating lymphocyte pool with those stored in the spleen. The spleen serves as an important source for IgM antibody, and these levels are diminished significantly after splenectomy. In addition, factors involved in activation of the complement system including properidin and tuftsin are produced in the spleen.[18]

Abnormal

Hyposplenism

Hyposplenism refers to decreased splenic function and phagocytic ability.[19] Acquired hyposplenia may be associated with a variety of conditions, and results in the finding of increased inclusion bodies in the peripheral smear as well as small erythrocyte membrane defects. In children, sickle cell disease is the most common cause of acquired hyposplenism, and is associated with a gradual loss of splenic function over several years.

In the normal neonate, developmental hyposplenia exists due to the immaturity of the white pulp. As a result, antigen processing is deficient, and intra-erythrocytic inclusions are common in the neonatal peripheral smear. Prematurity accentuates this normal developmental finding in the neonate.[20]

Hypersplenism

Hypersplenism refers to a state of increased splenic destruction and sequestration of preformed blood elements, in conjunction with a relative deficiency of the same blood element in the peripheral blood as well as increased production in the marrow.[21] This condition is most commonly acquired, and may or may not be associated with splenomegaly. Portal hypertension resulting in venous outflow obstruction is the most common cause of hypersplenism. Other associated conditions are listed in Table 96.1.

INDICATIONS FOR SPLENECTOMY

The main indications for splenectomy in children are listed in Table 96.2. Absolute indications for splenectomy are rare and splenectomy should be performed only after careful consideration.

Table 96.1: Conditions associated with hypersplenism
- Portal hypertension
- Splenic vein thrombosis
- Congestive heart failure
- Leukemia
- Felty syndrome
- Lupus erythematosus
- Sarcoidosis
- Amyloidosis
- Gaucher disease
- Niemann-Pick disease

Table 96.2: Indications for splenectomy in children
- Chronic Hemolytic anemias
- Hereditary spherocytosis
- Autoimmune hemolytic anemia
- Thalassemia intermedia
- β-thalassemia (with increasing transfusion requirements)

Chronic Thrombocytopenias
- Idiopathic thrombocytopenic purpura
- Thrombotic thrombocytopenic purpura (refractory to medical therapy)

Severe Hypersplenism
- Severe cytopenias, splenic infarction
- Myeloproliferative disorders
- Myeloid metaplasia
- Chronic myelogenous leukemia
- Congestive splenomegaly
- Storage diseases
- Parasitic diseases (schistosomiasis, malaria, leishmaniasis)

Primary Malignant Lesions of the Spleen
- Lymphoma
- Angiosarcoma

Splenic Lesions
- Cysts (congenital; post-traumatic; echinococcal)
- Hodgkin's disease

Trauma
- Hemodynamic instability secondary to splenic hemorrhage

Hematologic Disorders

Hereditary Spherocytosis

Hereditary spherocytosis is inherited as an autosomal dominant trait, and is a hemolytic anemia that occurs most commonly in caucasians. A cell membrane defect causes erythrocytes to be spherical rather than biconcave, rendering them more fragile and prone to destruction during their passage through the splenic circulation.[22] This condition typically presents as a mild chronic anemia with periodic exacerbations causing more severe anemia. On examination, the spleen is mildly enlarged, and firm. A peripheral blood smear reveals spherocytes, and laboratory findings include an elevated reticulocyte count, increased osmotic fragility, and a negative Coomb's test. Moderate to severe spherocytosis is an absolute indication for splenectomy, which results in complete resolution of the anemia in almost all cases. Spherocytosis persists after removal of the spleen, however the lifespan of erythrocytes returns to normal. Since postsplenectomy sepsis is more common in very young children, splenectomy for spherocytosis is usually delayed until the age of at least five years if the underlying anemia is not severe.[15] Most patients respond to medical therapy in this waiting period.

Sickle Cell Anemia

Sickle-cell anemia is a common hereditary hematologic abnormality, occurring in 1 in 625 live births in the United States.[23] This condition results from homozygous hemoglobin S resulting in polymerization and sickling of affected erythrocytes in conditions of hypoxia, acidosis, cold, and dehydration. Abnormal hemoglobin detected during electrophoresis is diagnostic of this condition. In most cases, the spleen is enlarged by six months of age as a result of increased phagocytosis of sickled erythrocytes which are less distensible and more readily destroyed during their passage through the splenic sinus, with its naturally hypoxic and acidotic environment. During acute splenic sequestration crises (ASSC), sudden trapping of blood in the spleen may be substantial, and cause rapid increase in the size of the organ. The volume of blood stored in the spleen during these crises may lead to hypovolemic shock. Older children who have experienced numerous vasooclusive crises have decreased splenic function and show evidence of splenic atrophy leading to functional autosplenectomy after approximately 10 years.[24] This results from fibrosis and scarring of the splenic parenchyma. In some cases, the spleen persists until adulthood.

The main indication for splenectomy is the development of (ASSC), which is the leading cause of death in sickle cell patients younger than 10 years of age. Patients with severe attacks should undergo splenectomy after recovering from a severe attack, since the risk of recurrence ranges from 40-50% and carries a 20% mortality rate. In most cases, transfusion requirements dictate the severity of the attack and the need for splenectomy. Partial or subtotal splenectomy is advocated in these patients since they are especially prone to developing postsplenectomy sepsis.[25]

Thalassemia

Thalassemias represent a heterogeneous group of hereditary hemoglobinopathies which vary in severity. Genetic defects range from partial to complete deletions of genes encoding for globin chains as a result of nucleotide deletions, insertions, or substitutions. The more severe forms are accompanied by diffuse deposition of iron in the splenic parenchyma which is engorged by destroyed abnormal erythrocytes. Hypersplenism results in further red blood cell sequestration and leads to increased transfusion requirements.[24] In severe cases with escalating transfusion requirements, partial or total splenectomy may be indicted. The rate of postsplenectomy sepsis in patients with thalassemias is high, approaching 15%.[26]

Idiopathic Thrombocytopenic Purpura

The etiology of idiopathic thrombocytopenic purpura (ITP) is unknown. Chronic ITP is mediated at least in part by IgG binding to platelet associated antigen resulting in phagocytosis by the reticuloendothelial system in the spleen.[27] Acute ITP, is a transient, more self-limiting form of this disorder, and is commonly treated with activity restriction, corticosteroids, and administration of intravenous gamma-globulin. Acute ITP most commonly occurs in children younger than 10 years of age following a viral illness. Symptoms are associated with thrombocytopenia, and include formation of petechiae, ecchymoses, perianal or oral bleeding, and intracranial bleeding.

Systemic corticosteroids increase the platelet count significantly in up to 80% of these patients. The mechanism is believed to be related to inhibition of phagocytosis as well as through stimulation of platelet production. Intravenous gamma-globulin binds to Fc receptors of the reticuloendothelial cells in the spleen, and inhibits phagocytosis. This treatment is usually reserved for cases refractory to steroids or in patients who are actively bleeding.

In 10-20% of patients with ITP, thrombocytopenia and associated symptoms last greater than six months. These patients are believed to have chronic ITP, and may also show improvement after administration of steroids and IV gamma-globulin. Approximately 20% of patients with chronic ITP will eventually require splenectomy due to medical treatment failure. In contrast, acute ITP almost always resolves after medical treatment, and splenectomy in those cases is only reserved for cases with severe bleeding complications. During surgery for ITP, a careful search for accessory splenic tissue must be conducted to avoid postoperative recurrences.[28]

Splenic Lesions

Abscess

Splenic abscess is rare in children and most commonly a result of an infected hematoma or pseudocyst.[29] It is most commonly seen in the immunosuppressed child who is at increased risk from seeding during bacteremia. Also, a splenic infarct resulting from a hemoglobinopathy may become secondarily infected. These patients show signs of sepsis, and complain of left upper quadrant pleuritic pain. The diagnosis is confirmed by CT scan. Solitary abscesses may be drained percutaneously, which allows identification of the organism and directed antibiotic treatment. Multiple, loculated abscesses sometimes respond to antibiotics alone. Empiric antibiotics should be aimed at the most likely organism–Salmonella species being most common in patients with hemoglobinopathies, and *Streptococcal* and *Staphylococcal* species most common in post-traumatic infection.[30] Immunosuppressed patients with multiple negative blood cultures are most likely to have a fungal infection. The indication for splenectomy is failure to respond to percutaneous drainage and antimicrobial or antifungal therapy.[31]

Tumors

Splenic tumors are rare. Hemangiomas are the most common benign tumor of the spleen, and splenectomy is indicated for large, symptomatic or bleeding tumors.

Other benign tumors include adenomas, hamartomas, fibromas, and dermoids all of which rarely require surgical intervention once diagnosed.[32] Angiosarcoma and lymphoma represent the two primary malignant tumors of the spleen in children. Most patients have disseminated disease once detected, and often present to the emergency department in hemorrhagic shock secondary to spontaneous splenic rupture. Lymphomas represent the most common malignant lesions of the spleen. In children, non-Hodgkin's lymphoma involving the spleen usually represents metastatic disease. Splenectomy is not indicated in these patients. In Hodgkin's disease, chemotherapy is now used in all stages of the disease in order to reduce the dose of radiation therapy. For this reason, laparotomy/splenectomy staging is much less commonly indicated, even in cases where the spleen is directly infiltrated by tumor.

Cysts

Splenic cysts can be classified as either congenital, pseudocysts (without epithelial lining), and parasitic.[33] Epidermoid cysts are the most common congenital variety. Pseudocysts usually arise after abdominal trauma, and are believed to result from the resolution of a subcapsular or intraparenchymal splenic hematoma. Small pseudocysts do not require further treatment; however, larger expanding pseudocysts should be followed by ultrasound and may be resected with spleen-preserving procedures with good results. Parasitic splenic cysts are rare, but may be caused by *E. granulosus* (Hydatid) or *echinococcus*[34] (Fig. 96.1). Splenectomy (either total or partial) may be required for large parasitic cysts. Smaller cysts may be enucleated in order to preserve splenic function (Fig. 96.2).

TRAUMA

Non-operative management of splenic trauma is a concept that was first introduced by pediatric surgeons in the 1960's who recognized the potentially life-threatening consequences of postsplenectomy sepsis. Today, this principle is widely accepted, and operative intervention in the management of splenic trauma is reserved only in cases where persisting and uncontrolled hemorrhage from the injured spleen is suspected to be the cause of hemodynamic instability.

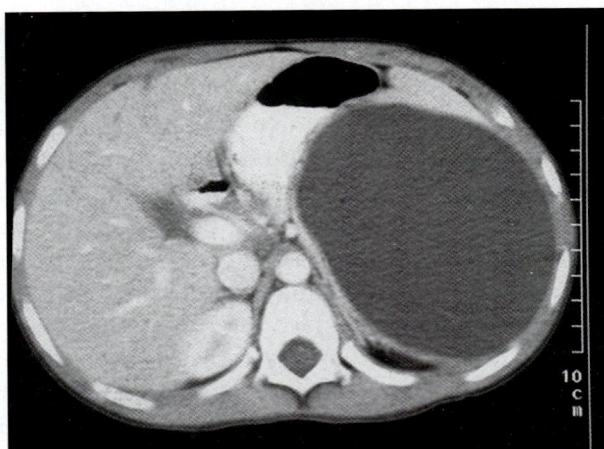

Fig. 96.1: CT Scan depicting a cyst in the spleen as a hypodense lesion *(courtesy: Dr Sandeep Agarwala, AIIMS)*

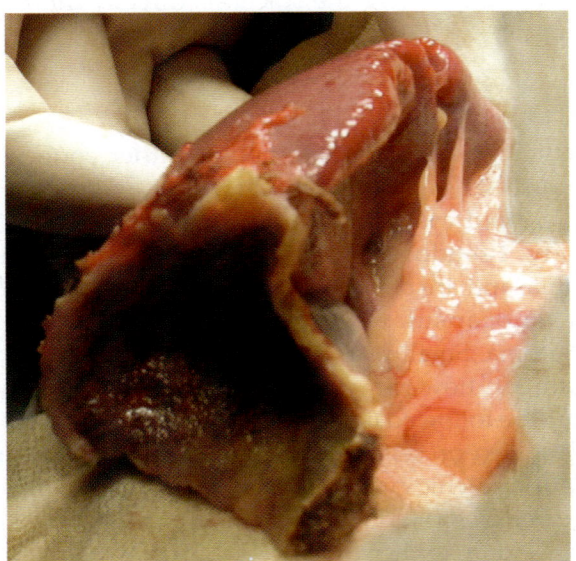

Fig. 96.2: Remaining pericyst after enucleated hydatid cyst of the spleen *(courtesy: Dr Sandeep Agarwala, AIIMS)*

that delayed secondary hemorrhage from the injured spleen is a very uncommon event, and such bleeding is almost always associated with a delay in diagnosis or an underlying pathologic condition such as a pseudoaneurysm of the splenic artery.[35] In addition, the incidence of associated hollow-viscus injury appears to correlate with the presence of hemodynamic instability, and not with the grade of splenic injury.[36]

Recently, the American Pediatric Surgical Association (APSA) Trauma Committee sought to define evidence-based guidelines for resource utilization in these patients.[37] A contemporary, multi-institution database of 832 children with isolated liver or spleen injuries was established and analyzed with the ultimate goal of standardizing treatment and promoting consensus among surgeons. Guidelines for intensive care unit (ICU) stay, length of hospital stay, use of pre- and postdischarge follow-up imaging, and length of physical activity restriction were proposed (Table 96.3).

In a follow-up study, these guidelines were prospectively applied to 312 patients at 32 pediatric trauma centers across North America.[38] The authors found that compared with the previously studied 832 patients, the 312 patients who had prospective application of the proposed guidelines had a significant reduction in ICU stay, hospital stay, follow-up imaging, and interval of physical activity restriction within each grade of splenic injury (Table 96.4). This study has led to the belief that safe early discharge from the hospital with fewer limitations on activity can be achieved in children who are hemodynamically stable regardless of the severity of injury to the spleen.

In cases when operation is unavoidable, partial splenectomy or a splenorrhaphy should be attempted if at all possible, particularly in younger children.

Despite the general agreement on a conservative, nonoperative approach, some disagreement exists on the acuity of care necessary for the child with an isolated injury to the spleen. Some pediatric surgeons have advocated the monitoring of children with moderate grade splenic injuries in the intensive care unit (ICU) in order to facilitate the early diagnosis of complications including delayed hemorrhage and associated hollow visceral injury. The validity of this approach has been questioned by others who believe

Table 96.3: Proposed guidelines for resource utilization in children with isolated spleen or liver injury[36]

CT Grade	I	II	III	IV
ICU Days	None	None	None	1 day
Hospital stay	2 days	3 days	4 days	5 days
Predischarge imaging	None	None	None	None
Postdischarge imaging	None	None	None	None
Activity restriction	3 weeks	4 weeks	5 weeks	6 weeks

Table 96.4: Impact of guidelines on resource utilization and activity restriction in children with isolated spleen or liver injury[37]

	Retrospective 1995-1997	Prospective 1998-2000	p-value
CT Grade I:			
Mean ICU stay (days)	0.93	0.12	< 0.0001
Mean hospital stay (days)	4.28	2.15	< 0.0001
Mean activity restriction (weeks)	5.05	3.77	< 0.04
Follow-up imaging (%)	34.4	7.3	< 0.001
CT Grade II:			
Mean ICU stay (days)	1.07	0.14	< 0.0001
Mean hospital stay (days)	5.25	2.73	< 0.0001
Mean activity restriction (weeks)	6.29	4.27	< 0.0001
Follow-up Imaging (%)	46.3	8.9	< 0.001
CT Grade III:			
Mean ICU stay (days)	1.62	0.38	< 0.0001
Mean hospital stay (days)	6.53	3.76	< 0.0001
Mean activity restriction (weeks)	7.58	5.71	< 0.0001
Follow-up Imaging (%)	54.1	10.9	< 0.001
CT Grade IV:			
Mean ICU stay (days)	2.02	1.02	< 0.0001
Mean hospital stay (days)	7.17	5.36	< 0.0006
Mean activity restriction (weeks)	9.42	6.98	< 0.004
Follow-up Imaging (%)	51.8	23.3	< 0.001

OPERATIVE TECHNIQUES

The technique used in splenectomy varies, largely depending on the diagnosis and the indications for the operation. The importance of splenic salvage has been emphasized, however, splenectomy continues to be the operation of choice for certain disorders. Laparoscopic techniques have gained popularity recently and have presented the surgeon with another option for the operative approach to this organ.

Open splenectomy is performed with the child in the supine position and the stomach decompressed with a nasogastric tube. The operation may be performed through either a midline incision or a left upper quadrant transverse incision extended to the flank. A midline incision is appropriate in cases where the operation is being performed for trauma or as part of a staging laparotomy for Hodgkin's disease. A thorough search for accessory spleens should be conducted during elective splenectomy in patients with hemolytic anemias to prevent recurrence of the disease postoperatively.

In cases of splenic trauma, all efforts should be taken to at least partially preserve the spleen. This can be accomplished more effectively after division of the lateral peritoneal reflection which allows for delivery of the spleen into the surgical wound where splenic repair and salvage can be attempted. Total splenectomy following trauma should only be performed in cases of extreme fragmentation, where the blood supply is entirely interrupted, or when the patient's hemodynamic status precludes an attempt at splenic salvage. Whether splenic fragment autotransplantation should be considered as an alternate therapy in this latter circumstance remains controversial.

In cases of marked splenomegaly, embolization of the splenic artery and its branches preoperatively can be utilized as a means to reduce the size of the organ, and make attempts at open or laparoscopic removal possible or at least safer.

POSTSPLENECTOMY SEPSIS

Postsplenectomy sepsis (also referred to as overwhelming postsplenectomy infection OPSI) is the most feared complication of splenectomy, particularly in children. Morris and Bullok[39] were the first to propose that splenectomy increases the risk of infection, and this proposal was later verified by King and Schuler in 1952 who documented the clinical relationship between splenectomy and infection.[2] The risk of infection is significantly higher in patients undergoing splenectomy for a hematologic disorder.[40] Specifically, the incidence of overwhelming postsplenectomy infection approaches 15% in children with thalassemia compared to 1-2% in patients undergoing splenectomy after trauma. Considering all patients undergoing splenectomy, the incidence of overwhelming infection is approximately 4%, and carries a 50% mortality.[41] Typically, the infections are caused by encapsulated organisms, including *Pneumococci, Hemophilus influenzae B, Gonococci,* and *Escherichia coli.*[42] The predominance of infections with encapsulated organisms is attributed to the spleen being the major site of antibody production against these bacteria. For this reason, total splenectomy should be avoided when possible, especially in children younger than two years of age due to the high incidence of postsplenectomy sepsis in this group. In cases where elective surgery is indicted, polyvalent *Pneumococcal* and *H influenza B* vaccines should be administered preoperatively. The most effective way to prevent infection is to administer the vaccine 2 to 4 weeks before operation. In all patients, postoperative antibiotics should be administered prophylactically. Penicillin is the most widely prescribed antibiotic for prophylaxis against overwhelming postsplenectomy sepsis. The appropriate duration of prophylactic antibiotic therapy is controversial and ranges between two years and a lifetime. The risk of developing postsplenectomy infection decreases significantly two years after the operation. Education of patients and families about early recognition of postsplenectomy infection is vitally important. A patient who has undergone a splenectomy should be examined by a physician at the onset of any febrile illness. In cases where postsplenectomy sepsis is suspected, the early and liberal use of intravenous antibiotics and supportive treatment are essential for a good outcome.

REFERENCES

1. Virchow R. Weisses Blut und Milztumoren. Med Zeitung 1846;5:157.
2. King H, Shumacker H. Susceptibility to infection after splenectomy performed in infancy. Ann Surg 1952; 136: 239.
3. Fleischmajer R. Epithelial-mesenchymal interactions. Science 1967;157(795):1472-82.
4. Tavassoli M. Embryonic and fetal hemopoiesis: An overview. Blood Cells 1991;17(2):269-81.
5. Skandalakis PN, et al. The surgical anatomy of the spleen. Surg Clin North Am 1993;73(4):747-68.
6. Groom AC, Schmidt EE, MacDonald IC. Microcirculatory pathways and blood flow in spleen: new insights from washout kinetics, corrosion casts, and quantitative intravital videomicroscopy. Scanning Microsc 1991;5(1): 159-73; discussion 173-74.
7. Herman PG. Microcirculation of organized lymphoid tissues. Monogr Allergy 1980;16:126-42.
8. Phoon CK, Neill CA. Asplenia syndrome: insight into embryology through an analysis of cardiac and extracardiac anomalies. Am J Cardiol 1994;73(8):581-87.
9. Freedom RM. The asplenia syndrome: a review of significant extracardiac structural abnormalities in 29 necropsied patients. J Pediatr 1972;81(6):1130-33.
10. Sty JR, Conway JJ. The spleen: development and functional evaluation. Semin Nucl Med 1985;15(3):276-98.
11. Balaji KC, et al. Splenogonadal fusion. J Urol 1996;156(2 Pt 2):854-56.
12. Rodkey ML, Macknin ML. Pediatric wandering spleen: case report and review of literature. Clin Pediatr (Phila) 1992;31(5):289-94.
13. Gayer G, et al. CT findings in congenital anomalies of the spleen. Br J Radiol 2001;74(884):767-72.
14. Peitgen K, Schweden K. Management of intermittent splenic torsion ("wandering spleen"): a review. Eur J Surg 1995;161(1):49-52.
15. Baccarani U, et al. Splenectomy in hematology. Current practice and new perspectives. Haematologica 1999;84(5): 431-36.
16. Coetzee T. Clinical anatomy and physiology of the spleen. S Afr Med J 1982;61(20):737-46.
17. Lockwood CM. Immunological functions of the spleen. Clin Haematol 1983;12(2):449-65.
18. Najjar VA. Tuftsin, a natural activator of phagocyte cells: an overview. Ann NY Acad Sci 1983;419:1-11.
19. Foster PN, Losowsky MS. Hyposplenism-a review. JR Coll Physicians Lond 1987;21(3):188-91.
20. Bridgen ML. Detection, education and management of the asplenic or hyposplenic patient. Am Fam Physician 2001;63(3):499-506, 508.
21. Peck-Radosavljevic M. Hypersplenism. Eur J Gastroenterol Hepatol 2001;13(4):317-23.
22. Tse WT, Lux SE. Red blood cell membrane disorders. Br J Haematol 1999;104(1):2-13.
23. Lonergan GJ, Cline DB, Abbondanzo SL. Sickle cell anemia. Radiographics 2001;21(4):971-94.
24. Samuels-Reid JH. Common problems in sickle cell disease. Am Fam Physician 1994;49(6):1477-80, 1483-86.
25. Hendricks-Ferguson VL, Nelson MA. Laparoscopic splenectomy for splenic sequestration crisis. Aorn J 2000;71(4):820-22, 825-28, 831-34; quiz 835-42.
26. Idowu O, Hayes-Jordan A. Partial splenectomy in children under 4 years of age with hemoglobinopathy. J Pediatr Surg 1998;33(8):1251-53.

27. Karpatkin S. Autoimmune (idiopathic) thrombocytopenic purpura. Lancet 1997;349(9064):1531-36.
28. Blanchette V, Freedman J, Garvey B. Management of chronic immune thrombocytopenic purpura in children and adults. Semin Hematol 1998;35(1 Suppl 1):36-51.
29. Losanoff JE, Kjossev KT. Re: Splenic abscess: report of six cases and review of the literature. Am Surg 2001;67(10):1014-15.
30. Ooi LL, Leong SS. Splenic abscesses from 1987 to 1995. Am J Surg 1997;174(1):87-93.
31. Arregui ME, Barteau J, Davis CJ. Laparoscopic splenectomy: techniques and indications. Int Surg 1994;79(4):335-41.
32. Hayes TC, et al. Symptomatic splenic hamartoma: case report and literature review. Pediatrics 1998;101(5):E10.
33. Urrutia M, et al. Cystic masses of the spleen: radiologic-pathologic correlation. Radiographics 1996;16(1):107-29.
34. Agarwala S, Bhatnagar V, Mitra DK, Gupta AK, Berry M. Primary tubercular abscess of the spleen. J Pediatr Surg 1992;27:1580-81.
35. Nagar H, Kessler A, Weiss J. Traumatic intraparenchymal splenic pseudoaneurysms in a child: nonoperative management. J Trauma 1997;43(3):552-55.
36. Nance ML, Keller MS, Stafford PW. Predicting hollow visceral injury in the pediatric blunt trauma patient with solid visceral injury. J Pediatr Surg 2000;35(9):1300-03.
37. Stylianos S. Evidence-based guidelines for resource utilization in children with isolated spleen or liver injury. The APSA Trauma Committee. J Pediatr Surg 2000;35:164-67; discussion 167-69.
38. Stylianos S. Compliance with evidence-based guidelines in children with isolated spleen or liver injury: a prospective study. J Pediatr Surg 2002;37:453-56. Comment in: Can J Surg 2004;47(6):458-60
39. Morris. The importance of the spleen in resistance to infection. Ann Surg 1919;70:513-17.
40. Bisharat N, et al. Risk of infection and death among post-splenectomy patients. J Infect 2001;43(3):182-86.
41. Altamura M, et al. Splenectomy and sepsis: the role of the spleen in the immune-mediated bacterial clearance. Immunopharmacol Immunotoxicol 2001;23(2):153-61.
42. Davidson RN, Wall RA. Prevention and management of infections in patients without a spleen. Clin Microbiol Infect 2001;7(12):657-60.

SECTION 6

Vascular Disorders

Hemangiomas

Richard G Azizkhan

Hemangiomas of infancy are the most common vascular tumors of childhood. They affect 1 in 10 Caucasian infants in North America and are less commonly seen in children of African or Asian descent.[1] Although review of the English-language literature published over the past four decades shows no population-based studies that specifically address hemangioma incidence in the Indian subcontinent, my personal experience in visiting medical centers throughout India indicates that these lesions commonly occur.

Hemangiomas of infancy usually present cutaneously in the cervicofacial region (60%), and may appear as focal, segmental, solitary or multiple lesions. They can also involve any anatomic site and may affect the extremities, thoracoabdominal walls and cavities, solid organs, hollow viscera, and brain.[2] Lesions undergo a phase of proliferation and subsequent gradual spontaneous regression. In light of this natural history, many smaller uncomplicated hemangiomas are best left untreated. Less common, lesions can cause function- or life-threatening complications or serious aesthetic concerns, having a serious impact on a child's quality of life. This chapter presents an overview of hemangiomas, describing recent insights into pathogenesis, complex clinical presentations, diagnostic approaches, and treatment strategies. I have prefaced my discussion with a concise nosologic summary of vascular anomalies.

NOSOLOGY OF VASCULAR ANOMALIES

In 1996, a consensus resolution of the International Society for the Study of Vascular Anomalies (ISSVA) designated a classification system of vascular lesions that is currently used worldwide by most experts in the field. Based on the pioneering work of Mulliken and Glowacki, this system comprises two categories of lesions—vascular tumors and vascular malformations (Table 97.1).[3] Within the category of vascular tumors, there are a number of distinct lesions, including hemangioma, kaposiform hemangioendothelioma (KHE), tufted angioma, pyogenic granuloma, and hemangiopericytoma.

Hemangiomas are the most common vascular tumor. They are typically observed at birth or during the first several weeks of life. They undergo an active period of growth characterized by endothelial proliferation and hypercellularity and a subsequent involutive phase that occurs over several years (Fig. 97.1A to D). In contrast, vascular malformations are structural anomalies believed to be caused by errors in vascular or lymphatic morphogenesis. They are subdivided according to their predominant channel type as capillary, venous, lymphatic, arterial, or combined lesions. Unlike hemangiomas, vascular malformations have normal levels of endothelial turnover, are present at birth, never involute, and grow commensurate with the child.

Despite the valiant efforts of the ISSVA to standardize the classification and nomenclature of vascular anomalies, the literature remains replete with outdated terminology that continues to hamper communication among specialists and often results in inappropriate management. Particularly important for clinicians to note, the term "hemangioma" is often misused to label a spectrum of vascular lesions with varying etiologies and natural histories. More specifically, lesions with large blood-filled spaces are sometimes incorrectly termed 'cavernous hemangiomas'; such lesions are generally venous or lymphaticovenous malformations.

Table 97.1: Distinguishing features of hemangioma of infancy and vascular malformations*

Hemangiomas	Vascular Malformations
Neoplasm	Congenital abnormality
30% visible at birth, seen as red macule; 70% become apparent during first few weeks of life	Present at birth, but may not be evident until months or even years later
Females more commonly affected (gender ratio of 3:1)	No gender predilection
Rapid postnatal growth followed by slow involution	Slow steady growth, with no involution; may expand secondary to sepsis, trauma, or hormonal changes
Endothelial cell hyperplasia	Normal endothelial cell turnover
Increased mast cells	Normal mast cell count
Multilaminated basement membrane	Normal thin basement membrane
No coagulation defects	Primary stasis (venous); localized consumptive coagulopathy
Angiographic findings: well-circumscribed, intense lobular-parenchymal staining with equatorial vessels	Angiographic findings: diffuse, no parenchyma Low-flow: phleboliths, ectatic channels High-flow: enlarged, tortuous arteries with arteriovenous shunting
Infrequent "mass effect" on adjacent bone; hypertrophy rare	Low-flow: distortion, hypertrophy, or hypoplasia High-flow: bone destruction, distortion, or hypertrophy
30% respond dramatically to corticosteroid treatment in 2 to 3 weeks	No response to corticosteroids or antiangiogenic agents
Immunopositive for biologic markers GLUT1, Fcγ RII, merosin, and Lewis Y antigen.	Immunonegative for these biologic markers

*Modified from RG Azizkhan. Vascular Lesions of Childhood, in Baker RJ, Fischer JE (Eds): Mastery of Surgery, Philadelphia, PA, Lippincott Williams & Wilkins;28. 2001

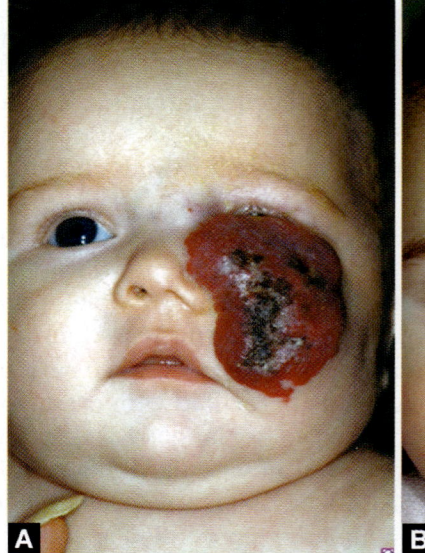
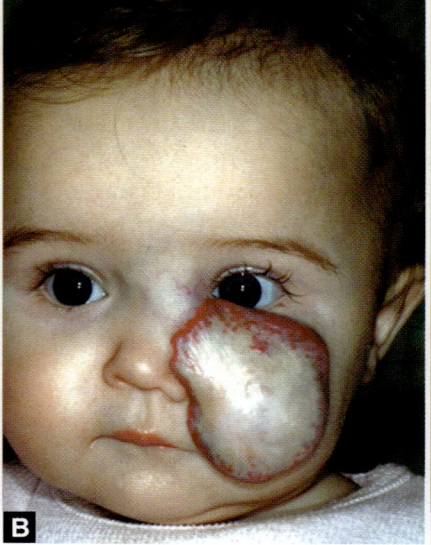
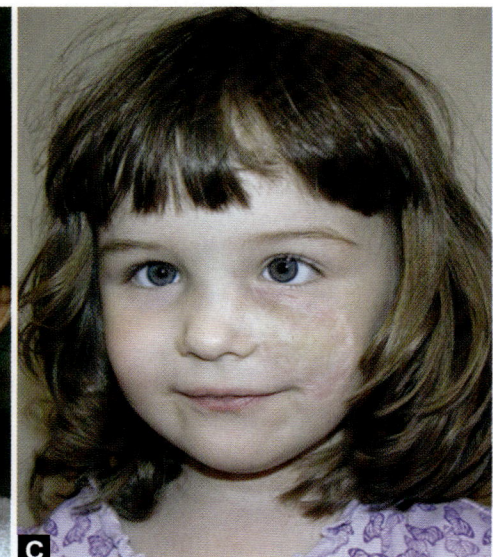

Figs 97.1A to D: Infantile hemangioma through several stages.
A. Early proliferative, **B.** Age 5 months, early involution and **C.** Late involution

HEMANGIOMAS OF INFANCY

Pathogenesis

Hemangiomas of infancy are benign vascular lesions that expand rapidly during infancy and gradually involute during childhood; tumor involution can last for up to 5 to 10 years. Expanding hemangiomas of infancy are composed of proliferating endothelial cells and large numbers of pericytes, mast cells, and fibroblasts.[4,5] As lesions spontaneously involute, apoptosis of endothelial cells increases and fibrofatty tissue gradually replaces the vascular network.

Although the molecular pathogenesis of hemangioma of infancy is largely unknown, over the past several years new insights have been gleaned from basic and translational research. Numerous investigations have focused on possible molecular factors that control the natural course of hemangiomas, and various cellular markers that distinguish the phases of hemangioma growth and regression have been identified. Studies of the cellular and molecular factors involved in lesion expansion indicate that endothelial progenitor cells are present predominantly in proliferating hemangiomas.[6] Endothelial progenitor cells coexpress the endothelial cell marker KDR and CD133-2, a stem cell-progenitor cell marker. Such findings demonstrate that endothelial progenitor cells comprise a cell population that plays a role in hemangioma expansion.[6] Studies with isolated hemangioma endothelial cells (EC) and whole lesions indicate that hemangiomas probably arise from uncontrolled clonal expansion of EC.[7,8] Both abnormal local cellular signals and somatic mutation in EC and/or pericytes have been proposed as triggers for EC proliferation.[8,9]

Proliferating hemangiomas have been shown to have increased expression of type IV collagenase, vascular endothelial growth factor (VEGF), and basic fibroblast growth factor.[10,11] In involuting hemangiomas, the high expression of basic fibroblast growth factor persists, while the level of expression of VEGF substantially diminishes. Also, as compared to proliferating lesions, involuting lesions show increased expression of apoptosis-associated proteins.[12] Gene-expression analysis comparing proliferating vs involuting has revealed that insulin-like growth factor 2 (IGF-2) is highly expressed during proliferation, but is substantially decreased during involution.[13]

Analysis of messenger RNA expression patterns of genes required for angiogenesis in hemangioma tissues and in hemangioma-derived EC reveal strong expression of the VEGF receptor family and the angiopoietin-Tie family (Tie-1, Tie-1, and angiopoietin 2), Tie-2 in particular, is increased in hemangioma tissues and hemangioma EC compared to normal EC, suggesting that the angiopoietin-Tie-2 system is a molecular regulator of hemangioma of infancy.[14]

Results of a number of studies aimed at determining possible mechanisms of hemangioma involution indicate that an immune-mediated process is involved.[15-18] DNA microarray analysis has identified indoleamine 2,3-dioxygenase as a potential modulator of the immune response in hemangiomas.[16] Indoleamine 2,3-dioxygenase messenger RNA is present in high levels in proliferating hemangiomas and decreases significantly during involution.

There is compelling evidence that infantile hemangioma derives from placental EC. North and colleagues have identified four markers of hemangioma vessels that are coexpressed in placental vessels; these EC markers include GLUT1 (a glucose transporter enzyme), merosin, Lewis Y antigen, and FCy-RIIb.[19,20] GLUT1 is strongly expressed in infantile hemangiomas, placentas, and the blood-brain barrier though not in normal surrounding vascular endothelium and not in vascular malformations (Table 97.2A and B). Other authors have reported hemangioma and placental vessel coexpression of type III iodothyronine deiodinase, indoleamine 2,3-deoxygenase, and IGF2.[13,15,21] With the exception of the central nervous system, no other tissue jointly expresses these markers. These studies raise the possibility that vascular precursor cells (angioblasts) aberrantly differentiate toward the placental vascular phenotype at sites of hemangioma development in the fetus.[22] An alternative possibility is that placental EC embolize into the fetal vascular system, becoming a source of hemangioma where they lodge and implant.[20] Corroborating evidence for a placental origin of hemangiomas is the 3-fold higher incidence of hemangiomas in infants born after transcervical chorionic villus sampling, which may cause placental injury and intravascular shedding of placental cells.[23] Data derived from a recent study using molecular profiling indicated a common genetic program between placental and hemangioma endothelium, further supporting the idea of a placental origin of

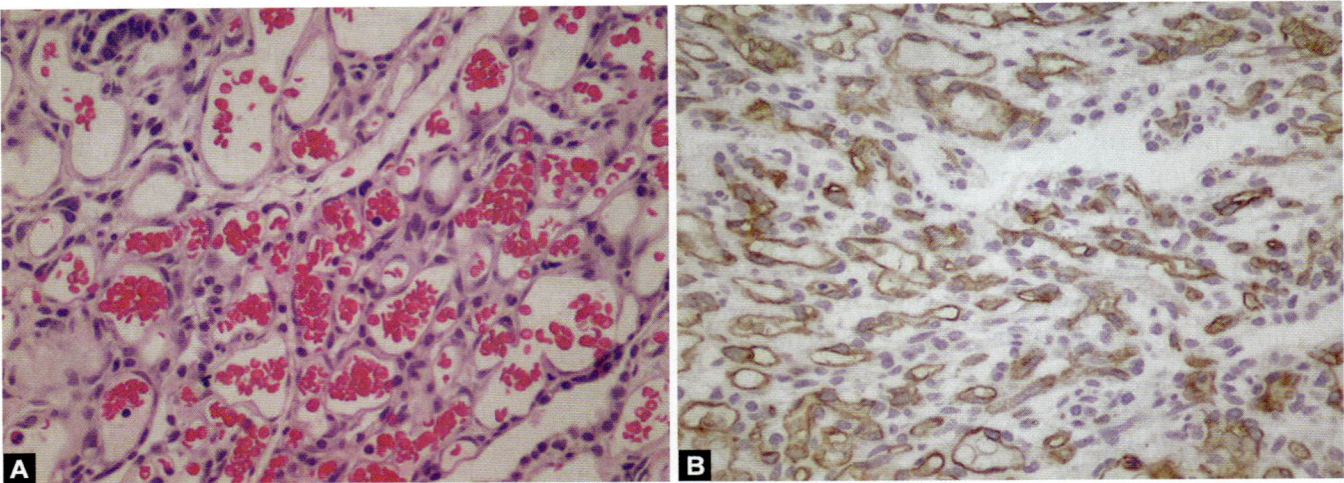

Figs 97.2A and B: A. Hematoxylin and eosin stained histological section of an infantile hemangioma
B. GLUT-1 staining (brown) of endothelial cells in an infantile hemangioma

hemangioma.[24] The positive expression of GLUT1 persists throughout the hemangioma life cycle, making this histochemical marker a valuable tool in distinguishing hemangiomas from other vascular tumors and from vascular malformations.

Dadras et al have shown that lymphatic endothelial hyaluronan receptor-1 (LYVE-1), a marker for both normal and tumor-associated lymphatic vessels, is strongly expressed in proliferating hemangiomas but absent in involuted lesions.[25] These authors propose that vessels from hemangiomas of infancy are arrested at an early developmental stage of vascular differentiation.

Presentation

Most hemangiomas of infancy present singularly. About one third of tumors are observed at birth, appearing as erythematous macules, some with a pale halo or a telangiectatic path. Most lesions, however, become evident during the first several weeks of life. Based on anatomic depth, lesions are categorized as superficial (50 to 60%), deep (15%), or combined (25 to 35%), with each of these categories showing a characteristic appearance. Superficial lesions are usually soft, red, and raised and only rarely telangiectatic. Deep lesions, which are sometimes difficult to distinguish from venous or lymphatic malformations, may show a spectrum of appearances and consistencies, ranging from soft and supple to raised and firmer warm masses that are bluish in color. Combined lesions appear as red dermal tumors with epidermal and dermal components, along with a subcutaneous mass that is either blue or flesh colored.

The proliferative phase of these tumors begins in the first few weeks of life and continues for 4 to 10 months. During this time lesions rapidly expand and the superficial component becomes more erythematous or violaceous. The proliferative phase of deep hemangiomas is typically longer, lasting for up to 2 years. Following this phase, the growth rate of lesions stabilizes and lesions grow in proportion to the child. This quiescent period is followed by an involuting phase during which hemangiomas become gray in color. This phase varies in duration, sometimes lasting as long as 5 to 6 years (Figs 97.3A and B). Maximum involution occurs in approximately 50% of children by age 5 years and in 90% of children by age 9 years.[26-28] In most patients, tumor regression results in restoration of normal skin; however, 20 to 40% of patients exhibit residual skin changes such as laxity, discoloration, telangiectasia, fibrofatty masses or scarring.

Ulceration

The most common complication of proliferating hemangiomas is ulceration (Figs 97.4A to E). This complication occurs in 10-15% of superficial lesions and usually leaves behind some degree of scarring.

Ulcerations can become infected and are often quite painful. In rare instances, they can lead to non-fatal hemorrhage. Lesions in perioral and perineal locations are especially prone to ulceration, with factors such as recurrent friction and moisture playing a role. Ulceration can significantly distort or even destroy a facial feature such as the eyelid, nose, ear, or lip.

PATTERNS OF PRESENTATION AND PROBLEMATIC ANATOMIC LOCATIONS

Hemangiomas that occur in developmental segments are termed "segmental" lesions. These lesions are less common than localized lesions and have a higher risk of being life or function threatening and of having associated structural anomalies. Large cervicofacial segmental lesions, especially those on the forehead, temple, upper cheek and around the periorbital area can be accompanied by a constellation of anomalies

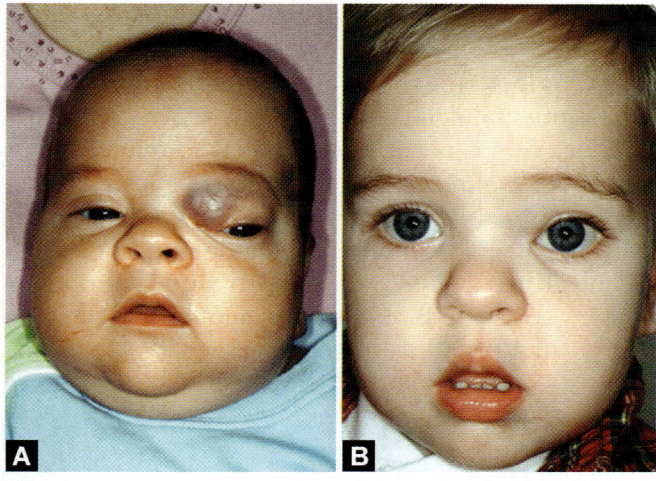

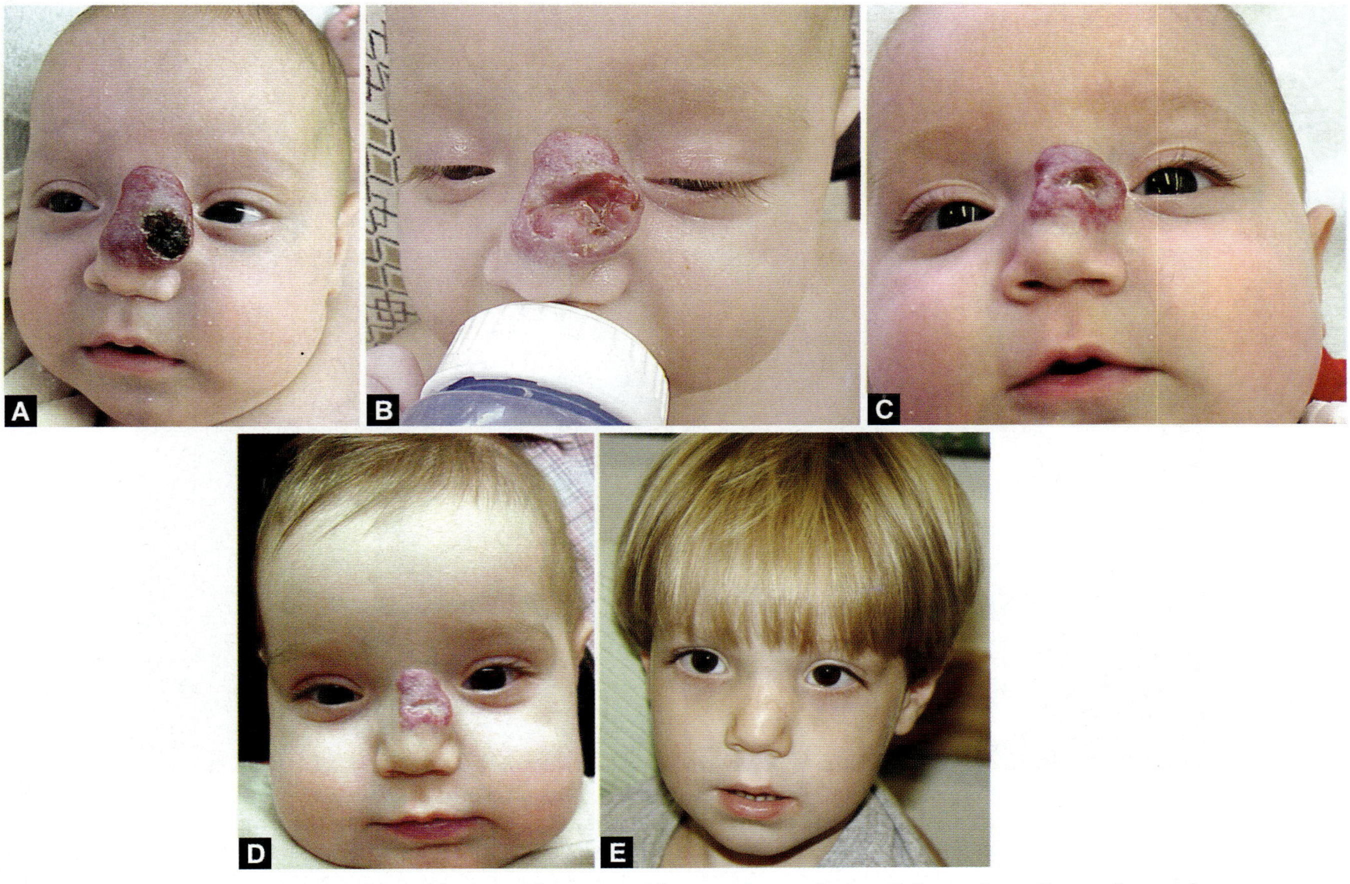

Figs 97.3A and B: A. Periorbital hemangioma in a 3 months old infant. **B.** Same child at age 4 with lesion almost completely involuted

Figs 97.4A to E: Infant with a significant nasal hemangioma. **A.** Age 2.5 months with crusting and ulceration starting. **B-D.** Healing of ulcer with partial involution over 18 months. **E.** Complete involution by age 3

that is referred to PHACES association.[29,30] This association is characterized by a group of anomalies, including posterior fossa brain malformations (e.g., Dandy-Walker malformation), hemangiomas that are typically plaque-like and segmental in the cervicofacial area, arterial abnormalities (especially of arteries supplying the face and central nervous system), cardiac and aortic arch defects (e.g. coarctation, aneurysms, and congenital valvular aortic stenosis), eye anomalies (e.g. optic atrophy, congenital cataracts, and retinal vascular abnormalities), and sternal clefts or supraumbilical raphes (Fig. 97.5A to E). More than 50% of these patients are affected by various neurologic sequelae, including seizures, stroke, developmental delay, and migraines.[31] When there is an index of suspicion, it is prudent to refer patients for an ophthalmologic examination, screening echocardiogram, and either magnetic resonance imaging (MRI) or magnetic resonance angiography (MRA). If a central nervous system abnormality is found on imaging, patients should undergo follow-up imaging every 3 months until 18 months of age.

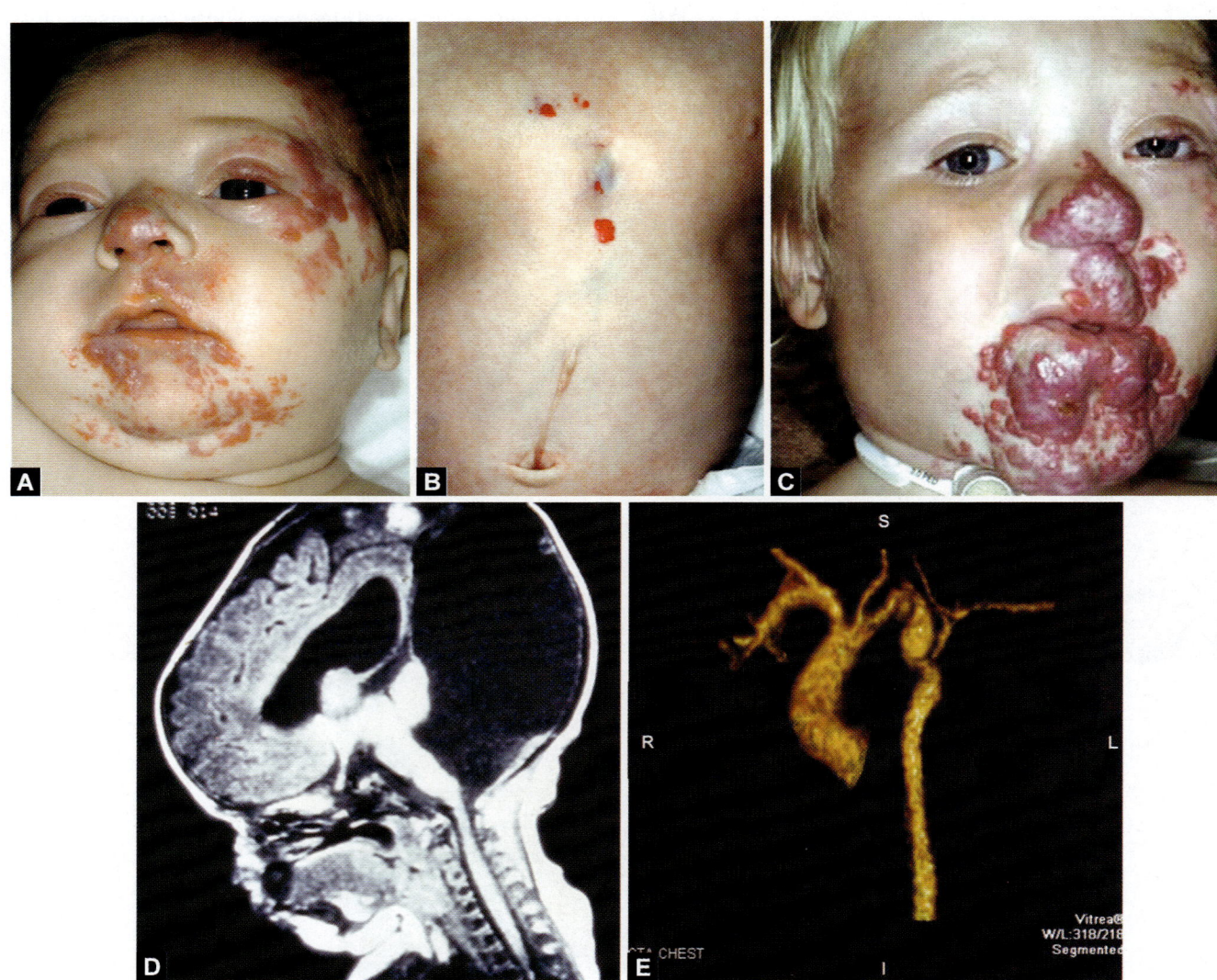

Figs 97.5A to E: Infant with PHACES association. **A.** At 4 weeks of age had subglottic airway involvement and obstruction. She required a tracheostomy and was treated aggressively with steroids. **B.** Supraumbilical median raphe and sternal cleft. **C.** Patient at 14 months; When patient was weaned of steroids, the lesions continued to grow. Weekly vincristine therapy was required to stabilize lesions. **D.** Posterior fossa Dandy-Walker cyst in a child with PHACES association. **E.** MRI 3 dimensional reconstruction of aortic arch coarctation of the in a child with PHACES association

In that 65% of patients with lesions that cover a beard distribution (i.e. the chin, jawline, and preauricular areas) have associated airway involvement, such patients should be closely followed and treatment should be initiated if airway involvement is suspected.[32]

Periocular and Orbital Hemangiomas

Periocular hemangiomas can involve the upper lid, lower lid, and or retrobulbar space; amblyopia is reported in 40-60% of cases.[33] Because of pressure from the hemangioma on the globe, astigmatism often occurs. Strabismic amblyopia occurs when a hemangioma affects the movement of extraocular muscles. Deprivation amblyopia occurs when there is partial or complete eyelid closure. When this occurs in the first few months of life, it can cause profound visual impairment. Periorbital hemangiomas that impair vision or create pressure on the globe require immediate treatment (Figs 97.6A to D). This may include medical approaches such as topical high-potency steroids, intralesional steroids, systemic steroids, or surgical resection. Ophthalmologic care such as patching the contralateral eye and monitoring the need for corrective lenses is imperative.

Tip of Nose, Lip and Ear Hemangiomas

Proliferation of hemangiomas on the tip of the nose can distort normal anatomy and cause splaying of the

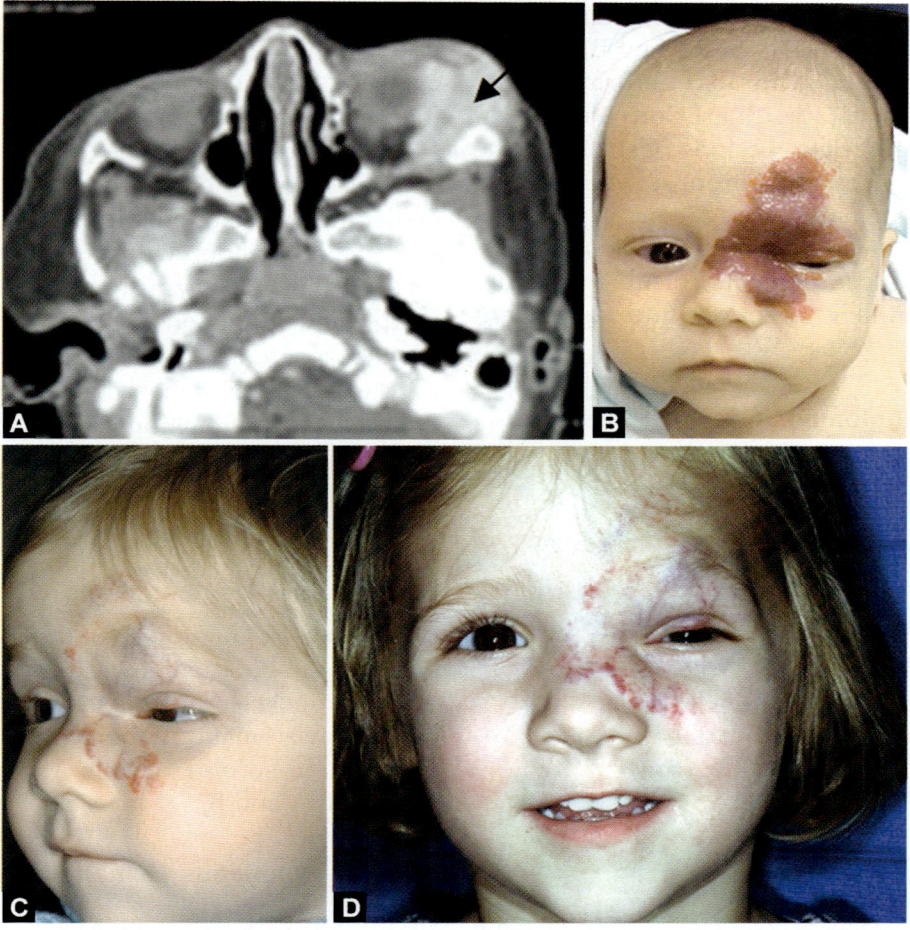

Figs 97.6A to D: A. Periorbital hemangioma with retro-orbital involvement as seen on CT scan. **B.** At 6 weeks patient was started on oral prednisolone and vision was preserved. Steroids were weaned off by 8 months of age **C.** At 18 months residual hemangioma can be seen. **D.** At 4.5 years of age slight left upper eyelid ptosis persists. This patient will have LASER treatment for residual surface lesions and an upper eyelid procedure to reduce ptosis

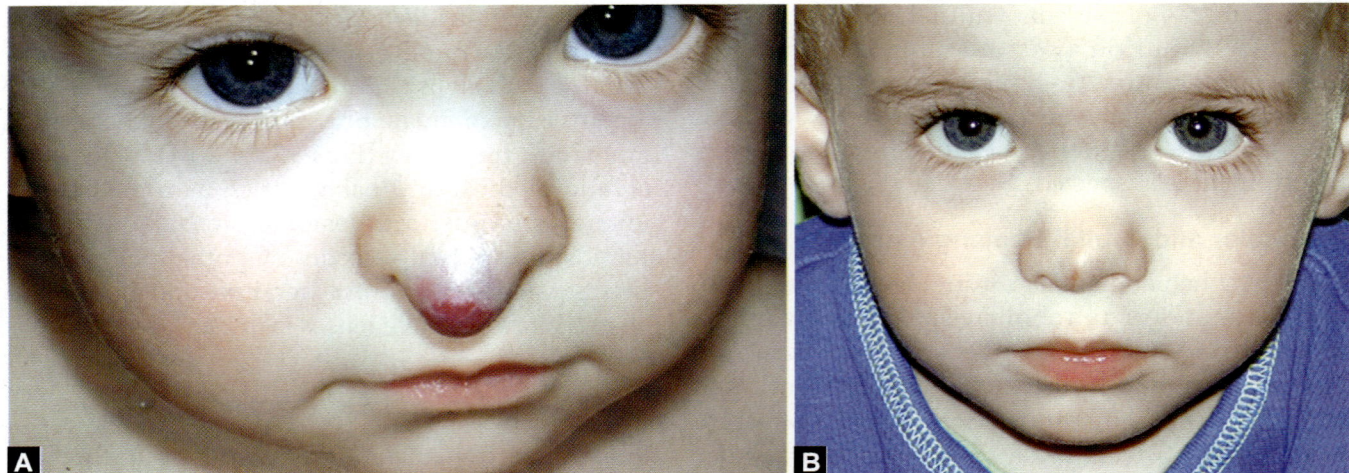

Figs 97.7A and B: A. Nasal tip hemangioma **B.** Post-resection at 20 months

nasal cartilage, resulting in what is referred to as "Cyrano nose" deformity (Figs 97.7A and B). Lesions on the pinna of the ear can also deform normal structures and result in ulceration with focal destruction of the auricle. Lesions obstructing the auditory canal can cause temporary conductive hearing loss. Lip hemangiomas frequently regress quite slowly, sometimes leaving residual skin changes. Additionally, lip ulcerations can result in feeding difficulties, secondary infection, and significant scarring (Fig. 97.8).

Subglottic Hemangiomas

Hemangiomas can occur anywhere within the tracheobronchial tree, however, they are most commonly seen in the subglottis. More than 50% of patients with subglottic hemangiomas also have cutaneous hemangiomas, which provide an indication for the presence of subglottic lesions.[34] Female infants are twice as likely to be affected as males. Most patients present during the first six months of life, and the earlier the presentation, the higher the likelihood that surgical intervention will be required.

Characteristic symptoms include progressive stridor and retractions. Diagnosis is made on rigid bronchoscopy, and though radiological evaluation (MRI with contrast enhancement) is indicated, it rarely demonstrates extension of the lesion beyond the confines of the subglottis. Lesions are typically asymmetric and usually covered by a normal smooth mucosa (Figs 97.9A and B).[34]

Lumbosacral Hemangiomas

Lumbosacral lesions can be associated with underlying spinal cord abnormalities (e.g., tethered spinal cord, lipomeningocele, and diastematomyelia) and with genitourinary malformations, including imperforate anus, recto-scrotal fistula, and renal anomalies (Figs 97.10A and B).

Multiple Cutaneous Hemangiomas

Up to 20% of affected infants have multiple cutaneous lesions, and such lesions increase the risk of visceral hemangiomas. The term "disseminated neonatal hemangiomatosis" is used to describe the uncommon

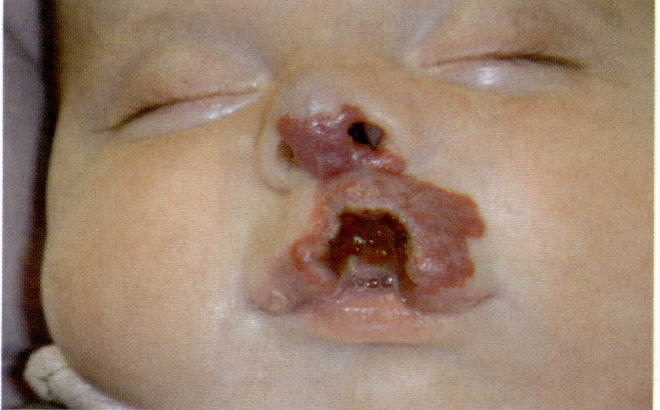

Fig. 97.8: Severe ulceration of upper lip hemangioma. This child will require reconstructive surgery when the lesion starts to involute

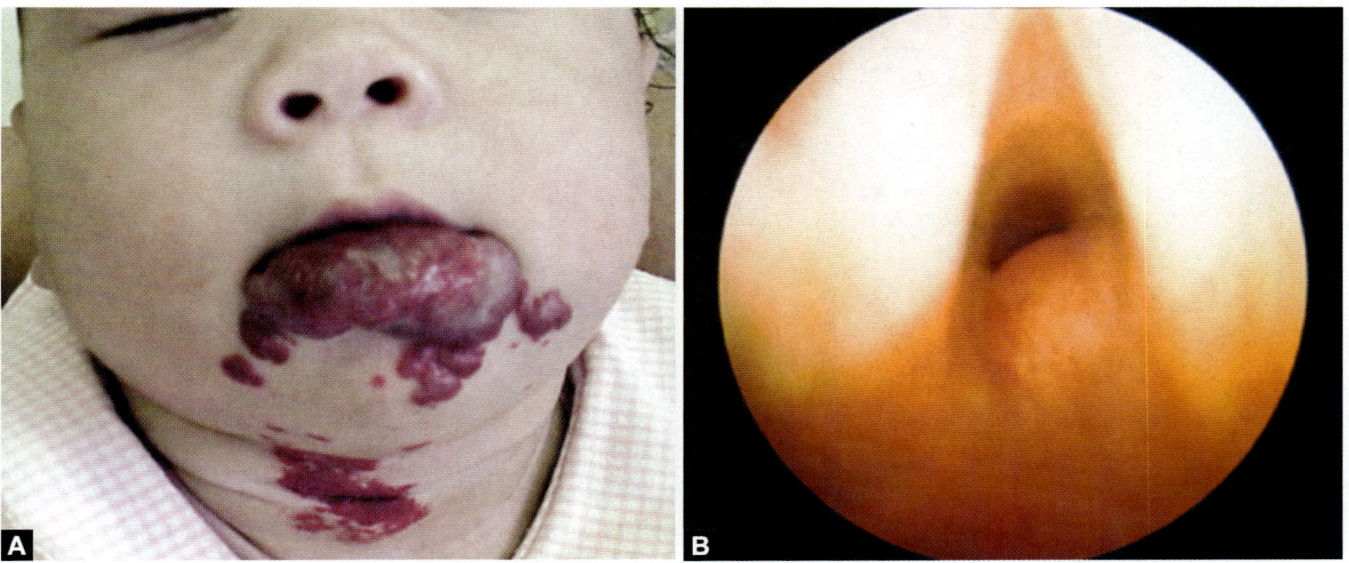

Figs 97.9A and B: A. Hemangioma in a "bearded distribution associated with a subglottic hemangioma. **B.** Direct laryngoscopy demonstrating subglottic involvement

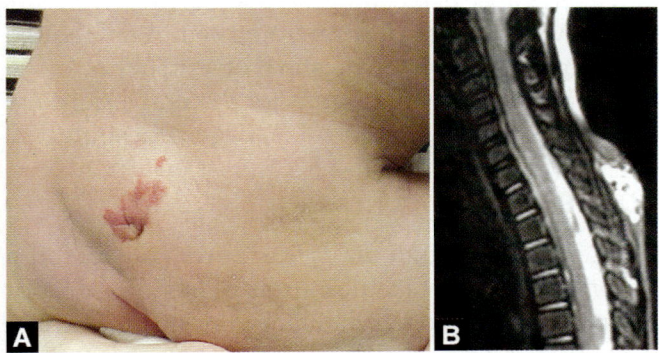

Figs 97.10A and B: A. Infantile hemangioma in the sacral region. **B.** MRI of the spine in a patient with a midline hemangioma. This study did not demonstrate any spinal anomalies

presentation of several to hundreds of small, multifocal cutaneous hemangiomas with associated visceral hemangiomas (Fig. 97.11). Most children have numerous hemangiomas, though no specific number of lesions must be present for systemic involvement to occur.

Visceral Hemangiomas

Symptomatic hemangiomas of the viscera are extremely uncommon. Lesions can occur anywhere in the gastrointestinal tract, though the liver is the most

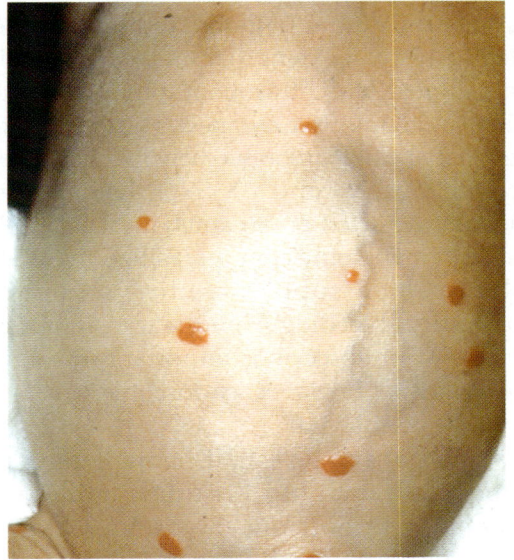

Fig. 97.11: Multiple hemangiomas in a neonate with hepatic hemangiomas

common visceral site. As mentioned above, the presence of multifocal cutaneous hemangiomas increases the likelihood of visceral lesions. Important to note, however, visceral lesions can exist without cutaneous involvement.

Hepatic hemangiomas follow a natural history similar to that of cutaneous lesions. Hepatomegaly, anemia, and high-output cardiac failure may be

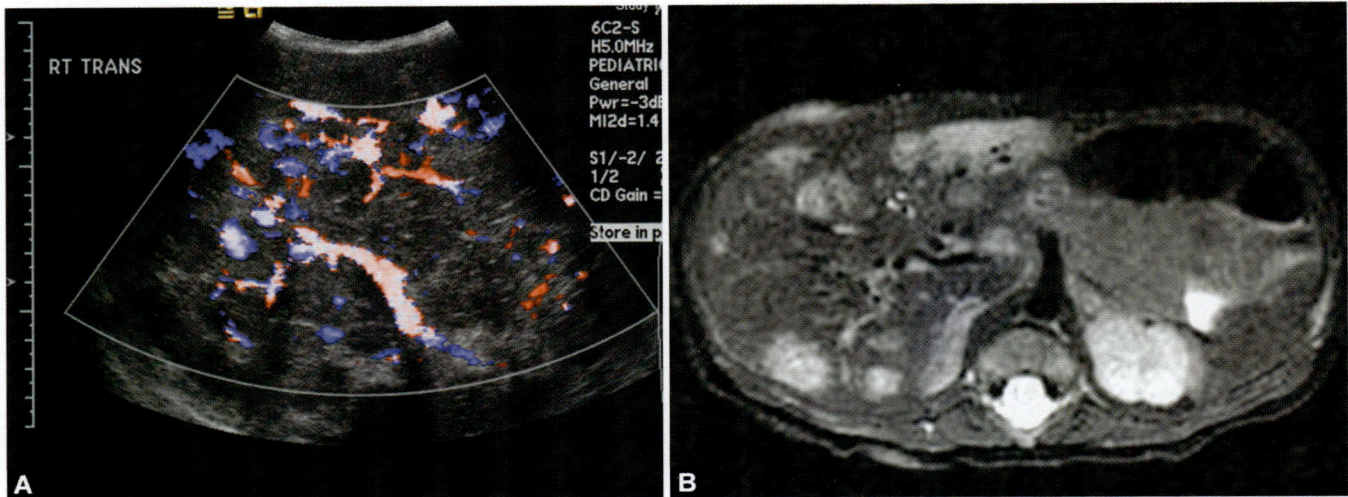

Figs 97.12A and B: A. Doppler US of the liver demonstrating high flow through multiple hepatic hemangiomas
B. MRI (T2 weighted image) demonstrating the multiple hepatic hemangiomas

present.[35] In severely affected patients, an abdominal compartment syndrome may arise from massive liver enlargement. In these patients, the diaphragms are elevated to such an extent that unassisted ventilation becomes impossible. Ultrasonography (US) of the liver in patients with multiple cutaneous lesions sometimes detects a hepatic hemangioma early in the proliferative phase (Fig. 97.12A and B). Such lesions are also occasionally detected on an antenatal US.[36,37] Rarely, a hepatic hemangioma may parasitize the duodenal or colonic blood supply, leading to significant gastrointestinal bleeding from the transmural tumor. In such cases, endoscopy is important in confirming the bleeding site; however, endoscopic hemostasis is unlikely to be achieved.

In some patients, a small hemangioma that is detected on imaging studies may remain asymptomatic throughout the proliferative phase, requiring no particular intervention. Such lesions warrant clinical vigilance and sequential US studies, with treatment reserved for patients in whom symptoms are apparent.

Hemangiomas of the stomach, small intestine, and colon are rare. As with liver lesions, they are often associated with multifocal cutaneous hemangiomas and become evident only when symptomatic. Mild to life-threatening gastrointestinal bleeding may occur, necessitating repeated blood transfusions. Since an intestinal hemangioma rarely bleeds after the proliferative phase has ended, such a lesion would not be a likely cause of bleeding beyond the first two years of life. Another possible presenting symptom, though less commonly seen, is intestinal obstruction.

Detailed treatment options for visceral lesions are presented in my discussion of management strategies.

CONGENITAL HEMANGIOMA

Congenital hemangioma is currently considered a distinct type of vascular tumor. Lesions do not resemble hemangiomas of infancy nor do they exhibit the same clinical behavior. In contrast to hemangiomas of infancy, congenital hemangiomas are fully 3-dimensional at birth. Lesions fall into two major subgroups: rapidly involuting congenital hemangioma (RICH) which regresses by 6 to 14 months of age, and noninvoluting congenital hemangioma (NICH).[38,39] Based on negative GLUT1 staining results, these lesions together comprise less than 3% of all hemangiomas seen in infancy.[19] They are occasionally diagnosed *in utero*.

Both RICH and NICH usually present as solitary lesions at birth and rarely coexist in a patient with a typical infantile hemangioma.[40] The most common location for RICH is on the limb, head, or neck. Most NICH occur in the head and neck, trunk, or limbs. These two tumor types share similar morphology and present with a violaceous color and with either fine or coarse telangiectasias. There is often a pale halo encircling the lesion, and in some lesions there is a central ulceration, linear scar, or central nodularity (Fig. 97.13A to C). Unlike infantile hemangiomas, RICHs leave behind a residual patch of thin skin with prominent veins and little, if any, subcutaneous fat. Both RICH and NICH exhibit fast flow on US and may show flow voids on MRI.[40] Both can be misdiagnosed as arteriovenous malformations.

Diagnostic Evaluation

Prenatal US has detected congenital hemangioma as early as the 12th week of gestation. Both congenital tumor types (RICH and NICH) initially exhibit fast flow by US and MRI.

The diagnosis of hemangioma of infancy is based on clinical presentation, history, and physical examination. Lesions exhibit varying degrees of compressibility to the limits of their underlying fibrofatty architecture. If lesions are complicated or if surgical intervention is necessary, additional investigation is generally required to determine the extent of involvement and to confirm the diagnosis. US with color flow Doppler is helpful in distinguishing hemangiomas from vascular malformations that may have a similar appearance. On US, hemangioma of infancy appears hypoechoic, well-defined, and heterogenous in texture, with small cystic and sinusoidal spaces. In most proliferating lesions, a fast-flow pattern is visualized by Doppler US.

Computed tomography (CT) can reveal the extent and involvement of the hemangioma. Additionally, it can be useful in differentiating hemangiomas from lymphatic malformations; however, it can only indicate qualitative differences in blood flow. In the proliferative phase, a hemangioma appears as a well-circumscribed tumor with homogeneous parenchymatous density and intense enhancement. In the involutive phase, it appears heterogeneous with distinct lobular architecture and large draining veins in the center and the periphery.

MRI and MRA are especially valuable in showing the extent of involvement with tissue planes as well as rheologic characteristics. Conventional angiography can provide information about the size of lesions and feeding vessels and can also differentiate hemangiomas from other vascular anomalies; nevertheless, it is reserved for patients who may undergo embolization or surgical intervention.

Differential diagnosis primarily includes other vascular tumors within the ISSVA classification system and malignant tumors such as infantile fibrosarcoma, rhabdomyosarcoma, neuroblastoma and angiosarcoma. Biopsy is indicated only when the diagnosis is uncertain or when the threat of malignancy must be excluded.

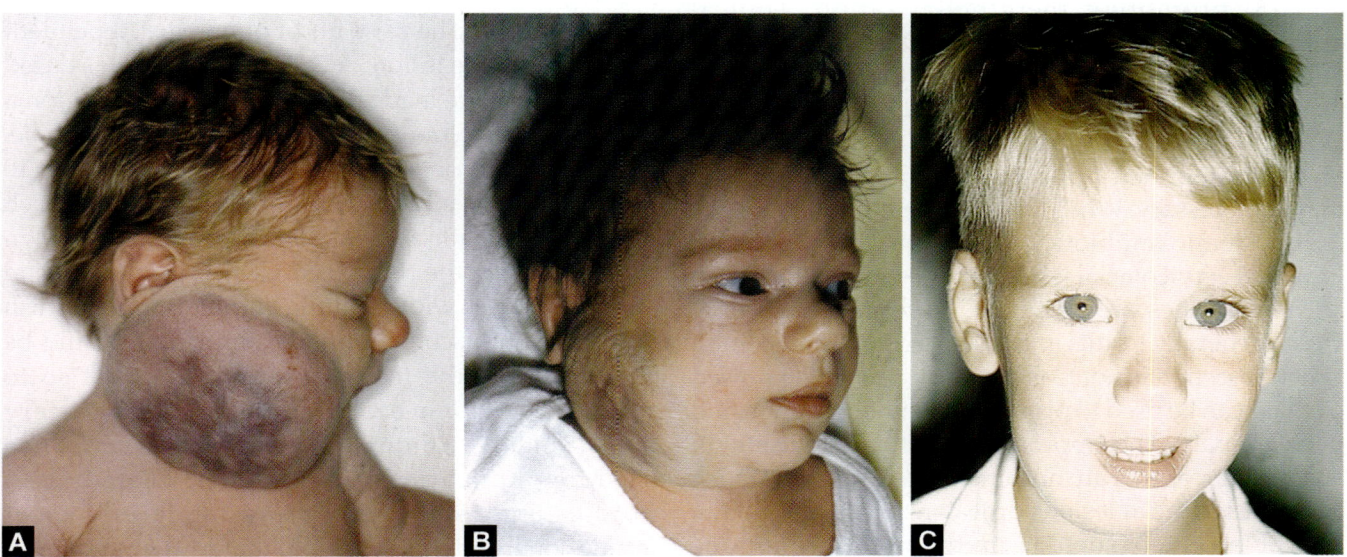

Figs 97.13A to C: Congenital hemangioma, **A.** At birth **B.** 6 months of age. **C.** Age 5

Management Strategies

As discussed, most uncomplicated hemangiomas spontaneously regress without the need for intervention. In some patients, however, rapidly proliferating lesions can cause a wide spectrum of complications, including infection, hemorrhage, necrosis, airway obstruction, loss of vision, and cardiac failure. As such, these patients almost always require multimodal therapy. Decisions as to possible intervention entail consideration of the size and location of the hemangioma, the presence of complications at diagnosis, the age of the patient, and the rate of tumor growth. Large segmental lesions and life-or function-threatening lesions are likely to mandate immediate treatment. In many patients, the possibility of permanent disfiguration or scarring warrants early intervention.

Therapeutic options include pharmacotherapy, chemotherapy, laser therapy, and surgical excision. Depending on anatomic location and severity of the lesion, these approaches are sometimes combined. Optimally, management strategies for complicated lesions should be individualized and collaboratively planned by a multidisciplinary team of clinicians with expertise in treating vascular anomalies.

Treatment of Ulcerations

The treatment of ulcerations should focus on (1) decreasing pain, (2) preventing secondary infections, and (3) promoting reepithelialization. Topical antibiotics are frequently used. Dressings such as DuoDERM® or Mepilex® that cover the ulceration can provide immediate relief of pain and promote healing. When ulcerations are painful, oral medications such as acetaminophen or acetaminophen with codeine may be necessary. When an associated cellulitis occurs, oral systemic antibiotics are given. Ulcerations on localized cervicofacial lesions and lesions on the trunk and extremities are amenable to surgical resection, which generally results in excellent cosmetic outcomes. When resection is not feasible or desirable, the pulsed dye lase can be used to promote reepithelialization and decrease pain. This approach is particularly useful in anatomic areas that are not amenable to resection, such as extensive facial lesions or lesions of the perineum. Newer products such as imiquimod, an immune modulator that stimulates endogenous interferon production, and becaplermin gel, which promotes wound healing, require further study to assess their usefulness in treating ulcerated hemangiomas.[41,42]

Pharmacotherapy

Corticosteroids

Corticosteroids are the first line of therapy for the management of complicated hemangiomas of infancy. These agents may be administered topically, intralesionally, or orally. High-potency topical agents such as clobetasol propionate (0.05%, applied twice daily) are useful in treating problematic localized craniofacial lesions.[43] Unlike orally administered systemic corticosteroids, these agents have only a limited degree of systemic absorption and are not associated with significant adrenal pituitary axis inhibition. One limitation, however, is that rapidly expanding lesions at the tip of the nose or upper lip may develop ulcerations in response to topical steroid application. Intralesional corticosteroids are effective in treating smaller localized, problematic lesions, particularly those in the periorbital region. Whereas some surgeons and ophthalmologists prefer to perform this procedure with the patient under general anesthesia, others prefer the use of a topical anesthetic on an outpatient basis. A long-acting steroid such as triamcinolone can be used together with a short-acting steroid such as cortisone acetate or betamethasone acetate, in a total volume that generally does not exceed 2.5 mL. The dose and volume are dependent on the size of the lesion. A 26-30 gauge needle is used and injections are made directly into the hemangioma in different directions through the same needle hole. Direct pressure is subsequently applied for 2 to 10 minutes to prevent bleeding. Although this approach is associated with a 70-90% response rate, a known complication is the risk of retinal artery embolization and thrombosis, with resulting blindness. To diminish this risk, funduscopic retinal examination should be performed as the lesion is slowly injected so to recognize evidence of imminent retinal artery involvement. Although we have observed some Cushingoid features in patients treated with intralesional steroids, the systemic effects of intralesional and topical steroid therapy have not been well studied.

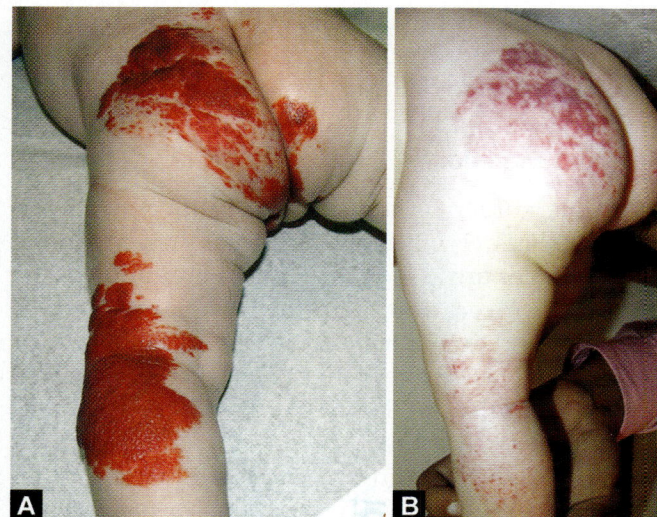

Figs 97.14A and B: A. Extensive hemangioma involving left buttock, leg and genitalia at 2 months of age. **B.** After 2 months of oral prednisolone there is significant regression and flattening of the lesion

Oral corticosteroids are commonly the first line of treatment for lesions that threaten life, limb, vital function, or significant tissues. As with intralesional corticosteroids, they are associated with a 70 to 90% response rate (Fig. 97.14A and B).[44,45] Although their specific mechanism of action is unclear, is believed to be an antiangiogenic effect that decreases endothelial cell expansion and causes endothelial cell apoptosis. Because there are no prospective randomized controlled studies that have investigated dosing or efficacy, current dosing strategies are based on retrospective studies. The general recommendation for oral steroids is a starting dose of 2 to 4 mg per kg daily of prednisolone as a single morning dose. Typically, an assessment of response is performed 2 weeks after this regimen is initiated. If the response is positive, this high dose is maintained for 4 to 6 weeks and then tapered over 4 to 6 months. Ranitidine or other antiacid medication is given concomitantly to diminish the risk of gastric irritation. For patients who undergo steroid therapy over an extensive period of time, some clinicians prescribe trimethoprim/sulfamethoxazole to prevent *Pneumocystis carinii*.

Reported short-term side effects of systemic steroids include irritability, gastric irritation, diminished linear growth and weight gain, nonsystemic fungal infections, and Cushingoid appearance and suppression of the hypothalamic pituitary axis.[46] Potential side effects of steroid use include immunosuppression, hypertension, significant but reversible suppression of the hypothalamic pituitary adrenal axis, hyperglycemia, ophthalmologic changes, myositis, osteoporosis, cardiomyopathy and neurologic changes.

Patients undergoing systemic glucocorticoid therapy should be monitored for potential side effects. Close monitoring of height and weight, blood pressure, developmental milestones, and adrenal suppression at the end of treatment should also be done. Live vaccines should not be given to these patients. If exposure to varicella occurs, a physician should be called immediately and the administration of VZIG should be considered. Patients should be seen for significant fevers and followed regularly. They should be instructed to increase their dosages during stresses related to illness or surgical procedures.

Chemotherapy

Vincristine

For patients who have failed or are unable to tolerate other medical therapies, chemotherapy with vincristine is an option. It interferes with mitotic spindle microtubules and induces apoptosis in tumor cells *in vitro*. Vincristine has a known side effect profile that includes peripheral neuropathy, constipation, jaw pain and irritability, electrolyte disturbances, and neurological problems. Because it is a vesicant, it is best delivered through central venous access. Only two studies have been reported pertaining to chemotherapy with vincristine following failed steroid therapy or significant complications from steroid therapy.[47,48] In one study, Enjolras and colleagues initiated vincristine in 10 patients with a mean age of 8 months and continued for a mean duration of 6 months.[47] Nine of 10 patients had a significant response; the remaining patient had a partial response. The average time to response was 3 weeks. Adams et al reported similar findings.[48]

Interferon-alpha

Interferon-α is an antiangiogenic agent that decreases endothelial cell proliferation by down-regulating basic fibroblast growth factor (bFGF). It is used as a tertiary therapy for life-threatening hemangiomas. Studies have reported the efficacy of interferon alpha-2a and interferon alpha-2b, showing a complete response rate ranging from 40 to 50% with doses between 1 and 3 million Units/m^2/daily.[49,50] Nevertheless, neurotoxicity resulting in spastic diplegia and other motor developmental disturbances has been reported with the use of all interferon preparations in 10 to 30% of patients. Moreover, some patients experience permanent spastic diplegia.[51] It is thus prudent for clinicians to conduct neurologic examinations prior to therapy and every month during the course of therapy. Laboratory evaluations should be done twice a month.

Laser Therapy

Laser treatment of hemangiomas has long been controversial. Although there is no substantial body of evidence indicating that pulsed-dye laser (PDL) therapy prevents the growth of hemangiomas or causes involution to occur significantly faster, it is commonly used to treat small lesions. The results of a prospective, randomized controlled study conducted Batta et al has shed light on this debate.[52] These authors compared outcomes of patients who underwent PDL laser therapy to those of patients who received observation alone. They found that the number of children whose lesions showed complete clearance or minimum residual signs at 1 year was not significantly different from the number in PDL-treated and observation groups. Moreover, PDL-treated infants were more likely to have subsequent skin atrophy and hypopigmentation. The only objective measure of resolution with PDL treatment was a more rapid decrease in hemangioma redness.

There are, however, a number of specific indications for PDL treatment. It is advocated for the treatment of ulcerated hemangiomas in that it decreases pain and promotes more rapid reepithelialization. The PDL is also effective for treating the residual telangiectasias that remain after lesion regression. In a small number of patients, particularly those with segmental lesions, ulceration may worsen after laser treatment.

Since the neodymium:yttrium-aluminum-garnet (ND:YAG) laser system has a greater depth of penetration than the PDL, several authors have reported its successful use in treating the deeper component of hemangiomas. The ND:YAG laser is also used for intralesional photocoagulation. Both the carbon dioxide (CO_2) laser and the erbium (ER:YAG) laser are useful for resurfacing wrinkled and scared skin following involution.

Surgical Excision

If feasible, surgery is indicated in a number of clinical circumstances: (1) when hemangiomas present a threat to function or are associated with complications (e.g., persistent ulceration, significant hemorrhage, or infection) and do not respond to pharmacotherapy or other less invasive alternatives; (2) when they have a high probability of leaving a bag-like fibrofatty residuum, such as seen in pedunculated hemangiomas; (3) when required to revise residual scars after lesions have involuted; (4) when lesions persist beyond a reasonable period of time or grow atypically; and (5) when there is a perceived emotional burden on the child or family and the lesion can easily be removed, leaving no significant cosmetic deformity. The timing of surgery remains controversial, particularly in regard to performing early surgery on disfiguring hemangiomas with post-involution outcomes that are difficult to predict. In such cases, the potential risks must be weighed against numerous factors, including the likely prognosis, the rate of involution, and parental expectations and desires. For example, nasal tip hemangiomas commonly require surgical intervention. They are usually medically managed in infancy with intralesional steroids for smaller lesions and systemic steroids for larger lesions. Staged resection should be contemplated in early childhood. If surgical excision is required to avoid the psychosocial consequences of a visible hemangioma, the operation should be performed during the preschool period, when the child is beginning to develop a defined body image.

The surgical approach is highly dependent upon the size and location of the hemangioma. Although lenticular excision enclosure is an established approach for localized lesions, the length of scarring is a major drawback (Fig. 97.15A and B). A particularly useful technique for localized lesions in most anatomic sites is circular excision and pursestring closure.[53] This technique can be used at any phase in the clinical course of a lesion. It reduces both the longitudinal and transverse dimensions and converts a large circular lesion into a small ellipsoid scar. No other excision and

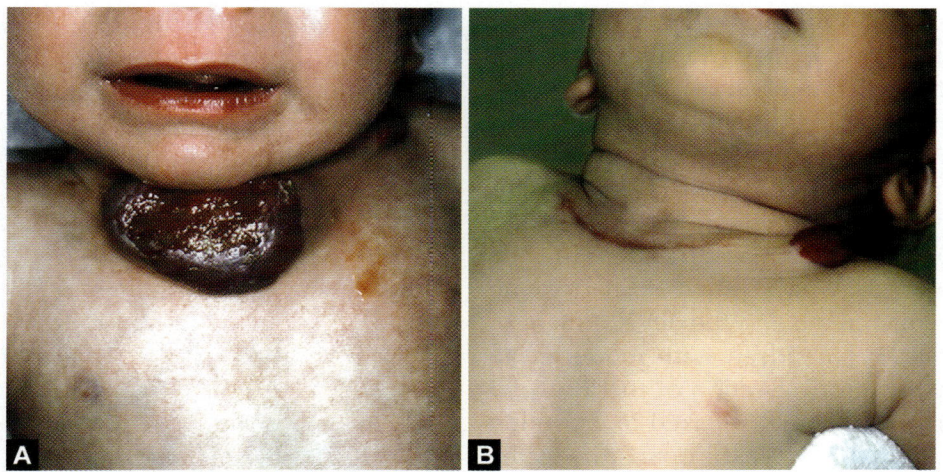

Figs 97.15A and B: A. Ulcerated hemangioma, **B.** Post-excision scar at 3 weeks

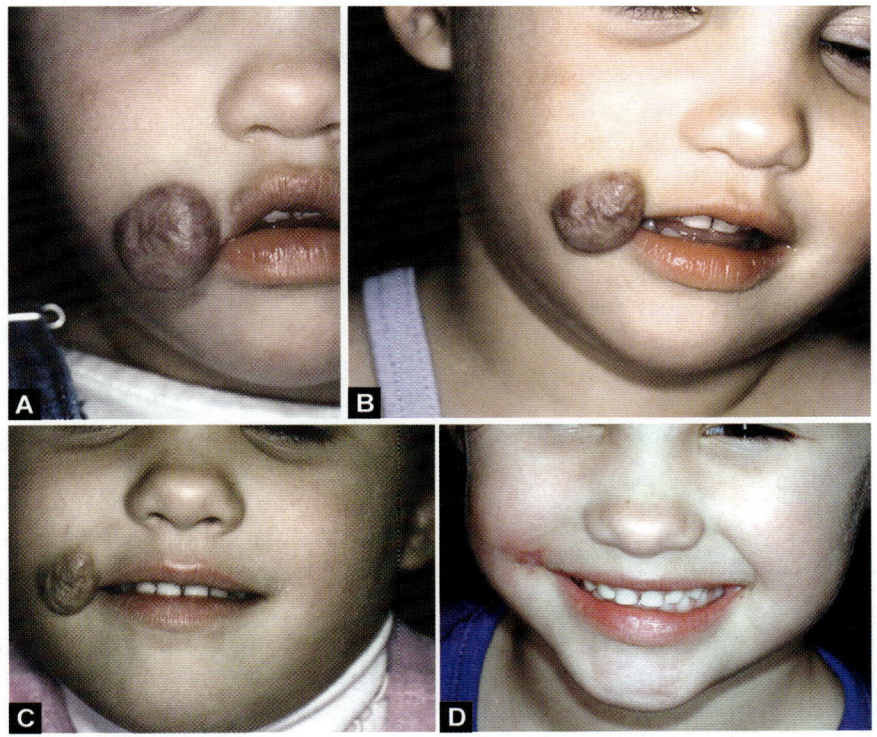

Figs 97.16A to D: Facial hemangioma **A.** 6 months of age **B.** 1.5 years of age with partial involution **C.** Residual lesion at age 3, **D.** Hemangioma excised and closed with purse string closure age 4. This photo was taken 1 year postoperatively

closure technique results in a smaller scar (Fig. 97.16A to D). Because normal skin and subcutaneous tissue are relatively lax, this technique is unlikely to result in significant distortion of surrounding structures. In addition, the scar can be readily revised and made even smaller or placed in desirable skin crease if necessary.

TREATMENT FOR SPECIFIC LESIONS

Subglottic Hemangioma

Traditional management of a subglottic hemangioma has thus been placement of a tracheostomy tube, with the expectation of decannulation between 1 to 2 years of age. In children with mild to moderate symptoms, high-dose systemic steroids may cause involution of the lesion and prevent the need for other surgical intervention; however, their prolonged use is strongly discouraged. Although a number of alternatives to tracheostomy placement have been used (e.g. intralesional steroids, prolonged intubation, CO_2 and KTP laser ablation, and microdebrider resection), they are associated with drawbacks such as inadequate removal of the hemangioma and the development of subglottic stenosis. For children with moderate to severe symptoms, surgical resection of the localized subglottic hemangioma is the preferred intervention of some surgeons. This is at least in part due to the association of subglottic hemangioma with mild to moderate congenital subglottic stenosis in the majority of cases. This approach permits removal of the hemangioma and simultaneous repair of the congenital subglottis stenosis if present. Segmental hemangiomas associated with subglottic hemangiomas are treated with systemic agents such as steroids or vincristine. Tracheostomy should be reserved for patients who fail medical therapy.

Parotid gland hemangiomas can be superficial and deep and can grow rapidly, causing extrinsic compression of the upper pharyngeal airway. These lesions can proliferate for up to 12 to 16 months and require systemic treatment if the airway is compromised.

Visceral Hemangiomas

Liver Lesions

Patients with asymptomatic liver hemangiomas detected on imaging studies should undergo both routine sequential physical examinations and imaging studies. Treatment should be reserved for patients in whom symptoms are apparent or there is significant liver enlargement (Fig. 97.17). Larger lesions or those causing heart failure require immediate treatment. Systemic corticosteroids are the preferred initial therapy; however, unresponsive lesions may necessitate the use of vincristine or interferon. For patients in whom heart failure persists or worsens, performing a hepatic arteriography may have to be considered. Embolization is likely to be useful when there are direct macrovascular shunts through the lesion. Both angiography and embolization are associated with significant rusks of injury to the

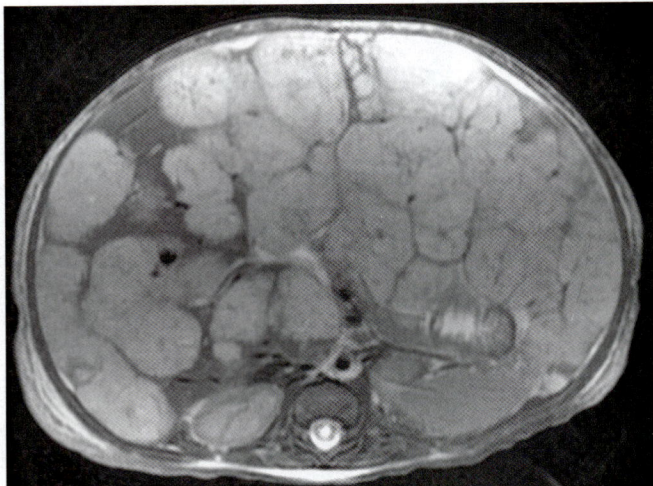

Fig. 97.17: MRI of an infant with extensive and diffuse intrahepatic hemangioma. This child had an abdominal compartment syndrome, high output cardiac failure and profound hypothyroidism

femoral access vessel or embolized visceral vessels, and should be performed only by an interventional radiologists who are highly skilled in using these techniques in infants.[35]

Surgical resection of the hemangioma is generally not indicated. Liver transplantation should be considered only when tumors are unresponsive to therapy, involve the entire liver, and are associated with unremitting abdominal compartment syndrome.[54] Many of these large lesions are associated with profound acquired hypothyroidism.[55] Some hemangiomas have been shown to express type 3 iodothyronine deiodinase, which inactivates circulating thyroid hormone; thyroid hormone may thus be destroyed by the tumor more rapidly than the thyroid can produce it. Such patients require large doses of exogenous hormone replacement. Since hypothyroidism may not develop until the hemangioma undergoes significant growth, repeated thyroid testing in the presence of such growth is indicated.

Other Lesions of the Gastrointestinal Tract

Treatment of hemangiomas of the stomach, small intestine, or colon is based on severity of symptoms, with gastrointestinal bleeding varying from mild to life threatening. If symptoms can be managed with persistent and aggressive blood replacement and pharmacotherapy, these are often the most prudent treatment strategies. Bleeding will diminish and cases after lesions enter the involution phase, which in many cases can be accelerated with angiogenesis inhibitors.

A small isolated hemangioma of the stomach or colon can be banded endoscopically, but this is not without risk of perforation or increased hemorrhage.[56] Occasionally, a focal lesion may be amenable to treatment with other endoscopic techniques such as multipolar thermocoagulation or argon plasma coagulation. For lesions visible by endoscopy, intralesional injection with corticosteroid may also be considered. Indications for excision include complications such as intussusception or obstruction, uncontrollable ulceration with hemorrhage or perforation, or infection. A surgical approach is not indicated when there is diffuse multifocal involvement of the gastrointestinal tract. Such lesions are more appropriately treated with corticosteroids, interferon alpha 2a, or other antiangiogenic agents.

Congenital Hemangiomas

In a patient with lesions that rapidly involute (RICH), observation is generally the first line of treatment. Involution may begin very early in the neonatal period, causing crusting and scaling on the surface of the lesion. Preventing ulceration is often accomplished by applying a petroleum-based emollient to the surface of the lesion several times daily. In patients in whom ulceration does occur, adherence to good wound care practices, pain control, and treatment of secondary infection is essential.[57] Once spontaneous tumor regression is complete, residual fibrofatty tissue and scarred skin can be excised to improve cosmesis.

Noninvoluting congenital lesions (NICH) require excision. For larger lesions, preoperative embolization may be required to reduce intraoperative bleeding.[57]

OTHER VASCULAR TUMORS

The classification of vascular tumors encompasses several other less commonly seen tumors, including kaposiform hemangioendothelioma, tufted angioma, and angiosarcoma.

Kasabach-Merritt Phenomenon and Kaposiform Hemangioendothelioma

Kasabach-Merritt (K-M) phenomenon is a coagulopathy characterized by profound thrombocytopenia (a platelet count of 300 to 50,000 per cubic millimeter) caused by platelet trapping and disseminated intravascular coagulation that leads to profound fibrinolysis and hypofibrinogenemia. Until the 1990s, this condition was mistakenly thought to be a life-threatening complication of some hemangiomas. However, it is now recognized as distinct from classic hemangioma and is associated primarily with kaposiform hemangioendothelioma (KHE), and far less commonly with tufted angioma.[58-61]

KHE is an aggressive vascular tumor, presenting at birth in about 50% of cases and usually appearing within the first year of life in most other cases (Figs 97.18A and B). The tumor is usually solitary and

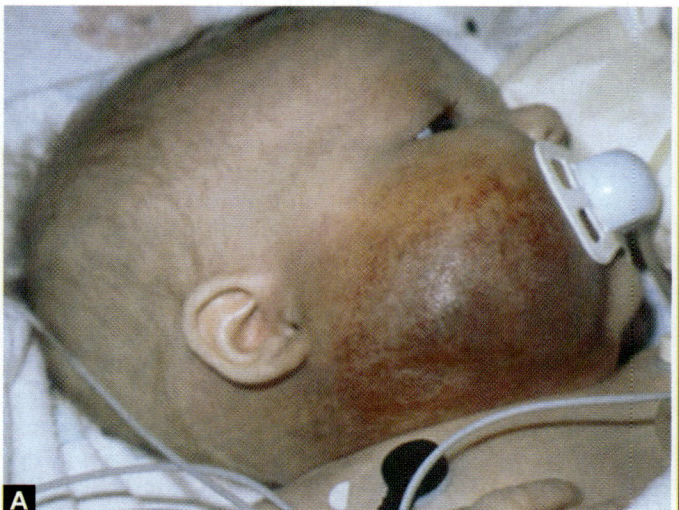
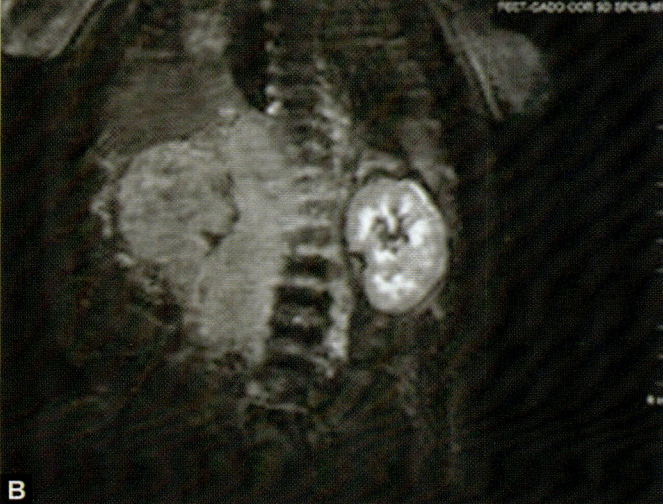

Figs 97.18A and B: A. Infant with kaposiform hemangioendothelioma (KHE) and Kasabach Merritt Phenomenon. **B.** MRI showing paraspinal involvement of KHE

multifocal lesions rarely occur. In contrast to hemangiomas of infancy, KHE has no female preponderance and typically occurs in the proximal arms and legs and the trunk (including the retroperitoneum); craniofacial lesions are uncommon. KHE is typically manifested as a plaque-like mass with a deep red-purple hue. It is associated with surrounding subcutaneous edema and induration, the degree of which depends upon the amount of trapped blood elements and the extent of intralesional bleeding in tissue. KHE does not completely regress and can involve adjacent muscle and bone, but does not metastasize. The mortality rate of this tumor is high, ranging from 20 to 37%, with bleeding being the primary cause of death.[59] Retroperitoneal involvement has been associated with a particularly poor outcome. A number of therapies have been reported in the treatment of K-M phenomenon, but none have been uniformly effective.[58-61] Treatment involves the use of steroids, interferon-alpha, antifibrinolytic agents, and chemotherapeutic agents, including cyclophosphamide, vincristine and actinomycin.

Tufted Angioma

Congenital and acquired tufted angioma usually present as an erythematous, slightly tender, indurated macule or plaque in a child younger than age 5. As with KHE, tufted angioma is typically located along the midline axis of the neck, upper trunk, and extremities. Unlike KHE, it is characterized by rounded nodules or tufts of densely packed capillaries and pericytes in the mid-dermis, which bulge into and compress large, thin-walled vessels at the periphery of the nodules. MRI imaging scans have demonstrated that tufted angioma invade the skin and subcutaneous fat and muscle.

Tumors exhibiting gradations between KHE and tufted angioma and containing elements of both lesions have been described. Since both can be associated with K-M phenomenon, they may represent variations of the same tumor.

REFERENCES

1. Mulliken JB, Fishman SJ, Burrows PE. Vascular anomalies. Curr Probl Surg 2000;37:517-84.
2. Mulliken JB, Fishman SJ. Vascular anomalies: hemangiomas and malformations. In O'Neill JA, Rowe MI, Grosfeld JL, et al (Eds) Pediatric Surgery, 5th edn. St. Louis, MO: Mosby 1998:1939-51.
3. Mullliken JB, Glowacki J. Hemangiomas and vascular malformations in infants and children: A classification based on endothelial characteristics. Plast Reconstr Surg 1982;69:412-22.
4. Gonzalez-Crussi F, Reyes-Mugica M. Cellular hemangiomas (hemangioendotheliomas) in infants. Light microscopic, immunohistochemical, and ultrastructural observations. Am J Surg Pathol 1991;15:769-78.
5. Nguyen VA, Furhapter C, Romani N, et al. Infantile hemangioma is a proliferation of beta 4-negative endothelial cells adjacent to HLA-DR-positive cells with dendritic cell morphology. Hum Pathol 2004;35:739-44.
6. Yu Y, Flint AF, Mulliken JB, et al. Endothelial progenitor cells in infantile hemangioma. Blood 2004;103:1373-75.
7. Boye E, Yu Y, Paranya G, et al. Clonality and altered behavior of endothelial cells from hemangiomas. J Clin Invest 2001;107:745-52.
8. Walter JW, North PE, Waner M, et al. Somatic mutation of vascular endothelial growth factor receptors in juvenile hemangioma. Genes Chromosomes Cancer 2002;33:295-303.
9. Bielenberg DR, Bucana CD, Sanchez R, et al. Progressive growth of infantile cutaneous hemangiomas is directly correlated with hyperplasia and angiogenesis of adjacent epidermis and inversely correlated with expression of the endogenous angiogenesis inhibitor, IFN-beta. Int J Oncol 1999;14:401-08.
10. Takahashi K, Mulliken JB, Kozakewich HP, et al. Cellular markers that distinguish the phases of hemangioma during infancy and childhood. J Clin Invest 1994;93:2357-64.
11. Chang J, Most D, Bresnick S, et al. Proliferative hemangiomas: analysis of cytokine gene expression and angiogenesis. Plast Reconstr Surg 1999;103:1-9.
12. Razon MJ, Kraling BM, Mulliken JB, et al. Increased apoptosis coincides with onset of involution in infantile hemangioma. Microcirculation 1998;5:189-95.
13. Ritter MR, Dorrell MI, Edmonds J, et al. Insulin-like growth factor 2 and potential regulators of hemangioma growth and involution identified by large-scale expression analysis. Proc Natl Acad Sci USA 2002;99:7455-60.
14. Yu Y, Varughese J, Brown LF, et al. Increase Tie2 expression, enhanced response to angiopoietin-1, and dysregulated angiopoietin-2 expression in hemangioma-derived endothelial cells. Am J Pathol 2001;159:2271-80.
15. Ritter MR, Morena SK, Dorrell MI, et al. Identifying potential regulators of infantile hemangioma progression through large scale expression analysis: a possible role for the immune system and indoleamine 2,3 dioxygenase (IDO) during involution. Lymphat Res Biol 2003;1:291-99.
16. Takikawa O, Yoshida R, Kido R, et al. Tryptophan degradation in mice initiated by indoleamine 2,3-dioxygenase. J Biol Chem 1986;261:3648-53.
17. Martinez M, Sanchez-Carpinetero I, North PE, et al. Infantile hemangioma: clinical resolution with 5% imiquimod cream. Arch Dermatol 2002;138:881-84.

18. Sauder DN. Immunomodulatory and pharmacologic properties of imiquimod. J Am Acad Dermatol 2000;43: S6-S11.
19. North PE, Waner M, Mizeracki A, et al. GLUT1: a newly discovered immunohistochemical marker for juvenile hemangiomas. Hum Pathol 2000;31:11-22.
20. North PE, Waner M, Mizeracki A, et al. A unique microvascular phenotype shared by juvenile hemangiomas and human placenta. Arch Dermatol 2001;137: 559-70.
21. Huang SA, Tu HM, Harney JW, et al. Severe hypothyroidism caused by type 3 iodothyronine deiodinase in infantile hemangiomas. N Engl J Med 2000; 343:185-89.
22. North PE, Waner M, Brodsky MC. Are infantile hemangiomas of placental origin? Ophthalmology 2002;109:633-34.
23. Burton BK, Schulz CJ, Angle B, et al. An increased incidence of haemangiomas in infants born following chorionic villus sampling (CVS). Prenat Diagn 1995;15:209-14.
24. Barnés CM, Huang S, Kaipainen A, et al. Evidence by molecular profiling for a placental origin of infantile hemangioma. Proc Natl Acad Sci USA 2005;102:19097-102.
25. Dadras SS, North PE, Bertoncini J, et al. Infantile hemangiomas are arrested in an early developmental vascular differentiation state. Mod Pathol 2004;17: 1068-79.
26. Fishman SJ, Mulliken JB. Vascular anomalies. A primer for pediatricians. Pediatr Clin North Am 1998;45:1455-77.
27. Enjolras O, Mulliken JB. Vascular tumors and vascular malformations (new issues). Adv Dermatol 1997;13: 375-423.
28. Drolet BA, Esterly N, Frieden IJ. Hemangiomas in Children. N Eng J Med 1999;341:173-81.
29. Frieden IJ, Reese V, Cohen D. PHACE syndrome. The association of posterior fossa brain malformations, hemangiomas, arterial anomalies, coarctation of the aorta and cardiac defects, and eye abnormalities. Arch Dermatol 1996;132:307-11.
30. Reese V, Frieden IJ, Paller AS, et al. Association of facial hemangiomas with Dandy-Walker and other posterior fossa malformations. J Pediatr 1993;122:379-84.
31. Burrows PE, Robertson RL, Mulliken JB, et al. Cerebral vasculopathy and neurologic sequelae in infants with cervicofacial hemangioma: report of eight patients. Radiology 1998;207:601-07.
32. Orlow SJ, Isakoff MS, Blei F. Increased risk of symptomatic hemangiomas of the airway in association with cutaneous hemangiomas in a "beard" distribution. J Pediatr 1997;131:643-46.
33. Kushner B. Infantile orbital hemangiomas. Int Pediatr 1990;5:249-57.
34. Rutter MJ. Evaluation and management of upper airway disorders in children. Sem Pediatr Surg 2006;15:116-23.
35. Fishman SJ, Fox VL. Visceral vascular anomalies. Gastrointest Endosc Clin N Am 2001;11:813-34.
36. Morris J, Abbott J, Burrows PE, et al. Antenatal diagnosis of fetal hepatic hemangioma treated with maternal corticosteroids. Obstet Gynecol 1999;94:813-15.
37. Marler JJ, Fishman SJ, Upton J, et al. Prenatal diagnosis of vascular anomalies. J Pediatr Surg 2002;37:318-26.
38. Boon LM, Enjolras O, Mulliken JB. Congenital hemangioma: evidence for accelerated involution. J Pediatr 1996;128:329-35.
39. Enjolras O, Mulliken JB, Boon LM, et al. Non-involuting congenital hemangioma: a rare cutaneous vascular anomaly. Plast Reconstr Surg 2001;107:1647-54.
40. Mulliken JB, Enjolras O. Congenital hemangiomas and infantile hemangioma: missing links. J Am Acad Dermatol 2004;50:875-82.
41. Hazen PG, Carney JF, Engstrom CW, et al. Proliferating hemangioma of infancy: successful treatment with topical 5% imiquimod cream. Pediatr Dermatol 2005;22:254-56.
42. Metz BJ, Rubenstein MC, Levy ML, et al. Response of ulcerated perineal hemangiomas of infancy to becaplermin gel, a recombinant human platelet-derived growth factor. Arch Dermatol 2004;140:867-70.
43. Cruz OA, Zarnegar SR, Myers SE. Treatment of periocular capillary hemangioma with topical clobetasol propionate. Ophthalmology 1995;102:2012-15.
44. Bartoshesky LE, Bull M, Feingold M. Corticosteroid treatment of cutaneous hemangiomas: how effective? A report on 24 children. Clin Pediatr (Phila) 1978;17:625, 629-38.
45. Brown SH Jr, Neerhout RC, Fonkalsrud EW. Prednisone therapy in the management of large hemangiomas in infants and children. Surgery 1972;71:168-73.
46. Boon L M, MacDonald DM, Mulliken JB. Complications of systemic corticosteroid therapy for problematic hemangioma. Plast Reconstr Surg 1999;104:1616-23.
47. Enjolras O, Breviere GM, Roger G, et al. Vincristine treatment for function- and life-threatening infantile hemangioma. Arch Pediatr 2004;11:99-107.
48. Adams DM, Orme L, Bowers D. Vincristine treatment of complicated hemangiomas. 14th International Workshop on Vascular Anomalies, Netherlands, June 2002.
49. Ezekowitz RA, Mulliken JB, Folkman J, et al. Interferon alfa-2a therapy for life-threatening hemangiomas of infancy. N Engl J Med 2992;326:1456-63.
50. Chang EA, Boyd A, Nelson CC, et al. Successful treatment of infantile hemangiomas with interferon-alpha-2b. J Pediatr Hematol Oncol 1997;19:237-44.
51. Barlow C F, Priebe C J, Mulliken JB, et al. Spastic diplegia as a complication of interferon Alfa-2a treatment of hemangiomas of infancy. J Pediatr 132 (3 Pt 1):527-30.
52. Batta K, Goodyear HM, Moss C, et al. Randomised controlled study of early pulsed dye laser treatment of uncomplicated childhood haemangiomas: results of a 1-year analysis. Lancet 2002;360:521-27.
53. Mulliken JB, Rogers GF, Marler JJ. Circular excision of hemangioma and purse-string closure: the smallest possible scar. Plast Reconstr Surg 2002;109:1544-54.

54. Daller JA, Bueno J, Gutierrez J, et al. Hepatic hemangioendothelioma: clinical experience and management strategy. J Pediatr Surg 1999;34:98-105.
55. Huang SA, Tu HM, Harney JW, et al. Severe hypothyroidism caused by type 3 iodothyronine deiodinase in infantile hemangiomas. N Engl J Med 2000;343:185-89.
56. Fishman SJ, Burrows PE, Leichtner AM, et al. Gastrointestinal manifestations of vascular anomalies in childhood: varied etiologies require multiple therapeutic modalities. J Pediatr Surg 1998;33:1163-67.
57. Krol A, MacArthur CJ. Congenital hemangiomas. Arch Facial Plast Surg 2005;7:307-11.
58. Enjolras O, Wassef M, et al. "Infants with Kasabach-Merritt syndrome do not have "true" hemangiomas." J Pediatr 1997;130(4): 631-40.
59. Haisley-Royster C. Enjolras O, et al. "Kasabach-merritt phenomenon: a retrospective study of treatment with vincristine." J Pediatr Hematol Oncol 2002;24(6): 459-62.
60. Kasabach H, Merritt K. "Capillary hemangioma with extensive purpura: Report of a case." Am J Dis Child 1940;59:1063-70.
61. Sarkar M, Mulliken J B, et al. "Thrombocytopenic coagulopathy (Kasabach-Merritt phenomenon) is associated with Kaposiform hemangioendothelioma and not with common infantile hemangioma." Plast Reconstr Surg 1997;100(6): 1377-86.

CHAPTER 98

Vascular and Lymphatic Anomalies

Robert Arensman, Jayant Agarwal, M Statter

ARTERIOVENOUS MALFORMATIONS

Classification and Pathology

Vascular malformations, are errors in morphogenesis and are populated by mature vascular endothelium, with normal endothelial turnover, and normal numbers of mast cells. These lesions are present at birth, though not always apparent, grow with the child and do not involute.

Vascular malformations need to be differentiated from hemangiomas. In a series, quantitative assessment of mast cells was done in cellulerly dynamic and adynamic vascular malformations.[1]

There was an increased number of mast cells in growing stages and during initial involution of strawberry hemangiomas that decreased in the later involuting stages.[1] However, the mean number of mast cells in cellularly adynamic lesions, i.e. port wine stains was 4.8, and in congenital arteriovenous malformations, it was 3.6, comparable to that in normal skin where the mean number of mast cells was 3.2.

Vascular malformations are further classified as capillary, venous, arterial (with or without fistula) or lymphatic anomalies.[2]

A recent revision of Mullikan and Glowacki's classification has broadened the category of vascular tumors of infancy to include hemangiopericytoma, pyogenic granuloma, tufted angioma, and kaposiform hemangioendothelioma.[3]

As in the case with hemangiomas, the terminology used to describe malformations has been very confusing. Many authors continue to use terms like port wine stain when describing capillary malformations. The incidence of arteriovenous malformations is 1-4%. Port wine stains, intradermal capillary malformations, are seen in 0.3% of newborns Figure 98.1. Approximately 25% of affected individuals have a positive family history of other vascular anomalies.[4] These lesions are found frequently on the face in the distribution of the trigeminal nerve. When associated with the trigeminal nerve there is an 8% incidence of ocular and central nervous system disorders. The variance in color of port wine stains is attributable to ectatic postcapillary venules.[5,6]

Presentation and Clinical Course

Unlike hemangiomas, malformations are present at birth and grow as the child grows. Table 98.1 outlines the clinical stages of a hemangioma (Figs 98.1 to 98.4) Table 98.2 gives the differences between a

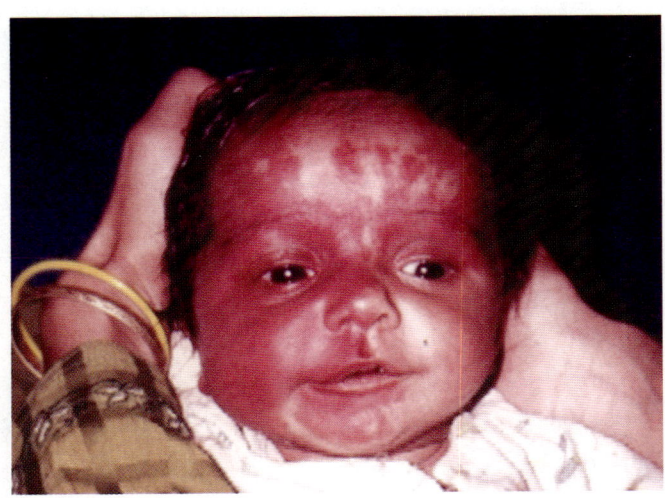

Fig. 98.1: Portwine stain

Table 98.1: Clinical stages of hemangiomas

Stage	Definition	Clinical appearance	Period
I.	Origin	Precursors: 1. Herald spot-pale patch, well-demarcated, nonelevated area, visible during crying 2. Small telangiectoria surrounded by a pale halo 3. Erythemaious patch	At Birth or in first four weeks of life
II.	Initial growth	1. Gradual appearance of closely packed pinhead lesions 2. Small red populea on the name area as the pale spot but not neccessarily limited to it.	2 weeks to 5 weeks
III.	Intermediate growth	1. Increase in area and thickness (sometimes rapidly) 2. Enlargement of bright red, tense lesion with irrgular surface patches and elevation above normal skin level	2 months to 10 months
IV.	Completed growth	Stationary period: 1. Raised, circumacribed, bright red, soft, lobubted (some-times even pedunculated), and compressible tumor 2. Becomes quiescent after reaching maximum size	5 months to 20 months
V.	Initial involution	1. Color fading from bright red to dull red or pink 2. Gray-white areas appear first on the previously bright red surface in the center of the hemangioma and gradually spread toward periphery 3. Lesion becomes solter and flatter 4. Ulceration, as a part of the involuting process posibly from injury or from intraluminal thrombus	5 months to 1.5 years
VI.	Intermediate involution	1. Gradual decreasing of thickness and volume 2. Flattening and softening of the entire area 3. Blanching, fibrosis, scarring, slightly wrinkted surface	1.5 years to 5 years
VII.	Completed involution	1. No residual skin changes 2. Variable degrees of atrophy, any wrinkles, a few telangiectatic vessels 3. Bag of loose, scarred skin with underlying lipomatous tissue	5 years to 16 years

Source: Reprinted with permission from pasyk ital quantitative evaluation of most cells in cellularly dynamic of adynamic vascular molformations, plast reconstr surg 1984;73:69

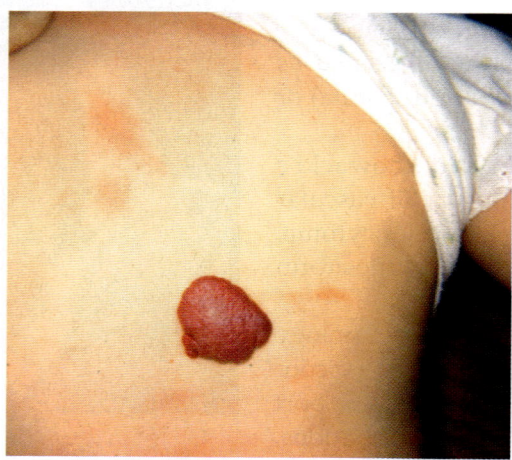

Fig. 98.2: Hemangioma on the back

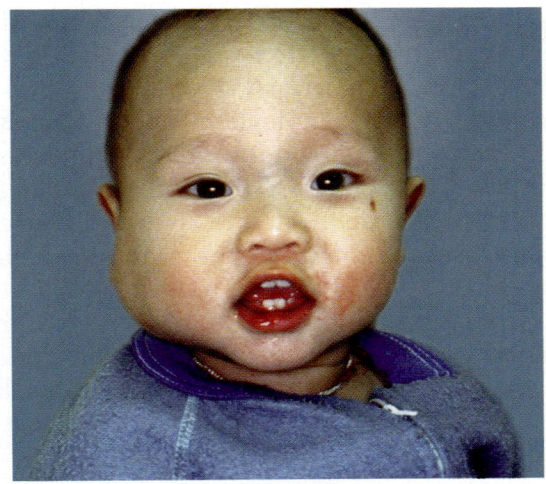
Fig. 98.3

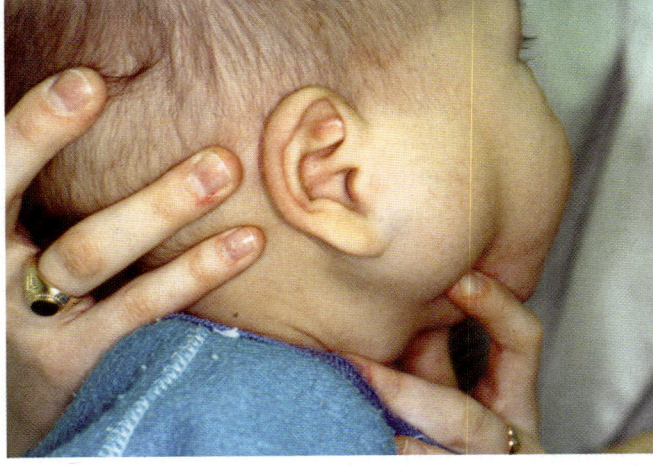
Fig. 98.4

Figs 98.3 and 98.4: Parotid hemangioma in infant. This lesion underwent involution without medical or surgical therapy

Table 98.2: Characteristics of vascular birthmarks

Hemangioma	Malformation
Clinical	
Usually nothing seen at birth 30% percent as red macule	All present at birth, may not be evident
Rapid postnatal proliferation and slow involution	Commensurate growth may expand as a result of trauma, sepsis, hormonal modulation
Female: male 3:1	Female:male 1:1
Cellular	
Plump endothelium, increased turn over	Flat endothelium, slow turnover
Increased mast cells	Normal mast cell count
Multilaminated basement membrane	Normal thin basement membrane
Capillary tubule formation in vitro	Poor endothelial growth *in vitro*
Hematological	
Primary platelet trapping: thrombocytopenia (Kasabach-Merritt syndrome)	Primary stasis (venous): localized consumptive coagulopathy
Radiological	
Angiographic findings: well-circumscribed, intense lobular-parenchymal staining with equitorial vessels	Angiographic findings: diffuse, no parenchyma Low-flow, pheboliths, ectatic channels High-flow: enlarged, tortuous arteries with arteriovenous shunting
Skeletal	
Infrequent "mass effect" on adjacent bone: hypertrophy rare	Low-flow: disortion, hypertrophy, or hypoplasia High-flow: destruction, distortion, or hypertrophy

(Modified from Mulliken JB: Classification of Vascular Birthmarks, In: Mulliken JB, Young AE, Vascular Birth Marks: Haemangiomas and Malformations. Philadelphia, WB Saunders, 1988, Ch 2, pp 24-37)[7]

hemangioma and malformation. One distinguishing feature of venous malformations is that they are emptied of blood with compression. The most important distinguishing feature is that malformations do not involute. Vascular malformations have no predilection for either sex and may demonstrate sudden growth secondary to trauma, infection or hormonal modulation. The appearance of malformations is dependant on the type of vessel involved. Venous malformations appear bluish and can be confused with subcutaneous hemangiomas. Vascular malformations are categorized based on the types of vessels involved (capillary, venous, arterial, lymphatic, or mixed) and flow characteristics. Arteriovenous malformations and fistulas are high flow lesions that present with pulsations, bruits, or thrills and can expand with rises in blood pressure.[7,8] The two types of congenital arteriovenous malformations are macrofistulas and microfistulas. Macrofistulas occur as solitary lesions in the head and neck and can result in distal ischemia. Microfistulas are usually multiple, occur in the lower extremity and do not cause distal ischemia. Low flow lesions are lymphatic, venous, capillary or combined. Doppler ultrasonography is useful in delineating microfistulas.[41] Vascular malformations on CT present as tissue heterogeneity. Magnetic resonance imagery (MRI) demonstrates both the extent of involvement within tissue planes and rheologic characteristics. During the proliferative phase, T1 and T2 weighted MRI images demonstrate a lobulated soft-tissue mass with feeding and draining vessels. Angiography can be utilized to define the anatomy and hemodynamics of these malformations and is utilized in patients requiring therapeutic embolization.[9]

In contrast to hemangiomas, arteriovenous malformations can be complicated by consumption coagulopathy. Stasis with dilated ecstatic venous channels precipitates the coagulopathy.

Port wine stains are intradermal capillary malformations that are present at birth and persist throughout life without regression. Sturge-Weber syndrome is the most common disorder associated with port wine stains. The port wine stain in Sturge-Weber is in the V_1 and V_2 distribution of the trigeminal nerve and is associated with leptomeningeal venous malformations, and atrophy and calcification of the underlying cerebral cortex. Consequently these patients may demonstrate mental retardation, focal motor seizures, hemiparesis, visual field defects and glaucoma.[10] It is recommended that children with facial port wine stain should undergo fundoscopic examination and CT scan. In addition, reflectance spectroscopy can delineate the level and degree of ectatic vessels and aids in the planning of laser therapy.[11]

Klippel-Trenaunay syndrome is a complex congenital malformation that may affect the upper or lower extremities, and less commonly the trunk, head or neck.[12] The three main components are varicosities and venous malformations, port wine stains, and hypertrophy of the bone and soft tissue. Venous drainage is abnormal because of persistent embryonic veins, agenesis, hypoplasia, vascular incompetence, or aneurysms of the deep veins. An important distinction is the absence of significant arteriovenous shunting.[13]

Treatment

Unlike hemangiomas, the endothelium of vascular malformations is not hyperplastic and exhibits normal turnover and is not susceptible to anti-proliferative treatments like steroids, interferon, or radiation/chemotherapy. Prior to surgical management of arteriovenous malformations any underlying consumptive coagulopathy should be treated. The treatment of venous malformations includes elastic compression garments for lower extremity lesions with analgesia for pain control. Sequential compression devices must be used with caution because of the risk of embolism. Intervention is mostly indicated with large lesions or with venous malformations of the head and neck. Lesions of the head and neck often involve neural structures and resection may be difficult. Good results have been reported with percutaneous injection of the sclerosing agent sodium tetradocyl sulfate at doses of 2-4 ml.[14] Others report favorable results with injection of 95% ethanol, however alcohol should be used with care since it can pass through arteriovenous shunts into normal tissues causing necrosis.[15] Cavernous sinus thrombosis has also been seen with injection of sclerosing agents therefore low doses are recommended. Ethibloc has been used with good results. It is biodegradable and more viscous than ethanol and less likely to diffuse into nearby tissues.[14-15] The argon, YAG, and nd:YAG lasers have all shown good results particularly with intraoral lesions. Repeated treatments may be necessary because these lesions tend to recur after photocoagulation.[16,17] The treatment of choice for port wine stains is laser photocoagulation. The flashlamp-pumped pulsed-dye laser has been used to successfully lighten these lesions.[4,9,18]

Management of Klippel-Trenaunay syndrome is primarily nonoperative. Those patients with patent deep veins can be considered for excision of symptomatic varicose veins and venous malformations.[12,13] Preoperative evaluations should include MRI and contrast venography.

LYMPHANGIOMAS

Classification and Pathology

Lymphangiomas are a heterogeneous group of benign malformations of the lymphatic system that consist of localized or generalized anomalous lymphatic channels and cysts. Lymphangiomas can present in any lymphatic bed and in order of decreasing frequency occur in the cervicofacial region, axilla, thorax, and extremities. There are two morphologic types, macrocystic and microcystic, which are often combined. Macrocystic lymphatic malformations are soft, large, smooth translucent masses under normal or bluish skin. Microcystic lymphatic malformations are firm, tiny cutaneous vesicles that permeate the skin and muscles and give the impression of brawny edema. Classification of congenital abnormalities of the lymphatic system has been based on pathology and on clinical presentation.[19]

Presentation and Clinical Course

Overall, lymphangiomas account for 6% of the benign tumors found in the pediatric population.[19] Both sexes are affected equally. Approximately 65% of lymphangiomas present at birth, and 90% appear by the second year of life. The size of a lymphatic malformation may increase due to intralesional hemorrhage, cellulitis, or increasing fluid accumulation noted with viral or bacterial infections. Pure lymphatic malformations or combined lymphaticovenous malformations, such as Klippel-Trenaunay syndrome, can be associated with soft-tissue and skeletal hypertrophy. Disfigurement is the principal reason patients seek medical attention. Spontaneous regression is rare, and malignant degeneration is unlikely.

History and physical examination usually suggest the diagnosis of lymphangiomas. The differential diagnosis includes lipoma, dermoid cyst, branchial cyst, thyroglossal duct cyst, teratoma, thyroid tumor, neurofibroma, and meningoencephalocele. Plain films are useful to evaluate the airway. Ultrasound and CT scan can determine whether the lesion is cystic or solid. MRI is useful to assess extension of the lesion (Figs 98.5 to 98.7).

Treatment

Surgical excision is indicated for lesions that interfere with function, cause major cosmetic disfigurement, or become easily infected. Lymphangiomas that obstruct the erodigestive tract may require aspiration, incision and drainage, tracheostomy, or feeding tube

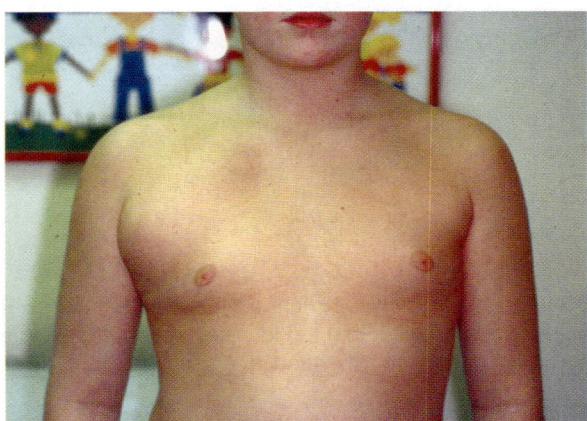

Fig. 98.5

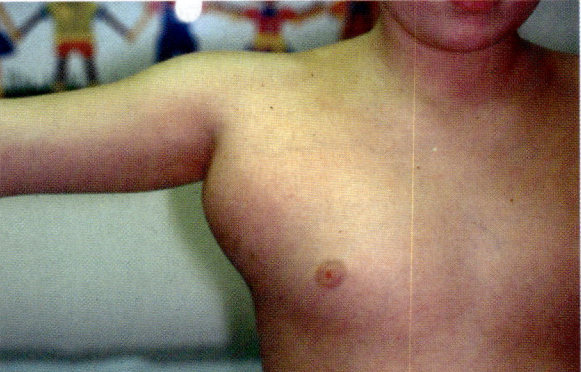

Fig. 98.6

Figs 98.5 and 98.6: Nine-year-old pitcher in baseball team with acute onset of right axillary mass

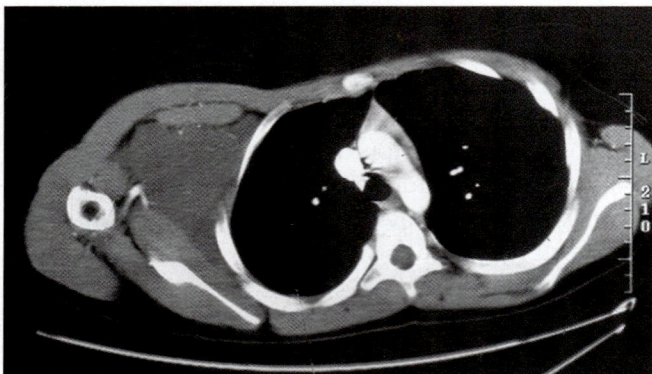

Fig. 98.7: CT scan of 9-year-old patient in Figures 98.5 and 98.6 demonstrates right axillary lymphangioma. There is no intrathoracic extension

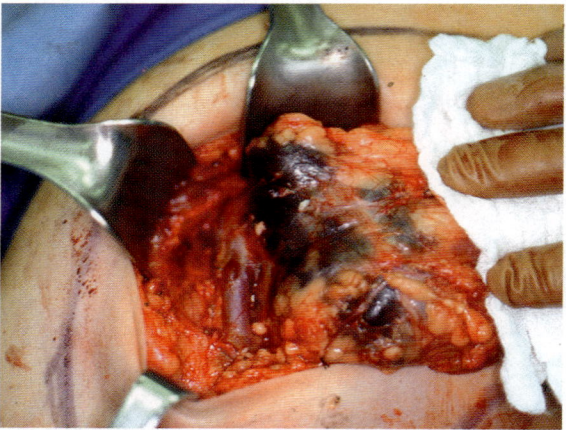

Fig. 98.8: Operative view of right axillary lymphangioma. The sudden increase in size that led to detection of the lesion was hemorrhage within the lymphangioma

placement. Aspiration or incision and drainage play a role in emergency decompression but are not considered definitive treatment. Complete resection is the goal of surgical therapy but because of the tendency to infiltrate and invest adjacent tissues and structures, resection of a lymphangioma is often incomplete (Fig. 98.8). Alqahtani et al in their 25-year retrospective study of 186 patients with 191 lesions performed complete excision in 77% of their patients with a 17% recurrence rate and minimal morbidity. It was concluded that observation with expectant management is safe and advisable in some cases to achieve a safer complete resection. Disadvantages of expectant management include possible complications such as hemorrhage, frequent follow-up, and the need for biopsy to rule out pre-malignant or malignant conditions. Expectant management is also advised initially for recurrent lesions; spontaneous regression was noted in 12% of patients who had a recurrence after initial complete excision. They also noted that the type of procedure and the site of the lesion were important factors in the recurrence rate. Neck lesions had a fairly low recurrence rate after complete excision (12%) and internally located lesions, other than head, trunk, and extremities, had the lowest recurrence. Aspiration, intralesional injection of bleomycin, Ethibloc, or OK-432, and laser excision were associated with high recurrence rates.[20]

CYSTIC HYGROMA

Presentation and Clinical Course

Cystic hygromas classically appear in the cervical, axillary, and inguinal areas. These macrocystic lymphangiomas are dysplasias that arise from the sequestration of lymphatic tissue that fails to communicate with the vascular tree. Grossly, these lesions are multilobular and multilocular cystic masses. Microscopically, the cyst wall consists of a single layer of flattened endothelium. In children afflicted with this condition, the cystic hygromas are present in 50-60% of infants at birth, and at least 90% are present by the end of the second year of life. They occur equally in males and females, except for inguinal hygromas, which are five times more common in males.[19]

The lymphovascular system begins to develop at the end of the 5th week of gestation, approximately 2 weeks after the cardiovascular system. There are 6 primary lymph sacs: 2 jugular sacs near the junction of the subclavian veins with anterior cardinal veins (the future internal jugular veins); 2 iliac lymph sacs; 1 retroperitoneal lymph sac near the root of the mesentery; and the cisterna chyli dorsal to the retroperitoneal lymph sac. The connection of the embryonic lymph system to the venous system is completed at 8 weeks gestation. Maternal-fetal ultrasound has allowed cystic hygromas to be identified early in gestation and to be followed. Nuchal cystic hygroma, when present at the time of a second-trimester scan, has a strong association with aneuploidy, 45X, trisomy 21 and trisomy 18. When a normal karyotype is present, the cystic hygroma may signal the presence of a single gene disorder such as Noonan syndrome, Robert's syndrome, or polysplenia syndrome. It is likely that many cystic hygromas associated with both Turner's and Noonan's syndromes regress; this regression may explain the webbed neck observed in children with these conditions.[21]

Cervical cystic hygroma presenting late in gestation, generally is not associated with hydrops or other anomalies. Patients should be advised about the prognosis according to category: (1) 1st trimester diagnosis with karyotypic abnormality-59% chance of poor outcome; (2) 1st trimester diagnosis without karyotypic abnormality-89% chance of reaching viability with dysmorphic sequelae occurring in 20%; (3) 2nd and 3rd trimester diagnosis (before 30 weeks) guarded; and (4) 3rd trimester diagnosis after 30 weeks gestation - good prognosis.[21] Seventy five percent of cystic hygromas are seen in the neck, 20% in the axilla, and the remaining 5% are distributed throughout the body in the mediastinum, retroperitoneum, and groin. The majority of cystic hygromas affecting the neck occur in the posterior triangle. Those occurring in the anterior triangle are often associated with intraoral lymphangiomas, and are the ones most prone to cause pharyngeal compression and airway compromise. The presenting complaint is a soft mass in the posterior triangle of the neck. They are transilluminant unless intracyst hemorrhage has occurred. The characteristic location and consistency of these lesions allow easy differentiation from other cervical masses.

Hayward et al reported 2 cases in which infants presented with congenital cervicothoracic masses. Both were initially diagnosed as having lymphatic malformations (cystic hygroma) based on history, physical findings, radiologic assessment and in one instance, biopsy. Subsequent excision showed both lesions to be congenital fibrosarcomas. These cases emphasize that rare congenital tumors can mimic the clinical and radiological appearance of the relatively common lymphatic malformation. The authors concluded that a congenital lesion that does not fit the classic history and physical findings of a vascular or lymphatic anomaly should be imaged radiologically and biopsied.[22]

Lymphatic malformations generally grow at a rate proportionate to that of the child. These lesions can enlarge suddenly due to infection or intralesional bleeding. Of all cervical hygromas, 2-3 % are associated with mediastinal extension. All patients with cervical cystic hygromas should have a preoperative chest X-ray to determine mediastinal involvement.[19] (Figs 98.9 and 98.10).

Treatment

Prenatal ultrasound and MRI provide information regarding compression and obstruction of the fetal airway by neck masses.[23] This information is useful in determining if a controlled delivery with ex utero intrapartum treatment is necessary. The EXIT (ex utero intrapartum treatment) procedure was designed initially for reversal of tracheal occlusion performed in fetuses with severe congenital diaphragmatic hernias. This procedure ensures a stable fetal

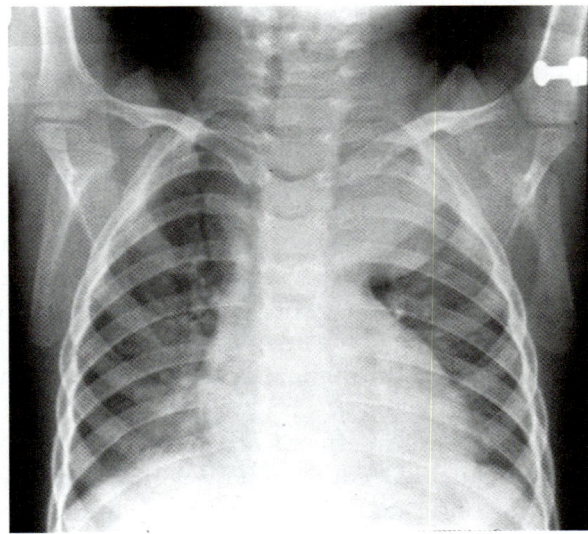

Fig. 98.9: CXR showing mediastinal extension of a cystic hygroma

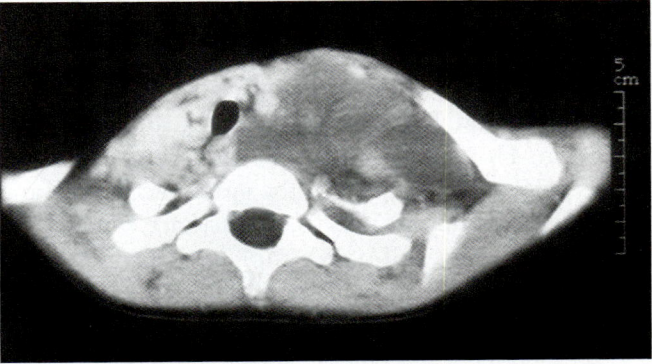

Fig. 98.10: CT scan showing mediastinal extension of a cystic hygroma

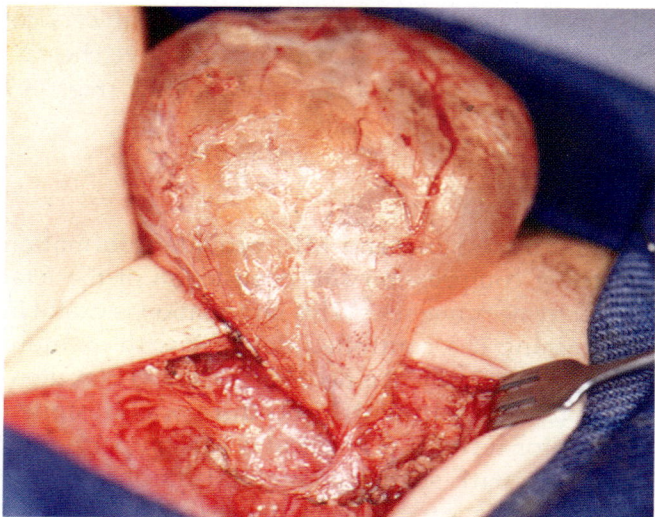

Fig. 98.11: Operative view of cystic hygroma

hemodynamic environment on uteroplacental bypass and has been applied to the management of fetal neck masses. This procedure has proved successful in establishing an airway in patients with potentially catastrophic airways. During the EXIT procedure, deep inhalational anesthesia is used to maintain uterine relaxation and preserve uteroplacental gas exchange. The duration of placental support required will vary according to the interventions performed on the fetus, e.g. endotracheal intubation or tracheostomy.[24]

Excision is the treatment of choice and the only effective available treatment (Fig. 98.11). Operative treatment is indicated whenever one of these lesions is encountered because of the risks of spontaneous infection, progressive growth leading to disfigurement with extension into uninvolved areas, and the possibility of airway obstruction and dysphagia. A cystic hygroma is not a malignant neoplasm and normal structures should not be sacrificed in the course of the operation. Postoperative complications include infection, Horner's syndrome, recurrent laryngeal nerve palsy, and damage to the spinal accessory and marginal mandibular nerves. Recurrence rate of 10% is expected as a result of incomplete excision.[19]

REFERENCES

1. Pasyk KA, Cherry GW, Grabb WC, Sasaki GH. Quantitative evaluation of mast cells in cellularly dynamic and adynamic vascular malformations. Plast reconstr surg 1984;73:69-77.
2. Stal S, Hamilton S, Spira M. Hemangiomas, lymphangiomas, and vascular malformations of the head and neck. Otolaryngol Clin North Am 1986;19:769-96.
3. Drolet BA, Esterly NB, Frieden IJ. Hemangiomas in children. N Engl J Med 1999;341:173-81.
4. Tan OT, Sherwood K, Gilchrest BA. Treatment of children with port-wine stains using the flashlamp-pulsed tunable dye laser. N Engl J Med 1989;320:416-21.
5. Persky MS. Congenital vascular lesions of the head and neck. Laryngoscope 1986;96:1002-15.
6. Pickering JW, Walker EP, Butler PH. The facial distribution of port wine stains on patients presenting for laser treatment. Ann Plast Surg 1991;27:550-52.
7. Mulliken JB. Classification of Vascular Birthmarks. In Mulliken JB and Young, AE (Eds.) Vascular Birthmarks: Hemangiomas and Malformations. Philadelphia: Saunders, 1988.
8. Mulliken JB, Glowacki J. Hemangiomas and vascular malformations in infants and children: A classification based on endothelial characteristics. Plast Reconstr Surg 1982;69:412-22.
9. Burrows PE, Laor T, Paltiel H, Robertson RL. Diagnostic imaging in the evaluation of vascular birthmarks. Dermatol Clin 1998;16:455-488 . Enjolras O, Mulliken JB. The current management of vascular birthmarks. Pediatr Dermatol 1993;10:311.
10. Enjolras O, Riche MC, Merland JJ. Facial port-wine stains and Sturge-Weber syndrome. Pediatrics 76:48-51, 1985.
11. Tang SV, et al. In vivo spectrophotometric evaluation of normal, lesional, and laser-treated skin in patients with port-wine stains. J Invest Dermatol 1983;80:420-23.
12. Stringel G, Dastous J. Klippel-Trenaunay syndrome and other cases of lower limb hypertrophy: Pediatric surgical implications. J Pediatr Surg 1987;22:645.
13. Gloviczki P, Stanson AW, Gunnar BS et al. Klippel-Trenaunay syndrome: The risks and benefits of vascular interventions. Surgery 1991;110:469-79.
14. Woods JE. Extended use of tetradecyl sulfate in treatment of hemangiomas and other related conditions. Plast Reconstr Surg 1987;79:542-49.
15. Goldman MP, et al. Sclerosing agents in the treatment of telangectasia. Comparison of the clinical and histologic effects of intravascular polidocanol, sodium tetradecyl sulfate, and hypertonic saline in the dorsal rabbit ear vein model. Arch Dermatol 1987;123:1196-01.
16. Sexton J, O'Hare, D. Simplified treatment of vascular lesions using the argon laser. J Oral Maxillofac Surg 1993;51:12-16.
17. Rebeiz E, et al Nd-YAG laser treatment of venous malformations of the head and neck: An update. Otolaryngol. Head Neck Surg 1991;105:655-61.
18. Garden JM, Polla LL , Tan OT. The treatment of port-wine stains by the pulsed dye laser. Arch Dermatol 1988;124:889-96.

19. Arensman RM, Statter MB. Vascular and Lymphatic Anomalies of Childhood. In Nyhus LM, Baker RJ, and Fischer JE (Eds.) Mastery of Surgery. Boston: Little, Brown, and Company 1997.
20. Alqahtani A, Nguyen LT, Flageole H, et al. 25 years' experience with lymphangiomas in children. Journal of Pediatric Surgery 1999;34:1164-68.
21. Trauffer MP, Anderson CE, Johnson A, et al. The natural history of euploid pregnancies with first-trimester cystic hygromas. American Journal of Obstetrics and Gynecology 1994;170:1279-84.
22. Hayward PG, Orgill DP, Mulliken JB, et al. Congenital fibrosarcoma masquerading as lymphatic malformation: report of two cases. Journal of Pediatric Surgery 1995;30:84-88.
23. Katharn N, Bulas DI, Newman KD, et al. MRI imaging of fetal neck masses with airway compromise: utility in delivery planning. Pediatric Radiology 2001;31:727-31.
24. Bouchard S, Johnson MP, Flake AW, et al. The EXIT procedure: experience and outcome in 31 cases. Journal of Pediatric Surgery 2002;37:418-26.

Picibanil (OK-432) in Lymphangiomas

DK Gupta, Shilpa Sharma

Lymphangioma is an entity caused due to anomalous lymphatic channels that are in close proximity to the vital structures like major vessels and nerves. Surgical excision in toto is associated with a high risk of damage to the facial nerves that leaves behind a disfigured face that is not acceptable by the patient as well as the surgeon. This has led to development of alternative methods of treatment of which OK-432 is one. The other aspects of management of lymphangiomas have been discussed in the previous chapter.

LAUNCH OF OK-432

OK-432 was launched after its approval for cancer by the Japanese Ministry of Health and Welfare in 1975, and was approved by this Ministry for the additional indication of lymphatic malformation in 1995.

OK-432 contains Lyophilized powder of Streptococcus pyogenes (A group, type 3) Su strain cells treated with benzylpenicillin. As components of culture medium in the manufacturing process, materials derived from bovine heart, bovine skeletal muscle, bovine bone marrow, bovine fat tissue, bovine connective tissue, and bovine milk, and materials derived from porcine heart, porcine pancreas, and porcine stomach are used. It was recognized as a potent biological response modifier.[1]

OK-432 IN LYMPHANGIOMA

In 1986, Professor Shuhie Ogita* used OK-432 in cystic lymphangioma and published their results in 1987.[2] (Fig. 99.1). Most of the published work on the use of OK-432 in lymphangioma has been accredited to him.[3-6]

MECHANISM OF ACTION IN LYMPHANGIOMA

The local administration of this product into lymphangioma induces inflammatory reactions, causes the induction of macrophages and induces the production of cytokines such as TNF. All inflammation mediated cytokines are involved. OK-432 increases the permeability of endothelial cells. This series of events accelerates the excretion of lymph, thus reducing the size of lymphatic vascular lumen (humans). The sclerosis of the cyst wall causes decreased production of cyst fluid and increased permeability of the endothelial cells causes increased collateral lymph drainage. The seepage of fluid thus causes shrinkage of the cyst. There is a difference in the response rate between cystic and cavernous lymphangiomas (Fig. 99.2). Figure 99.3 depicts the mechanism of action.

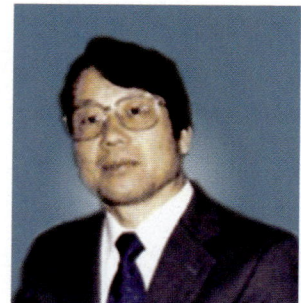

Fig. 99.1: Late Shuhei Ogita

---

*This chapter is dedicated to Late Dr Shuhei Ogita, the man who is credited with the use of OK-432 in pediatric lymphangioma

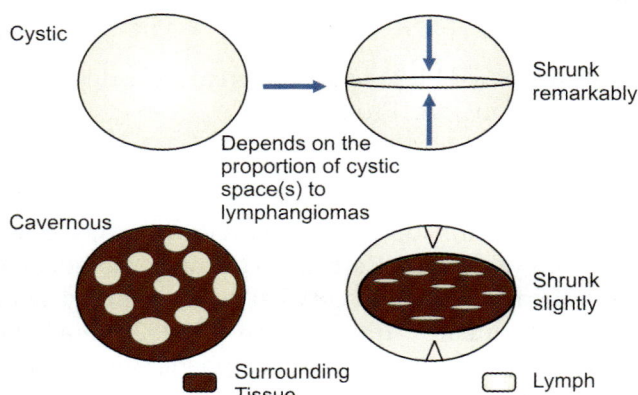

Fig. 99.2: The response rate in cystic lymphangiomas is much better than in cavernous lymphangiomas *(Courtesy: S. Ogita, Kyoto, Japan)*

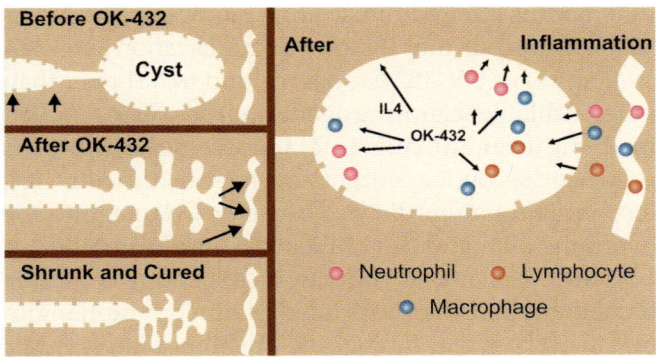

Fig. 99.3: OK-432 Therapy: Results and speculation *(Courtesy: from S. Ogita, Kyoto, Japan)*

Dosage and Administration of OK-432 for Treatment Lymphatic Malformation

OK-432 is suspended in isotonic sodium chloride solution to prepare 0.05-0.1 KE/ml solutions. As a general rule, the dosage equals the amount of aspirated fluid collected from lymphatic malformation. The maximum dosage is 2 KE/injection. The dosage may be adjusted depending on the patient's age and symptoms. In this context, generally, 1-5 KE Picibanil injection is enough for a course of treatment per lymphatic malformation patient. [1.0 KE (Klinische einheit/clinical unit) = 0.1 mg (dried bacterial cells)] It is usually supplied in 1 KE vials of OK-432, and the 5 vials/box package. The expiration date is two years from production.

Some have given the injection under ultrasonography guidance to yield good response without complications. Depending on the size, location, and anatomical relationship of the airway while others have even used general anesthesia.[7,8]

PRECAUTIONS

Due to the known sensitivity toward OK-432, it is advisable to start treatment with a low dose and gradually increase the dose while monitoring the patient's condition.

As shock may rarely occur, the patients or their relatives should be well informed and a consent taken before administration. Facilities for emergency care should be available to ensure that patients can be treated immediately after the onset of shock. It is advisable to perform a skin test with a diluted solution of benzylpenicillin before the administration of this product. During administration, the general condition of patients should be closely monitored. If any abnormalities are observed, the administration should be immediately discontinued and appropriate measures taken.

OK-432 is a preparation of whole bacterial cells that are incapable of growing in any culture media, and is to be administered repeatedly. Therefore, it should be administered with care while monitoring for the onset of adverse reactions. The dose should be minimized and the patient carefully observed since postinjection local swelling may cause a compression of the trachea or stridor (especially injection into the neck).

The injection should not be injected at innervated sites. If insertion of the injection needle evokes intense pain, or if blood flows back into the syringe, the needle should be withdrawn immediately and injected at a different site. Intramuscular injection to infants and children should be kept to the absolute minimum. After administration of OK-432, the patient should be carefully monitored. After a drug-free period, OK-432 should be administered with care starting with a low dose. The risk of malign diseases has to be excluded before the commencement of the Picibanil treatment.[9]

CONTRAINDICATIONS

OK-432 is contraindicated in patients with a history of shock caused by OK-432 or benzylpenicillin. A history of hypersensitivity to OK-432 or other penicillin antibiotics is a relative contraindication. OK-432 should be administered carefully in patients with cardiac or renal diseases or in patients with a personal or familial predisposition to allergic reactions such as bronchial asthma, rash or urticaria.

ADVERSE REACTIONS

The reported adverse reactions during treatment of Lymphangioma include swelling and redness, fever, pain and tenderness. The major abnormal laboratory values were increased WBC in 64% and increased CRP in 71.8%.

Major Adverse Reactions

1. *Shock:* Since shock may occur, patients should be closely monitored. If any abnormalities are observed, the administration of this product should be discontinued and appropriate measures taken.
2. *Interstitial pneumonia:* Since interstitial pneumonia may occur or be exacerbated, patients should be closely monitored. If abnormalities such as fever, cough, dyspnea and abnormal chest X-ray findings, are observed, the administration of this product should be discontinued and appropriate measures taken (e.g. administration of adrenocorticotropic hormone).
3. *Acute renal failure:* Since acute renal failure may occur, patients should be closely monitored. When abnormalities such as increased BUN or creatinine, or decreased urinary output are observed, the administration of this product should be discontinued and appropriate measures should be taken.
4. Delayed shock occuring up to several hours after high-dose administration by intralesional or intracavity injection has been reported.

Minor Adverse Reactions

When the following adverse reactions are observed, appropriate measures such as dosage reduction or discontinuation should be taken.

Hypersensitivity– Purpura, Itching, rash, local reactions

Regional– Pain, swelling/redness, feeling of warmth, induration.

Fever

General– malaise, headache, arthralgia.

Hematologic– Leucocytosis, Thrombocytosis, increased CRP, anemia

Hepatic– Increased enzymes

Gastrointestinal– Anorexia, nausea,/vomiting, diarrhea, etc.

Renal– Increased BUN, increased creatinine, decreased urinary output, etc. Proteinuria.

RESULTS

The application of OK-432 (Picibanil) has been described as safe and effective primary method for sclerotherapy of benign cervical cysts by many with excellent results.[9-11] Intralesional OK-432 therapy is effective for most unresectable lymphangiomas.[3] Local swelling should be anticipated, especially when treating lesions near the upper airway.[10]

The rate of effectiveness in treating patients of lymphangioma with 0.5 KE/10 ml or 1.0 KE/10 ml, two months after administration has been reported as 53-75.5% and six months after administration as 85.4%.

The use of OK-432 has been found to be better than other available sclerosing agents that has often resulted in disfigurement due to extensive scarring, thus rendering secondary surgery even more difficult.[7] The local inflammation did not cause any damage to the overlying skin and did not lead to scar formation.[3]

There are many reports of excellent cosmetic outcome.[12] Some authors have grouped lymphangiomas according to radiological appearance into 4 types: single cystic, macrocystic microcystic, and cavernous.[13]

In a series of 128 patients with lymphangioma treated with OK-432, the effectiveness was 90.9%, 100%, 68.0%, and 10.0% for single cystic, macrocystic microcystic, and cavernous types respectively.[13] Thus they recommended OK-432 injection therapy alone for single cystic, and macrocystic types and surgical excision after pretreatment with OK-432 for microcystic and cavernous types.[13]

Cystic lymphatic vascular malformations are benign lesions that can cause disfigurement and functional impairment.[14] Complete surgical resection is often difficult, and clinical recurrence is common.[14] Sclerotherapy has been used as an alternative to excision. OK-432 is an excellent treatment for patients with macrocystic lymphatic malformations. However, it is ineffective for microcystic lesions.[14]

86% of patients with predominantly macrocystic lymphangiomas had a successful outcome in a multi institutional study.[15]

AIIMS EXPERIENCE WITH PICIBANIL[16,17]

From 1996 to 2001, 54 patients were treated with OK-432. Of these, 47 cases had the cystic variety of lymphangioma. The age range was between day 1 of life upto 10 years.

The investigations done prior to injection of OK-432 included an ultrasound and a CT Scan or MRI. A cavitogram was done to see the presence of hemangiomatous component. The response was described as excellent: Complete Response, Good : > 50% response, Fair : < 50 % response and Poor : no response. The site of the lymphangioma is given in Table 99.1.

Response

There was an onset of fever that started after 6 hours of injection and lasted for 2-4 days. There was local inflammatory reaction with pain and local erythema that subsided in few days. If there was no response to the first dose, a repeat dose was given on the seventh day. If there was local inflammatory response that was seen in 80 % cases, the dose was repeated, if necessary, after 6 weeks. A maximum of 3 doses was given. The adverse reactions noted is given in Table 99.2.

Results

At 4 weeks after treatment, 16 cases had excellent results (Fig. 99.4). At 8 weeks after treatment, 21 cases had excellent results. At 24 weeks after treatment, 37 cases had excellent results. One patient was lost for follow up.

The best results were seen for single large cystic lymphangioma with a response rate of 80-100%. A poor response was noted in the multicystic variety, cases that were postsurgery, if there was hemangiomatous component or a history of other sclerosants previously.

Conclusions

The response is better if OK-432 is used as an initial therapy. when used as a secondary therapy for postoperative lesions, only 36% showed response. Surgical adhesions prevent diffusion of OK-432 throughout the lesion. No special problems encountered during surgery following failure of OK-432. The advantages over other Selerosants is that there was no skin damage or scar formation.

RARE SITES

Other rare sites where OK-432 has been used for lymphangioma include Orbital and perineal area.[18,19]

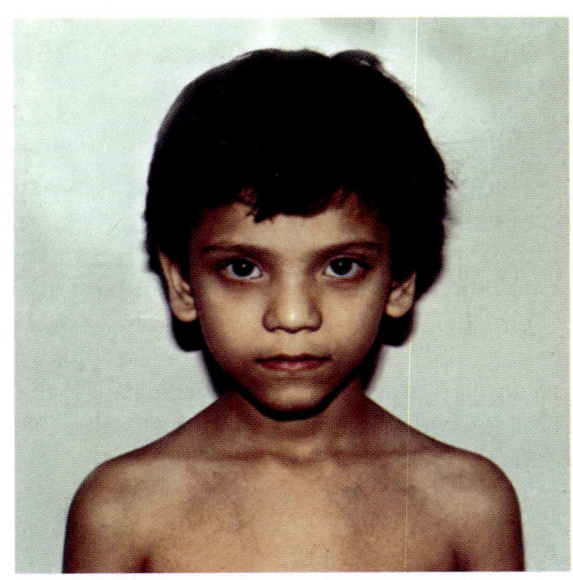

Fig. 99.4: Complete cure of a right cervical lymphangioma after OK-432

Table 99.1: Site of lymphangiomas for OK- 432: N = 54	
Head and neck	31
Cheek, submandibular	13
Axilla, upper arm	2
Interscapular region	3
Breast	1
Nape of neck	2
Tongue and floor of mouth	2

Table 99.2: Adverse reactions noted with OK-432	
Swelling and redness	85 %
Fever	84 %
Local pain	14 %
Tenderness	10 %
Induration	4.3 %
Leucocytosis	64 %
Vesicle formation, Ulceration	Rare
Hypersensitivity, skin rashes	0.18%
Nausea, Malaise, Anorexia	Rare and well tolerated

Orbital Lymphangioma

Surgical excision of orbital lymphangiomas is difficult, and almost always incomplete due to the diffusely infiltrative pattern of these tumors. Successful use of intralesional OK-432 administration to treat two children (1 and 3 years old) with intractable hemorrhagic proptosis due to orbital lymphangiomas has been reported. In both cases, intracystic administration of 0.05 mg of OK-432 in a 1 ml volume resulted in a successful outcome. The adverse effects were minor (mild transient fever and lid swelling), and rebleeding and intraocular pressure elevation did not occur. Proptosis and eyelid swelling gradually improved over 1 month, and completely resolved within 3 months of treatment. Although this drug concentration is higher than in previous reports, there were no major adverse effects.[18]

OTHER DISEASES WHERE OK-432 HAS BEEN USED

Malignancy

OK-432 has been used to prolong survival in patients with gastric cancer or primary lung cancer in combination with chemotherapy, reduction of cancerous pleural effusion or ascites in patients with gastrointestinal cancer or lung cancer, head and neck cancer (maxillary cancer, laryngeal cancer, pharyngeal cancer, and tongue cancer) and thyroid cancer that are resistant to other drugs.[20] Local injection of OK-432 has been reported to be effective as a palliative therapy for recurrent carcinoma esophagus.[21] An 85-year-old man with a massive recurrent tumor of mediastinum 3 years after esophagectomy for squamous cell carcinoma of the intrathoracic esophagus was given endoscopic local injection of OK-432 and lived for two years and three months after recurrence without severe side effects.[21]

Ranula

Intracystic injection therapy with OK-432 is relatively safe and can be used as a substitute for surgery in the treatment of ranulas.[22-24] It has been used both in intraoral type and plunging type of ranula. Aspirated mucus of ranula was replaced with an equal volume of OK-432 solution.[23,24]

Thoracic Duct Cyst

OK-432 therapy has been successfully used for a cervical thoracic duct cyst.[25]

Warts

Warts, recalcitrant to various treatment, including cryotherapy, have been successfully treated with OK-432 injection.[26] The injection has been given both subcutaneously and intralesionally.[26] Complete clearing of the warts has been reported in 75% patients.

Chronic Wound Healing Impairment

OK-432 has been used effectively for the treatment of chronic wound healing impairment. It was used successfully in a 13-year-old girl who suffered a polytrauma with a displaced fracture of the sacrum which required neurosurgical decompression of the sacral plexus that led to a seroma with recurrent fistulation postoperatively.[27] OK-432 was instilled into the wound.[27]

Ganglia

OK-432 injection has also been used as a safe, convenient, and effective alternative to surgical treatment for either symptomatic or recurrent ganglia.[28]

Simple Renal Cysts

Percutaneous treatment of simple renal cysts with OK-432 sclerotherapy was found to be a safe, effective and minimally invasive procedure in a series of 20 patients with 25 symptomatic or large simple cysts.[29] The average reduction was 93.0%. Complete and partial resolution occurred in 44.0% and 52.0% cysts, respectively. Renal pain improved in all patients, regardless of complete or partial resolution. Minor complications occurred in 3 patients, 2 developed leukocytosis and 1 had mild fever following aspiration and sclerotherapy.[29]

Dislocation of the Temporomandibular Joint

Dislocation of the temporomandibular joint has also been treated injection of OK-432 as a sclerosing agent.[30]

Experiment

The author has experience of creating cholangitis-induced liver damage in rats by intraductal injection of OK-432, and studying the response of oral, low-dose methotrexate.[31]

REFERENCES

1. Ishida N, Hoshino T. A Streptococcal Preparation as a Potent Biological Response Modifier OK-432 (ed 2). Amsterdam, The Netherlands, Excerpta Medica, 1985; 60-62.
2. Ogita S, Tsuto T, Tokiwa K, et al. Intracystic injection of OK-432: a new slerosing therapy for cystic hygroma in children. Br J Surg 1987;74:690-91.
3. Ogita S, Tsuto T, Deguchi E, Tokiwa K, Nagashima M, Iwai N. OK-432 therapy for unresectable lymphangiomas in children. J Pediatr Surg 1991;26(3):263-68; discussion 268-70.
4. Ogita S, Tsuto T, Nakamura K, et al. OK-432 therapy in 64 patients with lymphangioma. J Pediatr Surg 1994;29:784-85.
5. Ogita S, Tsunoda A, Okabe I, et al. Phase III study on OK-432 therapy for lymphangioma in children. J Jpn Soc Pediatr Surg 1995:31:1-8.
6. Ogita S, Higuchi K, Kimura O, et al. Therapia con OK-432 en lingangiomas de lengua. Revista Cirugia Infantil 1998; 8: 145-48 (Spanish).
7. Claesson G, Gordon L, Kuylenstierna R. A revolutionary Japanese method for treatment of lymphangioma. Lakartidningen 1998;95:2074-77.
8. Schmidt B, Schimpl G, Höllwarth ME. OK-432 therapy of lymphangiomas in children. Eur J Pediatr 1996;155: 649-52.
9. Knipping S, Goetze G, Neumann K, Bloching M. Sclerotherapy of cervical cysts with Picibanil (OK-432). Eur Arch Otorhinolaryngol 2007;264:423-27.
10. Laranne J, Keski-Nisula L, Rautio R, et al. OK-432 (Picibanil) therapy for lymphangiomas in children. Eur Arch Otorhinolaryngol 2002;259:274-78.
11. Luzzatto C, Lo Piccolo R, Fascetti Leon F, et al. Further experience with OK-432 for lymphangiomas: Pediatr Surg Int 2005;21:969-72.
12. Peral Cagigal B, Serrat Soto A, Calero H, Verrier Hernández A. OK-432 therapy for cervicofacial lymphangioma in adults. Acta Otorrinolaringol Esp 2007; 58:222-24.
13. Okazaki T, Iwatani S, Yanai T, et al. Treatment of lymphangioma in children: our experience of 128 cases. J Pediatr Surg 2007; 42:386-89.
14. Peters DA, Courtemanche DJ, Heran MK, Ludemann JP, Prendiville JS. Treatment of cystic lymphatic vascular malformations with OK-432 sclerotherapy. Plast Reconstr Surg 2006; 118:1441-46.
15. Giguere CM, Bauman NM, Sato Y, et al. Treatment of lymphangiomas with OK-432 (Picibanil) sclerotherapy: a prospective multi-institutional trial. Arch Otolaryngol Head Neck Surg 2002; 128:1137-44.
16. Gupta DK. Efficacy of sclerosing agents in vascular malformations with special reference to role of OK-432. Lecture delivered in Indo-Japan Symposium on Lymphangiomas AIIMS, New Delhi, 1998.
17. Gupta DK. Experience with OK-432 in Pediatric lymphangiomas. Lecture delivered at Clinical Grand Round on congenital vascular malformations at AIIMS, New Delhi, 2002.
18. Yoon JS, Choi JB, Kim SJ, Lee SY. Intralesional injection of OK-432 for vision-threatening orbital lymphangioma. Graefes Arch Clin Exp Ophthalmol 2007 ;245:1031-35.
19. Ahn SJ, Chang SE, Choi JH, Moon KC, Koh JK, Kim DY. A case of unresectable lymphangioma circumscriptum of the vulva successfully treated with OK-432 in childhood J Am Acad Dermatol 2006; 55:S106-07.
20. Uchida A, Micksche M, Hoshino T. Intrapleural administration of OK-432 in cancer patients: Augmentation of autologous tumor killing activity of tumor-associated large granular lymphocytes. Cancer Immunol Immunother 1984;18(1):5-12.
21. Ryutokuji T, Miura A, Izumi Y. A case of recurrent esophageal cancer treated by local injection of OK-432 for 8 months and the patient survived for 2 years and 3 months. Gan To Kagaku Ryoho 2007;34:1988-90.
22. Fukase S, Ohta N, Inamura K, Aoyagi M. Treatment of ranula wth intracystic injection of the streptococcal preparation OK-432. Ann Otol Rhinol Laryngol 2003; 112:214-20.
23. Roh JL. Primary treatment of ranula with intracystic injection of OK-432. Laryngoscope 2006; 116:169-72.
24. Rho MH, Kim DW, Kwon JS, Lee SW, Sung YS, Song YK, Kim MG, Kim SG. OK-432 sclerotherapy of plunging ranula in 21 patients: it can be a substitute for surgery AJNR Am J Neuroradiol 2006;27:1090-95.
25. Miwa T, Tatsutomi S, Tsukatani T, Ito M, Furukawa M. OK-432 therapy for a cervical thoracic duct cyst. Otolaryngol Head Neck Surg 2007; 136:852-53.
26. Inui S, Asada H, Wataya-Kaneda M, Miyamoto T, Itami S, Yoshikawa K. OK-432 therapy for recalcitrant warts. J Dermatol 1997; 24:301-05.
27. Fasching G, Sinzig M. OK-432 as a sclerosing agent to treat wound-healing impairment. Eur J Pediatr Surg 2007; 17:431-32.
28. Hotta T, Kawashima H, Endo N. A painful large ganglion cyst of the ankle treated by the injection of OK-432. Mod Rheumatol 2007;17:341-43.
29. Choi YD, Cho SY, Cho KS, Lee DH, Lee SH. Percutaneous treatment of renal cysts with OK-432 sclerosis. Yonsei Med J 2007; 48:270-73.
30. Matsushita K, Abe T, Fujiwara T. OK-432 (Picibanil) sclerotherapy for recurrent dislocation of the temporomandibular joint in elderly edentulous patients: Case reports. Br J Oral Maxillofac Surg 2007; 45:511-13.
31. Alladi A, Gupta DK, Gupta SD. Evaluation of the protective effect of methotrexate on OK432-induced liver injury in a rat model. Pediatr Surg Int 2003; 19:96-99.

SECTION 7

Pediatric Neurosurgery

CHAPTER 100

Hydrocephalus

DK Gupta, Shilpa Sharma

HISTORICAL BACKGROUND

Hydrocephalus has been described by Hippocrates, Galen, and by early medieval Arabian physicians, who believed that this disease was caused by an extracerebral accumulation of water.[1] Historically, hydrocephalus has been treated by primitive and totally ineffective measures like venesection, tight head bandages, leeching and purgatives. These methods have now been condemned. Evacuation of superficial intracranial fluid in hydrocephalic children was first described in detail in the tenth century by Abulkassim Al Zahrawi. In 1744, LeCat published findings on a ventricular puncture. Effective therapy required aseptic surgery as well as pathophysiological knowledge—both unavailable before the late nineteenth century. In 1881, Wernicke performed a sterile ventricular puncture and external CSF drainage. These were followed in 1891 by serial lumbar punctures (Quincke) and in 1893, by the first permanent ventriculo-subarachnoid-subgaleal shunt (Mikulicz), which was simultaneously a ventriculostomy and a drainage into an extrathecal low pressure compartment. Diversion of the cerebrospinal fluid (CSF) from head into various body cavities was first attempted as early as 1898 and almost all known body cavities have been tried for the same though none seems to be perfect for the purpose.

Between 1898 and 1925, lumboperitoneal, and ventriculoperitoneal, -venous, -pleural, and -ureteral shunts were invented, but these had a high failure rate due to insufficient implant materials in most cases. Ventriculostomy without implants (Anton 1908), with implants and plexus coagulation initially had a very high operative mortality and were seldom successful in the long term, but gradually improved over the next decades.[1] In 1949, Nulsen and Spitz implanted a shunt successfully into the caval vein with a ball valve. Between 1955 and 1960, four independent groups invented distal slit, proximal slit, and diaphragm valves almost simultaneously. Around 1960, the combined invention of artificial valves and silicone led to a worldwide therapeutic breakthrough. After the first generation of simple differential pressure valves, which are unable to drain physiologically in all body positions, a second generation of adjustable, autoregulating, antisiphon, and gravitational valves was developed, but their use is limited due to economical restrictions and still unsolved technical problems. At the moment, at least 127 different designs are available, with historical models and prototypes bringing the number to 190 valves, but most of these are only clones. In the 1990s, there was a renaissance of endoscopic ventriculostomy, which is now widely accepted as the method of first choice in adult patients with aquired or late-onset, occlusive hydrocephalus; in other cases the preference remains controversial.

Hydrocephalus is an entity that has till date no satisfactory treatment in terms of cure and long-term good outcome. The indications for surgical intervention with the insertion of a shunt, the shunt related complications and the ultimate long-term prognosis are still far from satisfactory.

DEFINITION

Hydrocephalus is defined as the dilatation of the cerebral ventricle/s due to accumulation of fluid under pressure caused by an imbalance of CSF production and absorption. This does not include conditions where there is excessive accumulation of CSF within the cranial cavities due to decrease of the cerebral substance resulting in an increase in ventricular size, as in patients with cerebral atrophy (hydrocephalus ex vacuo).

INCIDENCE

The condition is not uncommon with an estimated incidence of infantile hydrocephalus around 3-4 per 1000 live births.[2] Congenital hydrocephalus comprises about 30% of all congenital malformations of the nervous system and is often associated with spina bifida and meningomyelocele (70 %).

PHYSIOLOGY OF CSF FORMATION

The choroid plexus appears as a mesenchymal invagination of the roof of the ventricles at 35 days of gestation. CSF circulation begins at 50th day of gestation.

The amount of CSF is around 150 ml in adults and the amount of CSF produced is 20 ml/hour irrespective of age amounting to around 500 ml/day. 65-80% of this fluid is produced by choroid plexus and 15-30% is secreted by ependymal surfaces of ventricles and arachnoid membranes. Small amount is produced from the brain itself through the perivascular spaces surrounding the blood vessels entering the brain. The rate of CSF production is around 0.02 ml/minute in neonates and the total "ventricular" CSF volume varies between 5-15 ml.

CSF is formed by the choroid plexuses of the lateral, third and fourth ventricles by an active transport process, across the endothelium of capillaries in the villous processes of the choroid plexus.[3] Each villus is lined with a single layer of cuboidal epithelium and has a central stromal core. The apical tight junctions represent the blood-CSF barrier. Na-K ATPase located in the microvilli extrudes sodium ions into the ventricles which osmotically draws water along with it. Na^+ transport is balanced by counter transport of K^+ and/or H^+ ions.[4] Carbonic anhydrase catalyses the formation of bicarbonate inside the cell, with the H^+ ion being fed back to the Na^+ transporter as a counter ion in exchange of K^+.

Acetazolamide and furosemide are diuretics that also decrease secretion of CSF at the level of the choroid plexus.

Carbonic anhydrase catalyzes a reversible reaction in which carbon dioxide becomes hydrated and carbonic acid dehydrated. Acetazolamide is a noncompetitive reversible inhibitor of enzyme carbonic anhydrase, which catalyzes the reaction between water and carbon dioxide, resulting in protons and carbonate. This carbonic anhydrase inhibition in central nervous system retards abnormal and excessive discharge from CNS neurons and thus decreases CSF secretion by choroid plexus (Fig. 100.1). Acetazolamide is also a weak natriuretic which noncompetitively inhibits carbonic anhydrase in the proximal convoluted tubule, preventing the reabsorption of bicarbonate and the excretion of hydrogen ions. The paucity of hydrogen ions in the tubular fluid for exchange with sodium ions prevents the reabsorption of filtered sodium. Hence, an alkaline diuresis rich in sodium and bicarbonate results in hyperchloremia (normal ion gap).

Various osmotic agents like glycerol also have ICP-lowering effects. The solute must be relatively restricted in its entry across the blood brain barrier. An osmotic gradient is necessary to draw water from the brain cell to the site of higher osmolality, the plasma. Once the solute has reached equilibrium in plasma and brain cell, the intracellular volume returns to its initial state and the intracranial pressure returns, to its initial level.

Mechanism of action proposed for Furosemide for lowering ICP include; lowering cerebral sodium uptake, affecting water transport into astroglial cells by inhibiting cellular membrane cation-chloride pump, and decreasing CSF production by inhibiting carbonic anhydrase.

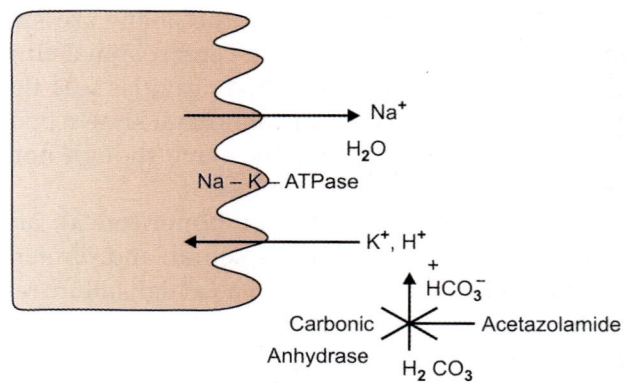

Fig. 100.1: Diagrammatic depiction of mechanism of action of acetazolamide

Furosemide, a loop diuretic is a potent, short acting natriuretic which inhibits sodium reabsorption in the medullary portion of ascending limb of the loop of Henlé by blocking the sodium-potassium-chloride ($Na^+K^+2Cl^-$) cotransporter. This leads to the excretion of 30% of the filtered sodium, as the sodium concentration in the distal nephron is increased; moreover, the sodium concentration in the renal medullary interstitium and peritubular capillaries is decreased, impairing the concentrating ability of the countercurrent multiplier mechanism. The co-dependent reabsorption of calcium and magnesium are inhibited. Potassium and hydrogen ion exchange for sodium in the distal convoluted tubule is increased. Loop diuretics also increase and redistribute renal blood flow and have a systemic venodilatory effect.

CSF FLOW

The CSF secreted in the lateral ventricles passes into the 3rd ventricle and then along the aqueduct of Sylvius into the fourth ventricles. It then passes out of the fourth ventricle through two lateral foramina of Luschka and the midline foramina of Magendie into the Cisterna Magna (Fig. 100.2).

This is continuous with the subarachnoid space that surrounds the entire brain and spinal cord. From the subarachnoid space, the CSF is absorbed into the large sagittal venous sinus and other sinuses by multiple arachnoid villi projecting into the sinuses. Transependymal CSF absorption into capillaries and the lymphatic channels associated with cranial nerves also act as alternate channels for CSF absorption. The optic nerve, the olfactory nerve sheaths and the choroid plexus have also been demonstrated as probable sites of CSF flow and absorption.[1]

The rate of CSF absorption is pressure dependent over a wide physiologic range. CSF formation is independent of pressure whereas the CSF absorption increases linearly after 6.8 cm H_2O pressure.[1] The formation and absorption rates become equal beyond 11.2 cm H_2O pressure. The CSF formation does not diminish significantly until the cerebral perfusion pressure is markedly reduced. It is the change in resistance to CSF absorption that determines CSF pressure and progression of the hydrocephalus. Ongoing research has continued to improve our understanding of the cerebral water circulation and is starting to provide insight into the pathogenesis and potential treatment options of this common group of disorders.[5]

PATHOPHYSIOLOGY

Regardless of the etiology, obstruction of CSF pathways results in a wide spectrum of changes that depend on the age of the patient and the expansibility of skull as well as the duration of the hydrocephalus.

Ventricular enlargement is caused by undamped pulsewave generated by the choroid plexus. The subarachnoid channels are the first CSF compartments to dilate and reduce CSF pressure. Later with progressive dilatation of the subarachnoid channels, the increase in CSF pressure is transmitted to the ventricular system resulting in ventriculomegaly. Ventricular enlargement causes displacement of the primary cerebral arteries and a reduction in the caliber and number of the secondary and tertiary vessels, causing diminished blood flow and ischemia.[6]

Ventriculomegaly causes changes throughout the cerebral cortex and affects the periventricular white matter. The deeper cortical layers are more affected than the superficial laminae, some of these changes may be permanent. Raised intracranial pressure (ICP) increases ventricular size in a newborn child as the brain is incompletely myelinated and the parenchyma is soft and pliable.

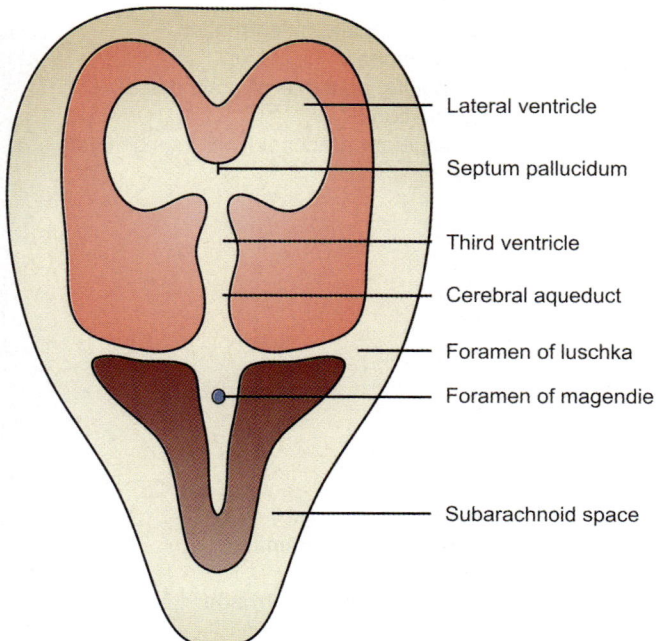

Fig. 100.2: Schematic representation of CSF flow pathways

The effects of raised ICP on the developing brain include:
1. Atrophy of white matter.
2. Stretching and denuding of ependymal epithelium with formation of ventricular diverticula.
3. Spongy edema of the brain parenchyma surrounding the ventricles.
4. Fenestration of the septum pellucidum
5. Thinning and elongation of the interhemispheric commisure.
6. Fibrosis of choroid plexus.

The atrophic process in hydrocephalus involves primarily a destruction of the axons, secondary loss of myelin and chronic astrogliosis. Neurons are selectively spared as grey matter enjoys a more luxuriant blood supply. Thus cerebral mantle thickness is not a reliable prognostic criterion in hydrocephalus. White matter ischemia and periventricular edema can cause porencephalic cavities. Porencephalic cavities and disappearance of the tertiary branches of the anterior and middle cerebral arteries represents irreversible brain damage. CSF drainage has a beneficial effect only till the stage when edema of the white matter and enlargement of the extracellular spaces begins.

ETIOLOGY AND CLASSIFICATION (TABLE 100.1)

Genetic Factors

The most common inherited form of hydrocephalus, X linked hydrocephalus is characterized by mental retardation, adducted thumbs and spastic paraplegia.

Environmental

The incidence of congenital hydrocephalus was more in mothers who received oral contraceptives in first trimester and in families with parental consanguinity.

Table 100.1: Causes of Hydrocephalus

Non-communicating	Communicating

Lesions that obstruct the ventricular system
1. Congenital lesions
    Aqueductal stenosis (0.5-1/1000 live births)
    i. Gliosis
    ii. Forking
    iii. True narrowing
    iv. Septum
    v. X-linked acqueductal stenosis in males
 	
Atresia of foramina of Luschka and Magendie (Dandy-Walker cyst) [2-4/1000 live births]
Atresia of foramen of Monro
Arnold-Chiari malformation
Skull base anomalies
Intrauterine infections
Toxoplasmosis
CMV infection
(b) Neoplastic
    i. Benign intracranial cyst
    ii. Vascular malformation
    iii. Tumors – Medulloblastomas, ependymomas, astrocytomas, craniopharyngiomas
2. Acquired lesions
 	
Aqueductal stenosis (gliosis)
Ventricular inflammations and scars-ventriculitis
Intraventricular hemorrhage Space occupying lesions- neoplastic, masses
	Lesion that obstruct the subarachnoid space
	1. Congenital lesions
	    Arnold-Chiari malformation
	    Encephalocele
	    Dandy Walker malformation
	    Leptomeningeal inflammation
	    Lissencephaly
	    Congenital absence of arachnoidal granulations
	    Incompetent arachnoid villi benign cysts
	
	2. Acquired lesions
	    Leptomeningeal inflammation
	    i. Meningitisii
	    ii. Subarachnoid hemorrhage
	    iii. Chemical arachnoiditis
	    iv. Particulate matter neoplastic
	    v. Posterior fossa tumors platybasia

Hydrocephalus, depending on the site of obstruction, is classically described as:

(i) *Non-communicating:* Blockage of CSF pathway at or proximal to the outlet foramina of the fourth ventricle (Figs 100.3A and B). In non-communicating hydrocephalus CSF flow can take place via the blood vessel adventitia and extracellular space of the cortical mantle to reach the subarachnoid space on the brain surface. These alternate pathways are established with time and lead to an equilibrium between CSF production and absorption.

(ii) *Communicating:* Obstruction located in the basal subarachnoid cisterns, subarachnoid sulci or arachnoid villi (Figs 100.3A and B).

Hydrocephalus can arise as a result of:
1. Obstruction of CSF pathways
2. Impaired venous drainage
3. Overproduction of CSF.

Impaired Venous Drainage

(i) Thrombosis of sinuses, jugular vein or superior *vena cava*
(ii) Tumor invading the sinuses
(iii) High flow arterio-venus malformation.

Overproduction of CSF

(i) Choroid plexus   :   Papilloma
                      :   Carcinoma
(ii) Hypervitaminosis A

In a nationwide survey conducted in Japan to assess the etiology and associated conditions of prenatally and postnatally diagnosed congenital hydrocephalus, destructive cystic lesions, holoprosencephaly, and agenesis of the corpus callosum were found significantly predominant in fetal hydrocephalus.[7] Arachnoid cyst was somewhat predominant in infantile hydrocephalus.[7]

CLINICAL PRESENTATION

There may be a positive history of congenital hydrocephalus in the family or an history of fever in the first trimester or if the child has other associated congenital anomalies like myelomeningocele or spina bifida. There may even be an obstructed labor due to giant hydrocephalus in the fetus.

The signs and symptoms related to hydrocephalus depend on the age of the patient, causative factor, associated malformations and the severity and progression of the disease. Baby may have a big head with no symptoms at all while others may have normal sized head with severe headache.

Infant

The infant with hydrocephalus presents with large head, a full or a bulging anterior fontanelle, poor feeding and lethargy (Fig. 100.4). The anterior fontanelle is examined in the upright position or at a

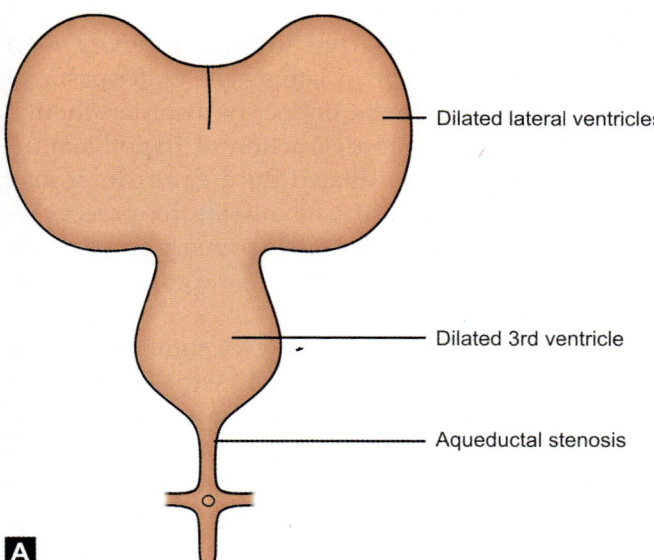
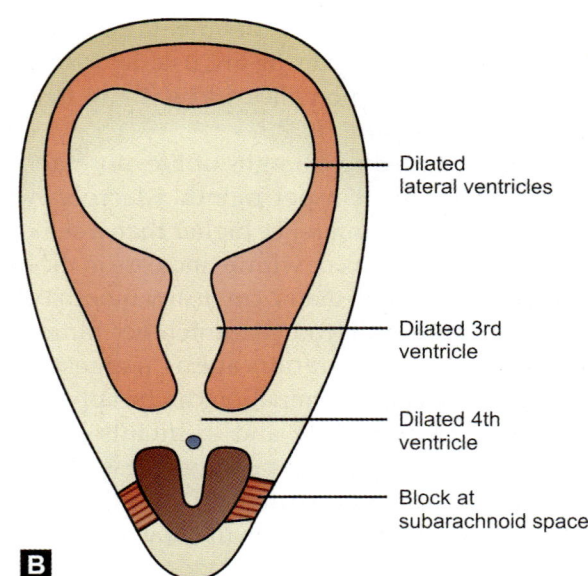

Figs 100.3A and B: Site of block to CSF flow determines nature of hydrocephalus **A.** Non-communicating, **B.** Communicating

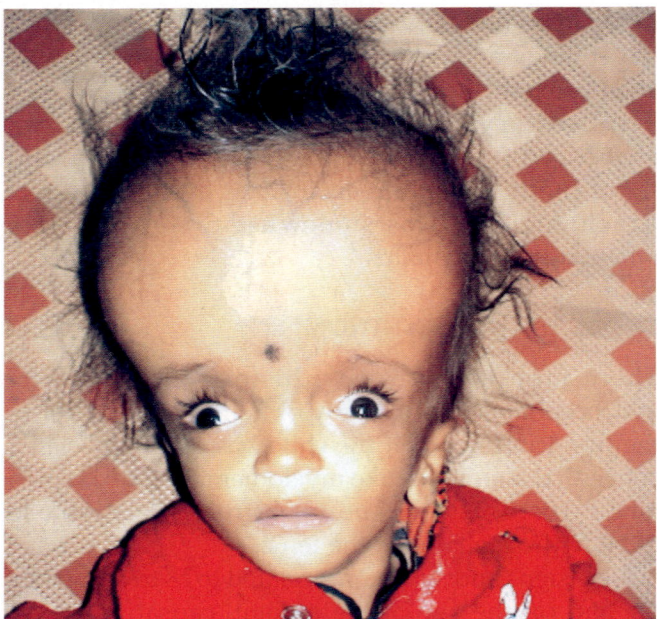

Fig. 100.4: A child with hydrocephalus with shiny veins over the scalp

45° incline. The infant may have sutural diastasis particularly the squamo-parietal suture. This suture should close early after birth and its diastasis after birth suggests presence of hydrocephalus. The other signs of hydrocephalus include thin scalp with visible veins, Parinaud's phenomenon (sun set sign caused by pressure on the tectal plate) and Macewan's sign (cracked pot resonance). Vascular lesions can be suspected if cranial bruits are audible. The infant will have delayed milestones and difficulty in head control. Apneic bouts and bradycardia are usually associated with posterior fossa anomalies and with an increase in intracranial pressure (ICP).

During the first three months of life, normal head growth velocity is 2 cm per month. Macrocrania is defined as head circumference higher than 2 standard deviation above normal, or with an increase in the head circumference by more than 2 cm in any month before the fusion of sutures. Head circumference more than 97th percentile for gestation age is suggestive of hydrocephalus. Transillumination can be appreciated in cases of hydrancephaly and in infants less than 9 months of age with a cerebral mantle less than 1cm. Bobble head doll syndrome with forward and backward nodding movements may be seen. Cranial nerve palsies especially lateral gaze palsy (VI nerve involvement) and stridor may also be seen in infants. Visual tracking disorders seen in hydrocephalus could be caused by oculomotor palsy. There may also be cortical blindness as a result of stretching of the optic radiations by the lateral ventricles. The discrepancy between head and chest circumference may suggest hydrocephalus. Normally the head measures about 1 cm more than the chest circumference until late in the first year when it reverses. An older child upto 2 years of age may present as an irritable child with alteration in the development of intelligence, affecting verbal capabilities more than nonverbal ones.

Older Child

The inability of the fused cranium to expand causes the older children more than 2 years of age, to have a more acute presentation. The triad of severe headache, vomiting and lethargy is commonly seen. The headache at first sporadic may become persistent and severe enough to awaken the child from sleep. It may be accompanied by typically early-morning abdominal pain with nausea and vomiting. Visual disturbances and papilledema is commonly seen in children unlike infants. Delayed motor and cognitive development and subtle behavioral changes are noted. A mild spastic diplegia with positive Babinski sign can also be elicited. A decline in school performance as well as memory loss may be seen. The presence of frank neurological signs usually reflects a primary pathologic condition. The other indicators of hydrocephalus include decreased active leg motion, poor placing and positive support reflexes. Gait disturbance may occur in late stages with spasticity involving the lower limbs. Endocrine disorders though rare may occur due to distraction of hypothalamus and pituitary stalk by dilated third ventricle. It may be in the form of obesity, small stature, precocious puberty, adiposogenital atrophy, primary amenorrhea or diabetes inspidus. Seizures are a common presentation due to raised ICP.

The shape of the skull may give some clue to the cause of the hydrocephalus. The expansion of the supratentorial compartment with a small posterior fossa, is characterisitic of Aqueductal stenosis while the ballooning of the whole head with predominance of posterior fossa is suggestive of the Dandy – Walker syndrome.

The sunset sign is most commonly seen in acqueductal obstruction in juxtaposition to the mesencephalic tectum.

DIFFERENTIAL DIAGNOSIS

1. Familial big head or constitutional macrocrania
2. Hydrancephaly–Transillumination may be marked in hydrancephaly
3. Subdural fluid–Hygroma, Hematoma, Effusion
4. Brain edema
   - Toxic, e.g. Lead encephalopathy
   - Endocrine, e.g. Galactosemia
5. Gigantism
6. Achondroplastic dwarfism
7. Leukodystrophy, e.g. Alexander's disease
8. Lysozymal disorders
9. Aminoaciduria
10. Thickened skull, e.g. Thalassemia, cranioskeletal dysplasia.

INVESTIGATIONS

The investigations are done to establish the diagnosis, evaluate the etiology of hydrocephalus and assess the progress with treatment. From a pediatric surgeon's point of view, based on the history and clinical examination, it is vital to judge whether the hydrocephalus has an infective origin or not. If there has been a history of meningitis associated fever in the past, an infective pathology is suggested.

Ultrasonography

Routine prenatal ultrasonography is an effective measure for antenatal detection of hydrocephalus.[8-10]

A transfontanellar ultrasound is the first investigation for an infant with accessible anterior fontanelle, being simple and noninvasive way of visualizing the ventricular dilatation. It can pick up the size of the ventricles as well as the presence of debris in infected cases. It is also useful for follow up screening. Ultrasonography is less accurate for evaluating posterior fossa anomalies, vascular lesions and neoplasms. The foramen magnum has been suggested as an alternative window besides the anterior fontanelle to evaluate posterior fossa lesions.

Doppler Studies

Doppler USG studies are very informative to assess the severity of the hydrocephalus by measuring the flow resistance index.

Transcranial doppler flow studies have shown a correlation between intracranial pressure and resistive indices in the middle cerebral artery and anterior cerebral artery. The normal mean resistive index in a newborn is 0.75 and found to be significantly higher in hydrocephalics (0.80).[11] The resistive index returns to normal after an effective shunt surgery.

PET scanning has shown that cerebral blood flow and regional cerebral metabolic rate of oxygen values indicate decreased metabolic activity in the developing hydrocephalic brain.[12] The values increase following shunt surgery.

Trans-systolic time (TST) is a new Doppler index used to evaluate intracranial pressure.[13] TST is the width of the systolic peak at the level of the mean of the peak systolic and end diastolic velocity. An increase in intracranial pressure results in a decrease in TST and vice versa.

Fundus Evaluation

This is an important tool to assess severity of the raised intracranial pressure. This is especially good for follow up for cases kept on medical management. It is useful in older children as a screening tool and may defer the repeated CT scan examination done during follow up. Changes on fundal examination are an indication for shunt placement for a patient on medical management. Fundus changes may occur in the form of papilledema, temporal pallor and primary optic atrophy.

Papilledema is a, non-inflammatory passive swelling of the optic disk, produced by raised intracranial tension. It occurs as a result of interrupted axoplasmic flow in the optic nerve due to transmitted elevated cerebrospinal fluid pressure in the subarachnoid space around it. This in turn causes venous congestion. Papilledema is one of the causes of "disk-edema", and they are not synonymous.

As a rule, papilledema does not develop if the optic nerve has already become atrophic, in congenital absence of arachnoidal sheath and in opto chiasmatic arachnoiditis or other forms of basal meningitis due to tuberculosis, etc.

Any intra-cranial tumor may induce papilledema. It is most evident with tumors in the posterior fossa which obstruct the aqueduct of Sylvius, and least with pituitary tumors. The site of the tumors is, thus, more important than its nature, its size and rate of growth.

The Ophthalmoscopic features in the different stages of the disease are:

(a) *Early papilledema:* Earliest change is disc hyperemia and dilated capillaries. Blurring of disc margins, spontaneous venous pulsation is absent (this may be absent in 20 % of normal population.) Splinter hemorrhages at or just off the disk-margin.

(b) *Established papilledema:* Disk margins become indistinct and central cup is obliterated. Disc surface is elevated above the retinal plane (more than + 3D (1mm) with direct ophthalmoscope). Peripapillary edema.[Paton's lines, present temporal to the disk]. Venous engorgement. Flame-shaped hemorrhages and 'cotton-wool' spots around the disk. Hard exudates in radiating pattern around the macula, [macular star]

(c) *Chronic papilledema:* Disk edema resolves, but margins are blurred. Hemorrhagic and exudative components gradually resolve. Optik disk appears pale like a champagne cork. White spots–corpora amylacea may be seen on the disk.

(d) *Atrophic papilledema* : Peripapillary retinal vessels are attenuated and sheathed. Dirty-white appearance of the optic disk, due to reactive gliosis-leading to secondary optic atrophy.

CSF Evaluation

CSF examination is warranted only if an infective pathology is suspected. CSF examination for protein and cell content is important prior to shunt placement in post meningitic hydrocephalus. Fat laden cells are indicative of brain damage in post infection states and can also be evaluated by CSF examination.[14] Experimentally, CSF biogenic amine, myelin basic protein, lactate:pyruvate ratio and cyclic nucleotide levels have all been used as indicators of cerebral injury implying progressive hydrocephalus.

Computed Tomography

CT scanning is useful to evaluate macrocrania or signs of raised intracranial pressure for comparisons during the course of the disease. The cause and site of obstruction can usually be defined and with contrast enhancement tumors as well as vascular lesions can be visualised. Dilatation of the temporal horns is a sensitive indicator of raised intracranial pressure. The presence of periventricular edema or ooze suggests high intracranial pressure but this sign may be absent in cases of shunt failure associated with high intracranial pressure. CT scan imaging gives a quantitative assessment of ventricular dilatation and its topography (Figs 100.5A and B). Aqueductal stenosis can be appreciated with dilatation of the lateral ventricles and third ventricle without dilatation of the fourth ventricle. Presence of periventricular lucency representing egression of fluid from the ventricles is an important sign (Fig. 100.6). CT scan also helps to differentiate other causes of macrocrania like hydrancephaly and also identify cases with leucodystrophy that give a picture of dilated ventricles simulating hydrocephalus (Figs 100.7 and 100.8).

The earliest sign of neonatal or infantile hydrocephalus is dilatation of occipital horns and atria of the lateral ventricles, followed by blunting of the dorsolateral angles of the ventricles above the caudate nuclei and the thalami.[15] The diagnosis of hydrocephalus is established when the bifrontal ventricular width expressed as a percentage of the brain width (ventricle skull ratio (VSR)) exceeds 35 percent. Calcification in tumors or periventricular cytomegalovirus inclusions and toxoplasmosis can be diagnosed (Figs 100.9A and B). The risk of repeated CT Scans for these children has been studied. The mean effective dose, lens dose and brain dose to children over 6 months of age were 1.2 mSv, 52 mGy and 33 mGy, respectively, and the corresponding doses to younger children were 3.2 mSv, 60 mGy and 48 mGy. The effective dose per CT examination varied by a factor of 64.[16] However, since the threshold for radiation-induced damage is not known with certainty, alternative modalities such as US and MRI should be used whenever possible.[16]

Magnetic Resonance Imaging

MRI is considered by some as the investigation of choice as it enables a pathophysiological approach to understanding the hydrodynamic disorder through the analysis of CSF fluid and the volumes of different intracranial components. MR measurement of total intracranial CSF volume may function as the "Gold standard" when making comparisons is time. The axial, coronal and saggital images available with MRI provide a more exact position and extent of the

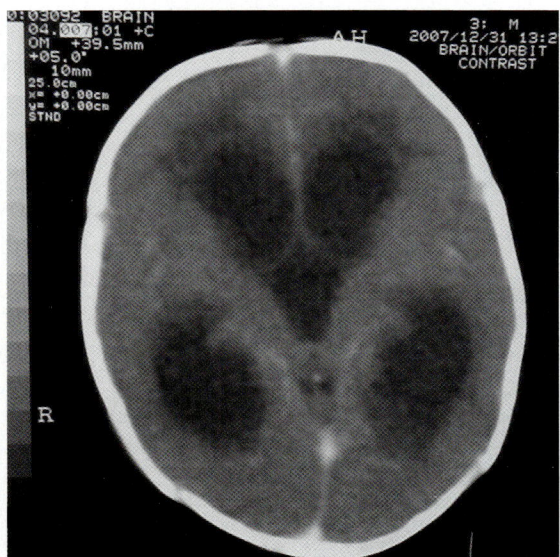

Fig. 100.5A: NCCT head of a child with congenital hydrocephalus showing dilated lateral and third ventricles

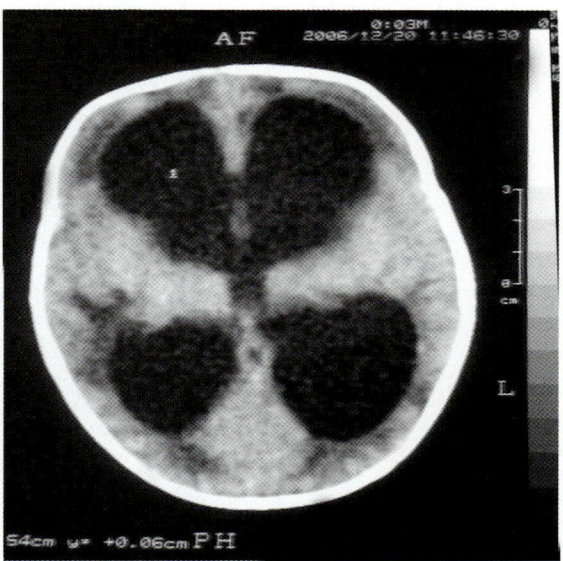

Fig. 100.5B: CT scan of a child showing dilated lateral and third ventricles. The fourth ventricle was also dilated suggestive of communicating hydrocephalus

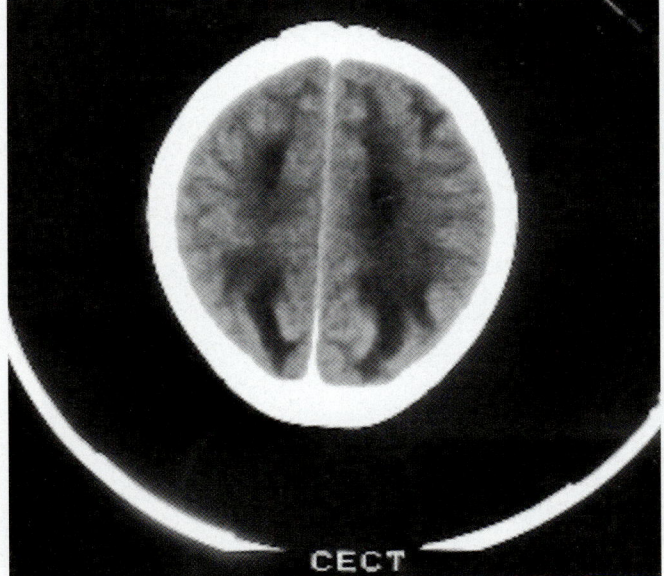

Fig. 100.6: CT scan of a child showing presence of periventricular lucency representing egression of fluid from the ventricles

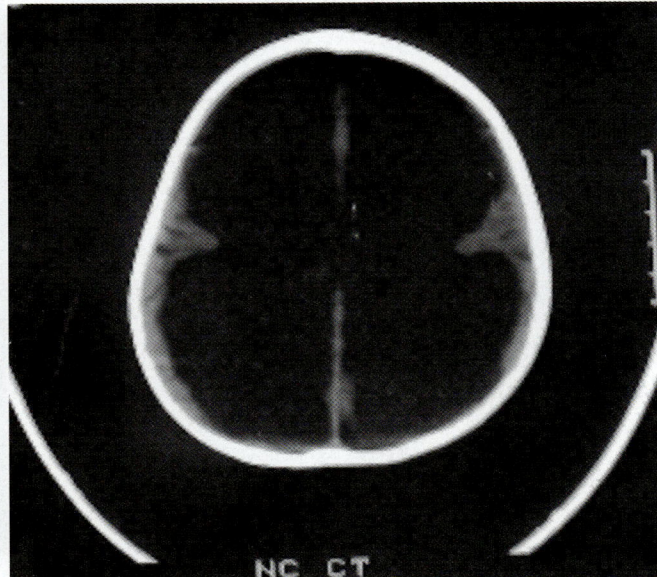

Fig. 100.7: CT scan of a child showing very poor cortical tissue and almost the whole cranial cavity filled with cerebrospinal fluid suggestive of hydrancephaly

lesion (Fig. 100.10). More subtle findings such as white matter pathology and dysmorphic anatomy can be demonstrated. The advent of magnetic resonance angiography has made it the ideal investigation to evaluate vascular lesions. Phase contrast cine magnetic resonance imaging technique is used to study CSF flow dynamics and is particularly useful to evaluate CSF flow following third ventriculostomy. The diagnosis of acqueductal stenosis made earlier by exclusion can now be confirmed on a 2D cine phase contrast MR.[9,17] MRI can also locate small tumors in the upper cord and brainstem which may be missed on a CT scan.

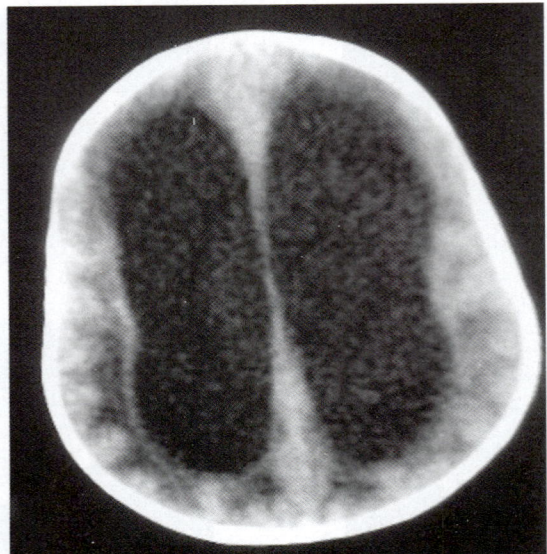

Fig. 100.8: CT scan depicting leucodystrophy

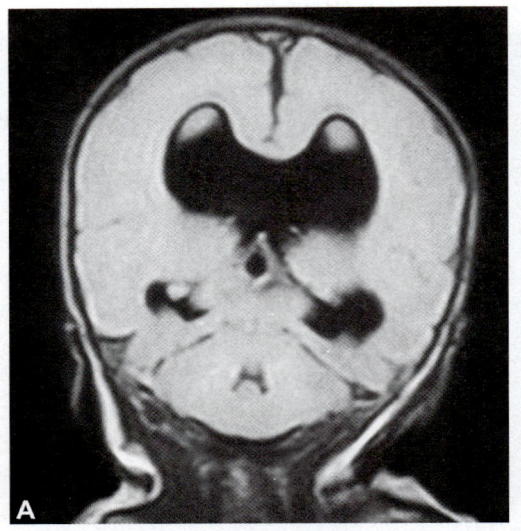
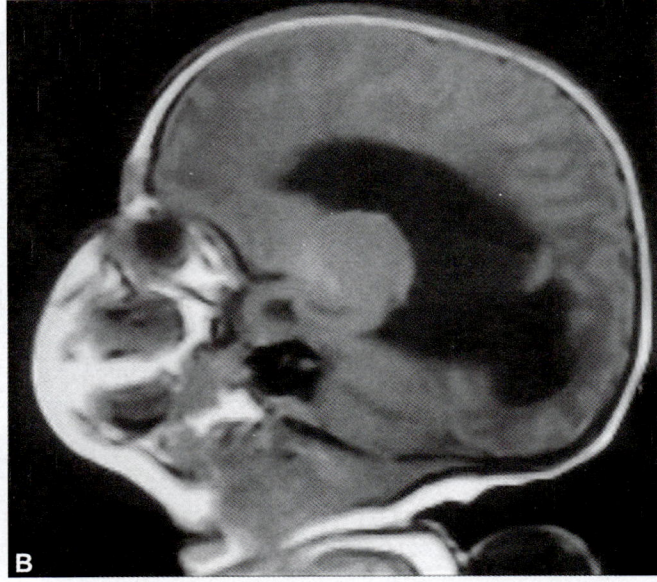

Figs 100.9A and B: MRI scan of a child with lumbar meningomyelocele and hydrocephalus.
A. Coronal section **B.** Sagittal section

ICP Measurement

This investigation is not recommended as a diagnostic tool in children. It is an invasive technique and may be performed in children only preoperatively in the operating room to measure the ventricular pressure and thereby decide the type of shunt required. In normal pressure hydrocephalus ICP monitoring showed that children who benefited with shunt placement demonstrated plateau waves and episodic increases in ICP during REM sleep. Progressive hydrocephalus is suggested if ICP monitoring shows prolonged pressure waves, frequent short term waves and augmented pulsatile indices which basically imply poor ventricular compliance.[18]

Noninvasive ICP monitoring involves assessment of ICP via a transducer placed over the anterior fontanelle. Recently it has been demonstrated that

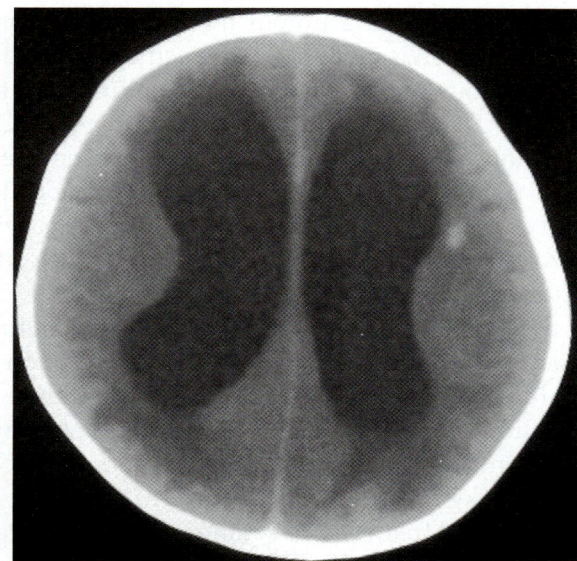

Fig. 100.10: CT scan of a child showing dilated ventricles and a calcified locus in the right cerebral hemisphere

tympanic membrane displacement correlates well with intracranial pressure and this can severe as an easy, noninvasive method to measure intracranial pressure.[19]

Proton Magnetic Resonance Spectroscopy

It has been studied that premature infants and neonates with hydrocephalus have elevated lactate, glutamine and alanine concentrations compared with age-matched controls.[20] Proton magnetic resonance spectroscopy has been reported to be of limited value in predicting outcome in infants with hydrocephalus. However, this test may be useful in identifying subsets of hydrocephalic neonates that, in fact, have severe neurologic disease and poor prognosis. Patients with dramatically reduced N-acetyl-aspartate and elevated Lac had poor neurologic outcome and were found to have neurologic disease that had not been identified with prior diagnostic tests.[20]

Ventriculography

It has been used previously for differentiating communicating and non-communicating hydrocephalus. Neutral Phenosulfonaphthalein dye was injected into the lateral ventricles, and if the chemical was recovered within 20 minutes from the spinal subarachnoid space it was termed as 'Communicating'. Ventriculography and cisternography were used for evaluating patients with suspected ventricular loculation and for mass lesions extrinsically compressing the ventricular system. The role of these investigations has diminished following the advent of same and no invasive investigations like ultrasonography, CT scanning and MRI imaging.

GOALS OF MANAGEMENT

The management of a patient with hydrocephalus would depend upon the rate of progression of the hydrocephalus and the etiology of the hydrocephalus. The goals in treatment of hydrocephalus include decreasing the intracerebral pressure to safe levels, allowing the increase in the volume of brain parenchyma to maximize the child's neurological development, minimizing the likelihood of complications, detect and aggressively treat any complications and maintain the integrity of CSF pathways to prevent ventricular cooptation and preserve the potential for life without shunt dependency.

ANTENATALLY DETECTED HYDROCEPHALUS

Congenital hydrocephalus may be diagnosed as early as 13 weeks of gestational age by USG and amniotic fluid tap. The treatment of antenatally detected hydrocephalus has been a subject of controversy in the past. The incidence of associated anomalies with antenatally detected hydrocephalus is very high and many of these anomalies can be missed on antenatal sonography. In utero, ventricular drainage had been reported two decades earlier between 1982 and 1985. This procedure did not gain popularity as the procedure related mortality rate was 10%, 53% had severe deficits and gross developmental delays while 12% were moderately handicapped. There has been a high rate of complications associated with the ventriculo-amniotic shunt and need for multiple revisions secondary to dislodgement and blockage. Serial cephalocentesis requires multiple punctures and does not allow consistent reduction of intracerebral pressure. The overall mortality in fetuses with antenatally detected ventriculomegaly is around 70% while only 50% of the survivors show normal intellectual development. It has been found that fetus who had demonstrable ventriculomegaly *in-utero* were managed postnatally by shunt insertion quite effectively. In modern day practice, *in-utero* surgery for hydrocephalus has no role. The authors feel that fetal interventions should not be advocated for hydrocephalus if the baby is to be delivered alive and with a fairly mild to moderate hydrocephalus that does not interfere with the delivery of the baby.

MEDICAL MANAGEMENT

Medical management is beneficial for slowly progressive hydrocephalus. The goal in treating hydrocephalus medically is to decrease ventricular size and decrease the intracranial pressure to normal levels with fewer side effects than that associated with shunt surgery. Also to stabilize the patient so that a shunt is not required or to temporize the patient until a shunt can be done more safely. The modes of medical therapy are removal of CSF, by decreasing CSF production, by decreasing cerebral water content and increasing CSF absorption. In the past head wrapping was also used with the principal being that CSF absorption increases with ICP. By this method, ICP's of 500-700 mm water could be generated that could lead to transependymal CSF absorption.

The potential for spontaneous arrest of hydrocephalus exists in infants because of the linear increase in CSF absorption seen with increase in ICP.

Medical treatment is advocated as the initial line of management for all cases of hydrocephalus due to the growing reservations against shunt surgery. Shunt insertion represent a life time commitment to an imperfect device that may require frequent revisions. Conditions associated with a treatable etiology fair well with medical treatment alone. Hydrocephalus associated with hypervitaminosis A, if treated appropriately after diagnosis will resolve with medical management alone. Appropriate antibiotics are added if there is evidence of infection leading to ventriculitis or meningitis.

Pharmacological agents like Acetazolamide 50-100 mg/kg/day, Glycerol 2 mg/kg every 6 hours and Isosorbide 2-3 gm/kg are used for medical treatment. Some authors have also used Furosemide 1 mg/kg/day, but the authors do not advocate its routine use. As the mechanisms of action of these drugs are different, these can be given in a cyclic manner at 3-4 hour intervals to maintain high efficacy of the drugs with minimal doses.

Acetazolamide is a potent inhibitor of carbonic anhydrase which is involved in the active secretion of water and ions by the choroidal epitehlium into the ventricles. Furosemide also inhibits choroidal CSF production. The inhibiting action of furosemide is around 10-100 fold less than acetazolamide but the overall decrease in CSF production is the same as with acetazolamide. This suggests alternate undefined sites of action of furosemide. Both the drugs can reduce CSF flow by 50-60% at sufficient doses.[21] Acetazolamide also acts by causing preferential vasoconstriction of choroidal arteries. There is a high incidence of metabolic acidosis especially in the newborns and small infants with acetazolamide doses if given above 60-75 mg/kg/day. In that case, this should be recognized and treated well in time by either reducing the dose or stopping the same temporarily. There has been some concern regarding the toxicity of high dose of the acetazolamide on myelin.

Authors had an unusual experience with the prolonged use of acetazolamide. This was the case of post-spina Bifida Hydrocephalus and had been on acetazolamide for almost 6 months after surgery. Baby was hospitalized for running continuous low grade fever of 2 month duration with loss of weight and milk intake. There was no evidence of raised ICT. Baby was investigated in detail but no cause could be found. Electrolytes remained normal. Finally, it was decided to stop the medical management (Acetazolamide) and insert the VP shunt. Once the shunt was inserted, fever disappeared with in hrs and remained so thereafter. It was possibly due either to dehydration disturbing the cellular transport mechanism or affecting the temperature control system in the brain. Furosemide is also known to cause metabolic alkalosis and nephrocalcinosis and should be considered in selected cases in addition to acetazolamide and not as a substitute to it.

Osmotic diuretics decrease the brain water content by increasing the outflow of water from the interstitial space into the capillaries. The transependymal CSF flow in hydrocephalus can be then cleared by osmotic diuretics. Additionally there may also be a small flow of water back into the choroidal capillaries from the ventricles as a result of osmotic gradient. These agents are not effective if there is little residual brain parenchyma to extract water from. Osmotic diuretics are effective temporarily in reducing ICP but prolonged use can lead to a rebound effect with an increase in interstitial water. Isosorbide, mannitol, urea and glycerol are the common agents which have been used and can be given orally. Isosorbide is a sorbitol derivative.

Hyaluronidase, urokinase, streptokinase and tissue plasminogen activator have been used experimentally to lyse fibrin blocking the subarachnoid villi following hemorrhage. Steroids decrease the inflammatory response following subarachnoid hemorrhage and meningitis but do not inhibit fibroblast proliferation. Head wrapping that was done previously was believed to increase the ICP and hence increase in transependymal CSF absorption to cause a decrease in ventriculomegaly. It is no more recommended in the scientific world.

Presently, acetazolamide and glycerol are the most frequently used agents in pediatric patients for the effective medical management of hydrocephalus.

Postpyogenic Meningitis Hydrocephalus

Meningitis is the most common cause of acquired hydrocephalus which produces obstruction to CSF flow usually at the subcrachnoid level. The incidence of hydrocephalus following meningitis ranges between 1-5%. Intrauterine viral infection with cytomegalovirus, rubella, mumps, varicella and parainfluenza are also responsible for congenital obstructive hydrocephalus of the noncommunicating variety. *Toxoplasma gondii* is a cause of congenital infection and presents as hydrocephalus, chorioretinitis and intracranial calcification in the newborns.

The early use of antibiotics in the treatment of local infection of the middle ear and paranasal sinuses has decreased the incidence of meningitis secondary to these infections.[1] Presently blood borne infections are the primary cause of meningitis and the organism involved depends on the age of the patient. The commonly involved organisms include *E. coli*, *Staphylococcus aureus*, gram negative enteric bacilli in neonates and babies upto 3 months, and *Hemophilus influenzae*, *Pneumococcus*, *Meningococcus*, *Streptococcus* and *Staphylococcus aureus* in older children.

In the acute stages of meningitis the subarachnoid space is engorged with pus and the leptomeninges are hyperemic and edematous. The exudates of *streptococcal* and *pneumococcal* infection accumulate over the cerebral convexities whereas meningococcus exudates aggregate at the base. In meningitis secondary to Hemophilus, the exudate is copious and diffuse. In the chronic stage there is fibroblast proliferation and the subarachnoid space is gradually obliterated by an adhesive scar. Communicating hydrocephalus results secondary to obliteration of the subarachnoid space but the 4th ventricle outlet may also be blocked leading to noncommunicating hydrocephalus as well.

Post-tubercular Meningitis Hydrocephalus

Tubercular meningitis is the commonest manifestation of CNS tuberculosis and constitutes almost half of the cases of childhood tuberculosis.[22,23] Communicating hydrocephalus may result due to blockage of basal cisterns by the tuberculous exudate in the acute stage and adhesive leptomeningitis in the chronic stage. Non-communicating hydrocephalus may be caused by blockage of the acqueduct or outlet foramina of the fourth ventricle.

Intraluminal subependymal tuberculoma or a plug of ependymal exudate may also block the acqueduct. The meningeal exudate may also cause circumferential compression of the brainstem and cause acqueductal obstruction. Tubercular meningitis may be associated with damage of lenticulostriate vessels, vessels of the circle of Willis and the middle cerebral artery in the sylvian tissue. There may be damage to cranial nerves 2nd, 3rd, 4th, 6th and 7th leading to multiple cranial nerve palsies.

Fungal meningitis can lead to hydrocephalus in up to 20% of cases if early and aggressive treatment is not instituted. Communicating hydrocephalus is an ominous complication and has an associated mortality of around 50-70%.

Posthemorrhagic Hydrocephalus in the Premature Infant

Hydrocephalus following intraventricular hemorrhage (IVH) is still one of the most serious complications of premature birth.[24] Posthemorrhagic hydrocephalus is secondary to a fibrous thickening of the meninges with an obliterative arachnoiditis and obstruction of CSF flow through the normal subarachnoid pathways. An acquired acqueductal stenosis can also occur because of cellular debris and red blood cells. The predisposing factors for intra ventricular hemorrhage leading to hydrocephalus include preterm neonates less than 1500 gm, respiratory distress syndrome, vigorous resuscitation, rapid volume expansion, soda bicarbonate administration, hypoxemia, hypercarbia and acidosis. The diagnosis may be picked up on a routine cranial ultrasound performed on postnatal day 2 or 3 followed by a repeat examination during the second postnatal week to screen preterm neonates of ≤ 1500 gm or less than 34 gestational weeks. Post-hemorrhagic hydrocephalus presents with increasing occipito frontal head circumference, tense anterior fontanelle, lethargy, feeding difficulty, bradycardia and ventilator dependency the other manifestations include SIADH, persistent metabolic acidosis, abnormal eye movements and hypertonia. Diagnosis is confirmed on ultrasonography or documentation of raised intracranial pressure.

The ultrasonographic grading of intraventricular hemorrhage is as follows:

Grade I : Germinal matrix hemorrhage;
Grade II : Blood in lateral ventricles, no dilatation of ventricle;
Grade III : Blood in ventricles with ventricular dilatation ;
Grade IV : Hemorrhage with parenchymal involvement.

Cases with Grade I and II are managed with observation alone. For higher grades the treatment is begun with medical management with acetazolamide (50-100 mg/kg/day) and furosemide (2 mg/kg/day) with careful electrolyte and acid base status monitoring. Ventricular taps or the insertion of ventricular catheters with reservoir for repeated tapping have been advocated in the past. There role is not much as there is a risk of porencephaly. Flexible ventriculoscopes for irrigation, evacuation of blood or to lyse intraventricular septations, have also been tried to decrease the need for shunt surgery. Children with posthemorrhagic hydrocephalus are more likely to become shunt independent on follow up though the ultimate prognosis would depend on the grade of intraventricular hemorrhage.

Ventriculoperitoneal shunt surgery cannot be carried out early and permanent dependence on a shunt is associated with several serious complications. Streptokinase has been used, based on the hypothesis that multiple blood clots in the cerebrospinal fluid (CSF) are the initial cause of posthemorrhagic ventricular dilatation and lysis of clots could reopen the pathways of circulation and re-absorption of CSF.[24]

No information on the effect of intraventricular streptokinase on disability is available. There is cause for concern about meningitis and secondary intraventricular hemorrhage, but numbers are insufficient to quantify the risks. On comparing intraventricular streptokinase with conservative management of post-hemorrhagic ventricular dilatation, the numbers of deaths and babies with shunt dependence were similar in both groups. Thus it has been concluded that intraventricular fibrinolytic therapy with streptokinase, given when post-hemorrhagic ventricular dilatation is established, should not be recommended for neonates following IVH. A conservative approach with CSF drainage applied only to symptomatic raised intracranial pressure seems appropriate.[24]

Emergency Temporary Treatment

Temporary treatment measures like external drainage and repeated percutaneous taps are only to be condemned due to a high risk of infection. Their use has been only to tide over the crisis in a moribund baby in emergency unfit for anesthesia or to wait till the infection subsides with the help of antibiotics prior to shunt placement. Instillation of thrombolytic agents has been tried for intracranial hemorrhage though the results have been the same with or without this treatment.

SURGICAL MANAGEMENT

A shunt operation is the most commonly performed surgery for Hydrocephalus. The studies by Young have demonstrated that a cerebral mantle of 2.8 cm is adequate to achieve normal MPQ status in follow up.[25] It is believed that the goal for treating a child with hydrocephalus is to achieve a cerebral mantle of 3.5 cm by the age of 5 months. Cases diagnosed to have removable etiological factors mandate other appropriate procedures. These include radical resection of a mass lesion, or correction of a malformation.

The various shunt procedures include:
- Ventriculoperitoneal shunts
- Ventriculoatrial

- Ventriculopleural
- Lumboperitoneal
- Ventriculocisternostomy (Torkildsen operation).

A recent development that is slowly gaining popularity is the "Third Ventricultostomy".

Indications for Shunt Insertion

It is difficult to outline the definite indications for the shunt surgery in children with hydrocephalus. Many of them can still be managed with medical decompression therapy while others may have too advanced a disease and may not benefit from any surgery. A broad based clinical approach is advisable. Commonly the indications for shunt surgery include:
a. Rapidly progressive hydrocephalus, uncontrolled with medical management even after 3-6 months therapy.
b. Symptomatic patients with established hydrocephalus, and raised ICP.
c. Head size > 2SD above normal at initial presentation.
d. Evidence of falling MPQ values during follow-up.
e. Evidence of papilledema and features of raised ICP like peri-ventricular ooze on CT scan.
f. Child develops serious side effects with medical management.
g. Hydrocephalus is caused by postnatal causes– post-meningitic, once infection is under control.
h. The value of the cortical mantle is very confusing in deciding in favour or against the shunt surgery. Patients even with the paper thin mantle can have normal intelligence while children with thick cortical mantle may not be so. In general, cortical mantle of ≤ 1 cm on initial radiological investigation or thinning of the cortical mantle on follow-up studies suggest the need for surgical intervention.

Contraindications for Shunt Surgery

1. Ventriculitis
2. Acute intraventricular hemorrhage
3. Hydrocephalus due to treatable obstructive lesions
4. Extreme brain pathology
5. Ventriculomegaly without elevated ICP
6. Asymptomatic nonprogressive hydrocephalus
7. Established irrecoverable optic atrophy with gross hydrocephalus.

SHUNT SYSTEMS

There are a many kinds of shunts available and there is no ideal one. The choice of the shunt depends upon the characteristics of the patient and the choice of the surgeon. The system characteristics that minimize shunt failure include a one piece system, a non-flanged ventricular catheter, a proximal non-slit valve and open ended distal tubing. The surgeon should adapt to using a particular type of shunt so that he may be aware of that particular shunt properties and would be well conversant in handling the complications that develop with it in the postoperative period. Most shunts are made of silicon (medical grade silastic) material. The advantages include flexibility, non-immunogenicity and blood does not clot to its inner surface and hence lesser chance of early obstruction.

All ventricular drainage systems feature three components (Fig. 100.11):
(i) A ventricular catheter
(ii) A one–way valve
(iii) Distal catheter.

Ventricular Catheter

They provide direct access to the ventricle and are placed via a twist drill (burr hole) and are made of sialastic material and are impregnated with barium for radiographic visualization. The tip may be a right-angled catheter with multiple tip perforations, a right-angled catheter with a molded, in-line reservoir

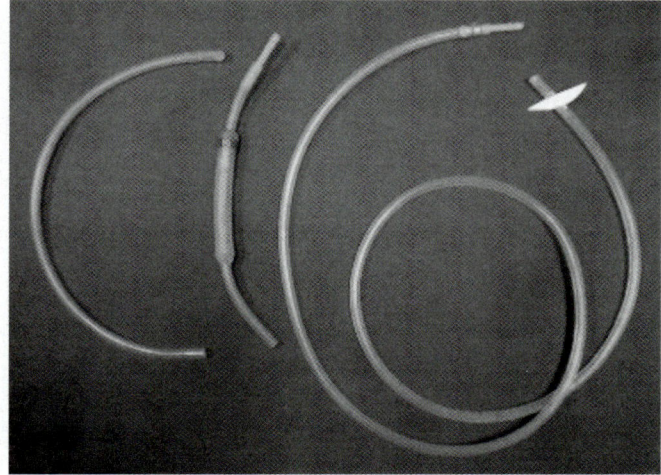

Fig. 100.11: The usual three parts of a shunt system include: a ventricular catheter, a one–way valve and a distal catheter (Upadhyaya shunt)

and multiple tip perforations, a grooved tip design or a flanged tip design. Although a straight catheter gives maximum flexibility vis-a-vis desired length, it requires some type of connection to the remainder of the system. The right-angled catheter although fixed in terms of functional length connects to the rest of the system via its side arm, eliminating possibility of ventricular catheter separation and migration into the enlarged ventricles. It also allows a valve or flush chamber to be placed any where in the system.

Valves

Two types of valves are currently available, e.g. differential pressure valves and the newer variable resistance flow regulated valves.

Differential Pressure Valves

They provide constant resistance and allow CSF flow when the proximal hydrostatic pressure exceeds valves present closing pressures.

Closing pressures are generally used for valve identification. The valves can be divided according the closing pressures as;
1. *Low pressure (20-40 mm H_2O) shunt:* The valve opens when CSF pressure rises even marginally over the normal range. It is used for normal pressure hydrocephalus. This type of shunt is not used commonly. There is always an inherent disadvantage that it might over drain the ventricles causing subdural hygroma, specially if the patient happened to be the newborns.
2. *Medium pressure (40-70 mm H_2O) shunt:* This is the most commonly used shunt to reduce the intracranial pressure and decompress the ventricles. However, the CSF pressure is never brought to normal.
3. *High pressure (80 – 100 mm H_2O):* This shunt valve opens at high CSF pressure. The indication to use the high pressure system, is acute obstructive hydrocephalus so that the fluid is drained slowly against resistance to avoid sudden decompression.

Differential pressure valves come in four designs:
a. Holter valve (Slit)
b. Hakim valve (ball-in-cone)
c. Upadhyay (Diaphragm), Pudenz valve, Chhabra, Ceredrain
d. Miter valve

- *Holter valve (Slit):* It is the simplest valve type. When the pressure builds up inside the tubing, the slit is forced open and CSF is allowed to flow outward. The pressure at which the valve open is determined by thickness of tubing wall. The advantage is easy placement and accessibility. It can be placed anywhere in the shunt system and do not require direct connection to the ventricular catheter. This allows for valve replacement without manipulation of ventricular catheter. However, it is bulky. It can be easily blocked by turbid fluid and debris.
- *Hakim valve (Ball-in-cone):* Similar to the Holter valve but differs in its mechanism. A synthetic ruby ball is held in place by a stainless steel spring. Depending on CSF flow rate, the ball moves back and forth within the cone under the control of calibrated spring. It is less vulnerable to obstruction by viscous, proteinaceous CSF and particulate matter.
- *Upadhyaya (Diaphragm), Pudenz valve, Chhabra, ceredrain:* Upadhyay shunt has a diaphragm valve above and a slit valve at the lower end (Figs 100.12 and 100.13). Pudenz valve utilizes a thin diaphragm against a seat to control flow. It is usually designed to attach directly to a ventricular catheter so that it is "seated" in a burr hole. Horizontal type constitutes the Chhabra shunt. Upadhyay shunt and Ceredrain (Sri Chitra shunt) also work on the same principle.
- *Miter valve:* It is constructed from two thin sheets of silicon rubber that are bound together at one end and open at the other to regulate pressure. Each leaflet act as a spring so that, as the pressure increases at the inlet end, the leaves are pushed apart.

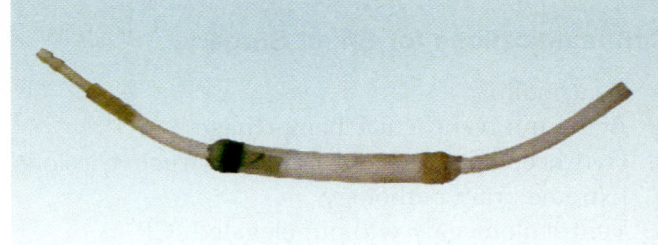

Fig. 100.12: Shunt chamber of Upadhyaya shunt with an operculum diaphragm valve near the ventricular end of the chamber

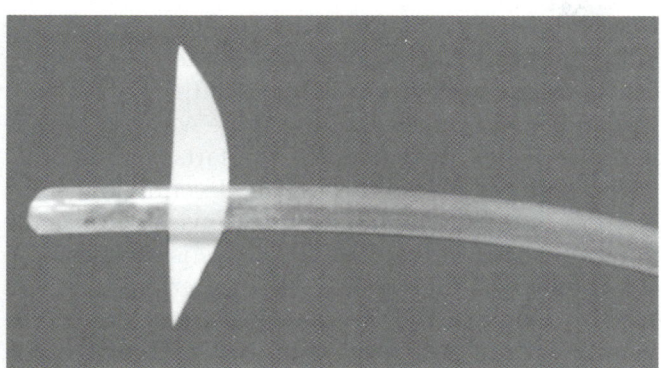

Fig. 100.13. The terminal part of lower end of an Upadhyay shunt assembly depicting the slit valve that opens to CSF pressure flow. The smooth blind end (not conical) can also be appreciated as a solid tube filled with silastic material for about 5mm to prevent intestinal perforation

Variable Resistance Flow Regulated Valves

These valves take care of over-drainage by varying valve resistance and keeping CSF flow constant. They are two types:
a. *OSV valve (Orbis-Sigma valve):* The valve resistance of this valve varies by changing the cross sectional area of the valve outlet area depending on the hydrostatic inlet pressure.
b. *Delta valve:* This is a simple diaphragm valve coupled with an antisiphon device. Two silicon leaflets cover the outlet port. This unit acts as a differential pressure valve but when negative pressure is in the distal tubing (i.e. when the patient is in erect posture), suction on the distal diaphragms occlude the outlet ports preventing CSF flow.

Programmable valves have been successfully put in preterm and term babies (< 2 months of age). The valve settings can be readjusted at different pressure levels as required. Several external adjustments of the valves apparently avoided several surgical shunt revisions.[26]

Distal Catheter

It is similar to ventricular tubing. It may come open-ended or closed end with a slit valve. It may have a metal spring or be made of heavier guage silicone to prevent kinking.

Additional Devices

- *Flush Chambers and reservoirs*: The basic tripartite shunt system consisting of a ventricular catheter, a unidirectional valve and a distal catheter does not allow access to the ventricular CSF. At times, it may be necessary to withdraw CSF for culture or administer antibiotic, chemotherapeutic agent or radiographic contrast medium directly into the ventricle. For direct ventricular instillation, reservoirs or flush chambers can be added to shunt system.
- *On-off device*: Can be used to provide intermittent shunting or to access shunt function.
- *Shunt filter*: It is used when ventricular obstruction is caused by tumor. The filter serves to stop the dispersal of tumor cells throughout the body via the distal shunt tubing.
- *Antisiphon device*: This is another approach to the problem of ventricular over drainage. The device closes when there is negative pressure within the shunt tubing, acutely raising resistance to CSF flow and preventing ventricular over drainage.

SHUNT INSERTION

Each surgeon adopts to a particular type of shunt and adopts a method most suitable for its insertion. The equipment used for shunt insertion also varies from surgeon to surgeon however the principles of strict asepsis and avoiding skin contact of the shunt to prevent contamination with staphylococcous epidermidis remain the same. It is also better to use the system with a minimum number of connections to avoid the postoperative complications.

Procedure for Placing the Upadhyaya's Shunt

Preoperative preparation includes combination of antibiotics (covering the gram-positive and gram negative organisms), shaving the head, removing the oil from scalp, cleaning the ears and the skin creases in the neck and behind the pinna, and painting of the part with betadine or mercurochrome a day before the surgery. The patient, like any other neurosurgical procedure, deserves high attention to be put as the first case in the list observing strict aseptic precautions. Insertion of Upadhyaya's ventriculo-peritoneal shunt, requires at least three skin incisions – in scalp, neck and abdomen. The shunt assembly is checked for its patency and placed in saline with antibiotic solution. Any contact of the shunt assembly with skin should be avoided as much as possible.

Positioning the Patient

It is the right ventricle which is used for shunt insertion routinely. However, it is only occasionally that the left ventricle would be utilized for shunt insertion either as a first choice (if it is too much enlarged) or the right ventricle is not available for use (bleeding, adhesions, sclerosis, localized infection). The right hemisphere is preferred because most commonly it is the non dominant hemisphere. The patient is placed supine with the head turned to the left, with suitable roll/s placed between the scapulae and the neck so that the neck is extended and rotated on the thorax. Care should be taken that the ventricular end, the distal end and the shunt tract, are all in a single straight line to prevent unwanted injuries and kinking. External ear should be temporarily plugged. The pinna is brought forward and strapped in front of the tragus to assist in cleaning the area behind it.

Skin Incision

Curvilinear skin incision, about 4-5 cm in length, is planned over the most prominent part of the scalp to expose standard burr hole site, to allow passage of shunt catheter from the scalp incision to the abdomen with only one additional intermediary incision in the neck to negotiate a curve and avoid any injury to the thorax, permitting final seating of the shunt away from the incision line.

Insertion of Ventricular Catheter

The ventricular catheter which has multiple holes near its end (and with the suitable sized stylet in situ) should be placed in the frontal horn, keeping the direction of the tip of the ventricular catheter towards the nasion while inserting the catheter. The tip of the catheter should be away from the choroid plexus. The stylet is withdrawn gradually while keeping the catheter inside the ventricular system. The CSF pressure is noted and the catheter is clamped to avoid CSF loss. To minimize blockade with choroids plexus, late fractures, disconnections and tethering of the shunt in the subcutaneous tissue, it is advisable to insert an additional length of the shunt for about 2-3 cm beyond the level of the "give way feel" in the choroids plexus or when the CSF starts coming out.

The catheter is placed in the lateral ventricle ideally, anterior to the foramen of Monro. This is because the anterior extent of the choroid plexus is present upto this foramen and it is believed that anterior placement would decrease the incidence of blockage of the ventricular catheter by the choroid. The two accepted approaches used are:
1. Parieto-occipital placement into the frontal horn of the lateral ventricle.
2. The more direct anterior approach through the frontal lobe at the area of the coronal sutures.

The posterior placement is sited 3 cm above and behind the tip of the ear or approximately around 2-3 cm lateral to the highest point of the occiput. From the posterior parietal site, catheter should be aimed at the glabella in both the axial and sagittal planes. The advantages of this approach are (i) shorter subgaleal tunnel for the external catheter (ii) longer ventricular segment for drainage. The disadvantages include the potential damage to the visual cortex if the lateral ventricles are grossly dilated and the cortex is thinned out.

The anterior approach is sited 3 cm lateral to the saggital suture and just anterior or posterior to the coronal suture and the brain cannula is directed towards the inner canthus of the ipsilateral eye. The advantages of the anterior approach are shorter distance through the brain parenchyma and better chances of achieving correct positioning.

The disadvantage of the anterior approach is that the catheter has to travel a longer distance subgaleally and as the child grows there is traction and risk of damage or disconnection. CSF is usually encountered at a depth of 2-4 cm in children. The CSF pressure may be measured at this point to decide the type of shunt to be placed. Once free flow is ensured, catheter is snapped into a right-angled clip that prevents kinking at the burr-hole and secured with a silk ligature. The extracranial portion of the shunt system is pulled taut from the abdominal end to eliminate kinks. The valve with the shunt assembly must come to rest on the surface of the skull.

Insertion of Distal Catheter

Abdomen is opened along the right sub-costal, (or alternately by a right paramedian or midline incision) upto the peritoneum. In the abdomen, a subcutaneous tunnel is created about 2 cm proximal to the skin incision. This tunnel is also created along the subgaleal plane above the pericranium, over the clavicle upto the peritoneum. An introducer may be passed from the abdominal side. This guides the distal shunt tubing from the subgaleal space into the abdomen. The distal tube is then placed into the abdominal cavity. The length of the distal tube left in abdomen is usually about 4-6 inches and placed either over the right dome of the liver with a gentle curve or deep in the pelvis to minimize omental adhesions. The wound is finally closed in layers, with the peritoneum around the catheter.

Connection of the Shunt Assembly

The shunt assembly is connected with the connectors. Care should be taken that the valve overlies the mastoid bone so that it can be felt to check its function.. One of the connectors is fixed to the pericranium.

SHUNT COMPLICATIONS

Complications Related to Ventricular Related End

1. Shunt infection[27-29]
2. Shunt Obstruction (Ventricular end, valve, distal end)
3. Shunt disconnection or fracture
4. Shunt migration
5. Overdrainage — Slit ventricle syndrome
6. Subdural/Extracerebral CSF collections
7. Craniosynostosis
8. Seizures
9. Penumocephalus
10. Isolated ventricle syndromes.

Complications Related to Peritoneal End

1. Inguinal hernia and hydrocele
2. Ascites
3. Pseudocyst formation[30]
4. Intestinal volvulus and obstruction
5. Bowel perforation, bladder perforation[31]
6. Peritonitis.

Shunt Infection (10-20% of Shunt Insertions)

This is the most important complication of shunts and difficult to establish (Fig. 100.14). Unequivocal evidence of shunt infection requires demonstration of the organism on Gram staining or culture from material in, on, or around the shunt, or from fluid withdrawn from the shunt. Shunt infection occurring within the first 2 months after surgery are usually caused by skin flora and indicate poor surgical aseptic technique. Infection occurring after this period are caused predominantly by Gram-negative bacilli. The risk factors for shunt infection include young age with relatively immature immune system and vulnerability of the skin, poor skin hygiene, long duration of operation, presence of CSF leak and increased number of OT personnel.

Acute shunt infection presents with fever, redness around the skin incision or the shunt tract and in later stages discharge of pus from the incision. Chronic infection may present with exposure of the shunt, CSF leak from the incision site or frank signs of meningitis. The diagnosis may be supported with leukocytosis and CSF examination. Gram staining will confirm the diagnosis 95% of cases.

Ventriculoperitoneal (VP) shunt is one of the commonest procedures in neurosurgical practice. A significant problem encountered in shunt procedures is infection, with infection rate ranging from 2 to 27%, often with poor outcome.[29] Shunt associated infections are most frequently (65%) caused by coagulase

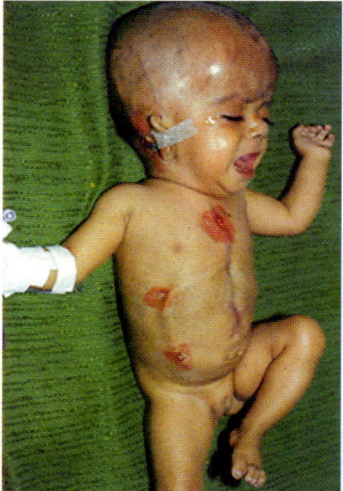

Fig. 100.14: An infant with an infected right ventriculoperitoneal shunt

negative Staphylococcus (CoNS).[27,28] Gram-negative bacteria are the next most frequent pathogens,. *Pseudomonas aeruginosa*, *E. coli* and *Klebsiella pneumoniae* accounting for 19-22% of cases.[29] Most of the infections occur within 30 days of the shunt procedure.[29]

Shunt infection has been defined as isolation of the organism from the ventricular fluid, shunt tube, reservoir, and/or blood culture along with the clinical signs and symptoms suggestive of shunt infection or malfunction like fever, peritonitis, meningitis, signs of infection along the shunt tract, or nonspecific signs and symptoms of headache, vomiting, change in mental status, or seizures.[29] Fever and vomiting have been reported as the most common clinical symptoms. Altered sensorium, abdominal tenderness and seizures were less common manifestations.[29] In gram positive shunt infections, majority of the organisms are commensals of the skin, a result of direct wound contamination during surgery.

The treatment depends upon the severity of the infection. If the CSF is turbid, more active treatment is initiated. The site of infection is to be identified. If the tract of the shunt is infected and there is leakage, removal of the shunt is warranted.

The treatment options include:

1. Antibiotics alone. It is useful in shunts infected with organism such as *Hemophilus influenzae*, meningococcus and gonococcus. Failure of the fluid to clear within 48 to 72 hours should prompt removal of the shunt equipment. Antibiotic treatment is recommended for a duration of 2-3 weeks and preferably the same antibiotic should be instilled intraventricularly at least once daily.
2. Antibiotics, with shunt removal and the immediate replacement with a new shunt, if the ventricular CSF is relatively sterile but the shunt taps have been positive for culture (suggestive of shunt colonization). It contemplates the need for a subsequent operation.
3. Shunt removal combined with antibiotic treatment is an alternative method to treat shunt infection. However, this requires to be supplemented with the adequate medical decompression (acetazolamide, glycerol, furosemide, alone or in combination). If the CSF leak is persisting from the shunt tract or the ventricular system is grossly infected with the positive CSF cultures, then an external ventricular drainage is preferred. This should be achieved preferably with a new shunt catheter discarding the previous one in place. This procedure is ideal and carries the highest cure rate once the shunt is found to be infected and not being cured by antibiotics alone. Many of these children with repeated surgeries in the past, produce gradually reducing amount of CSF each day suggestive of developing ventricular sclerosis or the status of the arrested hydrocephalus. These children may not require a shunt at all in future as they may well be managed with the medical decompression alone.
4. Shunt removal combined with antibiotic treatment, interval external ventricular drainage and shunt placement on the opposite site once the CSF is clear. This is the preferred procedure in children who would require shunt drainage once the infection has been cleared however, the ventricular system used so far has multiple loculi with septae due to previous surgeries and the repeated infection. Even if the shunt has been placed effectively, it may fail to drain the ventricular system effectively. Thus the choice for placing the shunt on the opposite virgin site to drain larger surface area of CSF production.

Besides, a 30-40% mortality reported in some series with shunt infection, the survivors risk psychomotor retardation as a result of the infection and alteration in CSF circulation.

Shunt Obstruction

It may be a proximal or the distal obstruction.

(a) *Proximal Shunt obstruction:* This is the most common cause of shunt obstruction in pediatric age group. It can be blocked by adherent choroid plexus, by debris, embedding of proximal catheter in periventricular ependymal and neural tissue or blood in the ventricular system which occludes the catheter lumen, by brain tissue adherent to the catheter, or in certain cases by another pathologic process such as tumor tissue growth around the catheter tip. The decision for shunt revision is based on clinical as well as radiological findings and has to be prompt. In three piece systems the neck connector is opened to check and confirm the blocked end. At surgery, the ventricular catheter may be tethered to the choroid plexus and in such a situation saline irrigation may be tried to free it.

The ventricular catheter obstruction is diagnosed by observing no flow or only a drop or two of the CSF exiting from the isolated ventricular catheter. It should be removed and replaced by a new catheter. Sometimes, the catheter may be struck and attempts to remove can cause intraventicular bleeding which may be difficult to control. Gradual traction on the catheter or cauterization of the plexus by using ventricular stylets may be considered in these situations. If the CSF is blood tinged, it is imperative to wait for in 3-5 minutes to allow the blood to form a clot. The clot gravitates to the recumbent portion of the ventricle and the shunt tubing floats to the superior portion of the ventricle. A formed clot, hence does not obstruct the ventricular catheter whereas fresh continuing bleeding does as it clots within the tubing. Persistent flow of fresh blood is an indication for exteriorization. It is best to use the same shunt tract, unless loculated, in revisions of the ventricular catheter.

(b) *Distal obstruction:* With the advent of silastic catheters, this complication is rare. The common causes are malposition of the catheter that typically results from placement of the distal end into pre-peritoneal fat rather than the peritoneal cavity proper and low-grade peritoneal infection by anerobic organisms, causing encystment and loculation of the peritoneal contents around the catheter tip, leading to pseudocyst formation and shunt obstruction. Other rare causes of distal shunt malfunction include distal slit valve occlusion by debris, migration of the tip of peritoneal catheter into an area where absorption is limited, e.g. hernial sac, embedding in the wall of the bowel, shortening of the catheter as the child grows and the catheter pulling out of the peritoneum.

Shunt Over Drainage

CSF flow through a valve can be represented as $F = DP/R$, where F = CSF flow rate, DP = Differential pressure and R = Resistance of valve. In upright position, an additional factor, 'H' = Gravity is added to overall system, so that the equation becomes $F = DP/HR$. Therefore, erect posture can lead to complication like slit-like ventricles and possibility of proximal shunt obstruction, low pressure headaches and subdural hematomas.

Over drainage phenomenon is directly responsible for several complications like orthostatic hypotension, subdural CSF collections, slit ventricle syndrome, and loculation of ventricles. This complication can be minimized by addition of Siphon-resistive devices to the shunt systems.

Slit Ventricle Syndrome

The term slit ventricle syndrome is applied to a subset of shunt dependent patients who develop chronic, recurring headaches associated with features of raised intracranial pressure in the presence of persistent small slit like ventricles. The incidence of this syndrome ranges between 0.9-3.3%.[32] Its hallmark is presence of definite elevation of ICP which may be as high as 50 to 60 cm H_2O in the face of small ventricle on CT scan.

Children with this syndrome often have functioning shunts throughout the period of rapid head growth, and their skulls are thus tightly configured to underlying brain with very little CSF space over the convexities. Any event which subsequently elevates CSF pressure even for brief periods such as viral infections will result in ICP rise that is not buffered by extraventricular CSF displacement as in the patient without shunts and symptoms associated with sustained rise in ICP develops.

Pathogenesis and Proposed Mechanisms

1. CSF over drainage due to siphoning effect of the peritoneal catheter.
2. Periventricular fibrosis.
3. Intermittent proximal catheter malfunction.
4. Decreased intracrainal compliance and intracranial hypotension.

Clinical Features

The patient presents with chronic, intermittent and recurrent headaches with or without vomiting. Minor viral illnesses may precipitate the headache and patients with chronic intracranial hypotension may have headaches with increased activity and in an upright position. The symptoms in this disorder are much more prominent than the signs which can be elicited. Papilledema is rare though venous pulsations in the retina are diminished during symptomatic periods. An examination will confirm the shunt chamber is filling slowly. Bradycardia, obtundation and hypertension are ominous and late signs.

Diagnosis

A CT scan done during the symptomatic period and compared to a baseline scan shows unchanged ventricular size. A radionuclide shunt patency study will confirm normal CSF flow and rule out partial shunt obstruction. ICP monitoring with a portable monitor is useful to record periods of increased ICP or intracranial hypotension which can then be correlated with the patients symptoms.

Treatment

1. Patients with mild symptoms associated with a systemic stress and unchanged CT scan from baseline are treated with corticosteroids and acetazolamide.
2. Shunt revision is indicated for patients with increased ventricular size or evidence of shunt obstruction. While revising such a shunt, a care must be taken not to allow the CSF to drain out. Rather, the proximal catheter is revised by dilating the ventricles with 10-15 of saline prior to the removal of the old catheter and insertion of a fresh ventricular catheter is done via the old shunt tract.
3. In patients with severe headaches, normal shunt function and dangerously high ICP levels, "cranial expansion" is an alternative. Craniotomy with morcellation of the posterior calvarium from the coronal suture to the inion and laterally to the squamosal suture is the preferred procedure.
4. Treatment of symptomatic intracranial hypotension requires addition of an antisiphon device to the shunt assembly with or without upgrading of the shunt to a higher valve pressure. The antisiphon device counteracts the siphoning action of the hydrostatic pressure of a fluid column between the head and the abdominal cavity.

Shunt Disconnections and Dislodgements

A disconnection is diagnosed frequently by palpating the shunt apparatus and detecting a gap in the tubing.[33] The gap may be distended by fluid collection and the presence of a lump over the shunt tubing may be the initial complaint of the parents or the patient.

This discontinuity can be confirmed by X-rays which may reveal discontinuity if it was a barium impregnated shunt. The neck is a common site of such fractures because of the frequent movements leading to the material fatigue and routine wear and tear. Due to slow leakage of the CSF in the neck, a pseudo sheath may be formed around around the shunt tubing. This may be draining the CSF to the abdominal cavity, albeit not satisfactorily, if the lower end of the shunt is blocked and not able to drain it effectively.

The most frequent cause of shunt disconnection is the improper use of connectors distal to the valve apparatus. To avoid repeated disconnections, all distal revisions of peritoneal shunts entail the replacement of the entire tubing distal to the cranial valve.

Tubing can also crack secondary to trauma and to deposition of calcific deposits around the subcutaneous tubing as it ages. Skiagrams may show the discontinuity of the shunt. In questionable cases of shunt malfunction, radioisotope study can be performed by injecting small volume of radioisotope usually 0.5 to 1 ml into the shunt reservoir while occluding the distal valve to direct the isotope into the ventricles.

Valve incompetence is rarely a cause of shunt dysfunction and can be ruled out by meticulous testing before shunt placement. Though, it is believed that a high CSF protein content predisposes to shunt obstruction, many studies have shown that there is no direct correlation between the incidence of shunt dysfunction and CSF protein content.

Seizure disorders can be secondary to shunt malfunction or secondary to ventriculitis following a shunt injection. There have been many studies which have demonstrated EEG abnormalities in shunted patients who could develop an epileptogenic focus after surgery.[34] Routine use of anticonvulsant therapy is not required but high risk patients with intraventricular hemorrhage and porencephalic cysts require serial EEG evaluation following a shunt especially during the first 2-4 years.

Subdural hygromas are seen in patients with gross hydrocephalus associated with cortical atrophy following CSF diversion. Subdural hematomas and effusions are usually asymptomatic but may cause focal neurological deficits due to midline shift. Extracerebral CSF collections usually recur after aspirations or simple drainage. Definitive treatment has to be directed towards increasing the intraventricular pressure relative to the subdural space. Temporary ligation of the shunt system or drainage of the extracerebral CSF collection into the shunt system below the level of the valve of the ventricular catheter, are the available options.

Pneumocephalus occurs in patients because of air entering through the enlarged congenital bony and dural defects after a shunt has decompressed the ventricles and the tamponade effect of the brain on these defects is lost. These patients are difficult to treat because the site of air ingress is unusually located and difficult to diagnose in the presence of CSF diversion.

Perforation of a viscus, bowel can happen rarely and after dislodgement may come out of the abdominal wound, anus or vagina. Spontaneous bowel perforation can present with shunt infection or obstruction. The shunt is replaced or externalized till the infection clears and the perforation repaired.

Craniosynotosis is another reported complication of CSF shunting and is seen frequently with the use of a low pressure valve. In most cases besides the cosmetic effect there is no restriction in brain growth. Cephalocranial disproportion is another rare complication of shunting in which there is cerebellar and brainstem herniation into the upper spinal canal. This is believed to be due to secondary craniosynostosis causing herniation of the brainstem to accommodate the growing brain.

Shunt Revision

When a part of the shunt system becomes non-functional, exploration of that end with repair or replacement is known as shunt revision.

Shunt Dependency and Independency

Recurrence of symptoms in individual once the shunt is blocked is known as shunt dependency. If the symptoms do not occur in the patient even in the presence of a blocked shunt, it is known as shunt independency. However, there is a dictum that "once a shunt, always a shunt". Even if the shunt is not needed in routine life, it should be left in situ so that it could serve the purpose if the need be.

VENTRICULOATRIAL SHUNT

Ventriculoatrial shunts are less preferred to ventriculoperitoneal shunts as the severity and consequences of the complications are more frequent and more serious with the use of vascular shunts.[35] Peritoneal shunts required fewer revisions and proximal revisions are more common unlike vascular shunts which require distal revisions more often. The second major advantage of VP shunts is that, unlike VA shunts, an unlimited length of distal catheter can be left behind to accommodate to catch up with the growth of the child and lessen the incidence of distal catheter revisions. However, there are conditions in which the peritoneum cannot be used like previous abdominal surgery with adhesions, unrecognized cryptic infections leading to recurrent pseudocyst formation and chemical content of the CSF may be irritating to the peritoneal surface as in post-hemorrhagic hydrocephalus.

Ventriculoatrial shunts are thus less performed with the absolute indication being a premature infant with necrotizing enterocolitis. The confluence of facial with internal jugular vein is exposed by incising the skin and either retracting the anterior border of sternocleidomastoid laterally or going in between the sternal and the clavicular head of the same muscle. Either the facial or the internal jugular vein is used. If the facial vein is preferred, then it is ligated proximally and the atrial catheter is passed through the facial vein into the internal jugular and into the right atrium. Alternately, if the internal jugular vein is to be used, then it is first isolated from the carotid sheath between two stay sutures. The vein is ligated proximally and the catheter is then inserted distal to it with a small incision to reach the atrium. Catheter is fixed with another suture around the internal jugular vein including the catheter. Alternately, a purse string suture is applied in the anterior wall of the internal jugular vein and about a 2 mm incision is made in its center. The atrial catheter is then negotiated through the incision into the internal jugular vein to reach the atrium. The purse string suture is then tightened making sure not to obliterate the lumen of the catheter, thus maintaining the blood flow to the heart along the side of the catheter.

Several techniques have been utilized to control catheter tip placement in the atrium. These include fluoroscopic control, catheter tip filled with 3% normal saline and used as ECG electrode ('p' wave becomes biphasic at entry into the atrium) and trans-esophageal ECHO that is the simplest. The simplest way is to measure the distance between the sternal notch and the xiphisternum. The atrial catheter equal to the length of the "upper one third of this distance" would be enough to place the same in the atrium from the sternal notch.[36] This coincides with the upper border of the fourth intercostal space.

The disadvantages include frequent revisions due to growth of the child, migration into it ventricle, cardiac arrhythmias and embolization into pulmonary artery. The other complications include mural thrombosis, endocarditis, cardiac tamponade secondary to right artrial perforation, superior *vena cava* obstruction, pulmonary hypertension, cor pulmonale and shunt nephritis.

LUMBOPERITONEAL SHUNTS

This is a good site for the placement of the shunt between the theca space in the lumbar region and the peritoneal cavity in patients with communicating hydrocephalus. The common indications for the lumboperitoneal shunt include CSF leaks following the MMC repair (not responding to the medical therapy), pseudotumor cerebri and CSF fistulas at the base of the skull.

The major advantages of this site are that it preserves the integrity of the CSF path ways and does not cause secondary acqueductal obstruction. Lumbar shunts are less likely to cause collapse of the cortical mantle than that seen with the VP shunts. The ventricular walls do not collapse around the catheter and this decreases the incidence of blockage. This procedure can also be performed percutaneously using a Touhy needle.[37] The disadvantages related to this procedure are associated risks of chronic symptomatic cerebellar tonsilar herniation, kyphoscoliosis due to arachnoiditis and nerve root damage.

INTRACRANIAL SHUNTING

(a) Ventriculoventricular shunting - Cannulation of the acqueduct of Sylvius has been performed after suboccopital craniotomy for the treatment of acqueductal stenosis. In occlusion of one of the foramina of Monro, an open cannulation has also been attempted.
(b) Ventriculocisternostomies.
 (i) Third ventriculostomy–This was proposed by Dandy in 1922. This may be performed either by an open or closed technique. Nowadays perforation of the floor of the III ventricle is performed by ventriculosopic techniques. Stereotactic guided puncture of the lateral ventricles is done either through the sub frontal or subtemporal approach. The ventriculoscope is passed through the lateral ventricles to the floor of third ventricle and an opening is made in the floor of third ventricle and communicating the ventricles to subgaleal space.

Although ventriculoperitoneal shunt remains the treatment of choice for many children with hydrocephalus, advances in endoscopic technology have greatly expanded the treatment options for these patients. For selected patients with obstructive hydrocephalus, endoscopic third ventriculostomy and other endoscopic techniques offer substantial advantages over shunt surgery, with a higher success rate being reported in the recent series. As with any surgical procedure, appropriate patient selection is critical to successful outcomes.[38]

Ventriculostomy has been reported as an effective treatment in cases of obstructive hydrocephalus that is caused by aqueductal stenosis and space-occupying lesions.[39] Early clinical picture after the operation plays an important role in predicting patient's outcome after endoscopic third ventriculostomy.[39] In cases of intraventricular tumors, in addition to ventriculostomy, biopsy was performed that successfully helped the patient management.

The disadvantages are the patient has to be reoperated if the opening gets blocked. However, the chance of shunt related infection is abolished in this procedure.

The overall results (shunt-independent patients with clinical remission or improvement) who had undergone endoscopic third ventriculostomy for obstructive hydrocephalus was very good in 87.1%.[40] As postoperative failures occur early, clinical and radiological control studies, particularly in the first year after the neuroendoscopic procedure, have been recommended. Simultaneous endoscopic third ventriculostomy and ventriculoperitoneal shunt group has also been recommended as the first choice of action for the hydrocephalic patients less than 1 year old.[41] The success rate was 83.9% in the endoscopic third ventriculostomy plus ventriculoperitoneal shunt group and 68.9% (31 of 45) in the ventriculoperitoneal shunt only group. The complications; like infections and obstructions were much less in the endoscopic third ventriculostomy plus ventriculoperitoneal shunt group.

(ii) Torkildsen procedure–This is a redundant procedure now and had involved the cannulation of both the lateral ventricles into the cisterna magna. The Ventricular catheter cannulates the lateral ventricle via occipital burr hole and the distal catheter is placed into the cervical subarachnoid space following a cervical laminectomy. The indication is obstruction of third ventricle or aqueduct of Sylvius. It is not to be considered as an alternative to a ventriculoperitoneal shunt.

(iiii) Fourth ventriculocisternostomy–This procedure has been attempted to treat the Dandy Walker cyst by establishing communication between the fourth ventricle and the perimedullary and pontocerebellar cisterns.

NORMAL PRESSURE HYDROCEPHALUS

Normal pressure hydrocephalus (NPH) may be defined as a state of chronic hydrocephalus in which the prevailing CSF pressure has returned to a physiologic range but in which a slight pressure gradient is moderate, the ventricles enlarge gradually, accompanied by a slow, progressive wasting of the white matter. In well compensated cases, the ventricles may not continue to enlarge, but the existing pressure gradient is sufficient to keep the CSF system inflated and results in a sustained stretching of neurons and associated fibers. This circumstance cannot be regarded as normal.

In normal pressure hydrocephalus, also known as occult hydrocephalus, there is dilatation of the ventricles without the rise in the ICP.

A salient pathologic feature of normal-pressure hydrocephalus is an incomplete block of the CSF pathways. This permits compensatory changes of occur, which, in time, retard the hydrocephalus process and equilibrate CSF pressure to within a normal range. Whereas the majority of cases of NPH involve an obstruction of the distal subarachnoid pathway, approximately 20 percent of the cases are of the noncommunicating type. The most common cause of communicating NPH are head trauma, meningitis and subarachnoid bleeding. Noncommunicating types are most often seen in patients with aqueductal stenosis and/or the Arnold-Chiari malformation.

The clinical syndrome of normal-pressure hydrocephalus is insidious and is characterized in adults by the classic triad of dementia, incontinence, and a disturbance of gait. Since the syndrome is disarmingly free of overt symptoms, and because signs of increased intracranial pressure are generally absent, the diagnosis can go undetected for a prolonged time. The differential diagnosis includes all the presenile and senile dementias, post-tramatic cerebral atrophy, and cerebral arteriosclerosis. CT scan shows the enlargement of the ventricles with the periventricular lucency along with Sylvian fissures. The MRI scan shows decreased cerebral flow. Treatment is the insertion of the low pressure VP shunt. In a study, the caudate and corpus callosum ROI measurements revealed diminished caudate nuclei volume in the NPH group.[42]

Gait abnormalities are the early clinical symptom in normal pressure hydrocephalus, and the subjective improvement in gait after the temporary removal of CSF is often used as an indication to perform shunt surgery.[43] There are significant, quantifiable changes in gait after CSF drainage that corresponds to improvement after shunt surgery for patients with NPH.

ARRESTED HYDROCEPHALUS

Arrested hydrocephalus is a state of chronic hydrocephalus in which the CSF pressure has returned to normal and in which the pressure gradient between the cerebral ventricles and brain parenchyma has been dissipated. Under these conditions, the size of the cerebral ventricles remains stable or decreases, new neurological signs do not appear and there is evidence of advancing psychomotor development with increasing age. This definition is consistent with the findings in patients with surgically treated hydrocephalus.

Spontaneous arrest of hydrocephalus is most likely to occur when the CSF obstruction is incomplete and when the block is distal (extraventricular) rather than proximal (intraventricular). Patients with this diagnosis should be followed for at least 1 year with periodic neurological examinations. IQ test and CT or MRI scans to rule out the insidious development of normal-pressure hydrocephalus. It is important to point out that if the hydrocephalic process is truly arrested, continuing damage to the brain ceases and, in the case of children, normal developmental processes such as myelinization and neuronal maturation resume. Clinically, these changes are manifested by resumption of psychomotor development, albeit as a subnormal level. It is my personal opinion that spontaneously arrested hydrocephalus is not an optimal physiologic state is the cerebral ventricles are significant enlarged, and if it can be established on the basis of clinical and neuroradiological evidence that this is not due to cerebral atrophy. Under such circumstances, consideration should be given to a ventricular shunting procedure.

ASSOCIATED CONGENITAL ANOMALIES

The various anomalies of the posterior fossa include Arachnoid and Neuroepithelial cysts, Dandy-Walker malformation, Isolated fourth ventricle, Pulsion diverticulum and Mega cisterna magna and ex-vacuo states.[44]

Arachnoid Cysts

These arise by a splitting of the arachnoid membrane and are lined by fibro-connective tissue. About 30-40% of arachnoid cysts arise in the posterior fossa and present with signs and symptoms of increased intracranial pressure secondary to hydrocephalus or direct mass effect. Neuroepithelial cysts resemble arachnoid cysts but are lined by cuboidal to columnar epithelium. Surgery is recommended only if the child is symptomatic or the cyst shows evidence of expansion. A cysto-peritoneal shunt using a low pressure valve is an accepted initial procedure. Cyst excision or decompression into the subarachnoid space is recommended by some neuro surgeons in view of the high rate of proximal shunt dysfunction and non obliteration of many cysts despite providing a drainage.

Dandy-Walker Malformation

This is characterized by the presence of a dilated fourth ventricle and enlarged posterior fossa and complete or partial agenesis of the vermis. Dandy-Walker malformation comprises of a triad of hydrocephalus, posterior fossa cyst and absence of cerebellar vermis. There is atresia of foramen of Magendie and Luschka. It is associated with hydrocephalus in 65% of cases.

MRI is the best diagnostic investigation which classically shows a large posterior fossa with an elevated torcula and complete or partial absence of the vermis. This syndrome is associated with hydrocephalus and agenesis of the corpus callorum. About 20% of the patients are asymptomatic. Most present with signs and symptoms related to the associated hydrocephalus and only a few have symptoms related to the cyst itself. Till last decade excision of the cyst membrane along with shunt was the treatment of choice. From the last decade, only a shunt is the treatment preferred. The lateral ventricle or the cyst has been drained by a ventriculo or cysto peritoneal shunt. It is now recommended that the shunt should be placed in the cyst and not in the lateral ventricles. Upto 40% of such patients require the other CSF space to be subsequently drained. With the advent of third ventriculostomy various authors now advocate an initial cystoperitoneal shunt followed by a third ventriculostomy if needed. With a recognized need for a second decompression surgery, some surgeons advocate an initial combined cysto-ventricular drainage using a Y connector, placed proximal to the shunt valve.

The outcome depends on the associated anomalies and over 50% of children with the Dandy-Walker complex perform satisfactorily at school provided the hydrocephalus is well controlled.

Isolated Fourth Ventricle

Patients of hydrocephalus adequately decompressed by a shunt can develop secondary acqueductal stenosis as a result of chronically diminished flow through the acqueduct. Some of these patients may develop an enlarged 4th ventricle and present with a mass lesion in the posterior fossa, nystagmus, lower cranial nerve palsy or bradycardia. Patients with posthemorrhagic or a post inflammatory hydrocephalus and Chiari II malformation are predisposed to developing an isolated fourth ventricle. In the absence of a Chiari II malformation, ventriculostomy is a viable alternative. Patients with a Chiari II malformation require cannulation of the 4th ventricle preferably under CT guidance to avoid injury to vital structures.

Chiari Malformations

The various types of Chiari Malformation described are:

Type – I   Caudal displacement of cerebellar tonsils below the plane of the foramen magnum
Type – II Caudal displacement of the cerebellar vermis fourth ventricle, and lower brain stem below the plane of the foramen magnum. Commonly associated with myelodysplasia
Type – III Caudal displacement of the cerebellum and brain stem into a high cervical meningocele
Type – IV Cerebellar hypoplasia (not a type of cerebellar hernia)

Only patients with type-II Arnold-Chiari malformations have associated hydrocephalus and require shunts (Fig. 100.15).

Meningomyelocele (MMC) and Hydrocephalus

About 80% of all infants with myelomeningocele either concomitant hydrocephalus or develop the same within the first few weeks after MMC surgery. More distal the lesion, more the chance of developing the hydrocephalus. Clinical features of hydrocephalus become apparent within 1 to 2 weeks of MMC repair. A regular monitoring of the head size in the postoperative period is mandatory to note the progress of hydrocephalus. A medical therapy is first instituted with acetazolamide and Glycerol. If the hydrocephalus remained uncontrolled on ultrasonography, surgical intervention is recommended.

There is much controversy about the timing of the MMC repair and the shunt in a patient who has both the MMC and the hydrocephalus at the time of presentation. In patients with hydrocephalus having a tense fontenella and raised ICP, it is better to drain the hydrocephalus before resorting to MMC repair. However, simultaneous surgery can also be performed for both the MMC and the hydrocephalus with some added risks of infection. Similarly, a shunt inserted before the MMC repair may allow the infection to ascend up from the surgery site to the ventricles due to suctioning effect of the VP shunt. Similarly, in the similar case if the excision of the sac is done first, to be followed by the shunt surgery, then there is a risk of persistent leak at the MMC repaired site.

PROGNOSIS

Natural History

Approximately 50% of untreated patients die.[45] The remaining 50% survive with so-called arrested hydrocephalus. Of these, 11-18% have normal cognitive and neurologic findings.

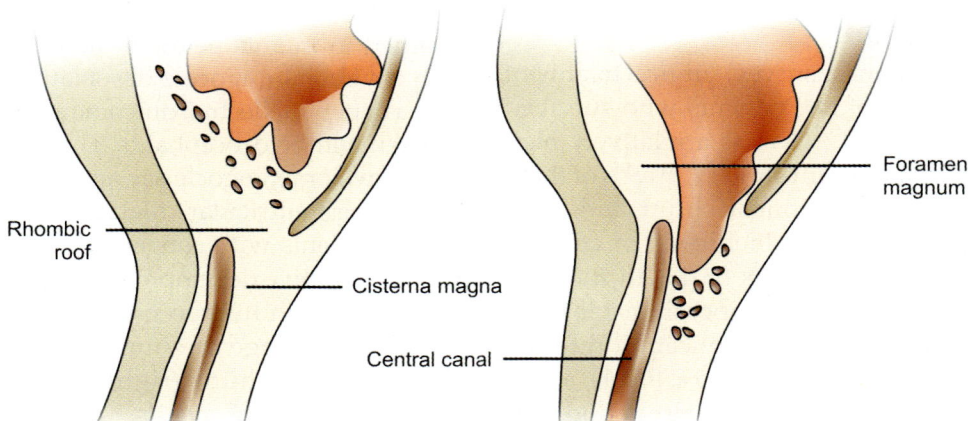

Fig. 100.15: A sagittal depiction through the craniocervical junction. The rhrombic roof bulges towards cisterna magna during fetal age. The choroid plexus has migrated intraventrically and caudally displaced cerebeller vermis

Course of the Disease

The course of the hydrocephalus is quite variable and depends on a complex interplay of factors such as patient age at the time of presentation, severity of symptoms, degree of dilatation, presence or absence of infection and associated abnormalities.

The etiology of the hydrocephalus affects the morbidity. Hydrocephalus following brain injuries affect the cognitive functions more than those by obstructive pathologies. Prenatal hydrocephalus is considered to have a poor prognosis with only 1/3 having an intelligent quotient (IQ) of above 80. The rate of progression also has a impact on development. Slowly progressive hydrocephalus may be asymptomatic with a normal IQ inspite of papery thin cortical mantle. About 1/3 of these patients with gradually progressing hydrocephalus will go into a state of arrested hydrocephalus in their life time. Mortality of patients with hydrocephalus associated with other congenital abnormalities is 80% within the first 5 years of life. The average life time of a shunt varies in different case series though it has even been reported to be as high as 73 months.

The rate of cardiac malformations has been reported to be higher in the group without neural tube defects (p = 0.015).[46] The morbidity has been reported to be higher in the group with neural tube defects, possibly due to the higher number of surgical interventions in the central nervous system.[46] However, the mortality was higher in the group without neural tube defects, possibly due to the presence of other associated malformations, especially congenital heart disease.[46]

In a nationwide Japanese survey, surgical treatment was performed in 341 of 380 patients who survived the early neonatal period.[47] This is a relatively high incidence of performing shunt surgery. 91.9% of these underwent ventriculoperitoneal shunt and 2.8% ventriculoatrial shunt.[47] The incidence of complications after the first shunt was 55.4% in the programmable and 61.6% in the non-programmable valve groups.[47] The types of shunt complication differed significantly between these groups (p < 0.001), as the incidence of shunt infection and malfunction was lower in the programmable valve group. Clinical outcome was generally better with later delivery stage during gestation (p < 0.02). The clinical outcome was statistically significantly better in term patients who underwent early shunt placement than in those who underwent late shunt placement (p < 0.05).[47] A mathematically model of survival to study the prognosis of a newly inserted shunt in pediatric or adult patients with hydrocephalus has been reported.

Shunt survival rates calculated with this model in children and adults were calculated for 1 year (64.2 and 80.1%, respectively), 5 years (49.4 and 60.2%, respectively), and the median (4.9 and 7.3 years, respectively).[48]

LONG-TERM FOLLOW-UP RESULTS

Mortality in hydrocephalus patients is usually related to the etiology and associated conditions. Most published series report long-term survival (50-90%) in surgically treated patients.[49,50] Patients with myelomeningocele associated hydrocephalus have a higher mortality rate as compared to isolated congenital hydrocephalus. Patients with vascular shunts have a significantly higher morbidity and the mortality than those with peritoneal shunts (19% vs 11%).[51] The natural history of untreated hydrocephalus is dismal and only 20% of patients survive till adulthood.[45] to IQ has been correleted cortical mantle thickness as[52]:

- Patients with cortical mantle thickness with < 2 cm. remain uneducable.
- Patients with the cortical mantle thickness between 2-3 cm develop an IQ < 100.
- Patients with cortical mantle thickness more than 3 cm have normal IQ.

The best functional results after shunt surgery are obtained in infants below 5 months of age. Patients with myelomeningocele associated hydrocephalus have a better intellectual outcome as compared to other children with hydrocephalus. This is probably related to the myelomeningocle sac acting as a reservoir and preventing ventricular dilatation before birth. Only 38% of patients with congenital hydrocephalus have normal cognitive development.[53] The factors affecting nonverbal IQ in hydrocephalus are associated brain malformation, age at shunt surgery, antiepileptic drugs, side of shunt (right better than left) and associated perinatal insults.

The care of children with hydrocephalus requires a multimodality approach. Early treatment and regular follow-up can ensure a favourable outcome in these children. A follow-up CT scan for at least

3 years or so with no increase in the ventricle size and the shunt lying blocked, would suggest that the hydrocephalus has achieved a state of arrest and the shunt is no more needed. However, in normal circumstances the shunt is not removed unless the surgeon feels that the shunt has really been unnecessary. Some patients manage with their shunts well, however, others would require many revisions, as many as 20 revisions in their life time. Each revision may be associated with deranged brain function. Many children have been achievers in their personal and family life including sports but it has been observed that number of children leading such quality of life decreases with age, especially after the age of 20-25 years. It is estimated that about 1,50,000 shunt units are marketed in USA alone with billions of dollar expenditure each year. In developing countries like India, an inexpensive shunt developed by Prof P Upadhyaya has been used regularly in the author's institution since 1970, costing now about USD 25 only. It has been used in over 2000 children with hydrocephalus of different etiologies, including the postmeningitic and tubercular hydrocephalus with gratifying results.[54] Patients with shunt hydrocephalus need to be kept under constant supervision of the experts so that the timely help could be provided in case the patient develops shunt related complications, which are in any case not infrequent.

RECENT ADVANCES

- To detect possible ultrastructural alterations of the lateral ventricles, choroid plexus (responsible for the CSF production) have been studied in rats that were submitted to an intracisternal injection of 20% kaolim (hydrated aluminum silicate) for hydrocephalus induction.[55]
- Newer shunt devices (Saply SV8): In this system the pressure valve is situated externally over the skin and patient manipulates the pressure valve as per his symptoms.
- Endoscopic laser ablation of choroid plexus: Recently the endoscopic laser ablation of choroid plexus has been done in cases of idiopathic hydrocephalus and the choroids plexus hyperplasia.
- Gentian Violet impregnated shunts to reduce the incidence of shunt infection and the shunt colonization with *Staph. albus*.
- Barium impregnated shunts for visualization of the shunt assembly by imaging. This is especially useful to demonstrate if the shunt assembly has either fractured or one of its ends has migrated and lost in the peritoneal cavity or the heart chambers.

IDIOPATHIC CHILDHOOD HYDROCEPHALUS

Magnetic resonance imaging with flow quantification has been done in idiopathic childhood hydrocephalus.[56] It was found that in children with hydrocephalus, the cerebral blood inflow was normal, but the superior sagittal sinus (SSS) and straight sinus outflows were reduced by 27% and 38%, respectively, when compared with the measurements in control group (p = 0.03 and 0.002).[56] These findings suggest that approximately 150 ml of blood per minute was returning via collateral channels from that portion of the brain drained by the SSS, and 60 ml/minute was returning from collaterals in the deep venous territory. This has been correlated with idiopathic intracranial hypertension seen in adults and it has been elucidated that the same venous pathophysiological process may be operating in both conditions. Whether or not the ventricles would dilate, may depend on the differences in brain compliance between adults and children.[56]

REFERENCES

1. Aschoff A, Kremer P, Hashemi B, Kunze S. The scientific history of hydrocephalus and its treatment. Neurosurg Rev 1999;22(2-3):67-93; discussion 94-95.
2. Gupta DK, Dave Sumit. Hydrocephalus. In Text book of Neonatal Surgery, Ed.DK Gupta, Modern Publishers, New Delhi, 2000; 67:434-50.
3. Milhorat TH. Choroid plexus and cerebrospinal fluid production. Science 1969;166:1514-16.
4. Pollay M, Hisey B, Reynolds E, et al. Chroid plexus Na+/K+ - activated adenosine triphosphatase and cerebrospinal fluid formation. Neurosurgery 1985;17(5):768-72.
5. Brodbelt A, Stoodley M. CSF pathways: a review Br J Neurosurg 2007;21(5):510-20.
6. De SN. A study of the changes in the brain in experimental internal hydrocephalus. J Pathol Bacteriol 1950;62:197-99.
7. Moritake K, Nagai H, Miyazaki T, Nagasako N, Yamasaki M, Tamakoshi A. Nationwide survey of the etiology and associated conditions of prenatally and postnatally diagnosed congenital hydrocephalus in Japan Neurol Med Chir (Tokyo) 2007;47(10):448-52; discussion 452.
8. Gupta DK, Sharma S, Gupta M. Outcome of antenatally referred congenital surgical anomalies – a Pediatric Surgeon's Perspective. Journal of Surgical specialties 2007; 1(1), 6-11.

9. Gupta DK. Editorial, Prenatally diagnosed surgical malformations – who should decide next? Journal of Indian Association of Pediatric Surgeons 2006;11(1):7-9.
10. Sharma Shilpa, Gupta DK. Discrepancies between the Antenatal and Postnatal Diagnosis of Pediatric Surgical Conditions. Journal of Indian Association of pediatric surgeons 2006;11:183.
11. Hill A, Volpe JJ. Decrease in pulsatile flow in the anterior cerebral artery in infantile hydrocephalus. Paediatrics 1982;69:4-7.
12. George AE, deLeon MJ, Miller J, et al. Positron emission tomography of hydrocephalus. Metabolic effects of shunt procedures. Acta Radiol 1986;369:435-39.
13. Hanlo PW, Peters RJA, Gooskens RMJM, et al. Monitoring intracranial dynamics by transcranial doppler - a new doppler index: Transsystolic time. Ultrasound in Med and Biol 1995;21(5):613-21.
14. Chester DC, Emery JL, Penny SR. Fat laden macrophages in cerebrospinal fluid as an indication of brain damage in children. J Clin Pathol 1971;24:753-55.
15. Gilles FH, Gilles EE. Hydrocephalus in the neonate, infant and child. In: Disorders of the Developing Nervous System: Diagnosis and treatment, edited by HJ Hoffman and F. Epstein. Blackwell Scientific Publication 1986;541.
16. Holmedal LJ, Friberg EG, Børretzen I, Olerud H, Lægreid L, Rosendahl K. Radiation doses to children with shunt-treated hydrocephalus. Pediatr Radiol 2007;37(12):1209-15.
17. Flodmark O. Hydrocephalus. In: BICER series on diagnostic imaging: Paediatric Radiology, edited by Harwood Nash DC, Petterson H. Merit communications. 1992;63-77.
18. DiRocco C, Mclone DG, Shimogi T, et al. Continuous intraventricular cerebrospinal fluid pressure recording in hydrocephalus children during wakefulness and sleep. J Neurosurg 1975;42:683-86.
19. Moss SM, Marshbanks RJ, Burge DM. Long term assessment of intracranial pressure using the tympanic membrane displacement measurement technique. Eur J Paediatr Surg 1991;1:25-26.
20. McNatt SA, McComb JG, Nelson MD, Bluml S. Proton magnetic resonance spectroscopy of hydrocephalic infants Pediatr Neurosurg 2007;43(6):461-67.
21. Shinnar S, Gammon K, Bergman EW, et al. Management of hydrocephalus in infancy: use of acetazolamide and furosemide to avoid cerebrospinal flud shunts. J Paediatrics 1985;107:31-37.
22. Udani PM. Neurotuberculosis. In: Puri RK, Sachdev HPS, (Eds). Tuberculosis in children, Delhi, Indian Pediatrics, 1994;143-87.
23. Dastur HM, Pandya SK, Rao YC. Aetiology of hydrocephalus in tubercular meningitis, Neurology (Bombay) 1972;Suppl: 73.
24. Whitelaw A, Odd DE. Intraventricular streptokinase after intraventricular hemorrhage in newborn infants Cochrane Database Syst Rev 2007;17;(4):CD000498.
25. Young HF, Nulsen EF, Weiss MH, et al. The relationship of intelligence and cerebral mantle in treated infantile hydrocephalus. IQ potential in hydrocephalic children. Paediatrics 1973;52:38-41.
26. Martínez-Lage JF, Almagro MJ, Del Rincón IS, Pérez-Espejo MA, Piqueras C, Alfaro R, Ros de San Pedro J. Management of neonatal hydrocephalus: feasibility of use and safety of two programmable (Sophy and Polaris) valves. Childs Nerv Syst 2007;9 [Epub ahead of print].
27. Bhatnagar V, George J, Mitra DK, Upadhyaya P. Complications of cerebrospinal fluid shunts Indian J Pediatr. 1983;50:133-38.
28. Bhatnagar V, Mitra DK, Upadhyaya P. Shunt related infections in hydrocephalic children . Indian Pediatr 1986;23;255-57.
29. Sarguna P, Lakshmi V. Ventriculoperitoneal shunt infections. Indian J Med Microbiol 2006;24:52-54.
30. Sharma Shilpa, Gupta DK, Sharma SP, Gopal SC, Gangopadhyay AN. Pseudo cyst formation following ventriculo peritoneal shunt: report of 2 cases and review of literature. Journal of Indian association of pediatric surgeons 2004;9:87-91.
31. Zhou F, Chen G, Zhang J. Bowel perforation secondary to ventriculoperitoneal shunt: case report and clinical analysis. J Int Med Res. 2007;35(6):926-29.
32. Epstein F, Lapras C, Wisoff JH. 'Slit ventricle syndrome': Etiology and treatment. Pediatr Neurosci 1988;14:5-10.
33. Sharma Shilpa, Gupta DK. Intraventicular migration of an entire VP Shunt. Indian Pediatr. 2005;42:187-88.
34. DiRocco C, Janelli A, Pallini R, et al. Epilepsy and its correlation with cerebral ventricular shunting procedures in infantile hydrocephalus. J Pediatr Neurosci 1985;1:255-57.
35. Little JR, Rhoton AL, Mellinger JF. Comparison of ventriculoperitoneal and ventriculo atrial shunts for hydrocephalus in children. May Clin Proc 1972;47:396-99.
36. Selman WR, Spetzler RF, Wilson CB, et al. Percutaneous lumboperitoneal shunt: Review of 130 cases. Neurogsurg 1980;6:255-59.
37. Rohatgi M, Goulatia RK. A new technique for accurate placing of the tip of the atrial catheter in ventriculo-atrial shunt operations for hydrocephalus. Acta Neurochirurgica 1976;33:167-72.
38. Sandberg DI. Endoscopic management of hydrocephalus in pediatric patients: a review of indications, techniques, and outcomes. J Child Neurol. 2008;23:550-60.
39. Rezaee O, Sharifi G, Samadian M, et al. Endoscopic third ventriculostomy for treatment of obstructive hydrocephalus. Arch Iran Med 2007;10(4):498-03.
40. Gangemi M, Mascari C, Maiuri F, Godano U, Donati P, Longatti PL. Long-term outcome of endoscopic third ventriculostomy in obstructive hydrocephalus. Minim Invasive Neurosurg 2007;50:265-69.
41. Shim KW, Kim DS, Choi JU. Simultaneous endoscopic third ventriculostomy and ventriculoperitoneal shunt

41. for infantile hydrocephalus. Childs Nerv Syst 2008;24: 443-51.
42. DeVito EE, Salmond CH, Owler BK, Sahakian BJ, Pickard JD. Caudate structural abnormalities in idiopathic normal pressure hydrocephalus. Acta Neurol Scand 2007;116 (5):328-32.
43. Williams MA, Thomas G, de Lateur B, Imteyaz H, Rose JG, Shore WS, Kharkar S, Rigamonti D. Objective Assessment of Gait in Normal-Pressure Hydrocephalus. Am J Phys Med Rehabil 2008;87(1):39-45.
44. Mapstone TB. Congenital CSF anomalies of the posterior fossa. In. Pediatric Neurosurgery. Surgery of the developing nervous system, edited by William R. Cheek, Saunders Company 1994;234.
45. Laurence KM, Coates S. The natural history of. hydrocephalus. Arch Dis Child 1962;37:345-62.
46. Schlatter D, Sanseverino MT, Schmitt JM, Fritsch A, Kessler RG, Barrios PM, Palma-Dias RS, Magalhães JA. Severe fetal hydrocephalus with and without neural tube defect: a comparative study Fetal Diagn Ther. 2008; 23(1):23-29. Epub 2007 Oct 9.
47. Moritake K, Nagai H, Miyazaki T, et al. Analysis of a nationwide survey on treatment and outcomes of congenital hydrocephalus in Japan. Neurol Med Chir (Tokyo). 2007;47:453-60; discussion 460-61.
48. Stein SC, Guo W. A mathematical model of survival in a newly inserted ventricular shunt. J Neurosurg 2007; 107:448-54.
49. Hirsch JF. Consensus: long term outcome in hydrocephalus. Child's Nerv Syst 1994;10:64-69.
50. Lumenta CB, Skotarczak U. Long term follow-up in 233 patients with congenital hydrocephalus. Child's Nerv Syst 1995;11:173-75.
51. Keucher T, Mealy J. Long term results after ventriculoatrial and ventriculo-peritoneal shunting for infantile hydrocephalus. J Neurosurg 1979;50:179-86.
52. Mapstone TB, Rekate HL, Nulsen FE, et al. Relationship of CSF shunting and IQ in children with myelomeningocele: a retrospective analysis. Childs Brain. 1984;11: 112-18.
53. Roseau GL., McGullough DC, Joseph AL. Current prognosis in fetal ventriculomegaly, J. Neurosurg 1992;77: 551-55.
54. Upadhyaya P, Bhargava S, Dube S, Sundaram KR, Ochaney M. Results of ventriculoatrial shunt surgery for hydrocephalus using Indian SAhunt valve: evqaluation of intellectual performance with particular reference to computerized axial tomography. Prog Pediatr Surg 1982; 15:209-22.
55. Tirapelli DP, Lopes Lda S, Lachat JJ, Colli BO, Tirapelli LF. Ultrastructural study of the lateral ventricle choroid plexus in experimental hydrocephalus in Wistar rats Arq Neuropsiquiatr. 2007;65:974-77.
56. Bateman GA, Smith RL, Siddique SH. Idiopathic hydrocephalus in children and idiopathic intracranial hypertension in adults: two manifestations of the same pathophysiological process? J Neurosurg. 2007;107:439-44.

CHAPTER 101

Encephaloceles

AK Mahapatra, GD Satyarthee

DEFINITION AND HISTORICAL ASPECTS ON ENCEPHALOCELES

Encephaloceles are congenital disorders characterized by protrusion of brain or meninges out of the cranial cavity through defect in the skull. Depending on the content or herniation, it may be cranial meningoceles or meningoencephaloceles. When herniated brain contains a part of the ventricle, the condition is called hydroencephaly. Thus, encephalocele is a generic term used to describe above mentioned congenital cranial abnormalities.

According to Emery and Kalhan, the first medical report on encephalocele dates back to 16th Century, however, deformity like encephalocele was first illustrated in medieval art and archaic sculpture. It was Ritcher et al, who first described a case of nasal encephalocele in 1813 (Fenger).[1,2] Heinecke in 1882 classified encephalocele (Fenger) depending on herniation tract.[2] In 1903, Stadfeldt first coined the term frontoethmoid encephalocele (Bumenfeld and Skolink).[3] Brower and de Veer in 1934 termed nasal encephaloceles as Rhinoencephaloceles.[4] Suwanwela and Suwanwela in 1972 proposed a morphological classification of sincipital encephaloceles.[5] Tessier in 1976 described different facial clefts and correlated them with the congenital deformities.[6]

The incidence of encephaloceles is less common than spinal dysraphism, being 1 per 3000 to 10,000 live birth.[7-10] Overall occipital encephaloceles are more prevalent than anterior encephaloceles. In western countries occipital encephaloceles constitute 80 to 90 percent of all encephaloceles.[10,11] However, higher incidence of anterior encephaloceles is reported from Thailand, Indonesia, India, Papua New Guinea and Africa.[5,11-15] The incidence of anterior encephalocele reported from the West is 1 per 35000 to 40,000 live birth.[15-17] Basal encephaloceles are rare.[18-21] Authors have encountered 5 cases of intranasal encephaloceles in their series of 65 cases.[21]

CLASSIFICATION OF ENCEPHALOCELES (TABLE 101.1)

Encephaloceles have large number of classifications based on several aspects of the encephalocele i.e. site of cranial defect, visibility of encephalocele from outside and the size of the encephalocele.[22-26] Encephaloceles are classification as occipital, parietal, frontal, nasal and nasopharyngeal type. Suwanwela and Suwanwela put forward the morphological classification of sincipital encephaloceles.[5]

Anterior encephaloceles (Table 101.2) again have many classifications. Heinecke, in 1882, classified the encephaloceles (a) sphenopharyngeal, (b) Spheno-orbital and sphenomaxillary types (quoted by Fenger) depending on hernial tract.[2] Mesterton in 1885, classified anterior encephaloceles into (a) Nasofrontal, (b) Nasoethmoidal and (c) Nasoorbital types. In 1965 Bumemfeld et al classified encephaloceles as (a) transethmoidal, (b) trans-sphenoidal, (c) spheno-ethmoidal and (d) Sphenomaxillary.[3] Suwanwela et al proposed the morphological basis classification of sincipital encephalocele.[5] The bony defects involving inner and outer tables of the skull are enumerated in Table 101.3.

EMBRYOLOGY

Anterior neuropore closes around 24th day of gestation. Developmental neural tube defects have

Table 101.1: Classifications of encephaloceles

A. **Based on origin**
  1. Congenital
  2. Acquired
     - Postoperative, post-traumatic, post-irradiation
B. **According to the size**
  1. Small encephalocele
  2. Giant encephalocele
C. **According to the content**
  1. Cephalocele
  2. Encephalocele
  3. Meningo-encephalocele
  4. Cranial meningocele
  5. Hydroencephalomeningocele
D. **Based on visibility of encephalocele**
  1. Overt
  2. Occult
     - Intranasal
     - Intraorbital
     - Intratemporal
  3. Intradiploic
E. **According to the locations**
  1. Anterior encephaloceles (Frontoethmoidal) or (Sincipital)
  2. Occipital, or suboccipital encephalocele
  3. Basal
     - Transsphenoidal
     - Transethmoidal
     - Intranasal
     - Spheno-oribital
     - Transtemporal
  4. Cranial vault
     - Frontal
     - Parietal
     - Temporal
     - Through anterior or posterior fontanel
F. **Encephalocele as a part of complex syndrome such as**
  1. Chiari III – Malformation
  2. Knobloch syndrome
  3. Morning glory Syndrome
  4. Walker-Warburg Syndrome (WWS)

Table 101.2: Different classification of anterior encephaloceles

Authors	Year	Types
Heinecke	1882	1. Sphenopharyngel 2. Spheno-orbital 3. Sphenomaxillary
Mesterton	1885	1. Nasofrontal 2. Nosoethmoidal 3. Naso-orbital
Bumenfeld and Skolnik	1965	1. Transethmoidal 2. Transsphenoidal 3. Sphenoethmoidal 4. Sphenomaxillary

Suwanwela and Suwanwela	1972	1. Frontoethmoidal
		  – Nasofrontal
		  – Nasoethmoidal
		  – Naso-orbital
		2. Interfrontal
		3. Sphenomaxillary

Tessier	1976	1. 14 Clefts

Mahapatra et al	1995	1. Frontoethmoidal
		  – Nasofrontal
		  – Nosoethmoidal
		  – Naso-orbital
		2. Interfrontal
		3. Transethmoidal
		4. Sphenoethmoidal
		5. Transsphenoidal
		6. Orbital encephaloceles

been attributed either to the primary failure of closure of neural tube, or neural tube rupture after its closure. Severe forms like an encephalus, and cranioschisis may point to an earlier effect, may be in early neurulation stage. The unfused cephalic end of the neural fold, or defective closure of anterior neuropore may communicate to amniotic cavity, when skin, cranium and dura fail to cover neural tissue. However, the above hypothesis does not explain the occipital or sincipital encephaloceles with healthy skin cover and the absence of cranial dysraphism.[1] Gardner's hydrodynamic theory does not explain the well formed skin cover and lack of cranial dysraphism, as it is usually the case with encephaloceles.[27] Neuroschisis theory proposes bleb formation over the neural tube, which on healing gets adherent to cutaneous ectoderm, this can explain the formation of encephalocele.

Various etiological factors have been incriminated in the formation of encephalocele.[17,28-31] Willamson et al[86] postulated viral antigen following maternal infection in the early phase of pregnancy.[17] Hypervitaminosis, irradiation, hypoxia, hyperthermia and salicylates have also been reported to cause encephalocele in experimental animals.[18,28,32] Moerman et al, postulated a band of amniotic adhesion resulting in formation of encephaloceles.[30] Leong et al postulated the displacement theory for occipital encephalocele, which also corresponds to the area of anterior neuropore.[19]

Table 101.3: Sites of bony defects at the skullbase and outer defect over the facial skeleton			
	Type of encephalocele	At the skull-base	In the face
1.	Nasofrontal (Glabellar)	Between ethmoid and frontal bone, in front of crista Galli	At the junction of frontal and nasal bone
2.	Nasoethmoidal (Anterior Nasal)	-do-	At the junction of nasal bone and nasal cartilage
3.	Nasoorbital (Nasolacrimal)	-do-	Between frontal process of maxilla and lacrimal bone
4.	Transethmoidal (Nasopharyngeal)	-do-	No outer defect (Encephalocele in naso-pharynx or in nasal cavity)
5.	Trans-sphenoidal (Intrasphenoidal)	Through the body of sphenoid or sphenoid sinus	No outer defect
6.	Interfrontal	—	Through metopic suture or anterior fontanel

Anterior encephaloceles result due to failure of anterior neuropore, which is located in front of the foramen caecum of anterior cranial fossa floor, just ahead of crista galli, which is the junction of the ethmoid bone and frontal bone. In the early embryonic life, failure of closure of anterior neuropore results in herniation of neuroectodermal tissue, interposed between the mesodermal elements, which later develops into ethmoid frontal bones.[33,34] Various theories have been put forward for the development of anterior encephaloceles. Geoffrey et al proposed the adhesive theory, while Wiese et al suggested the primary mesodermal failure theory leading to defective bone formation resulting in formation of anterior encephalocele.[35,36]

ASSOCIATED PATHOLOGY

A number of systemic abnormalities (Table 101.4) may be associated with encephaloceles.[27,37-40] Musculoskeletal defects, the "morning glory syndrome (progressive hormonal and visual disturbance progressive), and the Knobloch syndrome (skin defect and visual problems).[38]

CLINICAL PRESENTATION

Swelling at Birth

Patients with encephaloceles are born with a swelling on the scalp at birth, the location depends upon type, which may or not be visible. The shape, size and contents of the encephaloceles are variable. In occipital encephalocele, a globular swelling is noticed over the occipital bone in midline, which may be sessile or pedunculated.[20,29] The size of encephalocele is independent of the amount of herniated neural tissue. Although most encephaloceles transilluminate brilliantly as they contain clear CSF, a large amount of gliosed brain within them may reduce the degree of transillumination.

Table 101.4: Systemic abnormalities associated with encephaloceles

1. Craniofacial abnormalities
   – Microcephaly
   – Cleft lip cleft palate
   – Micrognathia
   – Microcephaly
   – Hair Collar sign

2. Vertebral and spinal cord anomaly
   – Klippel-Feil deformities
   – Vertebral abnormalities
   – Spina bifida
   – Diastematomyelia

3. Ophthalmological anomaly
   – Visual disturbances
   – Vitreoretinal degeneration
   – Retinal detachment
   – Myopia

4. Cardiovascular and respiratory system anomaly
   – Dextrocardia
   – Septal defects
   – Patent ductus arteriosus
   – Pulmonary hypoplasia

5. Urinary system anomaly
   – Renal agenesis
   – Renal hypoplasia

6. Miscellaneous   – Polydactyly

Size of Encephalocele and Relation with Size of Head

Size of the head is usually small[41,42] and depends on the amount of herniated brain tissue. Occasionally the size of the encephaloceles may be very large. Encephaloceles with diameters larger than the diameter of head of the patient.[3,4,43-45] are called giant encephaloceles. Typically the head looks smaller than the size of the encephalocele causing difficulty in nursing. Over the years the authors have encountered 4 patients with giant encephaloceles, 3 in occipital and one in frontal area. Giant encephaloceles contain a large amount of brain tissue and can cause considerable problems during closure.

Location of Encephalocele

Site of encephaloceles (Fig. 101.1) is frequently occipital or suboccipital.[20,26,29,46] Ten percent of the encephaloceles are located anteriorly (Fig. 101.2).[5,11,41] Rarely encephaloceles could be in frontal, temporal, parietal, transethmoid, intranasal, or orbital region (Fig. 101.3) (Table 101.5).[9,11,14,18,42,44,47-51]

Visibility of Encephalocele

Patients with frontoethmoid encephalocele present with swelling over the root or the bridge of nose since birth.[5,14,15,24,52] Those with nasopharyngeal, transsphenoidal, and sphenoethmoidal encephaloceles do not have an obvious external swelling and may present with nasal obstruction causing difficulty in breathing, CSF rhinorrhea, or recurring attacks of meningitis.[8,14,20,24,32,43,50,53-55] Often a suspicion of encephalocele becomes evident when a patient with intranasal encephalocele presents to an Ootolaryngologist as a nasal polyp and it is inadvertently biopsied or operated leading to development of CSF rhinorrhea.[13,14,24,43,54] Rarely, encephaloceles may present in mouth through a cleft palate.[9]

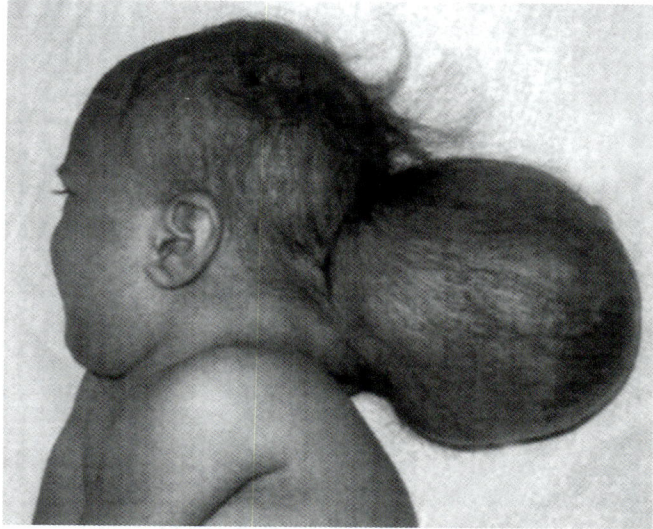

Fig. 101.1: Clinical photo of occipital encephalocele

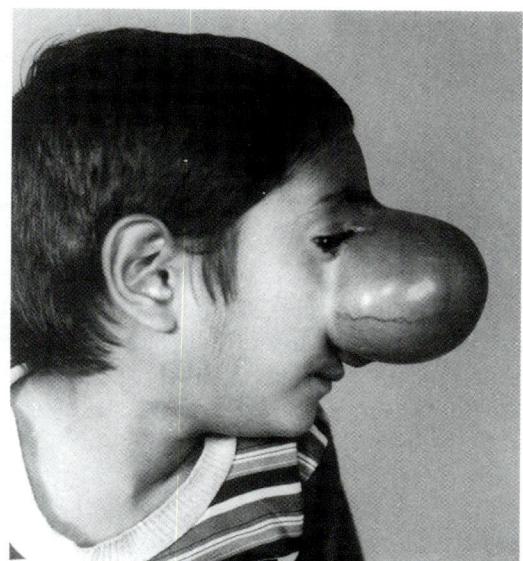

Fig. 101.2: Clinical photograph of a patient with anterior encephalocele

Table 101.5: Locations of anterior encephaloceles at AIIMS (n= 75) (1972-1996)

Types of encephalocele	Number
1. Frontoethmoidal	
– Nasofrontal	4
– Nasoethmoidal	52
– Nasoorbital	7
2. Nasopharyngeal	6
3. Orbital	6
Total:	75

Local Deformities

Proptosis may be caused by orbital encephaloceles. It could be a part of nasoorbital encephalocele when there is proptosis along with hypertelorism.[14-16,37,47,51,52,56,57] Orbital encephaloceles could also be a part of neurofibromatosis, when there is

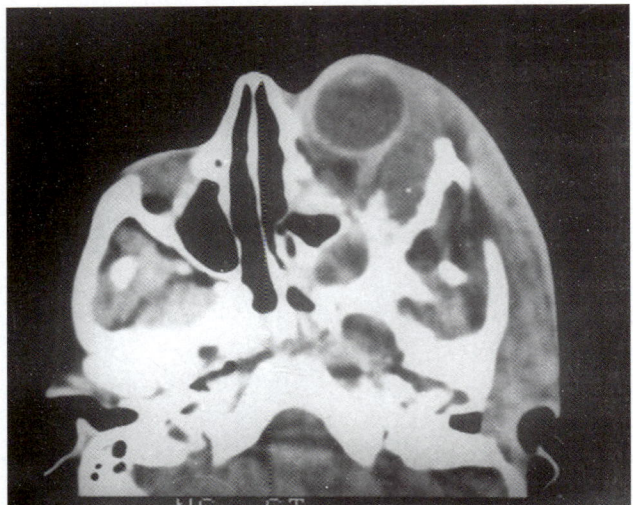

Fig. 101.3: CT scan of a patient with Lt. orbital encephalocele showing Lt. sided proptosis

absence of wing of the sphenoid bone.[56] The proptosis is positional, and disappears on assuming a supine position.

Anterior Encephalocele

It can be subdivided into following sub-groups (Fig. 101.4)

a. *Nasoethmoid type:* Also called *Long nose encephalocele* is the commonest type of sincipital encephalocele constituting 85% of anterior encephalocele.[16,32,52,58] The inner cranial defect lies in front of crista galli in the floor of anterior cranial fossa. The facial defect lies at the junction of the nasal bone and nasal cartilage (Fig. 101.5).[15,59] The frontal process of maxilla and nasal bone form the anterosuperior part of the sac, and the postero-inferior wall is formed the nasal cartilage and nasal septum. The lateral part of the sac extends into the orbit and presents at the inner canthi causing bilateral displacement orbit and the eye ball laterally, downward and produces severe degree of hypertelorism. The neck of the encephalocele is also very long. The swelling causes widening of the nasal bridge and pushes the tip of the nose typically downward, thus producing a markedly elongated the nose.[12,15,60]

b. *Nasofrontal type:* Also called glabellar or frontonasal encephalocele and is relatively rare (Fig. 101.6).[10,14,26,61] The internal bone defect is

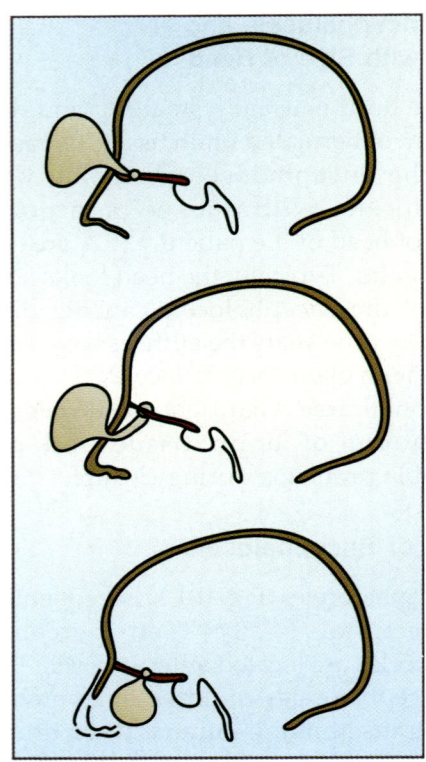

Fig. 101.4: Diagram showing site of brain herniation (a) Nasofrontal (b) Nasoethmoidal (c) Nasopharyngeal. In all inner defect in cribriform plate and outer defect. In (a) at nasion, in (b) between the nasal bone and nasal cartilage in (c) not visible from outside swelling in nasopharynx

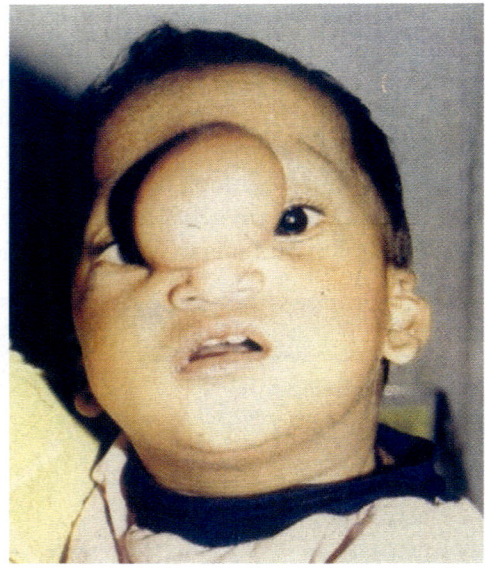

Fig. 101.5: A clinical photo of a patient with Nasoethmoid type of frontoethmoidal encephalocele with gross hypertelorism

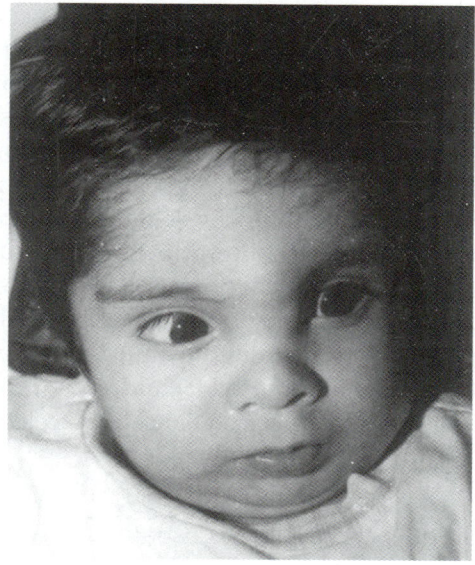

Fig. 101.6: A clinical photograph of a 2 years girl with Nasofrontal encephalocele, swelling at nasion

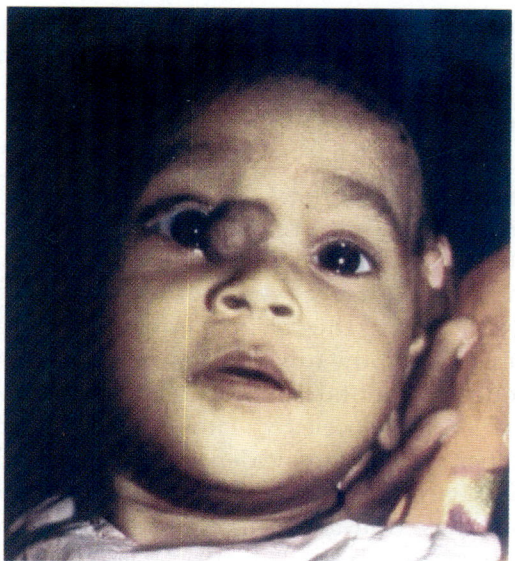

Fig. 101.7: Clinical photograph of a child with unilateral Naso-orbital encephalocele

present in front of the crista galli with is round or oval shaped. Usually crista galli project into the defect and forms the posterior margin of bone defect. Anterior cranial fossa is deep. The fascial bone defect lies at the junction of nasal bone and frontal bone. Patient may or may not have hypertelorism. However, maxilla, nasal bone and nasal process of maxilla are normal.

c. *Naso-orbital type:* A rare form of frontoethmoidal Encephalocele.[5,15,32,61] Among the reported 75 cases of anterior encephaloceles, the authors have noted 7 of them (Table 101.5). The inner skull defect is located in front of crista galli and the outer fascial defect is present between the frontal process of maxilla and lacrimal bone. Frontal process of maxilla forms the anteromedial whereas lacrimal bone forms the posterior lateral boundaries of the sac. Outer swelling appears at the inner canthus of the eye. It may either project unilateral or bilaterally. The eyeball and the inner canthi are pushed downward and laterally (Fig. 101.7). Thus, all these patients invariably have some degree of hypertelorism, which will require correction. Nose and nasal bones are normal.

d. *Trans-sphenoidal encephaloceles:* This is the rarest from of encephalocele.[9,36,42,53,62] Pollack et al reviewed 8 case of trans-sphenoidal and transethmoid encephaloceles.[63] The Bony defect is present over the roof of the sphenoid sinus. Thus, the encephalocele may come through the sella or through planum sphenoidale and enters into the sphenoid sinus and nasopharynx. Patients may present with history of CSF rhinorrhea, endocrine disturbances and rarely visual disturbances.[62,64]

Rare Clinical Features (Table 101.6)

Hypertelorism

Hypertelorism is a common finding in anterior encephalocele.[6,8,15,16,24,37,57,60] This type of encephalo-

Table 101.6: Clinical presentation in patients with anterior encephaloceles at AIIMS, (n=75)	
Clinical Finding	Number of patients
Swelling over the nose or at inner Canthus	63
Hypertelorism	60
Proptosis	12
CSF rhinorrhea	10
Meningitis	6
Nasal obstruction	6
Mental retardation	4
Neurofibromatosis Type I	3
Leaking encephalocele	3
Cleft palate	1

cele have a higher incidence of hypertelorism.[24,61] Rarely, maxillary and zygomatic bone abnormalities, neurofibromatosis and 13-15 triosmy have been reported.[65]

Mental Retardation and Other Neurological Deficits

1. Mental retardation: Severity of mental retardation depends upon the degree brain damage in encephalocele. Suwanwela et al reported a higher incidence of mental retardation in patients with anterior encephalocele.[15,57] However, in the authors series there was a low incidence.[24,25,61] Children with occipital encephaloceles may present with poor cry and suckling due to herniation of cerebellum and brainstem into the sac.[29,31] Increased tone in limbs and defective temperature regulation indicate a poor prognosis.

2. Smell and visual abnormalities: Defects of smell and vision are rarely discussed. It is logical to have smell abnormalities in patients with frontoethmoidal or sphenoethmoidal encephaloceles. In cases of unilateral nasoorbital encephaloceles with paramedian anterior fossa defect, smell is likely to get preserved in one side.[25] Visual abnormalities may be due to herniation of occipital lobe into occipital encephalocele, chiasmal abnormality in transsphenoidal encephalocele, compression of optic nerve by an orbital encephalocele, associated hydrocephalus, or rarely vitreoretinal degeneration.[39,51,56,66]

3. Associated Syndromes: Few rare syndromes are associated with encephaloceles. **"Knobloch syndrome"** was deserved by Knobloch and Layer in 1971.[39] The syndrome is transmitted by autosomal recessive inheritance and characterized by vitreoretinal degeneration with retinal detachment, high myopia and encephalocele. **"Morning glory syndrome"** is a condition, characterized by nasal encephaloceles associated with progressive hormonal and visual problems.[38] The basal encephaloceles are in the form of transsphenoidal or sphenoethmoidal type. Because of pituitary involvement, deficiency of growth hormone and ADH patients present with polyuria, polydipsia and dwarfism. **"Von Vos-Cherstvoy syndrome"** is another clinical entity described by Von Voss et al in 1979.[67] The syndrome is characterized occipital encephalocele, phocomyelia, along with cerebellar anomalies transmitted by autosomal recessive gene. The upper limb abnormality more often due to defect in radius. The other associated anomalies involve face, heart, lungs, urogenital system, gastrointestinal system and include thrombocytopenia. Lubinnsky et al in 1994 reported 4 cases and a review the literature on this subject.[67] Walker–Warburg Syndrome (WWS) is a lethal, complex syndrome involving of the CNS and the eyes, and is genetically transmitted by autosomal recessive gene. Martinez et al reported 9 children with WWS, 8 children of them had occipital encephaloceles.[68]

INVESTIGATIONS

Diagnosis of encephalocele is usually made clinically, except in rare cases where encephaloceles is not visible externally. A large number of factor influence the treatment and ultimate prognosis.[16,20,32,38,41,69] These includes hydrocephalus, associated CNS anomalies, facial deformity and associated systemic abnormalities. Assessment of all the above factors needs proper radiological, genetic and hormonal assessment.

Plain X-ray

Shows a soft tissue mass and a circular smooth bone defect depending on the site of the encephalocele. It may show nasopharyngeal soft tissue mass or displacement of nasopharyngeal region in sphenoidal or nasopharyngeal encephalocele.[9,42,53,63] In sincipital encephaloceles, X-ray skull shows deformity of orbits and hypertelorism and enlargement of orbit in intraorbital encephaloceles. There may be hypoplasia of anterior or middle fossa.[18,47,51,53,56,70]

Carotid Angiograms and Pneumoencephalograms

Have been used as investigations in the past.[41,71,72] Suwanwela et al reported the value of ventriculography in patients with anterior encephaloceles.[72] in assessment of communication between CSF pathway with encephalocele sac. Similarly cerebral angiography delineates the intracranial vasculature including sagittal and transverse sinus. In a large number of cases there may be abnormalities of dural venous sinuses.[73]

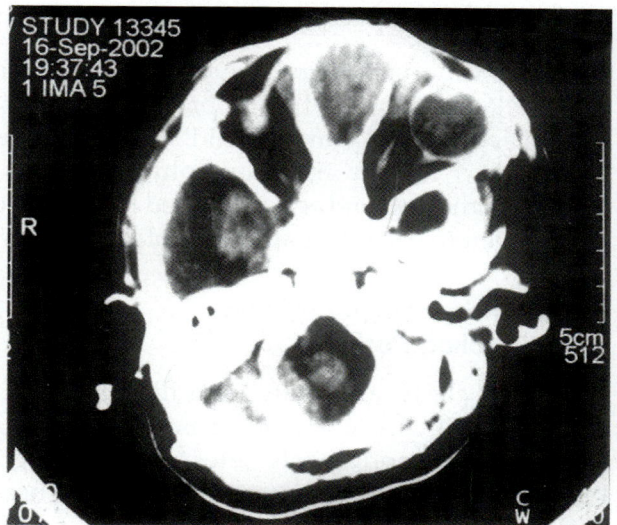 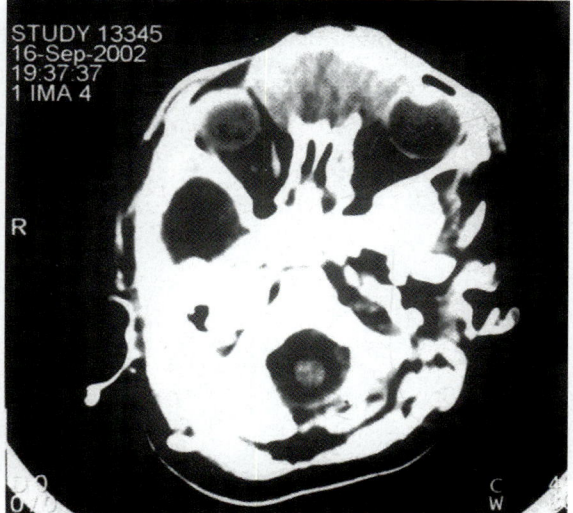

Figs 101.8A and B: CT scan axial slicer show frontoethmoidal encephalocele

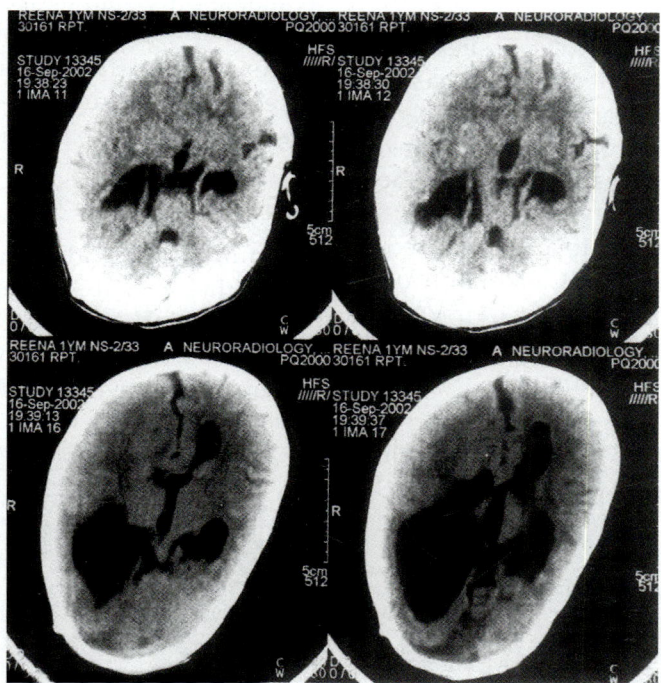

Fig. 101.9: CT scan axial cuts showing partial agenesis of corpus callosum and porencephalic cyst

Computerized Tomography and Magnetic Resonance Imaging

CT and MRI scans are the commonly used modalities to evaluate craniocerebral anomalies including encephalocele.[8,32,37,61,63,74] (Fig. 101.8). There are only few reports dealing with MRI.[32,73,74] CT scan helps in evaluation of dilation of ventricular system and CSF pathway. The bone window can delineate the contents of encephalocele and the bony defect in the skull base.[8,25,55,73-75] Hydrocephalus is commonly associated with posterior encephaloceles. However, in anterior encephaloceles association of hydrocephalus is reported in 10-15% cases.[8,16,32,33,37,41] CT scan is also helpful in detection of associated CNS anomalies like agenesis of the corpus callosum (Fig. 101.9) and porencephalic cysts.[21,37,40,62] In cases of transethmoidal

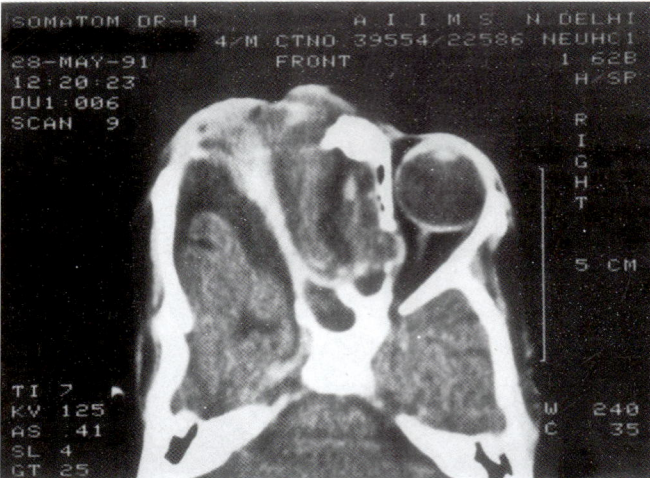

Fig. 101.10: CT scan in a case of orbital encephalocele show absence of Lt. sphenoid wing and brain tissue in orbit

or transsphenoidal encephaloceles, a soft tissue density mass in the sinuses and bone defect in skull base are well visualized.[8,9,15,50,55] In orbital encephaloceles the relation to the eyeball and optic nerve can be established (Fig. 101.10). The bone window may show a sphenoid wing defect. Recently, metrizamide CT cisternography has been used in cases of occult encephalocele.[76] Three-dimensional CT scans are used for evaluation of basal defect (Fig. 101.11A).[32,74] MRI helps in soft tissue delineation (Fig. 101.11B), diagnosis of Chiari malformation and syringomyelia.[21,32,73,74]

Isotope Studies

Are sometime useful in diagnosis of encephalocele.[43,55,72] Yoshimoto et al reported trans-ethmoid encephalocele in a 2 year old child, who had bacterial meningitis.[55] Isotope cisternography confirmed the CSF rhinorrhea. Anand et al suggested Isotope studies for preoperative surgical approach planning.[1]

Electroencephalography and Visual Evoked Potential

May show electrical activity from the content of the sac. However, little attention is usually paid in assessing encephalocele electrophysiological. Recently, visual evoked potentials have been used to assess occipital lobe and anterior visual pathway function.[77] Surprisingly, not much literature is available on visual evoked potentials. The ability to obtain VEP from the sac indicate presence of occipital cortex within the sac, absence of visual evoked potentials may suggest defect in visual cortex or dysplasia of optic pathway.[7,29]

TREATMENT

The aim of surgical therapy of encephalocele is to excise the hernial sac, repair the dural defect after putting back the herniated brain into cranial cavity. Sometime it may not be possible to push the brain into the cranial cavity. Then the choice is to either excise

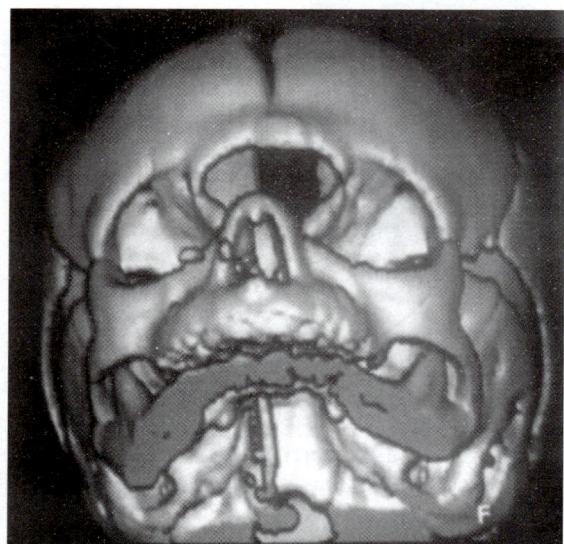

Fig. 101.11A: 3D CT scan of skull base showing defect in anterior fossa in a child with frontoethmoidal encephalocele

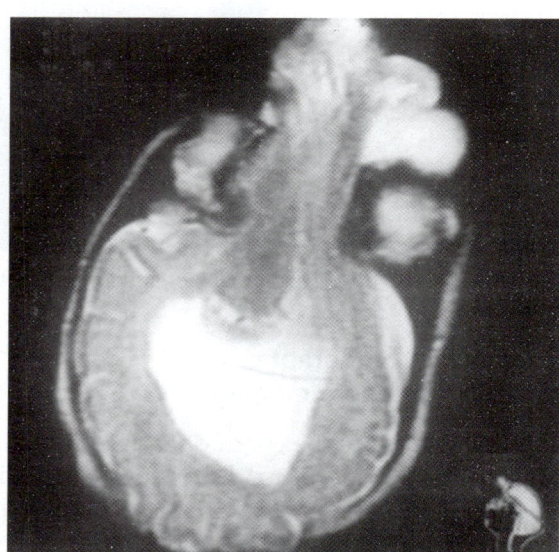

Fig. 101.11B: MRI scan T_2 weighted image showing large frontoethmoidal encephalocele with single ventricle

part of the brain or to give support to the brain in an extracranial space. Sometimes, in a patient with leaking encephalocele associated with hydrocephalus, shunt surgery may stop CSF leak and allows skin to heal. A large number of children with occipital and anterior encephalocele require CSF shunt diversion.[21,32,77]

Except for the situation with CSF leak, fortunately most of the encephaloceles are with good skin cover, and an immediate or emergency surgery is not required.[78,79] Surgery can be delayed for weeks and months depending on the condition of the neonate. Surgical procedure becomes simple, when an encephalocele sac has a small cranial defect, narrow neck, small sized and with very little or no herniated brain tissue inside the sac.

SURGERY OF OCCIPITAL ENCEPHALOCELE

Occipital encephalocele without brain herniation can be operated easily, however, when the sac contains cerebrum, cerebellum, and brainstem, surgery may be harmful and it is better to avoid an operation.[20,71,77] Large number of authors have reported a poor outcome in patients with microcephaly with large volume of neural tissue within the sac.[29,46] Some authors have treated the occipital encephalocele in special way.[34,46,66] Gallo described a technique for the management of a giant occipital encephalocele where an extracranial compartment is created by utilizing a fine tantalum mesh to enclose the herniated brain for the protection.[46]

Patients with occipital encephalocele are operated in a prone position, with controlled ventilation and closed temperature monitoring. In patients with large encephalocele aspiration of CSF prior to incision in, helps in dissecting out the sac. For a circular encephalocele with small occipital bone defect, a transverse incision is ideal. Patients in whom the encephaloceles extend above and below the posterior fossa need a vertical incision. The sac is separated out from the skin flap. Care must be taken to identify the contents of the sac. Sometimes brainstem and occipital lobe are present in the sac (Fig. 101.12). Rarely, sagittal sinus, torcula and transverse sinus are in the vicinity of the sac. It is always preferable to preserve the neural tissue. The dural defect can be repaired by using pericranium as graft. In neonates and infants no attempt should be made to cover the bone defect by graft.[68] In older children with large cranial defect, the autogenous bone graft or acrylic plate may be used for the closure (Figs 101.13A and B).

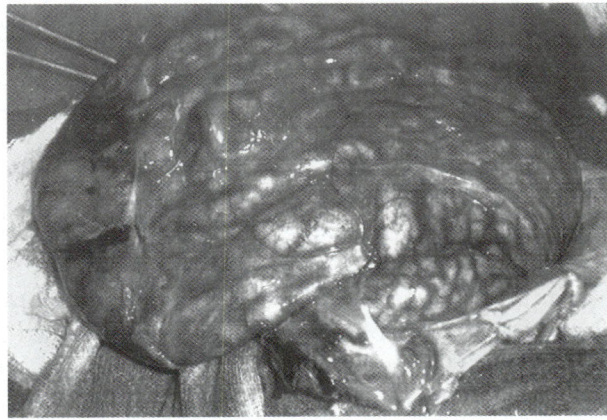

Fig. 101.12: Intraoperative photograph of a patient with giant occipital encephalocele show large volume of parieto-occipital lobe in the sac

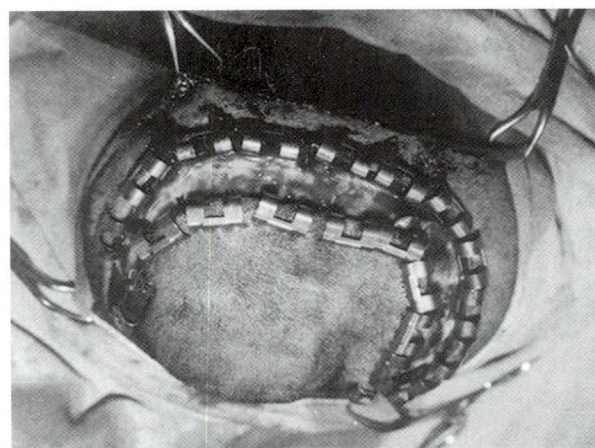

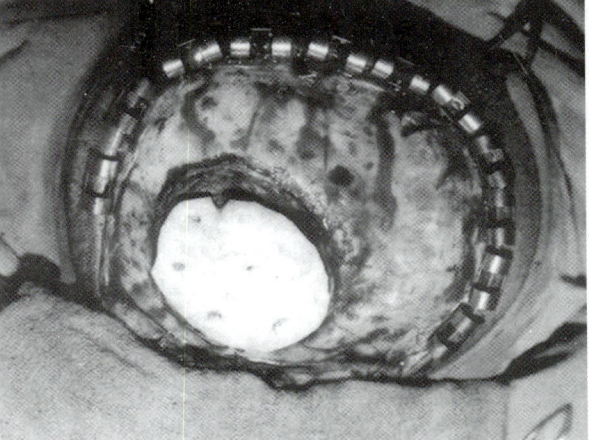

Fig. 101.13A and B: Intraoperative photograph showing bone grafting following excision of occipital encephalocele

Postoperatively patients may develop CSF leak, acute hydrocephalus and meningitis. Patients where shunt is not performed prior to encephalocele repair may need CSF diversion procedure subsequently. External ventricular drainage is the only alternative in patients with meningitis. Once the meningitis is adequately controlled, a ventriculoperitoneal shunt is advisable.

PROGNOSIS IN PATIENTS WITH OCCIPITAL ENCEPHALOCELES

Large number of factors can influence the outcome, including, site, size of the encephalocele, amount of the brain herniated into the sac, presence of brainstem, occipital lobe, cerebellum, with or without dural sinuses and presence of hydrocephalus.[7,27,46,66-68] One of the most important prognostic factor is the associated brain and systemic anomalies.[19,26,31,46,66,67] Overall, the long-term outcome in occipital encephalocele is not encouraging.

ENCEPHALOCELES THROUGH THE CRANIAL VAULT

Encephaloceles through the cranial vault are rare. They may be through frontal, parietal or temporal bones. Encephaloceles can occur through anterior or posterior fontanel. Parietal or interparietal encephaloceles are probably the most common encephaloceles of the cranial vault. Interparietal encephaloceles are difficult to treat and have poor prognosis.[41,27] Only 15% of these patients have normal mental development, while the rest have mental and physical abnormalities. Treatment in patients with small parietal encephaloceles is not difficult. Patients with large skull defect need cranioplasty. In several occasions, when there is a large cranial defect. To cover the large cranial defect the authors have used spilt autogenous outer table grafts (Fig. 101.13), using Aesculap or Midas Rex drill.

Temporal encephaloceles are less common.[41,80,81] They constitute 1% of all encephaloceles. Rarely, temporal encephalocele may develop following radiation.[18] Clyde and Stechison reported a temporal encephalocele presenting with CSF rhinorrhoea.[80] They repair the temporosphenoidal encephalocele with vasularised split calvarial graft.

TREATMENT OF ANTERIOR ENCEPHALOCELES

The main aim of the management of the anterior encephalocele is to repair the dural defect and to correct the bony deformities. Unfortunately a vast majority of patients have facial abnormality and associated hypertelorism.[12,16,32,52,60] Sometimes the malformation may be complex. The associated facial deformity plays an important role in final corrective surgery.[4] The cosmetic outcome depends upon the experience of the surgeon.

One stage repair of encephalocele along with the correction of facio-orbital deformity is a long procedure and requires on an average 6-8 hours of surgery.[6,12,16,24,25,32,60] Hence, the age of patient at the time of surgery must be such that the child should be able to stand a long surgical procedure. In our centre, we prefer the surgery when the child is over 8-10 months old.[12,24,32,61,82] Early surgical repair is ideal, as the bones being thin can be easily moulded. Early surgery also prevents CSF leak and risk of meningitis.

A Ventriculoperitoneal shunt procedure prior to definitive corrective surgery prevents postoperative CSF leak in patients having hydrocephalus. One stage correction of craniofacial deformity is ideal.[6,8,12,15,16,24,37,83] The factors that influence the surgery are, type of encephalocele, degree of hypertelorism, degree of nasal deformity, and associated CSF leak or meningitis. Tesier, popularized the concept of one stage repair.[6] Sometime, in a small child with CSF leak, two stage procedure may have to be carried out.[24,61] Large numbers of authors have reported good results with one stage craniofacial correction.[12,16,23,24,52,79] Recently Mahapatra et al and Mahapatra have reported craniofacial surgery in new born with good results.[78,79]

One Stage Surgical Correction Involves Following Steps

1. Bifrontal craniotomy, frontoorbital osteotomies.
2. Medial advancement of orbit, after excising the extra bone is the midline, to correct the hypertelorism.
3. Initial part of surgery deals with delineation of neck of encephalocele, followed by excision of herniated gliosed brain.
4. The dural defect is closed by dural graft, either by suturing or by using biological glue.

5. The type of correction of hypertelorism depends upon degree of the hypertelorism. In case of mild hypertelorism, excision of soft tissue in medial canthus and fixing the medial canthi to nasal bone may suffice.[24,61] Sometimes, nibbling of bone at the medial canthi followed by reconstitution of medial canthus by canthal stitch corrects the hypertelorism.[12,61]
6. Over correction of hypertelorism is important, as a significant amount of soft tissue may still be left in the medial canthus at the end of the operation. The aim is to achieve an inner canthal distance of 25 mm. Sometimes, a classical Tessiers operation may not be necessary. Recently, Mahapatra[21,25,32] reported advancement of medial half of the orbit medially and placing a supraorbital bone graft on either sides. By above procedure the operating time can be reduced by an average of 90-100 minutes.
7. Reconstruction of the nose is also a very important step in correction of anterior encephaloceles.[6,12,16,32,79] Nose deformity is maximum in patients with nasoethmoid type of anterior encephalocele. Extra skin over the encephalocele has to be excised.
8. The bridge of the nose is reconstructed either by using rib or split calvarial graft.[6,12,24,79] Overall cosmetic correction is satisfactory in our experience (Figs 101.14A and B).

Sometimes, to achieve a cosmetically excellent result, several small plastic surgical procedure may be necessary depending on the need of an individual patient, to correct nasal deformity or to excise extra skin or soft tissue at the medial canthi. This is basically because of cosmetic acceptance depends upon socioeconomic status and age of the patient. In girls the need for a better cosmetic result is more. An important postoperative problem following anterior encephalocele repair is, CSF leak leading to meningitis (Table 101.7). Large number of children develop transient CSF rhinorrhoea, which Stops within few days. Small number of patients require a thecoperitoneal shunt. In our series of 65 patients there was one postoperative mortality.[21]

PROGNOSIS IN PATIENTS WITH ANTERIOR ENCEPHALOCELES

Anterior encephalocele has a better overall prognosis than occipital encephalocele.[11,21,32,68,75,79] Presence of hydrocephalus in occipital encephalocele makes the prognosis poorer.[29,46] In absence of hydrocephalus or

Table 101.7: Postoperative complications in 75 cases of anterior encephalocele treated at AIIMS (1972-1996)

Complications	Numbers
Wound infection	5
CSF rhinorrhea	15
Meningitis	4
Infection of bone graft	1
Mortality	2

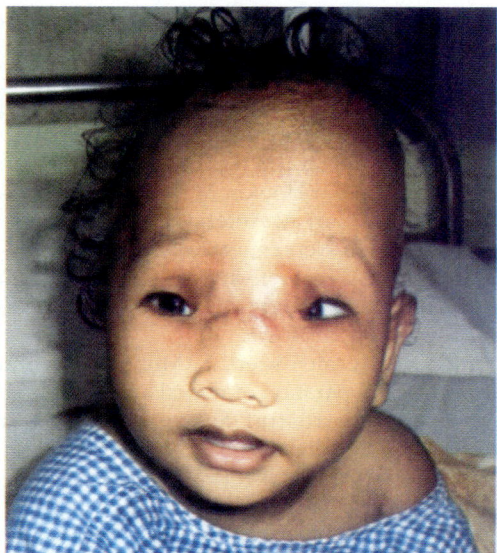

Fig. 101.14A: A 15 months old boy with Nasoethmoid encephalocele and gross hypertelorism

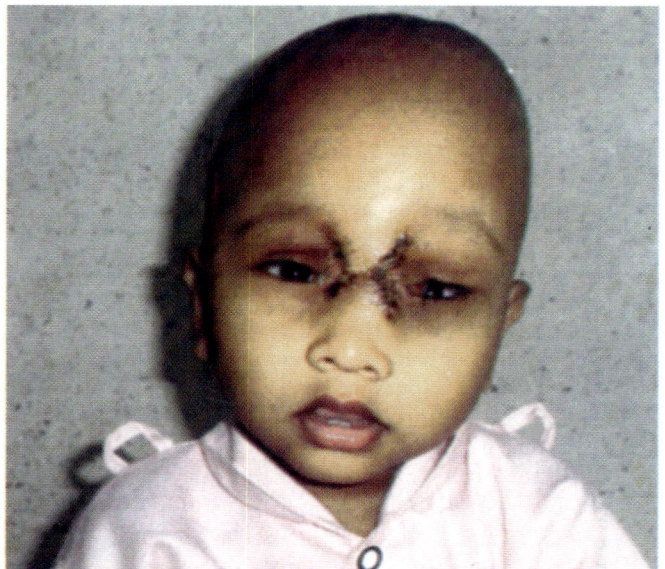

Fig. 101.14B: Postoperative photograph of the patient (Fig. 14A) showing correction of hypertelorism

meningitis, a large number of children are a have normal intellectual development.[21,23,24,32,75] Cosmetic deformities can be corrected with appropriate craniofacial surgery. Thus, overall outcome in children with anterior encephaloceles are more favourable as compared to occipital encephaloceles.

REFERENCES

1. Emery JL, Kalhan SC. Pathology of exencephalus. Dev Med Child Neurol Suppl 1970;22: 51-64.
2. Fenger C. Basal herniation of brain. Am J Med Sci 1895;109:1-17.
3. Bumenfeld R, Skolnik EM. Transnasal encephaloceles. Arch Otolaryngol 1965;82:527-31.
4. Browder J, deVeer JA. Rhinocephalocele. Arch Path (Chicago) 1934;18:646-59.
5. Suwanwela C, Suwanwela N. A morphological classification of sincipital encephalomeningocele. J Neurosurg 1972;36:201-11.
6. Tessier P. Anatomical classification of facial craniofacial and lateral facial clefts. J Maxillo facial Surg 1976;6:69-75.
7. Caviness VS, Evrad P. Occipital encephaloceles. A pathological and anatomical analysis. Acta Neuropath (Berlin) 1995;32:245-55.
8. Kalangu K. Anterior encephaloceles. Child's Nerv System 1990 ;6: 283 (Abstract).
9. Lewin ML. Sphenoethmoidal encephalocele with cleft palate. Transpalatal versus transcranial repair. Report of two cases. J Neurosurg 1983;58:924-31.
10. Sharma RR, Mahapatra AK, Pawar SJ, Thomas C Ismaily M. Transsellar trans-sphenoidal encephalocele: Report of two cases. J Clinic Neurosci 2001;9:189-92.
11. Nakamura T, Grant JA, Hubbard RE. Nasoethmoidal meningoencephalocele. Arch Otolaryngol (Chicago) 1974;100:62-64.
12. Dhawan IK, Tandon PN. Excision repair and corrective surgery for frontoethmoidal encephaloceles. Child's Brain 1982;9:126-36.
13. Izquierdo JM, Gil-Carcedo L. Recurrent meningitis and transethmoidal intranasal meningoencephaloceles. Dev Med Child Neurol 1988;30:248-51.
14. Luyendijk W. Intranasal encephaloceles. A survey of Neurosurgically treated cases. Psychiat Neurol Neurochir 1969;72:272-78.
15. Suwanwela C, Sukabate C, Suwanwela N. Frontoethmoidal encephalocele. Surgery 1971;69:617-25.
16. David DJ. New perspective in management of severe craniofacial deformity. Ann Roy Col Surg (England) 1984;66:270-79.
17. Williamson AP, Blattner RJ, Robertson GG. The relationship of viral antigen to virus induced defects in chick embryo. Newcastle disease virus. Dev Biol 1965;12:498-519.
18. Lalwani AK, Jackler RK, Harsh GR, Gutt FY. Bilateral temporal bone encephaloceles after cranial irradiation: a case report. J Neurosurg 1993;79:596-99.
19. Leong AYS, Shaw CM. The pathology of occipital encephalocele and a discussion of the pathogenesis. Pathology 1979;11:223-34.
20. Lober J. The prognosis of occipital encephaloceles. Develop Med Child Neurol Supp 1967;13:75-86.
21. Mahapatra AK. Anterior encephaloceles: A study of 65 cases. Indian Journal of Paediatrics 1997;64:699-704.
22. Barreto E, Barbosa J, Telles C. Anatomical classification of anterior encephaloceles. Arg-Neuropsiquia 1993;51:107-11.
23. David DJ. Cephaloceles: classification, Pathology and management a review. J Craniofacial Surg 1993;4:192-202.
24. Mahapatra AK. Frontoethmoidal encephalocele. A study of 42 patients. In: Skull Base Anatomy, Radiology and Management. Samii M (Eds) S Karger Basel 1994;220-23.
25. Mahapatra AK. Anterior encephaloceles. In: Progress in Clinical Neurosciences. S.Venkataraman and MM Mehndiratta (Eds) Naresh Press, New Delhi 1995;10: 293-306.
26. Smith Mt, Huntingon HW. Inverse cerebellum and occipital encephalocele. A dorsal fusion defect uniting the Arnold-Chiari and Dandy Walker spectrum. Neurology 1977;27:246-51.
27. Gardner WJ. The dysraphic status from syringomyelia to an encephaly. Amsterdam Excerpta Medica 1973.
28. Cawdell-Smith J, Upfold J, Edwards M, Smith M. Neural tube and other developmental anomalies in the guinea pig following maternal hyperthermia during early neural tube development. Teratog-Carcinog-Mutagen 1992;12: 1-9.
29. Karch SB, Urich H. Occipital encephaloceles: A morphological study. J Neurol Sci 1972;15: 89-112.
30. Moerman P, Fryns JP, Vandenbergh K, et al. Constrictive aminotic bands, amniotic adhesions and limb-body wall complex: discrete disruption sequences with pathogenetic overlap. Ame J Med Genet 1992;42:470-79.
31. Padget DH, Lindenberg R. Inverse cerebellum morphogenetically related to Dandy Walker and Arnold-Chiari Syndrome. Bizarre malformed brain with occipital encephalocele. John Hopkin Med J 1972;131:228-46.
32. Mahapatra AK, Suri A. Anterior encephalocele : a study of 92 cases. Paed Neurosurg 2002;36:113-18.
33. Hoving EW, Vermeji-keers C Frontoethmoidal Encephaloceles, a study of their pathogenesis. Paed Neurosurg 1997;27:246-56.
34. Hoving EW, Vermeji-keers C, Mommaaikienhuis AM, Hartwig NG. Separation of neural and surface ectoderm after closure of rostral neuropore. Anat Embryol 1990;83:453-63.
35. Gisselson L. Intranasal form of encephaloceles. Acta Otolaryngol 1947;35:519-31.
36. Wiese GM, Major MC, Ludwing GK, et al. Transsphenoid meningoencephaloceles. J Neurosurg 1972;36:475-78.

37. Hanich A, David DJ. Frontoethmoidal meningo-encephalocele classification and associated features. Child's Nervous Sys 1990;6: 283(Abstract).
38. Morika M, Marubayashi T, Masamitsu T. Basal encephaloceles with morning glory syndrome and progressive hermonal and visual disturbances. Case report and review of literature. Brain Dev 1995;17:196-201.
39. Seaver LH, Joffe L, Spark RP, et al. Congenital scalp defect and vitreoretinal degeneration redefining the Knobloch syndrome. Ame J Med Genet 1993;46:203-08.
40. Van Nouhuys JM, Bruyn GW. Nasopharyngeal transsphenoidal encephaloceles. Craterlike hole in optic disc and agenesis of corpus callosum; pneumocephalographic visualization in a case. Psychiat Neurol Neurochir 1964;67:243-58.
41. French BN. Midline fusion defect and defects of formation. In Youman's Neurological Surg. 2nd Eds WB Sunder Comp Philadelphia 1982;8:1236-380.
42. Modesti LM, Glasauer FE, Terplan KL. Sphenoethmoidal encephalocele. A case report with review of the literature. Childs Brain 1977;3:140-53.
43. Anand VK, Melvin FM, Reed JM, Parent AD. Nasopharyngeal gliomas: diagnostic and treatment consideration. Otolaryngol Head Neck Surg 1993;109:534-39.
44. Cartwright MJ, Eisenberg MB. Tension pneumocephalus associated with rupture of a middle fossa encephalocele. Case report. J Neurosurg 1992;76:292-95.
45. Mulliken JB. A large frontoethmoid encephalomeningocele: case report. Plast Reconstruct Surg 1973;51:592-95.
46. Gallo AE Jr. Repair of giant occipital encephalocele with microcephaly secondary to massive brain herniation. Child's Nerv System 1992;8:229-30.
47. Leene CRJr, Malome JF. Orbital presentation of an ethmoidal encephalocele. Arch Ophthalmol 1970;83: 445-47.
48. Berlit P, Rakicky J, Tornow K. Primary intranasal encephalocele: a rare cause of bacterial meningitis. Acta Neurol Scand 1992;85:404-07.
49. Dodge HW Jr, Love JG, Kernohan JW. Intranasal encephalomeningocele associated with cranium bifidum. Arch Surg (Chicago) 1959;79:87-96.
50. Love GL, Richi AP. Intranasal encephalocele masking as a polyp in an adult patient. Arch Otolaryngol 1983;180: 420-21.
51. Chouhan BS, Parmar IPS, Bhatia JN. Anterior orbital meningoencephalocele. Am J Opthalmol 1969;68:144-46.
52. Jacob OJ, Rosenfeld JU, Watters DA. The repair of frontal encephalocele in Papua new guinea. Aust Nz J Surg 1994;64: 856-60.
53. Lau BP, Newton TH. Sphenopharyngeal encephaloceles. Radiol Clin Biol 1965;34:386-93.
54. Copty M, Vervet S, Langeller R, et al. Intranasal meningoencephalocele with recurrent meningitis. Surg Neurol 1979;12:49-52.
55. Yoshimoto Y, Nogachi M, Tsutsumi Y. A case of transethmoidal encephaloceles. No shinkei Geka 1992;20:249-54.
56. Fargaeta JS, Menezo JL, Borde M. Posterior orbital encephalcoele with anophthalmos and other brain malformation. Case report. J Neurosurg 1973;38:215-17.
57. Suwanwela C. Geographical distribution of frontoethmoidal encephalocele. Brit J Prev Soc Med 1972;26: 193-98.
58. Tandon PN. Meningoencephaloceles. Acta Neurol Scand 1970;46: 369-83.
59. Sekerci Z, Iyigun O, Baris S, et al. Transnasal (Transethmoidal) encephalomeningocele. Case report. Neurosurg Rev 1995;18:123-26.
60. Whatmore WJ. Sincipital encpehalomeningoceles. Brit J surg 1973;60: 261-70.
61. Mahapatra AK, Tandon PN, Dhawan IK, Khazanchi RK. Anterior encephalocele: A report of 30 cases. Childs Nerv Syst 1994;10:501-04.
62. Abiko S, Aoki H, Fudaba H. Transsphenoidal encephaloceles report of a case. Neurosurgery 1988;27:933-36.
63. Pollock JA, Newton JH, Hoyt WP. Transsphenoidal transethmoidal encephalocele. A review of clinical and roentgenologic features in 8 cases. Radiol 1968;90:442-53.
64. Hayashi T, Utsahomiya H, Hashimoto T. Transethmoidal encephaloceles. Surg Neurol 1985;24:251-55.
65. Miller JQ, Selden RF. Archinencephaly, encephalocele and 13-15 trisomy syndrome with normal chromosome. Neurology (Minneap) 1967;17:1087-91.
66. Hutchison JW, Stovring J, Turner PP. Occipital encephalocele with holoprosencephaly and aqueductal stenosis. Surg Neurol 1979;12:331-35.
67. Lubinnsky MS, Kahler SG, Speer IE, et al. VonVos – Cherstvoy syndrome: a variable perinataly lethal syndrome of multiple congenital anomalies. Ame J Med Genet 1994;52:272-78.
68. Martinez-Lage JF, Garcia-Santos JM, Poza M, et al. Neurosurgical management of Walker Warburg Syndrome. Childs Nervs Syst 1995;11:145-53.
69. Onuigbo WIB. Encephaloceles in Nigerian Igbos. J Neurol Neurosurg Psychiat 1977;40:726.
70. Haverson G, Bailey IC, Kiryabaice WM. The radiological diagnosis of anterior encephaloceles. Clin Radiol 1974;25:317-22.
71. Gilmor RL, Kalsbeck JE, Goodman JM, et al. Angiographic assessment of occipital encephalocele. Radiology 1972;103:127-30.
72. Suwanwela C, Poshyachinda V, Poshyachinda M. Isotope cisternography and ventriculography in frontoethmoidal encephalocele. Acta Radiol (Diag) Stockholm 1973;14: 5-8.
73. Castillo M, Quencer RM, Dominquez R. Chiari III malformation: Imaging features. Am J Neuro Radiol (AJNR) 1992;13:107-13.
74. Gudinchet F, Branelle F, Duvoisin B, et al. The value of CT and MRI in the assessment of basal encephalocele in children. Schweiz-Runalsch med-Prax 1992;81: 1196-201.

75. Turgut M, Ozcan OE, Benli K, et al. Congenital nasal encephalocele: a review of 35 cases. J Craniomaxillofacial Surg 1995;23:1-5.
76. Colqutoun IR. CT cisternography in the investigation of cerebrospinal fluid rhinorrhoea. Clin Radiol 1993;47:403-08.
77. Engel R, Buchan GC. Occipital encephaloceles with and without visual evoked potentials. Arch Neurol 1974;30:314-18.
78. Mahapatra AK, Dev EJ, Krishnan A, Sharma RR. Craniofacial surgery in leaking encephalocele in a newborn: A case report. Child Nerv Sys 2002;17:626-28.
79. Satyarthee GD, Mahapatra AK. Leaking frontonasal encephalocele in a neonate. J Clinic Neuroscien 2002:14.
80. Clyde BL, Stechison MT. Repair of temporosphenoidal encephalocele with vasularised split calvarial cranioplasty: technical case report. Neurosurgery 1995;36:202-06.
81. Nagulich I, Bovuce G, Georgevichz. Temporal meningocele. J Neurosurg 1967;27:433-48.
82. Mahapatra AK, Gupta PK, Dev EJ. Posterior fontanel Giant encephalocele. Paed Neurosurg 2002;5:36.
83. Rahman Naimur. Nasal encephalocele: Treatment by a transcranial operation. J Neurol Sci 1979;42:73-85.

CHAPTER 102

Microcephaly

Shilpa Sharma, Veena Kalra

Microcephaly is a common situation in pediatric practice.[1] The clinician has to first confirm presence of microcephaly, distinguish primary and secondary microcephaly, identify microcephaly as distinct from craniosynostosis, evaluate family for a possible familial microcephaly and lastly probe into etiology of pathologic microcephaly. The clinician must clearly identify all neurological and systemic associations to determine the cause and appropriately counsel the family. A thorough evaluation of influence on development, neurological deficits and intelligence is warranted. The variations of norms of head size in the population should also be addressed to in drawing clinical conclusions.

DEFINITION

Microcephaly denotes an occipitofrontal circumference (OFC measured around forehead and occipital protuberance) as two or more standard deviations below the mean for the individuals age gestation gender and race (below the 2nd percentile).

The definition of microcephaly inadvertently includes 1.9% of normal children who have a head circumference below 2 SD of mean. At term the average neonate has an average head circumference of 33.5-35 cm and the brain averages about 12% of the body weight. At one year age the OFC is 45 cm and is almost 950 grams. In clinical practice serial measurement of head circumference and comparing the serial head circumference profile to norms is a very useful clinical parameter because a deviant OFC warns of an abnormal brain. It may be important to remember that patients may have normal neurological function and intellectual abilities even with a small sized brain.

In general however the brain size -OFC-IQ have a good correlation in normal subjects. Only 14% of subjects with an OFC below 2 standard deviations below the means had IQ above 100, while in 70% the IQ ranged between 71-80, only 10.5% had an IQ below 70. If growth was concurrently affected 13.3% had IQ below 70.

The OFC correlates strongly with the intracranial volume. Factors that determine the OFC are thickness of the scalp, the thickness of the calvarial bones, the ability of the cranial sutures to expand, and most importantly the volume of the intracranial contents. The intracranial contents are comprised by brain volume, CSF in ventricles and subarachnoid spaices, blood volume in the intracranial vessels and any space-occupying lesions.

ETIOLOGY

Microcephaly may be caused by a teratogen, a chromosomal abnormality, or a genetic defect (Table 102.1).

A small brain volume is the most common cause of microcephaly except in cases of premature sutural fusion. Extremely preterm birth is associated with adverse neurodevelopmental sequelae. Head circumference has been used as a measure of brain growth (Figs 102.1A and B). In a study on 227 preterm infants, a strong correlation was noted between head circumference and brain volume at term.[2] There was no significant relationship between head circumference and white or gray matter abnormalities on MRI. The microcephaly increased from 7.5% at term to 29.7% at 2 years.[2] Brain volume is a determinant of head size at term. Microcephaly is associated with a

Table 102.1: Common causes for microcephaly

Infection	Chromosomal
Cytomegalovirus	Down syndrome
Rubella	
Varicella	Aneuploidies
Acquired immunodeficiency syndrome	Syndromic microcephalies
Toxoplasmosis	**Malformations**
Syphilis	Atelencephaly
Drugs	Lissencephaly
Alcohol	
Antiepileptic	**Trauma**
Anticancer drugs	
Corticosteroids	
Anoxia/ischemia	**Perinatal metabolic/ endocrine imbalances**
Generalized cerebral anoxia	Hypoglycemia
Irradiation	Hypothyroidism
Hereditary	Hypopituitarism
Normal variation in OFC, asymptomatic	Hypoadrenocorticism
Mendelian pattern	
Craniosynostosis	**Malnutrition**
Heredofamilial degenerative diseases	
Miscellaneous syndromes factors	**Prenatal maternal illness or pregnancy**

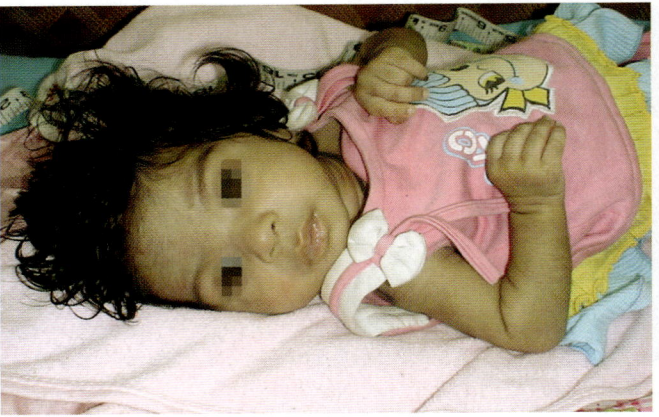

Fig. 102.1A: A three months old female child presenting with spastic diplegia and dysmorphic facies had microcephaly. There was history of delayed developmental cry. The sibling also had similar history of asphyxia, delayed cry and epilepsy. A. genetic cause needs to be ruled out

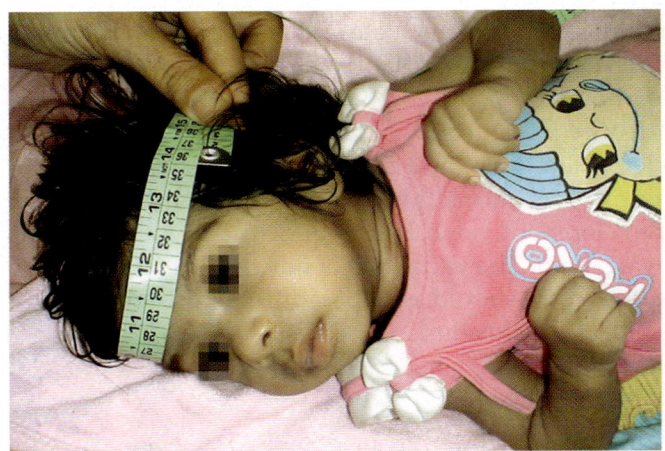

Fig. 102.1B: The head circumference was 35 cm at three months age. Note the upper limb and clenched fists. There was no social smile and eye fixation

reduction of brain tissue volumes, especially deep nuclear gray matter, which suggests a selective vulnerability. Poor postnatal head growth in preterm infants becomes more evident by 2 years and is strongly associated with poor neurodevelopmental outcome and cerebral palsy.[2]

An abnormally small brain results from anomalous development in the first 7 gestational months (primary microcephaly) or from an insult after 7 months of gestation, perinatal period or in infancy when it is termed secondary microcephaly. The earlier the insult the greater the potential of microcephaly. Primary microcephaly results from anomalies of neuronogenesis and migration due to genetic or early detrimental influences.

In vivo studies suggest that many forms of microcephaly result from defects in the control of cell fate: precocious formation of neurons during early developmental stages produces deficiencies in progenitor cells at later stages of neurogenesis, resulting in an overall small cerebral cortex.[3]

Malformations of cortical development caused by disruptions at various stages are increasingly recognized as an important cause of developmental delay especially with the emergence of high resolution imaging.[4] Disorders of neurogenesis give rise to microcephaly (small brain) or macrocephaly (large brain). Disorders of early neuroblast migration give rise to periventricular heterotopia (neurons located along the ventricles), whereas abnormalities later in migration lead to lissencephaly (smooth brain) or subcortical band heterotopia (smooth brain with a band of heterotopic neurons under the cortex). Abnormal neuronal migration arrest give rise to over migration of neurons in cobblestone lissencephaly. Lastly, disorders of neuronal organization cause polymicrogyria (abnormally small gyri and sulci).[4] Identification of various gene mutations has not only given us greater insight but also an understanding of the processes involved in normal cortical development.[4]

Genetic factors determine much of the normal variation in brain size and hence OFC, and thus usually result in primary microcephaly. Many errors of chromosomal morphology and aneuploidies translocations, trisomies, nondisjunctions, and duplications — cause a small, defective brain. In genetic microcephalies the migration anomalies include lissencephaly, pachygyria, polymicrogyria and corpus callosum defects. Heterotropias are commonly recorded. Primary microcephaly can be transmitted as autosomal dominant, autosomal recessive or even in X linked manner. Various genetic loci have been identified of which a common one is on 8 p chromosome. In some families migration defects, visuo-retinal abnormalities or spasticity in varying combinations may be observed. Associated dysmorphisms lead to identification of the various syndromes. Other genetic disorders, such as neurofibromatosis I and achondroplasia generally cause large brains.

Microcephalic osteodysplastic primordial dwarfism type II is a specific disorder characterized by severe intrauterine and postnatal growth retardation, acquired microcephaly, cerebrovascular abnormalities, progressive bone dysplasia, and a characteristic face.[5] Genetic malformations of the cerebral cortex are an important cause of neurological disability in children.[6] The genes implicated in these disorders are essential for normal cerebral cortical development. Therefore, identifying these genes and studying their functions will help us further the understanding of the normal biological mechanisms of brain development. Lissencephaly and microcephaly are two groups of disorders that have been intensely studied and several causative genes within each group have been identified. Type I (classical) lissencephaly is characterized by a smooth-appearing brain with a lack or severe reduction of normal gyri. Three of its identified causative genes (LIS1, DCX and TUBA1A) are related to microtubules, which are essential for neuronal migration in the developing cerebral cortex. Microcephaly vera is a form of microcephaly with four responsible genes reported to date. Three of them (ASPM, CENPJ and CDK5RAP2) localize to the mitotic centrosome, and one (MCPH1) is implicated in cell cycle checkpoint regulation and DNA damage response. This suggests that abnormalities of neural progenitor cell division are fundamental to the pathogenesis of microcephaly vera. These genes for microcephaly vera are also suggested to have played a role in evolutionary volume expansion of the human cerebral cortex. Genetic studies of lissencephaly and microcephaly have been very fruitful in providing novel insights into various aspects of human cerebral cortical development.[6]

A network of DNA damage response mechanisms functions co-ordinately to maintain genomic stability and ensure cellular survival in the face of exogenous and endogenous DNA damage.[7] Microcephaly, representing reduced brain size, is a feature common to a diverse range of DNA damage response -defective disorders. Microcephaly is most likely caused by loss (increased cell death) or failure of the developing neuronal stem cells or their progenitors to divide suggesting a fundamental role for the DNA damage response in maintaining proliferative potential in the developing nervous system.[7]

Microcephaly may be associated with a normal contour of the skull or an abnormal shaped head. In the latter situation focal anatomical lesions of the brain, e.g. porencephaly, hemimegalencephaly or abnormalities of the overlying bones like craniosynostosis may need to be excluded.

Craniosynostosis may be simple, i.e. single suture fusion or compound. It may be an isolated phenomenon or part of a dysmorphology, genetic or chromosomal syndrome.

Intrauterine infections with the TORCH-S complex, varicella, HIV can all result in microcephaly. The associated perinatal events and associated clinical features IgM Ab against specific agents in the perinatal period and identification of HIV infection can all provide diagnostic pointers.

Irradiation during the first two trimesters of pregnancy can result in microcephaly. Irradiation of less than 1uGY is safe. The risk is proportional to the amount of radiation. Hypoxia is one of the important and commonly encountered insults, severe hypoxia can result in permanent sequelae.

Chronic maternal exposure to alcohol, coccaine smoking have been recognized as incriminative. Additionally drugs such as antiepileptic drugs, corticosteroids, antineoplastic agents may result in microcephaly besides other teratogenic consequences. Maternal phenylketonuria, if untreated may also result in a microcephalic neonate.

ANTENATAL DIAGNOSIS

There are cases of antenatal diagnosis of microcephaly but the diagnosis is usually based on ultrasound examination.[8] The diagnosis may not be correct in some cases especially in twins.[9] It is not always possible to differentiate between the normal and the abnormal by ultrasound. In borderline cases ultrasound has the advantage that it can point out the need for extra careful post-natal examination of the infant. Thus complementary examination should be performed and the results obtained should be studied critically, confirmed by repeated examinations and integrated into the whole clinical picture.[8]

Modern ultrasound equipments allow a detailed investigation of the fetal brain from a very early stage of development.[10] Congenital anomalies involving the central nervous system can be accurately predicted. These include hydrocephalus, holoprosencephaly, cephaloceles, porencephaly, hydranencephaly, and microcephaly.

The antenatal diagnosis of microcephaly is most commonly made in the third.

Trimester or rarely in the second trimester.[11] Biometric measurements of the head of three or four standard deviations below the mean are suggestive of microcephaly.[11] Antenatal ultrasound diagnosis of isolated microcephaly is difficult.[12] Other malformations must be safely excluded. The presence of associated intracerebral calcification suggests antenatal congenital infectious encephalopathy and may warrant medical termination of pregnancy.[13]

Prenatal detection of lissencephaly by high-resolution ultrasound has also been reported.[14] To confirm the diagnosis, a fetal blood sample may be obtained to look for any chromosomal abnormality.

The sibling recurrence risk was 19% in a series of 29 isolated cases of microcephaly and 9 families with recurrent microcephaly, which reflects the high incidence of autosomal recessive microcephaly in this series.[15] The most frequent, affecting 5 sib pairs, was associated with spastic quadriplegia, seizures, and profound mental handicap.[15] Infants with congenital microcephaly are mentally and motorially severely retarded and thus if the diagnosis can be confirmed antenatally, termination may be advised.[12] It is estimated that 20-35% of idiopathic microcephaly is hereditary. Thus after the birth of such a case, subsequent pregnancies should be monitored ultrasonographically in order to facilitate early antenatal diagnosis and genetic counseling.[16]

APPROACH TO THE MICROCEPHALIC INFANT

The detailed clinical history of antenatal, natal and perinatal events is extremely important. Details of pregnancy, maternal health, drugs specially antiepileptics, corticosteroid antineoplastic agents, chronic narcotic agent use and toxins is relevant. The nutritional history must be ellucidated despite the common knowledge that nutritional deficit spares the brain. The OFC of siblings should be recorded. History of microcephaly in the family in at least 2 generations should be carefully enquired as genetically inherited microcephaly often run in families. Familial microcephaly needs to be excluded before investigating for other causes. Genetic microcephaly may also be associated with other phenotypic abnormalities and thus justifies a good systemic examination. The critical dysmorphology evaluation examination should not miss facial dysmorphism, skeletal asymmetries, somatotype of the individual and growth abnormalities. Specific syndrome characteristic features should be carefully looked for. On examination the sutures, sutural ridging of the skull and the shape of the skull help, distinguish microcephaly and the small head size resulting from craniosynostosis. The diagnosis of the symptomatic, familial microcephaly is confirmed by absence of risk factor for pathologic microcephaly.

Investigations to exclude craniosynostosis include X-ray skull, CT scans including bone window examination to evaluate sutures. In all such patients special investigations may be required. A simple fundus examination to look for papilloedema is warranted. Specific chromosomal studies and molecular diagnostic are necessary in specific circumstances. Serological tests for intrauterine infections are non contributory at the age at which patients present.

The approach to nonfamilial microcephaly is dependent upon consideration of common causes (Table 102.1).

Hereditary microcephalies may be observed as an isolated familial occurrence or as part of various syndromes. If the infant is dysmorphic a karyotyping is useful to distinguish chromosomal, e.g. Down's from non chromosomal syndromic microcephalies.

Repeated and severe hypoglycemia may also predispose to permanent brain damage and microcephaly. Associated endocrinopathies may need exclusion specially if there are associated thyroid, pituitary or adrenal dysfunction pointers.

Chronic malnutrition may also contribute, calorie deficits, early trace element deficiency, e.g. zinc may have microcephaly besides growth failure.

OUTCOME

In general, life expectancy for individuals with microcephaly is low and the prognosis for normal brain function is poor. The prognosis varies depending on the presence of associated abnormalities. The prognostic significance for intellectual impairment is more likely to be accurate when the head circumference is 3 SD or more below the mean for dates. Microcephaly was associated with delayed development but did not influence final seizure outcome in a series of 94 infantile epileptic encephalopathies.[17]

REFERENCES

1. Kalra V. Pediatric neurology—need for development. Indian Pediatr 1983;20(4):231-33.
2. Cheong JL, Hunt RW, Anderson PJ, et al. Head growth in preterm infants: correlation with magnetic resonance imaging and neurodevelopmental outcome. Pediatrics 2008;121:e1534-40.
3. Chae TH, Walsh CA. Genes that control the size of the cerebral cortex. Novartis Found Symp 2007;288:79-90;discussion 91-98.
4. Pang T, Atefy R, Sheen V. Malformations of cortical development. Neurologist 2008;14(3):181-91.
5. Galasso C, Lo-Castro A, Lalli C, et al. Neurologic Aspects of Microcephalic Osteodysplastic Primordial Dwarfism Type II. Pediatr Neurol. 2008;38(6):435-38.
6. Mochida GH. Molecular genetics of lissencephaly and microcephaly. Brain Nerve 2008;60(4):437-44.
7. O'Driscoll M, Jeggo PA. The role of the DNA damage response pathways in brain development and microcephaly: Insight from human disorders. DNA Repair (Amst) 2008 [Epub ahead of print].
8. Sejean S, Turpin JC, Quarre MC, Tournaire M. Antenatal microcephaly. A contribution of ultrasound. Twelve cases J Gynecol Obstet Biol Reprod (Paris) 1981;10:699-709.
9. Chadwick JM, Gilmore DW, Herbert WW. The problem of antenatal diagnosis of microcephaly by ultrasonography in twin pregnancy. Aust N Z J Obstet Gynaecol 1983;23:244-47.
10. Pilu G, Rizzo N, Orsini LF, Bovicelli L. Antenatal recognition of cerebral anomalies Ultrasound Med Biol 1986;12(4):319-26.
11. Rees AE, Bates A, Clarke H. Cerebellar hypoplasia in the second trimester associated with microcephaly at birth. Ultrasound Obstet Gynecol 1995;5(3):206-08.
12. Litschgi M. Prenatal ultrasonic diagnosis of severe congenital microcephaly Geburtshilfe Frauenheilkd. 1986;46(4):250-52.
13. Samson JF, Barth PG, de Vries JI, et al. Familial mitochondrial encephalopathy with fetal ultrasonographic ventriculomegaly and intracerebral calcifications. Eur J Pediatr 1994;153(7):510-16.
14. Saltzman DH, Krauss CM, Goldman JM, Benacerraf BR. Prenatal diagnosis of lissencephaly. Prenat Diagn. 1991;11(3):139-43.
15. Tolmie JL, McNay M, Stephenson JB, Doyle D, Connor JM. Microcephaly: genetic counselling and antenatal diagnosis after the birth of an affected child. Am J Med Genet 1987;27(3):583-94.
16. Jaffe M, Tirosh E, Oren S. The dilemma in prenatal diagnosis of idiopathic microcephaly. Dev Med Child Neurol 1987;29(2):187-89.
17. Kalra V, Gulati S, Pandey RM, Menon S. West syndrome and other infantile epileptic encephalopathies—Indian hospital experience. Brain Dev 2002;24(2):130-39.

CHAPTER 103

Spina Bifida

DK Gupta, Shilpa Sharma

The history of spina bifida stretches back to ancient times, though the plight of an infant born with an open neural tube defect has improved significantly only recently that too only in developing countries that can provide an insurance cover for rehabilitation.

The intellectual evolution of neurological spine surgery had originated in the golden age of Greece with the founding of the Alexandrian School way back in 300 BC. In the 1950s, John Holter, an engineer, developed the first effective differential pressure valve to control hydrocephalus for his son who was born with spina bifida.[1] This was at that time perceived as the ultimate answer to the problems of a child with spina bifida. In the 1960s, worldwide, the birth of an infant with spina bifida was treated as an emergency. Open neural tissue was surgically covered regardless of the time of day or night. Ventricular atrial shunts were installed to control hydrocephalus. The early mortality rate decreased rapidly, almost reversing the previous 90% mortality to a survival rate of 80%. The shunt brought with itself further problems not anticipated. In the 1970s, the main problems were incontinence, paraplegia, and scoliosis coupled with the new problems of shunt malfunction, infection, and mental retardation. John Lorber, a neurologist in England, led the drive to control the problem.[2] Selection criteria were developed based on the perceived quality of life expected for the infant. Children selected for nontreatment were not allowed to survive. The mortality rate climbed to 70%, and this method of caring for the newborn with spina bifida was adopted worldwide.

However, a prospective study performed between 1975 and 1979 on the outcome of 100 children with spina bifida treated aggressively from birth clearly demonstrated that the selection criteria were not valid predictors of the functional outcome for the child.[3] Lorber's selected population was not more functional than the unselected aggressively treated group. The only difference was the number of survivors in the selected group was much fewer. Thus the controversy remains till date and the management polies adopted differ from place to place.

The term spina bifida was mentioned way back in 1645 by Dr Nicolaes Tulp to define certain congenital malformation of the spine associated with overt cystic protrusion and some of the content of vertebral canal.[4]

DEFINITION

Spina bifida is a neural tube defect where the vertebral and/or spinal cord of the fetus fails to develop properly and results in varying degrees of permanent damage of the spinal cord and nervous system, usually accompanied by hydrocephalus. The damage usually occurs within the first 4 weeks or pregnancy. The various synonyms are spina bifida cystica, spina bifida occulta, myelomeningocele, spinal dysraphia.

INCIDENCE

The incidence of spina bifida has been estimated at 1-2 persons per 1000 population, with certain populations having a significantly greater incidence based on genetic predilection.

A decrease in incidence has been noted as a result of improved maternal nutrition and antenatal diagnosis with elective termination. Wider availability of maternal alpha-fetoprotein and more refined high resolution ultrasonography have given the parents an option to terminate the pregnancies. The incidence is

0.7 to 1 in 1000 live births in US, 1 in 750 live births in Canada and 0.2 in 1000 in Japan. Spina bifida aperta is at least 7 times greater than the occult. The risk factor in a mother with previously affected children is 40-50 in1 000 that rises to 100 in 1 000 with two such children. The recurrence rate usually after the birth of one affected sibling is 5%.

The chance of producing dysraphic child after the birth of two affected children increases two fold to 10%. The improved outcome with better medical care, and possible prevention of myelomeningocele with the use of folic acid has a direct impact on the recurrence risks. Originally myelomeningocele was considered to be a polygenic disorder, but later studies have shown that a recurrence risk in affected parents is only 1%. Despite this, a sufficiently high recurrence risk for parents, one of whom is affected with myelomeningocele, or a mother with one affected child warrants a therapy of 5 mg of folic acid 3 months prior to planned pregnancy.

EMBRYOLOGY

The primitive streak that appears at the caudal end of the embryo in stage 6 between day 13-15 of gestation elongates cranially. The Hensen's node is at the cranial end of the primitive streak. The epiblast cells migrate through the primitive groove and form the endoderm and mesoderm (gastrulation) during stage 6. As the primitive streak regresses the notocord is formed which has a central canal (Fig. 103.1). The notocord induces the overlying ectoderm to form the neural plate as a slipper shaped plated of thickened ectoderm in the middorsal region in front of the primitive gut. The lateral ends of the neural plate form neural folds that fuse in the midline to form the neural tube (neurulation – stage 8-12, 18-27 days). The formation of the neural tube starts from the cervical region and proceeds cranially and caudally. At both ends fusion is delayed and cranial and caudal neuropores temporarily form open connection between lumen of the neural tube and amniotic cavity. The final closure of the cranial pore occur on 23rd-25th day, caudal neuropore closes on 25th-27th day.

The superficial ectoderm fuses in the midline and mesenchymal cells migrate between the neural tube and skin to form the meninges, neural arches and muscles.

By day 27, the caudal end of the neural tube blends into the caudal cell mass. Small vacuoles form in the caudal cell mass, which coalesce and eventually connect with the central canal of the cord by a process called canalization. The distal spinal cord then involutes (retrogressive differentiation) to form the filum terminale and the differential growth causes the conus medullaris to ascend. The conus lies at the L 2-3 interspace at birth and reaches the adult position (L1-2) by 3 months of age.

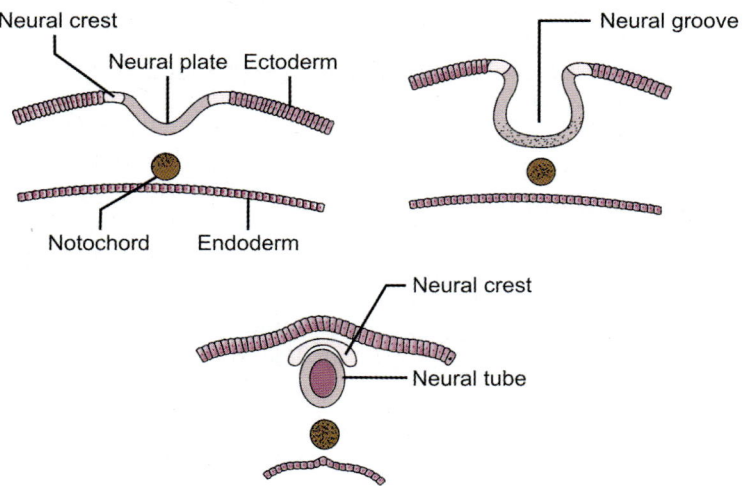

Fig. 103.1: Embryological development of the neural tube

Theories on Embryogenesis of Neural Tube Defects

a. *Simple nonclosure:* This theory postulates that the normal process of neural fold formation and closure is interrupted in a localized area leading to a NTD.
b. *Overgrowth and nonclosure:* The overgrowth of the neural epithelial cells interfere with the normal folding and neural tube formation.
c. *Reopening:* This theory states that the neural tube reopens after closure as a result of degenerative changes at the junction of the ectoderm and neural tissue.
d. *Overgrowth and reopening:* The overgrown dorsal caudal neural plate is exposed after normal closure has taken place.
e. *Primary mesodermal insufficiency:* The mesodermal defect is the primary event that leads to the neural tube defect.
f. A unifying hypothesis for hydrocephalus, Chiari malformation, syringomyelia, anencephaly and spina bifida has been proposed recently.[5] It proposes that hydrocephalus is caused by inadequate central nervous system venous drainage. Any volume increase in the central nervous system can increase venous pressure. This occurs because veins are compressible and a CNS volume increase may result in reduced venous blood flow that has the potential to cause progressive increase in cerebrospinal fluid volume. Obstruction to CSF flow causes localised pressure increases, which have an adverse effect on venous drainage. The Chiari malformation is associated with hindbrain herniation, which may be caused by low spinal pressure relative to cranial pressure. When spinal injury occurs as a result of a Chiari malformation, the primary pathology is posterior fossa hypoplasia, resulting in raised spinal pressure. It is proposed that hydrocephalus may occur as a result of posterior fossa hypoplasia, where raised pressure occurs as a result of obstruction to flow of CSF from the head to the spine, and cerebral injury with raised pressure occurs in anencephaly by this mechanism. It is proposed that the mesodermal growth insufficiency influences both neural tube closure and central nervous system pressure, leading to dysraphism.

ETIOLOGY

I. Unknown
II. *Multifactorial:* These include a combination of various causes.
III. *Genetic:* The genetic and familial risk of first born being affected is 1 in 250 but increases to about 1 in 20 or 1 in 25 in next pregnancy.
Polymorphism in UCP2 (uncoupling protein-2) gene
- Deranged myo-inositol, glucose and zinc metabolism in fetus.
- Polymorphism of the 5, 10-methylenetetra-hydrofolate and methionine synthase reductase gene. The risk of recurrence is around 3-5%.
IV. *Viral infection:* Influenza infection in the childhood
V. *Birth order:* Higher in 1st and 2nd born
VI. *Geographical variation.*
VII. *Vitamin deficiency:* Folic acids association seen with vitamin A deficiency in the experimental animals.
VIII. *Chemicals:* Trypan blue
Solanine present on the skin of potatoes (in experimental animal).
Smoking during peri conceptional period and pregnancy
IX. *Environmental:* Alcohol, drugs like Carbamazepine and Valproate.
X. Malnutrition.
XI. *Others:* Relation with maternal age and seasonal variation have all been implicated as etiologic factors.

ROLE OF FOLIC ACID

Folic acid supplementation has been demonstrated to reduce the prevalence of myelomeningocele. Studies of serum RBC cell levels of folic acid and its absorption in women who have borne children with myelomeningocele suggests that there is an increased need for folic acid by these women. An alternative explanation to the deficiency theory may be the action of Pterin aldehyde, a known contaminant of commercially produced folic acid. Pterin aldehyde inhibits xanthine oxidase that in turn produces free radicals. Free radicals are known to injure tissues. By reducing the free radical load at the high energy site, folic acid may impart and protective effect. It has been suggested that changes in prevalence of anencephaly and spina bifida surrounding folic acid fortification

(Period 3) could be part of preexisting trends.[6] The UK Food Standards Agency Board conducted a research on options to increase folate intake in women of reproductive age in order to reduce the risk of neural tube defect (NTD) affected pregnancies. Only a minority of participants knew about a link between spina bifida and folic acid, and these tended to be women with young families. In this research, mandatory fortification was the preferred option.[7] The risk of recurrence is around 1-3% and it is mandatory that mothers with one affected child are started on 5 mg tablet of folic acid daily at least three months prior to a planned pregnancy to prevent recurrence in the next pregnancy. It may be stressed that the amount of folic acid incorporated in the iron tablets/capsules (available in the market, and usually prescribed during pregnancy) is not sufficient enough to prevent spina bifida.

CLASSIFICATION

Spina Bifida Occulta

- Radiological
- Clinical
  - Extradural,
  - Intradural with or without surface stigma,
  - Intramedullary.

Spina Bifida Aperta

- Meningocele
- Meningomyelocele or myelomeningocele
- Myelocele – (Myeloschisis/Rachischisis)
- Neuroenteric canal.

Spina Bifida Occulta

Spinal bifida occulta is a mild form of dysraphism that is not accompanied by extrusion of the contents of vertebral canal. It is usually a radiological diagnosis. The defect is in the spinous process and/or associated posterior neural arch and is usually in the lumbar spine at one level only. Manifestations are less severe and diagnosis are missed until a definite and often irreversible orthopaedic or urologic syndrome develop. The cutaneous manifestations are present in half of the cases that act as sentinel for malformations of bone and nervous tissue deep beneath the skin surface. In order of decreasing frequency, these include lipoma, hypertrichosis (hairy patch) dermal dimple or sinus. Pigmented macules, vascular nevus and tail like cutaneous appendage. A pilonidal sinus usually terminates extradurally, but those occurring cephalad to the lumbosacral region should be reviewed with high index of suspicion and should be evaluated to exclude intraspinal pathology. These patients may be completely asymptomatic for years and operative interventions are usually not needed for asymptomatic cases. However, some of them may present in infancy and childhood with progressive neurological deficit (bladder dysfunction, clawing of toes, pees caves, spasticity, shortening of a limb and trophic ulcers).

Spina Bifida Aperta

Meningocele: Is a cystic lesion occurring due to herniation of the covering of the cord through a bifid neural arch that may be skin covered. The contents are only cerebrospinal fluid covered with meninges and skin. The dura is some times very thinned out and fluid contents are visible. The neural tube is fully developed There is usually no associated neurological deficits and poses no emergency unless it is thin walled with impending rupture.

Occasionally, there are double menigoceles in the same child, usually one in the cervical or the occipital region and the other in the lumbar area.

Myelomeningocele: A myelomeningocele or meningomyelocele is a parchment membrane covered lesion that in addition to CSF and meninges also contains the neural plaque which is usually an abnormal conus medullaris (Figs 103.2A and B). The duramater and skin are deficient over the posterior aspect of the defect but the cord is still protected by the pia arachnoid. The visible abnormal tissue is usually covered by a reactive response that consists of gliosis and dysplastic axons and cell bodies. At rostral end of the sac, the spinal cord can be traced as it exits from the spinal canal: caudally may end within the meninges, extend out as a thickened filum or penetrate the spinal canal to continue. Multiple healthy nerve roots may be present on the ventral surface of placode.

In addition, there are nerve roots present that end blindly to the lateral and dorsal dural encasement. The interior of the sac is frequently honeycomb by arachnoid strands and at least one or two anomalous vessels, usually veins are present. There is usually

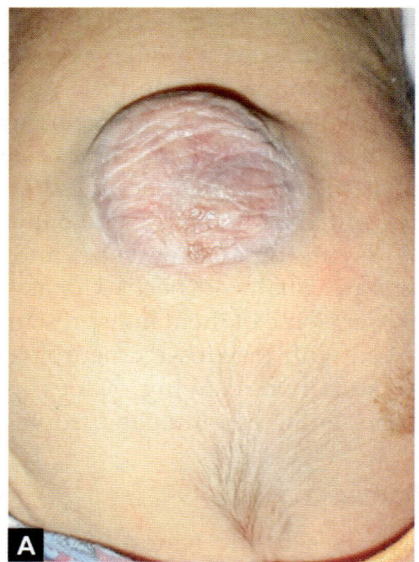

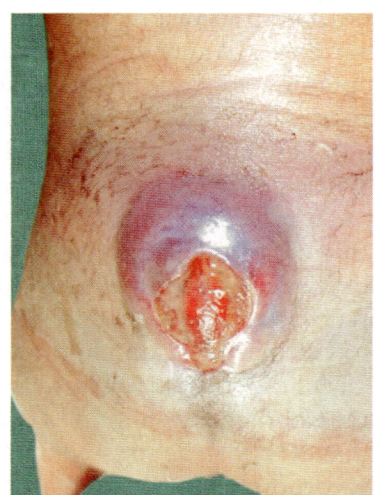

Fig. 103.3: Rachischisis with open neural tube defect

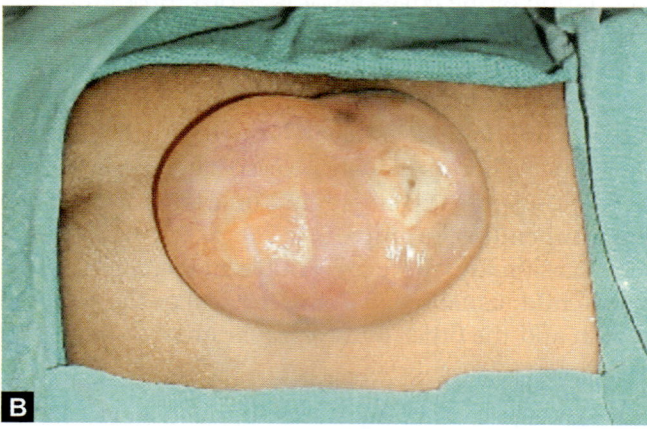

Figs 103.2A and B: A. Lumbar meningomyelocele in a patient with parchment like membranous covering **B.** Large lumbosacral meningomyelocele with thin membrane cover, ulcerations and the weakness of legs. The defect was large and the sac was tense, requiring urgent surgical intervention

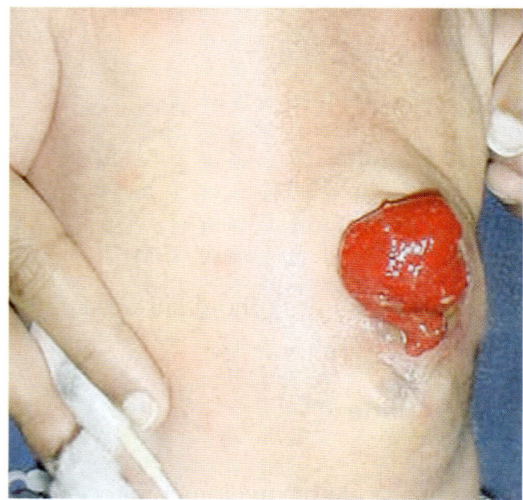

Fig. 103.4: Neuroenteric canal with intestinal mucosa, bilateral paresis, neurogenic bladder and bowel, associated with hydrocephalus

evidence of myelodysplasia and diastematomyelia. The neurologic deficit depends the upon the level of the defect that is usually lumbar or lumbosacral.

Associated hydrocephalus is noted in 75-90% patients and neurological deficits are common. Myelomeningocele is the commonest lesion.

Rachischisis refers to a large filleted neural placode with open central canal without any encasing meninges (Fig. 103.3). The dura is deficient and stops at the margin of the defect. The lesion is usually oblong with open central canal constituting a median furrow and crossing the thoracolumbar junction. Early hydrocephalus and severe neurological deficit are present. Myelodysplasia and diastematomyelia are common. There is evidence of intrauterine muscles paralysis leading to CDR talipes arthrogryposis. If left untreated, it is usually not compatible with life.

Neuroenteric canal: During embryogenesis, the neuroenteric canal connects the neurotube with the york sac, the structure that later develops into the midgut. The neuroenteric canal should close during development. Neuroenteric canal is a rare malformation that results from persistence of the embryonic neuroenteric canal that allows the content of the gut to flow into the spinal central canal and causes infection (Fig. 103.4).

PRENATAL DIAGNOSIS

Screening for spina bifida may be done by assessing maternal serum AFP levels at 16-18 weeks gestation. A raised value suggests a neural tube defect with a sensitivity of 75% only and is not expected in skin covered lesions. Elevated amniotic fluid AFP and acetylcholinesterase measurement also suggests NTD but false positive results can be expected. Fetal ultrasonography may visualize the spinal placode or splaying of the posterior elements or vertebral anomalies.

Positive test needs to be reconfirmed after about a week. A single high value is not be relied. Ultrasound is making rapid technical advancements. Minor variations in the frontal bones of the fetuses and compression of the malformed and caudally displaced cerebellum can be interpreted as the lemon and the banana sign. There are direct and indirect signs of neural tube defects on ultrasound. Fetal spine is ossified by the 16-17 week of gestation. In the coronal plane the normal posterior ossification centers are seen as two parallel lines of discrete echoes that normally widen in the cervical region and converge in the lumbosacral region. Disruption of smooth alignment of the spinal segments may be seen. There may be failure to see the normal, gradual craniocaudal narrowing of the spinal canal and disruption of the intact integument overlying the spine. The most reliable feature of spina bifida is the splaying of the posterior elements of the spine in the axial plane.

In 1986, Nicolades and associates described two signs, the so called Lemon and the Banana sign. *Lemon Sign* refers to the concave contours of the frontal bones, the cause of which is unknown. One fact of the lemon sign is that, it is known to disappear in many fetuses as the gestational age progressed. The *Banana Sign* refers to the anterior curving of the cerebellar hemispheres (like a banana), with simultaneous obliteration of the cisterna magna and has proved to be a *specific sign* for spina bifida. It is also a sonographic manifestation of *Chiari malformation*.

Indirect signs of myelomeningocele are more easily detected and include the banana sign (elongated appearance of the cerebellum secondary to the Chiari malformation) and the lemon sign (inward appearance of the frontal bones). The lemon signs detects 80% of NTD as compared to 93% with the banana sign.

The earliest antenatal diagnosis of a case of spina bifida in the upper thoracic spine with an accompanying meningocele was suspected at 8 weeks' gestation via transvaginal sonography as a subtle angulation or "step" in the posterior contour of the embryo; this may be attributed to kyphosis, which often accompanies this condition.[8] This was confirmed at 13 weeks' gestation via 3-dimensional sonography.[8]

Ventriculomegaly is assessed by measuring the transverse diameter of the lateral ventricular atrium Ventriculomegaly (> 10 mm lateral ventricular atrium diameter) is usually more common after 24 weeks of gestation. Ventriculomegaly is reported to occur in 70-80% of myelomeningocele, however literature reports that the ventriculomegaly varies with gestational age, with a prevalence of only 44% before 24 weeks of age, compared with 94% after 24 weeks of age. USG helps to establish the precise duration of pregnancy and direct demonstration or exclusion of the neural tube defect. Together with amniocentesis, USG detects 96-100% of defects.

Fetoscopy is direct visualization of the fetus for birth anomalies. The main source of alphafetoprotein in the amniotic fluid is fetal urine. Alphafetoprotein is synthesized from normal embryonal liver cells, yolk sac and intestinal tract. The normal value is 25 microgm/ml between 14-16 wks or gestation and increases upto 10 times in dysraphic fetus. The causes of false negative reports are skin covered lesions and amniotic fluid samples taken late in pregnancy. The increase in alphafetoprotein in neural tube defects is due to direct communication between CSF and amniotic fluid in open defects. Though not specific marker, it is recommended for woman at high risk of having a child with neural tube defects. High Field MRI can document anatomy of a fetus thus helps in intrauterine surgical repair. These screening programs have allegedly decreased the frequency of spina bifida cystica if the affected parents agree for medical termination of pregnancy.

Upto 14% of fetuses with NTD detected in the 2nd trimester have associated trisomy 13 or 18 and therefore, it is mandatory to do a chromosomal analysis prior to taking a decision regarding further management. Cesarean section or continuation of pregnancy is contraindicated in presence of chromosomal abnormality, associated anomaly, advanced hydrocephalus, flat lesion at or below plane of the back and absent knee and ankle movements.

CLINICAL FEATURES

The lesion is covered with a sterile dressing immediately after birth. The child is placed in a prone or a lateral recumbent position (Fig. 103.5). Evaluation of the degree of neurological deficit, child's functional level and the associated hydrocephalus, orthopedic, genitourinary problems, head circumference, shape are all noted at repeated intervals by different observers to avoid any bias.

The sensory examination requires that the child be relaxed and quiet or even sleeping. The cutaneous dermatomes are stimulated sharply from distal to proximal until one identifies the dermatome that produces facial or upper extremity response characteristic of pain.

The motor examination begins with sharp or painful stimulation of the torso or the upper extremity with observation for voluntary motion below the level of the lesion. Hip flexion and knee extension requires innervation of L1-L3, and adduction requires the innervation of L2-L4. Hip abduction, extension, and knee flexion requires the presence of L5-S2. The sensory level is usually one or two segment higher than the anticipated motor level.

More than 90% of myelomeningocele have a neurogenic bladder. A history of constant leakage of meconium and of urine implies a state of future incontinence. Not all cases require surgery. The anomaly is associated with serious postoperative morbidity, a strict selection criteria is followed.

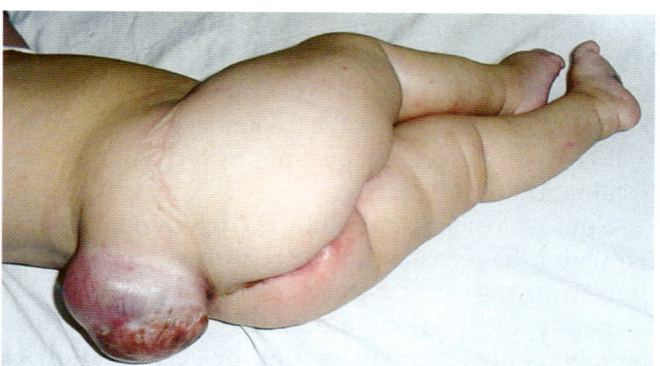

Fig. 103.5: A five months old boy with large lumbosacral meningomyelocele, weak legs, patulous anus and neurogenic bladder. The baby is nursed in lateral position

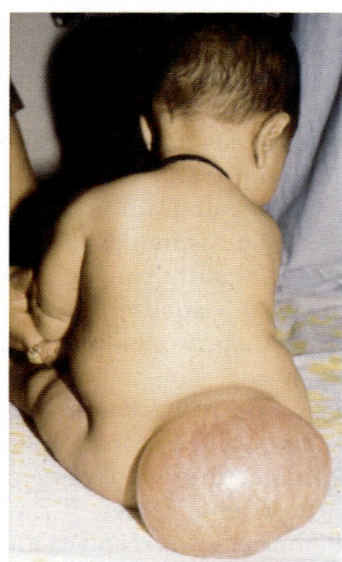

Fig. 103.6: A large very tense lumbosacral meningomyelocele with neurogenic bladder and bowel and weak legs. Surgery was performed only for easy nursing. Postoperatively baby developed hydrocephalus, could not be managed with drugs and required shunt surgery

CLINICAL EXAMINATION

General Assessment

General assessment is done to rule out associated anomalies or chromosomal anomalies (club feet, congenital heart disease, cleft palate, hernias, congenital dislocation of the hips, genitourinary abnormalities).

Local Examination

The meningomyelocele is examined as a swelling (Fig. 103.6). The size, extent, location, underlying defect, consistency, fluctuation and transillumination to assess the amount of neural tissue in sac is elicited. A cervical meningomyelocele has a better prognosis than a lumbosacral meningomyelocele (Fig. 103.7). The presence of scoliosis or kyphosis and laxity of surrounding skin to plan surgery is examined. Evidence of rupture / impending rupture, CSF leak or infection are noted. The extent of marginal epithelialized dura is noted. The level of the defect, size of neural plate and size of membrane covering are noted. A sacral meningomyelocele needs to differentiated from a sacrococcygeal teratoma (Fig. 103.8).

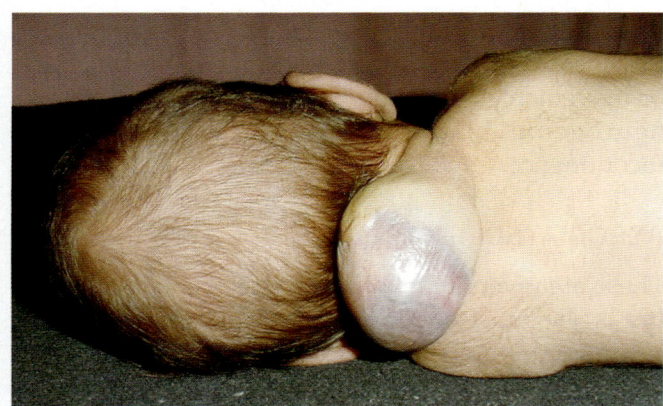

Fig. 103.7: A cervical meningomyelocele covered with parchment epithelium

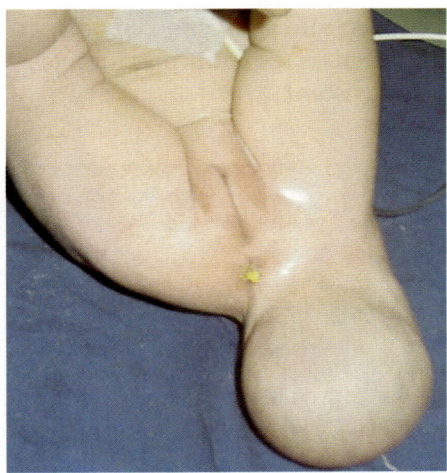

Fig. 103.8: A six months old girl with large sacral meningocele filled with CSF with no neurological deficits. The lesion needs to be differentiated from sacro-coccygeal teratoma

Table 103.1: Nerve roots involved for the various movements	
Motor examination	Nerve roots
1. Hip flexion	L1-3
2. Hip adduction Knee extension	L2-4

3. Hip abduction
   Hip extension
   Knee flexion
	L5-S2

4. Plantar flexion	S1

Evaluation of Other Regions

Lower limb power, tone and reflexes: There is usually flaccid paralysis with lumbosacral meningomyeloceles. In cervical/and some of the thoracic lesions there may be features of spasticity. Deformities of the foot and evidence of flexion contractures. Note grade of muscle power by stimulating upper abdomen or chest. The lower lesion, the more restricted is the neurologic deficit. In less than 10% cases, the lesion is present in sacral region. The nerve involved at the various joints for the associated movements is given in Table 103.1. Lesion at or above the thoracolumbar junction may have flaccid paraplegia without hip dislocation or deformity. The involvement of lower lumbar segments may have preserved hip flexors and abductor but weak/absent extensors and abductor with no useful function at knee or ankle as well as dislocation at this joint is common because opposed muscular activity at the hip. Cases of low myelomeningocele may present with deficits below the knee or involvement of only the ankle or movements of distal foot. The movements can be observed by the response to pulling or extension of extremities.

Spine: Widened pedicles may be felt in the region of spina bifida. Visible and palpable prominent laminae are usually scattered at the lateral margin of the defect. Associated kyphosis, lumbar lordosis, telescoping and scoliosis may be looked for. Congenital dislocation of hip (Paralytic type) may be associated. The feet may have Talipes equinovarus or Calcaneo valgus. Knee joint deformities in the form of arthrogryposis may be present.

Hydrocephalus: The initial head circumference is measured. The size and tension of the anterior fontanelle are noted. The amount of separation of the skull sutures especially squamo-parietal sutural diastasis and prominent scalp veins are looked for. The eyes are examined for sunseting of the eyes and VI cranial nerve palsy. The nature of the cry is observed.

Lower cranial nerves and brainstem function: Look for regurgitation, difficulty in feeding, stridor, apnea, hypotonia which suggests a significant chiari malformation (poor prognostic factor).

Bladder and bowel: The anocutaneous refex and bulbocavernous reflex are elicited. The bladder and kidneys are palpated. A patulous anus is suggestive of fecal incontinence (Fig. 103.9). The expressibility of the bladder is noted and the urinary stream is observed. The excoriation in the peritoneal area is suggestive of urinary incontinence (Fig. 103.10). It is important to note that if one leg is normal, bladder function can be expected to be normal. The bladder and bowel involvement is due to autonomic system involvement. If there is flacid involvement, there is urinary and fecal incontinence, rectal prolapse and a palpable bladder. In the presence of a palpable bladder, there is dribbling of urine which increases on crying or movement. If there is spastic involvement, there is neurogenic bladder, megacolon and urinary incontinence.

ASSOCIATED ANOMALIES

These are given in detail in Table 103.2. Hydrocephalus is the most common associated anomaly. It is secondary to sylvian aqueduct stenosis, as well as Chiari Malformation. In the skull, craniolacunia, small post fossa with enlarged foramen magnum and low attachment of tentorium may be seen. The vertebral defect may extend beyond the obvious region of myelomeningocele. In telescoped spinal axis, the head seems to impacted on the trunk and lumbar spine seem almost non coexistent.

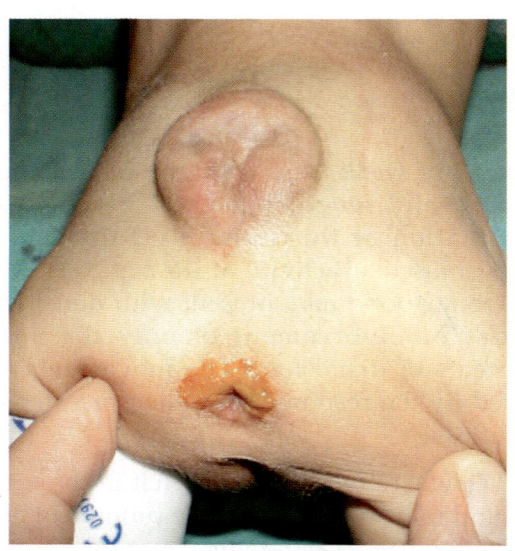

Fig. 103.9: A two months old baby with infected and tethered meningomyelocele in lumbosacral region with weak legs, patulous anus and neurogenic bladder

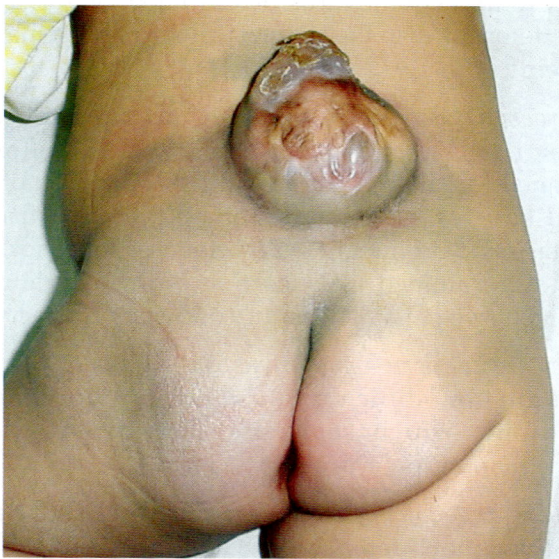

Fig. 103.10: A six months old baby with lumbosacral meningomyelocele, neurogenic bladder and bowel and weak legs. The surgery was performed only for social reasons. The baby developed hydrocephalus postoperatively that could be managed with medical decompression therapy

Table 103.2: Associated anomalies in myelomeningocele
1. Hydrocephalus 80-90%
2. Chiari malformation–nearly 100%   • Clinically significant – 10-20%
3. Brain–   • Micropolygyria   • Cerebellar dysgenesis   • Corpus callosum agenesis   • Cysts
4. Vertebral anomalies–   • Fusion defect   • Hemivertebrae   • Butterfly vertebrae   • Widened inter pediculate distance   • Telescoped spinal axis
5. Rib anomalies – absent, bifurcation or duplication
6. Scoliosis / kyphosis (30%)
7. Genitourinary   • Undescended testes   • Vesicoureteric reflux   • Hydronephrosis   • Hypospadias   • Horseshoe kidney   • Renal agenesis   • Urethral diverticulum   • Bladder exstrophy   • Posterior urethral valve
8. Club feet
9. Hydromyelia, 'second lesion'
10. Others–cardiovascular anomalies, cleft palate, congenital dislocation of hip, hernias, Diaphragmatic hernia, esophageal atresia, TOF, ARM

Pathogenesis of Cerebral Malformations in Human Fetuses with Meningomyelocele

In fetal SBA, neuroepithelial/ependymal denudation in the telencephalon and the aqueduct can occur before Chiari II malformation and/or hydrocephalus. Since denuded areas cannot re-establish cell function, neurodevelopmental consequences could induce permanent cerebral pathology.[9]

INVESTIGATIONS

1. Swab culture: of the surface and its content for prophylaxis against meningitis and ventriculitis
2. X-ray spine
   - Multisegment canal widening
   - Anterior or posterior fusion defects
   - Hemivertebrae
   - Block vertebrae
   - But features are not essential for early treatment decision
3. X-ray skull:
   - Craniolacunia
4. CT Skull:
   - Features of hydrocephalus
   - Expansion of lateral ventricle with minimal dilatation of hook shaped frontal and expanded occipital horns.
   - Mild to moderate dilatation of 3rd ventricle
   - Scalloping of petrous bone
   - Prominent cercebellar vermis.
5. USG skull
   - Coronal views–teardrop appearance of the ventricle.
   - Apparent ablation of interhemispheric fissure.

MANAGEMENT

Fetal Surgery

Fetal repair of myelomeningocele in utero has been attempted to decrease the risk of neurological deficits as a result of trauma or amniotic fluid exposure. This is currently done in very few centers who believe that it can reverse some effects of spinal birth defects and ultimately decrease paralysis and brain damage and improve the quality of life. The disadvantages include bleeding, infection and some times even the life threatening side effects caused from drugs used during fetal surgery to control premature labor. However, the authors have treated a baby who had got the fetal surgery done for spina bifida, with quite a bad scar, residual meningocele sac, neurological deficit and tethered cord.

Cesarean section becomes necessary for further deliveries. Virtually all fetuses are born prematurely, increasing the chances of complications. Although surgical closure of this anomaly is usually performed in the early postnatal period, an estimated 330 cases of intrauterine repair have been performed in a few specialized centers worldwide.[10] It was hoped prenatal intervention would improve the prognosis of affected patients, and preliminary findings suggest a reduced incidence of shunt-dependent hydrocephalus, as well as an improvement in hindbrain herniation. However, the expectations for improved neurological outcome have not been fulfilled and not all patients benefit from fetal surgery in the same way.[10]

In future, refined, risk-reduced surgical techniques and new treatment options for preterm labor and preterm rupture of the membranes are likely to reduce associated maternal and fetal risks and improve outcome, but further research will be needed.[10]

Collagen biomatrices can be used for intrauterine coverage of an experimental spina bifida and can preserve the architecture of the spinal cord.[11] Neurological outcome is not different between fetuses with their spinal cord covered and fetuses with uncovered cords.[11]

Initial Assessment

A detailed family history is taken for previous history of CNS anomalies, number of pregnancies and abortions and age of parents including chances of future normal pregnancies. A history of drugs or viral infections during pregnancy especially in the 1st month is also elicited. The management depends upon the age and general condition at presentation, level and magnitude of defect, presence of infection or CSF leak, status of lower limbs and sphincters, presence of hydrocephalus and socio-economic status of parents and family history. The prognosis in terms of ambulation, mental development and continence is explained to the parents. The need for shunt surgery in upto 75-80% cases with its associated complications and revisions need for urological and bowel treatment with repeated follow up and surgical intervention, chances of secondary tethered cord are explained.

The parents should ultimately decide regarding the management, but it is the duty of the surgeon to give the correct picture in detail. Also, it must be remembered that not all untreated children die and may present later with a far worse neurological status. A few of them may require surgery of the large sac for better nursing care. Active treatment is withheld if the patient already has gross hydrocephalus and significant neurologic impairment who after closure of defect develop meningitis and ventriculitis. Active treatment is also withheld in presence of Kyphosis/Scoliosis clinically evident at birth, severe cerebral birth injury/intracranial hemorrhage and other congenital defects, e.g. cyanotic heart disease, Mongolism and or serious GU malformation.

Elective early treatment is widely accepted with improvement in the quality of survival. The results of early operation without selection have been disheartening. A large number of survivors are mentally retarded and physical handicaps. The social life of the involved family is adversely affected. If the child survives by the age of 6 months and if it appears likely that will continue to live, a decision could then be made afterwards.

Timing of Operation

If a decision is made for surgery, then under favorable conditions, it should be done as soon as possible to decrease the risk of meningitis and to prevent possible drying of the sac and damage to neural structure. Immediate surgery is warranted in presence of rupture/imminence of rupture of the sac. Progressive hydrocephalus is not a contraindication for surgery provided a shunting procedure is done early to prevent irreversible brain damage with subsequent mental retardation.

The operation should be delayed in the presence of an already infected/ulcerated lesion, until the infection is controlled and the ulcer is healed. This should include to (cover the sac with sterile gauze soaked in saline, daily baths with soap and water and antibiotics. If meningitis has already set in, intravenous antibiotics should be given before operating upon the lesion. Unless the hydrocephalus is rapidly progressive, it may be better to defer the shunt surgery until 4-6 weeks of age as there is high incidence of complications (obstruction of ventricular end of shunt and shunt dependence) if shunt is done before 1 month of age. Also there is no significant increase in proportion of retarded children by such judicious delay.

If the hydrocephalus is rapidly progressive, primary treatment of hydrocephalus is indicated to decrease the size of sac, promote healing of the infection and prevent post repair CSF leak.

PREOPERATIVE CARE

Besides maintaining normothermia and the standard neonatal care, these children have to be nursed prone. The lesion is covered with sterile and saline soaked dressings. A deep head ring may be helpful for nursing. Preoperative antibiotics are used routinely in anti-meningitic doses.

Operative Treatment

The goals of an early operative treatment in a neonate with an open myelomeningocele are:
1. Preserving all viable neural tissue.
2. Water tight closure of the dura.
3. Reconstituting the normal anatomic environment.
4. Minimizing the chance of infection or preventing ascending infection of the neural axis.

The threat of superficial infection of the placode increases after the 72 hours of birth, thus a surgery at that time increases the risk of meningitis, ventriculitis, and an increase in the deficit. It is important to identify the neural placode, intermediate epithelial layer, skin, and the pia-arachnoid and the dura to achieve a complete skin closure, and to prevent any leakage of CSF.

Principles of Operation

The patient is positioned in the prone position with a roll under the pelvis and a folded towel under the chest to keep the abdomen free for respiration. An elliptical incision is given after planning the adequacy of the skin to cover the defect. The sac is mobilized from the skin and subcutaneous tissues and neck delineated. The use of bipolar coagulation and optical loupes are advisable. The central membrane and placode are separated by sharp dissection from the sac. The cord is detethered by dividing arachnoid adhesions and epithelial elements trimmed from the placode. The neural placode retubularized by 7-0 sutures on the pia-arachnoid tissues. The dura is dissected from the sac and areolar tissue and closed with continuous

5-0 prolene or Vicryl. Fascial flaps are used to cover the dura. Wide mobilization of the skin and subcutaneous tissues is done in all directions till closure is possible without tension. Closure of subcutaenous tissue and skin is done and a pressure barrier dressing is applied.

POSTOPERATIVE CARE

Routine antibiotics are given. The baby is nursed prone or in a lateral recumbent position. Hydrocephalus associated with myelomeningocele is attributed to aqueduct stenosis. About 15% of patients with myelomeningocele are born with clinical signs of hydrocephalus, but 80% develop hydrocephalus in late infancy with myelomeningocele.

Mannitol is given for 3 doses followed by oral diamox (50-100 mg/kg/day) the next day. The head circumference is monitored and serial ultrasound is done for hydrocephalus. The diagnosis is confirmed by a CT scan or an ultrasound scan and a shunt (preferably a VP shunt) is inserted. A watch is kept for Chiari malformation complications. The postoperative neurological status is monitored. The CSF leak is managed by increasing the dose of acetazolamide, repeated aspirations from the subcutaneous plane, pressure dressings and CSF shunting (lumbotheco-peritoneal). Barrier dressing is done at all times to prevent any source of infection from the perineum.

Postoperative Complications

1. *Worsening neurological deficit:* Occasionally worsening of the neurological function may be seen after the closure that may be preventable with a little caution. One should not splash betadine on to the neural placode, which is best rinsed with warm jets of plain saline and not subjected to any mechanical scrubbing. One should not cut the membrane too medially into the neural tissues causing bleeding and loss of function. One should cauterise the bleeding edges with a bipolar cautery, set at its lowest current. The lower part of the placode should be inspected for the presence of a neurulated cord, caudal to it, to rule out a segmental neural placode.

   Mild fever is not unusual. This is usually due to the presence of blood in the CSF in the post-operative period. This does not result in neurological deficits. However, the presence of intradural hematoma or an ongoing bleeding should be suspected if the neurological deficit has appeared a few hours later after the surgery. An urgent MRI scan may be indicated and an urgent re-exploration is helpful.

2. *Wound Dehiscence:* It is common to have erythema along the either side of the wound. Sometimes the flaps may look deep red to purple as a result of venous stasis. The predisposing factors include a state of cortisol mediated catabolic stress and poor feeding due to associated hydrocephalus, postoperative ileus, Chiari malformation, and prematurity. There may be tension at the suture line in cases with a large sac. An untreated kyphosis may add a vertical vector to the stretching of the wound.

3. *Wound infection:* The infection rate is about 1-5%. The prolonged catabolic phase after surgery certainly interferes with the newborn's white cell function and immunity. Also because IgA does not cross the placenta, infections with enteric bacteria are common. Local factors predisposing to infection are, a large sac with a redundant multiply folded membrane surrounding the placode.

   Intradural infection is usually primary. Because most of the organisms are gram negative enteric bacteria, systemic signs of sepsis are usually present within the first 24 hours of surgery. In the neonates these signs are non specific. The infant shows poor feeding, lethargy, ashen complexion, and mottled blotches (livido reticularis) over the trunk. Hypothermia, low TLC often less than 4000 cells / mm, and a very high band count are suggestive of sepsis. A ventricular tap to obtain CSF for bacteriological examination may be done, and treatment started according to the sensitivity pattern.

   If the infection is confined to the extradural space, the wound becomes red, hot, and fluctuant on day 5-7. The surrounding skin may be edematous. The untreated subcutaneous infection passes on to the dura. A red fluctuant wound should be aspirated for purulent material that may be sent for culture.

4. *CSF Leak:* CSF leaks are more common in large myelomeningocele. Also since more than 80% of

myelomeningocele are associated with hydrocephalus, increased CSF pressure poses a risk of leak. CSF leaks occur most commonly during the 4th postoperative day. A slight fluctuation under the skin flaps during the first few postoperative days is likely due to collection of blood and CSF, and if the closure is strong this transdural seepage is self limiting. A large transdural leak presents as a rapid accumulation of a bulging fluctuancy in the wound, usually at 5-6 days after closure. Spontaneous closure of such a leak is not hopeful.

The best preventive measure is a meticulous watertight closure of the dura. It is preferable to use a 7-0 prolene on an atraumatic needle. Immediate integrity of the closure is tested by two Valsalva manoeuvres held at a peak pressure of 40 cm H_2O for 2 seconds. If the lateral dura is too tenuous the lumbosacral fascia and the periosteum overlying the incomplete neural arches is mobilised. Fascia Lata is the most suitable graft material. Lastly even the best closure cannot withstand a high CSF pressure when hydrocephalus develops. Good judgement dictates that progressive hydrocephalus in the first 2 weeks of life should be promptly treated with an external ventricular drainage.

MULTIDISCIPLINARY CARE

Counseling of the family should begin immediate with explanation of the problem and potential difficulties to be encountered. A social worker may be helpful for guiding the family for education requirements and vocational trainings.

A paediatric urologist determines the degree of sphincter impairment, bladder dysfunction, arterial reflux, infection and begins clean intermittent catheterisation. Bowel management programs are easily achieved by supplementing proper nutrition, by using laxatives. The pediatric orthopedist evaluates the spine for scoliosis, neurogenic clubfoot, and neurogenic hip dislocation.

Most children born with spina bifida have normal renal function. If left untreated, more than half of these children will have serious renal deterioration by age 5 secondary to neurogenic changes of the bladder.[12] Renal development should follow a normal course when close evaluation and intervention are undertaken during the newborn period and toddler years. As children age, attention is directed to quality-of-life issues, such as the establishment of urinary and bowel continence. Teenagers face the responsibility of understanding their medical condition and should begin to assume responsibility for their own care with eventual transition to the adult health care system.[12]

In children with spinal dysraphism such as myelomeningocele the relation between muscle mass and body composition varies considerably. Therefore, it is difficult to evaluate the relevance of renal function assessments done with serum creatinine. Since serum cystatin C has been suggested to be independent of body size and composition, this evaluation was compared to chromium(51) edetic acid clearance.[13] Cystatin C values were within the normal range in all patients, while chromium(51) edetic acid clearance was reduced in 10.[13] Using chromium(51) edetic acid clearance as a gold standard, children with spinal dysraphism and slightly to moderately reduced renal function may remain undiagnosed if cystatin C is used for evaluation.[13] Robotic-assisted laparoscopic surgery has been applied to creating both an appendicovesicostomy and an antegrade continent enema colon tube in a 9-year-old female with a neurogenic bladder and bowel secondary to myelomeningocele.[14]

The majority of patients can be dry for urine by the time they go to primary school if they have been treated from birth onward for detrusor overactivity. As the upper urinary tract changes predominantly start in the first months of life, they should be treated right from birth by clean intermittent catheterization and pharmacological suppression of detrusor overactivity with imipramine. Urinary tract infections, when present, need aggressive treatment, and in many patients, permanent prophylaxis is indicated. Later in life, therapy can be tailored to urodynamic findings. Children with paralyzed pelvic floor and hence urinary incontinence are routinely offered surgery around the age of 5 years to become dry. Rectus abdominis sling suspension of the bladder neck is the first-choice procedure, with good to excellent results in both male and female patients. In children with detrusor hyperactivity, detrusorectomy can be performed as an alternative for ileocystoplasty provided there is adequate bladder capacity.[15] Bladder augmentation, artificial sphincter and perineal urethrostomy are other options that may be required depending on the case. Wheelchair-bound patients can manage their bladder more easily with a continent catheterizable stoma on top of the bladder. This stoma provides them extra privacy and diminishes parental burden. Bowel management is done by retrograde or antegrade enema therapy. Concerning sexuality, special attention is needed to address expectations of adolescent patients. Sensibility of the glans penis has been reported to be restored by connecting the ilioinguinal nerve with the dorsal nerve of the penis in the majority of patients.[15]

Management of bowel continence has been given in the chapter on bowel management.

Orthopedic Management

Orthopedic management is required for correction of the deformity and maintenance of the correct position as well as for obtaining the greatest possible degree of mobility and self sufficiency. Early correction enables prevention of the further disuse deformities and contracture. Conservative measures like casting and brace are usually contraindicated because of risk of causing skin breakdown in the presence of sensory deficit or existing deformity. Recurrence is likely if muscle imbalance is present. Muscle balance may be achieved by tendon transfer or lengthening, denervation or excision of overactive muscle and correction of the deformity by osteotomies. The ideal time is between 6 months to 2 years. For lumbar lordosis and scoliosis, a multiple wedge osteotomy and fusion is done.

For hip flexion contracture, anterior hip release or iliopsoas transfer with or without osteotomy are done. For hyper extension deformity of the knee joint, serial plaster casting in the position of flexion to prevent elongation of the quadriceps may be done. Flexion deformity of the knee is treated by Hamstring tendon transfer. Orthopedic devices are given for CTEV.

LONG-TERM OUTCOME

Patients with spina bifida exhibited more problems than both published norms and a local comparison group of healthy children in metacognition but not behavior regulation.[16] More shunt-related surgeries and history of seizures predicted poorer metacognitive abilities. Adolescents and young adults with spina bifida who smoked were 10 times more likely to report being sexually active and women were 2.3 times more likely to be sexually active than men.[17] Participants with urinary incontinence were less likely to be sexually active. Women without hydrocephalus were significantly more satisfied with life than women with hydrocephalus.[17] Adolescents and young adults with spina bifida were only slightly satisfied with life and sexual activity was only associated with life satisfaction among women.[17] Survival to adulthood for people with Spina Bifida now exceeds 85% due to improvements in medical and surgical management. Rates remain lower than expected for community participation, healthy lifestyle choices, employment and independent living. The importance of transition programming to help adolescents with disabilities prepare for adult life roles is now understood.[18] Both the transition to adulthood and the transfer of care to adult care clinics are important and distinct components of spina bifida lifespan care.[18]

With multidisciplinary approach, the survival rates are approaching 95% in the first 2 years of life. The most common cause of death is related to hindbrain dysfunction (73%). Around 10% have mild dysfunction, with inspiratory stridor, 9% have moderate dysfunction with inspiratory stridor and periodic apnea, and 13% have severe dysfunction with periodic apnea and GER. The natural history of this hind brain dysfunction appears to be that of gradual improvement. An Arnold Chiari malformation can cause severe symptoms, such as choking, stridor, becoming clinically significant in only 10-32% of these conditions. Leakage of the CSF after closure of an myelomeningocele is reported as high as 17%. Most of these leaks close down spontaneously.

Children with myelomeningocele and no evidence of ventriculitis develop normal intelligence. Children with hydrocephalus who are treated aggressively have near normal IQ. Success with walking is subject to many factors. To stand erect requires a level of motor function at L3, motor function at L4-L5 is necessary for walking. As children age, their body weight may exceed the increase in their motor strength, creating difficulties in walking. However with better care about 80% of patients are able to walk. Sexual development and function requires motor ability at the level of S2-S4. Patients have a variable level of sexual development. Psychosocial problem is one of the greatest obstacles in children with myelomeningocele. Therefore, a co-ordinated and a comprehensive treatment plan should be charted out.

SPINA BIFIDA OCCULTA

Spina bifida occulta is present with an incidence of about 2-3% in the general population as a bony defect in the L-S region without any neurological symptoms. However, only a few of them are likely to develop symptoms and gait changes much later in life. Over 60% patients with hypertrichosis would have an associated diastematomyelia, a fibrous cartilaginous, or more commonly a bony spicule separating the spinal cord into hemicords can occur as an isolated defect or in association with either myelomeningocele or lipomyelomeningocele.

TETHERED CORD SYNDROME (TCS)

The entity "Tethered cord syndrome" is a result of interference with normal cephalad migration of spinal cord during the disproportionate growth of the vertebral column. The fixation is due to abnormally thickened filum terminale tethered to the inner surface of dorsal dura mater. TCS refers to a group of lesions in which the spinal cord is fixed to a structure like a lipoma, vertebra, dura or skin and abnormal stretching of the cord results in progressive neurological damage.

In 1981, Yamada and associates adopted the term tethered cord syndrome to designate two groups of patients (i) Patients with tethered cord and (ii) Patients who harbour any structures that may cause viscoelasticity of the filum terminale to be ineffective in protecting the cord which could be a tumor, occult myelomeningocele, arachnoiditis or a bony spur.

Primary TCS or occult spinal dysraphism includes lesions that are not associated with an open neural tube defect or trauma (Table 103.3). Secondary TCS includes lesions that occur due to prior arachnoiditis, surgery or trauma.

Functional and Metabolic Impairment in TCS

The interlacing fibres of neurones, glia, pia, blood vessels in the spinal cord provide some resistance against traction in the longitudinal direction of the cord. If the viscoelasticity is sufficient to stretch the spinal cord the viscoelasticity of each structure protects neurones and glia from disruption and helps to maintain normal function to a certain degree. If the spinal cord is stretched to a level beyond this inherent viscoelastic resistance neuronal function may be disrupted. In brief, experimental studies of cord tethering and laminectomy and dural opening, various correlations between experimental results and clinical observations have been made:

1. Cord tethering produces excessive tension within the spinal cord and can result in metabolic derangement and histologic changes.
2. Oxidative metabolism is impaired in the spinal cord under tension. The severity of neuronal dysfunction parallels the degree of impairment in the oxidative metabolism.
3. Blood flow decrease and glucose metabolic impairment also contribute to cytochrome reduction. Blood flow increases are reported with post surgical improvement in neurological status.
4. Irreversible damage can occur with sudden stretching of the already chronically stretched TCS.

Table 103.3: Classification of tethered cord syndrome

a. Primary
- Dermal sinus
- Diastometamyelia
- Lipoma/lipomyelomeningocele
- Tumors
- Tight filum terminale
- Neurenteric cysts
- Anterior meningocele

b. Secondary
- Arachnoiditis
- Retethered spinal cord syndrome
- Trauma

Primary TCS

Cutaneous markers like midline dimples, dermal sinuses, nevi, hemangiomas, hairy patch (Fawn's tail), lipoma, gluteal assymetry or split-buttock crease and small areas of thinned out epidermis are pointers towards an occult spinal lesion (Figs 103.11 to 103.13B). However, 20-40% patients may not have any cutaneous marker.

Clinical Features Associated with TCS

a. Cutaneous markers
b. Symptoms
- Pain -Back, legs
- Lower limb fatigue, weakness
- Scoliosis, Lordosis, Kyphosis

- Abnormal gait
- Delayed toilet training
- Recurrent UTI
- Recurrent meningitis
- Progressive foot deformity
- Sudden neurologic deficit due to trauma or postural change.

The symptoms may be broadly divided into two, orthopedic symptoms or urologic symptoms. The orthopedic symptoms include asymmetry of legs due to predominant unilateral diminished muscle bulk, short foot, often inverted with high arch and clawed toes, variable sensory loss and trophic ulcer present on sole. The deep tendon reflexes in the involved extremity may be absent in the presence of extensor plantar response.

Kyphosis and scoliosis may be present. The urologic symptoms include frequent bed wetting or incontinence present or UTI.

In a study to evaluate presence of spinal cord abnormalities in 176 patients with functional urinary and bowel problems out of which 88 children had radiographic evidence of spina bifida occulta and 88 were age-and sex-matched controls. Magnetic resonance images were obtained in all patients and evaluated for spinal cord abnormalities. Sacral ratios were calculated on the basis of plain radiographs.[19]

Among children with functional bowel and urinary problems, there was no statistically significant difference in the prevalence of abnormal spinal MR imaging findings in those with radiographic spina bifida occulta and an age- and sex-matched control group. Spina bifida occulta was thus not shown to be a reliable indicator of spinal cord structural abnormalities.[19]

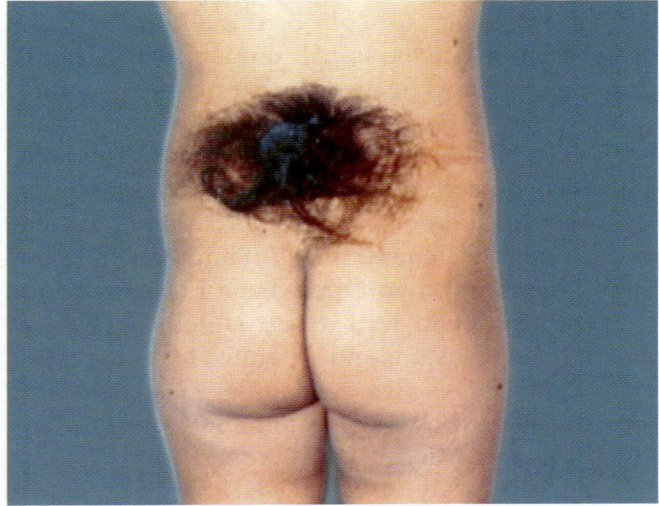

Fig. 103.11: Spina bifida occulta with a tuft of hair on the back. The child had diastematomyelia on investigating with an MRI

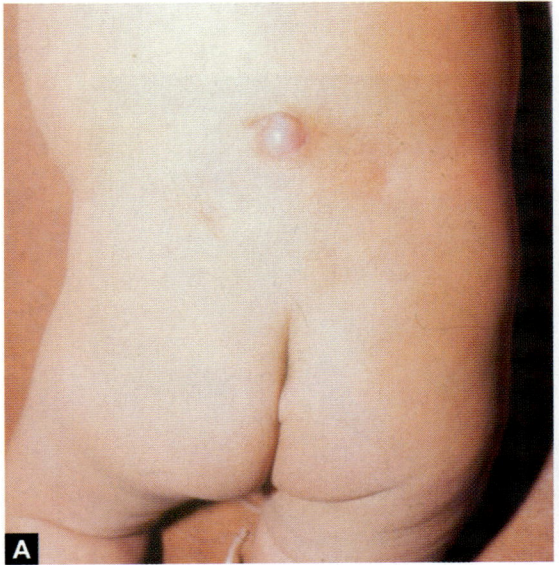
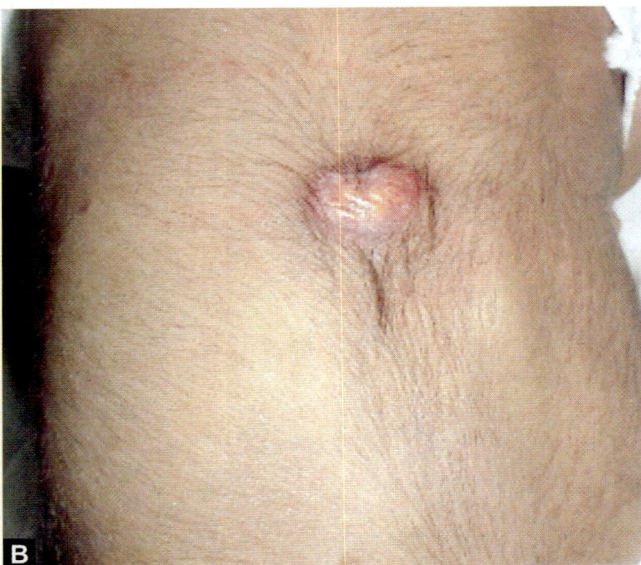

Figs 103.12A and B: A. Spina bifida occulta—atretic meningomyelocele
B. A newborn with an atretic meningomyelocele with parchment skin membrane cover

Investigation

All children with suggestive symptoms and those with cutaneous markers should be evaluated completely. Current recommendations also include children with the VACTERL association, cloacal exstrophy and imperforate anus. The basic investigation to assess the spinal anomaly is MRI. During follow up and in presence of symptoms, Urodynamic study may be helpful to study the urological status. Somatosensory evoked potentials have also been studied.

Treatment

The treatment of TCS involves surgical release and excision of the tethering lesion. It is presently the consensus that detethering should be carried out at diagnosis even in the absence of symptoms. Since a number of studies have reported neurological damage in infancy, the current recommendation is for prophylactic repair at 3-6 months of age.[18] It is believed that up to 90% of patients with TCS will develop deficits which are irreversible if left untreated. The surgical risk of a new deficit is around 2%.

The principles of surgical treatment include removal of the abnormal tissue to reconstruct the dural sac. Vigorous toilet is needed to remove any debris or blood that can cause secondary TCS. Lipomyelomeningoceles do not need to be totally resected but should be debulked. In SCM, all tethering bands need to be resected and a single dural tube is reconstructed. The filum terminale should be identified in all cases and sectioned if it appears to contribute to the pathology. Intraoperative motor evoked potential and EMG monitoring is vital to prevent operative trauma to viable nerve roots.

DIASTEMATOMYELIA

Diastematomyelia (or split cord malformation) is a condition in which the spinal cord is split in a sagittal plane forming two hemicords that may be separated by a spur (Figs 103.13A and B). This lesion is seen more frequently in girls and is most commonly associated with a hairy patch (Fawn's tail) on the overlying skin. Over 60% of patients with hypertrichosis have an underlying Diastematomyelia. Pang has classified these lesions into two types. Type I is the classical Diastematomyelia with two hemicords lying in separate dural sheaths and separated by a bony spur. Type II consists of two hemicords in a single dural sheath separated by a thin sagittal fibrous spur. This lesion was earlier termed as diplomyelia.

Embryologically, it is believed that these lesions result due to a defect in gastrulation where there is either a localized duplication of the notochord or persistence of the neuroenteric canal causing a split notochord. Mesenchymal elements interpose between

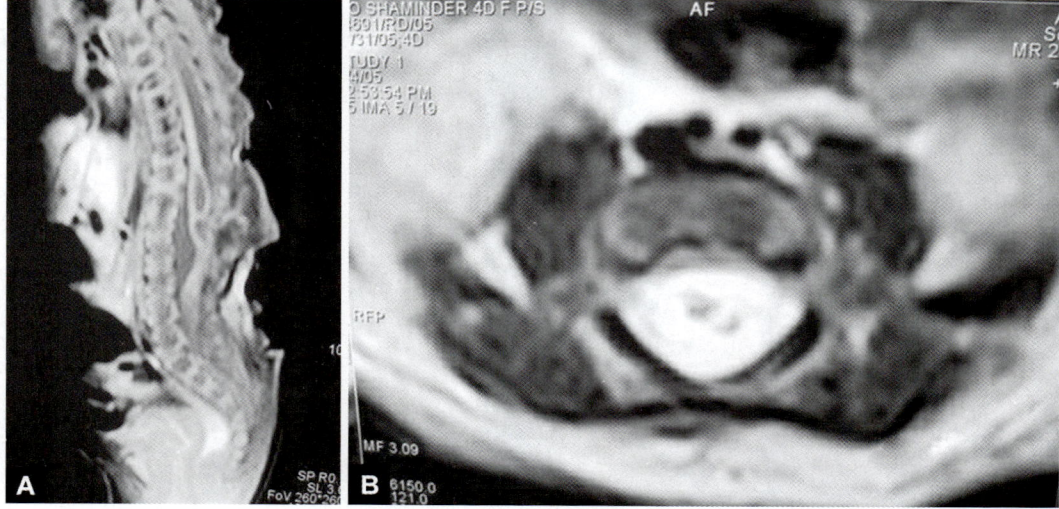

Figs 103.13A and B: MRI in sagittal section **A.** Axial section **B.** Diastematomyelia with a low cord, syringomyelia and an intradural lipoma. The patient had a sinus extending from skin, vertebral anomalies, scoliosis and a bony lesion under skin

the split notochord and lead to the development of the lesion. Surgical treatment consists of laminectomy, complete dethering of the cord with excision of the bony spur and division of the tight filum-terminale if warranted.

LIPOMYELOMENINGOCELE

Lipomyelomeningocele usually present as a swelling in the lower back that is well covered with a healthy skin. It has to be differentiated from extramedullary lipoma and from the fat in the filum terminale. The subcutaneous component of the lipoma extends through the dural defect due to a premature dysjunction of the cutaneous and neuroectoderm. The spinal cord is low lying and tethered by the lipoma and closely resembles the neural plate seen in myelomeningocele. The dural attachment, which has surgical significance, is attached to the edges of the neural plate just dorsal to the entry of the dorsal nerve roots. The intra medullary component of the lipoma grows with the child and causes spinal cord compression as well. The term lipomyelomeningocele is actually a misnomer in that it suggests herniation of neural elements through a spina bifida defect into a meningeal sac. Chapman has classified lipomyelomeningocele into dorsal and caudal variant. A third transition form has also been described.

Spinal lipomas have thus been classified into:
a. Dorsal variant were the fatty tissue lies dorsal to the neural plate and nerve roots. These often present as subcutaneous masses which may be asymmetric. The pia and dura are fused along the lateral interface with sensory roots emerging just anterior to this line of fusion, as a result neither the sensory nor the motor roots lie within the lipoma.
b. Caudal variant which is located at the transition of the cones and filum terminale. Here the fatty tumour may replace the filum. The normal roots lie ventrally but may lie within the lipoma also.
c. Transitional form which is an admixture of the dorsal and caudal variants.

Pathogenesis

Abnormal function of the spinal cord and roots during embryogenesis may result in permanent damage manifesting at birth, as seen in myelomeningocele. Local mass effect from the fatty tissue may be cause several dysfunction. Finally symptoms may be produced by the traction on the cord. Early in the embryonic period there is progressive ascent of the conus within the spinal canal owing to the faster growth of the vertebral bodies compared to the spinal cord. If the cord is tethered to the spinal canal there is loss of mobility of the conus during spinal flexion and extension and decreased cord pulsations as demonstrated by MR imaging.

Manifestations

Manifestations are those of tethered cord syndrome and patients present with one or more of the syndromes.

1. *Cutaneous Syndromes:* The cutaneous abnormalities, which are indicative of an underlying lipoma, are situated on or near the midline in the lumbosacral region. The most common finding is a skin covered fatty mass which is usually indicative of an underlying intradural lipoma (Figs 103.14 and 103.15). A hemangioma in the lumbosacral region is highly suggestive of underlying spina bifida. Another striking feature is a hairy patch (hypertrichosis) also known as the Fawn's Tail. This always occurs in the midline, occurring as a diamond shaped patch. Dimples, sinus tracts, skin tags, or even appendages are associated with lipomyelomeningocele. A current are of controversy is the radiological investigation of the infant with a dimple overlying the coccyx. Such abnor-

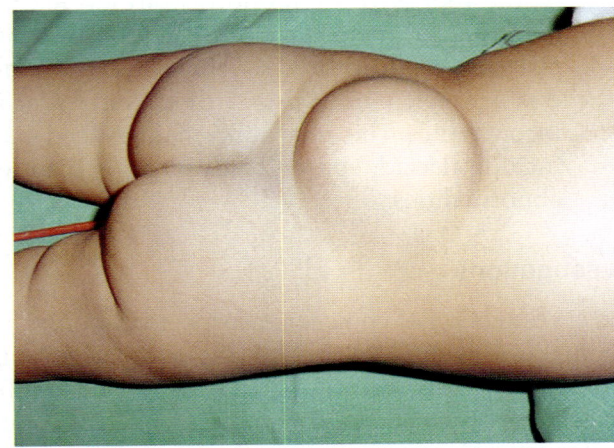

Fig. 103.14: A two years old girl with lipomeningomyelocele associated with low anorectal malformation (Anovestibular long fistula). Colostomy was done at birth followed by mini PSARP later

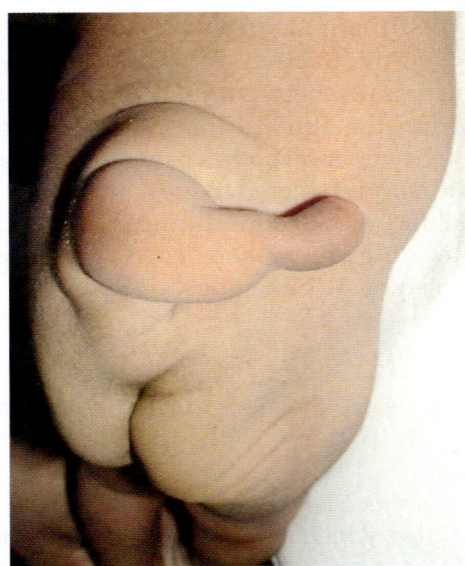

Fig. 103.15: Spina bifida with large bony defect and an attempt on caudal twinning

malities are extremely common and rarely associated with symptoms. Imaging should be done only if the dimple is rostral to the level of the coccyx or if there are associated problems such as orthopedic or the urological abnormalities.

2. *Neurological manifestations:* Motor dysfunction becomes apparent only after the child begins to walk.
3. *Orthopedic manifestations:* Most frequent finding is the unilateral/bilateral cavovarus deformity of the foot with or without limb leg length discrepancy. There may be claw toe, or scoliosis.
4. *Urologic manifestations:* Abnormal voiding pattern with new onset of urinary/fecal incontinence. The other abnormalities seen may include flaccid, spastic or dysynergic bladder abnormalities.

Investigations

The investigation of choice of a suspected lipomyelomeningocele is the MRI in both sagittal and coronal planes. Fatty tumors are readily visualised on T1 images as areas of increased signal intensity. The conus is often low. The primary consideration from the surgical perspective is inferring the presence of tethering from an abnormally low conus and the mechanism of tethering. In typical cases MRI suggests either a dorsal or an caudal insertion of the fatty mass. Additionally presence or absence of Syriax or a terminal hydromyelia is readily apparent.

Surgery

All children with radiographically demonstrated lipomyelomeningocele should be operated upon preferably in the first 6 months of life. The goals are to:
1. Untether the cord from the lipoma, filum terminale, or both
2. Remove the lipoma, or a dermoid cyst causing compression of the spinal cord.
3. Excise the dermal sinus completely.
4. Avoid damage to the nerve roots.
5. Reconstruct the dural canal, to prevent the CSF leakage, often requiring a dural patch graft.
6. Reduce the bulk of the subcutaneous lipoma, excise an area of hypertrichosis, and achieve a tension free anastomosis.
7. Approximate the skin and the subcutaneous surfaces liberally to avoid formation of the dead space allowing postoperative collection.

Complications

Major postoperative complications have been CSF leaks (14%). A persistent subcutaneous collection/frank leak requires re-exploration. A external spinal drainage catheter carefully inserted above the laminectomy defect is useful in protecting the closure following re-exploration. The incidence of a permanent neurological defect after the initial surgery is around 3-6%.

Retethering

Although the neurological and urologic status of a patient with a lipomyelomeningocele should remain stable after a successful surgery, any significant deterioration in a patients status (e.g. new onset incontinence, pain, or progressive weakness), should provoke a search for a cause. Possible ones being hydromyelia, re-tethering, infection, or an unrecognised diastematomyelia superior to the operated lipomyelomeningocele.

Hydromyelia if noted on a preoperative scan should be addressed at the same time of surgery by a terminal ventriculostomy. If a symptomatic hydromyelia recurs, treatment is by a syringopleural/ syringoperitoneal shunt. An association between terminal syringomyelia and tethered cord syndrome has been recognized. However, it has been suggested that tethered cord release alone may be sufficient to improve preoperative symptoms and the terminal syringomyelia may be an associated phenomenon that does not mandate separate treatment.[20]

The incidence of retethering is 10%. It is possible that virtually all patients retethering within a few weeks of surgery, but the dorsal reattachment is at a higher level and thus the symptoms are relieved. The onset of new pain/neurological deficit/urological signs prompt a repeat MRI of lumbosacral spine. Immediate postoperative MR imaging scans in successfully untethered patients continue to show a low lying conus and a dorsally displaced spinal cord and therefore these findings neither confirm/rule out retethering in postoperative period. It has been suggested that ultrasound evaluation through the laminectomy defect is helpful in this situation. The finding of prominent pulsations of the spinal cord is reassuring that retethering has not taken place. Another technique helpful is the prone supine metrizimide CT myelography. It has been a policy to recommend re-exploration in any patient in whom significant radicular pain develops regardless of the radiological studies. The techniques include;

1. Use of dural graft.
2. Use of stay sutures.

Successful reuntethering can be done in 90% of patients.

DERMOIDS AND DERMAL SINUS TRACTS OF THE SPINE

A midline cutaneous pit or dimple above the intergluteal crease is present in all children with a dermal sinus. There may be associated cutaneous manifestations as discussed above. The most common location is the lumbosacral region. Family history is unusual and there is a small male preponderance. Although all midline skin pits above the intergluteal fold must be assumed to communicate intraspinally, those below the top of the intergluteal crease are blind sacrococcygeal dimples. They are seen in nearly 5% of newborns. Dermal sinuses provide a portal for infection. Meningitis or intraspinal abscess occurs in nearly half of all cases. The most common organisms are the *Staph aureus* and *E coli*. Nearly all patients with dermal sinuses have intact neurological function at birth. Rapid neurological deterioration suggests infection within dermoid tumors adjacent to the conus or adherent within the cauda equina. An unusual presentation of dermoid tumors is recurrent episodes of sterile meningitis caused by contact of the spinal fluid with irritative dermoid or epidermoid elements.

Dermal Sinus Tract

These lesions are seen mainly in the lumbosacral region (usually above S2 level) and extend from a caudal skin level to a rostral intra-spinal level (Fig. 103.16A). Besides tethering, a dermal sinus tract is suggestive of intraspinal dermoids and epidermoids. There is also a significant risk of epidural abscess or meningitis. The lesion can be differentiated from benign sacral dimples by their location and by applying caudal traction on the skin below the lesion which causes the skin lesion to elongate.

Radiological Diagnosis

Dimples below top of the intergluteal crease require no investigation other physical examination probe insertion is not justified traction tests of skin movement may suggest the cephalad or caudal path of a sinus tract. The usefulness of plain radiographs may be limited because of immature calcification in children less than 18 months of age (Fig. 103.16B). Ultrasound readily demonstrates the subcutaneous tract, intraspinal inclusion tumors and diminished cord pulsations. Fine section axial CT images with sagittal reconstruction following intrathecal contrast defines bony landmarks and tract attachment to distal neural elements invasive contrast studies have largely been replaced by MRI which visualises in three dimensions the extraspinal tract path, inclusion tumors and other malformations associated with spinal cord tethering.

Surgery

An elliptical skin incision excising the sinus opening, is dissected circumferentially to the fascial defect. Laminectomy is performed over the intact arch and the tract is followed in epidermal space up to the point of entry through dura. The dura is opened

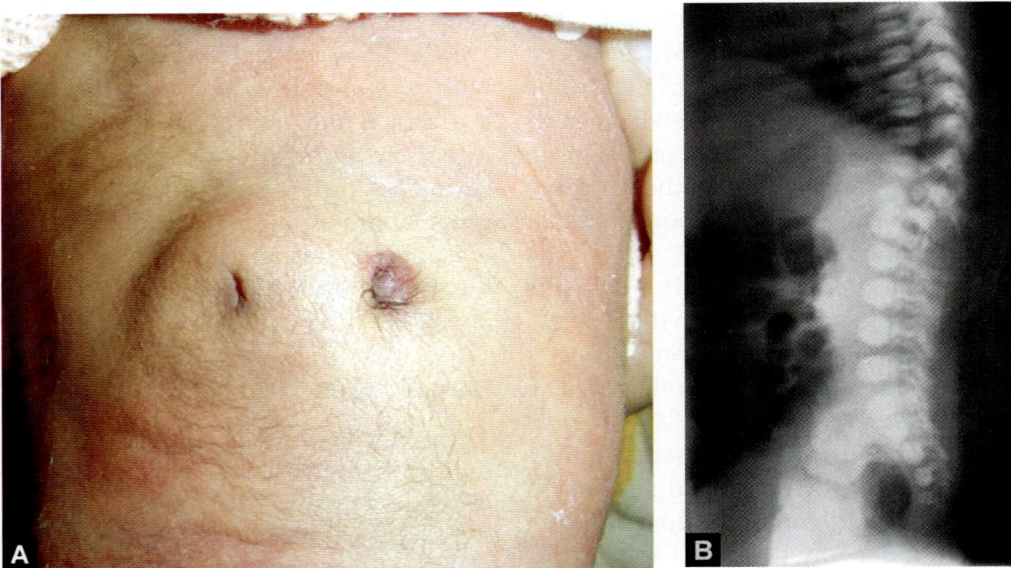

Figs 103.16A and B: **A.** Newborn with antenatally diagnosed spina bifida occulta, with a discharging dermal sinus. **B.** Skiagram of the spine in lateral view

circumferentially around it, the tract is followed further down and divided flush with the neural elements. Any associated dermoid cyst or the tumor is also excised. The filum is divided if thickened. The dura is then repaired watertight.

TIGHT FILUM TERMINALE

The tight filum terminale refers to patients with features of tethered cord syndrome associated with a short and thickened (> 2 mm) filum terminale. The filum often contain fat and fibrous tissue and the conus is below L2 level in 80-90% cases.

REFERENCES

1. Nulsen FE, Spitz EB. Treatment of hydrocephalus by direct shunt from ventricle to jugular vein. Surg Forum 1952; 399-403.
2. Lorber J. Results of treatment of myelomeningocele: An analysis of 524 unselected cases with special references to possible selection of treatment. Dev Med Child Neurol 1971;13:279-303.
3. McLone DG. Treatment of myelomeningocele: Arguments against selection, in Little JR (ed): *Clinical Neurosurgery*. Baltimore, MD, Williams and Wilkins 1986;359-70.
4. Mellick, Sam A. Nicolaes tulp of amsterdam, 1593-1674: anatomist and doctor of medicine. Proceeding of the 2006 cowlishaw symposium anz journal of surgery. 2007;77:1102-09.
5. Williams H. A unifying hypothesis for hydrocephalus, Chiari malformation, syringomyelia, anencephaly and spina bifida. Cerebrospinal Fluid Res 2008;5:7.
6. Besser LM, Williams LJ, Cragan JD. Interpreting changes in the epidemiology of anencephaly and spina bifida following folic acid fortification of the US grain supply in the setting of long-term trends, Atlanta, Georgia, 1968-2003. Birth Defects Res A Clin Mol Teratol 2007;79: 730-36.
7. Tedstone A, Browne M, Harrop L, et al. Fortification of selected foodstuffs with folic acid in the UK. consumer research carried out to inform policy recommendations J Public Health (Oxf) 2008;30:23-29.
8. Lulla C, Hegde A, Shah J, Sheth J. Early antenatal diagnosis of spina bifida presenting with a "step" in the posterior contour of an 8-week embryo. J Clin Ultrasound 2008;36:384-86.
9. de Wit OA, den Dunnen WF, Sollie KM, et al. Pathogenesis of cerebral malformations in human fetuses with meningomyelocele. Cerebrospinal Fluid Res 2008;1;5:4.
10. Fichter MA, Dornseifer U, Henke J, et al. Fetal spina bifida repair—current trends and prospects of intrauterine neurosurgery Fetal Diagn Ther 2008;23:271-86.
11. Eggink AJ, Roelofs LA, Feitz WF, et al. Delayed intrauterine repair of an experimental spina bifida with a collagen biomatrix. Pediatr Neurosurg 2008;44:29-35.
12. Joseph DB. Current approaches to the urologic care of children with spina bifida. Curr Urol Rep 2008;9(2): 151-57.
13. Abrahamsson K, Jodal U, Sixt R, et al. Estimation of Renal Function in Children and Adolescents With Spinal Dysraphism. J Urol 2008;179(6):2407-09.

14. Lendvay TS, Shnorhavorian M, Grady RW. Robotic-assisted laparoscopic mitrofanoff appendicovesicostomy and antegrade continent enema colon tube creation in a pediatric spina bifida patient. J Laparoendosc Adv Surg Tech A 2008;18:310-12.
15. de Jong TP, Chrzan R, Klijn AJ, Dik P. Treatment of the neurogenic bladder in spina bifida. Pediatr Nephrol 2008;23:889-96.
16. Brown TM, Ris MD, Beebe D, et al. Factors of biological risk and reserve associated with executive behaviors in children and adolescents with spina bifida myelomeningocele. Child Neuropsychol 2008;14:118-34.
17. Cardenas DD, Topolski TD, White CJ, et al. Sexual functioning in adolescents and young adults with spina bifida. Arch Phys Med Rehabil 2008;89:31-35.
18. Mukherjee S. Transition to adulthood in spina bifida: changing roles and expectations. ScientificWorldJournal. 2007;7:1890-95.
19. Nejat F, Radmanesh F, Ansari S, et al. Spina bifida occulta: is it a predictor of underlying spinal cord abnormality in patients with lower urinary tract dysfunction? J Neurosurg Pediatrics 2008;1:114-17.
20. Beaumont A, Muszynski CA, Kaufman BA. Clinical significance of terminal syringomyelia in association with pediatric tethered cord syndrome. Pediatr Neurosurg 2007;43:216-21.

SECTION 8

Head and Neck Surgery

Craniosynostosis

M Bajpai

Craniosynostosis is a congenital defect that causes one or more sutures on an infant's skull to close earlier than normal. The premature closing of a suture leads to an abnormally shaped head. During the first year, the brain more than doubles its size and attains 60% of its adult weight. Except for the uniqueness of the cranial vault sutures, the brain growth could be pathologically restricted with irreversible damage caused to it by mounting intracranial pressure. In the past, the sutures were thought to be sites of active growth that push the cranial plates apart, but further investigation has shown their role to be passive. In response to the rapidly enlarging brain, bone is deposited along the edges of the sutures and the epicranium while resorption occurs along the dural surface.

Normally the cranial sutures are patent at birth and progress in early infancy to a yielding fibrous union that allows continuation of appositional bony growth. By 6 years of age, the cranium has attained 90% of its adult size, but complete solid sutural bony union does not occur until at least the 5th decade. Should a suture close prematurely, however, growth is arrested in a direction perpendicular to the fused suture, whereas compensatory expansion occurs in a parallel plane to the affected suture (Virchow's law). The resulting distortion of the skull depends on the suture or sutures that are closed.

The two subdivisions of craniosynostosis have important genetic and long-term growth implications. In general, the malformations of the non-syndromic subset occur sporadically, whereas the syndromic ones have a hereditary component. Furthermore, after surgical correction, normal craniofacial development is the rule for the non-syndromic patients, whereas those with syndromal attributes do not fare so well.

NONSYNDROMIC CRANIOSYNOSTOSIS

The overall incidence of nonsyndromic premature stenosis of cranial sutures has been stated to be 1 in 1000 live births. These figures include all forms of single suture fusion with the sagittal being most commonly affected and unilateral coronal, metopic, and lambdoidal areas following in frequency. Bilateral fusion of the coronal as well as multiple suture involvement also occurs.

Based upon the suture involved, the following deformities present clinically:

Scaphocephaly (Boat shaped)

The sagittal suture is partially or wholly fused; when fusion is complete, there is often external bony overgrowth extending in the midline from lambda to bregma. Sometimes there is overgrowth on the internal surface (Fig. 104.1). X-ray of the skull in an anteroposterior (AP) view shows sagittal suture fusion (Fig. 104.2).

Plagiocephaly (Unilateral coronal suture fusion)

The affected coronal suture shows synostosis in its lateral segment. In young infants, the medial end of the suture is usually patent. In cases older than 6 months the synostosis is usually total and extends up to the anterior fontanelle, which may be small or even absent. There may then be no external trace of the suture, or it may be seen as a shallow groove like a

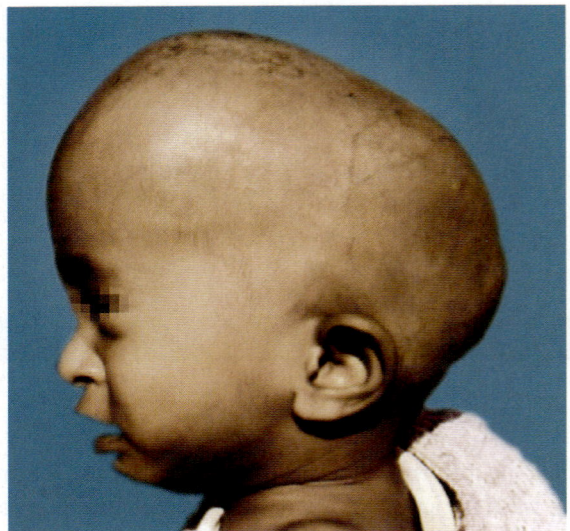

Fig. 104.1: *Scaphocephaly* (Boat shaped) – sagittal suture involvement

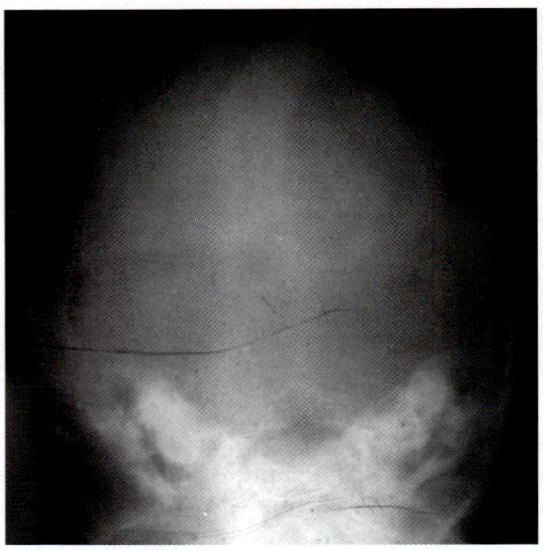

Fig. 104.2: X-ray skull (AP view) – showing sagittal sutural fusion

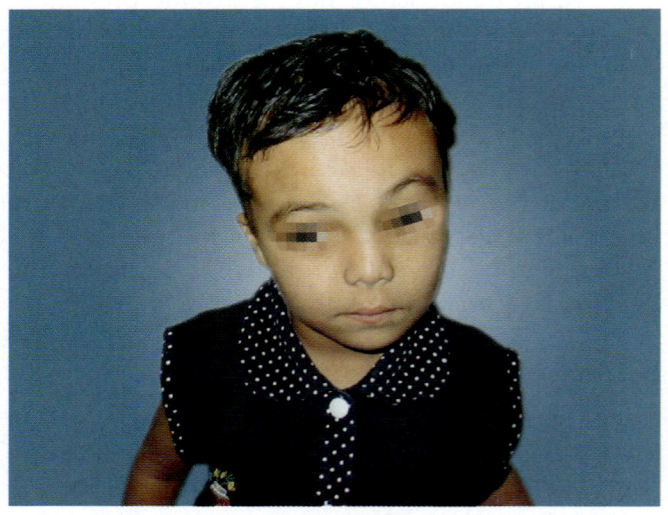

Fig. 104.3: *Plagiocephaly* (Oblique) – unilateral coronal suture involvement

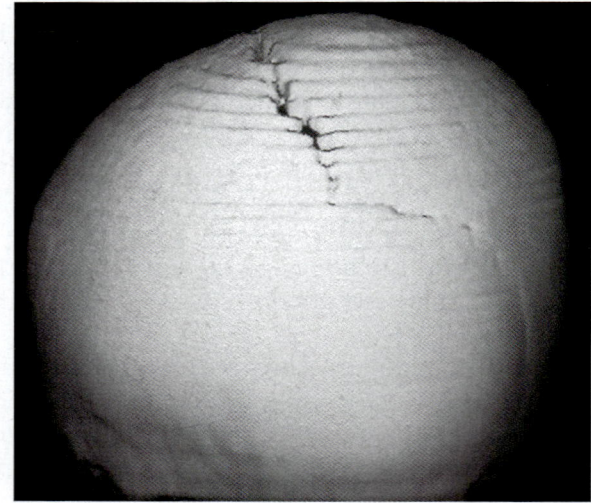

Fig. 104.4: 3-D CAT scan of skull showing right coronal suture fusion

constriction ring in the bone (Fig. 104.3). Sutural fusion can be seen on a plain X-ray or a 3-D CAT scan of the skull (Fig. 104.4).

Brachycephaly
(Short–bilateral coronal suture fusion)

When both coronal sutures are involved the forehead becomes fore-shortened antero-posteriorly (Fig. 104.5).

The diagnosis can be confirmed by X-ray skull (Fig. 104.6) and 3-D CAT scan.

Trigonocephaly
(Triangular-metopic sutural fusion)

Premautre fusion of the metopic suture is usually most evident above the glabella, and may be incomplete or absent in the region of the anterior fontanelle. There

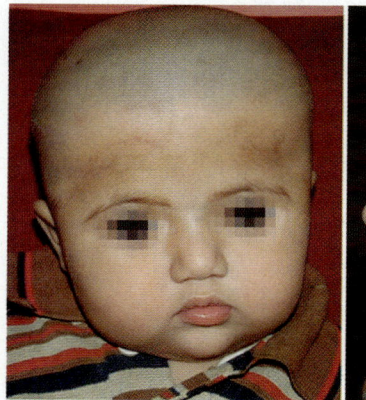 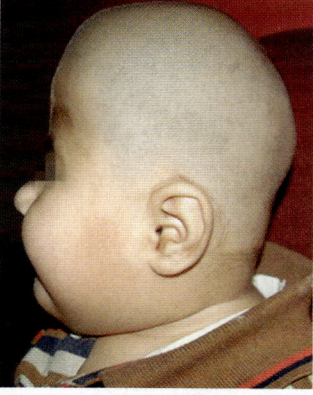

Fig. 104.5: *Brachycephaly* (Short) – bilateral coronal suture involvement

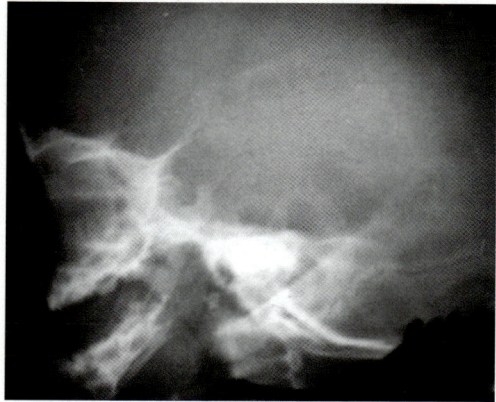

Fig. 104.6: X-ray skull (Lateral view) – showing coronal suture fusion

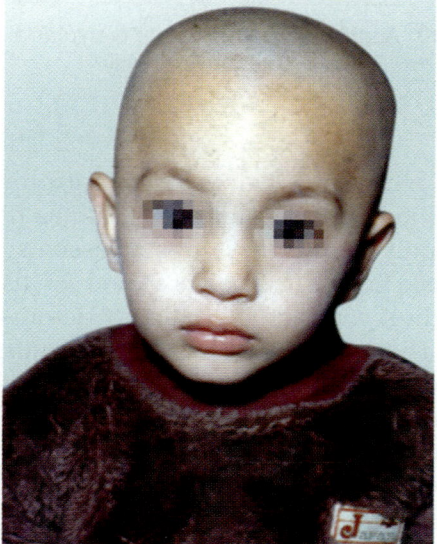

Fig. 104.7: *Trigonocephaly* (Triangular) – metopic suture involvement: note hypotelorism (Closely set orbits)

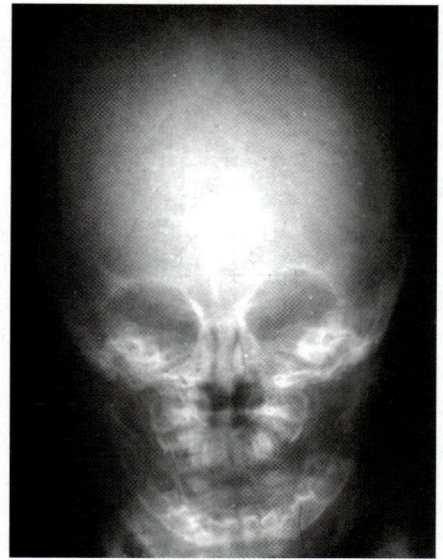

Fig. 104.8: X-ray skull (AP view) – showing metopic suture fusion

is often a marked bony overgrowth on the inner surface of the frontal bone at the lower end of the synostosis (Fig. 104.7). X-ray of the skull (Fig. 104.8) or 3-D CAT scan is unmistakable.

SYNDROMAL CRANIOSYNOSTOSIS

In contrast to nonsyndromic fusions, syndromal craniosynostoses behave differently and have genetic implications and pattern of inheritance have been established for these malformations. Crouzon's syndrome is the most commonly seen syndromal craniosynostosis anomaly, and its incidence has been estimated as being as high as 1 in 10,000 births. The inheritance pattern is autosomal dominant with almost complete penetrance.[1]

Crouzon's Syndrome

Mid-face hypoplasia, parrot beak nose, lateral canthal dystopia, hypertelorism (Broad set orbits) and relative mandibular prognathism characterize the defect (Fig. 104.9). High arched palate is also an associated finding. The typical skull deformity is brachycephalic, though other head shapes are seen. Exorbitism is a cardinal sign. It is often very marked, and may endanger sight.

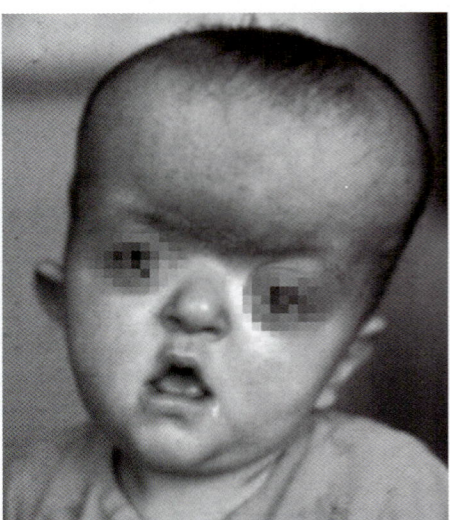

Fig. 104.9: Crouzon's syndrome – Note mid-face hypoplasia, parrot beak nose, Lateral canthal dystopia and hypertelorism (Broad set orbits). High arched palate is also an associated finding

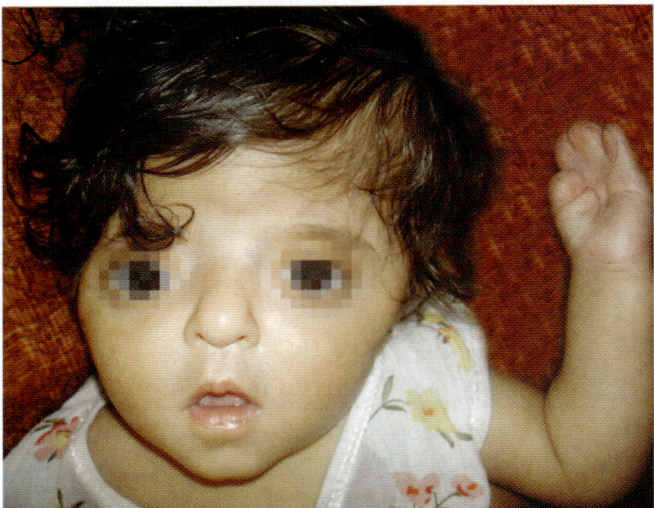

Fig. 104.10: Apert's syndrome – Note craniofacial deformity along with polysyndactyly

Apert's Syndrome

Also termed as acrocephalosyndactyly, the incidence of this anomaly has been estimated to be 1 in 1,60,000 live births. Exorbitism, midfacial retrusion with maxillary constriction, and pseudomandibular prognathism, as in Crouzon's syndrome, are present. The exorbitism is more moderate and asymmetric. The face also is transversely flattened. The distance between the orbits is greater. The cranial deformity is almost always associated with premature fusion of the coronal sutures, though the skull base is also involved. The Apert's syndrome is distinguished from other acrocephalosyndactylies by the severity of the syndactyly, which involves bony fusion of the phalanges of at least the index, middle, and ring fingers (Fig. 104.10). The inheritance mode is autosomal dominant, although occurrence tends to be sporadic. As with Crouzon's syndrome, a genetic defect has been identified.[2]

Others

More than 50 syndromes associated with craniosynostosis have been described in addition to the most common Crouzon's and Apert's syndromes. Because they are few in number, their frequency is not well established. Pfeiffer's, Carpenter's and Saethre-Chotzen syndromes belong to this group and are distinguished by broad toes and thumbs (Pfeiffer's), Preaxial polysyndactyly with soft tissue syndactyly of shortened fingers (Carpenter's), and soft tissue webs between the second and third digits (Saethre-Chotzen) are seen. These malformations are also transmitted in an autosomal dominant manner except Carpenter's syndrome, which is autosomal recessive. The rare Kleeblattsschadel (cloverleaf skull) anomaly is not easily forgotten. The skull cap assumes a trilobular configuration with a protruding vertex and bulging temporal regions (see Fig. 104.12).

MULTIPLE SUTURE INVOLVEMENT

Oxycephaly or Turricephaly (Figs 104.11 and 104.12)

Oxycephaly– has been defined as a deformity in which the head is abnormally high and conical. The vertex appears pointed whether viewed from the side or from the front in a case of typical oxycephaly. Depending on the part of the cerebral capsule first involved, the deformity process can also involve the coronal suture.

Cloverleaf Skull

This deformity (triphyllocephaly) appears to be a nonspecific consequence of multiple sutural fusion: a

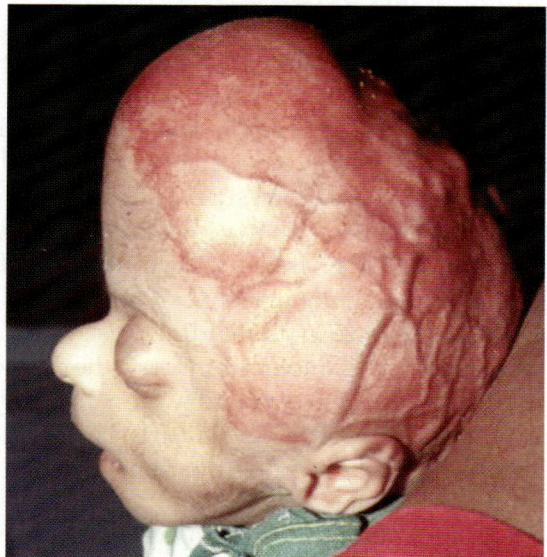

Fig. 104.11: Acrocephaly/ turricephaly or oxycephaly – multiple suture involvement

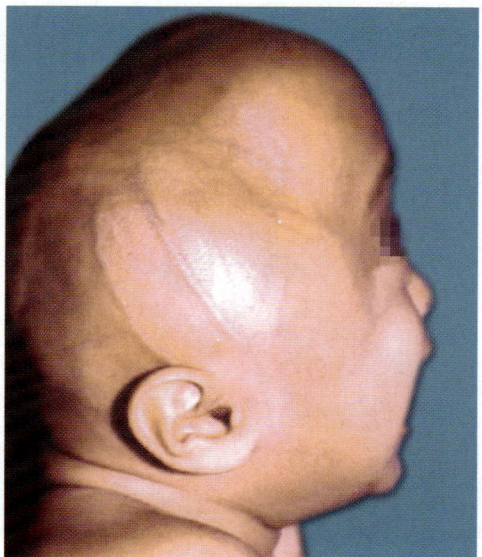

Fig. 104.12: Clover leaf skull – multiple suture involvement

constriction ring develops in the lambdoid-squamosal zone and allows disproportionate bulging in the frontal and temporal bones. Seen from in front, the head looks trilobular (Fig. 104.12). There is almost always associated hydrocephalus. Less severe forms of this condition may exhibit a pointed oxycephalic appearance.

DIAGNOSIS

Diagnosis of craniosynostosis can be established in most instances on clinical examination alone because of the characteristic deformation of the skull cap and evidence on palpation of a ridge formed by the fused suture. Plain X-rays of the skull in different views should be taken to help confirm the clinical impression. A radiographic linear opacity replaces the wormian lucency of a patent suture. For unilateral coronal synostosis, a classic 'Harlequin' eye sign formed by the elevated ipsilateral lesser wing of the sphenoid can be seen on a postero-anterior skull film. Computed tomography (CT) scans are usually not diagnostically helpful unless reformatted in three-dimensionally (Figs 104.13 and 104.14). Detailed psychological assessment, ophthalmic evaluation for evidence of raised ICT and dental examination should be carried out.

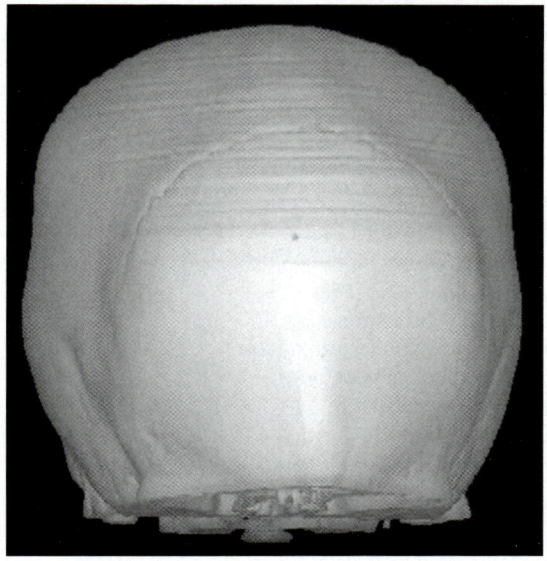

Fig. 104.13: 3-D CAT scan of skull in trigonocephaly

DIFFERENTIAL DIAGNOSIS (TABLE 104.1)

Muscular torticollis, cervical spinal abnormalities and favored sleeping positions can produce positional distortions. The sutures are patent in these conditions. Treatment should be focused primarily on the cause of positional deformities.

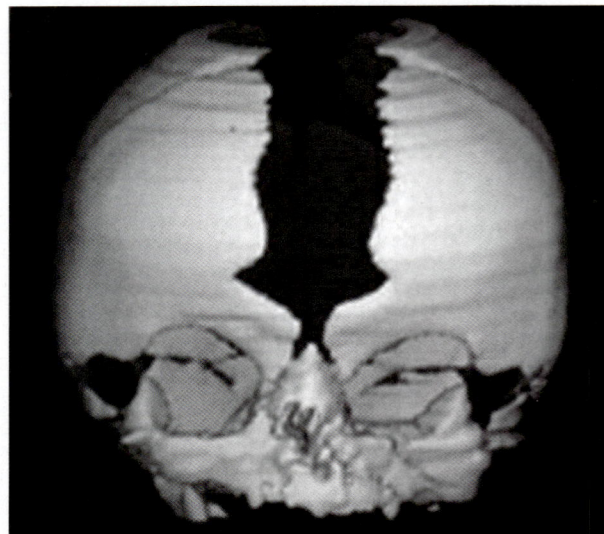

Fig. 104.14: 3-D CAT scan of skull in brachycephaly

Table 104.1: Differential diagnosis of craniosynostosis

- Primary microcephaly
- Hydrocephalus–sutural fusion secondary to decompression and overlapping of bones
- Postural plagiocephaly

Table 104.2: Investigations

- Skull radiograph–Antero-posterior, lateral, Towne's and basal views
- CAT scan– 3 dimensional
- Ophthalmological examination
- Psychological assessment
- Genetic evaluation
- Dental evaluation
- Clinical photograph

Positional posterior plagiocephaly, when viewed from the vertex, has an oblique orientation of the skull cap, and the ear on the affected side is pushed anteriorly and away from the flattened posterior side. In contrast, true unilateral lambdoidal synostosis produces a trapezoid deformity with the ipsilateral ear being drawn toward the defective suture. It is critically important to distinguish positional deformations from those caused by true craniosynostosis.

Investigative workup for these patients has been summarized in Table 104.2.

SURGICAL MANAGEMENT

Non-syndromic craniosynostosis should be corrected because of the severe distortion reflected onto the face. Other reasons address possible functional problems that the condition might cause, all of which are related to increased intracranial pressure. Thirteen percent of infants with single suture synostosis have elevated pressures and 42% of those with multiple sutural involvement. Visual impairment can occur but is rare when only one suture is prematurely fused.

Before the era of craniofacial surgery, the classically accepted method of treatment was a linear strip craniectomy of the pathologic suture. The incidence of refusion and continued deformation, however, was disappointingly high.[3]

To take advantage of the rapidly expanding infant brain, early intervention is advised. Most centers favor the period of 3 to 6 months of age; others wait until after the sixth postnatal month. Early correction produces superior results than late intervention, in the long-term.

Because of disappointment with the strip craniectomy techniques, the principles of treatment have constantly evolved. Regardless of the type of craniosynostosis, emphasis has been directed toward releasing the affected suture and immediately restoring normal architecture by repositioning and recontouring the deformed bones.[4,5]

Initial enthusiasm to the benefits offered by rigid fixation provided by using biocompatible plates and screws, has not sustained. Subsequently, their use on a growing skull cap found the devices being translocated from the epicranium onto the dura.

Partial Calvariectomy and Onlay Periosteoplasty

Partial calvariectomy and harvesting the periosteum is an alternative technique. In this procedure, not only the involved sutures are removed but the adjacent deformed bones are also excised after separating and preserving the periosteum. Towards the end of the procedure this harvested periosteum is laid down as an onlay over the exposed dura (Figs 104.15 and 104.16). Subsequently, neocalvarium is formed by the periosteum according to the contour of growing brain. (Figs 104.17 to 104.20).

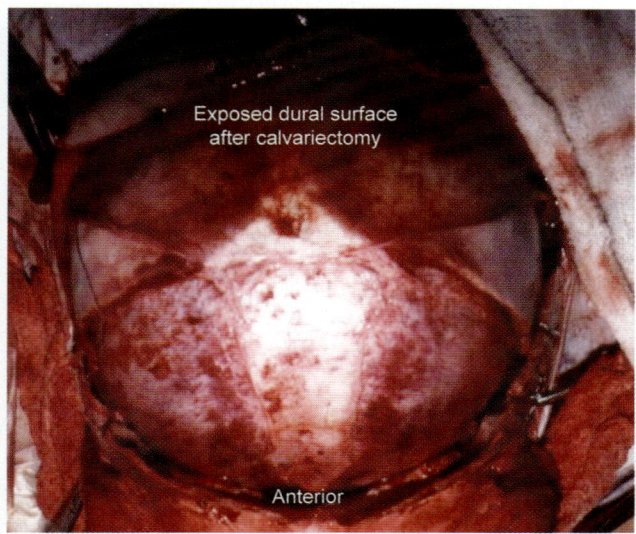

Fig. 104.15: Intraoperative photograph-exposed dura after partial calvariectomy

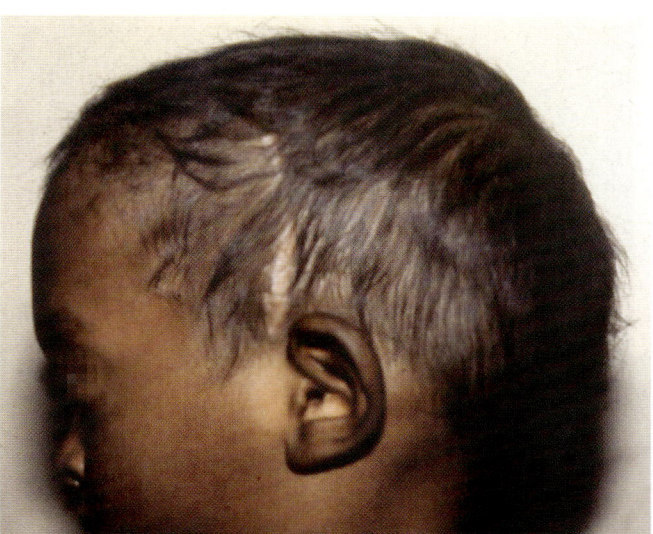

Fig. 104.17: Same child as in Fig. 104.1– one year after surgery

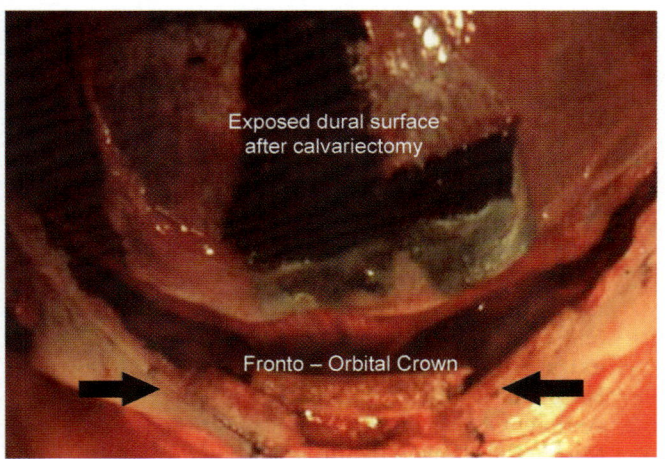

Fig. 104.16: Intraoperative photograph– placement of fronto-orbital 'crown'

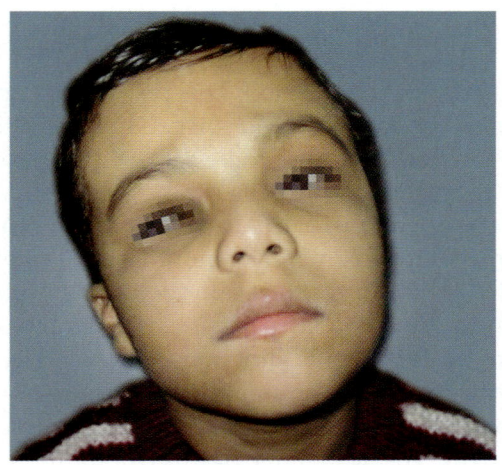

Fig. 104.18: Same child as in Fig. 103.3– eight months after surgery

The surgical management of all the syndromic craniosynostosis malformations generally falls into three chronologic stages. In contrast to the non-syndromic variety, in this group normalization of facial growth is not realized after surgical intervention. Treatment is directed at the immediate problem. Thus, a phased approach is used. Elements that must be addressed are release of elevated intracranial pressure caused by the premature suture closure, compromise of the airway by severe midfacial retrusion, and protection of the corneas because of the exorbitism. During the first year of life, the synostotic suture is released as well as a fronto-orbital advancement (Figs 104.15 and 104.16). This frees the rapidly expanding brain, more normal calvarial contours are achieved, and the corneas are offered more protection.

Treatment plans and timing may vary according to experience and preference. A second operation is performed around the sixth year of life when the orbits and skull cap have attained 90% of their adult size. If the forehead is of normal shape, the classic LeFort III midfacial advancement is used to bring the entire midface forward. The maxilla is deliberately placed in an overcorrected anterior position as future

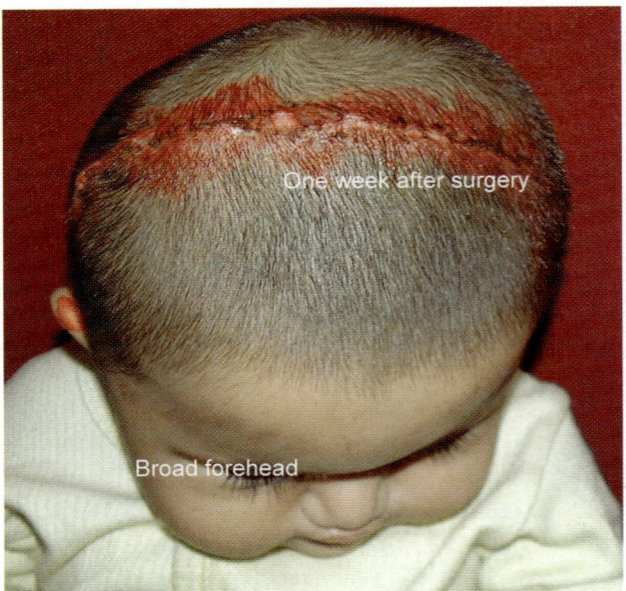

Fig. 104.19: Same child as in Fig. 103.5– one week after surgery

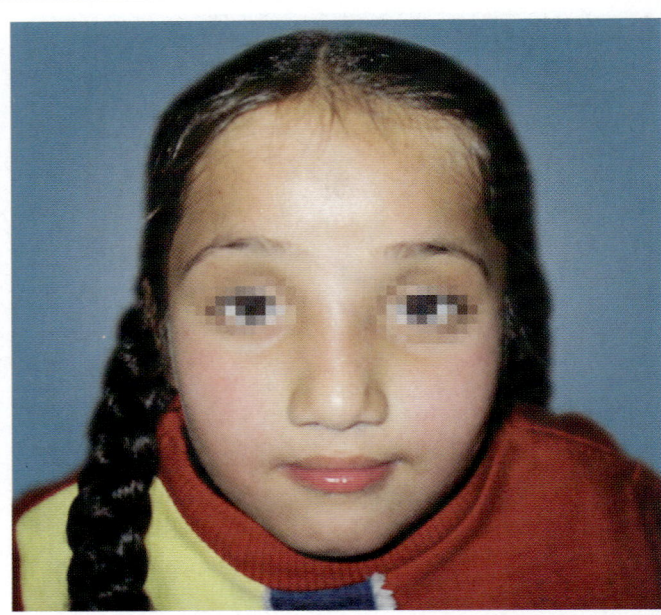

Fig. 104.20: Same child as in Fig. 103.5– six years after surgery

midfacial growth is be limited. This positioning opens the crowded nasopharynx and corrects the exorbitism.

If the forehead is found to be recessed, as is often the case, two alternative paths can be followed. As a preliminary operation, a fronto-orbital advancement is performed. Approximately 6 months later, a LeFort III is added. This approach is safer because sterility is maintained by separating a clean intracranial procedure from the contamination introduced by the subsequent extracranial midfacial advancement.

The other approach is the monobloc frontofacial advancement. The advantage of this technique is that only one operation is required to reposition the forehead.

When orbital hypertelorism is present, a facial bipartition procedure can be added to either the LeFort III or frontofacial monobloc advancement. This procedures is particularly indicated in correcting the flattened forehead and midface that is typical of patients with Apert's syndrome.

The final stage must await the completion of facial growth. After presurgical orthodontic alignment of the teeth, the pseudomandibular prognathism is corrected with a LeFort I (maxillary) advancement. A simultaneous advancement osseous genioplasty is frequently required to correct the retruded chin.

REFERENCES

1. Carinci F, Pezzetti F, Locci P, Becchetti E, Carls F, Avantaggiato A, Becchetti A, Carinci P, Baroni T, Bodo M Apert and Crouzon syndromes: clinical findings, genes and extracellular matrix. J Craniofac Surg 2005;16(3): 361-68. Review.
2. Andrew OM Wilkie, Sarah F Slaney, Michael Oldridge, Michael D Poole, Geraldine J Ashworth, Anthony D Hockley, Richard D, Hayward, David J David, Louise J Pulleyn, Paul Rutland, Susan Malcolm, Robin M Winter and William Reardon. Apert syndrome results from localized mutations of FGFR2 and is allelic with Crouzon syndrome. Nature Genetics 1995;9:165-72.
3. Shillito J Jr, Matson DD. Craniosynostosis: a review of 519 surgical patients.Pediatrics 1968;41(4):829-53.
4. Mohr G, Hoffman HJ, Munro IR, Hendrick EB, Humphreys RP. Surgical management of unilateral and bilateral coronal craniosynostosis: 21 years of experience. Neurosurgery 1978;2(2):83-92.
5. Marchac D, Renier D. Faciocraniosynostosis: from infancy to adulthood. Childs Nerv Syst. 1996;12(11):669-77.

Cleft Lip and Palate

Peter AM Raine

Facial clefts have been recognized and recorded in medical writings from the earliest times.[1] Their occurrence has been attributed to many weird and wonderful causes, but stigmatization and victimization of sufferers was common place until relatively recently. The first attempt at repair by surgery was noted in a Chinese text from 390 BC.[2] Concepts of the lip cleft as simply a split or dehiscence led to early attempts at direct edge to edge closure by cautery, pinning and stitching.

The gradual elucidation of cleft anatomy, and recognition of the importance of failed fusion processes, allowed a more refined definition of the requirements for corrective surgery.[3] The advent of anesthesia made possible more comprehensive efforts at the re-alignment of distorted and displaced cleft structures and brought about the introduction of many novel and clever developments and variations on the theme of tissue mobilization and flap design by eminent surgeons of the day.[4-7] Follow-up of patients from infancy to adulthood emphasized the important role of growth in outcome of cleft repair and identified those repairs which facilitated normal growth and those which impaired it. Some initially promising designs were therefore discarded so that current surgical approaches both observe closely the anatomical defect and also respect the potential for interference with growth potential.

EMBRYOLOGY

The development of facial anatomy takes place from about the 5th week of gestation as frontonasal and maxillary processes become apparent. Growth downwards of the median and two lateral processes of the frontonasal process defines the central lip and palate and the future nares—the prolabium and premaxilla. Growth forwards and inwards of the lateral maxillary process defines the maxilla. Fusion of these processes (Fig. 105.1) and in growth of mesoderm unite the upper jaw by about the 8th week of fetal life forming the primary palate.[8] Failure of this fusion process leads to the common form of clefting (i.e. in the line of the philtral ridge and between lateral incisor and canine teeth) and failure of ingrowth of mesoderm into the central part of the frontonasal process leads to the rare form of midline cleft. The range of highly unusual facial clefts categorized by Tessier (1976) are explained by variations and aberrations of this relatively simple fusion model.[9]

From 8 weeks onwards, the formation of the secondary palate continues by growth of palatine

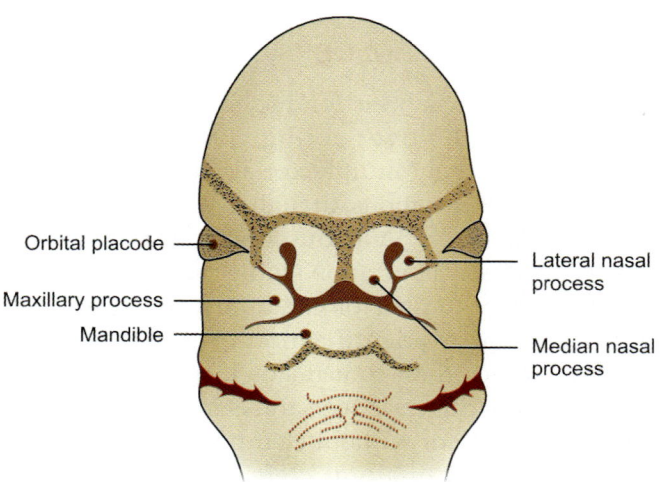

Fig. 105.1: Fusion of embryological facial processes at about week 8

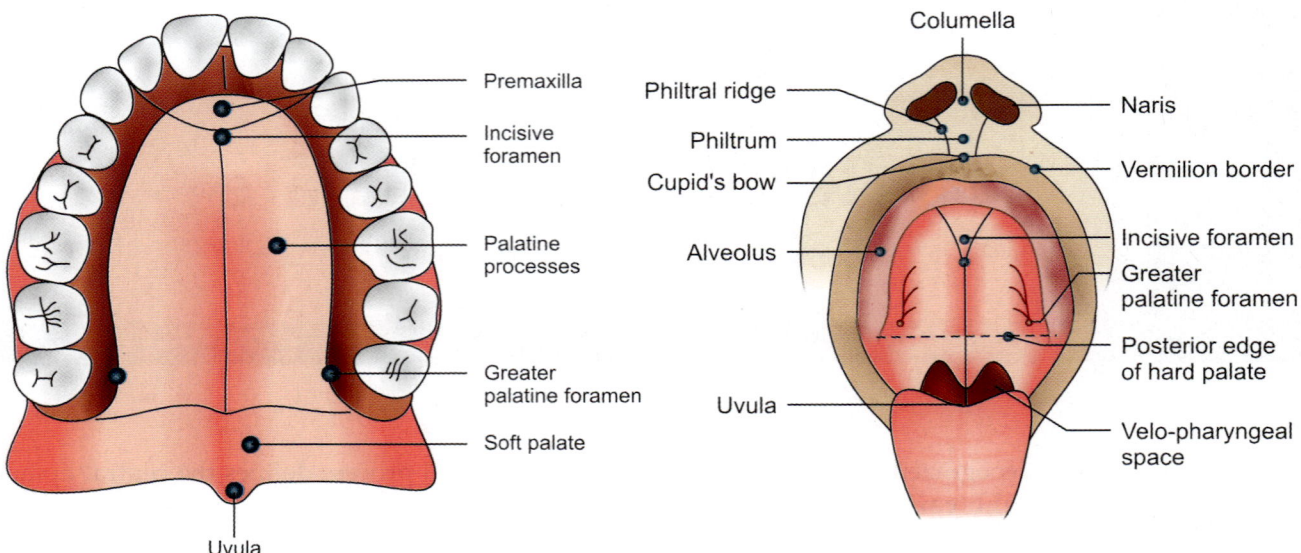

Figs 105.2 and 105.3: Anatomical landmarks of midface and palate

processes inwards from each maxillary process. These plates or shelves move from a more vertical to a transverse orientation where they come into contact, adhere and fuse from anterior (incisive foramen) to posterior to form the hard and soft palates. In front of the incisive foramen, fusion between palatine processes and premaxilla forms part of the primary palate behind the alveolus. The fusion processes are complete by 12 weeks of intrauterine life (Figs 105.2 and 105.3).

GENETICS AND ETIOLOGY

Much research has been conducted into the etiology of clefts and the over-riding conclusion is that causation is largely multifactorial and due to gene-environment interactions, though monogenic patterns are recognized.[10,11] Various investigations using linkage analysis, association studies and gene probes into the large number of candidate genes and loci generally lead to identification of genetic predisposition rather than to a major locus.[12] A familial pattern of inheritance is seen and is more pronounced for cleft lip with or without cleft palate than for cleft palate alone. In bilateral cleft lip and palate, an incidence of up to 18.5% is found in first degree relatives.[13] The risk of recurrence for further siblings following presentation of an index case is approximately 4%, rising to 10% if two siblings are affected and up to 15% if both sibling and parent are affected. There is no sex-linked genetic influence. Though most genetic patterns are autosomal recessive, occasional autosomal dominant inheritance emerges as in the van der Woude (1954) syndrome consisting of lower lip pits in association with cleft lip (Fig. 105.4).[14] A relatively recent and common association of cleft with 22q11 chromosome deletion is described as part of the Di George spectrum and presents as the velo-cardio-facial syndrome.[15] The syndrome has a wide phenotypic spectrum (Fig. 105.5)

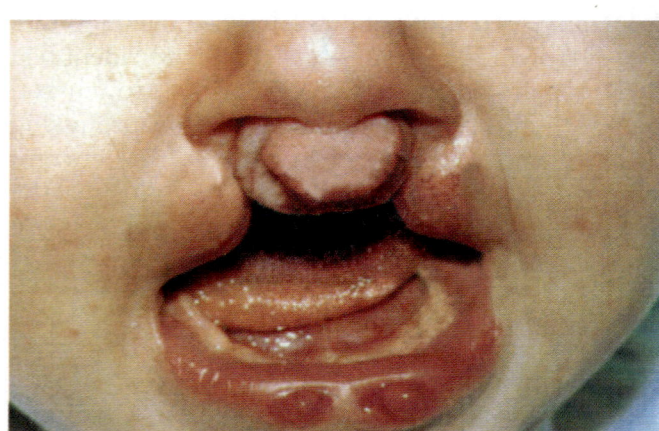

Fig. 105.4: Lower lip pits with bilateral cleft lip and palate (van der Woude's syndrome)

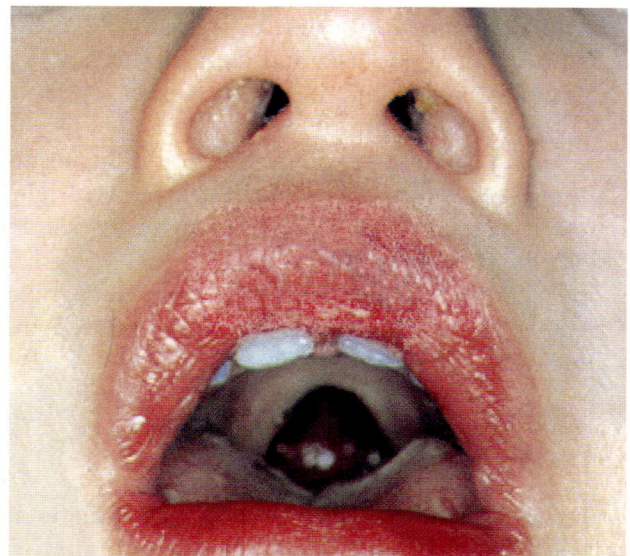

Fig. 105.5: Secondary palate cleft. Broad nasal tip and flat upper lip in velocardiofacial syndrome

that has been described in detail but early diagnosis of the syndrome can be reached by fluorescence *in situ* hybridization (FISH) test.[16,17] An association has been described between CL (P) and the transforming growth factor alpha locus, which may offer further clues to etiology.[18]

The geneticist requires taking a full and detailed family history in order to assess risks accurately and to establish the counseling process.[19] Throughout the patient's care pathway, teamwork is essential and all members need an appreciation of the origins and etiology of clefts.[20] The pediatric nurse, who plays a major role in the care of child and family and in education of parents, must base advice on a sound understanding of underlying genetic and etiological factors.[21] The high incidence of associated anomalies has major implication for genetic counseling.[22]

Environmental and exogenous factors are also implicated in cleft pathogenesis although interactions and multifactorial effects make unequivocal identification difficult. Inferences drawn from clinical studies and observations and from experimental animal work point to some of the following as teratogenic agents:

- Drugs such as thalidomide, phenytoin, aminopterin, paracetamol, retinoids and folate antagonists;[10]
- Dietary factors such as vitamin deficiency;
- Alcohol intake during pregnancy which may not necessarily be dose related[23]
- In utero infection
- Excess fetal flexion in utero associated with oligohydramnios
- Irradiation in utero

The common link between genetic and environmental influences on cleft formation and a key to the pathogenesis of clefting is thought to lie in the process of epithelial breakdown and fusion which depends on changes in enzymes in the extracellular matrix.[24]

EPIDEMIOLOGY AND INCIDENCE

Studies on epidemiology of cleft lip and palate have continuing importance partly because of the lack of full understanding of the etiology. The very detailed studies from Denmark starting with the work of Paul Fogh-Andersen which included twin studies, have been fundamental to this.[25,26] Various registers such as EUROCAT (European Register of Congenital Anomalies and Twins) collect and assess information about prevalence, incidence and associations of clefts and gradually increase the knowledge base.

The incidence of cleft lip and palate ranges from 1:1000 to about 2.2:1000.[13,27-29] Scandinavian data are possibly most reliable and give an incidence of about 1.7:1000. There is usually a greater incidence of cleft lip and/or cleft palate (CL/P) than cleft palate alone (isolated cleft palate, CP).

CP is commoner in girls and CL (P) is commoner in boys: there is a slight male preponderance (60%) for all clefts.[30] The left side is affected significantly more commonly than the right and there are geographical and racial variations with a lower incidence in black than white races. More clefts are reported in still than in live births.[28,31] CP is associated with socioeconomic deprivation and an important increased risk (1.5) is noted with maternal cigarette smoking during pregnancy.[25,32] Annual frequency variations may suggest environmental influences.

ASSOCIATED ANOMALIES

The incidence of associated anomalies with facial clefts is as high as 50%[22] and well over 300 syndromes in which orofacial clefting is a part have been defined.[33] It is essential that each newborn is examined carefully and extensively particular for skeletal, central nervous system and cardiac defects.[22] Low birth weight, preterm newborns and newborns with bilateral clefts have a higher risk of associated anomalies and should be especially carefully screened.[34] Both minor (e.g. external ear deformity) and major, life-threatening (cardiac, esophageal atresia) anomalies demand recognition before prognosis and treatment planning.

The associated anomalies and syndromes include:
- Chromosomal anomalies: Trisomy 13, 18 and 21
- Pierre Robin syndrome (or sequence) in which the cleft palate is associated with a small mandible (micrognathia) (Fig. 105.6). This leads to respiratory and feeding problems.[35,36]
- Treacher Collins syndrome (facial dysostosis) shows a typical facial appearance of down-slanting palpebral fissures, coloboma and ectropion of the lower eyelids due to maxillary hypoplasia associated with cleft palate and mandibular hypoplasia. Inner ear anomalies lead to deafness.
- Stickler syndrome has a phenotype of flat nasal bridge and midface in association with cleft palate and myopia, which carries a risk of retinal detachment and consequent blindness. The syndrome is autosomal dominant.
- Goldenhar syndrome is better known as the oculo-auriculo-vertebral syndrome and is a spectrum of malformations including cervical spinal fusion, external ear anomalies, epibulbar dermoid, mandibular hypoplasia and cleft (Fig. 105.7). The hemifacial syndrome, in which facial asymmetry is pronounced, is variant of this.
- Van der Woude syndrome is important in alerting to an autosomal dominant pattern of cleft inheritance. Lower lip pits present in association with the cleft;
- The velo-cardio-facial syndrome is now recognized as part of the Di George syndrome related to a 22q11 chromosomal deletion.[15,16]

TERMINOLOGY, CLASSIFICATION AND RECORDING

The terms used in description of orofacial clefts are various and, although some are self-explanatory, others are less clearly defined.[37] They include:
- Primary and secondary palate
- Pre-alveolar, alveolar and post-alveolar
- Complete and incomplete
- Unilateral and bilateral
- Hard palate, soft palate and submucous clefts.

Some terms, such as "isolated cleft palate", are confusing: either a cleft of the palate only, as opposed to lip and palate, or a cleft of the palate without any other anomaly could be implied.[38] The terms "syndromic" and "non-syndromic" better describe cleft palate with or without other anomalies.

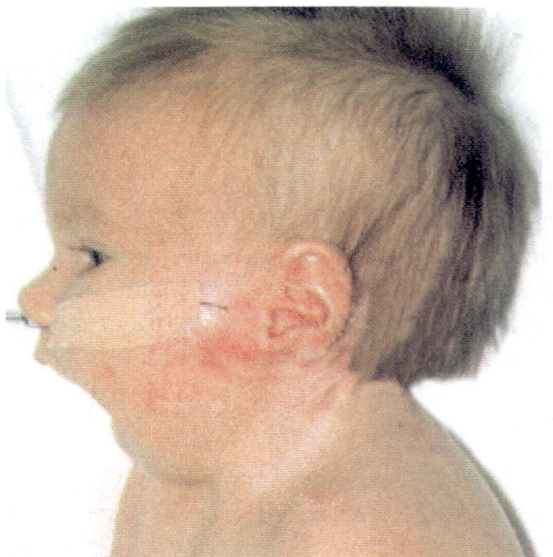

Fig. 105.6: Severe micrognathia and cleft palate in Pierre Robin sequence

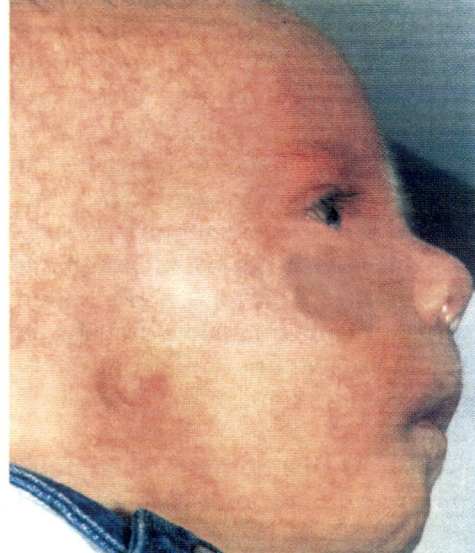

Fig. 105.7: Absent external ear, micrognathia and cleft in Goldenhar syndrome

Four groups of cleft type were defined by Veau (1928) in his classification:[39]
- Cleft of soft palate only
- Cleft of hard and soft palate to incisive foramen (the secondary palate)
- Complete cleft of soft palate. Hard palate, alveolus and lip on one side
- Complete cleft on both sides.

However, this does not include clefts of the lip and alveolus only (the primary palate).

Kernahan and Stark (1958) developed a more detailed, descriptive classification based on the use of the embryological concepts of primary and secondary palate:[40]

- Clefts of the primary palate only;
  - Unilateral, complete/incomplete
  - Median, complete/incomplete
  - Bilateral, complete/incomplete
- Clefts of the secondary palate only;
  - Complete/incomplete/submucous
- Clefts of both primary and secondary palate;
  - Unilateral, complete/incomplete
  - Median, complete/incomplete
  - Bilateral, complete/incomplete

A diagrammatical form of cleft recording (Fig. 105.8) was introduced by Kernahan and developed by Millard (1976) to allow greater definition of detail and has been further enhanced and modified to allow recording of minor morphological differences and variations of the lip deformity.[41,42] This has the additional advantage of suitability for computer storage and potential for subsequent analysis.[43]

Photography affords an objective method of recording the cleft appearance and is used from birth and throughout the child's clinical course. Reproduction of a standard image presents difficulties and relies as much on the experience and expertise of the photographer as it depends on technical aspects such as use of a grid.[44] Capture of a satisfactory image may be achieved best when the child is anaesthetized for surgery.[45] Recently, work has been done on 3D photographic recording linked to computerized data storage, which holds out the promise of accurate analysis of facial growth in clefts and the effects of surgery on growth.

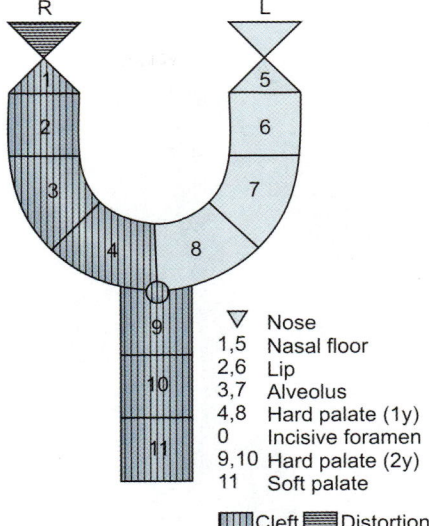

Fig. 105.8: "Striped Y" diagram for recording of cleft anatomy

ANATOMICAL AND CLINICAL FEATURES OF CLEFTS

Lip and Alveolar Cleft

In the lip the cleft line follows the philtral ridge on the lateral margin of the philtrum (Fig. 105.9) from the middle of the nostril sill to the peak of the cupid's bow of the vermilion border. The abnormal muscle insertions of the broken ring of the circumoral muscles causes marked displacement and distortion of the anatomical features but, although some degree of hypoplasia of tissues occurs, there is no significant loss or absence of tissues (Fig. 105.10). Some of the factors leading to aberration of both soft tissues and bone/cartilage structures are therefore:
- Inherent abnormality of growth centers in the orofacial complex;
- Asymmetry and imbalance of muscle forces in the cleft area;
- Absence of the restraining forces of normal lip structures;
- Misplaced pressure of the tongue in the cleft area.

In the dynamic situation of facial movements of smiling, blowing or whistling, the insertion of interrupted circumoral muscle sphincter into the cleft margins at the base of the ala and the columella leads to a prominent bulge or bunching of muscle fibers. The cleft edges show progressive thinning of the

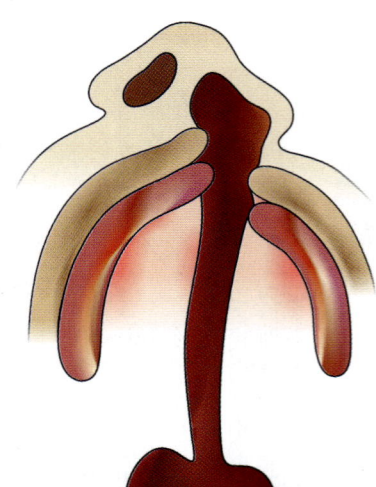

Fig. 105.9: Left complete cleft lip and palate

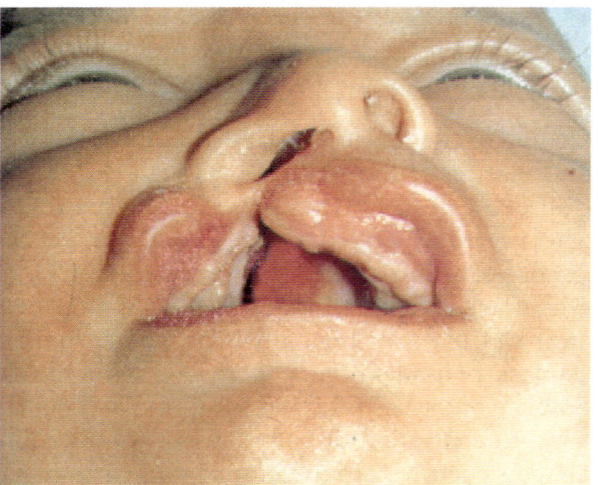

Fig. 105.10: Right cleft lip and palate

The normal regular arch of the maxilla is replaced in the cleft case by greater and lesser maxillary segments, which are misaligned. The line of the cleft at the alveolar margin is between the lateral incisor and canine teeth. The greater maxillary segment is more prominent and the premaxilla is rotated into an anterior position with the midline displace towards the non-cleft side. The lesser segment tends to collapse into the cleft. The absence of symmetrical soft tissue and muscular restraining forces fails to mold a normal arch. In addition to asymmetry, there is relative hypoplasia of the lesser segment with decreased height or vertical shortening of the maxilla.

Bilateral cleft lip may present a symmetrical appearance but also may display disproportion of the two sides and a displaced midline (Fig. 105.11). The premaxilla and prolabium can rotate around a vertical axis and also tilt markedly upwards with the effect of foreshortening the columella. While growth of the premaxilla may be excessive, the prolabium may be relatively deficient and is devoid of muscle tissue. There is no buccal sulcus between premaxilla and prolabium. In complete bilateral clefts the nasal tip may be central and the alae and nostrils symmetrical and equal although wide and flattened. However, when there is a difference in degree of cleft between the sides - one complete and one incomplete - marked asymmetry and deviation of structures from the midline arises. The presence of even a minimal skin bridge - Simonartz bar - limits extent of deviation and asymmetry (Fig. 105.12).

vermilion border of the lip as they run towards the deficient and cleft nasal sill. The columella is misaligned due to the offset position of the nasal spine and comes to lie in a plane canted away from the vertical toward the horizontal. In turn the nasal septum is deviated from the midline and the lower lateral alar cartilage of the cleft side is splayed out and looses its "C" shape. The medial and lateral crurae of the cartilage are attached on either side of the cleft respectively to the base of the septum and the alar base in the region of the nasal vestibule.

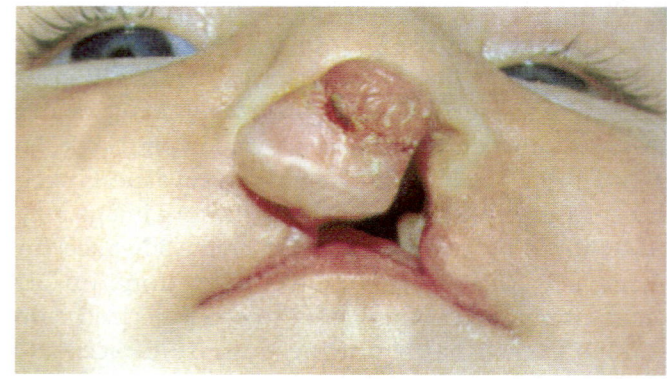

Fig. 105.11: Bilateral cleft lip and palate with marked displacement and rotation of premaxilla

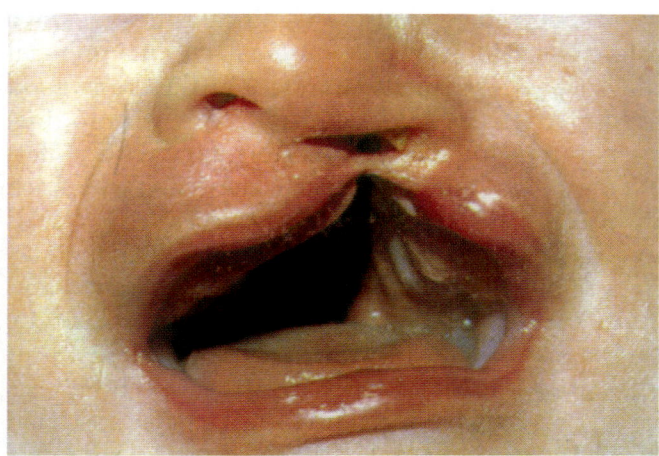

Fig. 105.12: Left cleft lip and palate with Simonartz bar

Palate Cleft

The line of a unilateral cleft of lip and palate is through the alveolus and primary palate to the position of the incisive foramen and then in the midline of the bony hard palate and soft palate ending with a bifid uvula. The cleft extends into the nasal cavity on the cleft side of the nasal septum but on the non-cleft side there is fusion of the palatine process of the maxilla to the nasal septum. The palatine process on the cleft side is usually deficient and is displaced cephalad into the nasal cavity. The lower and middle turbinate bones intrude into the cleft and may be more prominent because of marked mucosal edema and hypertrophy. The principle blood supply to the palate tissues is the greater palatine artery, which emerges through the palatine foramen in the bone just medial to the position of the posterior molar teeth. At the posterior edge of the hard palate the muscles of the soft palate, levator palati and tensor palati — are inserted into the bone instead of uniting and fusing in the midline raphe. This abnormal muscle orientation is evident as a ridge in the soft palate tissue running obliquely forwards and medially into the hard palate margin. The hemi-uvula is drawn into a lateral position on each side. The absence of a complete sphincter encompassing the palate (velum) and the posterior pharynx causes failure of velopharyngeal closure (incompetence) and is responsible for typical cleft palate or nasal speech tone.

In a complete bilateral cleft of primary and secondary palate, the premaxilla has no maxillary attachments and shows unrestrained forward growth. The free lower border of the vomer and nasal septum is prominent in the midline of the cleft and the lateral palate processes are often displaced into the nasal cavity alongside the vomer. The cleft soft palate tissues are drawn into a lateral position and the muscle may be deficient.

An isolated secondary palate cleft may involve only the soft palate or both hard and soft (Figs 105.13 and 105.14). A complete secondary cleft extends posteriorly from the incisive foramen and the relative positions of the palatine processes and the vomer are better preserved than in a complete primary/secondary cleft. Incomplete clefts include lesser degrees of hard palate cleft, simply a notch at the posterior margin of the hard palate, or soft palate cleft only. The shape of the defect may conform more to a "U" than a "V" especially in conjunction with a small mandible (micrognathia) in the Pierre Robin sequence. The sequence possible starts with hypomandibulism, which causes the developing tongue to intrude into the space of conjunction of palatine process and vomer and interfere with the normal fusion. Soft palate cleft may be muscular only with intact mucous membrane on oral and nasal surfaces–so-called submucous cleft palate (SMCP) (Fig. 105.15). The anatomical/clinical features consist of a notch in the posterior edge of hard palate, a midline grey, translucent zone, oblique muscle prominence and a bifid uvula but may be difficult to define and lead to delayed diagnosis.

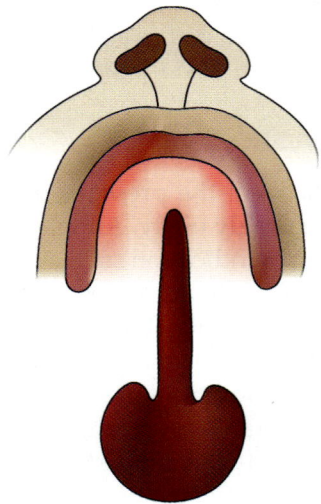

Fig. 105.13: Cleft of secondary -hard and soft -palate

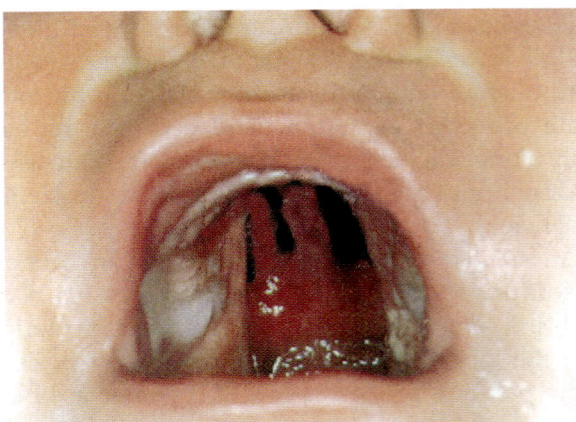

Fig. 105.14: Moderately wide secondary cleft palate with exposed vomer

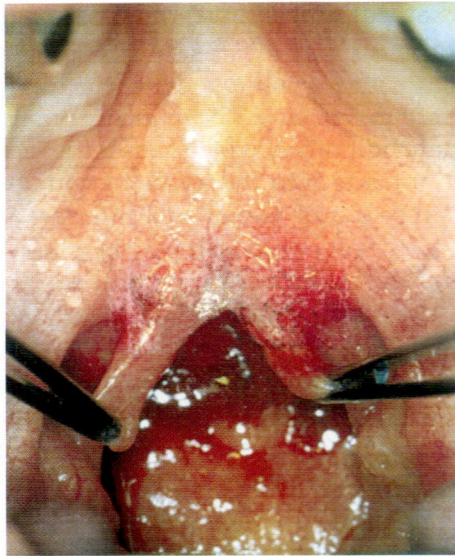

Fig. 105.15: Submucous cleft palate showing bifid uvula and central lucency of muscle dehiscence

PRENATAL DIAGNOSIS

Prenatal diagnosis of the presence of a facial cleft is becoming increasingly likely. Anomaly scanning may detect clefts but an indication such as previous family history, risk factors or hydramnios may be the stimulus to careful inspection of fetal craniofacial anatomy. Other anomalies also increase the index of suspicion and detection rate for craniofacial abnormalities and will also lead to fetal karyotyping.

Whilst in utero detection does not necessarily confer specific benefit on the fetus or neonate, the parents have the advantage of up to 80% detection rate though there is also a significant false positive rate.[46] Detailed counseling in the event of a prenatal diagnosis is extremely important and there is good evidence of the major benefit of psychological preparation for the birth of an infant with a cleft anomaly - 85% felt that prenatal counseling was much more helpful than postnatal counseling.[47] Full evaluation and counseling may be especially important in Pierre Robin sequence where concurrent cardiac anomalies (20%) and abnormal karyotype (10%) are more common.[48] Careful ultrasound evaluation is needed to give an accurate prognosis based on where the fetus/neonate fits in the spectrum of the Pierre Robin sequence. The potential for much greater clarity of definition of fetal craniofacial anatomy from in utero magnetic resonance imaging (MRI) is now gradually becoming evident.

Informed parental choice regarding continuation or termination of the pregnancy and consideration of the option of early neonatal surgery follow directly from in utero diagnosis.[49] However, prenatal diagnosis raises difficult practical, moral and ethical issues at a sensitive time for prospective parents and complex medicolegal questions such as "wrongful life" potentially follow from decisions made prenatally.[50] Fortunately, normal pregnancy and term delivery of a healthy baby are the usual sequelae.

It is well known that in utero surgery may produce virtually scarless healing and recent experiments have confirmed that both scar formation and growth are better following in utero than neonatal cleft surgery in an ovine model.[51,52] A large body of research continues into the potential for fetal surgery for clefts though the work is complicated by the natural history of a significant association of other anomalies and high consequent fetal loss in animal models.[53,54]

PRESENTATION

The cleft usually comes to notice first at birth or at the time of routine newborn examination. To this end it is important that those performing routine examinations are familiar with the need to visualize the palate on intraoral examination. It is also important that attending staff are trained to cope with the inevitable anxiety and concern which recognition of a congenital anomaly raises, and can provide initial answers and appropriate reassurance based on a basic knowledge of facial clefts. This should include the immediate risks and an outline of the plan of management. Early and definitive consultation with a member of a cleft team—specialist nurse, surgeon, orthodontist, speech therapist – follows and affords an opportunity for detailed discussion of residual concerns and of the planned treatment program. The parents should be helped towards an understanding of the nature of clefts and to a realistic expectation of outcome. Unreasonable doubts and anxieties can be allayed but false reassurance must be avoided. Further counseling to deal with genuine concerns may be arranged. The course of cleft management stretches throughout childhood and adolescence into early adult life and cannot be guaranteed to be smooth. The full cooperation and patience of the parents is needed to achieve the best outcome for the patient.

Respiratory Problems

Airway obstruction due to relative micrognathia, abnormal tongue position and retained oropharyngeal secretions is a potential immediate postnatal risk for all babies with a cleft. Routine measures to clear the newborn's airway by suction will be sufficient to avert problems in most cases but readiness to take further steps is required. These include drawing the tongue forward with an instrument if necessary, placing the baby in the more favorable ventral suspension position, or airway intubation. More major problems are associated with Pierre Robin sequence.[35,55]

Pierre Robin Sequence

Respiratory distress and feeding difficulty associated with a small mandible was reported by Pierre Robin (1934) particularly with reference to feeding of the infant in an upright (orthostatic) position.[56] A cleft palate was not an essential or invariable association though it is often present. The commonly noted U-shaped (as opposed to V-shaped) cleft may be caused by the upward displacement between the palatine shelves of a normal sized tongue in a small oropharynx resulting in failure of fusion. The poor support for the tongue allows it to slip (glossoptosis) posteriorly while increased respiratory efforts produce greater negative pressure and draw the tongue further into the pharynx compounding the problem of obstruction. This vicious and life-threatening cycle can be interrupted by insertion of a nasopharyngeal tube to relieve the suction effect. This sequence is not always recognized at an early stage and examination such as polysomnography may help in defining the respiratory problem.[57] Strategies for managing upper airway obstruction in Pierre Robin sequence include:

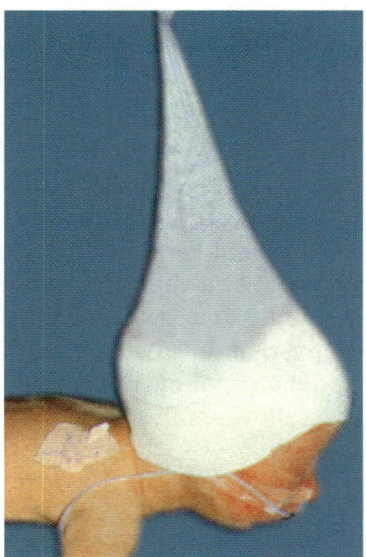

Fig. 105.16: Ventral suspension of infant with respiratory difficulty due to micrognathia

- Insertion of an oral (McGill) airway to control tongue position
- Ventral suspension with neck extension to open airway maximally (Fig. 105.16)
- Nasopharyngeal tube positioned with tip in pharyngeal airway to prevent development of negative pressure;[58,59]
- Endotracheal intubation, which may be exceedingly difficult due to the anterior position of the larynx relative to the tongue
- Tracheostomy, which may be preferable if long-term airway protection is needed, but it carries other risks.

An alternative to intubation of the airway is mechanical displacement of the tongue into a forward position by tongue suture, lip/tongue anastomosis or transmandibular wire suspension of the tongue. These techniques however, carry risks of infection, bleeding and tissue damage and are not wholly reliable.

It is essential that careful monitoring be maintained for any baby with upper airway obstruction to detect any signs of decompensation or secondary cardiac effects. Blood gas analysis, electrocardiography and echocardiography will show warning signs of hypoxia and hypercapnia and cardiac enlargement and failure due to pulmonary hypertension and corpulmonale.[60] Failure to control these consequences may precipitate hypoxic damage with psychomotor impairment and potential fatal outcome.[36] With growth of the infant the respiratory problem lessens which appears to be due to catch-up in jaw size in some cases but this does not always occur and the mandible/maxilla relationship may remain unchanged.[61] It is clearly essential that adequate, or even enhanced, nutritional intake is assured throughout this period.

Feeding and Growth

Feeding normally from the breast may present no problem at all to a baby with CL+/-P and, unless breathing problems preclude it, a trial of breast-feeding should certainly be allowed if the mother wishes. Similarly, feeding from a normal bottle and teat may well be possible despite the cleft. However, normal sucking may be prevented by inability to seal the lips around the nipple or teat and by inability of the tongue to compress either against the palate. Negative suction in the hypopharynx may not be possible because of velopharyngeal incompetence and attempted feeding may cause respiratory distress due to incoordination and entry of milk into the nasopharynx. About 25% of babies have significant feeding problems reflected in poor weight gain and those with Pierre Robin sequence are especially disadvantaged.[62] The lag in weight gain may continue beyond the first months despite a relatively normal birth weight and a deficiency of growth hormone in some cases has been postulated.[63] Growth delay (both weight and height) is more evident in infants with syndromic than non-syndromic clefts and in cleft palate than cleft lip, but catch up usually occurs following cleft palate repair by 2 years of age:[64] short stature, however, tends to be a persisting feature of syndromic cleft patients.

At the first sign of feeding difficulty help and advice and suggestions for feeding strategies should be offered to the mother.[65,66] A variety of modified teats is available ranging from a specific cleft palate teat (Nuk Medical Services) to lamb's teats, flanged teats and double teats (Fig. 105.17). The Haberman feeder (Fig. 105.18) allows delivery of milk at a variable rate without requiring the baby to suck.[67] Prosthetic plates and obturators can be developed to occlude the cleft and aid sucking and may be incorporated into an extra-oral appliance to realign the maxillary segments.[68]

If feeding difficulty is complicated by respiratory problems and the baby shows signs of failing to thrive, tube feeding is indicated. A nasogastric tube is a short-term solution but may increase pharyngeal secretions and pulmonary aspiration. Persisting trouble is best helped by a percutaneous endoscopic gastrostomy tube insertion but the possibility of associated gastro-esophageal reflux should be considered. Thickened feeds using Carobel (Cow and Gate) or Gaviscon (R and C) less readily reflux but fundoplication and gastrostomy is needed in a few cases. A calorie intake of at least 100 cals/kg/24 hr is required and should be exceeded if energy demands are increased by respiratory effort, pulmonary disease, cardiac disease or pyrexia.

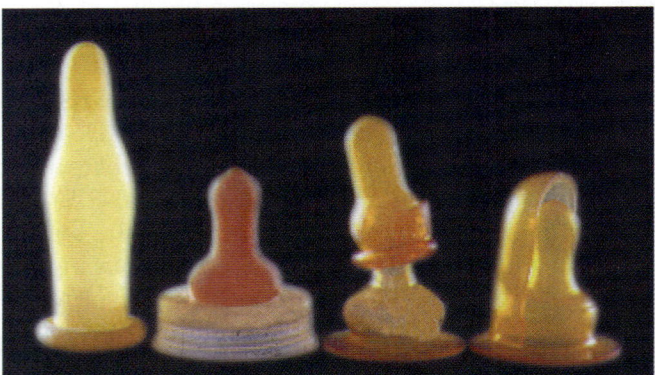

Fig. 105.17: Variety of modified feeding teats

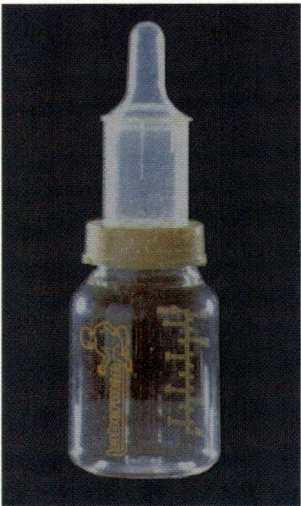

Fig. 105.18: Haberman feeding bottle

Submucous cleft palate (SMCP) is frequently missed at birth despite an incidence of about 1: 1,200.[69] As a large proportion are asymptomatic, this is not a great problem.[70] However, some do not come to light until the child presents with hypernasality, relative unintelligibility of speech and possibly Eustachain tube dysfunction at nursery or early primary school age.[71] Initial referral may be to an otolaryngologist on suspicion of obstruction due to enlarged adenoids or tonsils, but examination reveals the features of an SMCP. There is, of course, a strong contraindication to adenoidectomy in this circumstance.[70] Confirmation of the SMCP may be sought in detailed speech assessment and demonstration of velopharyngeal inadequacy and can be documented in the cooperative patient using lateral videofluoroscopy of palate movement or nasoendoscopy. The latter investigation shows a characteristic abnormality of the dorsal convexity on palate movement and a coronal, as opposed to circular, pattern of velopharyngeal closure.[72]

PRESURGICAL ORTHODONTICS

The disruption of continuity of the maxillary arch in complete unilateral and bilateral clefts allows the maxillary segments to assume markedly misaligned and asymmetrical positions. The consequences for primary surgery and later jaw development are considerable and have led to various strategies to realign segments.[73] Simple techniques using gentle sustained pressure from elastic strapping to more comprehensive attempts to mold both alveolus and nasal structures have been devised; however, alveolar realignment must not occur at the expense of excessive maxillary collapse inwards and an intraoral plate may be needed to prevent this.[74,75] A further benefit may be seen in improved sucking and feeding and assumption of a more normal tongue position, which is helpful in later speech development. In addition, some parents may derive psychological benefit from the recognition that active steps are being taken to help their child's problems.[76]

Whilst evidence for long-term improvement in arch formation is sparse, there is no doubt that surgery for lip repair and primary rhinoplasty is facilitated.[77-79] The best outcomes are achieved when orthodontic management is continued through to the time of eruption of the permanent dentition.[80] Although many technical and surgical advances have been made in orthodontic management of the cleft patient, objective evidence of improved outcomes from controlled, randomized studies is generally lacking.[81]

In practice, close cooperation between orthodontist and cleft surgeon is needed to decide on precise timing of lip closure once optimal molding has been achieved. Recording of cleft shape using plaster models before, during and after surgery allows assessment of progress in individual cases.

PREOPERATIVE PREPARATION

Preparation for the surgical procedure of lip and palate repair includes the full preoperative assessment and consent procedures necessary for all surgery in infants and children. Points of specific relevance in for satisfactory cleft surgery are:
- Adequate weight gain
- Hemoglobin above 10 gm/100ml
- Bacteriological swab of oral cavity to exclude pathogens (e.g. hemolytic streptococcus)
- Consideration of blood grouping/cross-matching (e.g. for severe cleft palate).

Close cooperation and understanding between anesthetist and surgeon are necessary as the airway is shared and the potential for ventilatory/respiratory problems is thereby greater. The anesthetist will normally wish to use a reinforced preformed endotracheal tube to minimize risks of tube compression and to give the surgeon the maximum degree of access. The surgeon is responsible for ensuring that peroperative bleeding does not track into the lower airway by adequate hemostasis and packing: a non-cuffed endotracheal tube is normally used for young infants and affords less protection to the lower airway against ingress of secretions. Laryngeal spasm, related to immediate postoperative irritation from blood, is potentially fatal. In experienced hands, anaesthesia in less sophisticated surroundings using basic techniques without access to advanced equipment and monitoring can be made very safe with a carefully derived protocol and close attention to detail.[82]

CLEFT LIP REPAIR

The timing of cleft lip repair has been a matter for debate. Protagonists have argued the case either for

an immediate neonatal repair or for repair at about 3 months of age.[83,84] It is agreed that repair in the first month or two is inadvisable for reasons including the neonate's natural drop in hemoglobin and lowered immune defenses at this stage. Factors to balance in considering the optimum age for repair are:
- Wound healing and subsequent scarring
- Technical ease or difficulty of repair
- Psychological effect on the mother and baby
- The effects of surgery on subsequent growth
- The presence or absence of other anomalies.

Whilst wound healing is undoubtedly better after operation in the early newborn period, the advantage of preoperative surgical orthodontics is lost and technical difficulty may be greater. Careful selection is necessary for early newborn repair to screen out significant associated anomalies and the maternal/newborn bonding process is interrupted. The parents' coping strategies may be enhanced by the psychological lift of immediate repair of the defect or, conversely, by the necessity of coming to terms with the unrepaired defect for a longer period prior to repair.

The success of the policy of a particular cleft unit with respect to age of repair may depend more on implementation and explanation of that policy than on the chosen age of repair. The most common age for repair of the lip, which is the best compromise between the various considerations, is approximately 3 months.

The repair of the lip attempts to achieve a series of objectives embracing:
- A scar which is inconspicuous and orientated to reproduce the missing philtral line
- A vermilion line with peaks of equal height and a balanced cupid's bow
- A central vermilion tubercle of the lip
- A nasal sill equal in width to that of the non-cleft side
- Repositioning of the lateral alar cartilage to correct the tip, dome and ala of the nose
- Restoration of the columella to a central, vertical position
- Reorientation of the orbicularis oris muscle to restore muscle function
- A buccal sulcus to allow lip movement.

In summary, a symmetrical, balanced, scarless normally functioning nostril and lip is the acme of the cleft surgery.

The earliest and simplest lip repairs involved straight line closure with little respect for the displacement and distortion of anatomical features. Subsequent efforts to realign and balance these features were typified by techniques such as rectangular flap and triangular flap but unsatisfactory scars ensued (Fig. 105.19).[85,86] A major leap forward was made by Millard (1960) who devised the rotation/advancement flap technique upon which most subsequent refinements have been based.[87,88]

Many technical points play a part in achieving satisfactory, reproducible primary lip repairs. Detailed assessment and precise planning of each repair includes silastic models, measurements and marking of all skin incisions - usually with methylene blue dye. Infiltration of tissues with 1:200,000 adrenaline with 0.5% Marcaine (Astra) both reduces bleeding, which helps to keep a clear operating field, and also minimizes the need for general anesthesia, which speeds postoperative recovery. Bipolar diathermy aids in maintaining clear vision and ensuring meticulous repair. Fine instruments and sutures (6/0, 7/0) and magnification are needed to achieve precise apposition of mucosa, muscle and skin (Figs 105.20 and 105.21).

Attention has been drawn to the need to avoid any interference with important growth sites in the midface in the repair of cleft lip. Scarring in the area of the vomer and premaxillary suture, in particular, might subsequently impede the development of the dentoalveolar structures.[89] Emphasis is also placed on the careful definition and reconstruction of the circumoral muscle complex so as to achieve restoration of function and hence optimal growth.[90] Some of the best outcomes of the primary lip repair have resulted form the recognition that the cleft nose correction can be performed as an integral part of the repair rather than as a second stage. Repositioning and elevation of the lower lateral alar cartilages can achieve a correction of the nasal tip and realignment of the nostril rim thereby avoiding the drooping appearance which is an obvious stigma of cleft repair, whilst preserving the potential for nasal growth into adolescence.[91-93]

Bilateral cleft lip repair introduces the additional difficulty of the excessive forward displacement of the premaxilla. Presurgical orthodontics may reduce the position to one where lip repair can be achieved without significant tension but this is not always the case. In extreme situations a unilateral repair may be

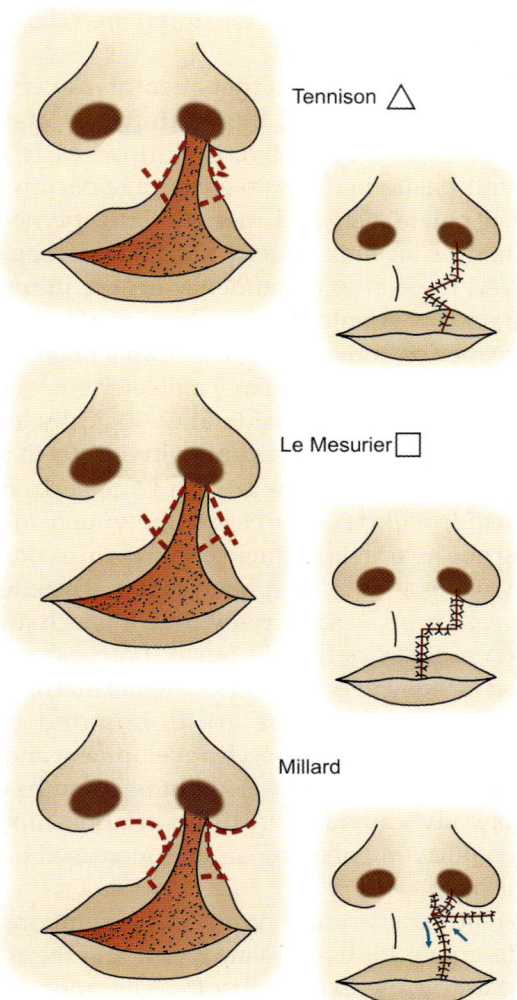

Fig. 105.19: Diagram showing Tennison, Le Mesurier and Millard cleft lip repairs

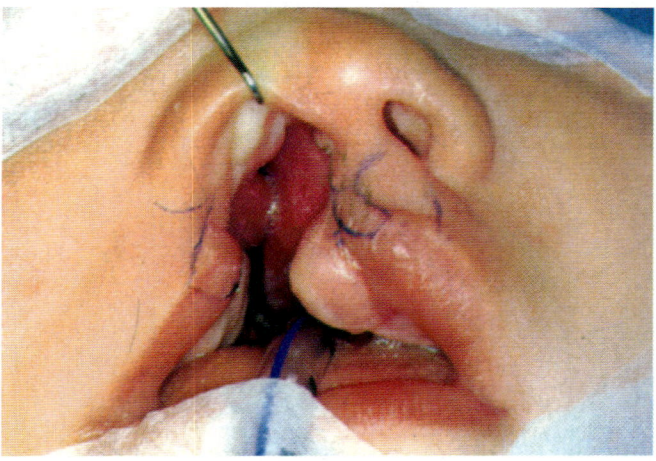

Fig. 105.20

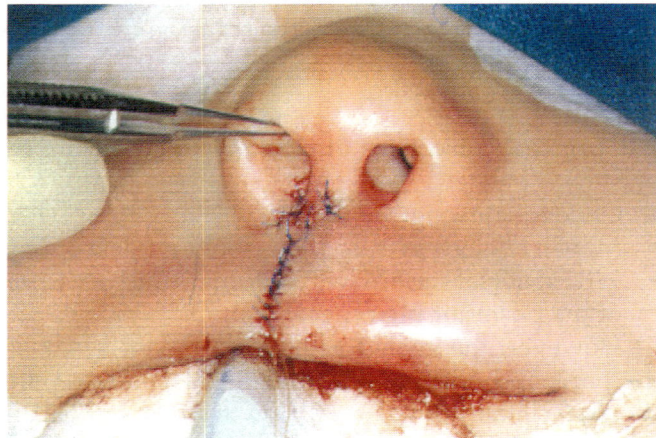

Fig. 105.21

Figs 105.20 and 105.21: Operative photographs showing markings for Millard repair and completed procedure

performed initially with a simple lip adhesion on the contralateral side to attempt to maintain a central position of the premaxilla. However, simultaneous is bilateral repair is the gold standard and preferred option. Before the significance of growth centers was fully understood, a set-back of the premaxilla by vomerine osteotomy and resection was used to achieve a satisfactory lip appearance initially, but gross mid-face hypoplasia and reverse dental bite developed subsequently. The lessons from unilateral lip repair may be imported with modifications into the bilateral operation.[94,95] A good functional result depends on realigning and establishing continuity of the orbicularis oris muscle and on creating a buccal sulcus between premaxilla and prolabium. In addition, a good cosmetic outcome follows from some narrowing of the often wide prolabium (Fig. 105.22), alar correction and development of the columella.[96]

Recovery from operation is usually rapid. Blood transfusion is rarely needed and feeding can be started from breast or bottle within a few hours and certainly by the following day — this may well be a better way of settling the baby and relieving strain on the repair than the use of sedation. Discharge from hospital will be on the second or third postoperative day and the non-absorbable monofilament sutures will be removed on about the fifth day.

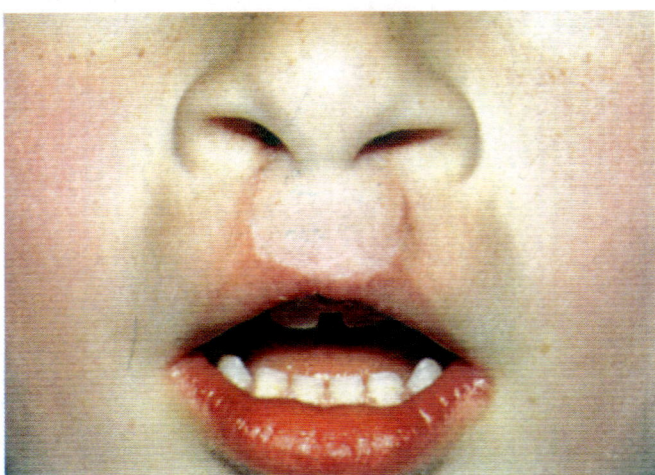

Fig. 105.22: Repaired bilateral cleft lip with excessively wide prolabium

CLEFT PALATE REPAIR

The principle objectives of cleft palate repair are to produce a palate:[97]
- Of adequate length
- Mobile enough to close the velopharyngeal space
- Whose dorsal surface will conform to the curvature of the posterior pharyngeal wall.

However, the goals for the outcome of repair of the hard and soft palate differ: hard palate repair should facilitate normal facial growth whilst soft palate repair aims to allow velopharyngeal competence.[98] An essential step in achieving the latter aim is the repositioning and reconstruction of the levator veli palatini sling by detaching the muscle insertions from their aberrant attachment to the posterior hard palate.[99] Lengthening of the soft palate and improved function of levator and tensor muscles may then permit adequate soft palate movement and velopharyngeal closure.

The timing of cleft palate repair is governed by various factors identified as:
- The size of the child and of the child's jaw, influencing access for the surgeon
- The effect of the age at palate repair on speech development
- The effect of age at palate repair on subsequent palate growth[100]
- The effect of repair on the nasal airway
- The effect of repair on Eustachian tube function and middle ear development.
- Changes in the width of the unrepaired cleft palate with time alone.

It is generally accepted that attempts at very early palate repair are vitiated by the difficulty of access, though some surgeons have performed early repair of the soft palate in order to encourage narrowing of the hard palate cleft and thereby limit the need for mobilization at subsequent hard palate repair.[101] However, there is some tendency for the unrepaired cleft to narrow spontaneously. Any interference with the mucoperiosteum and soft tissue attachments of the facial skeleton is liable to have a deleterious effect on bone growth and this consideration logically leads to delay in palate operations; unrepaired clefts in adults show excellent maxillary growth.[102] Speech, on the other hand, will develop best if the young infant is making noises and reproducible sounds in a consistent way by using an intact, repaired palate. The effects of palate repair on nasal airway and Eustachian tube function are less definable but in both cases better function is likely to occur with more normal anatomy.

These considerations are dominated by the advantage of improved speech development and, with this in mind, palate repair at about 6-9 months of age is widely advocated.[84,103] A direct relationship exists between delayed palate repair and increased nasality of speech.[104,105]

A great variety of techniques and operations have been described for hard palate repair and these differ principally in the extent of soft tissue mobilization advocated to perform repair without excessive tension. Simple lateral peri-alveolar releasing incisions and mucoperiosteal bipedicle flap elevation allows midline cleft closure (Fig. 105.23). More mobility and easier closure can be achieved using a flap based only on a greater palatine artery posterior pedicle but maxillary growth may be affected to a slightly greater degree. The two techniques show very similar results with an overall need for repeat velopharyngeal surgery in about 15% which rises to 23% for severe clefts.[104] The soft palate muscle is normally repaired synchronously using an intravelar veloplasty technique or a double reversing Z-plasty to reconstitute the levator/tensor muscle sling.[106]

The Furlow operation for soft palate repair is based on retroposition of the levator/tensor complex and lengthening of the palate by Z-plasty in two layers which are not superimposed (double reversing) and

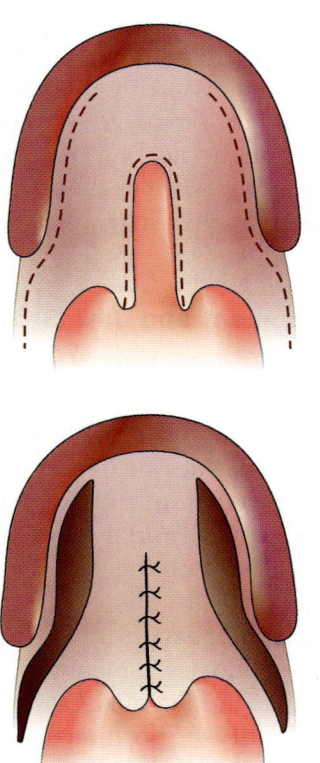

Fig. 105.23: Diagram of Langenbeck secondary palate repair

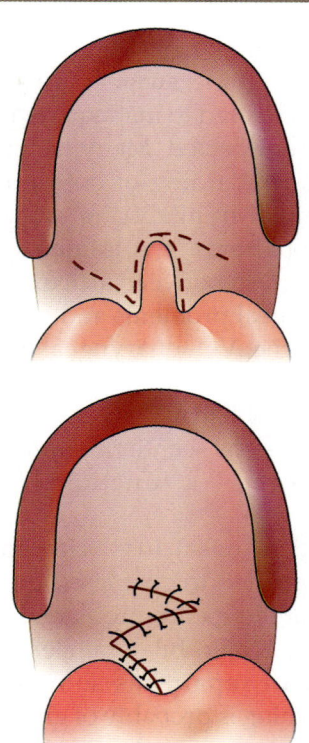

Fig. 105.24: Diagram of Furlow soft palate repair

is therefore a secure and reliable closure (Fig. 105.24). In comparison with intravelar veloplasty there is a reduced need for subsequent pharyngoplasty.[107]

Submucous cleft of the palate requires muscle repositioning and repair despite the intact mucosal layers and apparent palate continuity.[108] The Furlow repair gives a high level of successful outcome unless the initial velopharyngeal gap is large — greater than 8 mm.[109]

In cleft palate surgery, the postoperative appearances are not helpful in predicting the functional outcome. Velopharyngeal functional outcome relates to severity of cleft but it has also been shown that there is a learning curve for each surgeon and a correlation between higher volume operators and a reduced need for secondary procedures.[110] The overall assessment of outcome after cleft palate surgery requires long-term follow-up including review of speech, hearing, dental development and maxillary/mandibular arch relationship. The need for secondary surgery depends on these parameters.

ASSESSMENT AND OUTCOME

The whole area of assessment of outcome from the management of cleft lip and palate is complicated by the wide range of treatment strategies, the complexity of the issues relating to outcome and the relatively long duration required for an assessment of final outcome. The perennial debate goes on about whether early repair aimed at producing the best speech results or later repair aimed at allowing optimal maxillary growth ultimately give the better functional and aesthetic outcome. Resolution requires randomized controlled trials to determine the issue from scientific study.[111] The need for detailed audit has been advocated not only to resolve matters of treatment protocols but to look at the important question of whether centralized services with relatively high volume operators lead to better outcomes.[112] Such an extensive study was established to look at all aspects of cleft management in the UK and has reported in detail.[113]

Speech

Following cleft palate surgery an initial residual speech problem related to inadequate velopharyngeal function is to be expected. Many factors are involved in this and understanding of both normal and cleft speech is essential in analyzing and measuring the individual components.[114] A trained speech therapist is able to distinguish between articulatory, dysphonic and velopharyngeal problems and concentrate on the predominant issue. Velopharyngeal inadequacy itself has various aspects, which may each contribute to the overall speech problem:[115]

- Insufficiency — as seen in the unrepaired cleft
- Incompetence — a functional or neurogenic problem
- Mishearing — nasal loss with specific sounds sometimes related to deafness.

The extent of the speech problem is generally more severe for more major, bilateral clefts and, although the technique of repair has some bearing on the outcome, the timing is probably of greater significance-earlier repair producing better results.[116,117] The principle in speech therapy management, however, is to start early in all cases with assessment and therapy with the goal of establishing normal speech by school age.[118] In addition to standard listening and recording methods, the therapist may use:

- Lateral videofluoroscopy of palate movements
- Nasoendoscopy to observe directly palate movement during speech
- Anemometry to assess airflow through the nose during speech.

Up to 20% of cleft palate patients will not achieve satisfactory articulation and nasal tone even with extended speech therapy and will go on to consideration for secondary surgery.[119,120]

Hearing

A degree of otitis media is common in children with cleft palate — unrepaired or repaired and the risk of conductive deafness should be borne in mind by teachers and specialists.[121] Formal audiometric evaluation should be performed regularly by a trained specialist and it must be recognized that a hearing loss of more than 15 decibels will compound the speech problems for cleft palate patients.[122,123] The management of the middle ear problem includes simple measures such as use of decongestants and antibiotics and also myringotomy and tympanostomy tube insertion for adequate ventilation.

The acquisition of language is a complex process depending not only on hearing but also on cognition and communication and it is notable that there is a significant delay in the early years for cleft palate patients.[124]

Dental Development and Jaw Growth

The care of the dentition starts at an early stage for the cleft patient with attention to adequate fluoride intake and good dental hygiene. The primary dentition may show abnormalities of dental development in addition to the problem of missing teeth at the cleft site. Hypoplastic, bigeminal (double) and supernumerary teeth are seen but generally do not warrant attention other than hygiene. As the permanent (second) dentition appears from age 7/8, attention is paid to alignment and assessment is made of the need for bone grafting to the alveolus. Orthopantomograms are needed to identify the position of unerrupted teeth and plan management fully. The restorative dentist has an important role in dealing with residual dental problems in an effort to achieve a symmetrical arch of well-aligned teeth which protects not only dental hygiene but also jaw function.[125]

Detailed assessment of the outcome of dental management and jaw growth uses an index (the Goslon index) for defining the dental relationships at the stage of early permanent dentition.[126] The need for later orthognathic surgery to establish satisfactory cosmetic appearance, jaw relationship and dental bite may be as high as 25% and is not entirely dependent on the nature of the cleft.[127]

SECONDARY SURGERY

Following initial repair of the cleft lip and palate, consideration of further (secondary) surgery is indicated in a number of situations including:

- Unsatisfactory cosmetic appearance of lip or nose
- Inadequate velopharyngeal function
- Residual cleft of alveolus and primary palate.

Lip and Nose

Current techniques of primary repair aim at as complete a correction as possible and avoidance of revision surgery. However, nasal asymmetry and persistent displacement of alar cartilages may warrant repositioning.[128,129] The deleterious effects on subsequent growth are always borne in mind. More minor scar revisions to improve the vermilion line can be performed at any stage without detriment.

Velopharyngeal Function

If adequate function is not achieved after initial palate repair and speech therapy, it is not likely that a further intravelar repair will be successful. In this circumstance a pharyngoplasty, incorporating both the velum and posterior pharyngeal wall tissue, is preferable. The principal techniques use either:
- A posterior pharyngeal flap which swings forward to anchor into the velum[130] or
- A sphincter formed by reorientation of palato-pharyngeus muscles, which offers a more dynamic solution.[131,132]

Both techniques produce excellent results in reducing velopharyngeal incompetence and there is no clear consensus for preference.[133]

A residual fistula in the line of palate repair is not necessarily symptomatic, but if nasality of speech or fluid loss through the nose is noted, fistula repair will be indicated. Direct closure using local flaps is simplest but, if deficiency or scarring is significant, tissue may be imported from buccal mucosa or tongue.

Alveolar Cleft

The cleft of alveolus is often not closed with primary surgery but remains open to allow maxillary growth to proceed. Following maxillary realignment just prior to eruption of secondary dentition, bone grafts (usually from iliac crest) are placed in order to provide a matrix for dental eruption and alignment and to retain maxillary position.[134]

PSYCHOLOGICAL ISSUES

It is obvious that a congenital abnormality as central to an individual's image and perception as a craniofacial anomaly is liable to have a significant effect on a young person's development. There is indeed wide awareness of the many psychological issues that confront not only patients with craniofacial anomalies but also their parents, and much research has been undertaken.[135] Up to 40% of children are known to have major problems such as learning disorders and difficulties with social competence.[136] It is important to recognize that patients and parents often have different perceptions about outcome, both in clinical and psychological terms and therefore to consider the opinions of both in reaching conclusions about management.[137] There is a need for early assessment of the psychological component of disability related to craniofacial clefts and for introduction of appropriate guidance, advice and counseling. Training in social skills at a young age may help the individual to circumvent later difficulties. Continuing multicenter research aims to define the psychological and social problems associated with craniofacial anomalies and to devise strategies for minimizing risks to patients.

ORGANIZATION OF CLEFT SERVICES

There is no doubt that management of the patient with a cleft requires teamwork of a high order. Many different disciplines are involved in delivering the total "package of care" and this must be presented to the patient and parents in an integrated, logical and timely manner. This is best achieved in the context of a multidisciplinary clinic[112] and this would generally include:
- Cleft surgeon
- Orthodontist
- Speech therapist
- Otolaryngologist
- Geneticist
- Specialist nurse
- Audiometrician
- Dentist
- Pediatrician
- Psychologist.

Some team members require dedicated and highly specialized training while others bring the more general skills of their specialty. It is increasingly recognized that, in order to draw together and capitalise on the expertise of a team, a support network embracing skills in the following fields is helpful:
- Clerical/administrative
- Audit
- Medical illustration
- Information technology
- Research.

A recent national survey has emphasized all these aspects of cleft care and has also highlighted the fact that concentration of experience in fewer centers performing a higher volume of work is more likely to fulfil the above objectives.[138]

REFERENCES

1. Perko M. The history of treatment of cleft lip and palate. Progr Pediatr Surg 1986;20:238-51.
2. Boo Chai K. An ancient Chinese text on a cleft lip. Plast Reconstr Surg 1966;38:39.
3. Fergusson W. On hare-lip and split palate. Lancet 1864; June 25: 719-24.
4. McGregor IA. The treatment of cleft lip and palate. Scot Med J 1959;4:276-99.
5. Watson ACH (a). The cleft palate dilemma: speech or beauty. J R Coll Surg Edinb 1980;25:425-35.
6. Wallace AF. A history of the repair of cleft lip and palate in Britain before World War ll. Ann Plast Surg 1987;19:266-75.
7. Millard DR. Cleft craft: the evolution of its surgery. Little, Brown Boston 1976.
8. Stark RB. Development of the face. In Transactions of the 5th Internat Congr Plast Reconstr Surg Butterworths, Melbourne 1971.
9. Tessier P. Anatomical classification of facial, craniofacial and laterofacial clefts. J Maxillofac Surg 1976;4:69-92.
10. Houdayer C, Bahuau M. Orofacial cleft defects: inference from nature and nurture. Annales de Genetique 1998;41:89-117.
11. Schutte BC, Murray JC. The many faces and factors of orofacial clefting. Hum Mol Genet 1999;8:1853-59.
12. Holder SE. Cleft lip- is there light at the end of the tunnel? Arch Dis Child 1991;66:829-32.
13. Jensen BL, Kreiborg S, Dahl E, et al. Cleft lip and palate in Denmark 1976-1981: epidemiology, variability and early somatic development. Cleft Palate J 1988;25:258-69.
14. Van der Woude. Fistula labii inferioris congenita and its association with cleft lip and palate Am J Hum Genet 1954;6:244-56.
15. Ryan AK, Goodship JA, Wilson DI, et al. Spectrum of clinical features associated with interstitial chromosome 22q11 deletions; a European collaborative study. J Med Genet 1997;34:798-804.
16. Goldberg R, Motzkin B, Marion R, et al. Velo-cardio-facial syndrome: a review of 120 patients. Am J Med Genet 1993;45:313-19.
17. Tobias ES, Morrison N, Whiteford ML, et al. Towards earlier diagnosis of 22q11 deletions. Arch Dis Child 1999;81:513-14.
18. Sassani R, Bartlett SP, Feng H, et al. Association between alleles of the transforming growth factor alpha locus and the occurrence of cleft lip. Am J Med Genet 1993:50; 565-69.
19. Mosher G. Genetic counseling in cleft lip and palate. Ear Nose Throat J 1986;65:330-36.
20. Thornton JB, Nimer S, Howard PS. The incidence, classification, etiology, and embryology of oral clefts. Semin Orthod 1996;2:162-68.
21. Bender PL. Genetics of cleft lip and palate. J Ped Nursing 2000:15;242-49.
22. Stoll C, Alembik Y, Dott B, et al. Associated malformations in cases with oral clefts Cleft Palate Craniofac J 2000;37: 41-47.
23. Munger RG, Romitti PA, Daack-Hirsch S, et al. Maternal alcohol use and risk of orofacial cleft birth defects Teratology 1996;54:27-33.
24. Kerrigan JJ, Mansell JP, Sengupta A, et al. Pathogenesis and potential mechanisms for clefting. J R Coll Surg Edinb 2000;45:351-58.
25. Christensen K. The 20th century Danish facial cleft population — epidemiology and genetic-epidemiological studies Cleft Palate Craniofac J 1999:36;96-104.
26. Fogh-Andersen P. Inheritance of Harelip and Cleft Palate. Arnold Busck, Copenhagen 1942.
27. Womersley J, Stone DH. Epidemiology of facial clefts. Arch Dis Child 1987;62:717-30.
28. Fitzpatrick DR. Personal communication 1991.
29. Derijcke A, Eerens A, Carels C. The incidence of oral clefts: a review. B J Oral Maxillofac Surg 1996;34:488-94.
30. Owens JR, Jones JW, Harris F. Epidemiology of facial clefting. Arch Dis Child 1985;60:521-24.
31. Vanderas AP. Incidence of cleft lip, cleft palate and cleft lip and palate amongst races: a review. Cleft Palate J 1987;24:216-25.
32. Chung KC, Kowalski CP, Kim HM, et al. Plast Reconstr Surg 2000:105;485-91.
33. Cohen MM, Bankier A. Syndrome delineation involving orofacial clefting. Cleft Palate J 1991;28:119-20.
34. Hagberg C, Larson O, Milerad J. Incidence of cleft lip and palate and risks of associated malformations. Cleft Palate Craniofac J 1998;35:40-45.
35. Williams AJ, Williams MA, Walker CA, et al. The Robin anomalad (Pierre Robin syndrome) - a follow-up study. Arch Dis Child 1981;56:663-68.
36. Caouette-Laberge L, Bayet B, Larocque Y. The Pierre Robin sequence: review of 125 cases and evolution of treatment modalities. Plast Reconstr Surg 1994;93;934-41.
37. Watson ACH (b) in Eds. Watson ACH, Edwards M. Advances in the management of cleft palate. Churchill Livingston, Edinburgh 1980.
38. Aylsworth AS. Genetic considerations in clefts of the lip and palat. Clin Plast Surg 1985;12:533-42.
39. Veau V. Etude anatomique du bec-de-levre unilateral totale. Ann d'Anat Path 1928;601:50-60.
40. Kernahan DA. A new classification for cleft lip and palate. Plast Reconstr Surg 1958;22:435-41.
41. Larson M, Hellquist R, Jakobsson OP. Classification, recording and cleft palate surgery at the Uppsala Cleft

Palate Centre Scand. J Plast Reconstr Hand Surg 1998;32:185-92.
42. Smith AW, Khoo AK, Jackson IT. A modification of the Kernahan "Y" classification in cleft lip and palate deformities. Plast Reconstr Surg 1998;102:1842-47.
43. Friedman HI, Sayetta RB, Coston GN, et al. Symbolic representation of cleft lip and palate. Cleft Palate Craniofac J 1991;28:252-60.
44. Vegter F, Hage JJ. Standardized facial photography of cleft patients: just fit the grid. Cleft Palate Craniofac J 2000;37:435-40.
45. McNulty E. Photography of the cleft palate. J Biol Photo 1988;56:20-21.
46. Hafner E, Stermoste W, Scholler J, et al. Prenatal diagnosis of facial malformations. Prenat Diagn 1997;17:51-58.
47. Davalbhakta A, Hall PN. The impact of antenatal diagnosis on the effectiveness and timing of counseling for cleft lip and palate. Br J Plast Surg 2000;53:298-301.
48. Hsieh Y-Y, Chang C-C, Tsai H-D, et al. The prenatal diagnosis of Pierre Robin sequence Prenat Diagn 1999;19:567-69.
49. de Ponte FS, Bottini DJ, Maggi E. Prenatal diagnosis: evolution in craniofacial surgery J Craniofac Surg 1998;9:190-95.
50. Blumenfeld Z, Blumenfeld I, Bronshtein M. The early prenatal diagnosis of cleft lip and the decision-making process. Cleft Palate Craniofac J 1999;36:105-07.
51. Hallock GG. In utero cleft repair in A/J mice. Plast Reconstr Surg 1985;75:786-90.
52. Stelnicki EJ, Lee S, Hoffman W, et al. A long-term, controlled-outcome analysis of in utero versus neonatal cleft lip repair using an ovine model. Plast Reconstr Surg 1999;104:607-15.
53. Mehrara BJ, Longaker MT. New developments in craniofacial surgery research. Cleft Palate Craniofac J 1999;36:377-87.
54. Lopoo JB, Hedrick MH, Chasen S, et al. Natural history of fetuses with cleft lip. Plast Reconstr Surg 1999;103:34-38.
55. Edwards JRG, Newall DR. The Pierre Robin syndrome reassessed in the light of recent research. Br J Plast Surg 1985;38:339-42.
56. Robin P. Glossoptosis due to atresia and hypotrophy of the mandible. Am J Dis Child 1934;48:541-47.
57. Wilson AC, Moore DJ, Moore MH, et al. Late presentation of upper airway obstruction in Pierre Robin sequence. Arch Dis Child 2000;83:435-38.
58. Heaf DP, Helms PJ, Dinwiddie R, et al. Nasopharyngeal airways in Pierre Robin syndrome. J Pediatr 1982;10:698-703.
59. Masters IB, Chang AB, Harris M, et al. Modified nasopharyngeal tube for upper airway obstruction. Arch Dis Child 1999;80:186-87.
60. Dykes EH, Raine PAM, Arthur DS. Pierre Robin syndrome and pulmonary hypertension. J Pediatr Surg 1985;20:49-52.
61. Vegter F, Hage JJ, Mulder JW. Pierre Robin syndrome: mandibular growth during the first year of life. Ann Plast Surg 1999;42:154-57.
62. Jones WB. Weight gain and feeding in the neonate with cleft lip: a 3-center study. Cleft Palate J 1988;25:379-84.
63. Seth AK, McWilliams BJ. Weight gain in children with cleft palate from birth to 2 years. Cleft Palate J 1988;25:146-50.
64. Lee J, Nunn J, Wright C. Height and weight achievement in cleft lip and palate. Arch Dis Child 1997;76:70-72.
65. Clarren SK, Anderson B, Wolf LS. Feeding infants with cleft lip, cleft palate or cleft lip and palate. Cleft Palate J 1987;24:244-49.
66. PashayanHM, McNab M. Simplified method of feeding infants born with cleft palate with or without cleft lip. Am J Dis Child 1979;133:145-47.
67. Haberman M. A mother of invention. Nursing Times 1988;84:52-53.
68. Samant A. A 1-visit obturator technique for infants with cleft palate. J Oral Maxillofac Surg 1989;47:539-40.
69. Moss ALH, Jones KJ, Pigott RW. Submucous cleft palate in the differential diagnosis of feeding difficulties. Arch Dis Child 1990;65:182-84.
70. Moss ALH, Pigott RW, Jones KJ. Submucous cleft palate. BMJ 1988;297:85-86.
71. Abyholm FE. Submucous cleft palate. Scand J Plast Reconstr Surg 1976;10:209-12.
72. Garcio-Velasco M, Ysunza A, Hernandez X, et al. Diagnosis and treatment of submucous cleft palate: A review of 108 cases. Cleft Palate J 1988;25:171-73.
73. Sierra FJ, Turner C. Maxillary orthopedics in the presurgical management of infants with cleft lip and palate Ped Dent 1995;17:419-23.
74. Georgiade NG, Mason R, Riefkohl R, et al. Preoperative positioning of the protruding premaxilla in the bilateral cleft patient. Plast Reconstr Surg 1989;83:32-38.
75. Grayson BH, Cutting CB. Presurgical nasoalveolar orthopaedic molding in primary correction of the nose, lip, and alveolus of infants born with unilateral and bilateral clefts. Cleft Palate Craniofac J 2001;38:193-98.
76. Friede H, Katsaros C. Current knowledge in cleft lip and palate treatment from an orthodontist's point of view. J Orofac Orthoped 1998;59:313-30.
77. Shaw WC, Semb G. Current approaches to the orthodontic management of cleft lip and palate. J R Soc Med 1990;83:30-32.
78. Sullivan PG. Early pre-surgical treatment of the cleft palate patient. J R Soc Med 1990;83:90-93.
79. Winters JC, Hurwitz DJ. Presurgical orthopedics in the surgical management of unilateral cleft lip and palate. Plast Reconstr Surg 1995;95:755-64.
80. Moore RN. Orthodontic management of the patient with cleft lip and palate. Ear Nose Throat J 1986;65:356-67.
81. Long RE, Semb G, Shaw WC. Orthodontic treatment of the patient with complete clefts of the lip, alveolus, and palate: lessons of the past 60 years. Cleft Palate Craniofac J 2000;37:533-37.
82. Hodges SC, Hodges AM. A protocol for safe anaesthesia for cleft lip and palate surgery in developing countries. Anaesthesia 2000;55:436-41.

83. Desai SN. Cleft lip repair in the newborn baby. Ann R Coll Surg Eng 1990;72:101-03.
84. Asher-McDade C, Shaw WC. Current cleft lip and palate management in the United Kingdom. Br J Plast Surg 1990;43:318-21.
85. le Mesurier AB. Method of cutting and suturing the lip in complete unilateral cleft lip. Plast Reconstr Surg 1949;4:1-12.
86. Tennison CW. The repair of the unilateral cleft lip by the stencil method. Plast Reconstr Surg 1952;9:115-20.
87. Millard DR. Complete unilateral clefts of the lip. Plast Reconstr Surg 1960;25:595-605.
88. Trier WC (a). Repair of unilateral cleft lip: the rotation advancement operation. Clin Plast Surg 1985;12:573-94.
89. Friede H. Growth sites and growth mechanisms at risk in cleft lip and palate Acta Odont Scand 1998;56:46-51.
90. Adcock S, Markus AF. Midfacial growth following functional cleft surgery. Br J Oral Maxillofac Surg 1997;35:1-5.
91. McComb HK, Coghlan BA. Primary repair of the unilateral cleft lip nose: completion of a longitudinal study. Cleft Palate Craniofac J 1996;33:23-31.
92. de la Torre JI, Gallagher PM, Douglas BK, et al. Repairing the cleft lip nasal deformity. Cleft Palate Craniofac J 2000;37:234-42.
93. Schendel SA. Unilateral cleft lip repair-state of the art. Cleft Palate Craniofac J 2000;37:335-41.
94. Black PW. Bilateral cleft lip. Clin Plast Surg 1985;12:627-41.
95. Trier WC (b). Repair of bilateral cleft lip: Millard's technique Clin Plast Surg 1985;12:605-25.
96. Mulliken JB. Repair of the bilateral complete cleft lip and nasal deformity - state of the art. Cleft Palate Craniofac J 2000;37:342-47.
97. Pigott RW. Objectives for cleft palate repair. Ann Plast Surg 1987;19:247-59.
98. LaRossa D. The state of the art in cleft palate surgery. Cleft Palate Craniofac J 2000;37:225-28.
99. Dellon AL. Are we selling the cleft palate short? Ann Plast Surg 1988;21:399-400.
100. Muir IFK. Maxillary development in cleft palate patients with particular reference to the effects of operation. Ann Roy Coll Surg Eng 1986;58:63-67.
101. Yonkers AH, Moore GF. Surgical management of clefts. Ear Nose Throat J 1986;65:368-75.
102. Lambadusuriya SP, Mars M, Ward CM. Sri Lankan cleft lip and palate project: a preliminary report. J R Soc Med 1988;81:705-09.
103. Sommerlad BC. Surgical management of cleft palate: A review. J R Soc Med 1989;82:677-78.
104. Marrinan EM, LaBrie RA, Mulliken JB. Velopharyngeal function in nonsyndromic cleft palate: relevance of surgical technique, age at repair, and cleft type. Cleft Palate Craniofac J 1998;35:95-100.
105. Nandlal B, Tewari A, Utreja AK, et al. Effects of variation of the timing of palatal repair on nasality of speech in complete cleft lip and palate children. J Ind Soc Pedod Prev Dent 1999;17:146-49.
106. Furlow LT. Cleft palate repair by double reversing Z-plasty. Plast Reconstr Surg 1986;78:724-36.
107. Gunther E, Wisser JR, Cohen MA, et al. Palatoplasty: Furlow's double reversing Z-plasty versus intravelar veloplasty. Cleft Palate Craniofac J 1998;35:546-49.
108. Pensler JM, Bauer BS. Levator repositioning and palate lengthening for submucous clefts. Plast Reconstr Surg 1988;82:765-69.
109. Seagle MB, Patti CS, Williams WN, et al. Submucous cleft palate: a 10 year series. Ann Plast Surg 1999;42:142-48.
110. Witt PD, Wahlen JC, Marsh JL, et al. The effect of surgeon on velopharyngeal function and outcome following palatoplasty: is there a learning curve? Plast Reconstr Surg 1998;102:1375-84.
111. Molsted K. Treatment outcome in cleft lip and palate; issues and perspectives. Crit Rev in Oral Biol and Med 1999;10:225-39.
112. Habel A, Sell D, Mars M. Management of cleft lip and palate. Arch Dis Child 1996;74:360-66.
113. Sandy JR, Williams AC, Bearn D, et al. Cleft lip and palate care in the United Kingdom; the Clinical Standards Advisory Group (CSAG) study. Part 1: background and methodology. Cleft Palate Craniofac J 2001;38:20-23.
114. Wyatt R, Sell D, Russell J, et al. Cleft palate speech dissected; a review of current knowledge and analysis. Br J Plast Surg 1996;49:143-49.
115. Trost-Cardamone JE. Coming to terms with velo-pharyngeal incompetence: a response to Loney and Bloem. Cleft Palate J 1989;26:68-70.
116. Seyfer AE, Simon CD. Long-term results following the repair of palatal clefts: a comparison of three different techniques. Plast Reconstr Surg 1989;83:785-90.
117. Grobbelaar AO, Hudson DA, Fernandes DB, et al. Speech results after repair of the cleft soft palate Plast Reconstr Surg 1995;95:1150-54.
118. Kuehn DP, Molloer KT. The state of the art: speech and language issues in the cleft palate population. Cleft Palate Craniofac J 2000;37:348.
119. Myklebost O, Abyholm FE. Speech results in cleft lip and palate patients operated on with a von Langenbeck palatal closure. Scand J Plast Reconstr Surg 1989;23:71-74.
120. Enemark H, Boland S, Jorgensen I. Evaluation of unilateral cleft lip and palate treatment: long-term results. Cleft Palate J 1990;27:354-61.
121. Grant HR, Quiney RE, Mercer DM, et al. Cleft palate and glue ear. Arch Dis Child 1988;63:176-79.
122. Garcia RG, Burton EH, Norris TW. Audiological management of the patient with cleft palate Ear Nose Throat J 1986;65:342-45.
123. Gould HJ. Hearing loss and cleft palate: the perspective of time. CPJ 1990;27:36-39.
124. Jocelyn LJ, Penko MA, Rode H. Cognition, communication, and hearing in young children with cleft lip and palate and in control children; a longitudinal study. Pediatrics 1996;97:529-34.
125. Kantorwicz GF. Role of the restorative dentist in the management of cleft palate patients: discussion paper. J R Soc Med 1990;83:29.

126. Mars M, Plint DA, Houston WJB, et al. The Goslon yardstick: a new system of assessing dental arch relationship in children with unilateral clefts of lip and palate. Cleft Palate J 1987;24:314-22.
127. DeLuke DM, Marchand A, Robles EC, et al. Facial growth and the need for orthognathic surgery after cleft palate repair: literature review and report of 28 cases. J Oral Maxillofac Surg 1997;55:694-97.
128. Cronin TD, Denkler KA. Correction of the unilateral cleft lip nose. Plast Reconstr Surg 1988;82:419-31.
129. Pigott RW. Aesthetic considerations related to repair of the bilateral cleft lip nasal deformity. B J Plast Surg 1988;41:593-607.
130. Argamosa RV. The pharyngeal flap. in: Kernahan DA, Rosenstein SW (Eds.) Cleft lip and palate: a system of management. Williams and Wilkins, Baltimore 1990; 263-69.
131. Jackson IT. Sphincter pharyngoplasty. Clin Plast Surg 1985;12:711-17.
132. Orticochea M. Physiopathology of the dynamic muscular sphincter of the pharynx. Plast Reconstr Surg 1997;100:1919-23.
133. Sloan GM. Posterior pharyngeal flap and sphincter pharyngoplasty: the state of the art. Cleft Palate Craniofac J 2000;37:112-22.
134. Eppley BL, Sadove AM. Management of alveolar cleft bone grafting - state of the art Cleft Palate Craniofac J 2000;37:229-33.
135. Pope AW, Speltz ML. Research on psychological issues of children with craniofacial anomalies; progress and challenges. Cleft Palate Craniofac J 1997;34:371-73.
136. Endriga MA, Kapp-Simon KA. Psychological issues in craniofacial care: state of the art. Cleft Palate Craniofac J 1999;36:3-11.
137. Turner SR, Thomas PWN, Dowell T, et al. Psychological outcomes amongst cleft patients and their families. Br J Plast Surg 1997;50:1-9.
138. Williams AC, Bearn D, Clark JD, et al. The delivery of surgical cleft care in the United Kingdom. J R Coll Surg Edinb 2001;46:143-49.

CHAPTER 106

Neck Anomalies

B Mukhopadhyay, SK Mitra

Neck masses, sinuses and fistulae are a frequent occurrence in pediatric surgical practice. By recording detailed history, careful clinical examination, by understanding the embryology of branchial arches and anatomy of its derivatives, the surgeon may arrive at a proper diagnosis on clinical grounds in most of the cases.

CONGENITAL LESIONS

The pharyngeal region, because of its complexity and its phylogenetic significance, has received more attention from embryologists than have most other regions of the body. Von Bear first described the clefts of the human embryo.[1,2] Von Acherson related cervical cysts to anomalous closure of the clefts.[1,2] Phylogenetically, the branchial apparatus is related to gill slits. In fish and amphibians, these structures are responsible for the development of the gills (Branchia is Greek for gills). The word pharyngeal is often substituted for branchial, because humans do not develop gills.

At the fourth week of embryonic life, the development of 4 branchial (or pharyngeal) clefts results in 5 ridges known as the branchial or pharyngeal arches (Fig. 106.1). They contribute to the formation of various structures of the head, neck and thorax. The fifth and the sixth arches are believed to be rudimentary (Fig. 106.2).[3] The second arch grows

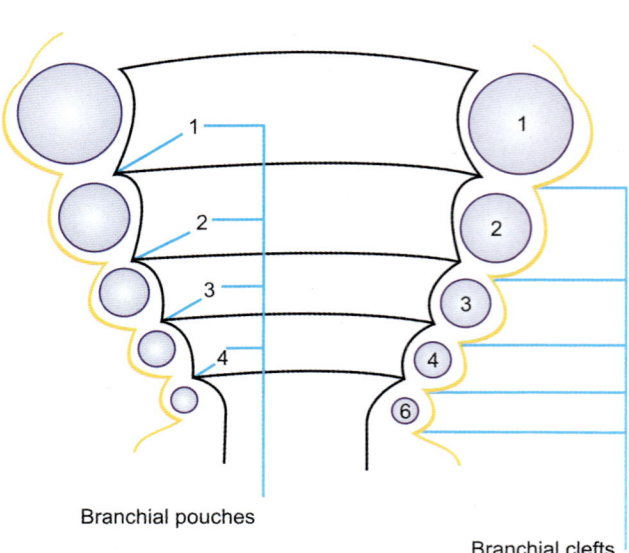

Fig. 106.1: Branchial arches and clefts

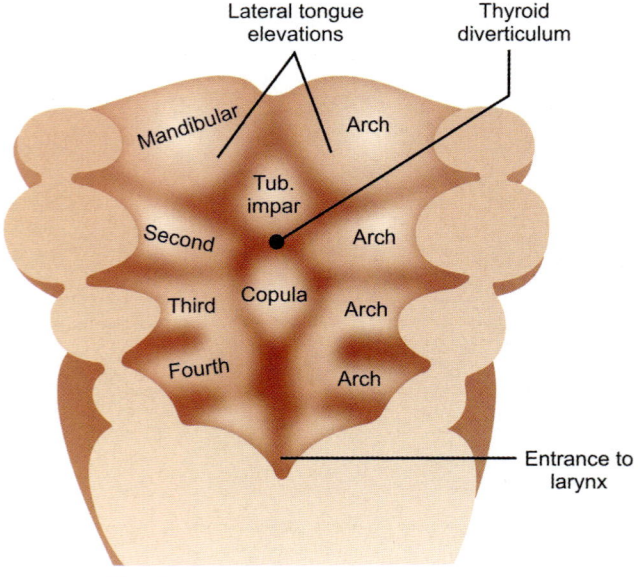

Fig. 106.2: Embryogenesis of branchial structures and thyroid

caudally and ultimately covers the third and the fourth arches. The buried clefts become ectoderm lined cavities which normally involute around 7th week of development. If a portion of the cleft fails to disappear completely, the entrapped remnant forms an epithelium lined cyst with or without a sinus tract to the overlying skin.

Cystic and Fistular Remnants of the Branchial Apparatus

Different types of cysts, sinuses and fistulae can arise from the incomplete obliteration of embryonic spaces of transitory branchial apparatus of the embryo.

First Cleft Defects

The earliest classification of first branchial cleft defects was published by Arnot in 1971 and was primarily based on the anatomical location of the defect.[4] In a simpler classification proposed by Olsen et al, a first branchial cleft anomaly need only be labeled as a cyst, a sinus or a fistula.[5] This classification was designed to facilitate preoperative decisions about surgical approach. Anomalies of the first branchial cleft have been reported to be around 8 to 10%.[6,7] It has been reported that cystic lesions are more common in adults and fistulas and sinuses are more commonly seen in children.[5,8] The patient may present as a preauricular swelling or sinus, as a mass in the external auditory canal or as a discharge from the ear (Fig. 106.3). The internal openings for both the sinuses or fistulae are found to terminate along any portion of the external auditory canal with antero inferior bony – cartilaginous junction being the most common site.[5] When a patient requires repeated incisions and drainage procedures in the pre auricular region or parotid region, one should suspect the possibility of a first branchial cleft anomaly.[9] The investigations like sonogram, CT scan or MR imaging are of limited value.[10,11] Various conditions like inflammatory lymphadenitis, dermoid cysts, cystic hygroma, hemangioma, lymphoma are to be differentiated from first branchial cleft anomaly. Operation can be done only after the infection has been controlled. During surgery the anomalous tract may run lateral to,[12] medial to or even directly through the main trunk of the facial nerve.[12,13] The surgeon must be aware also that the tract may involve the middle ear.[5] Recurrence

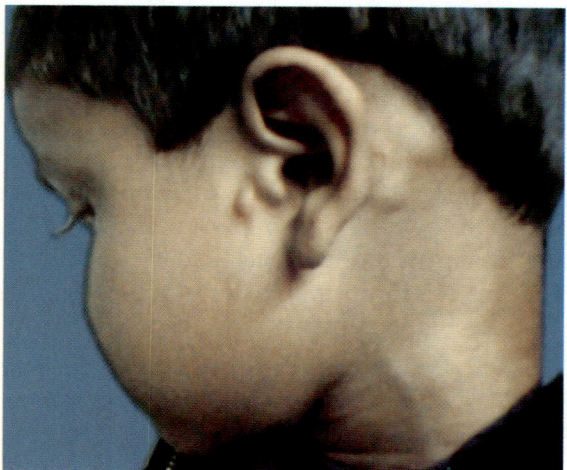

Fig. 106.3: Preauricular cyst

is uncommon after complete excision.[14] Higher incidence of recurrence have been reported in patients with pre-existing fibrosis from prior infections and surgery.[10]

Congenital Auricular Pits

They represent ectodermal folds sequestrated during the fusion of the six tubercles. These pits or sinuses are lined by skin and are usually only few millimeters deep but they may be longer, tortuous and branched. They appear to be bilateral in 33% of patients and when unilateral, more common on the left side.[15] These sinuses may be familial. They are said be associated with congenital nasal fistulae and with deafness and branchial cleft anomalies in the same pedigree.[16] Preauricular pits and sinuses are present from birth and most of the time there is history of recurrent infection.

Prior infection increases the difficulty of complete surgical excision and increases the risk of recurrence.[17] Complete surgical excision of the sinus tract up to temporalis fascia should be done. During excision, one should search for branches from the main tract. Recurrence rate as high as 42% has been reported particularly in the presence of multiple branches.[18]

Cervicoaural Fistulae, Sinuses and Cysts

Cervicoaural fistula represents the persistence of the ventral end of the first branchial cleft (the external auditory canal represents the dorsal end). It is lined with skin and extends from the neck below the ear to the styloid process and carotid sheath and open into the external auditory canal. In some cases the tract reaches the canal but does not actually open into it. The tract usually passes over the facial nerve (a component of the second arch) but may also pass under the nerve. The anomaly usually presents as a swelling below the ear or as an infected sinus. Treatment consists of complete excision of the sinus tract or cyst. It is important to note that the facial nerve may be displaced upward or downward by the anomalous tract and must be identified to prevent injury to the facial nerve.[19,20]

Second Cleft and Pouch Defects

Sixty seven to ninety percent of all branchial anomalies are due to defects of the second branchial cleft and pouch.[21] Most complete branchial fistulae derive from the ventral portion of the second branchial cleft and pharyngeal pouch. Typically the external opening is in the lower third of the neck on the line of the anterior border of the sternocleidomastoid muscle. The fistula courses through the subcutaneous tissues, the platysma and penetrates the deep fascia to reach the carotid sheath. Above the hyoid bone, the tract turns medially beneath the stylohyoid and the posterior belly of digastric muscle. It passes in front of the hypoglossal nerve, between the internal and external

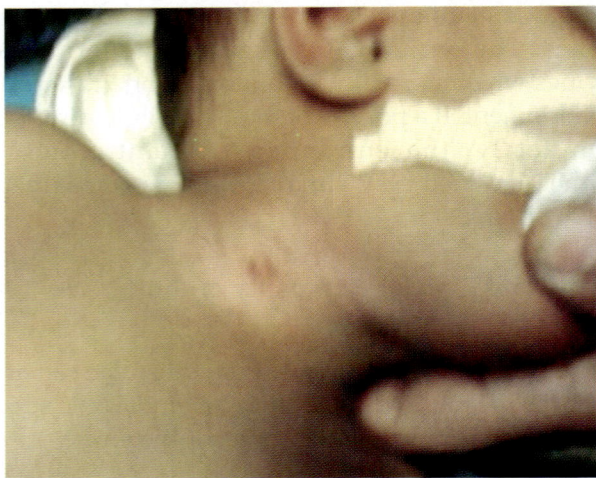

Fig. 106.5: Branchial sinus right side

carotid arteries and over the glossopharyngeal nerve, deep to the stylohyoid ligament, to enter the pharynx as a slit on the anterior side of the upper half of the posterior pillar of the fauces (Fig. 106.4). Occasionally, the opening is in the supratonsillar fossa or even in the tonsil itself.

The branchial sinus or fistula is usually noticed at or shortly after birth (Fig. 106.5).[22] In one series, 78% of second arch sinuses and fistulae were diagnosed at the age of 5 years.[10] Mucous discharge from the sinus opening along the anterior border of sternomastoid muscle between the hyoid bone and the supra sternal notch is the classical presentation.[23] A complete fistula from the external skin to the tonsillar fossa is rare.[10] Bilateral branchial sinuses are occasionally encountered.[10] Family history is positive in as high as 6% of patients.[10] In approximately 5% of patients, there is associated preauricular sinus.[10] Most authors believe that the role of preoperative imaging in second arch defects is not helpful.

Excision of the whole tract is the only curative method. The tract should be excised with an adequate amount of supporting stroma to increase the likelihood that all epithelial tissue is removed. The step ladder technique is often used to gain surgical access to the entire tract. In addition to recurrence, transient injury to hypoglossal nerve has been reported.[21]

Sinuses Opening at the Surface

External sinus tract are rare. They usually arise from the anterior border of the sternocleidomastoid muscle and terminate in a cystic dilatation.

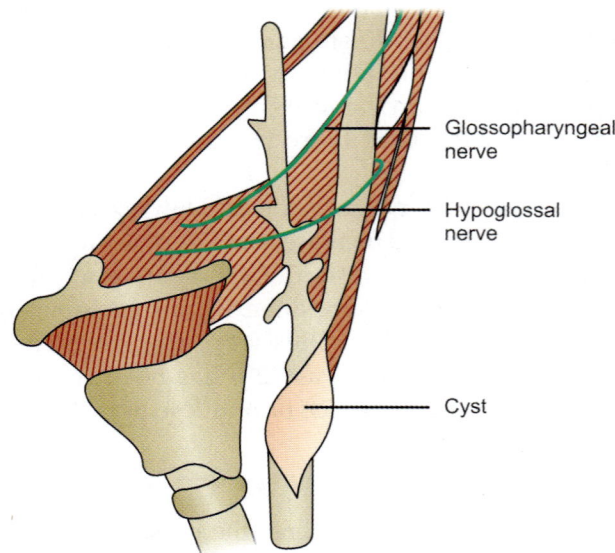

Fig. 106.4: Nerves related to branchial sinus

Neck Anomalies

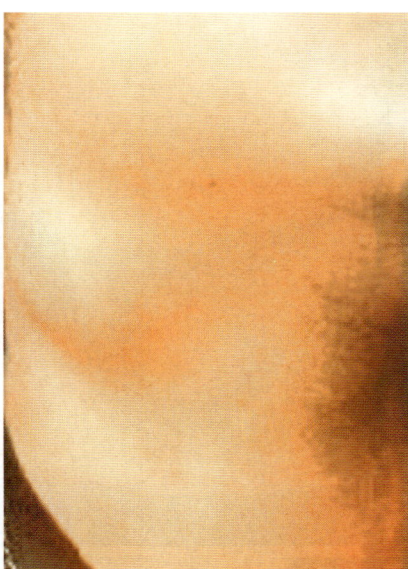

Fig. 106.6: Branchial cyst

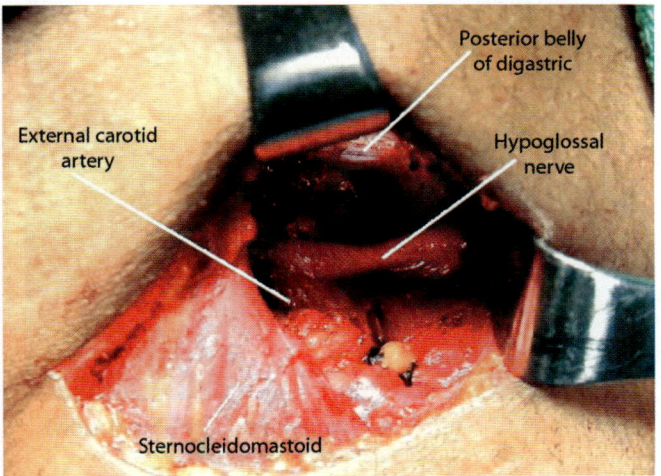

Fig. 106.7: Operative picture after removal of branchial cyst

Cysts

The deepest of the second pouch cysts are rare and present as swellings that bulge into the nasopharynx. They are derived from the dorsal portion of the second pouch. Branchial cleft cysts are three times more common than branchial fistulae.[23]

They tend to present at a later age than fistulae or sinuses, usually in the second decade of life.[22,24] The incidence of bilateral lesions is reported as 2%.[25] Most of the patients present with a painless, smooth lump typically located along the upper third of the anterior border of the sternocleidomastoid muscle (Fig. 106.6).[22] The patient may present with infection, pain and pressure symptoms like dyspnoea or dysphagia.[26] An infected cyst may progress to frank abscess formation, rupture leading either to sinus formation or recurrent cyst formation. The treatment of branchial cyst is to complete surgical excision with preservation of surrounding neurovascular structures (Fig. 106.7). Recurrence ranging from 3 to 21% has been reported.[27] With higher incidence in patients with history of previous surgery. Infection and prior operation cause adhesions and distortion of tissue planes, which may lead to higher chances of recurrence and increased risk of damage to adjacent nerves and vessels.[22]

Third Cleft and Pouch Defects

Complete fistulae of the third cleft and pouch are not known to occur. Cysts lying deep to the internal carotid artery and intimately associated with the vagus nerve are probably remnants of the third cleft or pouch. The incidence of third branchial anomalies is 2 to 8% and fourth branchial arch anomalies 1 to 2% of all branchial anomalies.[28]

A complete third arch and pouch fistula starts at the pyriform fossa of the hypopharynx and pierce the thyroid membrane. The tract would pass superficial to the hypoglossal nerve, deep to the glossopharyngeal nerve and the internal carotid artery and then pierce the platysma to exit in the lower neck in line with the anterior border of the sternocleidomastoid muscle. The termination of the anomalous tract at the thyroid gland near the superior parathyroid gland suggest fourth pouch origin. Fourth pouch anomalies are diagnosed mostly in childhood and 97% of them occur on the left side.[29] The lesion may present even in neonates as lateral neck cysts or abscess with associated obstructive airway symptoms.[30] The diagnostic evaluation centers on determining the presence of a sinus tract originating from the pyriform fossa. Plain X-ray may show air inside the cyst. Flexible fiberoptic nasopharyngoscopy is very helpful. Other investigations which are also helpful to localize the sinus opening are direct laryngoscopy and pharyngo esophagogram. The role of CT scan is also helpful. Complete excision including the piriform fossa attachment is the treatment of choice.

Thyroglossal Cyst and Sinus

Thyroglossal cysts are tubuloembryonic cysts formed due to persistence of the thyroglossal duct. During 4th to 7th week of intrauterine life, the thyroid diverticulum develops at the base of the tongue near foramen cecum and descends in the midline. The tract passes ventral to the 2nd arch mesenchyme from which hyoid develops and may arch anteriorly around the body of the hyoid bone. Normally the tract is obliterated once the thyroid gland reaches its final position. Persistence of the tract leads to the development of cysts which may be located anywhere along the line of descent of the thyroid gland.

Positions of the Cysts

Thyroglossal duct cyst never have a primary external opening because embryologically the tract does not reach the surface of the neck. Ectopic thyroid tissue is identified within the thyroglossal duct remnant in about 62% of patients.[31] The diagnostic features of thyroglossal cysts are midline swelling which move on swallowing and on protrusion of tongue. However, 10 to 42% of patients, cysts are located laterally and frequently to the left.[32,33] Nearly 50% of the thyroglossal cysts present in the first 2 decades of life.[32] Most of the cysts present in the midline (Fig. 106.8A,B). Majority of the patients present as cyst and remainder may present with sinus, either due to spontaneous rupture after infection or following incision and drainage. Anatomically, the cyst may be adjacent to the hyoid bone (60%), above the hyoid bone (24%), below the hyoid bone (13%) and intralingual (8%) (Fig. 106.9).[32] The different conditions which need to be differentiated from thyroglossal cyst are subhyoid bursitis (does not move up on protrusion of tongue but most of the time difficult to differentiate clinically), sublingual dermoid (does not move on swallowing and on protrusion), midline lipoma, enlarged lymph node. Carcinoma arising from the thyroglossal cyst is rare. Allard reported an age range from 6 years to 81 years with a mean age of 39.2 years.

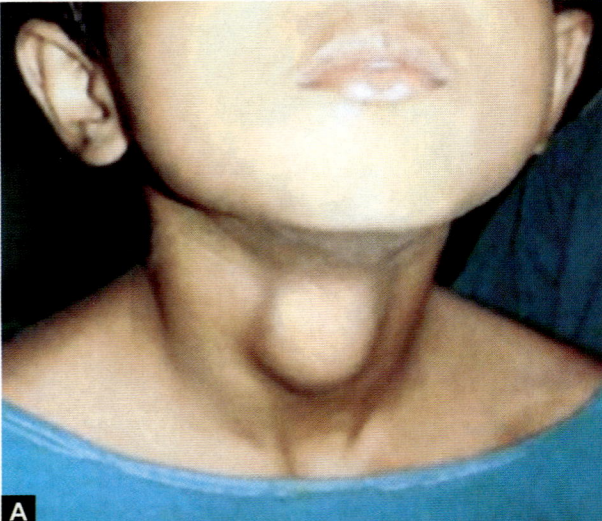
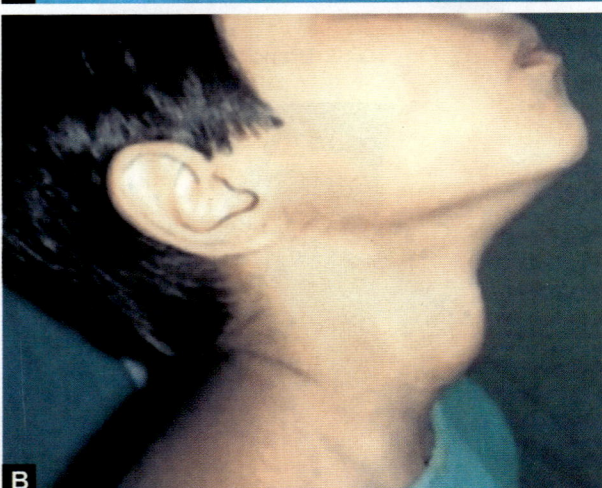

Figs 106.8A and B: A. Thyroglossal cyst (Front view) **B.** Thyroglossal cyst (Lateral view)

Investigation

Preoperative evaluation of a thyroglossal cyst includes a thorough clinical examination, thyroid function test usually TSH estimation. La Rouere MJ et al recommended several criteria for doing thyroid scan in thyroglossal cyst particularly if there is suspicion of an ectopic thyroid tissue or a palpable mass within the cyst.[34] Ultrasonography is being used quite frequently. While fine needle aspiration cytology is frequently done in thyroid nodule, it has not been evaluated for thyroglossal cyst.[35]

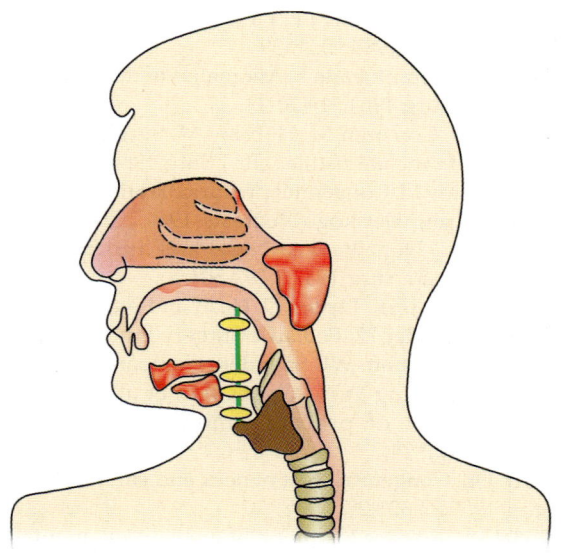

Fig. 106.9: Various positions of the thyroglossal cyst

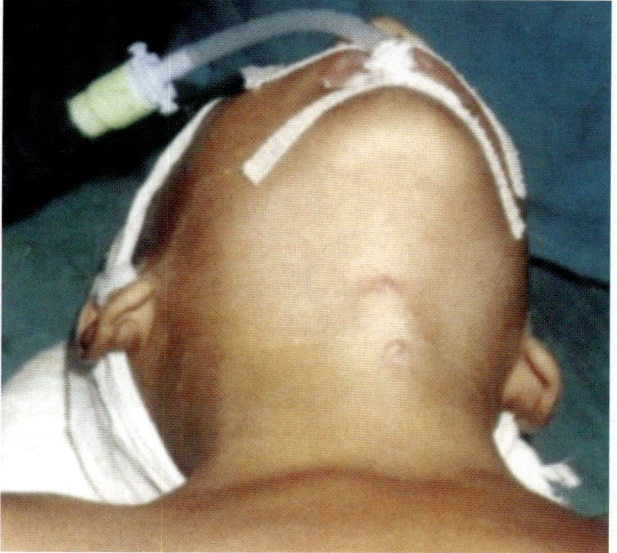

Fig. 106.10: Thyroglossal sinus

Surgical Treatment

Complete excision of the cyst and the sinus tract is the treatment of choice (Fig. 106.10). Sistrunk first described the classical procedure of excision of the tract along with a core of tissue around it and central portion of the body of the hyoid bone.[36] Recurrence rate of 5 to 7% have been reported but the rate is high if the adjacent hyoid is not excised.[32,33]

Ethanol Injection Sclerotherapy for Thyroglossal Cyst

There are reports of treating thyroglossal cyst with ethanol injection sclerotherapy.[37,38] Injection is given under sonographic guidance. Following selection criteria are met before injection:
1. Cytologic studies show that the lesion is benign.
2. Cystographic studies indicate that there is no extravasation.
3. A monocystic lesion is present.

The result is reported to be satisfactory.[39]

Dermoid Cyst

Dermoid cyst result due to entrapment of epithelium during the closure of branchial arches.[40,41] Most common differential diagnosis is the thyroglossal cyst and the correct diagnosis is made during surgery. Dermoid cyst contains hair follicles, sebaceous glands, connective tissue and other epidermal appendages.[42] Complete excision along with the capsule is curative.

Cervical Thymic Cyst

Thymic swelling may present as lump and pain in the neck.[43] Nests of thymic tissue may be found along the descent of the thymic primordia from the angle of the mandible to the mediastinum. Mediastinal extension is seen in 50% of cervical thymic cysts.[44]

Ultrasound and CT scan are both helpful investigations for diagnosis and planning for surgical management.[45] Surgical excision is the treatment of choice.

Ranula

The word Ranula means Frog's belly (Ranula is very soft and bluish in color simulating frog's belly. The word Rana means frog).

Ranula is a retention cyst arises due to partial obstruction of the sublingual salivary gland.[46] The cyst is lined by columnar or cuboidal epithelium and contain mucoid fluid. The patient presents with a cystic swelling on the undersurface of the tongue (Fig. 106.11). It is bluish in color due to the presence of sublingual veins. Fluctuation is positive and the cyst is brilliantly transilluminant. When localized inside the

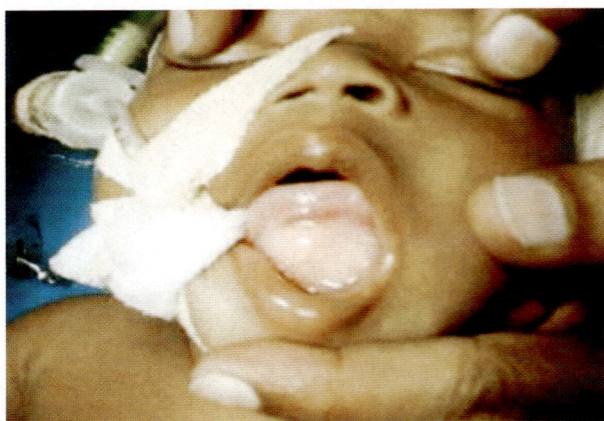

Fig. 106.11: Ranula

oral cavity, it is termed as simple ranula. When the ranula extends into the neck from the oral cavity along the posterior border of Mylohyoid, it is called a plunging or complex ranula. This lesion lacks a true epithelial lining.[47] Marsupialization of the cyst is the most common performed for ranula.[48] Plunging ranula may be excised either orally or combined intraoral and cervical approach.[48] Excision of the cyst along with the ipsilateral sublingual salivary gland has been shown to decrease the rate of recurrence.

REFERENCES

1. Mandell DL. Head and Neck Anomalies related to the Branchial Apparatus. Otolaryngologic Clinics of North America 2000;33(6):1-19.
2. Simpson RA. Lateral cervical cysts and fistulas. Laryngoscope 1969;79:30-59.
3. Nancy P, Aumount GC, Bobin et al. Fistulae of the fourth endobranchial pouch. Int J Pediatr Otorhinolaryngolo 1988;16:157-65.
4. Arnot RS. Defects of the first branchial cleft. S Afr J Surg 1980;9:93-98.
5. Olsen KD, Maragos NE, Weiland LH. First branchial cleft anomalies. Laryngoscope 1980;90:423-36.
6. Clevens RA, Weimert TA. Familial Bilateral Branchial cleft cysts. Ear Nose Throat J 1995;74:419-21.
7. O' Mara W, Amedee RG. Anomalies of the branchial apparatus. L La State Med Soc 1998;150:570-73.
8. Doi O, Hutson JM, Myers NA, et al. Branchial remnants: A review of 58 cases. J Pediatr Surg 1988;23:789-92.
9. Mc Rae RG, Lee KJ, Goertzen E. First branchial cleft anomalies and the facial nerve. Otolaryngol Head Neck Surg 1983;91:197-202.
10. Ford GR, Balakrishnan A, Evans JNG, et al. Branchial cleft and pouch anomalies. J Laryngol Otol 1992;106:137-43.
11. Randall P, Royster HP. First branchial cleft anomalies. Plast Reconstr Surg 1963;31:497-506.
12. Belenky W M, Medina J E. First branchial cleft anomalies. Laryngoscope 1980;90:28-39.
13. Crymble B, Braithwaite F. Anomalies of the first branchial cleft. Br J Surg 1964;51:420-23.
14. Miller PD, Corcoran M, Hobsley M. Surgical excision of first cleft branchial fistulae. Br J Surg 1984;71:696-97.
15. Shcherbatov I I. Congenital preauricular fistulae. Voprosy Otorinolaring Detskogo Vozrasta 1964;2:55-64.
16. Brunner H, Donelly WA. Nasal and auricular fistulae. Plast Reconstr Surg 1947;2:497-504.
17. Waldhausen JHT, Tapper D. Head and Neck sinuses and masses, Chapter 72: Pediatric Surgery Edited by Ashcraft KW, third edition, WB Saunders Company, 2000;987-99.
18. Currie AR, King WW, Vlantis AC, et al. Pitfalls in the management of pre auricular sinuses. Br J Surg 1996;83:1722-24.
19. Stark DB. Congenital tract of neck and ear. Plast Reconstr Surg 1959;23:621-27.
20. Ronald P, Royster HP. First branchial cleft anomalies. A not-so-rare and potentially dangerous condition. Plast Reconstr Surg 1963;31:497-506.
21. Agaton-Bonilla FC, Gay-Escoda C. Diagnosis and treatment of branchial cleft cysts and fistulae. A retrospective study of 183 patients. Int J Oral Maxillofac Surg 1996;25:449-52.
22. Chandler JR, Mitchell B. Branchial cleft cysts, sinuses and fistulas. Otolaryngol Clin North Am 1981;14:175-86.
23. Procter B, Procter C. Congenital lesions of the head and neck. Otolaryngol Clin North Am 1970;3: 221-48.
24. Chinoh EH, Pham VH, Cooke RA, et al. Aetiology of branchial cysts. Aust N Z J Surg 1989;59:949-51.
25. Maran AGD, Buchanan DR. Branchial cysts, sinuses and fistulae. Clin Otolaryngo 1978;l 3:77-92.
26. Androulakis M, Johnson JT, Wagner RL. Thyroglossal duct and second branchial cleft anomalies in adults. Ear Nose Throat J 1990;69:318-22.
27. Deane S A, Telander RL. Surgery for thyroglossal duct and branchial cleft anomalies. Am J Surg 1978;136: 348-53.
28. Choi SS, Zalzal GH. Branchial anomalies: A review of 52 cases. Laryngoscope 1995;105: 909-13.
29. Miller D, Hill JL, Sun C, et al. The diagnosis and management of pyriform sinus fistulae in infants and young children . J Pediatr Surg 1983;18:377-81.
30. Burge D, Middleton A. Persistent pharyngeal pouch derivatives in the neonate. J Pediatr Surg 1983;18:230-34.
31. Li Volsi VA, Perzin KH, Savetsky L. Ectopic thyroid (including thyroglossal duct tissue). Cancer 1974;34: 1303-15.
32. Allard RHB. The thyroglossal cyst. Head and Neck Surg 1982;5:134-46.
33. Pollock WF. Cysts and sinuses of the thyroglossal duct. Am J Surg 1966;122:225-29.
34. La Rouere MJ, Drake AF, Baker SR, et al. Evaluation and management of a carcinoma arising in a thyroglossal duct cyst. Am J Otolaryngol 1987;8:351-55.

35. Hilgar AW, Thompson S D, Smallman L A, et al. Papillary carcinoma arising in a thyroglossal duct cyst : A case report and literature review. J laryngol Otol 1995;109:1124- 27.
36. Sistrunk WE. The surgical treatment of cysts of the thyroglossal tract. Ann Surg 1928;71:121-22.
37. Yasuda K, et al. Treatment of cystic lesions of the thyroid by ethanol instillation. World J 1992;16 (5):958-61.
38. Fukumoto K, et al. Ethanol injection sclerotherapy for Baker's cyst, thyroglossal duct cyst, brachial cleft cyst. Ann Plast Surg 1994;33(6):615-19.
39. Monazani F, et al. Percutaneous aspiration and ethanol sclerotherapy for thyroid cyst. J Cli Endocrinol Metab 1994;78(3):800-02.
40. McAvoy JM, Zuckerbraun L. Dermoid cysts of the head and neck in children. Arch Otolaryngol 1976;102:529-31.
41. Gold BC, Skeinkopf DE, Levy B. Dermoid , epidermoid and teratomatous cysts of the tongue and the floor of the mouth. J Oral Surg 1974;32:107-11.
42. Reede DL, Whelan AM, Gengeron RT. C T of the soft tissue structures of the neck. Radiologic Clinics of North America 1984;22(1):239-50.
43. Nguen Q, Tar M de, et al. Cervical thymic cyst: Case reports and review of literature. Laryngoscope 1996;106:247-52.
44. Jones JE, Hession B. Cervical thymic cysts. Ear Nose and Throat J 1996;75(10):678-80.
45. Quick CA, Lowell SH. Ranula and the sublingual salivary glands. Arch Orolaryngol 1977;103:397-400.
46. Khafif RA, Schwartz A, Friedman E. The plunging ranula. J oral Surg 1975;33:537-41.
47. Roediger WE, Kay S. Pathogenesis and treatment of plunging ranulas. Surg Gynaecol Obstet 1977;144:862-64.
48. Baurmash HD. Marsupialization for treatment of oral ranula : A second look at the procedure. J Oral Maxillofac Surg 1992;50:1274-79.

CHAPTER 107

Torticollis

DK Gupta, Manish Pathak, Shilpa Sharma

Torticollis is a Latin word. Torti, meaning twisted, and Collis, meaning neck. Torticollis refers to twisted position of neck. Congenital torticollis is the most common cause of torticollis. Incidence is about 0.4% of all births.[1-2] Right side is affected more commonly than the left side (60%).[3] Two to eight percent of cases have bilateral involvement.[1,2,4]

ETIOLOGY

Torticollis is broadly divided into two types, congenital and acquired (Table 107.1). Congenital or idiopathic spasmodic torticollis is the most common cause of torticollis. It is due to the tightness or shortening of sternomastoid muscle on one side. The etiology of acquired torticollis is varied. It includes cervical hemivertebrae, strabismus, retropharyngeal abscess, posterior fossa tumor, and severe gastroesopharyngeal reflux (Sandifer's syndrome). Acquired torticollis may also occur due to acute atlantoaxial subluxation of the joint during tonsillectomy.

There are various theories to explain the etiology of congenital torticolllis.
1. Intrauterine embryopathy[5]
2. Intrauterine compression—according to this theory intrauterine compression of neck leads to sternomastoid fibrosis.[6-8]
3. Traumatic delivery—20-30% of patients with torticollis are delivered by breech delivery. According to this theory traumatic delivery leads to muscle injury with hemorrhage and fibrous replacement of the sternomastoid muscle.[6-11]
4. Neoplastic— there is little or no evidence to support this theory.

None of the theory is able to answer all the questions. Presence of mature fibrous tissue in sternomastoid tumor of neonates indicates that the process of fibrous replacement of muscle starts in the intrauterine period only.[5,12]

PATHOPHYSIOLOGY

The common histological finding is the fibrous replacement of the muscle bundles. Endomycial fibrosis with fibrous encasement of individual muscle bundles leads to muscle atrophy.[5] Sernat et al studied biopsy of the sternocleidomastoid muscle in children with idiopathic torticollis.[13] They noted extensive fibrosis and nonspecific myopathic changes, i.e.

Table 107.1: Etiology of torticollis

A. Congenital torticollis (sternomastoid tumor/fibrosis)	Commonest
B. Acquired torticollis	
1. Cervical hemivertebrae	Confirmed by plain radiograph
2. Imbalance of ocular muscles	Squint manifests on passive straightening of neck
3. Retropharyngeal abscess	Acute; dysphagia, dyspnea
4. Atlantoaxial subluxation	Acute; may occur following tonsillectomy
5. Posterior fossa tumor	Frozen neck
6. Gastroesophageal reflux	Sandifer's syndrome

cytoarchitectural alteration, necrosis, and focal inflammation, mainly in the sternal head of the muscle. The atrophic changes were noted predominantly in the clavicular head. The ultrastructural studies done by Mickelson et al using electron microscope revealed a marked increase in interstitial collagen deposition.[14] Features of immobilization degeneration were also noted with nearly complete loss of myofibrils. Histology has also demonstrated that the fibrous tissue even at neonatal age is mature.[5,12] The maturity of fibrous tissue at neonatal age indicates that the process of fibrosis had started during the intrauterine period. Sternomastoid fibrosis may prevent the engagement of head during delivery. Thus the high incidence of breech delivery (~20-30%) may be the result of sternomastoid fibrosis rather than being the cause.[6,8]

CLINICAL FEATURES

Sternomastoid torticollis may present as sternomastoid tumor in about two-third of cases, other one-third of the patients have fibrosis but no tumor. Typically this mass or misnomerly called as the tumor, is not present at the time of birth, but is noted at 3-6 weeks of age.[2,4] The tumor is hard and painless. The swelling is located within the substance of the sternomastoid muscle, usually in the middle. Size of the tumor varies from 1-3 cm. In the other group of patients, though, the mass is not palpable but a thickened sternomastoid muscle can be palpated along its whole length.

The infant has the characteristic posture; head is rotated to the opposite side of the tumor and tilted towards the ipsilateral shoulder. Older children compensate the head tilt by elevating the ipsilateral shoulder. This maneuver helps them to keep the eyes horizontal.

On clinical examination restricted movement of neck to the ipsilateral side of the involved muscle can be noted. Infant is made to lie at the edge of couch. Assistant holds the shoulders firmly against the surface. Examiner stands behind the patient and tries to rotate the head on either side. Movement of head on ipsilateral side is restricted due to the fibrotic shortening of muscle. When examining the patient with torticollis, one should always do the complete physical examination including palpation of cervical spine, ophthalmological, and neurological examination.

CLASSIFICATION

There are various classifications based either on clinical findings or on ultrasonographic findings.[10,15-17]

Clinically Torticollis can be Classified into Three Types

1. Palpable sternomastoid tumor.
2. Muscular torticollis (thickening and tightness of the sternocleidomastoid muscle).
3. Postural torticollis (torticollis but no tightness or tumor).

Classification On the Basis of Ultrasonography

Hsu TC et al divided congenital torticollis into four types.[17]

Type I.   A fibrotic mass in the involved muscle;
Type II. Diffuse fibrosis mixing with normal muscle;
Type III. Diffuse fibrosis without normal muscle in the involved muscle; and
Type IV. A fibrotic cord in the involved muscle.

The patients of type IV are most likely to require surgery.

The severity of the torticollis can be graded according to the degree of deficits in passive rotation of the neck.

INVESTIGATIONS AND DIFFERENTIAL DIAGNOSIS

Most of the times clinical examination is sufficient to make the diagnosis (Figs 107.1A and B). Ultrasonography may not be required for diagnosis but it helps in predicting the likelihood of spontaneous resolution of torticollis.[3,16-20] The qualitative and quantitative changes in the ultrasound image of sternocleidomastoid have been found to correlate significantly with the severity of rotational deficits of the neck. Ultrasonographic imaging can be used for monitoring the progress of torticollis longitudinally.[16]

Magnetic resonance imaging and computed tomography can also give the similar information but rarely required.[20,21]

Cervical hemivertebrae can also cause torticollis. Cervical spine abnormality can be detected by inspection or palpation. Plain radiographs of neck (antero-posterior and lateral) can confirm the diagnosis.

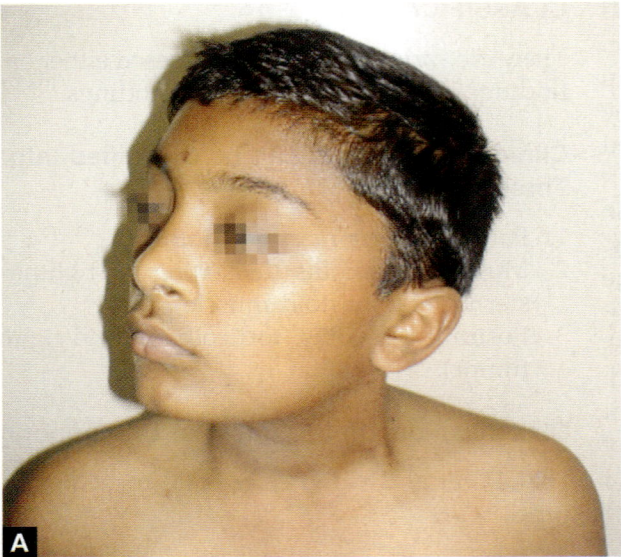 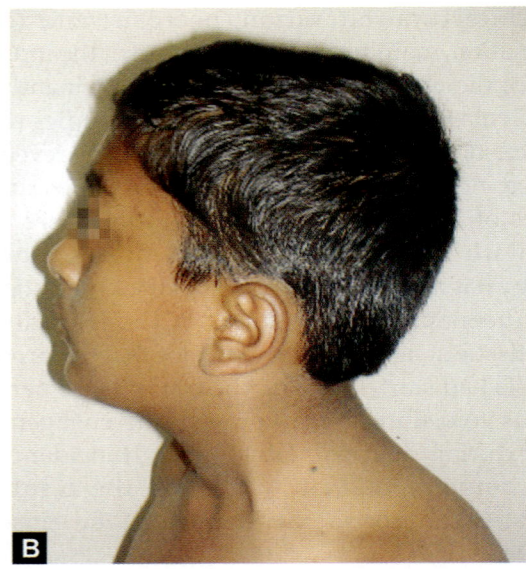

Figs 107.1A and B: **A.** Clinical photograph of a boy with torticollis, **B.** Lateral view of the same showing the taut muscle

Posterior fossa tumor can cause frozen neck with torticollis. Even the passive straightening of neck is not possible. Patient may have features of lower cranial nerve palsy. Computed tomography or magnetic resonance imaging of brain is required.

A patient with imbalance of ocular muscles can also present with torticollis. On passive straightening of neck, strabismus gets manifested.

Severe gastroesophageal reflux can cause spasmodic torticollis (Sandifer's syndrome).[22] Excessive regurgitation of feeds, recurrent episodes of respiratory tract infection, failure to thrive, and supra-esophageal symptoms, i.e. asthmatic features may be present. Barium swallow, radionuclide study and a 24 hour pH monitoring would help in confirming the diagnosis.

Retropharyngeal abscess can also cause head tilt. Patient has fever, difficulty in swallowing and respiration.[23] Lateral radiograph of neck can show soft tissue shadow.

Atlantoaxial subluxation and postural torticollis are the other differentials.[24,25]

NATURAL HISTORY AND SECONDARY EFFECTS

Spontaneous resolution with or without manual stretching has been reported in upto 90% of cases.[10,15,19] Various factors have been proposed to affect the rate of resolution of torticollis. These factors include the clinical type, passive rotation deficit of the neck, side of involvement, difficulties with the birth and age at presentation.[15,26]

Persistent torticollis can cause secondary effects like plagiocephaly, facial hypoplasia, and scoliosis. Small infants have soft head.[26-33] Due to the fixed position of head, a flattening of the ipsilateral occiput and the contralateral forehead, occurs. As the torticollis resolves or child adopts sitting position, plagiocephaly also has tendency to resolve. It may persist in few patients.

Flattening of the ipsilateral face occurs due to prolonged immobilization of face by fibrotic sternomastoid. The degree of hemihypoplasia can be determined by the angle between the plane of eyes and the plane of the mouth. Facial hemihypoplasia is reversible if surgical correction of torticollis is done early. The severity of the abnormality can also be recorded by measuring the distance between the outer angle of eye and the ipsilateral angle of mouth and comparing the same with the opposite side.

Older children compensate the persistent torticollis by elevating the ipsilateral shoulder. This maneuver helps them to keep the eyes aligned. Compensatory cervical and thoracic scoliosis can also occur.

TREATMENT

As majority of patients show spontaneous resolution conservative management is employed initially.

Whether physiotherapy expedites the resolution or not is controversial.[34] If the baby presents within the first few weeks after birth, a regular message with a baby oil is advised and may be helpful in making the fibrosis soft. The torticollis may resolve completely within few months, provided the theapy has been instituted early and effectively. The message should be done regularly at least twice a day for about 5-10 minutes each time over the weeks. This may not be effective if the baby is already more than 3 months of age more, possibly by then the fibrosis has already been established.

In older infants, a physiotherapy schedule may be started. Even if it does not help in resolution it definitely make the parents feel that something is being done for their infant. Parents are explained and advised to do regular neck exercises. The infant is made to lie with the shoulders brought out at the edge of couch. One person holds the shoulders firmly against the surface. Other person stands behind the patient and try to rotate the head on either side. This gentle maneuver is done twice a day. Parents may be asked to keep the toys on the ipsilateral side to encourage the infant to rotate his neck to the affected side. Though the usefulness of physiotherapy is questionable but it is safe. It also allays unnecessary parental anxiety by keeping them involved.[7,15,25] Some surgeons prefer to give a trial of botox injection in recalcitrant torticollis before resorting to surgery. Botox injection may be helpful in tight but non-fibrotic sternocleidomastoid muscle.[35,36]

Operative Treatment

The aim of surgery is not only to correct and even the deformity but also to prevent the serious irreversible complications of torticollis, specially the facial deformities.

Indications[15,37]

1. Persistent torticollis beyond 12-15 months of age
2. Persistent torticollis with progressive secondary effects, i.e. facial hemihypoplasia, scoliosis.

Operative Technique

The procedure is performed under general anesthesia. Child is placed supine with a folded towel under shoulders and head rotated to the other side so as to keep the ipsilateral side of neck up. A transverse

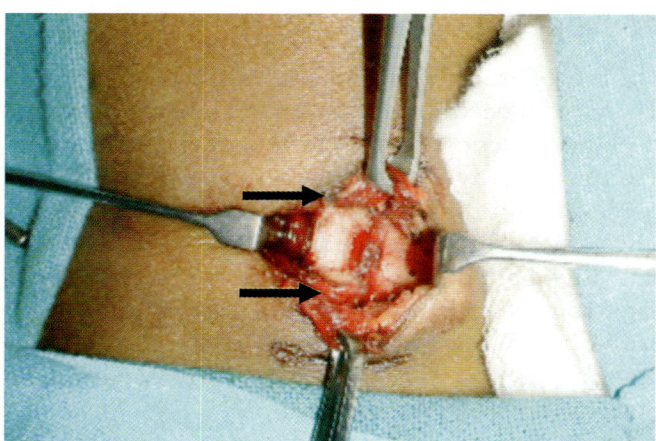

Fig. 107.2: Operative photograph in a case of torticollis, the fibrosed muscle is divided

incision is made about 1 cm above the sternal and clavicular heads of the sternomastoid muscle or over the most fibrotic part of the muscle. The platysma is divided along the skin incision. Muscle is mobilized all around to avoid any inadvertent injury to the underlying major vessels and other structures. The muscle is best divided at its lower end (Fig. 107.2). Although division at upper end, mid-portion, or at both ends have been described.[5,38-41] Both the heads of the muscle are divided using diathermy. Use of diathermy and careful ligation and division of larger superficial veins should be done to avoid any hematoma formation. Deep cervical fascia of neck, anterior and posterior to the sternomastoid muscle, is also divided to obtain optimal result. The neck is over stretched and a careful inspection and palpation of the neck is performed for any residual tightness. If required, division of the deeper structures is also done but with great care. Any injury to the internal jugular vein, external jugular vein, the carotid artery, accessory nerve, or the fibers of the cervical plexus, which may also be involved in the process of fibrosis, must be avoided. With the successful release, the two ends of the muscle go apart for a variable distance. The ends of the sternomastoid muscle are not sutured. Hemostasis is ensured and wound is closed in layers. Endoscopic tenotomy of muscle also has been described.[42-44]

Histological investigations have shown that there is a transition zone from fibrous tissue to normal muscle. It has been recommended to excise a margin of 1-2 mm on each side of fibrous tissue to avoid recurrence (Lehmann recommendations).

POSTOPERATIVE CARE

The procedure can be performed as a day-care surgery. There is no need for any postoperative restriction of neck movement. The success of surgery depends on the preoperative preparation of patients and the parensts with the commitment to learn and practice physiotherapy. Physiotherapy is started in the postoperative period as soon as the patient is pain free.[33] Full range of neck movement can usually be achieved within one week of surgery. Facial hemihypoplasia and plagiocephaly has the tendency to resolve slowly once the torticollis has resolved.[45]

COMPLICATIONS

1. Injury to the internal, external jugular vein, carotid artery, accessory nerve, fibers of the cervical plexus.
2. Hematoma formation.
3. Recurrence of symptoms specially if the surgery has been done in older children. The reported incidence of recurrence is, however, less than 3%.

In the Author's experience at the tertiary care level institute, only a few babies would present in the neonatal period, and most of these are with the cervical tumor. A local message is helpful in those newborns who present only with muscle fibrosis and without the tumor. Majority of these would present during and after infancy, with established torticollis and deformity of the face. The vertebral anomalies are found only occasionally. The post surgical results, combined with pre and postoperative physiotherapy are gratifying.

REFERENCES

1. Jaber MR, Goldsmith AJ. Sternocleidomastoid tumor of infancy: two cases of an interesting entity. Int J Pediatr Otorhinolaryngol 1999;47(3):269-74.
2. Kumar V, Prabhu BV, Chattopadhayay A, Nagendhar MY. Bilateral sternocleidomastoid tumor of infancy. Int J Pediatr Otorhinolaryngol 2003;67(6):673-75.
3. Lin JN, Chou ML. Ultrasonographic study of the sternocleidomastoid muscle in the management of congenital muscular torticollis. J Pediatr Surg 1997;32(11):1648-51.
4. Tufano RP, Tom LW, Austin MB. Bilateral sternocleidomastoid tumors of infancy. Int J Pediatr Otorhinolaryngol 1999;51(1):41-45. Review.
5. Jones PG. Torticollis in Infancy and Childhood. Springfield, IL: Charles C. Thomas; 1969.
6. Sherer DM. Spontaneous torticollis in a breech-presenting fetus delivered by an atraumatic elective cesarean section: A case and review of the literature. Am J Perinatol 1996;13(5):305-07. Review.
7. Demirbilek S, Atayurt HF. Congenital muscular torticollis and sternomastoid tumor: results of nonoperative treatment. J Pediatr Surg 1999;34(4):549-51.
8. Davids JR, Wenger DR, Mubarak SJ. Congenital muscular torticollis: sequela of intrauterine or perinatal compartment syndrome. J Pediatr Orthop 1993;13(2):141-47.
9. Cheng JC, Tang SP, Chen TM. Sternocleidomastoid pseudotumor and congenital muscular torticollis in infants: a prospective study of 510 cases. J Pediatr. 1999;134(6):712-16.
10. Cheng JC, Tang SP, Chen TM, Wong MW, Wong EM. The clinical presentation and outcome of treatment of congenital muscular torticollis in infants—a study of 1,086 cases. J Pediatr Surg 2000;35(7):1091-96.
11. Hsieh YY, Tsai FJ, Lin CC, Chang FC, Tsai CH. Breech deformation complex in neonates. J Reprod Med 2000;45(11):933-35.
12. Macdonald D. Sternomastoid tumour and muscular torticollis. J Bone Joint Surg Br 1969;51(3):432-43.
13. Sarnat HB, Morrissy RT. Idiopathic torticollis: sternocleidomastoid myopathy and accessory neuropathy. Muscle Nerve 1981;4(5):374-80.
14. Mickelson MR, Cooper RR, Ponseti IV. Ultrastructure of the sternocleidomastoid muscle in muscular torticollis. Clin Orthop Relat Res 1975;(110):11-18.
15. Cheng JC, Wong MW, Tang SP, Chen TM, Shum SL, Wong EM. Clinical determinants of the outcome of manual stretching in the treatment of congenital muscular torticollis in infants. A prospective study of eight hundred and twenty-one cases. J Bone Joint Surg Am 2001;83-A(5):679-87.
16. Cheng JC, Metreweli C, Chen TM, Tang S. Correlation of ultrasonographic imaging of congenital muscular torticollis with clinical assessment in infants. Ultrasound Med Biol 2000;26(8):1237-41.
17. Hsu TC, Wang CL, Wong MK, Hsu KH, Tang FT, Chen HT. Correlation of clinical and ultrasonographic features in congenital muscular torticollis. Arch Phys Med Rehabil 1999;80(6):637-41.
18. Tang SF, Hsu KH, Wong AM, Hsu CC, Chang CH. Longitudinal follow-up study of ultrasonography in congenital muscular torticollis. Clin Orthop Relat Res 2002;(403):179-85.
19. Tatli B, Aydinli N, Caliskan M, Ozmen M, Bilir F, Acar G. Congenital muscular torticollis: evaluation and classification. Pediatr Neurol 2006;34(1):41-44.
20. Entel RJ, Carolan FJ. Congenital muscular torticollis: magnetic resonance imaging and ultrasound diagnosis. J Neuroimaging 1997;7(2):128-30.
21. McGuire KJ, Silber J, Flynn JM, Levine M, Dormans JP. Torticollis in children: can dynamic computed tomography help determine severity and treatment. J Pediatr Orthop 2002;22:766-70.

22. Deskin RW. Sandifer syndrome: a cause of torticollis in infancy. Int J Pediatr Otorhinolaryngol 1995;32:183-85.
23. Hasegawa J, Tateda M, Hidaka H, Sagai S, Nakanome A, Katagiri K, Seki M, Katori Y, Kobayashi T. Retropharyngeal abscess complicated with torticollis: case report and review of the literature. Tohoku J Exp Med 2007;213:99-104.
24. Tonomura Y, Kataoka H, Sugie K, Hirabayashi H, Nakase H, Ueno S. Atlantoaxial rotatory subluxation associated with cervical dystonia. Spine 2007;32:E561-64.
25. Hicazi A, Acaroglu E, Alanay A, Yazici M, Surat A. Atlantoaxial rotatory fixation-subluxation revisited: a computed tomographic analysis of acute torticollis in pediatric patients. Spine 2002;27:2771-75.
26. Emery C. The determinants of treatment duration for congenital muscular torticollis. Phys Ther. 1994;74:921-29.
27. Ferguson JW. Cephalometric interpretation and assessment of facial asymmetry secondary to congenital torticollis. The significance of cranial base reference lines. Int J Oral Maxillofac Surg 1993;22:7-10.
28. Yu CC, Wong FH, Lo LJ, Chen YR. Craniofacial deformity in patients with uncorrected congenital muscular torticollis: an assessment from three-dimensional computed tomography imaging. Plast Reconstr Surg 2004;113:24-33.
29. Hollier L, Kim J, Grayson BH, McCarthy JG. Congenital muscular torticollis and the associated craniofacial changes. Plast Reconstr Surg 2000;105:827-35.
30. Chate RA. Facial scoliosis from sternocleidomastoid torticollis: long-term postoperative evaluation. Br J Oral Maxillofac Surg 2005;43:428-34.
31. Chate RA. Facial scoliosis due to sternocleidomastoid torticollis: a cephalometric analysis. Int J Oral Maxillofac Surg 2004;33:338-43.
32. Keller EE, Jackson IT, Marsh WR, Triplett WW. Mandibular asymmetry associated with congenital muscular torticollis. Oral Surg Oral Med Oral Pathol 1986;61:216-20.
33. Arslan H, Gündüz S, Subaþi M, Kesemenli C, Necmioðlu S. Frontal cephalometric analysis in the evaluation of facial asymmetry in torticollis, and outcomes of bipolar release in patients over 6 years of age. Arch Orthop Trauma Surg 2002;122:489-93.
34. Cheng JC, Chen TM, Tang SP, Shum SL, Wong MW, Metreweli C. Snapping during manual stretching in congenital muscular torticollis. Clin Orthop Relat Res 2001;384:237-44.
35. Joyce MB, de Chalain TM. Treatment of recalcitrant idiopathic muscular torticollis in infants with botulinum toxin type A. J Craniofac Surg 2005;16:321-27.
36. Do TT. Congenital muscular torticollis: current concepts and review of treatment. Curr Opin Pediatr 2006;18:26-29. Review
37. Sönmez K, Türkyilmaz Z, Demiroðullari B, Ozen IO, Karabulut R, Baðbanci B, Baþaklar AC, Kale N. Congenital muscular torticollis in children. ORL J Otorhinolaryngol Relat Spec 2005;67:344-47.
38. Wirth CJ, Hagena FW, Wuelker N, Siebert WE. Biterminal tenotomy for the treatment of congenital muscular torticollis. Long-term results. J Bone Joint Surg Am 1992;74:427-34.
39. Stassen LF, Kerawala CJ. New surgical technique for the correction of congenital muscular torticollis (wryneck). Br J Oral Maxillofac Surg 2000;38:142-47.
40. Gürpinar A, Kiriþtioðlu I, Balkan E, Doðruyol H. Surgical correction of muscular torticollis in older children with Peter G. Jones technique. J Pediatr Orthop 1998;18:598-601.
41. Chen CE, Ko JY. Surgical treatment of muscular torticollis for patients above 6 years of age. Arch Orthop Trauma Surg 2000;120:149-51.
42. Burstein FD, Cohen SR. Endoscopic surgical treatment for congenital muscular torticollis. Plast Reconstr Surg 1998;101(1):20-24; discussion 25-26.
43. Burstein FD. Long-term experience with endoscopic surgical treatment for congenital muscular torticollis in infants and children: A review of 85 cases. Plast Reconstr Surg 2004;114:491-93.
44. Swain B. Transaxillary endoscopic release of restricting bands in congenital muscular torticollis—a novel technique. J Plast Reconstr Aesthet Surg 2007;60(1):95-98. Epub 2006 May 11.
45. de Chalain TM, Katz A. Idiopathic muscular torticollis in children: the Cape Town experience. Br J Plast Surg 1992;45:297-301.

SECTION 9

Pediatric Surgical Specialities

Common Eye Problems in Children

Supriyo Ghose, Sanjeev Nainiwal

There are certain milestones in ocular development during neonatal life, infancy, and at least up to 5 years of age, which are important to appreciate, even though visual acuity assessment may be fraught with difficulties.

Generally speaking, all ocular disorders would present to the pediatrician with one or more of the following: history of injury, pain, red eye, watering swelling, a squint or diminution of vision.

Before actually seeing the eye, it is important to have a proper history (such as the exact nature of the injury) as accurate an assessment of the vision as possible (careful observation for both eyes separately, with a proper Snellen's chart in the older and co-operative child), and a quick examination of the adenxal structures. Noting such details would be of great help in the initial diagnosis and treatment, and their first hand recording would afford a lot of useful and reliable information to the ophthalmologist, if the patient has to be referred later.

Examination of an eye after injury should be undertaken with great caution, especially after a suspected perforating injury. Forcible examination is dangerous, as the eye may suffer further damage, and the intraocular contents may be lost. The lids may be gently retracted and held against the bony orbital margins, which sometimes may require sedation or a general anesthetia.

Ocular examination of pediatric age group is actually a challenge to the clinicians, which requires expertisation. To effectively handle common ocular problems, the pediatrician must have some basic ophthalmic equipment (good torch with focal illumination, cotton swab-sticks, eye pads and dressings, and preferrably a magnifying device such as a loupe, and an ophthalmoscope). Common drugs must be available, as topical anesthetic agents (2 and 4% xylocaine), antibiotic drops and ointments, mydriatics (phenylephrine drops 2.5 and 5%), and fluorescein paper strips (fluorescein solutions are often contaminated by Pseudomonas). Cycloplegics are not necessary normally to dilate the pupils for a good fundus examination, and drugs like topical atropine, which viciate the pupillary findings, should preferrably be avoided unless the ocular condition demands it. Tropicamide 0.5 and 1 percent may be useful.

CONGENITAL ANOMALIES

As for congenital abnormalities anywhere in the body several teratogenic factors have been implicared congenital anomalies of the eye, operating pre or perinatally. These teratogens include physically chemical, mechanical, drugs and poisons (including vasoconstrictors), inflammations and fevers and the (noxious) treatments thereof, malnutrition, and of course irradiation. Any such factor operating very early in intrauterine life in the first 6-8 weeks may produce organogenetic deformities as anophthalmos, microphthalmos, congenital cystic eye, and even cyclopia. These deformities often present with other ocular and systemic associations. Several lesser anomalies of differentiation may be the result of noxious influences later on in intrauterine development.

Congenital Cataract

Congenital cataract (Fig. 108.1) is associated with intra-uterine infections (rubella, toxoplasmosis), antenatal malnutrition (zonular cataract), metabolic disease

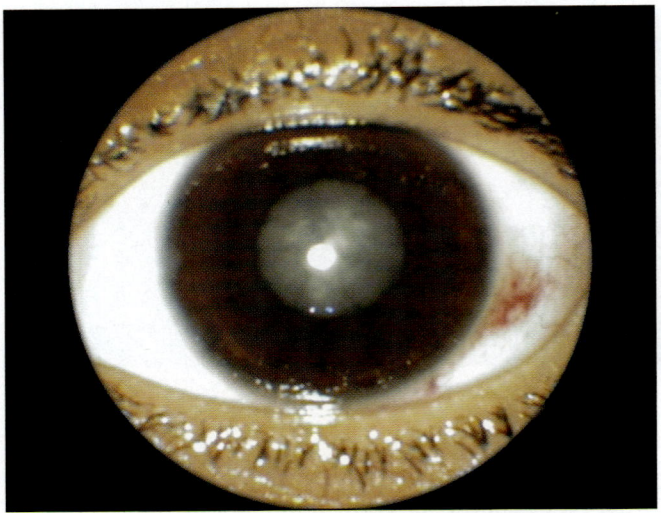

Fig. 108.1: Total congenital cataract

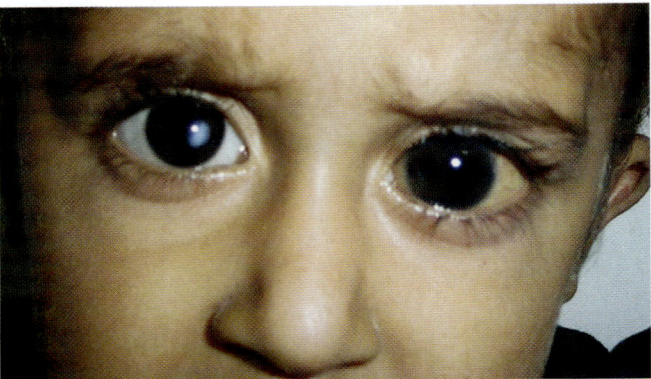

Fig. 108.2: Congenital glaucoma

(galactosemia, hypocalcemia), chromosomal anomalies (down syndrome), ocular malformations (microcornea, nystagmus, megalocornea, keratoconus, pigmentary retinitis), mental retardation and various cutaneous, neurological, musculoskeletal and endocrine disorders (diabetes mellitus, hyperparathyroidism). Cataract may develop secondary to eye disease such as trauma, retrolental fibroplasias, uveitis and glaucoma. Marfan's syndrome and homocystinuria may be typically associated with ectopia lentis. Cataracts in children may be hereditary and familial, and require early referral for proper management and visual rehabilitation.

The management of congenital cataract is a semi-emergency because during infancy not only does the cataract blur the retinal image but it also disrupts the development of the visual pathways in the control nervous system. In addition to a complete ophthalmic examination, A and B scan ultrasonography should be performed to record the axial length and assess the posterior segment. Visual acuity should always be recorded. Indication for surgery for congenital cataract is lenticular opacity > +2.5 mm or visual acuity of + < 6/18. Unilateral cataracts should be operated as early as the child becomes medically fit with minimal risk of anesthesia, but must be operated before 3 months of age to prevent amblyopia. In bilateral cataracts, both the eyes must be operated and the optical corrections should be given. Intraocular lens, can be implanted if the child is 2-3 years of age. Antiamblyopia therapy should be given and continued till both eyes have got an equal vision and preferably up to the age of 7 years.

Acute Glaucoma

Acute glaucoma as typically described in adults, is usually not seen in children. Up to 3 years of age, congenital (or secondary) glaucoma manifests by progressive enlargement of the globe (buphthalmos), hazy cornea, watering, photophobia, and poor vision (Fig. 108.2). After 3 years of age, the eye loses its stretchability, and glaucoma does not manifest with buphthalmos. A suspicion of glaucoma definitely warrants an immediate referral. Intraocular inflammation, metabolic disorders like homocys-tinuria and tumors like retinoblastoma, may manifest as secondary glaucoma.[1]

Congenital Ptosis

Classification

- Simple
- Associated with superior rectus underaction
- Associated with blepharophimosis syndrome
- Associated with synkinesis
- Marcus Gunn phenomena
- Misdirected third nerve

Assessment

1. Good Bell's phenomena and normal corneal sensation are absolute prerequisites for proceeding to ptosis surgery.

2. If the above is intact then we proceed to:
   i. Assessment of visual acuity
   ii. Correction of amblyopia
   iii. Correction of strabismus
   iv. Correction of other lid abnormalities (coloboma, ankyloblepharon).
3. If Bell's phenomena and corneal sensations are not normal then crutch glasses with appropriate refractive correction and amblyopia treatment if required is instituted.
4. Assessment of ptosis
   I. Measurement of palpebral aperture
      a. The upper lid covers 2 mm of the superior cornea
      b. Beyond 2 mm, a droop of ≤ 2 mm comprises mild ptosis
      c. A droop of 3 mm comprises moderate ptosis
      d. A droop of ≥ 4 mm comprises severe ptosis.
   II. In cases of bilateral ptosis, the final position of the lid at surgery is kept such that it covers 2 mm of the superior cornea bilaterally.
   III. In cases of unilateral ptosis the droop in the ptotic eye is aligned according to the position of the lid in the fellow normal eye.
   IV. Absence of lid crease or a furrow in the infra brow area indicates poor levator action.
   V. Any significant head tilt/torticollis has to be assessed.
   VI. In cases of unilateral ptosis, retraction in the fellow eye has to be assessed.
5. Assessment of LPS action:
   – Normal   –   12-15 mm
   – Good   – ≥ 8 mm
   – Fair   –   5-7 mm
   – Poor   – ≤ 4 mm

   The LPS action is always measured after occluding the action of frontalis muscle after asking the patient to gradually look upwards from downgaze to upgaze. In a patient not cooperative for assessment of the LPS action, we perform the lliff's test, i.e. we evert the upper lid of the child. A spontaneous reinversion of the lid indicates fair to good LPS action and hence levator resection can be performed.
6. Presence of synkinesis
   i. Marcus Gunn phenomena – Mild ≤ 2 mm
                              Moderate 3 mm
                              Severe ≥ 4 mm
   ii. Misdirected third nerve – Assessment of hypotropia/Ocular motility disorder/abnormal lid movements, etc.
7. Drug test
   i. Phenylepherine test – This is to determine preoperatively the effectivity of the Fasanella Servat procedure. If it is positive, then the surgeon can proceed with the tarsoconjunctivomullerectomy.
   ii. Tensilon test – This is to rule out myasthenia gravis which is an important cause of acquired ptosis.

Acquired Ptosis

- Neurogenic (Third nerve palsy, Horner's syndrome)
- Myogenic (Myotonic dystrophy, myasthenia gravis)
- Aponeurotic/Senile
- Traumatic.

In cases of acquired ptosis, the assessment of the ptosis and levator action would be similar to that done for congenital ptosis. In addition, other associated examination would include:

- Assessment of higher mental function and a complete CNS examination (Third nerve palsy/Horner's syndrome).
- Examination of the pupil (Third nerve palsy/Horner's syndrome/traumatic).
- Examinatin of the ocular motility and strabismus (Thrid nerve palsy/Horner's syndrome ophthalmoplegias/myasthenia).
- A high lid crease indicates levator disinsertion (Aponeurotic/traumatic).
- Assessment of the orbital rim surrounding the lid (Traumatic).
- The tensilon test is an absolute must in every case of acquired ptosis.
- Clinical test rule out myasthenia gravis in the form of the lid hopping signs, cogan's lid twitch signs can be undertaken.

- Other tests in the diagnostic armamentarium of myasthenia gravis in the form of repetitive nerve stimulation test, and electromyography can be performed. EMG can also be used to diagnose ocular myopathies.

Surgical treatment of acquired ptosis is undertaken only if the ptosis is stable for 6 months or more. The type and extent of surgery almost commensurates with the extent of surgery done in cases of congenital ptosis. In acquired ptosis, generally the accepted end point of the correction is mild under correction.

Pseudoptosis

- Associated with Anophthalmos/Microphthalmos/Phthisis
- Associated with hypotropia
- Associated with dermatochalasis.

Treatment of pseudoptosis aims towards the treatment of the primary cause of the condition.

The assessment of ptosis is thus aptly elucidated by the following acronym.

- D – Drop
- E – Excursion (LPS action)
- S – Superior rectus function (Strabismus)
- T – Tensilon tests (Other drug test)
- I – Iliff's Sign (LPS action)
- N – Nerves (Corneal sensation, Bell's phenomena)
- Y – Yawn (Synkinesis)
  - Lid crease / Fold
  - Brow position.

Surgical Management of Ptosis

- Age at which ptosis surgery is performed is usually at about 3 years of age when proper assessment of visual acuity, strabismus, ptosis, levator action, other lid abnormalities and Bell's phenomena can be performed correctly. Surgery is indicted in the pre-school age so as to obviate any psychological trauma that the child may suffer after he begins social interaction at school.
- Surgery is indicated prior to this if there is significant sensory deprivation amblyopia present due to the ptosis and significant torticollis present.
- An infant whose pupils are completely occluded by the lid (No reflects seen on distant direct ophthalmoscopy) would require immediate ptosis surgery.
- Assess for the skin fold in the lid as this is an indicator for fair to good levator action and hence LPS resection can be performed. In case of marked frontalis overaction and a chin elevated head posture, a frontalis sling surgery is indicated.

Surgical Protocol

Mild Ptosis (Unilateral/Bilateral)

i. Good LPS action
   a. Positive phenylephrine test
      - Fasanella servat's procedure
   b. Negative phenylephrine test
      - Fasanella Servat's Procedrue
      - LPS resection (11-14 mm)
ii. Fair LPS action
      - LPS resection (14-17 mm)
iii. Poor LPS action
      - Hypothetical situation. If present, supramaximal LPS resection (< 23 mm) can be attempted.

Moderate Ptosis (Unilateral/Bilateral)

i. Good LPS action
      – LPs resection (14-22 mm)
ii. Fair LPS action
      – LPS resection (14-22 mm)
iii. Poor LPs action
      – Frontalis sling surgery
      – Supramaximal LPS resection (< 23 mm).

Severe Ptosis

i. Bilateral
   a. Good/Fair LPS action
      – LPS resection (23 mm)
   b. Poor LPS action
      – Frontalis sling surgery
ii. Unilateral
   a. Good/Fair LPS action
      – LPS resection (< 23 mm)
   b. Poor LPS action
      – Levator excision of normal eye with bilateral sling surgery (Beard's method)
      – Bilateral sling surgery without excision of the levator of the normal eye (Callahan's method).

Marcus Gunn Phenomena

It is usually, commonly seen in the left eye. It is associated with superior rectus underaction in 75% cases.

i. Mild
   - Mild MG phenomena does not affect the surgical management of the patient which is planned according to the protocol mentioned above.
ii. Moderate/Severe
   - Levator excision and bilateral sling surgery.

Indications for Sling Surgery

i. Severe/Moderate ptosis with poor LPS action
ii. Moderate/Severe Marcus Gunn phenomena
iii. Blepharophimosis syndrome (Fig. 108.3)
iv. Failed LPs resection/Other ptosis procedure
v. Misdirected third nerve phenomena
vi. Total third nerve palsy
vii. Temporary sling procedure in children.

Indications for Fasanella Servat Surgery

i. Mild congenital ptosis with good LPS action
ii. Ptosis in Horner's syndrome
iii. Postcataract surgery blepharoptosis
iv. Steroid induced ptosis

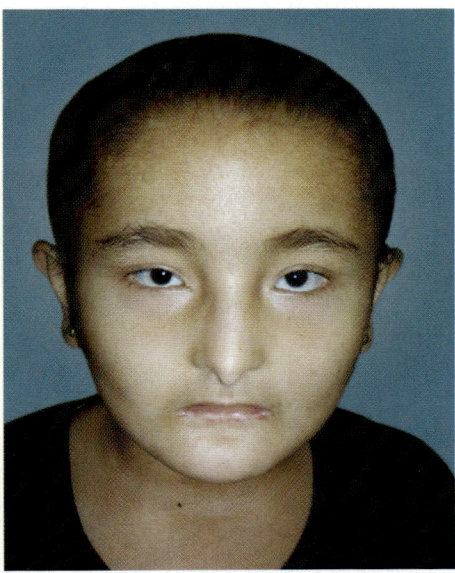

Fig. 108.3: Blepharophimosis syndrome

How much Levator to Resect?

There is no exact rule. However, for the sake of some guidelines, the following protocol may be followed (Fox).

i. If levator action is 2 mm or less, no levator resection is performed.
ii. If levator action is less than 5 mm, over correct 2-3 mm, i.e. at least 20 mm
iii. If the levator action is 6-9 mm, correct full, i.e. up to 16 mm of the levator is resected, more if the levator is of poor quality.
iv. If the levator action is 10-12 mm, the ptosis is under corrected. No more than 8-11 mm is resected. The horns are not cut.

Strabismus (Squint)

Early detection and treatment of squint is very important since significant improvement in the vision of the deviated eye and good binocular vision cannot be achieved if proper therapy is not undertaken as early as possible and not later than 5 years of age. Some degree of occasional squint may be normal in the first few moths of infancy, since binocular vision is not well developed. If squint persists beyond 2 to 3 months of age, an ophthalmologist should be consulted. A false impression of convergent squint (pseudostrabismus) may be given by epicanthal folds with a wide bridge of nose.

Concomitant squint accounts for most cases. There is no muscle paralysis but the muscles fail to act in coordination. The degree of deviation is the same irrespective of the direction of gaze. In noncomitant (paralytic) squint resulting from ocular muscles paralysis, the eyes deviate most on turning in the direction of the paralyzed muscle. Diplopia may develop and to avoid it, the child learns to suppress the vision in the affected eye. Abnormal head posture may also develop.

The treatment of concomitant squint consists of cycloplegic refraction and corrective lenses, drugs such as cycloplegics or miotics, patching of the normal eye for determind periods to prevent image suppression and amblyopia in the deviating eye, orthoptic exercises and surgery, singly or in combination. Timely referral is vital-children do not "grow out " of squint.

Involuntary ocular rhythmic movements (nystagmus) should also be referred early for complete investigations.

PHYSICAL AND CHEMICAL TRAUMA

Foreign Body

A conjunctival foreign body should be located and easily removed. It is not quite so, easy when the foreign body is lodged in the upper tarsal conjunctiva in the subtarsal sulcus, as this requires the eversion of the upper lid.

A corneal foreign body should be gently removed with wet swab or spud. If find difficulty, apply antibiotic ointment and refer promptly.

A suspected intraocular foreign body should be immediately referred for investigations and urgent management to the eye casualty (Fig. 108.4).[2]

Chemical Injuries

Chemical injury to the external eye is one of the common problems presenting to the eye casualty that may vary in severity from mild irritation to complete destruction of the ocular surface epithelium, corneal opacification, loss of vision, and rarely loss of the eye (Fig. 108.5).[3] Most of the victims are young patients and children who become exposed to chemicals during industrial accidents, at home, and in association with criminal assaults. The offending chemical may be in the form of a solid, liquid, powder, mist or vapor. At the home, most injuries result from detergents, disinfectants, solvents, cosmetics, drain cleaness, oven cleaners ammonia, bleach and other common household alkaline agents. Because their more frequent presence in household cleaning agents and in many building materials, alkali injuries occur more frequently than acid injuries. Some of the worst chemical injuries result when strong alkalies (lye) or acids are used as assaultive weapons.

Alkalies increase the pH of tissues, which causes saponification of fatty acids in cell membranes and ultimately cellular disruption. Acids cause coagulative necrosis of the tissue proteins on contact. This denatured and precipitated tissue protein forms a barrier for the chemical (acid) and prevents its further penetration into deeper tissues thereby decreasing damage vis a vis alkalies. This is the reason how acide solutions tend to cause less severe damage than alkaline solutions.

The most important step to deal with such situation is to give immediate and copious irrigation to the ocular surface, for at least 30 minutes, preferably with normal saline or Ringer's lactate solution.[3] However, if both (Saline and Ringer lactate solution) are not available at the moment, simple tap water can be used. A topical anesthetic (4% xylocaine) may be instilled into the eye prior to the irrigation, which may help in putting eyelid speculum or retractor. Double eversion of the eyelid can visualize the foreign bodies in the forneies, and make their removal easy. Irrigation should be continued until the pH of the conjunctival sac normalizes, that may be checked easily with a pH strip (Litmus peper). After emergency treatment patient should be evaluated thoroughly. The next

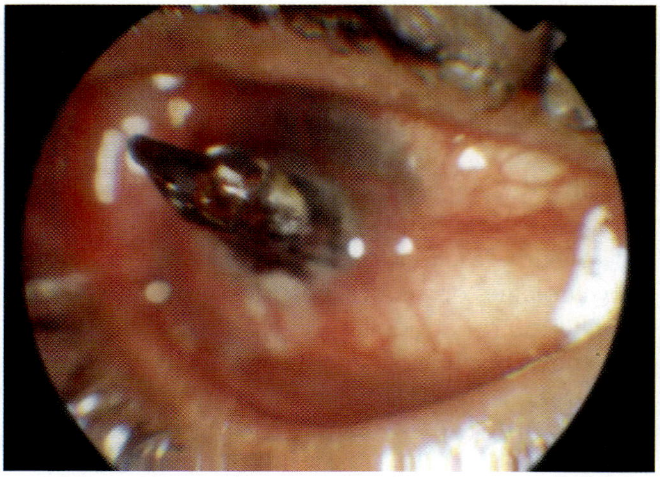

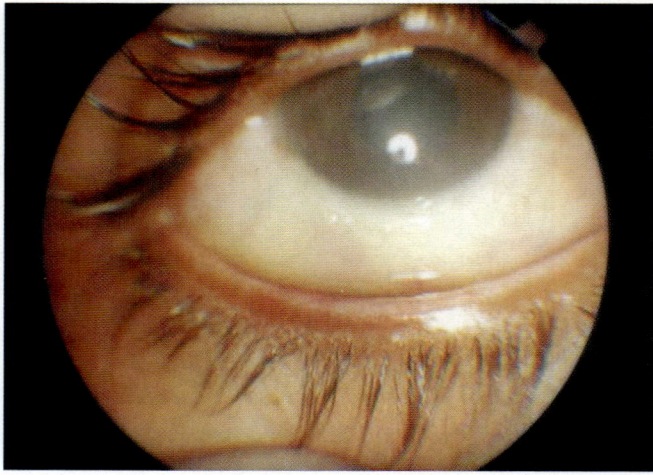

Fig. 108.4: Large intraocular foreign protruding from the eye

Fig. 108.5: Acute chemical injury

phase of therapy for the chemical injury should be directed towards decreasing inflammation, controlling intraocular pressure (IOP), limiting sterile keratolysis and promoting recpithelialization.

Thermal Burns

Thermal burns should be treated on conservative lines and efforts should be made to protect the cornea. Explosive injuries by fireworks, crackers and bombs may cause serious damage to the eyes. Ocular fireworks injuries are much more severe and dangerous in children than adults.

Blunt Injury

A ball, stone, fist, stick, slingshot, gullidanda, fireworks, etc can cause blunt ocular trauma. Blunt injuries are potentially very dangerous. If the child has significant hyphema, he or she should be administered hypotensive agents as glycerol, diamox (acetazolamide) or intravenous mannitol to reduce the chances of rise of intraocular pressure and corneal blood-staining (Fig. 108.6). Mobilization is avoided to prevent the occurrence of rebleed in the eye. The visual prognosis is guarded, as many more complications may or will take place. Referral without delay is advocated after primary treatment.

Penetrating Injury

Penetrating eye injury is a major cause of ocular morbidity and leading cause of monocular visual loss.

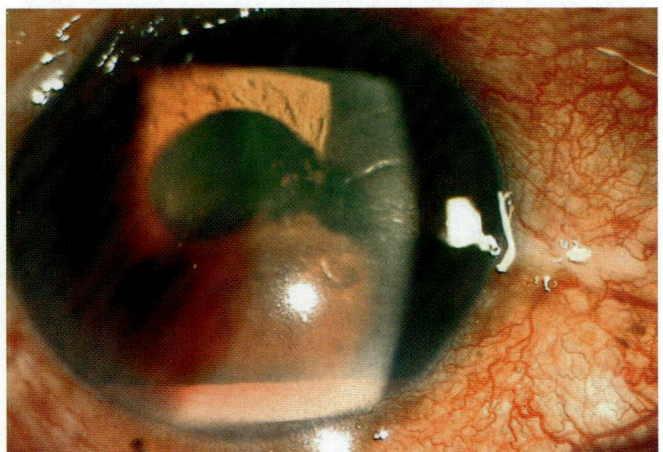

Fig. 108.6: Post blunt injury hyphema

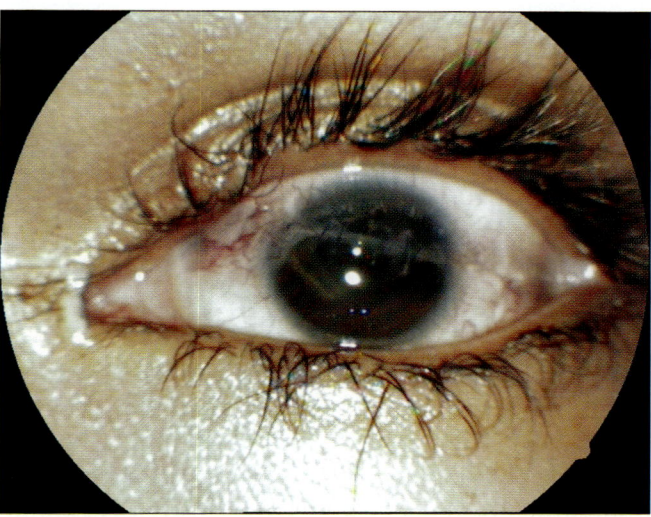

Fig. 108.7: Repaired penetrating eye injury

It is one of the most important surgical ocular emergencies in children and demands urgent treatment (Fig. 108.7). Bandage the eye and refer immediately for proper examination and repair under general anesthesia, with the operating microscope. From management point of view, penetrating trauma can be divided into anterior and posterior ocular trauma. Though a general ophthalmic surgeon can repair most of the anterior segment trauma, it is important that posterior segment trauma cases should be urgently referred to the vitreoretinal surgeon. An extensive injury may sometimes necessitate excision of the globe. The possibility and dangers of sympathetic ophthalmia should always be borne in mind. Lid lacerations also require prompt repair, and canalicular injuries have to be adequately managed.

Corneal Abrasion

Corneal abrasion can be very painful with marked photophobia. Trivial injuries may abrade the corneal epithelium as with edges of paper, leaves, twigs, toys and fingernail scratches, etc., and the area of epithelial denudation can be easily demonstrated by fluorescein staining. The treatment is almost the same as for an ulcer, except that atropine is not routinely indicated, and a 24-hour firm pad and bandage is very beneficial in promoting epithelial healing. Analgesics are useful, but topical anesthetics should be used minimally or not at all in view of their epitheliotoxic properties.

1246 Pediatric Surgery—Diagnosis and Management

Table 108.1: Differentiating features between conjunctivitis, corneal ulcer, iridocyclitis and acute ACG

Features	Conjuctivitis	Corneal Ulcer	Iridocyclitis	Acute ACG
Cornea	Clear	Ulcer, hazy	May be hazy	Hazy
Pupil	Normal	Often miosed	Miosed	Middilated and vertically oval
Anterior chamber	Normal	Usually normal	May be deep	Shallow
Congestion	Conjunctival	Ciliary	Ciliary	Ciliary
Intraocular tension	Normal	May be high	Low may be normal or high	Very high
Vision	Normal	Reduced	Reduced	Reduced

Subconjunctival Hemorrhage

Subconjunctival hemorrhage is another common alarming sign for the patient and the parents (Fig. 108.8). The cause should be elicited, as severe coughing (whooping cough), straining, minor local trauma, hemorrhagic conjunctivitis and rarely vitamin C deficiency. More serious entitites such as head injury, fractures, and deeper trauma must be kept in mind. Rarely, a small subconjuctival hemorrhage may be overlying a small scleral intraocular perforation, which may be an intraocular foreign body. Small tears of the conjuctiva may result from injury.

Red Eye

A red eye is by and large the most common ocular problem to be seen, and a differential diagnosis has been made between the not so serious conjunctivitis and the more grave conditions of corneal ulcer, iridocyclitis and glaucoma (Table 108.1). However, acute glaucoma as typically described in adults is not usually seen in children.[4]

Corneal Ulcer

Corneal ulcer is defined as breach in corneal epithelium along with the underlying infiltration.[5] It is one of the most significant causes of ocular morbidity around the world (Fig. 108.9). Corneal ulcer presents with a typical corneal picture ciliary congestion, and may be iridocyclitis. It demands immediate attention. Swabs should be sent for culture and sensitivity (preferably from ulcer edge scrapings). Local hygiene should be maintained and start on topical antibiotics (systemic coverage also if required) and topical atropine, application of heat, systemic supportive therapy and if necessary, ocular hypotensive agents as acetazolamide to prevent impending perforation. Steroids should by and large be avoided. Children should be discouraged from touching the eye, if necessary, mechanical restraint, as by a hollow cardboard cylinder over the elbows, may have to be resorted to.

A history of trauma or a corneal foreign body may be evident. Injury with vegetable matter may lead to a fungal corneal ulcer, more recalcitrant to therapy and requiring specific antifungal measures.

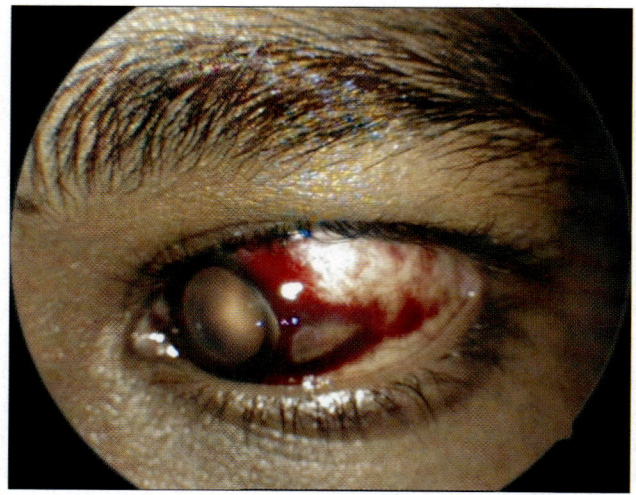

Fig. 108.8: Subconjunctival hemorrhage

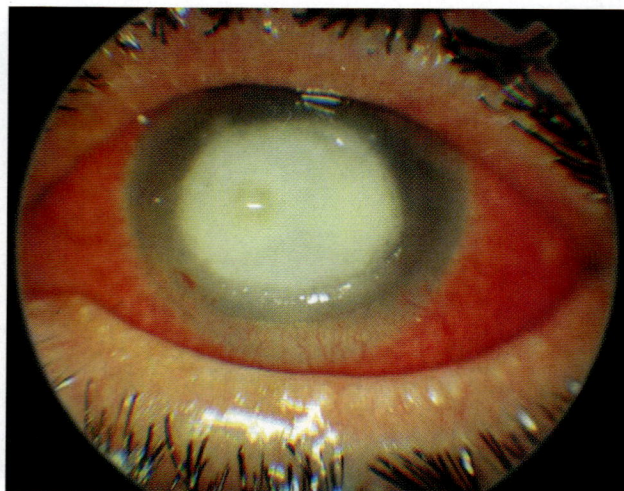

Fig. 108.9: Corneal ulcer

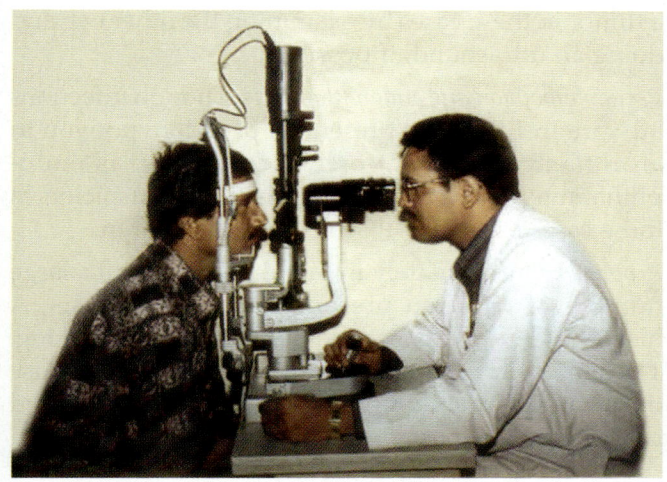

Fig. 108.10: Slitlamp biomicroscopic examination

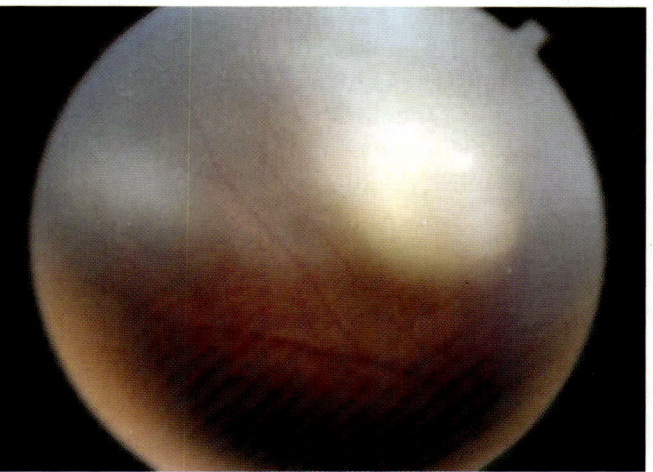

Fig. 108.11: Retinoblastoma

A herpetic corneal ulcer may exhibit a typical dendritic figure on fluorescein staining, and may be associated with herpes simplex lesions elsewhere as on the lips, nose and genitalia (Fig. 108.10). Recurrences may be associated with lowering of body resistence. Antiviral therapy topically is indicated to start with. The corneal sensations diminish in this condition, as they also do in keratomalacia.

If the Bowman's membraine is damaged in a corneal ulcer a corneal opacity will result on healing. Early institution of therapy would restrict the opacity to a minimum, and reduce the chances of corneal blindness. Nonhealing or progression of the ulcer, or the appearance of a hypopyon merits urgent referral. Early xerophthalmia should be talked most energetically before full-blown keratomalacia develops with irreparable loss of vision.

NEOPLASTIC DISORDERS

Retinoblastoma

A typical "Cat's eye" reflex or leucocoria is a well-known feature of retinoblastoma (Fig. 108.11).[6-7] However, many other congenital and acquired conditions may produce an identical pupillary reflex such as retinal dysplasia, retinal vascular folds, persistent hyperplastic primary vitreous (PHPV), retinal detachment, retained intraocular foreign body, endophthalmitis, cataract, uveitis, Coats' disease, and retrolental fibroplasias (RLF) or retinopathy of prematurity (ROP). Retinoblastoma is usually associated with neovascularization, high intraocular tension features of bilateral involvement, optic nerve extension with distant metastases, and hereditary predisposition. Besides the pathognomic yellowish white reflex, retinoblastoma may present with a squint, red eye pain and secondary glaucoma. These children should be immediately referred for further investigations and management, because delay may adversely affect survival. In spite of various imaging modalities, the differential diagnosis during the early stage may be difficult, and the exact diagnosis may be possible only after histopathological examination of the enucleate eye. Earlier radical treatment modalities, as enucleation are giving way to eye salvaging procedures of cryotherapy, chemoreduction and lens-sparing techniques of modern radiotherapy.

Retinoblastoma (RB), as we all know, is one of the commonest intraocular malignancies in children. Though this is not a common condition, it is one of the few life-threatening conditions that present to an ophthalmologist. A timely diagnosis could thus save the life of the child. Now, with the advent of newer therapeutic modalities like laser, chemotherapy and radiotherapy, an early diagnosis and the use of combination therapy can result in preservation of vision thus avoiding enucleation. The goal of RB therapy now is to save the life and preserve the vision.

How not to miss the diagnosis of Retinoblastoma?

The commonest presentation of retinoblastoma is leucocoria in a child aged 1-5 years. In a typical case it may not be so difficult to make the diagnosis.

However, given the grave consequences of a missed or delayed diagnosis, it is prudent for us ophthalmologists to maintain a high index of suspicion so as to pick up the all the cases at the earliest. The clinical features together with the investigations can correctly establish the diagnosis in most cases.

Age: Though RB commonly presents between 18-24 months, in our country we often find children presenting at a later age. A word of caution: RB can present in neonates and also in older children (7-8 years) so one should be careful to rule it out in all cases of leucocoria.

Family history and genetics: RB is said to be familial in 25-30% but in Indian conditions we are not always able to elicit a positive family history. One should look for regressed lesions in the parents of bilateral cases and ask for a history of deaths in early childhood in the family. Also, screening of siblings (aged less than 5 years) of all cases should be done, whether unilateral or bilateral. Though the genetic abnormality is identifiable in some cases, chromosomal analysis may not be practical in our scenario since it is expensive and the results take a long-time.

Leucocoria: Leucocoria, unilateral or bilateral, is by far the commonest presentation of RB. There may be overlying engorged vessels or calcification visible. There is a long list of differential diagnosis of leucocoria usually clubbed a 'pseudoglioma'. The ones likely to cause a diagnostic dilemma are PHPV, organized vitreous hemorrhage, endophthalmitis and Coat's disease in older children. The associated anterior segment findings may help, in the form of microcornea in PHPV and a low tension in endophthalmitis. Raised IOP, ectropion uveae, rubeosis and pseudohypopyon are all pointers to a tumor in the eye.

Squint: Any squint in a child warrants a fundus examination with dilated pupils. A macular tumor causing the squint can be picked up even with a cursory indirect ophthalmoscopic examination so there is no excuse for telling the parents to bring the child back for squint surgery later, without seeing the fundus.

Secondary glaucoma: If the parents miss the initial leukokoria, RB can present as secondary glaucoma with an opaque cornea. Therefore, one should rule out a tumor in these cases by examining the other eye and doing an ultrasound, if possible.

Pseudohypopyon and endophthalmitis: Though infections are rare in RB, it can present as pseudohypopyon in an inflamed eye and/or masquerading as endophthalmitis. One needs a high index of suspicion in these cases especially if seen in older children.

Proptosis: Unfortunately in India, there are still a large number of children presenting with proptosis. A history of leucocoria may sometimes be forthcoming. Though orbital cellulitis is still the commonest cause of proptosis in children, tumors like orbital RB and rhabdomyosarcoma should be kept in mind.

How to Investigate a Case of Suspected Retinoblastoma?

Investigations in RB are aimed at confirming the diagnosis and establishing extent of disease both for the prognosis and therapy decisions.

Ultrasonography: USG is an important tool in establishing the diagnosis of RB. RB is usually seen as a mass lesion of moderate–high internal reflectivity, arising from the retina. There may be an overlying detachment visible. Calcification, characterized by spikes of 100% reflectivity, is seen in 90% cases and is diagnostic of RB. Optic nerve involvement and scleral infiltration may also be picked up. USG monitoring of tumor height is important when the patient is on chemoreduction.

CT Scan: On CT scan, RB is seen as a moderately attenuating mass lesion with calcification. Extraocular spread in the from of optic nerve or scleral infiltration and/or intracranial extension is well demonstrated. CT scan is required for radiotherapy planning as well.

MRI: MRI is not as useful in the diagnosis of RB except in cases where vitreous hemorrhage/exudative retinal detachment is suspected. Though calcification is not so well demonstrated, the soft tissue visualization is better especially in case of chiasmal involvement.

Special Investigations

In most cases the diagnosis can be clinched with the above-mentioned clinical features and investigations. In certain cases where the diagnosis is difficult, like leucocoria without calcification, non-responsive uveites/vitritis in children older age groups, etc. some special investigations may be indicated like Fine

Needle Aspiration Biopsy (FNAB) done under indirect ophthalmoscopic guidance and with an experienced cytopathologist.

PROPTOSIS

Proptosis of the eye may be due to orbital cellulitis, orbital tumor (hemangioma, rhabdomyosarcoma, glioma, leukemic infiltration, extraocular extension or retinoblastoma, neuroblastoma, etc.) orbital hemorrhage, vascular malformations, and other rarer causes (Fig. 108.12).

The exposure of the eye should be prevented by oily drops (suspensions) and ointments, and if necessary, by a tarsorrhaphy, to prevent the avoidable and tragic complication of exposure keratitis and severe corneal ulceration with resulting blindness.

The above principle of corneal protection extremely important, but often forgotten management of a semicomatose or unconscious. The cornea should always be protected by an oily film especially if a pad and bandage has to be applied though a pad is better avoided unless there is actual keratitis.

INFLAMMATORY DISORDERS

Uveitis

Uveitis is defined as inflammation of the uveal tissue (i.e. iris, ciliary body and choroid), which is the major source of blood supply to the eye.[8] The etiology of uveitis may be infectious, infestations, trauma, neoplastic disorders or inflammatory reactions secondary to immune disorders. It can be classified based on the anatomical location of the disease process in the eye, its mode of onset and the etiology involved (Table 108.2).

Clinical features of uveitis are produced by an inflammatory response to the etiological factor (i.e. infections, trauma, malignancies, autoimmune process, etc). The chemical mediators of the acute stage of inflammation include serotonin, complement and plasmin. Leukotrienes, kinins and prostaglandins modify the second stage of the acute response through antagonism of vasoconstrictors. Polymorphonuclear leukocytes, eosinophils, and mast cells may all

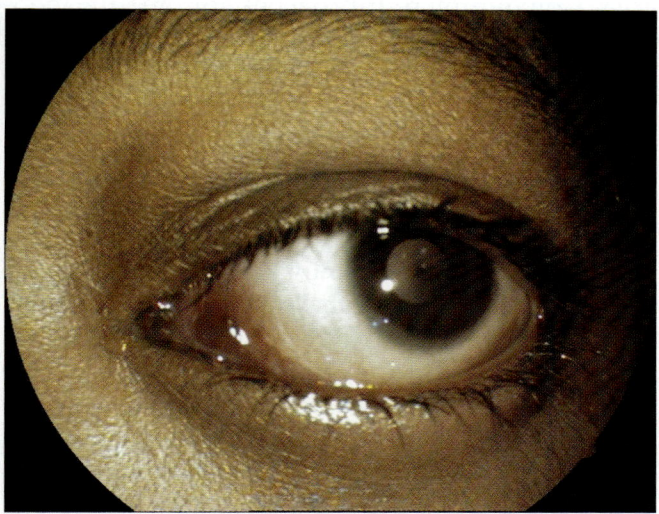

Fig. 108.12: Proptosis

Table 108.2: Classification of uveitis

Type of uveitis	Features
A. Anatomical location	
i. Anterior uveitis	Inflammation of the iris and anterior part of ciliary body (pars plicata)
ii. Intermediate uveitis	Predominantly inflammation of the posterior part of ciliary body (pars plana) and extreme periphery of the retina
iii. Posterior uveitis	Inflammation located behind the posterior border of the vitreous base
iv. Panuveitis	Inflammation of the entire uveal tract
B. Clinical classification (based on mode of onset and duration)	
i. Acute uveitis	Sudden symptomatic uveitis that persists for 8 weeks or less
ii. Chronic uveitis	Usually asymptomatic uveitis of insidious onset persists for > 3 months
C. Based on the etiology involved	
i. Exogenous uveitis	Uveitis secondary to external injury to the uveal tissue or invasion of microorganisms from outside
ii. Endogenous uveitis	Uveitis due to microorganisms or other agents from within the patient.

contribute to signs of inflammation but the lymphocyte is, by far, the predominant inflammatory cell involved in uveitis in the inner eye.

Uveitis usually present with blurred vision, floaters, pain, redness, photophobia and/or lacrimation.[8] Blurred vision may be because of refractive error (e.g. myopic or hyperopic shift due to macular edema, hypotony, or change in lens position), or opacities in the visual axis from inflammatory cells, fibrin or protein in the anterior chamber, keratic precipitates, or secondary cataract. Pain in uveitis results from acute onset of inflammation of the iris, secondary glaucoma or ciliary body spasm. Photophobia and increased lacrimation present when iris, cornea or irisciliary body complex is involved. However, occasionally uveitis may be discovered on a routine ophthalmoscopic examination in an asymptomatic patient.

The signs of uveitis in the anterior portion of the eye include keratic precipitates (KP) cells, flare, fibrin, hypopyon, pigment dispersion, pupillary miosis, iris nodules and synechial, both anterior and posterior. In the intermediate anatomical area of the eye, there may be vitreal inflammatory cells and vitreal stands.

Signs of the posterior segment (posterior two-thirds) of the eye include retinal or choroidal inflammatory infiltrates, perivascular inflammatory cuffing, retinal pigment epithelial hypertrophy or atrophy, and atrophy or swelling of retina, choroid or optic nerve head. Retinal or choroidal signs may be unifocal, multifocal or diffuse. The uveitis may be diffuse throughout the eye (panuveitis) or appear dispersed with spill over from the area to another (e.g. toxoplasmosis).

The morphological features present in uveitis are of importance in relation to give clues to diagnose the specific cause of uveitis, though; sometimes laboratory evaluation is required for corroboration.

Generally speaking the treatment of uveitis ranges from case to case. Some patients may need simple observation however; others may require medical or surgical intervention. Medical therapy usually includes topical or systemic steroids along with the cycloplegics. In few cases immunosuppressive therapy may also be required. Treatment should be tailored to the individual patient and adjust according to the response. The treating clinician should also keep in mind and consider the patient's systemic involvement and other factors such as age, immune status, and tolerance for side effects of the drugs.

Surgical therapy for uveitis may include paracentasis or vitreous biopsy for diagnostic evaluations to rule out neoplastic or manage the particular complications of uveitis (e.g., cataract extraction, trabeculectomy or other glaucoma surgery to control the IOP and vitrectomy for dense vitreous membranes). As a general rule, before performing cataract surgery in such cases, the eye should be quiet for at least 3 months.

Treatment modalities for diseases involving the posterior segment of the eye have been limited by the lack of effective delivery of the drug to the affected area. Conventional approaches for treating non-infectious inflammatory diseases affecting the posterior segment are topical steroid administration, peribulbar steroid injections and systemic steroid and cytotoxic agent administration.

Topical medication does not provide high enough concentrations of the drug for it to be effective in treating posterior uveitis. Peribulbar steroid injections have the advantage of minimizing the systemic side effects while maximizing the local effects. Though this method of treatment may be efficacious it requires repeated intervention and is not desirable for long-term therapy. Also, the local toxicity may be increased due to the regional concentration of the drug immediately after administration. Systemic steroid administration requires high doses to be effective in treating posterior segment diseases. More importantly, these concentrations are associated with debilitating systemic side effects. Similarly, systemic toxicities are also dose limiting for cytotoxic agents.

The novel new technique of intravitreal sustained release drug delivery was first devised to treat CMV retinitis in AIDS patients, in the form of a gancyclovir implant. The intravitreal steroid implant for recurrent noninfectious posterior uveitis is based on the same principle. This mode of therapy has the advantage of maintaining therapeutic levels in the target tissue with minimum systemic exposure and consequently minimum systemic toxicity.

The intravitreal steroid implant for uveitis contains the corticosteroid, fluocinolone acetonide. This form of medication was chosen as it could be prepared in a form concentrated enough to fit into the device and provide the duration needed for long-term delivery of steroid. The implant has a polymer coating of PVA and silicone designed to release efficacious levels of the drug inside the eye over an extended time period.

Appropriate patient selection is very essential to ensure favorable results. Only those patients with a history of recurrent intermediate or posterior uveitis treated repeatedly with oral or peribulbar steroids should be considered for this mode of treatment. Those patients showing a tendency towards steroid induced glaucoma should be excluded.

The placement of the implant involves a minor surgical procedure. The device is implanted at the pars-plana region after making an appropriate sclerotomy and secured with the help of non-absorbable sutures.

The intravitreal steroid implant could offer an alternative treatment option for diabetic macular edema and age related macular degeneration.

Orbital Cellulitis

Orbital cellulitis is defined as infection of the orbit (Fig. 108.13). It is one of the few ophthalmic emergencies, which can have severe systemic implications besides causing loss of vision, if appropriate management is not instituted in the right time.[6]

Orbital cellulitis is more common in children, and more severe in diabetics and immunocompromised patients. Patients typically present with history of unilateral pain, redness and proptosis of recent onset, often in the seasons when allergies are more prevalent. The patient looks obviously sick, and is usually febrile. This is in contrast to, say, rhabdomyosarcoma and retinoblastoma where the general condition is relatively unaffected till later on in the disease. The common causative organisms of cellulitis are *Staph. aureus, Streptococcus, H. influenzae*, anaerobic bacteriae like *Bacteroides*. Fungi and *Mycobacterium tuberculosis* may be the culprits in recalcitrant cases. Mucor is typically found in diabetics. The microbes usually spread to orbit from infected paranasal sinuses, lids and rarely from infected tooth, pyoderma, CNS and penetrating trauma. Diminution of vision in orbital cellulitis is usually due to optic nerve involvement, which reflects poorer prognosis–the other common cause is exposure keratopathy due to proptosis. Both these poles of the eye have to be taken care of adequately and in time.

Routes of Infection

1. *Sinus:* Secondary sinusitis is the commonest cause. Ethmoid sinus is the most frequently responsible sinus due to the very thin wall of this sinus.
2. *Trauma:* Post-traumatic orbital cellulits is seen secondary to an injury that also damages the orbital septum. It is commoner if a foreign body is retained within the orbit.
3. *Surgery:* This is rare but may complicate a retinal or an orbital surgery.
4. It may also be seen as an extension from adjacent structures, e.g. secondary to a panophathlmitis or a dental infection, very rarely due to dacryocystitis.
5. In our country, it is not uncommon to see cases of very advanced retinoblastoma or rhabdomyosarcoma which present with a cellulitis like picture. This is not true cellulitis, but rarely there may be superadded infection.

On local examination, unilateral axial proptosis is seen which is later noncompressible. The lids are tense and inflamed; conjunctiva is diffusely congested. An equal decrease in ocular movement in all directions is a reliable sign to exclude the possibility of only a preseptal cellulitis where ocular movements are usually preserved; here also, a reactionary postseptal (orbital) edema induced through the still intact septum could also produce features overlapping an actual

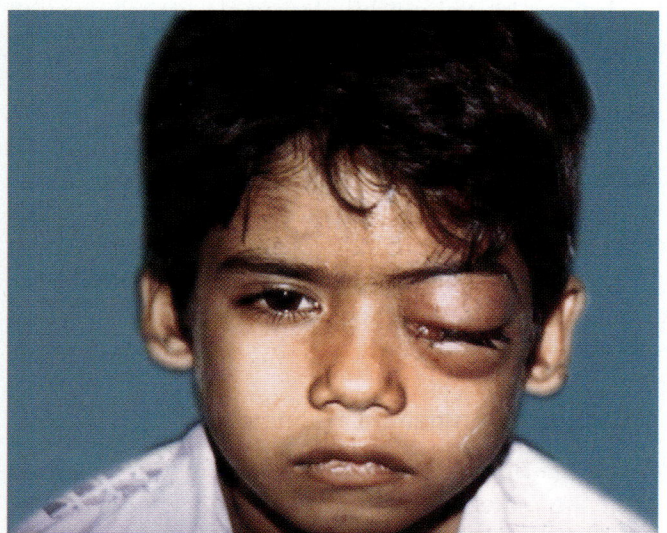

Fig. 108.13: Orbital cellulitis

orbital cellulitis—the reverse is also true. Examination of the disks and both pupils, although often difficult because of tense lid edema and irritable state, can throw light on optic nerve involvement. Checking the sensation of the skin distributed by ophthalmic division V(1) of trigeminal nerve is essential as it is affected in superior orbital fissure syndrome (paralysis of III, IV, V(1) and VI cranial nerves + dilated pupils + proptosis + ptosis). Associated diminution of vision may indicate optic nerve involvement (Orbital Apex Syndrome). Paralysis of VI cranial nerve and congestion of conjunctival and retinal vessels of the other eye are the early signs of cavernous sinus thrombosis, a dreaded complication of orbital cellulitis. ENT, CNS and evaluation of other systems should be done to find the focus of infection.

The patient has to be promptly admitted for further management. Pain relief should be the first consideration. Orbital ultrasonography can provide valuable information regarding pus pockets, etc. CT scan of orbit, head and paranasal sinuses confirms the diagnosis, and aids in deciding further management and also prognosticating. Hemogram, TLC, DLC, baseline renal function tests and blood sugar levels should be done. Gram stained smears and KOH smears can provide important clues regarding causative organisms and hence, can guide initial antimicrobial therapy. Pus (if any) should be obtained for culture and sensitivity testing before starting antimicrobial therapy. Blood cultures are useful in management but rarely positive after antibiotics have been started even in suboptimal dosage. Antimicrobials should always be given intravenously, at least 2 drugs, and in at least twice the normal dosage. Our protocol of empirical treatment at the center includes:

1. Injection amoxycillin (any suitable semi-synthetic penicillin) 1 gm IV 6 hrly (50-100 mg/kg/day in 4 divided doses) after samples taken form sensitivity testing, and a skin test (Vancomycin used in cases of sensitivity to penicillin).
2. Injection amikacin (or any suitable amnioglycoside) 250 mg IV 8 hrly (20 mg/kg/day in 3 DD) given along with above.
   Suitable cephlosporin and/or ciprofloxacin to be considered as second line of defence Ceftriaxone (100 mg/kg/d in 2 divided doses) + Vancomycin (40 mg/kg/d in 2 doses).
3. Injection metronidazole 500 mg IV 8 hrly (30 mg/kg/day in 3 DD), and even antifungal or antitubercular treatment wherever indicated.
4. Corneal lubricants in prevention/management of exposure keratopathy and
5. Multivitamins are to be prescribed too.

Intravenous antibiotics should be continued till an afebrile period of at least 4 days with subsidence of symptoms and signs. Oral antibiotics are started, continued at home thereafter, and stopped appropriately during follow-up. Antimicrobial therapy should of course be modified according to culture and sensitivity reports.

On reviewing the patient, following parameters should be carefully recorded:
1. Visual acuity.
2. Proptosis (quantitated by Hertel's exophthalmometer).
3. Limitation of ocular movements (with diplopia charting when required).
4. Exposure keratopathy.
5. Pupillary reactions.
6. Contralateral VI cranial nerve.
7. Temperature monitoring (for fever).
8. Neck rigidity/mental status.

Orbital abscesses and large subperiosteal collections should be drained. Small subperiosteal abscesses are known to respond to medical therapy alone. Paranasal sinuses, if containing pus, should also be drained by the otorhinolarnygologist, along with the orbital drainage. Help from other specialists, as neurosurgeons, should be sought whenever felt necessary.

Initial presentations may not predict the final outcomes, either functional or cosmetic. Despite the advent of more potent antimicrobials, orbital cellulitis still remains a potential killer especially with virulent and resistant strains inadequately treated. Otherwise, the results are satisfactory, unless the optic nerve or cornea is involved early.

Chlamydia Ophthalmia Neonatorum

Chlamydia ophthalmia neonatorum may be acquired from the maternal birth passage and have a longer incubation period than the earlier more common gonococcal ophthalmia. Proper diagnosis and aggressive therapy are necessary. Trachoma is still widely prevalent in our country, and manifests mostly in the upper palperbral conjuctiva with follicles and scarring later with cicatrzation. An early diagnosis and tretment prevents serious complication of blinding trachoma.

Membranous Conjunctivitis

Diphtheritic conjunctivitis is associated with true membrane formation Pseudomembranes may form in other bacterial infections and also in Stevens-Johnson syndrome. It may be dangerous to peel off the membrane, as toxins may be released with grave consequenes. A pinkish white elevation appearing at the limbus in the bulbar conjunctiva, could be a phlycten with engorged conjunctival vessels clustering around its base. Phlyctenular keratoconjunctivitis is believed to be an allergic response to tubercular or other bactierial protines often associated with undernutrion and poor health. Treatment consists of topical steroid/ NSAID therapy. A systemic tubercular focus should be ruled out and respiratory infections looked for.

The presence of congested nodules on the sclera is suggestive of episcleriris, or the more severe condition of scleritis (usually with associated underlying uveitis). Episclertis and scleritis should be differentiated from acture conjunctivitis by their more localized nature and presence of pain and tenderness.

MISCELLANEOUS DISORDERS

Vitamin A Deficiency

Conjunctival xerosis and Bitot spots are not emergencies perse, but they may be the forerunners of keratomalacia. Most pediatricians in developing countries are familiar with the grim picture and hopeless visual prognosis of keratomalacia. The treatment consists of administraion of systemic vitamin A, topical and systemic antibiotics, atropine ophthalmic ointment and warm compresses. Vitamin A 100,000-200,000 IU is given orally daily for 2 successive days if the child does not have any diarrhea, otherwise a water dispersible preparation of vitamin A is administered by intramuscular route. This dose should be repeated 2-4 weeks later. The nutritional status and education of these children should be improved. The condition must be identified early before irreversible damage to the eyes has taken place. The alarming magnitude of nutritional blindness in the country can be reduced by vitamin a prophylaxis with suitable short-term, medium-and long-term measures. Besides xerophthalmia, diffuse or focal corneal haze can occur due to several causes; congenital, traumatic, inflammatory (intrauterine or postnatal), neoplastic, degenerative, allergic and metabolic (mucopolysaccharidoeses) disorders.

Night blindness most commonly occurs due to vitamin A deficiency. Pigmentary retinal degeneration (retinitis pigmentosa) as in Laurence-Moon-Bardet-Biedl (LMBB) syndrome and other uncommon hereditary conditions may also produce night blindness.

REFRACTIVE DISORDERS

Hyperopia (Hypermetropia, Far-sightedness)

Moderately severe hyperopia may cause headache reading difficulty and even squinting. Hyperopia with symptoms may require correctional glasses after cycloplegic refraction.

Myopia (Near-sightedness)

In congenital myopia, children are born with high myopia and one or both parents are often myopic. Usually myopia develops between the age of 5 and 15 years because of rpid growth of the eyes. They have few early symptoms, and the detection is often made at school or on routine visual testing. Associated astigmatism may lead to eye fatigue, headache and blepharitis. Corrective glasses (or contact lenses) after cycloplegic refraction should be prescribed for constant use, and the child is encouraged to wear them all the time for distance as well as for near.

Astigmatism (Inability for Point Focus)

A mild degree of astigmatism is common. Red eyes, recurring blepharoconjunctivitis, stye and chalazia often indicate the presence of astigmatism. Eye strain (asthenopia), pain in and around the eyeballs, headache, and nausea may occur. Astigmatism may be associated with hyperopia or myopia. If the vision is not subnormal and there are no symptoms, glasses may not be required, but in case of either, correction should be ordered for constant use after cycloplegic refraction.

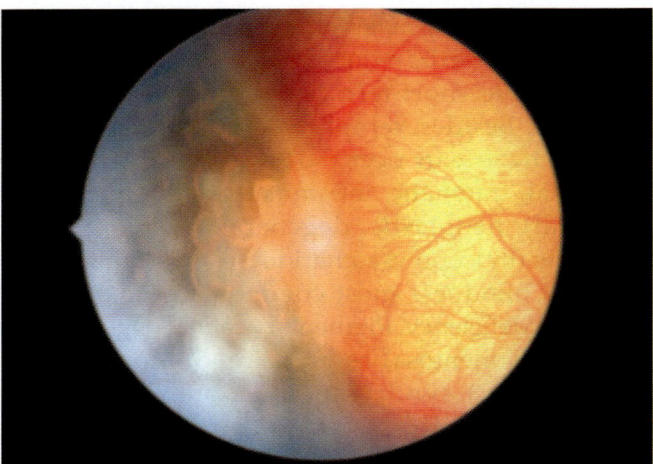

Fig. 108.14: Retinopathy of prematurity

Retinopathy of Prematurity

The development of retrolental fibroplasias (or retinopathy of prematurity) is probably related to exposure of preterm low birth weight (LBW) infants to high concentrations of oxygen above 40 percent because of the immaturity of the retinal vasculature in these premature eyes.[9,10] Initially, there is vasoconstriction of retinal vessels. Later the vessels dilate and become tortuous. Hemorrhages occur along the blood vessles. Retinal detachment may occur. Neovascularization and vitreous opactieis may be seen at the junction of the detached retina with the normal reina (Fig. 108.14). Organization of vitreous and formation of retrolental membranes follow (retrolental fibroplasias). The eye becomes small with marked visual loss. The anterior chamber becomes shallow. Myopia and strabismus are common. The progression of disease may be arrested at any stage Prevention of the condition is important and depends upon the use of minimal oxygen concentration for least possible time with careful monitoring.

Watering

Watering may be because of inflammation, infections foreign bodies, ENT problems, uveitis, glaucoma, and nasolacrimal obstruction. It can be one of the major causes of anxiety to the parents of a neonate. Persistent watering from one or both the eyes in infants should lead to the suspicion of blockage of the nasolacrimal duct with congenital dacrocystitis. The regurgitation of mucopus from the puncta on pressure over the lacrimal sac clinches the diagnosis of dacryocystitis. The discharge should be sent for culture and antibiotic sensitivity. The mother should be advised to massage the sac firmly twice a day, clean the discharge, and instill an appropriate antibiotic as drops. The associated rhinitis should be controlled and the nose kept dry so as to facilitate the opening up of the blocked nasolacrimal duct. The child may be referred for further management to an ophthalmologist. The probing and syringing of the nasolacrimal duct should preferably not be delayed beyond six months of age, though many infants do undergo spontaneous resolution by one year of age with proper conservative treatment.

Even though a congenital obstruction of the nasolacrimal duct and the ensuing dacryocystitis remains one of the prominent causes of watering in the younger patients, one should always keep in mind other important sight threatening entities such as congenital glaucoma and corneal disorders.

Lid Disorders

Lid edema is not uncommon, and it is an alarming sign. It may be due to allergy (topical medications), or due to an insect bite. The loose areolar tissues of the lids allow considerable swelling to occur. Conservative treatment is quite satisfactory. A swelling in the lid may be neoplastic in nature. Injury around the lids and a black eye may be associated with lid edema. Systemic causes of lid edema should be excluded.

Stye (hordeolum externum), a painful tender erythematous infection of the hair follicle of eyelashes, and furuncles may also produce lid edema. The temptation to express the pus should be avoided, as it may lead to development of lid abscess.

A chalazion is a painless granulomatous nodule of the Meibomian tarsal glands in the eyelid. It may start as an acute hordeolum internum, at which stage it may be aborted with timely hot fomentation, antibiotic drops and massage. Once established, a chalazion may require incision and curettage as an elective procedure. Causes of eyestrains as refractive errors and orthoptic problems need to be ruled out in styes, chalazia and blepharitis, especially if recurrent. Squamous and especially ulcerative blepharitis require energetic treatment. Associated dandruff should also be managed. Vaccinial and herpetic blepharitis are known to occur.

Others

Some congenital lid conditions require early surgical intervention such as congenital coloboma with corneal exposure (Goldenhar's syndrome), and severe ptosis, Entropion (congenital or trachmomatous) and distichiasis may require correction if the cornea is endangered. Congenital ectropion is rare, but the more common ciccatricial type necessitates repair by skin grafting.

Congenital craniofacial and CNS disorders such as hydrocephalus, microcephaly, mental retardation cerebral palsy (to maximize head control) encephalocele, meningomyelocele, and craniosynostosis often produce significant ocular features. Corneal exposure and early papilloedema constitute virtually emergency situations for the pediatrician and the pediatric surgeon.

Some inborn errors of metabolism such as homocystinuria (subluxated lens) and galactosemia (cataract), albinism, lipidoses, chromosomal aberrations, Marfan's syndrome (ectopia lentis), Weil-Marchesani syndrome with spherophakia and "inverse" glaucoma (responding to dilation of pupils), and phakomatoses can also produce urgent ocular situations.[1] Color vision defects are often hereditary and are not yet amenable to any treatment, except eugenics.

Sudden diminution of vision in children may be associated with serious neurological disease, like meningitis and encephalitis and may occur due to optic neuritis, or brain damage (cortical blindness). The importance of careful evaluation of pupillary reflexes cannot be overemphasized. Prompt empirical treatment with systemic corticosteroids and antibiotics along with specific therapy may save the vision. Parenteral administration of vitamins B1 B6 and B12 (as injection. Triredisol-H) may be of some help. In a child with poor vision, common conditions like refractive errors (high myopia) and amblyopia (blunting of vision following sensory visual deprivation due to squint, anisometropia, corneal opacities, cataract, etc.) should be ruled out Other causes of sudden visual deterioration in children include demyelinating and convulsive disorders, vascular lesions, migraine and iatrogenic reasons due to the toxic effects of drugs. Functional blindness may occur in adolescent children and simple tests for visual malingering may help the clinician.

PREVENTION

Of all the ocular problems in childhood, injuries, infections and malnutrition form the major bulk, and all are largely preventable. It is hoped that programs for better nutrition, sanitation, dietary education, and control of infectious diseases especially diarrheal disorders will reduce the incidence of blinding malnutritions. Prophylactic administration of vitamin A to preschool children can eradicate blindness due to vitamin A deficiency. The current recommendations by the Government of India are to administer first dose of prophylactic vitamin A 100,000 IU at 9 months (along with measles vacination) followed by second dose of 200,000 IU around the age of 15-18 months (along with first booster of DPT/OPV) and three more doses at an interval of every 6 months.

Children should be discouraged from playing with pointed objects and sharp toys. The hazards of arrows, airguns, catapults and fireworks should be highlighted through the mass media. Eyes are precious and must be protected both at work and play. The teachers should be well informed to teach preventive and promotive aspects of eye health care of the students.

Gonococcal ophthalmia neonatorum can be prevented by prophylactic topical instillation of either silver nitrate 1 percent or erythromycin 0.5 percent ophthalmic ointment to newborn babies at risk. The erythromycin prophylaxis provides additional protection against eye infections due to chlamydiae. However, if the eye damage has occurred, the earlier it is effectively managed, the better are the chances for salvaging useful vision. Injuries and inflammation of other parts of the body may heal with minimal or no side effects, but the delicate ocular tissues are greatly compromised by the reparative process leading to serious cosmetic and visual handicaps.

REFERENCES

1. Kalra BR, Ghose S, Sood NN. Homocystinuria with bilateral absolute glaucoma. Indian Ophthalmol 1985;33:195-97.
2. Nainiwal K Sanjeev K, Talwar D. The investigations and localization of intraocular foreign body. Monthly Bulletin of Delhi Ophthalmological Society DOS Times, December 2000;6(6): 21-27.
3. Nainiwal K Sanjeev, Dada VK. Acute Chemical Injury: Approach to Management. Monthly Bulletin of Delhi Ophthalmological Society DOS Times, 2001;7 (5): 20-23.
4. Ghose S, Kalra BR. Red eye–a common problem in children. Indian J Pediatr 1982;49:751-59.
5. Nainiwal K Sanjeev. Bacterial Corneal Ulcer: Approach to Management. Monthly Bulletin of Delhi Ophthalmological Society DOS Times, August 2001;7(2):30-33.
6. Ghose S, Seth V, Singhal V, et al. Diagnostic problems in leucocoria. Indian Ophthalmol 1983;31:233-37.
7. Verma N, Ghose S, Sekhar GC. Ultrasonic evaluation of retinoblastoma. Jap Ophthalmol 1984;28:222-29.
8. Garg SP, Nainiwal K Sanjeev, Krishnan Suma, Tewari Hem K. Uveitis: Current concepts and management. Monthly Bulletin of Delhi Ophthalmological Society DOS Times, December 2002;8(6):21-23.
9. Kumar Harsh, Nainiwal Sanjeev, Singh Ujwala, Azad Rajvardhan, Paul VK. Examination stress induced by screening for retinopathy of prematurity. J Paediatr Ophthalmol Strabismus. 2002;39(6):349-50.
10. Nainiwal K Sanjeev. Retinopathy of Prematurity-"FOCUS". Monthly Bulletin of Delhi Ophthalmological Society DOS Times 2001; 7 (1): 3-10.

CHAPTER 109

Pediatric Otolaryngology

RC Deka, DN Jha

In this chapter, a special emphasis is laid on the pediatric otolaryngologic emergencies and their management as would be of interest to the pediatric surgeons.

I. THE EAR

ACUTE OTITIS MEDIA (AOM)

Acute otitis media is the most common bacterial infection in children and the most frequent indication for medical or surgical therapy. Known risk factors are young age, male gender, bottle feeding, crowded living conditions, smoking in the home, heredity and a variety of associated conditions such as cleft palate, immunodefeciency, ciliary dyskinesia, Down syndrome and cystic fibrosis.[1]

AOM is typified by the symptoms and signs of acute infection (fever, pain, red bulging tympanic membrane). The pathophysiology of AOM is the result of bacterial entry into the middle ear. This entry is due to an abnormally patent (compliant) eustachian tube. The bacteria commonly implicated in the infection are *Streptococcus pneumoniae, Hemophilus influenzae, Branhamella catarrhalis, Streptococcus pyogenes* and *Streptococcus aureus*.[1] Viruses have been recovered from the middle ear in 20% of early cases and in some cases as the sole agent, but more often with pathogenic bacteria.[2,3]

Antibiotic therapy is the mainstay for treatment of AOM. A 10-day treatment is the usual course prescribed. Amoxicillin is the first line drug of choice, but if the inflammation does not show signs of response, then the initial agent is discontinued and a second line drug (e.g. Cefaclor or amoxicillin-clavulanate is used. Because of the frequent association of OM and upper respiratory tract infection, the use of a nasal decongestant to open the airway may be helpful. Antihistamines should be avoided because their atropine-like effects leads to drying of secretions.

Myringotomy promptly relieves severe pain in cases of AOM, but adds little to either remission of infection or clearence of middle ear effusion in cases of AOM treated with amoxicillin-clavulanate.[4,5] In complicated cases of AOM as in facial paralysis, meningitis, or other central nervous system event, myringotomy should be done without delay to prompt drainage and collect material for culture.

Untreated or incompletely treated cases of AOM leads to infection spreading and causing mastoiditis or a frank abscess. Infection may cause meningitis, intracerebral abscess, labyrinthitis or facial nerve paralysis.

CHRONIC SUPPURATIVE OTITIS MEDIA (CSOM)

Tubotympanic Type

This variety usually follows a benign course and is virtually always a complication of acute otitis media where there is a persisting perforation in the tympanic membrane. This usually starts in early childhood and is a common entity. The persisting or recurring infection in the middle ear cleft spreads via the eustachian tube which is shorter and more horizontal in young children. The edges of the perforation get epithelised in due course and then the child is likely to have persistent or recurrent discharge secondary to upper respiratory tract infections. The infection may also result from bacteria gaining access to the middle ear cleft via the external auditory canal. The children present with mucopurulent discharge which is intermittent or occasionally persistent. Examination confirms the presence of central perforation. In all the cases the nasal cavities, the nasopharynx and pharynx must be examined because the source of infection may be found in the upper respiratory tract. The common causes are in the infected tonsils, adenoids or the sinuses. Hearing tests including tuning fork tests and pure tone audiometry usually reveals the presence of conductive deafness. Radiography of the mastoids would reveal a cellular mastoid, but if the infection has been long standing then it may be sclerotic. Treatment includes eliminating upper respiratory tract infection first. The ear is cleaned under direct vision (preferably under a microscope) and the patient advised to use antibiotic ear drops active against gram negative infections such as *Pseudomonas Pyocyanea* or *B. Proteus*.[6] The patients should be warned not to get water into their ears while washing or swimming . If the child gets a cold, then he should not blow his nose as this may cause massive movement of nasal discharge up the eustachian tube into the middle ear. If there is bilateral perforation causing severe hearing handicap, then Myringoplasty is advised, otherwise this surgery is usually done at our center when the child has attained 15 years of age when the eustachian tube function has stabilised.

Atticoantral Type

In this type of infection the bone of attic, antrum or mastoid process is involved as well as the mucosa of the middle ear cleft. An erosion of the bone may extend to adjacent vital structures by direct spread or via osteothrombo phlebitis causing intratemporal complications (facial nerve palsy, labyrinthitis, sensorineural hearing loss) or intracranial complications (meningitis, intracranial abscess, lateral sinus thrombosis).

Cholesteatoma

Cholesteatoma consists of a sac of keratinizing squamous epithelium surrounded by granulation tissue. The granulation tissue on the outside of the sac produces lysozymes and this gradually erodes the ossicles, ear drum and the mastoid bone. In children cholesteatoma tends to be more aggressive and destructive.

The symptoms and bacteriology are very similar to those of tubotympanic otitis media. The discharge however is purulent rather than mucopurulent and frequently very foul smelling. Deafness is usually present and may vary from trivial to profound depending upon the involvement of the ossicular chain and the inner ear. If granulations or polyps are present, bleeding from the ear my be noticed.

On examination the discharge is very offensive to smell and is scanty in amount. The deep retraction pocket is usually seen in the attic or the postero-superior quadrant area of the tympanic membrane. Hearing tests may usually reveal varying levels of conductive deafness, but if the inner ear is involved then sensorineural deafnes may be seen. Radiography of the mastoid may reveal a cholesteatoma cavity as an area of translucency with a clearly outlined bony margin. Surgery is the mainstay of treatment of this condition. The basic aims of the surgery are to make the ear safe, dry and if possible to improve hearing.[7] If the residual hearing is present then a modified Radical Mastoidectomy is done, but if there is no cochlear reserve then a Radical Mastoidectomy is done.

OTITIS MEDIA WITH EFFUSION (OME)

OME is one of the commonest chronic otological conditions of childhood. It results from alteration of the mucociliary system within the middle ear cleft where serous or mucoid fluid accumulates in association with a negative pressure. The pressure change is almost invariably caused by a malfunction of the eustachian tube. Although there are no signs of inflammation, bacteria can be cultured from the effusion in almost 50% of cases. Chronic Otitis media with effusion is usually present in children with cleft palate.[8] I frequently occurs in association with chronic upper respiratory tract infection and conditions affecting the nose and sinuses. The condition occurs in childhood as an overt or covert hearing loss presenting as educational or behavioral problem.[9,10] In younger children it may present as speech and language delay or as an articulation defect. Treatment varies widely and is dependent on the duration and severity of the problem. Mild forms of the disease resolve spontaneously. Unilateral effusion as is expected is less detrimental to normal childhood development than bilateral effusion. Topical and systemic vasoconstrictors, antihistaminics, antibiotics and systemic steroids have been tried, but none has been established as a proven modality or treatment. If there is persistent otitis media with effusion, a myringotomy and insertion of ventilating tube (grommet) is recommended.

DEAFNESS IN CHILDREN

An attempt should be made to diagnose hearing impairment in children as early as possible.[11] For acquisition of speech, the important years of life are the first 2 years and hence it is vital that children born with a significant loss should be identified before reaching the age of 1 year. If a definite diagnosis is made, then a hearing aid can be fitted from as early as 3 months of age.

Hearing assessment can be made by:
 i. *Distraction Techniques:* At the age of about 6-7 months a normal baby will search for the source of sound by turning his head towards the noise. A fairly accurate assessment can be made of the child's hearing thresholds at a variety of frequencies. Beyond the age of 1 year, voice distraction techniques can be used.
 ii. *Conditioning Techniques:* At the age of 2-5 years the child can be taught to make some simple movement in response to sounds. When the child has been conditioned, an accurate assessment of hearing loss is possible and actual audiograms can be plotted.
 iii. *Pure Tone Audiometry:* Most children between the ages of 4-5 years can be persuaded to co-operate so that pure tone audiogram can be obtained.
 iv. *Impedance Audiometry:* This test is essential to indicate the status of middle ear conducting mechanism.
 v. *Brainstem Evoked Response Audiometry:* This test is now widely used to estimate hearing thresholds in children. In a neonate it can be performed when the child is sleeping or after a feed. Once the infant is 3 months old, sedation can be given. Surface electrodes are applied to the mastoid, vertex and forehead and the auditory stimulation is by 2000 or 4000 broad band click or tone bursts. The response is recorded and the intensity reduced until the N5 wave disappears. The V wave form is normally seen 6 or 7 msec after the stimulus, depending on the age of the child.[12]
 vi. *Electrocochleography:* In this test an insulated needle electrode is inserted through the tympanic membrane to lie on the promontary. A series of clicks or tone bursts are used. The number varies from the size of response from 64-512 or more. The threshold is estimated by identifying the action potential and reducing the intensity of auditory stimuli until the action potential is no longer seen.

The types of deafness can be classified as:
1. *Congenital Conductive Deafness:* The complicated embryology allows for a great variety of congenital malformations involving the pinna, the external meatus, the tympanic membrane, the middle ear cavity and the ossicles. Important among them are the defects in the external meatus which prevent sound waves from reaching the tympanic membrane and the abnormalities of the ossicular chain which interfere with the transmission of sound to the inner ear. With a bilateral meatal atresia, surgery should be considered and the accepted age for this is between 18 months and 2 years of age.
2. *Sensorineural Deafness:* Sensorineural hearing loss should be identified as early as possible and hearing aids may be fitted as early as 3 months of age. If the child is detected to have a profound hearing loss not benefiting by a hearing aid, then a cochlear implant is advisable.[13] This device is implanted in the temporal bone in the post-auricular region, with the electrodes being introduced in the cochlea via the promontary or the round window. The device is switched on 6 weeks later when the surgical wound has healed. Vigorous rehabilitation is employed for a period of 6 months to several years for the device to be effective.

II. THE NOSE

DEVELOPMENTAL ABNORMALITIES

1. Choanal Atresia occurs in 1 in 5000-8000 live births.[14] Of these 50% have associated anomalies whereas the rest have isolated anomalies. About 65-75% of these anomalies are unilateral, whereas the rest are bilateral.[15] Patients with long standing unilateral nasal obstruction and discharge may not present until later in life, whereas those with bilateral atresias present as new born with cyclic

cyanosis relieved on crying. Bilateral atresia is an emergent situation as the neonates are obligate nose breathers. An oropharyngeal airway should immediately be inserted to save life. Choanal atresia can simply be diagnosed by passing a catheter through the nose into the nasopharynx or by flexible endoscopy. Computed tomography is the radiographic procedure of choice which can show the nature and thicknenn of the constricting membrane. Surgical repair of choanal atresia involves transnasal, transpalatal, transantral and transseptal approaches.

2. *Encephaloceles and Gliomas:* An encephalocele is a herniation of cranial contents through a defect in the skull. It may include meninges only termed as meningocele, or it may involve brain and meninges, termed as meningoencephalocele. A glioma is thought to be an encephalocele that has lost the intracranial connection although 15% remain attached to the central nervous system via a fibrous stalk. Diagnosis is confirmed both by CT scan and MRI. The definitive management is surgical and a neurosurgical consultation is mandatory.

EPISTAXIS

The commonest cause of epistaxis is either from external trauma or from picking of the nose. Most epistaxis originates from the Little's area, not only because of the highly vascular nature of this region but also because inspired air tends to be directed onto it causing undue drying and crusting. When this is removed, some of the mucosa is also removed with it causing bleeding. Other common etiologies include upper respiratory tract infections, foreign bodies, tumors, disorders of blood vessels and clotting mechanisms. First aid measures include sitting the patient forwards and pinching the nostrils tight. Ice is sucked and put over the forehead until the bleeding stops. The simplest method to stop bleeding is to insert a pledget of cotton wool soaked in adrenaline solution into the nostril. If bleeding persists, an anterior or a post-nasal pack may need to be inserted.

THE CATARRHAL CHILD

Nasal catarrh and history of frequent colds are commonly encountered conditions in general practice. Certain factors that predispose to the condition are:

i. *Environment:* Hygiene, overcrowding, illness in the family and general nutritional factors and environmental pollution are contributing factors.
ii. *Viral Infections:* There are two main types of respiratory viruses. The first type enters the cells of the respiratory tract where they multiply to cause respiratory infections, and among these are the influenza and the parainfluenza viruses, the adenovirus, the respiratory syncytial virus and the rhinovirus. The second type enter the respiratory cells where they cause no local damage but spread by the blood stream to give rise to exanthemata such as measles, rubella, varicella, etc.
iii. *Allergy:* Allergy is frequently hereditary in origin, and the child of two atopic parents stands a 75% chance of producing symptoms of nasal allergy.
iv. *Nasal Polypi:* In children, unilateral polypi is more common requiring surgery. Multiple bilateral ethmoidal polypi are rare in children and if seen, a search for mucoviscidosis should be made.
v. *Vasomotor Rhinitis:* This is as common in older children as it is in adults. The turbinates appear congested and hypertrophied and do not have the pallor of the allergic turbinate. The major complaint is that of nasal obstruction, but persistent rhinorrhea with or without sniffing is not common.
vi. *Immotile Cilia Syndrome:* Children with recurrent unexplained chest infections or chronic obstinate nasal catarrh may have this problem. Detailed investigation is needed to diagnose this condition.

SEPTAL DEVIATION IN CHILDREN

Trauma to the nose of the fetus can occur in the mother's womb or during delivery because of the pressure effects as the fetus passes through the birth canal.[16] The new-borns to be tested for nasal septal deformity should undergo external nasal examination.[17] They should also undergo the test for tip instability, cotton wool test, metal plate test, and examination by a small auriscope and strut.

Nasal septal deviation occurs more frequently in childhood, although it occurs at any age due to trauma.[18] Due to the deviation, eustachian tube and middle ear functions are also affected. Septoplasty in childhood does not produce any untoward events in terms of developmental delay of the nose and face.

Though deviation of the septum has a greater chance of recurring after surgery, the results of septoplasty in children are fairly satisfactory.

SINUSITIS IN CHILDREN

Chronic sinusitis among patients referred for evaluation has a peak incidence of approximately 3 years of age followed by gradual tapering. The variables that cause chronic and recurrent sinusitis are: (1) Inflammatory problems such as upper respiratory tract problems and allergies, (2) Mechanical obstruction include adenoid hypertrophy, nasal polyps, foreign bodies and choanal atresia, (3) Systemic diseases such as cystic fibrosis, immotile cilia syndrome and immune deficiencies. The anterior ethmoids, Frontal sinuses and Maxillary sinuses drain into the area known as the ostiomeatal complex. If this area is obstructed because of anatomic deformity or mucosal edema, the cilia do not function normally. Secretions accumulate and the patient is predisposed to recurrent or chronic sinusitis.

Symptoms of sinusitis vary with the age of the patient and the severity of infection. Young patients often have nasal congestion, cough, and anterior purulent rhinorrhea as primary symptoms. Older children do not have anterior discharge as the primary symptom, but may complain of sore throat or post-nasal drip. The most consistent symptoms are nasal airway obstruction, purulent nasal discharge, headache, irritability and coughing both in the day and night.

Anterior rhinoscopy (can be effectively done by the otoscope) and Nasal endoscopy (only older children may allow) is done to examine the nasal cavity. CT has become the standard for diagnosing the extent and severity of chronic sinusitis.

Bacteriology: Acute and recurrent sinusitis is usually caused by *S. pneumoniae, M. catarrhalis,* and *H. influenzae.* Brook found increased anaerobic bacteria in patients who had symptoms that lasted longer than 3 weeks.[19] The most common anaerobes were *Peptococcus, Peptostreptococcus* and *Bacteroids*; the most common aerobes identified were α- *Hemolytic Streptococci,* and *Staph aureus.*

Treatment: Medical treatment includes antibiotics, effective amongst them are Amoxicillin with clavulanate potassium and second generation cephalosporins such as Cefuroxime axetil. Antibiotics are given for 10-14 days in acute sinusitis and for a period of 3-4 weeks for chronic sinusitis.

Endoscopic Sinus Surgery: Preservation of normal structures and mucosa is especially important in pediatric population because the sinuses are small and still developing. Surgery should be considered only after appropriate medical management, including several courses of long term (4-6 weeks) broad spectrum antibiotics and probably nasal corticosteroid sprays have proved unsuccessful.

III. THE THROAT

TONSILS AND ADENOIDS

The tonsils are grouped as secondary lymphatic organs. It has been suggested that tonsillar hypertrophy is a physiological process, indicating B-lymphocyte proliferation, while sunken atrophic tonsils indicate a collapse of the B-cell activity and a 'collapse' of the defence process. It may therefore be that small atrophic tonsils are more often the seat of infection of a chronic sort.

Indications for Tonsillectomy

1. Recurrent acute tonsillitis (more than 6 episodes per year or 3 episodes per year for more that or equal to 2 years).
2. Recurrent acute tonsillitis associated with cardiac valvular disease or recurrent febrile seizures.
3. Chronic tonsillitis that is unresponsive to medical therapy and associated with halitosis, persistent sore-throat, and tender cervical adenitis.
4. Peritonsillar abscess and tonsillitis associated with abscessed cervical nodes.
5. Obstructive sleep apnea and sleep disturbances.

Adenoid hypertrophy or chronic adenoiditis may cause significant problems requiring adenoidectomy in situations in which the tonsils themselves are not diseased and are not contributing to the symptomatology.

ADENOIDECTOMY

Adenoid hypertrophy or chronic adenoiditis may cause significant problems requiring adenoidectomy in situations in which the tonsils themselves are not diseased and not contributing to symptomatology.

Indications for Adenoidectomy

1. Purulent adenoiditis.
2. Adenoid hypertrophy associated with chronic otitis media with effusion, chronic recurrent acute otitis media, chronic otitis media with perforation and otorrhea or chronic tube otorrhea.
3. Adenoid hypertrophy associated with excessive snoring and chronic mouth breathing.
4. Sleep apnea or sleep disturbances.
5. Adenoid hypertrophy associated with cor pulmonale, failure to thrive, dysphagia and speech abnormalities.
6. Craniofacial growth abnormalities and occlusion abnormalities.

STRIDOR AND AIRWAY MANAGEMENT

Stridor is an abnormal or unwanted noise made by turbulent airflow in the airway. Not every child with stridor requires endoscopy because a thorough history and a limited physical examination can in some conditions (e.g. mild laryngomalacia) provide sufficient diagnostic probability to avoid initial endoscopy. The common causes are listed below:

I. Nasopharyngeal causes of airway obstruction
   A. Neonates
      1. Neonatal rhinitis
      2. Choanal atresia or stenosis
      3. Craniofacial abnormalities
      4. Micrognathia
   B. Children
      1. Allergic rhinitis
      2. Adenoiditis
      3. Adeno-tonsillar hypertrophy
      4. Foreign bodies
II. Laryngeal causes of airway obstruction
   A. Neonates
      1. Laryngomalacia
      2. Intubation trauma
      3. Reflux laryngitis
      4. Laryngotracheal stenosis
      5. Vocal cord palsy
   B. Children
      1. Croup (Laryngotracheobronchitis)
      2. Hemangiomas
      3. Papillomatosis
      4. Intubation trauma
      5. Vocal cord palsy
III. Tracheal causes of airway obstruction
   A. Neonates
      1. Tracheobronchomalacia
      2. Tracheal stenosis
      3. Vascular compression
   B. Children
      1. Foreign bodies
      2. Tracheal stenosis.

Stridor at birth is unusual and generally denotes fixed congenital narrowing (e.g. a laryngeal web, subglottic stenosis, tracheal narrowing).[20] Dynamic conditions such as laryngomalacia and congenital vocal cord palsy become evident in the first few weeks of life. A gradually increase in severity of stridor or airway compromise implies growth of an obstruction which may be luminal as in a subglottic hemangioma or extrinsic as with a mediastinal mass. Hoarseness suggests a laryngeal lesion such as laryngeal papillomatosis but also occurs in vocal cord palsy. Inspiratory stridor is caused by extrathoracic obstruction such as larynx or high trachea; bronchial obstruction causes expiratory stridor.

Endoscopy should be done for diagnosis and flexible endoscopes afford a comprehensive view of the lesion with very few risks. Once the airway is stabilised, then rigid endoscopy can be undertaken with a view to diagnose and treat the offending pathology.

The management has to be emergent. If chronic hypercarbia is present then oxygen is useful in the management of airway obstruction. Intravenous corticosteroids are beneficial in croup. Inhaled corticosteroids have a similar effect.

Intubation is increasingly being used as an alternative to tracheotomy in acute airway obstruction, partly because of technologic advances in anesthesia and partly because of the realisation that even short term pediatric tracheostomy is not without complications. Sometimes intubation may fail and then tracheostomy has to be done to secure the airway.

Vocal Cord Palsy

Vocal cord paralysis is rare in children. Central lesions are more often associated with bilateral cord palsy and peripheral lesions with unilateral palsy.[21] Congenital vocal cord palsy typically presents in the first month of life.[22] Stridor, cyanosis and apnea are the most frequent symptoms of bilateral paralysis; unilateral paralysis usually presents with dysphonia. Infants with unilateral vocal cord paralysis requiring tracheostomy can usually be decannulated following growth of the airway, between 1 and 2 years of age without further surgical intervention even if paralysis persists. In patients with bilateral vocal cord paralysis, vocal cord lateralization can improve the airway permanently and permit decannulation when spontaneous recovery of function does not occur.

Subglottic Hemangioma

The usual age of presentation is 6 weeks and is nearly always in the first 6 months of life. The most common symptom is stridor, often initially intermittent and misdiagnosed as recurrent croup but usually progresses to become constant, may be inspiratory or biphasic and is exacerbated by crying or upper respiratory tract infections. The diagnosis is made by direct laryngoscopy. The classical appearance of the tumor is pink or bluish sessile mass arising from the lateral wall of the subglottis and often extending to involve the subglottis. Airway maintenance is bypassing the obstruction by a tracheostomy. Systemic corticosteroids, carbon dioxide laser vaporization, Interferon α-2A and selective embolization are some of the recommended modalities of treatment.

Respiratory Papillomatosis

Recurrent respiratory papillomatosis is characterised by benign, non keratinizing, squamous papillomas that may be sessile or pedunculated, multiple and are typically recurrent. They have a predilection for the squamo-ciliary junctions of the airway. The disease is caused by epithelial infection with human papilloma virus (HPV) types 6 and 11.[23] Peak age incidence is between two and five years of age. Presenting symptoms may vary from hoarseness, abnormal cry to frank stridor. Carbon dioxide laser vapourization is the preferred modality of treatment. Adjuvant therapy like podophylum and photodynamic therapy have also been used. Tracheostomy for airway maintenance may be required in severe cases, though the disadvantage is that the chances of stomal seeding by the papillomas is very high. Human leukocyte interferon has a well documented benefit in respiratory papillomatosis.[24]

FOREIGN BODIES OF THE AIRWAY AND ESOPHAGUS

Airway foreign bodies pose a diagnostic and therapeutic challenge to the pediatric otolaryngologist. Foreign body aspiration mimics other conditions of the airway causing stridor and hence a high index of suspicion is required to come to a diagnosis. The introduction of rod-lens telescope in the 1970s greatly improved the visualisation of bronchoscopic foreign body removal. Up to 25% of patients with airway or esophageal foreign bodies are less than 1 year of age.[25] Vegetable matter is seen in approximately 80% of the airway foreign bodies. The most common esophageal foreign bodies are coins.[26]

Most airway foreign bodies become lodged in the bronchi because their size and configuration allow passage through the larynx and trachea. Larger foreign bodies may become impacted in the larynx or trachea causing at times complete obstruction, which is a dire emergency. Most esophageal foreign bodies become impacted in the cervical esophagus, just below the cricopharynx.[25]

Complete airway obstruction resulting from a foreign body is an absolute emergency. The Heimlich maneuver is of a great help in this situation. For children less than 1 year back blows and chest thrusts are recommended. Children older than 1 year require gentle abdominal thrusts when supine. Older children are positioned standing, sitting, or recumbent for the Heimlich maneuver.

Foreign body aspiration is suspected when the victim develops acute choking, gagging, and paroxysms of severe coughing with respiratory distress. Neck and chest radiography should be done to identify the location of the foreign body. The basic principles of endoscopic foreign body has not changed since the days of Chevalier Jackson.[27,28] The type and size of the endoscope depend upon the age of the patient and the location of the object. Foreign body removal is done under general anesthesia. Extraction of sharp or pointed objects can be very challenging. Locating the point is crucial. Usually the tip of the pointed object engages the mucosa, causing object to tumble and proceed with the point trailing. The endoscope is aligned parallel to the long axis of the esophagus or the airway to minimise the likelihood of damage to the surrounding mucosa. During extraction, the object is at first moved distally to disengage the point.

Pneumonia and atelectasis are the most common complications after bronchial foreign body removal. Esophageal perforation is a grave but a very real complication in the attempt to remove foreign body from the esophagus.

Prevention is ideal, with increased education of parents on age appropriate foods and household objects and strict industry standards in the manufacture of toys.

REFERENCES

1. Bluestone, et al. Frequency of bacteria isolated from middle ear effusions of children from the United States, Finland, Japan and Denmark. Ann Otol Rhinol Laryngol 1990;99 (Suppl 149):42.
2. Klein BS, Dollete FR, Yolken RH. The role of respiratory syncytial virus and other viral pathogens in acute otitis media. J Pediatr 1982;101:16.
3. Deka RC. Acute Otitis media. Indian Pediatr 1996;33(10):832-36.
4. Roddey OF Jr, Eagle R Jr, Haggerty R. Myringotomy in acute otitis media, JAMA 1966;197:849.
5. Englehard D, et al. Randomised study of myringotomy, amoxicillin/clavulanate, or both for acute otitis media in infants, Lancet 1989;2:141.
6. Deka RC, Kacker SK. Chronic otitis media- a clinical and bacteriological study, Eye Ear Nose Throat Month 1975;54(5):198-201.
7. Deka RC. Surgery of middle ear cholesteatoma, Editorial, Indian Journal of Otolaryngology 1999;5(3):115-19.
8. Stool SE, Randall P. Unexpected ear disease in infants with cleft palate, Cleft Palate Journal 1967;4:99-103.
9. Deka RC. Middle ear effusion; its management. Indian Pediatr 1994;31(6):631-33.
10. Deka RC. Otitis Media with effusion in children. Pediatric Audiology in India (Proceedings of the seminar on Pediatric Audiology, 29-30 January 1994. Published by ORSA, AIIMS, New-Delhi; 1997;76-79.
11. Deka RC. Management of hearing impaired children. Indian Pediatr 1993;30(8):1977- 80.
12. Deka RC. Auditory Brainstem evoked responses in Infants and Children. Indian J Pediatr 1992;59:361-66.
13. Deka RC. Cochlear Implantation Surgery in children. Indian Journal of Otology (in press), 2001.
14. Persig W. Surgery of choanal atresia in infants and children: historical notes and updated reviews, J Pediatr Otorhinolaryngol 1986;11:153.
15. Duncan NO, Miller RA, Catlin FI. Choanal atresia and associated anomalies: the CHARGE association. Int J Pediatr Otorhinolaryngol 1988;15:129.
16. Sooknundun M, Kacker SK, Bhatia R, Deka RC. Nasal septal deviation: effective intervention and long term follow-up, International Journal of Pediatric Otorhinolaryngology 198612;65-72.
17. Deka RC, Kacker SK. Septoplasty in children, Indian Journal of Otolaryngology 1990;42:39-40.
18. Bhatia R, Deka RC, Kacker SK. Diagnosis of septal deformities in new-borns. Indian Journal of Otolaryngology 1987;39:18-19.
19. Brook I. Bacteriological features of chronic sinusitis in children, JAMA 1981;246:967.
20. Pedraza Pena LR, Rodriguez Santana JR, Sifontes JE. Neonatal stridor: a life threatening condition. PR Health Sci J 1994;1:33.
21. Katz HP, Askin J. Multiple hemangiomata with thrombopaenia: an unusual case with comments on steroid therapy. Am J Dis Child 1968;115:151.
22. deGaudemar I, et al. Outcome of laryngeal paralysis in neonates: a long term retrospective study of 11 cases. Int J Pediatr Otorhinolaryngol 1996;4:101.
23. Mounts P, Shaw KV, Kashima H. Viral aetiology of juvenile and adult onset squamous papilloma of the larynx. Proc Natl Acad Sci USA 1982;79:5425-29.
24. Haglund S, et al. Interferon therapy in juvenile laryngeal papillomatosis, Arch Otolaryngol Head Neck Surg 1981;107:327.
25. Crysdale WS. Esophageal foreign bodies in children: 15 years review of 484 cases. Ann Otol Rhinol Laryngol 1991;100:329.
26. Hawkins DB. Removal of blunt foreign bodies from the esophagus. Ann Otol Rhinol Laryngol 1990;99:935.
27. Jackson C, Jackson CL. Vertebral magnets for removal of foreign bodies from the air and food passages. Ann Otol Rhinol Laryngol. 1949;58:55-60
28. Jackson CL. Foreign bodies in the bronchi and esophagus in children and adults. Ann otolaryngol Chir Cervicofac. 1955;72:179-82.

CHAPTER 110

Pediatric Larynx and Trachea

Abhinit Kumar, Suresh C Sharma

HISTORY OF LARYNGOLOGY

In India, Charaka Samhita (Circa AD 100) and Susruta (Circa AD 300) mentioned remedies for disorders of the voice. The earliest mention of the larynx is by Aristotle (Circa 350 BC).[1]

Sir William Macewin in 1878 was first to intubate the larynx for purposes of general anesthesia in a 55 years age old man, although anesthesia through a preliminary tracheotomy tube was advocated by Trendelenburg in 1869 (Davison MHA 1965).

EMBRYOLOGIC DEVELOPMENT (FIGS 110.1 TO 110.6)

The first evidence of respiratory system appears at three weeks of embryonic stage as a median pharyngeal groove or respiratory diverticulum (RD). The respiratory diverticulum (RD) is a ventral outpouching of the foregut lumen that expands into respiratory primordium (RP). The site of the origin of the RD is called the primitive pharyngeal floor which eventually develops into the infraglottic region of the adult larynx. It is separated from the pharyngeal floor by a segment of foregut originally described by Aaw –Tun and Burdi as the primitive laryngopharynx that eventually becomes the supraglottic larynx.[2]

At approximately 24 days of embryonic age, respiratory pulmonary primordium divides into right and left lobes (Fig. 110.4). The respiratory primordium descends in a proximal to distal sequence. Once the outgrowth of the lung bud begins, the digestive and

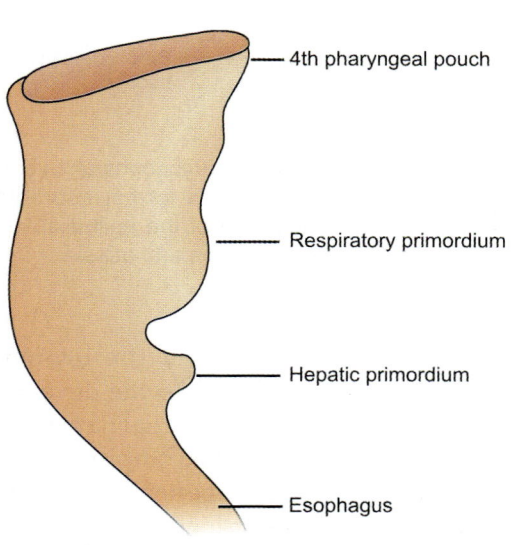

Fig. 110.1

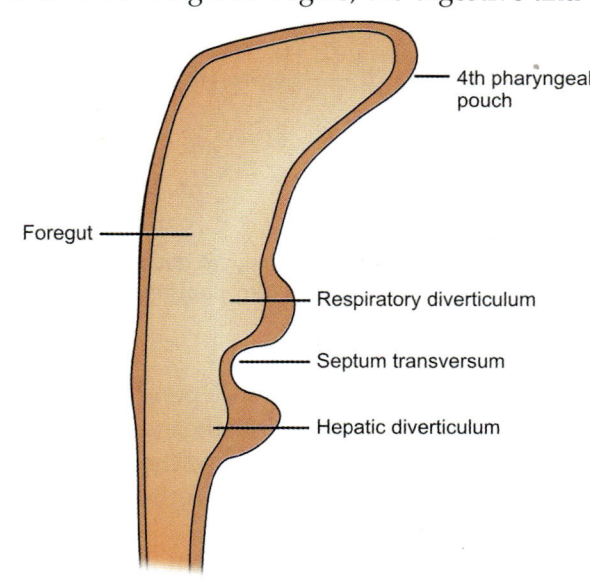

Fig. 110.2

Figs 110.1 and 110.2: Shows respiratory diverticulum as a ventral outpouching of the foregut lumen, which expands into respiratory primordium

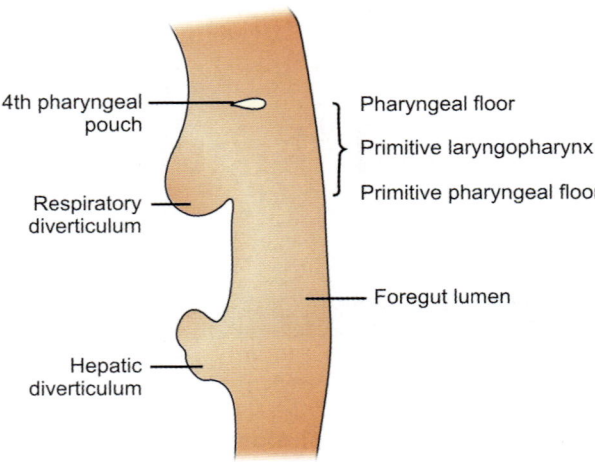

Fig. 110.3: Showing primitive laryngopharynx, a segment of foregut between 4th pharyngeal pouch and primitive pharyngeal floor (infragottis)

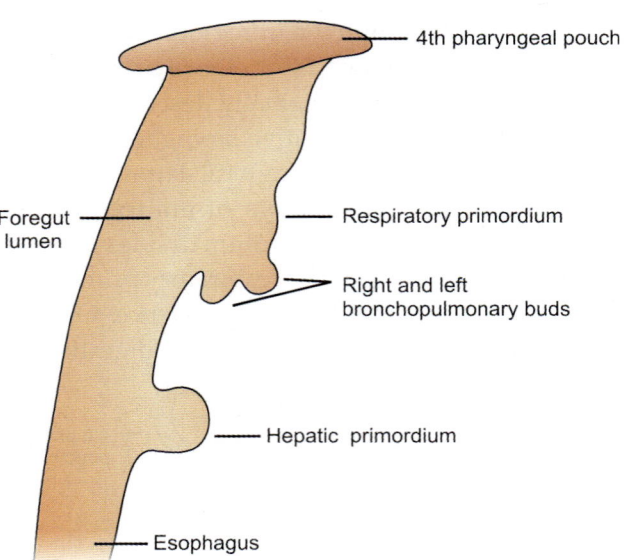

Fig. 110.4: At approximately 24 days, the respiratory primordium divides into right and left lobes

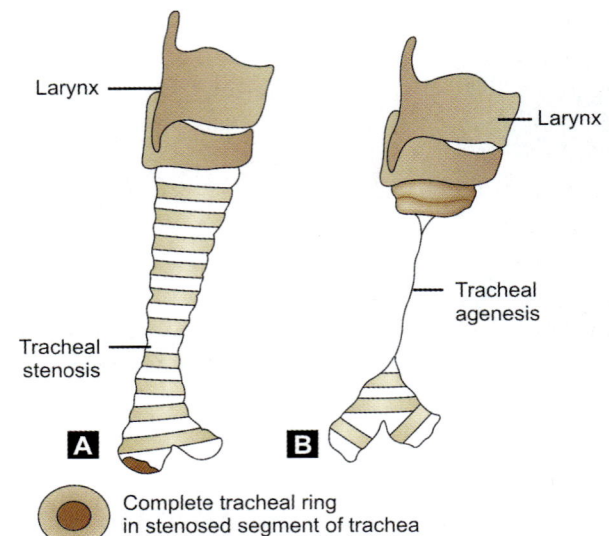

Figs 110.5 A and B: Vascular compromise of trachea shows **(A)** tracheal stenosis with complete tracheal rings and **(B)** tracheal agenesis

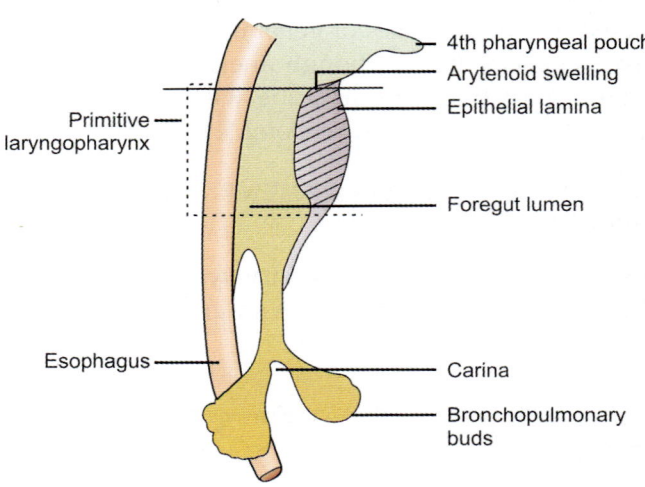

Fig. 110.6: Compression of primitive laryngopharynx ventrally gives rise to epithelial lamina, which forms, supraglottic structures. Incomplete recanalization of the epithelial lamina give rise to supraglottic and glottic webs and atresia

respiratory tubes pursue independent courses. The lung bud grows caudally into the mesenchyme ventral to the foregut. The mesenchyme that lies between the respiratory and digestive tubes constitutes the tracheoesophageal septum.[3]

In subsequent stages the right and left lung buds are more evident, and the trachea becomes identifiable. Angiogenesis begins in the mesenchyme and serves to mark off the esophagus from the bronchial investment. Vascular compromise to the developing esophagus may cause esophageal atresia or tracheoesophageal fistula. Vascular compromise to the trachea may cause tracheal agenesis or tracheal stenosis with complete tracheal rings. These anomalies are associated with relatively normal laryngeal and pulmonary development because the insult is limited to the region of the developing trachea. The hypopharyngeal eminence and arytenoid swelling appear in the floor of the pharynx. The inlet of the embryonic larynx is identifiable.

At 33 days of embryonic stage, the primitive laryngopharynx is seen. It develops from the foregut segment extending from the fourth pharyngeal pouch above to the infraglottis below. The superior laryngeal nerve can be identified. Lobar buds are present and esophageal and bronchial territories are differentiated from each other by capillary plexus. The ventral portion of primitive laryngopharynx becomes compressed bilaterally by the mesoderm of laryngeal cartilages, muscles and branchial arch arteries. Eventually, obliteration of the ventral lumen of the primitive laryngopharynx occurs to give rise to the epithelial lamina.[4] The epithelial lamina which later form laryngeal structures recanalize from dorsocephalic to ventrocaudal direction. The last portion to recanalize is at the glottic level. Incomplete recanalization can give rise to supraglottic and glottic webs and atresia.[4]

ANATOMY OF PEDIATRIC LARYNX AND TRACHEA

The larynx acts as both an air conduit and a protector of lower airway during swallowing.

Characteristics of Pediatric Airway

Apart from being smaller in size than adult, it is different in following aspects.

Infants are obligatory nasal breather. Hence, conditions with nasal obstruction, such as choanal atresia or stenosis can cause severe respiratory difficulty.

Tongue in an infant is proportionately bigger in size and occupies a larger volume of the oral cavity. Position of larynx is higher in infants than adults.

The tip of infant epiglottis corresponds with the junction of first and second cervical vertebra. This high position helps the infant to use its nasal airway to breathe while sucking (Fig. 110.7).

The pediatric airway axis has greater curvature than in the adult. This is of some relevance during intubation, laryngoscopy and bronchoscopy (Figs 110.8A and B).[5]

The connective tissue composing the infant larynx are more pliable than adult. This causes tendency of

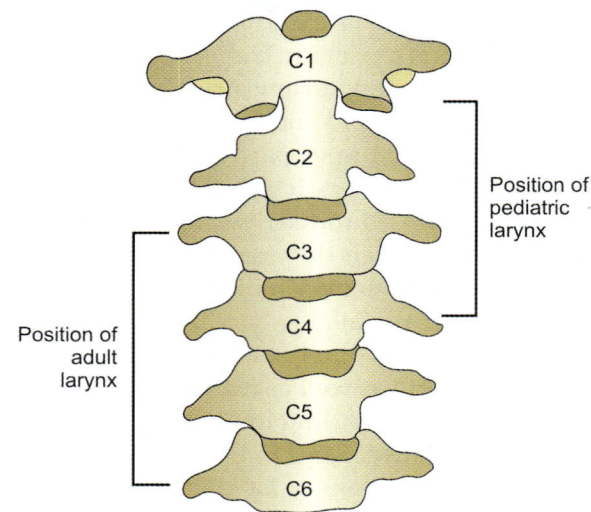

Fig. 110.7: Relative position of pediatric and adult larynx

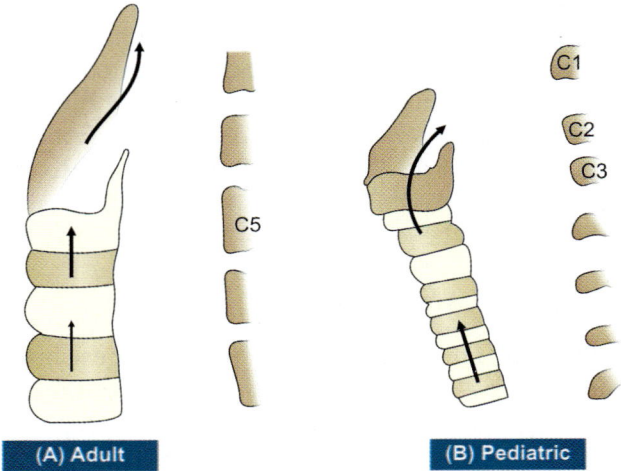

Figs 110.8A and B: The pediatric airway axis in comparison with adult airway axis

soft tissues to be sucked with negative intraluminal pressure. The classic example is larygomalacia (during inspiration) and tracheomalacia (during expiration). The cricothyroid ligament is relatively short, making emergency cricothyrotomy extremely difficult.

The mucosa of laryngeal inlet is lax; hence inflammation causes rapid formation of edema. The narrowest part of infant larynx is subglottis measuring 3.5 mm in diameter, than adult where it is glottic region. There are multiple glandular tissues in the region of aryteriod cartilage and saccule is relatively large.[6]

Relationship among hyoid-, thyroid- and cricoid cartilage is different in infant. It is important to identify them before proceeding to any airway surgery. There is no gap between hyoid and thyroid cartilage, infact hyoid overlaps the upper part of thyroid cartilage, obscuring the thyroid notch. The shape of thyroid cartilage is more rounded, without a prominent midline vertical ridge (laryngeal prominence); the cricoid cartilage is not prominent; the cricothyroid membrane is very small.

Unlike the adult, the neonatal subglottic cavity extends posteriorly as well as inferiorly an important fact to be considered during intubation.

Trachea is relatively small in relation to the larynx in the neonate. The walls of the trachea are relatively thick and the tracheal cartilages are relatively closer together. The ability to resist external compression is also less in infant trachea. The trachea commences at the upper border of sixth cervical vertebra, a relationship conserved with growth, it bifurcates at the level of the third or fourth thoracic vertebra.

The larynx, which is an air passage, a sphincteric device and an organ of phonation, extends from the tongue to the trachea. Above, it opens into the laryngopharynx and forms its anterior wall; below, it continues into the trachea.

LARYNGEAL FRAMEWORK

Skeleton of larynx is formed by cartilages, interconnected by ligaments and fibrous membranes. Muscles provide movement. Hyoid bone, though not a part of the larynx, is intimately related with it.

Laryngeal Cartilages

The thyroid, the cricoid and the greater portions of the arytenoid cartilages are composed of hyaline cartilage. The corniculate, cuneiform, epiglottic cartilages and the apices of the arytenoid cartilages are composed of elastic fibrocartilage and don't undergo calcification (Figs 110.9A and B).

Cricoid Cartilage

The cricoid (cricos = "ring" Greek) is the only cartilage which forms a complete ring in the larynx. It is the skeletal foundation of the larynx, attached below to the trachea and articulated by synovial joints to the thyroid cartilage and two arytenoids. It consists of a narrow anterior arch, and a broad flatter posterior lamina.

Thyroid Cartilage

The thyroid cartilage (Thyrus = "shield" Greek) is the largest laryngeal cartilage. It consists of two quardilateral laminae, which are joined anteriorly to form an obtuse angle of 110 degrees in an infant, posteriorly they diverge. The posterior borders being prolonged as slender horns, the superior and inferior cornu. On the external surface of each lamina lies the oblique line, which runs downwards and forwards from the superior thyroid tubercle to the inferior thyroid tubercle, to which are attached the

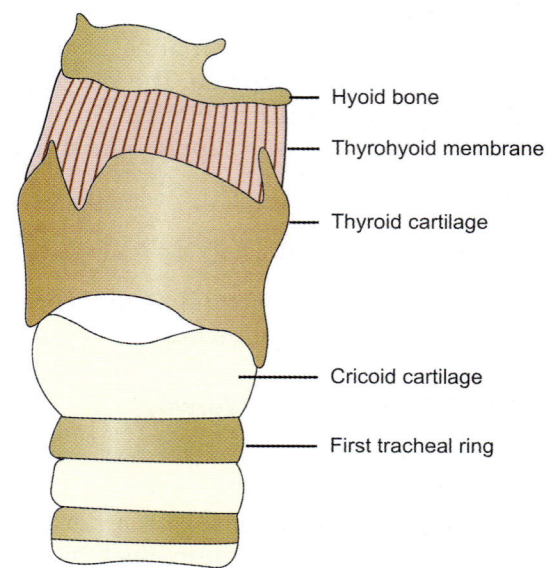

Fig. 110.9A: Laryngeal framework

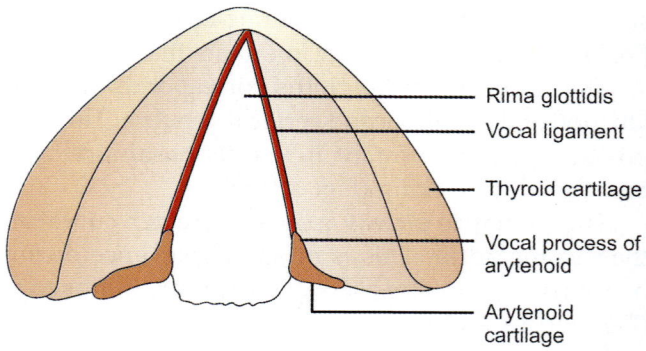

Fig. 110.9B: Transverse section through larynx

sternothyroid, thyrohyoid and the thyropharyngeus part of the inferior pharyngeal constrictor.

The superior border gives attachment to thyrohyoid membrane. The inferior border provides attachment to cricothyroid ligament anteriorly.

The posterior border of each lamina receives fibers of stylopharyngeus and palatopharyngeus. The superior cornu provides attachments to lateral thyrohyoid ligament. The inferior cornu articulates on the side of the cricoid cartilage.

A narrow, rhomboidal, flexible strip, the intrathyroid cartilage, lies between two laminae and joined by fibrous tissue in infancy.

Arytenoid Cartilage

Arytenoid cartilages, are pyramidal in shape, present on each side, on the superior surface of cricoid, posterolaterally. The lateral angle called muscular process gives attachment to the posterior cricoarytenoid muscle behind and the lateral cricoarytenoid in front. The anterior angle called vocal process provides attachment to the vocal ligament. The arytenoids have low mass, thus allow for rapid abduction and adduction in less than 0.1 second.

Epiglottic Cartilage

Consists of elastic fibrocartilage is connected by the thyroepiglottic ligament to the back of laryngeal prominence just below the thyroid notch. Its sides are attached to the arytenoid cartilages by aryepiglottic fold. Anteriorly, the mucosa over it forms a median glossepiglottic and to lateral glossoepiglottic folds. Vallecula is a depression on both sides of the median glossoepiglottic fold with no function in humans.

There are two pairs of synovial joints in the laryngeal framework—one for the cricoid and inferior horn of the thyroid cartilage and one for the arytenoids and cricoid.

Laryngeal Ligaments and Membranes

Extrinsic Ligament

Thyrohyoid membrane bridges the gap between the upper part of thyroid cartilage and the hyoid bone. It is fibroelastic membrane, thicker in median and lateral parts. It is pierced on both sides by superior laryngeal vessels and nerves.

Intrinsic Ligaments

There is fibroelastic membrane, beneath the laryngeal mucosa. Its upper part called *quadrangular membrane* extends between arytenoid and epiglottis. Its lower larger part forms well defined cricothyroid ligament, connecting thyroid, cricoid and arytenoid cartilages (Fig. 110.10).

Rima glottidis or glottis is a space between vocal folds anteriorly (constitute three fifth of it anteroposterior length) and between arytenoids posteriorly. It is the narrowest part of the larynx in adult.

Subglottis– Lined by respiratory epithelium, its walls are made up of cricothyroid ligament above and cricoid cartilage below. Subglottis forms the narrowest part of the larynx in pediatric age.

Trachea– It begins at the level of the cricoid cartilage and usually bifurcates at the level of the sternal angle. There are 18 to 22 cartilaginous rings in the human trachea. The only complete cartilaginous ring in the normal airway is the cricoid cartilage of the larynx. The remainder of the rings is C-shaped, connected posteriorly by the fibroaerolar connective tissue and smooth muscle fibers oriented transversely. The lumen of the trachea is lined by a mucosa consisting of a thin lamina propria and a ciliated pseudostratified columnar epithelium. Goblet cells and some small subepithelial glands are interspersed among the columnar cells. Scattered lymphoid elements are also

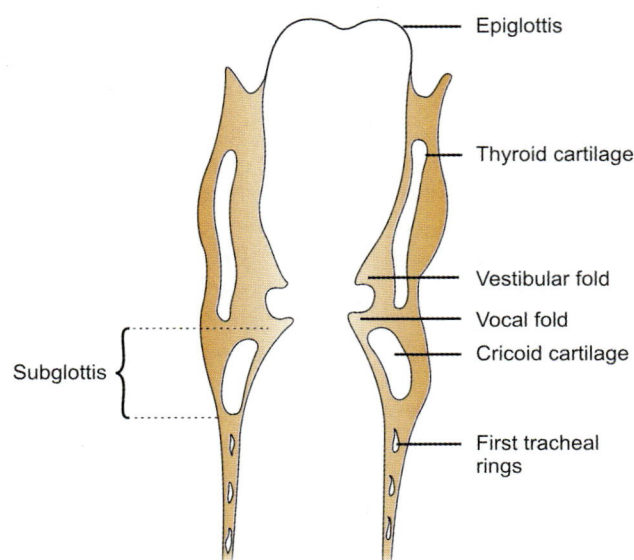

Fig. 110.10: Coronal section of laryngeal cavity

present within the lamina propria. The right bronchus is usually more in line with the tachea and wider and shorter than the left. However, in children the left bronchus is less horizontal than in the adult, hence the incidence of foreign bodies in the two bronchi is approximately equal.

Laryngeal Musculature

The muscles of the larynx can be divided into two groups (a) *Extrinsic* and (b) *Intrinsic*.
a. *Extrinsic muscles* connect larynx with the surrounding structures and are responsible for movement of the larynx as a whole, during phonation or swallowing. They include thyrohyoid, sternothyroid, inferior constrictor, stylopharyngeus, palatopharyngeus and salpingopharyngeus.
b. *Intrinsic muscles* connect the cartilaginous elements of the larynx. They are described in detail in Table 110.1.

Action of the Intrinsic Muscles

Among intrinsic muscles, only *posterior crico-arytenoids* open the glottis. They can be placed into three groups according to their action.
a. *Varying the rima glottidis:* Posterior cricoarytenoid opens the glottis. Lateral *cricoarytenoid* and *transerve arytenoids* close the glottis.
b. *Regulating tension in the vocal ligaments:* Cricothyroids, posterior cricoarytenoids, thyroarytenoids and vocales.
c. *Modifying the laryngeal inlet:* Oblique arytenoids, aryepiglottici and thyro epiglotti.

It is considered that tension of vocal folds determine the pitch of voice.

Laryngeal Vessels and Nerves

Larynx is supplied by a pair of superior and inferior thyroid arteries. Drainage is by the corresponding veins. Superior thyroid artery is a branch of external

Table 110.1: Origin and insertion of the intrinsic muscles of the larynx

	Muscle/Innervation	Origin	Insertion
1.	Cricothyroid (a) oblique part (Lower) (b) straight part (Superior) Ex. branch of superior Laryngeal nerve.	External surface of cricoid arch anteriorly	Inferior cornu and lower part of thyroid lamina
2.	Posterior cricoarytenoid Recurrent laryngeal nerve of vagus nerve (X)	Posterior surface of the cricoid lamina	Back of muscular process of the arytenoids of the same side
3.	Lateral cricoarytenoid Recurrent laryngeal nerve of vagus nerve (X)	Upper border of cricoid arch	Front of muscular process of the arytenoid cartilage of the same side
4.	Transverse arytenoids Recurrent laryngeal nerve of vagus nerve (X)	Single muscle attached to the back of the muscular process and adjacent lateral border of both arytenoids.	
5.	Oblique arytenoids Recurrent laryngeal nerve of vagus nerve(X)	Superficial to the transverse arytenoids, back of the muscular process of one arytenoids cartilage to the apex of the opposite one, some fibers form aryepiglottic muscle.	
6.	Vocalis Recurrent laryngeal nerve of vagus nerve(X)	Thyroid cartilage (posterior surface near midline)	Vocal process and oblong fovea of arytenoids cartilage
7.	Thyro-arytenoid Recurrent laryngeal nerve of vagus nerve(X)	Lamina of thyroid cartilage (medial surface near origin of vocalis)	Muscular process (anterior surface) of arytenoid cartilage
8.	Thyro-epiglottic part Recurrent laryngeal nerve of vagus nerve (X)	Lamina of thyroid cartilage (medial surface near origin of thyroarytenoid	Epiglottic cartilage (lateral margin)

carotid artery. Inferior thyroid artery is a branch of thyrocervical trunk, which is turn, is a branch of first part of subclavian artery. Superior thyroid vein drains into the left brachiocephalic vein.

Lymphatic system above the vocal folds drains into the deep cervical node near the bifurcation of the common carotid artery.

Lymphatic system below the vocal folds drains to lymph nodes, along inferior thyroid artery, in front of trachea and to the deep cervical nodes.

The lower trachea shares its supply with the esophagus from the bronchial arteries. The upper trachea is supplied by three branches from the inferior thyroid artery with fine collateral pathways between these branches. In mobilization of the trachea care is therefore taken to free the trachea anteriorly and posteriorly, leaving the lateral pedicle intact except for a short distance which is to be used in the anastomosis.[7]

Sensory supply above the vocal fold is by superior laryngeal nerve and below the vocal fold by recurrent laryngeal nerve.

SYMPTOMS AND DIAGNOSIS OF LARYNGEAL ABNORMALITIES

The larynx has three functions, respiration, protection of airway and phonation. The signs and symptoms of airway obstruction are dyspnea, air hunger, attacks of cyanosis, cough, increase respiratory rate, and retractions of the suprasternal, substernal, infraclavicular and intercostal regions.

The quality and type of the stridor may indicate the location of the anomaly. A high pitched crowing type of stridor, present only during the inspiratory phase of respiration indicate problem at larynx most of the time (supraglottic, glottic and subglottic). High pitched inspiratory stridor with low pitched prolonged expiratory phase (biphasic, double or to and fro strider) suggests main airway obstruction below the larynx (i.e. trachea). Low pitched inspiratory sound (stertor; snoring) is produced by obstruction above the level of larynx, i.e. nasopharynx, pharynx or soft palate.

Infants with airway obstruction often fail to thrive. Deglutition and respiration share a common pathway at oropharynx. Hence during feeding, there is aggravation of respiratory obstruction. Conversely, tachypnoea and prolongation of inspiration impede normal swallowing activity.

Weak feeble cry or aphonia suggests a glottic web or neurological dysfunction. Hoarseness, suggests changes in the structure and/or function of the vocal cords, may raise possibility of laryngeal inflammation, trauma, tumors or vocal cord immobility.

Severity of stridor/stertor is assessed clinically by its character, i.e. (continuous or intermittent, loudness) and associated features like cyanosis, shortness of breath, difficult or labored breathing and periods of apnea.

Symptoms of congenital stridor (laryngomalacia) may not develop immediately after birth. It may happen after a child get infection, or due to increased physical activity, he developed stridor in a compromised airway. Congenital causes of stertor on the other hand usually present soon after birth (e.g. choanal atresia)[8] (Tables 110.2 to 110.4).

Besides laryngotracheal abnormalities, it is important to exclude cardiac, neurological or systemic problems. Information concerning the birth history, previous intubations, surgery or similar episodes must

Table 110.2: Typical age at presentation for specific diagnosis	
Age	Likely Diagnosis
Birth	Choanal atresia Vocal cord paralysis Laryngeal webs and atresia
1-3 months	Laryngomalacia, Subglottic hemangioma Vocal cord paralysis with Arnold-Chiari malformation
Above 6 months	Papillomas Foreign body

Table 110.3: Differential diagnosis for respiratory distress	
a.	Inflammatory diseases Supraglottitis, croup, parapharyngeal retropharyngeal abscess.
b.	Trauma (Postintubation, caustic ingestion, sports related injury, laryngeal stenosis, tracheal stenosis, laryngeal paralysis)
c.	Foreign body
d.	Congenital malformation Laryngomalacia, vocal cord paralysis, subglottic hemangiomia, Subglottic stenosis
e.	Neoplasm (Oral, orpharyngeal and laryngeal) Laryngeal papilloma, thyroid tumors lymphangioma

Table 110.4: Non-airway – related causes of respiratory distress

a. Neuromuscular disorder including central nervous system depression, poliomyelitis and apnea of infancy
b. Cardiac disorders
c. Systemic toxicity

be elicited. Foreign body aspiration must be kept in mind especially in toddlers (age 2 or 3) presented with acute onset dyspnea. Esophageal foreign bodies in young children may compress the cervical airway and give respiratory symptoms.

PHYSICAL EXAMINATION

General Examination

A "hands off" approach with careful observation of the patient is very important. History with mother, regarding degree of obstruction during awake, asleep, during feeding and prone position is valuable. Skin should be examined for hemangioma, as 50% of children with subglottic hemangioma also have cutaneous hemangioma. Degree of respiratory distress is estimated by respiratory rate, stridor, air movement, supraclavicular and suprasternal retractions, indrawing of subcostal space, consciousness level and oxygen saturation (Table 110.5).[8] Reflex apnea, after coughing or during feeding, may indicate the presence of innominate artery compression of the trachea.[9] Chest wall deformities, like scoliosis, barrel chest, or pectus deformity may indicate lower airway obstruction.

Nose and Oral Cavity

Nasal patency is evaluated by cold spatula test or by bringing a whisp of cotton in front of nostril. A red rubber catheter should be passed to check choanal patency. Nasal examination may reveal septal deviation, septal hematoma or abscess, congenital cysts or swellings, nasal polyp and choanal atresia. Nasal cavity should be evaluated for presence of discharge, color of nasal mucosa to rule out infective or allergic rhinitis. Examination of the nasopharynx can be done by mirrors but nasal endoscopes either rigid or flexible are better option to rule out adenoidal hypertrophy, or tumors of the nasopharynx.

Examination of oral cavity and or pharynx should be done to rule out micrognathia or retrognathia (Treacher collins and Pierre Robin syndromes), macroglossia (Down's syndrome, Beckwith's syndrome), and tonsillar hypertrophy. Rare conditions, such as hypertrophy of lingual tonsil or thyroid, cystic hygroma, hemangioma, teratoma or branchial cleft cysts may be found.

Auscultation

Chest auscultation assesses symmetry and quality of breath sounds. Very quiet stertor or stridor is often audible only when stethoscope held close to the child's nose or open mouth.

Palpation

Palpation of the neck may reveal lymphadenopathy, congenital thyroid enlargement thymic tumors or cysts.

RADIOLOGIC EVALUATION OF THE UPPER AIRWAY

Frontal and lateral radiographs of the neck are usually taken, at the end of inspiration, with the head and neck extended and held in true lateral position. Radiographs of the upper airway should include all structures between the nasopharynx and the carina.

Table 110.5: Respiratory distress score[8]

	0	1	2	3
Respiratory rate	< 30	30-40	40-50	> 50
Strider	None	Rest	Severe	
Air movement	Normal	Slight decrease	Moderate decrease	Poor
Retractions	None	Nasal flaring	Retraction	Severe
Consciousness	Normal	Restless	Thrasing	Lethargic
O$_2$ saturation	95% on < 30%	90-95% on 30%	< 90% on < 30%	< 90% on.> 30%

Lateral Radiographs

For assessment of adenoidal size lateral radiograph should be taken with the mouth closed and not during swallowing to avoid overestimation of adenoidal size relative to the size of nasopharynx. Radiographically visible adenoidal tissue should never be seen in neonates but should be noted routinely in full term infants > 6 months of age.[10] Posterior nasopharyngeal masses in a child < 1 month of age are abnormal; the differential diagnosis should include teratoma, hemangioma neuroblastoma, and basilar encephalocele. Absence of adenoidal tissue in a child of > 6 months of age who had no prior surgery is also abnormal and indicates immunodeficient state.[10]

The classic radiographic finding in acute epiglottitis is the *thumb sign*. Normally, the epiglottis is thin in anteroposterior diameter, whereas inflamed epiglottis appears shorter and has an increased AP diameter. Besides in acute epiglottitis, there is obliteration of vallecular air-space, thickening of the aryepiglottic folds, distention of the hypo-pharyngeal airway and straightening or reversal of normal cervical lordosis.

Frontal radiographs of the neck provide the clearest evidence of the subglottic narrowing that is found in Laryngo tracheo-bronchitis.

Normal prevertebral soft tissue anterio-posterior thickness gradually decreases as the child grows older and should not exceed ¾ times the anteroposterior dimension of C4 in infants, or more than 3mm in older children. One of the most reliable signs of prevertebral space –occupying pathology is the loss of the normal step-off between air-filled pyriform sinuses and the upper airway resulting in an abnormal, straight vertical air-soft tissue interface in the prevertebral region.

Retropharyngeal abscess is one of the commonest causes of retropharyngeal mass in the pediatric population, which results from local or lymphatic spread of nasopharyngeal or inner ear infections.[11]

Frontal (AP) Radiographs

It is essential for evaluation of vocal cord contour and motion, the laryngeal ventricle, and the subglottic airway. Vocal cord granulation tissue and papillomas appear as non specific soft tissue densities outline by air. Symmetric or asymmetric loss of this "squared" configuration due to subglottic airway narrowing of at least 1 cm in length suggests the presence of congenital or acquired subglottic stenosis.

The most common cause of stridor in children is viral laryngotracheal bronchitis which produces a radiographic appearance like a sharpened pencil or a funnel, also called *steeple sign*. Steeple sign is also found in subglottic stenosis, acute epiglottitis, and as a sequel to prolonged intubations.[11,12]

The normal trachea is slight deviated towards right side due to presence of left aortic arch. A trachea that is completely midline is a significant and abnormal finding, suggesting a double aortic arch.[12]

Airway Fluoroscopy

Airway fluoroscopy is a noninvasive way of documenting dynamic changes in airway caliber and position during different phases of respiration.[11] Lateral fluoroscopy is used to document the inspiratory nasopharyngeal and oropharyngeal collapse in the sleep apnea lab. The inspiratory anterior and inferior buckling of aryepiglottic folds and the downward bending of the epiglottis is seen with laryngomalacia and the excessive expiratory collapse of the intrathoracic trachea in children with congenital or acquired tracheomalacia.[12]

Frontal fluoroscopy is used to assess the motion of the vocal cords and hemidiaphragms.[13] Anterior fluoroscopy is used as a supplemental technique for evaluating children suspected of foreign-body aspiration, in which chest X-rays are equivocal. Normally, the heart and mediastinum remain in the midline during all phases of respiration. If they shift during inspiration or expiration foreign body is suspected in the airway. This results due to atelectasis or post obstruction air trapping.

CONGENITAL ANOMALIES OF THE LARYNX AND TRACHEA

Congenital airway anomalies (CAA) comprise greater than 85% of the stridor cases in children < 2.5 years of age.[14]

A thorough analysis of the nature of the stridor, including its quality and timing, postural change, and association with feeding or crying is essential to evaluate any laryngeal lesion Fig. 110.11 outlines the diagnosis for stridor.

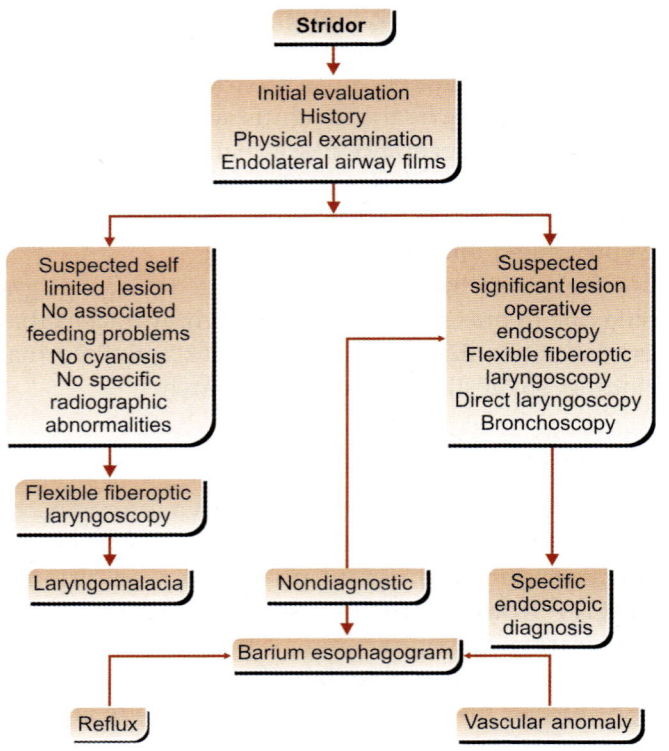

Fig. 110.11: Algorithm for the diagnosis of stridor

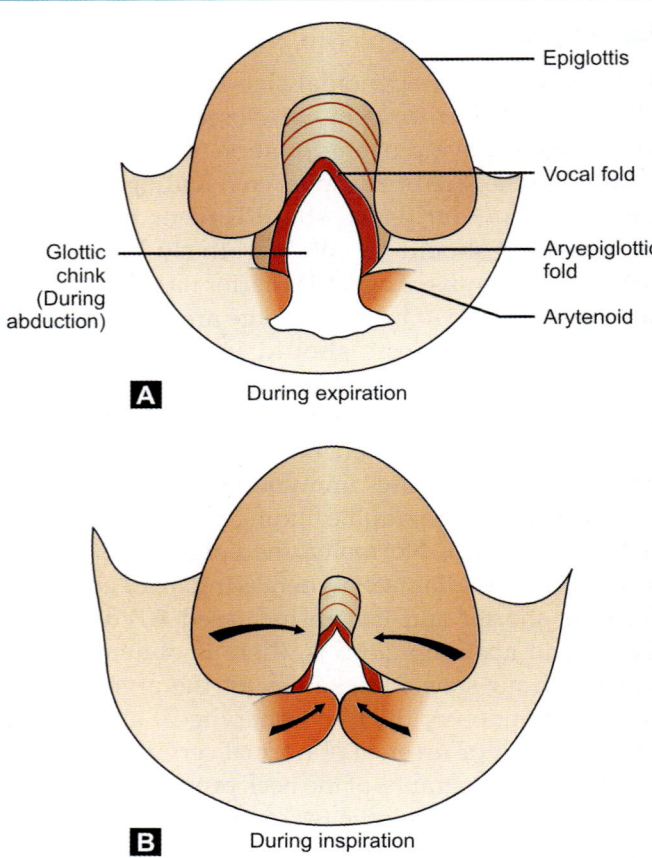

Figs 110.12A and B: Direct laryngoscopic view of larynx in laryngomalacia: **A.** during expiration **B.** during inspiration

High-voltage, soft tissue, anterior-posterior and lateral airway films may help localize the lesion. A barium esophagogram can detect external compression or a tracheoesophageal fistula (TEF). Computed Tomography or magnetic resonance imaging (MRI) is useful in defining vascular anomalies including vascular rings, pulmonary artery slings or aberrant innominate artery.

When stridor is not severe, flexible fiber optic endoscopy can be done, to establish the lesion. In severe cases, an awake flexible endoscopy is performed to assess cord mobility. When possible, the anesthesiologist should maintain spontaneous ventilation during general anesthesia. Sometimes, it is possible to assess the movement of vocal cords during recovery period of anesthesia.

LARYNGOMALACIA

Laryngomalacia is the most common congenital anomaly of the larynx and is defined as supraglottic collapse of the larynx during inspiration.[15] The stridor is inspiratory. The sound varies in pitch and is often coarse and jerky during inspiration, giving it a fluttering character. The stridor is mild in prone position and worsens with agitation. The cry is normal and cyanosis is absent. The onset of stridor is usually within the first few weeks of life, worsens with growth and increasing oxygen demands and then slowly resolves between 6 and 18 months of age.

The cause of laryngomalacia is suggested as either an intrinsic abnormality in the supraglottic larynx or a hypotonicity of the airway. Three abnormalities in the supraglottis have been described in laryngomalacia. An *omega*-shaped epiglottis, *short* aryepiglottic folds and *redundant bulky* arytenoids. Infants with gastroesophageal reflux disease (GERD) may be affected more severely by laryngomalacia. Airway symptoms often are improved with antireflux medications. Central neurological disorders associated with neuromuscular co-ordination difficulties are likely to exacerbate laryngomalacia.

Awake *flexible fiberoptic laryngoscopy* (FFL) confirms the diagnosis (Figs 110.12A and B). FFL evaluation should be postponed until the time of bronchoscopy if operative evaluation is warranted.

Watchful waiting is the treatment of choice, since majority of the patients improves by themselves. Holinger and Brown in a review of 650 patients with laryngomalacia, found that only two required surgical intervention because significant respiratory distress during feeding and need for hospitalization other studies have shown the incidence of severe laryngomalacia to be 5-22%.[16,17] These children have associated feeding difficulties, respiratory compromise, apnea or cor pulmonale and are candidates for surgical intervention, such as tracheotomy.

Several surgical techniques are described treatment. Use of laser is preferred. Surgical procedures include division of the aryepiglottic fold, partial amputation of the epiglottis, epiglottopexy with glossoepiglottic adhesion, removal of redundant supra arytenoid mucosa and lateral borders of the epiglottis, removal of the cuneiform and corniculate cartilages and the surrounding mucosa, and in extreme cases, tracheotomy. The most commonly recommended management appears to be endoscopic laser trimming and removal of the prolapsing aryepiglottic fold with cuneiform cartilage or division of a tight, short aryepiglottic fold (Fig. 110.13).

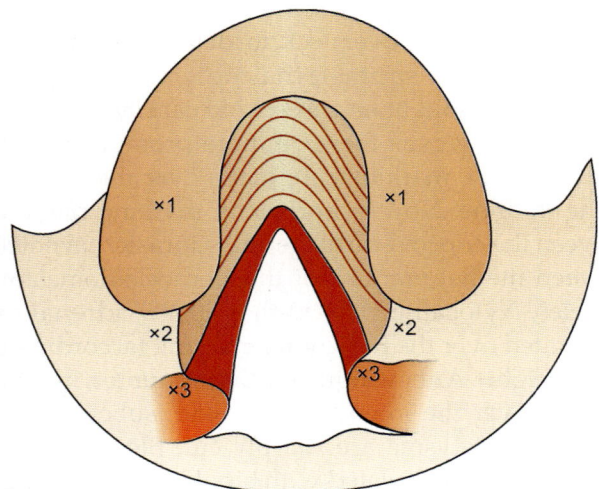

Fig. 110.13: Reduction of excess tissue is done at three points in laryngomalacia: 1. Lateral epiglotitis, 2. Aryepiglottic fold, 3. Arytenoid/corniculate cartilage

Differential diagnosis of laryngomalacia includes severe neurological impairment and pharyngeal and hypopharyngeal hypotonia. They may develop a chronic acquired flaccidity of the supraglottic larynx with similar symptomatology. Another condition, called pharyngolaryngomalacia[18] associated with complete supraglottic collapse during inspiration without shortened aryepiglottic folds or redundant mucosa and with accompanying pharyngomalacia. These patients don't respond with usual surgical intervention aimed for laryngomalacia. Some require tracheotomy and some may respond with bi-level positive airway pressure.

VOCAL CORD PARALYSIS

Vocal cord paralysis (VCP) accounts for 10% of all congenital laryngeal anomalies and is the second most common cause next to laryngomalacia.[19] VCP manifests early in life, and is without gender predilection. The majority is recognized before the age of two. Cohen et al, 1982, reported 100 children with VCP, 58% of whom presented within the first 12 hours of birth.[20]

Isolated unilateral or bilateral VCP is rare in the pediatric age group. Usually, it is only one manifestation of a multisystem anomaly. Although most frequently associated with central nervous system (CNS) malformations, VCP can be seen in conjunction with other congenital anomalies such as cardiovascular or pulmonary malformations. A higher incidence of other associated laryngeal malformations such as clefts or stenosis also has been reported.[21]

Etiology of VCP in children has been divided into two broad categories: congenital and acquired. The etiologies include Arnold-Chiari malformation or hydrocephalous alone, idiopathic and local trauma (including iatrogenic), birth trauma, and following bronchiolitis.[21]

Arnold-Chiari malformation is the most common cause of bilateral VCP in newborns. VCP in children with Arnold-Chiari malformation may be due to stretching of vagal nerve rootlets, altered vascular supply to the brain stem, dysplastic changes in the vagal nuclei, or a lack of afferent input from carotid bodies.[22] Prompt neurosurgical correction of the elevated intracranial pressure usually results in improvement. The return of stridor in a patient with a

VP shunt is often an indication of shunt malfunction and the need for revision.

Familial bilateral abductor vocal cord paralysis has been reported.[23] The cause of vocal cord paralysis is dysgenesis of the abductor portion of the nucleus ambiguous.

Bilateral abductor vocal cord paralysis in a neonate or infant presents with high pitched inspiratory stridor and evidence of airway compromise. The stridor may be *biphasic* and voice is usually *normal*. The respiratory compromise may be more obvious with increasing age due to the increased oxygen requirement. Unilateral vocal cord paralysis typically presents with a weak breathy voice and signs of aspiration, such a coughing, feeding difficulties and aspiration pneumonia. Usually there is no respiratory compromise.

Once suspected, the diagnosis of VCP requires endoscopic visualization of the larynx. The method of choice is flexible fiberoptic nasopharyngolaryngoscope (NPLS).[24] It provides an undistorted view of the larynx as compared with the view obtained when the base of the tongue is being lifted anteriorly with a rigid laryngoscope, is atraumatic, can be done bedside and a camera can be attached to provide the ability for playback in slow motion so that subtle abnormalities can be carefully analyzed. Ultrasound evaluation of larynx has been found to be an accurate, reproducible method for the evaluation of VCP in children.

Acoustic analysis of cry has shown to differentiate an abnormal cry from a normal cry in an infant with unilateral vocal cord paralysis.[25]

Management

Factors that influence management decisions include etiology of the paralysis, prognosis for recovery, unilateral or bilateral vocal cord involvement, length of impairment, severity of symptoms or associated conditions and existing facilities for monitoring the patient. Some suggest that in cases in which the potential for airway improvement is good, the airway should be secured with nasal tracheal intubation for at least 4 weeks before considering tracheotomy.[22]

The rate of spontaneous resolution of laryngeal paralysis, unilateral or bilateral, in pediatric population varies from 16 to 64%.[20,21,26] Recovery has been noted from 6 weeks to 5 years after the initial diagnosis. It is essential in children to observe them for reasonable period of time before any decision is made concerning irreversible laryngeal procedure.[27]

Surgical Procedure for Bilateral Abductor Vocal Cord Paralysis

Tracheotomy (Figs 110.14A to I)

When indicated, the initial surgical procedure of choice is tracheotomy. It is potentially reversible procedure, allowing time for potential spontaneous laryngeal recovery. Approximately 50 percent of children that need a tracheotomy for VCP require cannulation for more than 3 years.[20,21] Most physicians recommend waiting at least 12 months before an irreversible lateralization procedure is attempted.[28,21] Laryngeal electromyography can provide prognostic information about laryngeal nerve function and the potential for nerve recovery.[29]

Tracheostomy is done in pediatric age group under general anesthesia with spontaneous breathing. Airway is maintained by endotracheal intubation. If endotracheal intubation is not possible due to laryngeal stenosis, nasopharyngeal airway mask or ventilation or jet ventilation is used.

Patient is positioned in supine position with gentle neck extension. Too much extension of the neck causes risk of mediastinal contents (thymus, innominate artery, plura of lung) to shift to the lower neck area.

Neck is cleaned with antibiotic solution. Sterilized drapping done. Suction and cautery (monopolar and bipolar) are attached. Gentle palpation with pulp of index finger is done over neck, to identify the laryngeal framework and suprasternal notch. It is easy to identify the hyoid bone and cricoid cartilage over the neck with finger; as they are more prominent. With gention violet, markings are made over these points in the midline. Now, a horizontal marking made in between the criocoid cartilage and suprasternal notch, between medial margins of the sternocleidomastoid muscles. Xylocaine (1%) with 4,00,000 adrenaline; infilterated over the horizontal marking (according to body weight). After waiting for five minuntes, incision is made over the intended site. Skin, subcutaneous tissue and platysma are sharply cut. Bleeding from the margins is coagulated with bipolar cautery. Blunt, right angle retracters are placed on sides, and tissue is retracted gently towards own sides by the surgeon and

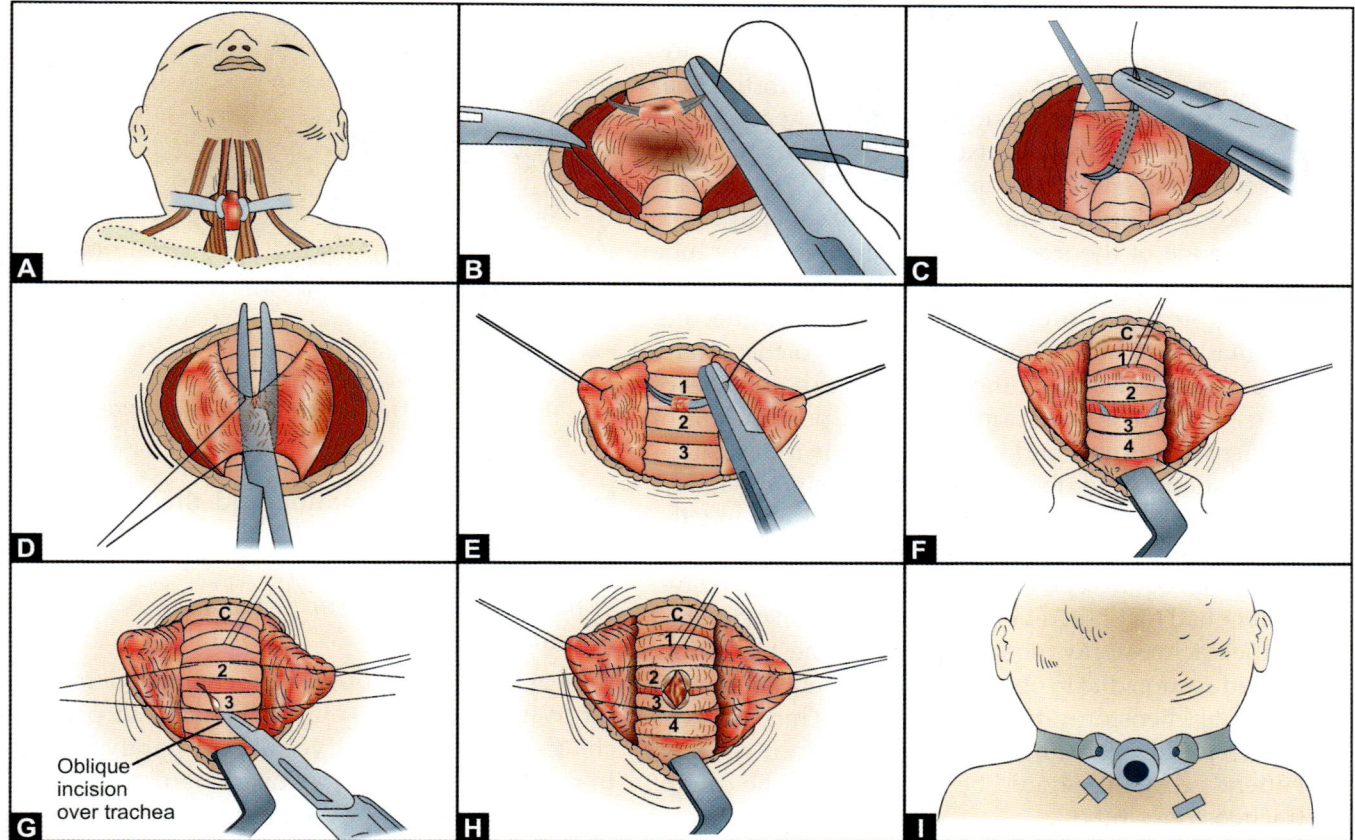

Figs 110.14A to I: Showing steps of tracheostomy

the assistant. Care should be taken, that retraction should be equal on each sides. Now tracheal positon is palpated with finger tips, to make sure that dissection is in right direction. Blunt dissection is done with artery forcep in the middle, along the direction of the trachea. Strap muscles are separated in the midline, and retactors are placed in new positions on both sides (Fig. 110.14A). Before further dissection, tracheal position is again checked because it is easy to displace the trachea inadvertently with retractors. Thyroid isthmus is visible after retraction of strap muscles. Thyroid isthmus is retracted with single hook retractor, superiorly or it may be ligated and cut (Figs 110.14B to D). Tracheal rings are visible beneath the thyroid isthmus. One percent xylocaine solution is taken in a 5 ml syringe with 24 gauze needle (Fig. 110.14E). Needle is inserted into the trachea, and aspiration done with syringe. (Fig. 110.14E) Air bubbles comes into the synringe if needle is into the right place (i.e. trachea). This technique is helpful in locating the trachea in revision cases, where fibrosis makes trachea less identifiable. In a small child, tracheal rings are very soft and can be mistaken for esophagus with a feeding tube or carotid artery. 2-0 or 3-0 silk sutures are placed around tracheal rings (2nd or 3rd) in a vertical diretion, around the proposed site of tracheostomy (Fig. 110.14F). These sutures are used as traction for the tracheal wall incision. This maneuver also prevents injury to the posterior membranous tracheal wall.

With 11 number sharp blade with B.P. handle oblique incision is made over anterior wall of trachea from below upwards, to prevent damage of mediastinal structure (Fig. 110.14G). Tracheal wall is not excised in children, as done in adult. The ends of stay sutures are brought outside the skin incision on either side and fixed over neck skin with tapes (Fig. 110.14H). It helps in initial period of tracheostomy tube placement (Fig. 110.14I). Stay sutures are removed after one week later following the first tracheostomy tube change. Appropriate size of tracheostomy tube is chosen and its tip is lubricated with xylocain gelly. Now, tracheostomy is gently retracted with the help of silk thread on both sides. Endotracheal tube is clearly seen into the trachea if child is intubated and or ventilating gases are coming out of it. Anesthetists is asked to withdraw the endotracheal tube, upto the upper edge of the tracheostoma. Tracheostomy tube is placed through the tracheostom. Without disturbing the endotracheal tube position, it is disconnected. Ventilation is now done through the tracheostomy tube. Anesthetist check the air entry on both sides of lungs. After confirmation of proper positioning of tracheostomy tube, endotracheal tube is removed.

Tracheostomy tube is secured in position with 1.0 silk and tape. Loose sutures are placed around the tracheostoma, and dressing done. Care of tracheostomy is required postoperatively. In initial few days, patient had lot of secretions, due to irritation of trachea by the tracheostomy tube and previous chest infection; pooled section due to obstruction. Frequent suctioning of the tracheostomy tube is required. Tracheostomy tube should be changed, at least once in a week. Patient's relatives should be taught about the care of tracheostomy tube.

Points to remember during tracheostomy:
- Patient neck should be extended.
- Incision should be adequate, so that tracheal positon can be palpated each time before blunt dissection.
- Do not resect the anterior wall of trachea, only make oblique incision to prevent post-decanulation problem.

Lateralization Procedures

It can be divided into two broad categories: (1) static or vocal cord lateralization techniques and (2) *dynamic* or *reanimation* techniques. Static techniques employ excision of laryngeal tissue (vocal cord or the arytenoids cartilage or and mechanical lateralization of the vocal cord. Surgical widening of the glottis must balance voice and airway patency. The lateralization of the vocal cord can be accomplished using a transoral arytenoidectomy mobilization technique or with an open laryngofissure technique. Laser arytenoidectomy or cordectomy is relatively difficult in children in comparison to adult because of its small size. Also there are higher rate of later failures in children

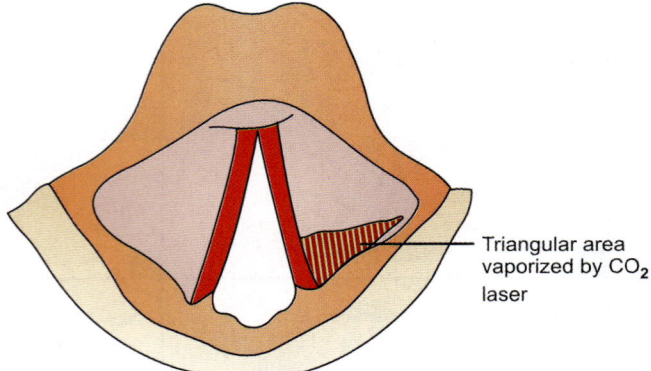

Fig. 110.15: Transverse partial laser cordectomy

because of scar formation and the smaller glottic diameter in children.

Transverse Partial Laser Cordectomy (Ventriculotomy)

It is performed through suspension microlaryngoscopy using the CO_2 laser has shown promise in children with bilateral vocal cord paralysis (VCP).[27] In this technique, a posterior triangular wedge of the posterior one-third of the paralyzed true vocal cord, false cord, and ventricle is delineated. The dissection is carried out laterally to the level of thyroid cartilage, with vertical extension from the level of the false vocal cord to the immediate undersurface of the true vocal cord (Fig. 110.15).

Reanimation Techniques

It include phrenic nerve to recurrent laryngeal nerve anastomosis, phrenic nerve to posterior cricoarytenoid muscle, and omohyoid nerve muscle pedicles. It is still a theoretical and experimental approach to VCP in children.

Unilateral Laryngeal Paralysis

Children usually adjust well to persistent, unilateral vocal cord paralysis with little sequelae. It is uncommon for a child with unilateral laryngeal paralysis to require a tracheostomy. Laryngeal augmentation procedures and thyroplasty techniques are not indicated in infants and young children. When unilateral vocal cord paralysis contributes to poor voice production, the treatment of choice remains speech therapy.[22]

SUBGLOTTIC STENOSIS

Subglottic larynx is the region extending from the insertion of the conus elasticus into the free edge of the vocal cords above to the inferior margin of cricoid cartilage below. Subglottic stenosis could be due to *congenital* or *acquired* causes.

Congenital Subglottic Stenosis

It is the third most common congenital laryngeal anomaly after laryngomalacia and vocal cord paralysis. However, it is the most common congenital laryngeal abnormality causing serious respiratory obstruction and requiring a tracheotomy in infants. By definition, congenital subglottic stenosis exists when this anatomic area has a diameter of less than 4 mm in a full term newborn or less than 3 mm in a premature infant, in the absence of endotracheal intubation or other apparent cause. It may also be a component of the acquired stenosis seen after prolonged neonatal intubation. Subglottic stenosis may be associated with other congenital anomalies, such as vocal cord paralysis or Down's syndrome.

Congenital subglottic stenosis is due to a defect in the development of the conus elasticus or cricoid cartilage. The most common abnormality is generalized circumferential stenosis of the cricoid cartilage (Fig. 110.16).

It may present with various degrees of symptomatology ranging from minimal airway obstruction to severe airway obstruction at birth.

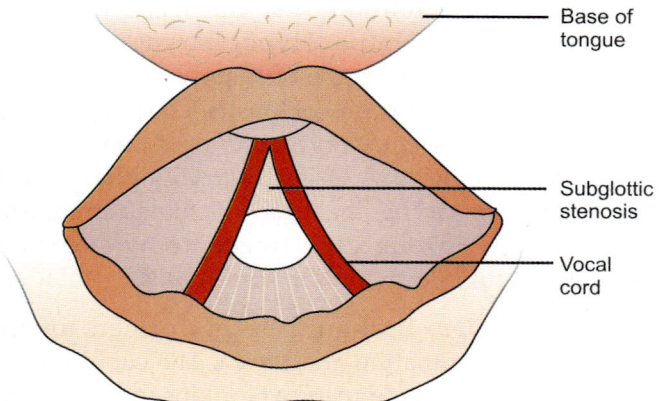

Fig. 110.16: Endoscopic view of larynx with area of subglottic stenosis

Recurrent croup is another common presentation for congenital subglottic stenosis. It affects males twice as often as females. The usual symptoms are biphasic stridor and a weak cry from the decrease in airflow.

Lateral and anteroposterior radiograph may help in diagnosis. Patients have a classic *hourglass* narrowing or *squared-off* configuration on this portion of the airway in an anterior posterior cervical airway radiograph. Flexible fiberoptic laryngoscopy should be performed to rule out other glottic or supraglottic pathology, such as vocal cord paralysis or laryngomalacia. Endoscopy under general anesthesia is necessary to confirm the diagnosis, plan further therapy and evaluate for other coexistent lesions. Typically, the larynx should admit an endotracheal tube that allows an air leak of 20 cm of water pressure or less around the tube.

Most children with congenital subglottic stenosis don't require any open operation. The child should receive aggressive medical therapy during upper respiratory infections to avoid intubation or tracheostomy. Severe cases may require tracheostomy or laryngotracheal reconstruction using costal cartilage grafting for expansion of the subglottic airway.[28]

Acquired Subglottic Stenosis

Acquired subglottic stenosis is a complication of medical therapy and is generally more severe. Endotracheal tube intubation is the most common cause.[1] Other causes are external trauma, high tracheostomy, cricothyroidotomy, infections, burn, tumor and dystrophic cartilage.[30]

In children, the subglottic region is prone to injury from endotracheal tube intubation, because, (1) Complete circular cartilaginous ring at cricoid, prevents outward extension of edema, (2) Lining epithelium (pseudostratified ciliated columnar) is delicate and tends to get traumatized easily, (3) Subglottic mucosa has loose areolar tissue that allows edema to develop easily and quickly, and (4) The subglottic region is the narrowest part of the pediatric airway.[31]

The pathophysiology is well described. The endotracheal tube causes pressure necrosis at the point of interface with tissue, leading to mucosal edema and ulceration. This causes mucociliary stasis leading to secondary infection and perichondritis. Healing occurs by secondary intention with granulation tissue proliferation and deposition of fibrous tissue in the submucosa. Primary healing of laryngeal injury is hindered by the presence of loose and mobile subglottic mucosa, poor blood supply of the cartilage, and constant motion of the larynx associated with swallowing and neck movement.[32]

Duration of intubation is the most important factor in the development of laryngeal stenosis.[33] Premature infants tolerate more prolonged intubation (weeks rather than days)[33] due to relative immaturity of the laryngeal cartilage, rendering it more pliable and the high location of the neonatal larynx with its posterior tilt and funnel shape. To prevent stenosis in children, the tube size should allow an air leak at 20 cm water pressure if possible. Polymeric silicone and polyvinyl chloride are considered safest materials for prolonged intubation. Nasogastric tubes can cause pressure necrosis and cricoid chondritis. Coexistence of endotracheal and nasogastric tubes may increase laryngeal complications.[33] Besides, systemic factors and nursing care also affect the outcomes.

Diagnosis

History and Physical Examination: In acquired subglottic stenosis, symptoms usually occur 2 to 4 weeks after the original insult. There is biphasic stridor. Symptoms gradually progress with increasing respiratory difficulty, dyspnea and air hunger. The cry and voice may not be affected till the true vocal cords are involved. Dysphasia and feeding abnormality with recurrent aspiration and pneumonia can occur. Auscultation should be performed to assess air entry, and of the anterior part of the neck to look for restricted air movements at a particular level of the upper airway.

Radiologic Evaluation

Radiography helps assess the exact site and length of the stenotic segment, especially for totally obliterated airway (Fig. 110.17). Also, the lower tracheal air column and the bronchial air column should be evaluated for the possibility of further distal lesions. Xeroradiography (selenium-coated charged plate is used) has a better tissue—air interface and therefore enhances the edge and better documents soft tissue details than does computed tomography (CT). CT

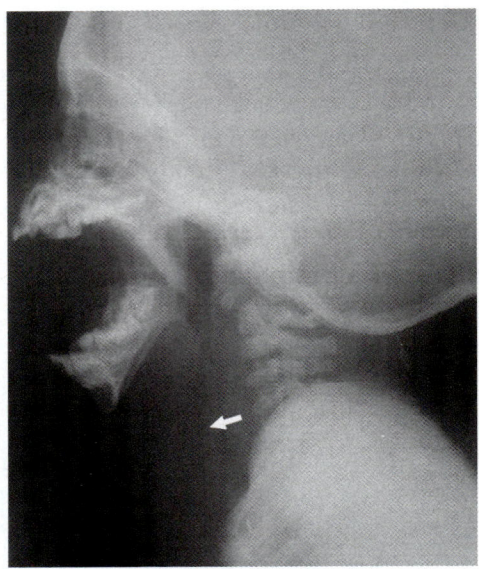

Fig. 110.17: X-ray soft tissue neck, lateral view, showing subglottic stenosis

examination may be used to determine the degree of loss of cartilaginous support of the cricoid. MR imaging of the neck and chest is required for suspected coincidental vascular lesion. In presence of swallowing or feeding disorders a modified barium swallow is essential.[30]

Endoscopic Evaluation

Flexible Endoscopy: Vocal cord function, as well as general dynamic motion of the larynx, may be evaluated in the awake patient if possible. Examination should include both nares, the hypopharynx, supraglottis and glottis. Hypopharyngeal visualization assesses the degree of hypopharyngeal tone and degree of hypertrophy of tonsils. The supraglottis is assessed for edema, erythema, or a cobblestone appearance suggestive of gastrolaryngopharyngeal reflux, and for laryngomalacia.[34] Flexible retrograde tracheoscopy through the tracheotomy site may provide useful information in some cases.

Rigid Endoscopy: It should be performed under spontaneous ventilation anesthesia. The subglottis, if patent is best evaluated using a Hopkins rod telescope of appropriate size, with the determination of site (anterior, posterior, and circumferential), maturity, length, and consistency of the obstruction (Table 110.6). When assessing vocal cord function it is important to realize that laryngeal neuromuscular function changes with growth. Very young infants may exhibit laryngeal dyskinesia and transient unexplained vocal cord paralysis, including paradoxic vocal cord movements.[34]

Evaluation of Gastroesophageal and Gastrolaryngopharyngeal Reflux

Presence of gastroesophageal reflux (GER) and gastrolaryngopharyngeal reflux (GLPR) is likely to play a role in the development and exacerbation of subglottic stenosis and may affect adversely the successful outcome of laryngotracheal reconstruction (LTR). Treatment should be done simultaneously.

Functional Endoscopic Evaluation of Swallowing

Dysfunctional feeding may complicate airway reconstruction by increasing the risk of aspiration postoperatively. This can be assessed by
1. Videofluoroscopic swallowing studies (VSS),
2. Functional endoscopic evaluation of swallow (FEES).

Pulmonary Function Test

Maximum inspiration and expiration flow rates, flow volume loops, or pressure flow loops show characteristic changes in upper airway stenosis and can be used to compare the postoperative results with preoperative values.

Voice Analysis

Psychoacoustic evaluation and acoustic analysis of the voice may be used to establish the degree of vocal abnormality before surgery and compare it after surgery.

Table 110.6 Grading of Subglottic stenosis[35]	
Grade	Percentage of laryngeal lumen obstruction
I	< 70%
II	70 to 90%
II	> 90% identifiable lumen present
IV	Complete obstructon; no lumen present

Management

Selection of the proper therapy should be individualized according to pathologic findings, patient age, degree and consistency of stenosis.

Patient with mild obstruction may be observed. If patient develops respiratory infection, it should be treated aggressively with antibiotics, and steroids. If airway symptoms continue or worsens, then surgical intervention is required.

Tracheostomy

Usually done below the stenotic segment. Smallest tube that permits adequate ventilation should be used. This allows air leakage to occur to avoid injury to the tracheal mucosa and simultaneously preserve phonatory potential. In cases of congenital subglottic stenosis, the cricoid may grow and allow decanulation within 2 years. The child with severe subglottic stenosis may be completely tracheostomy dependent. Mortality rates in children with complete subglottic stenosis and tracheostomy is very high (from 5 to 24%). Hence, most authors propose some type of intervention to allow decanulation.

Endoscopic Management

Dilatation

Usually performed with round, smooth dilators. We use red rubber dilators (Rouch). Dilators are kept on warm water for few minutes to become softer. The maximum size of dilator to be used depends upon the expected size of lumen of subglottis, according to age of the patient. After the procedure, *mitomycin-C* is applied over the raw area for few minutes. *Corticosteroids* are also used locally or systemically after the dilatation. *Balloon dilatation* has also been used in subglottic stenosis in children. Dilatation is not recommended for mature, firm stenosis or cartilaginous stenosis.

Scar Excision: Endoscopic scar excision is done with microcauterization, cryosurgery, serial electrosurgical resection and CO_2 laser. CO_2 laser is more popular because of its precision and minimal damage to healthy areas. The laser is helpful in early or mild subglottic stenosis. Laser techniques have been refined

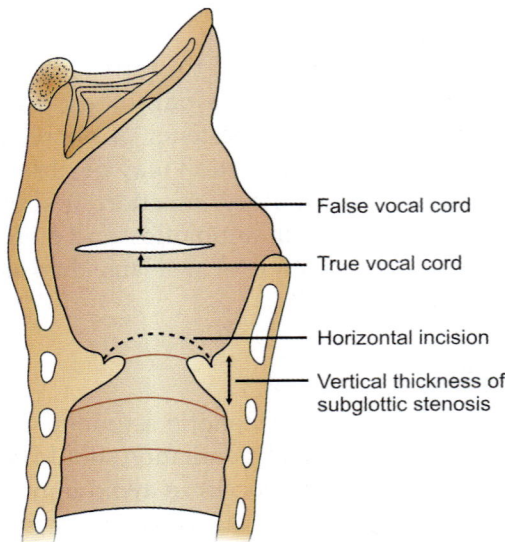

Fig. 110.18: Lateral view of larynx and subglottis showing vertical thickness of subglottic stenosis and horizontal incision in the proximal aspect of the stenosis

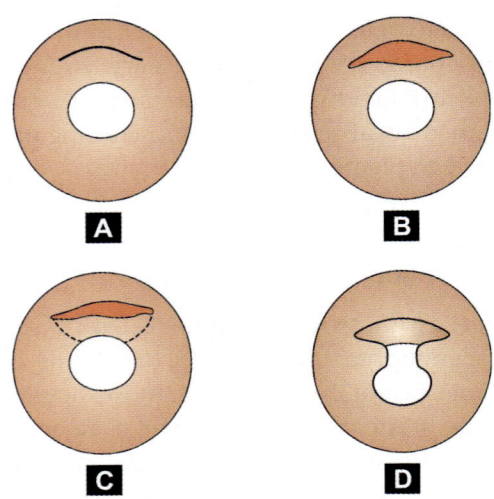

Figs 110.19A to D: A. Horizontal incision made with laser in the superior portion of the scar, **B.** Submucosal flap raised, and scar is vaporized with the laser proceeding distally in the subglottis, keeping in the submucosal plane, **C.** Vertical mucosal cuts are made, **D.** Inferior based microtrapdoor mucosal flap replaced in their position after underlying scar was vaporized

to excise scar tissue using serial microtrapdoor flaps, preserving airway mucosa (Figs 110.18 and 110.19A to D).

Cases involving circumferential subglottic scarring, scarring of the interarytenoid area, vertical scar extending more than 1 cm, or tracheomalacia should not be treated with endoscopic management alone and usually require open surgical repair. Endoscopic management is also contraindicated if laryngeal framework is significantly deficient.

External Surgical Reconstruction

There are two broader groups of surgical options that are available for laryngotracheal reconstruction externally—expansion surgery with or without prolonged stenting and resection surgery with or without prolonged airway management. Usually grades III and IV lesions require external methods.

Expansion of the laryngotracheal airway can be done in various ways.
1. Splitting the stenosed anterior segment of cricoid lumen and associated upper few rings of trachea if stenosis is primarily involving the anterior subglottic area.
2. Combined laryngofissure and posterior cricoid division for persistent posterior glottic pathology or primarily posterior subglottic pathology.
3. Combination of the above procedure.

Anterior cricoid split operation has been used for congenital subglottic stenosis (Fig. 110.20). Criteria for patient selection are:[30]
1. Extubation failure on at least two occasions secondary to subglottic laryngeal pathology.
2. Weight of the patient should be greater than 1500 gm.
3. Off ventilator support for at least 10 days before procedure.
4. Supplemental oxygen requirement less than 30%.
5. No congestive heart failure for at least 1 month before procedure.
6. No acute respiratory tract infection.
7. No antihypertensive medication for at least 10 days before the procedure.

Complications of anterior cricoid split and ICU management include malposition of the endotracheal tube, accidental extubation, persistent tracheocutaneous fistula, and subcutaneous edema.

Various types of grafts; autologus costal cartilage (Figs 110.21A to E), ear cartilage, free thyroid cartilage

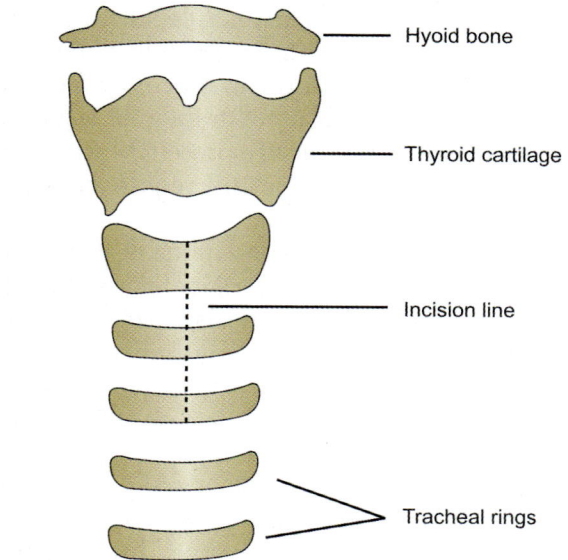

Fig. 110.20: Anterior cricoid split, showing vertical incision through anterior cricoid cartilage and upper two tracheal rings

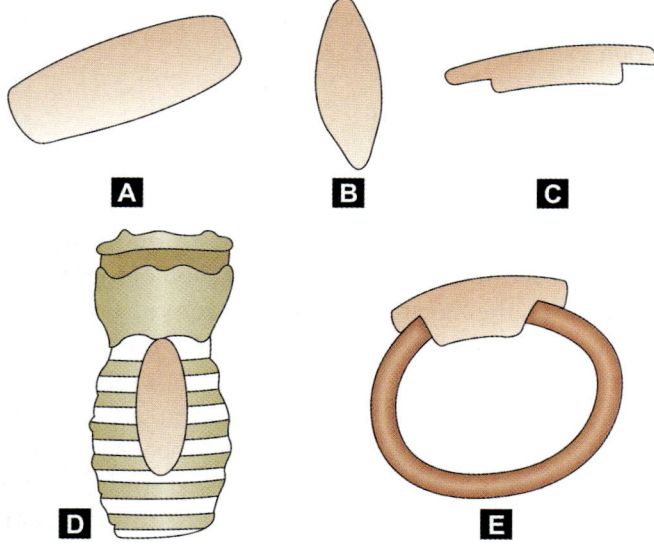

Figs 110.21A to E: Repair of subglottic stenosis, using costal rib Cartilage **A.** Rib cartilage harvested, **B** and **C.** Trimmed to fit into subglottic space, **D** and **E.** Rib cartilage into its position

grafts, composite nasal cartilage grafts, hyoid bone – muscle flap, free hyoid bone has been described. The purpose of graft is to augment the lumen and or to support the laryngotracheal framework, if deficient. In children, autologus costal cartilage is the graft material of choice. Cartilage grafts are contraindicated in unstable diabetic patients and patients on continuous steroid therapy.[30]

Stents: Stents are usually used after reconstruction of the chronic stenosis. Stents counteract scar contractures and promote a scaffold for epithelium to grow. It prevents disruption during physiological movement of larynx and trachea, e.g. swallowing and coughing. In single stage laryngotracheal reconstruction, endotracheal tube is used as a stent for 7-14 days. Short-term (4-6) weeks) stenting is useful in mild subglottic stenosis. Long-term (more than 2 months) stenting is indicated for severe or complete subglottic stenosis, for poor graft stability, or with placement of most posterior cricoid graft.[36]

Selection of the proper stent is done, keeping in mind, the *material* and its *size*. The *location* of the stenosis and *duration* to be kept is also very important.. A variety of stents have been used, including *finger cots*, (made from surgical gloves), Montgomery *T-tubes, polymeric silicone sheet rolls*, and *Aboulker* prosthesis. Silastic sheeting in "Swiss roll" exerts a constant gentle pressure during healing but is associated with excessive granulation tissue formation. The Cotton-Lorenz stent, a variation of the aboulker stent, is the stent of choice in children in western countries. At All India Institute of Medical Sciences, we use Montgomery silicon T-tube because it is easily available here.

Montgomery T Tube is made up of silicon, is soft with little tissue reaction. It is self secured and allows normal respiration and speech.

Cotton-Lorenz stent is available in various sizes (from 7 to 16 mm outer diameter). It is made of highly polished polytef, which is harder, provides better support, is more inert than silicone, and does not adhere to tissue. A laryngofissure may be required because the superior tip of the stent should be inserted at the level of the superior edge of the arytenoid.[34] Stent may be fixed using a Hollinger tracheostomy tube (Figs 110.22A and B).

Single Stage Laryngotracheal Reconstruction

This implies the use of cartilage grafts to obtain stability of the reconstructed airway and compress the prolonged stenting period of traditional methods into a briefer period endotracheal intubation.[28,37] It is indicated primarily in subglottic stenosis without significant obstructions in the trachea or significant tracheomalacia.[30] It may include all types of cricoid

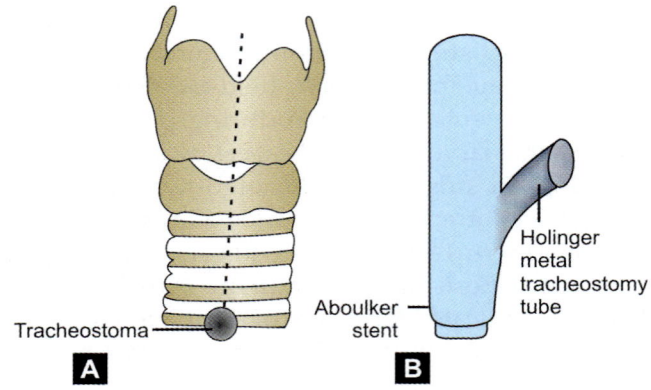

Figs 110.22A and B: A. Division of larynx and trachea from superior thyroid notch to tracheostoma, **B.** Holinger metal tube wired to Aboulker prosthesis

division, and in most cases these divisions are stabilized by use of a cartilage graft.[30] The optimal time for intubation varies from 7 to 10 days for anterior cartilage graft alone to 12-14 days if posterior graft is used as well. Patients with significant craniofacial or vertebral anomalies are usually excluded. Children weighting more than 4 kg and greater than 30 weeks gestation have a greater chance for successful extubation and eventual airway patency.[37]

Cricotracheal Resection with Thyrotracheal Anastomosis

The results are superior due to complete resection of the stenotic segment with restoration of a lumen using a normal tracheal ring, preservation of normal laryngotracheal support structures and full mucosal lining thus minimizing or preventing granulation tissue and restenosis. Due to absence of widening of anterior commissure by graft, voice quality is good in cricotracheal resection anastomosis. Cricotracheal resection is used when the stenosis is entirely subglottic or upper tracheal with a normal lumen of at least 10 mm below the glottis.

SACCULAR CYSTS AND LARYNGOCELE

Laryngeal saccule is a pouch that opens into the laryngeal sinus ascends laterally between vestibular fold and thyroid cartilage, occasionally reaching the cartilage's upper part. Normally secretions from the saccule lubricate true vocal cords. Laryngocele is an abnormal dilatation of saccule, is filled with air and communicates with internal laryngeal lumen; whereas saccular cyst is filled with thick, mucoid fluid, and usually doesn't communicate with internal laryngeal lumen. These children typically present with stridor that begins soon after birth and 20% require emergent airway intervention.[38]

Soft tissue lateral radiography of the neck shows a cyst in all cases. CT may be helpful in determining the extent of these lesions. The diagnosis can be confirmed only at the time of direct laryngoscopy. Surgical management of saccular cysts include endoscopic marsupilization using CO_2 laser or with sharp dissection, aspiration and incision drainage. There is high recurrence after endoscopic marsupilization in comparasion to excision via laryngofissure

Laryngoceles typically cause intermittent symptoms during acute inflammation or infection. For internal laryngocele treatment usually is not required, although endoscopic deroofing can be done if symptomatic. External and mixed laryngocele require open excision (Figs 110.23A to C).

LARYNGEAL CLEFTS

Posterior laryngeal cleft is rare and is frequently missed. They can involve the entire tracheoesophageal spectrum or be isolated to the posterior larynx. It is due to arrested medial fusion of the lateral aspects of the laryngo-tracheal groove. Posterior laryngeal clefts may be an isolated anomaly or associated with other congenital anomalies, e.g. VATER association (vertebral, anal, tracheal, esophageal and renal anomalies), tracheoesophageal fistula, esophageal atresia, cleft lip and palate, congenital heart defects (transposition of great vessels), gastrointestinal anomalies (Imperforate anus, rectal stenosis, meckel's diverticulum), genitourinary anomalies (hypospadias, hypoplastic kidneys), subglottic stenosis, Hamartomas, G syndrome (Opritzfrias syndrome), Pallister-Hall syndrome or BBB syndrome (hyperterolism – hypospadias syndrome).[39]

Depending on the extent of the cleft, the cardinal presenting feature, especially with oral feeding, is aspiration, which causes choking, and cyanosis. Stridor is unusual, when present; it is usually caused by tracheobronchial obstruction from aspirated secretions. There may be radiographic evidence of

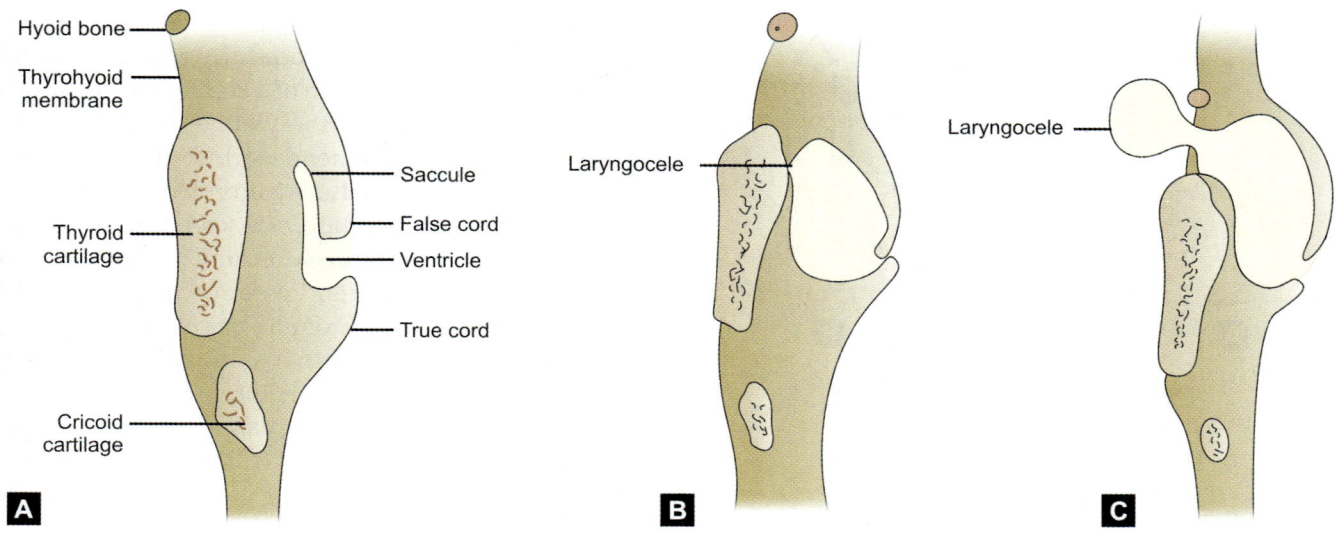

Figs 110.23A to C: Coronal section of larynx at the level of saccule showing
A. Normal anatomy, B. Internal laryngocele, C. Combined laryngocele

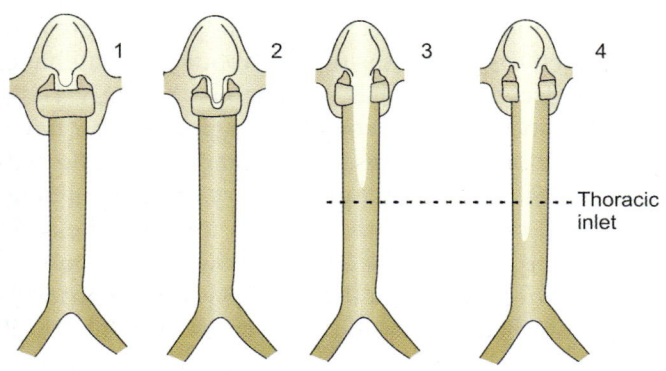

Fig. 110.24: Classification of four types of cleft larynx
(Benjamin and Inglis)

aspiration pneumonitis. *Benjamin and Inglis (1989)* classified *type I* as a supraglottic interarytenoid cleft above the vocal cords, *type II* as a partial cricoid cleft, *type III* completely involving cricoid with or without extension into part of the tracheal esophageal wall and *type IV* as a laryngotracheal esophageal cleft (Fig. 110.24).[40]

For definitive diagnosis, careful direct microlaryngoscopy and esophagoscopy is required. Findings may be missed easily during evaluation, hence a laryngeal probe should be used to separate the redundant mucosa between the arytenoids and palpate for a possible cricoid defect. The diagnosis can also be confirmed by examining the patient under general anesthesia. The typical finding is that despite the endotracheal being *in situ* the whole length of vocal cord is visible and the tube appears partly or completely buried between the arytenoids.

A 93% mortality rate is associated with laryngotracheal esophageal clefts with significant intrathoracic involvement. A 43% mortality rate however is associated with clefts limited to the laryngeal region. Surgical repair must be undertaken in all cases of symptomatic posterior laryngeal cleft.[39]

Repair of laryngeal cleft can be done, depending upon severity, through endoscopic, anterior laryngofissure, lateral cervical or thoracotomy approach. To improve results of surgery in severe cases, use of interposition tibial periosteum graft, and extracorporeal membrane oxygenation have been described (Figs 110.25A to D).

LARYNGEAL WEBS AND ATRESIA

Laryngeal web, subglottic stenosis and congenital laryngeal atresia result from different degrees of failure of the epithelium's resorption during the seventh and eighth weeks of intrauterine development. Webs occur primarily at the level of the glottis. Other types include the posterior glottic web, causing interarytenoid vocal cord fixation, subglottic webs, which may occur with or without cricoid cartilage involvement and subglottic stenosis; and very rarely supraglottic webs. Complete

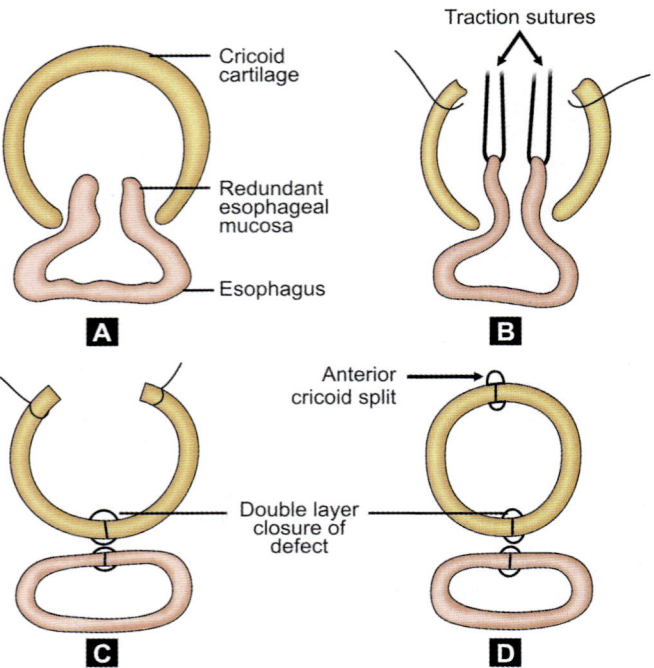

Figs 110.25A to D: Repair of cleft larynx through anterior approach

atresia is the rarest of these lesions and causes immediate respiratory obstruction at birth unless there is a concomitant tracheoesophageal fistula or if the obstruction is relieved by tracheostomy.

Majority present with an abnormal cry or voice, respiratory distress, and stridor. Laryngeal webs always should be considered in children with a congenital history of hoarseness and recurrent coup presenting before 6 months of age.[39] Many patients have associated abnormalities of other systems, principally of the upper respiratory tract, most often subglottic stenosis (Benjamin B 1998).

The diagnosis of laryngeal webs or atresia is made by fibreoptic laryngoscopy or direct endoscopy under general anaesthesia. A lateral radiograph or xeroradiogram may give valuable information about the anterior thickness of the web, the presence or absence of congenital subglottic stenosis and the site of a subglottic we. CT scan is advisable to assess involvement of laryngeal skeleton.

Surgical management includes endoscopic management versus open laryngotracheal reconstruction.[39] Small limited webs may be treated endoscopically by dilatation, microsurgical excision or laser excision. Recurrence after the surgery can be prevented by staging the procedure, repeated use of dilators, endoscopic insertion of a keel, or using sutures through the cut edge of the web. A thick anterior laryngeal web or one extending into the subglottic space requires a tracheostomy followed by a laryngofissure and insertion of a keel at the anterior commissure or laryngofissure and possible costal cartilage graft and stents. Posterior interarytenoid webs alone usually don't require any kind of surgery, unless associated with other congenital anomaly (subglottic stenosis, dysmorphic facies or midface hypoplasia). Most patients are managed with watchful waiting or tracheostomy with subsequent decanulation after 3 to 5 years.

SUBGLOTTIC HEMANGIOMA

Hemangiomas are only present at birth 30% of the time, with the majority presenting within the first few weeks or months of life.[39] About 80-90% will present within the first 6 months of life. About 50% will have lesions elsewhere, usually cutaneous. Yet only 1-2% of children with cutaneous hemangiomas also have subglottic hemangiomas. Females are more affected than males (2:1). The natural history of hemangioma is one of rapid growth for 8-18 months (i.e. the *proliferative phase*) followed by a slow regression (i.e. the *involutive phase*) over the next 5-8 years. About 50% show complete regression by 5 years and 70% by 7 years. One case of malignant transformation of a subglottic hemangioma has been reported.

The lesion is usually localized to the subglottic region on one side as a sessile, fairly firm and compressible pink, red or bluish lesion that is poorly delineated from the surrounding tissues. However, if there is any doubt about the diagnosis, biopsy should be performed.[39] With precautions taken to maintain the airway in the unlikely event of excessive bleeding. Preoperative fluoroscopy or anteroposterior radiographs of the neck may demonstrate an asymmetric subglottic narrowing, however tumours or subglottic cysts may also present with the same radiographic characteristic. Besides airway obstruction, subglottic hemangiomas associated with compound hemangioma or multiple large lesions may be associated with high cardiac output failure or

Kasabach-Merritt syndrome resulting from platelet sequestration and destruction as well as consumptive coagulopathy.

For symptomatic patients management options include tracheostomy, laser ablation using CO_2 or potassium titanyl phosphate (KTP) laser, external beam radiation, radioactive gold grain implantation, cryotherapy, sclerosing agents, corticosteroids therapy, (systemic or intralesional injection), open surgical excision and interferon alpha -2α.[39] Tracheotomy allows the tracheal lumen to enlarge with growth of the child and giving the hemangioma an opportunity to involutes spontaneously. However, tracheostomy may have to remain in place for 3 to 4 years and has associated morbidity (tube obstruction, language delay and mortality). Radiotherapy has a cure rate of 93%, but the risk of secondary malignancies and often more acceptable alternatives now preclude their general use. The most common intervention is CO_2 laser ablation. However, 20% subglottic stenosis rate following laser excision has been reported in a large series of cases.[41]

Corticosteroid therapy is considered by some authors as an alternative method of managing airway hemangiomas, either alone or in conjunction with laser therapy. Ohlms et al (1994) suggest the use of interferon alpha -2α when traditional therapeutic modalities such as steroid and laser therapy fail, and especially when subglottic hemangioma is massive.[34]

Open surgical excision has also been advocated. This technique may be used when airway obstruction is significant enough to require a tracheostomy.

MISCELLANEOUS ABNORMALITIES OF LARYNX

Bifid Epiglottis

Bifid epiglottis is a rare laryngeal anomaly may be associated with other laryngeal abnormalities or congenital syndromes. Patients with bifid epiglottis should undergo an endocrine evaluation because of the possibility of associated hypothyroidism or hypothalamic abnormalities.[39] The presenting symptoms are usually feeding difficulties owing to aspiration and respiration compromise owing to enfolding of the two epiglottic halves. In cases of severe airway obstruction, surgical management is necessary that includes tracheostomy and amputation of epiglottis.

Cri du Chat Syndrome

It is due to partial deletion of the short arm of chromosome 5. The newborn infant has a cry similar to that of a cat's mew. There is a characteristic congenital high-pitched stridor. Classically, upon inspiration, the vocal cords of these patients have a narrow diamond-shaped appearance. On phonation, the posterior part of the larynx shows an open triangle, probably caused by paralysis of the interarytenoid muscle. Other associated abnormalities include microcephaly, hypertelorism, generalized hypotonia, severe mental retardation and low-slung ears with a beak-like profile. In general, the prognosis is poor.

Cystic Hygromas (Lymphangiomas)

These are congenital developmental malformations of lymphatic vessels present at birth or within the first 2 years of life. Most commonly they involve the soft tissues of the lateral neck as diffuse, compressible, smooth, non tender masses. They are usually asymptomatic, sometimes compress tissues of the pharynx and larynx to produce airway obstruction. A cystic hygroma is virtually always a supraglottic mass. Aspiration or external excision of the bulk by laser or some other modality may be required.

CONGENITAL ANOMALIES OF THE TRACHEA TRACHEOMALACIA

Tracheomalacia is characterized by abnormal flaccidity of the anterior wall of trachea. Tracheomalacia is defined as collapse of the trachea during expiration, which results in greater than 10-20% obstruction of the airway. Primary tracheomalacia is a rare congenital deformity, caused by an inherent weakness of the cartilaginous ring (Figs 110.26A and B). Secondary tracheomalacia occurs as a result of extrinsic compression by a mass by vascular structure. It may be secondary to surgical intervention, such as tracheoesophageal fistula repair or by pressure from tracheostomy or endotracheal tube cuff.

Clinically, the patients exhibit *expiratory* stridor secondary to collapse of the anterior tracheal wall against the posterior membranous wall. Stridor may be present at birth, but often later on, when infant becomes more active. Patients may present with reflex apnea and recurrent pneumonitis secondary to their chronic obstruction.[42]

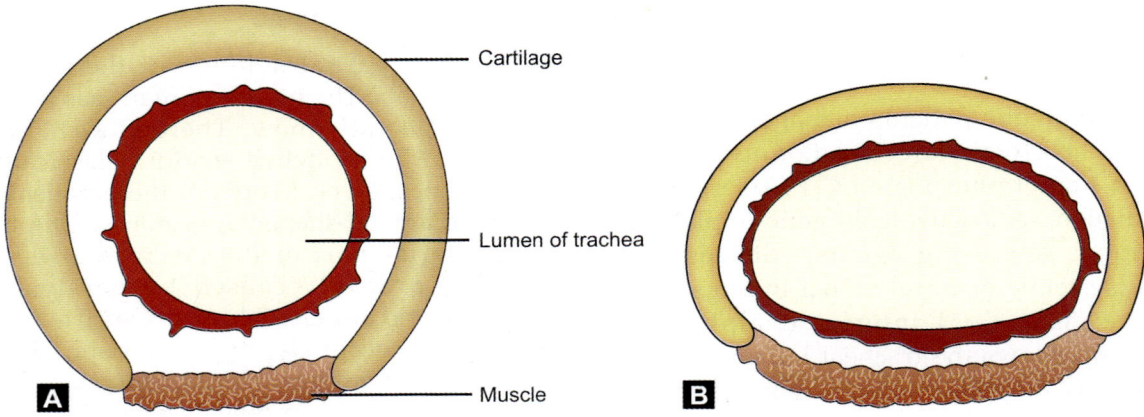

Figs 110.26A and B: A. Normal trachea with cartilage to muscle ratio as 4.5:1, **B.** Trachea in primary tracheomalacia with cartilage to muscle ratio as 2:1

Dynamic assessment of the tracheo-bronchial tree is needed to diagnose the luminal obstruction during expiration. Airway fluoroscopy (and rigid bronchoscopy) in normal condition and rigid bronchoscopy under spontaneous ventilation technique is helpful for that purpose. Barium swallow excludes any vascular compression. In cases of suspected vascular compression or cardiac anomalies contributing to tracheomalacia, MR imaging with contrast or MR-angio and echocardiography also may be warranted.[39]

Mild cases of tracheomalacia often resolve within the first 1 to 2 years of age.[39] In severe cases, it may be necessary to place a tracheostomy tube or stent the trachea during development. In cases of vascular compression of the trachea surgical decompression of the trachea may lead to significant improvement.[39] Surgical procedures, used to correct diffuse tracheomalacia include placement of internal stents, segmental resection, cartilage grafting of the trachea and external tracheal stents.[39]

VASCULAR COMPRESSION OF THE TRACHEA

Vascular rings completely encircle the tracheoesophageal region, whereas vascular slings are noncircumferential. Patients with vascular rings present earlier than vascular slings as more severe the compression, the earlier the symptoms present. Besides stridor, these patients are more prone to recurrent respiratory infections resulting from difficult clearing of secretions past the narrowed segment.

Innominate Artery Compression (Figs 110.27 and 110.28)

It is the most common cause of vascular compresssion of the tracheobronchial tree. Cases usually present within the first year of life. Signs and symptoms gradually disappear over months to years in most patients. Tracheal compression is more pronounced in the expiratory phase, often obliterating the tracheal lumen when the child coughs.[43]

Chest radiography or airway fluoroscopy may show persistent compression of anterior trachea at the thoracic inlet. The definitive diagnosis however may be made using rigid bronchoscopy.[39] Typically the compression is relatively short segment, located a few

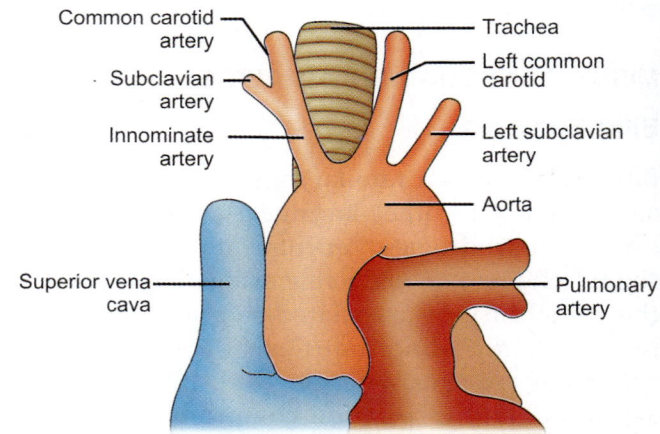

Fig. 110.27: Normal relations of great vessels to tracheobronchial tree

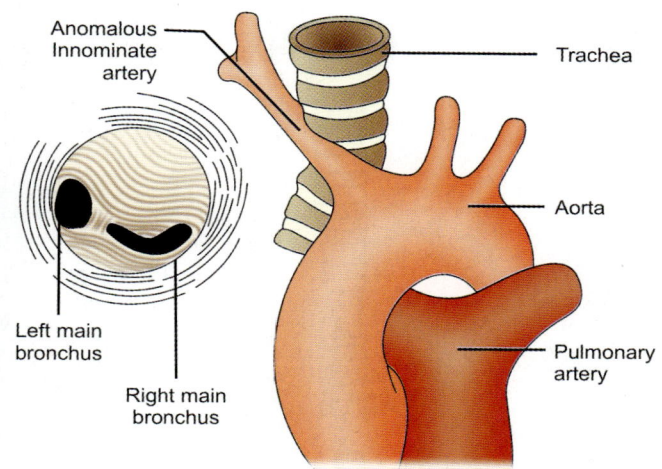

Fig. 110.28: Endoscopic appearance of tracheal compression by an anomalous innominate artery and the position of the artery in respect to the trachea externally

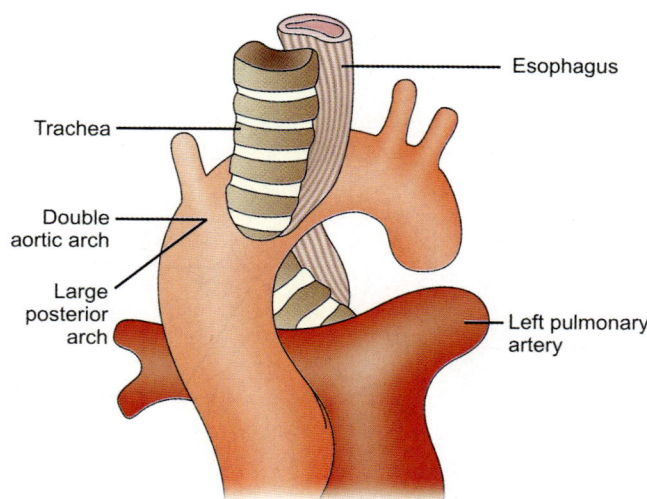

Fig. 110.29: Double aortic arch with a large (right) posterior arch

centimeters above the carina. Pressure with the tip of the bronchoscope may decrease the right radial and temporal pulses.[43]

In patients, with severe symptoms, aortopexy (where the innominate artery is suspended from the sternum to relieve compression over trachea) is indicated. The innominate artery may also be divided and reimplanted more proximal on the aorta to the right side so that it does not cross and compress the trachea.[39]

Double Aortic Arch

It is the second most common cause of vascular compression of the tracheobronchial tree. In most cases, the left arch is smaller and even atretic or non-patent in some cases (Fig. 110.29).[39] Bronchoscopy reveals anterior and posterior pulsatile compression of the trachea just above the carina, usually involving one or both main bronchi. Compression with bronchoscope does not affect the radial pulse. Management consists of division of the small arch.[44]

Anomalous Subclavian Artery

An aberrant right subclavian artery passes behind the oesophagus, causing dysphagia termed *dysphagia lusoria*.

Right Aortic Arch (Fig. 110.30)

With a right aortic arch, the aorta courses over the right bronchus, to the right of the trachea, curving downward to lie just right of the midline posteriorly. It can be similar to a vascular ring if a persistent ligamentum arteriosum or ductus arteriosum is present. Management consists of division of the

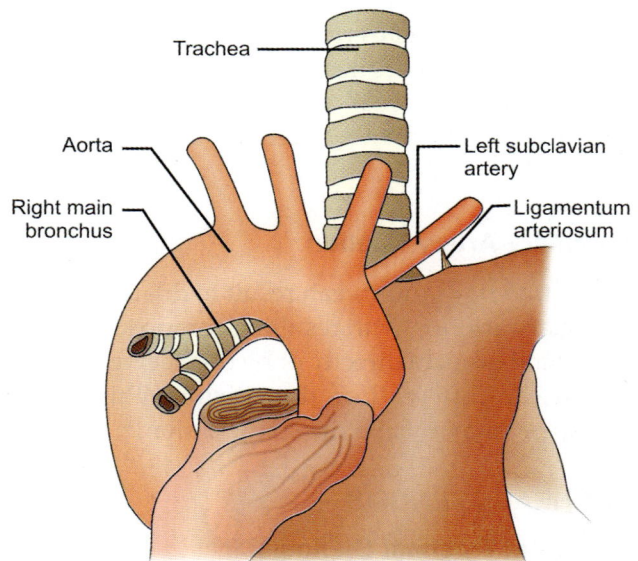

Fig. 110.30: Right aortic arch with a vascular ring formed by left subclavian artery and ligamentum arteriosum

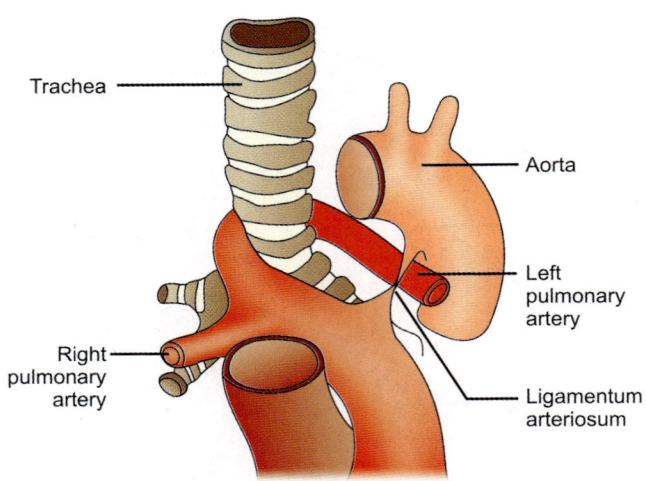

Fig. 110.31: Anomalous left pulmonary artery compressing right main brounchus

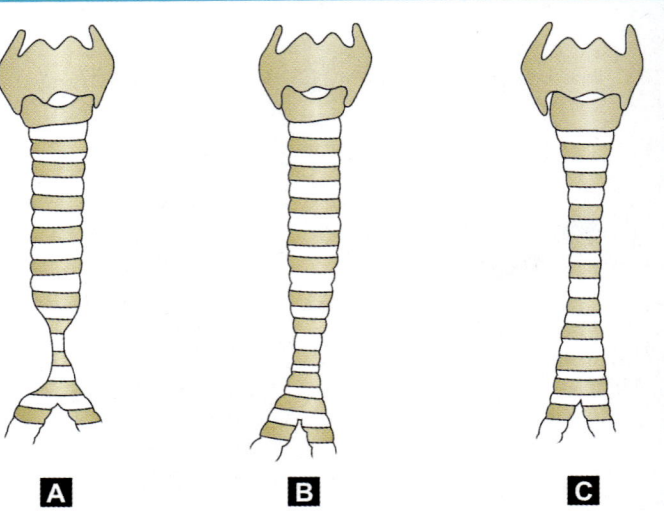

Figs 110.32A to C: Cantrell and Guild Classification of congenital tracheal stenosis **A.** Segmental stenosis, **B.** Funnel like stenosis, **C.** Generalized hypopasia

ligamentum arteriosum or ductus anteriosum to relieve the obstruction.[43]

Pulmonary Artery Sling (Fig. 110.31)

The anomaly results when the aberrant left pulmonary artery, arises from the right pulmonary artery, encircles the trachea and passes between the trachea and esophagus. It is often associated with congenital tracheal stenosis and complete tracheal rings. If the trachea is normal, there is usually marked compression of the right main branches. Surgical reanastomosis of the aberrant vessel may not relieve the respiratory symptoms unless the tracheal abnormality is addressed.[43]

Pulmonary Artery Dilation

Large left to right shunts can result in dilatation of the pulmonary arteries, with resulting compression of the trachea and bronchi directly or by displacing the aorta against the left wall of the trachea. Pulmonary arteriopexy may relieve the compression.[43]

TRACHEAL STENOSIS

Congenital Tracheal Stenosis

Three types of congenital tracheal stenosis have been described by *Cantrell and Guild in 1964*. (1) Segmental stenosis, (2) Funnel shaped stenosis and (3) Generalized hypoplasia (Figs 110.32).[43] The association of congenital tracheal stenosis with H-Type tracheo esophageal fistula, pulmonary hypoplasia, vascular ring, skeletal abnormalities, and subglottic stenosis has been established.

Presentation of symptoms depends upon severity of disease; some present at birth, whereas others develop symptoms months later. The usual presenting symptom is stridor, classically biphasic, if stenosis is located high within the trachea or primarily expiratory if located lower in the trachebronchial tree. Other signs and symptoms include wheezing, recurrent pneumonia, cyanosis, apnea and failure to thrive. A definitive diagnosis of tracheal stenosis usually is made by a combination of radiographic studies and rigid endoscopy. CT and MRI can be used in conjunction with endoscopy to identify intrathoracic relationships and associated anomalies. Endoscopy should be done under great caution; even minimal trauma to the stenotic segment may lead to edema and acute airway obstruction. In severe stenosis, evaluation is done under apneic technique using small 2.2 mm telescope. Passage of instrumentation through the stenosis should be avoided, unless definitive repair at that time.[39]

Treatment depends upon the severity of stenosis. Because, stenotic segments appear to grow faster than normal surrounding trachea, mildly symptomatic children may be treated by observation alone. Severe stenosis requires surgery. Short segment stenosis is treated with resection and anastomosis. For more diffuse lesions, tracheoplasty is done. These include; anterior tracheal split with pericardial patching or cartilage grafting, slide tracheoplasty and homograft tracheal transplantation. Mortality ranges from 20 to 80%.[43]

Aquired Tracheal Stenosis

Besides congenital causes, increased use of endotracheal intubation has resulted in increased incidence of tracheal stenosis athough the use of low pressure, high volume cuffed endotracheal and tracheotomy tubes has been shown to decrease the rate of tracheal stenosis.[45] Diagnosis and surgical management of tracheal stenosis remains a challenge. Success of any surgical procedure is predicted upon several elements—(1) Accurate topographic diagnosis of stricture(s), (2) Associated complicating factors, and (3) Appropriateness of the surgical philosophy in relation to the histopathology of induced changed.[45]

Tracheal stenosis caused by endotracheal intubation and/or tracheotomy can occur at any one or more of four predictable locations. (1) Strictures that occurred above the tracheotomy site were caused by a high tracheotomy, trauma to the anterior wall during tracheotomy, or intubation trauma. (2) At the level of the tracheotomy, inflammatory changes associated with infection, polyps or granulation tissue resulted in loss of cartilaginous support. (3) Granuloma formation or ulceration secondary to excessive cuff pressure below the tracheotomy site, while loss of cartilaginous support and circumferential stenosis were identified at the same level in the chronic stage of this disease. (4) At the tip of the endotracheal tube, excessive pressure against the anterior tracheal wall leads to granuloma formation and loss of cartilaginous support.

Diagnosis

Presentation of tracheal stenosis includes difficulty in extubation or decanulation, stridor (inspiratory and expiratory), atypical asthma, recurrent respiratory disease, poor weight gain and sometimes poor feeding.

Endoscopic evaluation with a rigid bronchoscope is the *most accurate* means of diagnosing tracheal stenosis and assessing its length, degree and character. The rigid bronchoscope can be placed above the stenosis while the smaller fibreoptic bronchoscope (1.9 mm outer diameter) is guided past the stenosis through the rigid bronchoscope. This arrangement allows for positive-pressure ventilation while one is examining the length and degree of distal stenosis.[46]

Associated aerodigestive anomalies such as laryngomalacia, laryngeal clefts, subglottic stenosis, tracheoesophageal fistula, hypoplastic and lung agenesis, severe gastroesophageal reflux, vascular compression when only complete tracheal rings are suspected or complete tracheal rings when only external vascular compression is noted.

Radiologic Evaluation

Lateral neck and the anteroposterior view under high kilovoltage with maximal inspiration and expiration is done. Fluoroscopy is useful in cases of suspected or proven tracheomalacia.

Barium esophagrams may show pharyngeal incoordination, vascular rings, pulmonary slings, occult tracheoesophageal fistulae and gastroesophageal reflux. Some advocate laryngotracheogram (using tantalum dust, Dionosil or suspension of 50% barium in isotonic Saline) to determine the length or thickness of the stenosis, its degree of airway occlusion, the distance between its upper edge and the free edge of the vocal cords or anterior commissure and determining the vocal cord fixation or paralysis. But there is a risk of life- threatening mucosal reaction to contrast material.

Airway fluoroscopy provides a dynamic view of the airway below the vocal cords to screen for isolated as well as synchronous lesions of the lower airway. They have a sensitivity of 80% for subglottic, 73 % for tracheal and 80% for bronchial sites of obstruction.[47] The main disadvantage is increased radiation exposure (10 rads).

Computed tomography and magnetic resonance imaging provide accurate evaluation of the airway. The contrast and spatial resolution of CT is superior to other cross-sectional imaging techniques such as MR imaging, and compares favorably to fibreoptic endoscopy.

Surgical Management of Tracheal Stenosis in Children

The surgical management of tracheal stenosis in children can be categorized as *endoscopic or open* techniques.

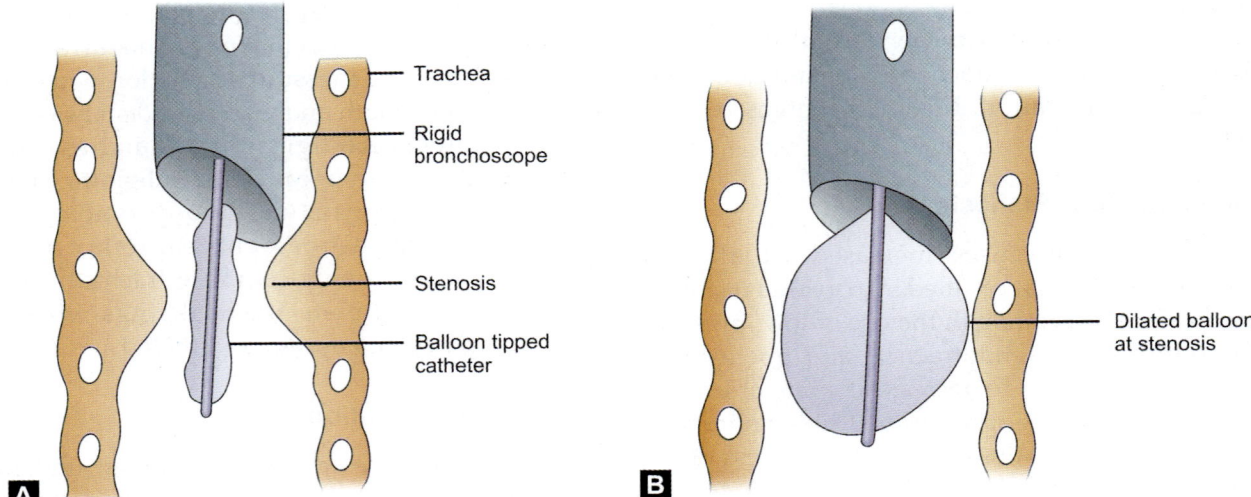

Figs 110.33A and B: Balloon dilatation of tracheal stenosis. Note that tip of rigid bronchoscope at the edge of stenosis prevent slipping of the balloon from the stenotic site

Endoscopic

Dilation by balloon or rigid dilators, laser vaporization of scar with or without intraluminal stent placement. Postoperative intraluminal granulation tissue can be controlled by endoscopic application of steroid or mitomycin-c.

Dilation

In cases of early, soft stenosis, before mature, firm stenosis has developed. Rigid dilation is done by *Jackson, maloney* or by red-rubber (rousch) rigid dilators. Balloon tracheoplasty is less traumatic (Figs 110.33A and B).

Laser Excision

Lesions most amenable are soft granulation and short segments of mature fibrosis. Laser excision of high grade stenosis sacrifices a significant amount of epithelium resulting in further contraction and restenosis of the airway. Preservation of the epithelial islands either by radial incisions and dilation or by elevation of mucosal flaps, followed by ablation of underlying fibrous tissue has been advocated for success. CO_2 laser, and KTP laser is used commonly for this purpose (Figs 110.34A to D).

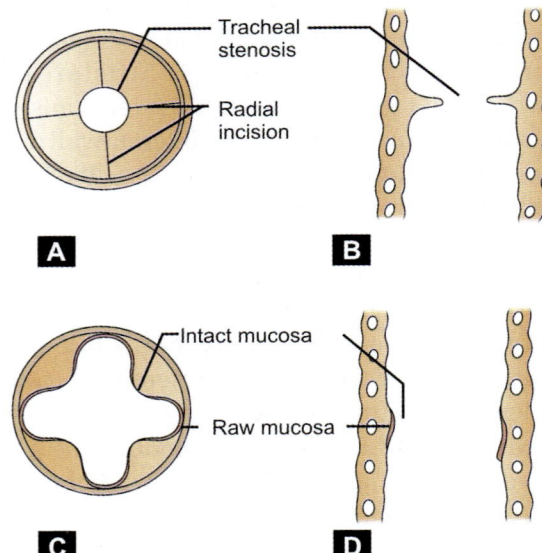

Figs 110.34A to D: A. Transverse section, showing stenosis and radial incision **B.** Sagittal section of trachea, **C** and **D.** Lumen of trachea after dilatation showing island of intact mucosa

Stents

For stenoses that are not suitable for segmental resection or expansion, in high surgical risks, after dilation of stenosis, or the likelihood of progression of the neoplastic stenosis. Generally airway stents can be subdivided into two categories – *metallic* and *silicone*. An important advantage of silicone stents is the relative ease of removal once no longer clinically necessary. Deaths have been reported during attempts at metallic stent removal.[48] Other problems associated with stents include obstruction, granulation tissue formation, infection malposition and perforation. In our Institute we use Montgomery silicone T-tube in pediatric age group.

A. *Open technique:* Various surgical techniques ranging from tracheoplasty to tracheal resection and reanastomosis can be used when conservative therapy fails or is deemed inappropriate.

B. *Tracheoplasty:* The common techniques are —1. Rib-cartilage tracheoplasty, 2. Pericardial tracheoplasty, 3. Tracheal autografts, 4. Slide tracheoplasty, and 5. Tracheal homografts.

Other materials proposed as augmentation patches for tracheoplasty are esophagus; solvent preserved dura, periosteum pulmonary homograft, aortic homograft cartilage from either chondral or auricular sources or omentum.

Rib Cartilage Tracheoplasty

Autologus cartilage derives its nutritional support though diffusion and can survive without a direct vascular supply. The approach to the trachea may be by cervical incision, thoracotomy or sternotomy, depending on site and extent of the stenosis. Physiologic gas exchange during tracheal reconstruction is maintained either by a previously placed tracheotomy or endotracheal intubation or by cardiopulmonary bypass. Rigid bronchoscopy is performed to identify the degree of stenosis and its proximal extent. After exposure of the trachea a 25 gauze needle is inserted in the midline of the anterior wall at the proximal end of the stenosis, guided by bronchoscopic visualization. A scalpel is used to open the anerior wall of the stenotic segment down through the distal end of the stenosis as identified by the bronchoscopic examination. The external appearance of the trachea can understimate the extent of the stenosis.[49] A segment of rib-cartilage is harvested from the sixth or seventh rib.[49] The perichondrium is preserved on the anterior surface of the rib graft and becomes the luminal surface of the airway. The graft is secured in place with interrupted stitches of nonabsorble monofilament suture. Care is taken to avoid exposure of any suture material to the lumen of the airway in an attempt to minimize the subsequent formation of granulation tissue. The endotracheal tube is again removed and repeat bronchoscopy is done to confirm the adequacy of the reconstruction and clear any retained secretions. The endotracheal tube is replaced, with the distal end of the tube positioned proximal to the distal end of the cartilage graft (Figs 110.35A to H).

During postoperative period, patient is kept under heavy sedation with the addition of muscle relaxants if necessary to minimize the motion of the endotracheal tube. Approximately 7-10 days after operation, the patient is returned to operation theatre for examination with rigid bronchoscope after removal of the endotracheal tube. If necessary, granulation tissue is removed. If the airway is believed to be stable and adequately healed, the patient is extubated. If the granulation tissue is believed to be excessive or if healing is judged inadequate, the endotracheal tube is replaced. This process is continued till extubation is successful.

Problems with cartilage (Rib) Tracheoplasty are granulation formation, difficult to achieve an airtight seal due to rigidity and displacement into the lumen.

Pericardial Patch Tracheoplasty

After a standard median sternotomy, pericardial patch is harvested from the diaphragmatic surface to the reflection of the pericardium at the great vessels. The patch is typically 4-6 cm in length and 2-3 cm in width. After cardiopulmonary bypass has been initiated an 11 blade is used to incise the trachea through the extent of the tracheal rings under bronchoscopic guidance. The pericardial patch is sutured in place using interrupted 6.0 vicryl suture. The suturing starts at the most inferior aspect of the incision adjacent to the carina and is carried superiorly. This helps to prevent collection of blood and secretions in the tracheobronchial tree clear. Then the endotracheal tube is reintroduced so that the tip of the tube is just above the carina. The endotracheal tube stents the patch open. Two small hemoclips are placed at the upper and lower aspects of the patch for radiographic identification of the patch location in the postoperative period. The patient is ventilated and weaned from cardiopulmonary bypass. Over the next week the patient is weaned from the ventilator and the patient is usually extubated 2-3 weeks following surgery (Figs 110.36A to C).

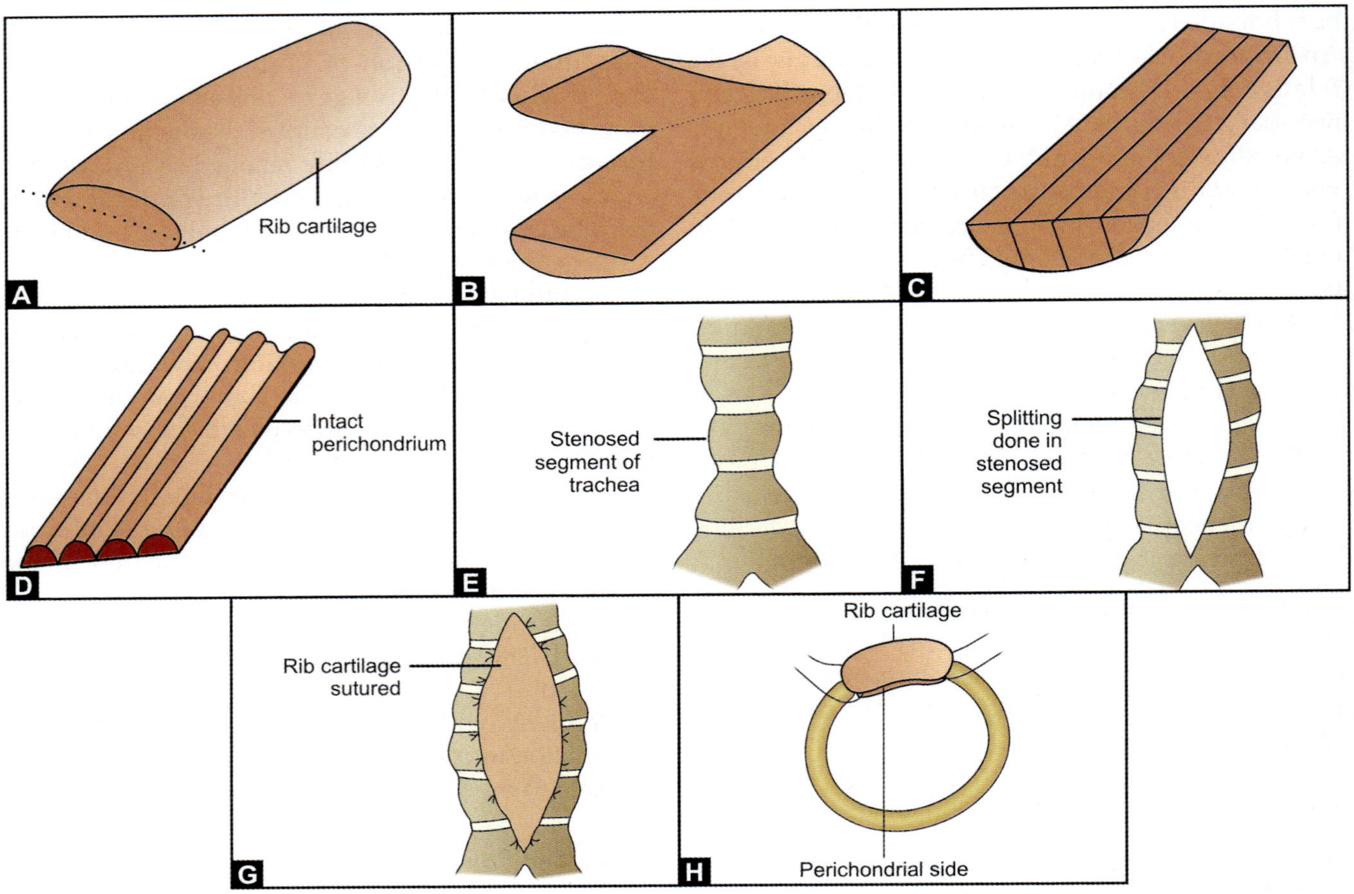

Figs 110.35A to H: A, B. The costal cartilage is longitudinally split, **C, D.** Longitudinal slits are made to obtain flexibility of the graft, **E to H.** Tracheoplasty in congenital tracheal stenosis using autologous rib cartilage

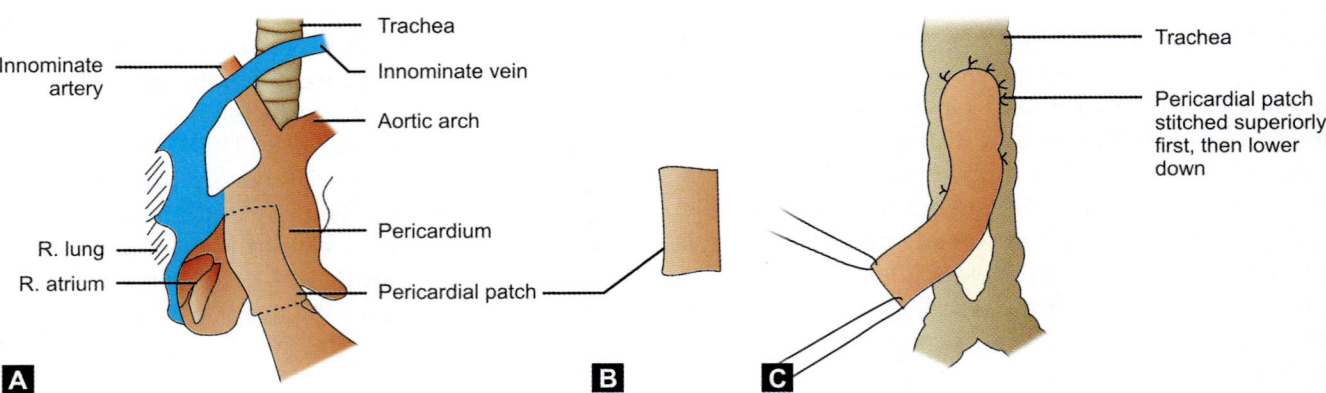

Figs 110.36A to C: A, B. Harvesting pericardial flap, **C.** Pericardial patch stiched over tracheal stenosis site

Advantages of pericardial tracheoplasty are; easy availability of pericardium, easy to obtain an airtight seal and its re-epithelialization with ciliated pseudostratified columnar epithelium. Mortality ranges from 17-47%. Long-term complications include prolonged hospital stay secondary to patch tracheomalacia, recurrent stenosis and exuberant granulation tissue particularly at the distal end of the trachea where the pericardial patch interfaced with the native trachea and carina.

Tracheal Autografts

The entire trachea is mobilized circumferentially. The anterior trachea is incised with a No. 11 blades through the extent of the complete tracheal rings. After this, an assessment is made as to how much trachea can be resected without causing excessive tension at the anastomosis. The excised midportion of the trachea is used as the free tracheal autograft. The two remaining ends of the trachea are anastomosed posteriorly with multiple 6.0 PDS suture, care being taken to keep the suture and knots out of the tracheal lumen. The corners of the harvested auto graft are trimmed and it is anchored in place with interrupted 6.0 PDS sutures (Figs 110.37A to C). If the tracheal auto graft is not sufficient, to augment the entire anterior opening in the trachea, then autologus pericardium is used to cover the remaining part (usually, i.e. superior part of the anterior tracheal opening). Tissell glue is used to seal the suture lines and the patch is checked for air leaks. Endotracheal tube is kept above the tracheal autograft for 7-10 days. Repeat bronchoscopy is done during this period, and during follow up for patency, and granulation tissue.

The advantages of tracheal autograft are— 1. The cartilage intrinsically maintains the tracheal contour, hence during postoperative period; endotracheal tube is kept above it. 2. Readily available. 3. Lined with respiratory epithelium and 4. Has potential for growth.

Complications reported with autograft are residual stenosis (21%), failure, granulation formation and operative mortality (7%).[50]

Slide Tracheoplasty

Long segment of stenosis is divided transversely in its midpoint, a vertical anterior incision made through the full length of the upper half of the stenotic segment and a corresponding vertical slit made posteriorly in the distal half of the divided stenotic segment (Figs 110.38A to D). The right angled corners where the

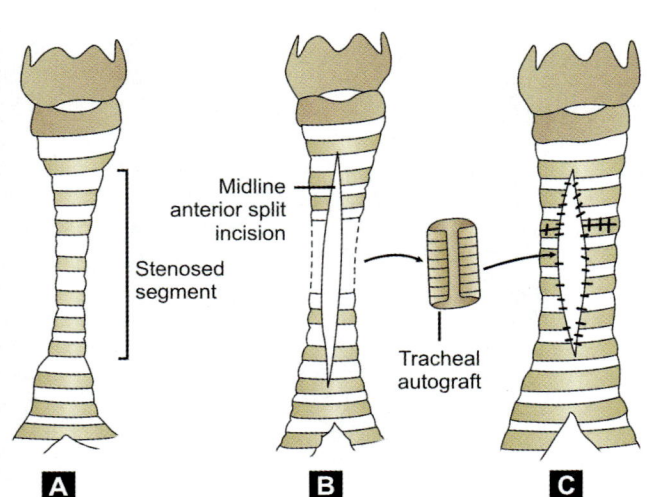

Figs 110.37A to C: Tracheal autograft: **A.** Congenital tracheal stenosis, **B.** Anterior trachea incised, throughout the extent of stenosis, and portion of stenosed trachea excised, **C.** End to end anastomosis with autologous tracheal autograft patch

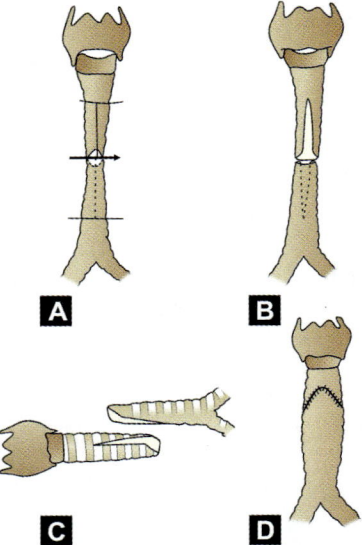

Figs 110.38A to D: Slide tracheoplasty: **A.** Trachea divided at the midpoint of the narrow segment, **B.** Tracheal ends were split longitudinally, **C.** Upper segment split anteriorly and lower segment split posteriorly, **D.** Reconstruction done with a wide lumen trachea

vertical incisions met the transverse incision were trimmed. The ends were slid together, doubling the circumference of the trachea. This resulted in a fourfold increase in cross-sectional area of the airway. The stenotic segment was shortened by half of its length. GrilloHC (1994) has modified it by incising the upper stenotic segment vertically posteriorly and the lower segment anteriorly for the full length of stenosis.[51]

Problems with slide tracheoplasty are exact identification of the midpoint of stenotic segment before the initial tracheal transection. After completion of sliding tracheoplasty the spring of the tracheal rings tends to form a *figure of the eight* contours in cross section in 9% cases.[52]

Tracheal Homograft

Cadaveric trachea is harvested, fixed in formalin, washed in thimerosal (methiolate) and stored in acetone. The stenosed tracheal segment is opened to widely patient segment proximally and distally. The anterior cartilage of the stenosed trachea is excised and the posterior trachealis muscle or tracheal wall remains. A temporary silicone rubber intraluminal Stent *(Dumon stent)* is placed and absorbable suture secure the homograft. Regular postoperative bronchoscopic treatment clears the granulation tissue. The stent is removed endoscopically after epithelialization over the homograft (Figs 110.39A to E). Advantages of tracheal homografts are nearly circumferential tissue for reconstruction, a carina that may be used for distal reconstruction and the procedure can be repeated if required. Ciliated columnar respiratory epithelium has been shown to cover the lumen of the homograft. However, growth potential is not known.

Presently, indications for tracheal homograft reconstruction are recurrent short segment upper tracheal stenosis and as a reserve for children in whom other alternative do not seem suitable.

Tracheal Resection and Reanastomosis

Indication for tracheal resection and reanastosmosis in children are– 1. Short segment (upto 30% of tracheal length).[52] 2. Presence of normal subglottic space. Some author feels that tracheal resection and anastomosis is the treatment of choice when feasible. Technically, the most important aspect of tracheal resection and anastomosis is providing a tension-free closure. Following endoscopy to outline the extent of the lesion, the dissection is kept to a minimum in order to

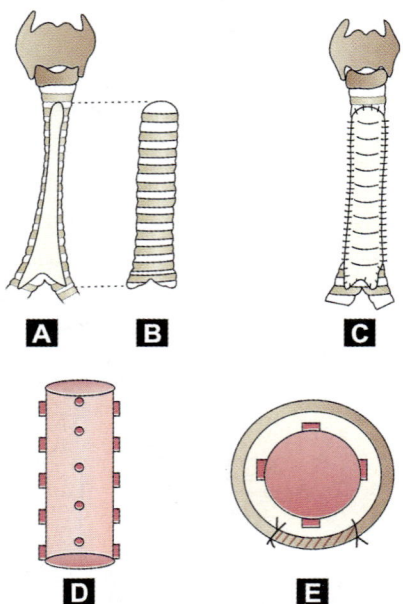

Figs 110.39A to E: A. The anterior part of trachea is removed leaving only the posterior tracheal wall and trachealis intact **B, C.** Homograft cut to size and sutured in place **D.** Dumon stent, **E.** Stent is placed to support the homograft internally until re-epithelialization has occurred

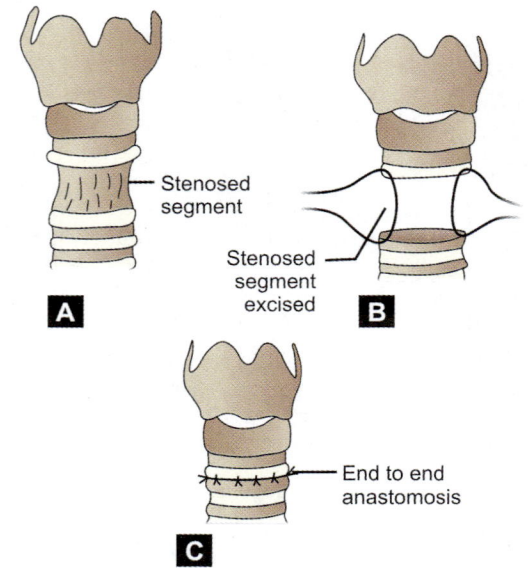

Figs 110.40A to C: Tracheal stenosis–resection and anastomosis

preserve the vascular supply to the trachea. It is crucial in dissecting around the trachea to dissect directly on the tracheal cartilage so as not to damage the recurrent laryngeal nerves. The head of the patient should flexed intraoperatively to help reduce tension during closure. Sutures (3-0 polyglactin, vicryl) are placed submucosally and tied extraluminally. In addition, four separate 2-0 polypropylene (prolene) sutures are interspersed along the anastomotic site to reduce tension on the anastomosis. It is important to maintain cervical flexion postoperatively, using a heavy suture extending from the chin to the chest. In children, sedation and, in some cases, neuromuscular paralysis is required for immobilization. After 24-48 hrs patients are weaned from the ventilator and extubated. Surveillance bronchoscopy is performed prior to extubation and prior to hospital discharge (Figs 110.40A to C). Results of tracheal resection and anastomosis are good.

REFERENCES

1. Fink BR. The brief history of ideas about the larynx in. The human larynx a functional study New York, Raven Pres, 1975;1-15.
2. Zaw – Tun HA, Burdi AR: Re-examination of the origin and early development of the human larynx, Acta Anat (Basel) 1985;122:163-84.
3. O'Rahilly R, Fabiola M. Respiratory and alimentary relations in staged human embryo (Chevalier Jackson Lecture). Ann Otol Rhinol Laryngol 1984;93(5):421-29.
4. Henick DH, Hoilger LD. Laryneal development in Holinger LD, Lusk RP, Green CG, (Eds): Pediatric laryngology and bronchoesophagolgy, Philadelphia Lippin Cott – Raven, 1997:1-17
5. Cote C, Todres ID. The pediatric airway in Ryan JF, et al. (Eds). A practice of anaesthesia for infants and children. Orlando, Grune and Stration 1985.
6. Pracy R. The infant larynx. J Laryngol Otol 1983;97:933-47.
7. Grillo HC. Reconstruction of the tracheal. Experience in 100 consecutive cases. Thorax 1973;28: 667-79.
8. Friedman EM: Evaluation of the child in respiratory distress in. Fried MP (ed). The larynx, a multidisciplinary approach, chapter -13 St Louis, Mosby 1996;137-41
9. Macdonald RE Fearon B. Innominate artery compression syndrome in children, Annals of Otology, Rhinology and Laryngology 1971;201:535-40.
10. Capitanio MA, Kirkpatrick JA. Nasopharyngeal lymphoid tissue Radiology 1970;96:389-91.
11. Zawin JK. Radiologic evaluation of the upper airway in Wetmore RF, Muntz HR and McGill TJ (eds): Pediatric otolaryngology Principles and practice pathways, Chapter –43, New York, Stuttgart.Theime 2000;689-736.
12. Strife JL. Upper airway and tracheal obstruction in infants and children; Radiol Clin North Am 1988;26:309-22.
13. John SD, Swischuk LE. Stridor and upper airway obstruction in infants and children. Radiographics 1992;12:625-43.
14. Zalzal GH. Strindor and airway compromise. Pediatr clin North Am 1989;36:1389-402.
15. Don McClurg FL, Evans DA: Laser laryngoplasty for laryngomalacia. Laryngoscope 1994;104;247-52.
16. Friedman EM, Vastola AP, McGill TJI, et al. chronic pediatric stridor, etiology and outcome. Laryngoscope 1990;100:277-80.
17. Fearon B, Eliss D. The management of long-term airway problems in infants and children. Ann Otol Rhinol Laryngol 1971;80;669-77.
18. Froechlich P, Seid AB, Denovelle F, et al. Disco-ordinate pharyngolaryngomalaria. Int J Pediatr Otorhinolaryngol 1997;39;9-18.
19. Dedo DD. Pediatric vocal cord paralysis, Laryngoscope 1979;89:1376-84.
20. Cohen SR, Birns JW, Geller KA, et al. Laryngeal paralysis in children a long term retrospective study. Ann Otol Rhinol Laryngol 1982;92:417-24.
21. Rosin DF, Handler SD, Potsic WP, et al. Vocal cord paralysis in children. Laryngoscope 1990;100:1174-79.
22. Grund fast KM, Harley E. Vocal cord paralysis, Otolaryngol clin North Am 1989;22:569.
23. Isaacson G, Moya F. Hereditary cogenital laryngeal abductor paralysis. Ann otol Rhinol Laryngol 1987;96: 701-04.
24. Hawkins DB, Clark RW. Flexible laryngoscopy in neonates, infants and young children. Ann otol Rhinol Laryngol 1987;96:81-85.
25. Gerber SE, Lynch CJ, Gibson WS. The acoustic characteristics of the cry of an infant with unilateral vocal cord paralysis. Int J Pediatr otorhinolaryngol 1987;13: 1-10.
26. De Gaudemar I, Rondaire M, Francois M, et al. Outcome of laryngeal paralysis in neonates: A long-term retrospective study of 113 cases, Int J Pediatr otorinolaryngol 1996;34; 101-10.
27. De Jong AL, kuppersmith RB, Sulek M, et al. Vocal cord paralysis in infants and children. Otolaryngologic clinics of North America 2000;33:131-49.
28. Cotton RT, Myer CM III, O'connor DM, et al. Pediatric laryngo tracheal reconstruction with cartilage grafts and endotracheal stenting. The single-stage approach. Laryngoscope 1995;105: 818-21.
29. Parnes SM, Satya Murtis S. Predictive value of laryngeal electromyography in patients with vocal cord paralysis of neunogenic origin. Laryngoscope 1985;95:1323- 26.
30. Cotton RT: Management of subglottic stenosis. Otolaryngologic clinics of North America 2000;33:111-30.
31. Holinger PH, Kutnick SL, Schild JA, et al. Subglottic stenosis in infants and children, Ann otol Rhinol Laryngol 1976;85:591-99.
32. Healy GB. An experimental model for the endoscopic correction of subglottic stenosis with clinical applications. Laryngoscope 1982;92;1103-15.

33. Zalzal GH, Cotton RT. Glottic and subglottic stenosis in Cummings CW, Fredrickson JM, Harker LA, et al (Eds). Otolaryngology head and neck surgery. Third ed, Vol 5, Chapter 18, St Louis, Mosby. 2000;303-24.
34. Ohlms LA, Jones DT, McGill TJ, et al. Interferon alfa-2α therapy for airway hemangioma. Ann Otol Rhinol Laryngol 1994;103:1-8.
35. Cotton RT. Pediatric laryngotracheal sterosis, J Pediatr surg 1984;19:699-704.
36. Zalzal GH. Rib cartilage graft for the treatment of posterior glottic and subglottic stenosis in children, Ann otol Rhinal Lanyngol 1988;97:506-11.
37. McQueen CT, Shapiro NL, Leighton S, et al. Single stage lanyngotracheal reconstruction. The Great Ormond Street experience and guidelines for patient selection. Arch Otolanyngol Head Neck Surg 1999;125:320-22.
38. Mitchell DB, Irwin BE, Bailey CM, et al. Cysts of the infant larynx, J Laryngol otol 1987;101:833-37.
39. Wiatrak BJ. Congenital Anomalies of the larynx and trachea, Otolaryngologic clinics of North America 2000;33:91-110.
40. Bejamin B, Inglis A. Minor congenital laryngeal clefts: Diagnosis and classification. Ann Otol Rhinol laryngol 1989;98:417-20.
41. Sie KC, McGill T, Healy GB. Subglottic hemangioma: Ten years experience with the carbondioxide laser. Ann Otol Rhinol Laryngol 1994;103:167-72.
42. Healy GB. Introduction to disorders of the upper airway in Wetmore RE, Muntz HR, McGill TJ, et al. (Eds) Pediatric otolaryngology, chapter 46 New York Thieme 2000; 763-74.
43. Healy GB and Cotter CS. Congenital disorders of the trachea in Cummings CW, Fredrickson JM, Harker LA, et al (Eds). Otolaryngology, Head and Neck Surgery 3rd edition vol –5 chapter 21 St. Louis Mosby. 1998;347-54
44. Cantrell JR, Guild HG. Congenital stenosis of the trachea. Am J Surg 1964;108:297-305.
45. Anand VK, Gilberto A, Warren ET. Surgical considerations in tracheal stenosis. Laryngoscope 1992;102:237-43.
46. Myer CM, Auringer ST, Wiatrak BJ, et al. Magnetic resonance imaging in the diagnosis of innominate artery compression of the trachea. Arch Otolaryngol Head Neck Surg 1990;116:314-16.
47. Rudman DT, Elmaraghy CA, Shiels WE, et al. The role of airway fluroscopy in the evaluation of stridor in children. Arch Otolaryngol Head Neck Surg 2003;129:305-309.
48. Filler RM, Forte V, Chait P. Tracheobronchial stenting for the treatment of airway obstruction. J Pediatr Surg 1998;33:304-11.
49. Jaquiss RDB, Lusk RP, Spray TL, et al. Repair of long-segment tracheal stenosis in infancy. J Thorac Cardiovasc Surg 1995;110:1504-12.
50. Backer CL, Mavroudis C, Dunham ME, et al. Intermediate term resutls of the free tracheal autograft for long segment congenital tracheal stenosis. J Pediatr Surg 2000;35: 813-19.
51. Grillo HC. Slide tracheoplasty for long-segment congenital tracheal stenosis. Ann Thorac Surg 1994;58:610-12.
52. Grillo HC, Wright CD, Vlahakes GJ, et al. Management of congenital tracheal stenosis by means of slide tracheosplasty or resection and reconstruction, with long-term follow-up of growth after slide tracheoplasty. J Thorac and Cardiovascular Surgery 2002;123:145-52.

CHAPTER 111

Orthopedic Problems in Children

Rajesh Malhotra

FEATURES OF THE PEDIATRIC MUSCULOSKELETAL SYSTEM

There are quite a few differences between the pediatric and the adult musculoskeletal system. The long bones in growing children contain the growth plate or the physis at both the ends, which contributes to longitudinal growth of the bone by the process of endochondral ossification (bone formation in preformed cartilage). The physis is an area of structural weakness and it often gets separated when injured.[1] Such epiphyseal/physeal injuries occur exclusively in the growing skeleton and can potentially cause disturbances of growth. Other disorders such as infections or tumors occurring in the vicinity of the physis may also compromise the longitudinal growth of the bone or may result in angular deformities.[2] Conversely, growth stimulation may occur in children following trauma (as in fracture shaft of femur or infection (growth stimulation due to hyperemia in the vicinity of growth plate).[3] The periosteum in children is loosely adherent to the bone in contrast to adults where it is densely adherent. Consequently, the pus originating in the medullary canal can travel to the surface of the bone through the Volkmann's canals and strip away the periosteum from the bone. This, coupled with the peculiar vascularity of the cortex in children where outer two thirds of the cortex is supplied by the periosteal vessels, results in avascularity of large segments of diaphyseal bone— the so-called "tubular sequestrum". Tumors from the medullary canal also can strip the periosteum and the triangular reactive bone formation at the corners where the periosteum is still attached to bone is called Codman's triangle.

The bones in children are porous as they are undergoing remodeling. These bones tolerate deformation better than the adult skeleton. Consequently children may have bent bones without fracture (Plastic deformation of bones), fracture of one cortex on the tension side when subjected to bending force (greenstick fracture) or buckling of the cortex when subjected to compression (Torus fracture).[4] The ligaments and capsular attachments are strong in children while physis or the porous bones are weak. Consequently, children sustain sprain of the ligaments or dislocation rarely, while the physeal injuries or avulsion injuries involving attachments of ligaments or musculotendinous structures are common.

Healing occurs rapidly in children and non-union is rare except in untreated avulsion fractures, displaced intra-articular fractures, fractures with inadequate bony contact due to soft tissue interposition, over-distraction (due to mal-treatment) or bone loss in compound fractures.

Malunion in children often corrects itself by remodeling.[5] Remodeling is most evident in children who are younger, when the deformity is close to the growth plate, when the plane of deformity is close to the growth plate and when the plane of deformity coincides with the plane of motion of the nearby joint. However, the remodeling does not correct rotatory malalignments and the abnormal tilt of the articular surface resulting from injury. The different regions of the pediatric bone have propensity for different pathologies. Infection has prediction for metaphysis. Other pathologies, which favor metaphysis, are simple bone cyst, osteochondroma and osteosarcoma. Epiphysis may be affected in chondroblastoma or the aneurysmal bone cyst while diaphysis is preferentially involved in Ewing's tumor.

CONGENITAL AND DEVELOPMENTAL CONDITIONS

Sprengel Shoulder

Scapula occupies a high cervical position in embryo. This is also evident by the nerve supply of the muscles acting on scapula (C3-5). During the development, the scapula descends down. Failure to descend results to a variety of abnormalities such as unilateral high scapula (sprengel shoulder) or Klippel-Feil syndrome where bilateral high scapulae are associated with fusion of cervical vertebrae and short neck.

Sprengel shoulder is the commonest congenital abnormality of the shoulder girdle (Fig. 111.1A). It is always associated with a fibrous or bony structure extending from supero-medial border of the scapula to the lower cervical vertebrae (Omovertebral Bar)[6] (Fig. 111.1B). The mild cases have no functional disability whereas severe cases may be associated with restriction of abduction at the shoulder joint.

Treatment of sprengel shoulder is done purely for cosmetic reasons.[7] Surgical treatment options range from extra periosteal resection of prominent supero medial border of the scapula with attached omovertebral bar to the repositioning of scapula inferiorly. Repositioning is a major undertaking and is reserved for patients with severe elevation of one scapula without wide spread congenital abnormalities.

The operation should not be delayed beyond the age of 5 or 6 years after which the secondary changes compromise the results.

Obstetric Birth Palsies

Brachial Plexus injury arising from obstetric injury to the newborn is the most important and serious injury. It commonly occurs in primigravida mothers with large babies after difficult deliveries. Fractures of clavicle and humerus may be associated. Most commonly the stretching of the brachial plexus is caused by an increase in the angle between the neck and the shoulder due to the forcible lateral flexion of the head to the opposite side. It is not uncommon for the upper limb to be completely paralyzed after birth. With passage of time, some muscles regain power and thereafter the arm assumes a characteristic deformity depending upon the resultant muscular imbalance. It is important to distinguish the traumatic brachial plexus neuropathy from osteomyelitis, septic arthritis or birth fractures as all these conditions can cause a pseudo paralysis of the extremity.

Erb-Duchenne Palsy (The Upper Arm Type)

It is the commonest palsy.[8] It is caused by excessive lateral traction on the emerging head at birth resulting in increased angle between head and shoulder. It involves 5th and 6th cervical nerve roots producing weakness of deltoid, biceps, brachialis and forearm supinators. As a result, the arm and forearm assume

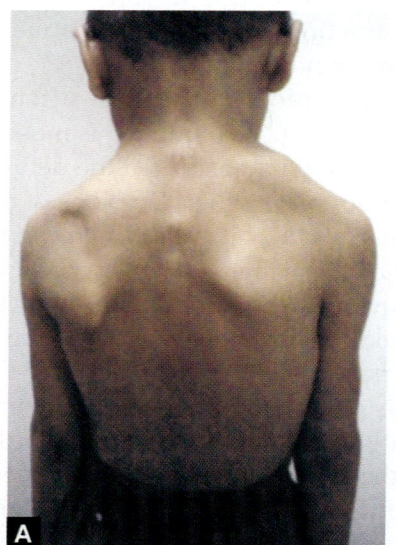 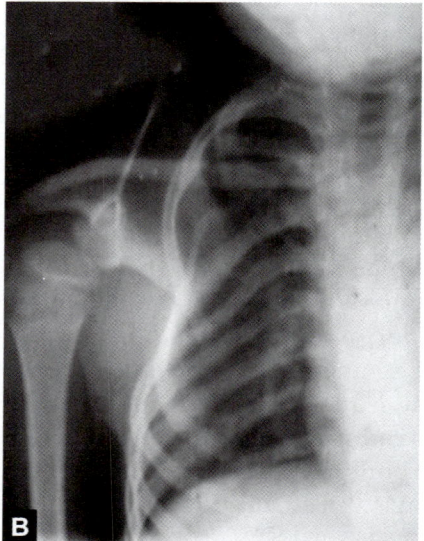

Figs 111.1A and B: **A.** Sprengel shoulder (Right) **B.** Skiagram of the same patient with right sprengel shoulder. Note the omovertebral bar

the characteristic posture of adduction and internal rotation at shoulder, pronation at forearm, extension at wrist and elbow and flexion of fingers (Policeman Accepting Tip).

There is usually a full range of painless motion at the shoulder. If there is no skeletal injury almost 20% cases recover completely. Adduction and internal rotation contracture develops in cases which do not improve and humeral head often subluxates posteriorly.

Treatment is expectant initially while waiting for recovery.[9] All joints of upper limb are moved through the full range atleast once a day to prevent stiffness. In refractory cases, exploration has no role, as the lesion is always a traction injury in continuity. Muscle transfers (L'Episcopo, Zachary) are described in these cases and the procedure essentially comprises of releasing latissimus dorsi and teres major (the deforming factors) and transferring them behind to the posterolateral aspect of proximal humerus where they serve as external rotators.[10]

In longstanding cases with complex secondary changes such as posterior subluxation of shoulder, external rotation osteotomy of the humerus can considerably improve function.

Klumpke's Palsy

Klumpke's paralysis affects the lower roots, C8 and T1. These patients have a flaccid hand with absence of grasp reflex in the involved extremity. The classic attitude of the limb reveals extension at the wrist and clawing of the fingers. Shoulder and the elbow are spared. Damage to the cervical sympathetic fibers may lead to Horner's syndrome. The prognosis in Klumpke's palsy is worse and it is often impossible to restore useful function.

Total Plexus Involvement

Involves all the roots of the plexus and the entire extremity is flaccid. The prognosis for recovery is very poor.

CONGENITAL AND DEVELOPMENTAL ABNORMALITIES OF THE CERVICAL SPINE

Klippel-Feil Syndrome (Brevicollis, Congenital Synostosis of the Cervical Vertebrae)

Klippel-Feil syndrome is the condition of congenital fusion of two or more cervical vertebrae caused by the failure of the normal segmentation of the cervical spine during the third to the eight weeks of gestation.

These patients have short neck, low posterior hairline, restriction of neck motion and frequently associated abnormalities such as scoliosis, genitourinary abnormalities, sprengel shoulder, deafness, ocular abnormalities, congenital heart disease and upper limb abnormalities (such as upper extremity hypoplasia, hypoplastic thumb, syndactyly, and supernumerary digits). Torticollis, facial asymmetry and webbing of neck (Pterygium colli) are also commonly associated with Klippel-Feil syndrome.[11]

Plain X-rays show vertebral synostosis with absent or hypoplastic disk spaces. Occipitalization of the atlas may be seen.

Treatment

Majority of these patients are asymptomatic. Patients are advised to avoid trauma to the cervical spine. When degenerative changes occur, conservative treatment is adequate for most patients. However, spinal fusion may have to be undertaken in selected unstable spines with spinal cord impingement. Treatment of cosmetic aspects of this deformity has met with limited success.

Torticollis (Congenital Muscular Torticollis, Congenital Wryneck)

This is the most common neck problem in childhood. It manifests in the first 6-8 weeks of life. The deformity is caused by the ischemia and contracture of the sternomastoid muscle ostensibly due to ischemia. Head is tilted to the involved side and the chin is rotated to the opposite side. A mass is usually palpable in the neck (sternomastoid tumor) within the first four weeks of life and usually disappears by four to six months. There is a preponderance of the right side involvement (in almost 85% cases). Congenital dislocation of the hip may be associated in 20% cases.

Clinically, the contracture of muscle is associated with typical deformity and reduced range of neck motion (Fig. 111.2). Contracted sternomastoid is prominent. Facial asymmetry (Plagiocephaly—flattening of the malar prominence and a lowering of the position of eye and ear on the involved side) is present in longstanding cases. The ipsilateral occiput is flattened. Mild dorsal compensatory scoliosis may be present.

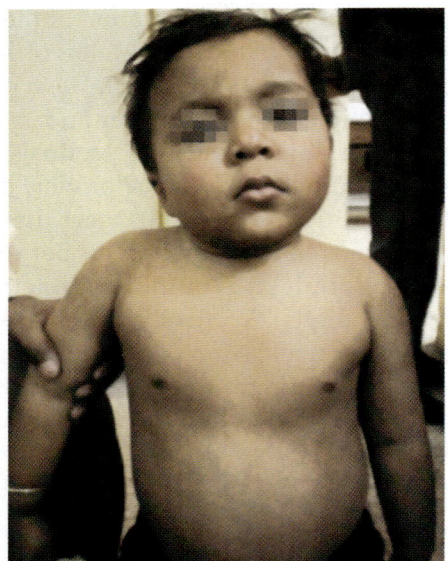

Fig. 111.2: Torticollis Right. Note that the chin is deviated to left and the occiput is rotated to right

Differential Diagnosis

Differential diagnosis includes congenital cervical spine abnormalities such as basilar impression, atlanto-occipital fusion, odontoid abnormalities, etc. Tuberculosis of cervical spine, fractures of the cervical spine, inflamed cervical lymph nodes, cervical disc prolapse, extraocular muscle imbalance and hysteria are the causes of acquired torticollis and must be differentiated from the congenital variety.

X-rays mare imperative to rule out bony causes of torticollis when suspected.

Treatment

The condition resolves spontaneously in about 90% patients within one year.[12] Surgery should be undertaken after 1 year if head tilt, facial asymmetry and restricted neck motion persist.

Surgery consists of release of clavicular head and Z-plasty of sternal head (for better cosmesis, to preserve 'V' of neck especially in female patients). Mastoid head may be released in older patients while bipolar release or Z-plasty may be indicated in longstanding deformity. Posterior auricular and spinal accessory nerves should be carefully protected during surgery at mastoid attachment.

Facial asymmetry and limitation of motion of more than 30° usually precludes good result. However, cosmesis can be expected to improve if surgery is done even as late as upto 12 years of age.

CONGENITAL CONDITIONS AFFECTING ELBOW

Congenital Radio-ulnar Synostosis

Is characterized by bony fusion/fibrous union between the proximal radius and ulna, placing forearm in pronated position. The synostosis may be limited to the proximal third of the radius and ulna (Fig. 111.3), or may be extensive.

The condition is often bilateral. It may be associated with the developmental dysplasia of the hip, clubfoot, chromosomal abnormalities or fetal alcohol syndrome (proximal radio-ulnar synostosis, bradydactyly and camptodactyly). Clinically the child presents with lack of the forearm rotations. Proximal dislocation of the radial head (anterior or posterior) may also be present.[13]

Treatment is difficult. Recurrences are common after surgery. Surgery should be considered if motion, function and potential growth of fused segments are interfered with. Osteotomies are performed through the fusion mass in younger children between the ages of 4 and 10 years for disabling pronation deformities. If bilateral, the dominant arm should be left pronated and the non-dominant arm is osteotomized distal to the fusion to achieve 20-30° of supination.

Congenital Absence of the Radius (CAR) (Radial Club Hand)

Is the most common long bone deficiency in the upper extremity. Disorders of the radial development lead to radial deviation of the hand, of males absent scaphoid and sometimes a hypoplastic thumb. Right hand is most commonly involved and the deformity is bilateral in 50% cases. Partial or complete absence

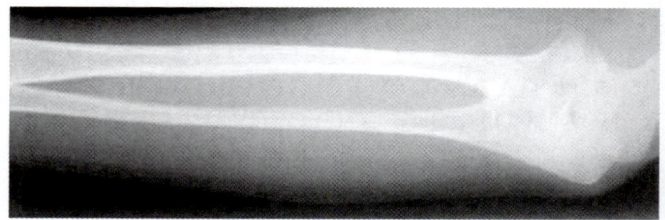

Fig. 111.3: Congenital radioulnar synostosis

of the radius, with or without adjacent hand deficiencies can be seen as an isolated finding or in association with several syndromes. Fanconi's syndrome and Vater syndrome should be considered when the radial dysplasia is bilateral. Fanconi's syndrome is an autosomal recessive disorder with pancytopenia, brown skin pigmentation, hip dislocation and aplastic thumb. The prognosis in these cases is poor.

VATER syndrome comprises of **v**ertebral anomalies, imperforate **a**nus, **t**racheo-**e**sophageal aplasia and **r**enal abnormalities. Other syndromes associated with CAR are thrombocytopenia (alongwith knee dysplasia), heart abnormalities (Holt-Oram-Lewis syndrome) and chromosomal abnormalities (trisomy 17). The terminal variety of CAR has absent radial ray and abnormalities of radial artery and median nerve; while the intercalary variety includes an absent radius with normal carpus and first ray.

The wrist in these patients is in radial deviation and flexion and the thumb may sometimes be rudimentary or absent (Fig. 111.4A).

Treatment consists of early splinting and passive stretching. Later, centralization of the distal wrist and hand over the ulna is performed[14] (Fig. 111.4B).

Pollicization is needed for the patient without a functional thumb. A stiff, nonfunctional elbow and associated medical problems are contraindications to the surgery.

CONGENITAL DISORDERS OF HAND

The cause of congenital hand disorders can be genetic (30%) or environmental (10%). However, almost in two third cases the cause is unknown. The congenital hand disorders can threaten the extremity (as in case of constriction bands), can cause tethering and disorders of growth (as in club hand), or can compromise appearance and function.

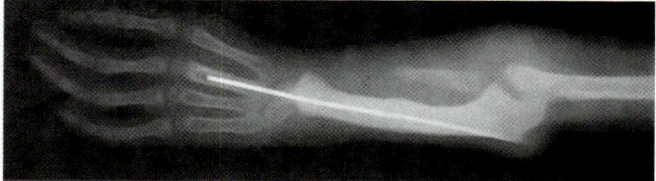

Fig. 111.4B: Congenital absence of radius treated by centralization of ulna

Syndactyly

It is one of the commonest congenital hand deformities. It involves ring and middle fingers most commonly. Syndactyly can be simple, involving only the skin or complex, involving the bones.[15] The fingers may be joined over the entire length of digits (complete) or over partial length (incomplete) (Fig. 111.5).

Syndactyly can be associated with several syndromes such as Apert's syndrome (syndactyly of all digits, mental retardation, skull and facial abnormalities), Poland syndrome and Streeter's dysplasia. Apert's syndrome is classically associated with acrosyndactyly (tips of the fingers are fused).

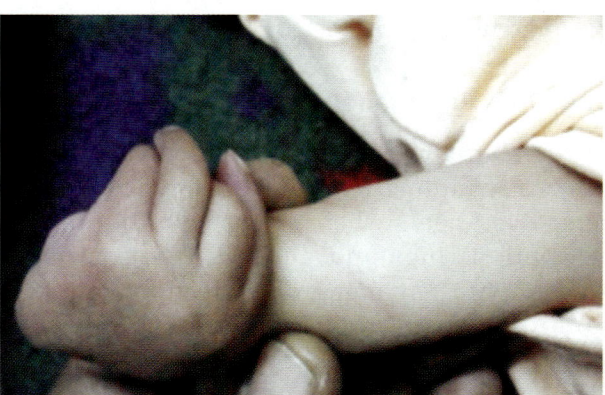

Fig. 111.4A: Congenital absence of radius. Note the absence of thumb

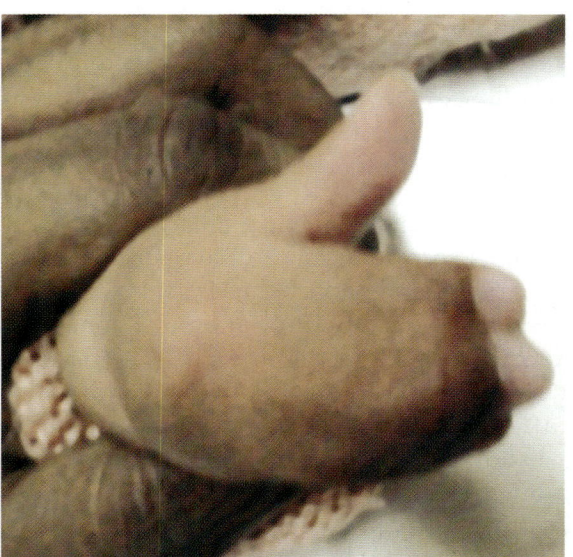

Fig. 111.5: Syndactyly affecting four ulnar digits of the right hand

Treatment is release, done between 18 months to 5 years of age. Skin grafting in usually required to cover areas of skin defect after release.

Polydactyly

Usually involves ulnar digits. It can be one of the three types:
a. Presence of only extra soft tissues;
b. Extra digit with its own bone, tendon and cartilage and
c. Complete with its own metacarpal. Polydactyly of thumb is usually associated with a generalised syndrome. The presence of a flail extra digit is treated by excision whereas the treatment of a separate digit is for cosmetic reasons.[16] The least developed digit is amputated; care must be taken to ligate neurovascular bundle and protect the ulnar collateral ligament.

Congenital Trigger Thumb

Congenital trigger thumb is caused by the stenosing tenosynovitis at A1 pulley. It presents with fixed flexion contracture of the thumb at birth and is often bilateral. It should be differentiated from the clasped thumb in which the flexion contracture is at IP as well as MCP joint of thumb and is caused by deficient extensors of the thumb. Trigger thumb can be left for one year when nearly 30% will resolve spontaneously. Splinting and passive stretching should be tried. Recalcitrant cases should be treated by surgical release of A1 pulley at the MCP joint.[17]

Macrodactyly

It is non-hereditary congenital enlargement of one or more digits corresponding to the distribution of one or more peripheral nerves; thus it is also called nerve oriented macrodactyly. It occurs most commonly in the territory of the median nerve. The enlargement affects distal part more than proximal and phalanges are affected more frequently than metacarpals (Fig. 111.6).

Joint stiffness is often present as is deviation of digits due to uneven overgrowth of the borders of the digits. Condition should be differentiated from cavernous hemangioma clinically (consistency and vascular examination) and radiologically. Treatment

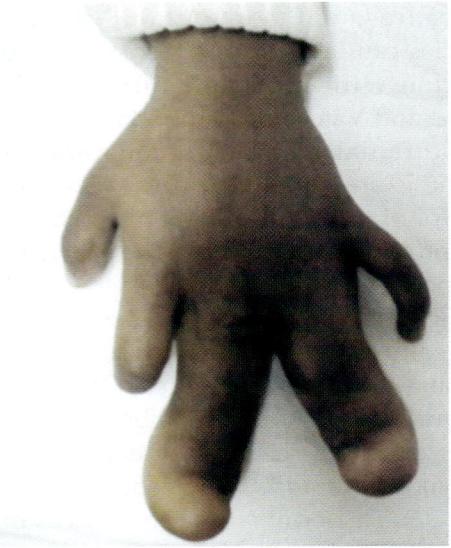

Fig. 111.6: Nerve oriented macrodactyly

is difficult and consists of reduction of the size of digit (osteotomies, defatting, epiphyseodesis) or amputation of the affected digit.[18]

Constriction Ring Syndrome (Streeter's Dysplasia)

It consists of congenital constriction ring/band affecting digits or more proximal part of limb. When severe these cause severe, lymphoedema or even amputation. Constriction rings are associated with club feet, syndactyly or acrosyndactyly (distal fusion of digits with cleft or separation proximally) and neurological abnormalities.[19] Treatment consists of early release of constriction rings with multiple, circumferential Z - plasties if the edema is gross.

Congenital Amputations

It can result either from failure of development or Streeter's syndrome. Amputations often involve only one or two fingers when associated with congenital constriction rings and good function is usually achieved with remaining digits. Amputation of the thumb, however, requires reconstruction with metacarpal lengthening, toe transfer or index finger pollicization. Complete absence of the hand in blind children is classically treated by a Krukenberg procedure, which involves creation of a radio-ulnar claw.

CONGENITAL AND DEVELOPMENTAL DISORDERS OF THORACOLUMBAR SPINE

Scoliosis

Scoliosis is an abnormal lateral curvature of the spine. It is a complex deformity with significant transverse and sagittal plane components.[20] The scoliosis can be classified into two main categories:

Non-structural

Non-structural or secondary scoliosis is caused by a number of conditions, which produce an apparent scoliosis without rotation of the vertebrae. There is no true, intrinsic spinal deformity in these cases. These conditions include poor posture, hysteria, limb length discrepancy, hip deformity spasm (sciatic scoliosis) and inflammatory conditions. Non-structural scoliosis is often mobile and disappears once the underlying disorder is treated.

Structural

Structural scoliosis is associated with rotation of the vertebrae, and is fixed. It is a true, intrinsic spinal deformity. Structural scoliosis can be further divided into various types depending on the etiology:

1. *Idiopathic* (without a primary cause) accounts for 85% of all cases. A genetic influence is strongly suggested in these cases. There is a female preponderance for curves (5:1) and a familial tendency. It is believed to be a sex-linked trait or autosomal dominant pattern with variable expressivity and incomplete penetrance.

    Idiopathic scoliosis is divided into three types depending on the age of the patient at the time of onset of scoliosis:
    a. Infantile (before 3 years of age)
    b. Juvenile (3 -10 years of age)
    c. Adolescent (from 10 years to skeletal maturity).
2. *Congenital:* Congenital scoliosis is caused by congenital bone malformation and the causes include diastematomyelia, hemivertebra, wedge vertebra, unilateral unsegmented bar, etc.
3. *Neuromuscular:* Neuromuscular or Paralytic scoliosis is caused by neuropathic causes (such as cerebral palsy, poliomyelitis, syringomyelia, spinal muscular atrophy, Fredrich's ataxia) or myopathic causes (such as arthrogryposis, muscular dystrophy).
4. *Neurofibromatosis*
5. *Mesenchymal disorders* such as Marfan's syndrome and Ehlers- Danlos syndrome.
6. *Trauma*
7. *Metabolic disorders* such as mucopolysaccharidosis
8. *Miscellaneous* (uncommon) causes such as bone dysplasias, extraspinal contractures, osteogenesis imperfecta, thoracic surgery, infections, tumors, etc.

Evaluation

Evaluation should establish the diagnosis assess the severity and allow the estimation of the potential for progression. These deformities are detected either incidentally on X-ray in early stages or are noticed by patient or the parents. History should provide information about the age of onset, progression and family history. Age at menarche is important for the female patients. History of pain is important as it points to an inflammatory or neoplastic cause for the scoliosis.

On physical examination, the initial screening should attempt to diagnose the constitutional disorders associated with scoliosis. The presence of café-an-lait spots suggests neurofibromatosis while body habitus in patients with Marfan's syndrome is characteristic. The patient presents with asymmetry in the level of the shoulders and waist crease. Scapula may be prominent on one side and inequality of breasts is present. The iliac crest is higher and more prominent on one side.

A rib hump is present posteriorly and it gets exaggerated on forward bending. The flexibility of the curve should be assessed by longitudinal traction and asking the patient to bend forwards. Balance of the spine should be assessed using a plumb line. Any paraspinal spasm or mass should be noted and tenderness over the spinous processes should be elicited. Leg length measurements should be taken for any discrepancy. A complete neurological examination should be performed in all cases.

Imaging

The radiographs of the spine (Lateral and AP views-errect and supine AP views in right and left bending positions) establish the extent, severity, rotation of vertebrae, presence of any bony abnormalities and

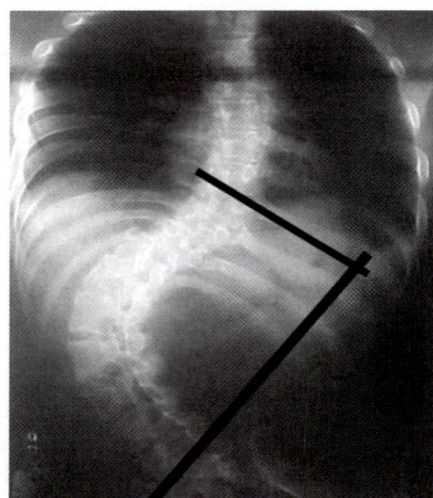

Fig. 111.7: Measurement of Cobb's angle

flexibility or correctability of the curve. Angle of the curve is measured by Cobb method (Fig. 111.7).

Mini Mehta's rib-vertebra angle difference is used to predict the progression of infantile idiopathic scoliosis (a difference of > 20° between the convex and concave sides is significant). Additional X-rays can be taken to establish the skeletal maturity or the skeletal growth remaining. Various methods used for the purpose are pelvis X-ray (Risser sign), ring apophysis of the vertebra and X-ray of the wrist for bone age.

Presence of certain danger signs (such as pain, left sided thoracic curve, stiffness and midline skin lesions) are indications for additional studies.

MRI may be indicated when spinal dysraphism, diastematomyelia, infection or tumor is suspected to be the cause of scoliosis.[21] Bone scan may be indicated in patients with stiffness and pain.

Pulmonary function test should be performed is all cases with curve measuring more than 60° to document decreased vital capacity.

The factors associated with poor prognosis are listed in Table 111.1.[22]

Treatment

The aims of treatment are to reduce the progression of curve, correct the curve and maintain the correction. Cosmesis is often the primary concern of the patient. Respiratory function usually does not improve after the surgery though the correction of the severe curve may check the deterioration of the respiratory function. Pain and neurologic problems are unusual and should be thoroughly investigated to rule out any intraspinal pathology. The following treatment modalities are commonly employed for the treatment of scoliosis.

Observation: A curve less than 20° in skeletally immature patients and less than 50° in mature patients is observed. Patients are asked to follow-up for clinical examination and radiographs every 4-6 months. If a curve in skeletally immature patient shows progression of more than 5°, these children are braced.

Exercises: Exercises are advised as an adjunct for the patients who are under observation or mature patients with less than 30° curve where the surgical treatment is not contemplated. Exercises are particularly useful for patients with obesity, back pain and exaggerated lumbar lordosis. Postural exercises, lateral bending and pelvic muscles exercises are commonly prescribed.

Orthosis: A curve more than 30° (but less than 45°) at the initial visit or more than 25° with documented progression in an immature patient is an indication for the brace treatment. The goal of brace treatment is to prevent progression of the curve. The spinal orthosis or brace is contoured to provide a corrective force to the spine while the child grows. Hence, the curve should be flexible and more than one year of skeletal growth should be remaining before the brace treatment can be instituted. Braces are not very effective for cervicothoracic curves. The following types of braces are commonly used:

i. *Milwaukee brace* or Cervico-Thoraco-Lumbo-Sacral Orthosis (CTLSO) is used for dorsal curves. It has adjustable supports made of steel and is distracted periodically. It has a chin support, which can cause deformation of teeth and malocclusion.[23] Hence careful supervision and orthodontic care is required. CTLSO is used in curves above D9 vertebra.

Table 111.1: Poor prognostic factors in scoliosis

- Female sex
- Onset before Menarche
- Positive family history
- Type of curve
  Severe curve
  Shorter curve
  Higher curve (e.g. Cervico-dorsal curves)
  Rigid curves

ii. *Boston brace* or Thoraco-Lumbo-Sacral Orthosis (TLSO) is used for thoraco-lumbar or lumbar curves. This type of brace has polypropylene shell, which is contoured to provide corrective force to the spine. It does not have the chin support. TLSO is used in curves below D9 vertebra. The braces are worn 23 hours a day till skeletal maturity and then are weaned off.

Contraindications to brace treatment are:
  a. Curve more than 40°
  b. Non-compliant patient
  c. Thoracic lordosis; and,
  d. Less than one year of growth remaining. Considerable guidance, direction and emotional support is required to the patient and family to ensure compliance with brace treatment.

iii. *Plaster:* Localiser casts are applied on special tables where head and pelvic traction reduce the curve. POP jacket is applied to maintain the correction.

Alternatively, hinged casts are applied with turnbuckle, which allows gradual correction of the deformity.

iv. *Electrical treatment:* Electrical stimulation of paraspinal muscles has been described to correct the scoliotic curve but has been shown to be less effective than brace treatment.

v. *Halo-Pelvic traction* is effected through adjustable steel rods fixed to the pelvis through a hoop with pins passing through the ilium and to skull using halo ring. Gradual distraction of these steel rods gradually corrects the curve.

vi. *Operative treatment:* Operative treatment is indicated for thoracic curves more than 40°, progressive curves and curves which fail the brace treatment. Curves, which are not cosmetically deforming especially when congenital, can be fused *in situ* when they show progression. Usually a posterior spinal fusion is done but when the posterior elements are deficient, anterior fusion using a rib graft can be done. The extent of fusion is decided by extent of the curve and must include neutral or non-rotated vertebrae on either end of the curve. Surgical stabilization often has to be supplemented with corrective instrumentation.

Various anterior (Zielke, Dwyer, Kaneda Anterior Spinal System-KASS) and posterior (Harrington, Luque, CD, Hartshill, Moss Miami) instrumentation systems are available to correct the scoliotic curves.[24] The newer instrumentation systems provide segmental fixation, which is more secure and derotate the curve to provide improved cosmetic results.

Spondylolysis and Spondylolisthesis

Spondylolysis implies a break in the pars interarticularis resulting in the loss of bony continuity between the superior and inferior articular processes. Condition occurs most commonly at L5 vertebra. Spondylolysis is believed to be the results of non-union of stress fracture. Spondylolysis is commonly seen in athletes who undergo hyperextension stress activities (gymnasts, football linemen). There is also high incidence among soldiers with heavy backpacks and Eskimos. Other causes of defect in the pars interarticularis are infection, trauma, tumor, congenital or developmental defects.

Spondylolysis can be asymptomatic or may present with activity related back pain in preadolescent or adolescent children.[25] Pain may radiate to buttock or thigh. Physical examination reveals spasm in paravertebral muscles and hamstrings and flattening of the lumbar lordosis. The neurological examination is usually normal.

Radiographs, (especially oblique views) are helpful in visualizing the pars defect, which is seen as a "*Collar*" (break) in the neck of "*Scotty dog*". Bone scan is extremely useful investigation for screening in a child with back pain before the plain radiographs show the bone defect. CT Scan can help in identifying the pars defect.

Treatment of spondylolysis is restriction of activities (especially hyperextension), stretching, abdominal strengthening and spinal flexion exercise and bracing for severely symptomatic patients. Severe unrelenting pain may need L5 - S1 fusion rarely.

Spondylolisthesis implies an anterior displacement of the vertebral column on a lower vertebra resulting from spondylolysis, articular process malformation or elongation of the pars interarticularis (Fig. 111.8). The condition is seen most commonly as anterior slippage of L5 vertebra over S1. Spondylolisthesis is classified, depending on etiology, into dysplastic, isthmic, degenerative, traumatic and pathologic. The severity of slip is graded according to the percentage of the superior anteroposterior extent of the vertebra below

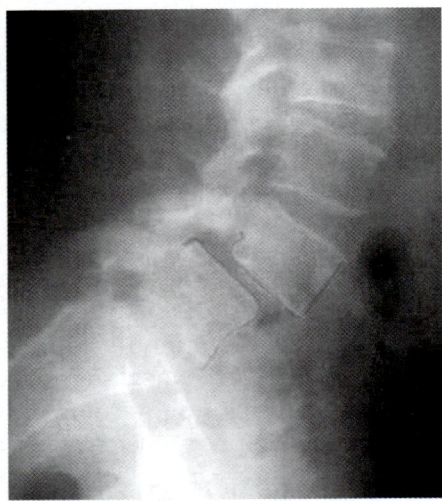

Fig. 111.8: Grade II spondylolisthesis L4-L5

by which the vertebral column has slipped forward; Grade I is 0-25% slip, Grade II is 25-50% slip, Grade III is 50-75% slip, Grade IV is 75-100% slip while grade V is > 100%, i.e. spondyloptosis when the vertebra above slips completely and comes to lie in front of the vertebral body below.

Spondylolisthesis occurs commonly around the adolescent spurt and progression occurs during 10-15 years of age (degenerative and pathologic varieties present late). Patients may be asymptomatic but low back pain or L5 radiculopathy may develop. A prolapsed intervertebral disc is commonly seen one level above the listhesis. Examination reveals restricted forward flexion of hips and back, hamstring tightness, flat buttocks (due to vertical sacrum) and lumbosacral kyphosis with compensatory hyper lordosis of lumbar spine. A pelvic waddle gait may be seen. Palpation of lumbosacral junction may reveal a step and an attempt to press spinous process from side to side elicits pain (due to loose lamina). Female patients may present with obstetric problems due to reduced anteroposterior dimensions of the pelvis.

Treatment

The goals of treatment are pain relief, return to activity and prevention of deformity. Grade I and II slips are treated with observation especially if they are asymptomatic. Symptomatic grade I and II slips are treated by restriction of activities, brace and physical therapy. Surgical treatment is required when patient is unresponsive to conservative treatment, shows progression of slip (especially in skeletally immature patient), when the patient has neurological deficit or when a severe degree of spondylolisthesis exists. Surgical treatment consists of *in situ* posterolateral fusion (from tip of transverse process to alae of sacrum—transalar fusion) from L4 to S1.[26] Decompressive procedures, such as laminectomy (for radiculopathy or cauda equina), or Gill's procedure (removal of loose lamina) are required for neurological deficit. Gill's procedure (operculectomy) alone is contra indicated in children as it can lead to rapid worsening of the slip. Decompression in adults is combined with posterolateral fusion or pedicular screws and segmental fixation. The availability of modern instrumentation has made it possible even to reduce the slip and fix it in the reduced position. Surgical fusion should always be combined in these cases to control pain and progression.

CONGENITAL AND DEVELOPMENTAL DISORDERS OF THE HIP

Developmental Dysplasia of Hip (DDH)

The term DDH is used to include dysplasia without subluxation, subluxatable hip and the dislocated hip. This spectrum has been identified because of the fact that a hip normal at birth may become dysplastic in early months of life. Congenital dislocation of hip may be teratologic (occurs at 12-18 weeks of intrauterine life) or typical (occurs in perinatal period). Teratologic dislocations are characterized by severe deformity of both the acetabulum and proximal femur.

Incidence of congenital dislocation is 4-10 per 1000 live births with considerable racial variation. DDH is more commonly associated with intrauterine crowding (other uterine packing problems such as metatarsus adductus, torticollis and calcaneovalgus are commonly associated), breech presentation (10× higher incidence), hyperextension at knees, oligohydramnios, twins and ligamentous laxity.[27] Genetic predisposition is known and the disease often has a familial pattern (Polygenic inheritance with 10% incidence in cases with positive family history). Postnatal factors are also involved in causation especially when infants are carried in a position of extension and adduction at the hips or in a cradle board.

Almost 60% of cases of congenital dislocation of hip (CDH) are first born and it affects females more frequently than males (6:1). The left hip is more commonly affected (60%) while 20% cases are bilateral.

CDH is often associated with diseases like Ehlers-Danlos syndrome, Larsen's syndrome, myelomeningocele, arthrogryposis, etc.

Pathology

CDH is characterized by marked laxity of hip joint capsule. Acetabulum is often shallow and maldirected. The proximal femur has a small ossific nucleus, which appears late. There is excessive proximal femoral anteversion and coxa valga. Labrum is inverted into the joint. The capsule may have an hourglass constriction often caused by a tight iliopsoas tendon traversing the front of the hip joint. Ligamentum teres is hypertrophied. The hip joint is filled with pulvinar, the hypertrophic fibrofatty tissue.

Diagnosis

Every newborn should be screened for signs of hip instability. CDH is diagnosed most commonly in infants by positive *Barlow test* and *Ortolani's test*.

Barlow's Test

It is a provocative test to detect a dislocatable or subluxatable hip. Adduction and axial loading (or depression) of the femur dislocates the hip.

Ortolani's Test

It is a reduction maneuver for a dislocated hip in a newborn. Elevation and abduction of the femur relocate the hip, often with an audible or palpable "clunk". The signs of DDH change with the infant's age. In a child older than 2 months of age, the best test is demonstration of reduced abduction (less than 60°), especially with hips flexed as the *Barlow and Ortolani's tests* may no longer be positive. In older children, there may be asymmetry of the gluteal, inguinal and thigh skin folds. Bilateral dislocations usually are associated with widened perineum. The limb is shortened and externally rotated. The greater trochanter on the affected side is higher. With the knees and hips flexed and feet together, the knee on the affected side is lower (*Galeazzi sign*). Telescoping is strongly positive.

When the child presents after walking, limp is the main complaint. Trendelenberg test is positive.

Radiographic Examination

Ultrasonography of hip should be obtained in infants with suspected CDH, as it is the most sensitive investigation in the newborn.[28]

Plain X-rays are useful in children over 3 months of age. The radiological features seen on plain radiographs are shown in Figure 111.9.
1. Delayed appearance of femoral ossific nucleus on the affected (left) side. (Normally appears by 6-12 months. Compare with opposite side).
2. Lateral and superior migration of proximal femur
3. Shenton's line is broken
4. Increased acetabular slope (Acetabular index > 40°).

Arthrography is useful in diagnosing mechanical blocks to reduction and in confirming shape and congruence of femoral head and the acetabulum. It can also be used post operatively for evaluation of the adequacy of reduction.

CT Scan is useful after ossification of femoral ossific nucleus, in children older than 6 months of age. Its real usefulness, however, remains in documenting concentric reduction when the patient is in a plaster cast.

MRI is now becoming popular as the investigation of choice before 6 months age when the proximal femoral ossific nucleus is still cartilaginous. It is useful to

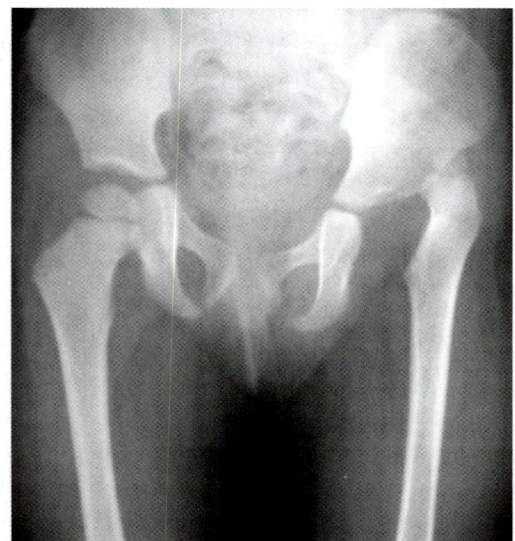

Fig. 111.9: Plain X-ray features of CDH

diagnose CDH as well as to confirm concentricity of reduction during treatment.

Treatment

The management of CDH is challenging.

The principle of treatment of dysplastic hip is to obtain and/or maintain reduction to allow for normal development and it should be achieved as early as possible. Treatment of CDH is categorised according to the age of presentation.

Birth to 3 Months of Age

Instability in neonatal period often resolves spontaneously persistent instability is treated by gentle manipulation and reduction. The reduction is maintained in a Pavlik harness or *von Rosen* splint. Splintage should be continued for duration of twice the age of infant with a minimum of 2 months.[29]

Three Months to Eighteen Months of Age

Children with CDH in this age group are initially treated conservatively. Traction may be continued at home to overcome hip contractures.

Closed reduction under anesthesia with adductor tenotomy if necessary and spice cast is the treatment of choice. Hip spica cast is applied in 110° flexion and *safe zone abduction* (30-60°) and 10-20° internal rotation. The spica cast is kept for 6 months. A single cut CT scan may be done to confirm reduction where plain radiographs look doubtful. Occasionally open reduction may be necessary in a child older than one year if closed reduction fails or when extreme positioning is required to maintain reduction, thus subjecting the femoral head to the risk of avascular necrosis.

Eighteen Months to Three Years

Operative treatment is usually necessary in this age group. Pelvic osteotomy is often performed at the same time to correct acetabular dysplasia. Open reduction, usually by anterolateral approach is required. Femoral varus derotation osteotomy may sometimes have to be done in cases with excessive femoral anteversion.[30] Postoperatively patient is kept in spica cast for 6 -12 weeks followed by abduction splint for 6-12 weeks.

Between 3 to 6 Years of Age

Children in this age group need open reduction along with an acetabular osteotomy to improve shape of the acetabular and/or coverage of the femoral head as the capacity for acetabular remodeling is diminished by this time. After 4 years of age, acetabular osteotomy is preferred to femoral osteotomy. Figure 111.10 shows the neurovascular structures to be considered while performing an acetabular osteotomy.

Most commonly performed acetabular osteotomy is Salter's osteotomy which is useful for mild to moderate acetabular dysplasia. Salter's osteotomy improves anterior (20-30°) and lateral (10-15°) coverage. Other pelvic osteotomies performed for CDH are Pemberton osteotomy, Steele (triple innominate) osteotomy, Sutherland (double innominate) osteotomy, Wagner (dial) osteotomy and Ganz osteotomy. Figures 111.11A and B show the relationship of neurovascular structures to the sites of Salter, Pemberton, Chiari and anterior Iliac (done for exstrophy of bladder) osteotomies.

In older children (above 5 years) with bilateral CDH, no surgical treatment should be attempted in view of poor results. Unilateral cases, however, can be salvaged with Chiari osteotomy or acetabular augmentation by shelf procedure (Staheli) (Fig. 111.12).

CONGENITAL AND DEVELOPMENTAL ANOMALIES OF THE KNEE

Bow Legs and Genu Varum

Normally infants have symmetric bowing of the legs which starts changing to genu valgum or knock knees after the age of 1.5 years and evolves completely into knock knees by 2.5 years. The valgus then gradually reduces to physiological valgus by 4 years.

Thus, genu varum in children less than 2 years of age is physiological and needs no treatment.

Pathological conditions, which can cause genu varum and/or bow legs include internal tibial torsion, osteogenesis imperfecta, rickets, trauma, osteochondromas and Blount's disease.

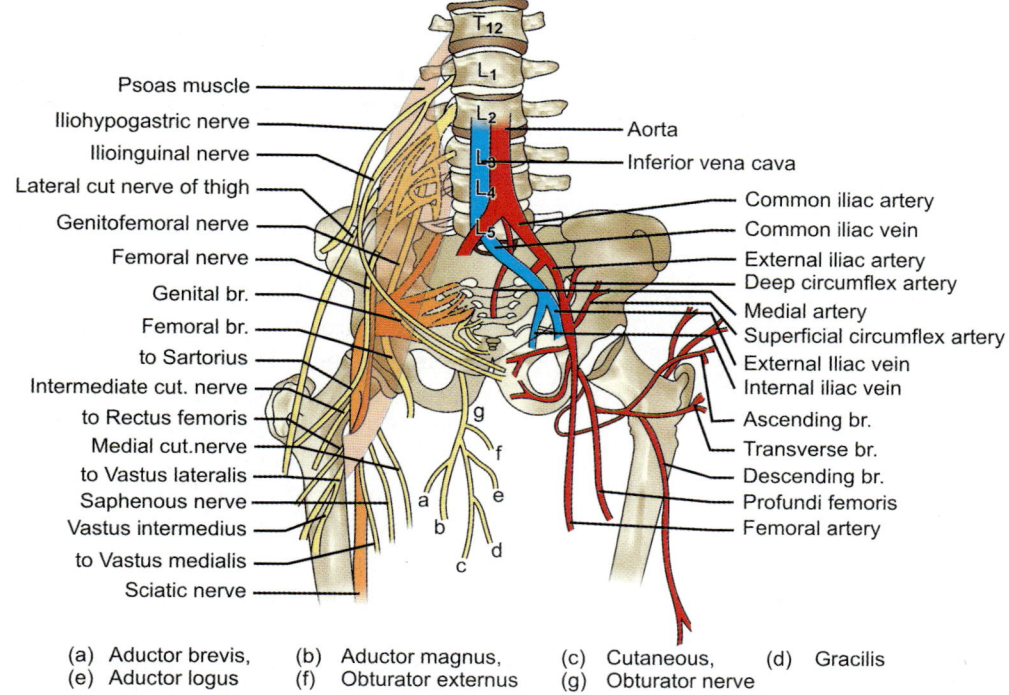

Fig. 111.10: Important structures to be considered while doing pelvic osteotomies

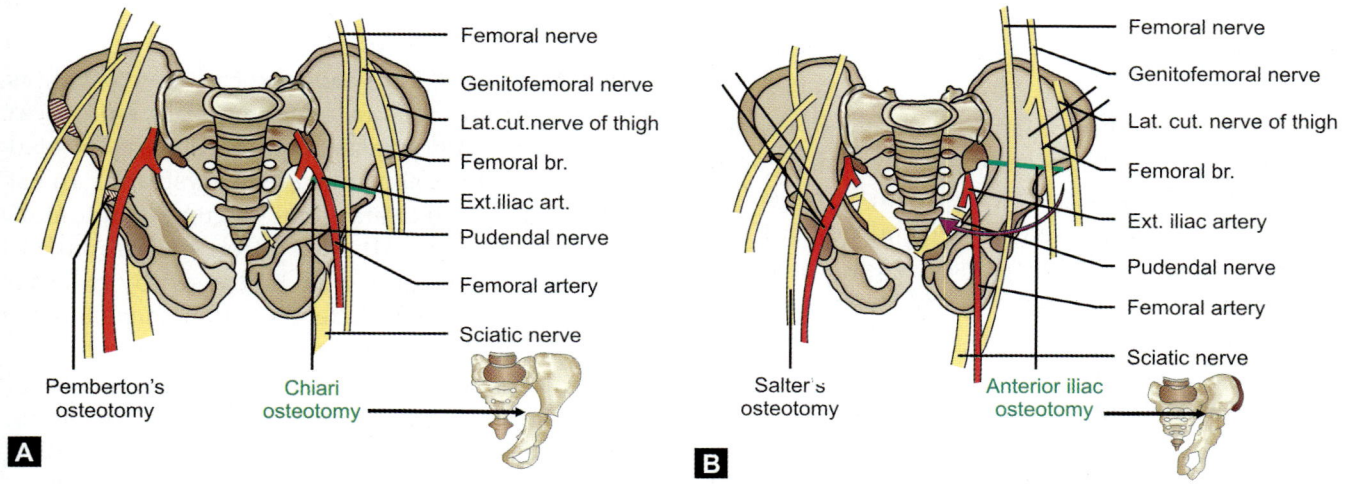

Figs 111.11A and B: Some commonly performed pelvic osteotomies and important structures to be considered

Internal Tibial Torsion

Internal tibial torsion leads to apparent bow legs or genu varum when the child walks with the knees forward and the feet rotated externally. Examination reveals internal tibial torsion. Most cases resolve by 4 years of age. Apparent bow leg deformity disappears with resolution of tibial torsion.

Blount's Disease (Tibia Vara)

Is a disease of unknown etiology that causes progressive bowing of the leg due to a disorder of the posteromedial tibial physis. It is particularly common in blacks and hispanic, obese male children. The disease can occur as early as 2-3 years of age. The disorder can be unilateral (in adolescents; less severe

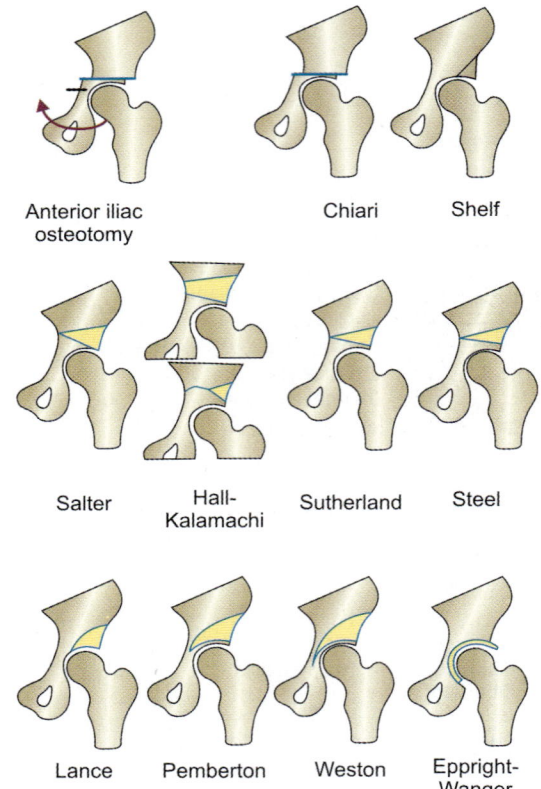

Fig. 111.12: Various types of acetabular osteotomies performed for congenital hip dysplasia and exstrophy of the bladder

variety) or bilateral (in infants; more severe variety). Diagnosis is based on radiographs which show decreased medial tibial physeal growth with resultant metaphyseal-diaphyseal angle abnormality.[31] Drennan's metaphyseal-diaphyseal angle is measured between a line joining metaphyseal beaks and a line perpendicular to the long axis of the tibia. An angle more than 11° is abnormal.

Later on, radiographs show distortion of medial articular surface and fusion of the physis. A progressive angular deformity develops as the lateral growth plate continues growing while the medial side is tethered. The characteristic defect on the posteromedial part of tibial articular surface is best shown by *Siffert-katz* sign (rocking in flexion of knee) and also on arthrography.

Treatment of Blount's disease is based on the age and stage of the disease. Mild cases may spontaneously improve. Severe cases need tibial osteotomy to realign the extremity and reduce the load on medial tibial plateau.[32] Osteotomy can be performed in the metaphyseal areas of tibia, intraepiphysealy or at both the sites.[33] Physisplasty and cartilage autografting are the latest techniques being used.

Rickets

It may lead to bow legs due to development of soft bones, which bow with the load of weight bearing.

Children with hypophosphatemic rickets (x-linked dominant) are often short and have bilateral symmetric bowing of legs. Treatment is with phosphates and massive doses of vitamin D supplements but it has little effect on bowing. Surgical correction may be required if the bowing is severe.

Treatment of Genu Varum is reassurance in cases with physiological genu varum. Other cases should be investigated for underlying pathology. Bracing (*Mermaid Splints*) was tried in the past but has been given up now. Surgical treatment is needed if the intercondylar distance at the knee is more than 8 cm. A tibial osteotomy below the tibial tubercle with removal of lateral based wedge and fibular osteotomy is the procedure performed.

Genu Valgum

Children between 2-6 years age can have a valgus angle of up to 15° as a normal physiological phenomenon. Pathological genu valgum is associated with trauma, infection, renal osteodystrophy (most common cause of bilateral genu valgum), and tumors (osteochondromas). It may often be idiopathic. Apparent genu valgum may be caused by external tibial torsion though the latter condition is uncommon. Genu valgum, if severe, may be associated with recurrent dislocations of patella (due to increased Quadriceps - "Q" angle - formed between a line joining ASIS to middle of patella and another line joining middle of patella to tibial tuberosity) and flat foot.

Conservative treatment with shoe wedges (mermaid) splints and braces is ineffective. Surgery should be considered if the tibiofemoral angle (angle between the long axis of tibia and the long axis of femur) is more than 15-20° or the inter-malleolar distance is more than 10 cm. Hemiepiphysiodesis or stapling of medial epiphysis can be done for severe deformities before completion of growth. A supracondylar medial close wedge femoral osteotomy can be done at any age to correct the deformity. Care should be taken to avoid injury to common peroneal nerve by stretching while correcting severe genu valgum deformities.

Bowing of Tibia can be of Three Types

Posteromedial

It is commonly associated with calcaneovalgus foot as both arise from abnormal uterine positioning. Spontaneous correction is the rule and tibial osteotomy is not indicated.

Anteromedial Bowing

It is typically caused by congenital absence of fibula with or without the absence of lateral rays. It is the most common congenital skeletal deformity in the leg. It is commonly associated with ankle instability, equino-varus foot, tarsal coalition and femoral shortening. Significant limb length discrepancy (LLD) is commonly associated with this disorder. A Syme's amputation is often performed in these cases in view of severe LLD.

Anterolateral Bowing of Tibia

Commonest cause of anterolateral bowing is the congenital pseudarthrosis of the tibia. About 50% patients have associated neurofibromatosis.[34] Dysplasia, sclerosis and cystic changes are seen in the tibia. Ipsilateral fibula is also commonly affected. Congenital pseudarthrosis is classified into 6 types of Boyd.

Boyd Classification of Congenital Pseudarthrosis of Tibia:

- *Type I:* Anterior bowing and defect in tibia.
- *Type II:* Anterior bowing and hourglass constriction of tibia. Fracture develops before 2 years of age.
- *Type III:* Intraosseous cyst gives rise to fracture which occasionally is seen at birth.
- *Type IV:* Sclerotic bone leads to stress fracture.
- *Type V:* Associated with dysplastic fibula.
- *Type VI:* Intraosseous neurofibroma/schwannoma.

Clinical Features

- Anterolateral bowing of the tibia ± fibula
- Patient presents with pseudarthrosis usually by 2 years of age (sometimes at birth)

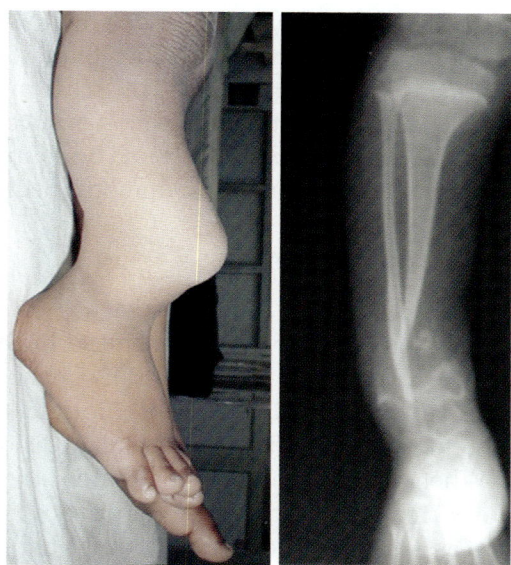

Fig. 111.13: Clinical and radiological features of Type V congenital pseudarthrosis of tibia

- Limb length discrepancy (sometimes marked)
- Varus deformity of the ankle
- Characteristic location of the pseudarthrosis is at the junction of middle and lower thirds of the leg (Fig. 111.13).

All children with any variety of this disorder need treatment. If anterolateral bowing is present without fracture, protective bracing is indicated. Corrective osteotomy of anterolateral bowing should not be done because it often leads to pseudarthrosis. McFarland posterior bypass grafting may be used in high risk patients (Sclerotic bone, hourglass constriction of tibia).

Prognosis is worse in children with a fracture at a younger age, especially before 3 years. The tendency to fractures decreases with age. If the first tibial fracture occurs at or after 8 years of age, it may heal following plaster immobilization with or without bone grafting. Principles of treatment of pseudarthrosis of tibia are excision of pseudarthrosis, correction of deformity and rigid internal fixation. Autogenous bone grafting is often added to the osteosynthesis. The various procedures used include McFarland bypass grafting; Boyd's double onlay graft, fragmentation and IM nailing and, IM nail with onlay graft.[35] Vascularized fibular graft (on pedicle or free) and Ilizarov methods have been used with some success in the treatment of pseudarthrosis. However, repeated failed attempts at reconstruction and/or marked (more than 18 cms) limb length discrepancy are indications for amputation. Surgical treatment is not often successful in this condition and the parents should be counselled about the ultimate need for an amputation if necessary.

Congenital and Habitual Dislocation of Patella

Congenitally dislocated patella presents at birth. The primary defect lies in the vastus lateralis (muscle and fascia), vastus intermedius and the iliotibial band. These structures are contracted and result in dislocated patella. When the patella stays dislocated, the knee does not extend from the flexed position.[36] The treatment is surgical release of iliotibial band and lateral retinaculum, mobilisation and recession of vastus lateralis from patella along with excision of any fibrotic bands in vastus lateralis or intermedius. Vastus medialis is transferred distally and laterally.

Habitual dislocation of patella is a condition where patella dislocates every time the knee is flexed and reduces with extension. Patients often present with a clicking sensation on flexion and extension of the knee. The child may keep the knee flexed and patella permanently dislocated because of the pain.

Palpation of the patella, which is displaced laterally, clinches the diagnosis. An ossified patella in an older child makes the diagnosis straightforward on X-ray of the knee. In cases with severe tightness, the tibia may be subluxated laterally on X-rays.

Treatment is release of the tight lateral structures and proximal realignment of the extensor apparatus by distal and lateral advancement of vastus medialis muscle. Other procedures, which can be performed in a skeletally immature patient, are Campbell's procedure (lateral retinacular release along with a medial capsular flap which is passed around the quadriceps tendon to pull it medially. The flap is then sutured upon itself), Galeazzi procedure (semitendinosus tendon is used to pull the patella and patellar tendon medially), and Roux-Goldthwait procedure (lateral half of patellar tendon is detached and reattached medial to the medial half).[37] In a skeletally mature patient with an increased Q angle, distal realignment procedures (such as Hauser's procedure-osteotomy of the tibial tuberosity and its transfer distally and medially) with or without proximal realignment procedures should be done.

Congenital Dislocation and Subluxation of the Knee

The spectrum of congenital dislocation and subluxation of knee includes, in the order of increasing severity, congenital hyperextension, congenital subluxation and congenital dislocation.[38]

Hyperextension is frequently normally present at birth in breech babies but may also be present along with subluxation and dislocation.

Subluxation is more common than dislocation. Difference from dislocation can be appreciated on X-rays. The subluxated knee may have up to 20-40° of flexion. The prognosis is better than congenital dislocation.

Congenital dislocation is characterized by anterior displacement of tibia on femur with complete loss of contact between the two. The tibia is usually internally rotated and often laterally displaced. Associated congenital anomalies may be present in 60% of patients with congenital dislocation of the knee. Children with arthrogryposis multiplex congenita often have associated dislocation of knee.

Children with congenital hyperextension/dislocation of knee should be thoroughly evaluated for congenital dislocation of hip.

Treatment of hyperextension and subluxation should begin soon after birth and consists of manipulation (passive flexion of knee) followed by plaster cast. Casts are changed every week till 90° flexion is achieved. Splintage is continued after that to prevent recurrences.

Dislocated knee is treated by open reduction and release of contracted quadriceps and its lengthening by V-Y plasty. Anterior capsule is released and collateral ligaments are freed if required. The knee is reduced and flexed to 90° and immobilised.[39]

Prognosis of knee dislocations, which need open reduction, is not good and movements more than 90° flexion are seldom obtained.

Osgood Schlatter's Disease is the osteochondritis or fatigue failure of the tibial apophysis of the tubercle in a growing child due to traction by extensor mechanism.

Clinically, it presents typically in a 10-15 year old boy. Symptoms vary from mild ache at the tubercle to severe pain. Pain is worse during climbing up or down the stairs, running or jumping. There may be a soft tissue swelling over the tibial tubercle due to the formation of a bursa. Tibial tubercle is tender on palpation.

Radiological examination shows soft tissue swelling anterior to the tubercle and thickening of the patellar tendon. Fragmentation and irregularity of the tibial tubercle apophysis is seen in older children. Often separate free fragments of bone due to heterotopic formation are seen anterior and superior to the tubercle.

Treatment in most cases is expectant, as the disease is self-limiting. Most cases resolve spontaneously around 15 years of age when fusion of the tubercle occurs.

When symptoms are severe and interfere with patient's activities, immobilization in a cylinder cast for 6-8 weeks may allow the patient to return to the normal activities. Very rarely, late excision of the separate ossicles may be required with peg grafting and therapeutic fusion of the tibial tuberosity apophysis (Bosworth procedure).

Popliteal Cyst (Baker's Cyst)

Popliteal cyst is a synovial cyst which arises from the semimembranosus bursa, from joint capsule or from underneath the medial head of gastrocnemius. In children it most typically arises from semimembranosus bursa, is filled with gelatinous fluid and has a lining of fibrous tissue, synovial cells and/or inflammatory cells. In children the swelling is always lateral to the semitendinosus. Popliteal cyst is usually asymptomatic but very large cysts can cause discomfort. The cyst always transilluminates unlike a vascular anomaly or a tumor. They often resolve. The treatment is expectant and the surgery is seldom required in children.

Quadriceps Contracture

Quadriceps contracture commonly occurs following intramuscular injections in quadriceps during childhood. The other causes of quadriceps contracture are congenital, arthrogryposis multiplex congenita, chronic osteomyelitis of femur, fracture shaft of femur and scarring due to surgery. Clinically, the patient has wasting of quadriceps and limitation of flexion and inability to squat.

Treatment in most cases should begin with physiotherapy. Resistant cases require excision of cicatrized muscle and V-Y plasty of the quadriceps.

CONGENITAL AND DEVELOPMENTAL DISORDERS AFFECTING FOOT

Clubfoot

Clubfoot (Congenital Talipes Equino Varus: CTEV) is a congenital foot deformity, which includes components of equin. The disorder occurs in 1/1000 live births and affects males twice as commonly as females. Half the cases are bilateral. Multiple factors are implicated such as genetic (polygenic inheritance), persistence of fetal positioning, primary germ plasm defects, neuromuscular factors, mechanical factors (twins, malposition in utero) and drugs.

Pathology

The foot is small and the calf is hypotrophied. The equinus deformity occurs at the ankle, the inversion at the subtalar joint and adduction and supination of the forefoot occurs at the midtarsal joints. Deformities are due to underdeveloped and contracted soft tissues on the medial, posterior and plantar aspect of the foot.

The talus is most deformed and its anterior part is deviated medially and in plantar direction. Talonavicular joint is dislocated and navicular is displaced medially. Cuboid is often subluxated medially. The calcaneus is small and rotates through the subtalar joint in a medial direction and inverts (varus tilt). The talus and calcaneus are more parellel in three planes.[40]

Clinically, the deformity is present at birth. The typical equinus, varus and adduction deformities are present in varying severity and flexibility (Fig. 111.14). It is not possible to manipulate the foot into normal position. A simple test for equinus is based on the observation that in normal newborns, the dorsum of the foot can be brought up to touch the skin. Failure to achieve this suggests the presence of the equinus deformity.

A child who starts walking on the clubfoot deformity (neglected clubfoot) develops callosities on the lateral border of the foot. Genu valgum and genu

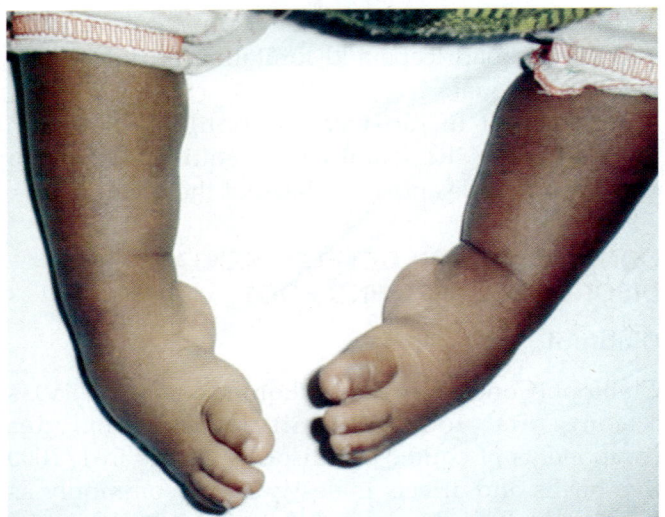

Fig. 111.14: Congenital talipes equino varus

recurvatum deformities may be associated in these patients.

Associated congenital abnormalities such as spina bifida, hip dysplasia and knee deformities should be ruled out in these patients.

Radiological examination reveals increased lateral tibiocalcaneal angle (> 120° due to equinus), decreased lateral talocalcaneal angle (< 35°; normal 35-50°) and anteroposterior talocalcaneal angle (< 20°: normal 20-40°) - both due to hindfoot varus. Talo - first metatarsal angle on AP film (normally zero) suggests talo-navicular dislocation.[41]

Treatment

Treatment objective of management is to correct the deformity and retain mobility. The foot should be plantigrade and have a normal weight bearing area satisfactory appearance and child should have ability to wear normal should be started immediately after diagnosis. Treatment in postnatal period consists of corrective manipulation and casting. The order of manipulation for correction of deformities is adduction, heel varus and lastly, equinus. Casts are changed every one to two weeks for 3 months.[42] The corrected foot is then held in a cast or brace (Denis Browne splint) till the child starts walking when he is advised to wear CTEV shoes. The non-operative treatment advocated by Ponseti is currently very popular and good results have been shown in several series.

Surgical treatment is required if the deformity does not respond to conservative treatment or if the CTEV has been neglected (A neglected CTEV is said to exist when the child starts walking on the deformity without any prior treatment).[43]

The most commonly done surgery for CTEV is Postero-Medial Soft Tissue Release (PMSTR). Contracted soft tissues to the posterior, medial and plantar aspects of the foot are released to correct the deformity. It can be done as early as 4 months of age but is often recommended at 8-9 months of age because of the following reasons:

a. Release in a very small foot in a very young child is technically quite difficult, as the structures in the foot are very small.
b. A very small foot may be difficult to hold in a plaster after surgery so maintenance of correction may be difficult.
c. A child who is close to the age of standing and weight bearing at the time of surgery can start walking soon afterwards. The walking on a corrected foot stimulates the near normal growth of foot bones and soft tissues.

PMSTR can be done by a posteromedial (Turco) or Cincinnati incision.

Following structures are released:
a. Posteriorly:
Tendo achilles (Z - plasty)
Capsule of ankle joint and subtalar joint
Posterior talofibular and calcaneofibular ligaments
b. Medially:
Tendons–
- Tibialis posterior
- Abductor hallucis muscle
- Sometimes FDL and FHL
c. Superficial medial release of the subtalar joint:
- Superficial deltoid (calcaneotibial and tibio-navicular)
- Calcaneonavicular (spring) ligament talona-vicular ligament dorsally
d. Deep medial release:
Bifurcate ligament (Calcaneonavicular and calcaneocuboid)
Talocalcaneal interosseous ligament
Capsule of talonavicular (medial, dorsal and plantar), naviculocuneiform, cuneiform - first metatarsal and medial side of subtalar joint.

e. Plantar structures:
   Plantar fascia (origin)
f. Lateral structures:
   Lateral talonavicular capsule and dorsal calcaneocuboid joint (if required).

After surgery, the correction is maintained in a plaster for 3 months followed by CTEV shoes.

CTEV shoes are specially modified shoes for patients who have undergone correction (casting or surgery) for clubfoot. These shoes have no heel, broad toe box, straight medial border and 3/16 inch raise on the outer side of sole.

1. *Tendon transfers* are required for cases which occur or relapse due to weakness of evertor (peroneii) muscles with resultant invertor overaction. Tibialis anterior or posterior tendon is transferred to cuboid to supplement evertor action. Tendon transfers are done after 5 years of age (when the patient can comply with muscle reeducation program) in a supple foot that is otherwise corrected.
2. *Evan's Procedure:* Evan's procedure is done for children between 4 - 8 years of age. It comprises of shortening of lateral column of the foot by wedge resection of calcaneocuboid joint.

Salvage operations are required for resistant or residual deformities of the foot.

Forefoot adduction is treated by Heyman-Herndon tarsometatarsal joints capsulotomies in younger children and by metatarsal osteotomies when the deformity becomes rigid in older children.

Heel varus is treated by modified Dwyer's osteotomy, which comprises of close wedge osteotomy on lateral aspect of calcaneus. However, it has the disadvantage of further reducing the size of an already small calcaneus.

Triple arthrodesis is done in skeletally mature children (>12 years of age) for neglected feet, significant residual deformity or for overcorrected planovalgus deformity. Appropriate wedges are removed from the talonavicular, calcaneocuboid and talocalcaneal joints to correct the deformities. Plaster cast immobilisation is continued after surgery for three months.

Triple arthrodesis is not done before twelve years of age because the bones are cartilaginous. A large amount of cartilage has to be removed, the growth of the foot is affected and the fusion is difficult to achieve.

Correction of rigid, recurrent, residual and/or multiply operated scarred clubfoot or clubfoot with poor overlying skin (or unstable scars) is possible by external fixator (Joshi's External Skeletal Stabilization-JESS or Ilizarov external fixation). The principle of correction by external fixator is one of differential distraction (both sides of the deformity are distracted-concave more than convex) to correct the deformities. After correction the foot should be immobilized in corrected position for 8 -12 weeks.

Calcaneovalgus Deformity

Calcaneovalgus deformity presents at birth with dorsiflexion and eversion of the foot. The condition is often bilateral.

This is an innocuous condition and most cases resolve spontaneously by the end of first year. Calcaneovalgus should be differentiated from congenital vertical talus. In the latter condition the calcaneum is in equinus and the hindfoot is rigid. In calcaneovalgus, the calcaneum is dorsiflexed (i.e. in calcaneus) and the hindfoot is supple. Parents can be reassured and told to gently manipulate the foot into corrected position.

Congenital Vertical Talus (Congenital Convex Pes Valgus)

Congenital vertical talus presents with rocker bottom foot deformity at birth. The deformity is usually associated with other anomalies, syndromes (Nail-patella syndrome, multiple pterygium syndrome, Marfan's syndrome, arthrogryposis), chromosomal abnormalities (trisomy 13-15 or 18) or with neuromuscular problems (e.g. spina bifida).

Pathology

Calcaneus is in equinus and rotated posterolaterally. Talus is plantarflexed and rotated medially. Head of the talus is palpable medially. Navicular is dislocated dorsolaterally. Cuboid is subluxed dorsally and laterally on calcaneus. Soft tissues on the posterior, anterior and lateral aspect of ankle are contracted.

Clinically, the patient has equinus and valgus at the hindfoot while the forefoot is dorsiflexed and abducted.

Differential diagnosis of congenital vertical talus is calcaneovalgus deformity of the foot.

Radiologically, there is increased talocalcaneal angle on AP and lateral X-rays. On lateral film, calcaneus is in equinus and talus is plantarflexed. A stress lateral view with forced plantar flexion differentiates congenital vertical talus from flexible hindfoot valgus. Talometatarsal alignment is restored in flexible deformity while it remains disturbed in congenital vertical talus as navicular remains dislocated.

Treatment

Treatment during the first 3-4 months is stretching of dorsolateral soft tissue by manipulation followed by casting (Plaster is applied in the position of clubfoot deformity).

Surgery is done for children over 4 months of age and consists of one stage soft tissue release in children up to 2½ years of age. Contracted posterior, anterior and lateral structures are released. Talonavicular joint and calcaneocuboid joints (if dislocated) are reduced and fixed with K-wire. Tibialis anterior is transferred to the neck of the talus if neurogenic imbalance is present.

Other Procedures

- Grice Green extra-articular subtalar arthrodesis can be done in children who are 4-6 years old
- Children over 3 years of age with severe deformities due to neuromuscular causes may need excision of navicular.
- Triple arthrodesis is required in patients who are over 12 years old.

Pes Planus (Flatfoot)

Pes planus is the condition when the longitudinal arch of the foot is low or non-existent. The foot is pronated, the navicular is prominent and the heel is in valgus. Flatfoot can be flexible or rigid. The rigid flatfoot remains flat in sitting, standing and in tiptoe standing positions of the foot. The flexible flatfoot, on the other hand, is flat only on standing. Etiology of the flatfoot is unknown but following pathologies are associated with flatfoot:
a. Congenital
b. Ligament laxity (Down's syndromes, Marfan's syndrome)
c. Muscle imbalance (as in poliomyelitis)
d. Tendo-Achilles contracture
e. Residual of calcaneovalgus foot
f. Congenital vertical talus (Rocker bottom foot)
g. Accessory navicular (Prehallux syndrome)
h. Tarsal coalition.

Rheumatoid arthritis and rupture of tibialis posterior tendon can lead to flat foot in later life.

Infantile Flatfoot

All infants have flatfoot and this is because of several reasons.
a. Normal longitudinal arch develops usually by 3 - 5 years.
b. Infants have ligamentous laxity thus, their arches collapse on weight bearing.
c. Infants have baby fat in the sole, which disappears by the age of 3 - 5 years. Hence, before 3-5 years, the arch may look flat even if it does not ultimately turn out to be flat foot.

Congenital hypermobile flatfoot is no longer considered an abnormality but a normal variant.

This is a genetic trait and is not considered to be an indication for treatment.

Accessory navicular syndrome is caused by a separate ossicle in the posterior tibial tendon adjacent to the navicular. The prominence of this bone may cause symptoms. Sometimes, this accessory bone receives anomalous insertion of tibialis posterior tendon along with the flattening of the longitudinal arch — the *"Prehallux Syndrome"*. The treatment is by padding and foot exercises. Occasionally excision of the accessory navicular may be required.

Clinically, the patient may be asymptomatic or may present with pain. Arch pain results from foot strain in severe cases with excessive use. Tight heel cords typically cause calf pain.

The patients with flatfeet also often present with uneven wear of the shoes; the inner side of sole wears more.

Radiologically, on the weight bearing lateral view of the foot, loss of arch is seen. The sagging can be at the talonavicular or naviculocuneiform joint. On the AP view, the talocalcaneal angle is increased.

Treatment of the pes planus is required only for the symptomatic feet. Shoes with good arch support and stretching for the tendo achilles contractures are useful measures. Medial navicular pad, Thomas heel (C and E: Crooked and Elongated Heel) consisting of medial heel wedge and longitudinal arch support is often used.[44] Surgery is required for persistent pain, excessive shoe wear problems or to address specific underlying condition (such as tendon transfer for paralytic conditions, triple arthrodesis for tarsal coalition or excision of accessory navicular).[45]

Surgical procedures for treatment of flatfoot can be soft tissue procedures (distal advancement of plantar calcaneonavicular ligament and posterior tibial tendon) or bony procedures (Talonavicular fusion, naviculocuneiform fusion, subtalar arthrodesis or triple arthrodesis).

Pes Cavus

Pes cavus is fixed equinus deformity of the forefoot on the hindfoot ("forefoot drop" for those who believe equinus can occur only at ankle) leading to accentuated longitudinal arch and contracture of the plantar soft tissues. Pes cavus is frequently associated with hindfoot varus and claw toes. Both calcaneus (calcaneocavus) and equinus (equinocavus) may be associated with pes cavus. Pes cavus can be idiopathic, familial or congenital. It can be caused by muscle imbalance (e.g. weak tibialis anterior with strong peroneus longus, paralysis of intrinsics, paralysis of triceps surae with strong long toe flexors) or by neuromuscular diseases (such as muscle dystrophy, peripheral neuropathies, myelomeningocele, diastematomyelia, Friedrich's ataxia, etc.).

Clinically, position of hindfoot, appearance of toes, flexibility of foot and muscle imbalance should be assessed. The patient has accentuated longitudinal arch and callosities under the metatarsal heads. Toes are curled and develop callosities on the dorsal aspect due to rubbing against the shoes.

Investigations for pes cavus must include muscle power examination, EMG/NCV, X-rays of the spine and the opinion of the neurologist.

Treatment is conservative in mild cases in the form of stretching, metatarsal pads and lateral wedge for the heel varus. Surgical treatment consists of Steindler's plantar release (release of contracted plantar fascia, muscles and ligaments), tendon transfer (long toe extensors to necks of metatarsals), dorsal wedge resection or Japa's V osteotomy of the tarsus, osteotomy of the calcaneus (Dwyer's lateral closing wedge) or triple arthrodesis.

Osteochondrosis

Osteochondritis can affect calcaneal apophysis (Sever's), navicular (Kohler's) or second metatarsal head (Freiberg's).

Clinically, the patient is an adolescent who complains of pain. X-rays show irregularity and fragmentation of the epiphysis/apophysis. Treatment is conservative and symptomatic with rest, NSAIDs and plaster cast if required.

BONE AND JOINT INFECTIONS

Introduction

Osteomyelitis often occurs in growing children and especially in lower limbs. Therefore, disabling sequelae such as partial or complete epiphyseal growth arrest with resultant deformities and limb length inequalities are common.

Acute Hematogenous Osteomyelitis

This is the infection of the bone and the bone marrow caused by blood borne organisms. It commonly affects children. Boys are affected more often than girls. *Staphylococcus aureus* (coagulase positive) is the commonest pathogen causing acute osteomyelitis. *E. coli* and Group *B streptococci* cause osteomyelitis in neonates. However, anaerobic infections may also be seen (*Peptococcus magnus,* bacteroides). Hemophilus influenzae commonly causes osteomyelitis in children three months to four years old.[46]

Metaphysis is the initial site of infection because it presents an extremely vascular area. Branches of nutrient artery provide network of vessels for zones of endochondral ossification in this area. Most vessels do not anastomose and terminate in venous sinusoids, i.e. they are end-arteries. They have hairpin bends, which leads to vascular congestion. Venous sinusoids are ideal bed for bacterial seeding. Large calibre of metaphyseal veins in children leads to marked slowing of blood flow and thus predisposes them to post-traumatic thromboses and colonization by blood borne bacteria. Also, trauma often localises to metaphysis and bacteremia may infect resultant hematoma. Metastatic infection may occur in spine following genitourinary infections by gram negative rods gaining access to spine via venous plexuses (Batson's plexuses) which lack valves and anastomose freely with segmental systemic veins and portal system.

Pathogenesis

Once infection occurs it spreads to adjacent cancellous bone and through cortex, via Haversian canals, to the periosteum. Periosteum reacts by forming new bone (involucrum) occasionally and may rupture. Infection leads to vascular compromise and leads to bone necrosis (sequestrum formation). Epiphyseal growth plate offers a barrier to spread of infection to the joint. However, intraarticular location of metaphysis may lead to spread of infection to joint. This is seen in hip (upper femoral), shoulder (upper humeral), elbow (radial neck) and ankle (distal fibular). Rarely, joint may be involved by pus tracking under the periosteum (outside the bone) and entering the joint.

Clinically, acute osteomyelitis is characterized by chills, fever, pain, erythema, swelling and tenderness. Empirical antibiotic treatment may mask the symptoms and delay diagnosis. The infection is most common in metaphysis of long bones, more frequently in the lower limbs. An effusion may be seen in an adjacent joint (sympathetic effusion). It is a sterile response and clinically the movements at joint are not restricted.

Investigations

The leukocyte count may be raised with neutrophilia. Erythrocyte sedimentation rate (ESR) and levels of C-reactive protein (CRP) are usually raised. Aspiration can help to diagnose infection, identify the organism and helps in choice of antibiotics.

Blood culture is rarely positive, often due to empirical antibiotic therapy initiated by primary physician.

Imaging

X-ray changes appear late and are non-specific. First 7-10 days may show muscular edema and obliteration of soft tissue (fat) planes. Periosteal reaction (elevation) is the earliest bone change and is seen at around 10 days. Demineralization of bone is seen at 10 - 14 days. Skeletal changes such as periostitis, sequestrum formation and involucrum formation take 3 - 6 weeks to appear.

Radionucleide Scans

Bone scans are useful in evaluating infection in the early stages of illness. Commonly used scans are:
  i. ^{99m}Tc diphosphonate scan-localizes vascularity and new bone formation.
     It may be negative in early period due to ischemia and necrosis. The scan is "Hot" in later phase.
 ii. Gallium 67 citrate-shows higher localisation in inflammation and is useful for spine infections.
iii. Indium 111-labelled leukocyte scan-localises neutrophils and is useful for extremities.

Ultrasound may localise deep-seated soft tissue swellings.[47] Magnetic Resonance Imaging (MRI) helps in diagnosis and defining the extent of the involvement.[48]

Differential Diagnosis

Osteomyelitis should be considered in differential diagnosis of all orthopedic afflictions with ambiguous clinical and radiographic findings. The parents often give the history of trauma but it should not allow the orthopedist to miss the septic process. It is extremely important especially in pediatric patients to rule out neoplastic lesions especially Ewing's sarcoma. The differential diagnosis of osteomyelitis is shown in Table 111.2.

Treatment

Management of infection in children is guided by several principles distinct from those, which apply, to adults. The children have greater healing potential, operative drainage is often required and the antibiotic selection is determined by the age concurrent illness and family situation (whether family is reliable).

Acute hematogenous osteomyelitis can be treated successfully with rest (splintage) and antibiotics if started early. Parenteral third generation cephalosporin or penicillinase resistant synthetic penicillin is drug of choice.[49] Choice of intravenous antibiotics should be decided by expected sensitivity of most

Table 111.2: Differential diagnosis of osteomyelitis
I. Tumors 　• Benign lesions 　　– Osteoid osteoma 　　– Osteoblastoma 　　– Eosinophilic granuloma 　• Malignant lesions 　　– Round cell tumors (especially Ewing's sarcoma) 　　– Lymphoma II. Inflammatory conditions 　• Septic arthritis 　　– Swelling and tenderness at the joint 　　– Any attempted movement at the joint is painful 　　– Aspiration of joint reveals pus 　• Rheumatic fever 　　– Insidious onset 　　– Less intense symptoms 　　– Differentiated from the osteomyelitis by fleeting arthritis III. Scurvy IV. Congenital syphilis (with syphilitic osteitis and periostitis) V. Trauma with fracture

likely pathogen, which may be modified if necessary, once culture report is available. The patient is monitored closely, clinically and with total and differential leukocyte counts. Intravenous antibiotics are continued till patient is afebrile. This is followed by oral antibiotics for a total of 6 weeks.

Surgical Treatment

Conservative treatment should be abandoned and patient operated when:
- The response to antibiotic is not rapid, which is evident by continuing fever, leucocytosis and severe pain ;
- Patient presents late (for drainage of pus and debridement of infected tissues).

Surgery consists of drainage of abscess. If no pus is found after incising the periosteum, holes should be drilled in the cortex to localise the site of infection. A window of cortex is removed to allow free drainage. Extensive curettage of medullary cavity should not be done routinely. Wound is closed over a drain, which is removed within few days to avoid secondary bacterial contamination.

Course

Complete resolution of acute hematogenous osteomyelitis is possible with early, effective, intravenous antibiotic therapy. Long-term morbidity occurs in almost one-fourth patients where the disease leads to chronic osteomyelitis. Chronic osteomyelitis and recurrences are more common in patients who are diagnosed late.

Neonatal Osteomyelitis

This is caused by hematogenous infection. The common organisms are Group-B *streptococcus* (commonest), *Staphylococcus aureus* and *Escherichia coli*. Group-B *streptococcus* is commonly found in vagina and infection occurs during delivery and commonly involves one bone. *Staph. aureus* and *E. coli* can cause polyostotic involvement in the newborns. Immunological incompetence of the newborn may delay clinical diagnosis in some patients due to absence of systemic symptoms. Combination of penicillinase resistant synthetic penicillin and third generation cephalosporin is the primary antibiotic regimen.

Subacute Osteomyelitis

It is primarily a radiological diagnosis. The condition most often involves femur and tibia. The patient may have pain without systemic / local signs or symptoms. It occurs following partially treated acute osteomyelitis. Total leukocyte count and blood cultures are often normal in this condition. ESR, radiographs and cultures from bone may help in making the diagnosis.

Brodie's Abscess (Bone Abscess)

This is a localized form of subacute osteomyelitis. The onset is insidious and systemic manifestations are mild or absent. Radiographic features consist of localized radiolucency usually seen in the metaphysis of long bones. It is typically elongated with well-demarcated margin and surrounded by reactive sclerosis.

Sequestra are always absent. A radiolucent tract may be seen extending from the lesion into the growth plate. (Bone abscess may cross the epiphyseal plate and extend into epiphysis unlike acute osteomyelitis). Epiphyseal osteomyelitis is caused exclusively by *Staphylococcus aureus*.

Differential Diagnosis

Brodie's abscess may mimic an osteoid osteoma radiologically and clinically. Presence of radiolucent tract from the lesion into the growth plate favors infection. When present in epiphysis, it should be differentiated from chondroblastoma.

Treatment

Treatment of Brodie's abscess in metaphysis includes surgical curettage. Epiphyseal osteomyelitis is treated with antibiotics. Drainage is indicated if pus is present.

Chronic Osteomyelitis

This may arise following inappropriately treated acute hematogenous osteomyelitis or inadequate surgical debridement of necrotic bone in exogenous osteomyelitis following trauma or surgery. The necrotic bone is walled off by periosteal new bone (involucrum) and fibrous tissue. Each cavity thus formed contains a piece of dead bone surrounded by granulation tissue (sequestrum) and harbors bacteria. Skin and soft tissues are often involved and get scarred, edematous and poorly vascularized. Fistulous tracts form sequestrum/sequestra may be extruded through the sinus tract. Cavities containing sequestra may remain quiescent for variable intervals. Periods of quiescence are often followed by acute exacerbations. If drainage persists over many years, epidermoid carcinoma may develop in 1% patients (may occur 30-40 years after original infection). A *Marjolin's ulcer* is ulceration developing in epidermoid carcinoma of sinus tract. Complications of chronic osteomyelitis are enumerated in Table 111.3.

Figures 111.15A and B. show sequelae of the osteomyelitis of humerus in a child.

Chronic osteomyelitis is rare in healthy adults. It is seen in immunosuppressed hosts, in the presence of major nutritional or systemic disorder, diabetics and in patients with peripheral vascular disease and IV drug abusers.

Table 111.3: Sequelae and complications of chronic osteomyelitis

- Acute exacerbation
- Pathological fracture
- Limb length discrepancy
- Shortening of bone (epiphyseal damage)
- Lengthening of bone (epiphyseal hyperemia)
- Angular deformities (Partial closure of epiphysis)
- Metastatic abscesses
- Contractures and joint stiffness
- Scarring of the skin
- Epidermoid (squamous cell) carcinoma of sinus tract
- Amyloidosis

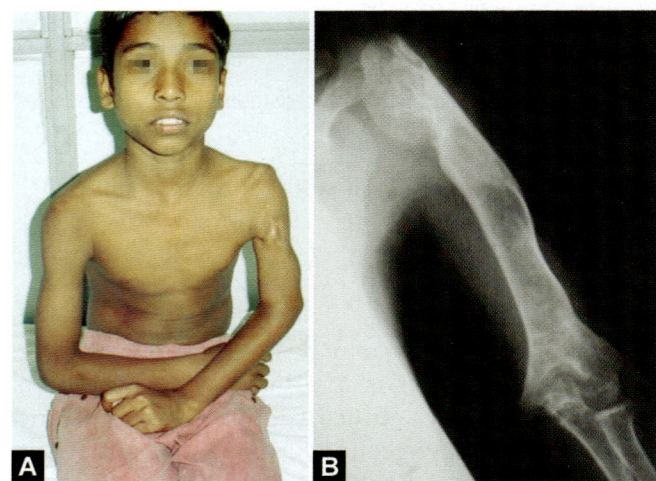

Figs 111.15A and B: Sequelae of the osteomyelitis of humerus in a child **A.** clinical picture; **B.** X-ray

Diagnosis

Diagnosis is readily made with presence of drainage and X-ray changes which include thickening and irregularity of bone, dense sequestrae surrounded by zone of lucency, cavities and radiolucent tracts in the bone and presence of involucrum (reactive periosteal new bone). Radionucleide studies may help in subtle cases without drainage. Attempt to isolate the offending organism should be made by taking cultures from deeper areas or cavity during surgery as drainage fluid has abundant contaminants. Bone scan (in the presence of implants) and Magnetic Resonance Imaging (MRI) (when implants are absent) are extremely valuable in establishing vascularity of segments of diaphysis with doubtful vascularity.

Treatment

Treatment consists of a wide range of procedures ranging from drainage of abscess and sequestrectomy to extensive debridement. The basic principles of surgical treatment of chronic osteomyelitis are:

Sequestrectomy and Saucerization

Debridement with excision of dead, necrotic, infected tissues and sequestrae (sequestrectomy) till bleeding surfaces of bone and removal of the sinus tracts is done. Dense reactive bone, though not necrotic, is removed, as it is often poorly vascularized. Deroofing of the osteomyelitis cavity (saucerization) is done to facilitate drainage.

Obliteration of the Dead Space

With an attempt to increase vascularity and promote healing by:
- Cancellous bone grafts/vascularised bone grafts
- *Antibiotic impregnated bone cement:* Polymethylmethacrylate (PMMA or bone cement) beads impregnated with antibiotics are used to obliterate dead space and provide high local concentrations of antibiotics without systemic ill effects. Antibiotics elute from beads within 2 weeks and their local antibiotic levels are insignificant by 6 - 8 weeks and the beads should then be removed
- *Surrounding muscle:* When antibiotic laden PMMA beads are not available local muscle flaps can be used to obliterate dead space.

Soft Tissue Coverage

It is often required. The various methods include:
- Skin grafting
- Local myocutaneous flaps
- Fasciocutaneous flaps
- Distant free flaps.

Garre's Chronic Sclerosing Osteomyelitis

It is an unusual form of osteomyelitis affecting diaphysis of long bones in adolescents. Anaerobes have been implicated as causative organisms. The disease is probably caused by organisms of low virulence and/or occurs in hosts with good resistance/immune response. The onset is insidious with localized pain and tenderness. Intense proliferation of periosteum occurs causing bony deposition, which is seen as dense progressive sclerosis on X-rays. Malignancy must be ruled out. Biopsy must be performed in cases where the diagnosis is doubtful. Surgery and antibiotics are ineffective in providing cure.

Sickle Cell Disease

Recurrent attacks of bone infection are common in sickle cell disease. Vascular insufficiency and bone infarcts are the underlying causes. *Staphylococcus aureus* is the most common causative agent, though salmonella may also be isolated. Patients with sickle cell anemia are ten times more susceptible to salmonella osteomyelitis as compared with normal population. Other diseases leading to ischemia and infection are Gaucher's disease (after biopsy) and osteopetrosis (Jaw osteomyelitis via tooth infection).

Osteomyelitis by Unusual Organisms

Syphilitic Osteomyelitis

Syphilis is a chronic systemic infection caused by treponema palladium.
Congenital Syphilis is transmitted from mother to infant. Osteochondritis, periostitis and osteitis are the typical features. Destruction at the medial aspect of the metaphysis of a long bone (Wimberger sign) is characteristic. It is most classically seen in tibia. In the late stages, involvement of tibia results in characteristic anterior bowing deformity known as "Saber-Shin" deformity.

Salmonella Osteomyelitis

It is mostly caused by serotypes other than *S. typhi*. It is common in sickle cell disease (but it is not the commonest organism causing osteomyelitis in sickle cell disease). It may occur in subjects without sickle cell disease. The bone affection occurs during convalescence 4 to 6 weeks after enteric fever. Diaphyseal involvement is common especially in femur. Vertebrae and ribs are also involved. Infection of tibia, fibula, humerus and clavicle has also been reported. Multiple sites of infection are commonly seen. After one to two weeks radiographs show multiple punched out destructive lesions throughout the metaphysis and diaphysis with extensive subperiosteal bone formation (massive involucrum) and irregular sclerosis.

Treatment

The treatment includes antibiotics (e.g. chloramphenicol, ampicillin or ciprofloxacin) for six weeks. Response to antibiotics is poor. Abscesses should be drained. A surprisingly good outcome may be seen without operative drainage. Recurrences are commonly seen.

Tubercular Osteomyelitis

Commonest involvement by tubercular osteomyelitis is in vertebral bodies. Metacarpals and phalanges (Tubercular dactylitis) are sometimes involved. Multiple bones may be involved and the affected bones become swollen and fusiform. The appearance is called *'spina ventosa'*. X-ray shows expansion of bone, rarefaction leading to cystic appearance and periosteal reaction. Tubercular dactylitis should be differentiated from enchondroma, rheumatoid arthritis and syphilitic dactylitis. In long bones, tubercular osteomyelitis involves metaphyseal regions. New bone formation does not occur except in vertebrae and in small bones of hands and feet. Juxta articular metaphyseal lesions may discharge into the adjacent joint and lead to tubercular arthritis. Treatment consists of antitubercular chemotherapy. Surgery (curettage of lesion) is indicated for juxta articular lesion to prevent arthritis of adjacent joint.

Infectious Arthritis

Relevant Anatomy

Orthopedic surgery is concerned mainly with synovial joints. Other types of joints are synostosis (bony), syndesmosis (fibrous) or synchondrosis/symphysis (cartilage). The ends of bones in synovial joint are covered with hyaline cartilage. Hyaline cartilage consists of chondrocytes embedded in matrix of collagen fibres and proteoglycans. Articular cartilage has zones like physis and a mineralization/calcification front at the junction between calcified cartilage and normal articular cartilage called *Tidemark*. Articular cartilage gets its nutrition by diffusion of metabolites from synovial fluid, as the cartilage has no neurovascular supply. The cartilage in adult cannot grow or repair itself. Defects resulting from injury are repaired by fibrocartilage or fibrous tissue.

Synovial membrane is a smooth, glistening membrane, which surrounds the joint cavity and produces synovial fluid. It has rich vascularity and cells specialized in phagocytosis and hyaluronic acid production. Synovial fluid is a dialysate of plasma with the addition of hyaluronic acid produced by synovial membrane. External to synovium, thick fibrous capsule surrounds the joint. Capsule has special thickenings to form ligaments of the joint. Nerve endings in the capsule transmit proprioception, pain and pressure sensation.

Pyogenic Arthritis

Source of Infection

Infection of the joint is most commonly caused by *Staphylococcus aureus*.

The bacteria can gain entrance in to the joint by following routes:

a. Hematogenous spread usually occurs from a distant focus of infection. It occurs most commonly in patients with underlying illness and immune deficiency. Chronic illnesses such as rheumatoid arthritis, intravenous drug abuse and local joint trauma may predispose adults to hematogenous infection.

b. Direct extension from adjacent focus of infection
- Infection in newborn and infants can extend from metaphysis to the joint by transphyseal vessels (which get obliterated after infancy).[50] Infection cannot cross the physis so septic arthritis is less common in children.
- Extension of metaphyseal osteomyelitis can occur where metaphysis is intra-articular, most commonly at hip. Other joints include shoulder (upper humeral epiphysis), ankle (distal fibular epiphysis) and elbow (radial neck).
- Contiguous soft tissue infection can extend and cause septic arthritis.
- Umbilical vein sepsis in newborn can lead to pyogenic arthritis.

c. Direct inoculation is seen following penetrating/open joint injuries and following diagnostic or therapeutic procedures (e.g. aspiration of joint fluid, intra-articular injections, arthroscopy). Femoral venipuncture may also lead to septic arthritis of hip in infants.

Prosthetic joint surgery is another source of direct inoculation.

Pathogenesis

The presence of bacteria in the joint incites an intense local reaction. The synovial membrane becomes hyperemic, edematous and proliferates. It produces purulent fluid containing markedly increased leukocytes. Articular cartilage gets destroyed by:
a. Proteolytic enzymes released by bacteria and disintegrating inflammatory cells.
b. Pressure necrosis by raised intra-articular pressure.
c. Interference with chondrocyte nutrition and
d. Invasion of matrix and enzymatic degradation by proliferating synovium.

Infection spreads to underlying bone and can destroy the growth plate resulting in limb length discrepancies and/or angular deformities in growing children. Infected synovial membrane eventually is replaced by granulation tissue. Marked distension of joint, destruction of cartilage, capsule and ligaments and spasm of the neighboring muscles may culminate in pathological dislocation of the joint (most commonly hip). In neglected cases, multiple discharging sinuses may form. The eventual outcome of the joint depends on the virulence of the organism, age of the patient and the state at which therapeutic intervention is done.

In newborns and infants, the femoral head is mainly cartilaginous and is rapidly destroyed by the infection. Marked destruction gives rise to a *hypermobile joint (Tom-Smith's Arthritis)* with exaggerated movements and marked shortening.[51] In young children the infection results in bony ankylosis. In adolescents and adults, the joint destruction by septic process may be followed by fibrous ankylosis.

Clinical Features

Pyogenic arthritis is usually monoarticular infection and most commonly involves hip in infants and young children and knee in older children and adults. The onset is acute with constitutional symptoms and high fever. Fever may sometimes be absent in infants. The child is apprehensive, anxious and anorexic. The chief complaint is swelling, pain and limitation of motion of involved joints. Affected joint is warm, erythematous, tender, distended and has reduced range of motion with pain on attempted movements. Spasm of surrounding muscles is often quite obvious. Patient holds the joint in the position of maximum capacity to reduce intra-articular pressure and thus minimize pain.

The position of maximum intra-articular volume of various joints is given in Table 111.4.

Laboratory investigations reveal leukocytosis with shift to the left and raised ESR and C-reactive protein. Blood culture may be positive in 50% patients with hematogenous septic arthritis.

Table 111.4: Position of maximum Intra-articular volume

Joint	Position
Hip	60° Flexion, 15° abduction and 15° external rotation
Knee	30-60° flexion
Ankle	15° plantar flexion
Shoulder	30-60° abduction
Elbow	30-60° flexion
Wrist	Neutral

Synovial Fluid Analysis

Evaluation of synovial fluid is critical for diagnosis and treatment of septic arthritis. Aspiration of joint fluid is done following an aseptic technique. Wide bore needle is used for aspiration and as much fluid as possible is removed from the joint (to decompress the joint). Aerobic and anaerobic cultures should be taken. Tubes containing heparin or EDTA should be used for collecting fluid for cell examination. In septic arthritis, the synovial fluid shows the following abnormalities (Table 111.5). These along with positive culture clinch the diagnosis.

Imaging Studies

Early X-ray changes may be subtle and comparison with opposite (normal) joint helps to distinguish subtle changes. An effusion with distension of capsule may appear as soft tissue swelling. The earliest bony change is rarefaction of bone. This is followed by erosion of juxta-articular bone. In later stages, joint space is

Table 111.5: Synovial fluid analysis in septic arthritis

Analysis	Normal	Septic arthritis
Color	Straw or clear yellow	Serosanguinous or purulent (Yellow-white, grey)
Volume	1- 4 ml	Increased
Clarity	Clear	Turbid
Viscosity	High (1" long string between thumb and forefinger)	Very low
Mucin clot	Good	Poor
Leukocytes (cells/ml)	< 300	> 50,000
Neutrophils	< 25%	> 80 %
Bacteria	Negative	Positive
Serum/synovial fluid glucose ratio	0.8-1.0 (20 mg/100 ml less than serum)	< 0.5 (50-100 mg/100 ml less than serum)
Protein (g/dl)	2	≤ 8
Culture	Negative	Positive

diminished due to destruction of articular cartilage. Bone scan, CT scan and MRI can help in early diagnosis in cases with ambiguous clinical signs.

Differential Diagnosis

Septic arthritis should be differentiated from acute osteomyelitis, hemophilia, gouty arthritis and tuberculosis.

Treatment

Septic arthritis should be treated as an emergency.

The principles of treatment are[51]:
1. Evaluation of pus
2. Sterilization of the joint
3. Prevention/Correction of deformity
4. Restoration of function

Evaluation of Pus

It is done to decompress the joint, clean it of enzymes and save the cartilage. Evaluation can be done by aspiration or arthroscopy. Hip joint is drained by posterior approach.

Sterilization of the Joint

Systemic antibiotics are started immediately, empirically based on suspected causative organism. They are changed if necessary after culture and sensitivity reports are available. Parenteral administration of high doses of antibiotics is continued till the constitutional symptoms subside. Once ESR comes down and the fever settles down, the oral antibiotics are started and continued for 4-6 weeks.

Splinting the Joint

Splinting provides rest expedites recovery and prevents/corrects the deformity.

Restoration of Function

The joint is mobilized to regain movement.

Sequelae of Septic Arthritis[52]

1. Ankylosis of joint: fibrous or bony.
2. Instability of joint/Hypermobile joint (Tom Smith arthritis), due to destruction of cartilaginous femoral head.
3. Pathological dislocation.
4. Complication of sepsis
   - Septicemia, even death
   - Metastatic abscesses
   - Osteomyelitis
5. Soft tissue contractures.
6. Epiphyseal damage
   - Limb length discrepancies — shortening/lengthening of bone
   - Angular deformities.

Tubercular Arthritis is a granulomatous infection caused by human or bovine strain of mycobacterium tuberculosis. It is very common in underdeveloped and developing countries. The increased incidence of HIV has given rise to increased incidence of tuberculous infection, multidrug resistant tuberculosis and tuberculosis by atypical organisms.

Pathology

The infection reaches the joint either by hematogenous route or rarely by spread from adjacent bone. Disease is usually synovial initially. Synovium proliferates and hypertrophies and gets studded with tubercles. Joint effusion follows. Tubercular granulation tissue covers articular cartilage as a pannus and destroys cartilage and subchondral bone. If untreated, necrotic material and synovial exudates perforate the capsule and form a cold abscess. Secondary pyogenic infection through the sinus tracts may further destroy the joint.

Clinical Features

Clinically, tuberculosis presents as monoarticular arthritis in children and young adults. Synovial thickening are readily effusion and appreciable in superficial joints such as knee. Marked muscle wasting is seen around the joint. The joint is held in position of deformity due to effusion and muscle spasm. Night cries and night sweats may be present. Fixed joint deformities develop in later stages due to destruction of cartilage and subchondral bone. Cold abscess and sinuses may be present in late stages.

Diagnosis

X-rays show increased joint space followed by rarefaction of bone as the earliest feature. Joint space narrowing occurs subsequently with destruction of cartilage. Reactive new bone is absent. Sequestrae are rare.

Blood examination shows anaemia and elevated erythrocyte sedimentation rate. Synovial fluid is straw coloured and has raised leukocyte count, low sugar content and forms poor mucin clot. Tubercular bacilli are rarely seen. Sometimes they can be cultured from synovial fluid. Synovial biopsy can confirm the diagnosis.

Treatment

Aims of treatment are eradication of disease, prevention and correction of deformities and preservation of joint functions. General measures consist of bed rest, balanced diet, pain relief and psychological support. Chemotherapy is usually started with 4 drugs HRZE (*INH, Rifampicin, Pyrazinamide and Ethambutol*) and if after three months, the response is good, it can be reduced to two HR. The total duration of therapy is 12-18 months. Traction in these patients relieves pain, counters spasm and prevents and corrects deformity at the joint. It also provides rest to the joint. Gentle active and passive exercises for mobilization of the joint should be started as soon as the disease activity has reduced and pain has abated. Surgical treatment may be required to confirm diagnosis, reduce disease load, improve vascularity (and hence penetration of chemotherapeutic agents), and correct deformities. Synovectomy and joint debridement are indicated when joint space is not compromised and useful range of motion is expected.

In markedly damaged and disorganized joints, arthrodesis in the functional position may be undertaken to eliminate pain, correct deformity and provide stable, functional joint.

Hemophilic Arthropathy

Hemophilia A is the commonest hereditary (sex linked recessive) coagulation disorder affecting 20 per 100,000 live male births and is caused by deficiency or malfunction of coagulation factor VIII. Hemophilia B (Christmas disease) is caused by lack of factor IX. Hemophilia C is a mild variety of disease caused by the deficiency of factor XI. It has autosomal dominant inheritance.

Normally very low serum levels of factor VIII are sufficient for adequate coagulation. Reduction of more than 75% in the serum levels (i.e. serum levels < 25% of normal) leads to perceptible clinical illness.[53] The disease is graded according to the severity of factor VIII deficiency into mild (serum factor VIII levels 5-25% of normal; moderate 1-5% and severe < 1%). Bleeding can be intraarticular, intrabursal or into the soft tissues. Repeated intra-articular bleeding leads to proliferative synovitis and extensive hemosiderin deposition.

Clinically, the disease presents with recurrent episodes of bleeding, especially in the joints. The disease usually presents in early childhood with discomfort, limitation of joint movement initially followed by pain and swelling. Contractures and deformities eventually occur. Knee is the most common joint involved followed by elbow, ankle, shoulder and hip. The affected joint is swollen, warm and painful to move and often confused with septic arthritis. Bleeding into ilicus can lead to femoral nerve palsy.

"Pseudotumors" are painless masses consisting of partially clotted blood surrounded by thick fibrous membrane resulting from juxta periosteal bleeding which mimic tumours clinically and radiologically.[54] They occur in 1-2% cases of hemophilia. They are commonly seen in lower limbs and pelvis. Pseudotumors can damage bone and muscles, can lead to infection or cause neuropathies.

Radiologic Features

Early stages show soft tissue swelling. This is followed by osteoporosis. Further damage to the joint is seen as bony changes (squaring of patella, widened intercondylar notch of femur and enlarged femoral condyles in the knee, formation of subchondral cysts), joint space narrowing and loss of articular cartilage. Osteophyte formation is seen.

Pseudotumors are seen as cystic expansile, lucent soft tissue swellings eroding the cortex. MRI is classical with low signal on T-1 weighted images and high signal on T-2 weighted images.

Ultrasonography is useful to diagnose the intramuscular bleeds.

Laboratory Investigations

Partial Thromboplastin Time (PTT) is elevated in hemophilia. Specified factor assays should be done to determine severity of the disease. Assays for factor VIII inhibitors (antibodies) should be done, as their presence is a contra-indication to any surgical intervention.

Blood for HIV should be tested in hemophiliacs as transfusion related AIDS is a well recognized complication of hemophilia (in up to 90% patients).

Treatment

Prophylaxis for hemophilia is extremely important and consists of avoidance of contact sports, physiotherapy and prophylactic administration of factor VIII whenever affordable.

Acute hemarthrosis is treated by splintage, compressive bandage, analgesics and replacement of factor VIII to bring the serum levels to 30-50% of normal. Aspiration of the joint to relieve pain and swelling is useful within the first 24 hours when the antibodies to factor VIII are absent in the serum.[55]

Fractures are usually managed conservatively in hemophilia with splintage/immobilization. Factor replacement is done for the first 48-72 hours.

Hemorrhage in the muscles is managed by immobilization, compression and factor VIII replacement. Medical synovectomy with radioactive phosphorus (32P) is useful for chronic hemophilic synovitis.

Surgical management of chronic hemophiliac arthropathy includes synovectomy, correction of soft tissue contractures, arthrodesis and total joint replacement. Pseudotumors need excision but can be treated with radiotherapy and/or factor replacement sometimes.

OTHER BONE AND JOINT DISORDERS

Legg-Calve Perthes Disease

Perthes disease is a non-inflammatory condition leading to deformity of the weight-bearing surface of femoral head. It arises as a result of repeated vascular insults leading to avascular necrosis of the proximal femoral epiphysis.[56]

The Perthes disease occurs between 4-8 years of age and is much more common in males (M:F = 4:1). Almost 10% cases are bilateral though usually not simultaneous. Perthes disease has a higher incidence among children with older parents, children of maternal smokers during pregnancy; breech delivery, low birth weight and delayed skeletal maturation.

Pathogenesis

Idiopathic avascular necrosis of the femoral head occurs followed by subchondral fracture, revascularization (by creeping substitution), and healing ossification processes. The disease is divided into avascular necrotic stage, fragmentation stage and reparative stage.[57] The process of necrosis and reconstitution takes about 2 years.

Clinical Features

Clinically, the disease varies in severity. Patient usually presents with limp with or without pain. Limping increases with activity and may be intermittent. Pain when present is usually in the groin, anterior thigh and sometimes in the knee. Sometimes the disease presents with synovitis with associated muscle spasm. Decreased range of motion is found in almost all patients and abduction and internal rotation are mainly restricted.

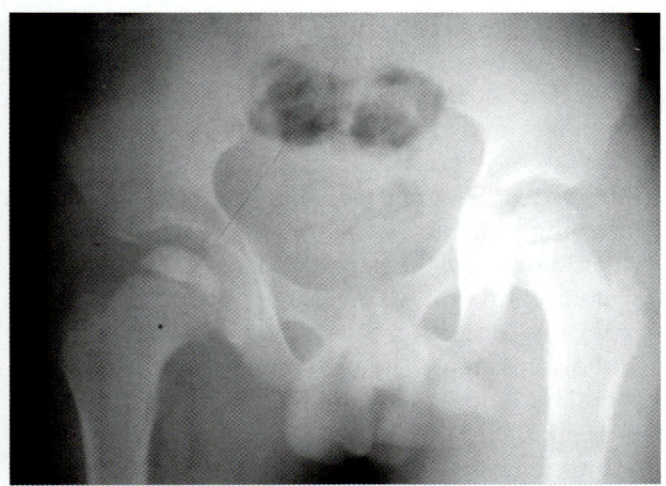

Fig. 111.16: Perthes' disease of right hip

Radiologically, the plain x-rays show increased joint space (because of increased cartilaginous growth) and subchondral lucency.[58] The femoral head shows increased density, fragmentation and is deformed (Fig. 111.16).

Based on plain radiographs, the extent of involvement can be graded according to the Catterall classification:[59]

a. *Group I:* Anterior head involvement (less than 1/2 femoral head affected) without any sequestrum or subchondral fracture.
b. *Group II:* Anterior and central half of head involved (more than 1/2 but less than 3/4th) with intact lateral margin. Sequestrum, subchondral fracture and anterolateral metaphyseal lesions are present.
c. *Group III:* Almost 3/4th of femoral head is involved including the posterior half of epiphysis - only posteromedial segment is spared. Large sequestrum forms along with subchondral fracture and diffuse metaphyseal changes.
d. *Group IV:* Entire head is involved.

Arthrogram can be used to assess containment of head and its deformity and subluxation.

Bone scan can be used to diagnose the condition early.

MRI is a non-invasive investigation, which is extremely useful for early diagnosis, and can differentiate between live and dead marrow.[60,61]

Differential Diagnosis

Perthes disease should be differentiated from transient synovitis, septic arthritis, blood dyscrasias (especially sickle cell disease), lymphoma, trauma, tumor and rheumatic fever. Bilateral cases must be differentiated from multiple epiphyseal dysplasia, spondyloepiphyseal dysplasia, pseudoachondroplasia, sickle cell disease and hypothyroidism.

Prognosis

Clinical and radiological prognostic factors have been recognized.

Clinical: Age more than 6-8 years, obesity, decreased range of movements especially presence of adduction contracture, and female sex are associated with poor prognosis.

Radiological *"Head at risk"* signs are identified as calcification lateral to the epiphysis, Gage's sign (V-shaped lucent area in lateral epiphysis and adjacent metaphysis), lateral subluxation, horizontal physis and diffuse metaphyseal reaction. The presence of these signs indicates impending extensive osteonecrosis of femoral head.

Uncovering of the femoral head by > 20% is a bad prognostic indicator.

Greater the Catterall group (more extensive the femoral head involvement) worse is the prognosis.

Treatment of Perthes disease is aimed at maintaining the sphericity of the femoral head and is based on the principle that hip mobility and containment of the femoral head within the acetabulum will lead to the best healing and remodeling of the avascular femoral head. Young patients (4 to 6 years age) with involvement of less than 50% of the head (Catterall I) are observed without active treatment. Catterall II group patients less than 6 years of age are observed if they have a good range of motion. Intermittent traction and active range of motion exercises are prescribed if there is limitation of movements. Aim of treatment of Catterall III and IV groups is to achieve good range of motion and containment. This can be achieved by orthotic devices (abduction braces) or surgery. Surgery can be Salter's innominate osteotomy or a femoral osteotomy.[62] These procedures are suitable only for those cases where there is no femoral head deformity. In group III and IV patients where the head is deformed or collapsed, no treatment is possible. Catterall V group patients older than 6 years are treated with traction and abduction bracing.

Slipped Capital Femoral Epiphysis (Adolescent Coxa Vara)

Slipped capital femoral epiphysis (SCFE) is a condition wherein the femoral neck displaces through the growth plate in anterior and superior direction while the femoral head remains in the acetabulum. The condition is caused by weakness of the perichondrial ring and the zone of hypertrophy in the growing growth plate. The exact cause is unknown. Various etiologies have been suggested including hormonal dysfunction.

The incidence of SCFE is 1-3 per 100,000. Males are affected more commonly than females (2.5:1). Almost 25% are bilateral. SCFE is common during 13-16 years age in males and 11-13 years in females. There is an increased incidence in overweight as well as slender tall patients, hypothyroidism, hypopituitarism, renal osteodystrophy hypogonadism, Down's syndrome and in the presence of a positive family history.

Classification

- An acute slip occurs suddenly.
- An acute on chronic slip presents with acute exacerbation of symptoms, which have been present for more than 3 weeks.
- A chronic slip is the one where history of symptoms is of more than 3 weeks' duration.

Pathogenesis

Slip occurs through the zone of hypertrophy and the displacement occurs due to body weight and muscle action.[63] Epiphysis displaces posteriorly and inferiorly while the neck displaces in anterior and superior direction. The leg rotates externally under the effect of these displacements. Progressive apparent coxa vara and shortening of the leg result.[64]

Clinical Features

Clinically the patient, usually between the age of 10 and 16 years presents with a history of chronic or intermittent pain of insidious onset in groin, thigh or medial knee associated with a limp. Patient may also present with acute pain after an injury with a history of intermittent pain previously (acute on chronic). In the acute phase, there is significant muscle spasm and synovitis with restricted range of motion. Gait is antalgic with externally rotated foot progression angle. There is decreased internal rotation, abduction and flexion. Hip flexion produces external rotation with knee pointing towards the axilla during flexion (other causes include coxa magna and gluteus maximus contractures. Severe cases may be associated with shortening of femur.

Radiologically the earliest changes are seen only on lateral X-ray. On AP view, a line along the superior neck does not intersect any part of epiphysis (Trethowen's sign). The medial and proximal part of femoral neck does not overlap the ischium (Capener's Sign).

Chronic changes are seen in longstanding cases and can be widening of physis, sclerosis, and ossification at the junction of medial femoral neck.[65] Narrowed joint space and osteopenia of femoral head are seen in chondrolysis.

Treatment in mild to moderate case is *in situ* pin fixation. A single pin or titanium screw is passed from close to base of neck anteriorly towards postero-inferiorly.[66] Patient is mobilized partial weight bearing with crutches for 6 weeks. Aim of pinning *in situ* is to prevent further progression of slip and to achieve early closure of physis.

Attempts to reduce the physis in longstanding cases leads to avascular necrosis.

In cases of severe slip primary epiphysiodesis is described as a method of treatment.

Compensatory transcervical and basal neck osteotomies are described to correct the deformities.[67] These procedures are technically demanding and associated with increased incidence of avascular necrosis. Contralateral hip should be closely observed till physeal closure. Prophylactic pinning is indicated only in cases with renal osteodystrophy, which are associated with increased incidence of bilateral slip.

Complications

Chondrolysis may be associated with forceful manipulation or after surgery when pin penetrates the head to enter the joint. Clinically, the patient presents with stiffness, severe pain and muscle spasm. Hemogram and other laboratory parameters are normal. Radiographs show joint space narrowing. Bone scan is positive with increased uptake in the region of acetabulum and femoral head. It may recover completely in 6-12 months but may cause degeneration or ankylosis of the joint. Treatment is traction, range of motion exercises, NSAID's and salvage operations such as arthrodesis or arthroplasty. Other complications are avascular necrosis and secondary osteoarthritis.

Transient Synovitis of Hip (Observation Hip, Toxic Synovitis, Coxitis Fugax)

Transient synovitis is a self-limiting condition seen in children between 3-5 years of age. Synovitis of the hip joint occurs without any obvious etiology.

The child presents with complaints of limp and pain in groin, anteromedial thigh or knee. The duration of symptoms varies from a couple of days to a fortnight. The affected hip is in attitude of flexion and external rotation. All the attempted movements are painful near the extremes. There may be history of sore throat, tonsillitis or low- grade fever. Leukocytosis and slight increase in sedimentation rate may be present. Radiographs are normal but may show soft tissue swelling in the region of gluteus medius, obturator internus and psoas. Aspiration of hip under aseptic conditions should be performed if differentiation from infective hip arthritis cannot be done.

Toxic synovitis must be differentiated from septic arthritis, tubercular arthritis, avascular necrosis of femoral epiphysis and Perthes disease.[68-70]

Treatment consists of bedrest and traction. Patient's symptoms quickly abate on elimination of weight bearing. Patients are mobilized when they have regained full, painless range of motion and can ambulate without pain and limp. If pain persists or recurs, pyogenic arthritis or avascular necrosis should be suspected. Even if the child becomes asymptomatic and returns to activity, a follow-up visit at 8-12 weeks should be advised to rule out avascular necrosis clinically and radiologically.

Elbow Disorders in Children

Little Leaguer's elbow is seen in adolescents involved in throwing activities, particularly Little League pitching in North America.

Little Leaguer's elbow results from the compressive forces at the radiocapitellar joint and distraction forces in the medial aspect of the elbow. Articular damage to the capitellum, ligamentous laxity of medial elbow ligamentous complex and ulnar nerve neuritis leading to tardy ulnar nerve palsy may result.

Clinically, the patient may present with medial and/or lateral elbow pain. Locking of elbow may occur in severe cases by the loose bodies formed by fragmentation of the capitellum. X-rays may show resorption and fragmentation of capitellum.

Treatment consists of change in throwing activities. Elbow should be splinted for rest and comfort. Arthrotomy or arthroscopy to excise the incarcerated loose fragment may be required.

Osteochondritis dissecans of the capitellum denotes osteochondral defect resulting from repetitive microtrauma or a vascular insult. In the elbow it most commonly involves capitellum (Panner's disease). Clinically the patient presents with pain and swelling over the lateral aspect of the elbow.

Radiologically, the plain X-rays show osteochondral fracture of the capitellum, intra-articular loose bodies and capitellar deformity. Treatment consists of rest and avoidance of throwing activities if fragment is intact and not separated.

Arthroscopic removal is indicated for intra-articular loose bodies. Drilling and bone grafting may help in selected cases.

Osteogenesis Imperfecta (Brittle Bone Disease)

This is one of the commonest heritable bone disorders (1: 20,000 births) characterized by fragility of bones but with wide variation in severity.

The disease is caused by abnormal collagen synthesis (failure of cross-linking) due to mutation in genes that produce type I collagen. Osteogenesis imperfecta is classified into four types:
- *Type I*: Mild
- *Type II*: Moderately severe
- *Type III*: Progressive deforming
- *Type IV*: Severe (often stillbirths).

Type I and II are autosomal dominant while Type III and IV are autosomal recessive.

Salient features are due to involvement of bones, teeth, ligaments or sclerae.

The condition is characterized by excessive fragility of bones, blue sclerae (Figs 111.17A and B), osteoporosis, excessive joint laxity, bowing of bones (Fig. 111.17C) and crumbling teeth or *dentinogenesis imperfecta*. Other features are herniae, deafness (both conductive and sensorineural), and undue ease of bruising with poor scar formation. Deformities, especially scoliosis, chest deformities, trefoil pelvis,

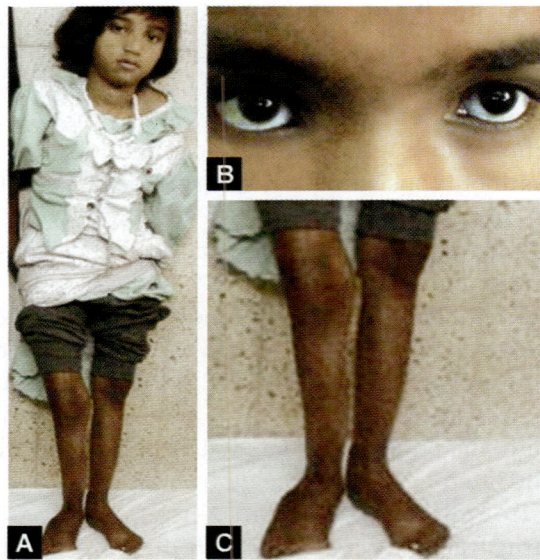

Figs 111.17A to C: A. Clinical picture of osteogenesis imperfecta; **B.** Blue sclerae and deformities of osteogenesis imperfecta; **C.** Note the bowing of bones

biconcave vertebrae and basilar invagination may be seen. X-rays show wormian bones in suture lines, beaded ribs, osteoporosis, thinned cortices and deformities due to malunited fractures. Metaphyses appear expanded. Occasionally a cystic or popcorn appearance is seen due to irregular (curliform) ossification adjacent to the epiphyseal metaphyseal region.

Hyperplastic callus is seen sometimes after fractures. Fractures unite readily and non-union is not a problem. The tendency to fractures reduces with age. The life expectancy can be normal in mild variety whereas severely affected subjects die before reaching adulthood.

Osteogenesis imperfecta (OI) should be differentiated from child abuse (battered baby syndrome). Children with OI have wormian bones, generalised osteoporosis, expansion of metaphysis and metaphyseal fractures (cf. diaphyseal fractures in child abuse) Histologically, there is increased diameter of haversian canals and osteocytic lacunae, increased number of cells and replicated cement lines.

Management comprises of prevention of fractures and correction of deformity whenever indicated. Soffield osteotomies (sheekh kabab bone with intramedullary fixation) are sometimes required for progressive bowing of long bones.[71]

UPPER EXTREMITY MUSCULOSKELETAL TRAUMA

Injuries of the Shoulder Region

Clavicle Fractures

Clavicle is the most often fractured bone in the body. Fortunately due to its intramembranous ossification origin, union is not a problem. Malunion, however, is quite common, as it is quite difficult to control the fracture fragments.

Clavicle fractures often occur in patient with other serious skeletal and extra-skeletal injuries.

Mechanism of Injury

Fractures of the clavicle are caused most often by an indirect injury as fall on the point of the shoulder or on the outstretched hand.[72,73] However, fractures of the clavicle may also result from the direct impact on the clavicle.

Classification

The fractures of clavicle are classified most commonly according to the location viz. fractures of the middle third (85% - including the fractures at the junction of the middle and the lateral thirds which is the commonest location), lateral third (10%) and medial third (5%) of the clavicle.[72,74] Fractures of the clavicle can also be classified as post-traumatic or pathologic (following radiation necrosis in patients with breast carcinoma); another way to classify these fractures would be displaced, undisplaced or greenstick (in children).

Evaluation

Patient with clavicular injuries should be assessed for vital functions and associated injuries. Usually patients with displaced fractures present with pain, deformity and shortening of the clavicle. The patient often supports the injured limb with the other hand. Patient resists any attempts to move the shoulder. Tenderness may be only elicitable sign in patients with undisplaced fractures.

Local bruising appears in cases that present a few days after the injury. A careful neurovascular examination must be done in all cases.

Imaging

A single anteroposterior projection of the shoulder is usually adequate imaging study in adults. However, superimposition of scapula and ribs may not allow adequate visualization of the clavicle. Cephalic angled view gets rid of the superimposition. Cephalad angulation of 15° visualizes lateral two thirds of the clavicle while the X-ray beam may have to be angulated 40° cephalad to visualize the medial third of the clavicle. X-rays confirm the diagnosis and reveal the location of the fracture and the degree of displacement of the fragments. The distal fragment typically sags downwards, forwards and medially while proximal end gets elevated (due to the pull of sternocleidomastoid). Fractures of the distal (or lateral) third of the clavicle are mostly undisplaced as the coraco-clavicular (especially trapezoid) ligaments remain attached to the proximal fragment and prevent its displacement while the acromioclavicular and conoid (lateral part of coraco-clavicular ligament) ligaments remain attached to the distal fragment.

In children the fractures of the clavicle may be very subtle and are difficult to diagnose. Any kinking of the cortical contour should raise the suspicion of clavicle fracture. Including both the shoulders on one film may help in comparison with the normal side.

Associated vascular injuries are rare but when present need angiography.

Management

Any associated injury takes precedence over clavicle fracture for management. The treatment for clavicle fracture is primarily conservative. For undisplaced fractures in children and in elderly, support is provided for the weight of the arm using a sling and these fractures unite readily.[75,76] Displaced fractures are treated with a figure of 8 bandage or commercially available braces applied with the shoulders braced backwards.[77,78] A triangular sling is given to the arm in addition. The aim of these methods is to reduce the overlap of fragments and anterior drift of the scapula around the chest wall as well as to relieve pain. Braces or the bandage has to be re-tightened every few days as it keeps on getting loose. Supports are discontinued as soon as the fracture site becomes non-tender.

Surgical treatment of clavicle fracture is indicated for associated vascular injuries, compound fractures or the displaced fractures of the lateral third of the clavicle with disruption of coraco-clavicular ligaments. Implants used for internal fixation of the clavicle include intramedullary pins or 3.5 mm reconstruction plate with screws.[79] External fixator may be applied for compound fractures.

Complications

Injury to the neurovascular structures (such as brachial plexus or the subclavian vessels) may occur rarely. Vascular injuries are managed by angiography, repair of the vascular injuries and internal fixation of the clavicle fracture. Closed neural injuries are treated expectantly while open injuries need exploration and repair.

Pneumothorax, other thoracic injuries or thoracic outlet syndrome can occur.

Malunion is the commonest complication. Offending and excessive callus may give rise to appearance of a bump under the skin.[79,80] Some remodeling occurs with time and there is no functional disability.[80]

Non-union is rare and reported in 1-5% cases. High-energy fractures, widely displaced fractures, open fractures and inadequate immobilization are commonly implicated caused. Only symptomatic non-unions need management with internal fixation and bone grafting. Shoulder joint stiffness may occur in the elderly. It is managed by physiotherapy to mobilize the joint.

Epiphyseal injury of proximal humeral epiphysis (Type II Salter Harris) occurs in adolescents (13-15 years of age) and is often displaced.[81] Closed reduction is performed by abduction, flexion and external rotation of the arm (*salute* position).[82] Open reduction and stabilization with K-wires is indicated in irreducible cases. Immobilization is continued for 4-6 weeks.

Elbow Injuries in Children

Elbow injuries account for 8-9% of all pediatric fractures. Elbow injuries in children are different from adults due to several peculiar anatomic features. The distal humeral bone is mainly cancellous and undergoing remodeling in children. This fact, along with the hyperextension possible in a pediatric elbow makes supracondylar fracture a very common fracture in this age group. In fact intercondylar fractures and elbow dislocations are much less common in children. Radial neck fractures (usually epiphyseal injuries) are much more common in children than radial head fractures. Medial epicondyle and lateral condyle fractures are other common fractures in children in this region.

Several ossification centers are present around elbow and they sometimes make diagnosis of a fracture difficult. It is always helpful to take radiographs of the opposite elbow for comparison. Average age of appearance of various secondary ossification centers around the elbow is (in order of appearance) **c**apitellum 1 year (6 months-2 years), **r**adial head 3 years (2-4 years), medial (internal) epicondyle 5 years (4-6 years), **t**rochlea 7 years (6-8 years), **o**lecranon 9 years (8-10 years), and lateral (**E**xternal) epicondyle 11 years (10-12 years) - **CRITOE**. Around 10-12 years of age the epiphyseal fuse to each other and to the metaphysis.

Supracondylar Fracture of Humerus

Supracondylar fracture of the humerus is the commonest fracture around elbow in children constituting about 69% of elbow fractures in children. Supracondylar fracture is usually a transverse fracture running just proximal to trochlea and capitellum. The fracture is common during 5-10 years of age and is rare in adults.[83]

Mechanism of Injury

Supracondylar fracture usually results from a fall on the out stretched hand. It can also be caused by direct injury as a fall on the point of the elbow.

Classification

Supracondylar fractures are of two types according to the mechanism of injury.

Extension type is caused by the force, which displaces the distal fragment (i.e. the lower end of the humerus) posteriorly. It is the common type and constitutes almost 97.7 % of the fractures. This is the type, which results from the fall on the out stretched hand.

Flexion type is caused by a force which displaces the distal fragment anteriorly. This type of supracondylar fracture constitutes about 2.3% of fractures.

Extension type of supracondylar fracture of the humerus is further classified by *Gartland* according to the degree of displacement.[84]

I. Undisplaced.
II. Displaced with intact posterior cortex.
III. Displaced without cortical contact.

Posteromedial displacement of distal fragment with varus angulation- more common.

Postero-lateral displacement of the distal fragment with valgus angulation.

The characteristic displacements in a supracondylar fracture in extension are posterior shift, medial/lateral shift, anterior angulation, posterior and medial tilt, internal rotation and overriding.

Evaluation

Patients present with a history of fall following which the elbow becomes painful and swollen. There may an obvious deformity and child is unable to move the elbow. Distal humerus is tender. The normal relationship olecranon and medial and lateral epicondyles is preserved. Dimpling of the skin over the anterior aspect of the distal arm suggests button holing of the spike of the proximal fracture fragment through the brachialis muscle and tethering the skin. Movements at the elbow are not permitted due to pain. Distal neurovascular examination must be performed in all cases.

In cases presenting late with severe swelling around the elbow, with or without encircling bandages, careful examination to rule out Volkmann's ischemia must be performed. Tense forearm, severe pain in the forearm, impairment of two point discrimination sense and pain on passive extension of fingers all suggest Volkmann's ischemia. It is important to note that radial pulse may still be palpable in the presence of established Volkmann's ischemia.

Imaging

Anteroposterior and lateral views of the elbow are usually sufficient to confirm the presence of fracture, type and degree of displacement and presence of comminution.

After the reduction the lateral and anteroposterior "shoot through" X-rays *(Jones view)* are taken to confirm the adequacy of reduction. The following facts should be remembered.

- A "fat pad" sign suggesting hemarthrosis often is the only indication of an undisplaced fracture.
- A minimally displaced fracture is discerned by extending the anterior humeral line distally. Normally, it divides distal humeral physis into anterior one third and posterior two thirds. Subtle posterior tilt of the distal fragment will diminish the fraction of distal physis anterior to the anterior humeral line.
- Sharp spike like appearance of proximal fragment suggests rotational deformity.
- Crescent shaped overlap between the distal humeral physis and olecranon on the lateral view suggests residual medial tilt, which may result in a cubitus varus deformity.

Treatment

Conservative treatment—Undisplaced fractures are treated in above elbow plaster slab in 1200° flexion at the elbow for 3 weeks.

Displaced fractures needing manipulative reduction include:

- Fracture with less than 50% bony contact
- Posterior tilt of the distal fragment by more than 15°
- Lateral or medial tilting of 10° or more
- Presence of rotational deformity
- Evidence of arterial obstruction in the presence of displacement and/or angulation of the fracture.

Technique of manipulative reduction of extension type fracture: The reduction is performed under general anesthesia. Radial pulse is palpated. Traction is applied to the forearm with the elbow in 20° of flexion while the assistant applies the counter-traction at the arm. The fracture fragments are disimpacted. The medial and lateral displacements are corrected and the elbow gently flexed to 120° with a hand on the radial pulse. Disappearance of radial pulse at any stage warrants a reduction in the flexion at the elbow till the pulse just returns. At this stage, pronating the forearm tightens the medial periosteal hinge in cases with medial tilt/lateral angulation (i.e. with varus deformity). Cases with lateral tilt/medial angulation (i.e. with valgus deformity) are managed with the forearm supinated.

Flexion of the elbow over 90° stretches the triceps over the fracture. Triceps than acts as an internal splint and stabilizes the fracture fragments.

Technique of manipulative reduction of flexion type fracture: Flexion type of supracondylar fractures are stable in extension. To reduce these fractures, traction is applied to the elbow in the flexed position to disimpact the fracture fragments. The elbow is then gradually extended and angulation reduced. An above elbow plaster slab is applied in 10° flexion for three weeks. At this time, the slab is removed and elbow is gently flexed.

Alternatively, Sultanpur method of reduction may be used where in a plaster cuff is applied to the arm extending upto the distal end of the proximal fragment. Once this sets the distal fragment is pushed back against this cast with elbow in about 110° flexion and the cast is quickly completed. This method avoids immobilizing the elbow in the extension, thereby reducing the risk of stiffness in this position. Stiffness of the elbow in extension greatly compromises function.

- *After care:* The plaster immobilization is continued for 4 weeks (slightly more in older children). Lack of the tenderness at the fracture site and the X-rays suggest union. Active elbow exercises are started at this stage. A sling may be worn for a few days and discarded as early as the patient is comfortable.
- *Percutaneous pinning:* If image intensifies is available and during reduction, it is discovered that the reduction is achievable but unstable, percutaneous pinning may be performed.[85] Two Kirschner-wires are used and both are introduced from the lateral side either parallel to each other or in a crossed manner. The ends of the wires are bent to avoid migration. The wires are removed after 3 weeks. Percutaneous fixation is also useful for flexion type of supracondylar fractures where it obviates the need for immobilization of the elbow in near extension.

- *Open reduction and pinning:* is used for irreducible fractures, cases where closed reduction cannot be maintained due to inability to flex elbow above 90° (due to severe swelling and disappearance of radial pulse) and in cases with an associated vascular injury.[86] A medial, lateral or anterior approach is used and the fracture is openly reduced and stabilized by crossed K-wires inserted from medial and lateral epicondyles (Figs 111.18A and B). K-wires are removed after 6 weeks.
- *Traction:* Skin (Dunlop) or skeletal (olecranon pin) traction is often useful in cases where the reduction is difficult to achieve or maintain due to significant soft tissue swelling or comminution of the fracture fragments.[87, 88] Traction is also indicated in cases with minimal circulatory impairment, when brachial artery exploration is not indicated.

Traction obviates the need for above 90° flexion at the elbow. Traction can be discontinued at 2-3 weeks and plaster slab can be applied till the fracture unites.

Complications

Vascular injury: Vascular injury is associated with less than 1% cases of supracondylar fractures. The vascular injury can be due to kinking over the proximal fragment, spasm of the vessel, extrinsic pressure by fracture hematoma and swelling, internal thrombus, internal tear, contusion of the vessel, partial or complete tear of the brachial artery.

Tethering of the skin overlying a prominent spike of proximal fragment in the absence of a palpable radial pulse suggests entrapment of the neurovascular bundle and is an indication for urgent exploration. Excessive swelling and bruising around elbow may suggest vascular injury. Other signs of vascular compromise should be looked for in these cases. Often the patient may present with Volkmann's ischemia or rarely frank gangrene of the fingers.

When a patient with vascular compromise is seen, all the encircling bandages are removed. Fracture is reduced by gentle manipulation and the radial pulse checked. If the radial pulse does not return the brachial artery is explored. Peroperatively, the local pressure on the vessel is relieved. The spasm of radial artery is relieved by local application of xylocaine or papaverine or by stripping the adventitia of the vessel, thus effecting sympathectomy. Spasm, which does not get relieved by these maneuvers, is possibly an intimal tear and needs expert vascular intervention. Laceration of the artery needs repair. The fracture should be openly reduced and stabilized with K-wires in all these cases. Acute Volkamann's ischemia is managed by urgent fasciotomy extending right from elbow distally up to the carpal tunnel. The wound is closed secondarily after 3-5 days or skin grafted.

Established cases of Volkmann's ischemic contracture are managed by physiotherapy and splintage when mild. Severe cases need excision of dead and fibrotic muscles correction of deformity (as by Maxpage flexor-pronator muscle slide or forearm/carpus shortening procedures) and restoration of function (using tendon or muscle transfers, nerve grafting).

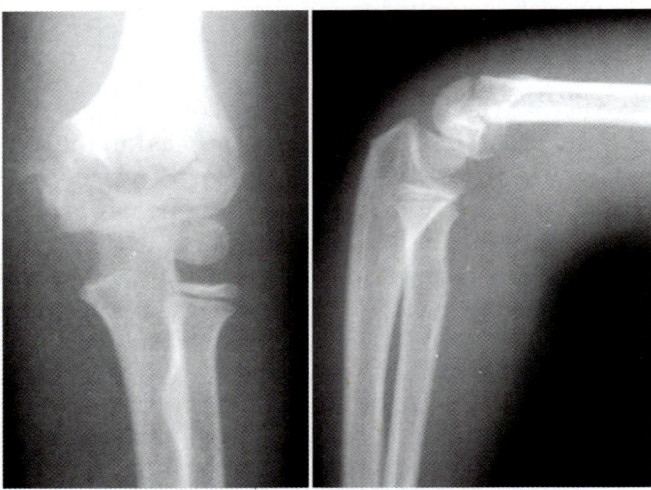

Fig. 111.18A: Lateral AP view of elbow showing supracondylar fracture of humerus

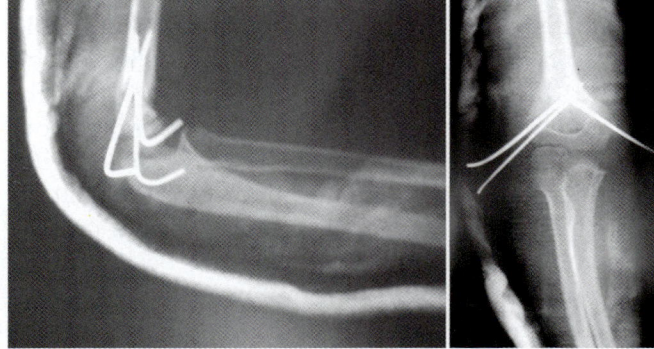

Fig. 111.18B: AP and lateral view of supracondylar fracture humerus stabilized by pinning

Nerve Injury: Nerve injury may be associated with 7% cases of supracondylar fractures of the humerus. The nerve injuries are commonly due to neuropraxia or axonotmesis and recover spontaneously. Radial nerve injury is most common and is seen in posteromedial type of fracture.[89] Median nerve is the next commonest and is involved in the posterolateral type of supracondylar fractures. Ulnar nerve is injured more commonly in flexion type of supracondylar fractures and in overhead skeletal traction. Nerve injuries are treated expectantly. However, if the recovery does not occur spontaneously, the nerve is explored.

Myositis ossificans: Myositis Ossificans is seen most commonly following massage (when fracture is set by osteopaths), repeated closed manipulations and open reduction sometimes, following open reduction.[90]

In the acute stage it presents with pain, swelling, erythema and stiffness. Serum alkaline phosphatase is often raised. On radiographs the calcific mass looks cloudy with ill-defined margins. Any intervention at this stage can aggravate the condition.

Mature myositis is quiescent clinically without attendant features mentioned above and looks well demarcated on radiographs. At this stage an excision of the myositic mass can be attempted if it is likely to improve range of motion at the elbow.

Malunion: Cubitus varus (Gunstock deformity) is the most common deformity following the supracondylar fracture of the humerus.[91] It occurs due to a combination of malunion in the three planes-coronal (medial tilt), sagital (posterior tilt) and horizontal (internal rotation of the distal fragment). The carrying angle at the elbow is reduced and patient has unsightly deformity. Radiographs show crescent sign and reduced Baumann's angle (angle between the line along lateral condylar epiphysis and a line perpendicular to the long axis of the humerus). Treatment is required only for cosmetic reasons. In case the deformity is cosmetically objectionable, it should be treated by lateral closed wedge osteotomy *(French osteotomy)* performed at least one year after the fracture after the remodeling is complete. Cubitus valgus occurs rarely, following the posterolateral type of fracture. This deformity is not cosmetically as objectionable as cubitus varus. A longstanding deformity, however, may result in tardy ulnar nerve palsy, which requires anterior transposition of the ulnar nerve.[92]

Stiffness of the elbow: Minimal loss of flexion is common even in the well-treated supracondylar fractures.[93] Severe stiffness may result in cases with myositis ossificans or when late open reduction is attempted (more than 5 days after injury).

Trans Condylar Fractures

These are type I epiphyseal injuries which usually occur in children less than 3 years of age.[94] Type II epiphyseal injury may occur in older children. The displacement is usually posteromedial. The radiographs confirm the injury and displacement. Treatment is by closed reduction and immobilization in flexion and pronation. Unstable reductions or irreducible fractures are managed by percutaneous or open pinning.

Fractures of the Medial Epicondyle

Fractures of the medial epicondyle are common between 8-14 years of age.[95] Almost 50% of fractures of the medial epicondyle are associated with elbow dislocations.

Mechanism of Injury

The medial epicondyle is fractured by a valgus pull with extension when it is avulsed by the flexor muscle mass and the ulnar collateral ligament.[96] Due to this mechanism, ulnar nerve injury is commonly associated.

Classification

Fracture of the medial epicondyle can be undisplaced or displaced (Fig. 111.19). Displacement can sometimes be intra-articular with the fragment trapped into the joint.

Evaluation

Patient presents with the history of forcible abduction at the elbow followed by pain and tenderness, on the medial aspect of the elbow. Bruising may be present over the medial sides. Ulnar nerve should always be tested.

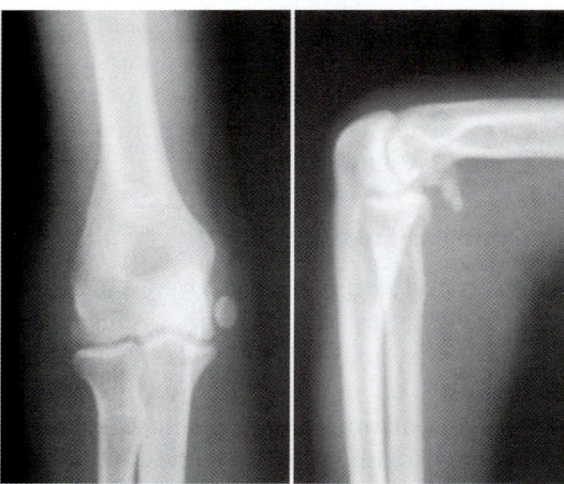

Fig. 111.19: Displaced fracture of medial epicondyle

Imaging

Anteroposterior and lateral views of the elbow should be taken. Radiographs of the opposite elbow taken for comparison can be extremely useful X-ray confirm the fracture and its displacement. Intraarticular displacement of medial epicondylar fragment should be suspected when the medial epiphysis is not seen in AP view in a child over 6 years age, when it is seen on the lateral film, and when the medial epicondylar fragment is seen at the level of the joint line.

Treatment

Conservative treatment is adequate when the fragment is displaced less than 2 mm. Above elbow plaster slab for 3 weeks followed by active exercises is adequate for all cases. Displaced fractures are treated by open reduction and K-wire fixation.

Intra-articular displacement of the medial epicondylar fragment is managed by manipulation under anesthesia. If this method fails, medial epicondyle is retrieved surgically and fixed to its bed using K-wire or soft tissue suture. K-wire is removed after 3 weeks.

The indications for surgery in fractures of medial epicondyle humerus are:
- Displaced fracture in individuals with athletic pursuits
- Acute post-traumatic ulnar nerve palsy and
- Acute incarceration of the medial epicondyle in the elbow joint with failed attempts at closed manipulation.

The methods of closed removal of the incarcerated fragment are as follows:
- *Robert's manipulative method:*[97] extension of elbow, supination of forearm, dorsiflexion of wrist and sudden hyperextension of the fingers causing tension on the common flexor origin may help in removal of the incarcerated fragment.[97] This is effective when done before 24 hours.
- Faradic stimulation has been used by some
- Distension of the joint by air/fluid may help in extraction.

Complications

1. Ulnar nerve injury is common in these fractures. Most ulnar nerve palsies in these injuries are lesions in continuity, i.e. neuropraxia.[98] Recovery usually begins within 3-6 weeks. Tardy ulnar nerve palsy may also occur long after these fractures.
2. Stiffness of the elbow may occur.
3. Weakness of forearm muscle (flexor-pronator group) may occur if a significantly displaced medial epicondylar fracture is left untreated.

Fracture of the Medial Condyle

This is a rare injury in children and is often missed. Injury is seen between 8-14 years of age. It is caused by an extension and valgus stress. The fracture is classified by Milch according to anatomical location as type I (fracture line passes through the apex of trochlea) and type II (fracture line passes through the capitello-trochlear groove).[99] Milch I is caused by impaction by radial head while Milch II is caused by impaction by olecranon. The fragment displaces anteromedially by pull of flexors and medial collateral ligament. Impacted or undisplaced fractures are treated in an above elbow cast. Displaced fractures, especially with rotation, are treated with open reduction and internal fixation. Complications include non-union with cubitus varus, delayed union and tardy ulnar nerve palsy.

Fracture of the Lateral Epicondyle

It is a very rare injury and is often missed as it is confused with the normal physeal line. The epiphysis usually appears at the age of 11 years and fuses 2-3 years later. Avulsion of the lateral epicondyle occurs following adduction stress. Comparison with radiographs of the opposite side is extremely helpful. If the displacement is less than 2 mm, the injury is treated in above elbow slab for 3 weeks. Greater displacements need open reduction and fixation with K-wire or soft tissue suture.

Fracture of the Lateral Condyle

The fracture of the lateral condyle occurs in 16.8% of elbow fractures and in 54.2% of physeal injuries around elbow. The injury is common between 4 to 8 years of age.

Mechanism of Injury

Extension and varus forces lead to avulsion of the lateral condyle. Lateral condylar fractures can also be caused by valgus stress over the elbow in which case it is fractured by shearing force.

The fragment is displaced by forearm extensors or the lateral ligament. Lateral condyle fractures are divided into two types according to Milch.[99] In type I, the fracture line extends lateral to trochlea through the capitello-trochlear groove. It is a type IV epiphyseal injury. In type II, the fracture line extends into the apex of the trochlea. It is a type II injury.

The lateral condyle fractures can also be classified as undisplaced, displaced or rotated.

Evaluation

Child presents with history of trauma followed by pain and swelling of the elbow. Tenderness is present over lateral aspect of the elbow. Crepitus may be present over the lateral aspect. Movements of the elbow are painfully restricted.

Imaging

Plain radiographs of the elbow confirm the diagnosis and degree of displacement of the fragment. Size of the fragment as visualized on the X-ray is much smaller than the real size of the fragment when encountered during the surgery due to the large cartilaginous component of the fragment.

Treatment

Undisplaced fractures are treated in above elbow cast for 4 weeks.[100] However, radiographs should be taken at weekly intervals to ensure that no late displacement of the fracture occurs.

For displaced fractures, especially with rotation conservative treatment is not effective. Open reduction and internal fixation with K-wires is recommended.[100] The blood supply to the fragment enters from the posterior aspect and this aspect of the fragment should not be stripped of the soft tissues. Following surgery above elbow cast is applied for four weeks. Active exercises are started at the end of this period.

Complications

- Delayed union or non-union is common in these cases.[101] Non-union leads to progressive cubitus valgus deformity and tardy ulnar nerve palsy.[102] The latter is treated by anterior transposition of ulnar nerve. Supracondylar osteotomy may be indicated sometimes to correct the deformity.
- Avascular necrosis of the fragment occurs in operated cases where excessive soft tissue stripping is done
- Premature physeal growth arrest may occur
- Lateral condylar overgrowth may be seen
- Myositis ossificans may occur
- Cubitus valgus occurs due to non union and/or epiphyseal growth arrest and can be progressive.

Pulled Elbow (Nursemaids Elbow; Guyrand's Elbow)

Pulled elbow occurs in young children (2-3 years old) due to ligamentous laxity. It is a hyperpronation injury, which leads to subluxation of radial head and partial displacement of the annular ligament. The parents give history of fall the child by holding his/her hands with forearm pronated. The child is often crying and refuses to use his upper limb, which hangs by the side of the body. Radiographs do not reveal any abnormalities and are not needed for diagnosis or treatment. Treatment consists of supination of the forearm with elbow flexed. The resumption of hand usage by the patient is immediate. No after care is required.

Fracture of Radial Neck

Fractures of radial neck occur in children. Metaphyseal compression is most common but often these injuries are type II epiphyseal injuries. These fractures may be associated with other injuries around elbow in almost half the cases.

Mechanism of injury

This injury is caused by fall on the outstretched hand.

Classification

Radial neck fractures can be undisplaced or displaced. Displaced fractures with the tilt of radial head from horizontal than 30° are treated differently from those with more than 30° tilt.

Evaluation

Patient presents with history of fall on the outstretched hand and pain in the elbow following that. There is tenderness over the lateral aspect of the elbow. Elbow and forearm movements are painfully restricted.

Imaging

Plain radiographs confirm the diagnosis and displacement of the fragment. Diagnosis is extremely difficult in a child younger than 3 years when radial head is not visualized on X-rays. High index of suspicion is required for diagnosis in these cases.

Treatment

Undisplaced fractures and with fractures less than 30° tilt of the radial head are treated conservatively in a plaster slab for two weeks.

Greater displacement is treated by manipulation to reduce the fracture under anesthesia. With the elbow extended a varus stress is applied to the elbow that one hand and the radial head is pushed into place with the fingers of the other hand. Failing manipulative reduction, open reduction is performed. The fracture is usually stable after reduction and is treated in a POP slab for two weeks. Transcapitellar wire into the head and neck of radius to fix the fracture has high rate of complications (breakage, migration of wire) and should be avoided.

Forearm Fractures

The radius and ulna are held together at the proximal and distal radio-ulnar joints, by annular ligament proximally, interosseous membrane along the length and the triangular fibrocartilage distally. These anatomical features do not allow only one forearm bone to fracture and shorten without disrupting either proximal or distal articulation between the two bones. The commonest fracture dislocation of this type is a fracture of ulna with dislocation of the radial head— the *Monteggia* fracture dislocation. A fracture of the shaft of radius associated with dislocation of inferior radio-ulnar joint is called *Galeazzi* fracture dislocation.

Fractures of the forearm bones are common in all age groups. In adults these fractures often result from the high-energy trauma, often with associated musculoskeletal and systemic injuries.

Mechanism of injury

Fractures of the radius and ulna can be caused by direct as well as indirect injury. Direct injury is commonly due to warding off blows, which commonly results in ulna fractures. These fractures are transverse and may be compound. Indirect injury occurs due to fall on outstretched hand and produces oblique or spiral fractures. *Monteggia* fracture dislocation can be the result of hyperpronation (indirect) or night stick (direct) injuries.

Classification

Forearm fractures are classified according to the location or configuration of the fractures. They are also characterized by the presence of dislocation of radio-ulnar or radio-humeral joints.

Monteggia fractures are classified into four types by *Bado*:[103]

Anterior type (Type I) has anterior dislocation of radial head with proximal third ulna fracture angulated anteriorly. This is the commonest type (60%).

Posterior type (Type II) has posterior dislocation of radial head with proximal third ulna fracture angulated posteriorly.

Lateral type (Type III) has lateral radial head dislocation with lateral angulation of proximal ulnar fracture.

Type IV proximal third both bone forearm fractures of the forearm with anterior dislocation of the radial head.

Monteggia Variants in Children

The injuries are considered to be the equivalent of the *Monteggia* fracture in children:

Type I: Plastic deformation of proximal 1/3rd of ulna.

Type II: Greenstick fracture of proximal 1/3rd of ulna.

Type III: Isolated radial head dislocation.

Type IV: Fracture of both bones forearm with radial fracture proximal to ulna.

Hume's fracture refers to the fracture of the proximal third of ulna with anterior dislocation of the radial head in children.

It should be remembered that in the proximal third fractures of the forearm bones, the proximal fragment of radius is supinated by biceps while the distal fragment is pronated by pronator teres and pronator quadratus. In the mid or distal third fractures the proximal fragment is in neutral position as the biceps and pronator teres are both attached to it.

Greenstick fractures in children are seen on X-rays as breech of only one cortex. *Torus fractures* caused by compression force are seen as buckling of the cortex in metaphyseal region.

Treatment

Conservative treatment is used in children, in undisplaced or minimally displaced fractures in adults, fractures in elderly and in patients in whom anesthesia or surgery is contraindicated. Manipulation under anesthesia is attempted in patients with displaced fracture, preferably under image intensifier and the forearm is immobilized in above elbow cast with elbow in 90° flexion for 12-16 weeks. Close follow up must be done for these patients, as there is a very high incidence of redisplacement. Weekly X-rays should be taken during the first 3 weeks and plaster checked for loosening or breakage. Undisplaced fractures can be managed by replacing the long-arm cast with a functional fracture brace with good interosseous moulding in the second week.

Monteggia fracture-dislocations are treated with open reduction and rigid internal fixation of ulna using AO 3.5 mm DCP. Radial head generally gets reduced spontaneously at this stage. Irreducible radial head is an indication for open reduction to address infolding of the annular ligament, entrapment of posterior interosseous nerve or incarceration of the radial head behind the lateral epicondyle. After surgery the limb is immobilized in above elbow cast in 110° flexion (to keep the anteriorly unstable radial head reduced) except in type II Monteggia where posteriorly dislocated head is stable in less than 90° (usually 70°) flexion after the reduction. The immobilization is discontinued after 6 weeks.

Galeazzi fracture dislocation: This consists of a fracture of the lower 1/3rd of the radius with dislocation of the distal radioulnar joint (DRUJ). It is often referred to as a fracture of necessity (c.f. lateral condylar physis injuries). This is because the fracture of distal radius are preferably immobilized in full pronation while the most common dislocation of the DRUJ is posterior which is stable only in full supination. The injury must therefore be treated with open reduction and internal fixation of radius (through an anterior approach using AO 3.5 mm DCP) and above elbow cast in supination for 6 weeks for the more common type with dorsal subluxation of ulna. Volar subluxation of ulna is treated with immobilization in pronation after internal fixation of the radius fracture.

Complications

1. Compartment syndrome may occur in patients with gunshot wounds, open fractures and fractures with vascular injury. High index of suspicion in needed for early diagnosis. Compartment pressures should be measured in doubtful cases. Early fasciotomy can preserve function.
2. Neurologic injury is otherwise uncommon in these fractures but posterior interosseous nerve palsy may complicate Monteggia fracture-dislocation.
3. Non-union is seen after conservative treatment if immobilization is ineffective or discontinued too

soon. Comminuted fractures and fractures which are not rigidly fixed at surgery are also prone to develop non-union. Treatment of non-union is autogenous bone grafting and rigid internal fixation.

4. Malunion is common with conservative treatment. It leads to deformity and restricted rotations. Severe malunion may warrant redoing the fracture followed by anatomical reduction and rigid internal fixation. Malunited Monteggia fracture-dislocations present with persistent radial head dislocation. Treatment includes ulnar osteotomy, plating after anatomic reduction and radial head excision in adults. In children, radial head should not be excised in order to avoid progressive instability at the elbow. Attempt should be made in these cases to openly reduce radial head and reconstruct the annular ligament using a fascial (*Bell-Tawse* procedure: fascial strip is taken from the tricipital fascia) or tendon graft.[104]

5. Cross union occurs in 3% cases and is common if the fractures are at the same level (most common in upper 1/3rd fractures) or are fixed by single incision allowing the fracture hematomas to communicate, if the fractures are caused by high-energy injuries, cases with infection, associated closed head injuries, if bone grafts are placed on the interosseous membrane during surgery and also following radial head excision. Cross union (proximal radio-ulnar synostosis) occurs more commonly following Monteggia fracture-dislocation.

6. Hardware related complications such as loosening, infection, breakage, etc.

7. *Missed associated dislocation:* Radial head dislocation is frequently missed when associated with proximal ulnar fractures. A useful clue is that normally in a lateral view of the elbow, throughout the range of flexion, a line along the longitudinal axis of the radius should always bisect capitellum.

Distal Radius Epiphyseal Injury

Distal radius epiphyseal injuries are common in adolescents. These are usually Salter Harris type II injuries and occur following fall on the outstretched hand. Diagnosis is easily made on radiographs. Anatomic reduction is mandatory for satisfactory results. Reduction should be done early. Displaced fractures are treated by manipulative reduction and below elbow Colles' plaster cast for 3-4 weeks. Growth disturbance is rare.

LOWER EXTREMITY MUSCULOSKELETAL TRAUMA

Fracture Neck Femur in Children

Fractures of femoral neck in children are treated with closed reduction and internal fixation using multiple Moore's or Knowle's pins. Surgery is done on the fracture table with the image intensifier. The fracture can be reduced in flexion or extension.

Reduction in Flexion

Traction is applied in the line of femur with the hip and the knee in 90° flexion and internal rotation at the hip. With the traction and internal rotation at the hip maintained, the hip is gradually extended and abducted. Reduction is checked under image intensifier/X-rays (Leadbetter tecnique).

Reduction in Extension

Traction is applied in the line of femur with hip and knee extended and 15-20° abduction and external rotation at the hip. The limb is firmly internally rotated fully to reduce the fracture and reduction checked under image intensifier/X-rays (Whitman technique).

Following reduction, the pins are inserted from the greater trochanter into the head of the femur. Pins should not cross the physis (Fig. 111.20).

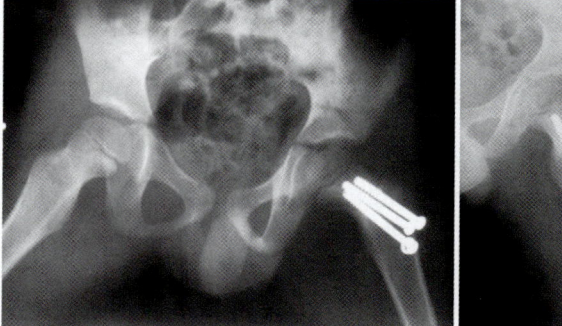

Fig. 111.20: AP and lateral views of fracture neck femur in a child stabilized by screws

The patients should be immobilized in a one and a half hip spica for 8-12 weeks following fixation.

If a femoral neck fracture is not treated, the femoral neck starts getting resorbed by the end of four weeks and marked up riding of greater trochanter occurs. Accurate anatomical reduction becomes impossible in these cases. The following methods of treatment are available for those cases which are neglected/detected after three weeks:

In children with neglected femoral neck fracture, an intertrochanteric valgus (or (abduction) osteotomy with internal fixation and or spica is the method of choice. Free fibular graft can be used across the fractures in these cases to provide fixation and enhance bone stock.

Fractures of the Femoral Shaft

Fractures of the femoral shaft result from severe injuries and are commonly associated with other serious injuries. The bone is enveloped by well vascularized musculature, which sustains considerable trauma in association with the shaft fracture. The compound femoral fractures are uncommon due to thick overlying soft tissue envelope. Considerable bleeding occurs from femur fracture and up to 1500-ml blood may be lost without any evidence of external bleeding.

Mechanism of Injury

Severe trauma, as in motor vehicular accidents, falls from height or natural calamities (as in earthquakes) leads to femoral shaft fracture. Bomb blast and gunshot wounds can lead to femoral shaft fractures along with severe injury to the soft tissues.

Pathological fractures of the femoral shaft occur commonly in association with various benign and malignant lesions located in the shaft.

Any patient with suspected femoral shaft fracture must undergo a quick assessment of vital parameters and resuscitation should be instituted immediately. Two wide bore no. 14 venflons must be used to access venous system and samples sent for blood group and cross matching, and hematocrit. Intravenous ringer lactate infusion should be started. Patient should be evaluated to rule out cranial, abdominal, thoracic and pelvic injuries.

Local examination reveals marked shortening, swelling and deformity of the thigh. The attempted movements are painful and the patient is unable to lift the leg. Any breech in the skin should be presumed to be an open fracture. Severely tense thigh should raise the suspicion of a compartment syndrome and warrants pressure measurement of the thigh compartments. A careful and detailed neurovascular examination of the extremity should be performed. Other skeletal injuries commonly associated with femoral shaft fracture should be looked for and include acetabular fractures, pelvic ring fracture, ipsilateral hip dislocation, patella fracture and ligamentous disruptions of the knee.

Imaging

Imaging for suspected femoral shaft fracture should include anteroposterior and lateral radiographs of the entire femur. Ipsilateral hip and knee X-rays must be taken to look for associated fractures. An anteroposterior view of pelvis must be taken in all patients with femoral shaft fractures as a screening tool for pelvic ring injury or acetabular fractures. An internal rotation view of the hip to visualize femoral neck is mandatory to rule out associated femoral neck fracture. Adduction of the proximal fracture fragment indicates associated posterior dislocation of the ipsilateral hip.

Treatment of Femoral Shaft Fractures

All patients with femoral shaft fracture are treated initially with resuscitation. Intravenous fluid infusion, blood transfusion and splintage. The femoral shaft fracture can be treated by both conservative as well as surgical means though surgical treatment has become the mainstay in recent times.

Conservative Treatment—Conservative treatment is the method of choice in infants and children.

Infants younger than 2 years are treated in the Gallow's or Bryant's traction.[105] Adhesive tape is applied on bilateral legs and traction rope through the tape is attached to an overhead point so that buttocks of the infant are just off the bed. Body weight acts to align the fragments and 3 weeks in this traction are sufficient to achieve union. This type of traction is

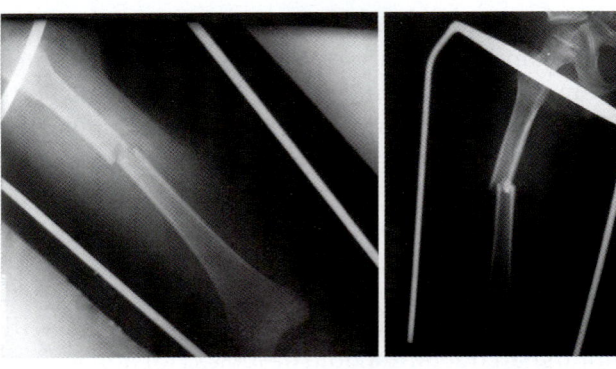

Fig. 111.21A: Lateral and AP view of femur showing shaft fracture

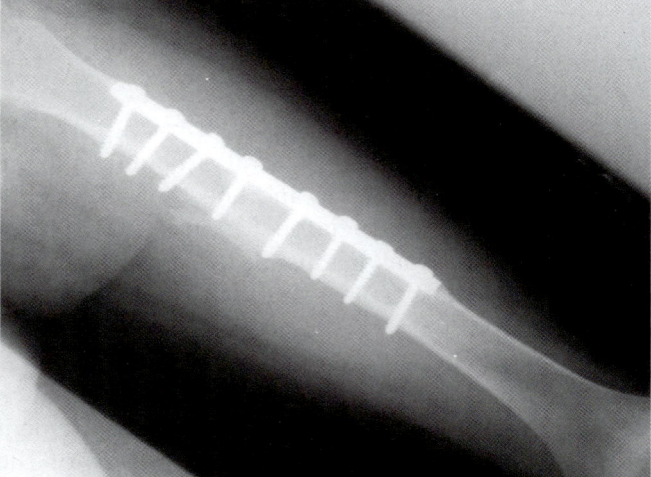

Fig. 111. 21B: Fracture stabilized by plating with union of fracture

contraindicated in older children as it can lead to compromise of the vascularity to the lower limbs.

Older children can be treated in fixed skin traction on Thomas splint or by sliding traction through an upper tibial (tensioned) Kirschner-wire with the thigh supported on a pillow. The fracture usually takes about 6 weeks to heal. Internal fixation with plating may be done in patients with polytrauma or floating knee (Figs 111.21A and B).

Distal Femoral Epiphyseal Injury

Separation of the distal femoral epiphysis (Type 3 Salter and Harris type) is a rare injury, which occurs in adolescents. Classically, the injury is sustained by a severe hyperextension force when the person is trying to ride on a cart while running after it. The epiphysis is displaced anteriorly and laterally and sharp spike of the proximal fragment can injure the popliteal artery. The diagnosis is evident on X-rays. The treatment is urgent closed reduction under anesthesia. The reduction may be stabilized by fixing the fragments using smooth Kirschner-wires. A long leg last is applied with knee flexed 60° for 6 weeks. The knee is mobilized at the end of this period and weight bearing started. The growth disturbance following the injury is uncommon.

Fractures of Tibia and Fibula

Fractures of tibia and fibula are the commonest long bone fractures. The spectrum of injuries causing these fractures ranges from repetitive cyclic stress loading leading to fatigue fractures to extreme high-energy injuries leading to severe disruption and loss of soft tissue structures and bone. Close to one fourth of all the patients may present as open injuries and soft tissue management is the key factor in the management of these fractures.

Mechanism of Injury

The commonest cause of the both bones fracture in children is the indirect injury where the foot is caught somewhere and the twisting force causes an isolated fracture of the tibia. Other causes are road traffic accidents, fall from height and other high-energy injuries. The type of injury determines the configuration of the fracture - torsion forces produce spiral fractures while direct injury (bending force) produces a transverse fracture. High-energy torsion and combinations of bending with torsion or compression lead to comminuted fractures.

Classification

Tibial and fibular fractures can be classified as closed or open. Open fractures are classified by Gustilo's classification.[106] No standardized classification for fracture pattern is available but a simple way is to classify these fractures into three types: simple (spiral, oblique or transverse), fractures with a butterfly fragment and comminuted (including segmental and crush) fractures.

Evaluation

Initial assessment includes vital function evaluation, examination for associated injuries and resuscitation. Other skeletal injuries in the affected extremity should be looked for. Local examination reveals deformity, which is readily apparent since tibia is mostly subcutaneous. The limb is shortened in cases with displaced fractures. Pain, tenderness and abnormal mobility is present at the fracture site. Soft tissues are inspected circumferentially for skin wounds, ecchymosis and any evidence of compartment syndrome. Neurovascular examination of the limb is extremely important and should be recorded.

Imaging

Anteroposterior and lateral radiographs are adequate for diagnosis and assessment of the fracture. It is imperative to include ipsilateral knee and ankle in the radiographs.

Treatment of Fractures of the Both Bones of the Leg

Treatment of fractures of the both bones of the leg is determined by the condition of soft tissues and location and configuration of the fracture and the nature of associated injuries. In treatment of fractures of both bones of the leg, fibula is ignored and treatment is planned mainly for the tibia fracture.

Conservative Treatment—Conservative treatment is the most commonly used method of treating fractures of the both bones of the leg in children. This method is applicable to closed fractures and grade I compound (skin opening < 1 cm, most likely from inside out) fractures. Rarely, fracture may have to be reduced under anesthesia. The fracture is then immobilized in an above knee plaster cast. Fractures where acceptable reduction is achieved are monitored with weekly check X-rays to detect redisplacement of the fracture. Accepted guidelines for reduction are atleast 50% cortical contact, varus/valgus up to 10°, anteroposterior angulation up to 10°, less than 10° rotational malalignment and less than 1 cm shortening. The immobilization is discarded after 6 to 8 weeks, once the radiological evidence of union appears.

REFERENCES

1. Ogden JA. Skeletal growth mechanism injury patterns. J Pediatr Orthop 1982;2:371-77.
2. Peters W, Irwing J, Letts M. Long-term effects of neonatal bone and joint infection on adjacent growth plates. J Pediatr Orthop 1992;12:806-10.
3. Edwardson P, Syversen SM. Overgrowth of the femur after fracture of the shaft in childhood. J Bone Joint Surg 1976;58B:339-46.
4. Sanders WE, Heckman JD. Traumatic plastic deformation of the radius and ulna: A closed method of correction of deformity. Clin Orthop 1984;188:58-67.
5. Giberson RG, Ivins JC. Fractures of the distal part of the forearm in children: Correction of deformity by growth. Minn Med 1952:35:744.
6. Cavendish ME. Congenital elevation of the scapula. J Bone Joint Surg 1972: 54-B;395.
7. Ross DM, Cruess RI. The surgical correction of congenital elevation of scapula. Clin Orthop 1977:125:17.
8. Wickstrom J. Birth injuries of the brachial plexus. Treatment of defects in the shoulder. Clin Orthop 1962;23:187-96.
9. Hardy AE. Birth injuries of the brachial plexus. J Bone Joint Surg 1981;63-B (1):98-101.
10. Leffert RD. Brachial plexus injuries. N Engl J Med 1974;291:1059-67.
11. Shoul ML, Ritvo M. Clinical and roentgenological manifestations of the Klippel-Feil syndrome. AJR 1972;68:369.
12. Ferkel RD, Westin GW, Dawson EG, Oppenheim WL. Muscular torticollis. A modified surgical approach. J Bone Joint Surg 1983;65-A,894.
13. Cleary JE, Omer GE. Congenital proximal radio-ulnar synostosis. Natural history and functional assessment . J Bone Joint Surg (Am)1985;67-A: 539-45.
14. Zaricznyj B. Centralization of ulna for congenital radial hemimelia. J Bone Joint Surg 1977;59-A: 694.
15. Bayne LG, Costas BL. Malformations of the upper limb. In: Morrissy RT (Ed): Lovell and Winter's Pediatric Orthopaedics. 3rd Ed. Philadelphia PA: JB Lippincott Co. 1990:577.
16. Temtamy S, Mckusick VA. Polydactyly. Birth defects 1978;14:364.
17. Dinham JM, Meggitt DF. Trigger Thumbs in children. J Bone Joint Surg 1974;56-B:153.
18. Boyes JG. Macrodactylism - A review and proposed management. Hand 1977;9:172.
19. Askins G, Ger E. Congenital constriction band syndrome. J Pediatr Orthop 1988;8:461.
20. Moen KY, Nachemson AL. Treatment of scoliosis. A historical perspective. Spine 1999;24:2570-75.
21. Bradford DS, Heithoff KB, Cohen M. Intraspinal abnormalities and congenital spine deformities. A radiographic and MRI study. J Pediatr Orthop 1991;11:36.

22. Weinstein SL, Ponseti IV. Curve progression in idiopathic scoliosis. J Bone Surg 1983;65-A;447.
23. Moe JH. Indications for Milwaukee brace non operative treatment in idiopathic scoliosis. Clin Orthop 1973;93:38.
24. Rhee JM, Bridwell KH, Won DS, et al. Sagittal plane analysis of adolescent idiopathic scoliosis: the effect of anterior versus posterior instrumentation spine 2002;27(21):2350-56.
25. Fredrickson BE, Baker D, Mc Hollick WJ, Yuan H, Lubicky J. The natural history of spondylolysis and spondylolisthesis. J Bone Joint Surg 1984;66-A:699.
26. Freeman BL III, Donati NL. Spinal arthrodesis for severe spondylolisthesis in children and adolescents: A long term follow up study. J Bone Joint Surg Am 1989;71:594-98.
27. Bennett JT, Mac Ewen GD. Congenital dislocation of the hip. Recent advances and current problems. Clin Orthop 1989;247:15.
28. Boeree NR, Clarke NMP. Ultrasound imaging and secondary screening for congenital dislocation of hip. J Bone Joint Surg (British) 1994;76-B:525.
29. Kalamachi A, Mac Farlane R 3rd. The Pavlik Harness: Results in patients over 3 months of age. J Pediatr Orthop 1982;2:3.
30. Galpin RD, Roach JW, Wenger DR, et al. One-stage treatment of congenital dislocation of the joint in younger children, including femoral shortening. J Bone Joint Surg 1989;71-B:734.
31. Langenskiold A, Riska EB. Tibia vara (osteochondrosis deformans tibiae). A survey of seventy - one cases. J Bone Joint Surg Am 1964;46:1405-20.
32. Schoenecker A, Johnston R, Rich MM, et al. Elevation of medial plateau of the tibia in the treatment of Blount disease. J Bone Joint Surg Am 1992;74(3):351-58.
33. Rab GT. Oblique tibial osteotomy for Blount's disease (tibia vara). J Pediatr Orthop 1988;8:715.
34. Morrissy RT, Riseborough EJ, Hall JE. Congenital pseudarthrosis of the tibia. J Bone Joint Surg Br 1981;63:367.
35. Dobbs MB, Rich MM, Gordon JE, et al. Use of an intramedullary rod for study. J Bone Surg Am 2004;86-A(6):1186-97.
36. Dewar FP, Hall JE. Recurrent dislocation of the patella. J Bone Joint Surg Br 1957;39:798.
37. Hall JE, Micheli U, Mc Namara GB Jr. Semitendinosus tenodesis for recurrent subluxation or dislocation of patella. Clin Orthop 1979;144:31.
38. Ooishi T, Sugioka Y, Matsumoto S, Fujii T. Congenital dislocation of the knee. Clin Orthop 1993;287:189.
39. Ferris B, Aichroth P. The treatment of congenital knee dislocation. Clin Orthop 1987;216:135.
40. Carroll NC. Pathoanatomy and surgical treatment of the resistant clubfoot. Instr Course Lectures 1988;37:93.
41. Simons SW. A standardized method for the radiographic evaluation of clubfeet. Clin Orthop 1978;135:107.
42. Noonan KJ, Richards BS. Nonsurgical management of idiopathic club foot. J Am Acad Orthop Surg 2003;11:392.
43. Goldner JL. Congenital talipes equinovarus-fifteen years of surgical treatment. Curr Pract Orthop Surg 1969;4:61.
44. Wenger DR, Maudlin D, Speck G, et al. Corrective shoes and inserts as treatment for flexible flatfoot in infants and children. J Bone Joint Surg Am 1989;71:800.
45. Gianninni BS, Caccarelli F, Benedetti MG, et al. Surgical treatment of flexible flat foot in children, a four-year follow up study. J Bone Joint Surg Am 2001:83(suppl 2): 73.
46. Morrey BF, Peterson HA. Hematogenous pyogenic osteomyelitis in children. Orthop Clin North Am 1975;6:935-51.
47. Abernethy IJ, Lee YC, Cole WG. Ultrasound localization of subperiosteal abscesses in children with late-acute osteomyelitis. J Pediatr Ortjhop 1993;13:766-68.
48. Boutin RD, Brossmann J, Sartoris DJ, et al. Update on imaging of orthopedic infections. Orthop Clin North Am 1998;29:41-66.
49. Gentry LO. Antibiotic therapy for osteomyelitis. Infect Dis Clin North Am 1990;4:485-99.
50. Chung SM. The arterial supply of developing proximal end of human femur. J Bone Joint Surg Am 1976;58: 961-70.
51. Kocher MS, Mandiga R, Murphy JM, et al. A Clinical practice guideline for treatment of septic arthritis in children. Efficacy in improving process of care and effect on outcome of septic arthritis of the hip. J Bone Joint Surg Am 2003;85:994-99.
52. Betz RR, Cooperman DR, Wopperer JM, et al. Late sequalae of septic arthritis of the hip in infancy and childhood. J Pediatr Orthop 1990;10:365-72.
53. Arnold WD, Hilgartner MW. Hemophilic arthropathy. Current concepts of pathogenesis and management. J Bone Joint Surg 1977;59-A:87.
54. Valderrama JAF de, Matthews JM. The hemophilic pseudotumor or hemophilic subperiosteal hematoma. J Bone Joint Surg 1965;47-B:56.
55. White GC II, McMillan CW, Blatt PM, Roberts HR. Factor VIII inhibitors: A clinical overview. Am J Hematol 1982;13:335.
56. Salter RB, Thompson G. Legg-Calve-Perthes disease. The prognostic significance of the subchondral fracture and a two-group classification of the femoral head involvement. J Bone Joint Surg 1984;66-A:479.
57. Inoue A, Freeman MAR, Vernon-Roberts B, Mizuno S. The pathogenesis of Perthes' disease. J Bone Joint Surg 1976;58-B:453.
58. Caffey J. The early roentgenographic changes in essential coxa plana: Their significance in pathogenesis. AJR 1968;103:620.
59. Caterall A. The natural history of Perthes disease. J Bone Joint Surg 1971;53-B: 37.
60. Bohr H. On the development and course of Legg-Calve-Perthes disease. Clin Orthop 1980;150:30.
61. Scoles PV, Yoon YS, Makley JT, Kalamachi A. Nuclear magnetic resonance imaging in Legg-Calve-Perthes disease. J Bone Joint Surg 1984; 66-A:1357.

62. Salter RB. The present status of surgical treatment for Legg-Perthes disease. J Bone Joint Surg 1984;66-A:961.
63. Speer DP. Experimental epiphysiolysis. Etiologic models of slipped capital femoral epiphysis. In, The Hip. Proceedings of the Hip Society. St Louis, Mosby, 1982; 68-88.
64. Crawford HB. Ten cases of marked slipping of the upper femoral epiphysis. Clin Orthop 1966;48:129.
65. Steel HH. The metaphyseal blanch sign of slipped capital femoral epiphysis. J Bone Joint Surg 1986;68-A:920.
66. Asnis SE. The guided screw system in slipped capital femoral epiphysis. Contemp Orthop 1985;11:27.
67. Irani RN, Rosenzweig AH, Cotler HB, Schwenther EP. Epiphyseodesis in slipped capital femoral epiphysis. A comparison of various surgical modalities. J Pediatr Orthop 1985;5:661.
68. Kocher MS, Zurakowski D, Kasser JR. Differentiating between septic arthritis and transient synovitis of the hip in children. An evidence based clinical prediction algorithm. J Bone Joint Surg Am 1999;81:1662-70.
69. Song J, Letts M, Monson R. Differentiation of psoas muscle abscess from septic arthritis of the hip in children. Clin Orthop 2001;258-65.
70. Zawin JK, Hoffer FA, Rand FF, et al. Joint effusion in children with an irritable hip: US diagnosis and aspiration. Radiology 1993;187:459-63.
71. Sofield HA, Millar EA. Fragmentation, realignment and intramedullary rod fixation of deformities in the long bones in children. J Bone Joint Surg Am 1959;41:1371.
72. Nordqvist A, Petersson C. The incidence of fractures of the clavicle. Clin Orthop 1994; 300:127-32.
73. Stanley D, Trowbridge EA, Norris SH. The mechanism of clavicular fractures. A clinical and biomechanical analysis. J Bone Joint Surg [Br] 1988;70:461-64.
74. Al-Etani H, D'Astous J, Letts J, et al. Masked rotatory subluxation of the atlas associated with fracture of the clavicle: a clinical and biomechanical analysis. J Bone Joint Surg [Am] 1998; 80:1477-83.
75. Andersen K, Jensen PO, Lauritzen J. Treatment of clavicular fractures. Figure-of-eight bandage versus a simple sling. Acta Orthop Scand 1987;58:71-74.
76. Stanley D, Norris SH. Recovery following fractures of the clavicle treated conservatively. Injury 1988;19:162-64.
77. Sankarankutty M, Turner BW. Fractures of the clavicle. Injury 1975;7:101-06.
78. Mullick S. Treatment of mid-clavicular fractures. Lancet 1967:499.
79. Kubiak R, Slongo T. Operative treatment of clavicle fractures in children: A review of 21 years. J Pediatr Orthop 2002;22(6):736-39.
80. Post M. Current concepts in the treatment of fractures of the clavicle. Clin Orthop 1989;245:89-101.
81. Burgos-Flores J, Gonzales-Herranz P, Lopez-Mondejar JA, et al. Fractures of the proximal humeral epiphysis. Int Orthop 1993;17:16-19.
82. Neer CS 2nd, Horowitz BS. Fractures of the proximal humeral epiphysial plate. Clin Orthop 1965;41:24-31.
83. Henrikson B. Supracondylar fracture of the humerus in children. Acta Chir Scand 1966; 369(suppl).
84. Gartland JJ. Management of supracondylar fractures of the humerus in children. Surg Gynecol Obstet 1959 109(2):145-54.
85. Wilkins KE. Supracondylar fractures: what's new? J Pediatr Orthop B 1997;6(2):110-16.
86. Reitman RD, Waters P, Millis M. Open reduction and internal fixation for supracondylar humerus fractures in children. J Pediatr Orthop 2001;21(2):157-61.
87. Agus H, Kalenderer O, Kayali C, Eryanilmaz G. Skeletal traction and delayed percutaneous fixation of complicated supracondylar humerus fractures due to delayed or unsuccessful reductions and extensive swelling in children. J Pediatr Orthop B 2002;11(2):150-54.
88. Prietto CA. Supracondylar fractures of the humerus. A comparative study of Dunlop's traction versus percutaneous pinning. J Bone Joint Surg (Am) 1979;61(3):425-28.
89. Sairyo K, Henmi T, Kanematsu Y, et al. Radial nerve palsy associated with slightly angulated pediatric supracondylar humerus fracture. J Orthop Trauma 1997;11(3): 227-29.
90. Kramhoft M, Keller IL, Solgaard S. Displaced supracondylar fractures of the humerus in children. Clin Orthop Relat Res 1987;(221):215-20.
91. Pirone AM, Graham HK, Krajbich JI. Management of displaced extension-type supracondylar fractures of the humerus in children. J Bone Joint Surg (Am) 1988;70(5):641-50.
92. Mitsunari A, Muneshige H, Ikuta Y, et al. Internal rotation deformity and tardy ulnar nerve palsy after supracondylar humeral fracture. J Shoulder Elbow Surg 1995;4(1 Pt 1):23-29.
93. Henrikson B. Supracondylar fracture of the humerus in children. A late review of end-results with special reference to the cause of deformity, disability and complications. Acta Chir Scand 1966;369(Suppl):1-72.
94. Moucha CS, Mason DE. Distal humeral epiphyseal separation. Am J Orthop 2003;32:497-500.
95. Wilson NIL, Ingran R, Rymaszewski L, et al. Treatment of fractures of the medial epicondyle of the humerus. Injury 1988;19:342-44.
96. Smith FM. Medial epicondyle injuries. JAMA 1950;142: 396-402.
97. Roberts NW. Displacement of the internal epicondyle into the joint. Lancet 1934;2:78-79.
98. Dias JJ, Johnson GV, Hoskinson J, et al. Management of severely displaced medial epicondyle fractures. J Orthop Trauma 1987;1:59-62.
99. Milch H. Fractures and fracture-dislocations of humeral condyles. J Trauma 1964;4:592-607.
100. Jakob R, Fowles JV. Observations concerning fractures of the lateral humeral condyles in children. J Bone Joint Surg 1975; 40:430-36.
101. Flynn JC, Richards JF. Non union of minimally displaced fractures of the lateral condyle of humerus in children. J Bone Joint Surg (Am) 1971; 53:1096-101.

102. Gay JR, Love JG. Diagnosis and treatment of tardy paralysis of the ulnar nerve. J Bone Joint Surg 1947;29:1087-97.
103. Bado JL. The Monteggia lesion. Clin Orthop 1967;50:71-86.
104. Bell-Tawse AJS. The treatment of malunited anterior Monteggia fractures in children. J Bone Joint Surg [Br] 1965; 47:718-23.
105. Holmes SJ, Sedgwick DM, Scobie WG. Domiciliary gallows traction for femoral shaft fractures in young children. Feasibility, safety and advantages. J Bone Joint Surg Br 1983;65:288-90.
106. Gustilo RB, Anderson JT. Prevention of infection in the treatment of one thousand and twenty-five open fractures of long bones: retrospective and prospective analyses. J Bone Joint Surg Am 1976;58:453-58.

CHAPTER 112

Conjoined Twins

Htut Saing, DK Gupta

Conjoined twins, one of the rarest congenital anomalies, have always fascinated the public, attracted intense media attention and challenged the surgeon caring for them. Even nature has pointed towards the existence of this entity in other living beings like plants and animals (Figs 112.1A and B). It is a rare opportunity for a pediatric surgeon during his or her professional career to encounter the challenge to separate conjoined twins. This chapter emphasizes the more common features of conjoined twins and their management.

HISTORICAL BACKGROUND

The earliest recorded case of conjoined twins is that of the 'Biddenden maids' born in England in 1110.[1,2] Bondeson who reviewed their history, also wrote about other cases of historical interest.[2] The first successful separation of omphalopagus conjoined twins by ligation of a small bridge of tissue at the level of the umbilicus has been attributed to Konig in 1689.[3]

The most famous conjoined twins were Chang and Eng, who were born in 1811 in Siam, as Thailand was previously called, giving rise to the misnomer Siamese twins. They were the first-born sons of a half-Chinese and half-Siamese mother and a Chinese father and were known in their native land as the Chinese twins. A narrow band of tissue measuring 3.5 inches across and 7.5 inches in circumference joined them at the epigastrium. Their mother noted that the junction was initially so short that the boys were always compelled to be face to face and in bed, they had to be lifted and placed in the desired position. As they grew, the union

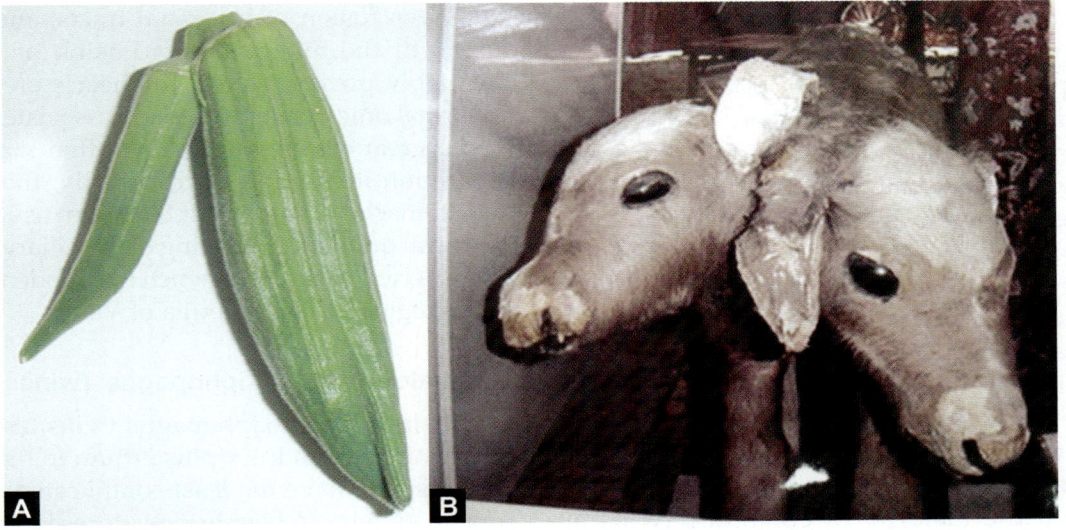

Figs 112.1A and B: Conjoined twins in nature: **A.** Lady finger, **B.** Photograph of a craniopagus twins in a calf displayed during the horse and cattle show, Lahore, Pakistan

gradually stretched so that they could stand side by side, and even back to back, and to turn themselves in bed, they rolled over one another.[4]

The twins emigrated to the United States and PT Barnum exhibited them in his circus shows. This resulted in conjoined twins being viewed as freaks. However, they were very popular and Chang and Eng became wealthy. They changed their family name to Bunker and married two sisters, English ladies 26 and 28 years of age, respectively. Chang and Eng retired as farmers in North Carolina and fathered 22 children between them.[1,5,6] On January 12, 1874, at the age of 63, following chest infection, Chang died. Eng refused to be separated, and he died 6 hours later, probably due to exsanguination through the conjoined bridge of tissue. The band of tissue which united Chang and Eng was found to be composed of some muscle with a thin bridge of liver tissue, a situation which would have allowed easy separation during life as well as after the death of Chang.

INCIDENCE AND ETIOLOGY

The exact incidence of conjoined twinning is unknown but is estimated to be approximately 1 in 50,000 deliveries. Since two-thirds are either stillborn or die soon after birth, the incidence ranges from 1 in 100,000 to 1 in 200,000.[7-10] In the Edmonds and Layde study from the United States, 40% of conjoined twins were stillborn, 35% survived only one day, and 25% survived long enough to undergo surgery.[10]

The etiology of conjoined twinning is unclear but is thought to be due to an aberration of the normal twinning process which occurs at about 20 days postovulation or a few days earlier.[11,12] Conjoined twins are monozygotic, monochorionic twins with identical chromosome patterns.[13] One theory suggests that complete separation of the inner cell mass within the chorionic vesical does not occur, and the resulting non-separated parts of the otherwise normal twins remain attached throughout development. Another theory is that the inner cell mass separates, but reunion occurs, giving rise to twins who are attached.[14] The high incidence of discordant anomalies unrelated to the site of union suggests that environmental influences may also play a role.[15,16]

Although the majority of conjoined twins are externally symmetrical, they can differ in size and personality, and have differences in energy metabolism.[17,18] Their viscera are usually neither similar nor mirror images of each other.

CLASSIFICATION OF CONJOINED TWINS

Symmetrical conjoined twins are classified according to the dominant anatomical area of union followed by the Greek root word "pagos", meaning —that which is fixed". This classification is informative and convenient for clinical use.[19] The five basic types are: thoracopagus, joined at the chest (40%); omphalopagus or xiphopagus, joined by the anterior abdominal wall with the union extending from the xiphoid process to the umbilicus (33%); pygopagus, joined at the buttocks (19%); ischiopagus, joined at the single pelvis (6%), and craniopagus, joined at the heads 2% (Figs 112.2A to H).[20] Ischiopagus twins are further grouped as ischiopagus bipus, tripus and tetrapus based on the number of lower limbs present. Recently, nomenclature based on the theoretical site of union has been proposed to facilitate identification of the pertinent anatomy of the twins.[21] However, this classification has not enjoyed widespread clinical use as yet.

Thoracopagus Twins

Thoracopagus twins are the most common type. They lie face to face, sharing varying degrees of fusion of the sternum, thoracic cage, diaphragm, and the abdominal wall down to the umbilicus (Figs 112.3A and B). Seventy-five percent have conjoined hearts, 50% have fusion of intestinal tracts, and 25% have fusion of the biliary tree.[22] Fusion of the liver is invariably present. When the hearts are joined, the abnormal union of ventricles and associated anomalies of the great arteries and veins often make surgical separation impossible. Occasionally, the esophagus and stomach are single, but the union usually starts in the distal duodenum. Joining of the biliary tree should be suspected particularly when the duodenum is single in the region of the Ampulla of Vater.

Omphalopagus or Xiphopagus Twins

Omphalopagus or xiphopagus twins also face each other, joined from the xiphisternum to the umbilicus. They usually have the least complicated union of all conjoined twins. A liver bridge is present in two-thirds of the cases. The peritoneal cavity of one may or may not communicate with that of the other. An

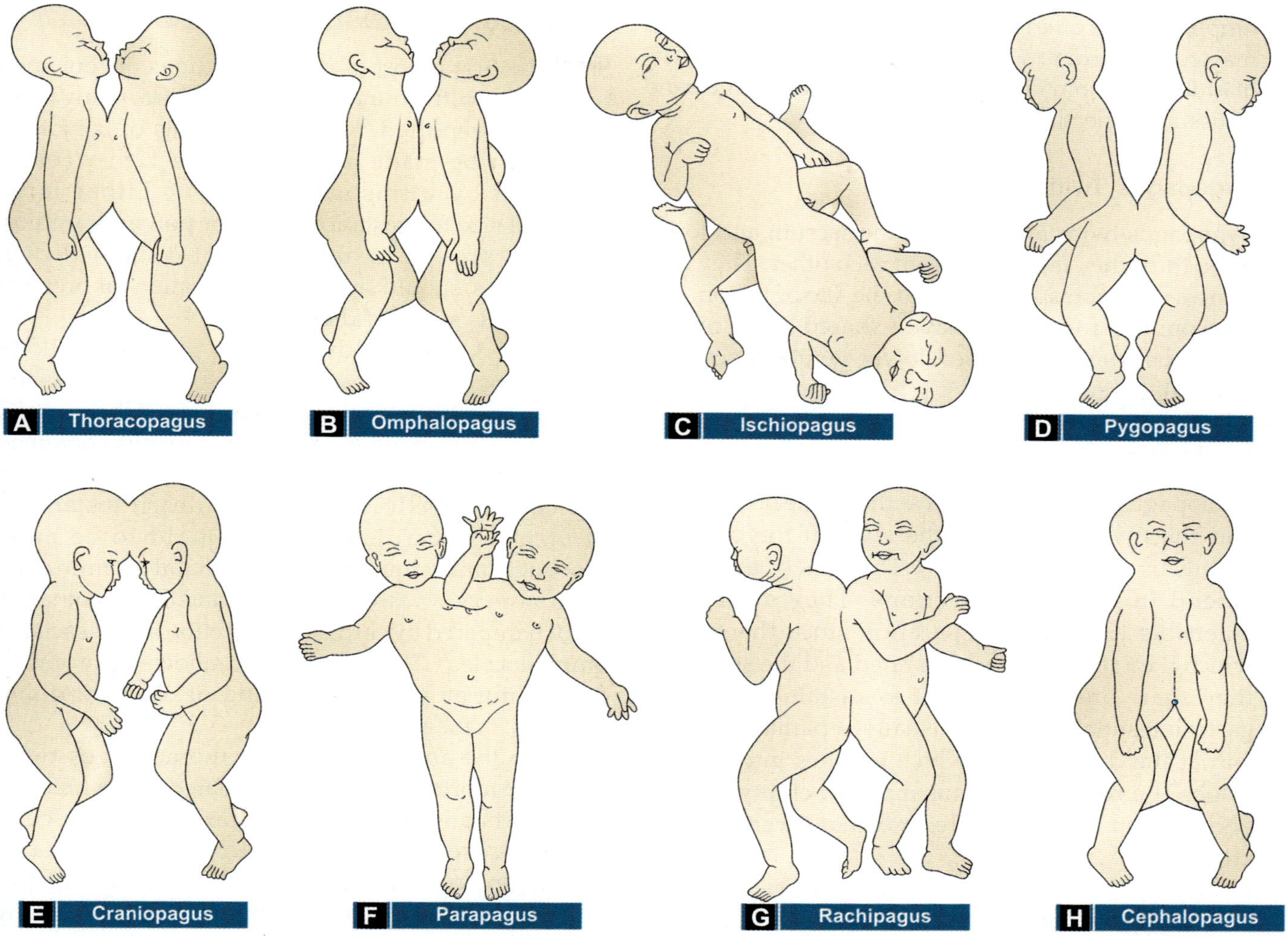

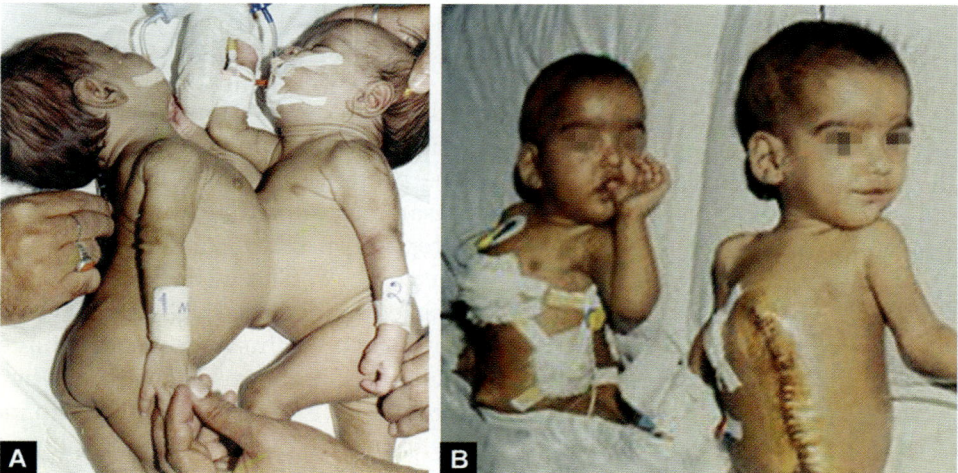

Figs 112.2A to H: Classification of conjoined twins

Figs 112.3A and B: A. Thoracopagus twins fused from the xiphisternum down to the umbilicus that were separated successfully **B.** The twins after separation omphalocele is often present. The single umbilical cord may contain from two to seven umbilical vessels. The bladders may join via each child's urachus in the band of tissue connecting the twins.

Pygopagus Twins

Pygopagus twins are joined at the sacrum and lower back; thus, they face away from each other. They may share a common spinal canal at the site of fusion, and it is common for them to have a shared lower rectum and anus, as well as fused lower genital tracts and external genitalia.

Ischiopagus Twins

Ischiopagus twins are united at the single bony pelvis, and the fusion begins at the level of the common umbilicus (Figs 112.4A to G). The axes of the bodies extend in opposite directions. They are mostly amenable to surgical separation since the organs, which they share, can be separated and the structures they share are not essential to sustain life. Upper gastrointestinal tracts are usually separate but often join at the distal ileum, which empties into a single colon. The rectum and anus may not empty into the perineum and may require proximal diversion soon after birth.

Craniopagus Twins

Craniopagus twins are rare. Joined at the heads, the union may be at the vertex, occiput or lateral parietal areas of the skull. The two brains may be connected by a bridge of neural tissue and have large intracranial vascular connections. Based on the location of the junction, the fusion of the brain tissue and the venous structures requiring interruption at operation, craniopagus twins have been reclassified.[23]

Asymmetrical Conjoined Twins

Unequal and asymmetrical conjoined twins in whom one is smaller and dependent on the other are called heteropagus conjoined twins. This type of twinning is extremely rare, occurring in about 1 or 2 per million live births.

PRENATAL DIAGNOSIS AND EVALUATION

Since the first report of *in utero* findings of conjoined twins using ultrasound in 1977 by Wilson, many cases have been reported.[24-29] The diagnosis of conjoined twins can be made as early as the 12th week of gestation by ultrasonography.[30,31] Either large maternal size for gestational age, or polyhydramnios, which is present in about 50% of conjoined twin pregnancies, should serve as an indication for prenatal sonographic study of the mother.

Detailed scanning during later pregnancy allows assessment of shared hearts and associated anomalies, such as an omphalocele. Echocardiography is useful in the prenatal evaluation of thoracopagus conjoined twins and the presence or absence of cardiac junction has been correctly determined in each instance.[32] *In utero* echocardiogram is thought to be more thorough and simpler than postnatal examination since more views can be obtained, and the examination is not hampered by cardiac conjunction and associated omphalocele.[32] This information allows appropriate counseling as well as planning of obstetrical and neonatal management.

Since the ability to separate thoracopagus twins and their mortality are directly related to the union of two hearts and the associated cardiac and vascular anomalies, reliable prenatal evaluation may play a significant role in deciding whether to consider termination of pregnancy. Computerized tomography (CT) and magnetic resonance imaging (MRI) have been introduced antenatally and provide additional detailed imaging.[33,34]

OBSTETRICAL MANAGEMENT

Although conventional hazardous vaginal delivery has been possible in many instances, particularly in the presence of a flexible connecting bridge, timely cesarean section in the presence of well-informed and prepared pediatricians and surgeons may improve survival.[35,36] The introduction of prenatal diagnosis has led to increased delivery by cesarean section and salvage of twins who would have succumbed if delivered by vaginal delivery.[37] When conjoined twin pregnancy is diagnosed, the pregnant mother should be transferred, with minimal delay and publicity to a center with special expertise or experience in

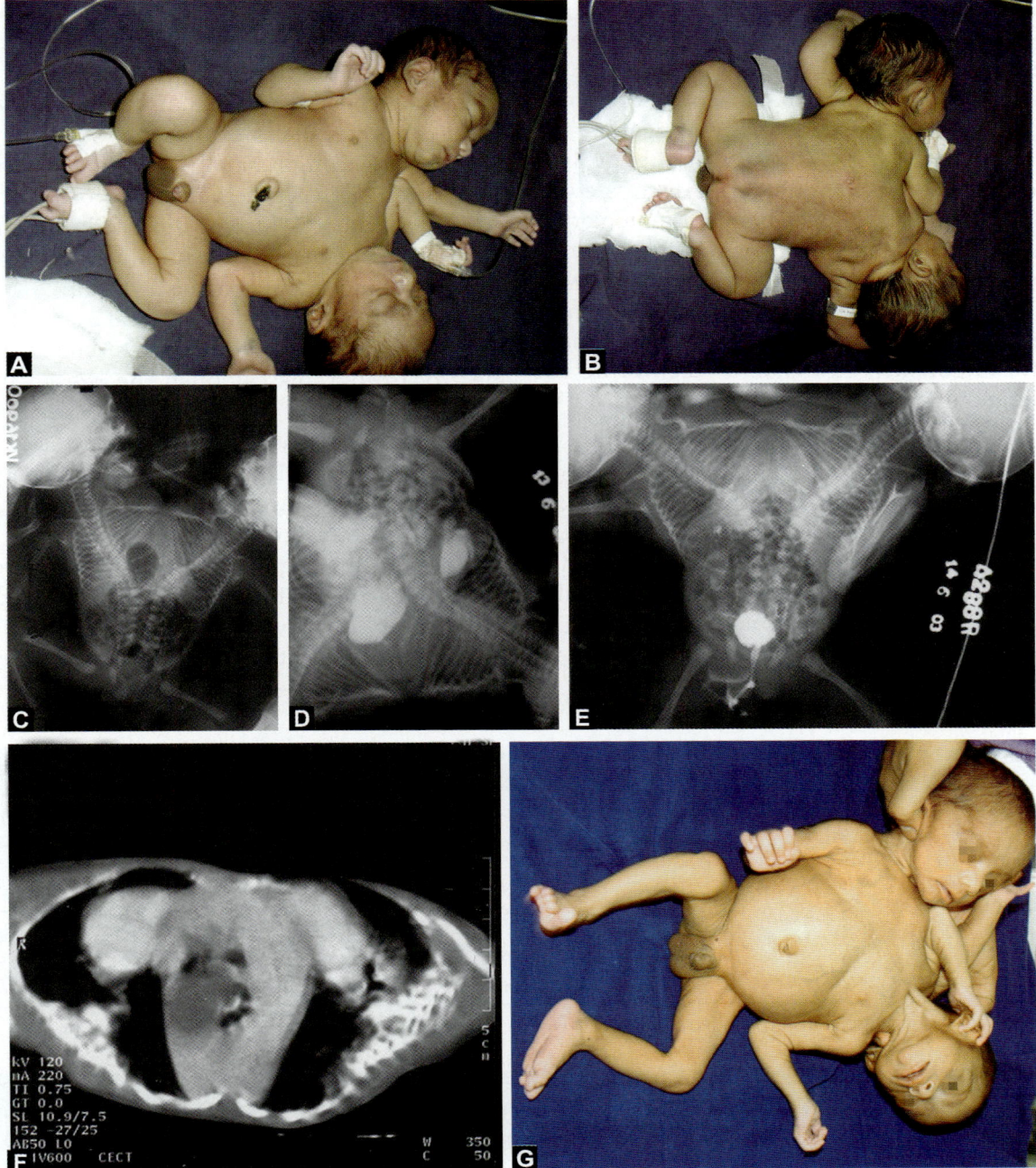

Figs 112.4A to G: Parapagus conjointed wins that were admitted at 12 hrs after birth by vaginal delivery. The combined weight was 3250 gm. There was early cyanosis in one twin that disappeared. The babies had normal feeding activity, **A and B.** The babies had two separate heads and upper chest, four upper limbs, lateral fusion with chest and abdomen, two vertebral columns, two legs, a single urinary outlet and a single bowel outlet, On investigation, there was a single liver with good uptake on HIDA, two hearts without any anomaly, four lungs; though compressed, two spines; each with a spinal cord, two each of stomach and duodenum but single distal colon and a normal single anus, **C.** Skiagram of the babies depicting two spines, **D and E.** On contrast study, the babies had two kidneys, 2 ureterus, but one urinary bladder and one urethra **F.** CT scan of the pelvis **G.** The parents were poor and not willing to undergo treatment. Thus the decision for separation was deferred

separation procedures. If prenatal transfer is not possible, early postnatal transfer of the twins should be arranged.

Appropriate perinatal management of conjoined twins has been outlined by many investigators.[16,27-29,32,33,35] If mothers with conjoined twins go into premature labor because of intrauterine distress, every effort should be made to stop labor in order to permit the fetuses to become as mature as possible to avoid respiratory distress syndrome. Amniocentesis with analysis of the lecithin/sphingomyelin ratio, which indicates when the fetus has achieved pulmonary maturity, is considered a useful technique for determining the timing of Cesarean delivery.[16]

POSTNATAL EVALUATION

Following initial resuscitation and physical examination, special investigations are essential, depending on the site and extent of union. Knowledge of potential visceral and bony unions in a particular set of twins serves as a useful guide to the choice of diagnostic imaging studies. Table 112.1 summarizes the possible visceral unions in different types of conjoined twins as described by Votteler.[20] Based on this information, appropriate diagnostic imaging studies can be performed (Table 112.2).

In thoracopagus twins, comprehensive evaluation of the cardiovascular system is mandatory. If this has not been assessed prenatally, it should be performed soon after birth since there is a possibility of an abnormality that is incompatible with life in one or both twins. The degree of separation of the two hearts is the most important prognostic factor.

Two separate pulses on physical examination and two independent QRS complexes on simultaneous electrocardiograms establish the presence of two separate hearts.[38] A single QRS complex on electrocardiography is present when the hearts are fused. The single QRS complex often appears in one twin as a mirror image of that seen in the similar limb leads of the other twin. Other non-invasive studies include echocardiography, which has been found to be extremely useful for cardiac evaluation, and MRI.[32] In addition, invasive angiographic studies will be necessary to delineate the intracardiac anatomy, blood flow, and anomalies of the great vessels.[39]

Table 112.1: Possible visceral unions in conjoined twins							
Type	Incidence[20] (%)	Heart and great vessels	Liver and biliary tract	Upper GI tract	Lower GI tract	GU tract	Nervous system
Thoracopagus	40	Yes	Yes	Yes	-	-	-
Omphalopagus	33	-	Yes	Yes	Yes	Yes	-
Pygopagus	19	-	-	-	Yes	Yes	Yes
Ischiopagus	6	-	Yes	Yes	Yes	Yes	-
Craniopagus	2	-	-	-	-	-	Yes

Abbreviations: GI-gastrointestinal; GU-genitourinary

Table 112.2: Diagnostic evaluation for conjoined twins											
	Plain XR	CXR	ECG	Echo	Cardiac cath	UGI	BE	IVU	LS	CT	MRI	Angio
Thoracopagus	√	√	√	√	√	√	–	–	√	√	√	–
Omphalopagus	√	√	√	√	√	√	√	–	√	√	√	–
Pygopagus	√	–	–	–	–	√	√	√	–	√	√	√
Ischiopagus	√	–	–	–	–	√	√	√	–	√	√	√
Craniopagus	√	–	–	–	–	–	–	–	–	√	√	√

Abbreviations: Plain XR-plain X-ray; CXR-chest X-ray; ECG- electrocardiogram; Echo- echocardiogram; Cardiac cath-cardiac catheterization; UGI-upper gastrointestinal series;
BE-barium enema; IVU-intravenous urogram; LS-radionuclide liver scan; CT-computed tomography; MRI-magnetic resonance imaging; Angio-angiography

Estimation of cross-circulation and admixture of the two circulatory systems is of practical importance since it allows the surgeon and the anesthetist to estimate the response to drug and anesthetics, or fluid and blood replacement. Spencer et al reported a technique of estimating the blood exchange from one twin to the other.[40] Radionuclide cardioangiography has also been used to estimate the degree of cross-circulation.[41] The rate of mixing due to cross-circulation is greatest in thoracopagus twins, especially in those with conjoined hearts or when there are significant vascular connections at the liver bridge or elsewhere.[42] Failure to recognize this or to take adequate preventive measures can result in the death of one twin.[43] The rate of cross-circulation in twins with less complicated unions is sufficiently low as to be of little clinical importance.

Thorough evaluation of hepatobiliary and pancreatic systems utilizing ultrasonography and radionuclide scans is extremely important. Instances in which the extrahepatic biliary tract is single and shared by both infants have been documented.[16,43-45] Since the majority of thoracopagus twins share a common liver, it is essential to ascertain whether the hepatic venous outflow drains into the inferior vena cava of the same side or not. Without hepatic drainage, survival after separation is not possible. Thorough investigations must be carried out before and during separation to determine the status of the liver, extrahepatic biliary tree, pancreas and duodenum.[46]

Depending on the level of junction, all forms of conjoined twinning except craniopagus, frequently share the gastrointestinal tract. In thoracopagus and omphalopagus twins, the junction can frequently be as high as the level of the duodenum.[43-45] However, in pygopagus and ischiopagus twins, the junction is usually at the terminal ileum, in the region of the Meckel's diverticulum. In these forms of twinning, imperforate anus may be present. The alimentary tract should, therefore, be carefully evaluated with contrast studies.

Urinary tract evaluation is particularly important in ischiopagus twins. It is done by ultrasound, intravenous urogram and cystography to obtain information on the function and number of kidneys, ureters and bladders. Further assessment of the genitourinary system is obtained with cystoscopy under anesthesia. Since most conjoined twins are female, the vagina should be assessed by ultrasound, vaginography and vaginoscopy. Whether or not the vaginas are duplex, the presence or absence of a cervix, a urogenital sinus and a hydrocolpus should be looked for. In males, proper evaluation of the penis and the scrotal contents is essential. If there is a possibility of gender change, discussion and consent of the parents must be obtained before surgery.

A thorough evaluation of the pelvis and the shared third lower limb by angiography is important in ischiopagus twins. CT and MRI are especially important to understand complicated bony unions and to visualize organ sharing in pygopagus and ischiopagus twinning. Large veins and arteries may communicate between the fused pelves in ischiopagus twins and knowledge of the blood supply to the shared limb will help in making a decision about limb salvageability and to which twin the limb should be given.[16,47,48] Conventional radiographs, CT with 3-D reconstruction, and MRI may be needed to evaluate the pelves, vertebral columns and the pelvic structures in ischiopagus and pygopagus twins. MRI, in particular, is becoming the preferred diagnostic tool, especially in the assessment of craniopagus and pygopagus twins.[46] Axial, coronal and sagittal views allow good assessment of neuroanatomy and pelvic floor muscles.

Craniopagus twins are assessed by CT scanning, digital substraction angiography, MRI and radionuclide scans. Electroencephalography, though often employed, does not help to determine cerebral connection but serves as a basis for future comparison.[49]

In complex forms of twinning such as ischiopagus tripus, evaluation of skin perfusion has been described by perfusion flurometry, which utilizes a specially designed light retransmission probe and a microcomputer to integrate photometric reception. This technique allows assessment of viability of large skin flaps required to close the abdominal wall and lower extremity.[50]

ETHICAL CONSIDERATIONS

Conjoined twins raise serious moral and ethical considerations.[51] Avoidance of publicity from the time of antenatal diagnosis, delivery, postnatal period of investigations and growth, surgical separation and after discharge, is the surgeon's responsibility. Transfer of conjoined twins immediately after delivery to centers with experience in surgical separation is desirable. Great care must be taken to protect the twins' and family's privacy and to resist all efforts by the media to create a "media circus".

The surgeon-in-charge must develop a close relationship with the family since many difficult decisions may lie ahead in the management of the twins. A careful and thorough preoperative evaluation must be performed before detailed discussions with the parents. The welfare of the conjoined twins should be paramount in discussions of investigations and management. Legal and ethical issues must be dealt with prior to emergent or elective separation. The survival of the twins, which is of great importance, must be balanced against the expected quality of life and the wishes of the parents. Where possible, consultations with surgeons familiar with the problems of separation of conjoined twins should be conducted.

It may become apparent that only one twin can survive the separation if there are conjoined hearts, or in situations where there is only one set of hepatic veins draining the liver. In twins with conjoined hearts, the question of sacrificing one twin so that the other may live is a difficult decision for both the family and the surgeon. It is important to understand that both twins would die without separation, and with separation, at least one life may be saved. It is the inherent anatomical conjunction rather than the complexity of the operation, which usually determines the outcome of separation. The Judeo-Christian attitude towards this subject is summarized in the Hastings Center Report.[52]

Thorough consultation with the parents is essential before decisions can be made on allocation of organs based on the data available. When there are no medical differences between the twins, management and allocation of organs must be individualized at separation. However, when one twin is obviously mentally or physically impaired, allocation should be directed toward the healthier twin to give this child as normal a life as possible.[53] Care must be taken to ensure the legal propriety of any course of action taken that may endanger the life of one twin at the expense of the other. Although life as conjoined twins would appear intolerable, there are historical as well as current examples of conjoined twins who have become relatively well-adjusted adults. Therefore, in certain situations, it may be wiser not to attempt separation.[54]

All discussions should take place in an atmosphere devoid of undue pressure from politicians, the curious, and the mass media that are out for sensationalism, as well as from inexperienced doctors or administrators who do not possess adequate knowledge of anticipated surgical procedures and results.

TIMING OF SURGICAL SEPARATION

Timing for separation should be decided on a case-by-case basis. Simple separations without life-threatening operative risks may be carried out at around three to six months of age. This allows for growth and physiological maturation of the infants, and before socialization begins. In addition, this reduces the time the parents are required to care for the conjoined twins before they grow large enough to become unwieldy and difficult to nurse as a conjoined pair of twins. For more complex separations, the timing may be delayed to around nine to twelve months. If the operation is delayed beyond one year, twins may have difficulty in developing an independent personality.

Emergency operations with or without separation of conjoined twins may be required before completion of diagnostic studies. Gans et al have proposed absolute indications for separation in the neonatal period.[55] An urgent operation is indicated when one twin is stillborn or unresponsive to resuscitation; if there are severe uncorrectable anomalies or clinical situations such as severe cardiac disease or advanced necrotizing enterocolitis in one twin which threatens the survival of the other; intestinal obstruction; respiratory failure; or if there is trauma to the connecting bridge, e.g. a ruptured exomphalus.[16,43,56-59] In cases of twins with significant cross-circulation, unless emergency separation is performed, the death of one twin is rapidly followed by that of the other, and is probably caused by 'exsanguination' of the live twin into the dead twin's circulation.[49]

PREOPERATIVE PLANNING

It is highly desirable that a team of experienced pediatric surgical specialists and anesthesiologists perform separation of conjoined twins. The separation should be a well-planned and rehearsed procedure.

While a single team of surgeons will perform the initial separation, the surgeon-in-charge must form a separate and complete team for each child, with appropriate specialists standing by to assist if needed. A multidisciplinary team should be organized comprising of surgeons, anesthesiologists, neonatologists and pediatricians, operating room and circulating nurses, and neonatal or pediatric intensive care nurses. Hematology and biochemical laboratories, the blood bank, respiratory therapists, physiotherapists and others should be informed well ahead of the planned separation.

Preoperative discussions should include diagramming of the positions and movements of the team, a review of the placement of the various equipment including two sets each of instruments, operating tables, anesthetic machines, ventilators, fluid and blood replacement pumps and stands, cardiovascular and temperature monitors, and warming equipment. The estimates of blood volume and cross-circulation should be conveyed to the team well in advance. The importance and method of estimating blood loss for both twins together initially and individually after separation must be emphasized and planned.

Rehearsal is mandatory in order to achieve coordination of personnel and to plan placement of equipment. Infant resuscitation mannequins of approximate size or even soft toys may be used. Color-coding of all tubes, drains, equipment and monitoring leads, is helpful in order to avoid confusion during the separation. Scrubbing and draping must be carefully practiced during the rehearsals since these aspects may be totally new to all except those who have experience in the separation of conjoined twins. The need for one or two operating rooms will be dependent upon the size of operating theatres in the hospital. While others have recommended the use of two operating rooms, the author has utilized only one operating theatre on each of the four occasions where separations were performed and found it to be totally acceptable and convenient.

ANESTHETIC MANAGEMENT

Anesthetic management of conjoined twins has been reported by several authors.[60-63] Similar to surgical teams, two experienced teams of anesthetists headed by the lead anesthetist and two complete sets of equipment are necessary for the separation. Because of the possibility of rapid cross-circulation and the anatomical configuration, the administration of anesthesia to conjoined twins may be difficult. The pharmacological effect of the drugs used will be dependent on the speed of cross-circulation and mixing between the twins and the distribution of the anesthetic agents in the tissues. Major shunting in most cases is venous. Hence, inhalation anesthetics given to one will have less effect on the other. Thiopentone, which has high tissue solubility, will also have little clinical effect on the other twin. Since succinylcholine is distributed to both vascular and extracellular compartments, its administration to one twin will produce a pharmacologic effect in the other twin as a result of cross-circulation. The degree of effect is also dependent on the dosage to weight ratio.[62]

Body temperature of the twins must be maintained throughout transport and during surgery so as to ensure physiological stability.[61] Hypothermia can be prevented by the use of warming mattresses and control of the room temperature. Warmed solutions for skin preparation can also be used. Adequate venous access for fluid and drug administration should be obtained before induction of anesthesia. Blood pressure, electrocardiogram, rectal temperature, chest sounds and pulse oximeter monitoring are essential. In order to prevent exsanguinating hemorrhage and hypovolemia, central venous catheters and additional venous lines will be essential in most cases for replacement of fluids, electrolytes, albumin and blood. Arterial canulation for direct arterial blood pressure monitoring, pH and determination of blood gas, and blood chemistry should be in place when twins with complex unions are separated. Prophylactic antibiotic cover will be essential according to standard surgical principles.

Intubation may be difficult in thoracopagus and omphalopagus twins since the children face each other and have cervical hyperextension. These children will need to be intubated with the children lying sideways. Placement of one twin above the other should be avoided in order to prevent draining of blood from the upper to the lower twin. In order to avoid overdoses due to cross-circulation, the weaker twin should be anesthetized first. Short-acting inhalation anesthetics with high concentration of oxygen, or induction by awake intubation while the other infant is maintained on preoxygenation is recommended.[16,64]

When endotracheal tubes, monitoring and intravenous lines are carefully secured, the esophageal stethoscope and nasogastric tubes can be inserted. Two teams of anesthetists and nurses can lift the twins into the air so as to allow total body sterile preparation and draping. While one operating nursing team is required for the initial part of the separation, two nursing teams are required once separation is accomplished. Blood loss in the initial stages of separation will be calculated as a shared loss by both twins, and if replacement is made, each twin will receive half the volume of calculated blood loss. After separation, replacement for each twin is decided individually. The rapidity and effects of cross-circulation must always be borne in mind during all intravenous infusions of fluids, electrolytes, blood or blood products and also during correction of acid/base imbalances.

SURGICAL CONSIDERATIONS

The type of major structures and organs, the severity of the required division and the nature of reconstruction anticipated will determine the surgical specialty teams and instruments. It is important for the lead surgeon to be present throughout the separation procedure to integrate the efforts of all team members and for approval of any deviations from the planned procedure. Specialty surgeons will be integrated into the separation when their expertise is needed.

The surgeon-in-charge must overcome two major technical problems. The first is to separate the shared structures leaving each child with a functioning residual whenever possible. The second is the closure of skin, muscle and bony defects at the site of union. It is beyond the scope of this chapter to review all the technical details of separation of different types of conjoined twins, which have appeared in the literature.[16,43,63,65-78] Therefore, only generalizations will be made.

Cardiovascular System

The separation of conjoined hearts is associated with extremely high morbidity and mortality. When there is evidence of conjoined hearts, surgeons planning to separate thoracopagus twins must be prepared to employ cardiopulmonary bypass and hypothermic circulatory arrest. The hearts may be connected at the atria or ventricles or both.[16,79,80] To date, there are no reports of successful separation of twins with conjoined ventricles. Though rare, successful separation in the presence of myocardial fusion at the level of atria has been reported.[68] Urgent separation and corrective surgery to save a healthier twin may be necessary in the presence of severe uncorrectable cardiovascular anomalies in one twin.[16] There may be complex cardiovascular malformations, which are not amenable to surgery.[16,79,81]

Hepatobiliary Pancreatic System

Almost all forms of conjoined twinning except craniopagus and pygopagus, have a shared liver. In cases where there is a small bridge of liver as seen in some omphalopagus twins, a relatively avascular cleavage plane can be found. For division of a relatively thicker hepatic bridge, the central area of the fused livers selected for division is first dissected free circumferentially so that penrose drains can be placed as tourniquets. A double row of large mattress sutures of absorbable material can be placed between the penrose tourniquets so that the division can be performed between them by traditional means. The use of an ultrasonic dissector is a definite advantage in the division of liver parenchyma with individual ligation of larger vessels and ducts, and fulguration of smaller vessels. Tissue glue may be applied to the raw surfaces but hemostasis should not depend on this method. The use of an argon beam coagulator can be an added advantage in controlling oozing from the raw liver surface.

Whenever the duodenum is shared proximally, it is likely that there is a single biliary tree. When there is a single extrahepatic biliary tree as determined by preoperative studies, an intraoperative cholangiogram may be necessary so that the twin with the ampulla can be given the entire extrahepatic biliary system while the other is left with a single hepatic duct, which may be drained externally or into a jejunal Roux limb.[43-45] If these twins share a pancreas, it is best left with the extrahepatic biliary tree. If two small pancreatic anlage are present, each infant should receive one.[16]

Omphalocele

Omphalocele is often present in omphalopagus and thoracopagus twins. If the sac is intact, a conservative approach is recommended and the sac allowed to epithelialize. If the sac ruptures and the evaluation is as yet incomplete, initial closure of the defect should be attempted and formal separation delayed.[82] However, in the hands of experienced surgeons, emergency separation is feasible.[16] It should be emphasized that unless life-threatening complications are present, emergency separation of the twins should not be performed when repairing a ruptured omphalocele or during surgery for intestinal atresia.

Gastrointestinal System

If intestinal atresia is present, it can be resected and primary anastomosis performed. A diverting enterostomy or colostomy may be an alternative temporary measure to treat atresia.

More commonly in thoracopagus and, less so, in omphalopagus twins, the second and third parts of the duodenum may be shared; the fourth part of the duodenum and the rest of the gastrointestinal tract are separate. It is also possible that sharing of the small bowel may begin at the second part of the duodenum and continue to the region of the Meckel's diverticulum. Ileocolonic or, in rare instances, only colonic sharing may also be present. Conjoined segments of intestine without obstruction may be left intact until formal separation, or separated earlier when indicated.[43,45,83] Fortunately, there is almost always a dual blood supply from each twin to the shared intestine. In case of colon sharing, it is preferable to give the ileocecal valve to one twin and the anus to the other twin.

Although initial correction of anorectal and genitourinary anomalies has been proposed, with the worldwide application of posterior sagittal anorectoplasty, it may be prudent to perform a diverting colostomy before attempting a definitive continence procedure in ischiopagus twins.[16,84,85] The use of a muscle stimulator to identify appropriate muscle groups to preserve bowel and bladder sphincter mechanisms is strongly advocated.

Genitourinary System

In ischiopagus and pygopagus twins, complex genitourinary and lower gastrointestinal fusions are common. The tripus variety is more likely to have major arterial communication than in the more symmetrical tetrapus variety.[47,71]

Although four kidneys and two ureters are usually present in ischiopagus twins, it is common to find that one ureter from each twin crosses the midline and empties into the bladder of the other.[16,17,57,86]

Two uteri, four ovaries and two sets of external genitalia on either side of a single anal opening are present in female ischiopagus twins. Frequently, vaginal anomalies and rectovaginal communications may be present. Halcomb et al has described the use of the urogenital sinus as a substitute bladder when the latter structure and a single bladder were present; a new vagina was also constructed.[87]

In male twins, although four gonads may be present, fusion of the genitourinary tract distal to the bladder is common. In cases with only one phallus, one twin can be reconstructed as a boy while the other as a girl using the available scrotal tissue to create the labia. Penile reposition of the abnormally sited penis will also be necessary.

Depending on the anomalies, a suprapubic catheter or vesicostomy may be necessary. Staged reconstructive procedures have proven to be the most rewarding. These include bladder augmentation, vaginal and genital reconstruction, and procedures to improve continence.[16,17,84,86]

Central Nervous System

Readers are referred to the excellent review by Winston and colleagues for details on this subject.[49] The spectrum of conjunction ranges from those with extensive fusion of cerebral tissue and venous sinuses to those with a limited area of attachment of skull bones and dura only. Winston's classification is based on the deepest shared structures and is the most practical.[15] In a review of surgically-separated twins by Hoyle, 37% of 27 craniopagus twins had a cerebral "connection" in the form of interdigitation of the two cortical surfaces or parenchymal continuity, resulting in a higher perioperative mortality as well as neurological morbidity of the survivors.[9] Parietal fusion is most frequent and is associated with deeper union.[88] Frontal and occipital unions have also been described. Because of the physical and mental handicaps associated with development in the conjoined state, surgical separation is considered to be justified even in high risk patients.[88,89]

The presence of a superior sagittal sinus for each cerebrum is a critical factor in separation.[90] Approaches to the venous anomalies have been developed.[49,91,92] The use of cardiopulmonary bypass, safe division and subsequent reconstruction of the superior sagittal sinus has been described.[93] Preoperative planning of skin flaps, mapping of vascular pedicles, and constructing models to evaluate skin cover have also been examined.[49,90,92] Successful limitation of the growth of the area of fusion by the use of an external constricter has also been reported.[90] Rotational flaps, skin grafts, tissue expanders, lyophilized human dural grafts and collagen sheets have been used to repair skin, skull and dura defects.[49,90,94]

Skeletal System

Orthopedic considerations, which are substantial and important particularly in ischiopagus twins, have been reviewed by Albert et al.[95] These considerations include three-dimentional visualization and evaluation of the problem, the separation of the pelvis, and the preservation and assignment of the shared limb to the appropriate twin. Postoperative care and procedures for the "shared" leg and the "normal" leg are essential. Other post-separation issues include deformities of the chest, congenital dislocation of the hip and knee, clubfeet, scoliosis and problems related to the shared and dystrophic limb.[95] Some pygopagus twins require neurosurgical and orthopedic involvement due to problems arising from sharing of the sacrum.

Abdominal Wall and Thoracic Cage

Reconstruction of abdominal and chest wall defects after separation of thoracopagus and omphalopagus twins can pose difficulties. In the absence of a sternum, forceful closure of this defect results in compression of the heart and cardiac decompensation. A variety of techniques to reconstruct thoracic cage defects have been utilized. These include flaps of the chest wall and artificial implants; chest wall of the nonsurviving twin; and more recently, the use of cryopreserved syngenic thoracic cage of a twin who died after separation.[96-101] To overcome the deficiencies in the skin and abdominal wall, silon chimney was used three decades ago followed by subcutaneous and intra-abdominal tissue expanders.[78,102-104] While the use of subcutaneous tissue expanders has gained popularity, intra-abdominal use is not as popular. Tissue expanders have also been used to facilitate the separation of craniopagus twins.

RESULTS OF SURGERY

In reviewing 47 pairs of surgically-separated thoracopagus twins, in 30 pairs with completely separate hearts, 41 patients (70%) survived; in five pairs with atrial connection only, one patient (10%) survived; in nine pairs with both atrial and ventricular connections, none survived; in three pairs of unknown type, two survived. The total survival rate was 47.9%.[96] The perioperative mortality rate for thoracopagus twins prior to 1975 was 55.6% (ignoring twins who were sacrificed to save the other). However, from 1980 to 1987, it decreased to 26%, a 32% reduction.[9]

The results of separation of omphalopagus and xiphopagus twins are very good. In a review of 11 sets of such twins some 25 years ago, 19 of 22 children survived.[64] However, the prognosis is worse when this type is associated with omphalocele. In 7 such sets treated between 1963 and 1981, four sets had rupture of omphalocele and one twin in three of the four sets died. Of the three sets with intact omphalocele, one twin from two of the sets also succumbed.[20]

It is not surprising that the outlook for pygopagus twins has been good since the joined structures usually are not necessary for life.[20,74,105,106] In most cases, both twins have survived the separation.

The separation of ischiopagus twins is complex since both the urinary and intestinal systems are joined. In addition, there is a single pelvic ring and often three lower limbs. In recent years, perioperative survival for ischiopagus twins has improved to about 90%; there is not much difference between tetrapus and tripus twins.[107] Votteler reviewed 12 ischiopagus separations from 1955 to 1981 in which one or both ischiopagus twins survived.[20] In another review of 17 sets of ischiopagus twins, 29 infants survived the separation; the remaining four died of a variety of causes.[108]

The severity of anatomical union of brain tissue and vasculature plays a major role in the success of separation of craniopagus twins. The overall perioperative mortality for craniopagus twins has been reported to be around 50%.[49] Votteler reporting on 22 sets of craniopagus twins, said eight of ten children with partial union survived, while only seven of twelve with total union lived.[20] Even among survivors, about half of the children have residual neurological deficits.

Major advances in antenatal and postnatal diagnostic investigations, refinements of surgical techniques and equipments, advances in anesthesia and intensive care, nutritional and rehabilitative support, and control of infection have all been responsible for a greatly improved outcome for conjoined twins, many of whom may have succumbed if they had been born a decade or two ago.

REFERENCES

1. Guttmacher AF. Biographical notes on some famous conjoined twins. Birth Defects 1967;3:10-17.
2. Bondeson J. The Biddenden Maids: A curious chapter in the history of conjoined twins. J Roy Soc Med 1992;85:217.
3. Konig G. Sibi invicem adnati feliciter separati. Ephemerid Natur Curios 1689;2:145.
4. Dragstedt LR. Siamese twins. Q Bull N West Univ Med Sch 1957;31:359-65.
5. Allen H. Report of an autopsy on the bodies of Chang and Eng Bunker, commonly known as the Siamese Twins. Trans Coll Physicians, Philadelphia, Third Series 1875;1: 3-46.
6. Luckhardt AB. Report on the autopsy of Siamese twins together with other interesting information covering their life, a sketch of the life of Chang and Eng. Surg Gynecol Obstet 1941;72:116-25.
7. Milham S Jr. Symmetrical conjoined twins: An analysis of the birth records of twenty-two sets. J Pediatr 1966;69: 643-47.
8. Hanson JW. Letter: Incidence of conjoined twinning. Lancet 1975;2:1257.
9. Hoyle RM. Surgical separation of conjoined twins. Surg Gynecol Obstet 1990;170:549-62.
10. Edmonds LD, Layde PM. Conjoined twins in the United States 1970-1977. Teratology 1982;25:301-08.
11. Benirschke K, Temple WW, Bloor C. Conjoined twins: Nosology and conjenital malformations. Birth Defects 1978;16:179.
12. Streeter GL. Formation of single ovum twins. Bul Johns Hopkins Hosp 1919b;30:235.
13. Zimmerman AA. Embryologic and anatomic considerations of conjoined twins. Birth Defects 1967;3:18-27.
14. Spencer R. Theorectical and analytical embryology of conjoined twins: Part I: Embryogenesis. Clin Anat 2000;13:36-53.
15. Winston KR. Craniopagi: anatomical characteristics and classification. Neurosurgery 1987;21:769-81.
16. O'Neill JA, Holcomb GW, Schnaufer L, et al. Surgical experience with thirteen conjoined twins. Ann Surg 1988;208:299-312.
17. Spitz L, Capps SNJ, Kiely EM, et al. Xipho-omphalo-ischiopagus tripus conjoined twins: successful separation following abdominal wall expansion. J Pediatr Surg 1991;26:26-29.
18. Powis M, Spitz L, Pierro A. Differential metabolism in conjoined twins. J Pediatr Surg 1999;34:1115-17.
19. Potter EL, Craig JM. Pathology of the Fetus and the Infant. 3rd edition. Chicago, Year Book Medical Publishers 1975.
20. Votteler TP. Conjoined twins, in Welch KJ, Randolph JG, Ravitch MM, et al. (Eds). Pediatric Surgery. Chicago, Year Book Medical Publishers 1986;771-79.
21. Spencer R. Anatomic description of conjoined twins: a plea for standardized terminology. J Pediatr Surg 1996;7: 941-44.
22. Nichols BL, Blattner RJ, Rudolph AJ. General clinical management of thoracopagus twins. Birth Defects 1967;3:38-51.
23. Bucholz RD, Yoon KW, Shively RE. Temporoparietal craniopagus: Case report and review of the literature. J Neurosurg 1987;66:72-79.
24. Wilson RL, Shaub MS, Cetrulo CJ. The antepartum findings of conjoined twins. J Clin Ultrasound 1977;5: 35-39.
25. Fagan CJ. Antepartum diagnosis of conjoined twins by ultrasonography. Am J Roentgenol 1977;129:921-22.
26. Morgan CL, Trought WS, Sheldon G, et al. B-scan and real time ultrasound in the antepartum diagnosis of conjoined twins and pericardial effusion. Am J Roentgenol 1978;130:578-80.
27. Vaughn TC, Powell LC. The obstetrical management of conjoined twins. Obstet Gynecol 1979;53:67-72.
28. D'Alton ME, Dudley DK. Ultrasound in the antenatal management of twin gestation. Semin Perinatol 1986;10:30-38.
29. Austin E, Schifrin BS, Pomerance JJ, et al. The antepartum diagnosis of conjoined twins. J Pediatr Surg 1980;15: 332-34.
30. Schmidt W, Heberling D, Kubli F. Antepartum ultrasonographic diagnosis of conjoined twins in early pregnancy. Am J Obstet Gynecol 1981;139:961-63.
31. Maggio M, Callan NA, Hamobka KA, et al. The first trimester ultrasonographic diagnosis of conjoined twins. Am J Obstet Gynecol 1985;152:833-35.
32. Sanders SP, Chin AJ, Parness IA, et al. Prenatal diagnosis of congenital heart defects in thoracoabdominally conjoined twins. N Engl J Med 1985;313:370-74.
33. Turner RJ, Hankins GD, Weinreb JC, et al. Magnetic resonance imaging and ultrasonography in the antenatal evaluation of congenital twins. Am J Obstet Gynecol 1986;155:645-49.
34. Barth RA, Filly RA, Goldberg JD, et al. Conjoined twins: Prenatal diagnosis and assessment of associated malformations. Radiology 1990;177:201-07.
35. Harper RG, Kenigsberg K, Sia CG, et al. Xiphopagus conjoined twins: A 300-year review of the obstetric, morphopathologic, neonatal and surgical parameters. Am J Obstet Gynecol 1980;137:617-29.

36. Gore RM, Filly RA, Parer JT. Sonographic antepartum diagnosis of conjoined twins: Its impact on obstetric management. JAMA 1982;247:3351-53.
37. Rudolph AJ, Michaels JP, Nichols BL. Obstetric management of conjoined twins. Birth Defects 1967;3:28-37.
38. Leachman RD, Latson JR, Kohler CM, et al. Cardiovascular evaluation of conjoined twins. Birth Defects 1967;3:52-65.
39. Freedom RM, Culham JAG, Moes CAF. The angiocardiographic approach to thoracopagus conjoined twins, in Freedom RM, Culham JAG, Moes CAF (Eds): Angiocardiography of congenital heart disease. New York, MacMillan 1984;655-63.
40. Spencer RP, Rockoff ML, Nichols Bl, et al. Radioisotopic flow studies in conjoined twins. Birth Defects 1967;3:120-22.
41. Mann MD, Coutts JP, Kaschula RO, et al. The use of radionuclides in the investigation of conjoined twins. J Nucl Med 1984;24:469-78.
42. Schnaufer L. Conjoined twins, in Raffensperger JG (Ed): Swenson's Pediatric Surgery. New York, Appleton and Lange 1990;969-78.
43. Saing H, Mok CK, Tam PKH, et al. Problems in the surgery of conjoined twins. Surgical Rounds 1987;10:81-96.
44. Lobe TE, Oldham KT, Richardson J. Successful separation of a conjoined biliary tract in a set of omphalopagus twins. J Pediatr Surg 1989;24:930-32.
45. Spitz L, Crabbe DCG, Kiely EM. Separation of thoraco-omphalopagus conjoined twins with complex hepato-biliary anatomy. J Pediatr Surg 1997;32:787-89.
46. Richardson RJ, Applebaum H, Taber P, et al. Use of magnetic resonance imaging in planning the separation of omphalopagus conjoined twins. J Pediatr Surg 1989;24:683-85.
47. Shapiro E, Fair WR, Ternberg JL, et al. Ischiopagus tetrapus twins: Urological aspects of separation and 10-year follow-up. J Urol 1991;145:120-25.
48. Macinski A, Lopatic HU, Wermenski K, et al. Angiographic evaluation of conjoined twins. Pediatr Radiol 1978;6:230-32.
49. Winston KR, Rockoff MA, Mulliken JB, et al. Surgical division of craniopagi. Neurosurgery 1987;21:782-91.
50. Ross AJ, O'Neill JA, Silverman DG, et al. A new technique for evaluating cutaneous vascularity in complicated conjoined twins. J Pediatr Surg 1985;20:743-46.
51. Pepper CK. Ethical and moral considerations in the separation of conjoined twins: Summary of two dialogues between physicians and clergymen. Birth Defects 1967;3:128.
52. Annas GJ. Siamese twins: killing one to save the other. The Hastings Center Report 1987;27-29.
53. Holcomb GW III, O'Neill JA Jr. Conjoined Twins, in Ashcraft KW, Holder TM (Eds): Pediatric Surgery. Philadelphia, WB Saunders Co. 1993;948-55.
54. Raffensperger J. A philosophical approach to conjoined twins. Pediatr Surg Int 1997;12:249-55.
55. Gans SL, Morgenstern L, Gettelman B, et al. Separation of conjoined twins in the newborn period. J Pediatr Surg 1968;3:565-74.
56. Saing H, Tam PK, Lau JT, et al. Advanced necrotizing enterocolitis: An indication for emergency separation of omphalopagus conjoined twins. Aust Paediatr J 1987;23:129-30.
57. Chen WJ, Chen KM, Chen MT, et al. Emergency separation of omphaloischiopagus tetrapus conjoined twins in the newborn period. J Pediatr Surg 1989;24:1221-24.
58. Graivier L, Jacoby MD. Emergency separation of newborn conjoined (Siamese) twins. Tex Med 1980;76:60.
59. Wong TJ, Lyou YT, Chee CP, et al. Management of xiphopagus conjoined twins with small bowel obstruction. J Pediatr Surg 1986;21:53-57.
60. Wong KC, Ohmura A, Roberts TH, et al. Anesthetic management for separation of craniopagus twins. Anesth Analg 1980;59:883-86.
61. Diaz JH, Furman EB. Perioperative management of conjoined twins. Anaesthesiology 1987;67:965-73.
62. Keats AS, Cave PE, Slatper EL, Moore RA. Conjoined twins-A review of anesthetic management for separating operations. Birth Defects 1967;3:80.
63. James PD, Lerman J, McLeod ME, et al. Anaesthetic considerations for separation of omphalo-ischiopagus tripus twins. Can Anaesth Soc J 1985;32:402-11.
64. Filler RM. Conjoined twins, in Oldham KT, Colombani PM, Foglia RP (eds): Surgery of Infants and Children: Scientific Principles and Practice. Phildelphia, Lippincott-Raven Publishers 1997;1763-71.
65. Kiesewetter WB. Surgery on conjoined (Siamese) twins. Surgery 1966;59:860-71.
66. Cywes S, Millar AJW, Rode H, et al. Conjoined twins - the Cape Town experience. Pediatr Surg Int 1997;12:234-48.
67. Grossman HJ, Sugar O, Greeley PW, et al. Surgical separation in craniopagus. JAMA 1953;153:201.
68. Synhorst D, Matlak M, Roan Y, et al. Separation of conjoined thoracopagus twins joined at the right atria. Am J Cardiol 1979;43:662-65.
69. Mestel AL, Golinko RJ, Wax SH, et al. Ischiopagus tripus conjoined twins: Case report of a successful separation. Surgery 1971;69:75-83.
70. DeVries PA. Separation of the San Francisco twins. Birth Defects 1967;3:75-79.
71. Eades JW, Thomas CG. Successful separation of ischiopagus tetrapus conjoined twins. Ann Surg 1966;164:1059.
72. Jayes PH. Plastic repair after separation of craniopagus twins. Br Med J 1964;1:1340.
73. Kling S, Johnston RJ, Michalyshyn B, et al. Successful separation of xiphopagus-conjoined twins. J Pediatr Surg 1975;10:267.
74. Koop CE. The successful of pyopagus twins. Surgery 1961;49:271.
75. Spencer R. Surgical separation of Siamese twins: Case report. Surgery 1956;39:827.

76. Wilson H. Surgery in Siamese twins: A report of three sets of conjoined twins treated surgically. Ann Surgery 1957;145:718.
77. Woolley M, Joergenson E. Xiphopagus conjoined twins. Am J Surg 1964;108:277.
78. Zuker RM, Filler RM, Lalla R. Intra-abdominal tissue expansion: An adjunct in the separation of conjoined twins. J Pediatr Surg 1986;21:1198-200.
79. Rossi MB, Burn J, Ho SY, et al. Conjoined twins, right atrial isomerism, and sequential segmental analysis. Br Heart J 1987;58:518-24.
80. Gerlis LM, Seo JW, Ho SY, et al. Morphology of the cardiovascular system in conjoined twins: Spatial and sequential segmental arrangements in 36 cases. Teratology 1993;47:91-108.
81. Edwards WD, Hagel DR, Thompson J, et al. Conjoined thoracopagus twins. Circulation 1977;56:491-97.
82. Walton JM, Gillis DA, Giacomantonio JM, et al. Emergency separation of conjoined twins. J Pediatr Surg 26:1337-40.
83. Poenaru D, Uroz-Tristan J, LeClerc S, et al. Minimally conjoined omphalopagi - a consistent spectrum of anomalies. J Paediatr Surg 1994;29:1236-38.
84. Hsu HS, Duckett JW, Templeton JM, et al. Experience with urogenital reconstruction in ischiopagus conjoined twins. J Urol 1995;154:563-67.
85. Ischitani MB, Egerton BW, Applebaum H. Conjoined twins, in Prem Puri (Ed): Newborn Surgery. Oxford, Butterworth - Heinemann 1996;470-74.
86. Chatterjee SK, Chakravarti AK, Deb Maulik TK, et al. Staging the separation of ischiopagus twins. J Pediatr Surg 1988;23:73-75.
87. Holcomb III GW, Keating MA, Hollowell JG, et al. Continent urinary reconstruction in ischiopagus tripus conjoined twins. J Urol 1989;141:100-02.
88. O'Connell JEA. Craniopagus twins: surgical anatomy and embryology and their implications. J Neurol Neurosurg Psych 1976;39:1-22.
89. Todorov AB, Cohen K L, Spilotro V, et al. Craniopagus twins. J Neurol Neurosurg Psych 1974;37:1291-98.
90. Gaist G, Piazza G, Galassi E, et al. Craniopagus twins. An unsuccessful separation and a clinical review of the entity. Childs Nerv Syst 1987;3:327-33.
91. Roberts TS. Craniopagus Twins, in Wilkins RH, Rengachary SS (eds): Neurosurgery. New York, McGraw-Hill 1985;2091-96.
92. Drummond G, Scott P, Mackay D, et al. Separation of the Baragwanath craniopagus twins. Br J Plast Surg 1991;44:49-52.
93. Cameron DE, Reitz BA, Carson BS, et al. Separation of craniopagus Siamese twins using cardiopulmonary bypass and hypothermic circulatory arrest. J Thorac Cardiovasc Surg 1989;98:961-67.
94. Shively RE, Bermant MA, Bucholz RD. Separation of craniopagus twins utilizing tissue expanders. Plast Reconstr Surg 1985;76:765-72.
95. Albert MC, Drummond DS, O'Neill J, et al. The orthopaedic management of conjoined twins: a review of 13 cases and report of 4 cases. J Pediatr Orthop 1992;2:300-307.
96. Chiu CT, Hou SH, Lai HS, et al. Separation of thoracopagus conjoined twins. A case report. J Cardiovas Surg (Torino) 1994;35:459-62.
97. Saing H, Mok CK, Lau JTK, et al. A method of repair of thoracic cage defects after separation of thoraco-omphalopagus twins. Pediatr Surg Int 1987;2:113-16.
98. Hisano K, Nakamura K, Okada M, et al. Separation of conjoined twins using chest wall prosthesis. J Pediatr Surg 1989;24:928-29.
99. Oberniedermayr A, Buhlmeyer K, Fendel H, et al. Report of operation on newborn thoracopagi, and of another inviable thoracopagus (in German). Z Kinder Chir 1968;6:162-74.
100. Cywes S. Challenges and dilemmas for a pediatric surgeon. J Pediatr Surg 1994;29:957-65.
101. Canty TG, Mainwaring R, Vecchione T, et al. Separation of omphalopagus twins: unique reconstruction using syngenic cryopreserved tissue. J Pediatr Surg 1998;33:750-53.
102. Pe-Nyun, Saing H. Thoracoomphalopagous conjoined twins of Burma. J Pediatr Surg 1972;7:691-95.
103. Ricketts RR, Zubowicz VN. Use of tissue expansion for separation and primary closure of thoracopagus twins. Paediatr Surg Int 1987;2:365-68.
104. Spitz L, Stringer MD, Kiely EM, et al. Separation of brachio-thoraco-omphalo-ischiopagus bipus conjoined twins. J Pediatr Surg 1994;29:477-81.
105. Voteller TP. Necrotizing enterocolitis in pygopagus twin. J Pediatr Surg 1982;17:555-57.
106. Cloutier R, Levassiur L, Copty M, et al. The surgical separation of pygopagus twins. J Pediatr Surg 1979;14:554-56.
107. Hoyle RM, Thomas CG. Twenty-three-year follow-up of separated ischiopagus tetrapus conjoined twins. Ann Surg 1989;210:673-79.
108. Doski JJ, Heiman HS, Solenberger RI, et al. Successful separation of ischiopagus tripus conjoined twins with comparative analysis of methods for abdominal wall closure and use of the tripus limb. J Pediatr Surg 1997;32:1761-66.

CHAPTER 113

Heteropagus Twinning

DK Gupta, Shilpa Sharma

Heteropagus conjoined twinning is a rare condition accounting for a small percentage of all the conjoined twins. However, it is treated more frequently by pediatric surgeons as it is a correctable anomaly with gratifying results.

The term heteropagus twinning is synonymous with parasitic, partial, incomplete or atypical asymmetrical, unequal twinning. Heteropagus twins display unequal duplication of features with varying degrees of development in each twin. It is usually characterized by an incomplete and parasitic dependent part, usually smaller than the well formed autosite.

Conjoined twins are symmetrical and predominantly seen in females. This may be due to the fact that a female zygote once formed is more likely to remain viable as compared to the male zygote which is likely to undergo ischemic atrophy. Heteropagus twins differ in several ways from symmetrical conjoined twins, including male preponderance, and usually no major connection of vessels, bowels, or bones.

Twinning occurs in approximately 1 of every 87 live births. Monozygotic twins account for one third of twin births. Conjoined twins account for 1% of monozygotic twins. The incidence varies from 1 in 50,000 to 1 in 200,000 live births. The stillbirth rate is 40-60%. The exact incidence of heteropagus twins is not known but it is estimated that they are seen at an incidence of 2-10% of all conjoined twins.[1,2] Some consider fetus in fetu to be a type of endoparasitic heteropagus twins and the external ones to be ectoparasitic Heteropagus twins.[3] If these are also included then the incidence is higher. Others consider it as a distinct entity or a special case of teratoma.

More cases are being reported now because of the routine use of fetal ultrasonography. The condition is probably more commonly reported from Indian and African populations.[1,4-10] Exact epidemiology across different races and nations is not known because of lack of reporting and facilities for prenatal diagnosis.

EMBRYOLOGY

Parasitic twins occur when a twin embryo begins developing *in utero*, but the pair does not fully separate, and one embryo maintains dominant development at the expense of the other. Unlike conjoined twins, one ceases development during gestation and is vestigeal to a mostly fully-formed, otherwise healthy individual twin. The undeveloped twin is defined a parasitic, rather than conjoined, because it is incompletely formed or wholly dependent on the body functions of the complete fetus. Conjoined twins are of the same sex, thus are most probably derived from monozygous twinning. Though incomplete cleavage of the embryo at two weeks of gestation is a plausible explanation for conjoined twins, it does not seem to hold true for parasitic twins. The exact etiology is thus not known. The complexity of the defect is variable with the number of functioning organs varying from case to case.[11]

Some ischemic insult has been suggested as the etiology behind the selective atrophy of the body structure of the parasite at an early gestational age.[4,12] The striking absence of structures other than the pelvis, lower limbs and pelvic organs except for the rudimentary hand seen in most cases of epigastric heteropagus twins may be due to the ischemic atrophy of the other structures of the body during the gestational development. Heteropagus twins thus develop when one component (autosite) is better placed so that it monopolizes the placental blood flow from the other member (parasite).

Rarely, DNA typing studies have even demonstrated dizygosity in a male parasitic twin. The unusual perpendicular orientation of the parasite to the autosite has been resembled to a mechanism observed in mares in which early fusion of two embryos is followed by resorption due to compromised embryonic polarity.[13]

It has been inferred that the event may be occurring much after the second week of intrauterine life based on angiography performed in one of authors cases that revealed the vascular supply to the parasite to arise from the left subclavian artery.[1] It passed under the skin bridge to supply the parasite aorta, which gave branches to all the organs of the parasite. Vasculogenesis during intrauterine life starts at 18 days, in the latter part of the third week, the intraembryonic blood vessels differentiate *in situ* from the angioblast cells of the intraembryonic mesoderm and establish secondary connection with the extraembryonic blood vessels.[14] By the 29th day the seventh intersegmental artery develops which is destined to form the subclavian artery. In this case, the arterial supply to the parasite was arising from the left subclavian artery of the autosite, therefore it is believed that the intrauterine event that leads to this malformation would have occurred only after the 29th day of intrauterine life.[1]

To date, the underlying disorder (whether genetic, metabolic or environmental) responsible for the development of this congenital malformation is not fully understood.[15] An apparent lack of an adequate arterial blood supply to the growing embryo can contribute to the etiopathogenesis by producing a local ischemic milieus during the critical phases of embryogenesis; damaging the normal sequence of cell differentiation and morphogenesis of the various tissues composing the craniofacial complex.[15] Impediment of the preprogrammed migration of neural crest cells to their end targets in the upper branchial arches has also been attributed to this.[15]

An omphalopagus parasitic twin has also been produced after intracytoplasmic sperm injection.[16]

CLINICAL FEATURES

In heteropagus twins, the dependent portion (parasite) is smaller than the host (autosite). Heteropagus twins are seen mostly in the males, though occasionally cases are reported in females.[17-19] The parasite may be attached to any portion of the body. Omphalocele is also present in most of the cases.[4,20] The most common type seen is the epigastric heteropagus twin, also known as Thoracopagus parasiticus.

In the epigastric heteropagus twinning, the parasite may have duplication of the pelvis and the pelvic organs such as complete urinary tract, external and internal genitalia.

The intestinal loops in the parasite are usually blind ending, not communicating with the autosite intestine.[1] Rarely, a duplicated bowel has been reported in the connecting stalk that ended blindly without any connection to the intestine of the autosite.[4] A case in which the parasite's bowel was connected to a Meckel's diverticulum of the autosite has been reported.[17,21] There is usually no bony connection between the autosite and the parasite in epigastric heteropagus twinning, though exceptions are not unusual. The vascular supply to the parasite may arise from the liver, left internal mammary, epigastric, umbilical, falciform ligament, left subclavian or/and local systemic arteries.[22] In most cases, the vascular supply to the parasite arises from the local systemic artery. Cardiac anomalies are common in autosites and should be evaluated.[20]

There is a great diversity in the organs and tissues described in the parasitic part.

A heteropagus parasitic twin presenting as a mass in the lumbosacral area with an additional limb, a pair of breasts with nipples and aerola, and an anus with a blind pouch has been reported.[19]

It is extremely rare to have bony fusions though it may be found occasionally. The pelvic bone and lower legs of the parasite were fused with the respective organs in the autosite.[18] The variations of epigastric parasitic twinning may include with a parasite with well developed lower trunk and pelvis with rudimentary lower limbs, and well developed upper extremities without shoulder girdles and thoracic cage apart from additional accessory.[6,22]

A rare case of epigastric heteropagus twinning in which the parasite presented with head, thorax, and a rudimentary heart has also been reported.[23] Rarely the parasite may have more organs. A parasite with a single lung, liver, stomach, intestine, pancreas, ovaries, a single kidney, and a bladder located in the abdominal and pelvic space of the autosite has been reported.[18]

A rare case of craniofacial microsomia in a partially developed, malformed heteropagus conjoined twin with complex involvement of bones, cartilage, teeth, salivary glands, auditory apparatus, cerebrum, cranial nerves, ocular neuroepithelium, cervical vertebrae and appendicular long bones has been reported.[15]

NOMENCLATURE

The terms endoparasitic twin has been used to describe the commonly seen external form of heteropagus twins.[3] Endoparasitic heteropagus twin has been used to describe fetus in fetu.

A rationale nomenclature for conjoined twins has been adopted worldwide.[24] The site of attachment of the parasite is referred to as Craniopagus (cranium); Thoracopagus (chest and upper abdomen); Omphalopagus (if heart is involved); Ischiopagus (ventral pelvis) and so forth. Additional terms suggested for identification are enumerating some parts such as di (two); tri (three); tetra, quadri (four) with brachius, pus, ophthalmia, otia and stoma referring to arms, legs, eyes, ears and mouth respectively.[1]

The same terminology may be adapted to heteropagus twins with addition of the word parasiticus after the initial name. Thus the term epigastric heteropagus may also be called as Thoracopagus parasiticus (Figs 113.1 and 113.2). However, about 70-80% of all heteropagus twins are inserted in the epigastrium thus the term epigastric heteropagus twin has gained wide popularity. In Epigastric Heteropagus twins, the dependent twin (parasite) is attached to the right or left upper abdomen of the dominant part (autosite).[25] Any deviation from the common form merits explanation.

Conjoined-parasitic twins united at the head are described as craniopagus or cephalopagus. Craniopagus occipitalis is the term for fusion in the occipital region; craniopagus parietalis is when the fusion is in the parietal region; craniopagus parasiticus is a general term for a parasitic head attached to the head of a more fully-developed fetus or infant.[26]

The term "acardiac amorphous parasitic twin" has been used to describe a cystic umbilical swelling

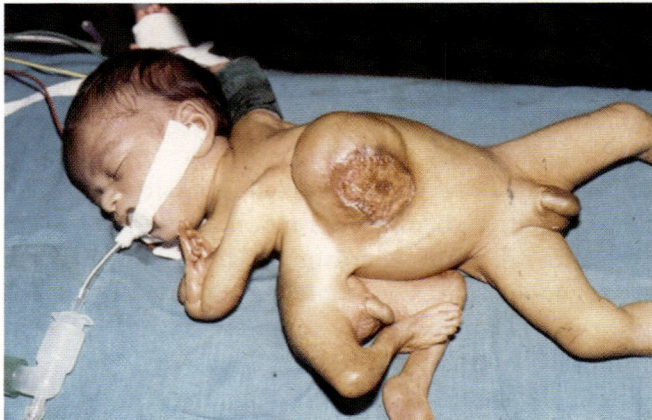

Fig. 113.1: Epigastric heteropagus in a pair of male twins with the omphalocele partially well covered with skin

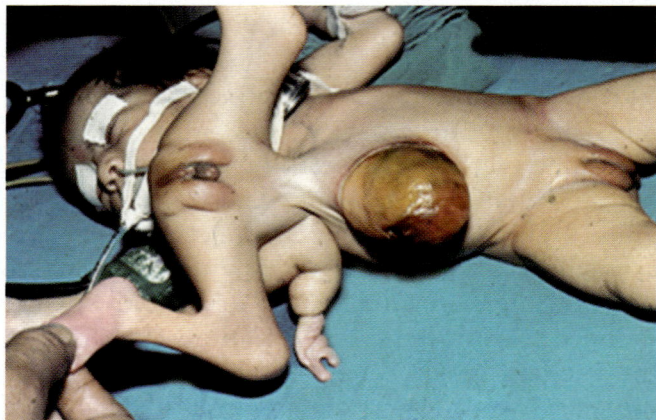

Fig. 113.2: Epigastric heteropagus in a pair of female twins with an omphalocele

covered mostly by skin and partly by amnion, resembling an early embryo-like structure with facial features and limb buds.[5] The deeper aspect was composed of large cystic and tubular structures and solid organs resembling liver and spleen.

The TRAP (twin-reversed arterial perfusion) sequence, results in an acardiac twin, a parasitic twin that fails to develop a head, arms and a heart. The resulting torso survives by leeching blood flow from the surviving normal twin by means of an umbilical cord-like structure, much like a fetus in fetu, except the acardiac twin is not enveloped inside the normal twin's body. Because it is pumping blood for both itself and its acardiac twin, this causes extreme stress on the normal fetus's heart. This twinning condition usually occurs very early in pregnancy.

INVESTIGATIONS

A proper evaluation at birth is necessary to establish the feasibility of separation. The separation is not an emergency and enough time may be spent in detailed investigations till all doubts are cleared.

Heteropagus twins may be suspected in the prenatal period with an ultrasonography and confirmed with a prenatal MRI.[27]

Skiagram of the baby helps to delineate the skeleton of the baby and the presence of bony structures in the heteropagus twin (Fig. 113.3).

A contrast enhanced computerized tomography (CECT) is helpful to delineate the anatomy of the autosite and the parasite. The tissue present in the skin bridge needs to be evaluated preoperatively, so as to prepare for the separation of the tissues shared in between the twins. A functioning kidney in the parasite will also be shown with evaluation of the ureteric and bladder anatomy.

A magnetic resonance imaging is also helpful to delineate the soft tissues and plan the surgical separation of the parasite especially in cases of abdominal wall defects.[25]

Barium Meal Follow through study may be useful to evaluate any connection between the autosite and the parasite intestines in epigastric heteropagus twins. It can be combined with the CECT scan to delineate the bowel anatomy.

Echocardiography is important to evaluate the associated congenital heart disease in the parasitic twins. Common associated anomalies are patent ductus arteriosus (PDA), ventricular septal defect (VSD) and atrial septal defects (ASD) and single ventricle.[20]

Chromosomal analysis may be performed to establish the karyotype of the twins. It will be helpful in understanding the embryopathy of the parasitic twinning.

Angiography is helpful in the exact delineation of the vascular anatomy of the autosite and the feeder vessel to the parasite. It helps establishing the anatomy and helps in the understanding of the embryopathy of this condition.

MANAGEMENT

Inspite of monstrous appearance, the parasite component of epigastric heteropagus can be separated successfully with minor surgery. This fact should be kept in mind during the intrauterine evaluation of these type of anomalies in order to avoid needless terminations.[22] Surgical excision of the parasite and repair of the abdominal wall defect in cases of omphalocele are usually successful.[20] If the skin cover is good, there is no urgency for the separation (Fig. 113.4). A proper evaluation leads to successful

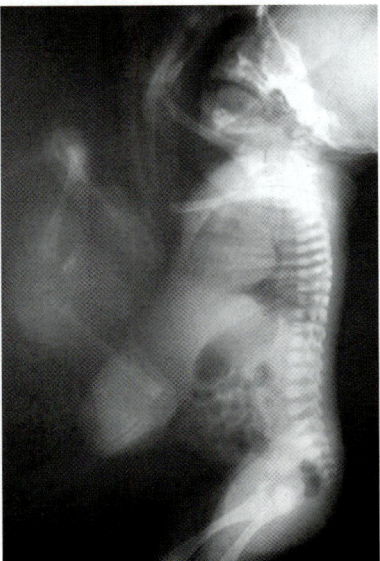

Fig. 113.3: Skiagram of the baby delineating the skeleton of the baby and the bony parts and soft tissue shadows of the heteropagus twin

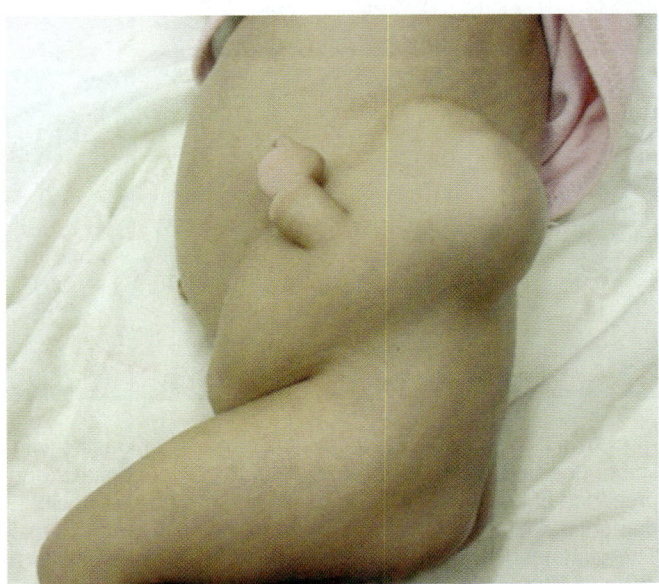

Fig. 113.4: An unusual case of heteropagus twinning with good skin cover

separation of the parasite from the autosite (Figs 113.5A to I). In the presence of an omphalocele with a thin sac, separation is expedited once the cardiac evaluation has been completed. The skin bridge should be carefully dissected, preserving all the vital tissues and securing the feeder vessel. Rarely, the autosite liver may be the content of the sac. The abdominal wall defect can be closed primarily wherever feasible, without any postoperative ventral hernia or else a silo or a ventral hernia is created. The omphalocele may also be managed conservatively by mercurochrome application after excision of the parasite.[6]

PROGNOSIS

The survival of the patient is adversely influenced by associated cardiac anomalies. Without a severe cardiac condition, the result is usually excellent.

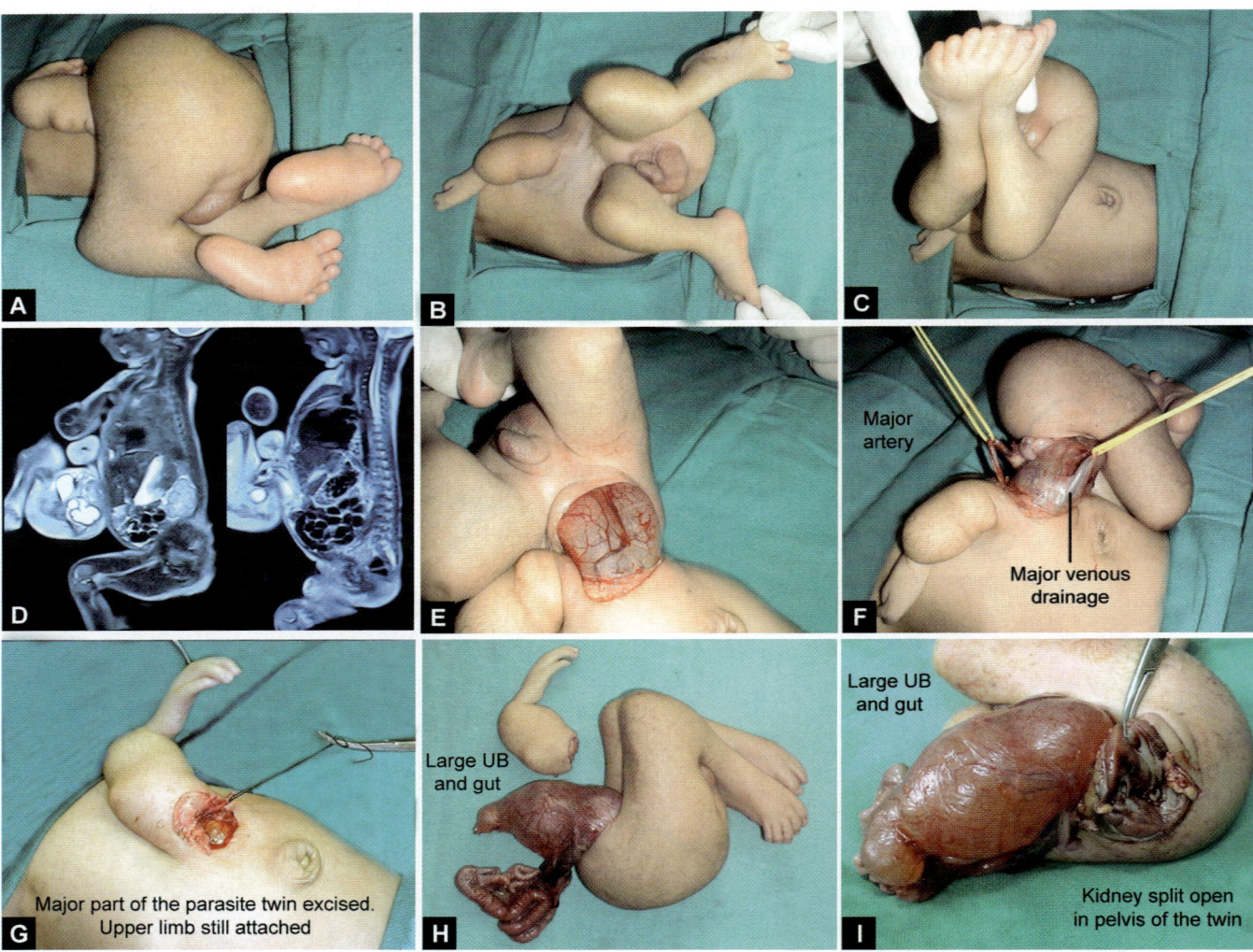

Figs 113.5A to I: **A-C.** A two days old parasitic epigastric twin presented with sepsis and palor. The parasitic twin had both lower limbs, one upper limb with three digits, external genitalia and used to pass urine occasionally. **D.** The CT scan demonstrated presence of bowel, kidney and bladder in the parasitic twin. Echocardiography showed double outlet right ventricle. DTPA scan demonstrated a functional kidney in the twin. **E.** Surgical excision was planned. The incision was given all around the junction. The distended bladder can be seen. **F.** The main vessels have been held in slings. **G.** The main part of the twin has been excised. The remaining upper limb can be seen with its vascular supply. Mass excised and defect repaired primarily. **H.** Parts of the excised parasitic twin including a large urinary bladder (UB) and gut. **I.** The split kidney of the parasitic twin can be seen (arrow).

Proper evaluation of the associated cardiac anomaly and its treatment is important for the successful outcome of the autosite. Cardiopulmonary failure has been reported as a cause of mortality.[20] There are not much reports on follow-up. A follow-up at 34 months has been reported with a healthy autosite.[25]

REFERENCES

1. Gupta DK, Lall A, Bajpai M. Epigastric heteropagus twins: a report of four cases. Pediatr Surg Int. 2001;17(5-6):481-82.
2. A T George, S Varkey, A Kalam, et al. Left over bowels: an unique complication in a surviving twin Postgraduate Medical Journal 2004;80:736-37.
3. Corona-Rivera JR, Acosta-León J, Velez-Gómez E, et al Unusual presentation of heteropagus attached to the thorax. J Pediatr Surg. 1997;32(10):1492-94.
4. Lall A, Gupta DK. Heteropagus (Parasitic) twins. In Textbook of Neonatal Surgery Ed DK Gupta, 2000; Chap 42:264-66.
5. Biswas SK, Gangopadhyay AN, Bhatia BD, et al. An unusual case of heteropagus twinning. J Pediatr Surg. 1992;27(1):96-97.
6. Chadha R, Bagga D, Dhar A, et al. Epigastric heteropagus. J Pediatr Surg 1993;28(5):723-27.
7. Borah HK. Epigastric heteropagus. Indian Pediatr. 1999 Mar;36(3):327.
8. Mahajan JK, Kumar D, Mainak D, Rao KLN. Asymmetric conjoined twins: Atypical ischiopagus parasite Journal of Pediatric Surgery 2002;37:E33.
9. Bhansali M, Sharma DB, Raina VK. Epigastric heteropagus twins: 3 case reports with review of literature. J Pediatr Surg. 2005;40(7):1204-08.
10. Jain PK, Budhwani KS, Gambhir A, et al. Omphalopagus parasite: a rare congenital anomaly. J Pediatr Surg 1998;33:946-47.
11. Cury EK, Schraibman V. Epigastric heteropagus twinning. J Pediatr Surg 2001;36:E11.
12. Hwang EH, Han SJ, Lee SJ, et al. An unusual case of monozygotic epigastric heteropagus twinning. J Pediatr Surg 1996;31:1457-60.
13. Logroño R, Garcia-Lithgow C, Harris C, et al. Heteropagus conjoined twins due to fusion of two embryos: report and review. Am J Med Genet. 1997;73(3):239-43.
14. William JL in Development of the vasculature, Human Embryology (2nd ed) Churchill Livingstone (1997).
15. Silbermann M, Bar-Maor JA, Auslander L. Craniofacial microsomia in a parasite of a heteropagus conjoined twin: a clinical and histopathologic evaluation. Head Neck Surg. 1984;6(3):792-800.
16. Fujimori, Shiroto T, Kuretake S, et al. An omphalopagus parasitic twin after intracytoplasmic sperm injection. Fertility and Sterility, 82(5):1430-32 K.
17. Eui HH, Seok JH, Jin SL, and Myo KL. A unusual case of monozygotic Epigastric Heteropagus twinning. J Pediatr Surg 1996;31:1457-60.
18. Kanamori Y, Tomonaga T, Sugiyama M, et al. Bizarre presentation of epigastric heteropagus: report of a case. Surg Today 2006;36(10):914-18.
19. Sathiakumar N, Ifere OA, Salawu SA, et al. Heteropagus: a case report. Ann Trop Paediatr 1988;8(1):38-41.
20. Tongsin A, Niramis R, Rattanasuwan T. Epigastric heteropagus twins: a report of four cases. J Med Assoc Thai. 2003;86 Suppl 3:S605-09.
21. Nasta R, Scibilia G, Corrao A, et al. Surgical treatment of an asymmetric double monstrosity with esophageal atresia. omphalocele and interventricular defect. J Pediatric surg 1986;21:60-62.
22. Karnak I, Ciftci AO, Büyükpamukçu N. Epigastric heteropagus: a case report with review of the literature. Eur J Pediatr Surg 1999;9(5):347-50.
23. Ribeiro RC, Maranhão RF, Moron AF, et al. Unusual case of epigastric heteropagus twinning. J Pediatr Surg 2005;40(3):E39-41.
24. Spencer R. Anatomic description of Conjoined twins: A plea for standardized terminology. J Pediatr Surg 1996;311:941-44.
25. Hager J, Sanal M, Trawöger R, et al. Conjoined epigastric heteropagus twins: excision of a parasitic twin from the anterior abdominal wall of her sibling. Eur J Pediatr Surg 2007;17(1):66-71.
26. Aquino DB, Timmons C, Burns D, Lowichik A. "Craniopagus parasiticus: a case illustrating its relationship to craniopagus conjoined twinning". Pediatric Pathology and Laboratory Medicine 1997;17(6):939-44.
27. Chen PL, Choe KA. Prenatal MRI of heteropagus twins. AJR Am J Roentgenol 2003;181(6):1676-78.

CHAPTER 114

Gynecological Problems in Children

Suneeta Mittal, Sonika Agarwal

The gynecological disorders of children, especially prior to puberty merit special consideration as these are far more difficult to diagnose and treat than in the adults. A knowledge of some of these disorders and their management is important as parents are frequently deeply alarmed by the diseases of sexual organs in children and some of these may have serious repercussions in later life. Adolescent and pediatric gynecology is now gaining importance with the awareness of the special issues involved pertaining to children.[1,2] Certain emergency situations may arise in adolescents like ectopic pregnancy and pelvic inflammatory disease.[3] A pediatric surgeon is required to understand these problems, though surgical intervention is only infrequently needed.

EMBRYOLOGY

Understanding the developmental anatomy is important as aberrations can result in several reproductive problems. Sex of the embryo is genetically determined at the time of fertilization. The development of gonads, internal genitalia and external genitalia takes place under the influence of Y chromosome and hormones. The gonads acquire male or female morphology from 7th week of development (Fig. 114.1).

The gonads develop from genital ridges formed by proliferation of the coelomic epithelium and condensation of the underlying mesenchyme. Primordial germ cells are derived from endoderm cells in the wall of yolk sac. These migrate along the dorsal mesentery of the hindgut and invade the genital ridges in the 6th week of development. Depending on the sex chromosome the gonads develop into either testis (XY) or ovary (XX).

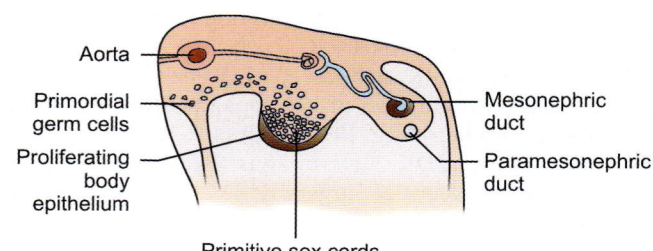

Fig. 114.1: Transverse section view of a 6-week embryo showing indifferent gonad and primitive sex cords

Internal genitalia develop from two pairs of the duct systems, which mature under the hormonal influence in the fetus. Both male and female embryos initially have both the genital ducts-the mesonephric and the paramesonephric ducts. Fetal testis produces an inducer substance, which causes differentiation and growth of the mesonephric ducts and inhibits the development of the paramesonephric ducts. Androgens stimulate the development of male genital organs. While in the absence of androgens the development takes place along female line. The mullerian inhibiting substance from fetal testes also plays an important role in genital differentiation. In the female embryo, the paramesonephric or mullerian ducts grow and develop into the internal genital organs in response to maternal and placental estrogens circulating in the fetus.

In the absence of male inducer substance and androgens the mesonephric duct system regresses. The paramesonephric ducts lie lateral to the mesonephric ducts (Fig. 114.2). The cranial part opens into the coelomic cavity, the middle part-crosses horizontally the mesonephric ducts and the caudal part lies

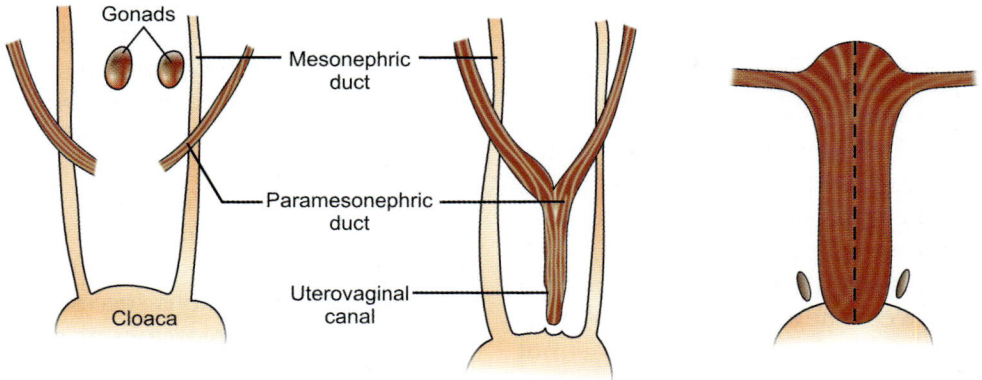

Fig. 114.2: Formation of uterovaginal canal

vertically alongside the duct from the other side. The two ducts fuse in the middle to form uterus, cervix and upper 2/3rd of vagina. The first two parts of paramesonephric ducts develop into the fallopian tubes. The lower 1/3rd of vagina is derived from the urogenital sinus (Fig. 114.3). Sinovaginal bulbs at the tip of paramesonephric ducts invade the urogenital sinus. The proliferation continues at the cranial end of the plate, thus increasing the distance between uterus and urogenital sinus. Lumen of vagina remains separated from that of the urogenital sinus by a thin tissue plate, the hymen.

Development of external genitalia takes place simultaneously. In the third week of development mesenchyme cells in the region of the primitive streak migrate to form cloacal folds around the cloacal membrane. Directly cranial to the cloacal membrane the folds unite to form the genital tubercle. In the sixth week, the cloacal membrane is subdivided into the urogenital and anal membranes. Genital swellings appear as elevations on either side of the urethral folds, forming scrotal swelling in the male and labia majora in the female. Genital tubercle elongates to form phallus in male fetus under androgenic influence. The external genitalia of the female forms under estrogenic influence. The genital tubercle elongates slightly to form the clitoris, the urethral folds remain unfused to form the labia minora and genital swellings enlarge to form the labia majora.

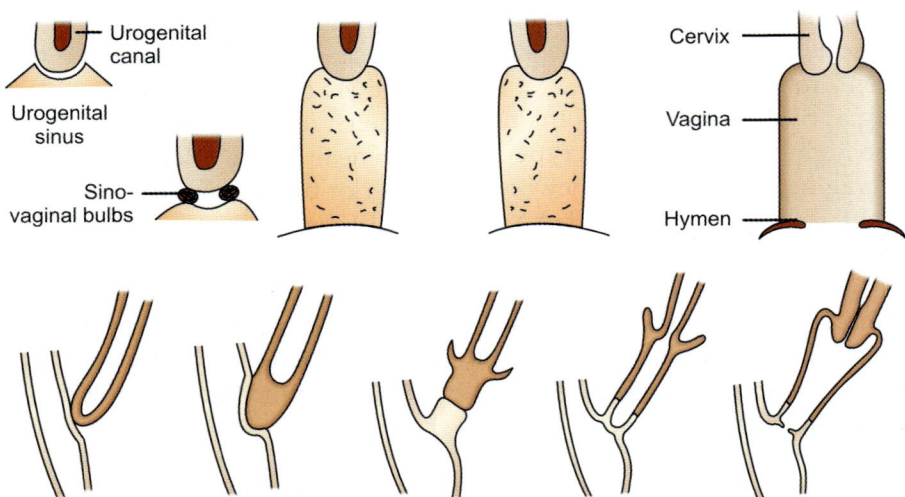

Fig. 114.3: Development of vagina

CLINICAL ANATOMY

The genitalia in a newborn undergo relatively few changes during the years of early childhood. The effects of maternal hormones on the genitalia of the newborn soon recede. The vulvar vestibule in the newborn infant is deeper and more anteriorly placed than in an adult. The labia majora do not actually develop as distinctive structures until late childhood. The perineal body is a thick, wedge-shaped mass of connective tissue between the anus and the vestibule. The mons pubis is a fatty pad over the symphysis, but does not acquire a rounded contour until late childhood. The labia minora which develop from the unfused urethral folds of the embryo, are relatively larger and thicker at birth and for several weeks thereafter, than in the older child or adult. The clitoris formed from the genital tubercle is also disproportionately larger and thicker at birth and for several weeks thereafter.

Separation of the labia minora exposes the urethral meatus and the hymen. In some infants a shallow urethral groove will be seen extending from the anterior margin of the urethral meatus to the base of the clitoris. The hymen is a thick membranous diaphragm, which, except for a central aperture of about 0.4-0.5 cm covers the opening of the vaginal canal. The thickness and succulence of the hymen reduces with the withdrawal of hormonal stimulation from the mother. Regressive changes in genitalia begin at birth and are usually complete by about two weeks. The resting phase of the genital growth usually lasts until the child is approximately seven years of age. The phase for the gradual growth of genitalia starts for most girls between 7 to 9 years of age.

The vaginal lining at birth is thick, soft, pink and moist and folded into high ridges and deep crypts by rugae. The length of vagina is 4-5 cm in the newborn. The external cervix of the newborn does not have the well-defined shape as in later life. The uterus undergoes marked hypertrophy under the effect of maternal placental hormones. The thick walled cervix forms the lower two-thirds of the organ and the corpus forms the upper third. The uterus rapidly regresses by about six months age to approximately half its weight at birth and remains infantile till puberty. A very rapid increase in uterine size occurs during premenarchial accelerated growth phase in response to estrogens. Growth of the upper segment is faster than cervix, but both progressively become larger during late childhood and acquire the adult size during the premenarchial growth phase.

Adolescence is characterized by maturation from a child to adult with an insidious beginning and end. All parts of biological system do not mature simultaneously; thus the process spans over a time period with puberty (anatomical change), menarche (functional change) and ovulation (endocrine change) occurring in a harmonious succession.

In recent years a precocious maturation of children is being noticed largely influenced by mass media exposure. This is more in terms of psychosocial maturation and may not be associated with proportionate physical maturation.

GYNECOLOGICAL EXAMINATION OF THE NEWBORN

Major anomalies of the external genitalia can be detected at birth. The baby should be placed on its back and having an assistant flex its thighs on its abdomen helps in exposing the genitalia.

The hymen, vulvar tissues, labia majora and minora, clitoris and urethra will be visible. Anomalies of the hymen, particularly imperforate hymen, can be discovered at birth. The opening is evident when the labia minora are separated and pulled gently posteriorly. If not evident as an orifice, the examiner can search by gently probing between the labia with the tip of no.14 French catheter. If the opening is not found it has to be differentiated whether it is an imperforate hymen - a thin shiny membrane or vaginal agenesis-vestibular tissues are thick and unyielding and there is a 'dimple' surrounded by an imperfectly formed hymen. Doubling of vagina is suspected if the hymeneal orifice is centrally divided by an antero-posterior band of tissue.

Clitoral enlargement in a newborn signifies congenital adrenal hyperplasia, excess of androgenic hormone treatment in the mother or intersex.

Digital palpation of the anorectal canal is part of the examination of a newborn.

Turning the baby onto its face and putting it in a knee-chest position makes it easier. If the child does not pass meconium the patency of the rectal canal is determined by gently inserting a soft rubber catheter to a point above that reached by the examiner's finger. Pelvic tumors are rare in newborn babies, but enough cases have been reported to warrant making recto-abdominal palpation a part of the newborn female examination.

EXAMINATION OF THE PREMENARCHIAL CHILD

In premenarchial age group the girls may present with complaints of discharge, redness or eruptions on the perineum and vulva, abdominal lump, vaginal bleeding, precocious development, urinary or rectal symptoms, etc.

Gynecologic examination of the premenarchial child is seldom difficult. Informed consent of the guardian is obtained as well as the child is explained about the examination. Cooperation of the child is important for satisfactory examination. For uncooperative children or children having perineal injury, it is better to conduct the examination under anesthesia. Habitus, built, gross congenital anomalies and hygiene are noted. Presence of secondary sexual characters—breast development, pubic and axillary hair is recorded. Having the child flex her thighs acutely on her abdomen offers better exposure. Examination can also be done in the Sim's or knee-chest position. Inspection is done after gently separating the labia and hygiene, excoriations, rashes or lesions are looked for and the patency of the hymen checked.

Vaginoscopy may be required to examine condition of vagina and cervix or to detect the presence of foreign body in the vagina. Proper inspection is important in girls with injury. Use of Huffman vaginoscope helps in visualization. A nasal speculum can also be used. Rectal and rectoabdominal palpation establishes the normalcy of the rectal canal and rectovaginal septum. Pelvic tumors or collections of blood or fluid can be detected on bimanual palpation.

EXAMINATION OF THE ADOLESCENT

Gynecological examination of an adolescent is no different than an adult, except that informed consent is a must. Adolescents are more uncooperative and shy than children are and proper explanation before examination is important. Special attention is paid to secondary sex characters, as well as any abnormality in puberty maturation. History of sexual activity may not be always forthcoming, but this opportunity can be utilized to educate the sexually active as well as other girls about sexual and reproductive health. This should include information about prevention of reproductive tract infections, including HIV/AIDS and contraception. It may be necessary to obtain specimen of discharge for microscopic examination and culture.

COMMON GYNECOLOGICAL PROBLEMS IN CHILDREN

Some of the commonly presenting gynecological disorders are discussed here.

The various gynecologic disorders in pediatric age group can be grouped as:
I. Congenital
II. Inflammatory
III. Traumatic
IV. Neoplastic
V. Endocrine
VI. Psychosomatic disorders

Congenital Disorders

Congenital Disorders Diagnosed in Utero

Conditions of the fetus requiring pediatric surgical consultation: With the use of routine screening by ultrasonography in pregnancy a majority of congenital malformations can be diagnosed during the prenatal period and require to be managed in consultation with pediatric surgeon to plan safe delivery and improve the neonatal outcome.

Ventriculomegly is one of the conditions diagnosed on basis of measurement of ventricular-hemispheric ratio and cortical mantle width. In a fetus with hydrocephalus intrauterine infections and chromosomal anomalies such as trisomy 13,18 and Turner's syndrome need to be ruled out. Based on the severity of affection termination or fetal surgery or early neonatal surgery is planned in consultation with the pediatric surgeon.

Urinary tract obstruction is found in one in 500-1000 pregnancy. Ultrasound helps in identifying unilateral/bilateral obstruction, bladder thickening/dilatation, renal echogenicity, ureteric dilatation, sex of fetus, other associated anomalies and amniotic fluid volume. The fetus is at a risk of pulmonary hypoplasia with bilateral obstructive nephropathy and oligohydramnios. Karyotype by cordocentesis helps to decide termination for abnormal fetuses. *In utero* treatment in early gestation with urethral obstruction has been tried by placing double pigtail vesicoamniotic shunt. If diagnosed late, most fetuses with significant nephropathy can be successfully managed after birth in collaboration with a pediatric surgeon and safe neonatal outcome achieved. Congenital diaphragmatic hernia is rare but appropriate management in the prenatal period and at birth can be life saving for the baby. *In utero* surgery to reduce development of pulmonary hypoplasia has been tried.

In gastroesophageal atresia and duodenal atresia diagnosed by ultrasound, pediatric surgeon's opinion is required and surgery in early neonatal period planned. Care after safe hospital delivery in a tertiary care center and practice of keeping the neonate on intravenous therapy, no feeding and nasogastric tube is important to prevent complications like aspiration and fluid-electrolyte imbalance.

Abdominal wall defects-gastrochiasis and omphalocele also require delivery to be planned after pediatric surgical consultation. Fetal karyotyping is essential in omphalocele where the association with chromosomal anomalies is as high as 60%. Labor induction, avoidance of emergency operation and quick transfer to the pediatric surgical unit for appropriate timing of neonatal surgery are important.

Congenital Disorders Detected after Birth

Anomalies of the hymen: Variations in size and number of fenestra and in thickness of the hymen are common. The hymen may be imperforate, cribriform, anteriorly displaced and septate. Two orifices in hymen may be associated with duplication of internal genitalia. Hymeneal anomalies are clinically important and require surgical correction, if they block the escape of vaginal discharge or menstrual fluid or cause coital problems.

Imperforate hymen may produce a mucocolpos in infancy and if not corrected before menarche, will cause a hematocolpos and hematometra when the girl starts to menstruate.[4] Symptoms are those related to pressure on the urinary tract, abdominal or pelvic lump and cyclical pain abdomen with failure to attain menarche. The girl may be brought to casualty with acute urinary retention. Inspection of the vulva reveals a bulging tense bluish membrane.

In a neonate this membrane may rupture spontaneously or may be incised to drain collected discharge and edges may be sutured with absorbable suture. In an adolescent girl a cruciate incision is given in the bulging membrane under general anesthesia and collected blood is sucked out. The child is nursed in Fowler's position to facilitate drainage and vaginal examination is deferred to a later date.

Anomalies of the Vagina

Anomalies of the vagina do not cause symptoms during infancy and childhood.

They present later when there is interference with menstruation. Double vagina and septate vagina are reported. Transverse vaginal septum occurs at any level above the hymen and needs surgical correction to widen the vagina and allow normal menstruation and coitus. To prevent stenosis of vagina, complete excision of septum is important and use of vaginal dilators may be required. In case of a high septum, vaginal advancement surgery is done to prevent restenosis. Longitudinal. vaginal septum does not interfere with menstrual flow, thus usually present later with dyspareunia or obstruction during labor. With uterine duplication, one side may be obstructed, and girl complains of severe pain during period due to hematometra on the obstructed side. Though uncommon, but this condition has often been misdiagnosed and mistreated, as menstruation occurs regularly from the normal side and girls continue to be treated for primary dysmenorrhoea. Endometriosis can occur due to retrograde menstruation.

Vaginal atresia due to complete or partial failure of canalization of the vaginal plate will also lead to hematometra and hematocolpos when the girl attains puberty. Vaginoplasty with amnion or split thickness skin graft is the treatment.

Mullerian agenesis is total agenesis of the uterus, vagina and cervix and vaginoplasty can help for coital function but these patients cannot menstruate or conceive. Most of these girls present with primary amenorrhoea. Some may get married young and report with apareunia.

Congenital vaginal cysts usually develop from occluded persistent fragments of the mesonephric ducts, from unfused portions of the paramesonephric ducts or from obstructed paraurethral ducts. Small cysts require no treatment; however, larger ones need to be excised.

Uterine Anomalies

These anomalies rarely cause problem in infancy and childhood. Bicornuate, septate, unicornuate uterus

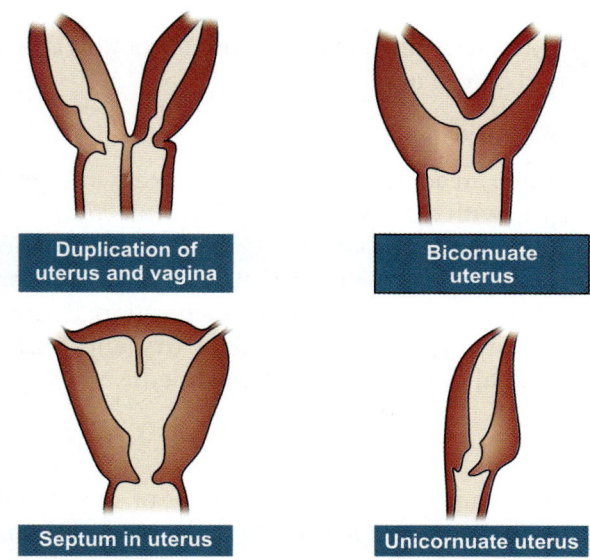

Fig. 114.4: Anomalies of the uterus

with rudimentary horn, uterus diadelphys, etc. all are associated with problems of conception and pregnancy complications (Fig. 114.4). Mullerian agenesis with congenital absence of vagina and uterus (Mayer Rokitansky Kustner Hauser Syndrome) manifests early with failure to menstruate. Approximately, 40% of these girls have associated urinary tract anomalies and 12% musculo-skeletal malformations. Endocrine and ovarian function as well as karyotype is normal. Ultrasound and laparoscopy are useful to differentiate this condition from isolated vaginal malformation.

A complex surgical procedure is required to create a new vagina in these girls. Vaginoplasty is usually carried out only when sexual function is desired, i.e. after the marriage has been fixed. Proper counseling is important and full co-operation of girl is essential to maintain the patency of neovagina by repeated use of vaginal dilators. Several tissues have been used for vaginal graft including split thickness skin graft from thigh, amnion, perineal skin, sigmoid loop, gracilis musculo-cutaneous flap or pelvic. peritoneum William's vulvoplasty my be done in selected cases to create a coital pouch.

Intersex

Intersexuality is the condition of imperfect sexual differentiation. Sex is Primarily determined by the sex chromosome supplied by the spermatozoa. The Y-chromosome gives the positive drive towards male sex differentiation and determines the gonadal development into a testis. In the absence of Y chromosome the gonad matures as ovary. If the chromosomal direction to the gonad is confused, ovotestes develop. When the chromosomal drive to the gonad is weak, hypoplasia of the gonad is likely, resulting in gonadal aplasia, hypoplasia or streak gonad.

Turner's syndrome is the classical syndrome associated with streak gonads, with a karyotype of 45 X0 or a mosaic. The primary cause is non-disjunction of the sex chromosomes. Triple X (47XXX) syndrome also results from non-disjunction and leads to problems of oligomenorrhea, secondary amenorrhea, infertility, genital hypoplasia and mental retardation. Klinefelter's syndrome (47XXY) is characterized by a tall eunuchoid figure with testicular and genital hypoplasia.

Maternal hormones during pregnancy cross the placenta but do not influence the sexual differentiation. If, however, the mother suffers from an androgenic tumor of the adrenal or ovary, congenital adrenal hyperplasia or she takes exogenous androgens the external genitalia of the female fetus can get virilized, the degree depending on the timing and strength of the influence. Progesterone is also weakly androgenic and synthetic progestogens when given to the mother for pregnancy support can sometimes virilize the female fetus.

Intrauterine adrenogenital syndrome is a familial disease transmitted by a recessive gene leading to inherent error in the biosynthetic process in the adrenal cortex, and elevated levels of androgenic hormones. Deficiency of adrenal cortical hormones further increases the output of ACTH causing bilateral adrenal hyperplasia. There is anomalous sexual differentiation of external genitalia in the female fetus including labial fusion, hypospadias and phallic enlargement. Congenital variety presents as ambiguous genitalia at birth, the acquired syndrome presents as stunted height, hirsutism, infertility, amenorrhea, voice change and clitoral hypertrophy at a later age. Diagnosis is based on elevated 17-hydroxy progesterone levels and testosterone with 46XX karyotype. Treatment is by dexamethasone to suppress adrenal hypertrophy and later in life correction of genital ambiguity and treatment for amenorrhea, hirsutism and infertility.

Intersex states can also result from androgen insensitivity leading to testicular feminization syndrome. This is an apparent female, with breast development, normal vulva and hairless skin, but the gonads are testes and karyotype is 46XY.

Of all these intersex disorders, the most significant is detection of ambiguous genitalia at birth. This requires immediate attention, as parents are keen to know the sex of the child. They should be counseled and sex assignment is delayed till complete evaluation is done.

Evaluation includes a history of similar disorder in family, maternal virilization and maternal drug intake. On labioscrotal and rectal palpation the presence of testes and uterus is determined respectively. Ultrasonography is also useful. Blood tests include measuring serum aldosterone, cortisol,[17] hydroxy-progesterone, LH and FSH levels and determining the karyotype. Electrolytes are also monitored till the diagnosis is established and treatment initiated. Sex assignment is not solely based on karyotype or gonad type but on what can be achieved subsequently. Female pseudohermaphrodites due to congenital adrenal hyperplasia are reared as females despite marked virilization, as it is possible to create a functional vagina, do clitoroplasty and even restore fertility in these girls. Male pseudohermaphrodites respond very well to androgen treatment, thus even when the testes is undescended and there is marked hypospadias, these children are brought up as males and surgical correction is done at a later age. Males with androgen resistance do not respond, to androgen treatment, thus should be brought up as females despite XY karyotype and with gonadectomy is done as soon as pubertal growth spert has taken place. Vaginoplasty is carried out as and when, the sexual function is desired.

Inflammatory Disorders

Inflammations and infections of perineal and vulvar skin is the most common problem that brings little girls to physicians.

Diaper Rash

Excess moisture, heat and poor hygiene can lead to infections due to fecal bacteria and urinary contamination in infants. Ammonia dermatitis is a major factor in causing diaper rash. Proper cleanliness, bathing and drying before applying talc helps in the treatment. Calamine ointment containing 1% erythromycin can be applied to the affected area. Diapers are sterilized by boiling and thoroughly rinsed and dried before use.

Perineal Dermatitis

This is often an acute inflammatory process in slightly older girls with a secondary pyogenic infection.

Nutritional disturbance, allergy or drug reaction can also lead to perineal dermatitis. Symptoms vary from itching, burning or pain on micturation. Perineal hygiene, keeping the affected area dry and topical antimicrobial ointment are the treatment.

Intertrigo

Intertrigo is an inflammatory disorder of skin, which occurs when skin surfaces of the vulva, buttocks and thighs are in apposition for a prolonged period. This can affect girls of all ages, but obese and diabetic are more prone to it. Friction produces erythema, maceration and inflammation. Secondary infection with bacteria or fungus may take place. Proper perineal hygiene, cleanliness in the crevices, talc application and topical antibiotic ointments is used. Sitz' bath and ointments with topical steroids also help.

Premenarchial Vulvovaginitis

Vulvovaginal inflammation with vaginal discharge is one of the most frequent disorders treated in a pediatric gynecologic clinic.

At birth babies have excess physiologic vaginal fluid and later it becomes blood—stained due to the withdrawal of maternal hormones. Discharge and bleeding disappear within 7-10 days and do not require any treatment.

Premenarchial girls are particularly susceptible to Vulvovaginitis due to thin vaginal lining and neutral pH. It is caused by bacterial, trichomonal, mycotic (candida) or viral infections and as reaction to medications, bubble baths or nylon undergarments, etc. Nonspecific vulvovaginitis is an infection of the vulvar and vaginal epithelium by pyogenic organisms secondary to poor hygiene, skin or urinary tract infections, foreign bodies in the vagina or sexual abuse. Discomfort, itching and discharge are usual presenting complaints. Burning sensation or irritation after voiding, stain on panties or vulvar redness may also bring the child for consultation. A sample of vaginal discharge is collected for wet smear, gram-stain and culture. For vaginal secretion sampling, compliance of the young patients has been studied and reported best with the otologic cotton swab.[5]

Porper perineal hygiene is the key factor in treatment along with treatment for the primary infection. Specific vulvovaginitis due to gonorrhea, chlamydia, hemolytic *streptococci*, hemophilus vaginalis, diplococcus pneumoniae, etc. need specific treatment. Trichomoniasis needs to be treated with metronidazole and candidal infection with clotrimazole or miconazole. Threadworm infections usually respond well to deworming by piperazine preparation or mebendazole suspension.

Labial Adhesions

Adherent or fused labia minora is a common pediatric gynecologic problem.

They occur most often in children between 1-6 years of age. Poor hygiene and inflammation lead to adhesions between the two labial surfaces due to the eroded epithelium. Lack of estrogen helps in adhesion formation. Labial adhesions are never present in a neonate, as maternal estrogen is protective. Sometimes parents bring the young girls suspecting that the sex of the child is changing. If labia are fused at birth the neonate should be evaluated for intersex problems. The treatment options available are:
a. Maintaining careful local hygiene and application of an estrogen ointment at bedtime for 14 days can separate the labial agglutination. Topical estrogen therapy has been found to be effective in treating persistent or recurrent labial agglutination.[6]
b. Gentle manual separation can be done easily as an out patient procedure. It is to be followed by local application of a soothing antibiotic cream to avoid adhesions
c. Surgical separation may be needed occasionally for dense adhesions recur. The mother should be instructed to maintain the genitalia clean and dry.

Traumatic Disorders

Injuries to the Genitalia during Childhood

Injuries usually occur as a result of fall on sharp or penetrating objects.

Many injuries are trifling in character, but few are life-threatening and require extensive reconstructive surgery. Physical or sexual assault may also lead to injuries. Most of the extensive hematomas or lacerations of vulva, vagina and urethra in young girls require proper resuscitation, examination under anesthesia, evacuation of hematoma and proper reconstructive surgery. However, we have noticed that healing in young girls with perineal injuries is very good even following extensive tissue damage. Repair needs to be done very patiently using atraumatic sutures, as the vaginal mucosa is very thin. Proper exploration for concomitant bladder and anorectal injury should be done. In very extensive cases prolonged bladder drainage or colostomy may be required. Maintenance of proper vulvar hygiene and use of broad-spectrum antibiotics is important for successful outcome.

For victims of sexual abuse screening for sexually transmitted infections including HIV is important. Postmenarchial girls should also be given emergency contraception.

Vaginal Foreign Bodies

Foreign bodies in the vagina although almost always considered a possibility in young girls presenting with mucopurulent fowl smelling or blood stained discharge, but are relatively uncommon. Bits of cloth, toilet tissue, pieces of toys are the common ones, which need to be removed at vaginoscopy. Profuse discharge and pain may necessitate removal under sedation or anesthesia. Antibiotics are given to take care of superadded infection. Hypercalciuria with microcrystals and urethral irritation has also been reported to cause genital bleeding in girls.[7]

Neoplastic Disorders

Benign Tumors of the Vulva and Vagina

Benign genital neoplasms occur very rarely in human females under 16 years of age. Epithelial inclusion cysts and paraurethral cysts are uncommon but can be found in any age group. Labial papillomas (skin tags) are asymptomatic and usually do not need surgical removal. Vulvar hydrocele or cyst of the canal of Nuck occurs as a cystic swelling of the distal closed end of a remnant of the processus vaginalis that extends into the labium majus. It requires surgical excision. Capillary hemangiomas of the vulva do not cause symptoms and do not require treatment. Many of them regress spontaneously over a period of 5-6 years due to thrombosis and fibrosis. Cavernous hemangiomas are however hazardous and require surgical ligation of the feeding blood vessel. Lipomas, myobastomas and teratomas of perineum are extremely rare.

Vaginal benign tumors include vaginal polyps, mullerian duct cysts and Gartner's cysts.

Malignant Tumors of the Vulva and Vagina

Most common tumors reported are mixed mesodermal tumors of the vagina. These malignancies are extremely rare in children and adolescents but are associated with a high malignant potential. Vaginal adenosis and adenocarcinoma occur in young girls with history of exposure to diethyl-stilbestrol (DES) *in utero*.

The most serious tumor in pediatrics age group is embryonal rhabdomyosarcoma, which progresses rapidly. Five-year survival has improved with combination chemotherapy—utilizing vincristine, actinomycin and cyclophosphamide.

Tumors of the Uterus, Tubes and Broad Ligaments

Benign tumors of the cervix include cervical papillomas and myomas. Uterine leimyomas have also been reported in young girls.

Carcinoma of the cervix has been rarely reported in girls below 16 years of age. Adenocarcinoma of the uterine corpus and mixed mesodermal tumors of the uterine corpus though extremely rare, have been reported in young girls. Management is similar to adults.

Ovarian Tumors in Children and Adolescents

Ovarian tumors constitute about 1% of all new growths in girls under 16 years of age. Despite their rarity, germ cell tumors of the ovary are the most frequent genital neoplasms during childhood and adolescence. Approximately 30% of all ovarian tumors in children and adolescents are benign cystic teratomas or dermoids. Simple cysts of follicular type may be found especially in the newborn and a very young child. Multicystic ovaries, polycystic ovarian disease, corpus luteal cysts and theca lutein cysts are the benign lesions in the ovary.

Malignant tumors include dysgerminomas, malignant teratomas, embryonal carcinomas and sex cord stromal tumors.

Dysgerminoma is relatively commoner in younger age than in the adult. Ten percent of all solid carcinomas of the ovary develop during the first two decades of life. The patient presents with pain and lump abdomen, anorexia, weight loss and abdominal distension due to ascites, etc. Estrogen producing tumors may cause precocious puberty, while, androgenic hormones may produce irregularity of menses, voice changes, hirsutism and clitoromegaly.

Treatment comprises of surgery, radiation and chemotherapy depending on the stage and type of malignancy. Fertility conservation is an important consideration in benign tumors and early stage cancers of the ovary. In tumors confined to one ovary, unilateral ovariotomy and wedge resection with biopsy from contralateral ovary is done. This is followed by radiation or chemotherapy depending on the stage.

Gynecological Consequences of Cancer Therapy in Children

A number of children with cancers like leukemia, lymphomas, CNS tumors and neuroblastoma are treated with surgery, radiation and/or chemotherapy that can affect their reproductive potential.

Surgery for CNS tumors can affect pubertal maturation. Resection of pituitary tumors can lead to endocrine dysfunction. Pelvic surgery for bladder or other tumors can also devitalize uterus or ovaries.

Ovaries in children are more resistant to radiation or chemotherapy than adolescents and adults, nevertheless, children receiving 3000 rads pelvic radiation can have permanent ovarian failure. In such children laparoscopic oophoropexy (fixing ovary out of radiation field) is currently being done routinely.

Ovarian suppression with long acting GnRH analogue has also been tried to reduce radiotoxicity.

Radiation to head can also affect pituitary hormones and result in gonadal failure. Most children surviving after acute lymphocytic leukemia suffer from growth failure.

Chemotherapy alone has very little effect on prepubertal ovary, thus most girls treated with combination chemotherapy have normal puberty.

Endocrine Disorders

The hormonal control of pubertal development begins in the hypothalamus by producing gonadotrophin-releasing hormone, which passes down the pituitary portal system to the anterior pituitary where follicle-stimulating hormone (FSH) is produced. This stimulates the development of Graffian follicles in the ovary, one of which ovulates as a result of luteinizing hormone (LH) surge at the appropriate stage of follicle development. These cyclical hormonal changes produce varying levels of oestrogen and progesterone leading to cyclical phases of the endometrial menstrual cycle.

The first sign of pubertal development is usually thelarche (breast growth) between the ages of 8 and 13 years. Growth in height occurs about the same time. Adrenarche (pubic hair development) usually follows next, and later the appearance of axillary hair and onset of menstruation (menarche).

Precocious Sexual Development

Sexual development must be considered precocious if there is breast and pubic hair growth before the age or 8 years and menstrual period before the age of 10 years.

The most common cause for this is constitutional precocious puberty, without any organic lesion being found. The signs of puberty usually appear in their correct order and the bone-age as well as the child's height are several years in advance of the chronological age.

Before labeling the condition as constitutional precocious puberty, the organic causes must be excluded. These include intracranial lesions, such as meningitis, encephalitis, cerebral tumours, third ventricle hamartoma or Albright's syndrome. MRI helps in detecting the CNS pathology. Less common is premature sexual development due to a feminizing tumor of the ovary. Treatment of cause, e.g. oophorectomy cures the girl. It may sometimes be partial precocious puberty with isolated breast development (excess estrogen only) or early pubic hair growth (adrenarche-with excess androgen alone). These usually require no treatment. Constitutional precocious puberty is treated with cyclic GnRH analogue injection 3.6 mg every 4 weeks, , cyproterone acetate 70-150 mg/m^2 orally or medroxy progesterone acetate 100-200 mg intramuscularly every 2-4 weeks.

Delayed Puberty

Absence of sexual maturation till 14 years of age is delayed puberty and absence of menstruation till 16 years is considered as primary amenorrhoea in a young girl.

Delayed puberty is commonly constitutional. Usually there is a family history of similar delay. Only reassurance and observation is required if investigations reveal no abnormality.

Delay in maturation may be due to primary gonadal failure (hypergonadotrophic hypogonadism) or hypothalamic-pituitary failure (hypogonadotrophic hypogonadism). In primary hypogonadism, estrogen level is low with high FSH and LH. This is seen in girls with gonadal dysgenesis, Turner's syndrome or following surgical removal of gonads. Hypogonadotrophic hypogonadism may occur secondary to CNS tumors, radiation or congenital hypothalamic defect. Anorexia nervosa and chronic illness can also delay the normal maturation. In both hypo and hypergonadotrophic hypogonadism cyclic estrogen replacement results in sexual maturation and withdrawal bleeds. Fertility is possible in hypogonadotrophic states, by ovulation induction using high doses of gonadotrophins.

Dysfunctional Uterine Bleeding

Early menstrual cycles are often irregular in their duration and amount of blood loss for some months after the onset of menarche, due to irregular ovulation. Such variation is within physiological limits, thus investigation and treatment are unnecessary. In girls presenting with excessive and irregular menstrual bleeding complications of early pregnancy and irregular oral contraceptive pill use should be excluded by careful history.

Reassurance and maintenance of menstrual chart along with mefenamic acid (500 mg TID) during menses is sufficient in majority. Puberty menorrhagia with heavy bleeding may necessitate hormonal therapy in some cases. Norethisterone (5 mg TID or QID) stops bleeding in few days. Subsequently cyclic treatment is given with combined pills for 2-3 cycles. Tuberculosis and blood coagulation disorders should be excluded as these may present as puberty menorrhagia. Iron therapy and dietary advice must also be given.

Irregular menstruation and oligomenorrhea or hypomenorrhea often result due to anxiety or stress of examination and emotional factors. These usually do not need any treatment except for protracted cases where tuberculosis should be ruled out. Thyroid disorders may also present as menstrual disturbances.

Dysmenorrhea

Anovular menstruation seldom causes pain. Dysmenorrhea is more common when regular ovulation is established. Some young girls take little discomfort at the time of periods in stride, while others feel extremely incapacitated by it. A significant number miss school due to pain. Exercise should be encouraged and the patient reassured. NSAIDS and mefenamic acid tablets (500 mg TID) are very helpful. Severe cases may require oral contraceptive pills to inhibit ovulation. An ultrasonographic scan of the uterus and ovaries should be done to exclude any organic pathology specially endometriosis or genital tract anomalies.

Amenorrhea and Hirsutism

The symptoms of secondary amenorrhea and hirsutism are both related to disorders in hormonal balance or due to specific organic cause. Primary amenorrhea needs to be evaluated if the girl has reached the age of 16 years without menarche or if secondary sexual development has not begun by age of 14 years. Secondary amenorrhea is the absence of menstruation for 6 months or longer in a girl who has previously had normal menstruation. These need detail gynecological and endocrinological investigation and management. Peripubertal polycystic ovary syndrome commonly manifests with oligomenorrhea, acne and hirsutism. Early identification and treatment is important to prevent long-term consequences.

Premenstrual Syndrome (PMS)

The premenstrual syndrome has been defined as menstrually related mood disorder that includes the cyclic occurrence of symptoms that are of sufficient severity to interfere with some aspects of life. Symptoms vary from tension, anxiety, anger, altered appetite, abdominal pain and bloating, weight gain, nausea, diarrhea, etc. Counseling, tranquilizers, pyridoxine and progesterone are used in the treatment.

Psychosomatic Disorders

Anorexia Nervosa and Bulimia Nervosa

This is a significant problem in affluent classes. The social climate as well as genetic, physiological or psychological vulnerability is there. In anorexia nervosa there is extreme weight loss which may lead to stoppage of menstruation. Bulimia is episodic binge eating of variable duration, which may be followed by a phase of anorexia nervosa. In anorexia there is loss of at least 25% of original body weight, while bulimia is usually associated with obesity. These disorders can be cured if treated early. Identification and correction of predisposing factors is important. Psychotherapy and reinforcement is often required.

CONCLUSION

Children and adolescents can present with a myriad of gynecological disorders. A knowledge of these is essential to prevent misdiagnosis and ensure proper management.

REFERENCES

1. Current world literature. Adolescent and pediatric gynecology. Curr Opin Obstet Gynecol 2005;17(5): 547-51.
2. Korczak DJ, MacArthur C, Katzman DK. Canadian pediatric residents' experience and level of comfort with adolescent gynecological health care. J Adolesc Health 2006;38(1):57-59.
3. Ahrendt DM, Roncallo PG. Emergencies in adolescents: management guidelines for four presentations. Pediatr Ann 2005;34(11):895-901.
4. Dadhwal V, Mittal S, Kumar S, Barua A. Hematometra in Postmenarchal adolescent girls. A report of two cases. Gynecol Obstet Invest 2000; 50(1):67-69.
5. Beolchi S, Mastromatteo C, Baietti M, et al. Vaginal swab in pediatric age. Pediatr Med Chir 2005;27(3-4):88-90.
6. Kumetz LM, Quint EH, Fisseha S, Smith YR. Estrogen treatment success in recurrent and persistent labial agglutination. J Pediatr Adolesc Gynecol 2006;19(6): 381-84.
7. Valcourt EE, Fleming NA, Weiler G. Hypercalciuria as a cause of genital bleeding in a 6-year-old girl. J Pediatr Adolesc Gynecol 2006 ;19(5):333-35.

CHAPTER 115

Ovarian Cysts

Shilpa Sharma, DK Gupta

Ovarian cysts in the pediatric age group are seen at two different peaks of age group, in the neonatal period and in the adolescent age. The cyst usually develops as a result of change in the hormonal milieu.

FETAL AND NEONATAL OVARIAN CYSTS

Ovarian cysts are most frequently diagnosed during the prenatal period due to routine antenatal ultrasonography. In the neonates, the ovarian cysts are rarely symptomatic. In absence of an antenatal ultrasonography, most of these cases would have passed unnoticed. More than 250 cases of antenatally diagnosed ovarian cyst had been reported till 1990. Though not all cases are reported yet, their number is increasing each year.[1,2]

The ovarian cysts in the fetus and the newborn develop due to the high level of fetal circulating gonadotropins, due to maternal estrogens and placental chorionic gonadotropins (HCG).[3] The HCG levels may be high in mothers with diabetes, Rh-iso-immunization and Toxemia.[4]

An immature hypothalamus-pituitary-ovarian feedback is thought to be responsible for gonadal hyperstimulation in severely premature fetuses. At birth, maturation of the central nervous system and regulation of anterior pituitary function lead to a negative-biofeedback mechanism decreasing hormonal stimulation and arrest of follicular maturation, and development.[4]

After birth the hormonal stimulation is withdrawn and the ovarian cysts that are small in size disappear spontaneously. However, the cysts that are larger (more than 4 cm. in size) do not disappear and are more likely to undergo complications.[5] The etiology of ovarian cysts varies with the developmental stage and hormonal milieu of the patient.[6]

CLINICAL FEATURES

Most ovarian cysts are unilateral, only rarely are they bilateral. Most of the Fetal and neonatal ovarian cysts are asymptomatic and are diagnosed in the antenatal period.

Rarely, the cyst may present as an abdominal lump. The newborn is usually asymptomatic despite the fact that the cyst may have already undergone complications like torsion, hemorrhage and adhesions with formation of bands.[3] A moderately sized cyst, especially with long pedicles is freely mobile in the abdomen and can reach up to the umbilicus, or even higher up without any difficulty. Occasionally the cyst may enlarge grossly, causing respiratory embarrassment, pressure over the inferior vena cava, bladder and the intestine and may simulate neonatal ascites.

COMPLICATIONS

1. Fetal ovarian cyst–Dystocia during delivery
2. Torsion of the cysts around the ovarian pedicle
3. Infarction
4. Autoamputation which may present as a wandering mass in the abdomen.[7]
5. Rupture. It may present as complicated ascites and a collapsed cystic structure in the abdomen.
6. Ascites
7. Hemorrhage
8. Infection
9. Respiratory embarrassment.[8]

10. Infertility in bilateral cases.
11. Compression of other viscera.[6]
12. Edema of the labia.

Most of fetal and neonatal cysts are simple cysts that involute during pregnancy or in the first months of life.[9,10] Torsion is the most common (50-78%) complication because the newborn ovary has a long pedicle and it is more common in cysts > 5 cm in diameter.[7]

Spontaneous hemorrhage into a fetal ovarian cyst is a serious complication and should be followed by serial ultrasound and Doppler assessments to reveal the development of fetal anemia, which should be managed by intrauterine blood transfusion.[11]

INVESTIGATIONS

Ultrasonography is the most useful and solely sufficient diagnostic modality for an ovarian cyst. Aspiration of the fluid in the cyst under ultrasonic guidance and analysis for high hormones levels (estrogens, progestins) is diagnostic.[12] Ultrasonographic evidence of torsion is described as an intracystic flocculation which typically is deposited on the sloping part of the cyst, and gives a characteristic liquid interface.[2] Antenatal ultrasonography reveals an echo-rare or echo-free area in the fetal abdomen.

Computerized tomography is indicated only if the diagnosis is in doubt, or a solid component is seen on ultrasonography.

DIFFERENTIAL DIAGNOSIS

The differential diagnosis includes the following:
1. Solid tumors with large cystic components. Granulosa cell tumor and cystadenoma have been reported as cystic lumps in the newborn. A fetal juvenile granulosa cell tumor has been diagnosed as a complicated ovarian cyst in the 32 nd week of pregnancy.[11]
2. Duplication bowel cyst (spherical type). The duplication cyst tends to have some intestinal symptoms. Most cystic duplication cysts are in relation to the small bowel and rarely with the left colon.
3. Urachal cyst. Mobility is very much limited.
4. Cyst of the renal origin. These can be easily differentiated on ultrasonography.
5. A small omental and the mesenteric cyst may be quite difficult to differentiate from an uncomplicated ovarian cyst.
6. Hydrometrocolpos presenting, as an abdominal mass is present in the midline, and extends deep into the pelvis. There may also be a single opening in the perineum and the symptoms of urinary obstruction may be present.
7. Occasionally, a duplex kidney with megaureter has also been mistaken for an ovarian cyst.[13]

MANAGEMENT

The management of fetal ovarian cysts is still controversial. Some studies suggest an aggressive management, while others opt for a conservative one. In general, most ovarian cysts are functional in nature and usually resolve without treatment, if small in size.[6]

Indications for Surgical Intervention

1. Patient is symptomatic.
2. If the diagnosis is in doubt.
3. Complex or functional cysts.
4. Cysts larger than 4 cm in the prenatal or newborn period and larger than 5 cm till one year of age.
5. The cyst persists longer than one year.

All surgical procedures for ovarian cysts should spare functional ovary as much as is technically possible.[5] Simple cysts should be fenestrated.

Complex or functional cysts should be excised, with preservation of the remaining ovary.[6]

The ovarian cyst, which is really small, can be left and observed regularly by serial ultrasonography.[9] The cut off size for conservative management with observation and reassessment by serial ultrasonography is taken by some as 4 cms and by others as 5 cm.[14,15] Involution of neonatal ovarian cysts occurs usually by 12 months.[16] Persisting cysts larger than 4 cm are prone to torsion.[16]

As the cyst involves almost whole of the ovarian stoma, oophrectomy is the procedure often required in most of the complicated cysts. Occasionally, if the ovarian stroma is seen uninvolved or found stretched over the cyst, a cystectomy or deroofing can be performed, preserving the remaining functional ovarian tissue (Fig. 115.1). In-patients with bilateral ovarian cyst or bilateral ovarian disease, every attempt

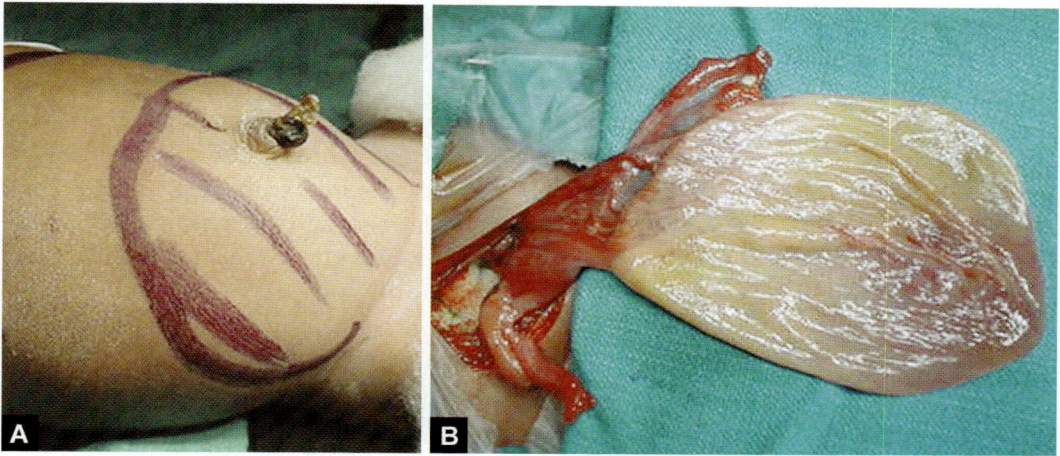

Figs 115.1A and B: **A.** A clinical photograph of a neonate with a large ovarian cyst, **B.** Operative photograph of the same. Showing the decompressed cyst

should be made to preserve whatever ovarian tissue can be salvaged (Fig 115.2). Failure to achieve this, would require a life long hormonal support.

Intrauterine intervention (needle aspiration) decompresses the cyst and is known thus to prevent complications and preserve ovarian functions.[12] Large cysts can also be decompressed if uncomplicated.[17] US-guided aspiration has been found quite safe and effective. The aspirations can be repeated also if the need be, for the salvage or decompression if the intrauterine ovarian torsion occurs.[16] Surgery should be reserved for patients with acute torsion, intestinal obstruction due to bands, adhesions and intestinal volvulus.[16]

In earlier reports, more liberal surgical intervention was advocated to prevent complication.[18] Neonatal cystic lesions may not always require therapy.[19] Nowadays surgical intervention is warranted in only about 50% of the cases. The most appropriate clinical approach in the management of benign feto-neonatal ovarian cysts is to adopt a wait-and-see policy, assessing the course of the condition by means of periodic ultrasound monitoring and intervene if the diagnosis remained in doubt.

In the authors experience most of the ovarian cysts seen during the neonatal period have presented with asymptomatic abdominal lumps. Most of these (60%) were found to have already undergone torsion, infarction, hemorrhage, or even auto-amputation, completely destroying the ovarian tissue.[3] The ovarian cysts were also found to have exudates and fibrotic bands attaching the same with the intestine loops. The

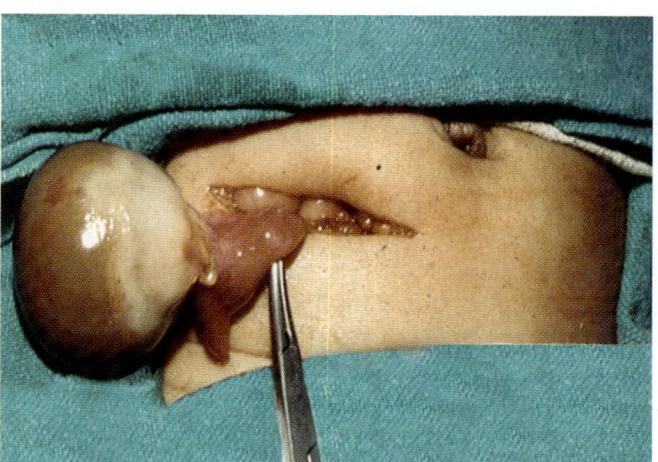

Fig. 115.2: Operative photograph of a patient with right ovarian cyst. The left ovarian tissue was poorly developed

bands can not be appreciated on ultrasonography. This may result in a serious complication in the form of intestinal herniation and volvulus, if the conservative treatment is followed. Thus, not only the large and complicated cysts, but all ovarian cysts, irrespective of their size, are best managed by surgery.

Laparoscopy has now become quite popular to treat ovarian cysts and the approach is favored by most pediatric surgeons who are in this field.[6] Aspiration, deroofing, cystectomy and salpingo-ophrectomy can all be performed, including the neonates, by laparoscope.[20] A complex ovarian cyst in a neonate has been successfully treated by laparoscopic-assisted transumbilical ovarian cystectomy procedure.[21]

Prenatally diagnosed complex ovarian cysts are most often managed surgically in an attempt to save the ovary.[22] Nevertheless, published surgical results show that most patients undergo oophorectomy or salpingo-oophorectomy.[22] Histologic analysis has suggested gonad maldevelopment as the origin of complex neonatal ovarian cysts.[22] Needle aspiration during the antenatal period, can help in regression of the large number of cysts, even those larger than 5 cm in diameter. In the meta-analysis of 420 cases, reported by Slodki et al, 89% cysts (25 out of 28) resolved with prenatal needle aspiration.[15]

PROGNOSIS

The prognosis of the majority of congenital ovarian cysts is good since they have a benign origin.[17] In about 50% cases, in which the cyst diameter was less than 4 cm, periodic ultrasound examinations have revealed a tendency towards spontaneous regression of the cysts.[17] In the other 50% casers, with a cyst diameter more than 4 cm, cystectomy is necessary due to subsequent complications (torsion, intracystic hemorrhage). In a series reported by Foiley et al, 8 out of 11 ovarian cysts which were simple at recognition, became complex by the time at birth, with an ovarian tissue loss in 54% cases.[23]

The meta-analysis of 420 fetuses with ovarian cyst reported by Slodki et al, showed that the majority of the ovarian cysts regressed (n-209, 50%) spontaneously and 98% of these were less than 5 cm in diameter. Surgical treatment was performed in 174 cases (41%) and 93% of these had ovarian cysts larger than 5 cm in diameter. Also, 145 cases (35%) cysts got complicated by torsion and intracystic hemorrhage requiring surgery.[15]

PERIPUBERTAL OVARIAN CYSTS

Ovarian cysts develop usually after puberty from the mature follicles when the ovaries become hormonally active. Most of these cysts are asymptomatic. Due to the widespread use of sophisticated and detailed diagnostic imaging, pediatric surgeons may encounter incidental ovarian masses on preoperative imaging obtained for abdominal pain, trauma or other indications, or at laparotomy or laparoscopy.[19]

Polycystic ovary syndrome (PCOS) appears to arise as a complex trait with contributions from both heritable and nonheritable factors.[24] Polycystic ovary syndrome is the most common endocrine disorder causing female infertility.[25]

Polygenic influences appear to account for about 70% of the variance in pathogenesis.[24] Congenital virilizing disorders; above average or low birth weight for gestational age; premature adrenarche, particularly exaggerated adrenarche; atypical sexual precocity; or intractable obesity with acanthosis nigricans, metabolic syndrome, and pseudo-Cushing syndrome or pseudo-acromegaly in early childhood have been identified as independent prepubertal risk factors for the development of PCOS.[24] During adolescence, PCOS may masquerade as physiological adolescent anovulation.[24] Intractable prepubertal obesity was recognized to culminate in early childhood pseudo-Cushing's syndrome or pseudo-acromegaly, which are manifestations of insulin-resistant hyperinsulinism, and to herald adolescent PCOS.[26] Functional ovarian hyperandrogenism is considered to be a form of polycystic ovary syndrome at adolescence. One of the earliest manifestations of PCOS is premature pubarche. Prepubertal girls with obesity or insulin resistance are also at risk to develop the full PCOS phenotype after puberty. In prepubertal girls who carry risk factors, including genetic polymorphisms and/or particular environmental factors, Functional ovarian hyperandrogenism or polycystic ovary syndrome could develop at a high rate.[27] Children with primary hypothyroidism generally have delayed sexual maturation and delayed puberty. Ovarian cysts have been reported in girls with longstanding uncompensated primary hypothyroidism.[28,29]

Anti-Müllerian hormone (AMH) is produced by the granulosa cells and reflects follicular development. Adult women with polycystic ovary syndrome (PCOS) have increased levels of AMH associated with an excessive number of growing follicles. Serum AMH concentrations are increased in prepubertal and peripubertal daughters of PCOS women, suggesting that these girls appear to show evidence of an altered follicular development during infancy and childhood.[30,31] An increased follicular mass is observed in these children that is established during early development, and persists during puberty.[31]

The phenotypes of the polycystic ovarian syndrome (PCOS) and congenital adrenal hyperplasia syndrome (CAHS) present a number of similarities.

The main symptoms of PCOS are obesity, menstrual disorders, hirsutism, and low fertility in which the pituitary and adrenal glands are spared. The CAHS is a group of various entities all characterised by different degrees of malfunction of the 21-hydroxylase (CYP21) enzyme that result in decreased levels of aldosterone and cortisol, and the hyperproduction of adrenal androgen hormones.[32] Metformin is an attractive option for induction of ovulation in PCOS patients, there is a need for more evidence related to its safety during pregnancy.[33]

McCUNE-ALBRIGHT SYNDROME

McCune-Albright syndrome (MAS) is characterized by gonadotropin-independent precocious puberty, café-au-lait spots on the skin and polyostotic fibrous dysplasia of bones. Ovarian cysts are common in peripheral precocious puberty in this Syndrome.[34] Gonadal hyperfunction is the most frequent endocrine dysfunction in females with McCune-Albright syndrome. Peripheral precocious puberty is usually the first MAS manifestation in children, characterized by episodes of hypersecretion of estrogens with a consequent reduction in gonadotropin secretion.

High estradiol level and low gonadotropins concentration as well as their level after GnRH administration suggest ovarian autonomy.[35,36] Scintigraphy, radiography and computed tomography scans may be helpful to delineate fibrous dysplastic bones.[35]

The clinical course of ovarian cysts is unpredictable due to episodes of hyperestrogenism typical of MAS ovarian hyperfunction. In persistent and recurrent large ovarian cysts with sustained estrogen hypersecretion and relevant clinical disturbances (increased linear growth and bone age maturation, vaginal bleeding and psychological disturbances) treatment is mandatory. Treatment of precocious puberty in MAS should be considered in patients with poor predicted adult height. Treatment of gonadotropin-independent precocious puberty in MAS with ketoconazole, cyproterone acetate or testolactone, an aromatase inhibitor, does not appear to be always effective in slowing bone maturation.[37] Tamoxifen, a selective estrogen receptor modulator has also been used with success for the management of advanced puberty and rapid bone maturation.[37]

Experimental courses of estrogen-blocking drugs may have insufficient or no therapeutic effects. In these cases and when molecular analysis is required to obtain MAS diagnosis as in isolated peripheral precocious puberty, surgery is the option.[34] Laparoscopy minimizes surgical intervention and facilitates obtaining tissue samples for molecular analysis, and sometimes relieves hyperestrogenism with the excision of hyperactive ovarian areas.[34]

TREATMENT OF PUBERTAL OVARIAN CYSTS

These cysts can be treated easily if the etiology is recognized. Identification of hypothyroidism in these girls obviates the need for extensive investigations.[29] The restoration of euthyroid state with thyroid hormone replacement has been associated with resolution of these cysts.

Autonomous functional ovarian follicle cyst is the most often cause of isosexual pseudoprecocious puberty.[38] Short period of observation is suggested because these cysts can resolve spontaneously.[38]

However, there are few cysts that require operative intervention that differs based on the size, type of lesion (cystic, solid or mixed) as well as the age of the child.[19] A solid ovarian mass in an adolescent requires appropriate evaluation to differentiate benign from malignant disease.[19] Pediatric dermoid cysts, adnexal torsion, ruptured lutein cysts, paraovarian cyst and serous cystadenoma require surgical intervention, though all these can be managed laparoscopically also.[39] Even the giant ovarian cysts can be treated successfully with the laparoscopic procedure.[40]

REFERENCES

1. Gupta DK, Lall A, Agarwal S, Mitra DK. Bilateral Ovarian cyst detected antenatally–A plea for In-Utero decompression. Jour Obst. Gynaecol of India 2002;52:113.
2. Meizner I, levy A, Katz M, Maresh AJ, Glezerman M. Fetal ovarian cysts: Prenatal Ultrasonographic detection and postnatal evaluation and treatment Am J Obstel Gynecol 1991;164:874-78.
3. Gupta DK, Lall A. Ovarian cyst in the Newborns. In Textbook of Neonatal Surgery Ed DK Gupta, 2000. Chap 78:521-22.
4. Oak Sanjay N, Parelkar SV, Akhtar T, Pathak R, Vishwanath N, Satish KV, Kiran R: Laparoscopic management of neonatal ovarian cysts. JIAPS; 2005;10:100-02.

5. Mizuno M, Kato T, Hebiguchi T, Yoshino H. Surgical indications for neonatal ovarian cysts. Tohuku J Exp Med 1998;186:27-32.
6. Brandt ML, Helmrath MA. Ovarian cysts in infants and children. Semin Pediatr Surg. 2005;14:78-85.
7. Chiaramonte C, Piscopo A, Cataliotti F. Ovarian cysts in newborns. Pediatr Surg Int 2001;17:171-74.
8. Widdowson DJ, Pilling BW, Cook RCM. Neonatal ovarian cysts:therapeutic dilemma!. Arch Dises in Childhood 1988;63:737-42.
9. Bagolan P, Giorlandino C, Nahom A, et al. The management of fetal ovarian cysts. J Pediatr Surg 2002; 37:25-30.
10. Ibrahim H, Lewis D, Harrison GK, et al Congenital ovarian cyst. J Perinatol. 2007;27:523-26.
11. Abolmakarem H, tharmaratnum S, Thilaganathan B- Fetal anemia as a consequence of hemorrhage into an ovarian cyst. Ultrasound obstet Gynecol. 2001;17:527-28.
12. Born HJ, Kuhnert E, Halberstadt E. Diagnosis of fetal ovarian cysts. Follow-up or differential diagnosis? Ultraschall Med 1997;18(5):209-13.
13. Rizzo N, Gabrielli S, Perolo A et al. Prenatal diagnosis and treatment of fetal ovarian cysts. Prenatal diagnosis 1989;9:97-104.
14. Kwak DW, Sohn YS, Kim SK, et al. Clinical experiences of fetal ovarian cyst: Diagnosis and consequence. J Korean Med Sci. 2006;21:690-94.
15. Slodki M, Respondek-Liberska M. Fetal ovarian cysts—420 cases from literature—metaanalysis 1984-2005. Ginekol Pol. 2007;78:324-28.
16. Kessler A, Nagar H, Graif M, et al. Percutaneous drainage as the treatment of choice for neonatal ovarian cysts. Pediatr Radiol. 2006;36:954-58.
17. Comparetto C, Giudici S, Coccia ME, et al. Fetal and neonatal ovarian cysts: what's their real meaning? Clin Exp Obstet Gynecol. 2005;32:123-25.
18. Croitoru DP, Aaron LE, Laberge JM, Neilson IR, Guttman FM. Management of complex ovarian cyst presenting in the first year of life. J Pediatr Surg 1991 26(12) 1366-68.
19. Hayes-Jordan A. Surgical management of the incidentally identified ovarian mass. Semin Pediatr Surg. 2005;14:106-10.
20. Esposito C, Garipoli V, Di Matteo G, De Pasquale M. Laproscopic management of ovarian cysts in newborns. Surg Endosc 1998;12:1152-54.
21. Prasad S, Chui CH. Laparoscopic-assisted transumbilical ovarian cystectomy in a neonate. JSLS. 2007;11:138-41.
22. Enríquez G, Durán C, Torán N, et al. Conservative versus surgical treatment for complex neonatal ovarian cysts: outcomes study. AJR Am J Roentgenol. 2005;185:501-08.
23. Foley PT, Ford WD, McEwing R, et al. Is conservative management of prenatal and neonatal ovarian cysts justifiable? Fetal Diagn Ther. 2005;20:454-58.
24. Rosenfield RL. Clinical review: Identifying children at risk for polycystic ovary syndrome. J Clin Endocrinol Metab. 2007;92:787-96.
25. Eggers S, Hashimoto DM, Kirchengast S. An evolutionary approach to explain the high frequency of the polycystic ovary syndrome (PCOS). Anthropol Anz. 2007;65:169-79.
26. Littlejohn EE, Weiss RE, Deplewski D, et al. Intractable early childhood obesity as the initial sign of insulin resistant hyperinsulinism and precursor of polycystic ovary syndrome. J Pediatr Endocrinol Metab. 2007;20: 41-51.
27. Siklar Z, Oçal G, Adiyaman P, et al. Functional ovarian hyperandrogenism and polycystic ovary syndrome in prepubertal girls with obesity and/or premature pubarche. J Pediatr Endocrinol Metab. 2007;20:475-81.
28. Indumathi CK, Bantwal G, Patil M. Primary hypothyroidism with precocious puberty and bilateral cystic ovaries. Indian J Pediatr. 2007;74:781-83.
29. Sharma Y, Bajpai A, Mittal S, et al. Ovarian cysts in young girls with hypothyroidism: follow-up and effect of treatment. J Pediatr Endocrinol Metab. 2006;19: 895-900.
30. Sir-Petermann T, Codner E, Maliqueo M, et al. Increased anti-Müllerian hormone serum concentrations in prepubertal daughters of women with polycystic ovary syndrome. J Clin Endocrinol Metab. 2006;91:3105-09.
31. Crisosto N, Codner E, Maliqueo M, et al. Anti-Müllerian hormone levels in peripubertal daughters of women with polycystic ovary syndrome. J Clin Endocrinol Metab. 2007;92:2739-43.
32. Robyr D, Llor J, Gaudin G, et al. Polycystic ovary syndrome and congenital adrenal hyperplasia: a different entity for comparable phenotypes? Rev Med Suisse. 2007;3(116):1595-6, 1598, 1600-01.
33. Kovo M, Weissman A, Gur D, et al. Neonatal outcome in polycystic ovarian syndrome patients treated with metformin during pregnancy. J Matern Fetal Neonatal Med. 2006;19:415-19.
34. Gesmundo R, Guanà R, Valfrè L, et al. Laparoscopic management of ovarian cysts in peripheral precocious puberty of McCune-Albright syndrome. J Pediatr Endocrinol Metab. 2006;19:571-75.
35. Wikiera B, Wawro J, Noczyńska A. Precocious puberty caused by McCune-Albright syndrome in a girl aged 6 years and 9 months. Endokrynol Diabetol Chor Przemiany Materii Wieku Rozw. 2006;12:63-67.
36. Matarazzo P, Lala R, Andreo M, et al. McCune-Albright syndrome: persistence of autonomous ovarian hyperfunction during adolescence and early adult age. J Pediatr Endocrinol Metab. 2006;19:607-17.
37. Sawathiparnich P, Osuwanaratana P, Santiprabhob J, et al. Tamoxifen improved final height prediction in a girl with McCune-Albright syndrome: patient report and literature review. J Pediatr Endocrinol Metab. 2006;19: 81-86.
38. Mitrovic' K, Zdravkovic' D, Milenkovic' T, et al. Ovarian cysts and tumors as the cause of isosexual pseudoprecocious puberty Srp Arh Celok Lek. 2006;134:305-09.
39. Takeda A, Manabe S, Hosono S, Nakamura H. Laparoscopic surgery in 12 cases of adnexal disease occurring in girls aged 15 years or younger. J Minim Invasive Gynecol. 2005;12:234-40.
40. Ates O, Karakaya E, Hakgüder G, et al. Laparoscopic excision of a giant ovarian cyst after ultrasound-guided drainage J Pediatr Surg. 2006;41:E9-11.

CHAPTER 116
Vaginal Anomalies and Reconstruction

Akshay Chauhan, Shilpa Sharma, DK Gupta

Vaginal anomalies can be present as a separate entity or may be associated with other anomalies like anorectal malformations. Misdiagnosis of vaginal anomalies is a common occurrence especially when present as separate entity.[1,2] It may be diagnosed as late as puberty or may present as infertility in older girls.[3,4] Adequate knowledge of the anatomical defect is essential for proper planning and reconstruction of the defect. Psychological counselling is also important in cases of absence of vagina. A good reconstruction at an early age with proper documentation of the defect is essential to prevent any gynecological mishap later in life.

The crux of treatment lies in a good follow-up and collaboration with a gynecologist at an early stage to help implement proper counselling that is required at the different stages of life.[5,6] Bowel vaginoplasty has now been used by various surgeons and has stood the test of time. For vaginal agenesis, a sigmoid vaginoplasty provides a functional self-lubricating neovagina.[7] Some authors have recommended reconstruction for absent vagina during adolescence because the local conditions are excellent and it allows adaptation of the anatomy to physical development.[7]

Frank's autodilatation, a nonsurgical method of creating a neovagina by recurrent dilatations requires long and often embarrassing self-catheterization which is often painful, and yields a vagina with limited length.[8] Surgical options are better accepted.

Laparoscopy sigmoid vaginoplasty for reconstruction of a vagina in patients with the Mayer-Rokitansky-Küster-Hauser syndrome has been reported.[8,9] For cases with associated anomalies, an early reconstruction during the definitive surgery is always preferred.[5] It is extremely important to establish an accurate neonatal diagnosis especially in cases of cloaca, drain the hydrocolpos when present, and avoid a persistent urogenital sinus.[5]

Patients born with persistent cloaca have a high incidence of gynecological problems at the onset of menses and in early adult life. Therefore, it is necessary to reassess these girls at early puberty by ultrasound/magnetic resonance imaging and vaginoscopy. Additional surgery may then be necessary to create a vagina for menstruation and sexual intercourse.[6]

Besides congenital anomalies, vaginal reconstruction may be required for, vaginal stenosis after treatment of pelvic tumors, severe vaginal scarring secondary to chronic inflammatory disease or as a secondary corrective surgery after failure gender surgery.

However, as each case is different, there is always scope for new innovations and experiments in the formation of a neovagina still continue.

CLASSIFICATION OF VAGINAL ANOMALIES

A classification of vaginal anomalies has been derived, which permits logical operative decisions. This tool allows the assignment of increasingly involved reconstructive operations to progressively more complex vaginal. Powell et al, categorize the vaginal anomalies as follows:[10]

Type A. Simple labial fusion
Type B. Distal urogenital sinus formation.
Type C. Distal vaginal atresia with proximal urethrovaginal fistula
Type D. Complete absence of the vagina

Based on the following anatomic classification, the following approaches to reconstruction can be recommended. For Type A (simple labial fusion), a midline division of the labia shows a normal hymenal ring and a normal or near normal urethral meatus. After division of the labia, the skin and mucosal layers are approximated to assure that the introitus remains open, creating a normal appearance. For Type B (distal urogenital sinus formation), a more extensive separation of the fused tissue is required. It is necessary to develop a posterior pedicle flap from the labioscrotal tissue, which then is sutured to the vagina, crating a satisfactory opening for the urinary and genital orifices. In those patients with Type C anomaly (distal vaginal atresia with proximal urethrovaginal fistula), a vaginal pull-through using a perineal approach is performed. Patients with Type D (complete absence of vagina), are rarely encountered. These patients will require a vaginal substitution of some kind discussed later.

The choice for and timing of vaginal reconstruction rests on precise anatomic evaluation. The complexity of vaginal reconstruction in the growing child and the essentiality of psychosocial adjustment to appropriate sexual identity and function mandate long-term comprehensive follow-up. Optimal care for each patient requires experience and continuity to take the child through diagnosis, surgical reconstruction, stressful adolescence, and into adulthood with full attention to anatomic, physiological, and psychological support.

Vaginal Agenesis

The female reproductive system is derived primarily from the müllerian or the paramesonephric ducts. In the absence of a fetal testis there is no production of androgen or mullerian inhibiting substance (MIS), and consequently the wolffian system regresses and the müllerian system is free to differentiate. Between the sixth and eight weeks of gestation, the paired müllerian ducts develop lateral to the wolffian ducts and then cross medially to fuse in midline. These fused müllerian ducts join the urogenital sinus at the müllerian tubercle. By the tenth week of gestation, the ducts form a single midline tubular structure called the uterovaginal canal. The lateral aspect of the müllerian ducts, which remain separate, ultimately become the fallopian tubes. The fused portion of these ducts, which thicken, become the fundus, body and cervix of the uterus. Complete absence or agenesis of the vagina, also known as Mayer-Rokitansky syndrome results from a disorder of the ureterovaginal canal or the vaginal plate. In 1829 Mayer and in 1838 Rokitansky first described autopsy specimens of mullerian dysgenesis in female subjects.[11,12] Subsequently Hauser et al described the frequent association of renal and skeletal anomalies.[13] The incidence of vaginal agenesis has been reported to vary from 1 in 4000 to 1 in 5000 live births. The patients are typically 46XX females with normal secondary sex characters who present with ancenorrhea. The association of congenital absence of vagina and anomalies of urinary system is very common.[14,15] Most common renal anomaly is agenesis of one kidney or ectopia of one or both kidneys. Fusion anomalies, such as horseshoe kidney and crossed renal ectopia, are also very common. The ureter may be defective, because of lack of wolffian duct, or because of inhibition, debilitation or duplication of the bud. Griffin et al have reported skeletal anomalies in approximately 12% of these patients.[15] Two-thirds of these patients have anomalies of spine, limb or rib. Six percent of skeletal malformations were of Klippel-Feil type. Duncan et al have suggested that this combination of malformations be called MURS association (müllerian duct aplasia, renal aplasia, and cervicothoracic somite association).[16]

SURGICAL PRINCIPLES FOR VAGINOPLASTY

Vaginal reconstruction is an extremely complex discipline due to wide diversity in vaginal anatomy and the commonly associated anatomical and functional abnormalities or the urogenital tract. Consequently no single reconstruction approach or combination of approaches can be applied empirically. Only an individualized approach can be expected to achieve the best possible outcome. This requires careful preoperative anatomical and functional evaluation, followed by extensive surgical planning based on the relative merits of surgical options. For a successful outcome of vaginal reconstruction in the setting of complex associated anomalies, adherence to several surgical principles is of paramount importance. The first principle is that all anticipated perineal reconstruction, including urethral, vaginal, and anorectal, should be done in a single stage.[17,18] To achieve single stage perineal reconstruction complete anatomical delineation is necessary before surgery, including ultrasound, a voiding cystourethrogram and endoscopy.[19,20] Some patients may benefit from computerized tomography or magnetic resonance imaging of the pelvis to delineate further anatomy, although these evaluations are not performed routinely.[22] Patients suspected of having neurovesical dysfunction require urodynamic studies because the resulting functional deficiency may significantly alter the surgical approach to reconstruction.[21]

The association of spinal cord disease must be carefully excluded. All children with associated anorectal or urogenital sinus anomaly should be screened by spinal ultrasound during infancy. After about the age of 6 months such children require magnetic resonance imaging, since vertebral calcifications precludes ultrasound transmission.

The second principle involves access for urethral catheterization. Since more than 50% of the patients require intermittent catheterization for neurovesical dysfunction, reconstruction must be performed to anticipate easy access. Accurate neourethral reconstruction is mandatory. The neourethra must have a smooth course and be well exteriorized to facilitate adequate intermittent catheterization. When the native urethra cannot be made to fulfill these criteria, the construction of a Mitrafanoff neourethra offers an excellent alterative.[22]

The third principle is that urinary tract reconstruction has a major role in cases of vaginal abnormalities. Ureteric reimplantation is frequently necessary.[23,24]

Of critical importance is the fourth principle of avoidance of overlapping suture lines, since they may result in fistula formation. Vaginal inlay flaps are especially important in the surgical correction of urogenital sinus, as demonstrated. Inlay flaps may be obtained from perineum, prepuce, or labia and all give excellent functional results. When vaginal reconstruction for cloacal anomalies is performed, the potential for overlapping suture lines with a neourethra is extremely high and can be readily avoided by rotating the neovagina 90°.

Since vaginal reconstruction of this type is performed early in childhood.[25] One must take every measure to ensure maximum growth potential of the neovagina, which is the fifth principle. Free grafts are to be avoided whenever possible. Vaginal inlay procedure (especially scrotum) and visceral substitution (usually colon or small bowel but occasionally bladder) are preferred for total creation of a neo vagina.[26] Vaginal substitution is a complex undertaking. The colon is commonly recognized as the intestinal segment of choice due to the low incidence of stenosis on long-term follow-up.[27] However, ileum has an important role when the colon is unavailable, as in genetically male infants with cloacal extrophy who undergo reconstruction to female gender. Ileum is also useful in cases of imperforate, when isolation of a colonic segment may devascularize the distal rectum by interrupting mesenteric collaterals. An alternate approach is the use of the distal end of rectum for vaginal replacement. Bladder substitution is an excellent substitute in some cases.

Meticulous follow-up is necessary to avoid stenosis and to ensure progressive enlargement of the vaginal vault to a degree appropriate with age. Routine dilatation, the sixth principle, is required to avoid stenosis.[28] Patient age at the time of reconstruction is important. Before age 3 years routine dilatation as relatively easy to achieve but after that age cooperation on the part of the child may prove difficult to obtain.

Children are best served by an exhaustive preoperative anatomical and functional evaluation followed by thorough preoperative parental counselling about realistic expectations and the need for continued cooperation and compliance. A coordinated approach to reconstruction, rather than a fragmented conceptual and reconstructive approach, is necessary to achieve optimal surgical restoration of anatomy and function in these children.

Vaginoplasty

Vaginoplasties have long been fraught with complications of poor cosmetics from abnormal location or size to more severe problems resulting in incontinence, or stenosis. These procedures continue to evolve, and current procedures have as their building blocks a few landmark techniques. In 1964, Fortunoff described a posteriorly based perineal flap, which is used nearly in all repairs today.[29] The most important advance came from Hendren and Crawford in 1969 when they defined the variable of anatomy of the confluence of the vagina with the urinary tract noting that the vagina may insert **proximal (suprasphincteric, high vagina)** or **distal (infrasphincteric, low vagina)** to the external sphincter

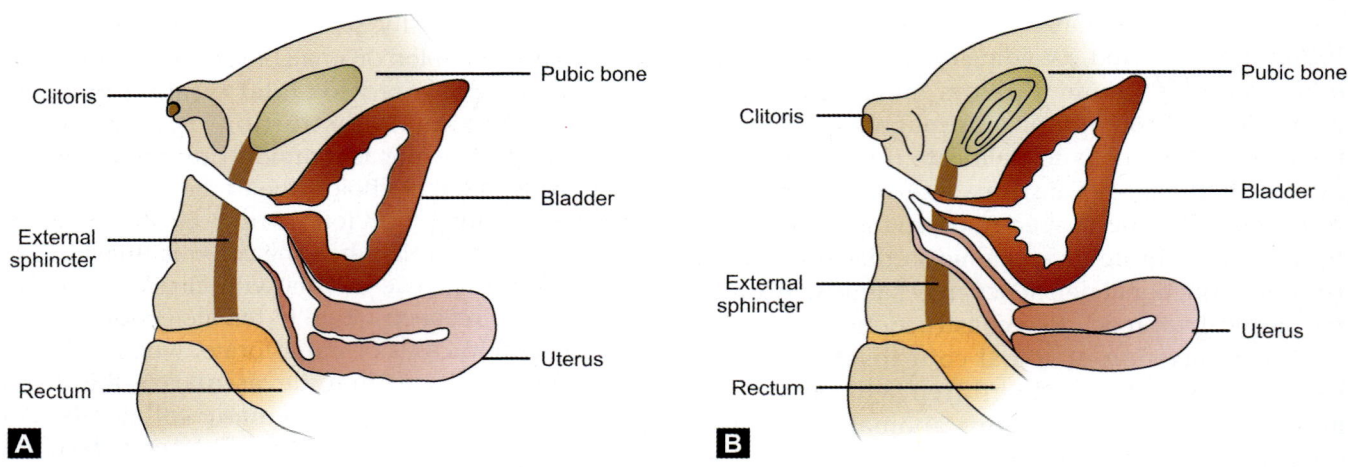

Figs 116.1A and B: Classification of vagina into high and low variety

(Figs 116.1A and B).[30] They also described the pull through vaginoplasty, which remains the basis of vaginoplasty for high confluence today.[31] Vaginoplasty is generally done by one of four procedures
1. Cutback vaginoplasty
2. Flap vaginoplasty
3. Pull-through vaginoplasty
4. Vaginal replacement.

APPROACH TO A LOW VAGINA

Cutback Vaginoplasty

The cutback vaginoplasty should be used in mild forms of labial fusion. Before any vaginal surgery is undertaken, the position of the vagina with respects to both the pelvic floor and perineal skin must be accurately determined from the genitogram, supplemented if necessary by endoscopy. When the vagina opens vary low, it may be laid open by a simple cutback, suturing the vaginal wall to the perineal skin with 6-0 absorbable sutures (Fig. 116.2). In most cases, however, a posteriorly based U flap will be necessary to ensure a tension free anastomosis, reducing the risk of postoperative stenosis.

Flap Vaginoplasty

The posteriorly based flap as an isolated procedure is applicable for only those with a low (infrasphincteric)

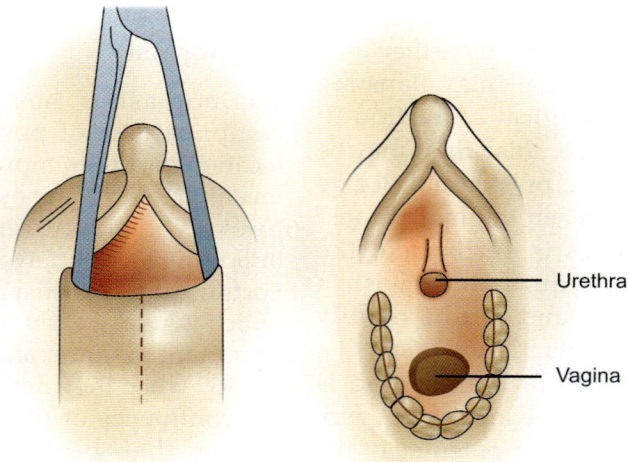

Fig. 116.2: Diagrammatic depiction of cutback vaginoplasty

confluence as it serves only to open the urogenital sinus more widely, not change the level of the confluence (Figs 116.3A and B). When used alone in those with a high confluence, a short hypospadiac urethra will result with the potential for vaginal voiding, stasis and even incontinence.

A urethral catheter is inserted. The posterior flap, which must be sufficiently long to reach the vagina without tension and wide enough to ensure a good blood supply, is elevated together with a generous covering of subcutaneous tissue. A plane is then developed in the midline immediately behind the urethra to expose the vagina. The posterior wall of the vagina is now widely opened in the same flap sutured down. The remainder of the flap is brought down using 6-0 absorbable sutures, the vulvoplasty is not previously carried out, is now completed. Ten days postoperatively the vagina is inspected under anesthesia and its caliber determined, separating any flimsy adhesions.

APPROACH TO A HIGH VAGINA

Reconstruction of the genitalia in severely virilized patient presents particular difficulties because the vagina has a high confluence and is often small.

Pull-through Vaginoplasty

First described by Hendren, it is used for high (suprasphincteric) confluence of vagina.[32]

A Fogarty catheter is first introduced endoscopically into the vagina to facilitate its identification during the dissection, and the balloon is inflated. A second catheter is placed in the bladder. The rectum is then cleaned by insertion of a Betadine soaked swab, which is retained for the duration of the procedure. Two U shaped perineal skin flaps, one based posteriorly and the other anteriorly (Figs 116.4A to F). These are elevated and the dissection continued, keeping strictly to midline until with gentle traction on the Fogarty the vagina can be felt in the depth of the field. A nerve stimulator is used at this point to identify the levator muscles and the external sphincter. The former is divided in the sagittal plane and the vaginal wall is stabilized with a series of 6-0 silk stay sutures. The Fogarty catheter is withdrawn. The vagina is then detached from the urethra and opened as widely as possible. The urethral defect is carefully closed transversely with interrupted 6-0 polyglycolic sutures. Using cautions blunt dissection the surgeon mobilizes the vagina from the back of the bladder and rectum. The anterior and posterior flaps are then brought down and sutured to the vaginal margins.

The mobilization of a high vagina is sometimes difficult particularly when there has been prior infection in a hydrocolpos. It may be then necessary to turn the child and free the vagina via a laparotomy from the back of the bladder.

Although this is the most commonly used technique, there are certain disadvantages to this technique.

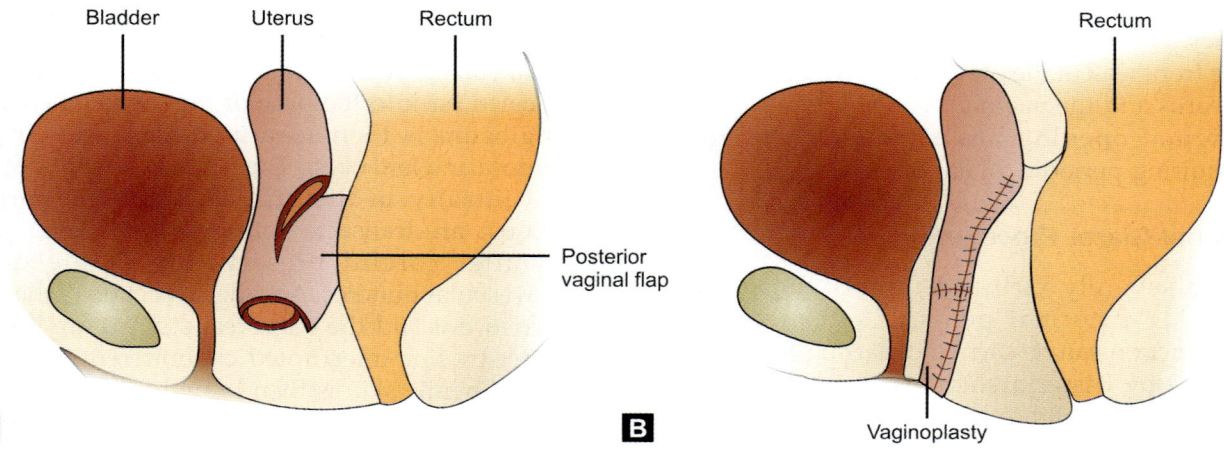

Figs 116.3A and B: Steps of posterior flap vaginoplasty **A.** Posterior flap created from vagina **B.** Vaginoplasty reconstructed

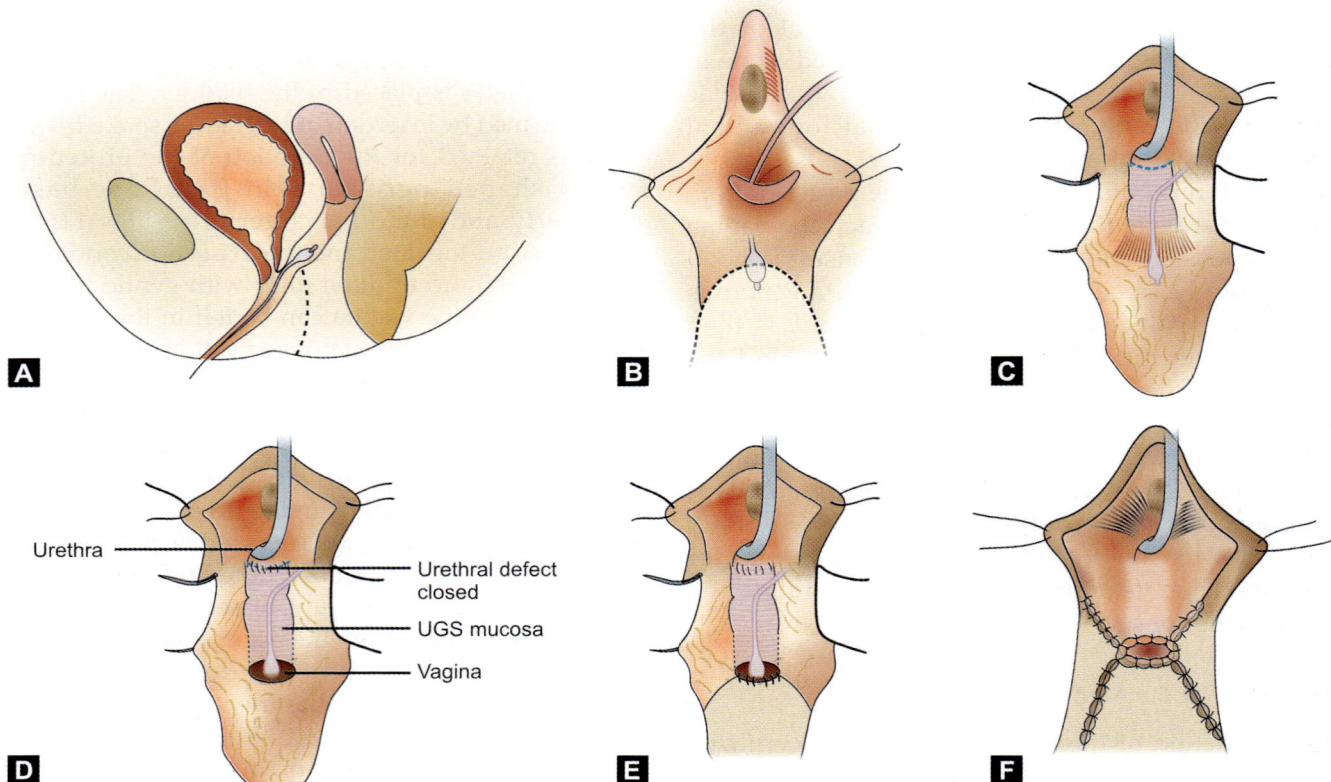

Figs 116.4A to F: Operative steps of Hendren's vaginal pull through. **A.** High confluence of vagina, **B.** Fogarty catheter placed endoscopically in vagina helps in identification of the vagina, **C.** Vagina is detached from the urethra, **D.** The urethral defect is closed transversely. The vagina is mobilized further, **E.** The posterior flap is sutured to the posterior vaginal wall, **F.** Completed Hendren's vaginal pull though

1. The vaginal introitus is located in the perineal wall far from the urethral meatus and the result is that of an isolated hole in the perineum.
2. There is no evidence of mucous lining is present in the front wall of the perineum between the urethral meatus and the vagina.
3. Vaginal opening has a tendency to stenose, requiring periodic dilatations.

Passerini-Glazel Procedure

For the severely virilized infant whose phallus resembles a normal penis, a satisfactory total reconstruction can be carried out using the technique described by Passerini and Glazel.[33] This procedure takes advantage of the sheath of penile skin, which is tubularized and brought up through the perineum to form the lower portion of the vagina, and provides a cosmetically pleasing midline strip of mucosa in vulva (Figs 116.5A to I).

The patient is positioned and prepared for both a perineal and an abdominal dissection, although the procedure can be carried out entirely from below. A circumferential incision is first made around the coronal sulcus, and the skin and subcutaneous tissue are peeled back to the base of the penis. The corpus spongiosum is then separated from the corpora cavernosa and laid open. The skin sleeve split dorsally and ventrally in the midline, and the corpora cavernosa are transected close to the inferior pubic rami after careful preservation of the dorsal neurovascular bundles. A wedge resection of the glans is carried out and the corporeal stumps are brought together by fine interrupted circumferential sutures. The split penile skin is then brought down on either side and sutured to the opened spongiosum. The resulting rectangular flap is rolled in with a running suture to form a composite tube that will serve as the lower portion of the vagina. The upper vagina is then exposed as in Hendren's operation and the

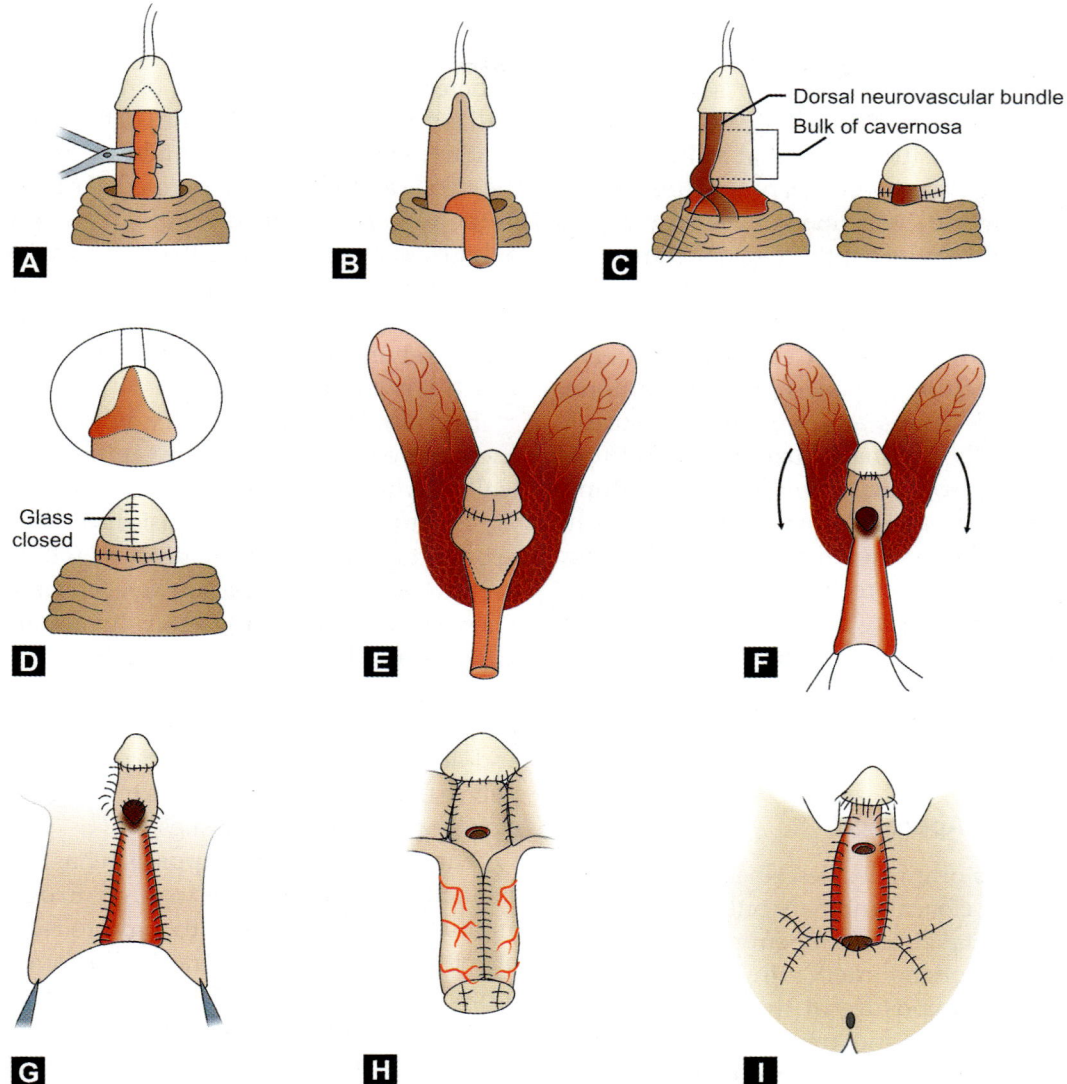

Figs 116.5A to I: Passerini – Glazel operation for one stage clitorovaginoplasty. **A.** The penis is degloved, the urethral plate and corpus spongiosum are separated from the corpora cavernosa, **B.** The corpus spongiosum is detached from the glans, **C.** The dorsal neurovascular bundles are mobilized on a generous strip of investing fascia and the bulk of corpora cavernosa is resected. **D.** A deep edge is excised from the ventral glans. The glans is closed and the corporeal stumps are approximated. The penile skin tube is cutback dorsally and ventrally, **E.** The skin flaps are elevated and the urethra and corpus spongiosum are incised. These are laid open, **F.** The dorsal flap is sutured to use base of the glans, **G.** The skin flaps are brought down and sutured to the lateral edges of the urethra, **H.** The composite flap is rolled into a tube with a running stitch, **I.** The upper portion of the vagina is now exposed. The skin tunnel is sutured to the vagina

anastomosis completed. Finally, the skin margins are brought together to complete the vulvoplasty.

Advantages

1. It allows clitorovaginoplasty to be completed in a single stage.
2. It preserves the neurovascular supply and allows an easy reduction clitoroplasty.
3. Since no vaginal dilatations are required, it can be carried out at any age.
4. Low risk of urethral meatal stenosis.
5. Construction of a vagina of appropriate size and position for the child.

A variant technique to the onestage clitorovaginoplasty in severely masculinized female pseudohermaphrodites is the anterior sagittal trans-ano-rectal approach (ASTRA).[34] With the patient placed in the prone position, after that a clitoroplasty is performed by the Paserini-Glazel procedure ASTRA permits to perform the dissection between the vagina and the urethra, the suture of the vaginal stump and the anastomosis between the neointroitus vaginalis and the vagina under direct vision. The anorectal sphincteric mechanism is divided in the anterior midline, and the rectum is opened just in the anterior rectal wall. This provides an excellent exposure to urogenital sinus. The vagina is then easily and fully separated from the urogenital sinus, the vaginal stump sutured and the anastomosis between the mucocutaneous cylinder (neointroitus vaginalis) and the vagina performed. The rectum, perineal body and the anterior sphincteric mechanism are then reconstructed. An anterior sagittal midline incision provides excellent exposure to the urogenital sinus and assures the preservation of the anorectal innervation and the sphincter mechanism.

Posterior Sagittal Approach

This approach was originally described for the rectal reconstruction of a cloacal anomaly but is adapted for repair of a urogenital sinus by opening the posterior and anterior walls of the intervening rectum.[35] This provides excellent exposure of the vagina and its insertion into the urethra and, provided the dissection is carried strictly in, the midline safeguards the pelvic nerves and the integrity of the pelvic floor musculature. Unless a perfect bowel preparation can be assured, a preliminary colostomy will be necessary.

A Fogarty catheter is first inserted in to the vagina endoscopically and the balloon inflated. A Foley catheter is inserted in to the bladder. With the patient in prone jack knife position incision is made extending from the tip of the coccyx anteriorly to the urogenital sinus opening. The dissection proceeds through the perineal body and fat until the muscle bundles of the levator muscle are visible. These are carefully identified by electrical stimulation and marked with long 6-0 silk sutures to facilitate accurate realignment at the end of the procedure. The posterior and anterior walls are then opened in the midline and the position of the vagina and its junction with the urethra determined by feeling for the presence of Fogarty catheter. The inferior aspect of the posterior vaginal wall is now marked with series of 6-0 silk stay sutures, gentle traction upon which allows the junction with the urethra to be clearly defined. The vagina is then detached, the urethral defect closed with fine polyglycolic sutures, and the vagina widely opened. Continuing gentle traction and blunt dissection in the surrounding connective tissues allow the vagina to be progressively mobilized towards the perineum to which it is sutured.

Because of the difficulty which is sometimes encountered in separating the vagina from the urethral wall, to which it may be fused for some distance above the confluence, it is often easier to carry out a total urogenital sinus mobilization in which the sinus, urethra, and the vagina are freed as a single unit.[36] These structures are progressively mobilized together down towards the perineum, where the redundant portion of the urogenital sinus is excised. After completion of the perineal anastomosis, the posterior and anterior rectal walls are closed in layers and the pelvic floor musculature is reapproximated prior to closing the superficial tissues.

The posterior sagittal approach has been beneficial for acquiring exposure to high urogenital sinus anomalies but it has been thought to require splitting of the rectum and temporary colostomy. Rink et al, have described a modification of this technique without division of the rectum.[37] This midline perineal prone approach has allowed excellent exposure of the high vagina even in infants. In their series of 8 patients with high vagina all reconstruction was done without difficulty and no patient required incision of the rectum or colostomy. This procedure did not preclude the use of a posteriorly based flap for vaginal reconstruction. While patients with low confluence can be treated with single posteriorly based flap vaginoplasty, those with higher confluence may benefit from a perineal prone approach to achieve adequate exposure for pull-through vaginoplasty. This prone approach to the high urogenital sinus anomaly can be performed without division of the rectum, provides excellent exposure of the high confluence even in small children and does not preclude the use of posterior flaps for vaginal reconstruction.

VAGINAL SUBSTITUTION

Improvements in the preoperative preparation, surgical techniques and postoperative management have made complex reconstruction of genital ambiguity possible. Efforts to create a viable vaginal substitute have been directed to improving cosmesis and functionality.

Timing of Surgery

Timing of surgery is crucial to the overall long-term success of the surgical approach utilized. If early surgery is contemplated (in infancy), then the tissue utilized should be one that will grow with the patient. Initial feminization(reduction clitoroplasty) with later completion of vaginal substitution may be undertaken with good results.

Non-surgical Technique

The only non-surgical technique reported is that of forceful dilatation of the perineal pit with a dilator over a protracted period of time to create a skin tube of adequate depth to permit intercourse.[38] While this technique obviates operative intervention it is only suited to those individuals with a deep vaginal dimple and who are adequately motivated.

Surgical Techniques

Vaginal substitution techniques can be broadly divided into those utilizing,
1. Skin flaps, including expanded skin
2. Bowel substitution
3. Other tissue substitutes.

SKIN FLAPS

Use of split thickness meshed skin graft, was first described by McIndoe.[39,40] A thin meshed skin graft is moulded around a Styrofoam or other mold and placed in cavity created between bladder and the rectum through a perineal incision. Once the graft has taken, the mold may be removed but early and repeated dilatation is required to prevent contraction and maintain size.[41] Hockel et al have proposed the use of the scalp as the donor site for vaginoplasty with split skin grafts.[42] Patients with a congenital absence of a vagina should also benefit from the obvious advantages, which made the scalp the preferred donor site in burn patients.[43]

Advantages of split thickness grafts:
- Adequate tissue readily available for reconstruction
- It is well accepted and widely taught surgical technique.

Disadvantages of split thickness skin graft: No potential for growth, therefore reconstruction should be delayed until puberty:
- Potential for "poor uptake"[41]
- Use of mold or other dilating method required[40]
- Dyspareunia may be noted
- Can undergo scarring and reduction in size over a period of time[42]
- May be site for development of malignancy.[44]

Results and complications of McIndoe procedure for vaginal agenesis have been presented in a large series by Buss et al.[41] During a 10 years interval, 50 patients with congenital absence of the vagina underwent McIndoe vaginoplasty. The mean duration of follow-up was 6.5 years. Two rectovaginal fistulas and one graft failure were among the complications that occurred. Five patients required additional reconstructive vaginal operations. Operative vaginoplasty was considered functionally successful by 40 of the 47 patients (85%) who responded to the survey, yet only 36 of these 40 (90%) had remained coitally active by the time of the survey. Recognizing the potential for complications, the need for long-term follow-up and care of the neovagina, and the less than perfect results achieved, they continue to consider the McIndoe operation as the procedure of choice for most patients with vaginal agenesis.

Modified McIndoe Procedure for Vaginal Agenesis

Ozek et al have proposed a modification of the original McIndoe procedure, by using a X incision instead of a straight-line horizontal or sagittal incision.[45] During the first postoperative week, a perforated Pyrex rigid mold was used. This was replaced with an unperforated mold at the end of the first week. Complications encountered included infection, total lack of skin graft take, stress urinary incontinence, partial graft loss, and vaginal stricture. All complications were treatable except the stress urinary incontinence, and the final results were satisfactory.

Full Thickness Skin Grafts

A full thickness skin graft from iliac crest has been used in the formation of a neovagina.[46] The potential risks and benefits of this procedure are similar to that with split thickness grafts. Donor site scarring and shrinkage may be greater with full thickness grafts.

The ideal operation for a young woman born without a vagina would be a one stage procedure, creating a functionally normal vagina without cosmetically unattractive scars, without the need for subsequent dilatation, stents or obturators. This goal can be achieved with a free flap vaginoplasty using a full thickness skin graft taken from the scapula region.[47] The blood supply of the graft is maintained by micro vascular anastomosis of the graft pedicles to vessels in the groin. This technique is demanding, and has the problems associated with the other forms of skin grafting, i.e. donor sites, shrinkage and appropriate take. Moreover, the operation is a major undertaking and needs to be performed by those with expertise in plastic surgery as well as in gynecology.

Myocutaneous Flaps

McGraw initially reported the use of a myocutaneous flap for the construction of neovagina.[48] This technique was initially designed for the use in patients who had exenteration performed for malignancy. Since then the gracilis myocutaneous flap has become very popular in recent years perineal reconstruction.[49-51] The basis of use of myocutaneous flaps is the fact that the blood supply for areas of skin is obtained from perforating vessels from the underlying muscle. A gracilis flap is the most commonly used tissue. The gracilis flap is the most superficial of the medial thigh muscles and is a weak adductor. It can be sacrificed without compromising leg functions or gait.[52] Its blood supply comes from a branch of profunda femoris and its nervous supply is from the obturator nerve that provides both motor and sensory innervation. For vaginal reconstruction, bilateral flaps are usually required. The flaps are raised and passed medially into the perineum. A skin tube is constructed from the two flaps and rotated medially in to the pelvis between bladder and rectum.[52] The tube is held in place with anchoring sutures to the periosteum of the symphysis and the levators.

In McGraws series of 22 patients, 6 suffered partial flap loss, while 1 patient suffered totally catastrophic loss of flap.[48] Thus about a third of the patients suffered some sort of flap embarrassment-an unacceptably high failure rate.

In recent years two techniques of vaginal reconstruction with sensate tissue have emerged. Song et al, have used bilateral flaps of labia majora and minora to create a neovagina.[53] In 14 patients with the longest follow-up of 10 years, soft, sensate, pliable vagina were created. A major disadvantage, however is the sacrifice of the labia majora and minora bilaterally, which scars and distorts the vulva. This technique also introduces hair bearing skin of the labia majore into the neovagina.

Wang et al, have described a fasciocutaneous flap from the medial upper thigh based on the suprafascial vascular plexus.[54] A partially sensate flap, measuring 20 × 9 cm, without using gracilis as a vascular carrier, could be raised to reconstruct the vagina and to close the perineal defects. However, this flap has a high incidence of flap loss owing to its precarious blood supply.

Wee et al, introduced the use of bilateral pudendal thigh flaps for total vaginal reconstruction.[55] The flap derives its blood supply from the posterior labial and perineal artery, which branches from the pudendal artery (Figs 116.6A to G). It retains its innervation from the pudendal labial branches of the perineal nerve, which arises from the pudendal nerve. The advantages of this procedure are:

1. It is a simple technique which can be completed in 2 to 2½ hours with little blood loss.
2. The blood supply of the flaps is reliable. This leads to early wound healing.
3. No stents are required, since the reconstructed vagina is stable.
4. The introduction of well vascularized flap tissue into the pelvic cavity after exenteration helps to obliterate the dead space.
5. The angle of inclination of the vagina is physiologic and natural.
6. The linear scars of the donor sites are well hidden in the groin crease and perineum.
7. The vagina is sensate, retaining the same innervation of the erogenous zones of the perineum and upper thigh.

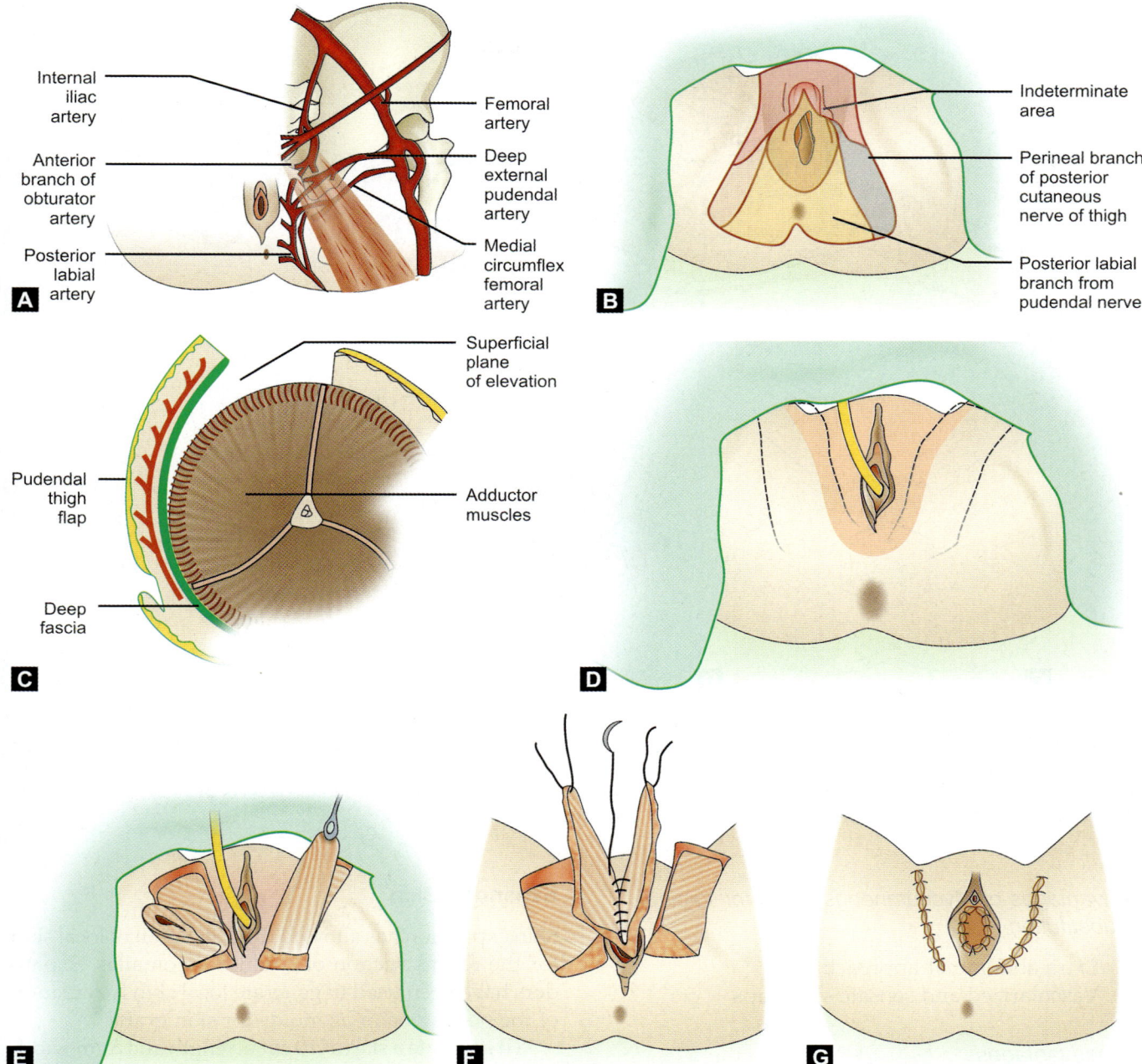

Figs 116.6A to G: Pudendal thigh myocutaneous flap. **A.** Arterial anastomosis over the proximal part of the adductor muscles, **B.** Innervation of the female perineum, **C.** The subfascial plane of the flap elevation is beneath the deep fascia of the thigh. The flap is arterialized throughout, **D.** Two incisions are marked, slightly curved and tapered flap on either side of the vulva, centered on the crease of the groin. The base in an adult is 6 cm wide, and the length may be upto 15 cm, placing the tip over the femoral triangle, **E.** Incision is made down to the deep fascia, the flap is raised, taking care to include the perimycium of the adduction muscles to avoid damage to the nerves in the flap. At the base of the flap, the skin is divided through the dermis to a depth of 1 to 1.5 cm to allow freedom of the flap. Tunnels are formed under the labia by dissecting from the pubic ramus. The flaps are passed under the labia with the flaps everted from the introitus, **F.** The paired flaps are sutured together in the midline to close the posterior wall of neovagina, **G.** At the apex, suturing is continued to approximate the anterior wall by bringing the lateral border together to form the vaginal tube

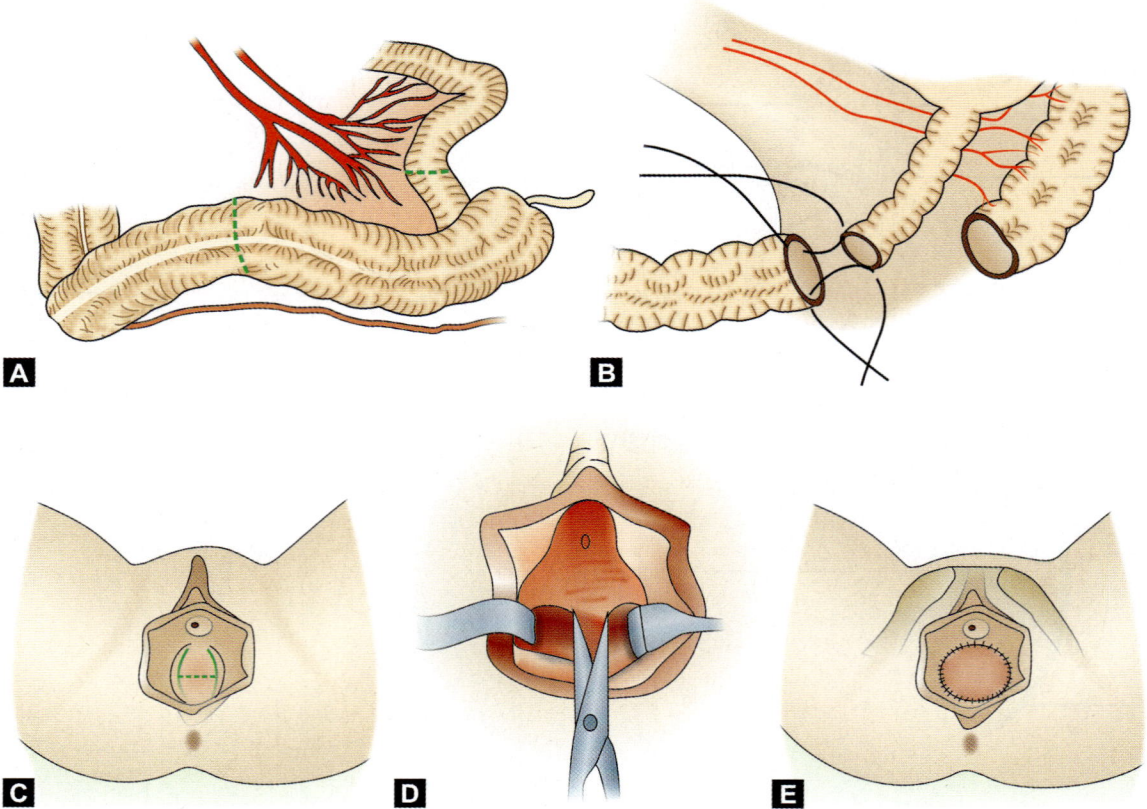

Figs 116.7A to E: Use of Bowel for vaginal substitution. **A.** Ileocolic artery is located to determine an adequately vascularized segment of bowel, **B.** Colon and terminal ileum are divided. Intestinal continuity is restored by ileocolic anastomosis, **C.** H-shaped incision is made at the site of the proposed neovagina, **D.** A space is created to the level of the vesicorectal pouch, **E.** The margin of the colon is sutured to the vulva with synthetic absorbable sutures

Advantages of Myocutaneous Flaps for Vaginal Substitution

- Extra-abdominal approach
- Vascularized and sensate skin flaps

Disadvantages

- No lubrication of vagina
- Reconstruction should be delayed until prior to start of sexual function
- Significant leg scarring that is cosmetically unappealing[56]
- Pain in the thigh region during intercourse
- May have prolapse of the neovagina.[56]

Expanded Skin

Skin expansion has allowed the utilization of local skin for the reconstruction of complex anomalies. Expanders have been used to generate local skin for creation of the neovagina or as molds for skin grafts.[57,58]

To generate a slap of 10 cm in length and 8 cm width a 250 ml capacity expander is required. Expanders with remote injection ports are used to prevent damage t the expander during filling. [57] The expander is inserted into a labial pocket via an inguinal incision . The remote port is inserted in a subcutaneous pocket above the pubic hairline. Two weeks following the placement expansion is initiated and continued weekly. Volume of the fluid injected in to the expander is dependent on the patients' tolerance to the discomfort. One week following complete expansion vaginoplasty is performed. In severe vaginal malformations, when the distance between the upper vaginal pouch and perineum is too long (6 cm or more), reconstruction of the vagina can be performed by long cutaneous flaps, obtained by the tissue expansion technique, as described by Belloli et al.[59] Dissection and anastomosis between the vaginal remnant and cutaneous tube is performed by the transtrigonal approach. Expanded labial skin-flap vaginoplasty has three main advantages: (1) it permits the construction of a large, soft, well-vascular zed neovagina using non-hair-bearing labial skin; (2) it obviates postoperative dilations and prevents delayed strictures; and (3) a transtrigonal approach permits an easy vaginal dissection and a careful, tension-free anastomosis.

Advantages of Skin Expanders

- Availability of large amounts of local skin for vaginal reconstruction
- Skin flaps are easy to rotate in to place
- No separate site for harvest of skin
- Procedure is performed extraperitoneally
- Does not contract or develop cicatrix since it is a full thickness, vascularized flap.

Disadvantages of Skin Expansion

- Significant deformity created by insertion of the expander, which needs to stay in place for 6-8 weeks
- Non-lubricated vaginal pouch
- May require periodic dilatation prior to the initiation of intercourse
- If hair bearing elements are part of the vaginal pouch, can lead to irritation
- Need to delay reconstruction until post-puberty, as segments do not grow over time
- Potential risk of infection of the tissue expander.

Vaginoplasty Using Deepithelialized Vulvar Transposition Flaps: The Grunberger Method

One of the most important criteria indicative of the long-term success of vaginal enlargement is the absence of postoperative contracture. Numerous procedures have been developed for reconstruction of an inadequate vagina. Some are technically complex techniques (myo- and fasciocutaneous flaps) with few postoperative complications of vaginal contracture, and others implement autografts with a greater tendency of tissue contraction. Grunberger et al, have described a method of vaginoplasty using deepithelialized vulvar transposition flaps to enlarge the width of narrow vaginas found mainly in cases of congenital adrenogenital syndrome-associated vaginal atresia, but also in cases of acquired vaginal atresia (surgery and radiotherapy-induced).[60] They used deepithelialized dermis from the labia majora to construct an enlarged vaginal entrance and cavity, a technique that is easy to learn and perform. The healing phase of this operation is free of tissue rejection, most likely because of the close embryologic relationship of the cornified, paravaginal squamous epithelium of the labia majora and the noncornified squamous epithelial lining of the lower third of the vagina. The epithelium of the graft loses its cornified layer and becomes nonhair-bearing; its cytology and histology mimic normal vaginal epithelium. Postoperative function and sexual contentment were reported to be satisfying.

Use of Autologous Buccal Mucosa for Vaginoplasty

Lin et al, studied the procedure and outcome of creating a neovaginal pouch lined with autologous buccal mucosa in patients with Mayer-Rokitansky-Kuster-Hauser syndrome.[61] The buccal mucosal wound completely healed 2 weeks after the operation and the neovaginal length and calibre were well formed. This was the first reported procedure of vaginoplasty using autologous buccal mucosa as graft material. The method is ideal in its simplicity, provides good cosmetic results, and improves the vaginal length of the patient.

BOWEL SEGMENTS

Various bowel segments have been used for vaginal substitution (Figs 116.7A to E). Intestinal segments have potential for growth along with the child and generally need less dilatation.[62] This allows performance of the procedure in infancy. Ileal, sigmoid, rectal, and hindgut segments have all been used. Preoperative bowel preparation is required and depending on the segments used, further cleansing with enemas or flushing is necessary.

Ileal Vaginal Substitution

Ileal vaginal substitution was initially described by Baldwin in 1904.[63] More recently Hanna described a modification of this approach with the use of a U shaped segment of the ileum combined with a perineal skin flap.[64] 15-20 cm of the ileum are used for this procedure. The ileum is opened on its antimesenteric edge and folded into a U shape. The medial edges of the limbs of the U age sutured together and then pouch is created by sewing the lateral edges to each other. This vaginal pouch is placed in a cavity created between the bladder and rectum and anastomosed to a perineal skin flap.

Cecal Vaginal Substitution

Use of the ileocecal region has the potential risk of vitamin malabsorption. Use of cecal segment has been suggested in patients who have had prior pelvic irradiation, in whom the sigmoid segment may be unsuitable for reconstruction.[27] An 8-10 cm cecal and ascending colon segment is harvested and rotated on its mesentery to bring it in to the perineum (Fig. 116.7).

Sigmoid Vaginal Substitution

Sigmoid colon is the most frequently used bowel segment for vaginal substitution, since a capacious vaginal cavity can be achieved without bowel reconfiguration.[27,65,66] Additionally the thick wall of the sigmoid makes its better suited for vaginal substitution. A 10-15 cm segment of sigmoid is harvested with its vascular supply and placed in a space between the bladder and rectum. The proximal end of the sigmoid is closed with a double layer technique. The distal end is brought out to the perineum and may be anastomosed to the opened rudimentary vaginal pit.[65]

Advantages

- Immediate availability of tissue for reconstruction
- Segments produce mucus and permit a lubricated passage
- Adequate caliber vagina can be created
- Usually no requirement for dilatation
- Will grow with the patient
- Sigmoid segment able to tolerate trauma of intercourse better than small bowel segments.

Disadvantages

- Distal prolapse may occur
- Frequent flushing of mucus required to prevent odor, inspissations and stone formation
- Are usually combined with labioplasty to improve cosmesis[64]
- Can develop ulcerative colitis[67]
- Malignancy.[68]

OTHER TISSUES USED FOR VAGINAL SUBSTITUTION

Human Amnion

Use of human amnion has been recommended to obviate the need for a donor site. This graft is used instead of skin modification of the McIndoe procedure.[69] Amniotic membranes are used as a graft on vaginoplasties. The amnion is not stripped from the chorion.[70] Excellent epithelialization with good functional results have been reported.[69,71] However, the potential for disease transmission from a third party has made this graft material less desirable for routine use. Early use of dilatation is recommended. An alternate tissue that has been suggested is the peritoneum and this will avoid some of the infectious problems of donor tissue.[72]

Bladder

In girls with a hypoplastic bladder who undergo creation of a neobladder, the residual bladder may be used for reconstruction of the vagina.[73]

Peritoneum

Vaginoplasty using pelvic peritoneum (Rothman's method) has been reported by Tamaya et al in 24 patients with congenital absence of the vagina.[74]

Additional Techniques

Apical Vaginal Extension

Incision into the vaginal pit in patients with congenital absence of the vagina leads to the potential space between the rectum and bladder. This space may be bluntly dissected and a posterior skin flap rotated in to this fossa. If a suitable mould is left in place the rotated flap of skin will act as a nidus for growth of new skin. The mould will need to be left in place for a greater period than that used with a skin graft. This technique has the potential risk for the mould to erode into the bladder over time.

Inferior Vaginal Extension

Williams described the creation of a pouch anterior to the vagina. This pouch when combined with a short vagina can permit intercourse.[75] A Uhaped incision is made around the posterior edge of the vulva and the skin edges are sewn to one another to create a pocket anterior to the penetration and this is a potential risk. Additionally the urethral meatus may be located so deep in the pouch that significant efforts need to be made to empty the pouch of urine following voiding.

RECENT ADVANCES

Total urogenital mobilization, a technique described by Pena is deemed to preserve the urogenital sinus blood supply and avoid ischemic complications.[36] This procedure is an effective technique for repairing short and long common channels, and a low surgical complication rate can be anticipated.[76] A modification of total urogenital mobilization by incorporating the mobilized urogenital sinus tissue that is a well vascularized flap into the repair rather than discarding it, has been found useful to create a mucosa lined vestibule, a posterior vaginal wall flap and an anterior vaginal wall flap.[77] The mucous fistula segment has also been used to create the neovagina in some cases thus obviating the need for a bowel anastomosis.[78]

A modified isolated ileal segment according to the Monti principle has also been reported in 6 patients to create the neovagina with excellent patient satisfaction and relatively low morbidity.[79]

A case of vaginal reconstruction using a flap from urinary bladder in a girl born with cloacal malformation and hemivaginas connected to the urinary bladder has been recently reported.[80] She had repeated urinary tract infection and vesicoureteral reflux. Urogenital reconstruction was performed at 14 months of age. After an initial posterior sagittal anorectoplasty. A part of the urinary bladder wall, which was connected to the vaginas, was used to lengthen the vagina so that the latter was able to pull down to the perineum.[80]

CONCLUSION

Multiple techniques have been described for vaginal substitution. The choice of surgical technique employed is based on the timing of reconstruction, indication for reconstruction, patient and parental motivation. Intestinal segments provide a lubricated vagina and are suited for early reconstruction. In patients that have later reconstruction tissue expansion or other skin flaps techniques are useful.

REFERENCES

1. Posner JC, Spandorfer PR. Early detection of imperforate hymen prevents morbidity from delays in diagnosis Pediatrics. 2005;115(4):1008-12.
2. Levitt MA, Peña A. Pitfalls in the management of newborn cloacas. Pediatr Surg Int 2005;21(4):264-69.
3. Sanders RM, Nakajima ST. An unusual late presentation of imperforate hymen. Obstet Gynecol 1994;83(5 Pt 2):896-98.
4. Patton PE, Novy MJ, Lee DM, Hickok LR. The diagnosis and reproductive outcome after surgical treatment of the complete septate uterus, duplicated cervix and vaginal septum Am J Obstet Gynecol 2004;190(6):1669-75;discussion 1675-78.
5. Peña A, Levitt MA, Hong A, Midulla P. Surgical management of cloacal malformations: A review of 339 patients. J Pediatr Surg, discussion 2004;39(3):470-79.
6. Warne SA, Wilcox DT, Creighton S, Ransley PG. Long-term gynecological outcome of patients with persistent cloaca. J Urol 2003;170(4 Pt 2):1493-96.
7. Khen-Dunlop N, Lortat-Jacob S, Thibaud E, et al. Rokitansky syndrome: Clinical experience and results of sigmoid vaginoplasty in 23 young girls. J Urol. 2007;177(3): 1107-11.
8. Lotan G, Mashiach R, Halevy A. Total endoscopic vaginal reconstruction in a case of Mayer-Rokitansky-Kuster-Hauser syndrome. J Laparoendosc Adv Surg Tech A 2005; 15(4):435-38.
9. Urbanowicz W, Starzyk J, Sulislawski J. Laparoscopic vaginal reconstruction using a sigmoid colon segment: A preliminary report. J Urol 2004;171(6 Pt 2):2632-35.
10. Powell DM, Newman KD, Randolph J. A proposed classification of vaginal anomalies and their surgical correction. Gynecol Oncol 1994;54(3):269-74.
11. Mayer CA. Uber Verdoppelungen des Uterus und ihre Arten, nebst Bemerkungen uber hasenscharte und Wolfsrachen. J Chir Auger 1829;13:525.
12. Rokitansky K. Uber die sogenannten Verdoppelungen des Uterus. Med Jahrb. Ost. Statt 1838;26:39.
13. Hauser GA, et al. Das Rokitansky-Kuster syndrome: Uterus biparitus solidus rudimentarius cum vagina solida. Gynaecologia 1967;151:11.

14. Fore Sr, et al. Urologic and genital anomalies in patients with congenital absence of vagina. Obstet Gynecol 1975;46:410.
15. Griffin JE, et al. Congenital absence of vagina. Ann Intern Med 1976;85:224.
16. Duncan PA, et al. The MURCS association: Müllerian duct aplasia, renal aplasia, and cervicothoracic somite dysplasia. J Pediatr 1979;95:399.
17. Nakayama DK, Snyder HM, Schaufer L, Ziegler MM, Tempelton JM, Duckett JW. Posterior sagittal exposure for reconstructive surgery for cloacal anomalies. J Pediatr Surg 1987;22:588.
18. Hendren WH. Repair of cloacal anomalies: Current techniques. J Pediatr Surg 1986;21:1159.
19. Jaramillo D, Lebowitz RL, Hendren WH. The cloacal malformations: Radiologic findings and imaging recommendations. Radiology 1990;177:441.
20. Hendren WH, Donahoe PK. Correction of congenital abnormalities of the vagina and perineum. J Pediatr Surg 1980;15:751.
21. Sheldon C, Cormier M, Crone K, Wacksman J. Occult neurovesical dysfunction in children with imperforate anus and its variants. J Pediatr Surg 1991;26:49.
22. Sheldon CA, Gilbert A. Use of the appendix for urethral reconstruction in children with congenital anomalies of the bladder. Durgery 1992;112:805.
23. Hendren WH. Urogenital sinus and anorectal malforamtions: Experience with 22 cases. J Pediatr Surg 1980;15:628
24. Parrot TS. Urologic implications of anorectal malformations. Urol Clin N Amer 1985;12:13.
25. Snyder H, McC III, Retik AB, Bauer SB, Colodny AH. Feminizing genitoplasty: A syntheses. J Urol 1983;129:1024.
26. Hendren WH. Reconstructive problems of the vagina and the female urethra. Clin Plast Surg 1980;7:207.
27. Hensle TW, Dean GE. Vaginal replacement in children. J Urol 1992;148:677.
28. Marshall FF. Vaginal agenesis. Clin Plast Surg 1980;7:175.
29. Fortunoff S, Edson M. Vaginoplasty technique for female pseudohermaphrodites. Surg Gynecol Obstet 1964;188:545.
30. Hendren WH, Crawford JD. Adrenogenital syndrome: The anatomy of the anomaly and its repair: Some new concepts. J Pediatr Surg 1969;4:49.
31. Rink RC, Adams MC. Feminizing genitoplasty: State-of-the-art. World J Urol 1998;16:212-18.
32. Hendren WH, Atala A. Repair of high vagina in girls with severely masculinied anatomy from adrenogenital syndrome. J Pediatr Surg 1995;30:91-94.
33. Pesserini-Glazel G. A new one stage procedure for clitorovaginoplasty in severely masculinised female pseudohermaphrodites. J Urol 1989;142:565-68.
34. Introduction of the anterior sagittal trans-ano-rectal approach (ASTRA) as a technical variation of the Passerini-Glazel clitoro-vaginoplasty: Preliminary results. Di Benedetto V, Di Benedetto A. J Urol 1998;159(3):1035-38.
35. Pena A, Filmer B, Bonilla E, et al. Transanorectal approach for the treatment of urogenital sinus: Preliminary report. J Pediatr Surg 1992;27:681-85.
36. Peña A. Total urogenital mobilization—an easier way to repair cloacas. J Pediatr Surg 1997;32(2):263-7;discussion 267-68.
37. Rink RC, Pope JC, Kropp BP, Smith ER Jr, Keating MA, Adams MC. Reconstruction of the high urogenital sinus: Early perineal prone approach without division of the rectum. Pediatr Surg Int 1997;12(2/3):168-71.
38. Frank RT. The formation of an artificial vagina without operation. Am J. Obstet Gynec 1938;35:1053.
39. McIndoe AH, Bannister JB. An operation for the cure of congenital absence of the vagina. J Obstet Gynaecol Br Emp 1939;45:590.
40. McIndoe A. The treatment of congenital absence and obliterative conditions of the vagina. Br J Plast Surg 1980;2:254.
41. Buss JG, Lee RA. McIndoe procedure for vaginal agenesis: Results and complications. Br J Plast Surg 1989;42(4):487-9.
42. Hockel M, Menke H, Germann G. Vaginoplasty with split skin grafts from the scalp: Optimization of the surgical treatment for vaginal agenesis. J Am Coll Surg 2003;196(1):159-62.
43. Duckett JW, Baskin LS. Genitoplasty for intersex anomalies. Eur J Ped 1993;152:S80-84.
44. Hopkins MP, Morley GW. Squamous cell carcinoma of the neovagina. Obstet Gynecol 1986;67(3):443-46.
45. Ozek C, Gurler T, Alper M, Gundogan H, Bilkay U, Songur E, Akin Y, Cagdas A. Modified McIndoe procedure for vaginal agenesis. J Urol 1998;160(1):186-90.
46. Morely GW, de Lancey JOL. Full thickness skin graft vaginoplasty for treatment of the stenotic or foreshortened vagina. Obstet Gynecol 1991;77:485-89.
47. Johnson N, Lilford RJ, Batchelor A. The free-flap vaginoplasty; a new surgical procedure for the treatment of vaginal agenesis. Arch Gynecol Obstet 1991;249(1):15-17.
48. McGraw JB, Massey FM, Shanklin KD, Horton CE. Vaginal reconstruction with gracilis myocutaneous flaps. Plast Reconstr Surg 1976;58:176-183.
49. Heath PM, Woods JE, Podratz KC, Arnold PG. Gracilis myocutaneous vaginal reconstruction. Mayo Clin Proc 1984;59:21.
50. Lagasse LD, Berman ML, Watring WG, Ballon SC. The Gynecologic Oncology Patient: Restoration of function and prevention of disability. In L McGowan (Ed): Gynecologic Oncology. New York: Appleton-Century-Crofts, 1978;398.
51. Lacey PM, Morrow CP. myocutaneous Vaginal reconstruction. In Morrow CP, Smart GE (Eds), Gynecologic Oncology. Berlin:Springer-Verlag,1986;255.
52. Soper JT, Larson D, Hunter VJ. Short gracilis myocutaneous flaps for vulvovaginal reconstruction after radical pelvic surgery. Obstet Gynecol 1989;74:823-27.
53. Song R, Wang X, Zhou G. reconstruction of the vagina with sensory function. Clin Plast Surgery 1982;9:105.
54. Wang TN, Whetzel T, Mathes SJ. A fasciocutaneous flap for vaginal and perineal reconstruction. Plast Reconstr Surg 1984;80:95.

55. Wee TK, Joseph VT. A new technique of vaginal reconstruction using neurovascular pudendal thigh flaps: A preliminary report. Plastic Reconstr Surg 1988;83:701.
56. Cain JM, Diamond A, Tamimi HK, Greer BE, Figge DC. The morbidity and benefits of concurrent gracilis myocutaneous flaps with pelvic exenteration. Obstet Gynecol 1989;74:185.
57. Patil U, Hixson FP. The role of tissue expanders in vaginoplasty for congenital malformations of the vagina. Plast Reconstr Surg 1992;90(3):487-91.
58. Johnson N, Batchelor A, Lilford RJ. Experience with tissue expansion vaginoplasty. Br J Obstet Gynecol 1991;98:564-68.
59. Belloli G, Campobasso P, Musi L. Labial skin-flap vaginoplasty using tissue expanders. J Pediatr Surg 1997;32(1):62-65.
60. Wierrani F, Grunberger. Vaginoplasty using deepithelialized vulvar transposition flaps: The Grunberger method. W Hum Reprod 2003 Mar;18(3):604-07.
61. Lin WC, Chang CY, Shen YY, Tsai HD. Use of autologous buccal mucosa for vaginoplasty: A study of eight cases. 2001;15(2):104-05.
62. Hitchcock RJI, malone PS: Colonovaginoplasty in infants and children. Br J Urol 1994;73:196-99.
63. Baldwin JF. The formation of an artificial vagina by intestinal transplantation. Ann Surg 1904;40:398.
64. Hanna MK. Vaginal construction. Urology 1987;29:272-75.
65. Wesley JR, Coran AG. Intestinal vaginoplasty for congenital absence of the vagina. J Pediatr Surg 1992;27:885-89.
66. Radhakrishnan J. Colon interposition vaginoplasty. A modification of the Wagner Baldwin Technique. J Pediatr Surg 1987;22:1175-76.
67. Hennigan TW, Theodorou NA. Ulcerative colitis and bleeding from a colonic vaginoplasty. Br J Obstet Gynaecol 1991;98(6):564-68
68. Ursic-Vrscaj M, Lindtner J, Lamovec J, Novak J. Adenocarcinoma in a sigmoid neovagina 22 years after Wertheim-Meigs operation. Case report. J Gynecol Surg 1992 Spring; 8(1):25-30.
69. Morton KE, Dewhurst CJ. Human amnion in the treatment of vaginal malformations. Br J Obstet Gynecol 1986;93:50.
70. Nisolle M, Donnez J. Vaginoplasty using amniotic membranes in cases of vaginal agenesis or after vaginectomy. Br J Urol 1992;70(5):554-57.
71. Morton KE, Dewhurst CJ. Human amnion in the treatment of vaginal malformations. J Pediatr Surg 1984;19(5):510-14.
72. Ashworth MF, Morton KE, Dewhurst J, Lilford RJ, Bates RG. Vaginoplasty using amnion. Br J Obstet Gynaecol 1986;93(1):50-54.
73. Sheldon CA, Gilbert A, Lewis A. Vaginal reconstruction: Critical technical principles. J Urol 1994;152:387-91.
74. Tamaya T, Imai A. The use of peritoneum for vaginoplasty in 24 patients with congenital absence of the vagina. Obstet Gynecol 1990;76(5 Pt 2):900-01.
75. Williams EA. Congenital absence of the vagina: A simple operation for its relief. J Obstet Gynecol 1964;71:511.
76. Leclair MD, Gundetti M, Kiely EM, Wilcox DT. The surgical outcome of total urogenital mobilization for cloacal repair J Urol. 2007;177(4):1492-95.
77. Rink RC, Metcalfe PD, Cain MP, Meldrum KK, Kaefer MA, Casale AJ. Use of the mobilized sinus with total urogenital mobilization. J Urol 2006;176(5):2205-11.
78. O'Connor JL, DeMarco RT, Pope JC 4th, Adams MC, Brock JW 3rd. Bowel vaginoplasty in children: A retrospective review. J Pediatr Surg 2004; 39(8):1205-08.
79. Trombetta C, Liguori G, Siracusano S, Bortul M, Belgrano E. Transverse retubularized ileal vaginoplasty: A new application of the Monti principle—preliminary report. Eur Urol 2005;48(6):1018-23; discussion 1023-24.
80. Chin T, Liu C, Tsai H, Wei C. Vaginal reconstruction using urinary bladder flap in a patient with cloacal malformation J Pediatr Surg 2007;42:1612-15.

Adrenal Disorders

Anurag Bajpai, PSN Menon

Adrenal gland is responsible for the production of glucocorticoids, mineralocorticoids and androgens, which regulate intermediary metabolism, fluid and electrolyte homeostasis and virilization respectively. Important pediatric adrenal disorders include defects in steroidogenesis, and excess and deficiency of individual hormones.[1] Early diagnosis and treatment of these conditions are important in preventing long and short-term morbidity and mortality.

PHYSIOLOGY AND METABOLISM

Effects of Adrenal Cortex Hormones

Adrenal cortex produces three important groups of hormones—the glucocorticoids, mineralocorticoids and androgens.[2] Cortisol, the major glucocorticoid hormone has an important role in intermediary metabolism leading to increased blood glucose levels and enhanced catabolism of proteins and lipids. Mineralocorticoids (aldosterone) act on the distal renal tubules and the collecting duct to promote sodium and fluid absorption. This leads to enhanced sodium absorption with increased excretion of other cations (potassium and protons).

The selectivity of action of adrenal steroids is determined at the level of hormone receptors. Mineralocorticoids act only on the type I steroid receptor while cortisol can act on both type I and II receptors. The inactivation of cortisol to cortisone by locally present enzyme 11β-hydroxysteroid dehydrogenase ensures that cortisol cannot interact with type I receptor. The importance of this regulation is emphasized by the presence of severe hypertension seen in patients with deficiency of this enzyme. In these patients cortisol is not inactivated and thereby acts on the type I receptor leading to apparent mineralocorticoid excess. Type II receptor is specific for cortisol and is responsible for glucocorticoid actions. Adrenal androgens play an important role in virilization. Dehydroepiandrosterone (DHEA) is the most abundant adrenal androgen while androstenedione is the most potent. In the peripheral tissues, these compounds can be converted to testosterone and estrogen.

Adrenal Steroidogenesis

Adrenal steroidogenesis is a multi-step enzyme pathway and is summarized in Figure 117.1. The adrenal cortex has been divided into various zones based upon histological and biochemical features. Different parts of adrenals have different biosynthetic capabilities due to the presence of specific enzymes. Zona glomerulosa, the outer most zone, synthesizes aldosterone while the zona reticularis and fasciculate synthesize both glucocorticoids (cortisol) as well as androgens (DHEA and androstenedione).

Regulation of Adrenal Steroidogenesis

Adrenocorticotropin (ACTH), a polypeptide secreted by the anterior pituitary, is the principle regulator of glucocorticoid and androgen synthesis. ACTH secretion is influenced by the circadian rhythm, corticotropin-releasing hormone (CRH) secreted by the median eminence of hypothalamus and serum cortisol levels. Release of ACTH also leads to release of melanocyte stimulating hormone (MSH), which is responsible for pigmentation seen in conditions with increased ACTH production such as primary adrenal insufficiency.

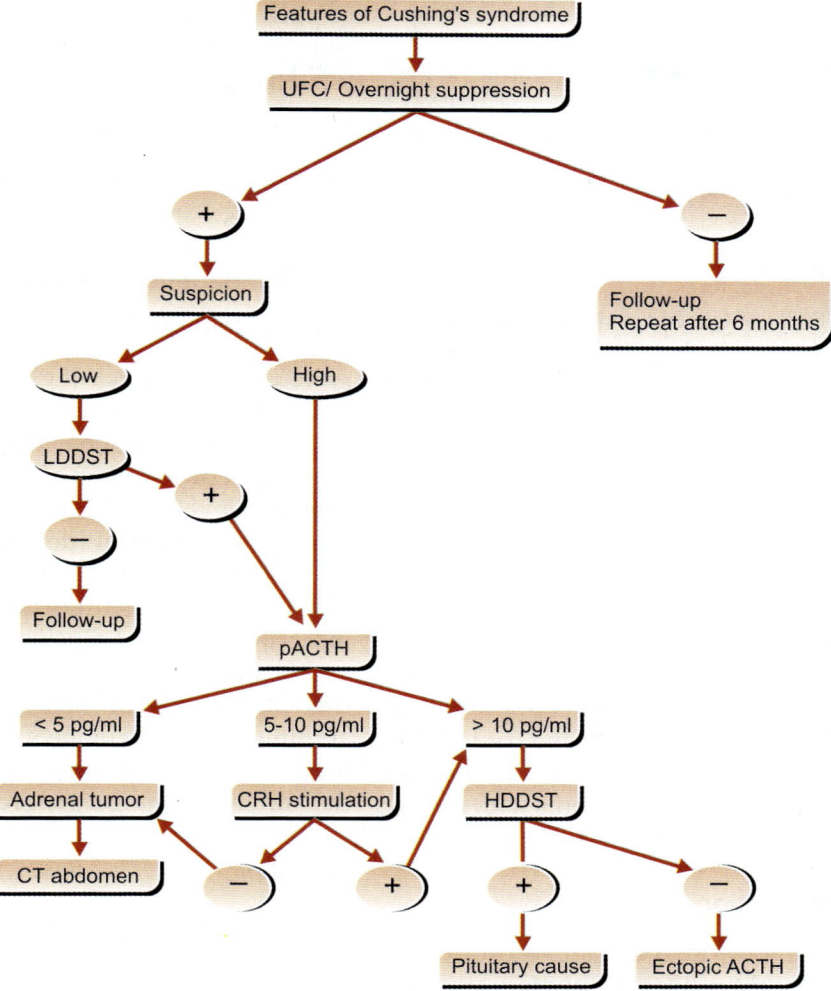

Fig. 117.1: Approach to Cushing's syndrome

Intravascular volume, serum potassium levels and renin-angiotensin system are the chief regulators of aldosterone synthesis. ACTH plays only a minimal role in aldosterone regulation. Patients with pituitary deficiency therefore do not present with salt wasting crisis, as aldosterone levels are normal.

DISORDERS ASSOCIATED WITH EXCESS OF ADRENOCORTICAL HORMONES

These disorders include conditions associated with excessive secretion of glucocorticoids, mineralocorticoids and adrenal androgens in isolation or in various combinations.

CUSHING'S SYNDROME (GLUCOCORTICOID EXCESS)

Cushing's syndrome, manifestation of hypercortisolism, is characterized by central obesity, proximal myopathy, glucose intolerance and hypertension. Most of these cases have features of androgen excess in the form of hirsutism, amenorrhea and virilization. The term Cushing's disease is reserved for those patients who have pituitary tumor as a cause of hypercortisolism while the constellation of clinical findings irrespective of etiology is described as Cushing's syndrome.

Etiology

Cushing's syndrome is a rare disease with a prevalence of 1-2/million general population. The exact prevalence in children is unknown but is lower compared to adults. Causes of Cushing's syndrome are summarized in Table 117.1.

ACTH Dependent Causes

Majority of cases (80%) of Cushing' syndrome in adults are related to increased levels of ACTH. However in children younger than 6 years adrenal causes are more common.

Pituitary Causes

Excessive secretion of CRH and ACTH are implicated in many cases of Cushing's syndrome. Most are associated with pituitary microadenoma but macroadenoma is found in some cases. In a few cases with bilateral adrenal hyperplasia, no cause is found despite meticulous investigations. It is important to differentiate Cushing's syndrome secondary to CRH stimulation from those due to ACTH excess, as resection of pituitary adenoma in patients with former is associated with high recurrence rates.

Ectopic ACTH Production

The syndrome of ectopic ACTH production is extremely rare in children. Extremely high levels of ACTH, hyperpigmentation and manifestations of Cushing's disease are important findings. Features peculiar to the tumors like flushing and diarrhea (carcinoid tumor) and episodic hypertension (pheochromocytoma) may suggest the diagnosis. In patients with malignancies and ectopic ACTH secretion classical features of Cushing's syndrome may not develop due to acute nature of the lesion and hypokalemic alkalosis with hypertension may be the presenting features.

ACTH Independent Causes

Adrenal Causes

Adrenal is the source of glucocorticoid excess in most children with Cushing's syndrome.[3] Adrenal carcinoma is commoner than adenoma and presents with rapid progression of clinical features and greatly elevated levels of DHEA and urinary ketosteroids. Patients with adrenal adenoma have on the other hand slower clinical course and mild elevation of these substances. Pigmented nodular hyperplasia is an important cause of Cushing's syndrome in children and is associated with normal adrenal imaging. This disorder has been associated with a variety of autoimmune and cutaneous defects. The presence of bilateral adrenal hyperplasia suggests ACTH dependent Cushing's syndrome.

Iatrogenic

Exogenous steroid intake is the commonest cause of Cushing's syndrome. Long-term treatment with any steroid leads to the condition. Drugs with high potency and prolonged half-life (dexamethasone) are more prone to toxicity than those with shorter half-life and lower potency (hydrocortisone). These patients can be identified by careful history. The diagnosis can be confirmed by normal serum and urinary levels of cortisol.

Clinical Features

Clinical features of Cushing's syndrome are summarized in Table 117.2. Features such as excessive

Table 117.1: Causes of Cushing's syndrome

1. ACTH dependent
   a. Hypothalamic- CRH producing tumor
   b. Pituitary-
      - Adenoma
      - Hyperplasia
   c. Ectopic ACTH/CRH production–
      Carcinoid tumor
      Pheochromocytoma
      Gastrinoma
2. ACTH independent
   a. Adrenal related–
      Adenoma
      Carcinoma
      Pigmented nodular hyperplasia
   b. Exogenous steroids

Table 117.2: Clinical features of Cushing's syndrome

- Central obesity
- Hirsutism
- Hypertension
- Striae (wide purple)
- Easy bruisability
- Proximal myopathy
- Polyuria

weight gain, hypertension and glucose tolerance are common but non-specific features of Cushing's syndrome. On the other hand hirsutism, central obesity, striae and proximal myopathy strongly indicate the need of evaluation for hypercortisolism. Children with constitutional obesity are most likely to be confused with Cushing's syndrome. They have generalized obesity, hypertension and high normal steroid excretion rates. These children are tall for their age and have advanced skeletal maturity. In contradistinction children with Cushing's syndrome have retarded somatic and skeletal development.

Diagnostic Evaluation

Diagnosis of Cushing's syndrome is complex and involves multi-step approach.[4] First step is to presumptively diagnose the disease using screening tests. Diagnosis is then confirmed using diagnostic tests. Once the diagnosis of Cushing's syndrome is established, further tests to diagnose the etiology are performed. Careful clinical evaluation forms an important part of such an approach. Hyperpigmentation suggests the possibility of excessive ACTH production (pituitary or ectopic tumor). Rapid progression with hirsutism indicates adrenal carcinoma while gradual progression is characteristic of pituitary adenoma. Features of CNS involvement and additional pituitary defects go in favor of pituitary lesions while hypertension out of proportion to other features indicates pheochromocytoma as a cause of ectopic ACTH production. The biochemical tests for evaluation of Cushing's syndrome are summarized in Tables 117.3 and 117.4.

Screening Tests

Twenty-four hour urinary cortisol is the best screening test for Cushing's syndrome and should be performed in all cases wherever it is possible. It provides accurate estimation of daily steroid production and has the advantage of being diagnostic at higher values. Its high sensitivity and specificity (95-100% and 98%) makes it superior to overnight suppression test, which has high sensitivity but low specificity (98% and 70%). Mid night cortisol is emerging as a simple measure of evaluating cortisol excess but is in experimental stages.

Table 117.3: Diagnostic modalities for Cushing's syndrome

Investigation	Protocol	Measurement	Positive	Comments
Screening UFC	24 hour urine collection	Free cortisol	> 70 µg/m2/day	Best screening test Diagnostic > 150 µg/m^2/day
Overnight suppression	Dexa- 15 µg/kg 11 PM	Cortisol 8 AM	> 5 µg/dl	Low specificity
Midnight cortisol	Sleeping 12 midnight	Cortisol	> 1.8 µg/dl	Less experience
Diagnosis LDDST	Dexa- 30 µg/kg/day q 6 hrly x 2 days	Cortisol 15 min later	> 5 µg/dl	Gold standard Less value now
LDDST and CRH test	LDDST followed by CRH 1 µg/kg iv	Cortisol 15 min later	> 1.4 µg/dl	Excellent test Limited experience
Etiology HDDST	Dexa- 100 µg/kg/day q 6 hrly x 2 days	UFC baseline and Post-dexa	< 10% of basal	Positive- microadenoma Negative- macroadenoma ectopic
ACTH	Random	ACTH	-	< 5 pg/ml- Adrenal >10 pg/ml- ACTH dependent
IPSS	Pituitary sampling	Petrosal: Peripheral ACTH	> 2	For pituitary localization
CRH test	CRH 1 µg/kg	ACTH basal and 30 min post-CRH	Increase > 35%	Adrenal versus pituitary cause

UFC- urinary free cortisol, Dexa- Dexamethasone, CRH- Corticotropin releasing hormone, LDDST- Low dose dexa suppression test, HDDST- High dose dexa suppression test, ACTH- Adrenocorticotropin, IPSS- Inferior petrosal selective sampling

| Table 117.4: Endocrine investigations in various forms of Cushing's syndrome ||||||
Condition	UFC	ACTH	CRH Test	HDDST	IPSS
Adrenal tumor	+	↓	-	-	-
Pituitary microadenoma	+	↑	+	+	+
Pituitary macroadenoma	+	↑	+	-	+
Ectopic ACTH secretion	+	↑↑	-	-	-
Exogenous steroids	-	↓	-	-	-

UFC- Urinary free cortisol, ACTH- Adrenocorticotropin, CRH- Corticotropin releasing hormone, HDDST- High dose dexamethasone suppression test, IPSS- Invasive selective petrosal sinus sampling

All patients with high index of suspicion but negative screening tests should be closely followed up with repeat biochemical evaluations in view of the possibility of periodic steroidogenesis.

Confirmatory Tests

High levels of urinary free cortisol (>150 µg/m²/day) are diagnostic of Cushing's syndrome and no other confirmatory test is required. In patients with lesser degree of elevation of urinary free cortisol who have low clinical suspicion, a confirmatory test is required. Low dose dexamethasone suppression test (LDDST) is based upon the principle that dexamethasone in low dose does not to suppress cortisol levels in patients with Cushing's syndrome while suppresses them in other causes of hypercortisolism. Some patients with pituitary microadenoma however show suppression by this test. These patients are responsive to stimulation with CRH. This has led to evaluation by CRH stimulation test after the standard LDDST. This test is emerging as the investigation for choice of confirming the diagnosis of Cushing's syndrome.

Etiological Diagnosis

Approach to diagnosis of Cushing's syndrome is presented in Figure 117.1. Initial step in etiological diagnosis is to distinguish ACTH dependent (hypothalamic-pituitary related and ectopic ACTH) causes from ACTH independent (adrenal) causes. Plasma ACTH levels are helpful in distinguishing ACTH dependent (ACTH > 10 pg/ml) from ACTH independent (ACTH < 5 pg/ml) cases. Cases with borderline ACTH levels (5-10 pg/ml) should be categorized by CRH stimulation test.

Spiral CT scan for adrenals should be performed in all patients with ACTH independent Cushing's syndrome. In patients with elevated levels of ACTH high dose dexamethasone suppression test (HDDST) and CRH stimulation test are helpful in differentiating pituitary adenomas from ectopic ACTH producing tumors. In cases with suspected pituitary tumors gadolinium contrast MRI followed by invasive petrosal sampling can be used to determine the location of the tumor. Imaging of adrenal and pituitary should ideally be performed only after the diagnosis of Cushing's syndrome is confirmed. This is to avoid confusion due to frequent occurrence of incidentalomas in both adrenals and pituitary.

Management

Surgery is the main modality of choice in Cushing's syndrome.[5] Medical management is important and recommended as a stopgap measure before surgery or when surgery is contraindicated (Fig. 117.2).

Adrenal Causes

Adenoma: Surgical resection is the treatment of choice. In most of these cases excessive secretion of cortisol suppresses the remaining adrenal tissue leading to adrenal insufficiency once the tumor is resected. This should be prevented by steroid replacement as done for stress conditions (discussed in adrenal crises states below).

Carcinoma: The outcome of these tumors is poor in view of highly invasive nature and high rates of metastasis. Adjunct treatment with chemotherapeutic agents like mitotane and cisplatinum has not improved the outcome in these patients.

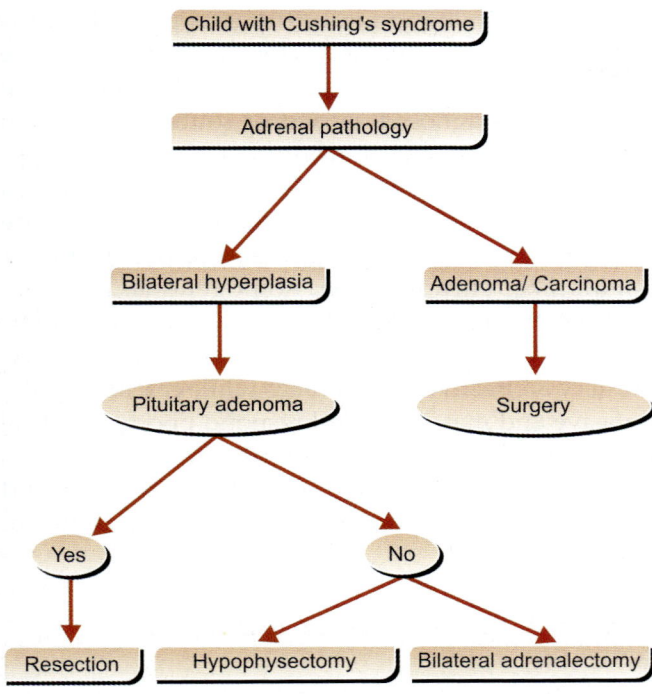

Fig. 117.2: Management of Cushing's syndromes

Pituitary Adenoma

Transsphenoidal resection of adenoma is the procedure of choice. It is important to rule out CRH dependent pituitary hyperplasia, as this is associated with high rates of recurrence after surgery.

Adrenal Hyperplasia without Pituitary Tumor

This condition is most likely due to undetectable pituitary tumors; ectopic ACTH secretion should however be ruled out by detailed evaluation. There is controversy regarding management of these cases. Bilateral adrenalectomy has been tried by some but has the problem of life-long replacement of corticosteroids and the high incidence of development of pituitary tumors (Nelson's syndrome). Hypophysectomy, the alternative to bilateral adrenalectomy, entails the risk of permanent hypopituitarism. The management of these patients remains highly unsatisfactory.

Medical Management

Anti-adrenal drugs (mitotane, ketoconazole, spironolactone) have been used as temporary measures in management of Cushing's syndrome. Cyproheptadine, a serotonin antagonist, has been found to be effective in management of Cushing's syndrome.

HYPERALDOSTERONISM

Excessive secretion of aldosterone is associated with hypertension and hypokalemic alkalosis.

Causes

The causes of hyperaldosteronism are summarized in Table 117.5. Pituitary tumors do not cause hyperaldosteronism as ACTH has minor role in aldosterone regulation. Most cases of hyperaldosteronism are due to increase in renin levels, which is a compensatory response to reduced intravascular fluid volume. Aldosterone secreting adrenal tumors are smaller compared to those associated with Cushing's syndrome or androgen excess. Bilateral adrenal hyperplasia can rarely present with features of aldosterone excess.

Clinical Features and Diagnosis

Hyperaldosteronism should be suspected in children with hypertension and hypokalemia. These children may present with features of hypokalemia in the form of muscle cramps and weakness (myopathy) and polyuria (impaired urinary concentration). Atrial natriuretic peptide is secreted in states of aldosterone excess. This provides escape from the fluid retaining

Table 117.5: Causes of hyperaldosteronism
1. Renin related
a. *Compensatory:* CHF/nephrotic syndrome/ascites
b. *Renal ischemia:* Renal artery stenosis
c. *Hypereninism:* Tumor
d. Bartter's syndrome (sodium/chloride channel defect)
2. Aldosterone related
a. Adrenal tumor
b. Adrenal hyperplasia
3. Apparent aldosterone excess
a. Glucocorticoid remediable aldosteronism
b. CAH- 11-hydroxylase deficiency, 17α-hydroxylase deficiency
c. 11β-steroid dehydrogenase deficiency
4. Psuedohyperaldosteronism
a. Constitutional activity of aldosterone receptor
b. Liddle's disease (Sodium channel defect)

effect of aldosterone. Patients with hyperaldosteronism thereby do not have edema unless complicating conditions like cardiac failure or renal dysfunction are present. These patients have borderline hypernatremia, marked hypokalemia, modest alkalosis and magnesium deficiency. Diagnosis of primary hyperaldosteronism requires the presence of diastolic hypertension, elevated and nonsuppressible aldosterone levels and low peripheral renin activity. Aldosteronomas should be differentiated from causes of apparent aldosterone excess mentioned in Table 117.5. Spiral thin slice CT scan should be performed in these patients considering the small size of most aldosteronomas.

Management

Hyperaldosteronism should be initially managed with salt restriction and anti-aldosterone agent spironolactone. Angiotensin convertase enzyme inhibitors are ineffective in these patients as renin-angiotensin system is already suppressed. Surgery is the treatment of choice for adrenal adenoma. Surgery however does not cause reduction of blood pressure in patients with bilateral hyperplasia. Surgery should thereby be performed only in those patients who have refractory hypokalemia.

ADRENAL ANDROGEN EXCESS

Congenital adrenal hyperplasia is the commonest cause of adrenal hyperandrogenism. Adrenal tumors associated with androgen excess are usually aggressive and have high rates of malignancy. They present with hirsutism, virilization and premature adrenarchae in girls and peripheral precocious puberty in boys. Elevated urinary levels of 17-keto steroids and serum levels of DHEA and androstenedione suggest the diagnosis. CT scan of the abdomen helps in localizing the tumor and also provides information regarding the extent of tumor spread. Treatment involves surgery in combination with radiotherapy and chemotherapy with antimitotic agent mitotane.

TUMORS OF THE ADRENALS

Adrenal cortical tumors present with excess secretion of glucocorticoids (Cushing's syndrome), aldosterone (hyperaldosteronism) or androgens (virilization). Rapid onset, young age and virilization points towards malignant tumor while slowly progressive features are suggestive of adenoma. A small proportion of adrenal tumors are diagnosed as part of routine abdominal imaging. These incidentalomas should prompt evaluation for adrenal excess (urine free cortisol, serum sodium and potassium and DHEA). If these tests are normal and imaging is suggestive of benign tumor (small size, encapsulated, homogenous, no calcification), the patient should be followed up by periodic imaging. Treatment of most adrenal tumors is surgery. Surgery is effective in adenomas while carcinomas are invasive and metastatic and respond poorly. Medical management with cyproheptadine (Cushing's syndrome), spironolactone (aldosteronoma) and ketoconazole (androgen excess) provide transient benefit.

ADRENAL INSUFFICIENCY (ADDISON'S DISEASE)

Insufficient synthesis or action of adrenal hormone can present as slowly progressive deterioration or salt wasting crises.

Causes

The causes of adrenal insufficiency are presented in Table 117.6. Pituitary deficiency is associated with preservation of mineralocorticoid function and does not lead to salt wasting. Adrenal hemorrhage, congenial adrenal hyperplasia and rapid tapering of corticosteroids are important causes of acute adrenal insufficiency. Autoimmune destruction and tuberculosis are the major causes of acquired adrenal insufficiency.

Clinical Features

Defect in steroid synthesis and congenital adrenal hypoplasia present in early neonatal period with polyuria, failure to thrive, recurrent vomiting and shock. Investigations reveal hyponatremia, hyperkalemia, metabolic acidosis, hemoconcentration and hypoglycemia. Acquired adrenal insufficiency presents with slowly progressive lethargy, vomiting, salt craving and fatigue. Adrenal insufficiency is manifest only after 90% of adrenal is damaged. Primary adrenal insufficiency is characterized by

Table 117.6: Causes of adrenal insufficiency
1. **Hypothalamic- pituitary related** 　a. Hypothalamic lesion 　b. Isolated ACTH deficiency 　c. Panhypopituitarism 　d. Suppression from steroid therapy/adenoma 2. **Adrenal related** 　a. *Defective steroidogenesis:* 21 hydroxylase deficiency, StAR deficiency, 3β-hydroxysteroid dehydrogenase deficiency 　b. *Anatomical defect:* Surgery, trauma, hypoplasia 　c. *Autoimmune destruction:* PGA I and II 　d. *Infection:* Tuberculosis, HIV, CMV 　e. *Hemorrhage:* Waterhouse Friderichsen syndrome, bleeding disorder 　f. *Genetic:* Adrenoleukodystrophy, Wolman's disease 3. **Drugs** 　a. *Increased steroid metabolism:* Rifampicin, phenytoin, phenobarbitone 　b. *Inhibition of steroidogenesis:* Ketokonazole, metyrapone, aminoglutethimide

hyperpigmentation due to elevated levels of MSH. Hyperpigmentation is present in sun-exposed areas as elbows, palmar creases and areas that are normally hyperpigmented as areolae and genitals. Features of hypoparathyroidism, hypothyroidism and diabetes mellitus suggest the diagnosis of polyglandular autoimmune syndromes (PGA I and II). Ectodermal dystrophy and chronic mucosal candidiasis are characteristic of PGA I.

Evaluation and Diagnosis

All patients suspected to have adrenal insufficiency should have urgent estimation of serum electrolytes and blood sugar. Basal levels of cortisol are low but can be in the low normal range. Rapid ACTH stimulation test (cortisol estimation 60 min after 0.25 mg of ACTH injection IM) is the best test for adrenocortical reserve. Serum cortisol levels lower than 15 µg/dl are suggestive of adrenal insufficiency. In patients with prolonged adrenal insufficiency long ACTH stimulation test (ACTH 1 mg/day IM for 3 days) is required for establishing the diagnosis.

Next step in evaluation of adrenal insufficiency is the estimation of ACTH levels. Elevated ACTH levels suggest primary adrenal pathology while low levels points toward pituitary defect. Further evaluation of primary adrenal insufficiency includes abdominal CT scan, estimation of anti-adrenal antibodies and workup for tuberculosis. Evaluation of hypothalamic-pituitary function (growth hormone stimulation test, FT4, LH, FSH and urinary specific gravity) is essential in patients with low ACTH levels.

Management

Initial management of salt wasting crises includes correction of shock by fluid boluses and management of hyponatremia and hypernatremia. Hydrocortisone should be administered immediately in a dose of 50 mg/m^2 followed by 100 mg/m^2/day. The patient should be started on twice maintenance fluids. Frequent monitoring of hemodynamic parameters, urine output and serum electrolytes are required. Once the child is hemodynamically stable hydrocortisone can be tapered gradually to a dose of 15-25 mg/m^2/day. Mineralocorticoids (fludrocortisone acetate 0.1 mg/day) should be added once the hydrocortisone dose is less than 50 mg/m^2/day.

Long-term management of adrenal insufficiency requires life long replacement of glucocorticoids and mineralocorticoids. The dose is regulated by clinical features and serum levels of cortisol and aldosterone. Parents should be educated about the need of increasing dose during periods of stress. Need of urgent medical attention in conditions of decreased oral intake and stress should be emphasized. The dose of glucocorticoid should be increased 2-3 times in conditions of minor stress (fever, mild infection) and 4-5 times in severe stress (severe infection, surgery). These doses should continue throughout the period of stress. Patients with pituitary deficiency do not require mineralocorticoid. Their glucocorticoid requirements are also lower than those with primary adrenal insufficiency.

CONGENITAL ADRENAL HYPERPLASIA

Congenital adrenal hyperplasia (CAH), a group of autosomal recessive defects in steroid synthesis, is characterized by deficiency of adrenocortical hormones on one hand and excess of steroid precursor on the other (Fig. 117.3). CAH is the commonest adrenal disorder in childhood.

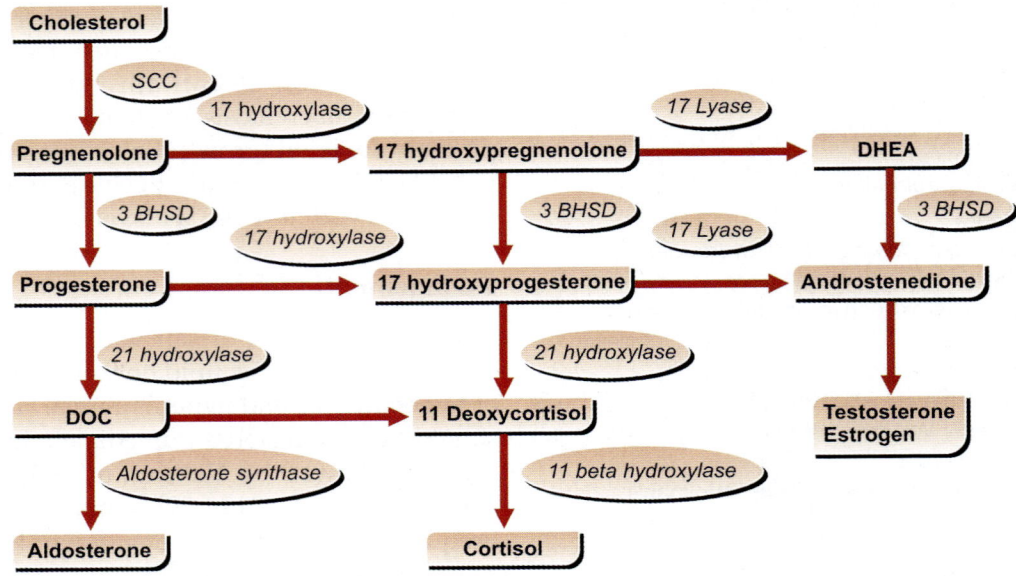

Fig. 117.3: Steroidogenic pathway

Types

The manifestations of CAH vary with the type of enzymatic defect.

21-hydroxylase Deficiency

21-hydroxylase deficiency is the commonest form of CAH accounting for 90% cases.[6] This disorder is associated with diminished synthesis of the hormones cortisol and aldosterone. Low cortisol levels stimulate ACTH synthesis. Elevated ACTH level causes accumulation of steroid precursors (DHEA, androstenedione and 17-hydoxy progesterone, 17OHP) prior to 21-hydroxylase. There is a wide variation in presentation of 21-hydroxylase deficiency ranging from acute life threatening salt wasting crises to virilization and premature adrenarche. These variations can be explained by different enzyme levels, which in turn depend upon the nature of mutation.[7] This disorder has been classified into three groups based on clinical features. These subsets are not separate disorders but are part of a spectrum and have significant overlap.

Classical Salt Wasting (CSW)

These patients have the lowest levels of 21-hydroxylase and present in the neonatal period with virilization. The level of virilization extends from mild clitoromegaly and labioscrotal fusion to the extreme levels where genitalia resemble that of a boy with cryptorchidism. Associated hyperpigmentation points towards the diagnosis of CAH. Diagnosis is delayed in boys as they lack specific clinical features. They present in the second week of life with failure to thrive, polyuria, hyperpigmentation, and shock. Early diagnosis is mandatory to prevent high rates of mortality. 21-hydroxyalse deficiency should be suspected in all neonates with ambiguous genitalia, polyuria, shock, recurrent vomiting and features of sepsis with negative septic screen. The diagnosis should be confirmed immediately by hormonal assay. If these are not available the child should be managed empirically in the lines of adrenal insufficiency.

Classical Virilizing (CV)

A subset of patients with classical 21-hydroxylase deficiency (25%) synthesizes enough aldosterone so as to prevent adrenal crises. These patients have features of androgen excess in the form of virilization in girls and peripheral precocious puberty in boys. Boys with this disorder have prepubertal testicular volume, a finding that differentiates them from those with central precocious puberty. Prolonged androgenic stimulation in untreated boys leads to triggering of central precocious puberty. These patients also have an increased incidence of ectopic adrenal rest tumors due to elevated ACTH levels. Testicular adrenal rests can mimic testicular tumors. The possibility of adrenal rests should be excluded by ultrasonogram and endocrine investigations before proceeding with invasive procedures like biopsy or surgical excision.

Non-classic (NC)

This disorder is associated with partial deficiency of the enzyme 21-hydroxylase. They present with mild hyperandrogenism in the form of premature adrenarche in girls and penile enlargement in boys. Aldosterone levels are normal and salt wasting is absent.

Diagnosis

Diagnosis of CSW is established by demonstration of extreme elevation of 17 OHP levels (10000-20000 ng dl, normal < 90 ng/dl) in the presence of clinical and laboratory features of adrenal insufficiency. In patients where therapy had been started empirically 17 OHP levels should be estimated 2 days after discontinuation of hydrocortisone. This should be done under hospital setting so as to monitor for adrenal crises. The 17 OHP levels are elevated in patients with CV and NC; the elevations are however not as high as in CSW. The best method of diagnosing these patients is the estimation of 17 OHP levels before and 60 min after an intramuscular injection of ACTH (0.25 mg). These values should be plotted against the standard nomogram that classifies the patients into CSW, CV, NC, carrier state or no disease.

Management

These patients require life long treatment.[8] Patients with CSW and CV should be treated with hydrocortisone (15-25 mg/m^2/day) and fludrocortisone (0.1 mg/day). Although features of aldosterone deficiency are absent in patients with CV, aldosterone therapy reduces the requirement of hydrocortisone by suppressing antidiuretic hormone (ADH) levels. Doses should be adjusted based on clinical (growth, cushingoid features and blood pressure) and laboratory parameters (17OHP 500-1000 ng/dl, androstenedione 20-50 ng/dl and normal serum electrolytes). Doses should be increased under stressful conditions as for adrenal insufficiency. Patients with NC variety do not require mineralocorticoid treatment. In adolescent girls and young women longer acting analogs of glucocorticoids (dexamethasone, prednisolone) can be used. These drugs should be avoided during periods of growth as they have significant growth-inhibiting activity.

Role of Surgery

Girls with CSW and CV present with ambiguous genitalia at the time of birth. These girls have normal uterus and ovaries and have the potential for normal reproductive function. They should be reared as girls. Pediatric surgical approach includes clitoral recession, labioscrotal reduction and exteriorization of vagina.[9] Single step procedures are replacing the cumbersome two-step procedure in most centers.

Adrenalectomy is emerging as a promising modality in the management of patients with CSW CAH. It has been observed that natriuretic steroid precursors antagonize the actions of aldosterone. Increased androgen production leads to growth retardation, enhanced skeletal maturity and virilization. Adrenalectomy helps in these patients by reducing the production of these substances.

Other Variants

Enzyme deficiencies other than 21-hydroxylase deficiency account for 10% of cases of CAH. Their clinical, laboratory features and management are summarized in Table 117.7. Patients with 11β-hydroxlase deficiency and 17α-hydroxylase deficiency present with hypertension and should be managed with hydrocortisone alone.[10] Deficiencies of StAR and 3β-hydroxysteroid dehydrogenase manifest as salt wasting crisis and require addition of mineralocorticoid. Virilization of 11β-hydrolase deficiency should be managed surgically as for 21-hydroxylase deficiency.

CONCLUSIONS

Adrenal disorders in children are associated with many short and long-term consequences. Appropriate diagnosis and management of these disorders require cooperation between neonatologists, pediatric surgeons and pediatric endocrinologists.

Table 117.7: Comparison of forms of CAH

Deficiency	Mineralocorticoid	Glucocorticoid	Androgen	BP	Ambiguity	Diagnosis	Treatment
21- Hydroxylase							
CSW	↓	↓	↑	↓	Female	17 OHP	HC and Flu
CV	n	n	↑	n	Female	17 OHP	HC and Flu
NC	n	n	↑	n	none	ACTH stimulation	HC
3βHSD	↓	↓	↓	↓	Male	↑Delta 5:Delta 4	HC and Flu
11- Hydroxylase	↑	↓	↑	↑	Female	DOC	HC
17- Hydroxylase	↑	↓	↓	↑	Male	18- hydroxy DOC	HC
StAR	↓	↓	↓	↓	Male	↓↓ Steroid precursors	HC and Flu

Min- Mineralocorticoid, Glu-Glucocorticoid, Sex- Sex Hormone, HC- Hydrocortisone, Flu- Fludrocortisone, CSW- Classical salt wasting, CV- Classical virilizing, NC- Non classical

REFERENCES

1. Migeon CJ, Lances RL. Adrenal Cortex: Hypo and hyperfunction. In: Lifshitz F, (Ed). Pediatric Endocrinology, 3rd Edn. New York, Marcel Dekker 1996;321-45.
2. New Mi, Rapaport R. The Adrenal cortex. In: Sperling MA, (Ed). Pediatric Endocrinology, 1st Edn. Philadelphia, WB Saunders 1996;281-14.
3. Williams HG, Dluhy RG. Diseases of the adrenal cortex. In: Fauci AS, Braunwald E, Isselbacher KJ, Wilson JD, Martin JB, Kasper DL, et al., (Eds). Harrison's Principles of Internal Medicine, 14th Edn. New York, McGraw Hill 1997;2035-57.
4. Meier CA, Biller MK. Clinical and biochemical evaluation of Cushing's syndrome. Endocrine Clin North Am 1997;26:741-61.
5. Orth DN. Cushing's syndrome. NEJM 1995;332:791-803.
6. Speiser PW. Congenital adrenal hyperplasia owing to 21-hydroxylase deficiency. Endocrine Clin North Am 2001; 30: 31-59.
7. Miller LW. Genetics, diagnosis and management of 21-hydroxylase deficiency. J Clin Endocrinol Metab 1993,78; 241-46.
8. Merke DP, Cutler GB. New ideas for treatment of congenital adrenal hyperplasia. ECNA 2001;121-35.
9. Schnitzer JJ, Donahoe PK. Surgical treatment of congenital adrenal hyperplasia. ECNA 2001;30:137-54.
10. Mathur R, Kabra M, Menon PSN. Diagnosis and management of congenital adrenal hyperplasia: Clinical, molecular and prenatal aspects. Natl Med J India 2001;14:26-31.

Childhood Obesity

Anurag Bajpai, PSN Menon

The incidence of obesity has seen a sharp rise in the past few years. The western hemisphere is faced with an epidemic of childhood and adolescent obesity with doubling of the prevalence of obesity in the pediatric age group over the last thirty years.[1-3] In India protein energy malnutrition remains the major nutritional challenge; economic disparity has led to the emergence of obesity as a pediatric health problem. Childhood obesity is associated with serious consequences such as coronary artery disease, hypertension and type 2 diabetes mellitus. This coupled with the observation that as many as 80% of obese adolescents become obese adults emphasizes the need of prevention and treatment of childhood obesity.

ASSESSMENT

Obesity implies excessive fat in the body and not merely excess weight. Body weight thus is not a reliable criterion for defining obesity. Long-term complications of obesity correlate best with body fat (specially visceral and intra-abdominal free fat) content. As methods of measuring body fat are cumbersome and expensive, clinical parameters are used as markers of obesity.

Body Mass Index (BMI)

BMI is the most widely used parameter to define obesity. It takes into account body weight as well as the height of the individual. It is calculated by the formula:

$$BMI = \frac{Weight(Kg)}{Height(m)^2}$$

Individuals above 18 years with BMI > 25 kg/m^2 are defined as at-risk for obesity while those with values > 30 kg/m^2 are diagnosed as obese. In view of the wide variation of BMI at different ages, age-specific cut-offs are used in the pediatric age group. Children with BMI > 85 percentile for age are considered at-risk for obesity while those > 95 percentile for age are labeled obese. BMI correlates well with intra-abdominal fat content on one hand and with complications of obesity on the other. There is however a problem in its sensitivity in that a few obese children are likely to be missed by these criteria. BMI also tends to overestimate the nutritional status of stunted children. Despite these shortcomings, BMI remains the most important anthropometric measure in evaluating a child for obesity.

Weight for Height

This parameter compares the child's weight to the expected weight for his/her height. Weight for height > 120% is diagnosed as obesity.

Skin Fold Thickness

Skin fold thickness measured over the subscapular, triceps or biceps regions is a reliable indicator for subcutaneous fat. Age specific percentile cut-offs should be used with values > 85 percentile being abnormal. WHO recommends combination of BMI and skin fold thickness for diagnosing obesity.

Waist-hip Ratio

This has been used as an indicator of intra-abdominal fat in adult populations. Its value in the pediatric age group has not been established. Values greater than 0.8 in women and 0.9 in men suggest obesity.

Precise Estimation of Body Fat

Bioelectric impedance studies are used to estimate skin fold thickness and body fat. Dual-energy X-ray absorptiometry (DEXA) provides accurate measurement of body fat but has the problem of radiation exposure. CT scan is helpful in delineating the distribution of fat in the body. MRI scanning is emerging as an excellent method of evaluating body fat stores without radiation exposure.

ETIOLOGY

In a vast majority of children with obesity, environmental and hereditary factors play the major role.[4] In only 5-10% cases endocrine, syndromic or CNS causes are implicated. The causes of childhood obesity are classified in Table 118.1 and summarized below.

Constitutional Obesity

Majority of children with obesity do not have an organic cause. These children grow normally and are tall for their age. They have proportional obesity and normal development. Important environmental influences include excessive calorie intake, sedentary life style, television viewing and playing computer games. It is important to identify this subgroup of children so as to avoid unnecessary investigations.

Endocrine Causes

Cushing's syndrome is characterized by central obesity, hypertension, striae and retarded skeletal maturation. Hypothyroidism is an extremely rare cause of isolated obesity. In most of these cases obesity is an additional feature to the other more prominent manifestations like short stature, developmental delay and coarse skin. In growth hormone deficiency and psuedohypoparathyroidism, growth retardation and hypocalcemia are dominant clinical features and obesity is a less prominent manifestation. It is important to emphasize that an endocrine cause of obesity is extremely unlikely in a child with normal height and skeletal maturation.

Genetic Syndromes

A variety of genetic syndromes have obesity as their major clinical feature. Klinefelter and Turner syndrome are readily identifiable by their clinical characteristics. Many of these syndromes are associated with hypogonadism or hypotonia (Prader-Willi, Carpenter, Laurence Moon Biedl-LMB).

Central Nervous System Causes

CNS insults in the form of surgery, radiation, tumors and trauma present with rapid onset obesity. These disorders are associated with excessive appetite, signs and symptoms of CNS involvement and other hypothalamic-pituitary defects. Children with features

Table 118.1: Causes of childhood obesity		
Genetic/ Familial	*Environmental*	*Endocrine*
	Decreased activity	Growth hormone deficiency
	Increased calorie intake	Hypothyroidism
	TV viewing	Cushing's syndrome
	Video games/computer use	Psuedohypoparathyroidism 1a
		Hyperinsulinism
		Hyperandrogenism
Genetic syndromes	CNS lesions	Miscellaneous
Pradder-Willi	Infection	Steroids
Lawrence-Moon-Biedel	Trauma	Anti-eliptetics
Carpenter	Surgery/radiation	Depression
Turner	Cranipharyngioma	Leptin deficiency
Klinefelter		
Alstrom		

Table 118.2: Constitutional versus pathological obesity

Feature	Constitutional obesity	Pathological obesity
Distribution	Generalized	Usually central
Height for age	Increased	Decreased
Bone age	Advanced	Retarded
Facial dysmorphism	Absent	May be present
Features of endocrinopathy	Absent	May be present

of CNS involvement and rapid onset obesity should therefore be evaluated by appropriate CNS imaging modality.

Miscellaneous Causes

There has been growing interest in the role of leptin in the pathogenesis of obesity. A 17 kd polypeptide secreted by the adipocytes, leptin acts on the hypothalamus to control appetite. Cases of obesity with documented leptin deficiency have been shown to respond to treatment with leptin. Treatment with corticosteroids and anti-epileptic agents leads to obesity as do psychological disorders like bulimia, depression and attention seeking behavior.

EVALUATION (FIG. 118.1)

Initial step in evaluation of a child with history of excessive weight gain is to confirm the presence of obesity using BMI and skin fold thickness. Next step is to determine whether obesity is constitutional or pathological (Table 118.2). History should include family history of obesity and its complications, clues to pathological cause and features of complications such as hypertension, diabetes and respiratory problems (Table 118.3). Examination should focus on features of endocrinopathy, dysmorphic syndromes and complications such as hypertension and acanthosis nigricans. Special emphasis should be given to sexual maturity and ocular examination, as they provide clues to specific etiology. Stretched penile length should be measured carefully, as in many cases of constitutional obesity penis may be buried in pubic fat giving a false impression of hypogonadism.

Investigations for obesity are decided based on the degree of obesity and associated complications. According to the expert group on clinical guidelines

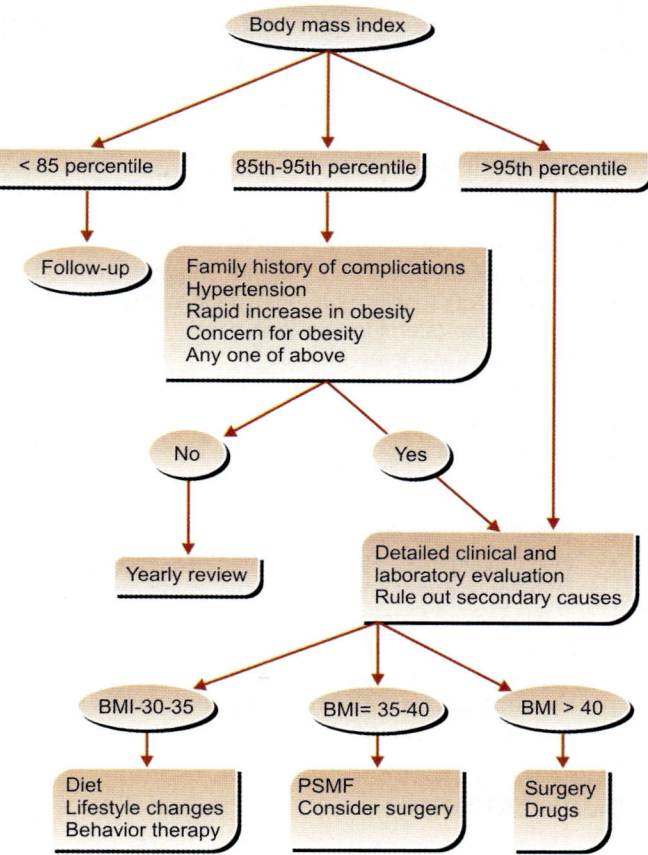

Fig. 118.1: Approach to a child with obesity

for overweight investigations are required for all children with BMI > 30 kg/m² (or > 95 percentile) and for those with BMI > 25 kg/m² (or > 85 percentile) associated with any one of the following:
1. Family history of cardiovascular complications/ type 2 diabetes
2. Rapid increase in obesity
3. Hypertension
4. Concern about obesity.

Evaluation should include blood sugar (fasting and postprandial), serum cholesterol, liver function tests and skeletal maturity evaluation. Complete lipid profile should be requisitioned if serum cholesterol level is >200 mg/dl once or >170 mg/dl on two occasions. Tests for endocrine causes (Urine free cortisol and FT4 / TSH) should be guided by clinical suspicion.

Table 118.3: Clinical evaluation of obesity

History
- Onset and progression of disease
- Appetite
- Growth and development
- Family history of obesity/ hypertension/ hyperlipidemia/ diabetes/ premature CAD
- Features of raised intracranial tension
- History of CNS infection/ trauma/ surgery/ radiation
- Features of Cushing's/ hypothyroidism/ hypoglycemia
- Drug intake (steroids, anti-epileptics)
- Features of diabetes mellitus
- Daytime somnolence/ sleep apnea

Examination
- Dysmorphism
- Polydactyly- LMB/Carpenter syndrome
- Developmental assessment
- Sexual maturity staging
- Visual evaluation - Retinitis pigmentosa- LMB syndrome
    Retinal degeneration- Carpenter syndrome
    Blindness- Alstrom syndrome
- Blood pressure
- Stretched penile length/ testicular volume
- Hypogonadism- Prader-Willi/ Carpenter/ LMB syndrome
- Acanthosis nigricans- Hyperinsulinism

COMPLICATIONS

Childhood obesity has multi-system effects and is associated with significant complications.

Cardiovascular

Obesity has been linked with hyperlipidemia, hypertension and premature coronary artery disease. Hypertension is associated with high cardiac output and increased sympathetic output and has been shown to respond to lowering of body weight. Hyperlipidemia is related more closely to visceral fat than subcutaneous fat and also responds to weight reduction.

Endocrine

Most important endocrine complication of obesity is insulin resistance. This presents as a spectrum of changes ranging from elevated insulin levels to impaired glucose tolerance to frank type 2 diabetes. A characteristic clinical feature is acanthosis nigricans, dark and rough areas on the exposed areas of skin including back of neck axilla and thigh. Syndrome X (hyperlipidemia, insulin resistance and obesity) is a well-known manifestation of obesity. Ovarian hyperandrogenism leading to premature adrenarchae and ovarian dysfunction has also been associated with obesity. Growth hormone deficiency and thyroid resistance though common are usually of no clinical consequence.

Respiratory

Obesity is associated with restrictive (decreased respiratory movements due to obesity) as well as obstructive pulmonary disease (fatty deposition in the airway). The most severe respiratory complication is the obesity-hypoventilation syndrome (Pickwickian syndrome) associated with hypoxia and features of cor pulmonale. In its milder form it is associated with snoring, irritability, hyperactivity and day time somnolence. Weight reduction leads to improvement in lung function.

Orthopedic

Obese children are prone to slipped femoral epiphyses, flat feet, Blount's disease (tibia vara) and early onset osteoarthritis.

Hepatic

Obesity has been linked with fatty changes in liver along with hepatitis resembling alcoholic liver disease. The incidence of cholelithiasis is greater in obese children and has been shown to increase with treatment for obesity.

MANAGEMENT

Management of childhood obesity is extremely difficult and unsatisfactory and rarely leads to long-term success. Diet, activity and behavioral measures are the cornerstones of therapy with intensive measures like drug therapy, severe dietary restriction and surgery reserved for morbid cases.[5]

Dietary Measures

Initial dietary measures for obesity includes mild caloric restriction and alteration in dietary habits. Intake of 1200-1800 calories depending upon the age of the individual with 30-40% restriction is recommended initially. Over-aggressive restriction of calorie and nutrition is associated with poor compliance and growth faltering. Apart from restricting calorie intake, efforts should be directed towards improving the nutritive value of the diet. Reduction in consumption of junk foods, carbonated drinks and saturated fat along with an increase in fiber, fruits and vegetable intake are helpful in improving body composition.

Intensive approaches to decrease dietary intake have also been tried. Regimens sparing protein (1.5-2 gm/kg/day for the expected body weight) with severe caloric restriction (750-1000 cal/kg/day) have been demonstrated to be effective over short periods of time (10-12 weeks). These Protein Sparing Modified Fast (PMSF) regimens fortified with micronutrients and vitamins lead to 0.5 kg/week reduction in body weight. They are too intensive for long-term use in pediatric population and require intense monitoring.

Lifestyle Modification

Increase in physical activity along with reduction in sedentary life-style is an important part of obesity management.[6] Swimming, running and playing outdoor games should be encouraged. Activities like TV viewing, videogames and internet surfing, which promote snack eating, should be restricted. Psychological and behavior therapy are also helpful. It is important to emphasize that dietary intake should not be increased in view of increased activity as this would offset the advantage of increased activity.

Drugs

Drug therapy is reserved for severe cases of obesity (weight for height >140%). Most of the anti-obesity drugs have not been tried extensively in children and thus cannot be recommended for routine use. Drugs used in obesity are summarized in Table 118.4. Stimulant drugs like amphetamines have been withdrawn due to high rates of dependency. Fenfluramine, a serotenergic agent, was withdrawn due to severe side effects like cardiac valvulopathies. Current medical treatment of obesity consists of drugs decreasing appetite through effects on neurotransmitters (sibutramine) and those interfering with absorption by inhibiting gastric enzymes (orlistast). Leptin (for those with leptin deficiency) and octreotide (for hypothalamic obesity) are promising approaches for sub-groups of children with obesity. The efficacy of pharmacological therapy for obesity has however been modest compared to surgery.

Surgery

Surgery for obesity is the last resort in treatment.[7] It is indicated for morbid obesity (BMI > 40 kg/m^2 or BMI > 35 kg/m^2 with complications of obesity) when other measures have failed. Experience with surgery for obesity in children is limited but has been shown to cause significant reduction in body weight (> 33% of pre-surgery weight) sustained for a period of 1 year. Surgery is the only modality with proven and sustained efficacy in the management of obesity. The various surgical techniques are summarized in Table 118.5. These have been described is detail in chap 119.

Table 118.4: Drug therapy for obesity

Drug	Mode of action	Efficacy	Side effects	Status
Fenfluramine	↑ Ser and Dopa ↓ appetite	Moderate	Pulmonary hypertension, cardiac valvulopathies	Withdrawn
Phentermine	↑ NE and Dopa ↓ appetite	Moderate	Insomnia, hypertension, arrhythmias, euphoria	Experimental
Sibutramine	↑NE, Dopa, Ser↓ Appetite	Mild	Anxiety, paresthesias, numbness	Experimental
Orlistat	Lipase inhibitor Malabsorption	Moderate	Vitamin deficiency, diarrhea, flatulence	Experimental
Leptin	↓ hypothalamic drive	High	–	Leptin deficient individuals
Octreotide	↓ insulin secretion	High	Gall stones, diarrhea, hypothyroidism, cardiac dysfunction	Hypothalamic obesity

NE-Norepinephrine, Dopa-Dopamine, Ser-Serotonin

Table 118.5: Surgical modalities for obesity

Surgery	Principle	Efficacy	Adverse effects	Status
Jejuno-ileal bypass	↓ Absorption, blind loop syndrome	Good	Hepatic dysfunction, renal calculi, RTA, Nutritional deficiency	Abandoned
Gastric bypass Roux-N-Y procedure	↓ Absorption ↓ Gastric emptying	Good	Stomal stenosis, Intussusception	Procedure of choice
Gastric balloon implantation	↓ Stomach capacity	Moderate	Resurgery	Experimental
Gastroplasty	↓ Stomach capacity	Moderate	Vitamin deficiency Late weight gain	Experimental

Jejuno-ileal Bypass

In this procedure a segment of proximal jejunum is anastomosed to distal ileum. The remaining portion of small intestine acts as a blind loop. This leads to decrease in absorption and thereby decreased caloric intake. Weight loss in this procedure is however greater than that achieved by resecting the same extent of the intestine indicating that the blind loop plays an important role in weight loss. The procedure is highly effective in lowering lipid levels in these patients. The initial enthusiasm of this procedure has however faded away due to the significant adverse effects including hepatic dysfunction and failure, renal dysfunction, renal calculi and multiple vitamin deficiencies. Most of these adverse outcomes are related to blind loop syndrome and bacterial overgrowth. Treatment with anti-anaerobic antibiotics like metronidazole is helpful in alleviating some of them. In view of these life-threatening complications, this procedure has been largely replaced by gastric bypass.

Gastric Bypass

These procedures take the advantage of decreased absorption without the limitation of blind loop. Roux-en-Y loop is the most commonly practiced procedure. A small portion of the stomach is anastomosed with a segment of jejunum 15-45 cm distal to ligament of Treitz. Proximal jejunum is re-anastomosed around 50-60 cm distal to gastrojejunostomy. This is the surgical technique of choice for treatment of obesity. The effects on weight loss are similar to jejunoileal bypass but the effect on lipid levels is less remarkable. Stomal stenosis and intussusception are important adverse effects.

Surgery to Decrease Gastric Capacity

Gastric balloon implantation and vertical band gastroplasty have been tried in adults aiming at decreased gastric capacity and thereby decreased caloric intake. The experience in these procedures in children is limited.

Other procedures like biliopancreatic bypass, jaw wiring and liposuction have not been used extensively in children and are not recommended for pediatric use.

CONCLUSIONS

Management of obesity is a therapeutic challenge and requires multi-disciplinary approach. In view of long-term complications drugs and surgery should be used for only morbid obesity where complications of the disease outweigh those of drug therapy or surgery. Under most of these circumstances surgical management is preferable to drug therapy.

REFERENCES

1. Alemzadeh R, Lifshitz F. Childhood obesity. In: Lifshitz F, ed. Pediatric endocrinology, 3rd Ed. Marcel Dekker, New York. 1996;753-74.
2. Epstein H, Myers MDF, Raynor HA, Saelens BE. Treatment of pediatric obesity. Pediatrics 1998;101 (Suppl):554.
3. Styne DM. Childhood and adolescent obesity. Pediatr Clin North Am 2001;48:823-54.
4. Diamond FB Jr. Newer aspects of the pathophysiology, evaluation, and management of obesity in childhood. Curr Opin Pediatr 1998;10:422-27.
5. Yanovski JA. Intensive therapies for pediatric obesity. Pediatr Clin North Am 2001;48:1041-53.
6. Himes JH, Dietz WH. Guidelines for overweight in adolescent preventive services. Recommendations from an expert committee. Am J Cin Nutr 1994;59:307-16.
7. Greenway FL. Surgery for obesity. Pediatr Clin North Am 1996;25:1005-27.

CHAPTER 119

Surgery for Pediatric Morbid Obesity

Reena Bhargava, Shilpa Sharma, Azad B Mathur

Obesity is a disease process with multiple etiologies influenced by genetics, culture, economics and psychological issues.[1] Identification of effective obesity treatment modalities continue to challenge, the medical community. Results from the American National Health and Nutrition Examination Survey demonstrate that approximately 65% of Americans aged 20 years of age or older are overweight (BMI > 25) and 31% are obese (BMI > 35) or morbidly obese (BMI > 40).[2] Amongst American children and adolescents, 21-24% are overweight and 10-11% are obese or morbidly obese.[3] 50-77% of children and adolescents who are obese carry their obesity into adulthood, thus increasing their risks of developing serious and often life-threatening conditions. The risk increases to 80% if one parent is obese.[2]

Obesity prevalence among children and adolescent is a serious health care issue all over the world.[4] Statistics in USA and UK is raising alarm and issues are discussed to address changes in lifestyle. The prevalence of childhood obesity in the UK continues to escalate with an estimated 1.3 million obese children forecast by 2010.[5] The developing countries with emerging economy are already seeing childhood obesity as a major health issue.

As the prevalence of obesity and obesity-related disease among adolescents increases, physicians are faced with the challenge of determining the best treatment strategies for affected patients. In order to determine who qualifies for bariatric surgery, a number of factors need to be considered. This includes patient comorbidities as well as a number of factors unique to overweight youths. The appropriate consideration of these factors preoperatively is important in order to increase compliance and decrease risk of adverse medical and psychosocial outcomes postoperatively.

WHAT IS OBESITY?

Obesity is a condition where weight has got to the point that it poses a serious threat to health. It is measured in terms of a person's body mass index, which is determined both by weight and height. BMI cut-off points have been agreed for obese and overweight adults, but for children the situation is more complex. A child's BMI varies with age, different cut-off points have to be used to define overweight and obese children depending on age (Table 119.1). A BMI of 25 or more is considered overweight; 30 or more, obese; and 40 or more, morbidly obese (Table 119.2, Fig. 119.1).

PATHOPHYSIOLOGY OF OBESITY

There is no denial of the fact that obesity is caused mostly because of imbalance in intake and consumption of calories. The current lifestyle is promoting less consumption of calories and easy availability of fast food loaded with calories is fuelling this epidemic of obesity all over the world.

Table 119.1: Calculating BMI	
Metric method	BMI = weight (kg) / Height (m)^2
Non-metric method	BMI = weight (pounds) x 703 / Height (inches)^2

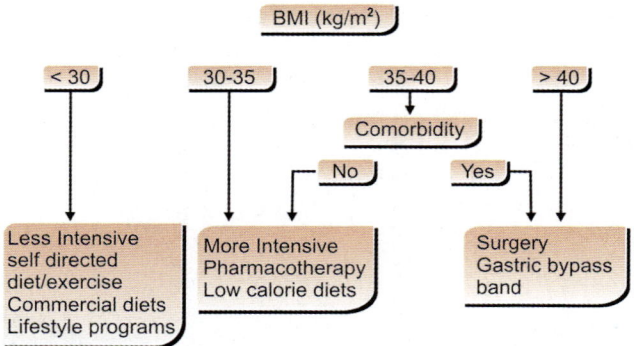

Fig. 119.1: Treatment algorithm for obesity

Table 119.2: Obesity classification		
Obesity Class		BMI (kg/m²)
Underweight		<18.5
Normal		18.5-24.9
Overweight		25.0-29.9
Obesity	I	30.0-34.9
	II	35.0-35.9
Extreme obesity	III	≥ 40.0

It is also important to understand that fat cells are no longer viewed as inert packets of energy, but they are two faced master minds of metabolism. It is now very well documented that there two types of "fat" cells and secrets hormones like leptin, and molecules called adipokines. The signals from 'fat' fat cells (in obese people) produce TNF α and make a circulating factor that makes other tissues resistant to insulin.[6] Obesity-related comorbid conditions in children and adolescents include:[7,8]

1. Hypertension
2. Impaired glucose tolerance
3. Diabetes mellitus
4. Hyperlipidemia
5. Obstructive sleep apnea
6. Cardiovascular disease
7. Degenerative joint disease
8. Gynecological and obstetric comorbidities.

ROLE OF BARIATRIC SURGERY IN CHILDREN AND ADOLESCENTS

The role of bariatric surgery in treating childhood obesity has been in flare recently.[9-11] As obesity has been referred to as a worldwide epidemic, there is an increasing trend towards Bariatric surgery even in children and adolescents worldwide.[7,12,13] It is considered as one of the most alarming public health issues facing the world today.[7] In North America, nearly one-third of the population is obese, and this figure includes children and adolescents who are likely to become obese adults. As obesity carries a great financial impact on society, treating morbidly obese patients with surgery may offer substantial economic savings.[14] Thus, early rather than later use of bariatric surgery in the treatment of extreme obesity has been recommended.[15] It has been found that adolescents undergoing bariatric surgery have a significantly shorter length of hospital stay compared to adults.[16]

In the US, extreme obesity affects approximately 9 million adults and 2 million children and is associated with both immediate health problems and later health risk, including premature mortality.[15] Increasing pediatric obesity is especially alarming because obesity is associated with significant medical and psychosocial consequences like cardiovascular, metabolic, hepatic complications and psychiatric difficulties.[17]

From 1997 to 2003, the estimated number of adolescent bariatric procedures performed nationally increased 5-fold in a series.[13] In another study, the population-based annual adolescent bariatric case volume varied little between 1996 and 2000 but more than tripled from 2000 to 2003.[16] Despite this trend, in this series, only 771 bariatric procedures performed in adolescents in 2003, representing fewer than 0.7% of bariatric procedures performed nationwide.[16]

Most hospitals that perform bariatric procedures on adolescents have limited experience with adolescent bariatric patients, although many of these hospitals have high overall bariatric volume (adolescents and adults).[13] Thus there are not much experienced pediatric bariatric surgeons. It has been suggested that bariatric surgery should be limited to selected adolescents in Institutional Review Board-approved research studies.[18]

INDICATIONS FOR SURGERY

To be considered for bariatric surgery, adolescents should have attempted and failed six months of

Table 119.3: Criteria for bariatric surgery in adolescents[19]
Adolescents being considered for bariatric surgery should:
Have failed 6 months of organized attempts at weight management, as determined by their primary care provider
Have attained or nearly attained physiologic maturity
Be very severely obese (BMI 40) with serious obesity-related comorbidities or have a BMI of 50 with less severe comorbidities
Demonstrate commitment to comprehensive medical and psychologic evaluations both before and after surgery
Agree to avoid pregnancy for at least 1 year postoperatively
Be capable of and willing to adhere to nutritional guidelines postoperatively
Provide informed assent to surgical treatment
Demonstrate decisional capacity

physician monitored weight loss attempts and have met certain anthropometric, medical, and psychologic criteria. Adolescent candidates should be morbidly obese, with BMI > 40 as defined by WHO (World Health Organization), have attained a majority of skeletal maturity: age 13 for girls and 15 years of age for boys, and have significant comorbidities that are amenable to improvement with bariatric surgery (Table 119.3).[19]

Current modalities for the treatment of morbid obesity include dietary modification, exercise, pharmacologic intervention and surgery. Indications for surgical weight loss are for the improvement or resolution of comorbid adverse health conditions present in many obese people. The term "morbid obesity" was developed to describe the significant morbidity associated with severe obesity including diabetes, sleep apnea, venous stasis, heart failure, deep venous thrombosis, pulmonary emboli, hypertension, degenerative arthritis, gallstones, hernias, and an increased incidence of ovarian, breast, prostate and colon cancer. Candidates for bariatric surgery have a BMI of greater than 35 in the presence of comorbidities or a BMI of 40 or greater in the absence of comorbidities.[20,21] Individuals with a BMI less than 35 are counseled on non-surgical methods of weight loss such as pharmacologic intervention, dietary modification, exercise, and psychotherapy.[21] International Pediatric Endosurgery Group has come up with following recommendations:[22]

- Be very severely obese (BMI 40) with serious obesity related comorbidities and; have attained nearly adult stature
- Have failed at least 6 months of organized conventional attempts at weight management
- Demonstrate commitment to comprehensive pediatric psychological evaluation both before and after surgery and agree to avoid pregnancy for at least one year postoperatively
- Be capable of and willing to adhere to nutritional guidelines postoperatively, and
- Have decisional capacity and provide informed assent for surgical management.

List of comorbid conditions is:

Serious comorbidity	Less serious comorbidity
- Type 2 diabetes mellitus	Weight related arthropathies
- Obstructive sleep apnea	Hypertension
- Pseudotumor cerebri	Dyslipidemia
- The venous stasis desease	
- Panniculitis	
- Urinary incontinence	
- Significant impairment in activity of daily living	
- Nonalcoholic fatty liver disease	
- Gastroesophageal reflux	
- Severe psychosocial distress	

For morbidly obese individuals, obesity surgery is the only proven method to lose weight and keep it off in long term, when all other therapies have failed. A recent study/meta-analysis of more than 22,000 patients has shown the mean percentages of excess weight loss was 61.2% for all patients and was 47.5% for patients who underwent gastric banding. Diabetes was completely resolved in 76.8% of patients and resolved or improved in 86.0%. Hyperlipiderniaimproved in 70.0%. Hypertension was resolved in 62.7%. Obstructive sleep apnea was resolved in 85.7%.[8]

- A person who has repeatedly tried and failed to lose weight with the aid of diets, exercise, behavior modification, or weight loss.

PREOPERATIVE COUNSELLING

The counselling should include discussion of the various options for treatment of obesity. The three main treatment modalities of childhood obesity are lifestyle interventions, medications, and bariatric surgery.[18] Primary prevention of childhood obesity is important. A trial of new medications including orlistat, sibutramine, and metformin can be offered to the older adolescents. The ultimate goal should be an improvement in health resulting in a reduction of life-threatening risk factors—A staged approach, emphasizing early intervention and lifestyle changes is important.[18] Continued behavioral intervention increases the likelihood of a sustained effect for up to 2 years. The various risks involved with the procedure should be discussed in detail with the patient. This should include the long-term side effects, such as possible need for reoperation, gallbladder disease, and malabsorption.

The need for lifelong medical surveillance after surgical therapy should be explained. The option of surgical treatment is a very serious decision and should be offered to patients who are morbidly obese, well informed, motivated and able to make a decision on their own. Patients with manifest psychopathology that affects an informed consent and long-term cooperation with follow-up should be excluded. Numerous parallels exist between obesity and addictive behaviors, including genetic predisposition, personality, environmental risk factors, and common neurobiological pathways in the brain.[17] A 5-10% reduction in weight can result in a 35% decrease in health risk. Obesity treatments should include counselling and behavioral approaches besides bariatric surgery.[23] Present medical and behavioral interventions for extreme obesity in adults and children rarely result in the significant, durable weight loss necessary to improve health outcomes, prompting a search for more aggressive measures.[15] Current evidence suggests that after bariatric surgery, adolescents lose significant weight and serious obesity-related medical conditions and psychosocial status are improved.[15] A decision to have surgical treatment requires an assessment of the risk and benefit in each case. The risks including association of iron deficiency following bariatric surgery should be well explained.[24]

Obese adolescent girls should be warned to use secure birth control methods during the period of postoperational weight loss.[25] This period of rapid weight loss could cause maternal malnutrition and may impair normal fetal development.

FACTORS IN PATIENT DECISION MAKING

The European guidelines for bariatric surgery clearly define criteria for operating children with morbid obesity. However, the appropriate technique for this age-group has not been identified yet. Gastric banding and Roux-enY bypass represent the standards, but they demand life-long tolerance of either an artificial device or significant malabsorption. The absence of significant nutritional deficiency, the continued adjustability, and potential reversibility of LAGB make it the safest, least invasive, and most effective surgical procedure to offer adolescents. However longer follow-up is required before universally recommending this procedure.

OVERVIEW OF BARIATRIC SURGERY

Obesity surgery stems from surgical weight loss identified in patients who underwent gastric and small bowel resections for treatment of diseases other than morbid obesity. Weight loss procedures have been performed based on malabsorptive techniques, restrictive techniques, and a combination of both. (Figs 119.2 to 119.5) Early attempts at weight loss procedures were based on properties of malabsorption via shortening the length of the digestive tract through which food travels.[26,27] The jejuno-ileal bypass was effective in achieving weight loss from the bypass of significant lengths of small bowel. Although effective in achieving weight loss, several complications of malabsorption ensued including socially limiting diarrhea, vitamin and protein deficiencies, arthritis, renal failure, liver failure and death.[21,28] These early malabsorptive operations should no longer be performed or recommended for surgical weight loss but rather reversed or converted to acceptable weight loss procedures when recognized.[21,28]

In the 1960's gastric bypass surgery was pioneered by Dr Edward Mason at the University of Iowa, emerging from observations of sustained weight loss after gastric ulcer surgery and stomach resection.[21]

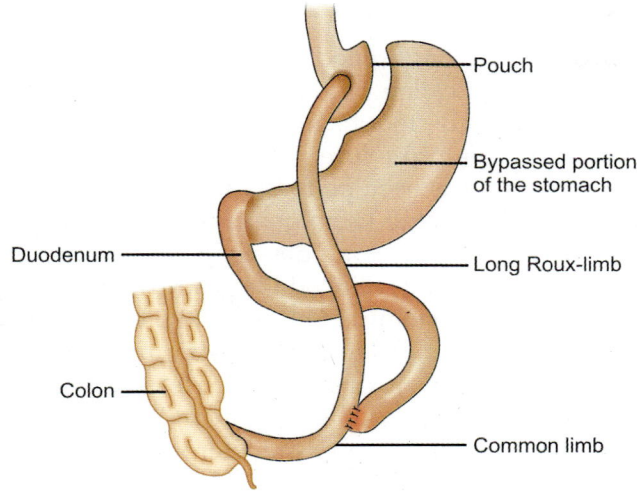

Fig. 119.2: Roux-en-Y gastric bypass procedure

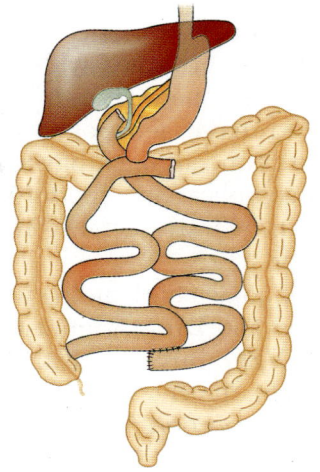

Fig. 119.3: Sleeve rectomus gastrotomy with duodenal switch with biliopancreatic diversion

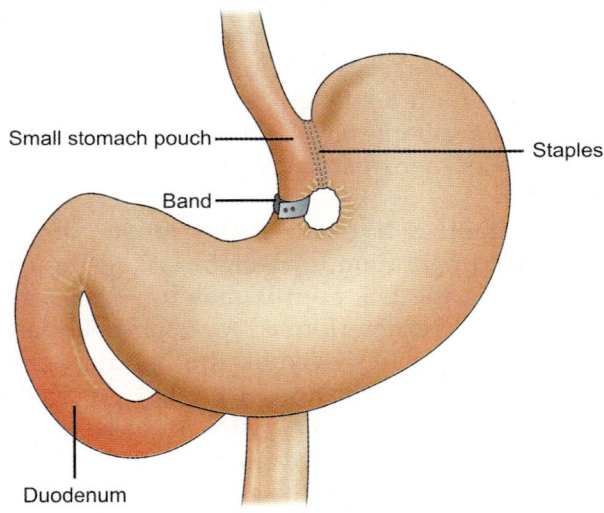

Fig. 119.4: Vertical banded gastroplasty

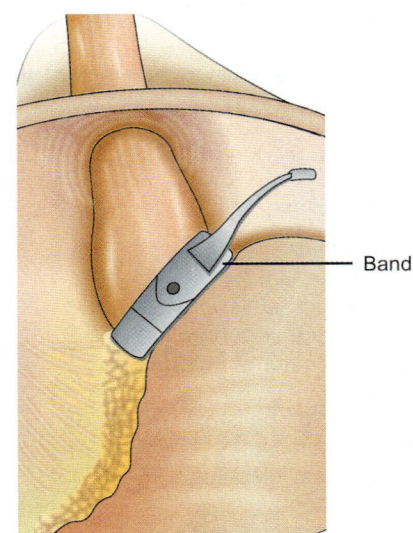

Fig. 119.5: Adjustable gastric banding

This procedure offered both components of weight loss surgery that have been previously used singularly; malabsorption and restriction. The complications from this Roux-en-Y gastric bypass (RNYGB) were less than those reported with the jejunoileal bypass and specifically did not include the severe malabsorptive side effects associated with earlier weight loss procedures.[21,29]

In 1982 the vertical banded gastroplasty (VBG) was first introduced.[30] The VBG procedure is a restrictive procedure limiting caloric intake by restriction of food volume (Fig. 119.4). The benefits of restrictive only procedures is that unlike their malabsorptive counterparts, there is a lesser likelihood of nutritional deficiencies, since absorption of nutrients is unaffected by the restrictive component of the surgery. Although effective in achieving weight loss, patients are counseled in avoidance of high caloric liquids that may lead to weight loss failures. VBG has fallen out of favor due to inferior long-term weight loss in comparison to the RNYGB.[31]

The first laparoscopic RNYGB was reported by Wittgrove et al in 1994.[32] The advent of minimally invasive surgery has helped place laparoscopic bariatric surgery at the forefront of general surgery. Complex procedures once performed with large incisions are being performed with equal safety and efficacy.[33] Patients benefit from minimally invasive RNYGB due to decreased post-operative pain, a decrease in the frequency of iatrogenic splenectomies, fewer wound complications, shorter hospital lengths of stay, and an overall decrease in mortality.[34-35] Tables 119.4 and 119.5)

Laparoscopic adjustable banding was approved for use by the Food and Drug Administration in 1991.[36] Analogous to VBG, this is a restrictive procedure which involves placement of an inflatable silastic cuff around the upper portion of the stomach.

CURRENT BARIATRIC SURGERY PROCEDURES RECOMMENDED BY INTERNATIONAL PEDIATRIC ENDOSURGERY GROUP (IPEG)

Table 119.4: Major Complications

Complications	Laparoscopic GBP (n = 79)	Open GBP (n = 76)	P Value
Gastrointestinal			
Anastomotic leak	1	1	
Gastric pouch outlet obstruction	0	1	
Hypopharyngeal perforation	1	0	
Jejunojejunostomy obstruction	3	0	
Pulmonary			
Pulmonary embolism	0	1	
Respiratory failure	0	1	
Gastrointestinal bleeding	1	0	
Wound infection	0	2	
Retained laparotomy sponge	0	1	
Total	6 (7.6%)	7 (9.2%)	.78*

GBP, Roux-en-Y gastric bypass.
*Fisher exact tests.

A study was performed by Nguyen et al on 155 patients. They performed a prospective randomized trial to compare outcomes, quality of life, and costs of laparoscopic vs open RNYGB. The table compares open vs laparoscopic major complications.

Various bariatric surgery procedurses described.[22,37,38] Here we will describe those commonly used for children and adolescents.

Roux-Y Gastric Bypass

This procedure has a good weight loss effectiveness and low complication profile, hence is considered as a "gold standard" to which all other procedures are compared. This procedure is favored in US centers. The operation has been performed both laparoscopic and open; the overall technique is the same. Mason, of the University of Iowa, developed gastric bypass and Ito (1967) first developed the gastric bypass with loop gastrojejunostomy.[27] Subsequently, he modified the procedure by creating the gastric bypass with lesser curve pouch of 50 ml. or less, a gastroenterostomy stoma of 0.9 mm and Roux-en-Y technique to avoid loop gastroenterostomy and the bile reflux which may ensue (Fig. 119.2).

Gastric bypass has stood the test of time, with one series of greater than 500 cases, followed for 14 years, maintaining 50% excess weight loss. The most common form of gastric bypass surgery is Roux-en-Y gastric bypass surgery. Here, a small stomach pouch is created with a stapler device, and connected to the distal small intestine. The upper part of the small intestine is then reattached in a Y-shaped configuration.

The gastric bypass is the most commonly performed operation for weight loss in the United States.[38] In the US, approximately 140,000 gastric bypass have been performed for almost 50 years, the gastric bypass has become the "gold standard" operation for weight loss in the US. An emerging factor in the success of gastric bypass surgery is following an established gastric bypass diet after surgery. Complications of gastric bypass are much less severe than those of intestinal bypass. The most serious acute complications include leaks at the junction of stomach and small intestine.

A comparison of complications between the laparoscopic and open Roux-en-y gastric bypass procedure has been outlined in Table 119.4[39] Brolin et al compared selected series of laparoscopic Roux-en-y gastric bypass procedure (Table 119.5).[40]

More recently, Capella and Capella reported a staple-line disruption rate of 22% in patients whose stomachs were stapled in-continuity using the TA90B and a reduction in that rate to 2% when the stomach was divided between two applications of that stapler. They recommend interposing a limb of jejunum as a

Table 5: Comparison of selected Series of Laparoscopic RY Gastric bypass

Parameter	Author				
	Lujan/Spain	Nguyen/US	Schauer	Biertho	DeMaria
Study type	Randomized	Randomized	Cohort	Cohort	Cohort
Approach	Lap/Open	Lap/Open	Lap	Lap	Lap
Operative time	186 vs 202*	225 vs 195*	260	–	198
Conversion	8%	2.5%	1.1%	2.0%	2.8%
Early morbidity	23% vs 29%	7.6% vs 9.2*	3.3%	4.2%	7.1%[†]
Late morbidity	11% vs 24%*	18.9% vs 15.2%	18.9%	8.1%	16.4%[†]
LOS. (mean)	5.2 vs 7.9*	4.0% vs 8.4*	3.6	3.0**	4.0
BMI range	36-80 kg/m^2	40-60 kg/m^2	35-68 kg/m^2	27-77 kg/m^2	40-71 kg/m^2

Mean operative time in munutes; LOS. in days
* Significant difference (P < 0.05) between laparoscopic and open
** Median LOS
† Extrapolated from separated morbidity data.

Brolin RE, in April 2004 compared previous randomized vs. cohort studies for laparoscopic RNYGB vs. open with regards to operative times, length of stay and early and late morbidities.[27]

serosal patch, and report no further occurrence of staple-line leaks. They advocate this modification of gastric bypass as the procedure of choice for treating morbid obesity with lowest rate of major complications.

Gastric bypass results in consistently greater sustained weight loss than from gastroplasty or gastric banding by altering resting energy expenditure, avoiding the observed reduction in resting energy expenditure usually found in persons restricting their dietary Intake.

Iron deficiency develops after gastric bypass for several reasons including intolerance for red meat, diminished gastric acid secretion, and exclusion of the duodenum from the alimentary tract. Menstruating women, pregnant women, and adolescents may be particularly predisposed toward developing iron deficiency and microcytic anemias after bypass surgery.[24]

Adjustable Gastric Banding

A constricting ring is applied completely around the fundus of the stomach, creating an hour-glass effect (Fig. 119.5). The ring has to be placed near the upper end of the stomach, just below the junction of stomach and esophagus. The silicone band can be adjusted by addition or removal of saline through a port placed just under the skin. This procedure can be performed laparoscopically, and is commonly called a "lap band."

An inflatable band connected to a small reservoir which is placed under the skin of the abdomen, through which the balloon can be inflated, thus reducing the size of the stoma, or deflated thus enlarging the stoma, has been described. Laparoscopic models have been developed that are associated with a short length of stay and a low frequency of complications. Since the hour glass configuration only constricts the upper stomach, with no malabsorptive effect, it acts as a pure restrictive operation. The favorable points are absence of anemia, dumping and malabsorption, while the disadvantages include the need for strict patient compliance., The Lap Band is freely available in the USA, been approved for use by the FDA. Laparoscopic adjustable gastric banding has been considered a procedure of choice for adolescent morbid obesity.[41]

When the Band is placed the balloon is empty, providing slight restriction to eating. Over the months following surgery, the balloon within the Band is gradually filled (outlet is tightened) to provide progressively increasing restriction matched to each patient, the balloon adjustment is accomplished using the access port (which is buried under the skin) to increase or decrease the amount of saline fluid contained in the balloon.

Advantages

1. Reduced the risk of surgery, especially important in obese patients.
2. There is no risk of leak or obstruction of the intestines.
3. Silastic substance even if it gets eroded has no tissue reaction.
4. The procedure is reversible.
5. The Lap Band aims to create slower and steadier weight loss Lap Band patients begin with a relatively loose Band that allows ongoing intake of nutrition, and the Band is gradually "tightened" according to the patient's weight progress and satiety symptoms. This approach aims to achieve a weight loss of 1-2 pounds per week, that continues upto or beyond 24 months after surgery.

Disadvantages

1. The band can get eroded into the stomach, become infected, or slip out of position.
2. Some patients have reported painful swallowing; reflux, or regurgitation. This may result from tightening the band too aggressively, and band deflation or removal is required.

Mean excess weight loss was 42% at 6 months and 60% at 1 year follow-up in a series with Lap Band in pediatric patients.[7] Patients are advised that weight loss is slower than that reported with RNYGB (47.5% vs. 61.6%. respectively).[42] Complications of band erosion and slippage have been reduced with improved techniques in band placement.[43] Gastric banding in adolescents has been reported as a safe, satisfactory and reversible weight reduction procedure with a mean preoperative BMI of 43 (35-61) kg/m^2 and mean postoperative BMI after 39.5 months follow-up as 30 (20-39) kg/m^2.[41]

Surgical Risks of Laparoscopic and Open Procedures

The risk of maintaining oneself in a morbidly obese state carries a high morbidity and mortality. This risk needs to be weighed against the risks of bariatric surgery which is a major operation whether performed laparoscopically or open. Those individuals who are at prohibitive risk for surgery in general are not candidates for weight loss surgery.

The overall morbidity resulting from bariatric surgery is reported as being in between 9.6-10%.[42,44,45] The resultant mortality has been reported as being between 0.1-1.5%.[42,44,46] Risks are stratified into those occurring early (within 24-48 hours) and those occurring late (after 48 hours). Improved outcomes are realized in the setting of qualified and experienced bariatric surgeons in conjunction with a qualified bariatric team composed of experienced surgeons, dieticians, exercise physiologists, mental health professionals and other support personnel.[47,48]

OUTCOME

No matter what therapy is chosen, the patient must be aware that success may depend on adherence and long-term follow-up.[49] Careful, lifelong medical supervision of adolescent patients who undergo a bariatric procedures will help in improving the outcome. Although there are numerous dietary guidelines for bariatric patients, most importantly, patients must consume 60-70 b of lean protein per day following operation. Supplementation of multivitamins, calcium, vitamine B_{12}, and iron in menstruating females must be provided after gastric bypass and to a lesser extent after banding. Ranitidine and ursodiol is also recommended for six months after surgery.[22]

The malabsorptive procedures lead to more weight loss than the restrictive procedures. A meta-analysis from UCLA reports the following weight loss at 36 months: Biliopancreatic diversion - 53 kg ,Roux-en-Y gastric bypass (RYGB) - 41 kg, Open - 42 kg, laparoscopic - 38 kg, Adjustable gastric banding - 35 kg and Vertical banded gastroplasty - 32 kg in adults.

Several recent studies report decrease in mortality and severity of medical conditions after bariatric surgery.

Complications from weight loss surgery are frequent including gastric dumping syndrome in about 20% (bloatedness and diarrhoea after eating, necessitating small meals or medication), leaks at the surgical site (12%), incisional hernia (7%), infections (6%) and pneumonia (4%). Mortality is low (0.2%).

EMERGING PROCEDURES AND FUTURE RESEARCH

A variation of the biliopancreatic diversion includes Duodenal switch. The part of the stomach along its graeture curve is resected. The stomach is "tubulized" with a residual volume of about 150 ml. This volume reduction provides the food intake restriction component of this operation. This type of gastric resection is anatomically and functionally irreversible. In 2003 a two stage BPD-DS was described consisting of laparoscopic sleeve gastrectomy as stage one of the procedure. There is increasing interest in this procedure among Pediatric Surgeons, but one should understand that currently, Laproscopic sleeve gastrectomy as a primary bariatric procedure is in its infancy because long term data are lacking. Randomized controlled trials are necessary to determine the outcomes and appropriateness of laparoscopic sleeve gastrectomy as a primary obesity operation.

Because of the evergrowing obesity epidemic, there is an increasing demand of procedures and industry is funding to find some new natural orifice transluminal endoscopic surgery (NOTES) procedures like endoluminal suturing and stapling devices. Other endoscopically delivered prostheses could be used to endoluminally bypass the stomach and proximal small bowel to effectively reduce the amount of food intake and the amount of nutrients absorbed.

The work of Dr V Cigaina of exogenous gastric electrical stimulation, has led to many randomized controlled trials throughout the world using various types of electrical stimulators.[50] To date these technologies have shown some promise, but the weight loss effectiveness seems significantly less potent than traditional bariatric procedures.

CONCLUSION

Bariatric surgery is one of several options for morbidly obese individuals seeking weight loss. Current data suggests marked improvement in co-morbidities from resultant weight loss. Although morbid obesity surgery is controversial in adolescents. Appropriate patient education includes dietary counseling, support group counseling, preoperative psychological, exercise and pulmonary evaluation, as well as, lifelong surgical follow-up. A well educated patient and established bariatric team is imperative for successful outcomes. The decision to undergo weight loss surgery should be made after consideration of all weight loss options and should involve patients, families, and clinicians.

REFERENCES

1. Obesity and Genetics: A public health perspective (February 2002) Center for Disease Control and Prevention.
2. Natinel Health & Nutrition Examination survey (NHANES) 1990-2000.
3. Trioano RP, Flegel KM: Overweight children and adolescents: description, epidemiology and demographics. Pediatrics 1998;101:497-504.
4. Kimm SY, Obarzanek E. Childhood obesity: a new pandemic of the millennium. Pediatrics 2002;110:1003-7.
5. Zanintto PW, Stamatakis H, Mindell E, et al. Forcasting Obesity to 2010. London: Department of Health, 2006.
6. Powell K. The two faces of fat. Nature 2007;447:525-27.
7. Al-Qahtani AR. Laparoscopic adjustable gastric banding in adolescent: safety and efficacy. J Pediatr Surg. 2007;42:894-7.
8. H.Buchwald, Y Avidor, M D Jensen et al Bariatric Surgery A Systematic Review and Meta-analysis. JAMA, October 13, 2004 – Vol 292, No 14, 1724-1737.
9. Jones N. Yes, there is a place for bariatric surgery (and paediatric surgeons) in childhood obesity. Arch Dis Child. 2008;93:354.
10. Inge TH. Childhood obesity—a problem of surgical proportions? Nat Clin Pract Gastroenterol Hepatol. 2008;5:180-1.
11. Shield JP, Crowne E, Morgan J. Is there a place for bariatric surgery in treating childhood obesity? Arch Dis Child. 2008;93:369-72.
12. Letonturier P. Obesity, a worldwide epidemic. Presse Med. 2007;36:1773-75.
13. Schilling PL, Davis MM, Albanese CT, Dutta S, Morton J. National trends in adolescent bariatric surgical procedures and implications for surgical centers of excellence: J Am Coll Surg. 2008;206:1-12.
14. Powers KA, Rehrig ST, Jones DB. Financial impact of obesity and bariatric surgery. Med Clin North Am. 2007;91:321-38, ix.
15. Inge TH, Xanthakos SA, Zeller MH. Bariatric surgery for pediatric extreme obesity: now or later?: Int J Obes (Lond). 2007;31:1-14.
16. Tsai WS, Inge TH, Burd RS. Bariatric surgery in adolescents: recent national trends in use and in-hospital outcome. Arch Pediatr Adolesc Med. 2007;161:217-21.
17. Acosta MC, Manubay J, Levin FR. Pediatric obesity: parallels with addiction and treatment recommendations. Harv Rev Psychiatry. 2008; 16:80-96.
18. Uli N, Sundararajan S, Cuttler L. Treatment of childhood obesity. Curr Opin Endocrinol Diabetes Obes. 2008;15:37-47.
19. Rodgers, Bradley M. MD Pediatrics Vol. 114 No. 1 July 2004, pp. 255-256
20. Lara MD, Kothari SN, Sugerman HJ. Surgical management of obesity: a review of the evidence relative to the health benefits and risks. Treat Endocrinol. 2005; 4(1):55-64.
21. MacGregor A, MD, CME director, ASBS, 2000.

22. www.ipeg.org , Guidelines for Surgical Treatment of Clinically Severely Obese Adolescents 2008.
23. Egger G. Helping patients lose weight—what works? Aust Fam Physician. 2008;37:20-3.
24. Love AL, Billett HH. Obesity, bariatric surgery, and iron deficiency: true, true, true and related. Am J Hematol. 2008;83:403-9.
25. Till HK, Muensterer O, Keller A, Körner A, Blueher S, Merkle R, Kiess W. Laparoscopic sleeve gastrectomy achieves substantial weight loss in an adolescent girl with morbid obesity. Eur J Pediatr Surg. 2008;18:47-9.
26. Buchwald H, Williams SE. Bariatric surgery worldwide 2003. Obes Surg. 2004 Oct; 14(9): 1157-64.
27. Buchwarld H, Buchwald JN. Evolution of operative procedures for the management of morbid obesity 1950-2000.
28. Griffen WO Jr, Bivins BA, Bell RM. The decline and fall of the jejunoileal bypass. Surg Gynecol Obstet. 1983 Oct; 157(4):301-8.
29. Hocking MP, Davis GL, Franzini DA, Woodward ER. Long-term consequences after jejunoileal bypass for morbid obesity. Dig Dis Sci. 1998 Nov; 43(11):2493-9.
30. Mason EE Vertical Banded Gastroplasty for Obesity. Archives of Surgery 1982; 117(5):701-6.
31. Sugerman HJ, Kellum JM Jr, DeMaria EJ, Reines HD. Conversion of failed or complicated vertical banded gastroplasty to gastric bypass in morbid obesity. *Am J Surg*. 1996 Feb; 171(2):263-9.
32. Kelvin D. Higa, MD; Keith B. Boone, MD; Tienchin Ho, MD; Orland G. Davies, MD. Laparoscopic Roux-en-Y Gastric Bypass for Morbid Obesity: *Arch Surg*. 2000; 135:1029-1033.
33. Wittgrove AC, Clark GW, Schubert KR. Laparoscopic Gastric Bypass, Roux-en-Y: Technique and Result in 75 Patients With 3-30 Months Follow-up. Obes Surg. 1996 Dec; 6(6):500-504.
34. Podnos YD, Jimenez JC, Wilson SE, Stevens CM, Nguyen NT. Complications after laparoscopic gastric bypass: a review of 346 cases. Arch Surg. 2003 Sep; 138(9):95-61.
35. Fried M, Peskova M, Kasalicky M. The role of laparoscopy in the treatment of morbid obesity. Obes Surg. 1998 Oct; 8(5); 520-23.
36. Ren CJ, Weiner M, Allen JW. Favorable early results of gastric banding for morbid obesity: the American experience. Surg Endosc. 2004 Mar; 18(3):543-6. Epub 2004 Feb 02.
37. www.asbs.org
38. Guidelines for Laparoscopic and Open surgical treatment of Morbid Obesity. American Society for Bariatric Surgery. Society of American Gastrointestinal Endoscopic Surgeons. Obesity Surgery 2000; 10: 378-9
39. Nguyen NT, Goldman C, Rosenquist C J, Arango A, Cole C J, Lee S Jand, Wolfe BM, Laparoscopic Versus Open Gastric Bypass: A Randomized Study of Outcomes, Quality of Life, and Costs. *Annals of Surgery. 234(3): 279-291, September 2001.*
40. Brolin RE Laparoscopic Verses Open Gastric Bypass to Treat Morbid Obesity. *Annals of Surgery. 239(4): 438-440, April 2004.*
41. Yitzhak A, Mizrahi S, Avinoach E. Laparoscopic gastric banding in adolescents. : Obes Surg. 2006;16:1318-22.
42. Buchwald H, Avidor Y, Braunwald E, Jensen MD, Pories W, Fahrbach Schoelles K. Bariatric surgery: a systematic review and meta-analysis. JAMA. 2004 Oct 13; 292(14):1724-37.
43. Hermann Nehoda, MD; Kathrine hourmont, MD; Tonja Sauper, MD; Reinhard Mittermair, MD; Monika Lanthaler, MD; Franz Aigner, MD; Helmut Weiss, MD. Laparoscopic Gastric Banding in Older Patients. Arch Sug. 2001; 136:1171-1176. Vol. 136 No. 10, October 2001.
44. Gastrointestinal Surgery for Severe Obesity. NIH Consensus Statement 1991 Mar 25-27; 9(1): 1-20.
45. Livingston EH. Procedure incidence and in-hospital complication rates of bariatric surgery in the United States. Am J Surg. 2004 Aug; 188(2):105-10.
46. Fernandez AZ Jr, Demaria EJ, Thicansky DS, Kellum JM, Wolfe LG, Meador J, Sugerman HJ. Multivariate analysis of risk factors for death following gastric bypass for treatment of morbid obesity. Ann Surg. 2004 May; 239(5):698-702; discussion 702-3.
47. Nguyen NT, Moore C, Stevens CM, Chalifoux S, Mavandadi S, Wilson S. The practice of bariatric surgery at academic medical centers. J Gastrointest Surg. 2004 Nov; 8(7):856-60; discussion 860.
48. Wadden TA, Sarwer DB, Womble LG, Foster GD, McGuckin BG, Schimmel A. Psychosocial aspects of obesity and obesity surgery. Surg Clin North Am. 2001 Oct; 81(5):1001-24.
49. Khaodhiar L, Apovian CM. Current perspectives of obesity and its treatment. Manag Care Interface. 2007;20:24-31
50. Current Problems in Surgery : Surgical Management of Morbid Obesity. DJ Tessier, J C Eagon, Vol 45 No 2 Feb 2008;45:2.

SECTION 10

Recent Advances

Molecular Genetics of Hirschsprung's Disease

Paul KH Tam, Mercè Garcia-Barcelo

Understanding how genes and other DNA sequences function together and interact with proteins and environmental factors is paramount to the discovery of the pathways involved in normal processes and in disease pathogenesis. In this respect, the study of the molecular basis of Hirschsprung's disease (HSCR) has made a marked contribution to the understanding of complex diseases which result from the interaction of two or more genes and/or gene-environment interactions.[1]

Hirschsprung's disease (HSCR) is a developmental disorder characterized by the absence of ganglion cells in of the lower digestive tract. Aganglionosis is attributed to a disorder of the enteric nervous system (ENS) in which ganglion cells fail to innervate the lower gastrointestinal tract during embryonic development. There is significant racial variation in the incidence of the disease, and it is most often found among Asians (2.8 per 10,000 life births).[2] HSCR has a complex pattern of inheritance and manifests with low, sex-dependent penetrance and variability in the length of the aganglionic segment. HSCR most commonly presents sporadically although it can be familial (approximately 20% of the cases) and is frequently associated with many other neurocristopathies and chromosomes abnormalities.[3]

The genetic complexity observed in HSCR can be conceptually understood in the light of the molecular and cellular events that take place during the ENS development in the embryonic stage. The ganglion cells of the fully developed ENS are derived from neural crest cells (NCCs) of the vagal, sacral and truncal regions of the neural tube.[4] During the colonization process, the NCCs have to adapt to a constantly changing intestinal environment that strongly influences their differentiation into enteric neurons.[5] The entire process is regulated by specific molecular signals from both within the neural crest and intestinal environment, and the success of the colonization of the gut depends on the synchronization and balance of the signaling network implicated.[6] DNA alterations in the genes codifying for the signaling molecules may interfere with the colonization process, and consequently represent a primary etiology for HSCR or other neurocristopathies. Since the range of interactions during the ENS development is large, the HSCR phenotype is variable, and may result from single severe mutations in a major gene encoding a crucial molecule or from accumulation of less severe mutations in several genes. The existence of non-clinically affected individuals carrying mutations in major genes invokes a compensatory effect by other genes. HSCR has become a model for oligogenic and polygenic disorders in which the phenotypes and mode of transmission result from interactions between different genes.

CLINICAL PRESENTATION AND CLASSIFICATION

The clinical presentation of HSCR is well documented. About 80% of HSCR patients can be diagnosed within the first few months of life presenting the following symptoms: (1) bilious vomiting; (2) enterocolitis-associated diarrhea; (3) difficulties in bowel movements; (4) progressive abdominal distension, and; (5) failure to pass meconium within the first 24 hours of life. Some patients show symptoms later in infancy or in adulthood with severe constipation, progressive abdominal distension, malnutrition and failure to thrive.[7]

The intestinal tract of HSCR patients can be categorized into three portions starting from the internal anal sphincter to the proximal part of intestinal tract: (1) aganglionic segment (segment without intrinsic nerves); (2) hypoganglionic segment (characterized by the reduced number of enteric ganglia), and (3) ganglionic segment (segment with enough number of enteormalric ganglia). HSCR patients are classified according to the length of the aganglionic segment into: short segment HSCR (SS-HSCR) (~80% of HSCR cases) and long segment HSCR (LS-HSCR) (~20% of HSCR cases). The rectosigmoid region acts as the boundary between LS-HSCR and SS-HSCR. LS-HSCR is defined as aganglionic segment extending to or beyond the proximal sigmoid colon, whereas, the remaining cases are grouped as SS-HSCR.[8]

Four other HSCR variants have also been reported: (1) total colonic aganglionosis (TCA) affecting the whole colon with or without the involvement of distal ileum[9]; (2) total intestinal aganglionosis characterized by the absence of enteric ganglia in the whole bowel;[10] (3) ultra short segment HSCR affecting the distal rectum below the pelvic floor and the anus, and (4) suspended HSCR, in which an aganglionic segment is proximal to the ganglionic part, however, the presence of this condition is still controversial.[8]

DIAGNOSIS

A diluted small intestine or proximal colon with empty rectum may be visible on a plain X-ray radiograph. On barium enema radiographs, a transition zone may be identified which serves as a diagnostic indicator of HSCR, especially when other radiographic features (such as barium retention and mixing of stool and barium) are also taken in to account. Barium enema radiography can also serve as a tool to roughly define the length of aganglionic bowel in SS-HSCR (Jamieson et al., 2004). Anorectal manometry of HSCR patients shows the failure of internal anal sphincter relaxation upon rectal distension.[11] Although contrast barium enema and anorectal manometry can help in HSCR diagnosis, there are drawbacks in these methods. It has been shown that the false-positive rate of HSCR diagnosis is high when using contrast barium enema, especially for LSA-HSCR cases and the anorectal manometry may not be reliable for < 12 months infant as the normal rectoenteric reflex is not yet present and the relaxation of internal anal sphincter may be masked by the contraction of external anal sphincter.[8,12] Therefore, full thickness rectal suction biopsy is a gold standard in HSCR diagnosis in most cases.

Rectal suction biopsy has high predictive value in HSCR diagnosis. The diagnosis can be confirmed by the absence of ganglion cells in myenteric plexus, the presence of hypertrophic nerve trunks and the elevated acetylcholinesterase (AChE) level in mucosa and submucosa.[7]

TREATMENT AND COMPLICATIONS

The treatment of HSCR is surgical and pull-through operations (Swenson, Duhamel and Soave operations) are commonly used nowadays. The basic principle of the pull-through operation is to remove the aganglionic intestinal segment and connect the ganglionic segment at the anus. One-stage operation is possible only in newborns with SS-HSCR if the colon is not yet dilated and there is not enterocolitis. If the child has enterocolitis and/or dilated colon, a colostomy should be placed. The pull-through operation should only be performed when the child recovers.[7]

Constipation, fecal incontinence, colonic rupture and Hirschsprung's disease associated enterocolitis (HAEC) are the major complications, in which, HAEC is the most common cause of HSCR-associated mortality. However, complications only occur in about 10% of HSCR patients after surgery.

THE GENETIC ETIOLOGY OF HIRSCHSPRUNG'S DISEASE

In 1886, the Danish pediatrician Harald Hirschsprung (1830–1916), described the disease as a cause of constipation in early infancy due to congenital dilatation of the colon. But it was not till the 1940's, when histological studies revealed absence of intramural ganglion cells of the myenteric and submucosa plexuses downstream the dilated colon (megacolon), that the primary pathology of the disease was discovered.[8]

The development of a pull-through surgical procedure by Swenson and Bill in 1948, made a major contribution to our understanding of the disease.[13] This innovative surgical technique enabled the disease to be treated with considerable success. The result was a far higher survival rate among patients, which created the conditions for the discovery of the familial transmission of the disease and the determination of its genetic nature. Additional evidence for a role of genetic factors in the pathology of HSCR was indicated by (i) an increased risk of recurrence for sibs of affected individuals compared with the population at large; (ii) an unbalanced sex-ratio; (iii) the association of HSCR with other genetic diseases, including malformation syndromes and chromosomal anomalies; and (iv) the existence of several animal models of colonic aganglionosis showing specific mendelian modes of inheritance.

In the late 1980s, the locus for multiple endocrine neoplasia (MEN) was assigned to chromosome 10q11.2.[14,15] The same locus was also identified as the cause of papillary thyroid carcinoma (PTC) and familiar medullary thyroid carcinoma (FMTC).[16-19] The cooccurrence of HSCR with multiple endocrine neoplasia type 2 (MEN2) and the observation of a deletion comprising the MEN2 locus in some HSCR patients, prompted the search for a HSCR gene in that chromosomal region.[20-21] Linkage analysis using chromosome 10 markers in HSCR families revealed a HSCR locus in the pericentromeric region of chromosome 10.[22,23] The observation of a HSCR-phenotype in mice with disrupted RET gene and the detection of RET germline mutations in HSCR families lead to the recognition RET as the cause of HSCR, almost a century after Harald Hirschsprung first described the disease.[24-26]

Subsequent studies lead to the identification of several genes implicated in the HSCR phenotype. To date, mutations in nine different genes (RET, GDNF, NRTN, PHOX2B, EDNRB, EDN3, ECE1, SOX10, ZFHX1B, and KIAA1279) have been detected in individuals affected with either isolated or syndromic HSCR (Table 120.1).[8-27] Most of these genes, genes encode protein members of important inter-related signaling pathways critical the development of enteric ganglia: the GDNF/RET receptor tyrosine kinase, the endothelin type B receptor and SOX10 mediated transcription. Nonetheless, RET is the major gene involved in all forms of HSCR, and its expression is critical for the normal development of the ENS.[28,29] Interaction between those signaling pathways governing the development of the enteric nervous system could therefore alter the expression of RET and influence the manifestation of the HSCR phenotype.[30-34] Similarly, yet unknown loci can modify RET expression and act as a disease promoting or suppressing genes. Common features to the mutations found in the HSCR genes are low and sex dependent penetrance (frequency of individuals carrying a mutation who develop disease as opposed to healthy carriers) and variable expression of the HSCR phenotype (variability in the length of the aganglionic segment and in the manifestation of associated anomalies). These characteristics are consistent with the expression of a HSCR gene subject to modification by other loci, perhaps as a result of cross-talk between signaling pathways.[35-36] In addition, phenotypic/genotypic assessment of the disease has become more difficult since a subset of the observed mutations in HSCR genes is also associated with several additional anomalies (syndromic HSCR).

Table 120.1: Genes involved in isolated or syndromic HSCR

Gene	Phenotype in patients with mutation/s
RET	Isolated HSCR or HSCR-MEN2/FMTC
GDNF	Isolated HSCR
NTN	Isolated HSCR
EDNRB	Isolated HSCR or WS4
EDN3	Isolated HSCR or WS4
ECE-1	HSCR with cardiac defects, craniofacial abnormalities and autonomic dysfunction
ZFHX1B	HSCR with Mowat-Wilson syndrome
SOX10	WS4
PHOX2B	Haddad Syndrome (CCHS + HSCR) Neuroblastoma/Neuroblastoma + HSCR
KIAA1279	Goldberg-Shprintzen sundrome (GOSHS)

RET RECEPTOR TYROSINE KINASE PATHWAY

The RET protein functions as a receptor for the Glial cell line-Derived Neurotrophic Factor (GDNF) family. Receptor-ligand interactions are mediated by RET co-receptors (GDNF-family receptors-α; GFRα).[37,38] Activation of the RET receptor by these neurotrophic factors is essential for the migration and differentiation of specific cell lineages of neural crest origin into enteric neurons.[24,39,40] The correct development of the ENS therefore depends on the ability of these neurotrophic factors to activate RET, on the ability of the RET receptor to transduce the signal, and on the competence of the intracellular machinery to elaborate a response (Figs 120.1 and 120.2).

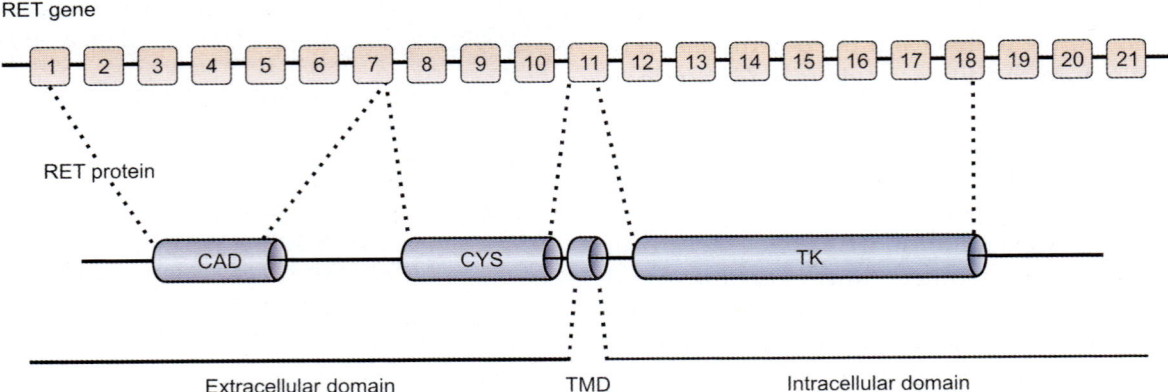

Fig. 120.1: Schematic drawing showing the RET gene and the RET protein receptor (adapted from[1]). Exons of RET gene are indicated with numbered boxes and dotted lines indicate the domains of the protein they encode. Different domains of RET receptor are indicated with cylinders. The extracellular part of RET contains cadherin domains (CAD) and the intracellular part of RET contains two tyrosine kinase domains (TK). TMD, transmembrane domain

RET PROTO-ONCOGENE AND HSCR

RET, also known as RET proto-oncogene, is composed of 21 exons that encode the RET receptor tyrosine kinase protein, a cell-surface molecule that transduces signals. Germline mutations in RET are responsible for four unrelated disorders in humans, HSCR, MEN2A, MEN type 2B and medullary thyroid carcinoma (MTC).[41] In PTC, RET rearrangements are the most commonly detected genetic alterations.

RET is a single-pass membrane protein with two main domains: extracellular (EC) and intracellular (IC). The extracellular domain contains a cadherin-like domain (CAD) and a large conserved cystein rich region (CYS).[42] The IC domain contains a typical tyrosine kinase domain (TK) (Fig. 120.1). The RET protein presents three isoforms of 1114 (RET51), 1106 (RET 43) and 1072 (RET 9) amino acids respectively, with distinct biological roles.[43,44]

Ligand and coreceptor complexes interact with the EC domain of two RET molecules inducing their homodimerization and tyrosine autophosphorylation. Once phosphorylated, the tyrosine residues (TK domain) serve as high affinity binding sites for various intracellular signaling proteins.[45] Activating mutations in the RET gene cause MTC, MEN2A and MEN2B, whereas inactivating mutations lead to Hirschsprung's disease.[46] A large number of RET mutations have been reported in HSCR patients. In general, RET gene mutations affecting the RET EC domain alter the folding of the protein impairing its maturation.[47,48] RET mutations affecting the RET TK domain abolish the kinase activity or interfere with the binding to intracellular signaling proteins.[48-50] Mutations in exons 20 and 21 of RET may affect the specific isoforms of the RET protein and modify their differential roles in signaling.[44] Mutations in any intron/exon boundary affecting the splicing consensus sequences can alter mRNA processing. Remarkably, silent mutations (i.e. the mutation does not result in an amino acid change in the protein) in any of the RET exons can also affect mRNA processing.[51] Unlike in MEN 2, RET mutations causing HSCR are, with a very few exceptions, scattered throughout the gene, affecting indiscriminately any part of the RET protein.[35] However, many RET mutations have not been functionally tested and is very difficult to discern between truly deleterious substitutions and non-deleterious ones. A recent study based on the alignment of the human RET protein with 12 orthologous sequences provides an insight on the prediction of the effect of the RET mutations.[52]

Mutations in the coding regions of RET and other HSCR genes (see below) only account for over 50% of the familial cases, and between 7 and 35% of the sporadic cases.[53-68] Intriguingly, genetic-linkage analyses in HSCR families keep implicating the 10q11 chromosomal region (RET locus) even though no RET coding regions can be found.[35,69] This, besides confirming the central role of RET in HSCR, also indicates that mutations in non-coding (regulatory)

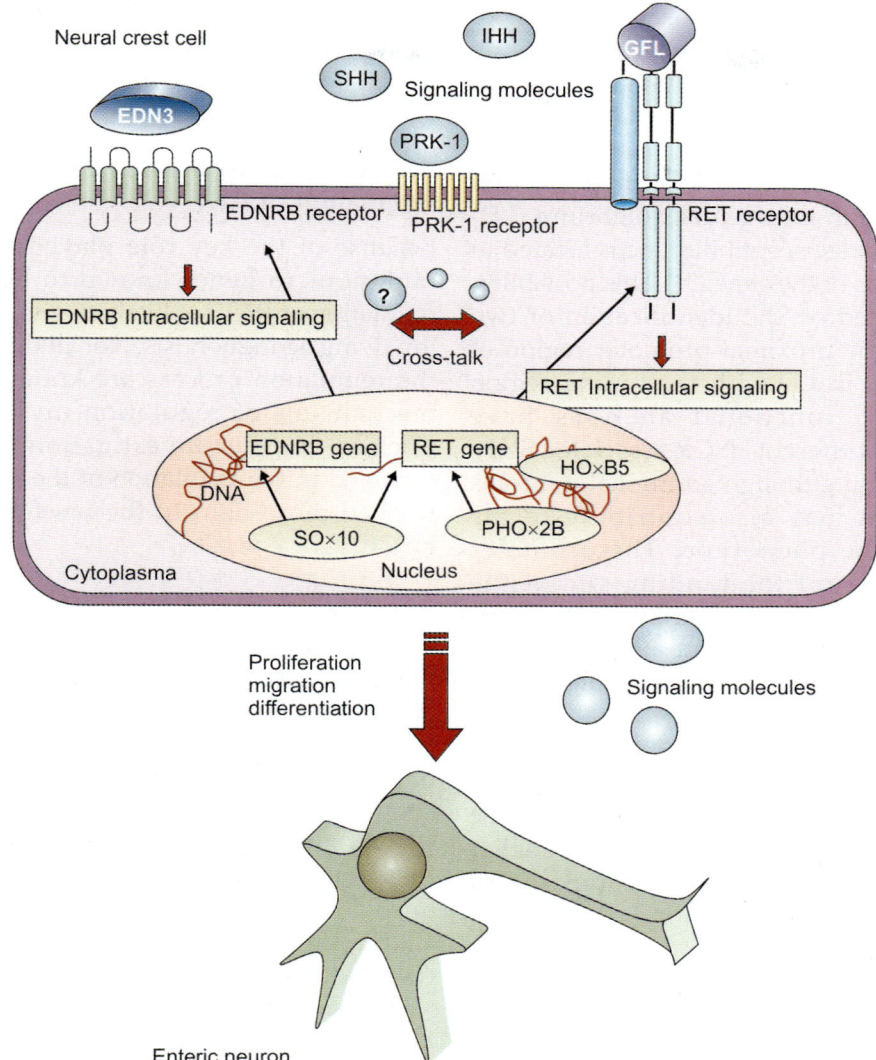

Fig. 120.2: Schematic representation of the network of interactions that govern the development of the enteric nervous system (adapted from[1]). Expression of the RET gene (regulated by transcription factors) leads to the formation of the RET protein which functions as a receptor for the Glial cell line-Derived Neurotrophic Factor family (GFL) through co-receptors (GFRA). Activation of the RET receptor by these signaling molecules of the gut environment activates the intracellular machinery necessary for the migration, proliferation and differentiation of specific cell lineages of neural crest origin into enteric neurons. Similarly, the EDNRB receptor is activated by EDN3 and initiates a series of events that will also regulate the development of the enteric nervous system in conjunction with the RET pathway. The Prok-1 pathway, thought to be involved in ENS development is also represented. Double head arrows indicated inter-relation between pathways. Question mark represents yet unidentified molecules members of the network (see modifying genes and interaction between signaling pathways section in the text)

regions RET remain to be found. Mutations in regulatory regions can alter the DNA binding sites of transcriptional regulators and reduce or abolish the expression of RET. In addition to RET mutations, a possible role in HSCR has been attributed to several single nucleotides polymorphisms (SNPs) of the RET gene since they have been found associated with the disease. Variant alleles of the RET coding-region polymorphisms are over-represented in HSCR sporadic patients.[70-73] The current data indicates that these RET specific SNPs, either singly or in combination (haplotypes), could act as modifiers by modulating the penetrance of mutations in other HSCR genes and possibly of those mutations in the RET gene itself.[32,74,75] They might also act as low penetrance alleles conferring risk of or protection against disease, or be in linkage disequilibrium (LD) with a yet unidentified susceptibility locus located in the regulatory regions of the gene.[76,77] This possibility has been corroborated by the identification of two polymorphisms in the proximal promoter region of RET and in intron 1 in LD with the coding region SNPs.[78-83] In vitro functional analyses have demonstrated a direct effect of HSCR-associated SNPs on the RET expression although additional cis/trans regulatory element may also contribute to the manifestation of the phenotype. The promoter polymorphisms disrupt the binding site of the transcription factor NK2,1. This gene has also been considered as a HSCR candidate gene and 3 mutations with possible damaging effect in the protein have recently been identified.[84]

Noteworthy, the overall frequencies of the HSCR-associated RET SNPs and haplotypes are significantly higher in Chinese, not only in patients but also in the general population, possibly explaining the higher incidence of HSCR in Asians when compared to Caucasians.[2,83,85]

GDNF Family Ligands and their Receptors (GDNF-family receptors-α; GFRα)

The relevance of RET signaling pathway in the ENS development and the phenotypic similarities between *RET*, *GDNF* and *GFRα-1* knock-out mice, prompted an extensive mutation screening of the genes encoding the GDNF family of ligands -GDNF, Neurturin (NTN) artemin (ARTN) and persepin (PSPN)- and of the genes encoding their coreceptors (GFR-α1-4) and adaptors.[24;86-88] However, mutations in those genes have been identified in a very small number of patients and generally co-segregate with mutations in RET.[89-93] None of the of mutations identified in the GDNF gene are likely *per se* to cause HSCR, although it is thought they can contribute to disease via interaction with other susceptibility loci.[94,95] Surprisingly, RET is virtually the only target of HSCR mutations in the RET signalling pathway. It is possible that homozygous mutations in the GDNF family of ligands were lethal, and that these ligands, particularly GDNF, may have other functions not mediated by RET, and therefore come under selective pressure against mutations.

HSCR Genes Involved in the Transcriptional Regulation of RET

Because of the key role played by RET in HSCR, mutations in genes known to be involved in the regulation of RET are likely to give rise to phenotypes involving aganglionosis. Not all the genes involved in the regulation process are known and the precise mechanisms of regulation involved also remain unclear. Further investigation on the molecules involved in the regulation of the RET gene is certain to shed more light to the mechanisms underlying HSCR.

SOX10

The SOX10 gene encodes a transcriptional regulator whose expression is essential for the development of cells in the neural crest cell lineage, including melanocites and enteric neurons. During the development of the ENS, the SOX10 protein physically interacts and cooperates with another transcriptional regulator (PAX3) to activate transcription of RET.[40,96,97] Importantly, SOX10 also interacts with EDNRB in mice.[98,99]

The significance of the SOX10 gene in HSCR was revealed through the study of a mouse model of HSCR (*Dom*) fortuitously generated at the Jackson Laboratory.[100] The molecular defect in *Dom* mice was a mutation in the SOX10 gene.[101-104] Heterozygous *Dom* mice presented with distal colonic aganglionosis and localized hypomelanosis of the skin and hair (features similar to those in Waardenburg's syndrome), which indicated that neural crest-derived melanocytes and enteric neurons were affected in SOX10 mutants. *Dom* homozygous mice were embryonic lethal.

In humans, heterozygous SOX10 mutations have been identified in patients with Waardenburg-Shah syndrome (WS4; HSCR type 2). Patients with WS4 display a combination of the features of Waardenburg syndrome (wide bridge of the nose, pigmentary abnormalities, and cochlear deafness) and Hirschsprung's disease.[101,105-111] SOX10 mutations also lead to Yemenite deaf-blind hypopigmentation syndrome and other myelin deficiencies.[112] To date, no SOX10 mutations have been found in patients presenting aganglionosis as an isolated trait. SOX10 is therefore unlikely to be major gene in isolated HSCR. Interestingly, and despite the absence of genetic mutations, abnormal SOX10 gene expression can be observed in aganglionic intestine of isolate HSCR patients.[111]

PHOX2B

The paired mesoderm homeobox 2B gene (PHOX2) encodes a transcription factor which is involved in the development of several noradrenergic neuron populations. In mice homozygous disruption of the PHOX2B gene results in absence enteric ganglia, a feature reminiscent of HSCR. Furthermore, there is no Ret expression in PHOX2B mutant embryos indicating that regulation of Ret by PHOX2B could account for the failure of the ENS to develop.[113,114] All these observations make the PHOX2B a candidate gene for HSCR. Interestingly, a chromosomal alteration involving the deletion of the PHOX2B locus has been described in a patient with syndromic HSCR (developmental delay, severe hypotonia, facial dysmorphism, and short segment aganglionosis).[115] This suggests that PHOX2B haploinsufficiency may predispose to HSCR. A SNP of the PHOX2B gene has been found to be associated with HSCR and importantly, the interaction between PHOX2B and RET HSCR-associated SNPs increase to susceptibility to HSCR.[116,117]

PHOX2B represents the first gene for which germline mutations predispose to neuroblastoma and is the major locus for congenital central hypoventilation syndrome (CCHS, Ondine's curse).[118-121] In particular, 25–30% of the CCHS patients are affected with aganglionosis (Haddad syndrome).[122] Intriguingly, both neuroblastoma and CCHS are frequently associated with HSCR.[8] Taken together these data support the contribution of PHOX2B to HSCR.

ENDOTHELIN TYPE B RECEPTOR PATHWAY

The endothelins are a family of three signaling peptides (EDN1, EDN2 and EDN3) that can act on two subtypes of G protein-coupled receptors, termed endothelin A and endothelin B receptors (EDNRA and EDNRB) (Fig. 120.2). The endothelins are synthesized as much larger proteins which are cleaved by the endothelin converting enzyme (ECE-1) to produce an active peptide. The human genes coding for these proteins are EDN1, EDN2, EDN3, EDNRA and EDNRB respectively.

The involvement of the endothelin type B receptor pathway in the pathology of HSCR was demonstrated when a targeted disruption of the mouse endothelin B receptor gene (EDNRB) resulted in an autosomal recessive phenotype with aganglionic megacolon and white spotting of the coat.[123] A targeted disruption of the mouse endothelin 3 ligand (EDN3) gene produced a similar recessive phenotype of megacolon and white coat spotting.[124] These findings indicated an essential role for the members of the EDNRB pathway in the development of two neural crest-derived cell lineages, enteric neurons and epidermal melanocytes. EDNRB signaling not only regulates migration of the ENS progenitors but can also modulate the response of NCCs to GDNF.[5,33] This provides evidence of interaction between two different pathways implicated in the pathogenesis of HSCR.

EDNRB Gene and HSCR

The occurrence of multiple cases of both isolated HSCR and WS4 in an inbreed old order mennonite community facilitated the mapping of another major HSCR susceptibility gene to the chromosomal region 13q22.[125,126] The gene identified on 13q22 was the endothelin type B receptor (EDNRB) which had a mutation that resulted in the W276C amino acid change in the protein. In contrast to the recessive, fully penetrant defects of the rodent model, this human mutation was neither fully dominant not fully recessive. The homozygous W276C mutation (CC) was more penetrant than the heterozygous (WC), and that penetrance was sex dependent. Individuals homozygous (CC) presented with WS4 features, while those with the heterozygous mutation (WC) presented with isolated HSCR. Furthermore, some family members with no W279C mutation were clinically affected. This implied the presence of additional predisposing genes among this closely-related group. In fact, a genetic modifier of HSCR found among the group was mapped to chromosome 21q21.[125] Subsequent EDNRB mutation analyses conducted on both isolated HSCR and WS4 patients revealed other EDNRB mutations with similar genetic behavior to W279C. Homozygous

EDNRB mutations were associated with WS4 and heterozygous mutations with isolated HSCR.[67;68;127-129-134] Overall, EDNRB mutations account for 5% of the isolated HSCR phenotype. Functional analyses of EDNRB missense mutations showed impairment of the intracellular signaling.[132,135,136] EDNRB mutations found this far, are mainly inherited from unaffected parents, and associated with short-segment aganglionosis.

EDN3 and ECE1 Genes

HSCR patients are being screened for mutations in the human EDN3 because of the HSCR-like phenotype presented by mice with disruption of the EDN3 gene. To the best of our knowledge, very few EDN3 mutations have been characterized in HSCR patients. With very few exceptions, heterozygous EDN3 mutations are associated with isolated HSCR and homozygous mutations with WS4.[103,137-140]

Another knock-out mouse model again provided evidence of the involvement of another member of the EDNRB pathway in HSCR.[141] The gene encodes the endothelin converting enzyme (ECE1), which cleaves the large inactive endothelins into smaller 21 amino acids active endothelins. Mice carrying an ECE1 null mutation (no protein is synthesized) present with craniofacial and cardiac abnormalities, absence of melanocytes and absence of the enteric neurons in the distal gut. This phenotype is similar to that presented by mice with mutations in the genes encoding other members of the EDNRB pathway (EDN3 and EDNRB). To date, only one mutation in the ECE1 gene has been found and the patient was affected with syndromic HSCR.[142]

As a general rule, severe homozygous mutations in genes involved in the EDNRB pathway are mainly associated with WS4 (absence of enteric ganglia and epidermal melanocytes, both neural crest cell derivatives). The association of homozygous mutations with WS4 and heterozygous mutations with isolated HSCR may indicate that melanocytes and enteric ganglia differ in sensitivity to the varying levels of EDNRB signalling.[30]

The restriction of aganglionosis to the distal colon in mice with EDNRB and EDN3 deficiency and the fact that HSCR patients with mutations in these genes mainly present with short segment aganglionosis indicated that the EDNRB signaling pathway is only required during the late states of the colonization of the colon.[143,144] However, it has recently been shown that the EDNRB signaling pathway is required for the colonization of both colon and small bowel.[33] The colonization process is subject to distinct spatial and temporal signaling requirements and at some stage, EDNRB signaling enhances the ability of the NCCs to migrate into the distal bowel.[5]

ZFHX1B (previously SIP1)

The observation of a translocation involving the ZFHX1B locus (2q22) in a patient with HSCR disease, microcephaly, mental retardation, epilepsy and characteristic facial appearance, led to the first documentation of ZFHX1B involvement in this syndromic form of HSCR.[145] Other chromosomal abnormalities involving 2q22 and mutations in the ZFHX1B gene are being described in patients with similar clinical features (recently named Mowat-Wilson syndrome) although not all of them present with aganglionosis.

ZFHX1B encodes a transcriptional repressor (SIP1, Smad Interacting Protein 1), which interacts with several members of the Smad family. Some Smad proteins act as transducers in signaling cascades critical to embryogenesis. It is not yet know how mutations in ZFHX1B may result in defects of the ENS, although it is tempting to speculate on a possible functional link between SIP1 and the signaling pathways currently known to be essential for the ENS development. As in SOX10, no mutations have been found in patients with isolated HSCR, and therefore ZFHX1B is unlikely to be major gene in non-syndromic HSCR.[146-148]

KIAA1279

By homozygosity mapping, a novel locus on 10q21.3-q22.1 for Goldberg-Shprintzen syndrome (GOSHS) was identified in an inbreed family. Phenotypic features of GOSHS in this inbred family included microcephaly, polymicogyria and mental retardation, as well as HSCR. Homozygous nonsense mutations were identified in the KIAA1279 gene at 10q22.1. This finding established the importance of KIAA1279[27] in both enteric and central nervous system development although the role of KIAA1279 is not yet understood. No mutations in this gene have been found in isolated HSCR patients.

MODIFYING GENES AND INTERACTION BETWEEN SIGNALING PATHWAYS

It has already been stressed that the successful colonization of the gut by the ENS precursors depends on a coordinated and balanced network of interacting molecules (Fig. 120.2). Conceivably, there should be a functional and genetic link among these molecules for them to interact. The mechanisms underlying these interactions may help to explain the complexity of the HSCR phenotype and resolve puzzling genetic observations, e.g. that in some cases more than one mutated gene is needed to produce the phenotype, while (conversely) healthy individuals exist with mutations in HSCR genes. Interaction between pathways requires not only coordination among the pathway members but also with those molecules that mediate their interaction.

The RET and EDNRB signaling pathways were initially thought to be biochemically independent. However, the case of an HSCR patient with a weak mutation in both RET and EDNRB whose healthy parents were heterozygous for one mutation implies interaction between these two pathways.[51] Some reports have also hinted the possibility of cross-talk between G-protein-coupled-receptors (EDNRB) and tyrosine kinase receptors (i.e. RET).[149] The genetic interaction between mutations in RET and EDNRB in HSCR was verified in 2002 in an association study conducted on 43 Mennonite family trios segregating the W276C mutation in the EDNRB described above.[32] The study demonstrated the join transmission of both, the W276C mutation in EDNRB and HSCR-associated haplotypes in RET in affected individuals. The combination of these two genotypes increased the penetrance of the mutation and therefore the risk to disease. Genetic interaction between *RET* and *EDNRB* pathways has also been demonstrated in mice.[32-34] The fact that two mutated genes are needed for the manifestation of the disease also implies functional interaction. EDN3 and GDNF seem to have a synergistic effect on the proliferation of the undifferentiated ENS progenitors and an antagonistic effect on the migration of differentiated enteric ganglia. It appears that EDN3 has a variable distribution along the developing gut with differential effects on processes regulated by the RET. It has been firmly established that the interaction between these signaling pathways controls ENS development throughout the intestine.[5,33] However, both pathways have to be integrated by additional molecules or "mediators". Protein kinase A has been suggested as a key component of the molecular mechanisms that mediate and link the RET and EDNRB signaling pathways[33] Also, in mice, SOX10 has been shown to act on both RET and EDNRB genes further linking these two signaling pathways.[96-99] Additional investigation is needed to identify all molecules members of these pathways/networks. This means that genes involved in the development of the enteric nervous system still await discovery, and that DNA alterations in multiple genes have the potential to combine and hinder a phenotype. Obviously, defective functioning of these still unknown "mediators" could modify the outcome of the development of the ENS. RET and EDNRB are central to the genesis of HSCR but little is yet known of the influence of variation in multiple genes or genetic background. Unknown loci (that could encode protein members of the RET and EDNRB pathways) can modify RET expression and act as a disease promoting or suppressing genes (modifiers). Therefore, the poor genotype-phenotype correlation in HSCR is due to the effects of multiple genes combined, including HSCR known genes and still unknown loci. A linkage study conducted on 12 HSCR families enriched for L-HSCR demonstrated linkage to RET in all but one family. However, 6 out the 11 families linked to RET, also showed linkage to the 9q31 locus. Interestingly, no severe *RET* mutations were detected in those 6 families. It was concluded that these 6 families harbored "weak" RET DNA alterations and that the effect of the 9q31 locus was required to produce the phenotype.[150] A genome-wide scan on 49 S-HSCR families detected linkage to three chromosomal regions, 10q12, 3p21 and 19q12. The 10q21 region corresponded to RET although causative RET mutations were present in only 40% of the linked families, again stressing the importance of variations in noncoding regions. Further analyses of the data demonstrated oligogenic inheritance of S-HSCR. The action of RET (10q12) and 3q21 and/or 19q12 seemed to be necessary and sufficient for the manifestation of S-HSCR. Since S-HSCR did not segregate in the absence of RET, the authors suggested that 3q21 and 19q12 loci are RET-dependent, therefore, modifiers of the RET expression.[35] A recent study on the 3p21 chromosomal region narrowed down a HSCR-associated region comprising three genes involved in neurological phenotypes. Follow-up studies on these genes are therefore warranted.[151]

These studies emphasize the central role of RET in all forms of HSCR (short and long) and explained the non-mendelian inheritance of the disease. Also, they suggest that the genetics of long-segment Hirschsprung's disease and short-segment Hirschsprung's disease may depend on the effects of the different RET modifiers.

OTHER HSCR CANDIDATE GENES

Mouse models and syndromes associated with HSCR provide insights into the genes that may share a common signaling pathway involved in the development of the ENS and therefore in the pathogenesis of HSCR. It is therefore logical to study the possible contribution of these genes to HSCR. This can be illustrated by the example posed by the Indian Hedgehog Gene (IHH). The Hedgehog gene family encodes a group of secreted signaling molecules that are essential for growth and patterning of many different body parts of vertebrate and invertebrate embryos.[152] In particular, IHH signaling controls growth of bones and is required for the proper development of the ENS and the intestinal stem cell proliferation and differentiation.[153] IHH mutant mice present with dilated colon with abnormally thin wall, and enteric neurons missing from parts of the small intestine and from the dilated regions of the colon. This HSCR-like phenotype is observed with an incomplete penetrance of 50%, which suggest that interaction with other factors will be required for full expression of the phenotype. These features are strikingly similar to those observed in HSCR patients. In humans, mutations in the IHH gene (2q33-35) are associated with congenital limbs malformations and other skeleton dysplasias some of which are also seen in some HSCR patients.[3,154,155] Nevertheless, IHH mutation analysis in over 60 HSCR patients with no mutations in the HSCR genes described so far, reveal no coding region mutations that could account for the disease.[156]

Similar results were obtained for the human L1CAM gene. This gene encodes the L1 cell adhesion molecule involved in the development of the nervous system.[157] Mutations in L1CAM are linked to a recessive form of congenital hydrocephalus.[158] The detection of L1CAM mutations in individuals with congenital hydrocephalus and HSCR and the fact that L1CAM maps to chromosome Xq28, (which could account for the higher penetrance of HSCR in males) encouraged the mutational screening of this gene in isolated HSCR patients.[159-161] Although no coding region mutations were identified, it was hypothesized that L1CAM-mediated cell adhesion may be important for the ability of ganglion cell precursors to populate the gut, and that the *L1CAM* gene could modify the effects of a Hirschsprung's disease-associated gene to cause intestinal aganglionosis.

Recently, using transgenic mouse technology, it has been shown that the transcription factor Hoxb5 may contribute to HSCR by interfering with the regulation of the RET gene. A fraction of HOXB5 mutant mice presented with reduction of ganglia (hypoganglionosis) and slow peristalsis and, occasionally, absence of ganglia. In addition Ret expression was markedly reduced or absent in neural crest cells and ganglia suggesting that HOXB5 may contribute to the etiology of Hirschsprung's disease.[162] In additional, HOXB5 SNPs were found associated to HSCR in humans. Taken altogether, these data also suggests a role for HOXB5 in HSCR.

Due to the current ambiguity regarding the role played by rare gene mutations it is important to perform exhaustive functional analysis in order to determine their association with the disease. Even so, the disease is likely to results from the combined effects of mutations or variants in many genes. The characterization of the gene network directing the development of the ENS may help in the identification of additional HSCR candidate genes. These genes may play a minor role in the expression of the disease, and they are likely to be modifiers of the already known HSCR major genes.

GENETIC COUNSELING

In isolated HSCR, a relatively precise recurrence risk tailored to individual families could be estimated based on the estimates provided by Badner.[163] The highest recurrence risk is for a male sib of a female proband with L-HSCR.[3] Nonetheless, the reduced penetrance of the HSCR mutations makes it difficult to rationally predict and assess the risk to disease. Genetic testing is only performed on a research basis, and due to the advances of the surgical management of HSCR, its utility is questionable.

As outlined earlier, mutations in the RET proto-oncogene are also the underlying cause of the inherited cancer syndromes MEN2A and MEN2B and FMTC. In HSCR patients, RET mutations are dispersed throughout the gene, while in MEN2A and FMTC patients, mutations are clustered in the cysteine codons of the RET extracellular domain (exons 10 and 11). Although HSCR and MEN2A are two different entities, occasionally they co-segregate in some families, and affected individuals carry a single mutations in exons 10 or 11. *RET*[164-168] Importantly, mutations identical to those found in MEN2A have been detected in HSCR patients with no clinical symptoms of MEN2A.[169,170] That means that some HSCR patients may be exposed to a highly increased risk of tumors. Where HSCR patients carry these tumor specific mutations, exploration of the family history of MEN2A and periodic screening for tumors is advisable. In families segregating both MEN2A and HSCR, RET gene testing, tumor screening, and prophylactic thyroidectomy is also warranted.

FUTURE DIRECTIONS

Although modern surgical procedures have already achieved a high success rate in the treatment of Hirschsprung's disease (HSCR), a better understanding of the mechanisms involved in the pathogenesis of this disease should enable doctors to prevent and diagnose it more easily and treat it even more effectively.

The major breakthrough in the study of the pathogenesis of HSCR has been the demonstration of the genetic and functional interaction between the RET and EDNRB signaling pathways and their establishment as key players in the development of the ENS. These important findings should lead to the study of the complete gene network that makes the genesis of the ENS possible. Regarding HSCR gene-discovery, genome-wide association studies and whole-genome sequencing of DNA of HSCR patients are currently underway. The challenge is using this newly-available genomic information to elucidate normal gene function, and determine how DNA alterations cause disease in humans. For obvious reasons, conducting gene or protein expression analyses for the study of HSCR and other human diseases that result from gene dysfunction during development is not feasible. Mice can provide access to the study of human genes and proteins that have an equivalent in mice. Scientists are now resorting to the isolation individual mouse cell types by making use of stem cell research. This has allowed the study the specific requirements of the gut neural crest stem cells (NCSCs).[33,171-172] A recent study has shown that Prokineticin-1 (Prok-1) can induce both proliferation and expression of differentiation markers of RET deficient mouse NCCs, suggesting that Prok-1 may provide a complementary pathway to GDNF/RET signaling during the ENS development. This indicates that Prok-1 crosstalks with GDNF/RET signaling and probably provides an additional layer of signaling refinement to maintain proliferation and differentiation of enteric NCCs.

If the behavior of the gut NCSCs is better understood, it may be possible to treat HSCR by transplanting NCSCs directly into the aganglionic gut. It will be intriguing to determine whether these NCSCs are able to mature and engraft in the forming gut and enhance bowel motility, and further research of this kind should yield new therapeutic approaches.

REFERENCES

1. Tam PK, Garcia-Barcelo M. Molecular genetics of Hirschsprung's disease. Semin Pediatr Surg 2004;13:236-48.
2. Torfs C. An epidemiological study of Hirschsprung's disease in a multiracial California population. Third International Meeting: Hirschsprung's disease and related neurocristophaties Evian, France 2004;1998.
3. Amiel J, Lyonnet S. Hirschsprung's disease, associated syndromes, and genetics: a review. J Med Genet 2001;38:729-39.
4. Burns AJ, Douarin NM. The sacral neural crest contributes neurons and glia to the post-umbilical gut: spatiotemporal analysis of the development of the enteric nervous system. Development 1998;125:4335-47.
5. Kruger GM, Mosher JT, Tsai YH, Yeager KJ, Iwashita T, Gariepy CE, et al. Temporally distinct requirements for endothelin receptor B in the generation and migration of gut neural crest stem cells. Neuron 2003;40:917-29.
6. Gariepy CE. Intestinal motility disorders and development of the enteric nervous system. Pediatr Res 2001;49:605-13.
7. Kessmann J. Hirschsprung's disease: diagnosis and management. Am Fam Physician 2006;74:1319-22.
8. Amiel J, Sproat-Emison E, Garcia-Barcelo M, Lantieri F, Burzynski G, Borrego S, et al. Hirschsprung's disease, associated syndromes and genetics: a review. J Med Genet 2008;45:1-14.
9. Wildhaber BE, Teitelbaum DH, Coran AG. Total colonic Hirschsprung's disease: a 28-year experience. J Pediatr Surg 2005;40:203-06.

10. Caniano DA, Ormsbee HS, III, Polito W, Sun CC, Barone FC, Hill JL. Total intestinal aganglionosis. J Pediatr Surg 1985;20:456-60.
11. de Lorijn F, Boeckxstaens GE, Benninga MA. Symptomatology, pathophysiology, diagnostic work-up, and treatment of Hirschsprung's disease in infancy and childhood. Curr Gastroenterol Rep 2007;9:245-53.
12. Dasgupta R, Langer JC. Hirschsprung's disease. Curr Probl Surg 2004;41:942-88.
13. Swenson O. Early history of the therapy of Hirschsprung's disease: facts and personal observations over 50 years. J Pediatr Surg 1996;31:1003-08.
14. Simpson NE, Kidd KK, Goodfellow PJ, McDermid H, Myers S, Kidd JR et al. Assignment of multiple endocrine neoplasia type 2A to chromosome 10 by linkage. Nature 1987; 328:528-30.
15. Mulligan LM, Kwok JB, Healey CS, Elsdon MJ, Eng C, Gardner E, et al. Germ-line mutations of the RET proto-oncogene in multiple endocrine neoplasia type 2A. Nature 1993; 363:458-60.
16. Grieco M, Santoro M, Berlingieri MT, Donghi R, Pierotti MA, Della PG et al. Molecular cloning of PTC, a new oncogene found activated in human thyroid papillary carcinomas and their lymph node metastases. Ann N Y Acad Sci 1988;551:380-81.
17. Grieco M, Santoro M, Berlingieri MT, Melillo RM, Donghi R, Bongarzone I, et al. PTC is a novel rearranged form of the ret proto-oncogene and is frequently detected in vivo in human thyroid papillary carcinomas. Cell 1990;60:557-63.
18. Donghi R, Sozzi G, Pierotti MA, Biunno I, Miozzo M, Fusco A et al. The oncogene associated with human papillary thyroid carcinoma (PTC) is assigned to chromosome 10 q11-q12 in the same region as multiple endocrine neoplasia type 2A (MEN2A). Oncogene 1989;4:521-23.
19. Donis-Keller H, Dou S, Chi D, Carlson KM, Toshima K, Lairmore TC et al. Mutations in the RET proto-oncogene are associated with MEN 2A and FMTC. Hum Mol Genet 1993;2:851-56.
20. Martucciello G, Bicocchi MP, Dodero P, Lerone M, Silengo M, Puliti A, et al. Total colonic aganglionosis associated with interstitial deletion of the long arm of chromosome 10. Pediatr Surg Int 1992;7:308-10.
21. Fewtrell MS, Tam PK, Thomson AH, Fitchett M, Currie J, Huson SM et al. Hirschsprung's disease associated with a deletion of chromosome 10 (q11.2q21.2): a further link with the neurocristopathies? J Med Genet 1994;31:325-27.
22. Angrist M, Kauffman E, Slaugenhaupt SA, Matise TC, Puffenberger EG, Washington SS et al. A gene for Hirschsprung's disease (megacolon) in the pericentromeric region of human chromosome 10. Nat Genet 1993;4:351-56.
23. Lyonnet S, Bolino A, Pelet A, Abel L, Nihoul-Fekete C, Briard ML et al. A gene for Hirschsprung's disease maps to the proximal long arm of chromosome 10. Nat Genet 1993;4:346-50.
24. Schuchardt A, D'Agati V, Larsson-Blomberg L, Costantini F, Pachnis V. RET-deficient mice: an animal model for Hirschsprung's disease and renal agenesis. J Intern Med 1995;238:327-32.
25. Romeo G, Ronchetto P, Luo Y, Barone V, Seri M, Ceccherini I et al. Point mutations affecting the tyrosine kinase domain of the RET proto-oncogene in Hirschsprung's disease. Nature 1994;367:377-78.
26. Edery P, Lyonnet S, Mulligan LM, Pelet A, Dow E, Abel L, et al. Mutations of the RET proto-oncogene in Hirschsprung's disease. Nature 1994;367:378-80.
27. Brooks AS, Bertoli-Avella AM, Burzynski GM, Breedveld GJ, Osinga J, Boven LG et al. Homozygous nonsense mutations in KIAA1279 are associated with malformations of the central and enteric nervous systems. Am J Hum Genet 2005;77:120-26.
28. Natarajan D, Marcos-Gutierrez C, Pachnis V, de Graaff E. Requirement of signalling by receptor tyrosine kinase RET for the directed migration of enteric nervous system progenitor cells during mammalian embryogenesis. Development 2002;129:5151-60.
29. Iwashita T, Kruger GM, Pardal R, Kiel MJ, Morrison SJ. Hirschsprung's disease is linked to defects in neural crest stem cell function. Science 2003;301:972-76.
30. McCallion AS, Chakravarti A. EDNRB/EDN3 and Hirschsprung's disease type II. Pigment Cell Res 2001;14:161-69.
31. Chakravarti A. Endothelin receptor-mediated signaling in Hirschsprung's disease. Hum Mol Genet 1996;5:303-07.
32. Carrasquillo MM, McCallion AS, Puffenberger EG, Kashuk CS, Nouri N, Chakravarti A. Genome-wide association study and mouse model identify interaction between RET and EDNRB pathways in Hirschsprung's disease. Nat Genet 2002; 32:237-44.
33. Barlow A, de Graaff E, Pachnis V. Enteric nervous system progenitors are coordinately controlled by the G protein-coupled receptor EDNRB and the receptor tyrosine kinase RET. Neuron 2003; 40:905-16.
34. McCallion AS, Stames E, Conlon RA, Chakravarti A. Phenotype variation in two-locus mouse models of Hirschsprung's disease: tissue-specific interaction between RET and EDNRB. Proc Natl Acad Sci U S A 2003; 100:1826-31.
35. Gabriel SB, Salomon R, Pelet A, Angrist M, Amiel J, Fornage M et al. Segregation at three loci explains familial and population risk in Hirschsprung's disease. Nat Genet 2002; 31:89-93.
36. Bolk S, Pelet A, Hofstra RM, Angrist M, Salomon R, Croaker D, et al. A human model for multigenic inheritance: phenotypic expression in Hirschsprungs disease requires both the RET gene and a new 9q31 locus. Proc Natl Acad Sci USA 2000;97:268-73.
37. Jing S, Wen D, Yu Y, Holst PL, Luo Y, Fang M, et al. GDNF-induced activation of the ret protein tyrosine kinase is mediated by GDNFR-alpha, a novel receptor for GDNF. Cell 1996;85:1113-24.

38. Treanor JJ, Goodman L, de Sauvage F, Stone DM, Poulsen KT, Beck CD et al. Characterization of a multicomponent receptor for GDNF. Nature 1996;382:80-83.
39. Pachnis V, Mankoo B, Costantini F. Expression of the C-RET proto-oncogene during mouse embryogenesis. Development 1993;119:1005-17.
40. Taraviras S, Marcos-Gutierrez CV, Durbec P, Jani H, Grigoriou M, Sukumaran M, et al. Signalling by the RET receptor tyrosine kinase and its role in the development of the mammalian enteric nervous system. Development 1999;126:2785-97.
41. Hofstra RM, Landsvater RM, Ceccherini I, Stulp RP, Stelwagen T, Luo Y, et al. A mutation in the RET proto-oncogene associated with multiple endocrine neoplasia type 2B and sporadic medullary thyroid carcinoma. Nature 1994;367:375-76.
42. Anders J, Kjar S, Ibanez CF. Molecular modeling of the extracellular domain of the RET receptor tyrosine kinase reveals multiple cadherin-like domains and a calcium-binding site. J Biol Chem 2001;276:35808-17.
43. Myers SM, Eng C, Ponder BA, Mulligan LM. Characterization of RET proto-oncogene 3' splicing variants and polyadenylation sites: a novel C-terminus for RET. Oncogene 1995;11:2039-45.
44. de Graaff E, Srinivas S, Kilkenny C, D'Agati V, Mankoo BS, Costantini F, et al. Differential activities of the RET tyrosine kinase receptor isoforms during mammalian embryogenesis. Genes Dev 2001; 15:2433-44.
45. Airaksinen MS, Saarma M. The GDNF family: signalling, biological functions and therapeutic value. Nat Rev Neurosci 2002;3:383-94.
46. Pasini B, Borrello MG, Greco A, Bongarzone I, Luo Y, Mondellini P et al. Loss of function effect of RET mutations causing Hirschsprung's disease. Nat Genet 1995;10:35-40.
47. Iwashita T, Murakami H, Asai N, Takahashi M. Mechanism of ret dysfunction by Hirschsprung's mutations affecting its extracellular domain. Hum Mol Genet 1996;5:1577-80.
48. Pelet A, Geneste O, Edery P, Pasini A, Chappuis S, Atti T et al. Various mechanisms cause RET-mediated signaling defects in Hirschsprung's disease. J Clin Invest 1998;101:1415-23.
49. Geneste O, Bidaud C, De Vita G, Hofstra RM, Tartare-Deckert S, Buys CH et al. Two distinct mutations of the RET receptor causing Hirschsprung's disease impair the binding of signalling effectors to a multifunctional docking site. Hum Mol Genet 1999; 8:1989-99.
50. Iwashita T, Kurokawa K, Qiao S, Murakami H, Asai N, Kawai K, et al. Functional analysis of RET with Hirschsprung's mutations affecting its kinase domain. Gastroenterology 2001;121:24-33.
51. Auricchio A, Griseri P, Carpentieri ML, Betsos N, Staiano A, Tozzi A, et al. Double heterozygosity for a RET substitution interfering with splicing and an EDNRB missense mutation in Hirschsprung's disease. Am J Hum Genet 1999;64:1216-21.
52. Kashuk CS, Stone EA, Grice EA, Portnoy ME, Green ED, Sidow A, et al. Phenotype-genotype correlation in Hirschsprung's disease is illuminated by comparative analysis of the RET protein sequence. Proc Natl Acad Sci USA 2005;102:8949-54.
53. Edery P, Pelet A, Mulligan LM, Abel L, Attie T, Dow E et al. Long segment and short segment familial Hirschsprung's disease: variable clinical expression at the RET locus. J Med Genet 1994;31:602-06.
54. Yin L, Barone V, Seri M, Bolino A, Bocciardi R, Ceccherini I et al. Heterogeneity and low detection rate of RET mutations in Hirschsprung's disease. Eur J Hum Genet 1994;2:272-80.
55. Angrist M, Bolk S, Thiel B, Puffenberger EG, Hofstra RM, Buys CH et al. Mutation analysis of the RET receptor tyrosine kinase in Hirschsprung's disease. Hum Mol Genet 1995;4:821-30.
56. Attie T, Pelet A, Edery P, Eng C, Mulligan LM, Amiel J et al. Diversity of RET proto-oncogene mutations in familial and sporadic Hirschsprung's disease. Hum Mol Genet 1995;4:1381-86.
57. Yin L, Seri M, Barone V, Tocco T, Scaranari M, Romeo G. Prevalence and parental origin of de novo RET mutations in Hirschsprung's disease. Eur J Hum Genet 1996;4:356-58.
58. Kusafuka T, Wang Y, Puri P. Mutation analysis of the RET, the endothelin-B receptor, and the endothelin-3 genes in sporadic cases of Hirschsprung's disease. J Pediatr Surg 1997;32:501-04.
59. Svensson PJ, Molander ML, Eng C, Anvret M, Nordenskjold A. Low frequency of RET mutations in Hirschsprung's disease in Sweden. Clin Genet 1998;54:39-44.
60. Inoue K, Shimotake T, Iwai N. Mutational analysis of RET/GDNF/NTN genes in children with total colonic aganglionosis with small bowel involvement. Am J Med Genet 2000;93:278-84.
61. Hofstra RM, Wu Y, Stulp RP, Elfferich P, Osinga J, Maas SM et al. RET and GDNF gene scanning in Hirschsprung's patients using two dual denaturing gel systems. Hum Mutat 2000;15:418-29.
62. Sancandi M, Ceccherini I, Costa M, Fava M, Chen B, Wu Y et al. Incidence of RET mutations in patients with Hirschsprung's disease. J Pediatr Surg 2000;35:139-42.
63. Julies MG, Moore SW, Kotze MJ, du PL. Novel RET mutations in Hirschsprung's disease patients from the diverse South African population. Eur J Hum Genet 2001;9:419-23.
64. Seri M, Yin L, Barone V, Bolino A, Celli I, Bocciardi R et al. Frequency of RET mutations in long- and short-segment Hirschsprung's disease. Hum Mutat 1997;9:243-49.
65. Li JC, Ding SP, Song Y, Li MJ. Mutation of RET gene in Chinese patients with Hirschsprung's disease. World J Gastroenterol 2002;8:1108-11.
66. Solari V, Ennis S, Yoneda A, Wong L, Messineo A, Hollwarth ME et al. Mutation analysis of the RET gene in

66. total intestinal aganglionosis by wave DNA fragment analysis system. J Pediatr Surg 2003;38:497-501.
67. Gath R, Goessling A, Keller KM, Koletzko S, Coerdt W, Muntefering H et al. Analysis of the RET, GDNF, EDN3, and EDNRB genes in patients with intestinal neuronal dysplasia and Hirschsprung's disease. Gut 2001;48:671-75.
68. Garcia-Barcelo M, Sham MH, Lee WS, Lui VC, Chen BL, Wong KK et al. Highly Recurrent RET Mutations and Novel Mutations in Genes of the Receptor Tyrosine Kinase and Endothelin Receptor B Pathways in Chinese Patients with Sporadic Hirschsprung's Disease. Clin Chem 2004;50:93-100.
69. Bolk S, Pelet A, Hofstra RM, Angrist M, Salomon R, Croaker D et al. A human model for multigenic inheritance: phenotypic expression in Hirschsprung's disease requires both the RET gene and a new 9q31 locus. Proc Natl Acad Sci USA 2000;97:268-73.
70. Borrego S, Saez ME, Ruiz A, Gimm O, Lopez-Alonso M, Antinolo G et al. Specific polymorphisms in the RET proto-oncogene are over-represented in patients with Hirschsprung's disease and may represent loci modifying phenotypic expression. J Med Genet 1999;36:771-74.
71. Fitze G, Schreiber M, Kuhlisch E, Schackert HK, Roesner D. Association of RET protooncogene codon 45 polymorphism with Hirschsprung's disease. Am J Hum Genet 1999;65:1469-73.
72. Ceccherini I, Hofstra RM, Luo Y, Stulp RP, Barone V, Stelwagen T, et al. DNA polymorphisms and conditions for SSCP analysis of the 20 exons of the ret proto-oncogene. Oncogene 1994;9:3025-29.
73. Garcia-Barcelo MM, Sham MH, Lui VC, Chen BL, Song YQ, Lee WS, et al. Chinese patients with sporadic Hirschsprung's disease are predominantly represented by a single RET haplotype. J Med Genet 2003;40:e122.
74. Fitze G, Cramer J, Ziegler A, Schierz M, Schreiber M, Kuhlisch E, et al. Association between c135G/A genotype and RET proto-oncogene germline mutations and phenotype of Hirschsprung's disease. Lancet 2002;359:1200-05.
75. Griseri P, Pesce B, Patrone G, Osinga J, Puppo F, Sancandi M, et al. A rare haplotype of the RET proto-oncogene is a risk-modifying allele in hirschsprung's disease. Am J Hum Genet 2002;71:969-74.
76. Borrego S, Wright FA, Fernandez RM, Williams N, Lopez-Alonso M, Davuluri R, et al. A founding locus within the RET proto-oncogene may account for a large proportion of apparently sporadic Hirschsprung's disease and a subset of cases of sporadic medullary thyroid carcinoma. Am J Hum Genet 2003;72:88-100.
77. Borrego S, Ruiz A, Saez ME, Gimm O, Gao X, Lopez-Alonso M, et al. RET genotypes comprising specific haplotypes of polymorphic variants predispose to isolated Hirschsprung's disease. J Med Genet 2000;37:572-78.
78. Fitze G, Appelt H, Konig IR, Gorgens H, Stein U, Walther W et al. Functional haplotypes of the RET proto-oncogene promoter are associated with Hirschsprung's disease (HSCR). Hum Mol Genet 2003;12:3207-14.
79. Sancandi M, Griseri P, Pesce B, Patrone G, Puppo F, Lerone M et al. Single nucleotide polymorphic alleles in the 5' region of the RET proto-oncogene define a risk haplotype in Hirschsprung's disease. J Med Genet 2003; 40:714-18.
80. Garcia-Barcelo M, Ganster RW, Lui VC, Leon TY, So MT, Lau AM et al. TTF-1 and RET promoter SNPs: regulation of RET transcription in Hirschsprung's disease. Hum Mol Genet 2005;14:191-204.
81. Burzynski GM, Nolte IM, Osinga J, Ceccherini I, Twigt B, Maas S, et al. Localizing a putative mutation as the major contributor to the development of sporadic Hirschsprung's disease to the RET genomic sequence between the promoter region and exon 2. Eur J Hum Genet 2004;12:604-12.
82. Burzynski GM, Nolte IM, Bronda A, Bos KK, Osinga J, Plaza M, I et al. Identifying candidate Hirschsprung's disease-associated RET variants. Am J Hum Genet 2005;76:850-58.
83. Emison ES, McCallion AS, Kashuk CS, Bush RT, Grice E, Lin S et al. A common sex-dependent mutation in a RET enhancer underlies Hirschsprung's disease risk. Nature 2005;434:857-63.
84. Garcia-Barcelo MM, Lau DK, Ngan ES, Leon TY, Liu T, So M, et al. Evaluation of the NK2 homeobox 1 gene (NKX2-1) as a Hirschsprung's disease locus. Ann Hum Genet 2008;72:170-77.
85. Garcia-Barcelo MM, Sham MH, Lui VC, Chen BL, Song YQ, Lee WS et al. Chinese patients with sporadic Hirschsprung's disease are predominantly represented by a single RET haplotype. J Med Genet 2003;40:e122.
86. Moore MW, Klein RD, Farinas I, Sauer H, Armanini M, Phillips H et al. Renal and neuronal abnormalities in mice lacking GDNF. Nature 1996;382:76-79.
87. Enomoto H, Araki T, Jackman A, Heuckeroth RO, Snider WD, Johnson EM, Jr. et al. GFR alpha1-deficient mice have deficits in the enteric nervous system and kidneys. Neuron 1998;21:317-24.
88. Shen L, Pichel JG, Mayeli T, Sariola H, Lu B, Westphal H. GDNF haploinsufficiency causes Hirschsprung-like intestinal obstruction and early-onset lethality in mice. Am J Hum Genet 2002;70:435-47.
89. Angrist M, Bolk S, Halushka M, Lapchak PA, Chakravarti A. Germline mutations in glial cell line-derived neurotrophic factor (GDNF) and RET in a Hirschsprung's disease patient. Nat Genet 1996;14:341-44.
90. Doray B, Salomon R, Amiel J, Pelet A, Touraine R, Billaud M et al. Mutation of the RET ligand, neurturin, supports multigenic inheritance in Hirschsprung's disease. Hum Mol Genet 1998; 7:1449-52.
91. Myers SM, Salomon R, Goessling A, Pelet A, Eng C, von Deimling A et al. Investigation of germline GFR alpha-1 mutations in Hirschsprung's disease. J Med Genet 1999;36:217-20.
92. Salomon R, Attie T, Pelet A, Bidaud C, Eng C, Amiel J et al. Germline mutations of the RET ligand GDNF are not sufficient to cause Hirschsprung's disease. Nat Genet 1996;14:345-47.

93. Ivanchuk SM, Myers SM, Eng C, Mulligan LM. De novo mutation of GDNF, ligand for the RET/GDNFR-alpha receptor complex, in Hirschsprung's disease. Hum Mol Genet 1996; 5:2023-26.
94. Eketjall S, Ibanez CF. Functional characterization of mutations in the GDNF gene of patients with Hirschsprung's disease. Hum Mol Genet 2002;11:325-29.
95. Borghini S, Bocciardi R, Bonardi G, Matera I, Santamaria G, Ravazzolo R et al. Hirschsprung's associated GDNF mutations do not prevent RET activation. Eur J Hum Genet 2002;10:183-87.
96. Lang D, Epstein JA. SOX10 and PAX3 physically interact to mediate activation of a conserved c-RET enhancer. Hum Mol Genet 2003;12:937-45.
97. Lang D, Chen F, Milewski R, Li J, Lu MM, Epstein JA. PAX3 is required for enteric ganglia formation and functions with SOX10 to modulate expression of C-RET. J Clin Invest 2000;106:963-71.
98. Zhu L, Lee HO, Jordan CS, Cantrell VA, Southard-Smith EM, Shin MK. Spatiotemporal regulation of endothelin receptor-B by SOX10 in neural crest-derived enteric neuron precursors. Nat Genet 2004;36:732-37.
99. Cantrell VA, Owens SE, Chandler RL, Airey DC, Bradley KM, Smith JR et al. Interactions between SOX10 and EDNRB modulate penetrance and severity of aganglionosis in the SOX10DOM mouse model of Hirschsprung's disease. Hum Mol Genet 2004,13:2289-301.
100. Lane PW, Liu HM. Association of megacolon with a new dominant spotting gene (Dom) in the mouse. J Hered 1984;75:435-39.
101. Southard-Smith EM, Angrist M, Ellison JS, Agarwala R, Baxevanis AD, Chakravarti A, et al. The SOX10(Dom) mouse: modeling the genetic variation of Waardenburg-Shah (WS4) syndrome. Genome Res 1999;9:215-25.
102. Southard-Smith EM, Kos L, Pavan WJ. SOX10 mutation disrupts neural crest development in Dom Hirschsprung mouse model. Nat Genet 1998;18:60-64.
103. Pingault V, Puliti A, Prehu MO, Samadi A, Bondurand N, Goossens M. Human homology and candidate genes for the Dominant megacolon locus, a mouse model of Hirschsprung's disease. Genomics 1997;39:86-89.
104. Herbarth B, Pingault V, Bondurand N, Kuhlbrodt K, Hermans-Borgmeyer I, Puliti A et al. Mutation of the Sry-related SOX10 gene in Dominant megacolon, a mouse model for human Hirschsprung's disease. Proc Natl Acad Sci USA 1998;95:5161-65.
105. Pingault V, Bondurand N, Kuhlbrodt K, Goerich DE, Prehu MO, Puliti A et al. SOX10 mutations in patients with Waardenburg-Hirschsprung disease. Nat Genet 1998;18:171-73.
106. Pingault V, Guiochon-Mantel A, Bondurand N, Faure C, Lacroix C, Lyonnet S, et al. Peripheral neuropathy with hypomyelination, chronic intestinal pseudo-obstruction and deafness: a developmental "neural crest syndrome" related to a SOX10 mutation. Ann Neurol 2000;48:671-76.
107. Pingault V, Girard M, Bondurand N, Dorkins H, Van Maldergem L, Mowat D et al. SOX10 mutations in chronic intestinal pseudo-obstruction suggest a complex physiopathological mechanism. Hum Genet 2002;111:198-206.
108. Touraine RL, Attie-Bitach T, Manceau E, Korsch E, Sarda P, Pingault V et al. Neurological phenotype in Waardenburg syndrome type 4 correlates with novel SOX10 truncating mutations and expression in developing brain. Am J Hum Genet 2000;66:1496-503.
109. Inoue K, Shilo K, Boerkoel CF, Crowe C, Sawady J, Lupski JR et al. Congenital hypomyelinating neuropathy, central dysmyelination, and Waardenburg-Hirschsprung disease: phenotypes linked by SOX10 mutation. Ann Neurol 2002;52:836-42.
110. Inoue K, Tanabe Y, Lupski JR. Myelin deficiencies in both the central and the peripheral nervous systems associated with a SOX10 mutation. Ann Neurol 1999;46:313-18.
111. Sham MH, Lui VC, Chen BL, Fu M, Tam PK. Novel mutations of SOX10 suggest a dominant negative role in Waardenburg-Shah syndrome. J Med Genet 2001;38:E30.
112. Bondurand N, Kuhlbrodt K, Pingault V, Enderich J, Sajus M, Tommerup N et al. A molecular analysis of the yemenite deaf-blind hypopigmentation syndrome: SOX10 dysfunction causes different neurocristopathies. Hum Mol Genet 1999; 8:1785-89.
113. Dubreuil V, Hirsch MR, Pattyn A, Brunet JF, Goridis C. The PHOX2B transcription factor coordinately regulates neuronal cell cycle exit and identity. Development 2000;127:5191-201.
114. Pattyn A, Morin X, Cremer H, Goridis C, Brunet JF. The homeobox gene PHOX2B is essential for the development of autonomic neural crest derivatives. Nature 1999; 399:366-70.
115. Benailly HK, Lapierre JM, Laudier B, Amiel J, Attie T, De Blois MC, et al. PMX2B, a new candidate gene for Hirschsprung's disease. Clin Genet 2003;64:204-09.
116. Garcia-Barcelo M, Sham MH, Lui VC, Chen BL, Ott J, Tam PK. Association study of PHOX2B as a candidate gene for Hirschsprung's disease. Gut 2003;52:563-67.
117. Miao X, Garcia-Barcelo MM, So MT, Leon TY, Lau DK, Liu TT et al. Role of RET and PHOX2B gene polymorphisms in risk of Hirschsprung's disease in Chinese population. Gut 2007;56:736.
118. Trochet D, Bourdeaut F, Janoueix-Lerosey I, Deville A, de PL, Schleiermacher G, et al. Germline mutations of the paired-like homeobox 2B (PHOX2B) gene in neuroblastoma. Am J Hum Genet 2004;74:761-64.
119. Perri P, Bachetti T, Longo L, Matera I, Seri M, Tonini GP et al. PHOX2B mutations and genetic predisposition to neuroblastoma. Oncogene 2005;24:3050-53.
120. Amiel J, Laudier B, ttie-Bitach T, Trang H, de PL, Gener B et al. Polyalanine expansion and frameshift mutations of the paired-like homeobox gene PHOX2B in congenital central hypoventilation syndrome. Nat Genet 2003;33:459-61.
121. Bachetti T, Matera I, Borghini S, Di DM, Ravazzolo R, Ceccherini I. Distinct pathogenetic mechanisms for PHOX2B associated polyalanine expansions and

121. frameshift mutations in congenital central hypoventilation syndrome. Hum Mol Genet 2005;14:1815-24.
122. Verloes A, Elmer C, Lacombe D, Heinrichs C, Rebuffat E, Demarquez JL et al. Ondine-Hirschsprung syndrome (Haddad syndrome). Further delineation in two cases and review of the literature. Eur J Pediatr 1993;152:75-77.
123. Hosoda K, Hammer RE, Richardson JA, Baynash AG, Cheung JC, Giaid A, et al. Targeted and natural (piebald-lethal) mutations of endothelin-B receptor gene produce megacolon associated with spotted coat color in mice. Cell 1994;79:1267-76.
124. Baynash AG, Hosoda K, Giaid A, Richardson JA, Emoto N, Hammer RE, et al. Interaction of endothelin-3 with endothelin-B receptor is essential for development of epidermal melanocytes and enteric neurons. Cell 1994;79:1277-85.
125. Puffenberger EG, Kauffman ER, Bolk S, Matise TC, Washington SS, Angrist M, et al. Identity-by-descent and association mapping of a recessive gene for Hirschsprung's disease on human chromosome 13q22. Hum Mol Genet 1994;3:1217-25.
126. Puffenberger EG, Hosoda K, Washington SS, Nakao K, deWit D, Yanagisawa M, et al. A missense mutation of the endothelin-B receptor gene in multigenic Hirschsprung's disease. Cell 1994;79:1257-66.
127. Attie T, Till M, Pelet A, Amiel J, Edery P, Boutrand L et al. Mutation of the endothelin-receptor B gene in Waardenburg-Hirschsprung disease. Hum Mol Genet 1995;4:2407-09.
128. Verheij JB, Kunze J, Osinga J, van Essen AJ, Hofstra RM. ABCD syndrome is caused by a homozygous mutation in the EDNRB gene. Am J Med Genet 2002;108:223-25.
129. Sakai T, Nirasawa Y, Itoh Y, Wakizaka A. Japanese patients with sporadic Hirschsprung: mutation analysis of the receptor tyrosine kinase proto-oncogene, endothelin-B receptor, endothelin-3, glial cell line-derived neurotrophic factor and neurturin genes: a comparison with similar studies. Eur J Pediatr 2000;159:160-67.
130. Amiel J, Attie T, Jan D, Pelet A, Edery P, Bidaud C et al. Heterozygous endothelin receptor B (EDNRB) mutations in isolated Hirschsprung's disease. Hum Mol Genet 1996;5:355-57.
131. Tanaka H, Moroi K, Iwai J, Takahashi H, Ohnuma N, Hori S et al. Novel mutations of the endothelin B receptor gene in patients with Hirschsprung's disease and their characterization. J Biol Chem 1998;273:11378-83.
132. Kusafuka T, Wang Y, Puri P. Novel mutations of the endothelin-B receptor gene in isolated patients with Hirschsprung's disease. Hum Mol Genet 1996; 5:347-49.
133. Kusafuka T, Puri P. Mutations of the endothelin-B receptor and endothelin-3 genes in Hirschsprung's disease. Pediatr Surg Int 1997;12:19-23.
134. Auricchio A, Casari G, Staiano A, Ballabio A. Endothelin-B receptor mutations in patients with isolated Hirschsprung's disease from a non-inbred population. Hum Mol Genet 1996;5:351-54.
135. Abe Y, Sakurai T, Yamada T, Nakamura T, Yanagisawa M, Goto K. Functional analysis of five endothelin-B receptor mutations found in human Hirschsprung's disease patients. Biochem Biophys Res Commun 2000;275:524-31.
136. Fuchs S, Amiel J, Claudel S, Lyonnet S, Corvol P, Pinet F. Functional characterization of three mutations of the endothelin B receptor gene in patients with Hirschsprung's disease: evidence for selective loss of Gi coupling. Mol Med 2001;7:115-24.
137. Svensson PJ, Von Tell D, Molander ML, Anvret M, Nordenskjold A. A heterozygous frameshift mutation in the endothelin-3 (EDN-3) gene in isolated Hirschsprung's disease. Pediatr Res 1999;45:714-17.
138. Bidaud C, Salomon R, Van Camp G, Pelet A, Attie T, Eng C et al. Endothelin-3 gene mutations in isolated and syndromic Hirschsprung's disease. Eur J Hum Genet 1997;5:247-51.
139. Edery P, Attie T, Amiel J, Pelet A, Eng C, Hofstra RM et al. Mutation of the endothelin-3 gene in the Waardenburg-Hirschsprung disease (Shah-Waardenburg syndrome). Nat Genet 1996;12:442-46.
140. Hofstra RM, Osinga J, Tan-Sindhunata G, Wu Y, Kamsteeg EJ, Stulp RP, et al. A homozygous mutation in the endothelin-3 gene associated with a combined Waardenburg type 2 and Hirschsprung phenotype (Shah-Waardenburg syndrome). Nat Genet 1996;12:445-47.
141. Yanagisawa H, Yanagisawa M, Kapur RP, Richardson JA, Williams SC, Clouthier DE, et al. Dual genetic pathways of endothelin-mediated intercellular signaling revealed by targeted disruption of endothelin converting enzymel gene. Development 1998;125:825-36.
142. Hofstra RM, Valdenaire O, Arch E, Osinga J, Kroes H, Loffler BM et al. A loss-of-function mutation in the endothelin-converting enzyme 1 (ECE-1) associated with Hirschsprung's disease, cardiac defects, and autonomic dysfunction. Am J Hum Genet 1999;64:304-08.
143. Leibl MA, Ota T, Woodward MN, Kenny SE, Lloyd DA, Vaillant CR et al. Expression of endothelin 3 by mesenchymal cells of embryonic mouse caecum. Gut 1999;44:246-52.
144. Sidebotham EL, Woodward MN, Kenny SE, Lloyd DA, Vaillant CR, Edgar DH. Localization and endothelin-3 dependence of stem cells of the enteric nervous system in the embryonic colon. J Pediatr Surg 2002;37:145-50.
145. Wakamatsu N, Yamada Y, Yamada K, Ono T, Nomura N, Taniguchi H et al. Mutations in SIP1, encoding Smad interacting protein-1, cause a form of Hirschsprung's disease. Nat Genet 2001;27:369-70.
146. Mowat DR, Croaker GD, Cass DT, Kerr BA, Chaitow J, Ades LC et al. Hirschsprung's disease, microcephaly, mental retardation, and characteristic facial features: delineation of a new syndrome and identification of a locus at chromosome 2q22-q23. J Med Genet 1998;35:617-23.
147. Garavelli L, Donadio A, Zanacca C, Banchini G, Della GE, Bertani G et al. Hirschsprung's disease, mental retardation,

characteristic facial features, and mutation in the gene ZFHX1B (SIP1): confirmation of the Mowat-Wilson syndrome. Am J Med Genet 2003;116A:385-88.
148. Cerruti MP, Pastore G, Zweier C, Rauch A. Mowat-Wilson syndrome and mutation in the zinc finger homeo box 1B gene: a well defined clinical entity. J Med Genet 2004;41:E16.
149. van Biesen T, Hawes BE, Luttrell DK, Krueger KM, Touhara K, Porfiri E, et al. Receptor-tyrosine-kinase- and G beta gamma-mediated MAP kinase activation by a common signalling pathway. Nature 1995;376:781-84.
150. Bolk S, Pelet A, Hofstra RM, Angrist M, Salomon R, Croaker D et al. A human model for multigenic inheritance: phenotypic expression in Hirschsprung's disease requires both the RET gene and a new 9q31 locus. Proc Natl Acad Sci USA 2000;97:268-73.
151. Garcia-Barcelo MM, Fong PY, Tang CS, Miao XP, So MT, Yuan ZW et al. Mapping of a Hirschsprung's disease locus in 3p21. Eur J Hum Genet 2008;16:833-40.
152. Murone M, Rosenthal A, de Sauvage FJ. Hedgehog signal transduction: from flies to vertebrates. Exp Cell Res 1999;253:25-33.
153. Ramalho-Santos M, Melton DA, McMahon AP. Hedgehog signals regulate multiple aspects of gastrointestinal development. Development 2000;127:2763-72.
154. Gao B, Guo J, She C, Shu A, Yang M, Tan Z, et al. Mutations in IHH, encoding Indian hedgehog, cause brachydactyly type A-1. Nat Genet 2001;28:386-88.
155. Hellemans J, Coucke PJ, Giedion A, De Paepe A, Kramer P, Beemer F et al. Homozygous mutations in IHH cause acrocapitofemoral dysplasia, an autosomal recessive disorder with cone-shaped epiphyses in hands and hips. Am J Hum Genet 2003;72:1040-46.
156. Garcia-Barcelo MM, Lee WS, Sham MH, Lui VC, Tam PK. Is there a role for the IHH gene in Hirschsprung's disease? Neurogastroenterol Motil 2003;15:663-68.
157. Faissner A, Kruse J, Nieke J, Schachner M. Expression of neural cell adhesion molecule L1 during development, in neurological mutants and in the peripheral nervous system. Brain Res 1984;317:69-82.
158. Van Camp G, Vits L, Coucke P, Lyonnet S, Schrander-Stumpel C, Darby J et al. A duplication in the L1CAM gene associated with X-linked hydrocephalus. Nat Genet 1993;4:421-25.
159. Parisi MA, Kapur RP, Neilson I, Hofstra RM, Holloway LW, Michaelis RC et al. Hydrocephalus and intestinal aganglionosis: is L1CAM a modifier gene in Hirschsprung's disease? Am J Med Genet 2002;108:51-56.
160. Okamoto N, Wada Y, Goto M. Hydrocephalus and Hirschsprung's disease in a patient with a mutation of L1CAM. J Med Genet 1997; 34:670-71.
161. Hofstra RM, Elfferich P, Osinga J, Verlind E, Fransen E, Lopez PJ et al. Hirschsprung's disease and L1CAM: is the disturbed sex ratio caused by L1CAM mutations? J Med Genet 2002;39:E11.
162. Lui VC, Cheng WW, Leon TY, Lau DK, Garcia-Bareclo MM, Miao XP, et al. Perturbation of HOXB5 signaling in vagal neural crests down-regulates ret leading to intestinal hypoganglionosis in mice. Gastroenterology 2008;134: 1104-15.
163. Badner JA, Sieber WK, Garver KL, Chakravarti A. A genetic study of Hirschsprung's disease. Am J Hum Genet 1990;46:568-80.
164. Borst MJ, VanCamp JM, Peacock ML, Decker RA. Mutational analysis of multiple endocrine neoplasia type 2A associated with Hirschsprung's disease. Surgery 1995;117:386-91.
165. Mulligan LM, Eng C, Attie T, Lyonnet S, Marsh DJ, Hyland VJ et al. Diverse phenotypes associated with exon 10 mutations of the RET proto-oncogene. Hum Mol Genet 1994;3:2163-67.
166. Reynolds LF, Eng C. RET mutations in multiple endocrine neoplasia type 2 and Hirschsprung's disease. Curr Opin Pediatr 1995; 7:702-09.
167. Cosma MP, Panariello L, Quadro L, Dathan NA, Fattoruso O, Colantuoni V. A mutation in the RET proto-oncogene in Hirschsprung's disease affects the tyrosine kinase activity associated with multiple endocrine neoplasia type 2A and 2B. Biochem J 1996; 314 (Pt 2):397-400.
168. Inoue K, Shimotake T, Inoue K, Tokiwa K, Iwai N. Mutational analysis of the RET proto-oncogene in a kindred with multiple endocrine neoplasia type 2A and Hirschsprung's disease. J Pediatr Surg 1999;34:1552-54.
169. Romeo G, Ceccherini I, Celli J, Priolo M, Betsos N, Bonardi G et al. Association of multiple endocrine neoplasia type 2 and Hirschsprung's disease. J Intern Med 1998;243:515-20.
170. Sijmons RH, Hofstra RM, Wijburg FA, Links TP, Zwierstra RP, Vermey A et al. Oncological implications of RET gene mutations in Hirschsprung's disease. Gut 1998;43:542-47.
171. Fu M, Lui VC, Sham MH, Pachnis V, Tam PK. Sonic Hedgehog regulates the proliferation, differentiation and migration of enteric neural crest cells in gut. Journal Cell Biology 2004;166:673-84.
172. Ngan ES, Lee KY, Sit FY, Poon HC, Chan JK, Sham MH, et al. Prokineticin-1 modulates proliferation and differentiation of enteric neural crest cells. Biochim Biophys Acta 2007;1773;536-45.

Duhamel's Pull-through Using Staplers

SN Oak, Prakash Agarwal

HISTORY

Bernard Duhamel first described his operation for Hirschsprung's disease in 1956.[1] This was described as a Modification of Swenson's procedure.[1-3] In the original procedure, a retrorectal approach was used, and a significant portion of the aganglionic rectum had to be left behind. The rationale for this operation was the ease of surgery, prevention of anastomotic leak and elimination of strictures. As no anterior rectal resection was involved sensory innervation was left undisturbed. The operative principle of this technique included minimal pelvic dissection, a wide but unsutured approximation (anastomosis) between aganglionic rectum and the pulled through ganglionic colon, a retrorectal approach, division of the internal anal sphincter and the preservation of anterior rectal wall.[3,4]

Duhamel devised this operation with an intention to apply this procedure earlier in infancy. However, the retention of the rectal spur, development of a rectal pouch, continuance of constipation, fecoloma impaction and incontinence were reported as the significant complications. This was followed by several modifications of Duhamel's procedure. Most of these modifications were centered around the elimination of the common wall of the rectal pouch "spur" and the effect of the stool filled blind rectal pouch (within the aganglionic rectal wall). Martin and Altemeier and Martin and Caudill described the technique to apply the clamps meticulously and eliminate the problem of rectal pouch completely.[5,6] Over the years, the surgeons have used many instruments like Kocher's forceps, crushing intestinal clamps and Lloyd-Davies crushing clamp to achieve the same purpose.[7] A modification of heavy Kocher's clamp was designed by Dr Irani and this has been in practice for nearly three decades. Dr Kittur designed a stainless steel clip having two prongs revetted at one end and free at the other. The free ends have a flange to accommodate a latex band when the two prongs are mated. The clip bears a pelvic curve and serrations to crush the opposing surfaces of the "spur".[7] Application of mechanical stapling device to the colorectal anastomosis and the simultaneous division of the common rectal was facilitated by Ikeda, Soper, Talbert and Ravitch.[8-10] This is the most commonly adapted technique for Duhamel's Pull through procedure these days and barring the cost of staplers, has several advantages including the convenience to the patient.

MANAGEMENT

The conventional management of Hirschsprung's disease is staged. There are reports of primary one stage pull through Soave or modified Duhamel's procedures without a diverting colostomy; still most of the centers worldwide confine themselves to a diverting colostomy as the first stage. Rectal biopsy confirms aganglionosis and a definitive pull through (modified Duhamel) is planned when the patient weighs 8-10 kg. The optimal age for the procedure is about 9-12 months.

With the help of a Proximate Linear Cutter device (TLC55), it is possible to perform the operation by the age of 6-7 months. Younger age does at times pose difficulty in accommodating Proximate Linear Cutter in the pelvis. Our preference of Duhamel's procedure is due to its technical ease, less morbid complications and preservation of sensory nerves and receptors along the anterior wall of rectum. The anterior pelvic extrarectal nerves to the bladder and ejaculatory mechanisms are also protected with the application of staplers, it is suggested that a definitive pull through can be done even without a diverting colostomy but in our series uptil now, we have always employed a proximal diverting stoma.

The child is anesthetized with an endotracheal general anesthesia. An epidural regional block is given to ensure postoperative analgesia. The child is catheterized with a size 8 Fr or 10 Fr indwelling Foley catheter. Abdomen is opened through a left lower quadrant curvilinear incision. On opening of the peritoneum, multiple seromuscular biopsies are taken from the zones of lowermost left normal colon, zone of transition and the distal most dilated part of bowel (Fig.121.1).The fold of peritoneum at the rectosigmoid junction is incised on either side and the rectum is mobilized. Ureters on both sides are identified and protected. The vascular supply to the aganglionic rectosigmoid is identified and divided. Anterior traction on the rectum allows an entry into retrorectal space. The space is explored by a blunt finger dissection and adequate tunnel is created to admit a retrorectal colon. This dissection is mostly carried down caudally and the finger is made to project in the posterior rectal wall at the anorectal junction. The proximal ganglionic colon is divided from the aganglionic intestine that will be resected later in the procedure. The mesenteric and the antimesenteric sides of colon are marked with different color stay sutures so that orientation can be secured at the time of pull-through.

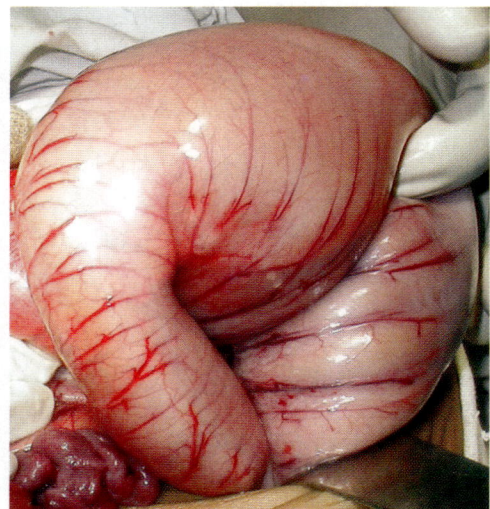

Fig. 121.1: Operative photograph depicting dilated bowel in Hirschsprung's disease

Attention is now directed towards the abdomen. The vessels are ligated proximally towards the root of the mesentery; keeping the mesenteric arterial arcades intact. Usually ligation of two vessels gives adequate length and pliability for the ganglionic colon and mesentery to be pulled through the retrorectal space. The vascularity of the distal most part of ganglionic colon is ensured, by confirming the presence of pulsations through the mesenteric arcades and the peristalsis of the segment, before ligating and cutting the taught vessels towards the root on mesentery. It is also essential not to keep the bulky mesentery near the bowel to be pulled through, otherwise accommodating this bulk in the retrorectal space becomes difficult.

A finger is now reinserted into newly created retrorectal tunnel and made to project in the posterior anorectal junction 1 cm above the dentate line. An electrocautery makes an incision at this level and an intestinal clamp or a grasper is passed through this incision to catch the ganglionic colon readied for pull through. It is easier to take two silk stay sutures at both lateral ends of this incised posterior rectal wall so that this wall of the spur does not retract upwards.

The grasper forceps introduced through the rent in the posterior rectal wall, is pushed upwards in the retrorectal tunnel, the ganglionic colon ready for pull through is held by the forceps and pulled through. This colon now appears at the anal verge (Figs 121.2A and B).

Mesenteric and antimesenteric borders must again be oriented and mesentery must be made to lie at 6 o' clock position. Color of the mucous membrane and fresh bleeding is confirmed. Pulled bowel is sutured (vicryl/PDS) full thickness into the anal zone from 3 o' clock to 9 o' clock position posteriorly and secured to anocutaneous junction. Thus, the rectum and the anterior wall of normal colon come to lie in close apposition and thus form a septum. From the perineal end, two red rubber tubes are passed, one each into the upper aganglionic bowel and the lower ganglionic bowel lumen through the anal opening.

A 3 cm transverse incision is now made in the anterior wall to the pulled through colon at the level of rectosigmoid junction. Two stay sutures are taken to hold the posterior wall of aganglionic rectum and anterior wall of pulled through colon at this newly made transverse incision. This forms the upper part of the "spur" to be cut.

1452 Pediatric Surgery—Diagnosis and Management

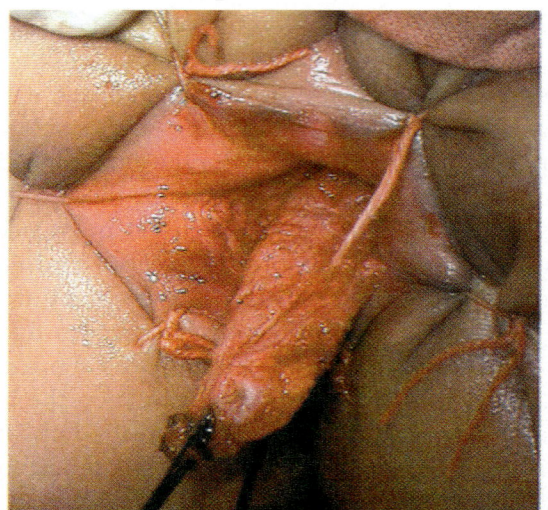

Fig. 121.2A: The ganglionated bowel is pulled the opening in the posterior rectal wall

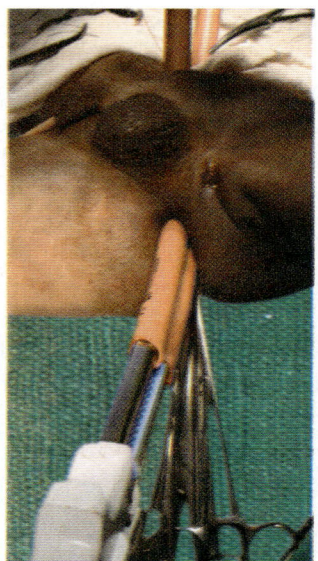

Fig. 121.3: Stapler being guided

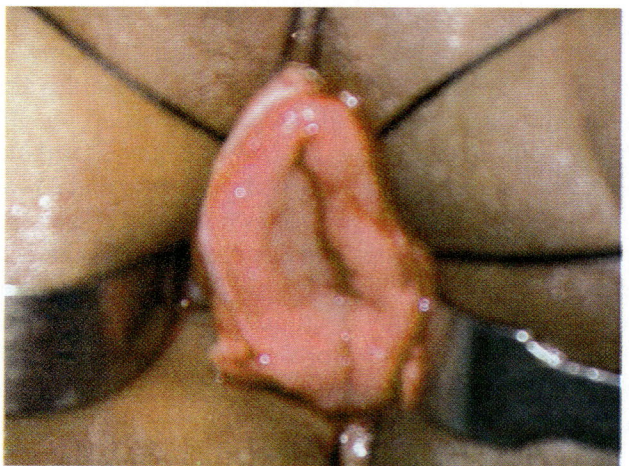

Fig. 121.2B: The pulled-through ganglionated bowel is oriented and anastomosed full thickness to the posterior rectal wall

confirm that the spur now lies in between the mated and locked halves of the cutter. The firing knob is now pushed ahead towards the locking lever all along the locking rib and returned back to its original return position in one single, smooth uninterrupted movement (Fig. 121.4). This movement brings the cutter into action and the spur is divided. At the same time, the staples are also fired from the cartridge and two parallel rows of staples create a longitudinal 5.5 cm of anastomosis between the rectum and the pulled colon. If the spur is too long, the apex of the spur may remain uncut. This can be easily divided with the help of an electrocautery and a colorectal anastomosis achieved by hand sewing with multiple

The red rubber catheters introduced from the anal end are now recovered at the abdominal end from the colon and rectum at the level of the upper end of 'spur'. Now a 55 mm Linear Cutter cartridge is chosen. Its orange colored staple retaining cap is removed and it is loaded on the cartridge half of TLC 55. Cartridge half of Proximate Linear Cutter is now railroaded with the red rubber tube in the posterior pulled through ganglionic colon (Fig. 121.3).

Anvil half is railroaded into anterior (upper) aganglionic rectum and inserted into the lumen. Both the halves are now made to project at the upper end; mated and the assembly is locked. The positioning of proximate linear cutter is now checked again to

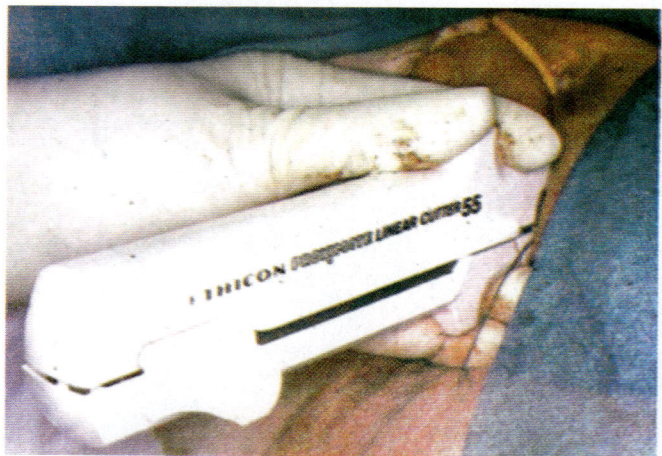

Fig. 121.4: Stapler being fired

interrupted 3-0/4-0 vicryl/PDS sutures. Alternatively a second TCR 55 mm cartridge can be fired from cranial end of spur to achieve cutting and suturing.

After the spur has been divided, the upper end anastomosis is completed between the rectum and the colotomy site at the rectosigmoid junction. This completely renders two bowels into one lumen and obviates the possibility of any residual rectal pouch.

A corrugated rubber drain is kept in the pelvis from abdominal side. Routinely there is no need to keep a retrorectal drain from the anal side. Seventy patients ranging from 6 months to 10 years have undergone this procedure during 1995-2002. The application of the Proximate Linear Cutter stapler device not only reduces the operation time but also ensures a stapled longitudinal anastomosis between the rectum and the pulled colon and provides an excellent hemostasis. Also, there is no bulky crushing clamp application which would otherwise stay in place for 5-7 days postoperatively, causing lot of inconvenience to the patient. Indwelling urinary catheter can be removed on 2nd postoperative day and the patients legs need not be tied together. The patient can therefore be ambulated on the second day.

It takes about 6-7 days for the opposing wall to get necrosed and natural adhesions to occur. We have recently modified our technique by using an Endo-Linear Cutter with a 45 mm length cartridge to crush the spur from anal end in patients with 5-6 months of age.

Patients who have internal diameter of rectum and the colon, smaller than the thickness of the locked assembly of Proximate Linear Cutter; we strongly recommend the use of Endo-Linear Cutter device. It is advisable neither to stretch nor to overdistend the bowel by forcing in the locked assembly to cut the spur.

Morbidity and mortality was assessed in 70 patients who had undergone modified Duhamel's pull-through with staplers. Episodes of enterocolitis were noted before and after colostomy and also before and after modified Duhamel's definitive procedure. Other complications noted included residual constipation, abdominal distension, and soiling.

Frank fecal incontinence was not seen in our series. Long-term problems of constipation, soiling and incontinence have been emphasized by Duhamel, Soave and Rehbein.[11-19] The various reported results for the Duhamel procedure are summarised in Table 121.1.

The potentials for sub optimal outcome are often associated with an anterior rectal pouch caused by a colorectal spur. Application of a Proximate Linear Cutter definitely reduces the percentage of sub optimal outcome. Constipation may also result from outlet obstruction caused by residual spasticity of the internal sphincter. Some of these patients would settle down with anal dilatation. Suggested explanations for sub optimal outcome after operation for Hirschsprung's disease include associated neuronal intestinal dysplasia significant neurological impairment and enterocolitis.[17,20,21]

Rectal achalasia is yet another reason which leads to increasing colonic inertia and ensuing symptoms of severe constipation. Modified Duhamel pull-through with staplers has also been employed in treating strictures and acquired aganglionosis following a Soave procedure.[20] Modified Duhamel's operation with Endo-linear cutter has also been used

Table 121.1: Outcome of Duhamel's procedure in various studies

Report	Patients	Outcome (Follow-up period < 6 years)
Hung[16]	198	100% Good Outcome
Duhamel[4]	270	3.7% constipation,
Marty[17]	91	100% continence
Foster[13]	43	12.1% Fecal soiling
Boemers et al[11]	11	100% asymptomatic 87% had lower urinary tract dysfunction.
Baillie CT et al[12]	91	Colonic Transit time was increased in recto sigmoid disease after pull through (80%). Satisfactory outcome (42%)
Yanagihara J et al[19]	36	Minimal anal bleeding due to GIA stapler– 6% Mild enterocolitis – 18%
Author's experience	70	2.8 % Constipation, 4.2 % Chronic Abdominal distension, 2.8 % Soiling. Lower urinary tract dysfunction 90% "Satisfactory" outcome 10%"Sub-optimal"outcome

as a primary definitive procedure in neonate and young infants.[22]

PRECAUTIONS WHILE STAPLING

1. Never force the halves of the instrument.
2. Halves must be properly mated.
3. Locking assembly must be checked before firing.
4. The septum (spur) to be cut must be included entirely within the firing range.
5. Staples are not designed to control bleeding from mesenteric vessels.
6. Inspect completeness of 'spur' cutting before closure of abdominal part of colorectal anastomosis.

PROBLEMS AND COMPLICATIONS OF STAPLERS

Mishaps are inherent in the use of devices as they are in all other aspects of surgery.

1. Technical failures
   a. Staples are not fired properly
   b. Many of the staples do not get engaged
   c. Stapler becomes locked, making their removal from the bowel difficult.
2. Staple-related bleeding.
3. Anastomotic leaks leading to pelvic abscess.

REFERENCES

1. Duhamel B. Une nouvelle operation pour le megacolon congenital: abaissement retrorectal et trans-anal du colon, et son application possible autraiteent de quelques autres malformations. Presse Med 1956;64:2249.
2. Duhamel B. Therapies Chirugicale infantile, Paris 1957.
3. Duhamel B. A new operation for the treatment of Hirschsprung's disease. Arch Dis Child 1960;35:38.
4. Duhamel B. Retrorectal and trans anal pull-through procedure the treatment of Hirschsprung's disease. Dis Colon Rectum 1964;7:455.
5. Martin LW, Altemeier WA. Clinical experience with a new operation (Modified Duhamel's procedure) for Hirschsprung's disease. Ann Surg 1962;156:678.
6. Martin LW, Perrin EV. Neonatal perforation of the appendix in association with Hirschsprung's disease; Ann Surg 1967;166:799.
7. Kittar D DK Clip. A new crushing instrument for use on Duhamel's Operation for Hirschsprung's Disease. Journal of Indian Assoc of Paed Surgeons 1997;2 (3+4):149-50.
8. Ikeda K. New technique in the surgical management of Hirschsprung's disease. Surgery 1967;61:503.
9. Soper RT. Surgery for Hirschsprung's disease, AORN J 1968;69.
10. Talbert JL, Seashore JH, Ravitch MM. Evaluation of a modified Duhamel operation for correction of Hirschsprung's disease. Ann Surg 1974;179:671.
11. Boemers TM, Bax NM, van Gool JD. The effect of Rectosigmiodectomy and Duhamel-type pull-through procedure on lower urinary tract function in children with Hirschsprung's disease. J Pediatr Surg 2001;36(3):453-56.
12. Baillie CT, Kenny SE, Rintala RJ, Booth JM, Lloyd DA. Long-term outcome and Colonic motility after the Duhamel procedure for Hirschsprung's disease. J Paediatr Surg 1999;34(2):325-29.
13. Foster P, Cowan G, Wrenn EL Jr. Twenty five years experience with Hirschsprung's disease. J Pediatr Surg 1990;25:531-34.
14. Hayashi A, Ishida H, Kamagata S, et al. Late complications of Hirschsprung's disease and anorectal manometry. Nippon Geka Gakkai Zasshi 1985;86:1290-92.
15. Heij HA, de Vries X, Bremer I, et al. Long term anorectal functions after Duhamel's Operation for Hirschsprung's disease. J Pediatr Surg 1995;30:430-32.
16. Hung W. Treatment of Hirschsprung's disease with a modified Duhamel-Grab Martin operation. J Pediatr Surg 1991;26:849-52.
17. Marty TL, Seo T, Matalk ME, et al. Gastrointestinal function after surgical correction of Hirschsprung's disease: long term follow-up in 135 patients. J Pediatr Surg 1995;30:655-58.
18. Tariq GM, Brereton RJ, Wright VM. Complications of endoanal pull through for Hirschsprung's disease. J Pediatr Surg 1993;26:1202-06.
19. Yanagihara J, Iwai N, Tokiwa K, Deguchi E, Shimotake T. Results of modified Duhamel operation for Hirschsprung's disease using the GIA stapler.
20. Langer JC. Repeat Pull through surgery for complicated Hirschsprung's disease: Indications, techniques and results. J Pediatr Surg 1999;34 (7);1136-41.
21. Moore S. W, Albertyn R, Cywes S. Clinical outcome and long term quality of life after surgical correction of Hirschsprung's disease. J Pediatr Surg 1996;31;1496-502.
22. Pierro A, Fasoli L, Keily EM, DraeD. Staged Pull-through for rectosigmoid Hirschsprung's disease is not safer than Primary pull through. J of Pediatr Surg 1997;32(3):505-09.

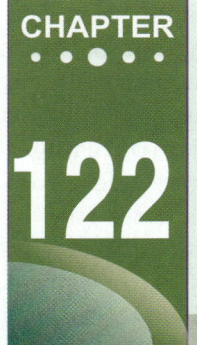

CHAPTER 122

Pediatric Laparoscopy

Anirudh Shah, Amar Shah

Laparoscopy as a diagnostic tool for abdominal viscera was recommended as early as 1901 by Kelling.[1] Almost 5 decades later, gynecologists were the first to use this technique. Laparoscopy was used as a diagnostic tool in the pediatric age group in the 1970's.[2-4] With advances in imaging however, the interest in diagnostic laparoscopy faded. It was only with the introduction of therapeutic techniques like cholecystectomy that surgeons started to take interest in the procedure. Previously an exploratory laparotomy was undertaken for diagnosis when simple investigative techniques or procedures were not adequate. In today's era, the indications for laparoscopy have remained the same as they were for laparotomy. A major advantage of laparoscopy however is that it therapeutic for most of its indications hence bringing about a significant reduction in the morbidity of the procedure.

INDICATIONS OF LAPAROSCOPY FOR ABDOMINAL PROBLEMS

- Acute abdominal pain
- Chronic abdominal pain
- Gastrointestinal bleeding
- Pathologies of the liver and biliary tree
- Oncology
- Trauma
- Ascites
- Determination of contralateral patent processus vaginalis in inguinal hernia
- Cryptorchidism
- Dysfunction of V-P Shunts or P-D catheters.

Laparoscopy in Acute Abdomen

Ruddock in 1937, described the use of laparoscopic surgery for acute abdomen. The benefits of the same were also described by Fahrlander (1969), Baerlocher et al (1973), Frangenheim (1974) and Sugarbaker et al (1975).[3,5-7] Acute abdominal symptoms can be secondary to inflammation, obstruction or strangulation.

Common Causes of Acute Abdomen

1. Constipation
2. Gastroenteritis
3. Acute appendicitis (Figs 122.1A and B)
4. Urinary tract infection.

Uncommon Causes of Acute Abdomen

1. Intussusception
2. Congenital obstruction
3. Adhesive obstruction
4. Strangulated inguinal hernia
5. Meckel's diverticulitis
6. Torsion of ovarian cyst (Fig. 122.2)
7. Acute Cholecystitis and Cholelithiasis
8. Nephrolithiasis
9. Pneumonia
10. Pancreatitis
11. Retroperitoneal hematoma
12. Paitonites (Fig. 122.3).

With a good history, clinical examination, relevant imaging and laboratory investigations most of the above mentioned pathologies can be diagnosed without laparoscopy. Laparoscopy only comes into picture when a speedy diagnosis cannot be made otherwise but should be made.

Diagnostic Laparoscopy in Acute Abdominal Pain

Diagnostic laparoscopy is most important when the possibility of acute appendicitis is raised. The diagnosis is many times difficult in view of the doubtful history and clinical presentation. Laboratory investigations like total and differential leucocyte count and imaging like ultrasound are often not conclusive in early appendicitis. More so a thorough examination of the abdominal cavity is not possible in the event of finding a so called 'negative appendix' through the small McBurney's incision. Judicious application of laparoscopy to patients with equivocal findings of appendicitis is helpful in reducing the negative appendicectomy rate and also the changes of missing a hidden but grave pathology. In a sick intensive care child or children with abdominal pain and severe underlying disease like diabetes mellitus, congenital or acquired immunopathy or nephrotic syndrome it may be sometimes difficult to put a finger on a single intra-abdominal pathology. Here too, diagnostic laparoscopy may play a vital role in excluding intra-abdominal disease. In children with colicky abdominal pain and a possible intestinal obstruction, a diagnostic laparoscopy helps to furnish a rapid and precise diagnosis. It can also be therapeutic in patients with congenital problems like internal herniation or volvulus around a vitello-intestinal duct remnant or acquired problems like adhesions from previous surgery.

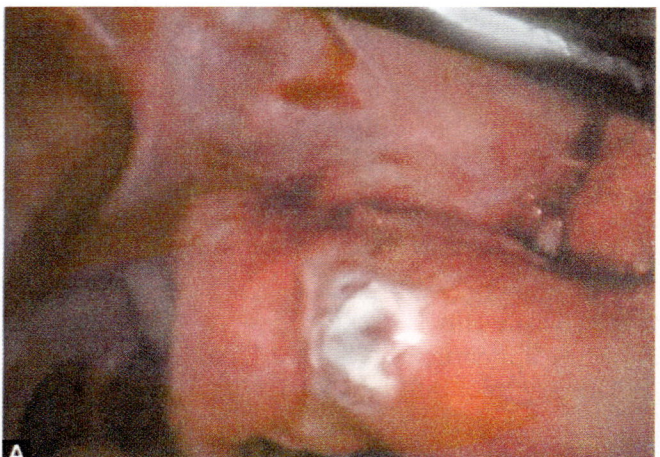 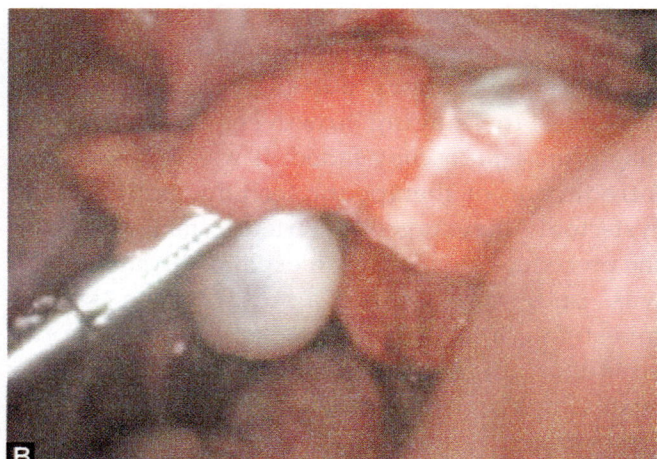

Figs 122.1A and B: Perforated appendicitis

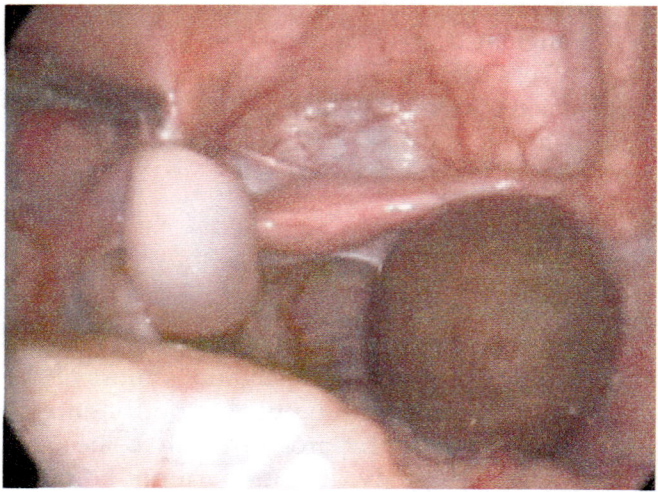

Fig. 122.2: Right torsion ovarian cyst

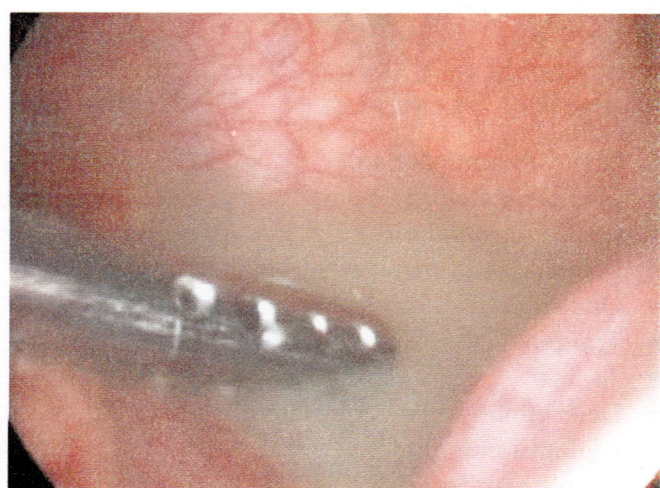

Fig. 122.3: Purulent peritonitis

Laparoscopy in Chronic Abdominal Pain

Laparoscopy is only one of the many diagnostic tools in children with chronic abdominal pain. At no means should laparoscopy replace a detailed history, careful clinical examination, selective additional imaging studies and laboratory investigations. The diagnostic yield of laparoscopy varies considerably from study to study. Leape and Ramenofsky (1977) in their initial series found no pathology in 11 out of 14 children.[8] However, in their subsequent series in 1980, 16 of their 33 patients were diagnosed to have pathology on laparoscopy. Waldschmidt subjected almost 50% of his cases with chronic abdominal pain to laparoscopy and found pathology in more than 99% of them.[9] Goldstein and Ozaksit et al found pathology in almost 90% of adolescent girls subjected to laparoscopy for chronic pelvic pain.[10]

A major problem of laparoscopy for chronic abdominal pain remains the interpretation of so called pathological findings and the question whether the finding is really responsible for the pain should always be asked. The matter of chronic appendicitis should certainly be addressed (Fig. 122.4). Does this exist and if so, what is the incidence. In a series of 660 children in which an identifiable cause for the chronic abdominal pain was found at laparoscopy. Waldschmidt diagnosed so called chronic recurrent appendicitis in more than half of them.[9] In contrast, in Utrecht, this diagnosis is hardly ever made.[9] There is also the difficult matter of postoperative adhesions (Fig. 122.5). After any surgery, there are always adhesions. The question is whether these are responsible for pain and if so, does adhesiolysis prevent recurrence of adhesions and complains. Complete disappearance of the symptoms after treatment of the pathological findings is probably the best indicator of whether the pathology found was really responsible for the complains although there may be significant placebo effect from the laparoscopy itself. Leape reported that 18 % were relieved of pain without any therapeutic action.[11] Goldstein experienced recurrence of the complains in 25 % of the adolescent girls after they had undergone laparoscopy.[10]

Laparoscopy in Gastrointestinal Bleeding

In the event of unclear gastrointestinal bleeding, laparotomy used to be the last resort when other diagnostic tools like upper and lower GI Endoscopy, radioisotope study or angiography fail to identify the exact localization of the bleeding. Children who are hemodynamically stable should have a laparoscopy before a formal laparotomy as a few causative conditions like Meckel's diverticulum, small bowel tumor, vascular malformation of the bowel wall, etc. can be diagnosed as well as treated laparoscopically (Fig. 122.6). In the event of a negative laparoscopy exteriorization of a bowel loop, subsequent enterotomy and introduction of a flexible scope can improve the diagnostic yield.[12]

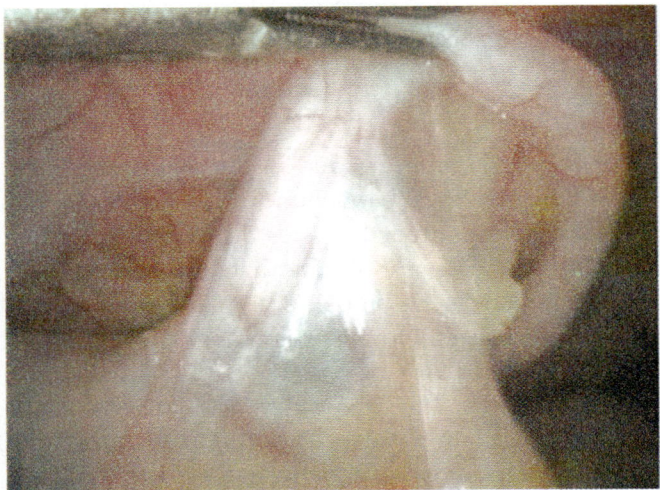

Fig. 122.4: Chronic appendicitis

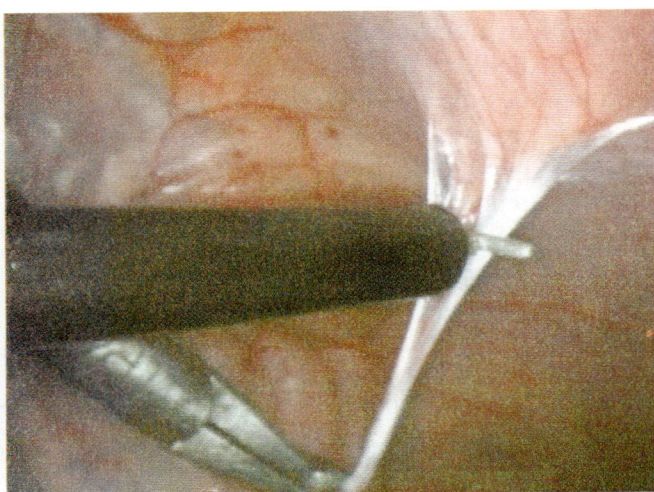

Fig. 122.5: Postoperative adhesions

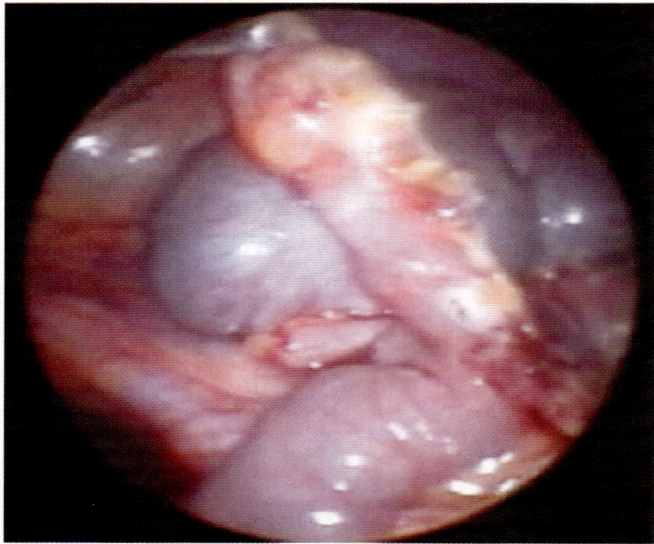

Fig. 122.6: Meckel's diverticulum

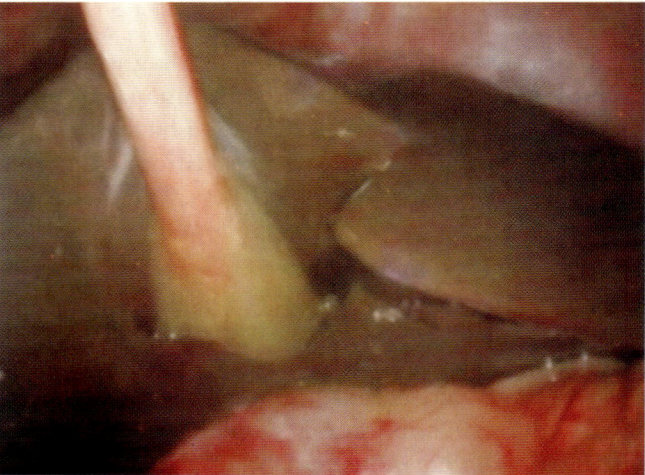

Fig. 122.7: Liver in neonatal hepatitis

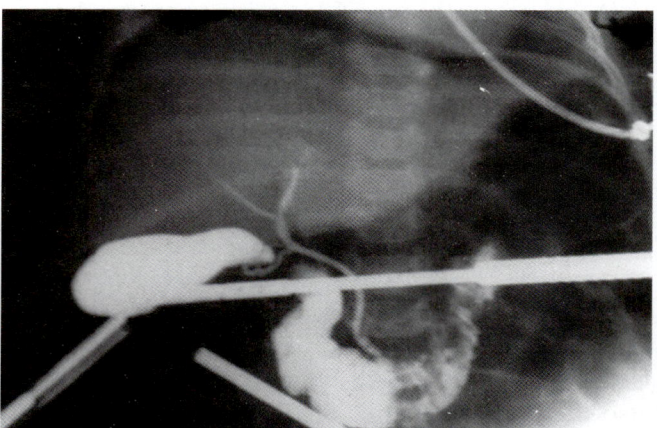

Fig. 122.8: Laparoscopic cholangiography

Laparoscopy in Pathologies of Liver and Biliary Tree

Neonatal Cholestasis

The diagnosis of a surgical cause is mandatory in any neonate who presents with conjugated hyperbilirubinemia. Surgically approachable cholestasis in the newborn or young infant include biliary atresia, choledochal cyst, inspissated bile syndrome (Fig. 122.7). In the event of dilated ducts, the diagnosis of extra hepatic biliary obstruction is easy. When the whole biliary tree is uniformly dilated with sludge in the gallbladder or bile ducts, the diagnosis of inspissated bile syndrome should be made. When the intra hepatic biliary tree is dilated, type 1 or 2 biliary atresia is present. In contrast, when neither the intra nor extra hepatic ducts are dilated, it is difficult to differentiate between type 3 biliary atresia and nonsurgical causes of cholestasis. In the year 1973, Gans and Bercy described laparoscopic cholangiography to differentiate between surgical approachable and medical causes of neonatal hyperbilirubinemia.[13] Nuclear scans do not have a high sensitivity for biliary atresia or neonatal hepatitis. In this scenario, laparoscopic cholangiography plays an important role in diagnosing children with biliary atresia preventing unnecessary exploration in the other group (Fig. 122.8).

Liver Biopsy

Liver biopsy is often needed in the diagnostic work up of liver diseases. Ultrasound guided liver biopsy or percutaneous liver biopsies are normally taken. However, in the event of a localized disease where a specific area must be biopsied, a laparoscopic biopsy may offer a solution to the problem. Direct inspection of the liver in case of a suspected disease is an additional advantage (Figs 122.9 and 112.10). In the event of coagulation disturbances, a laparoscopic liver biopsy is helpful as bleeding from the biopsy site can be controlled at the same time.

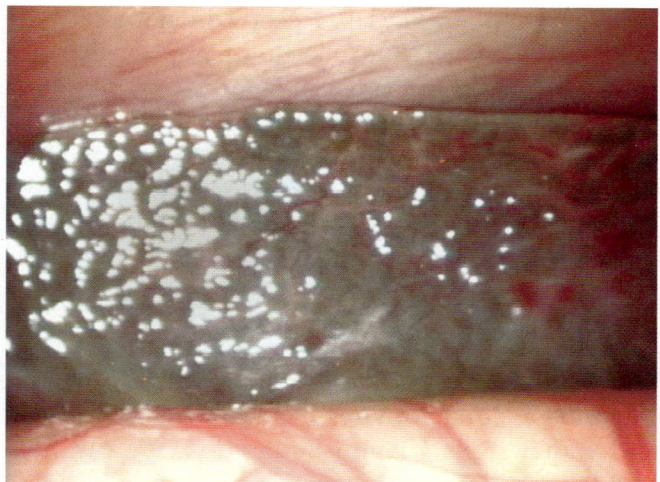

Fig. 122.9: Liver cirrhosis

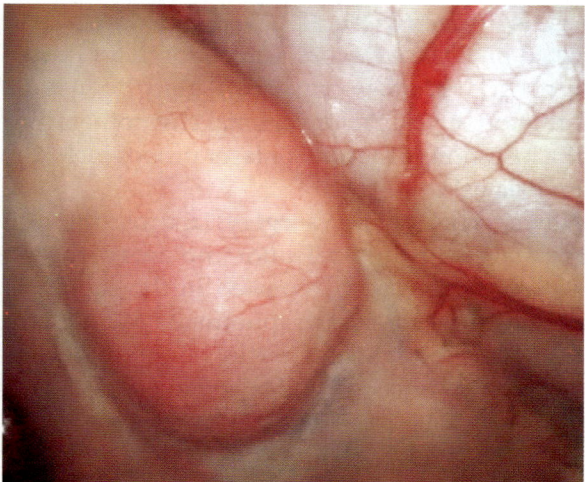

Fig. 122.11: Large abdominal lymphnodes

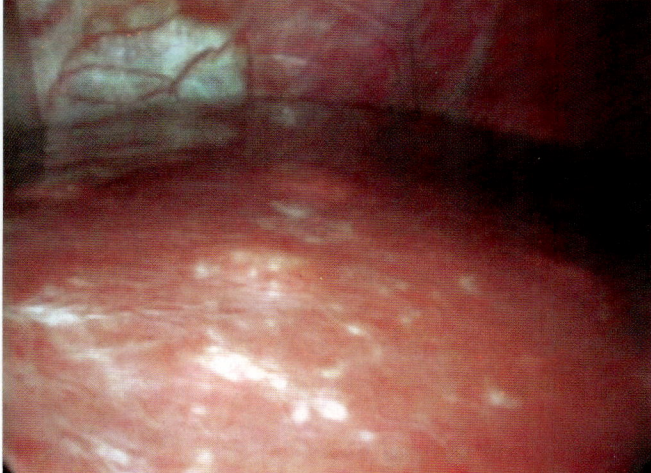

Fig. 122.10: Tuberculosis of liver

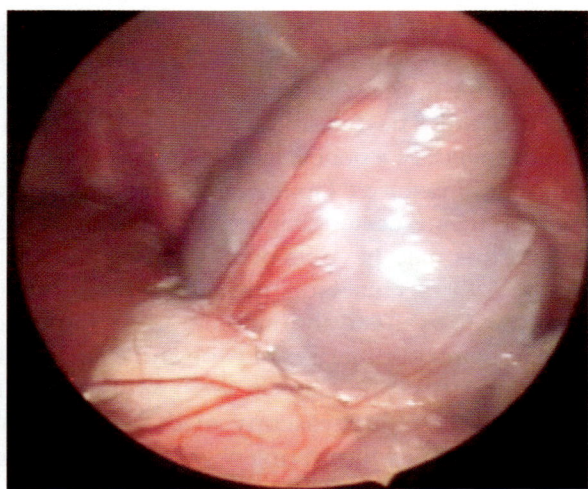

Fig. 122.12: Splenomegaly

Cholecystectomy

The overwhelming indication for laparoscopic cholecystectomy in children is the development of gallstones and related symptoms. Previously in many centers, it was reported that the majority of patients with gallstones developed them secondary to hemolysis. However, the trend towards non-hemolytic cholelithiasis seems to be increasing in recent years.

Laparoscopy in Oncology

The role of laparoscopy in pediatric oncology is still limited. At present, it is not included in the pediatric oncology protocols except for the Hodgkin's study HD96 in the German speaking countries.

Lymphomas

There are several reports on laparoscopic staging of Hodgkin's and non-Hodgkin's lymphoma (Figs 122.11 and 122.12).[14-18] Laparoscopy allows sampling of the lymph nodes and liver biopsy along with oophropexy in preparation for radiotherapy.

Other Malignancies

Laparoscopy is an ideal tool when a biopsy is essential before therapy is started or when residual or recurrent disease is suspected (Fig. 122.13). Holcomb et al (1995), reported on 60 laparoscopies in children for oncology purposes.[19] Laparoscopy can also be used for cannulation of vessels for regional chemotherapy and for the insertion of thermal or laser probes into tumors and metastasis.

However, as for open surgery, laparoscopic biopsy also upstages the tumor. Tumor implants at the site of laparoscopy have been reported in the sampling of both solid tumors and lymphomas.[20] Whole lymph nodes should be taken as far as possible to prevent metastasis. Specimen should be removed in a recipient bag.

Laparoscopy in Trauma

Assessment of blunt abdominal injury may be very difficult in children and especially in the event of polytrauma. Associated head injuries compromises consciousness making interpretation of the clinical picture difficult. The decision to open the abdomen is easy in the event of a penetrating trauma. To decrease the number of negative laparotomies in blunt trauma Root et al 1965, advocated diagnostic peritoneal lavage. However, this may have its own disadvantages.[21] In the early 1970's Heselson introduced diagnostic laparoscopy to evaluate abdominal trauma. However, this did not gain popularity.[22] Leape and Ramenofsky in 1977 and Austin and Gans in 1983, wrote about the role of diagnostic laparoscopy in the traumatized child.[8,23] The rapidly improving new imaging methods such as ultrasound and CT Scan in contrast to the then amateur technique like laparoscopy did not contribute to its use. However, due to technical improvements, a renewed interest in the use of laparoscopy in trauma has emerged. One must be cautious in laparoscopy in children with head injury as pneumoperitoneum increases the intracranial pressure. The key for success of laparoscopy in trauma is a stable patient, good equipment and an experienced surgeon.

Diagnostic Laparoscopy in Trauma

In Blunt Abdominal Trauma: In cases of multiple injuries, decreased consciousness, persisting equivocal abdominal signs, diagnostic laparoscopy can help exclude an unstable abdominal injury such as bleeding liver injury, mesenteric tear and splenic laceration. A negative laparotomy in such circumstances unnecessarily adds morbidity in the already compromised child.[24] Laparoscopy however still lacks wide popularity in the diagnosis of blunt abdominal trauma.

In Penetrating Trauma: Laparoscopy is an excellent diagnostic tool in looking for violation of peritoneum, diaphragmatic injuries in the case of penetrating trauma . Not every stab wound penetrates the abdominal wall or causes injury to the intra-abdominal viscera. Laparoscopy can help identify whether the peritoneum has been penetrated.[24,25]

Laparoscopy in Ascites

Ascites in children as it is in adults may be hepatic, renal, cardiac, pancreatic, gastrointestinal, infectious, neoplastic or gynecological. It could also be secondary to a congenital or acquired lymphatic cause. Laparoscopy is rarely indicated in children with ascites (Fig. 122.14). An exception may be lymphatic or cylous ascites where laparoscopy may be able to detect or even treat the leak. Intestinal lymphangiectasia can be very well diagnosed laparoscopically.[26]

Laparoscopy in Determination of Contralateral Patent Processus Vaginalis

In recent years few topics have raised as much controversy across the world as has the role of laparoscopy in the treatment of children with inguinal hernia (Fig. 122.15). A very high number of North

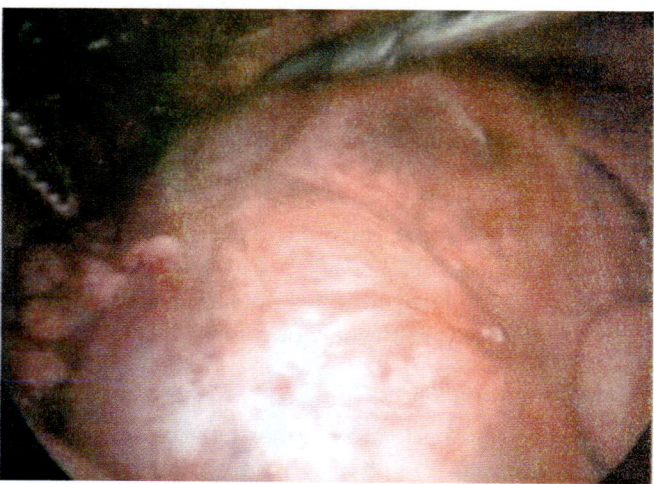

Fig. 122.13: Abdominal mass

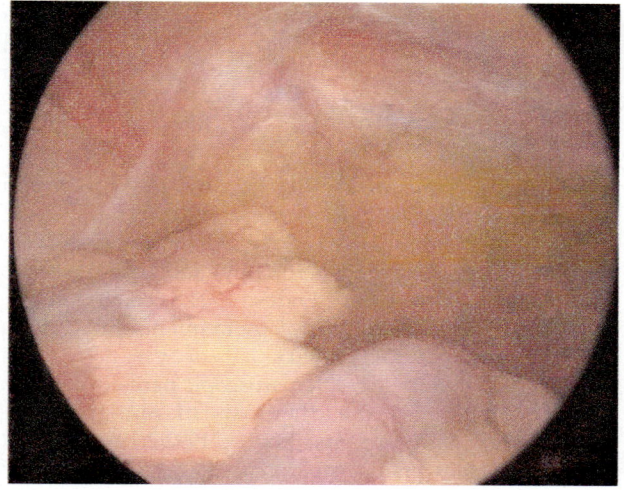

Fig. 122.14: Ascites

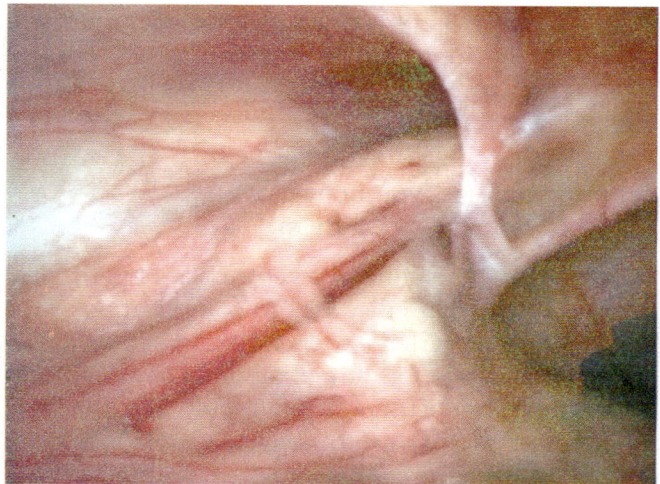

Fig. 122.15: Omentocele

American Pediatric Surgeons routinely explore the contralateral groin when operating children below the age of 2 years with inguinal hernias (Fig. 122.16). The reported incidence of contralateral patency is about 40%. However, the incidence of later development of a symptomatic hernia after unilateral hernia repair is only 10-20%. Studies need to be carried out to laparoscopically evaluate the characteristics of the contralateral ring in children undergoing surgery for inguinal hernia. This can help us predict which of these children have a high incidence of developing a contralateral hernia in the future.

Laparoscopy in Cryptorchidism

Cryptorchidism is one of the most frequent anomalies where laparoscopy has been used in today's pediatric practice. Testicular maldescent is not a uniform disorder but rather a spectrum of clinical situations in which it may not be possible to define the exact etiology, pathogenesis, prognosis and appropriate treatment in a single case. The aim however is to relocate the cryptorchid testis in the scrotum before onset of parenchymal damage. Early orchidopexy seems to reduce the risk of future infertility and also makes self examination and early pick up malignancy possible. It is generally believed that success after orchidopexy is related to the preoperative testicular position. Impalpable testis falls into one of the five categories:

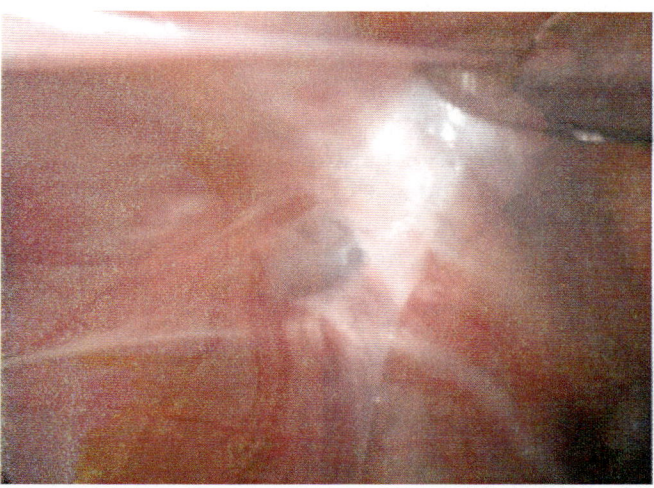

Fig. 122.16: Closed contralateral processus vaginalis

1. Absent gonad as a consequence of intrauterine torsion in the abdomen or in the inguinal canal (vanishing testis) or because of agenesis (rare).
2. Gonad present, but dysgenetic.
3. Normal testis present in the abdomen close to the internal ring and free to be mobilized into the inguinal canal (peeping testis).
4. Low abdominal testis.
5. High intra-abdominal testis.

Shah and Shah (1996) and Hrebinko and Bellinger (1993), studied children with undescended testis and found imaging studies to have a limited role in the pre-surgical evaluation of children with impalpable testes.[27,28] Laparoscopy gives an exact picture of the position of the impalpable gonad. Extensive groin and retroperitoneal exploration in these cases may be time consuming and possibly fruitless.

Laparoscopy in Dysfunction of V-P Shunts and P-D Catheters

Blind placement of either the ventricular or peritoneal end of the shunt predisposes to complications than when both are inserted under endoscopic control. The use of laparoscopy for intra-abdominal complications related to the venticuloperitoneal shunt like infection, blockage, obstruction and perforation has been advocated for almost two decades.[29-31] Combination of neuroendoscopy with laparoscopy optimizes the placement of venticuloperitoneal shunts and undoubtedly reduces complications related to shunt revisions by diminishing the incidence of distal obstruction. Moreover, the infection rate may further decline by using this almost no touch technique.

Laparoscopy has also shown to have a reliable role in the placement of peritoneal dialysis catheters in children. It provides a better catheter survival and trouble free dialysis in many series. The technique also allows a simultaneous partial to near total omentectomy which is crucial in preventing postoperative catheter occlusion. The approach also allows a clear inspection and prophylactic ligation of patent processus vaginalis to avoid hernia formation after commencement of peritoneal dialysis.

REFERENCES

1. Kelling, Uber Oesophagoskopie, Gastroskopie and Koelioskopie. Munch Med Wochenschr 1902;49:21-24.
2. Gans SL, Berci G. Advances in Endoscopy in infants and children. J Pediatr Surg 1971;6:399-405.
3. Frangenheim H. Die Stellung der Laparoskopie bei gynakologischen und chirurgischen Problemen im Kindesalter. Padiatr Forbild K Praxis 1974;39:71-78.
4. Gazzanagia AB, Stanton WW, Bartlett RH. Laparoscopy in the diagnosis of blunt and penetrating injuries to the abdomen. Am J Surg 1976;131:315-18.
5. Fahrlander H. Laparoscopy in abdominal emergencies. Germ Med Mon 1969;14:430-32.
6. Baerlocher C, Engelhart G, Farlander H. Die Notfall-Laparoskopie. Leber Magen Darm 1973;3:11-14.
7. Sugarbaker PH, et al. Preoperative laparoscopy in diagnosis of acute abdominal pain. Lancet 1975;1:442-44.
8. Leape LL, Ramenofsky ML. Laparoscopy in infants and children. J Pediatr Surg 1977;12:929-38.
9. Waldschmidt J, Bax NMA. Diagnostic Laparoscopy. In: Bax NMA, Georgeson KE, Najmaldin AS, Valla JS (Ed). Endoscopic Surgery in Children. Springer-Verlag, Berlin, 1999;137-54.
10. Goldstein DP, et al. New insights into the old problem of chronic pelvic pain. J Pediatr Surg 1979;14:675-80.
11. Leape LL, Ramenofsky ML. Laparoscopy in children. Pediatrics 1980;66:215-20.
12. Phillips E, Hakim MH, Saxe A. Laparoendoscopy (laparoscopic assisted enteroscopy) and partial resection of the small bowel. Surg Endosc 1994;8:686-88.
13. Gans Sl, Berci G. Peritoneoscopy in infants and children. J Pediatr Surg 1973;8:399-405.
14. Childers JM, Surwit EA. Laparoscopic para-aortic lymph node biopsy for the diagnosis of non-Hodgkin's lymphoma. Surg Laparosc Endosc 1992;2:139-42.
15. Lefor AT, Flowers JL. Laparoscopic wedge biopsy of the liver. J Am Coll Surg 1994;178:307-08.
16. Nord HJ, Boyd WP. Diagnostic laparoscopy. Endoscopy 1996;28:147-55.
17. Zornig C, et al. Staging-Laparoskopie beim Morbus Hodgkin. Stsh Med Wochenschr 1993;118:1401-04.
18. Coleman M, et al. Peritoneoscopy in Hodgkin Disease. JAMA 1976;236:2634-36.
19. Holcomb GW III, et al. Minimal invasive surgery in children with cancer. Cancer 1995;76:121-28.
20. Aractingi S, et al. Acalculous cholecystitis: the use of diagnostic laparoscopy. J Laparoendosc Surg 1995;5:227-31.
21. Root HD, et al. Diagnostic peritoneal lavage. Surgery 1965;57:633-37.
22. Heselson J, Peritoneoscopy in abdominal trauma. S Afr J Surg 1970;8:53-60.
23. Austin E, Gans SL. Laparoscopy for trauma. In: Gans SL (Ed) Pediatric Endoscopy. Grune and Stratton, New York, 1983;189-94.
24. Nagy A, Sutter M. Laparoscopy in abdominal trauma. In: Taterson-Brown S, Garden J (Eds). Principles and practice of surgical laparoscopy. Saunders, London, 1994;501-14.
25. Poole GV, Thomae KR, Hauser CJ. Laparoscopy in trauma. Surg Clin North Am 1996;76:547-56.
26. Fox U, Lucani G. Disorders of the intestinal mesenteric lymphatic system. Lymphology 1993;26:61-66.
27. Shah A, Shah A. Impalpable testes — Is imaging really helpful ? Indian Pediatr 2006;43:720-23.
28. Hrebinko RL, Bellinger MF. The limited role of imaging techniques in managing children with Undescended testes. J Urol 1993;150:458-60.
29. Lemay J-L, et al. Laparoscopic removal of the distal catheter of ventriculoperitoneal shunt (Ames valve) Gastrointest Endosc 1979;25:162-63.
30. Morgan WW Jr. The use of peritoneoscopy in the diagnosis and treatment of complications of ventriculoperitoneal shunts in children. J Pediatr Surg 1979;14:180-81.
31. Rodgers BM, Vries JK, Talbert JL. Laparoscopy in the diagnosis and treatment of malfunctioning ventriculoperitoneal shunts in children. J Pediatr Surg 1978;13:247-53.

CHAPTER 123

One Port Laparoscopically Assisted Appendectomy

Vadim Kapuller

The development of surgery knows number of "jumps" in its history; the last of which has been associated with progress of technology at the end of Twentieth century that gave us ability to perform traditional surgical manipulation through small incisions.

Laparoscopy that knows from early 80th has received fast progress with development of fiber optic technology and manufactures of surgical instruments.

Appendectomy is the most common intra-abdominal operation in western countries.[1] There are three approaches to perform this operation: open, laparoscopic, and in the last a few years the one port laparoscopically assisted appendectomy that has become more and more popular. Each of these approaches has its own advantages and disadvantages.

The traditional open approach is safe, cheap and fast; however, it has a higher morbidity, late complications (like bowel obstruction due to intra-abdominal adhesions) and worse cosmetic results. Although an experienced surgeon can perform an appendectomy through a small incision, the scar grows with the child, and in the future, this can cause an aesthetic problem. This fact may be very important in young girls and adolescents.

The laparoscopic approach has been widely adopted for this operation for its ability to reduce morbidity and hospital stay and obtain good cosmetic results.[2-8] This technique requires special technical skills, is more expensive and leaves three scars.[9] A new approach combines the benefits of both techniques: the appendix is extracted from the abdominal cavity by an operating laparoscope through one intra-umbilical incision, after which the operation is completed in the traditional open manner.[10-15]

Catheterization of bladder before the surgery is unnecessary, if the child has urinated recently. We use the operting laparoscope with long grasper (Fig. 123.1). The operation is performed under general anesthesia. The patient is placed in a supine position with slight

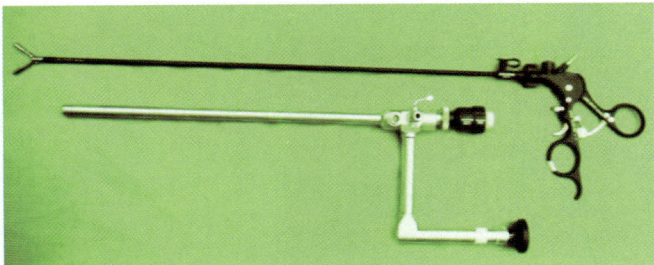

Fig. 123.1: The instruments used for the procedure

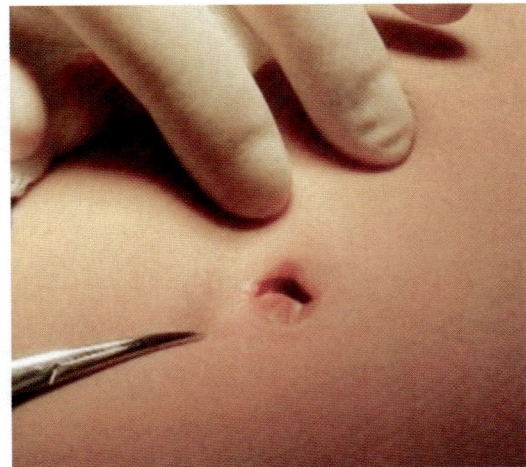

Fig. 123.2: The site of the incision for entry of the port is the umbilicus

left tilt. The pneumo-peritoneum is achieved by a 10 mm semi-lunar intraumbilical incision (Fig. 123.2) through which a Veres needle is placed (Fig. 123.3). A 10 mm trocar is inserted and an operating laparoscope is introduced (Fig. 123.4). The appendix is identified, grasped and removed through the intraumbilical incision (Fig. 123.5). The trocar is removed, and the operation is completed in the traditional open manner (Figs 123.6 to 123.9). Before the closure of fascia (Fig. 123.10) we put the trocar and laparoscope back for hemorrhage control, suction and wash out under direct vision. The skin is closed with an intradermal suture (Fig. 123.11).

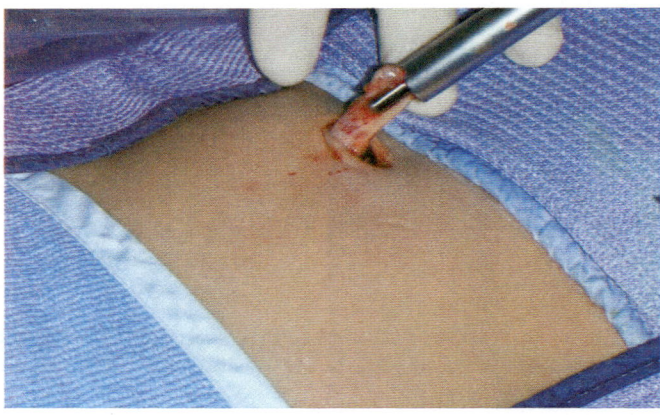

Fig. 123.5: The appendix is grasped and brought out through the umbilicus

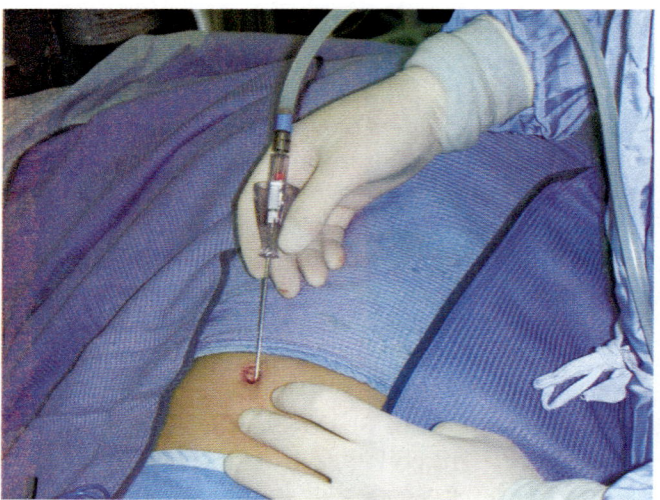

Fig. 123.3: The insertion of the Veres needle

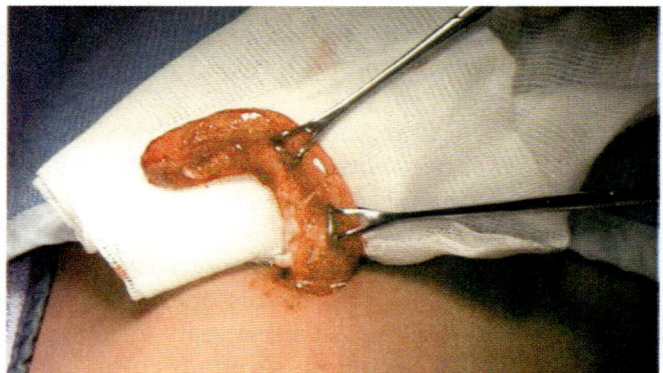

Fig. 123.6: The appendix is delivered in steps completely till the base is reached

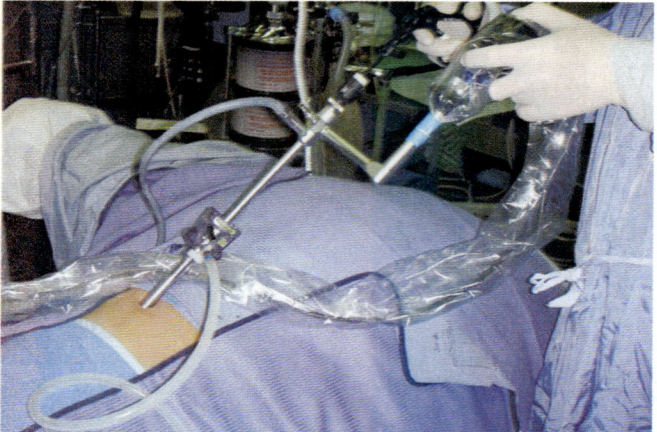

Fig. 123.4: The position of the surgeon is towards the left side of the patient and facing towards the caudal end in an oblique direction towards the right iliac fossa. The patient is put in a supine position with a slight left tilt and 20 degrees Trendelenberg position

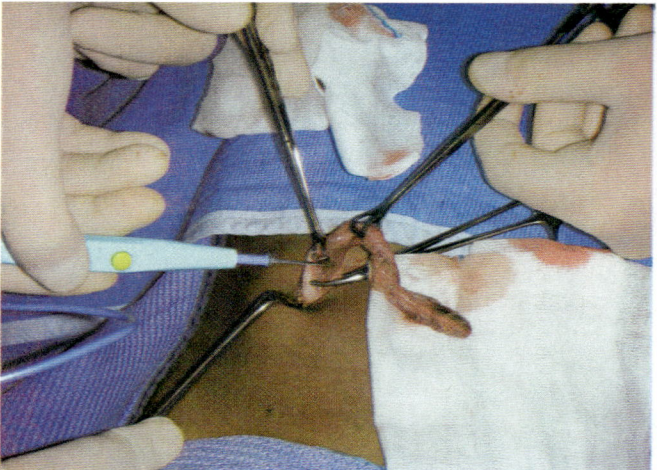

Fig. 123.7: The mesentery is divided in steps

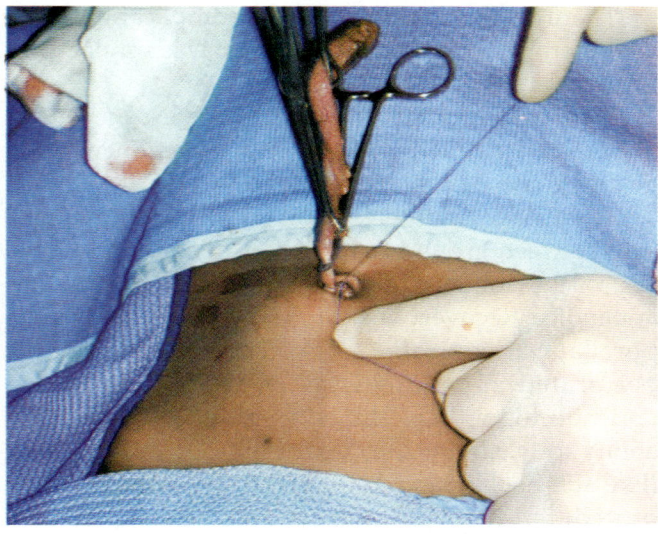

Fig. 123.8: Ligation of the base of the appendix

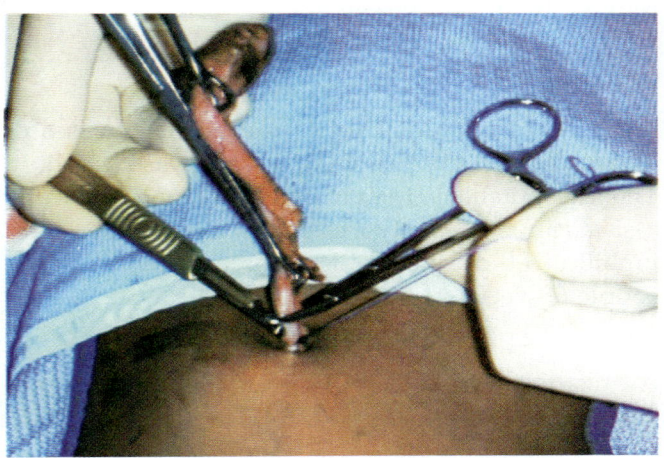

Fig. 123.9: Appendectomy in process

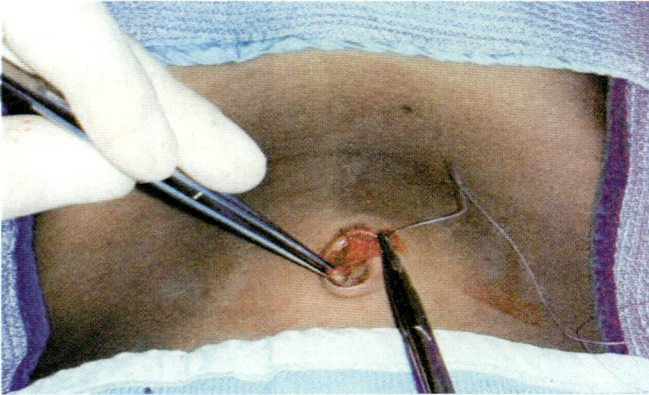

Fig. 123.10: Closure of the fascia

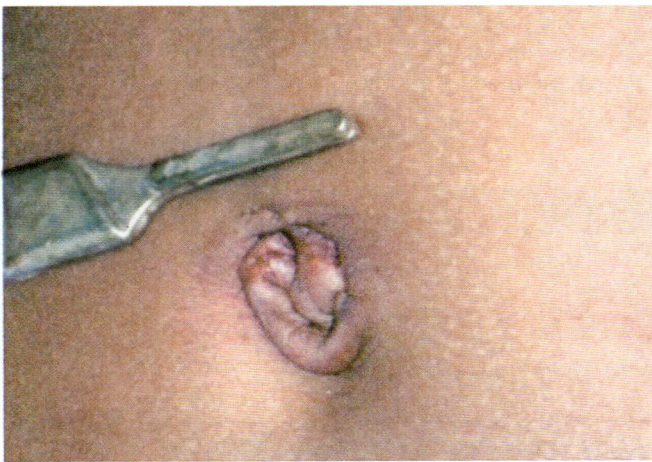

Fig. 123.11: The postoperative photograph showing the small periumbilical scar

Although the operation is simple and safe, not all the appendices can be managed by this manner. Short mesentery of the appendix may require insertion of additional 5 mm port for release of it. In case of extremely necrotizing appendix, when even slight traction can cause detachment of the appendix from its basis we advice not to hesitate convert this operation to open procedure. Additional reason for conversion is retrocaecal and/or subserotic localization, when appendix is not visualized. In some cases mobilization and removal of appendices through intraumbilical incision are difficult because of extremely short length or fixed caecum; if attempts to release the caecum are unsuccessful, the open procedure seems to be the best solution of this problem.

EXPERIENCE AT KAPLAN MEDICAL CENTER (JAN. 2006-MARCH 2007)

During the last 14 months, 106 appendectomies were performed in 61 boys and 45 girls.

There were 14 normal, 65 phlegmonous, 9 gangrenous and 18 perforated appendices (Table 123.1).

We operated on 67 children with acute appendicitis through one umbilical port (Group 3). Records of 33 (Group 1) and 6 children (Group 2), who underwent open and laparoscopic appendectomy respectively, were also evaluated (Table 123.2). Observations were made regarding intra- and postoperative complications, postoperative analgesic requirement, and postoperative hospital stay.

One port trans-umbilical laparoscopically assisted appendectomies were completed in 61 children; in 2 cases an additional 5 mm port was placed for release of the mesentery. Conversion to an open procedure was necessary in 4 cases: one of which had a very short appendix and fixed cecum, and the remaining three were retrocecal. In all of the retrocecal cases, the appendices were not visualized by the laparoscope (Table 123.2).

There were no intraoperative complications. The postoperative analgesic requirement was similar in all three groups.

Intra-abdominal collection that resolved after antibiotic treatment and wound infection were in groups 1 and 3 (Table 123.3).

There were no differences in postoperative hospital stay between groups 1 and 3 after one port and open approaches for normal, phlegmonous and gangrenous appendice. Recovery was almost twice as fast after one port laparoscopically assisted appendectomy for perforated appendicitis as compared with open appendectomy (Table 123.4), perhaps because of the ability to wash out sites which are difficult to access (like sub-hepatic and sub-phrenic areas) by an open procedure. Although recovery time was shorter with the one port group, this is not a randomized trial and therefore our conclusions must be confirmed (or refuted) by further research.

SUMMARY

Though a learning curve does exist in all cases of laparoscopy, in this method the curve was very short. The indisputable benefit of one port laparoscopically assisted appendectomy is cosmetic: the scar after intra-umbilical 1.0 cm incision is absolutely invisible after couple of weeks.

Table 123.1: Pathology

Appendix	Patients (%)
Normal	14 (13.2%)
Phlegmonous	65 (61.4%)
Gangrenous	9 (8.5%)
Perforated	18 (16.9%)
Σ	106 (100%)

Table 123.2: Types of surgery

Appendectomy	Patients
Open	33
Laparoscopic	6
One Port Lap. Assisted	67*
Σ	106

* 2 pts – additional 5 mm port,
4 pts – conversion to open procedure

Table 123.3: Complications related to surgery

Appendectomy	Discoloration	Wound infection	Intra-abdominal collection
Open (33 pts)		1 (3.03%)	1 (3.03%)
Laparoscopic (6 pts)	1 (16.6%)		
One Port Lap. Assisted (67)	4 (5.96%)	1 (1.49%)	1 (1.49%)
Σ	5	2	2

Table 123.4: Hospital stay related to surgery

	Open appendectomy	Laparoscopic appendectomy	One Port Lap. Assisted appendectomy
Normal	2.4		2.0
Phlegmonous	1.5	4.4	1.4
Gangrenous	4.6		4.4
Perforated	9	14	5.5

The one port laparoscopically assisted appendectomy is easy to perform, as one becomes familiar with the equipment and technique.

The procedure is safe and the postoperative course and cosmetic results are excellent.

One port trans-umbilical laparoscopically assisted appendectomy is a simple method that combines the advantages of minimally invasive surgery with the safe classical approach.

REFERENCES

1. Kokoska ER, Murayam KM, Silen ML, et al. A state-wise evaluation of appendectomy in children. Amer J Surg 1999;178;537-40.
2. Meguerditchian A-N, Prasil P, Cloutier R, et al. Laparoscopic appendectomy in children: a favorable alternative in simple and complicated appendicitis. J Pediatr Surg 2002;37:695-98.
3. Lavonius MI, Liesjarvi S, Ovaska J, Pajulo O, Ristkari S, Alanen M. Laparoscopic versus open appendectomy in children: a prospective randomised study. Eur J Pediatr Surg 2001;11:235-38.
4. Lejus C, Delile L, Plattner V, et al. Randomized single-blinded trial of laparoscopic versus open appendectomy in children: effects on postoperative analgesia. Anesthesiology 1996;84:801-06.
5. Lintula H, Kokki H, Vanamo K. Single-blind randomized clinical trial of laparoscopic versus open appendicectomy in children. Br J Surg 2001;88:10-514.
6. El Ghoneimi A, Vall JS, Limmonne B, et al. Laparoscopic appendicectomy in children: report of 1,379 cases. J Pediatr Surg 1994;29:786-89.
7. Gilchrist BF, Lobe TE, Schropp KP, et al. Is there a role for laparoscopic appendectomy in pediatric surgery. J Pediatr Surg 1992;27:209-14.
8. Sauerland S, Lefering R, Neugebauer EAM. Laparoscopic versus open surgery for suspected appendicitis. In: The Cochrane Library, Issue 1, 2002. Oxford: Update Software.
9. Little DC, Custer MD, May BH, et al. Laparoscopic appendectomy: an unnecessary and expensive procedure in children? J Pediatr Surg 2002;37:310-17.
10. Inoue H, Takeshita K, et al. Single-port laparoscopy assisted appendectomy under local pneumoperitoneum condition. Surg Endosc, 1994;8(6):714-16.
11. Kala Z, Hanke I, et al. A modified technique in laparoscopy-assisted appendectomy – a transumbilical approach through a single port. Rozhl Chir, 1996;75(1):15-18.
12. D'Alessio A, Piro E, et al. One-trocar transumbilical laparoscopic assisted appendectomy in children: our experience. Eur J Pediatr Surg 2002;12(1):242-47.
13. Pappelepore N, Tursini S, et al. Transumbilical laparoscopic-assisted appendectomy (TULAA): a safe useful alternative for uncomplicated appendicitis. Eur J Pediatr Surg 2002;12(6):383-86.
14. Suttie SA, Seth S, et al. Outcome after intra- and extra-corporeal laparoscopic appendectomy techniques. Surg Endosc, 2004;18(7):1123-25.
15. Meyer A, Preuss M, et al. Transumbilical laparoscopic assisted "one-trocar" appendectomy – TULAA – as an alternative operation method in the treatment of appendicitis. Zentralbl Chir 2004;129(5):391-95.

Robotic Pediatric Surgery

Aayed R Al-Qahtani

The introduction of laparoscopic techniques in the 1980s revolutionized surgery. It provided significant benefits for the patient (e.g. improved cosmetic effect, reduced postoperative pain, quicker recovery) and the health care system (e.g. quicker recovery times, shorter inpatient stay, earlier return to normal activity).[1] However, with conventional endoscopic instrumentation, there are substantial difficulties. Loss of wrist articulation, poor touch feedback, the fulcrum effect, loss of 3-dimensional vision, and poor ergonomics of the tools mean that only relatively simple procedures are truly widespread.[2,3] The promise of robotic assistance is to eliminate many of these impediments, with the concurrent enhancements of motion scaling and tremor filtration. It was suggested that, laparoscopic surgery is a "transitional" technology leading to robotic surgery.[4,5] The surgeon may now remotely teleoperate a robot in a comfortable, dexterous, and intuitive manner.

HISTORY OF ROBOTIC SURGERY

The word robot is derived from the Czech word robota, meaning "forced labor". Use of this term gained popularity after Karel Capek's play Rossum's Universal Robots in 1921, where a scientist discovers the secret of creating humanlike machines which later dominate the human race and threaten it with extinction. Since then, robots have taken on increasingly more importance in both imagination and reality.[6,7] It has evolved in meaning from dumb machines that perform menial, repetitive tasks to the highly intelligent anthropomorphic robots of popular culture.

The history of robotics in surgery begins with the Puma 560, a robot used in 1985 to perform neurosurgical biopsies with greater precision.[8,9] Three years later, the Puma 560 was used to perform a transurethral resection of the prostate.[10] The first surgical robot approved by the FDA was ROBODOC, a robotic system designed to machine the femur with greater precision in hip replacement surgeries.[6]

This concept of telesurgery became one of the main driving forces behind the development of surgical robots. In the early 1990s, several of the scientists from the NASA-Ames team joined the Stanford Research Institute (SRI). Working with SRI's other robotocists and virtual reality experts, these scientists developed a dexterous telemanipulator for hand surgery.

The US Army noticed the work on telesurgery, and it became interested in the possibility of decreasing wartime mortality by "bringing the surgeon to the wounded soldier-through telepresence.[6] With funding from the US Army, a system was devised whereby a wounded soldier could be loaded into a vehicle with robotic surgical equipment and be operated on remotely by a surgeon at a nearby Mobile Advanced Surgical Hospital (MASH). This system, it was hoped, would decrease wartime mortality by preventing wounded soldiers from exsanguinating before they reached the hospital. This system has been successfully demonstrated on animal models but has not yet been tested or implemented for actual battlefield casualty care.

Computer Motion, Inc. of Santa Barbara, CA, developed the Automated Endoscopic System for Optimal Positioning (AESOP), a robotic arm controlled by the surgeon voice commands to manipulate an

Table 124.1: Advantages and disadvantages of robot-assisted surgery	
Advantages	Disadvantages
3-D visualization	No haptic feedback
Seven degrees of freedom	Expensive
Improved dexterity	Needs set-up prior to each surgery
Elimination of physiologic tremors	The current robot is big and needs large space slim arms and small instruments (3 mm) not available yet
Elimination of fulcrum effect	3-D Visualization are not available in 5 mm telescope yet (working now on 8 mm telescope, 3-D)
Motion scaling	
Ergonomic positioning	
Tele-surgery improved hand-eye coordination	

endoscopic camera. Shortly after AESOP was marketed, Integrated Surgical Systems (now Intuitive Surgical) of Mountain View, CA, licensed the SRI Green Telepresence Surgery System. This system underwent extensive redesign and was reintroduced as the da Vinci surgical system. Within a year, Computer Motion put the Zeus system into production.

RATIONAL FOR ROBOTIC SURGERY

The robotic surgical systems provide unique advantages (Table 124.1) when compared with conventional minimally access surgery: (1) the surgeon holds control of a stable camera-telescope platform, eliminating the dependence from a camera assistant. In addition, having the fourth arm will give the surgeon the ability to control more than two arms allowing them to become their own assistant, (2) the surgical field is presented to the surgeon in a 3-D display, (3) the robotic instruments have articulations near the tip that increase the degrees of freedom to function more like a human hand (Fig. 124.1); (4) the computer eliminates hand tremor and the scale of motion is programmable; and (5) the console provides a more ergonomic operating position for the surgeon. All together, these computer-enhanced functions add precision and dexterity to the MIS surgeon, particularly when performing microsurgical procedures.[11] Further refinement of the computer motion enhancement has enabled the camera image to be synchronized with the beating of the heart in cardiac surgery, producing a virtual motionless cardiac image that allows coronary artery bypass surgery to be done without the need for cardiologic bypass.[12]

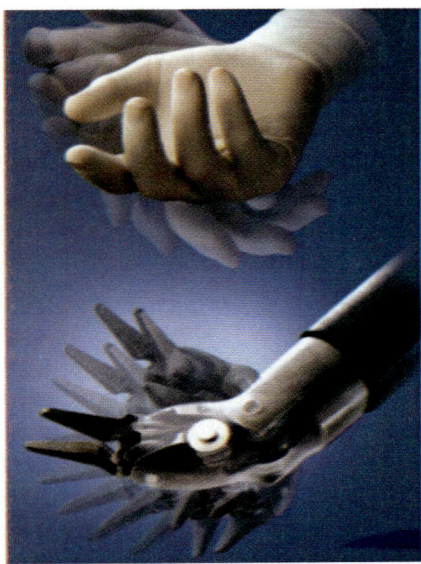

Fig. 124.1: Seven degrees of freedom (surgeon hand like)

Surgeons using robotic technology experience these benefits that indirectly extend to patients. They allow surgeons to offer minimally access surgery approaches to patients who would not have been considered for these approaches before robotic technology was available.[13,14] For example, performing laparoscopic surgery on small children and infants is difficult because of the challenge in performing laparoscopic anastomoses in small area. Fallopian tube reanastomosis is another example of a procedure that is very difficult to perform laparoscopically that can be performed more easily using robotics. Robotic technology also is transforming the surgical arena indirectly by changing surgical approaches, equipment, and instrumentation for nonrobotic procedures.[13] For example, robotics renewed manufacturers' interest in improving traditional laparoscopic instruments.[14] To ensure that the traditional laparoscopic approach is competitive with the robotic approach, manufacturers now are investing effort and money in developing truly innovative laparoscopic instrumentation.[14]

TYPES OF ROBOTIC SYSTEMS

A variety of classifications for defferent types of robots help to describe these heterogeneous devices. Robots can be characterized as automated arms, mobile devices, mills, or telerobotic devices. Additionally, they can be active, semiactive, or passive. Active devices are totally programmable and carry out tasks independently. Semiactive devices and passive robotic devices translate movements from an operator's or surgeon's hands into powered or unpowered movements of the robot arms. Surgical robots in use or research today include both active mills and semiactive telerobotic devices.

Passive robots function to hold a fixture at a desired location through which the surgeon introduces an instrument into an area of difficult access. The first passive robot appeared in 1985; was "Puma 560" used to guide drills and needles for intracranial biopsies.[8,9]

Semiactive robots are devices that combine the capability of some autonomous function with other actions carried out by the surgeon. One example is LARS (Laparoscopic Assistant Robotic System, Johns Hopkins University and IBM).[15,16] LARS is a robotic arm that has four degrees of freedom for positioning of video camera or retracting instruments and is fitted with sensors that monitor forces and torque. The arm is driven by the operator, but should the forces exceed the programmed safety thresholds (e.g. tissue resistance), the robot halts the motion until the operator corrects the position. The arm is mounted in a cart that is rolled to the side of the operating table. LARS has been used in experimental surgery only.

Synergistic robots are devices simultaneously powered by both the robot's engine and the surgeon. This hybrid platform establishes a partnership between the skills and experience of the surgeon and the geometric accuracy of a tireless machine. ACROBOT (Active Constraint Robot, Imperial College, London, UK) is an example of a synergistic robot ACROBOT was designed to cut bone with maximum precision and safety in preparation for knee replacement.[17] Another example of synergistic robot is the Steady Hand Robot (Johns Hopkins).[18] The Steady Hand Robot is a device under development with the purpose of enhancing the ability of the human hand to perform micromanipulations.

Active surgical robots are powered devices that can function with significant independence from the surgeon. These robots carry the greatest safety concerns and have been developed for specific purposes as follow:

CAMERA HOLDER ROBOTS

Robots for camera holding were the first active robots to be developed for commercial use. AESOP (Automated Endoscopic System for Optimal Positioning, Computer Motion, Inc.) and EndoAssist (Armstrong Healthcare, Ltd.) are the better-known robotic camera holder systems around the world.[19,20] AESOP was the first laparoscopic robot to gain approval by the US. Food and Drug Administration. This system is composed of a control computer, a power system, and an articulated, electromechanical arm for holding and maneuvering the telescope (Fig. 124.2).[19] The arm attaches to the operating table,

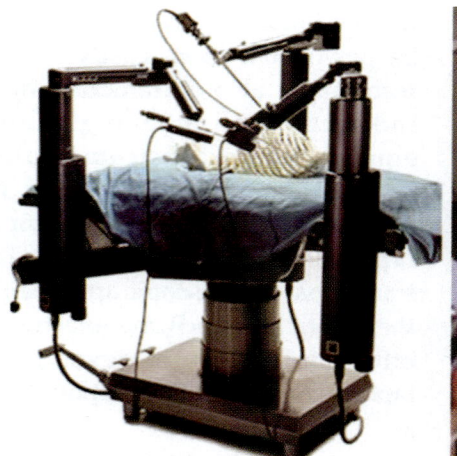
The Zeus surgical system

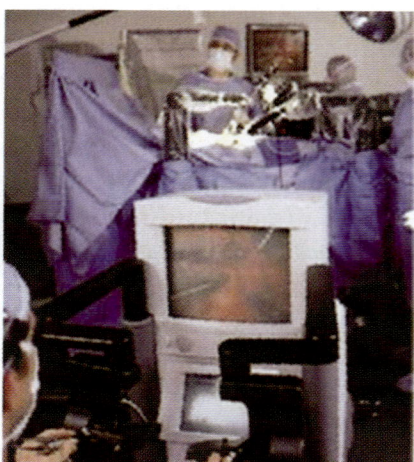
View from surgeon's console, Zeus

Fig. 124.2: Zeus system

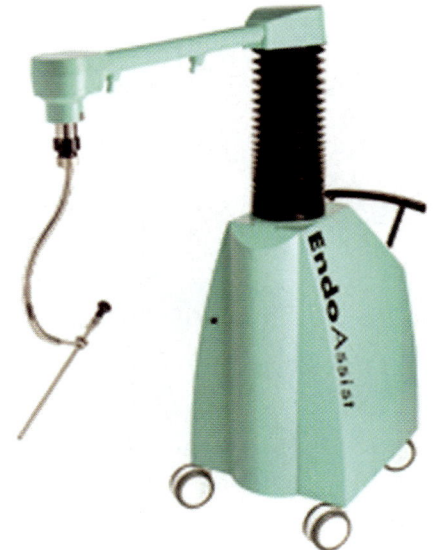

Fig. 124.3: EndoAssist

and its action can be controlled via foot pedals, hand controls, or a voice activation/recognition system. The voice activation platform has been the preferred technique.[21] The arm provides 7 degrees of freedom and centers at the point where the telescope enters the patient (e.g. abdominal or chest cavity). AESOP has been used extensively to assist in urologic (e.g. nephrectomy, prostatectomy), gynecologic (e.g. hysterectomy), gastrointestinal (e.g. cholecystectomy, colectomy, Nissen fundoplication), and thoracic (e.g. internal mammary artery) videoscopic operations.[22-24]

EndoAssist (Fig. 124.3) is another robot for camera holding that differs from AESOP in the commanding mechanism. EndoAssist is a head-mounted navigation system that allows the laparoscopic camera to follow the surgeon's head movements by tracking a headband sensor.[25] The robot is in active mode only when a foot switch is pressed by the surgeon. In active mode, any glance of the operator in one direction on the video monitor causes the camera to pan in the same direction (left/right, up/down, zoom in/out).

ORTHOPEDIC ROBOTS

One of the first active robots was designed for orthopedic surgery. Robodoc (Integrated Surgical Systems) has been developed for primary total hip replacement, revision hip replacement, and total knee replacement.[26,27] Robodoc is a computer-controlled mechanical arm capable of 5 degrees of freedom and force sensing in all axes. The tip of the arm holds a rotary bone cutter. Robodoc functions in coordination with a preoperative planning station, Orthodoc (Integrated Surgical Systems).[26-28] Orthodoc is a computer workstation that converts actual CT images of the patient to create a 3-D reconstruction of the joint to be replaced. Using computer modeling, the surgeon can choose the prosthesis (from a software library) with the best fit and can simulate the joint replacement (virtual surgery).

There are other computer-assisted robotic systems under development for different orthopedic applications that integrate image reconstruction and guidance; some examples include CASPAR, CRIGOS, and Loughborough manipulator.[29-31]

NEUROSURGERY ROBOTS

Minerva is a powered neurosurgery robot that functions under the guidance of a dedicated CT imaging system.[32] Specifically designed instruments loaded onto a rotary carrousel can carry out the entire operation without assistance from the surgeon.[32] Minerva was developed at the University of Lausanne and has not been commercialized.

NeuroMate (Integrated Surgical Systems) is a computer-assisted, image-guided device for stereotactic procedures in neurosurgery.[33,34] (NeuroMate also classifies as a semi-active robot).

PathFinder (Figs 124.4A and B) (Armstrong-Healthcare, Ltd.) is a powered, image-guided robot for accurate positioning of stereotactic instruments.[35]

CyberKnife (Accuray) is an advanced system for stereotactic radiosurgery in neurosurgery.[36,37] It can be used for any other parts of the body.[37]

UROLOGY ROBOTS

Probot (Mechatronics in Medicine, Imperial College) is a powered, image-guided, computercontrolled robot for Transurethral Resection of the Prostate (TURP).[38-39] The operation is completely performed by Probot under the supervision of the surgeon. The surgeon follows the progression of the procedure at the workstation and can adjust the cutting parameters or can stop the robot at any time.

1472   Pediatric Surgery—Diagnosis and Management

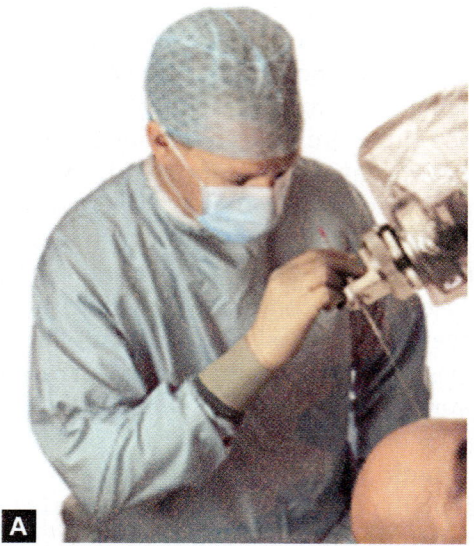
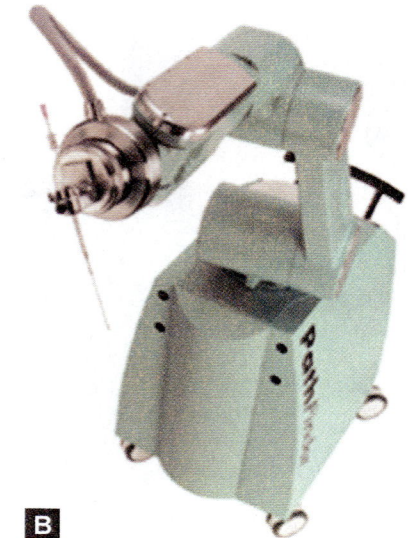

Figs 124.4A and B: Pathfinder

The RCM robot (Remote Center of Motion, Brady Urological Institute, Johns Hopkins University) was initially developed for percutaneous access of the kidney (PAKY), the device also has been referred to as the PAKY-RCM robot.[40,41] The low and flexible profile of the robot makes it compatible with CT scanners and C-arms in operating rooms.

MASTER-SLAVE ROBOTS

Master-slave robots are powered, computer-controlled devices that do not perform autonomous tasks but are completely governed by the surgeon, thus the term *master-slave* system where the surgeon is the "master" and the robot is the "slave". The master surgeon is seated at a control console (Fig. 124.5), and the slave robotic arm is located at the surgical field over the patient (Figs 124.6 and 124.7). They are also called *telemanipulators*, implying that the master and the slave are separated from each other by a distance but communicate through data cables. At the console, the surgeon observes the surgical field on a video display and actuates his or her hands not on traditional surgical instruments but on mechanical transducers (masters or joysticks) (Figs 124.8 and 124.9). The surgeon's motions are telecasted from the console to the robotic arms, which, in turn, manipulate instruments and the telescope (Figs 124.10 to 124.13).

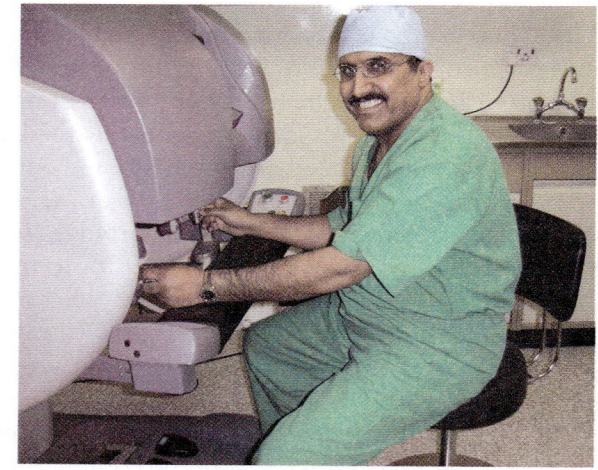

Fig. 124.5: The surgeon at the console

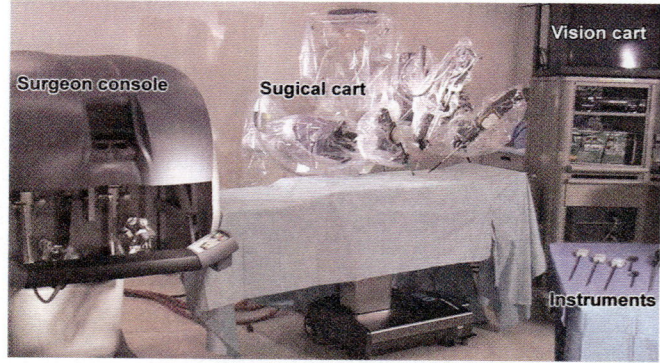

Fig. 124.6: da Vinci components

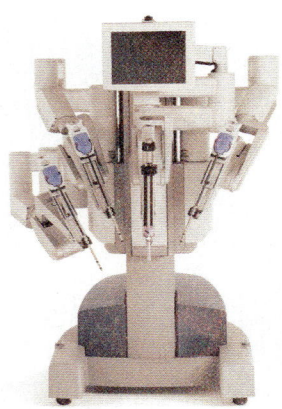

Fig. 124.7: Patient cart in da Vinci S with the 4th arm

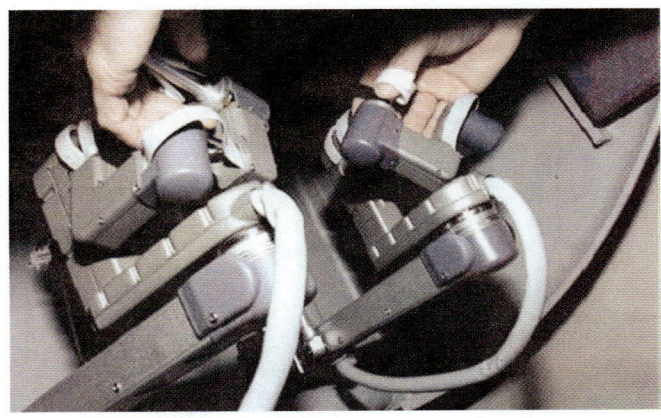

Fig. 124.9: Hand controls in the da Vinci robotic system

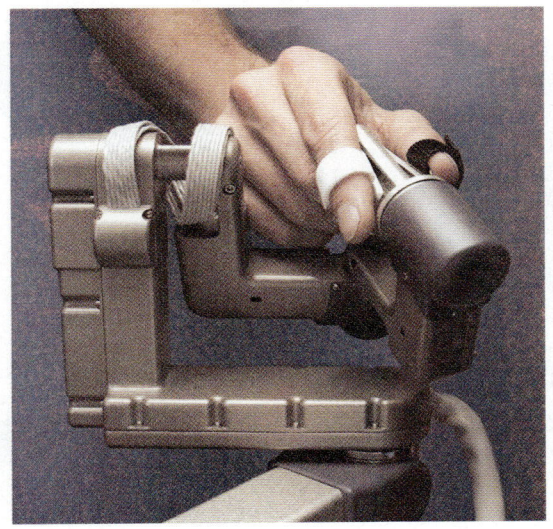

Fig. 124.8: Hand controls in the da Vinci robotic system

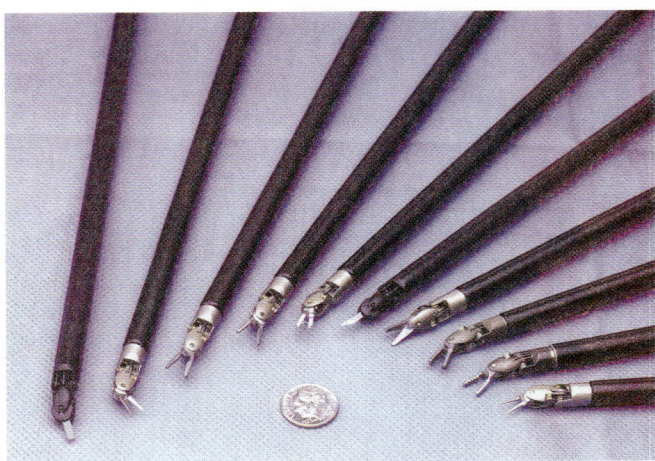

Fig. 124.10: 8 mm robotic instruments in da Vinci system

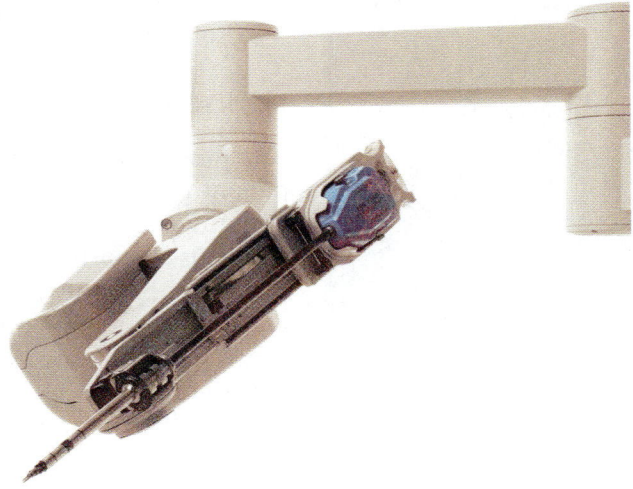

Fig. 124.11: Arm angled instrument

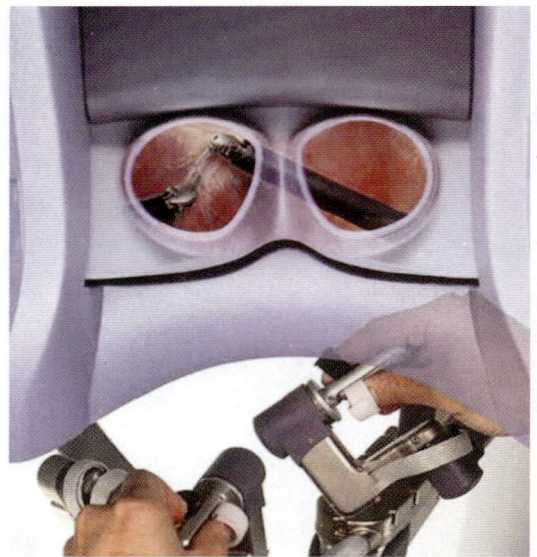

Fig. 124.12A: 3-D vision

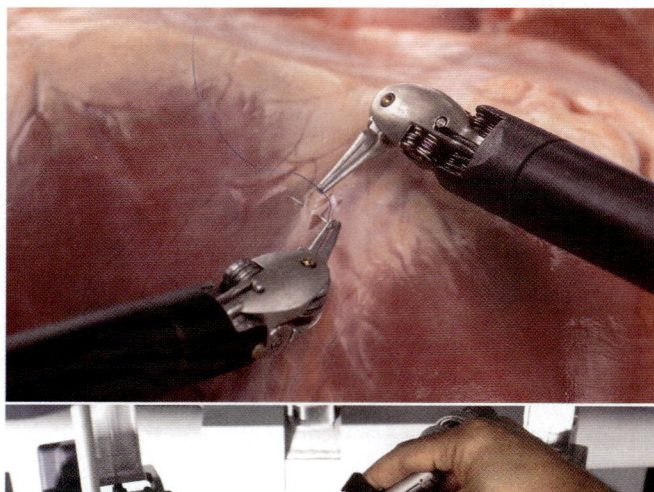

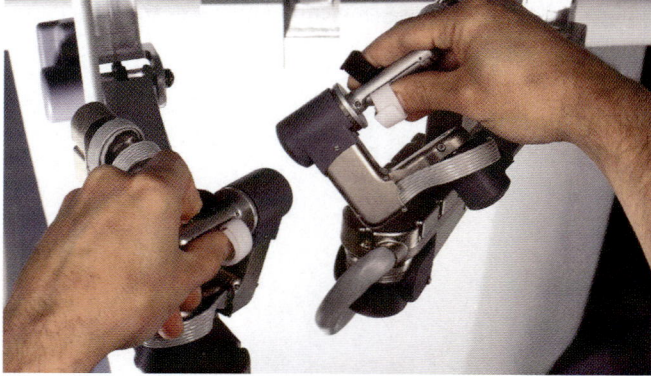

Fig. 124.12B: Surgeon hand manipulating the instruments with 3-D vision

The surgeon's console also holds commands for special functions (e.g. focusing, motion scaling) and accessory equipment (e.g. electrosurgical and ultrasonic units) (Fig. 124.14). The separation between master and slave

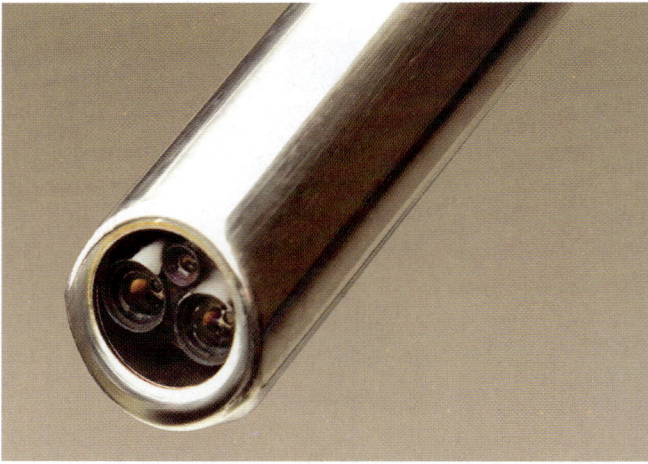

Fig. 124.13: Binocular endoscope in da Vinci robotic system

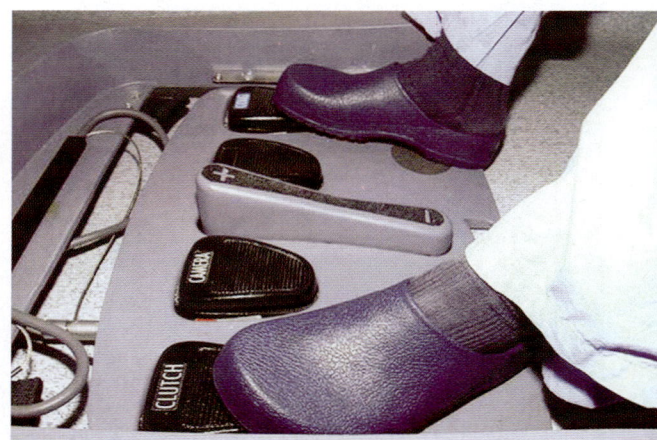

Fig. 124.14: Feet control

components may vary, from a few meters (e.g. inside the same operating room) to several kilometers apart (e.g. transatlantic operation).[42]

ROBOTIC PEDIATRIC SURGERY

Compared with the adult-sized patient, the pediatric patient poses additional challenges, such as smaller operative fields and more delicate tissues.[43] Pediatric surgeons are particularly interested in robotic surgery, because they apply minimally invasive techniques to a broader range of procedures than adult general surgeons, and because we would like to apply the benefits of this approach to complex procedures in smaller patients and even smaller anatomic areas. In the pediatric population, surgeons most often use some degree of visual magnification either in the form of standard loupes for open surgery or via a telescope.

Table 124.2: Robotic gastric banding in adolescent and children: The saudi experience		
	LAGB# 50	RAGB# 25
Female: male	27:24	14:11
Age (mean)	16	18
MBI (mean)	49	51
Comorbidites	67%	71%
Overall operating time mints (Mean)	50	73.5
Complications	10	4
LOS (days)	1	1
EWL in 6 months (mean)	42%	39%
Narcotic use (mean)	3 doses	3 doses

LAGB: Laparoscopic adjustable gastric banding,
RAGB: Robotic adjustable gastric banding,
LOS: Length of hospital stay,
EWL: Excess weight loss.

Currently robots are used on children to perform most procedures that can be done using minimally access surgery, including, cholecystectomy (Fig. 124.15), splenectomy (Fig. 124.16), fundoplication (Figs 124.17 and 124.18), Kasai procedure, choledochal cyst excision, and Heller myotomy.[44-49] At our own institution, between June 2002 and December 2006, we have used da Vinci robotic system to perform surgery on 115 patients ranging in age from 1 month to 19 years and in weight from 3 to 150 kg, including 34 Nissen fundoplications, 37 cholecystectomies, 25 gastric banding (Table 124.2, Figs 124.19 to 124.22), 5 imperforate anus, 5 splenectomies, 2 diaphragmatic hernia repairs (Morgagni), 2 Heller myotomies, 1 adrenalectomy, 2 interval appendectomy, and 2 liver cyst (one hydatid).

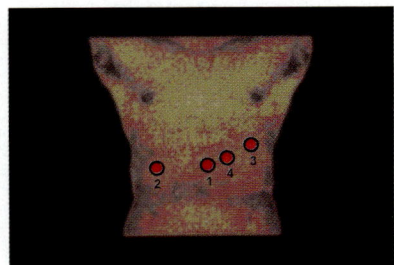

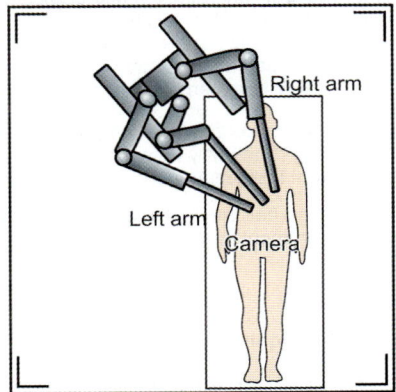

Surgical cart position
Surgical cart positioned next to right shoulder Camera arm positioned in line with anatomy and camera port. Camera arm "elbow" should point towards the foot of the bed

Procedure overview recommended port placement

- Camera port (12 mm) cannula in umbilicus

- Left instrument port (8 mm) right mid-clavicular line, one hand-breadth (10 cm) away from camera port; at the level of the umbilicus.

- Right instrument port (8 mm) left mid-clavicular line one hand-breadth (10 cm) away from camera port; one hand-breadth above the level of the umbilicus

- Accessory ports (5 mm) patient's left side; between camera port and left instrument port.

Instrument requirements

30° Endoscope, angled downward
wide-angle camera head
cardiac forceps
cautery hook
round tip scissors
large needle driver

Conventional laparoscopic suction/irrigation
Conventional laparoscopic grasper

Fig. 124.15: Robotic cholecystectomy set-up

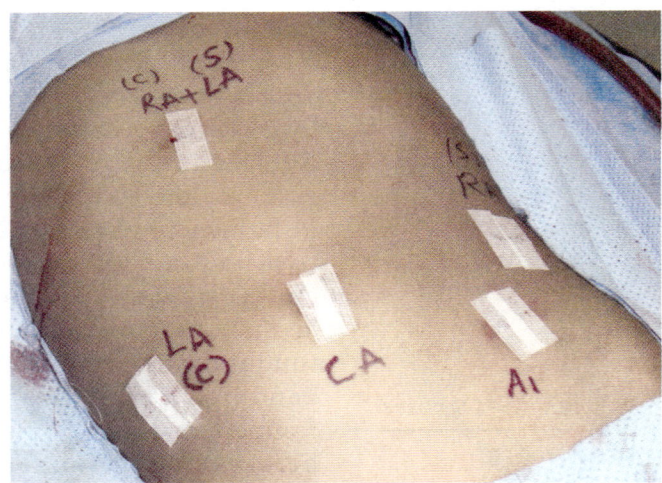

Fig.124.16: Port placement in combined robotic cholecystectomy and splenectomy (C = Cholecystectomy, S = Splenectomy, LA = left arm, RA = right arm, CA = camera arm, A1 = assistant port)

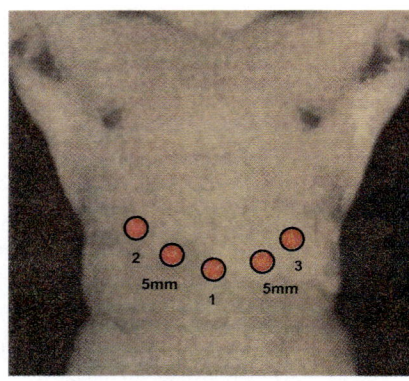

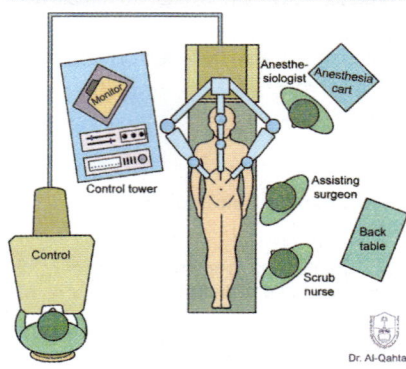

Surgical cart position

Surgical cart positioned next to left shoulder. Camera arm positioned in line with epigastric anatomy and camera port. Camera arm "elbow" should point towards the foot of the bed.

Procedure overview recommended port placement

- Camera port (12 mm):
Cannula in umbilicus

- Left instrument port (8 mm):
Right mid-clavicular line, 2-3 finger breadths below right costal margin; at least one hand-breadth (~10 cm) separation from camera port

- Right instrument port (8 mm):
2 figner breadths lateral to left mid-clavicular line; 2-3 finger breadths below left costal margin; at least one hand-breadth below left costal margin; at least one hand-breadth (~10 cm) away from camera port

Accessory ports (10 mm and 5 mm):
- 10 mm port half way between camera port and right instrument port

- 5 mm port half way between camera port and left instrument port.

Instrument requirements

30° Endoscope, angled downward
wide-angle camera head
2 cardiac forceps
cautery hook
2 large needle drivers
da Vinci™ ultrasonic shears
Conventional laparoscopic tissue graspers
Conventional laparoscopic suction / irrigation
Conventional laparoscopic clip applier
Liver retractor (optional)

Fig. 124.17: Robotic Nissen setup

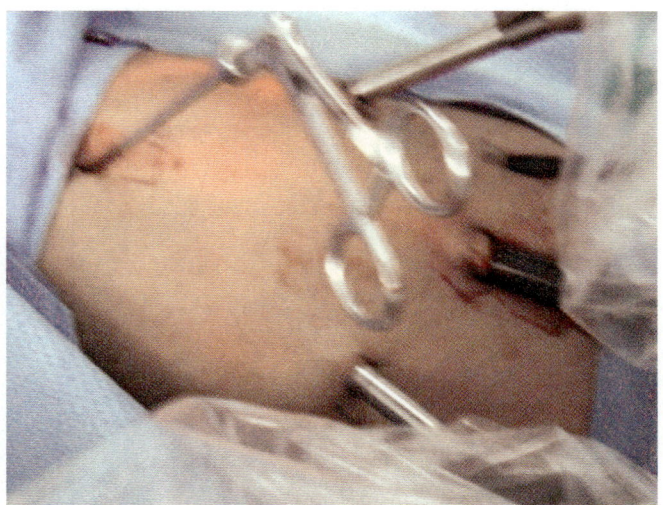

Fig. 124.18: Robotic Nissen, note the liver retractor in the epigastrium holding the diaphragm behind the liver

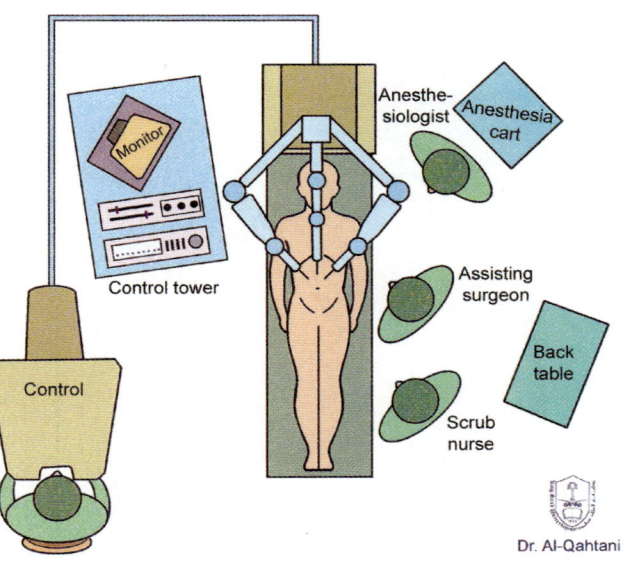

Fig. 124.19: Robotic gastric banding set-up

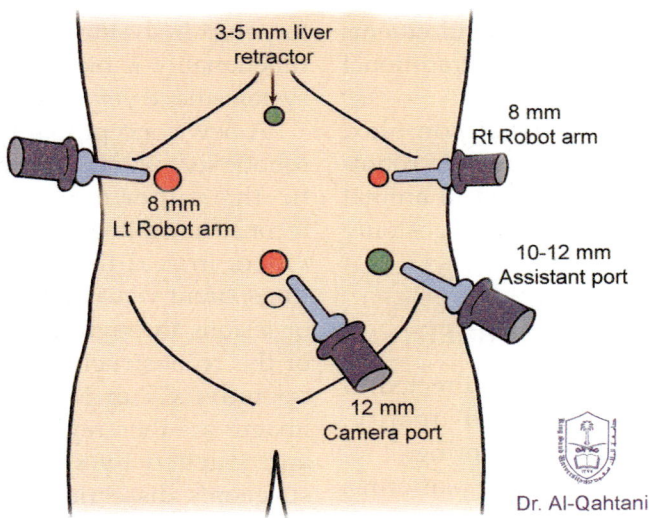

Fig. 124.20: Robotic gastric banding trocars placements

Current technology is primarily used to facilitate thoracoscopic pediatric procedures on extracardiac lesions, such as ligation of a patent ductus arteriosus and division of vascular rings.[50] Although some studies have reported intracardiac robotic surgery applications in adults, the current size of the robotic surgical systems available is a critical limitation in preventing their application in pediatric cardiac surgery patients.[51-55] In the field of pediatric urology, robotic assistance is described for nephrectomies, pyeloplasties, and appendicovesicostomies.[56-59] Lee and colleagues assessed the usefulness of robot-assisted laparoscopic pyeloplasty in children in a retrospective case-control study.[59] As experience increased, operative times improved, and the investigators noted a shorter mean length of stay as

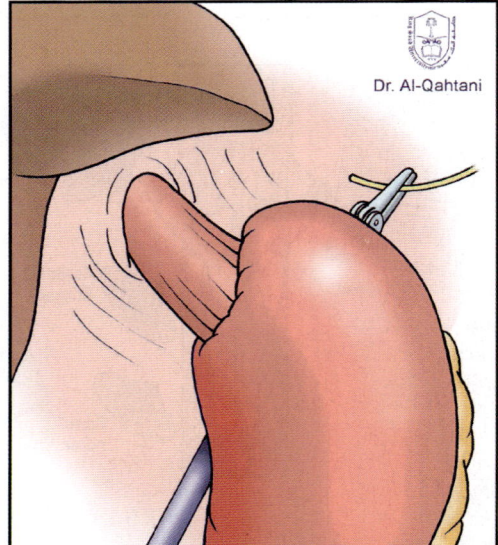

Fig. 124.21: Robotic gastric banding creating the retrogastric tunnel

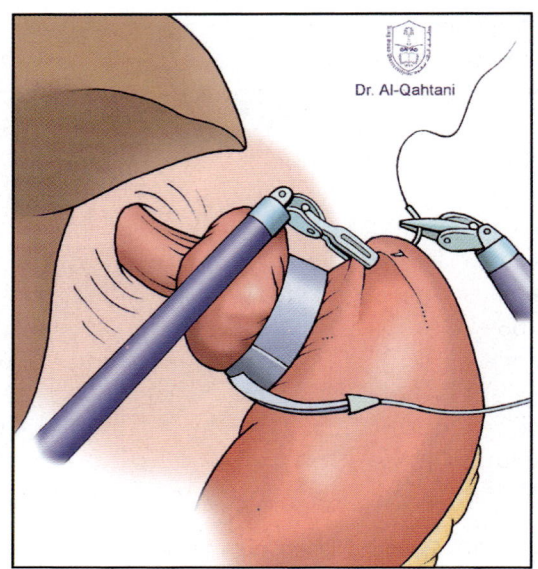

Fig. 124.22: The band in palce

well as significantly less total narcotic requirements in the robotic group as compared with the traditional open procedure.

Recently, successful robot-assisted complex, technically challenging procedures, such as robot-assisted fetal surgery, has been reported in animal models in addition to performing an esophagostomy and myelomeningocele repair.[60-67]

FUTURE DIRECTION IN ROBOTIC SURGERY

Future directions in robotic surgery are directed to development in haptics, augmented reality, miniaturization, telesurgery and telementoring.

Robotic devices with more-streamlined platforms, smaller instrumentation, and remote telementoring will all likely be a reality in the foreseeable future. Current and previously marketed telerobotic devices lack haptic or sensory feedback. While this technology has been the source of a great deal of research and funding, with numerous patents having been granted, it has not been applied clinically.[68] The potential to improve upon current technology by the addition of haptic feedback exists and will likely continue to be a source of additional research.

A major concern in robotic surgery is the cumbersome and unwieldy nature of robotic systems that require considerable space and additional time for setup. In the time-pressed operating room, compact functionality is highly desirable, and current robotic systems have yet to deliver in this regard.

A new concept that will add to the importance of robotic surgery is augmented reality (AR) which refers to the superimposition of 3D computerized reconstructed images onto a real patient's images and video, in real time.[69,70] This gives the surgeon a transparent visual anatomy of the internal structures or lesions through the overlying tissues. The source of the reconstructed images is often based on preoperative CT or MRI images. These reconstructed images are then registered onto anatomic landmarks and tracked by the computer according to the surgeon's dissection and camera movements. The images are displayed through either heads-up or headmounted displays. Most of the existing research on medical AR focused on neurosurgery, maxillofacial surgery or orthopedic surgery where bony landmarks provided constant reference points for image registration and tracking. Marescaux et al. recently demonstrated the use of AR in laparoscopic adrenalectomy although AR in general surgical and urological procedures are usually more challenging since the organs get deformed during surgical manipulation.[71]

Telesurgery refers to surgical procedures performed by a surgeon located at a remote location from the operating room via a telecommunication line. Telementoring refers to surgical guidance by a surgeon located remotely from the operating room where the procedure is performed. These capabilities have the potential for applications in the battle and disaster areas as well as guidance of surgeons in a different state or country less facile in specific complex surgeries. The first telesurgery was a laparoscopic cholecystectomy performed by surgeons in New York on a 68-year-old patient in Strasbourg, France on September 7, 2001.[42,72] Telementoring was shown to be feasible by surgeons in different continents between United States and Austria, Singapore and Thailand.[73-75] The future of telesurgery is limited by the availability of high bandwidth communication lines and lag time, cost of technology, ethical and liability issues and possible conflicts of jurisdictions between countries involved.

Another expected future work will focus on the continued development of miniature robots and its integration in Natural Orifice Translumenal Endoscopic Surgery (NOTES).

REFERENCES

1. Neugebauer E, Troidl H, Spangenberger W, Dietrich A, Lefering R. Conventional versus laparoscopic cholecystectomy and the randomized controlled trial. Cholecystectomy Study Group. Br J Surg 1991;78:150-54.
2. Diodato MD, Damiano RJ Jr. Robotic Cardiac Surgery: Overview. Surg Clin North Am 2003;83:1351-67.
3. Falk V, Diegler A, Walther T, Autschbach R, Mohr FW. Developments in robotic cardiac surgery. Curr Opin Cardiol 2000;15:378-87.
4. Satava RM. Emerging technologies for surgery in the 21st century. Arch Surg 1999;134:1197-202.
5. Ballantyne GH, Moll F. The da Vinci telerobotic surgical system: the virtual operative field and telepresence surgery. Surg Clin North Am 2003;83:1293-304.
6. Satava RM. Surgical robotics: the early chronicles: A personal historical perspective. Surg Laparosc Endosc Percutan Tech 2002;12:6-16.
7. Felger JE, Nifong L. The evolution of and early experience with robot assisted mitral valve surgery. Surg Laparosc Endosc Percutan Tech 2002;12:58-63.
8. Kim VB, Chapman WH, Albrecht RJ, Bailey BM, Young JA, Nifong LW, et al. Early experience with telemanipulative robot-assisted laparoscopic cholecystectomy using da Vinci. Surg Laparosc Endosc Percutan Tech 2002;12:34-40.
9. Kwoh YS, Hou J, Jonckheere EA, Hayati S. A robot with improved absolute positioning accuracy for CT guided stereotactic brain surgery. IEEE Trans Biomed Eng 1988;35:153-61.
10. Davies B. A review of robotics in surgery. Proc Inst Mech Eng 2000;214:129-40.
11. Hashizume M, Konishi K, Tsutsumi N, Yamaguchi S, Shimabukuro R. A new era of robotic surgery assisted by a computer-enhanced surgical system. Surgery 2002;131:S330-S33.
12. Mohr FW, Falk V, Diegeler A, Walther T, Gummert JF, Bucerius J, et al. Computer-enhanced "robotic" cardiac surgery: experience in 148 patients. J Thorac Cardiovasc Surg 2001;121:842-43.
13. A Chandra, ZD Frank. "Use of robotics in health procedures—Are we ready for it?" Hospital Topics 81 (Winter 2003) 33-35.
14. Lanfranco AR, Castellanos AE, Desai JP, Meyers WC, "Robotic surgery: A current perspective," Annals of Surgery 239 (January 2004) 14-21.
15. Stoianovici D. Robotic surgery. World J Urol 2000;18: 289-95.
16. Poulose BK, Kutka MF, Mendoza-Sagaon M, Barnes AC, Yang C, Taylor RH, et al. Human vs robotic organ retraction during laparoscopic Nissen fundoplication. Surg Endosc 1999;13:461-65.
17. Davies BL, Harris SJ, Lin WJ, Hibberd RD, Middleton R, Cobb JC. Active compliance in robotic surgery—the use of force control as a dynamic constraint. Proc Inst Mech Eng [H] 1997;211:285-92.
18. Taylor R, Jensen P, Whitcomb L. A steady-hand robotic system for microsurgical augmentation. Int J Robotics Res 1999;18:1201-10.
19. Sackier JM, Wang Y. Robotically assisted laparoscopic surgery: From concept to development. Surg Endosc 1994;8:63-66.
20. Yavuz Y, Ystgaard B, Skogvoll E, Mårvik R. A comparative experimental study evaluating the performance of surgical robots aesop and endosista. Surg Laparosc Endosc Percutan Tech 2000;10:163-67.
21. Allaf ME, Jackman SV, Schulam PG, Cadeddu JA, Lee BR, Moore RG, et al. Laparoscopic visual field: Voice vs foot pedal interfaces for control of the AESOP robot. Surg Endosc 1998; 12:1415-18.
22. Mettler L, Ibrahim M, Jonat W. One year of experience working with the aid of a robotic assistant (the voice-controlled optic holder AESOP) in gynaecological endoscopic surgery. Hum Reprod 1998; 13:2748-50.
23. Omote K, Feussner H, Ungeheuer A, Arbter K, Wei GQ, Siewert JR, et al. Self-guided robotic camera control for laparoscopic surgery compared with human camera control. Am J Surg 1999;177:321-24.
24. Merola S, Weber P, Wasielewski A, Ballantyne GH. Comparison of laparoscopic colectomy with and without the aid of a robotic camera holder. Surg Laparosc Endosc Percutan Tech 2002; 12:46-51.
25. EndoAssist. Prosurgics. Accessed July 16, 2007, from http://www.prosurgics.com/

26. Paul HA, Bargar WL, Mittlestadt B, Musits B, Taylor RH, Kazanzides P, et al. Development of a surgical robot for cementless total hip arthroplasty. Clin Orthop 1992; 57-66.
27. Robodoc. Integrated Surgical Systems. Accessed July 1, 2007, from http://robodoc.com/eng/robodoc.html
28. Orthodoc. Integrated Surgical Systems. Accessed July 1, 2007, from http://www.robodoc.com/eng/orthodoc.html
29. Siebert W, Mai S, Kober R, Heeckt PF. Technique and first clinical results of robot-assisted total knee replacement. Knee 2002;9:173-80.
30. Brandt G, Zimolong A, Carrat L, Merloz P, Staudte HW, Lavallee S, et al. CRIGOS: A compact robot for image-guided orthopedic surgery. IEEE Trans Inf Technol Biomed 1999;3:252-60.
31. Bouazza-Marouf K, Browbank I, Hewit JR. Robotic-assisted internal fixation of femoral fractures. Proc Inst Mech Eng [H] 1995;209:51-58.
32. Glauser D, Fankhauser H, Epitaux M, Hefti JL, Jaccottet A. Neurosurgical robot Minerva: First results and current developments. J Image Guid Surg 1995; 1:266-72.
33. Li QH, Zamorano L, Pandya A, Perez R, Gong J, Diaz F. The application accuracy of the NeuroMate robot—a quantitative comparison with frameless and frame-based surgical localization systems. Comput Aided Surg 2002;7:90-98.
34. NeuroMate. Integrated Surgical Systems. Retrieved July 26, 2007, from http://robodoc.com/eng/neuromate.html
35. Finlay PA, Morgan P. PathFinder image guided robot for neurosurgery. Prosurgics. Accessed July 16, 2007, from http://www.prosurgics.com
36. Adler JR Jr, Chang SD, Murphy MJ, Doty J, Geis P, Hancock SL. The Cyberknife: A frameless robotic system for radiosurgery. Stereotact Funct Neurosurg 1997;69:124-28.
37. CyberKnife. Accuray. Accessed July 20, 2007, from. http://www.accuray.com/cyberknife.html
38. The Probot. Mechatronics in Medicine—Imperial College. Accessed August 7, 2007, from http://www3.imperial.ac.uk/mechatronicsinmedicine/projects/theprobot
39. Arambula Cosio F, Davies BL. Automated prostate recognition. A key process for clinically effective robotic prostatectomy. Med Biol Eng Comput 1999;37:236-43.
40. The RCM Robot. URobotics Brady Urological Insititue, Johns Hopkins Medical Institutions. Accessed August 8, 2007, from http://urology.jhu.edu/urobotics/pub/2002-su-jendourol.pdf
41. Stoianovici D, Whitcomb LL, Anderson JH. A modular surgical robotic system for image guided percutaneous procedures. Lecture Notes in Computer Science, New York: Springer 1998:404-10.
42. Marescaux J, Leroy J, Gagner M, Rubino F, Mutter D, Vix M, et al. Transatlantic robot-assisted telesurgery. Nature 2001;413:379-80.
43. Fuchs KH. Minimally invasive surgery. Endoscopy 2002;34:154-59.
44. Dutta S, Woo R, Albanese C. Minimal access portoenterostomy: advantages and disadvantages of the standard laparoscopic and robotic techniques. Pediatr Surg Int 2006, in press.
45. Woo R, Le D, Kim S, Albanese C. Robot-assisted laparoscopic resection of a type I choldedochal cyst. J Laparoendosc Adv Tech 2006; 16:179-83.
46. Goh PMY, Lomanto D, So JBY. Robotic-assisted laparoscopic cholecystectomy. Surg Endosc 2002;16:216-17.
47. Lorincz A, Langenburg S, Klein MD. Robotics and the pediatric surgeon. Curr Opin Pediatr 2003;15:262-66.
48. Zhou HX, Guo YH, Yu XF, Bao SY, Liu JL, Zhang Y, et al. Zeus robot-assisted laparoscopic cholecystectomy in comparison with conventional laparoscopic cholecystectomy. Hepatobiliary Pancreat Dis Int 2006;5:115-18.
49. Chaer RA, Jacobsen G, Elli F, Harris J, Goldstein A, Horgan S. Robotic-assisted laparoscopic pediatric Heller's cardiomyotomy: initial case report. J Laparoendosc Adv Surg Tech 2004;14:270-73.
50. Le Bret E, Papadatos S, Folliguet T, Carbognani D, Pétrie J, Aggoun Y, et al. Interruption of patent ductus arteriosus in children: robotically assisted versus videothoracoscopic surgery. J Thorac Cardiovasc Surg 2002;123:973-76.
51. Wimmer-Greinecker G, Dogan S, Aybek T, Khan MF, Mierdl S, Byhahn C, et al. Totally endoscopic atrial septal repair in adults with computer-enhanced telemanipulation. J Thorac Cardiovasc Surg 2003;126:465-68.
52. Reichenspurner H, Damiano RJ, Mack M, Boehm DH, Gulbins H, Detter C, et al. Use of the voice controlled and computer-assisted surgical system ZEUS for endoscopic coronary artery bypass grafting. J Thorac Cardiovasc Surg 1999;118:11-16.
53. Torracca L, Ismeno G, Alfieri O. Totally endoscopic computer-enhanced atrial septal defect closure in six patients. Ann Thorac Surg 2001;72:1354-57.
54. Argenziano M, Oz MC, Kohmoto T, Morgan J, Dimitui J, Mongero L, et al. Totally endoscopic atrial septal defect repair with robotic assistance. Circulation 2003;108:II191 (suppl 1).
55. Suematsu Y, del Nido PJ. Robotic pediatric cardiac surgery: present and future perspectives. Am J Surg 2004;188:98S-103S.
56. Pedraza R, Palmer L, Moss V, Franco I. Bilateral robotic assisted laparoscopic heminephroureterectomy. J Urol 2004;171:2394-95.
57. Pedraza R, Weiser A, Franco I. Laparoscopic appendicovesicostomy (Mitrofanoff procedure) in a child using the da Vinci robotic system. J Urol 2004;171:1652-53.
58. Atug F, Woods M, Burgess SV, Castle EP, Thomas R. Robotic assisted laparoscopic pyeloplasty in children. J Urol 2005;174:1440-61.
59. Lee RS, Retik AB, Borer JG, Peters CA. Pediatric robot assisted laparoscopic dismembered pyeloplasty: comparison with a cohort of open surgery. J Urol 2006;175:683-87.
60. Hollands CM, Dixey LN. Robotic-assisted esophagoesophagostomy. Pediatr Surg 2002;37:983-85.

61. Hollands CM, Dixey LN, Torma MJ. Technical assessment of porcin enteroenterostomy performed with ZEUS robotic technology. J Pediatr Surg 2001;36:1231-33.
62. Malhotra SP, Le D, Thelitz S, Hanley FL, Riemer RK, Suleman S, et al. Robotic-assisted endoscopic thoracic aortic anastomosis in juvenile lambs. Heart Surg Forum 2002;6:38-42.
63. Aaronson OS, Tulipan NB, Cywes R, Sundell HW, Davis GH, Bruner JP, et al. Robot-assisted endoscopic intrauterine myelomeningocele repair: a feasibility study. Pediatr Neurosurg 2002;36:85-89.
64. Olsen LH, Deding D, Yeung CK, Jørgensen TM. Computer assisted laparoscopic pneumovesical ureter reimplantation a.m. Cohen: initial experience in a pig model. APMIS Suppl 2003;109:23-25.
65. Guillónneau B, Rietbergen JB, Fromont G, Vallancien G, et al. Robotically assisted laparoscopic dismembered pyeloplasty: a chronic porcine study. Urology 2003;61:1063-66.
66. Lorincz A, Knight CG, Langenburg SE, Rabah R, Gidell K, Dawe E, et al. Robot-assisted minimally invasive Kasai portoenterostomy: a survival porcine study. Surg Endosc 2004;18:1136-39.
67. Hollands CM, Dixey LN. Applications of robotic surgery in pediatric patients. Surg Laparosc Endosc Percutan Tech 2002;12:71-76.
68. Madhani AJ, Niemeyer G, Salisbury JK. The black falcon: a teleoperated surgical instrument for minimally invasive surgery. In: Proceedings IEEE/Robotics Society of Japan International Conference on Intelligent Robotic Systems 1998;2;936-44.
69. Tang SL, Kwoh CK, Teo MY, Sing NW, Ling KV. Augmented reality systems for medical applications. IEEE Eng Med Biol Mag 1998;17:49.
70. Shuhaiber JH. Augmented reality in surgery. Arch Surg 2004;139:170.
71. Marescaux J, Rubino F, Arenas M, Mutter D, Soler L. Augmentedreality- assisted laparoscopic adrenalectomy. Jama 2004;292:2214.
72. Marescaux J, Leroy J, Rubino F, Smith M, Vix M, Simone M, et al. Transcontinental robot-assisted remote telesurgery: feasibility and potential applications. Ann Surg 2002;235:487.
73. Lee BR, Caddedu JA, Janetschek G, Schulam P, Docimo SG, Moore RG, et al. International surgical telementoring: our initial experience. Stud Health Technol Inform 1998;50:41.
74. Lee BR, Png DJ, Liew L, Fabrizio M, Li MK, Jarrett JW, et al. Laparoscopic telesurgery between the United States and Singapore. Ann Acad Med Singapore 2000;29:665.
75. Lee BR, Bishoff JT, Janetschek G, Bunyaratevej P, Kamolpronwijit W, Cadeddu JA, et al. A novel method of surgical instruction: international telementoring. World J Urol 1998;16:367.

CHAPTER 125

Tissue Engineering: Present Concepts and Strategies

Amulya K Saxena

Medical or surgical procedures that have attempted to partially replace lost tissue, account for a large part of health care resources which exceed over $400 billion per year.[1] Replace like tissue with like tissue is a basic principle of surgery. However, certain congenital, posttraumatic, postablative, or even multiply operated deformities may be so severe that autologous tissue does not exist in sufficient quantity, or is difficult to obtain in order to achieve a favorable result (Fig. 125.1). Current therapeutic modalities to treat tissue or organ loss include total artificial or mechanical devices, biological processed tissues, transplanting organs from one individual into another, surgical reconstruction, autologous transfer of tissue to the diseased-site or supplementing metabolic products of the lost tissue.

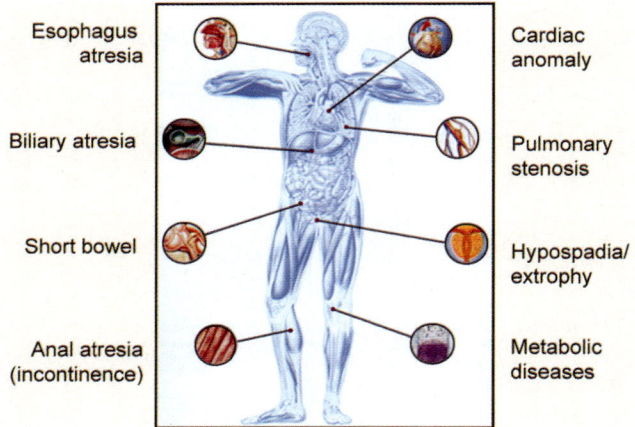

Fig. 125.1: While concentrating on the adult population the actual demand of tissues required in the pediatric population is being underestimated

Although these traditional forms of tissue replacement have rescued millions of patients and have improved countless lives, they suffer from problems of scarce supply, increased susceptibility to infection, immunologic rejection, as well as uncertain long-term interactions with the patients; and however still remain imperfect solutions. The problems are much more severe in the pediatric age group, since implantable mechanical devices do not grow as the child grows.

Tissue engineering is an interdisciplinary field which applies the principles and methods of engineering and the life sciences towards the fundamental understanding of structural and functional relationships in normal and pathological tissue and the development of biological substitutes to restore, maintain, or improve function.[2] Tissues that are engineered using the patients own cells, or immunological inactive allogenic or xenogenic cells have the potential to overcome current problems of replacing lost tissue function and offer new therapeutic options for diseases where currently no options are available. Tissue engineering technology can play a vital role in the future management of pediatric patients.[3] Tissues or organs absent at the time of birth, in congenital anomalies such as esophagus atresia, bladder extrophy and congenital diaphragmatic hernia to name a few, pose a serious challenge in surgical repair. The advances in prenatal diagnostics, that allow earlier detection of such anomalies, could give sufficient time to engineer the missing tissue or organs and have them fabricated for surgical replacement at the time of birth.

GENERAL STRATEGIES TO REPLACE TISSUE LOSS

The primary intention of all approaches in tissue engineering is the functional or structural restoration of tissue through the delivery of living elements which become integrated into the patient. Most of the techniques of guided tissue restoration developed during the last two decades have mainly been only cell based or only matrices based, however investigators in the rapidly emerging field of tissue engineering presently use a combination of both to achieve new tissue formation.

Cell and Cell Based Techniques

In cell based tissue engineering methods, isolated and disseminated cells are injected into the blood stream or a specific organ of the recipient. The cells transplanted using such injection methods will utilize the blood supply for nutrients and the ground substance provided by the host tissue as a matrix bed for attachment, reorganization and desired growth.[4] The cell injection approach avoids the complications of surgery, allows substitution of only those cells that supply the needed function, and permits manipulation of cells before infusion. This method might find applications in replacing lost metabolic functions however its application in replacing functions of structural tissues is severely limited.

Cell Encapsulation Techniques

In this concept for cell transplantation, the cells are cultured and encapsulated in a semipermeable membrane that isolates the cells from the body. However, at the same time the semipermeable membrane, which allows the diffusion of nutrients and wastes, prevents macromolecules such as antibodies, complement factors and immune cells from accessing the transplant. This application of this system has been successfully demonstrated in the production of a bioartificial liver, using xenogenic hepatocytes, as an extracorporeal liver support system and was effective in clinical trials for the treatment of acute liver failure.[5]

Tissue Engineering Using Open Systems of Cell Transplantation

The primary goal of the open system of cell transplantation is to engineer new tissues by having the transplanted cells in direct contact with the host with the intention to provide a permanent natural solution to the replacement of lost tissue. Cells for transplantation using this technique are attached to matrices consisting of natural materials or synthetic polymers and are then implanted into the host. These cell-polymers constructs then incorporates itself into the recepient's own tissue. In cell culture experiments it has been observed that dissociated mature cells tend to reform their original structures when given the appropriate environmental cues. This has been demonstrated by the formation of tubular structures by capillary endothelial cells in culture, as well as the formation of milk secreting acini by mammary epithelial cells *in vitro*.[6] Isolated cells also have the capability to reform their structure, however only up to a limited degree when placed as a suspension into the host. This is mainly due to the absence of an intrinsic tissue ground substance framework. Implantation of tissue in larger volumes is also severely restricted because diffusion limitations restrict interaction with the host environment for nutrition, gas exchange and waste elimination. Based on these observations, approaches to engineer tissue by attaching isolated cells to porous polymeric templates have been developed. The application and introduction of cell-polymer construct concept in the engineering of new tissue was to provide a structural foundation to support tissues undergoing constant remodeling, integration and restructuring (Fig. 125.2). Over the past two decades, a lot of research work has been done to design, develop and experimentally demonstrate the increasing advantages of polymer matrices based open cell system transplantation in the manufacturing of new tissues.

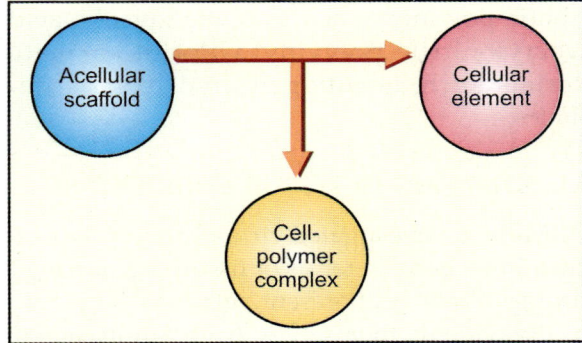

Fig. 125.2: Tissue engineering involves combining of cell along with biodegradable scaffolds to manufactures tissue or organs

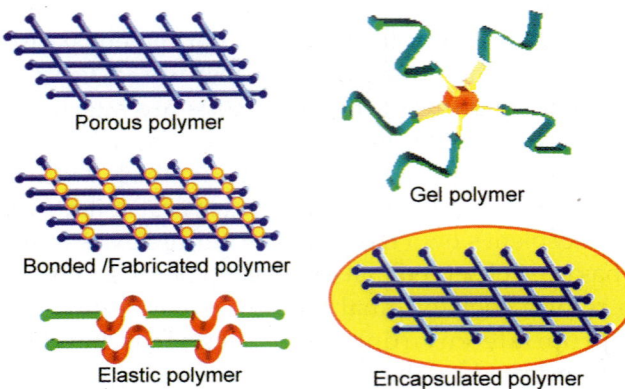

Fig. 125.3: Schematic representation of polymers showing the different structure and shapes required as demanded by the tissue generated

BIOCOMPATIBLE POLYMER MATRICES

Polymer matrices used in tissue-engineered devices need to be biocompatible and have been designed to meet the nutritional and biological needs of the cell populations involved in the formation of new tissue (Fig. 125.3). The next important feature is that the materials should also be resorbable so that they leave a complete natural tissue replacement. Furthermore, polymer matrices should be reproducibly processable into desired structures and shapes and be able to retain their shapes after implantation in the host. If desired, the material should promote the growth of cells to increase the mass of the tissue. Finally, the surface of the material should interact with the transplanted cells to allow retention of differentiated cell function. Materials on the other hand that do not possess the above properties or are nonresorbable carry a permanent risk of infection.[7] The most commonly materials being used as substrates or encapsulating materials in the field of tissue engineering are either synthetic polymers such as lactic-glycolic acid or polyacrylonitrile polyvinyl chloride, or natural materials such as collagen, hydroxyapatite, or alginates.

CELL SOURCING IN TISSUE ENGINEERING

Scientists have investigated virtually every tissue type in the human body in terms of tissue engineering. For clinical applications at present, cells have been derived from the patients themselves, from family members or close relatives, or other individuals. However, although this may be the most ideal source of cells, availability and accessibility may often be quite difficult. One approach to over come the cell-source difficulty could be isolation of human stem cells. Human stem cells can be proliferated through multiple generations and made to differentiate into the appropriate cell type. Recent studies have shown that stem cells derived from human embryonic blastocytes possessed these characteristics.[8] These stem cells identified, can be signaled to turn into different morphological cell types by changing the culturing conditions of the cells prior to implantation. Although there are a number of technical hurdles such as the need for pure stem-cell preparations, methods to reduce adhesion of cells during cell culture and processes to generate large number of cells to create tissue; work on stem cells involved in the creation of muscle, bone, and cartilage has demonstrated promising results in tissue engineering applications.

IN VITRO CULTURE SYSTEMS

Static Cell-Cultures

Early work in the field of tissue engineering was based on the use of standard static cell-culture conditions for the *in vitro* fabrication of tissues before implantation. However, there have been certain limitations to the exchange of nutrients and gases. These limitations are being overcome by advanced application of mechanical engineering expertise in the field of biotechnology by designing and producing dynamic cell culture systems, better known as bioreactors (Fig. 125.4).

Bioreactors

Bioreactors are dynamic cell culture systems that allow more control to generate larger volumes of cells when compared to conventional static-culture techniques. The flow of tissue culture medium and their mixing within bioreactors can be controlled to enhance mass transfer of nutrients, gases, and metabolites in order to regulate the size and structure of the tissue being generated.

PRESENT STATUS OF TISSUE ENGINEERING

Seeding of cells on 3-D biodegradable polymers in cell culture or flow bioreactor gave the opportunity to

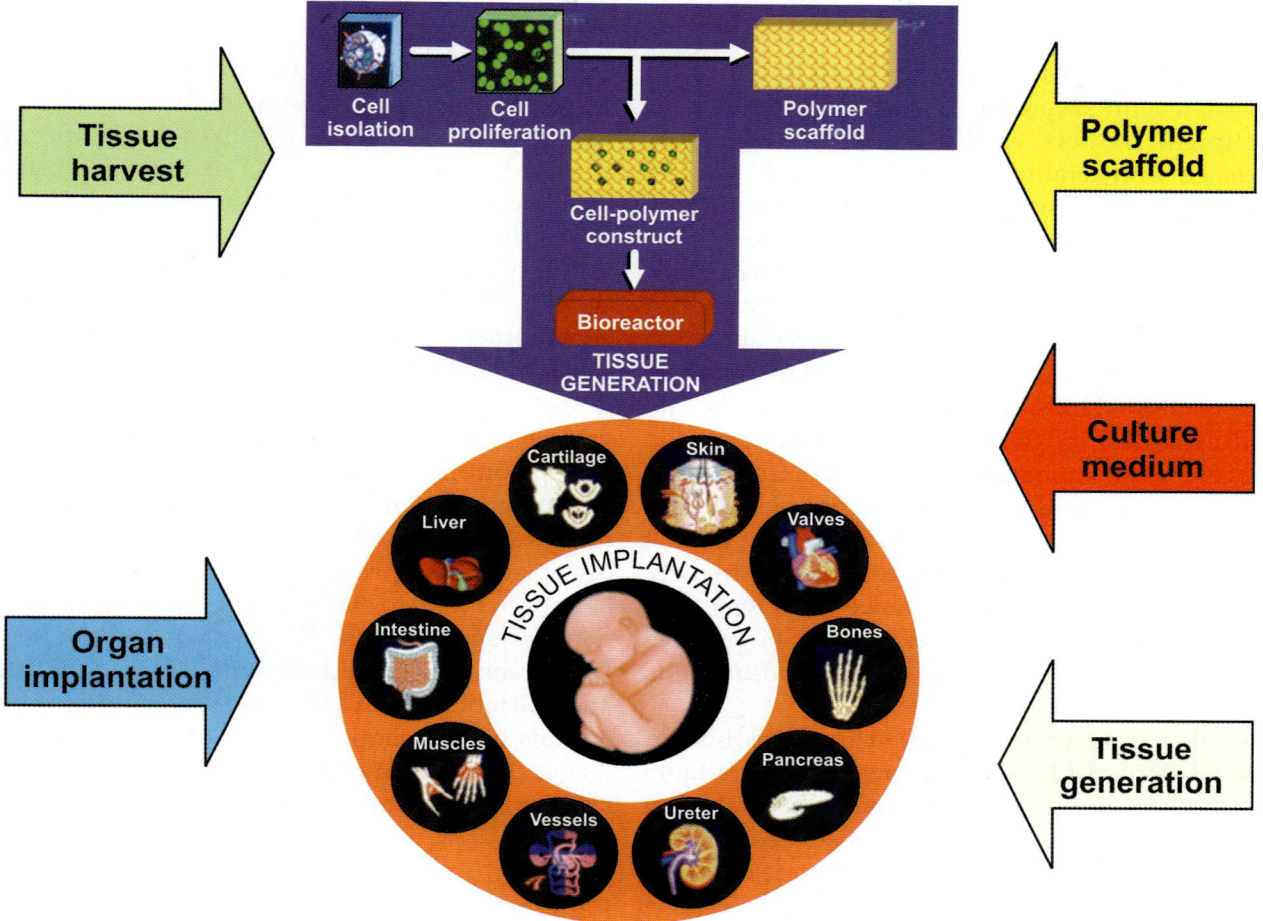

Fig. 125.4: Bioreactors are used to help cells integrate with the polymer scaffolds to generate new tissue

study tissue development, tissue regeneration, and tissue repair *in vitro*. Investigators have attempted to study the properties of almost all mammalian cell types under *in vitro* conditions. Implantation of the cell polymer constructs allows further study *in vivo*. Knowledge obtained from the different disciplines participating in active tissue engineering research has promoted the evolution of this new field from primary animal research to clinical trials. The present status of different structural and functional tissue has been described below:

Nervous System

Progress has also been reported in attempts to regenerate the peripheral nerve. Synthetic nerve guides, fabricated in the shape of tubes, have been found to aid the regeneration of nerves that have been injured and separated by gaps that are too wide for healing. The tubes help the regenerating nerve from scar infiltration and also direct the new regenerating axons towards their target. It has been also demonstrated in several animal models that synthetic guides composed of natural polymers and synthetic polymers have enhanced axonal regeneration *in vivo*.[9,10] The process of nerve regeneration has been further promoted by lining polymer membranes with Schwann cells.[11] Additionally, polymers have been also designed to slowly release growth factors that aid in the regeneration of the damaged nerve over longer distances.

Skin

Burn and burn related injuries are known to be associated with severe morbidity and mortality. In preclinical models, acellular dermis has been populated with keratinocytes and fibroblasts and has been tested as skin substitute.[12] Biosynthetic analogs of skin on the other hand have combined cultured skin cells with polylactic/polyglycolic fabric, collagen gels, and collagen-glycosaminoglycan (GAG) sponges to provide skin replacements. (Fig. 125.5) This approach involves the in vitro culture of keratinocytes obtained from small skin biopsies (1 cm^2) of burn patients. The rapid expansion of the keratinocyte population is achieved by cultivating keratinocytes on a feeder layer of irradiated fibroblasts (NIH 3T3) in association with certain media components. The advantage of this method is that it allows the graft to cover extremely large wounds; a disadvantage however is that a 3-4 week period is required for cell expansion. It is possible that cryopreserved allografts may help to address this problem.[13]

Another approach to fabricate skin, utilizes human neonatal dermal fibroblasts grown on degradable polyglycolic acid polymers. In this method selective cultures of dermal fibroblasts are inoculated into the porous reticulations of the substrate. In case of severe burn injuries involving all the skin layers, the graft is placed directly on the wound bed and a skin graft (cultured epidermal autograft) is placed above. This graft then organizes and vascularizes to form organized dermis like tissue. Furthermore, the addition of a dermal matrix to epithelial tissue engineered replacements adds the theoretical advantage of a thicker, more durable graft that more closely resembles the "gold standard" of split-thickness skin grafts.[14]

Liver

Donor shortfall for liver transplantations presents a severe challenge to clinicians worldwide. After tedious research it has been found out that a number of critical steps determine the success of hepatocyte transplantation. Simple manipulations such as sandwiching the cells between hydrated collagen gels have prolonged the secretion of albumin, transferrin, fibrinogen, bile acids and urea from cultured hepatocytes.[15] Furthermore, in order to maintain their differentiated function, hepatocytes must be attached to the polymer substrates, and also be implanted in vascular areas of the body so that a constant supply of hepatotrophic factors can be maintained.[16] These factors taken in to account, have demonstrated that tissue structures can be formed when hepatocytes have been placed on appropriate polymers. The hepatocytes have been found to maintain a distribution of filament network similar to the *in vivo* state and the hepatic tissue generated has also shown evidence of bile ducts and bilirubin removal.[17] Vast spectrum of investigations are presently being undertaken to enable larger transplantation of hepatocytes, as well as to prolong the cell viability, using various polymers.[18]

Pancreas

Diabetes mellitus affects a major part of the adult population worldwide (Fig. 125.6). Transplantation of grafts of isolated pancreas islets has been performed to tackle this problem, however despite immune

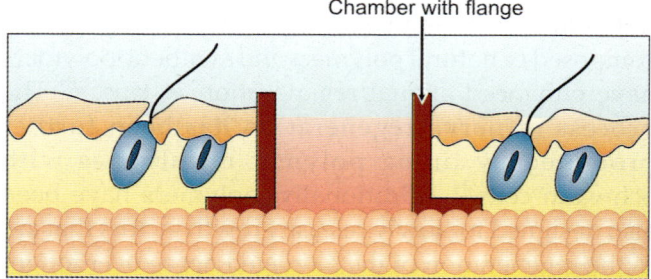

Fig. 125.5: The porcine chamber model is the optimal system to investigate skin tissue engineering since it provides well defined wounds of known depth and size

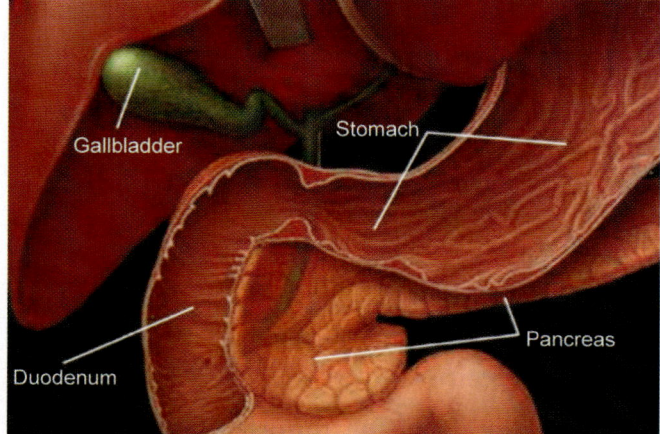

Fig. 125.6: The large prevalence of diabetes mellitus has catapulted the research in pancreas tissue engineering

alterations of the transplants no success has been reported in animal models. To overcome the problem of immunorejection and autoimmune rejection, the concept of immunoisolation has been advocated. This is achieved by enclosing the pancreatic islets by semipermeable and biocompatible membrane (bioartificial pancreas). The semipermeable membrane is impermeable to high molecular weight antibodies, but permeable to oxygen, glucose and internally generated hormones (insulin, glucagons, somatostatin, pancreatic polypeptides and other islet proteins).[19]

Urinary Tubular Structures

Replacement of the ureter, bladder, and urethra using parts of other organs for reconstruction, often leads to reflux, infection and dilatation of the upper urinary tract. Nonbiological or metal implants have been used to replace ureters but have largely failed due to poor biocompatibility, lack of peristalitic activity and deposition of salt on their surfaces. Since the urothelium has a good regenerative capability, the fabrication of urothelium-polymer constructs as implants for replacement therapy have been explored. Successful fabrication of the ureter and segmental ureteral replacement has been achieved using urothelial cells seeded onto polyglycolic acid polymer tubes.[20]

Esophagus

The application of the concepts of using tubular polymers has broadened from ureter replacements to the possible replacements of other tubular structures such as the trachea, esophagus and intestines. Copolymer tubes of lactic-glycolic acid used in a dog model as an esophageal replacement have shown encouraging results. The tubes were over time covered by connective and epithelial tissue and the dogs were able to drink freely and eat semisolid foods.[21] Further research using better designed copolymer tubes and cell seeding techniques could provide breakthrough for esophagus replacement and treatment for the management of malformations such as long-gap esophageal atresia.[22]

Small Intestine

In a similar approach, fetal intestinal cells have been seeded onto polymers tubes and have shown promising results in new intestinal tissue generation. The new intestinal epithelium engineered has demonstrated the presence of differentiated intestinal epithelium cells lining the tubes.[23] Histology has revealed the development of crypt-villus structures in the neointestine cells which have the functional capability to secrete mucous. Promising results emerging after the anastomosis of tissue-engineered neointestine to native small bowel, and its successful structural and functional integration, gives hope for the management of patients with short bowel syndromes.[24]

Cartilage

Research has been aimed at creating new cartilage based on collagen-glycosaminoglycan templates, isolated chondrocytes and chondrocytes attached to natural or synthetic polymers (Fig. 125.7). Articular cartilage is composed of a highly organized extracellular matrix, which consists mainly of type-II collagen and proteoglycan (chondroitin and keratan sulfate glycosaminoglycans) and a relatively sparse cell population of articular chondrocytes. The mechanical performance of articular cartilages is dependant on the architecture of its extracellular matrix and the ability of the constituent chondrocytes to maintain the matrix. The use of well-stirred bioreactors for cultivating chondrocytes on polymer

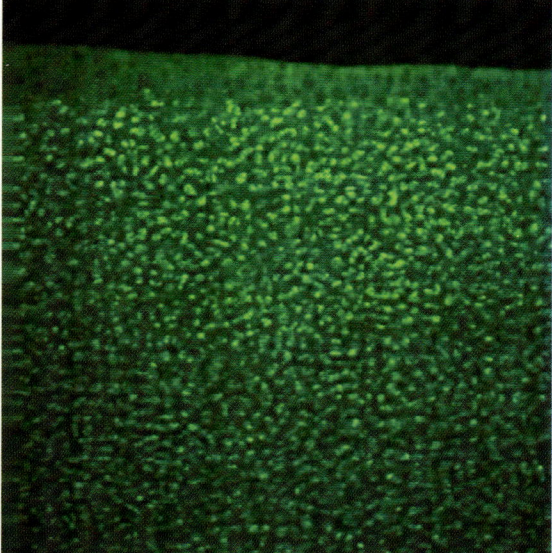

Fig. 125.7: Fluorescently stained cartilage cells suspended in a collagen matrix demonstrating engineered cartilage tissue

scaffolds *in vitro* may enable nutrients to penetrate the center of this nonvascularized tissue, leading to strong and thick implants.[25] Cartilages for replacement of various tissue such as nasoseptum, human ear cartilage as well as trachea replacement have been engineered. In the case of joint replacements, tissue engineered cartilages have been shown to induce the same lubricity, produce the same coefficient of friction, as well as absorb and dampen the joint forces settings of a normal articular cartilage.

Bone

Culture of seeded osteoblastic cells in 3-D osteoconductive scaffolds *in vitro* is a promising approach to produce an osteoinductive matter for the repair of bone defects.[26] Small phalanges and joints resembling the shape and composition of human phalanges have been successfully fabricated using periosteum, chondrocytes, and tenocytes seeded differentially onto biodegradable polymer scaffolds. To achieve this, the gross form of a composite tissue structure was constituted in vitro by assembling the parts and suturing them to create models of the phalanges. The sutured composite tissues were then implanted subcutaneously and resulted in the formation of new tissue after 20 weeks.[27]

Muscle

Skeletal muscle comprises approximately 48% of the body mass and is responsible for voluntary control and active movement of the body. Application of tissue engineering techniques and successful fabrication of skeletal muscle mass holds now a promising future for the restoration of 3-D contour as well as the loss of function for the affected part of the body.[28,29] In order to generate skeletal muscle tissue, myoblasts which are skeletal muscle tissue precursors, have been employed (Fig. 125.8). Myoblasts have been seeded onto polyglycolic acid porous polymers with successful generation of vascularized new skeletal muscle *in vivo*.[30]

Under cell culture conditions, myoblasts cultures have exhibited twitching movement on stimulation.[31] This exhibition of movement by myoblasts in culture is very important for the fabrication of new skeletal muscle which is not only a structural but more an important functional tissue.[32] Research is presently

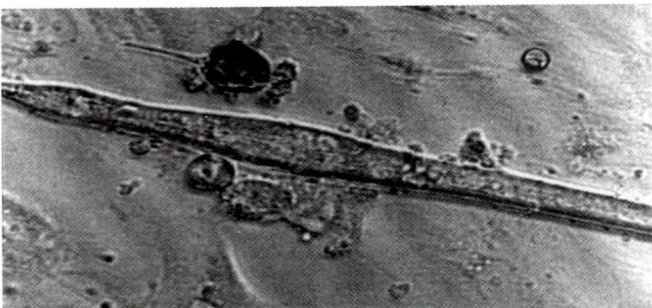

Fig. 125.8: Myoblasts (14 days old) used for muscle tissue engineering exhibit contraction and "twitching" in culture medium when stimulated

being carried out in improving the vascular infrastructure of the muscle to enable generation of larger muscle mass.[33] Gel polymers have also been successfully used for the transplantation of myoblasts.[34]

Heart Valves and Blood Vessels

Tissue engineering of heart valve was demonstrated using autologous myofibroblasts and endothelial cells harvested from the femoral artery of a lamb. The cells were expanded in culture and cell separation was performed using a fluorescent activated cell sorter. The myofibers were first seeded onto a polymer scaffold composed of polyglactin polymer mesh sandwiched between two polyglycolic acid meshes. The endothelial cells were seeded onto the polyglycolic acid meshes after a time lag of 7 days. The construct was trimmed to size and was implanted in the same lamb to replacing the right pulmonary leaflet. The polymer disappeared after 6 weeks of implantation leaving behind a leaflet histologically resembling the native pulmonary valvular architecture. The mechanical properties of the tissue engineered leaflet approached the natural parameters over time.[35] Grafts are also being designed from relatively inert materials (with heparin coatings) or with materials that interact with blood cells in a desirable way.

FUTURE ASPECTS AND RESEARCH

For the clinical success of tissue engineering numerous areas of research are critical (Fig. 125.9). Precise understanding of cell biology with emphasis on cellular differentiation, cell to cell interaction and

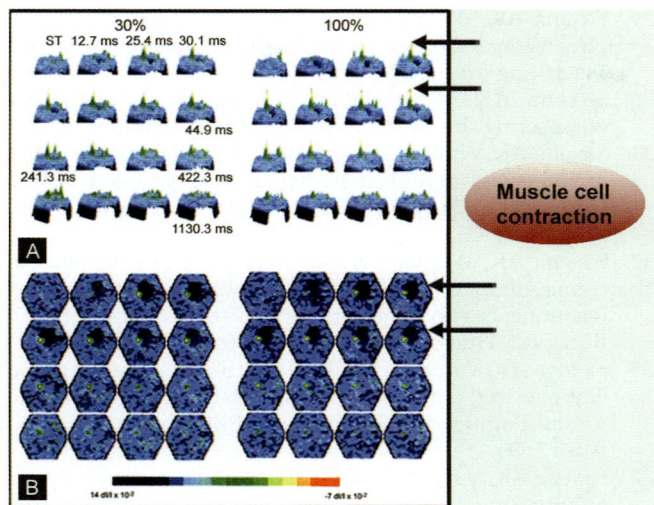

Fig. 125.9: It is important to demonstrate the functionality of the engineered tissue. Using nanoelectrodes tissue engineered skeletal muscle was stimulated and muscle contractions were recorded showing that engineered tissue posses the same characteristics as that of the original tissue

extracellular matrix formation will be of paramount importance. Cell sourcing, cell preservation and cryopreservation of cells, or establishment of cell banks, which are only possible for certain tissues at present must be made possible for other tissues in the future. Large-scale cell culture systems, capable of resolving the nutrient transport issue and allowing the proliferation of larger number of required cell types in vitro, must be designed. The continuous work performed in designing better polymers is another major area of study. Tissue engineering is a new technology, with profound benefits and an enormous potential that offers future promise in the treatment of loss of tissue or organ function as well as for genetic disorders with metabolic disorders.

REFERENCES

1. Langer R, Vacanti JP. Tissue engineering. Science 1993;260:920-26.
2. Skalak R, Fox CF (eds): Tissue Engineering: Proceedings of a workshop held at Granlibakken, Lake Tahoe, CA, February 26-29, 1988, New York, NY, Liss, 1988.
3. Saxena AK, Höcker H, Willital GH. [Present status of tissue engineering for surgical indications in children]. 116th Congress of the German Association for Surgery, Munich, Germany, April 1999.
4. Matas AJ, Sutherland DER, Steffes MW, et al. Hepatocellular transplantation for metabolic deficiencies: Decrease of plasma bilirubin in Gunn rats. Science 1976;192:892-94.
5. Rozga J, Podesta L, Le Page E, et al. A bioartificial liver to treat severe acute liver failure. Ann Surg 1994;219:538-46.
6. Folkman J, Haudenschild C. Angiogenesis in vitro. Nature 1980;288:551-56.
7. Christina AG: Biomaterial-centered infection. Microbial adhesion versus tissue integration. Science 1987;237:1588-95.
8. Thomson JA, Itskovitz-Eldor J, Shapiro SS, et al. Embryonic stem cell lines derived from human blastocytes. Science 1998;282:1145-47.
9. Madison R, da Silva CF, Dikkes P, et al. Increased rate of peripheral nerve regeneration using bioresorbable nerve guides and a laminin-containing gel. Exp Neurol 1985;88:767-72.
10. Stang F, Fansa H, Wolf G, et al. Collagen nerve conduits-assessment of biocompatibility and axonal regeneration. Biomed Mater Eng. 2005;15:3-12.
11. Guénard V, Kleitman N, Morrissey TK, et al. Syngeneic Schwann cells derived from adult nerves seeded in set guidance channels enhance peripheral nerve regeneration. J Neurosci 1992;12:3310-20.
12. Medalie DA, Eming SA, Tompkins RG, et al. Evaluation of human skin reconstituted from composite grafts of cultured keratinocytes and human acelllular dermis transplanted to athymic mice. J Invest Dermatol 1996;107(1):121-27.
13. Yannas IV, Burke JF. Design of an artificial skin. I. Basic design principles. J Biomed Mater Res 1980;14:65-81.
14. Tinois E, Tiollier J, Gaucherand M, Dumas H, et al. In vitro and posttransplantation differentiation of human keratinocytes grown on the human type IV collagen film of a bilayered dermal substitute. Exp Cell Res 1991;193:310-19.
15. Dunn JCY, Tompkins RG, Yarmush ML. Long-term in vitro function of adult hepatocytes in collagen gel sandwich configuration. Biotechnol Prog 1991;7:237-45.
16. Yarmush ML, Toner M, Dunn JC, et al. Hepatic tissue engineering. Development of critical technologies. Ann NY Acad Sci 1992;665:238-52.
17. Uyama S, Kaufmann PM, Takeda T. Delivery of whole liver-equivalent hepatocyte mass using polymer devices and hepatotrophic stimulation. Transplantation 1993;55:932-35.
18. Lin P, Chan WC, Badylak SF, et al: Assessing porcine liver-derived biomatrix for hepatic tissue engineering. Tissue Eng. 2004;10:1046-53.
19. Sullivan SJ, Maki T, Borland KM, et al. Biohybrid artificial pancreas: long-term implantation studies in diabetic, pancreatectomized dogs. Science 1991;252:718-21.
20. Koh CJ, Atala A. Tissue engineering for urinary incontinence applications. Minerva Ginecol 2004;56:371-78.
21. Grower MF, Russell EA Jr, Cutright DE. Segmental neogenesis of the dog esophagus utilizing a biodegradable polymer framework. Biomater Artif Cells Artif Organs 1989;17:291-314.

22. Lynen Jansen P, Klinge U, Anurov M, et al. Surgical mesh as a scaffold for tissue regeneration in the esophagus. Eur Surg Res. 2004;36:104-11.
23. Kim SS, Kaihara S, Benvenuto MS, et al. Effects of anastomosis of tissue-engineered neointestine to native small bowel. J Surg Res 1999;87:6-13.
24. Chen MK, Beierle EA. Animal models for intestinal tissue engineering. Biomaterials 2004;25:1675-81.
25. Freed L, Vunjak-Novakovic G, Langer R. Cultivation of cell-polymer cartilage implants in bioreactors. J Cell Biochem 1993;51:257-64.
26. Ohgushi H, Kotobuki N, Funaoka H. Tissue engineered ceramic artificial joint-ex vivo osteogenic differentiation of patient mesenchymal cells on total ankle joint for treatment of osteoarthritis. Biomaterials 2005;26:4654-61.
27. Isogai N, Landis W, Kin TH, et al. Tissue engineering of a phalangeal joint for application in reconstructive hand surgery. J Bone Joint Surg Am 1999;81:306-16.
28. Saxena AK, Marler J, Benvenuto M, et al. Skeletal muscle tissue engineering using isolated myoblasts on synthetic biodegradable polymers: preliminary studies. Tissue Eng 5:525-31.
29. Saxena AK, Willital GH, Vacanti JP. Vascularized three dimensional skeletal muscle tissue engineering. Biomed Mater Eng (in press).
30. Saxena AK, Willital GH. Skeletal muscle tissue-engineering. Int Med J Exp Clin Res 2000;6(4):18.
31. Saxena AK, Willital GH, Vacanti JP. Skeletal muscle tissue engineering: myoblast twitch recordings. 38th World Congress of Surgery, Vienna, Austria. August 1999, abstract 92, 23.
32. Saxena AK, Willital GH. Application of skeletal muscle tissue engineering for possible future management of incontinence. 4th European Congress of Pediatric Surgery, Budapest, Hungary. May 2001, abstract 17 (Pécs), 421.
33. Saxena AK, Vacanti JP, Willital GH: Skeletal muscle tissue engineering - in vivo studies. Pittsburgh Orthopaedic Tissue Engineering Symposium, Pittsburgh, PA, USA. April 1999.
34. Saxena AK, Vacanti JP, Willital GH. Skeletal muscle tissue engineering using pluronic gel polymers. Acta Chir Austriaca 2001;33:17-18.
35. Shinoka T, Breuer CK, Tanel RE, et al. Tissue engineering heart valves: Valve leaflet replacement study in lamb model. Ann Thorac Surg 1995;60:5513-16.

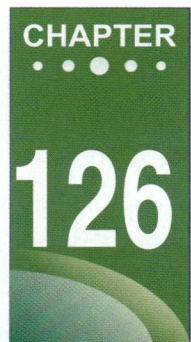

Stem Cell Therapy

DK Gupta, Shilpa Sharma

Stem cell research is today like an octopus expanding its tentacles into every field of medical science. Stem cells may hold the key to replacing cells lost in many diseases that are caused by loss of functioning cells.[1]

It is thus a type of cell-based therapy for treating diseases. Cell based therapies are also often referred to as regenerative or reparative medicine. In future, stem cells may become the basis for treating diseases such as Parkinson's disease, diabetes, and heart disease.

The 5th Annual Meeting of the International Society for Stem Cell Research focused on a number of issues, such as stem cell transplantation, tissue regeneration, biology of embryonic and adult stem cells of various species, regulation of stem cells epigenetic state and cancer stem cells.[2]

It has been felt that the twenty-first century will belong to regeneration medicine, with therapeutic applications of stem cells.[3]

STEM CELL

A stem cell is an undifferentiated cell in the body that in its original form has an undetermined function. However, the unique capability of this cell to form various tissues under definite signals received from the body, makes this cell an object of extensive research. Stem cells are unspecialized cells, can divide and renew themselves for long periods of time and become specific specialized cell types of the body.

HISTORICAL BACKGROUND

In 1981, researchers reported methods for growing mouse embryonic stem cells in the laboratory. Human embryonic stem cells have only been studied since 1998, when James Thomson at the University of Wisconsin-Madison isolated cells from the blastocyst, and developed the first human embryonic stem cell lines. At the same time, John Gearhart at Johns Hopkins University reported the first derivation of human embryonic germ cells from the primordial germ cells. Most of the knowledge about embryonic stem cells has emerged from in vitro fertilization technologies and basic research on mouse embryology.

After many years of isolating and characterizing stem cells, researchers are now exploring their utility for potential clinical applications (Fig. 126.1). Active stem cell research is going on with various animal models.

Autologous bone marrow stem cells have been used in various pilot studies for various disorders like cardiomyopathies, diabetes, bony disorders, biliary atresia and choledochal cyst (cirrhotic livers), spina bifida, multicystic kidney, cerebral palsy and muscular dystrophy.[4-6] At AIIMS, with the help of the centralized stem cell facility, various specialities including cardiothoracic, ophthalmology, endocrinology, surgery, orthopedics and pediatric surgery, have used stem cells in more than 500 patients now, including neonates and infants for various disorders since the last 4 years.[1,4-12]

AREAS OF RESEARCH

Today, scientists all over the globe are intensively studying the fundamental properties of stem cells, that is determining precisely how stem cells remain unspecialized and self renewing for many years; and identifying the signals that cause stem cells to become specialized cells. Stem cell research has been found beneficial in the following areas (Fig. 126.2).[13-34]

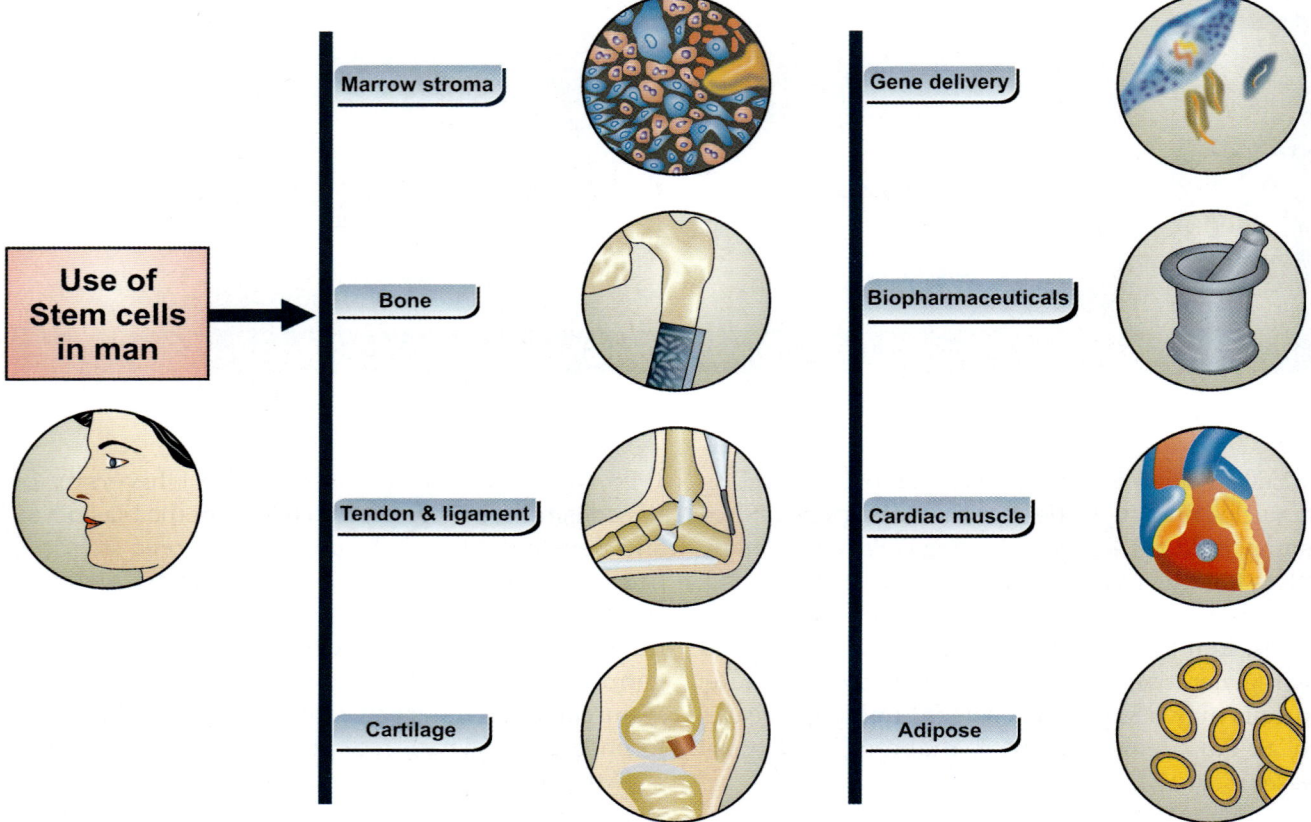

Fig. 126.1: Potential uses of stem cells

1. Alzheimer's
2. Parkinson's
3. Myocardial infarction
4. Stroke
5. Spinal cord injuries
6. Chronic liver cirrhosis
7. Sickle cell anemia
8. Leukemia
9. Non-Hodgkin's lymphoma and some other cancers,
10. Auto-immune diseases
11. Multiple sclerosis
12. Diabetes
13. Chronic heart disease
14. End-stage kidney disease
15. Liver failure
16. Cancer
17. Burns
18. Baldness
19. Infertility

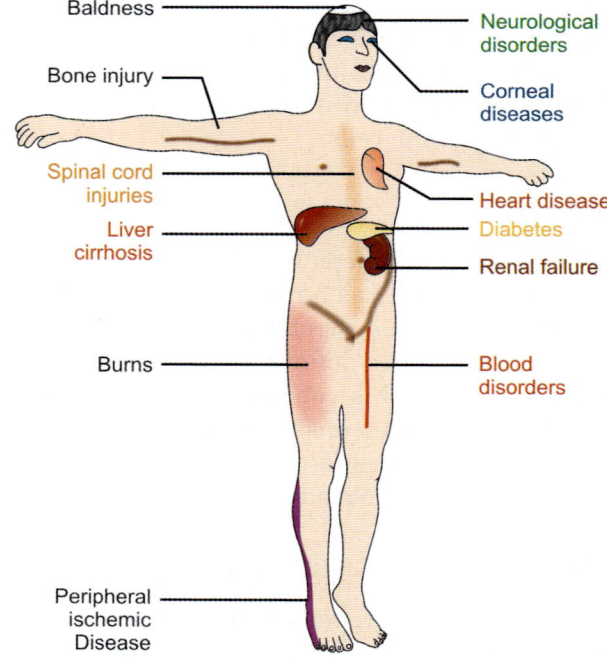

Fig. 126.2: Diseases that may be cured by stem cells

20. Lupus
21. Deafness
22. Diabetes.

CLASSIFICATION OF STEM CELLS BASED ON POTENTIALITY

Stem cells may be classified into three basic types according to the potentiality to transform into different cells. These include
1. *Totipotent Stem Cells:* These are capable of forming a completely new embryo that can develop into a new organism. A fertilized egg is totipotent. None of the stem cells used in research appear to have this capacity.
2. *Pluripotent Stem Cells:* These are unspecialized cells and have the potential to develop into any of the cell types found in an adult. Embryonic stem cells are pluripotent. Embryonic stem cells are able to renew themselves indefinitely in the laboratory and are therefore 'immortal'. Pluripotent stem cells from embryos and fetal tissue possess the ability to repair or replace cells or tissues that are damaged or destroyed by devastating diseases and disabilities.[1]
3. *Multipotent Stem Cells:* These have the potential to make a few cell types in the body.

SOURCES OF HUMAN STEM CELLS

Stem cells have been isolated from human embryos, fetal tissue, umbilical cord blood and also from "adult" sources. There are six major types of human stem cells, based on their source:

Adult Stem Cells

These are undifferentiated cells found among specialized or differentiated cells in a tissue or organ after birth and are capable of maintaining, generating, and replacing terminally differentiated cells (Fig. 126.3). Based on current research they appear to have a more restricted ability to produce different cell types and to self-renew. They are thus multipotent. In some adult tissues, such as bone marrow, muscle, and brain, a discrete populations of adult stem cells generate replacements for cells that are lost through normal wear and tear, injury, or disease. These cells produce new cells to replace old ones, such as blood, liver and nerve cells. Adult stem cells have been found in tissues that develop from all three embryonic germ layers.

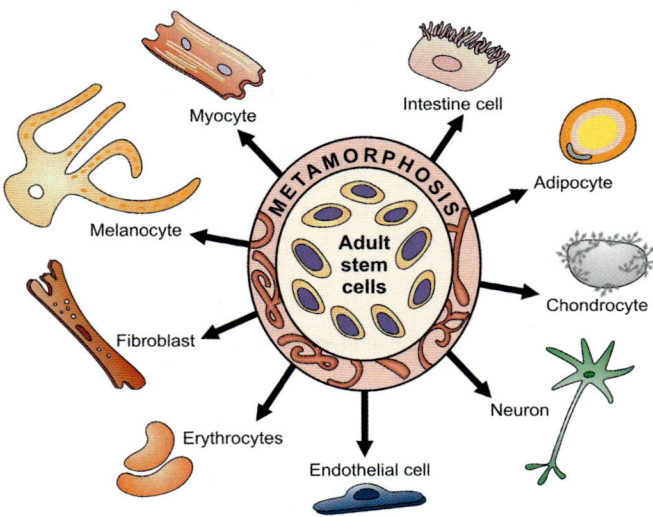

Fig. 126.3: Cells that can be derived from adult stem cells

They have been identified in brain particularly in the hippocampus, bone marrow, peripheral blood, blood vessels, skeletal muscle, epithelia of the skin and digestive system, cornea, dental pulp of the tooth, retina, liver, and pancreas.[1] In the adult skeletal muscle, satellite cells are the primary muscle stem cells, responsible for postnatal muscle growth, hypertrophy, and regeneration.

Umbilical Cord Blood Stem Cells

Non-embryonic stem cells can also be sourced from umbilical cord blood following birth (cord blood stem cells). These cells have properties similar to adult stem cells. Umbilical cord blood stem cells can also differentiate across tissue lineage boundaries into neural, cardiac, epithelial, hepatocytic, and dermal tissue.[35] Umbilical cord blood-derived stem cells offer multiple advantages over adult stem. cells, including their widespread availability, immaturity, which may play a significant role in reduced rejection after transplantation into a mismatched host and their ability to produce larger quantities of homogenous tissue or cells.[35]

Embryonic Stem Cells

These are collected from blastocyst, the inner cell mass of an early embryo (usually 5-6 days old) resulting in the destruction of the embryo (Figs 126.4 to 126.6).

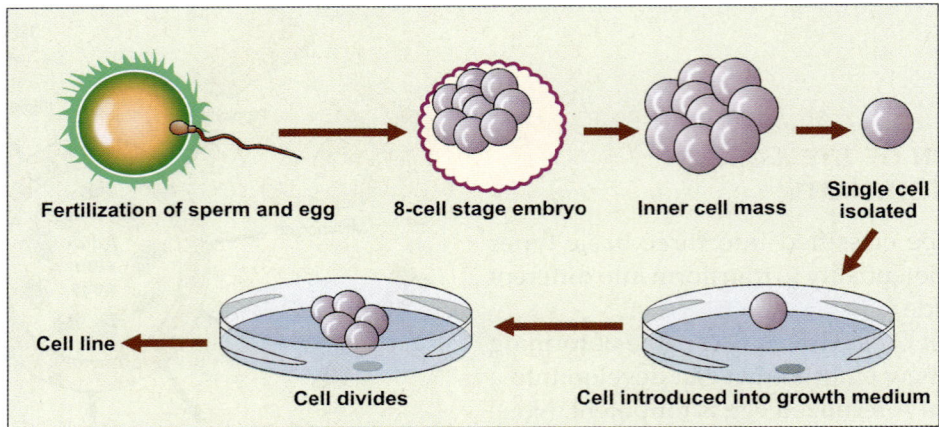

Fig. 126.4: The creation of a stem cell line from an embryo

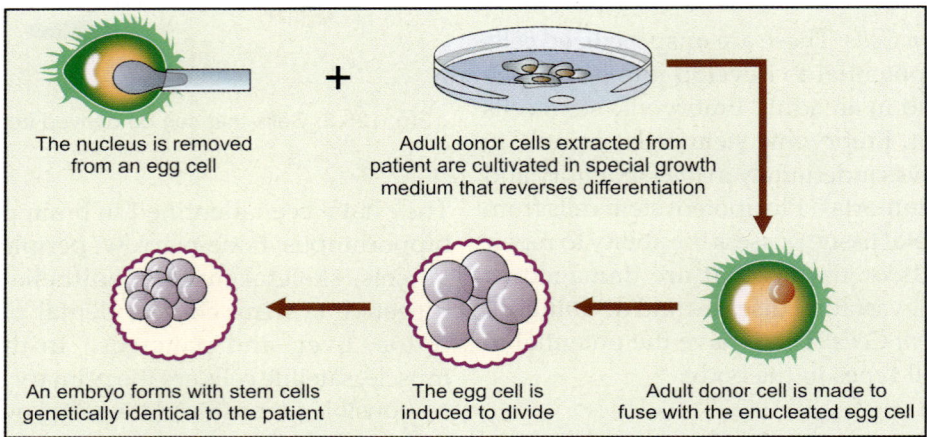

Fig. 126.5: The creation of a stem cell line from cloning

In a blastocyst, the stem cells in developing tissues give rise to the multiple specialized cell types that make up the heart, lung, skin, and other tissues. Once these cells are removed from the embryo, they can no longer give rise to a whole organism. They have the ability to form virtually any type of cell found in the human body.[36] They are pluripotent.

Germline

Embryonic germline stem cells are immature cells derived from the part of a human embryo or fetus that will ultimately produce sperm and egg cells (gametes). They are also pluripotent and their properties are similar to those of embryonic stem cells.

Amniotic Fluid Stem Cells

About 4 years ago, the discovery of amniotic fluid stem cells, expressing Oct-4, a specific marker of pluripotent stem cells, and harboring a high proliferative capacity

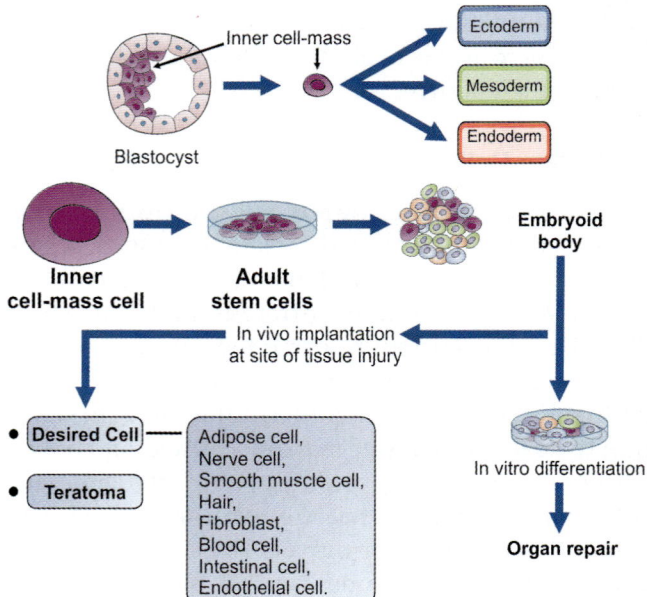

Fig. 126.6: Invitro and In vivo implantation of embryonic stem cells

and multilineage differentiation potential, initiated a new and promising stem cell research field. Since then, amniotic fluid stem cells have been demonstrated to harbor the potential to differentiate into cells of all three embryonic germlayers. These stem cells do not form tumors in vivo and do not raise the ethical concerns associated with human embryonic stem cells. Further investigations will reveal whether amniotic fluid stem cells really represent an intermediate cell type with advantages over both, adult stem cells and embryonic stem cells.[37] They can be used to generate clonal amniotic fluid stem cell lines as new tools to investigate molecular and cell biological consequences of human natural occurring disease causing mutations.[37] The amnion possesses advantages that the isolated cells can differentiate into all three germ layers; they have low immunogenicity and anti-inflammatory functions; and they do not require the sacrifice of human embryos for their isolation, thus avoiding the current controversies associated with the use of human embryonic stem cells.[38] Significant research has been done based on mesenchymal stromal cells isolated from various parts of the placenta or epithelial cells isolated from amniotic membrane.[39]

Placental Tissue

Placental tissue draws great interest as a source of cells for regenerative medicine because of the phenotypic plasticity of many cells types isolated from this tissue and the immunomodulatory properties of the cells that make it useful for future cell therapy-based clinical applications.[39]

Which Cells to Use?

Each of these is being used in active research, and all have the potential to treat disease in future. Most scientists feel research using embryonic cells being pleuripotent will be more fruitful. However, recently, it has been shown that some adult stem cells may be able to generate different tissues under the right conditions and this may increase their therapeutic potential.

Embryonic stem cells have a greater capacity for renewal. Their uncontrolled growth may lead to tumour formation that may restrict their use in cell-based therapies. Embryonic germ and adult stem cells do not form these tumors in culture, which may make them better alternatives for transplant tissue sources.

Thus, most scientists agree that it is important to continue to pursue research into embryonic stem and germ cells and adult stem cells. Embryonic stem cells have the potential to develop into organs and tissues (such as kidneys) that could replace diseased organs. This would help alleviate the shortage of organs and tissues available for transplantation.

Embryonic stem cells and adult stem cells are being compared in terms of their ability to proliferate, differentiate, survive and function after transplant, and means to avoid the immune rejection are being explored.

Adult Stem Cell Plasticity

Adult stem cell plasticity or trans-differentiation has been defined as the ability of some adult stem cells to be "genetically reprogrammed", given the right environment, into specialized cells that are characteristic of different tissues.

MESENCHYMAL STEM CELLS

Multipotent mesenchymal stromal cells (MSC) are a group of clonogenic cells present among the bone marrow stroma and capable of multilineage differentiation into mesoderm-type cells such as osteoblasts, adipocytes and chondrocytes.[40] These may also be isolated from various adult tissue sources.[41] Mesenchymal stem cells from adult marrow can differentiate in vitro and in vivo into various cell types, such as bone, fat and cartilage.[42]

Due to their ease of isolation and their differentiation potential, MSC are being introduced into clinical medicine in variety of applications and through different ways of administration.[40] Mesenchymal stem cells preferentially home to damaged tissue and thus may have therapeutic potential.[42]

Emerging evidence indicates that the class of single-stranded non-coding RNAs known as "microRNAs" also plays a critical role in the differentiation process.[41] Expression of unique microRNAs in specific cell types serves as a useful diagnostic marker to define a particular cell type.[41] MicroRNAs are also found to be regulated by extracellular signaling pathways that are important for differentiation into specific tissues, suggesting that they play a role in specifying tissue identity.[41]

In vitro data suggest that MSCs have low inherent immunogenicity as they induce little, if any, proliferation of allogeneic lymphocytes. Instead, MSCs appear to be immunosuppressive in vitro.[42] They inhibit T-cell proliferation to alloantigens and mitogens and prevent the development of cytotoxic T-cells.[42]

Mesenchymal stem cells have also been separated from umbilical cord vein. These gave rise to a population of adherent cells with a typical fibroblast-like morphology. Similarly to bone marrow-derived MSCs, they highly expressed CD29, HLA-ABC, CD166, CD105, CD73 and CD44, and were negative for any hematopoietic and endothelial markers (CD45, CD34, CD14 and CD144).[43] Functionally, these could differentiate into the osteoblast, adipocyte and chondrocyte.[43]

AUTOLOGOUS STEM CELL TRANSPLANTATION

This has been widely used for autoimmune diseases and lymphome

Autoimmune Diseases

In a study, of the 1,000 patients that received an autologous hematopoietic stem cell transplant as treatment for a severe autoimmune disease, the majority were cases of multiple sclerosis, systemic sclerosis, systemic lupus erythematosus, rheumatoid arthritis, juvenile idiopathic arthritis, and immune cytopenias.[44] Many patients have experienced long-term disease-free remissions and immune reconstitution studies have shown in some cases that a "resetting" of autoimmunity is possible.

There is a growing interest in the role and potential therapeutic application of mesenchymal stem cells in the immunomodulation of autoimmune diseases, as in the early experience with acute-graft-versus host disease.

Allogeneic stem cell transplantation is the treatment of choice for the majority of young patients with myelodysplasia who have a histocompatible donor (sibling or unrelated donor).[45]

Lymphoma

High-dose therapy (HDT) followed by autologous transplantation of hematopoietic stem cells (ASCT) is frequently performed in patients with lymphoma.[46] Patients with indolent or aggressive B-cell lymphoma may benefit from HDT/ASCT if considered as part of first-line therapy or at the time of relapse.[46]

ETHICAL ISSUES

All scientists are aware that they must undertake their work ethically and within the bounds of the law, and these can vary from country to country.

Harvesting stem cells from embryos involves lots of ethical issues. These differ in different societies. The idea of destruction of a potential human conflicts with religious and moral views in some societies. For others, the potential for this research to provide treatments and possibly cures for debilitating illnesses that have no cure and significantly impact on our way of life overrides this concern.

Opinions vary on what actually constitutes the beginning of life for a human :from the moment of conception, to a 14 day embryo, to a living baby at birth.

As life is considered by some to begin at conception so it may be considered criminal to sacrifice an embryo for experimental and research purposes.[47,48] Embryonic Stem Cells are derived from embryos that develop from eggs that have been fertilized in vitro and then donated for research purposes with informed consent of the donors. The main ethical conflict about Embryonic Stem Cells research is between the alleviation of human suffering that stem cell technologies may provide and the destruction of embryonic life that is involved in their extraction. With the autologous infusion, there are no ethical issues involved with the stem cell therapy. However, being a new therapy with no definite known long term results, it is being done only in selected institutes with full ethical clearance and with a special informed consent.

It is important to balance the harm that might be done against the potential good this research may provide for those suffering from debilitating diseases. In some countries like Australia, legislation states that no embryo may be created for the purpose of this research or to generate stem cell lines.

The embryonic stem and germ cells are obtained from either donated embryos not required for an IVF procedure that would otherwise be destroyed, or from pregnancies that were terminated for medical or social reasons.

While research with embryonic stem cells continues to generate considerable controversy, human umbilical stem cells provide an alternative cell source that has been more ethically acceptable and appears to have widespread public support.[35]

Prerequisites

1. Ethical issues should be solved well in advance.
2. Harvested stem cells from umbilical cord blood or embryos require proper cross matching and may lead to complications like graft versus host reaction

LIMITATIONS

1. The rare occurrence of adult stem cells among other differentiated cells.
2. There are difficulties in isolating and identifying the cells with molecular "markers".[49]
3. There are difficulties in growing stem cells in tissue culture.[50]
4. There are obstacles to organ construction using human stem cells. Stem cell-derived organs will be grown outside the human body and will therefore require some type of scaffolding during development. Such scaffolds are presently being developed incorporating human or animal stem cells.
5. The injection of undifferentiated embryonic stem cells into an adult and an uncontrolled proliferation may carry the risk of teratoma formation at any stage after stem cell therapy. To avoid this, undifferentiated embryonic stem cells must be eliminated before injection. Current cell-sorting technology is not yet efficient enough to do this. Understanding how tumor suppressor genes impinge on quiescent stem cell populations could provide us with a means of designing more effective therapies to reduce the frequency of stem cell-derived tumor growth that occurs following treatment.
6. There is a problem of immune rejection if there is a poor match between the cells of the embryo from which the embryonic stem cells are derived and the recipient.
7. Scientists still have to elucidate what prompts the stem cell to take up a specific function.
8. The disregulation of imprinted genes can be associated with tumorigenesis and altered cell differentiation capacity and so could provide adverse outcomes for stem cell applications. Although the maintenance of mouse and primate embryonic stem cells in a pluripotent state has been reported to disrupt the monoallelic expression of several imprinted genes, available data have suggested relatively higher imprint stability in the human equivalents.[51] Gene-specific differences have been demonstrated in the stability of imprinted loci in human embryonic stem cells and identify disrupted DNA methylation as one potential mechanism.[51]

STEM CELL CULTURE

Appropriate culture conditions are required for maintenance of signaling pathways and transcriptional networks to maintain murine and human embryos in a stable, pluripotent state.

Cultures of human pluripotent stem cells have active telomerase, which is an enzyme that maintains the length of telomeres and is important for cells to maintain their capacity to replicate.

In order to safely use stem cells or cells differentiated from them in tissues other than the tissue from which they were isolated, researchers will need purified clonal lines of adult stem cells. In addition, the potential for the recipient of a stem cell transplant to reject these tissues as foreign is very high. Modifications to the cells or the immune system, or both will be a major requirement for their use.

Evidence of structural, genetic, and functional cells characteristic of specialized cells developed from cultured human and mouse embryonic stem cells has been shown for pancreatic islet-cell like cells that secrete insulin, cardiac muscle cells with contractile activity, blood cells and nerve cells that produce certain brain chemicals.[1]

STEM CELL TRANSPLANTATION FOR NEURODEGENERATIVE DISEASES

Stem cell transplantation has the potential to improve function by replacing cells lost to the disease and reconstructing elements of neural circuitry or by providing support for host cells (e.g. by secretion of trophic factors).[33]

Other mechanisms, such as modulation of the immune system by bone marrow stem cell transplantation, pertinent to conditions such as multiple sclerosis, are emerging as therapies.[33] Using stem cells to provide trophic support places less stringent requirements on the cells and this is the area in which many of the first clinical studies are taking place.[33] There are real prospects of stem cell technology having a place in clinical management of neurodegenerative conditions, but directing the differentiation of stem cells towards the appropriate neural phenotype remains a challenge.[33]

RECENT RESEARCH

The spermatogonial stem cells can self-renew and generate a large number of differentiated germ cells. A balance between their renewal and differentiation in the adult testis is essential to maintain normal spermatogenesis and fertility. It has been demonstrated in adult mice that spermatogonial stem cells self-renewal could be controlled by glial cell-line-derived neurotrophic factor GDNF during the perinatal period of development while it is dependent on ERM, a transcription factor which is exclusively expressed in mature Sertoli cells, during the pubertal period.[52]

Granulocyte-macrophage colony stimulating factor (GM-CSF) is a hematopoietic growth factor involved in the generation of granulocytes, macrophages, and dendritic cells from hematopoietic progenitor cells.[53] Addition of Granulocyte-macrophage colony stimulating factor to adult neural stem cells in vitro increased neuronal differentiation in a dose-dependent manner as determined by quantitative PCR, reporter gene assays, and FACS analysis.[53]

Bone marrow stem cells may offer the potential for treatment of acute kidney injury.[34]

Neural stem cells may be used to investigate the molecular mechanisms involved in manganese developmental neurotoxicity.[54]

Cancer stem cells with genetic instability can be considered as 'the best vehicle with the best engine', a formidable challenge for the future development of new anticancer therapies.[55]

It has been reported that when transplanted into the denervated rat colon, neuroepithelial stem cells survived and could differentiate into neurons and glial cells in vivo thus could provide a promising cellular replacement candidate for enteric nervous system.[56]

An important area of research that links developmental biology and stem cell biology is understanding the development of the embryo and the various factors like genes, molecules, growth factors and nutrients that function during development. A new source discovery of adult stem cells, carotid body stem cells, which proliferate in response to hypoxia and generate neurons that secrete dopamine, may be useful in therapies for treating Parkinson's disease.[57,58]

The clinical scope of the use of stem cell therapy is expanding continuously. The pertinent areas include liver cirrhosis due to biliary atresia and severe forms of choledochal cysts and sclerosing cholangitis, spina bifida, Hirschsprung's disease, renal dysplasia, residual tumors, pancreatic insufficiency due to diabetes, following surgical resection (nesidioblastosis, tumors), neurogenic bladder and bowel.[59-61] The authors have used stem cells in cases of biliary atresia, meningomyelocele and anorectal malformation with incontinence (Figs 126.7A to C).

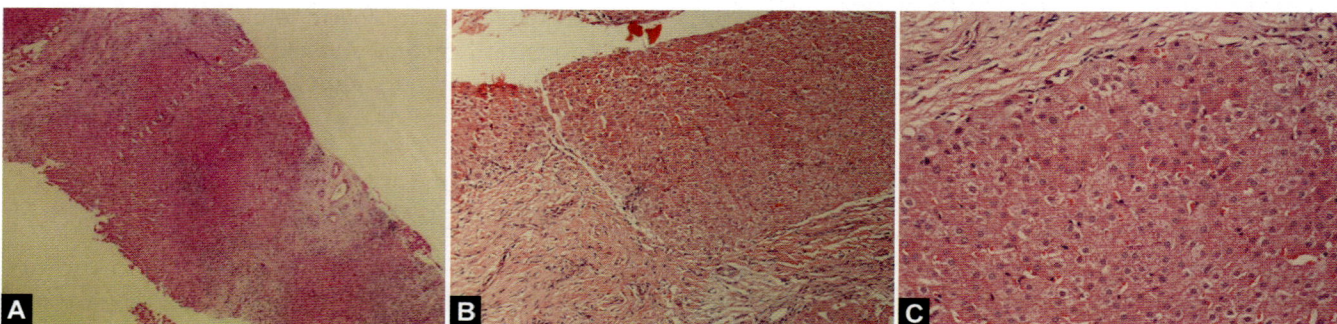

Figs 126.7A to C: A. Nodules and cirrhosis seen in aextrahepatic biliary atresia that presented at 6 months of age post Kasai's procedure with a cirrhotic liver. **B.** The same patient 17 months after stem cell injection had a liver biopsy showing near normal hepatocytes. **C.** The same slide seen in high power field

FUTURE APPLICATIONS

The application of stem cells to regenerative medicine could help the cure of a number of diseases that are affecting a large share of the population. Regenerative medicine is a new field based on the use of stem cells to generate biological substitutes and improve tissue functions, restoring damaged tissue with high proliferability and differentiability.[38]

Recent progress in the stem cell field includes clinically compliant culture conditions and directed differentiation of both embryonic stem cells and somatic stem cells.[62] With a growing understanding, stem cell biology, and spinal cord injury pathophysiology, stem cell-based therapies are moving closer to clinical application.[62]

An important issue is to find out how a cell begins to proliferate or differentiate. Genome reprogramming, both following nuclear transfer and cytoplast action, will likely highlight some of the molecular mechanisms of cell differentiation and dedifferentiation. In turn, these clues should be useful to the production of populations of reprogrammed cells that could develop into tissues or, in the future, into proper organs.[13] Cell lines that have been established will be useful for research into early human development. Embryonic stem cells might be 'programmed' to develop into neurones and then purified and injected into the brain to regenerate new tissues to replace those that are diseased.

The stem cell phenotype of human and murine ES cells has recently been shown to be maintained by a self-stabilizing network of transcription factors, NANOG, OCT4 and SOX2.[63] Aberrant activation of the ES transcription factor network elicited by increased dosage of an embryonic gene cluster at 12p including NANOG, together with additional genetic and epigenetic alterations, appears to be a crucial event in the genesis of testicular germ cell cancers.[63]

Laser-assisted isolation of the inner cell mass may be applied for the derivation of new human embryonic stem cells lines in a xeno-free system for future clinical applications.[64] These human embryonic stem cells lines can serve as an important model of the genetic disorders that they carry.[64]

Both adult neural stem cells and embryonic stem cells have shown the capacity to differentiation into multiple cell types of the adult nervous system.[65] However, there are significant challenges remaining, including the identification of signaling factors that specify cell fate in the stem cell niche, the analysis of intracellular targets and mechanisms of these extracellular signals, and the development of ex vivo culture systems that can exert efficient control over cell function.[65]

Applications of imaging techniques to visualize stem cells for monitoring, control and treatment of biological systems, in particular the brain, is at the forefront of investigations.[66]

Potential new drugs could be tested for their toxicology on tissues developed from stem cell lines. Stem cells are likely be used to develop specialized liver cells to evaluate drug detoxifying capabilities.

In a mouse model, local RT delivered to the left leg causes preferential accumulation of bone marrow mononuclear cells to the irradiated site, with maximum signal intensity observed at 7 days post-RT.[67] The combination of stem cell technology and tissue engineering has been investigated and offers promising avenues for myocardial tissue regeneration, and this shows great promise in future reconstructive surgery.[68] The genome and transcriptome of Embryonic Stem Cells have been extensively examined in order to decipher their self-renewal and differentiation mechanisms.[69] Epigenetic analysis reveals methylation patterns and microRNA profiles unique to Embryonic Stem Cells.[69]

Genetic engineering of adult stem cells from various sources with osteogenic genes has led to enhanced fracture repair, spinal fusion and rapid healing of bone defects in animal models.[70] Many authors are now discussing the potential of gene-enhanced tissue engineering to enter widespread clinical use.[70] Neural stem cells transplanted into the brain after neuronal ablation survive, migrate, differentiate and, most significantly, improve memory mouse model.[71] Oligodendrocytes derived from stem cells are being used to remyelinate axons following spinal cord injury.[72]

Bone marrow derived mesenchymal stem cells are pluripotent cells which can differentiate into osteogenic, adipogenic and other lineages. The number of bone marrow mesenchymal stem cells but neither phenotype nor differentiation capacities changes with age of rats.[73] Cellular therapies derived from embryonic stem cells have gained a renewed interest with the experimental demonstration that an embryonic stem cell line can be established from human blastocyst-stage embryos and prompted to differentiate into almost all types of cells present in the body including hematopoietic cells.[32] Embryonic stem cells show great potential and it may be technologically feasible to transplant differentiated embryonic stem cells and to cure various kinds of blood disorders.[32] The potential utility of embryonic stem cells for gene therapy, tissue engineering and the treatment of a wide variety of currently untreatable diseases has been recognized.[32]

Stem cells are already being explored as a vehicle for delivering genes to specific tissues in the body.[74-76] In future, antibodies could be developed against the targeted disease, tissues and tumors, tagged with the stem cells and infused locally for achieving the maximal benefit. Hardware also needs to be developed to inject the stem cells direct to the smaller vessels in the infants and newborns, without the need for surgery for therapy.

The major challenges faced by scientists today are to direct the differentiation of embryonic stem cells into specialized cell populations and to devise ways to control their proliferation once placed in patients.[1] More refined experimental work is needed to study the mechanism of action of stem cells but the hurdles lie in creating the exact environment experimentally as found in the clinical setup.[77-81]

REFERENCES

1. Gupta DK, Sharma S. Stem cell therapy - Hope and scope in pediatric surgery. J Indian Assoc Pediatr Surg 2005;10:138-41.
2. Romano G. Advances in the field of stem cell research. Drug News Perspect 2007;20:469-74.
3. Rowinski W. Future of transplantation medicine. Ann Transplant 2007;12:5-10.
4. Sharma S, Gupta DK, Venugopal P, Kumar L, Dattagupta S, Arora MK. Therapeutic use of stem cells in congenital anomalies-a pilot study. J Ind Assoc Pediatr Surg 2006:11:211-17.
5. Sharma S, Gupta D K, Kumar L, Dinda AK, Bagga A, Mohanty S. Are therapeutic stem cells justified in bilateral multicystic kidney disease? A review of literature with insights into the embryology. Pediatr Surg Int 2007;23: 801-06.
6. Airan B, Talwar S, Choudhary SK , Bisoi AK , Seth S , Mohanty S, Venugopal P. Application of Stem cells technology for coronary artery disease at the All India Institute of Medical Sciences, New Delhi, India. Heart Surgery Forum 2007;10:1-4.
7. Seth S, Narang R, Bhargava B, Ray R, Mohanty S, Gulati S, Kumar L, Reddy KS, Venugopal P. Percutaneous intracoronary cellular cardiomyoplasty for non-ischemic cardiomyopathy - Clinical and histopathological results: The first in man ABCD (autologous bone marrow cell in dialated cardiomyopathy) trial. Journal of the American College of Cardiology 2006:48 (11): 2350-51.
8. Mohanty S, Kumar L. CME on stem Cell Therapy. Indian Journal of Medical and Pediatric Oncology. 2006;27(1):46-48.
9. Seth S, Narang R, Bhargav Balram, et al Role of intra coronary injection of autologous mononuclear bone marrow stem cells in patients with chronic left ventricular dysfunction due to dilated cardiomyopathy or ischemic heart disease with open coronary arteries. Indian Journal of Medical and Paediatric Oncology, 2005;26(3);1-2.
10. Kumar A, Pahwa V K, Tandon R, Kumar Lalit, Mohanty Sujata. Use of Autologous Bone Marrow Derived Stem Cells for Rehabilitation of Patients with Dry Age Related Macular Degeneration and Retinitis Pigmentosa: Phase-1 Clinical Trial. Indian Journal of Medical and Paediatric Oncology 2005;26(l. 3); 12-14.
11. Bedi R, Kumar L, Bhutani M, Sharma A, Kochupillai V, Mohanty Sujata. Autologous peripheral blood stem cell transplantation: A study of engraftment kinetics. Indian Journal of Medical and Pediatric Oncology 2003;24(3):9-14.
12. Raju GMK, Guha S, Mukhopadhyay A, et al. Colony stimulating activity of fetal liver cells: Synergistic role of stem cell factor in bone marrow recovery from aplastic anemia. Journal of Hematotherapy and Stem cell research 2003;12:491-89.
13. Redi CA, Monti M, Merico V, et al. Stem cells. Endocr Dev 2007;11:145-51.
14. Weissman I. Stem cell research: paths to cancer therapies and regenerative medicine. JAMA 2005;294:1359-66.
15. Shah RV, Mitchell RN. The role of stem cells in the response to myocardial and vascular wall injury. Cardiovasc Pathol 2005;14:225-31.
16. Van Rhenen A, Feller N, Kelder A, Westra AH, Rombouts E, Zweegman S, et al . High stem cell frequency in acute myeloid leukemia at diagnosis predicts high minimal residual disease and poor survival. Clin Cancer Res 2005;11:6520-27.
17. Silani V, Corbo M. Cell-replacement therapy with stem cells in neurodegenerative diseases. Curr Neurovasc Res 2004;1:283-89.
18. Kang KS, Kim S, Oh Y, Yu J, Kim KY, Park H, et al. A 37-year-old spinal cord-injured female patient, transplanted of multipotent stem cells from human UC blood, with improved sensory perception and mobility, both functionally and morphologically: a case study. Cytotherapy 2005;7:368-73.
19. Sanberg PR, Willing AE, Garbuzova-Davis S, Saporta S, Liu G, Sanberg CD, et al. Umbilical cord blood-derived stem cells and brain repair. Ann N Y Acad Sci 2005;1049:67-83.

20. Brodie JC, Humes HD. Stem cell approaches for the treatment of renal failure. Pharmacol Rev 2005;57:299-313.
21. Ricardo SD, Deane JA. Adult stem cells in renal injury and repair. Nephrology (Carlton) 2005;10:276-82.
22. Mendez-Sanchez N, Chavez-Tapia NC, Uribe M. Hepatocyte transplantation for acute and chronic liver diseases. Ann Hepatol 2005;4:212-15.
23. Fujikawa T, Oh SH, Shupe T, Petersen BE. Stem-cell therapy for hepatobiliary pancreatic disease. J Hepatobiliary Pancreat Surg 2005;12:190-95.
24. Rasulov MF, Vasilchenkov AV, Onishchenko NA, Krasheninnikov ME, Kravchenko VI, Gorshenin TL, et al. First experience of the use bone marrow mesenchymal stem cells for the treatment of a patient with deep skin burns. Bull Exp Biol Med 2005;139:141-44.
25. Bukovsky A. Can ovarian infertility be treated with bone marrow- or ovary-derived germ cells? Reprod Biol Endocrinol 2005;15;3-36.
26. Pellicer M, Giraldez F, Pumarola F, Barquinero J. Stem cells for the treatment of hearing loss. Acta Otorrinolaringol Esp 2005;56:227-32.
27. Brolen GK, Heins N, Edsbagge J, Semb H. Signals From the Embryonic Mouse Pancreas Induce Differentiation of Human Embryonic Stem Cells Into Insulin-Producing {beta}-Cell-Like Cells. Diabetes 2005;54:2867-74.
28. Soria B, Roche E, Reig JA, Martin F. Generation of insulin producing cells from stem cells. Novartis Found Symp 2005;265:158-67; discussion 167-73, 204-11.
29. Bjorklund A. Cell therapy for Parkinson's disease: problems and prospects. Novartis Found Symp 2005; 265:174-86; discussion 187, 204-11.
30. Illei GG, Pavletic SZ. Blood stem cells as therapy for severe lupus. Expert Opin Biol Ther 2005;5:1153-64.
31. Docherty K, Bernardo AS, Vallier L. Embryonic stem cell therapy for diabetes mellitus. Semin Cell Dev Biol. 2007 Sep 11; [Epub ahead of print].
32. Srivastava AS, Malhotra R, Esmaeli-Azad B, et al. Prospects of embryonic stem cells in treatment of hematopoietic disorders. Curr Pharm Biotechno 2007;8(5):305-17.
33. Rosser AE, Zietlow R, Dunnett SB. Stem cell transplantation for neurodegenerative diseases. Curr Opin Neurol 2007;20(6):688-92.
34. Lin F. Renal repair: role of bone marrow stem cells. Pediatr Nephrol 2007 Nov 9.
35. Van de Ven C, Collins D, Bradley MB, et al. The potential of umbilical cord blood multipotent stem cells for nonhematopoietic tissue and cell regeneration. Exp Hematol 2007 Oct 17.
36. Wang L, Menendez P, Cerdan C, Bhatia M. Hematopoietic development from human embryonic stem cell lines. Exp Hematol 2005;33:987-96.
37. Siegel N, Rosner M, Hanneder M, et al. Stem Cells in Amniotic Fluid as New Tools to Study Human Genetic Diseases. Stem Cell Rev 2007 Oct 23; [Epub ahead of print].
38. Toda A, Okabe M, Yoshida T, Nikaido T. The Potential of Amniotic Membrane/Amnion-Derived Cells for Regeneration of Various Tissues. J Pharmacol Sci 2007 Nov 6; [Epub ahead of print].
39. Parolini O, Alviano F, Bagnara GP, et al. CONCISE REVIEW: Isolation and Characterization of Cells from Human Term Placenta: Outcome of the First International Workshop on Placenta Derived Stem Cells. Stem Cells 2007 Nov 8; [Epub ahead of print].
40. Abdallah BM, Kassem M. Human mesenchymal stem cells: from basic biology to clinical applications. Gene Ther 2007 Nov 8.
41. Lakshmipathy U, Hart RP. Concise Review: Micro RNA Expression in Multipotent Mesenchymal Stromal Cells. Stem Cells. 2007 Nov 8.
42. Le Blanc K, Ringdén O. Immunomodulation by mesenchymal stem cells and clinical experience. J Intern Med 2007;262(5):509-25.
43. Liu XD, Liu B, Li XS, Mao N. Isolation and identification of mesenchymal stem cells from perfusion of human umbilical cord vein. Zhongguo Shi Yan Xue Ye Xue Za Zhi 2007;15(5):1019-22.
44. Passweg J, Tyndall A. Autologous stem cell transplantation in autoimmune diseases. Semin Hematol 2007;44(4):278-85.
45. de Witte T, Suciu S, Brand R, Muus P, Kröger N. Autologous stem cell transplantation in myelodysplastic syndromes. Semin Hematol 2007Oct;44(4):274-77.
46. Schmitz N, Buske C, Gisselbrecht C. Autologous stem cell transplantation in lymphoma. Semin Hematol 2007;44(4): 234-45.
47. Devolder K. Creating and sacrificing embryos for stem cells. J Med Ethics 2005;31:366-70.
48. Murray TH. Ethical (and political) issues in research with human stem cells. Novartis Found Symp 2005;265:188-96; discussion 196-211.
49. Walczak P, Kedziorek DA, Gilad AA, Lin S, Bulte JW. Instant MR labeling of stem cells using magnetoelectroporation. Magn Reson Med 2005;54:769-74.
50. Check E. Stem-cell research: the rocky road to success. Nature 2005;437(7056):185-86.
51. Kim KP, Thurston A, Mummery C, et al. Gene-specific vulnerability to imprinting variability in human embryonic stem cell lines Genome Res. 2007 Nov 7; [Epub].
52. Dadoune JP. New insights into male gametogenesis: what about the spermatogonial stem cell niche? Folia Histochem Cytobiol 2007;45(3):141-47.
53. Kruger C, Laage R, Pitzer C, Schabitz WR, Schneider A. The hematopoietic factor GM-CSF (Granulocyte-macrophage colony-stimulating factor) promotes neuronal differentiation of adult neural stem cells in vitro. : BMC Neurosci. 2007 Oct 22;8(1):88.
54. Tamm C, Sabri F, Ceccatelli S. Mitochondrial-mediated apoptosis in neural stem cells exposed to manganese. Toxicol Sci. 2007 Oct 31; [Epub ahead of print].
55. Lagasse E. Cancer stem cells with genetic instability: the best vehicle with the best engine for cancer. Gene Ther 2007 Nov 8; [Epub].

56. Liu W, Wu RD, Dong YL, Gao YM. Neuroepithelial stem cells differentiate into neuronal phenotypes and improve intestinal motility recovery after transplantation in the aganglionic colon of the rat. Neurogastroenterol Motil. 2007 Aug 28[Epub].
57. Pardal R, Ortega-Sáenz P, Durán R, López-Barneo J. Glia-like Stem Cells Sustain Physiologic Neurogenesis in the Adult Mammalian Carotid Body. Cell 2007;131:364-77.
58. Kokovay E, Temple S. Taking neural crest stem cells to new heights. Cell 2007;131(2):234-36.
59. Kawashita Y, Guha C, Yamanouchi K, Ito Y, Kamohara Y, Kanematsu T. Liver repopulation: a new concept of hepatocyte transplantation. Surg Today 2005;35:705-10.
60. Vadivelu S, Platik MM, Choi L, Lacy ML, Shah AR, Qu Y et al. Multi-germ layer lineage central nervous system repair: nerve and vascular cell generation by embryonic stem cells transplanted in the injured brain. J Neurosurg 2005;103:124-35.
61. Choi BH, Zhu SJ, Kim BY, Huh JY, Lee SH, Jung JH. Transplantation of cultured bone marrow stromal cells to improve peripheral nerve regeneration. Int J Oral Maxillofac Surg 2005;34:537-42.
62. Coutts M, Keirstead HS. Stem cells for the treatment of spinal cord injury Exp Neurol 2007 Sep 12; [Epub].
63. Schulz WA, Hoffmann MJ. Transcription factor networks in embryonic stem cells and testicular cancer and the definition of epigenetics. Epigenetics 2007;2:37-42.
64. Turetsky T, Aizenman E, Gil Y, et al. Laser-assisted derivation of human embryonic stem cell lines from IVF embryos after preimplantation genetic diagnosis. Hum Reprod 2007 Nov 7; [Epub].
65. Robertson MJ, Gip P, Schaffer DV. Neural stem cell engineering: directed differentiation of adult and embryonic stem cells into neurons. Front Biosci 2008 Jan 1;13:21-50. [In press].
66. Dousset V, Tourdias T, Brochet B, et al. How to trace stem cells for MRI evaluation? J Neurol. Sci 2007 Oct 24; [Epub].
67. Bastianutto C, Mian A, Symes J, et al. Local radiotherapy induces homing of hematopoietic stem cells to the irradiated bone marrow. Cancer Res. 2007;67(21): 10112-16.
68. Wu KH, Mo XM, Liu YL, Zhang YS, Han ZC. Stem cells for tissue engineering of myocardial constructs. Ageing Res Rev 2007 Aug 31; [Epub ahead of print].
69. Zhan M. Genomic studies to explore self-renewal and differentiation properties of embryonic stem cells. Front Biosci 2008 Jan 1;13:276-83.
70. Betz VM, Betz OB, Harris MB, Vrahas MS, Evans CH. Bone tissue engineering and repair by gene therapy. Front Biosci 2008 Jan 1;13:833-41.
71. Yamasaki TR, Blurton-Jones M, Morrissette DA, et al. Neural stem cells improve memory in an inducible mouse model of neuronal loss. J Neurosci 2007;27(44):11925-33.
72. Rossignol S, Schwab M, Schwartz M, Fehlings MG. Spinal cord injury: time to move? J Neurosci. 2007;27(44):11782-92.
73. Tokalov SV, Gruener S, Schindler S, et al. A Number of Bone Marrow Mesenchymal Stem Cells but Neither Phenotype Nor Differentiation Capacities Changes with Age of Rats. Mol Cells. 2007;24(2):255-60.
74. Vats A, Tolley NS, Bishop AE, Polak JM. Embryonic stem cells and tissue engineering: delivering stem cells to the clinic. J R Soc Med 2005;98:346-50.
75. Atala A. Tissue engineering, stem cells and cloning: current concepts and changing trends. Expert Opin Biol Ther 2005;5:879-92.
76. Narbonne P, Roy R. Genes that affect both cell growth and polarity mediate stem cell quiescence. Front Biosci 2008;13:995-1002. {In press}.
77. Gupta DK, Sharma S, Venugopal P, Kumar L, Mohanty S, Dattagupta S. Stem cells as a therapeutic modality in pediatric malformations Transplant Proc. 2007;39:700-2 published as proceedings of the lecture delivered at 17th Annual conference of Indian Society of Organ transplant (ISOT), 2006. Ahmedabad.
78. Sharma Shilpa. Lecture delivered on Stem cell Use in Pediatric Surgery at Norfolk and Norwich Hospital, UK. November, 2005.
79. Gupta DK, Venugopal P, Shilpa Sharma, Lalit Kumar, Mohanty S, Arora MK, Gupta M, Malhotra A. Stem cell therapy in biliary atresia - as an Alternative to liver transplant - some hope and scope 25th Annual Conference of International Fetal Medicine and Surgery Society in Kona, Hawai .June 11-15, 2006.
80. Gupta DK, Venugopal P, Sharma Shilpa, Kumar Lalit, Mohanty S, Arora MK, Gupta M, Malhotra A. Application of Stem cells in Spina Bifida - Can it improve neurological status? 25th Annual Conference of International Fetal Medicine and Surgery Society in Kona, Hawai. 2006;11-15.
81. Gupta DK. Plenary Lecture delivered on Stem Cell Application in Pediatric Malformations during the International Conference on Hot Topics in Neonatology. Jeddah, February 2008;17-20.

CHAPTER 127

Nanotechnology: Technology to Revolutionize the Future of Medicine

Amit K Dinda

Nanotechnology, "the technology of nanoscale materials or devices", is a unique phenomenon in the recent scientific development that has revolutionized the advancement of medicine and galvanized almost every specialty of science engineering and business community. The ability to characterize, manipulate and organize matter systematically at the nanometer scale has resulted a revolution in science, engineering, and technology. The progress in nanotechnology is happening at an astonishingly rapid pace. It has dramatically altered the area of electronics as well as computing towards development of smaller and smaller chips with extraordinary processing power. In the therapeutic arena, nanotechnology promises to expand the repertoire of innovative systems, thereby revolutionizing health care modalities. At the same time, it is changing the relevance of the existing business model of drug discovery, medical imaging, laboratory diagnosis and other health sectors. The unique properties of nanosized material or devices are being utilized to develop complex intelligent and interactive systems which can be used at molecular level in innumerable areas of pathobiology.

Before we proceed to understand the application of nanotechnology in medicine we should go through the following definitions:

Nanotechnology is the technology of design, characterization, production and applications of structures, devices and systems by controlling shape and size at the nanometer scale.

Nanoscience is the study of phenomena and manipulation of materials at atomic, molecular and macromolecular scales, where properties differ significantly from those at larger scale.

Nanomedicine can be defined as application of nanotechnology in health care.

HISTORY OF NANOTECHNOLOGY

The idea of nanotechnology was born on December 29, 1959, in the annual meeting of American Physical Society, at the California Institute of Technology (Caltech), when Richard P Feynman (Fig. 127.1) delivered an invited talk entitled, *There is plenty of room at the bottom (http://www.zyvex.com/nanotech/feynman.html)*. The presentation and discussion was on the problem of manipulating and controlling things on a small scale. He asked the audience whether it would be possible to write the 24 volume of Encyclopedia Britannica on a pin head. Though it appeared to be science fiction at that time, it is reality in modern science.

Professor Feynman was awarded Nobel Prize in Physics in 1965. He was born in New York City on the 11th May, 1918. He studied at the Massachusetts

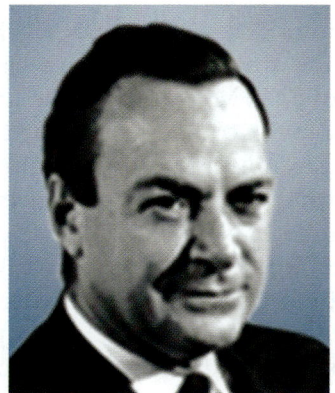

Fig. 127.1: Richard P Feynman

Institute of Technology where he obtained his BSc in 1939 and at Princeton University where he obtained his PhD in 1942. He was Research Assistant at Princeton (1940-1941), Professor of Theoretical Physics at Cornell University (1945-1950), Visiting Professor and thereafter appointed Professor of Theoretical Physics at the California Institute of Technology (1950-1959). He was Richard Chace Tolman Professor of Theoretical Physics at the California Institute of Technology when he received the Nobel Prize.

For more than a decade after the idea of miniaturization floated by Professor Feynman, there was hardly any scientific report in this area till 1974, when Norio Taniguchi first used the word "Nanotechnology" to refer to "production technology to get the extra high accuracy and ultra fine dimensions, i.e. the preciseness and fineness on the order of 1 nm (nanometer), 10^{-9} meter in length", in paper on ion-sputter machining.[1] In 1977, Professor K. Eric Drexler conceptualized "molecular nanotechnology" at Massachusetts Institute of Technology. In 1981, he published the paper entitled, "Molecular engineering: An approach to the development of general capabilities for molecular manipulation" in Proc. Nat.[1] Acad. Sci. USA.[2] The progress in nano-research got a tremendous boost with invention of Scanning Tunneling Microscope (STM) or scanning probe microscope which was of great help for characterization of nanoparticles. Gerd Binnig and Heinrich Rohrer developed the first working STM while working at IBM Zurich Research Laboratories in Switzerland in 1981. This instrument helped Binnig and Rohrer to win the Nobel Prize in physics in 1986. This year was also memorable as the first book entitled, "Engines of Creation: The Coming Era of Nanotechnology" by Professor Eric Drexler was published in the area of nanoscience and the atomic force microscope (AFM) was invented. In 1988, for the first time a ten-week course on "Nanotechnology and Exploratory Engineering" was taught at Stanford during the spring quarter. The first scientific journal in this area entitled, "Nanotechnology" was published in 1990. The book "Nanomedicine, Vol. I: Basic Capabilities" by Robert A, Jr. Freitas was published in 1999 which opened the gate of application of nanotechnology in health care and medicine. In the year 2000, President Bill Clinton, announced US. National Nanotechnology Initiative. The current decade witnessed an explosion of nano research world over. There is maximum increase in number of publications over last 10 years in this area.[3]

APPLICATION OF NANOTECHNOLOGY IN MEDICINE

Current applications of nanotechnology in medicine may be discussed under the following three headings:
A. Imaging
B. Clinical laboratory diagnosis
C. Drug and bio-molecular delivery system

Nanotechnology and Imaging

Imaging is one of the most important diagnostic tool in clinical medicine. The era of medical imaging started when Wilhelm Roentgen captured the first X-ray image of his wife's hand in 1896. Following the X-ray technology, a large number of non-invasive imaging technologies have been successfully developed and applied in clinical medicine as well as medical research including cell-molecular biology and drug discovery. Currently available methods of imaging are summarized in Table 127.1.

Application of nanotechnology may revolutionize the area of medical imaging. It can improve the current modalities like CT and MRI in terms of sensitivity and specificity as well as study of cellular functional alterations. It may help to develop fluorescence-based *in vivo* imaging systems. Now fluorescent nanoparticles can be developed which are resistant to photobleach. The nanoparticles have tremendous ability to enhance the contrast as well as visibility by conventional radiological techniques.

Among the various nanoparticle-based optical contrast agents, few appears to have potential for clinical application which include; quantum

Table 127.1: Commonly used non-invasive imaging techniques in clinical practice

Imaging technique	Detection method
Computed tomography (CT)	X-ray
Magnetic resonance imaging (MRI)	Magnetic field
Positron emission tomography (PET)	Gamma rays
Single photon emission computed tomography	Gamma rays
Ultrasonography	Ultrasonic waves

dots (QDs), gold nanoparticles, organically modified dye doped silica, up-converting phosphors and lanthanide-based contrast agents.

The development of quantum dots (QDs) for biological and biomedical applications is one of the fastest moving fields of nanotechnology today. The unique optical properties of these nanometer-sized semiconductor crystals make them an exciting fluorescent tool for *in vivo* and *invitro* imaging as well as for sensoric applications. QDs are fluorescent semiconductor nanocrystals, a few nanometers in diameter whose size and shape are precisely controlled by the duration, temperature, and ligand molecules used during synthesis. These are generally composed of II-VI and III-V elements.[4] Compared with conventional fluorophores, the nanocrystals have a narrow, tunable, symmetric emission spectrum and are photochemically stable.[5] Single QDs can be observed and tracked over an extended period of time (up to a few hours) with confocal microscopy, total internal reflection microscopy, or basic widefield epifluorescence microscopy.[6,7] Some of the most successful uses of QDs include immunofluorescence labeling of fixed cells and tissues; immunostaining of membrane proteins, microtubules, actin, and nuclear antigens; and fluorescence *in situ* hybridization on chromosomes or combed DNA.[7-12] Functionalized QDs like surface antibody tagged particles can be used to localize antigen *in vivo*. Thus in future techniques can be evolved for detection of early metastasis or staging of the cancers easily with non-invasive methods utilizing QDs. Rapid development in this area will change the face of medical practice in near future. Development of Cadmium sulphide nanoparticles, "Quantum Dots (QD)", with unique stable luminescent capability has helped to develop labeling and advanced imaging techniques for detection of very small quantity of marker molecules and even few microorganisms which can not be detected by conventional methods available at present. QDs bioconjugates raise new possibilities for studying genes, proteins and drug targets in single cells, tissue specimens and even in living animals and enable visualization of cancer cells in living animals. Though the concepts are feasible the main hurdle in utilizing QDs in diagnostic imaging is their toxicity.[13]

Due to the unique optical (colorimetric) properties, gold nanoparticles are now finding increased applications in the detection of biological systems.[14] Gold nanoparticle with less than 2 nm in diameter may be used as safe and better radiocontrast agent. Gold has higher absorption than iodine with less bone and tissue interference achieving better contrast with lower X-ray dose. Nanoparticles clear the blood more slowly than iodine agents, permitting longer imaging times.[15] However, safety issues related to systemic injection of gold nanoparticles as radiocontrast agent needs further study and confirmation.

Nanotechnology in Clinical Laboratory Diagnosis

The experimental applications of nanotechnology in laboratory and molecular diagnosis is expanding in such a rapid pace, it is beyond the scope of review in this chapter. However, some of the application with potential to be used in laboratory diagnosis may be enumerated as follows:
1. Nanotechnology for designing various biochips
2. Nano-barcode technology
3. Nanopore technology
4. Cantilever arrays
5. DNA micro-array for molecular diagnostics
6. Nanoparticle-based immunoassays
7. Resonance light scattering technology
8. Nanosensors

Within last few years, the biological and biomedical applications of micro- and nanotechnology (Biomedical or Biological Micro-Electro-Mechanical Systems [BioMEMS]) have become increasingly popular and have a potential for widespread use in a wide variety of diagnostics applications. The concept of "lab-on-a-chip" has become a reality today. Biochips, constructed with microelectromechanical systems on a micron scale, use micromanipulation, whereas nanotechnology-based chips are on a nanoscale acts on nanomanipulation.[16] The size of devices to move (levitate) tiny fluid droplets has been reduced by using micron scale diamagnets to create a magnetic micromanipulation chip, which operates with femtodroplets levitated in air.[17] The droplets used are 1 billion times smaller in volume than has been demonstrated by conventional methods. Thus, use of this technology of "lab-on-a-chip" would require micro- to nanoliter of sample for detecting different biomarkers, traces of toxic materials, signature molecules of virus or other infections. The size of this integrated "lab-on-a-chip" will be small enough to carry like a pen or watch and enable the patients to carry out the tests at any place and time of their choice. The day will come when there will be no need of samples to be sent to laboratory ushering the era of personalized medicine or medical care.

Nano-barcodes are submicrometer metallic barcodes with striping patterns prepared by sequential electrochemical deposition of metal ions. The differential reflectivity of adjacent stripes enables identification of the striping patterns by conventional light microscopy. This readout mechanism does not interfere with the use of fluorescence for detection of analytes bound to particles by affinity capture, as demonstrated by DNA and protein bioassays. Nanobarcodes can be used for SNP mapping and multiplexed assays for protein diagnostics.[18]

Biobarcode assay is another ultrasensitive method for detecting protein molecules. It relies on magnetic microparticle probes with antibodies that specifically bind a target of interest and nanoparticle probes that are encoded with DNA that is unique to the protein target of interest and antibodies.[19] Magnetic separation of the complexed probes and target followed by dehybridization of the oligonucleotides on the nanoparticle probe surface allows the determination of the presence of the target protein by identifying the oligonucleotide sequence released from the nanoparticle probe.

DNA-nanopore is formed by an individual DNA oligonucleotide covalently attached within the lumen of the alpha-hemolysin pore. The binding of single-stranded DNA (ssDNA) molecules to the tethered DNA strand causes changes in the ionic current flowing through a nanopore. The DNA-nanopores are able to discriminate between individual DNA strands up to 30 nucleotides in length differing by a single base on the basis of DNA duplex lifetimes substitution.[20] One of the example of use of this technology is the detection of a drug resistance-conferring mutation in the reverse transcriptase gene of HIV.

Mechanical detection for biochemical entities and reactions is an interesting method used through the use of micro- and nano-scale cantilever sensors on a chip. These cantilever sensors (diving board type structures) can be used in two modes, namely stress sensing and mass sensing. In stress sensing mode, the biochemical reaction is performed selectively on one side of the cantilever. A change in surface free energy results in a change in surface stress, which results in measurable bending of the cantilever. The bending of the cantilever can then be measured using optical means (laser reflecting from the cantilever surface into a quad position detector, like in an AFM) or electrical means (piezo-resistor incorporated at the fixed edge of the cantilever). In the mass sensing mode, the cantilever is excited mechanically so that it vibrates at its resonant frequency (using external drive, the ambient noise or other methods). The resonant frequency is measured using electrical or optical means, and compared to the resonant frequency of the cantilever once a biological entity is captured. The change in mass can be detected by detection of shift in resonant frequency, assuming the spring constant does not change. One of the main advantages of the cantilever sensors is the ability to detect interacting compounds without the need of introducing an optically detectable label on the binding entities. Detection of bacteria or viral agents and cancer marker like prostate specific antigen are some of the examples of use of this technology.[21,22]

DNA micro-arrays have become the most successful example of the merger between microelectronics technologies, biology, and chemistry. The techniques used to define patterns on semiconductor surfaces were utilized to construct arrays of single-stranded DNA. Once single strands of known sequences (capture probes) are placed at specific known sites on a chip surface, hybridization with molecules of unknown sequence (target probes) can reveal the sequence. There are two basic approaches to 'forming' the DNA arrays, namely optical (fluorescence) and electrical. This technique is being commercialized for detecting single nucleotide polymorphisms (SNPs), short tandem repeats (STRs), insertions, deletions, and other genetic mutations.[23]

Simple convenient method of preparation of bright, negatively or positively charged, water-soluble CdSe/ZnS core/shell nanocrystals (NCs) and their stabilization in aqueous solution has been developed.[24] Single NCs can be detected using a standard epifluorescent microscope, ensuring a detection limit of one molecule coupled with an NC, thus, increasing the sensitivity of the detection system. NC-antibody conjugates obtained by the method described can be used for specific detection of antigens in paraffin-embedded formaldehyde-fixed cancer tissue specimens.

Surface plasmon resonance (SPR) is an optical-electrical phenomenon involving the interaction of light with the electrons of a metal. The optical-electronic basis of SPR is the transfer of the energy carried by photons of light to a group of electrons (a plasmon) at the surface of a metal. The next-generation microarray-based SPR systems are designed to help researchers profile and characterize biomolecular interactions in a parallel format.[25]

Several nanomaterials are highly sensitive to chemical or biological alterations. The nano-scale sensors with immobilized bioreceptor probes that are selective for target analyte molecules are called nanobiosensors.[26] They can be incorporated into other technologies such as lab-on-a-chip to facilitate molecular diagnostics. They have potential for wide applications like detection of microorganisms in various samples, monitoring of metabolites in body fluids and detection cancer or genetic diseases. Various types of nanobiosensors may be fabricated. Boron-doped silicon nanowires (SiNWs) have been used to create highly sensitive, real-time electrically based sensors for biological and chemical species. The Ion Channel Switch (ICS™), a novel biosensor technology. It is based upon a synthetic self-assembling membrane, which acts like a biological switch that detecting the signaling the presence of specific molecules by triggering an electrical current. Virus particles are essentially biological nanoparticles. Herpes simplex virus (HSV) and adenovirus have been used to trigger the assembly of magnetic nanobeads as a nanosensor for clinically relevant viruses.[27] Sensing of Phage-Triggered Ion Cascade (SEPTIC), uses a nanowell device with two antenna-like electrodes to detect the electric-field fluctuations that result when a bacteriophage infects a specific bacterium and then identifies the bacterium. This method had a 100% success rate in detecting and identifying strains of E. coli quickly and accurately. Probes Encapsulated by Biologically Localized Embedding (PEBBLE) nanosensors consist of sensor molecules entrapped in a chemically inert matrix by a microemulsion polymerization process that produces spherical sensors in the size range of 20 to 200 nm.[28] These sensors are capable of real-time inter- and intra-cellular imaging of ions and molecules and are insensitive to interference from proteins. PEBBLE can also be used for early detection of cancer. Different optical biosensor devices are also developed based on surface plasma resonance and laser systems.[25,29] Nanoshell biosensors can enhance chemical sensing by 10 billion times. Gold nanoshells can be used for detecting sub-nanogram per milliliter quantities of immunoglobulins in saline, serum, and whole blood.[30] Optical nanosensor, based on singlewalled carbon nanotubes that modulate their emission in response to the adsorption of specific biomolecules, can be used as glucose sensor which may be an important tool for continuous blood glucose monitoring and development of real time biosensor-based therapy.[31]

Drug and Biomolecular Delivery System

In the journal Advanced Drug Delivery Reviews in 2004, the editorial by Vincent HL Lee chose the title as "Nanotechnology: challenging the limit of the creativity in targeted drug delivery". This is one of most popular and challenging field of nanomedicine and nanobiotechnology research.[32] Development of nanoparticle based targeting system for delivering the toxic anticancer drugs in the cancer cells is a reality now which reduces the systemic toxicity as well as more effective for cancer therapy. Here the nanoparticles are used as vehicle to carry anticancer drugs to the cancer cells. Thus, the logistics and the modalities of this kind of drug delivery system are completely different from the conventional chemotherapy and dosage. The first step for nanoparticle based delivery system to reach the cancer cell is to avoid trapping by the reticuloendothelial (RE) system (e.g. liver and spleen). Hydrophilic nanoparticles less than 100 nm in diameter are less trapped by RE system (Fig. 127.2).

Difference in the structures and functions of different types of cancers, poor blood flow due to irregular distribution of blood vessels, increased intratumoral pressure due to lack of functional lymphatic drainage at the cancer site allow poor transport and inadequate delivery of conventionally administered drugs and thus poor treatment modalities.[33,34] Also high doses of non-specific, highly cytotoxic anti-cancer drugs needed to achieve sufficient therapeutic concentrations at the site leads

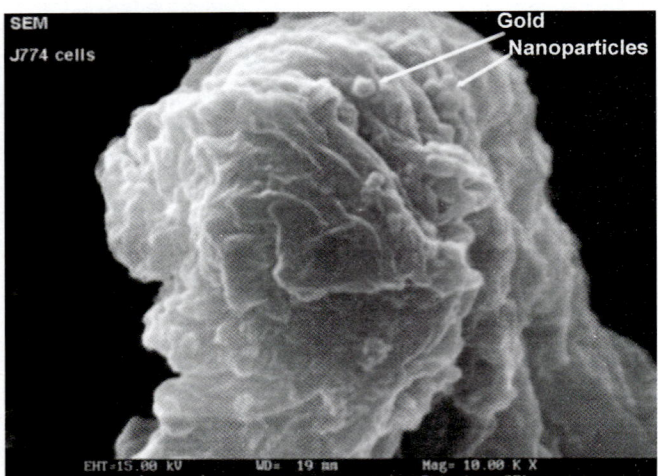

Fig. 127.2: Scanning electron micrograph of mouse macrophage (J774) cell engulfing 50 nm gold particles. The exposure of nanoparticles increases the surface ruffling of the cells with increased rate of phagocytosis

to severe side effects like nephrotoxicity, neurotoxicity, weight loss, hair loss, etc. Although radiotherapy and surgical removal of solid tumors are of interest in the current treatment methods, the undesired side effects due to chemotherapy and radiotherapy, development of multi-drug resistance cancer cells from the residual cells after the surgery are showing equally disappointing results.[34]

But targeted drug delivery systems (TDDS) in the form of small sized architectures as injectable preparations, like nanoparticles, liposomes, micelles, dendrimers and antibody targeted systems, which have been in current research compromise those above said critical requirements and reach therapeutic phase.[35] Especially targeted polymeric nanoparticulate carriers offer higher drug loading and programmable drug release properties depending upon the environmental conditions. Development of specific targeting of cancer cells avoiding normal cells is a major challenge. This requires targeting of cancer specific receptor or other molecules which has a high expression in cancer cells. For example, the overexpression of folate receptors only on the cancer cell surfaces, promises selective delivery of drug into the intracellular compartment.[36,37] We are in the process of developing folate conjugated nanoparticles for selective cytotoxic delivery for breast cancer (Fig. 127.3).

The nanoparticle based drug delivery system for cancer can utilize several issues related to cancer biology. The different systems that can be used may be enumerated as in Table 127.2.[38]

Targeted delivery through enhanced permeability and retention based on the concept of poorly formed defective vasculature in the tumor which are more leaky in comparison to vasculature in normal tissue. This is often associated with poor lymphatic drainage from tumor tissue resulting in enhanced permeation and retention effect (EPR effect).[39] The drug loaded nanoparticle may be sequestrated in the tumor due to EPR effect when injected in systemic circulation. This is a form of passive targeting.

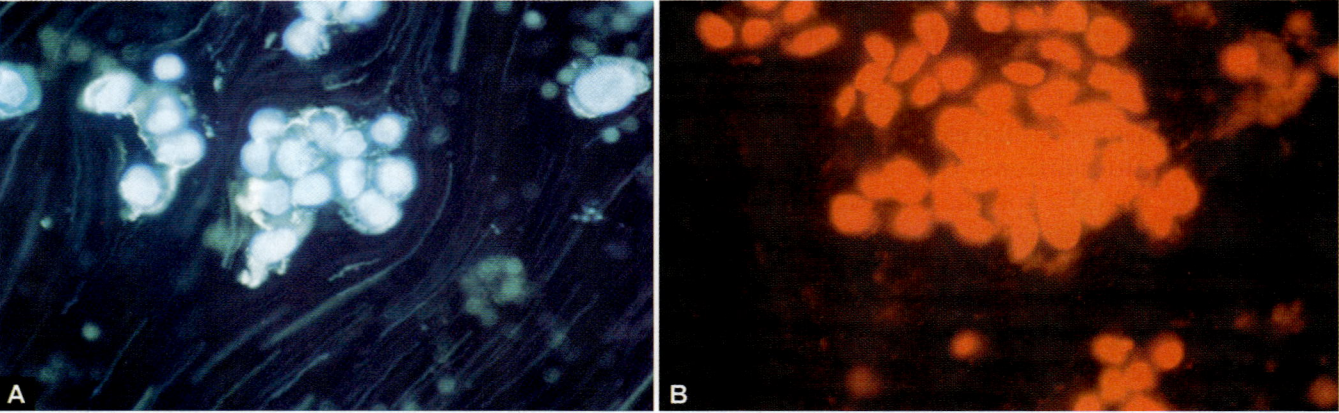

Figs 127.3 A and B: The MCF7 (Human breast cancer cell line) cells incubated for 6 hours *in vitro* with Doxorubicin loaded NIPAM nanoparticle without folic acid residue on the surface showing no nuclear fluorescence indicating no significant entry of the drugs in the cells: **A.** When these cells were incubated in same condition for same duration with similar nanoparticles with surface conjugation with phosphofolate there was marked nuclear fluorescence of Doxorubicin, **B.** Demonstrating specific folic acid receptor mediated targeting of breast cancer cells and efficacy of drug delivery by nanoparticles

Table 127.2: Different drug delivery systems
Drug delivery systems
1. Targeted delivery through enhanced permeability and retention
2. Tumor-specific targeting
3. Targeting through tumor angiogenesis
4. Targeting tumor vasculature

It is possible to target tumor specific antigen or other target molecule as mentioned earlier with nanoparticle. For example, Her-2 neu receptor of breast carcinoma can be targeted in case of Her-2 positive carcinomas. Similarly, CD20 may be targeted for B cell immunophenotype nonHodgkin lymphoma.[40]

Angiogenesis is a process vital to the continued expansion of a tumor mass. Some of the most prominent angiogenesis stimulatory molecules include vascular endothelial growth factor (VEGF), basic fibroblast growth factor, platelet-derived growth factor and certain matrix metalloproteinases. Some endogenous angiogenesis inhibitors are the interferon family (a, h and g), thrombospondin-1 and -2, certain tissue inhibitors of matrix metalloproteinases and protein fragments such as angiostatin and endostatin. During active tumorogenesis the turnover rate of endothelial cells increases up to 50 fold with the formation of a new vascular sprout.[41]

Because a vascularized tumor is capable of increased growth and is more readily able to metastasize, increasing amounts of research are focused on developing treatments to slow angiogenesis and limit tumor growth and dissemination. Nanoparticle based therapy to inhibit tumor angiogenesis is an active field of research and development which has a great therapeutic potential.

Targeting of tumor vasculature may be another mode of cancer treatment. Recent work has also shown that gene delivery may also be targeted to neovasculature by coupling lipid-based cationic nanoparticles to an integrin AVH-targeting ligand in tumor-bearing mice.[42]

Research activity aimed towards achieving specific and targeted delivery of anti-cancer agents has expanded tremendously in the last 5 years or so with new avenues of directing drugs to tumors as well as new types of drugs. Currently nanoparticle loaded drug like paclitaxel is available in India marketed by Dabur India Limited.

Innovative modality like burning of tumor tissue with injection of gold nanorod in the tumor followed by low power laser irradiation may be an important safe alternative to radiotherapy with much less side effects. We have developed such a system (Fig. 127.4).

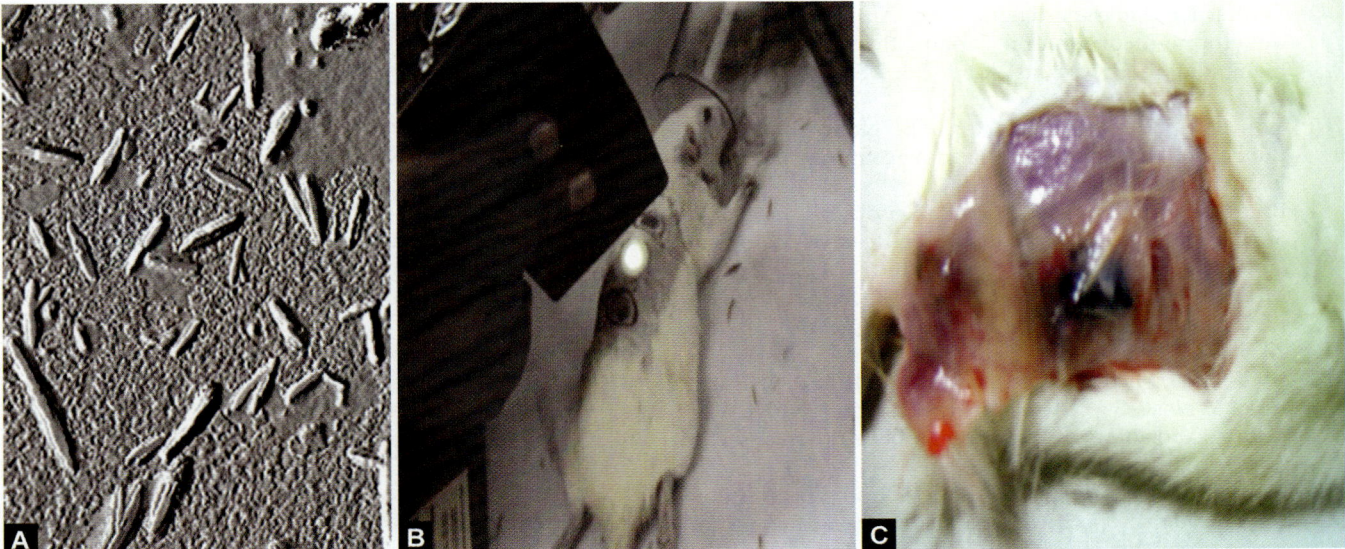

Figs 127.4 A to C: The Atomic Force Microscopy (AFM) photograph: **A.** of gold nanorods. The gold nanorods injection in the tumor followed by irradiation with low power laser, **B.** Caused production of intense heat due to alteration in surface plasma resonance of gold nanorods leading to burning of the impregnated tissue, **C.** This safer modality can be applied to solid tumor in place of radiotherapy

Apart from conventional drug targeting innovative methods like magnetic sensor based drug release system, temperature sensitive drug release and other biosensor based system are being developed with multi-functional nanoparticle. In near future it will be possible to replace conventional cancer therapy with these smart multifunctional targeted system with least systemic toxic effect and it may safer than many antibiotic therapy.

SUMMARY

Advances in nanotechnology are providing nanofabricated devices that are small, sensitive and inexpensive enough to facilitate direct observation, manipulation and analysis of single biological molecule from single cell. This opens new opportunities and provides powerful tools in the fields such as genomics, proteomics, molecular diagnostics, drug delivery and high throughput screening. Nanotechnology has potential advantages in applications in POC (Point-of-care) diagnosis: on patient's bedside, self-diagnostics for use in the home, integration of diagnostics with therapeutics and for the development of personalized medicines.

REFERENCES

1. Taniguchi. On the basic concept of 'Nanotechnology', Proc. ICPE, 1974;1:5-10.
2. Drexler KE. Molecular engineering: An approach to the development of general capabilities for molecular manipulation, Proc. Natl. Acad. Sci. USA 1981;78:5275-78.
3. Youtie J, Shapira P, Porter AL. Nanotechnology publications and citations by leading countries and blocs. J Nanopart Res 2008;960-66.
4. Bruchez M Jr, Moronne M, Gin P, Weiss S, Alivisatos AP. Semiconductor nanocrystals as fluorescent biological labels. Science 1998;281(5385):2013-16.
5. Michalet X, Pinaud FF, Bentolila1 LA. Quantum Dots for Live Cells, in vivo Imaging, and Diagnostics Science 2005;307(5709):538-44.
6. Lacoste TD. Michalet X, Pinaud F, Chemla DS, Alivisatos AP, Weiss S. Ultrahigh-resolution multicolor colocalization of single fluorescent probes. Proc Natl Acad Sci USA 2000;97:9461-66.
7. Michalet X, Lacoste TD, Weiss S. Ultrahigh-resolution colocalization of spectrally separable point-like fluorescent probes. Methods 2001;25(1):87-102.
8. Sukhanova A, Devy J, Venteo L, Kaplan H, Artemyev M, Oleinikov V, Klinov D, Pluot M, Cohen JH, Nabiev I. Biocompatible fluorescent nanocrystals for immuno-labeling of membrane proteins and cells. Anal Biochem 2004;324(1):60-67.
9. Xingyong Wu, Hongjian Liu, Jianquan Liu, et al. Immunofluorescent labeling of cancer marker Her2 and other cellular targets with semiconductor quantum dots. Nature Biotechnol 2003;21:41-46.
10. Akerman ME, Chan WCW, Laakkonen P, Bhatia SN, Ruoslahti E. Nanocrystal targeting in vivo. Proc Natl Acad Sci USA 2002;99:12617-21.
11. Bruchez M, Moronne M, Gin P, Weiss S, Alivisatos AP. Semiconductor nanocrystals as fluorescent biological labels. Science 1998;281:2013.
12. Xiao Y, Barker PE. Semiconductor nanocrystal probes for human metaphase chromosomes. Nucleic Acids Res 2004;32:28E.
13. Hardman R. A Toxicologic Review of Quantum Dots: Toxicity Depends on Physicochemical and Environmental Factors. Environ Health Perspect 2006;114:165-72.
14. Storhoff JJ, Lazarides AA, Mucic RC, Mirkin CA, Letsinger RL, Schatz GC. J Am Chem Soc 2000;122:4640.
15. Hainfeld JF, Slatkin DN, Focella M, et al. Gold nanoparticles: a new X-ray contrast agent. British Journal of Radiology 2006;79:248-53.
16. Jain KK. Nanotechnology-based lab-on-a-chip devices. Encyclopedia of Diagnostic Genomics and Proteomics. New York 7 Marcel Dekkar Inc 2005;891-95.
17. Lyuksyutov IF, Naugle DG, Rathnayaka KDD. On-chip manipulation of levitated femtodroplets. Appl Phys Lett 2004;85:1817-19.
18. Walton ID, Norton SM, Balasingham A, et al. Particles for multiplexed analysis in solution: detection and identification of striped metallic particles using optical microscopy. Anal Chem 2002;74:2240-47.
19. Nam JM, Stoeva SI, Mirkin CA. Bio-bar-code-based DNA detection with PCR-like sensitivity. J Am Chem Soc 2004;126:5932-33.
20. Howorka S, Cheley S, Bayley H. Sequence-specific detection of individual DNA strands using engineered nanopores. Nat Biotechnol 2001;19:636-39.
21. A Gupta, D Akin, R Bashir. Resonant mass biosensor for ultrasensitive detection of bacterial cells, Microfluidics, Biomems, and Medical Microsystems Conference at SPIE's Photonics West Micromachining and Microfabrication 2003 Symposium, San Jose, Ca. Jan. 27, 2003. Proceedings of SPIE, the International Society for Optical Engineering, 2003;4982:21-27.
22. A. Gupta, D. Akin, R. Bashir. Single virus particle mass detection using microresonators with nanoscale thickness. Applied Physics Letters 2004;84 (11):1976-78.
23. MJ Heller, An active microelectronics device for multiplex DNA analysis, IEEE Eng. Med. Biol. Mag. 1996;15(2):100.
24. Sukhanova A, Devy J, Venteo L, et al. Biocompatible fluorescent nanocrystals for immunolabeling of membrane proteins and cells. Anal Biochem 2004;324:60-67.
25. Haes AJ, Duyne RP. Preliminary studies and potential applications of localized surface plasmon resonance

spectroscopy in medical diagnostics. Expert Rev Mol Diagn 2004;4:527-37.
26. Cui Y, Wei Q, Park H, Lieber CM. Nanowire nanosensors for highly sensitive and selective detection of biological and chemical species. Science 2001;293:1289-92.
27. Perez JM, Simeone FJ, Saeki Y, Josephson L, Weissleder R. Viral-induced self-assembly of magnetic nanoparticles allows the detection of viral particles in biological media. J Am Chem Soc 2003;125:10192-93.
28. Cao Y, Lee Koo YE, Kopelman R. Poly (decyl methacrylate)-based fluorescent PEBBLE swarm nanosensors for measuring dissolved oxygen in biosamples. Analyst 2004;129:745-50.
29. Vo-Dinh T. Optical nanosensors for detecting proteins and biomarkers in individual living cells. Methods Mol Biol 2005;300:383-402.
30. Hirsch LR, Jackson JB, Lee A, Halas NJ, West JL. A whole blood immunoassay using gold nanoshells. Anal Chem 2003;75:2377-81.
31. Barone PW, Baik S, Heller DA, Strano MS. Near-infrared optical sensors based on single-walled carbon nanotubes. Nat Mater 2005;4:86-92.
32. Lee Vincent HL. Nanotechnology: challenging the limit of creativity in targeted drug delivery. Advanced Drug Delivery Reviews 2004;56:1527-28.
33. Jain RK. Delivery of molecular and cellular medicine to solid tumors. Adv Drug Del Rev 1997;26:71-90.
34. Moghimi SM, Hunter C, Murray JC. Long-circulating and target-specific nanoparticles: Theory to practice Pharmacol Rev 2001;53:283-318.
35. Jaracz S, Chen J, Kuznetsova LV, Ojima I. Recent advances in tumor-targeting anticancer drug conjugates. Bioorg Med Chem. 2005;13(17):5043-54.
36. Leamon CP, Low PS. Delivery of macromolecules into living cells: A method that exploits folate receptor endocytosis. Proc Natl Acad Sci USA 1991;88:5572-76.
37. Stefano GD, Lanza M, Kratz F, Merina L, Fiume L. A novel method for coupling doxorubicin to the lactosaminated human albumin by an acid sensitive hydrazone bond: synthesis, characterization and preliminary biological properties of the conjugate. Eur J Pharm Sci 2004;23:393-97.
38. Brannon-Peppas L, Blanchette J O. Nanoparticle and targeted systems for cancer therapy. Advanced Drug Delivery Reviews 2004;56:1649-59.
39. G. Sledge, K. Miller. Exploiting the hallmarks of cancer. the future conquest of breast cancer. European Journal of Cancer 2003;39:1668-75.
40. R. Abou-Jawde, T Choueiri, C Alemany, T Mekhail, An overview of targeted treatments in cancer, Clinical Therapeutics 2003;25:2121-37.
41. SB Fox, KC Gatter, R Bicknell. Relationship of endothelial cell proliferation to tumor vascularity in human breast cancer. Cancer Research 1993;53:4161-63.
42. JD Hood, M Bednarski, R Frausto, S Guccione, RA Reisfeld, R Xiang, DA Cheresh. Tumor regression by targeted gene delivery to the neovasculature. Science 2002;296:2404-07.

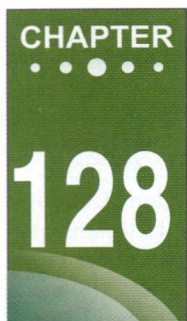

CHAPTER 128

Laser Applications in Pediatric Surgery

V Bhatnagar

Laser is an acronym which stands for *"Light Amplification by the Stimulated Emission of Radiation."* The surgical applications of laser were introduced in 1965 even though the phenomenon was first proposed by Einstien as early as 1917.[1,2] Today, lasers have added a new dimension to operative surgery because of greater precision, better hemostasis, lesser tissue damage and a diversity of uses.

BASIC PRINCIPLES

Laser energy is produced by the emission of photons from excited atoms. Photons are emission energy made up of electromagnetic waves released by atoms and these propagate with the speed of light (i.e. 300000 km/s). Under normal circumstances atoms are in the 'ground state' (i.e. the electrons orbit the nucleus in their respective designated orbitals). An atom gets 'excited' when a photon of energy strikes it (i.e. the electron moves from a lower to a higher orbital). The excited atom then releases a photon of energy in order to return to the ground state. This phenomenon is known as 'spontaneous emission'. Emission of energy can be 'stimulated' by striking already excited atoms with photons — the excited atoms then release identical photons and return to the ground state. Lasers work on this principle of stimulated emission. The energy of photons is directly proportional to the frequency and is indirectly proportional to the wavelength. Atoms can be excited by 'external energy' which could be in the form of absorption of light, collision with electrons, a chemical process, electricity or nuclear fission. The amplification is done in a resonator or 'laser medium' which could be liquid (*e.g. dye laser*), solid (*e.g. neodymium:yttrium-aluminium-garnet*) or gaseous (*e.g. argon, carbon dioxide*). The wavelength of the emitted beam varies with the medium (0.2-10.0 μ).[3,4] The laser beam is characteristically monochromatic (i.e. of a single frequency), coherent (i.e. the rays are spatially and temporally in phase) and collimated (i.e. the rays are parallel to each other).

LASER INTERACTION WITH TISSUES

The effects of laser on tissues can be photochemical, photothermal or photodecomposition. Surgical techniques mainly utilise the photothermal effects for vaporisation, cutting and coagulation (Table 128.1). The laser beam has to be absorbed for it to have the photothermal effect; if it is reflected, transmitted or scattered then it will not have the desired effect. The photothermal effect is governed by several factors including wavelength, mode of operation (pulsed or continuous), power density of the beam and the duration of exposure to the beam (Table 128.2). Generation of smoke, hemorrhage or charring result in scattering, reflection or absorption of the beam and hence the results may be undesirable. Photothermal effects are also modified by the presence of

Table 128.1: The photothermal effects on tissues

Tissue changes at different temperatures[7]

up to 45°C	No irreversible damage
over 45°C	Irreversible damage
45-60°C	Denaturation of enzymes
60-100°C	Coagulation of proteins
over 100°C	Drying of tissues
over 150°C	Carbonization of tissues
over 300°C	Vaporization of tissues

chromophores (e.g. hemoglobin, melanin, etc.) in the tissues and this phenomenon has been utilized for selective photoablation of tissues, e.g. the treatment of hemangiomas and port wine stains.[5,6]

The photothermal effect produces a characteristic lesion. A crater is formed at the centre of impact due to vaporization of the tissue. Immediately surrounding this crater is a zone of cellular coagulation produced by the diffusion of heat and surrounding this area is a zone of cellular edema. Focussed beams are used for cutting and defocussed beams are used for coagulation. The depth of injury will depend on the exposure time.[5,7]

There are numerous kinds of lasers but the majority are essentially research tools. The types of lasers which have applications in medical science for clinical purposes or research have been categorized as gas lasers (e.g. Argon, Carbon dioxide, Excimer), chemical lasers, dye lasers, metal vapor lasers (e.g. Copper), solid state lasers (e.g. Nd:YAG, Er:YAG, Ho:YAG), semiconductor lasers, etc.

LASERS WITH SURGICAL APPLICATION

CO_2

Carbon dioxide, nitrogen and helium are used as the medium in which excitation of nitrogen transfers the energy to carbon dioxide and helium returns it to the ground state. The emitted beam lies in the non-visible infrared range at 10600 nm (heat radiation). This laser is ideal for cutting because of the absorption coefficient and hence the tissue penetration is high and scattering within the tissues is low. 20-100 Watts power is usually sufficient for surgical uses.[7,8] However, a very major disadvantage is that it cannot be transmitted through fibreoptic systems and hence needs either an operating microscope or a hand held probe. It has found great applicability in laryngeal and vocal cord lesions. This laser was developed by Patel in 1964.[9]

Nd:YAG and Ho:YAG:

Neodymium atoms are used as the laser medium and are incorporated into a yttrium-aluminium-garnet crystal. The Nd:YAG laser emits a non-visible infrared beam of 1064 nm wavelength. Depending on the type of discharge lamp the laser can be continuous wave (cw) or pulsed (p) wave. The laser beam is delivered via a quartz fiber and this makes it ideally suited for endoscopic use. The surgical application of Nd:YAG laser is with 100 Watts power in the continuous mode. This is the most commonly used laser in surgical practice because of its versatility, it can coagulate blood vessels up to 2 mm, cut and vaporise tissues but the drawbacks are that it has a deeper tissue penetration and cause more tissue damage.[7,8] The Nd:YAG laser was developed by Johnson in 1962.[6]

Holmium

YAG laser is similar to the Nd:YAG laser but it has been found to be better for tissue ablation, renal stone removal and in dentistry. It has now taken over almost all the clinical applications of the Nd:YAG laser. The Ho:YAG laser can produce the same effects of the Nd:YAG laser with a lesser wattage and hence it is safer and less harmful to the surrounding tissues.

Argon

Argon ions are used as the laser medium. Two wavelengths are emitted - 488 nm in the blue light area and 514 nm in the green light area. The wavelength is close to the maximal absorption for melanin, myoglobin and hemoglobin and tissue penetration is only 1 mm. Hence, it is a very good laser for pigmentary disorders and vascular malformations. It can be delivered through a fibreoptic cable and therefore it can be used for endoscopic surgery. The Argon laser generates a lot of heat which needs to be dissipated by an effective cooling system.[7,8] It was introduced by Bennett in 1962.[10]

Dye

Fluorescing dyes, e.g. rhodamine, stilbene and coumarine are used as the amplifying medium. Using different dyes and pump sources this laser can be tuned within a wide spectral region extending from ultraviolet to near infrared and depending on the pump source it can be either pulsed or used as continuous wave. They can be delivered through fibreoptic cables and hence are useful in endoscopic applications particularly for lithotripsy procedures.[7,8]

KTP

When an Nd:YAG laser beam is passed through a potassium titanyl phosphate crystal, it results in a visible beam which has half the wavelength of the Nd:YAG laser beam and it can be delivered through a fibreoptic cable. Tissue penetration is approximately 1 mm deep and hence it is better for coagulation as compared to cutting.[7,8]

ORGANIZING A LASER SET-UP

Lasers can be extremely dangerous if they are not used properly or if basic precautions are not taken.

Lasers can damage eyes and skin and can cause fires and explosions. The laser beam can be reflected from shiny or smooth unpolished metallic surfaces. Hence, in addition to the safety measures for heavy electric equipment, it is very important to follow the basic precautionary steps specifically for lasers:

1. It is preferable to have a theatre dedicated for lasers. If that is not possible then the staff should be dedicated to the laser set-up so that the basic drill for safety measures is ingrained in them.
2. There should be adequate warning signals when lasers are in use. 'Casual' visitors to the operating room should be discouraged.
3. Laser glasses should be worn by everybody in the room where lasers are being used.[7,8]
4. Combustible material should not be used with lasers. Endotracheal/tracheostomy or other non-metallic tubes which are likely to be in the field of laser use should be adequately protected.

CLINICAL APPLICATIONS OF LASER IN PEDIATRIC SURGERY

Due to reduced blood loss the operative field is clean and thus lasers help in providing a high degree of surgical precision. The laser technology and the fact that it can have a fiberoptic transmission has given significant advantages and improved the results of surgery in a number of difficult areas and has also opened up possibilities for the treatment of conditions which were considered impossible or very hazardous:

1. Vascular malformations; cutaneous or those which can be reached by endoscopes.
2. Airway lesions; vocal cord nodules, laryngotracheal papillomas, tracheal diverticulum, tracheoesophageal fistula, choanal atresia.
3. Gastroenterological procedures; coagulation of upper or lower gastrointestinal bleeders.
4. Minimally invasive surgical procedures.
5. Resections of solid organs; hepatectomy, partial nephrectomy.
6. Urologic procedures; posterior urethral valves, urethral strictures, ureteroceles, bladder tumors and vascular malformations, lithotripsy.[11]
7. Neurosurgical procedures; choroid plexectomy, third ventriculostomy. Retinal surgery.

The photothermal properties of lasers have made it particularly useful in pediatric surgical practice because it provides a high degree of precision and reduces blood loss significantly.[8]

THE AIIMS EXPERIENCE

The Nd:YAG laser was commissioned at AIIMS in March 1997, and was in use till the very early 2000s. During this time it was extensively utilized by the general surgeons, plastic surgeons, urologists, gynecologists, ENT surgeons, gastroenterologists and of course pediatric surgeons. The author's experience is summarized in Table 128.3.

The main advantages of laser surgery are that it is bloodless, very precise, does not cause damage to surrounding tissue, there is no morbidity, there has

Table 128.2 : Factors governing use of Nd:YAG lasers[7]

	Power (Watts)	Distance (mm)	Exposure time (seconds)	Interval (seconds)	Mode
Coagulation					
Minor bleed	30-35	2-5	0.5-2.0	0.2	P
Major bleed	50	2-5	0.5	0.2	P
General	35	2-5	-	-	cw
Cutting	50-100	0.5	-	-	cw/p
Resection	100-120	0.5	-	-	cw

Type of use	Area of use	Lesion	N
Open surgical procedure	Surface lesions	A-V fistula, scalp	1
		Hemangioma, chest	1
		Tongue nodule	1
		Tongue lymphangioma	3
Endoscopy	Genitourinary tract	Posterior urethral valves[12,13]	47
		Ureterocele	2
		Urethral stricture	4
		Anterior urethral diverticulum	1
	Respiratory tract	'H' tracheo-esophageal fistula[14]	1
		Recurrent tracheo-esophageal fistula[14]	3
		Tracheal diverticulum[15]	2
		Tracheal papillomatosis	1

Table 128.3 : Nd:YAG laser applications in paediatric surgery

been no mortality and the majority of children have been treated as day care cases. It is particularly advantageous in the respiratory tract where congenital and recurrent tracheoesophageal fistulae can be treated endoscopically and without a major operative procedure, thus avoiding considerable morbidity and mortality (Figs 128.1A to C).

In posterior urethral valves and other urethral/bladder conditions the property that the laser can be transmitted through a fibre has been used very effectively. Since the laser does not have a deep tissue penetration and the tissue ablation is bloodless, the majority of urethral endoscopic surgery can be done

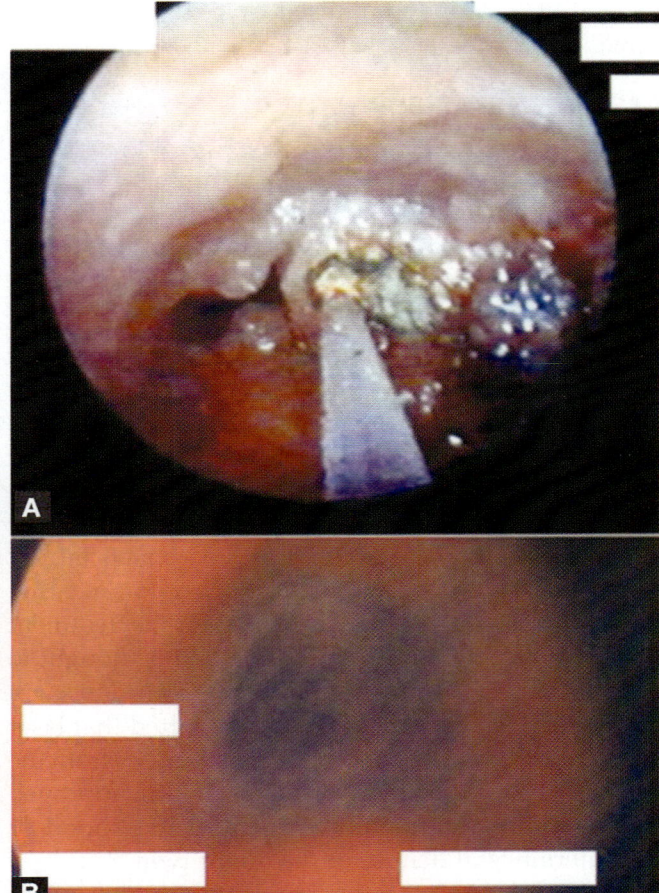

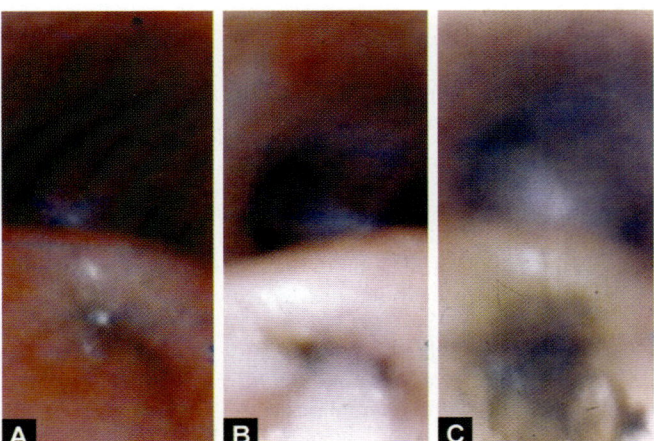

Figs 128.1A to C: A. Endoscopic view of 'H' type tracheo-esophageal fistula. **B.** Laser fiber in position inside the fistula. **C.** Following vapourization of the mucosa

Figs 128.2A and B: A. Endoscopic view of tracheal papillomas being vapourized using the laser fiber. **B.** Following the vapourization the trachea is clean

without postoperative catheterization and the patients can be discharged within a few hours of the surgery. Also, the risk of postoperative stricture formation is negligible.

Similarly, in tracheal lesions, e.g: papillomatosis, the lesions can be vapourized without damaging the surrounding tissues (Figs 128.2A and B). The only draw back is that tissue may not be available for histopathological examination. In tracheoesophageal fistulas, the mucosal lining of the fistula is vapourized thus allowing the fistula to close.

The initial expenditure on the laser machine and the set-up in an existing operation theatre complex is estimated to be approximately Rs. 50 lacs. Hence, considerable thought must be given to the type of laser which is required for the needs of the hospital and a central facility should be created. The recurring expenditure can be minimised by re-using the laser fibers.

LASER IN FETAL SURGERY

Lasers have been recently used in fetal surgery for indications that merit antenatal intervention to improve the prognosis. Anterior and posterior urethral valves have been fulgurated with laser beams.[16,17] Rarely, laryngeal webs have been fulgurated with a laser beam when diagnosed during the antenatal period. Though these conditions can be treated after birth, the condition in vogue today as a preferred indication for fetal laser treatment is twin-to-twin transfusion syndrome.

Twin-to-twin transfusion syndrome (TTTS) is a severe fetal condition that has regained attention since surgical endoscopic treatment proved beneficial.[18-20] Selective laser photocoagulation of communicating vessels technique has been described for the treatment of twin-twin transfusion syndrome that is thought to result from a net transfer of blood from the donor twin to the recipient twin.[18] It has been reported that laser coagulation of the arteriovenous anastomoses from the donor to the recipient first would result in an improved hemodynamic status and decreased likelihood of intrauterine fetal demise of the donor twin.[18]

Perinatal survival was significantly higher when treatment was performed in the early stages.[20] Twin weight discordance and donor fetus intrauterine growth restriction appear to improve after laser therapy for TTTS.[21] In a 5 year multicenter, prospective, randomized controlled trial with primary outcome variable as 30 day postnatal survival of donors and recipients, there was no statistically significant difference in 30-day postnatal survival between fetoscopic laser photocoagulation vs serial amnioreduction treatment for donors or recipients.[22] Most series report comparable results with laser photocoagulation and serial amnioreduction. However, some authors have reported that laser therapy is associated with better outcomes and less major neonatal morbidity.[23,24] The perinatal survival rate varies from 65-70%.[20,25]

The percutaneous technique has gained wide acceptance, with an acceptable risk of maternal morbidity but a significant risk of miscarriage (6.8-23%) or preterm rupture of the membranes (5-30%).[25] In a review of perinatal outcome of 1300 TTTS cases treated by laser from 17 publications, with a median perinatal survival rate of 57% (50-100%); brain lesions were present in 2-7% of the survivors at the age of 1-6 months.[25] Other complications reported include Pseudoamniotic band syndrome (1.8%) And TTTS cardiomyopathy in recipient survival.[22,26]

ACKNOWLEDGEMENT

This chapter was first published in Textbook of Neonatal Surgery, Ed., DK Gupta, Modern Publishers, New Delhi, 2000. It is being reproduced with kind permission of MBD publishers.

REFERENCES

1. Goldman L, Wilson R, Homby P, et al. Laser radiation of malignancy in man. Cancer 1965;18:533.
2. Rosomoff HL, Carroll F. Reaction of neoplasm and brain to laser. Arch Neurol 1966;14:143.
3. Dixon JA. Current laser applications in general surgery. Ann Surg 1988;207:355.
4. Stellar S, Polanyi TG, Bredemeier HC. Lasers in surgery. In, Laser Applications in Medicine and Biology. New York, Plenum Press 1974-241.
5. Berlein HP, Muller G, Waldschmidt J. Lasers in pediatric surgery. Prog Pediatr Surg 1990;25:5.
6. Unthank JL. Fundamental principles of surgical lasers. In, Weisberger EC (Ed). Lasers in Head and Neck Surgery. New York, Igaku-Shoin, 1991:1.
7. Tutorial: Laser in Medicine. Laser-Medizin-Zentrum, gGmbH, Berlin, 1992.
8. Azizkhan RG. Lasers in pediatric surgery. Surg Clin North Am 1992;72:1315.

9. Patel CKN, McFarlane RA, Faust WL. Selective excitation through vibrational energy transfer and optical master action in N_2-CO_2. Phys Rev 1964;13:617.
10. Bennett WR, Faust WL, McFarlane RA, et al. Dissociative excitation transfer and optcial master oscillation in NeO_2 and ArO_2 rf discharges [letter]. Phys Rev 1962;8:470.
11. Bhatnagar V. Laser application in paediatric urology. In, Gupta NP (Ed). Guidelines in Lasers in Urology. AIIMS, New Delhi 1997:55.
12. Bhatnagar V, Lal R, Agarwala S, Mitra DK. The technique of endoscopic laster fulguration of posterior urethral valves. J. Indian Assoc Paediatr Surg 1998;3:133-34.
13. Bhatnagar V, Agarwala S, Lal R, Mitra DK. Fulguration of posterior urethral valves using the Nd: YAG laser. Pediatr Surg Int 1999;15: under publication.
14. Bhatnagar V, Lal R, Sriniwas M, Agarwala S, Mitra DK. Endoscopic treatment of tracheoesophageal fistula using electrocautery and ND:YAG laster. J. Pediatr Surg 1999;34:464-67.
15. Bhatnagar V, Lal R, Agarwala S, Mitra DK. Endoscopic treatment of tracheal diverticulum following repair of esophageal atresia and tracheoesophageal fistula. J. Pediatr Surg 1998;33:1323-24.
16. Sago H, Hayashi S, Chiba T, et al. Endoscopic fetal urethrotomy for anterior urethral valves: a preliminary report Fetal Diagn Ther 2008;24(2):92-5.
17. Quintero RA, Shukla AR, Homsy YL, Bukkapatnam R. Successful in utero endoscopic ablation of posterior urethral valves: a new dimension in fetal urology. Urology 2000;55(5):774.
18. Quintero RA, Ishii K, Chmait RH, Bornick PW, Allen MH, Kontopoulos EV. Sequential selective laser photocoagulation of communicating vessels in twin-twin transfusion syndrome. J Matern Fetal Neonatal Med 2007;20(10):763-68.
19. Sepulveda W, Wong AE, Dezerega V, Devoto JC, Alcalde JL. Endoscopic laser surgery in severe second-trimester twin-twin transfusion syndrome: a three-year experience from a Latin American center. Prenat Diagn 2007; 27(11):1033-38.
20. Middeldorp JM, Sueters M, Lopriore E, et al Fetoscopic laser surgery in 100 pregnancies with severe twin-to-twin transfusion syndrome in the Netherlands. Fetal Diagn Ther 2007;22(3):190-94.
21. Chmait RH, Korst LM, Bornick PW, Allen MH, Quintero RA Fetal growth after laser therapy for twin-twin transfusion syndrome. Am J Obstet Gynecol 2008; 199(1):47.e1-6.
22. Crombleholme TM, Shera D, Lee H, et al. A prospective, randomized, multicenter trial of amnioreduction vs selective fetoscopic laser photocoagulation for the treatment of severe twin-twin transfusion syndrome. Am J Obstet Gynecol 2007;197(4):396.e1-9.
23. Rossi AC, D'Addario V. Laser therapy and serial amnioreduction as treatment for twin-twin transfusion syndrome: a metaanalysis and review of literature. Am J Obstet Gynecol 2008;198:147-52.
24. Middeldorp JM, Lopriore E, Sueters M, et al. Twin-to-twin transfusion syndrome after 26 weeks of gestation: is there a role for fetoscopic laser surgery? BJOG 2007;114:694-98.
25. Yamamoto M, Ville Y. Laser treatment in twin-to-twin transfusion syndrome Semin Fetal Neonatal Med 2007;12:450-57.
26. Winer N, Salomon LJ, Essaoui M, Nasr B, Bernard JP, Ville Y. Pseudoamniotic band syndrome: a rare complication of monochorionic twins with fetofetal transfusion syndrome treated by laser coagulation. Am J Obstet Gynecol. 2008;198:393.e1-5.

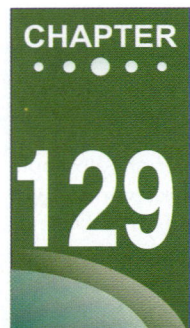

Pediatric Surgeon and the Computer

Gian Battista Parigi, Giacomo Parigi

The story goes that, some one hundred years ago, a Californian farmer approached for the first time a curious instrument called "telephone". Being the operator temporarily away he managed on his own: he scribbled few words on a sheet of paper, rolled it up and poked it into the receiver with all the gentleness typical of the rugged Westerner. Needless to say, his message encountered some problems getting through this new technological gadget: the same problems that many "computer greenhorns" likewise experience when sitting for the first time in front of the fiendish instrument. Hence the funny stories of people using as a "cup-holder" the sliding driver for CD/DVD, or searching desperately for the key "ANY" - among the various CTRL, INS, DEL, ALT keys - to comply with the message "press 'any' key to continue".

As a sort of retaliation to the binary system being at the basis of the computer science, understanding only "0" or "1", "on" or "off", "true" or "false", it seems that the feeling of the common people towards "the computer" splits in only two definite and mutually uncommunicative groups: the one of "computer-addicts" - sharing with their instrument a feeling dangerously near to the romantic love - and the one of "computer-convicts" - curtailing their approaches to the intimately hated machine at the very minimum exacted by the circumstances.

Physicians in general and pediatric surgeons in particular can be as well roughly divided in these two groups. "Computer-addicts" will forejudge this chapter absolutely elementary if not definitely useless, while "computer-convicts" will expect something esoteric, dealing with topics fully unrelated to their daily job, and hence again definitely useless. In spite of that, what follows presumes to present an overview - basic but hopefully not too sketchy - of the extremely various ways in which a physician in general and a pediatric surgeon in particular can interact with a computer, offering to the "addicts" some remarks and tricks of interest, to the "convicts" some hints and incitement to brave the unappreciated but, all things considered, indispensable tool.

In order to explain as clearly as possible the subject this chapter will be divided in three main parts, dealing respectively with the computer used as "standalone" (i.e. as a single, isolated apparatus not connected with others), with the computer used as an element of the hospital information system (the so-called "Intranet") and eventually with the computer acting as a way to navigate the fascinating world of Internet. It must be emphasized again that this subdivision is aimed merely to schematize the matter and hasn't any substantiation in the general practice (the same computer can obviously be used as standalone and to access Internet). Every part will be subdivided in paragraphs with a question as a heading, just to emphasize the practical layout of this chapter trying to give some answers to the many questions that computer technology can raise. At the end of the chapter two appendices will help: (1) to wriggle out of the jungle of computer science technicalities and acronyms (terms described in this glossary are followed in the text by an asterisk); (2) to avoid some computer-related troubles.

STAND ALONE

What is a computer?

A computer is an electronic apparatus structurally similar to a TV set, a HiFi player, a mobile phone that simply has been designed to perform different tasks.

As all machines, it has no discretional capacity whatsoever: paradoxically, a computer is a rather "stupid" machine understanding only two statuses, "on" or "off", "passage" or "non passage" of electricity in a circuit. These statuses can be expressed also with the digits "1" (on) or "0" (off), that constitute the so-called "binary system", by which an infinite set of numbers can be written using only "bits" (Binary digITS, 0 and 1). Arranged in blocks of 8 bits, called "bytes", these numbers are used to draw sets of instructions enabling the computer to perform an enormous amount of activities. These instructions are listed in sequences (named "algorithms" from the name of the Arab mathematician Muhammad ibn Musa al Khuwarizmi, who lived in Baghdad in the first half of IX century), structured according to arithmetical and logical rules into different sets of instructions named programs, each one intended for a particular task. Thus, although apparently quite different from each other, activities of a computer can basically be traced back to computing and rearranging at a terrific speed. For example, simple numerical data used to express figures, letters, pictures, sounds, etc.

Tangible components of a computer system are defined the hardware, while intangible programs that let the hardware work are called the software.

From where computers evolved?

Modern computers are the evolution of a long series of computing machines, dating back from the Babylonian abacus of the X century BC through the "Pascaline" designed by B Pascal in 1642, the punched cards ideated in 1887 by H Hollerith and used in the 1897, USA, census operations, until the first electronic computer realized in 1946 by JW Mauchly and JP Eckert at the Moore School of Electrical Engineering of the University of Pennsylvania for the negligible sum of well over 5 millions US$ (!). The ENIAC (Electronic Numerical Integrator and Computor - sic!) was able to perform 100 operations per second through 20 registers of 10 digits, 18,000 thermionic valves, 70,000 resistors, 10,000 capacitors and 6,000 switches for a total RAM of 18 Kbytes. It was not exactly an handy tool: hosted in a 200 m^2 university gym needing an heavy air-conditioning for the huge amount of heat produced by the valves, 30 mt long and 2.5 mt wide, it weighed 35 tons and consumed 140 kW. Wiring of the ENIAC was so complex that it wasn't at all unusual to find a dead bug short-circuiting two valves thus causing whimsical effects: hence the word "debugging" used till now to mean search and correction of hidden mistakes and faults ("bugs"!) in computer programs.

Trying to foresee the future of computers, the journal "Popular Mechanics" in 1969 optimistically observed "While ENIAC has 18,000 valves and weighs 30 tons, future computers will have only 1,000 valve and will possibly weigh only one ton and half". Invention of transistor - instead of the huge thermionic valve - and of silicon technology for microcircuitry - instead of the many km of electrical wiring needed by the ENIAC - altered just a bit this prediction: the Pentium Pro processor hosts 5.5 millions of transistors in an area of 306 mm^2 (2×1.5 cm) with an external cache of 31 millions of bytes. To visualize the hectic pace kept by computers' evolution-schematically represented in Tables 129.1 and 129.2 — it has been observed that first computers were computing in milliseconds, modern ones in nanoseconds: ratio between the two time units is the same than the one between two years and a minute! If aeronautics had the same evolution, today a Boeing 737 would cost less than 500$ and could complete the round-the-world flight in 20 minutes consuming 20 litres of kerosene. All this well justifies the observation that, after agricultural and industrial revolution, computer science revolution is the third fundamental revolution of mankind civilization.

How many types of computers do exist?

There are many categories of computers, subdivided according to the computing power and the utilization. This distinction can sometimes be rather vague, but some reference categories can be indicated:

Supercomputer

It's an elaboration system planned to obtain extremely high calculation powers. Until the early 90's those computers were just built with more sophisticated hardware than common computers. Today, instead, most of them are based on hundreds of thousands of calculation units not much more powerful than a good personal computer working together. Due to the current speed of the technological development in computer science and microprocessors field, they

Table 129.1: Historical evolution of computers

Generation	Years	Models processors	Notes
0	1941-1944	Z3 (Destroyed in a air raid)	Built by Konrad Zuse, with recycled telephonics parts
1°	1945-1960	ENIAC, EDSAC, EDVAC (Electronic Discrete Variable Automatic Computer), UNIVAC	John Von Neumann
2°-Transistors	1959-1964	IBM 7030 "Stretch" (world's fastest computer until 1964)	Fortran language
3°-Integrated circuits	1964-1971	IBM 360	Clock 4 MHz
	1971-1977	Intel 8080, Cray 1 supercomputer	VLSI - first microprocessor
3°-PC	1977-1981	Apple II (1977), Xerox Star (1981) IBM-PC (1981), Intel 8086	DOS operating system
	1984	Apple Macintosh	Mac OS (birth of icons, and of "user-friendly" Operating systems)
	1985		Windows 1.0
	1991	Intel 386	Linux (first totally "open source" Operating system)
4°	1995	Pentium PRO	

Table 129.2: Computers' Performances in time

Year	Computer	Generation	Dimensions (m³)	Power consumption (watt)	Performances (sums/sec)	Memory (kbyte)	Price (1996 US$)	Price / UNIVAC performances
1951	UNIVAC	1°	28	124,500	1,900	48	4,996,749	1
1964	IBM 360/50	2°	1.68	10,000	500,000	64	4,140,257	318
1965	PDP-8	3°	0.23	500,000	330,000	4	66,071	13,135
1976	Cray-1	3°	1.62	60,000	166,000,000	32,768	8,459,712	51,604
1981	IBM-PC	3°PC	0.03	150	240,000	256	4,081	154,673
1991	HP900 mod. 750	3°	0.06	500	50,000,000	16,384	8,156	16,122,356
1995	Pentium Pro	4°	0.06	500	400,000,000	65,536	3,200	239,078,908

usually loose the "Super" prefix after few years from their birth.

Mainframe

Those are big computers used in government administrations, large companies, banks, wherever a centralized running of a huge data processing network system is needed. Mainframes are direct successors of the first large computers, and still maintain their basic structure with a central machine linked with several secondary terminals.

Workstation

Direct consequence of the minicomputer (an appliance midway from a PC and a Mainframe), it's considered like a more powerful version of a PC, engineered for a specific task and provided with purpose-built software. They are often present in research laboratories and in universities, used for heavy duty calculations or for advanced graphical purposes (virtual sets, multimedia editing, movie special effects, etc.).

Personal Computer (PC)

This term, once a trademark of IBM, denotes the computer we are used to have at home or in office, used for one of the many tasks mentioned afterwards. Put on the market in 1981, the PC was designed for the use in small companies or as a home gadget whose tasks were rather obscure ("recipes archive" was one of the suggested uses!). So minimal was IBM confidence in this new product that they didn't even bother to develop a dedicated operating system. It was in fact adopted a system already present on the market, the MS-DOS written by a small software house called MicroSoft, owned by a young man on his early twenties bound to become the richest man in the world, Bill Gates.

In the slowly developing market of the PC the MS-DOS established itself as the standard; computers working with this system were called "IBM compatibles", while all machines working with other operating systems were soon turned out the market. Only exception to this rule was represented by the Macintosh (or "Mac") produced by the Apple Computers since 1984 and still present on the market with the iMac and PowerMac. The Mac, although similar to the PC, is not usually defined as such, considering this term as synonymous with "IBM compatible". Most of the PC are "assembled" computers, i.e. computers realized assembling parts produced by different manufacturers, while the Macs, as well as the laptops, are only branded goods: for this reason the former are cheaper than the latter.

Among PC there is another classification related to the shape and dimensions of the computer:
- "Desktop" is defined a computer with horizontal box; originally all computers were as such, while now there are more diffused models with vertical box, the "Tower Computers", occupying less space on the desk or positioned on the floor. There are the sizes, minitower, miditower and fulltower (or Bigtower) according to the number of the appliances hosted inside.
- Portable computers (Laptop) are suitable for users needing to move around with their computer at hand; an internal battery with some hours of autonomy allows using the computer also during transfers. To maintain this autonomy it is advisable to let the battery go completely flat at least once a week. Laptops can be used also on the airplanes once the permission is obtained from the crew. In recent models, more and more lights and thins, are also known as "Notebooks".
- PDA (Personal Digital Assistant) once known as "Palmtops" or "Pocket PCs", are the evolution of the pocket electronic notebooks able to perform some basic computer functions such as Internet navigation, e-mailing, word processing in addition to the normal notebook functions (schedule, phonebook, reminder, calculator). Usually endowed with both keypad and touch screen, and small enough to stay in one hand, they implement most of the functions of a PC and all the functions of a cellular phone. It's easy to imagine why they are one of the most promising branch of modern informatics.

How does a computer work?

Basically, a computer is an instrument that receives data, process and stores them and as a result gives back the processed data. To do so it needs devices to introduce the data and to give them out, the so-called input/output devices (I/O); systems to memorize these data (disk drives, streamers, etc.) and finally a central core where these data are processed, usually contained in a desktop or tower case. All devices not pertaining to this central core are defined "peripherals".

Let's remove the cover of our desktop and have a look inside it (if you want really do that, remember beforehand to pull out the plug!). In a basic setting you will find on the back slots for add-on cards and a power supply with a transformer and its cooling fan, on the front the sliding holder for the CD/DVD and some USB ports, in the middle a large printed circuit board that houses all the circuitry, called the motherboard. The motherboard contains the CPU, the real "brain" of the computer that executes instructions of the various programs and supervises the functioning of all the system, as well as other chipsets, cache memory and BIOS. Directly attached to the motherboard or, more often, through separated expansion cards we will also find connections to the various I/O devices that allow the computer to interact with the outer world (pediatric surgeons among it!): display adapter card for the monitor, video acquisition cards for retrieving images from a recorder or a TV set, audio card for the recording or reproduction of sounds and music, SCSI cards to control devices needing particular speed in data transfer, etc.[1]

The Central Processing Unit (CPU)

The CPU is a microprocessor (Intel compatible for the Microsoft Windows system, Motorola compatible running MacOs operating system) whose internal activity is synchronized by an electric signal, called clock, made by extremely rapid impulses each one corresponding to one elementary operation. Speed of the clock is measured in MegaHertz (MHz) or, more recently, in GigaHertz (GHz): the higher the value of the clock the faster the computer. CPU speed doubles approximately every 12 to 18 months (Moore's law): the fastest CPU now available, with a clock of 3 GHz, is able to perform some 3 billions operations per second. A CPU is composed by: (a) a control unit; (b) an arithmetic/logic unit (ALU); (c) a work memory, divided in two parts, one smaller not transient and one bigger whose contents disappear when the computer is switched off. The first is called ROM (Read Only Memory) and contains the basic routines for the functioning of the computer. It runs the boot program at the switching on and controls at the lowest level all the components and peripherals of the computer. This part of the memory maintains its contents unchanged, when the computer is switched off and cannot be modified by the user to avoid unfortunate troubles. The remainder of the memory, called RAM (Random Access Memory) can on the contrary be read and written, and is the memory where are the data temporarily store under processing and the instructions of the program used for that particular process.

For example, to write a letter the CPU loads a program used for typing (word processor), receives the input from the keyboard, converts letters in numerical code (usually ASCII), arranges the report according to the instructions of the word processor and stores temporarily what results in the RAM. When the user launches the order to "save" his work, the letter is copied from the volatile memory of the RAM to the permanent memory of the hard disk or removable device such as a pen drive. Hence, the fact that, in the event of a blackout while working with a computer, the data contained in the RAM and not yet saved on a disk are lost. Why then not to give up the RAM and to work directly on a disk? Because writing/reading from the RAM is enormously quicker than writing/reading from a disk (some hundreds of thousands times quicker). RAM capacity is measured in MB; the last generation of operating systems (like Windows XP, old Linux, or Mac OS X 10.4 "Tiger" for Apple Macintosh) worked with RAMs of 128 to 512 MB. At now, most of the common PCs have 1 GB RAMs (512 MB at least are needed to run the base versions of the last OS, like Leopard, successor of Tiger, and Windows Vista), that, thanks to the dual channel technology, can easily be extended to 3-4 GB in about 20 minutes of do-it-yourself on the insides of your computer. If this capacity is not enough to contain all the needed data, the CPU runs an operation called "swap", by which part of the content of the RAM is temporarily copied on a disk and then retrieved when needed, thus freeing some space in the RAM. Obviously this time-consuming operation is more often required when the RAM is scanty, and then the bigger the RAM (within certain limits) the quicker the computer.

RAM dimension and CPU speed are precisely the two main parameters in defining a computer performance.

Mass Storage Devices

Mass storage devices can be divided in four main categories:

I. Magnetic Disks

Those are disks in which data are memorized magnetizing their surface by a writing/reading head. Data can be written and cancelled as many times as desired without wearing the support. Magnetic disks are nevertheless volatile: a huge magnetic field can destroy in few seconds the entire content, therefore they must be kept well away from possible sources of magnetic field (magnets, power supply transformers, electrocardiographs, etc.).

The hard disk (HD) is the permanent memory of the computer, where programs, data and documents are stored. HD are manufactured in two technologies, EIDE and SCSI: the latter are faster but a bit more expensive. The HD is the only major component with moving parts subject to failure: being the storage of an often invaluable amount of data and documents, is strongly advisable to back up all critical data in some other removable media to be kept in a safe place, away from excessive heat, humidity or magnetic fields. The best solution is to have a second hard disk, external to the PC, with independent electric input and to be connected via an USB port; available are also compact external hard disks, smaller than the standard external HD, not needing an independent power supply but powered directly through the USB port. Hard disks capacity is measured in GB: models now available have usually up to 250 GB (billions of bytes) of capacity for the internal disks, and up to the incredible capacity of one TeraByte (a thousand GB, or one thousand billions of bytes!) for the external ones.

II. Removable Memory Devices

Removable memory devices such as floppy disks, zip disks and LS-120 and Jaz disks, in wide use till few years ago, have been totally superseded by the USB flash drives.

They are flash memory data storage devices integrated with a USB connector, typically small, lightweight, removable and rewritable. (USB Memory card readers are also available, whereby rather than being built-in, the memory is a removable flash memory card housed in what is otherwise a regular USB flash drive). USB flash drives offer potential advantages over other portable storage devices, particularly the floppy disk. They are more compact, faster, hold more data, are more reliable due to their lack of moving parts, and have a more durable design. Additionally, it has become increasingly common for computers to ship without floppy disk drives. USB ports, on the other hand, appear on almost every current mainstream PC and laptop. With nothing being mechanically driven in a flash drive, the name is something of a misnomer. It is called a "drive" because it appears to the computer operating system (and the user) in a manner identical to a mechanical disk drive, and is accessed in the same way. An account on all technical details can be found at the site http://en.wikipedia.org/wiki/USB_flash_drive.

III. Optical Disks

These are disks in which memorization is done through a laser beam that "carves" the shiny surface, thus becoming dull. Usually they are of the WORM type (write once read many), although now are available disks (CD-RW) that can be re-written for a limited number of times (due to the low cost of the standard disk, their use is not advisable; moreover, they have been largely ousted by pen drives).

CD-ROM: They are exactly the same disks used for music recording, typically contain 650 MB (corresponding to 74' recording) and are very cheap. They can be read in dedicated drives, marked 20x, 32x, 52x: these numbers indicate the reading speed of the disk, being 1x the reading speed of the standard audio CD. Masterizers drives are used to write on an empty CD: writing on a CD is a delicate operation that cannot be interrupted for any reason, otherwise all the CD will be spoiled.

Mini CD are CD with reduced diameter (8 cm) and contain up to 180 MB or 21'. Are compatible with standard CD drives, except for the drives loading through a slot and not with a sliding holder.

DVD externally identical to a CD, can hold from 9 to 17 GB. In addition to be used to store digital movies, they can be used as well for storing large amounts of data; the only problem is that a definite standard does not exist yet. To be read a DVD requires an appropriate drive (normal CD drives cannot read a DVD, while a DVD drive can read a normal CD).

IV. Magneto-optical Disks (MOD)

Magneto-optical disks are magnetical disks that can be written only at high temperature with a laser beam, and cannot be erased by magnetic fields. They are scarcely diffused, being ousted by the CD-ROMs, and are used mostly for the storage of large amounts of data in safety conditions.

Input/Output (I/O) Devices

To interact with a computer the pediatric surgeon, as well as all other users, needs devices to input data and to retrieve results. I/O devices, listed in Table 129.3, are connected with the motherboard by special "sockets" called ports. Ports are divided in parallel (LPT) with 25 holes and "serial" (COM) ports with 9 holes; before connecting a new I/O device to a port the system must be switched off. Keyboard and mouse can be connected through special PS/2 ports or more often through an USB port, used also to accommodate digital cameras, printers, scanners, etc.; to plug / unplug a device into an USB port there is no need to switch the computer off.

- Keyboard is usually connected to a PS/2 special port. It can have 101 or 104 (Windows adapted) keys, divided in four groups:
  1. Function keys (F1, F2, etc.), placed in the upper row, their exact function depends from the

Table 129.3: Input output devices

Input only

	by human operator	by instruments
Keyboard	touch-screen	impulse counters (ECG, scintiscans)
Joystick	touch-pad	position encoders
Mouse	scanner	A/D converters
Trackball	voice input devices	Links (serial links Data Set and Data Terminal RS-232 IEEE-488 realising a LAN)
Light-pen	video input devices (webcam)	

Output only

Monitor	Printer
Plotter	Loudspeakers
Masterizer	

Input and Output

Removable memory devices	CD ROM/DVD drive
Modem	Net expansion card

program used in that moment. The F1 key in almost all programs is used as the "help" key, opening a file giving instructions on how to use the program itself. Its use is strongly advised when approaching a program little known.

2. *Alphanumeric keys* in addition to the standard keys (such as in a typewriter) there are the modifying keys CTRL ("Control") and ALT ("Alternate") that, together with the SHIFT key, are used to modify the function of other keys, according to the program used in that moment

3. *Number keypad* located on the right side of the keyboard, is a simple duplication of the numeric keys (on the second upper row), for user's convenience. To this purpose the "BLOC NUM" key, located on the left upper hand corner of the number keypad, must be pressed (warning light on).

4. *Cursor keys* between alphanumeric and number keypads are located the keys used to shift cursor and pages. In some keyboards cursor keys are included in the number keypad; to be used as such the "BLOC NUM" toggle key must be off (warning light off).

- Monitor is the main interface between user and computer. The most diffuse type is probably still the cathode-ray tube, the same as old television screen, but it's been slowly replaced, as it becomes more and more obsolete, by (Liquid Crystal Display (LCD). In a computer's monitor, images are composed by a grid of dots, each one called "pixel". The highest the number of pixels, the highest the sharpness of the screen images; today's LCD screens support resolutions from 800 × 600 to 1920 × 1080 pixels, and even further for special applications.

- Printers can be divided in three main categories:
  1. *Dot impact printers:* old type printers, totally outdated because slow, noisy and of poor quality results.
  2. *Laser printers: They share technology with photocopiers:* fit for high volume of prints because it is quick and noiseless, and with results of the highest quality. More expensive than dot impact printers, particularly if color printers.
  3. *Inkjet printers:* Slower but cheaper and smaller than laser printers, they work spraying an extremely thin jet of ink on the paper, giving a print of good quality although slightly less than laser printers. The best solution when colour print is requested.

Plotters are a particular type of printers using ink nibs to draw on wide size sheets.

- For what purposes a computer can be used?

It is quite difficult to enumerate the ways in which a computer, also if used just as a standalone, can be useful for a pediatric surgeon. Very schematically we can identify some basic activities:

a. Text processing (word processor)
b. Images processing and CAD
c. Calculations (spread sheet)
d. Data recording and retrieving (database)

Each one of these tasks needs a dedicated program: it is well outside the scope of this chapter to elaborate how to use each one of them, and therefore we will give only some elementary advice. The first one is condensed in a famous acronym, reading RTM (Read the Manual), or in a more gross version, RTFM (we leave to the reader's fertile imagination realizing what the F stands for!). In other terms, before loosing time and hopes trying to get out from a program seemingly mocking you, have a look at the manual. Almost all programs are provided with an on-line help, which typically can be opened by pressing the F1 key; some sophisticated on-line help programs allow to directly formulate a question, while others are more schematic. For people starting from scratch it is advisable to read beforehand some written instructions: far better are the simple booklets explaining just the basics, available in all specialized bookshops, rather than the ponderous tomes sometimes enclosed in the program package.

Basic programs are now often sold in comprehensive packages including a word processor, a spreadsheet, a database, etc. Characteristic of these packages is that fundamental instructions, as well as the graphic presentation of the commands, are the same in various applications so as to simplify their learning and use. For example, in all MS-Office environment applications, pressing simultaneously the keys "Ctrl" and "C" (Ctrl+C) after selection of a text or an image copies it in the computer memory, Ctrl+X cuts the selected items (deletes and copies in the memory; this item remains in the memory until a new item is overwritten or the computer is switched off), Ctrl+V retrieves what has been copied and paste it somewhere else (also in a different file), Ctrl+Z undoes the last action made, etc.

Text Processing

Special programs, called word processors (such as MS Word), convert the computer in a very sophisticated typewriter, able to page up, to correct wording, to change font, to store for further use, etc. every kind of writing, from the scientific paper to the discharge report of a patient. Standard forms for informed consent, clinical and operative reports, instructions for parents can thus be compiled and stored, and then retrieved, modified and printed as required by the particular case.

Using a word processor some very simple tricks must be kept in mind: the text must be written continuously, without pressing the return key at the end of every line but only at the end of the paragraph; the setup of the text (font, dimensions of letters, italics, etc) must not be adapted manually line by line, but rather once for all resorting to the "styles" already present as default in the program or personally adapted (e.g. "title", "normal text", "caption", "table", etc.). Every paragraph can then be linked to one of these different "styles", according to need; every modification in the "style" will modify automatically the entire file.

Images Processing and CAD

The market offers plenty of programs for images processing, to be used for various tasks. Most useful for pediatric surgeons are programs: (1) to frame and store clinical images, taken directly in the theater or in the ward by a digital camera or a standard camera, to be then digitized with a scanner (e.g. Photoshop); (2) to prepare presentations for a congress or a lecture, either in slides or directly through a LCD beamer (e.g. Power Point). For pediatric surgeons involved in teaching and lecturing, it is highly advisable to build up a virtual library of such images, framed and stored in appropriate indexed files, to be retrieved for inclusion in presentations easily changed and adapted according to the needs. While preparing presentations, it is recommendable to avoid busy slides with crowded tables, long texts, showy colors (eventually illegible); ideal is considered a text no longer than six lines of seven words each per slide.

A particular field of image processing is represented by the computer-aided design (CAD), a software realized for professional design and planning, as well as for virtual reality applications. Through this technology, computers are able to reproduce objects and situation with astonishing three-dimensional realism. In pediatric surgery, CAD has been used to develop a virtual model of an infant's body wall, stomach, and hypertrophied pylorus as well as laparoscopic cannulas and two experimental sets of retractable hook for laparoscopic treatment of hypertrophic pyloric stenosis.[2] Tridimensional visualization and computer-assisted operational planning based on CT data are being increasingly used for difficult operations in adults, and an initial experience with 3D-visualized MRI with volume rendering in planning pediatric abdominal surgery has been described,[3] as well as a computer-assisted navigation system in pediatric intranasal surgery, realized utilizing a wireless passive marker system that allows the calibration and tracking of virtually any instrument, adapted to children and used during pediatric endoscopic sinusonasal surgery.[4]

Calculations

"Computers" draw their name from making calculations, or computing; that actually was their first task, and the conquest of the moon would have been impossible without computers. It is rather unlikely that pediatric surgeons will need to undertake this kind of calculations, but a "spreadsheet" will turn out to be rather useful to them in many ways. With this term is defined a program (e.g. MS Excel) presenting an array of squares, called "cells", arranged in rows and columns identified respectively by a number and a letter, exactly as in the warships game. Cells can be linked each other by a mathematical, logical or statistical formula, and a number input in a cell will automatically change the content of all linked cells. For example, a spreadsheet can be programmed so as the input of weight and height of a patient will give as output body surface, caloric needs, quantity of intravenous drips and drugs' dosages. This latter task is particularly helpful in the running of complex multidrugs protocols, such as in pediatric oncology. Moreover, spreadsheets are indispensable in the everyday administrative management of a clinical ward, particularly if the DRG system is adopted (DRG encoding is elaborated by a specific software called *grouper*). As an added benefit, most spreadsheet programs include also utilities for standard statistical data elaboration; if a more elaborated statistical analysis is required, the market offers plenty of sophisticated software such as the one in use in our Center, MedCalc (www.medcalc.be).

Data Recording and Retrieving

French term for "computer" is "ordinateur", i.e. "orderer", "sorter", thus emphasizing one of the earlier tasks given to computers, to store huge amount of data and to sort them according to a particular order (alphabetical, chronological, etc.) with special programs named "databases" (e.g. MS Access). These data are grouped in logical sets, named "files", each one divided in single entities named "records", each one in turn subdivided in different parts named "fields". For example, patients' archive of a hospital can be divided in one "file" per department, each single patient's data collected in a "record" containing various "fields" (name, date of birth, diagnosis, etc.). Former paper archives were formed by file-cards ("records") arranged according only to a single field, and to have the same amount of data arranged in two different ways implied to double literally each file-card. A typical example was that of libraries, needing an author catalogue and a subject catalogue, arranged in two different cardholders, the more awkward to use the many file-cards were contained. On the contrary, a computer database can record an almost unlimited number of data, which can be quickly retrieved according to each one of the fields by which records are composed. On this subject, it is advisable not to exceed in the number of fields per record (say, 50 to 100 maximum), not to slow the data processing. If a higher amount of fields per record is required, it is better to create two different files with two parallel sets of records linked by a shared field. For example, if I need to record 300 different parameters for each patient included in a trial (rather complex a trial, I must admit!), it is better to split these parameters in two or three subgroups and to store the data in two or three different files, with the name of the patient acting as a shared field in all three sets of records. A database allows unsophisticated numerical elaboration of the contained data; for more complex calculations it is possible to export the relevant fields of a database into a spreadsheet, having higher calculus power and flexibility.

Databases are meant to store and retrieve data put in manually (patients' records, scientific experiment results, addresses of colleagues, etc.). Moreover, the computer allows retrieving data already gathered and digitized in form of electronic encyclopedias, medical treatises, MedLine collection of medical abstracts, anatomical atlases, interactive dictionaries, etc. Typically these data are multimedial, i.e. composed not only by text but also by pictures, videos, sounds, and are contained in a CD-ROM whose sophisticated internal architecture allows condensing in a single disk the equivalent of up to one or two dozens of volumes. The most attractive feature presented by this system of data retrieving is the possibility to carry along in a compact DVD case the equivalent of a small library, at hand - with a laptop available - almost everywhere.

On top of these basic, general activities computers can intervene in so many other medical fields to foster the creation of a scientific society devoted to this very issue, the International Society for Computer Aided Surgery (http://www.iscas.net/), with the mission to encourage scientific and clinical advancement of computer-aided surgery and related medical interventions throughout the world. According to the statutes, the scope of Computer Aided Surgery encompasses all fields within surgery, as well as biomedical imaging and instrumentation, and digital technology employed as an adjunct to imaging in diagnosis, therapeutics, and surgery. A quick survey of some of the papers published on the last available issue [13 (2), 2008] of the society's journal, Computer aided surgery, published six times a year in simultaneous print and online edition, can offer a rough idea of the front-line researches on this field: "Providing metrics and performance feedback in a surgical simulator", "Virtual reality-enhanced ultrasound guidance: A novel technique for intracardiac interventions", "Surgery with cooperative robots", "Multimodal virtual bronchoscopy using PET/CT images", "Electromagnetic navigation improves minimally invasive robot-assisted lung brachytherapy", and so on. Quite a long way from the "recipes archive" before mentioned.

INTRANET

The term of "Intranet", clearly derived from the one of "Internet", describes the informatics technology system of a definite and restricted area, such as for example a factory or an office block. In medical field it defines the connecting system of all the components of the so-called Hospital Information System (HIS) (Fig. 129.1).

Conventional organization of medical services currently relies on paper documents as a storage medium of clinical data and on physical transport of the information (sheets of paper) as a communication system. In this traditional framework, the patient acts as "deliveryman of himself", first moving himself as a source of medical information (for example, going to the radiologist for a chest X-ray) and then moving the medical information he generated (bringing back the radiograph to the ward). Obviously this system

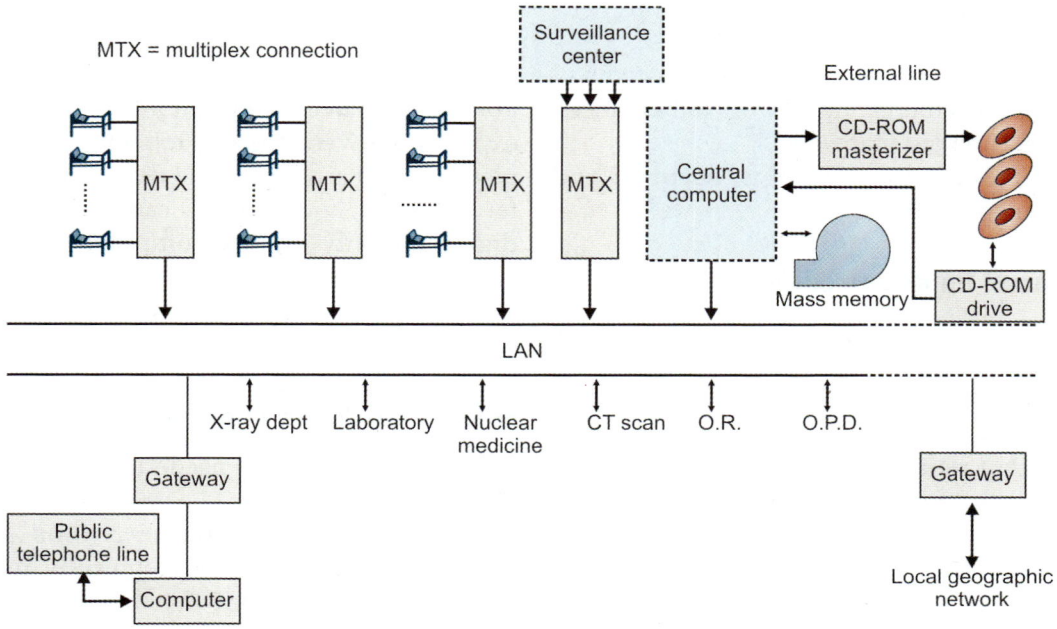

Fig. 129.1: Schematic representation of a hospital information system (HIS)

implies delays, nuisances for the patient, difficulties in data storage and retrieval: all troubles that pediatric surgeons working in a hospital know well.

HIS aims to realize a computerized system in which information are as digitally formalized as possible and therefore amenable to be treated with computer technology. In detail: (a) a computerized clinical management system (biomedical data input, case sheets); (b) a patient accommodation management system and a hospital administrative system; (c) an integration of all hospital services (biomedical, administrative, accommodation) through dedicated hardware and software linking all hospital departments.

What can a Medical Intranet be used for?

A fully operational HIS is expected to perform a good array of different tasks, such as:
1. Computer-based patient records.
2. Optimal utilization of all hospital structures.
3. Transmission of biomedical data in real time.
4. Better assistance and monitoring of the patient.
5. Home assistance via telemedicine apparatuses.
6. Computerized database of general archives of the hospital data.
7. Computerized lecture halls for training of medical and paramedical personnel.
8. External gateways for connection to Internet - Medline.
9. Computer-assisted diagnosis/Expert systems.
10. Management of emergency network (ambulances, helicopters, first aid teams, etc.).
11. Building Automation Systems, security and power management systems.

Computer-based Patient Records

Medical computing allows realizing an electronic case sheet (including history, surgical report, daily report, lab results, digitalized X-rays, etc.). The system can also aid clinicians in the areas of billing, documentation, reporting, and data retrieval. Value-added features like decision support and event monitoring facilitate patient outcome, decrease health care costs and allow improved administration. Problems in security and confidentiality of clinical data introduced in the system must be always carefully considered.[5] Time-saving for redaction of a computerized discharge letter and a surgical report was quantified respectively from 66 and 37 to 24 and 14 minutes ($p < 0.0001$).[6] Computer technology includes bar code-based electronic positive patient and specimen identification systems, utilized to reduce identification errors in the daily management of laboratory specimens. A 3-year study conducted in a pediatric oncology hospital showed a significant reduction in the median percentage of mislabeled specimens, with a decline from 0.03% to 0.005% ($P < 0.001$).[7]

Computer-assisted Diagnosis/Expert Systems

Ability of computers to deal easily with huge amounts of data has fostered the development of plenty of programs intended to enhance the diagnostic capabilities of many electromedical tools, urodynamics, rectal or anal manometry among many others.[8-10] These programs are usually part of a HIS, but can run also on a standalone computer. Also the sophisticated image-processing possibilities offered by computers has been extensively utilized in various pediatric surgical fields, such as computer-assisted analysis of lung area in infants with CDH, advanced-stage neuroblastomas, tumor volume determination, hepatic hilar bile ducts in biliary atresia, ischemic injury to the gut, etc.[11-15]

Expert systems, intended as a computer program able to suggest directly a diagnosis once acquired a sizeable amount of patient's clinical data, have been extensively studied and implemented in the last years but recently have fallen a bit into disuse. This because expectations were possibly too optimistic: variables to be taken into account while diagnosing a disease are far too many, and only few can be fully expressed in digits, the only input a computer can understand. Nevertheless, research in this field is still in progress, although no experiences are recorded in pediatric surgery.[16]

What is needed to implement an intranet?

Hardware components needed to realize practically a HIS are:
1. *Communication infrastructure or Local Area Network (LAN)*: A LAN can be technically realized with wired transmission (twisted pair or coaxial cable), fiberoptic cable or radio link (mobile phones). The more reliable medium for a LAN is considered to

be fiberoptic linkage, allowing a transmission speed up to 20 MB per second.
2. *Data I/O terminals acting as sources/destinations of information.* Radiology dept. with scanners or digital radiological equipment, laboratory instruments with digital output of results, admissions office, theater, nuclear medicine dept. etc.
3. *Patient monitoring devices:* ECG, oxymeter, thermocouple for temperature check, etc.
4. *Data Management Center:* running and maintenance of the HIS, data storing and management.
5. *External gateway:* Connection with the external network → Intranet - Internet linkage.

INTERNET

In the 1960's, the coldest years of the cold war, a nightmare facing military intelligence was a complete breakdown of a centralized communication network in the aftermath of a nuclear holocaust. The notion of creating several nodes of super computers that convey each other through standard telephone lines was thus developed and realized in the USA: ARPANet, the Advanced Research Project Agency Network (1969). It was a distributed network, without a centralized and vulnerable branch point but with all nodes equally able to put through all information sending the data in small packages that would meet at the other end of the line, in order to stand a nuclear attack and to be able to run on also after the destruction of part of the system. This technical solution was so brilliant, particularly for its modular structure allowing a simple and quick development of the system, that soon after many other networks were established, essentially for military and research purposes.

In the 1980's the networking was already so extended that ARPANet architects realized the need of using a uniform protocol of communication and regrouping data packages, to allow the different networks to "understand" each other and to guarantee the interchangeability of communication: it was thus created the Transmission Control Protocol / Internet Protocol (TCP/IP). This protocol immediately became the international standard for all networks in the meanwhile developing in many countries, thus allowing the development of a worldwide network using the same modular architecture and the same "language", named precisely Internet. Its potentiality in terms of real-time transmission, extent of audience, unrestrainable contents was dramatically tested in 1991 during the attempted coup d'état in the former USSR. With Gorbachev under arrest and the KGB having censored the press and cut off all radio and phone communication lines with the rest of the world, the RelCom, a small factory in Moscow connected via e-mail to the Internet - and therefore to hundred of thousands people, at that time, turned out to be the only link with the outer world. A handful of people, sending in Internet hourly messages disclosing what was going on, was able to defeat the powerful KGB which paradoxically had its headquarters few hundred meters away from a networked computer, a unknown weapon destined soon to change the world.

In the same years (1989-1991) at the CERN laboratories in Geneva, Switzerland, Tim Berners-Lee and coworkers were developing the World Wide Web (www), the ultimate and most versatile resource of the Internet, used to publish information that can reach and be accessed in almost every corner of the planet, organized in sets of one to hundreds of pages each, called sites. In 1993, there were 130 sites available, in 1994 some 3,000, in 1998 10,910,997; in 2002 the total number of webpages available in Internet sites, well over 6 billions, exceeded the number of people on the whole Earth! Total number of Internet users grew in parallel, now reaching more than a billion people scattered from Afghanistan to Zimbabwe (first and last world country in alphabetical order), as detailed in Table 129.4.[17]

Today, Internet is so deeply intermingled with everyday life's events that we can assume it as a reliable gauge of their overall impact. A dramatic example of that is shown in Fig. 129.2, plotting internet performance the 11th of September 2001. Few minutes after 9:00 a.m., New York time, a sudden drop in Internet reachability was recorded, due to the enormous amount of people crowding the Net trying to find there in real time a clue on what was going on. The first stroke sensibly decreased Internet performance, but within one hour the shock was deaden and the Net was running again smoothly: a further brilliant proof, if yet needed, of Internet's intrinsic strength.

Table 129.4: Some data about Internet diffusion (June 2007 est.)						
Country	Internet users 2002 (x 1000)	Internet users 2007 (x 1000)	x-fold increase 2002 / 07	total population (x mln)	% internet users on the country population	Internet hosts
Afghanistan	3	535	178.3	31.88	1.68%	27
India	5,000	60,000	12.0	1129.86	5.31%	2,306,000
Italy	19,250	28,855	1.5	58.14	49.63%	4,117,000
USA	166,000	208,000	1.3	301.15	69.07%	3,950,000
Zimbabwe	30	1,220	40.7	12.31	9.91%	15,500
World	513,000	1,018,057	2.0	6602.22	15.42%	188,729,200

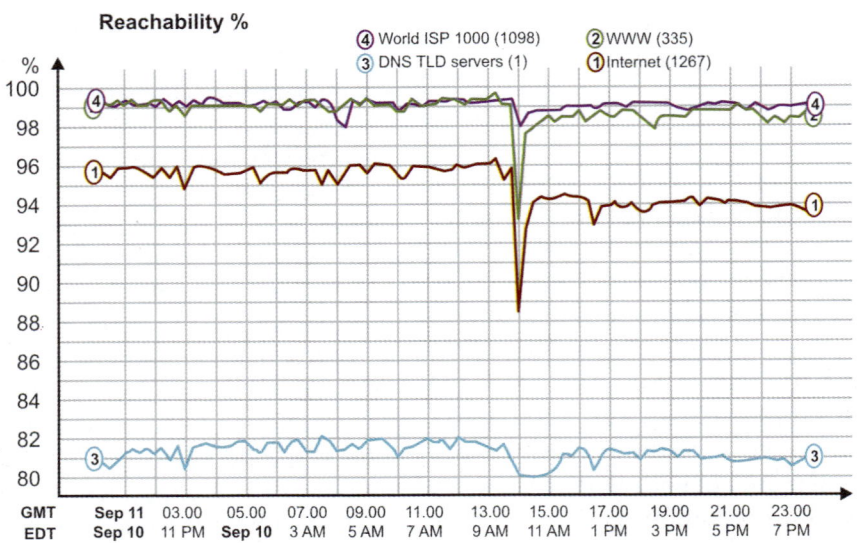

Fig. 129.2: Internet reachability the 11th September, 2001

But Internet presents also a dark side: web involvement in our lives is so deep to induce even behavioral changes, particularly among children and adolescents that, according to a recent Italian study, spend on the Net an average of 22 hours/month for children, with a jump to 87 hours/month for adolescents.[18] A new psychopathology has been described, the Internet Addiction Disorder, particularly affecting nightly users of the Net, diminishing patients' individual quality of life and disabling their time control.[19] Mental impact can be so devastating to induce the so-called "Net suicide": suicide pacts that are prearranged between strangers who meet over the Internet. Japan has one of the highest "Net suicide" rates in the world, particularly among adolescents: as many as 60 people a year have died of this method and the numbers continue to rise.[20]

What do I need to get connected with internet?

To gain access to Internet you will need a telephone line or a wireless connection, hardware, software, and a service provider.[21]

Telephone line should be an ISDN or DSL dedicated line allowing a faster communication with the service provider and the use of the telephone while connected to the internet (ISDN) or a 24 over 24 hours link with the provider without interfering with the telephone (DSL). Usual telephone lines on twisted pair are painstakingly slow in connection.

Wireless connection: A wireless LAN or WLAN is a wireless local area network, which is the linking of two or more computers - one of which is the server of the service provider - without using wires. WLAN utilizes spread-spectrum or OFDM modulation technology based on radio waves to enable communication between devices in a limited area, also known as the basic service set. This gives users the mobility to move around within a broad coverage area and still be connected to the network. For the home user, wireless has become popular due to ease of installation, and location freedom with the gaining popularity of laptops. Public businesses such as coffee shops or malls have begun to offer wireless access to their customers; some are even provided as a free service. Large wireless network projects are being put up in many major cities.

Hardware is exactly the computer described before under "standalone", simply supplemented with a modem providing the telephone line communication or with an expansion card connecting the computer to a LAN, or else with an internal antenna to link to the WLAN. Modems can be external (hosted in a box to be connected to the computer through a port) or internal, located on a slot into the computer box; the former is easier to check and to maintain, the latter less cumbersome. There are four modem types in commerce nowadays: (1) *Analogic modems* have a working speed from 14 to 56 KB per second - Kbps -; obviously, the cheaper the modem the slower the transmission. It should be however noted that, before buying an expensive, fast modem, the maximum workload of the telephone line must be checked (it's useless to have a 56 Kbps modem and a line allowing only 14 Kbps). Connection to the telephone line through the modem is controlled by dedicated software included in the standard package of an OS. (2) *ISDN modems* can reach 128 Kbps, reduced to 64 Kbps when the telephone line is used simultaneously. (3) *DSL modems* can run from 640 KBPS to 100 MBPS, and are the most common way of access to the net, together with wireless. (4) *GPRS/EDGE/UMTS/HSDPA modems* are usually integrated on last generation cellular phones.

Software needed to navigate the web is known as web browser. Web browsers are in essence a navigational aid for moving around and between the various nodes and links of the WWW; actual Internet trend is to concentrate all current utilities in a single program. Some web browsers are non-graphic like Lynx, and graphical like: Mosaic, Mozilla and MS Internet Explorer, with these latter being the leading companies.

Internet service providers (ISP) are either private or universities based. The service provider will give access to the Net using a local or toll-free telephone number. Some may include web space with the monthly rate offer, while a university-based ISP usually provides service for a nominal or none rate. To select a provider it's a must to consider various factors: (1) Does it directly own a server? (2) Which bandwidth has it? The higher the bandwidth, the faster the access to the web; (3) Does it offer a technical service "on line" 24 over 24 hours 365 days a year? (4) How many users per modem does the provider have?

Once chosen the ISP, it will provide detailed instructions for the connection, usually on a CD-ROM containing also the web browser to be installed on the computer. The computer is thus ready to connect with Internet.

What can an Internet be used for?

Basically, tools offered by Internet to the pediatric surgeon are:[22,23]
1. E-mail
2. Discussion lists
3. File transfer/ USENET/TELNET
4. WWW
5. Long-distance education
6. Telemedicine.

E-mail

This abbreviation stands for electronic mailing: this possibly is the most useful resource offered by Internet, allowing sending mail (composed by text, images, videoclips, etc) through the net in an extremely convenient and fast way. It takes on average 2 to 8 minutes for messages to reach another computer node at the antipodes for the cost of a local phone call. With e-mail is possible to consult colleagues on a clinical problem, send a draft of paper for peer revision, take part to long-distance CME programs, participate to discussion lists, etc.[24]

An e-mail address is composed by the username (one single or more words separated by dots), the ampersand @ (the typical symbol marking e-mail addresses, introduced first in 1972 by Ray Tomlinson), the ISP and the domain name separated by one or more dots. For example, e-mail addresses of the author are gbparigi@unipv.it or gbparigi@smatteo.pv.it for office use and gbparigi@hotmail.com for private use. In these, "gbparigi" is the username, followed by the @ characterizing the e-mail, the ISP name, indicating respectively the University of Pavia (unipv), the "S Matteo Hospital" of Pavia (smatteo.pv), a commercial ISP (hotmail), and finally the domain name separated by a dot (.it for Italy or .com for commercial). While choosing a username it is advisable to pick up something easy to spell and to remember (think about a friend asking your address through a mobile phone in a noisy road !).

E-mailing will soon become an essential tool in medical research, teaching medical students, clinical practice, postgraduate studies, although the lack of a traditional peer-review process and author identification might prevent e-mail text from being taken as authoritative.[25] Another problem raised by e-mail communication in the medical environment is related to important questions of legal, ethical, and professional propriety. This new technology is not free from potential associated hazards, and policies and practices that mitigate its weaknesses must be sought for.[26]

Discussion Lists

A discussion list is a list of e-mail addresses of people sharing the same interest and wishing to keep in touch via Internet (members of a society, alumni of a college, chocolate lovers, Star Trek Theologians -not joking! etc). Curiously, the first discussion list developed among scientists was called the Science-Fiction list.[27] Messages posted by authors to the list or discussion group are automatically mailed to all subscribers.

Free software is available to adhere or to build up a new list: Listserv, Majordomo, Yahoogroups, with this latter being the most diffuse with some 2,652,614 groups already created as per March 2008 (www.groups.yahoo.com). Environmental motivations have created an informal code of conduct known as "netiquette" (net-etiquette), dealing with politeness in replying along with accessibility, identification of the author and social responsibility (a full list of netiquette rules can be found at http://www.dtcc.edu/cs/rfc1855.html). Problems to avoid once joined a discussion list are: not signing, replying to the whole group when answering privately to one person, including the entire text of the received message when replying.

List servers for different surgery and pediatric sub-specialties exist: NICU-Net, PICU-Net, cardiology, gastroenterology, neurology, emergency medicine, critical care, pediatric pain, etc.[28] A popular list among Pediatric Surgeons worldwide is the Paediatric Surgery List, developed in July 1995 by Tom Whalen, Chief of Pediatric Surgery at Robert Wood Johnson Medical School in New Jersey. Scopes of the list are discussion of difficult clinical cases, technical tricks and options, exchange of ideas, consensus on management, career opportunities, referral of patients to other parts of the world, meetings and all possible topics dealing with the development of our specialty. The list is intended for pediatric surgeons and interested general surgeons and residents; technical problems imposed to close the original list of 1057 members, exchanging in 7 years 15285 "clinical" messages, in a new one - Pedsurg 2006 - for the moment joining 324 pediatric surgeons throughout the world.[23] The list can be freely joined by sending a message to Pedsurg 2006-subscribe @yahoogroups.com. While posting messages to the list it is paramount to remember: (1) not to betray privacy; (2) to be extremely wary in identifying patients; (3) to back comments with published citations; (4) not to waste the carrying capacity of the Net (bandwidth) with heavy attachments such as pictures; (5) not to post unsolicited advertising (spamming); (6) to identify clearly the author. The inclusion of e-mail and address at the end of a message represent a legal signature for all aspects of the law.[29] Disclaimers notice stating the medico-legal responsibility behind frequent response to complex medical problems are being asked for to list server administrators.[30]

File Transfer/USENET/TELNET

File transfer provides the unique opportunity of retrieving archives from public file libraries, with free software also available (FTP). Downloading of data into the hard disk of the computer is very straightforward.

USENET is a news discussions system distributed among hosts worldwide. News articles are grouped into newsgroups, which cover almost any topic one can imagine.

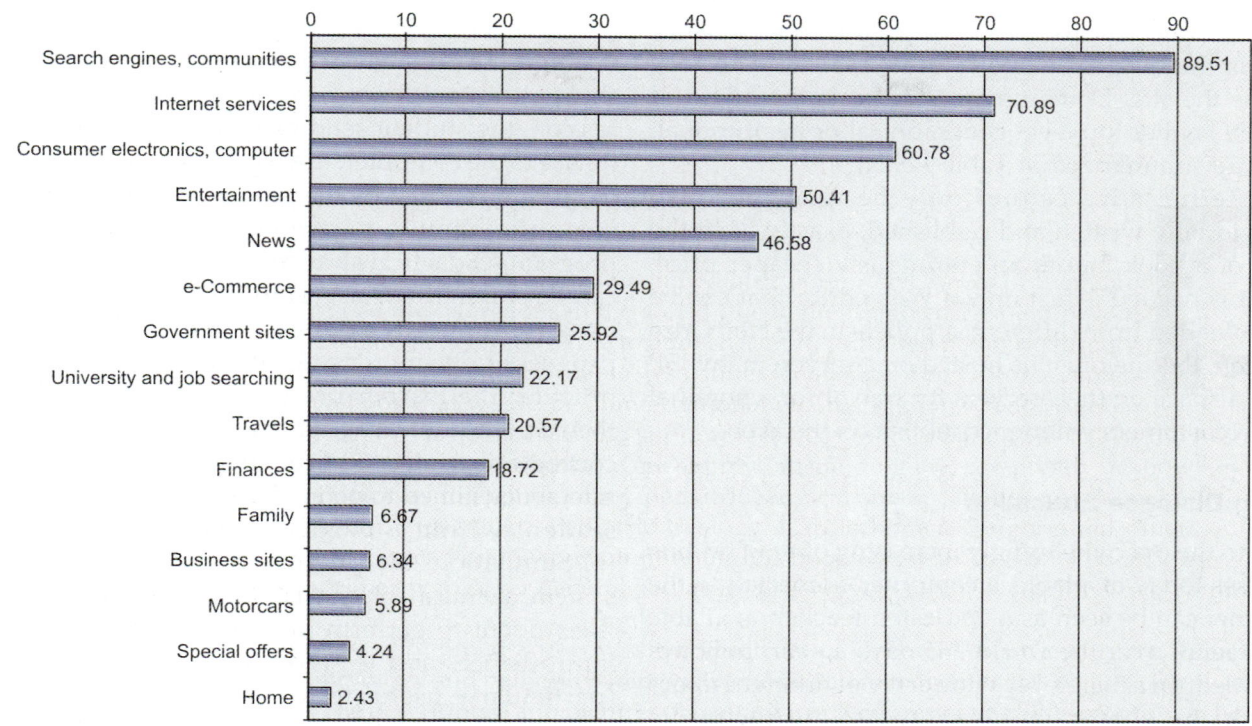

Fig. 129.3: Internet sites categories most visited in Italy - Percentage on the total of Internet navigators (28.8 mln) in Italy - December 2007 Ac-Nielsen/Net ratings

TELNET is a term referring to both the protocol and the terminal emulator that allows the user to connect across the Internet and to log onto another computer as if he was connected directly.

WWW

The www — known also as "The Web" - can be seen as an enormous and continuously expanding library, composed not by books but by "sites". As a book, a site is composed by pages (webpages), written in a particular language (HTML - its successor has already been proposed, the XML), consisting of all one medium, such as text, or including multiple media such as graphics, sounds, animation, and video. As a book, every site is identified by a "title", known as uniform resource locator (URL), that actually is a unique numerical address, composed by four blocks of up to 3 digits each, divided by a dot. Contrary to a book, the Web is fully interactive, allowing the user to buy a good while visiting a commercial site or to try one's fortune while entering a virtual casino. Just to give a very rough idea of the fields of interest of Web users, Fig. 129.3 shows the Internet sites categories most visited in Italy in 2007 expressed in percentage on the total of Internet navigators.

The most attractive feature of the Web is the possibility to jump from one page to another one (to "navigate" or "surf the Web"), in the same site or in another one, through links to other URL. Links are identified by a text underlined or in a different color, where the cursor of the pointer device changes (usually assuming the shape of a pointing hand) as though sensing an executable movement. By either clicking the device or hitting the return key, Internet "navigator" will be moving to that link, addressing in few seconds to a site that can physically be hosted in a computer located in the most remote spot in the world but nevertheless connected to the Net.

URL essential ingredients are protocol, site name, domain and directory, divided by slash or dots. For example, the address of the Medline service named "Entrez" at the National Library of Medicine of the National Institutes of Health is: http://www.ncbi.nlm.nih.gov/PubMed/.http:// is the protocol name; ncbi.nlm.nih the name of the site, in this case composed by the different acronyms of the involved organisms; gov is the domain name; /PubMed/ the directory inside the site. Domain names indicate the origin of the site, either top level geographical or institutional, and are summarized in Table 129.5.

Internet sites cannot only be read, but also individually written and published, exactly as in the case of a book, but at an enormously cheaper price. What is needed is just only a Web editor that can be downloaded from different suppliers in the Net. Once written, the site must be hosted on a server; many ISP allot a space on their servers for free or for a nominal fee to customers willing to publish on the Web.

Long Distance Education

Due to the overwhelmingly increasing offer of on-line courses today available, a computer connected to the Internet can be seen as a dedicated teacher, available for free all over the world 365 days a year, holidays included, on a incredibly wide array of different topics taught by some among the most authoritative academics available. This is the so-called Computer Assisted Instruction (CAI), otherwise described as Computer Assisted (Based) Learning (CAL/CBL) or Computer Based Education / Training (CBE/CBT).

These terms define a teaching system in which the user has the possibility to learn in an interactive way through a computer program. In a CAI teaching session, the student send messages through an input device to the computer: these messages can be answers to questions posed by the program, or requests to the computer about a particular topic covered by the program. Didactical strategies envisaged for the CAI can be summarized as: (1) tutorial: teaching goes on as a simulated dialogue, with questions of progressively increasing difficulty; (2) Drill and practice: the teacher presents a traditional lecture, then a computer program trains the student on the concepts presented; (3) Evaluation: student/computer interaction aimed to define areas of competence of the student within a particular field of knowledge; (4) Simulation: the program simulates a particular system, chemical, physical or biological, thus allowing the student to perform procedures through various input devices and to study the results of his action (particularly useful in teaching videolaparoscopic techniques); (5) Problem solving: aimed to teach the procedure to analyze and solve a particular problem (e.g. a clinical case), deepening student's knowledge by applying rules progressively more sophisticated for the solution of the simulated problem.

Among the tools offered by long distance education deserves a mention the largest encyclopedia now available on Internet, Wikipedia, that in its English version describes today some 2,279,919 articles (http://en.wikipedia.org/wiki/Main_Page); noticeable also the offer of 1800 on-line free courses given by the Massachusetts Institute of Technology (http://ocw.mit.edu), from "Aeronautics and Astronautics" to "Writing and Humanistic studies", or the one by Yale University (http://open.yale.edu) offering free and open access to seven introductory courses taught by distinguished teachers and scholars.

In a more specific medical field, it is possible to follow CME accredited long-distance teaching programs, sometimes offered for free such as Medscape (http://www.medscape.com), challenges subscribers with complex clinical cases to be solved.

This possibility of building a purpose-specific Internet site, with all its interactive features, offers to pediatricians and to pediatric surgeons a still largely unexplored field of creativity, such as the Internet-based interactive asthma educational and monitoring

Table 129.5: Domain names

gov	government	only agencies of the USA Federal government
com	commercial	used for commercial entities, particularly if present in more than one country
edu	educational	limited to US educational institutions (4 years colleges and universities)
mil	military	Self explaining
net	network resources	holding the computers of network providers, network node computers
org	organizations	miscellaneous for organizations not fitting anywhere else, such as non government organizations
int	international	for organizations established by international treaties or international databases
eu	europe	European Union official sites and organizations
.af	Afghanistan.... ..through....	National domains, always composed by two letters and derived from the international Country code (.in for India)
.zw	..Zimbabwe	

program, used in Taiwan in the management of asthmatic children, or the Internet-based protocol developed at Stanford to facilitate a multicenter trial for the surgical treatment of necrotizing enterocolitis.[31-32]

Telemedicine

The possibility of sending through Internet all clinical data that can be digitized (X-rays, CT, MRI, PET, scintiscans, echocardiograms, intraoperative photographs, histologic images, etc.), as well as real time video and audio technology (clinical rounds, lectures, videolaparoscopic procedures, etc.) has ushered the development of the so called Telemedicine.[33,34] This technologic tool allows to consult in real time specific experts in the subspecialties of childcare, even if in the other corner of the world; to train and guide surgical trainees by experts without their physical presence; to link hospitals and research centers in virtual multi-campuses; to link rural health clinics and central hospital, or physician to hospital for transfer of patient information; to distribute programs for public education on health care issues; to resort on video and satellite relay to train health care professionals in widely distributed or remote clinical settings, etc. Added benefits are improved access to areas in needs of health service, reduced cost of travelling, reduced professional isolation, improved quality of the care given. Development of the infrastructure needed along with cost containment issues are two of the problems faced by this technological advance; nevertheless, telemedicine is bound to become soon an integral part of the health care of children and the training of pediatric surgeons.[35]

How to find an e-mail address on the Internet?

The easiest way to get an email address is simply to get someone to mail you first and to record his address on your list: but this is not always possible, and then some of these tricks can help.
1. *Consult a paper directory:* Bookshops were used to sell Internet directories, and some of these include interesting and useful email addresses. This technique can work well if you want a commercial email address.
2. *Consult an on-line directory:* The InterNIC directory and database at http://www.internic.net is a 'directory of directories' that lists all the widely used public access on-line directories. Useful for anyone looking for commercial or educational email contacts.
3. *Consult an on-line archive:* Doing a web search on someone's surname can turn up some surprisingly useful leads, as can searching through the Usenet archives. If someone has posted to Usenet, his e-mail address will be included in Usenet mailing lists.
4. *Mail: postmaster@...* If you know the name of the organization where the person has an e-mail account, you can mail the postmaster there and you'll often get their full address by return.

How to find a particular site in the Web?

We have just compared Internet to an immense public library accessible from anywhere: unfortunately such a wealth of information has not any index or table of contents. Therefore finding something on the Web when one doesn't know exactly where to look can be a time-consuming task, if not frustrating at all due to the huge amount of rubbish present in the Web. A survey on the evolution of Internet use in health care based on the experience of 1129 healthcare professionals applying the medical Net showed that the main obstacle encountered was the lack of time (56.14%), and that the most burdening shortcoming of e-health experienced is the time-wasting information searches (58.89%).[36] Not without a reason the new Internet produced job for retrieving information is called "data mining"!.

User's ingenuity can sometime be helpful in figuring out the possible address of the requested site: for example, searching for the site of the American Academy of Pediatrics, one could try writing "www" (the Web mark), then a dot ".", the acronym of the Society "aap", again a dot and eventually the domain name "org" (organization): "www.aap.org" will actually take this fortunate "netter" (= the one who navigates in the Net!) to the requested site. Unfortunately this procedure does not always works: searching for the Journal of American Medical Association under "www.jama.org" you will be taken to the site of Japan Automobile Manufacturers Association! (Try better under www.jama.ama-assn.org).

Solution of this problem was sought for since the very beginning of the Web: some extensive indices and catalogues were created, such as Gopher, Veronica, WAIS and Archie, but the tumultuous evolution of the Web made soon outdated these indexes. New search tools were thus devised, aiming at retrieving in few seconds a more or less complete list of URL responding to definite key words introduced by the user: the so-called "search engines".

Unfortunately most of these search engines are completely non-discriminatory about the information they index. This inability to discriminate the quality of information is exacerbated in technical domains, where the source and prestige of information take on added importance. In the health care field, for example, information from peer-reviewed journals, followed by that from health sciences universities and government agencies, is valued much higher than other information. Postings not signed by an author or not subject to peer review are unlikely to be used for educational purposes or to make serious clinical decisions. For this very reason some search engines specialized in medical field have been created: unfortunately again, also the number of search engines - both general and specialized in medical field - grew exponentially (up to the incredible number of 9,608,000 and 499,500 respectively, according to a ... search made through a search engine!). To address the reader in this pandemonium of information, we will suggest some sites among the most reliable.

General Search Engines

Search engines are giant computer systems that search the web automatically and collate the results into a useable index of web addresses (URL). This index can be browsed in a variety of ways. Some search engines use a keyword system - you specify the words you want to find on the web, and the search engine returns a list of relevant web addresses. Note that it's not just the addresses that are searched - the text of the pages is searched as well, so if the word you are looking for is embedded deep inside a web site, you'll get the URL of the page that contains it, not the main 'welcome mat' URL for the rest of the site.

Search engine indexing can be performed either automatically through a robot or manually through redaction of thematic indexes: the former system is more inclusive, the latter more selective. Thematic indexes, known also as category searchers, catalogues or directories, are links to information sources organized in hierarchical trees.

Indexing Robots

Altavista (www.altavista.com)
Offers a great quantity of hits in any search, excellent options for advanced search and allows the use of wildcards. Utilities Advance, Compact and Detailed turned out to be really useful.

Hotbot (www.hotbot.com)
Search engine created by the magazine Wired (USA); is a great indexer. The best rival of Altavista, its advanced search is as easy but with less quantity of addresses. If properly utilized can offer an extensive guide of shareware. Its homepage is not impressive: better to use it with Super Search for more refined searches.

Lycos (www.lycos.com)
Search is quick and allows searches advanced and rather exhaustive, although not always satisfying. Some utilities are somewhat puzzling.

Metacrawler (www.metacrawler.com)
A meta-search engine, originally developed in 1994 at the University of Washington, that searches simultaneously some other search engines such as Google, Yahoo! Search, MSN Search, Ask Jeeves, About, MIVA, LookSmart and more. The site, owned and operated by InfoSpace Network, is particularly indicated for searches of unusual terms.

Thematic Indexes

Excite (www.excite.com)
Sorts out a good deal of addresses but does not number them. Offers a lot of interesting features, but using them is a bit disappointing. Allows reducing the search field with key words or sentences and obtaining good results with titles and abstracts. Needs to be used jointly with Power Search.

Google (www.google.com)
The largest human-edited directory on the web, searching the Web, Usenet, and images. The core of the system is represented by software developed at Stanford University, PageRank™, able to classify web sites in order of importance. One of Google's main

features is the high search speed, due partly to the search algorithm and partly to the high number of PC networked. The system is fancy enough to give, together with the results of the search, also the time needed to complete it (just as a curiosity, to retrieve 87,900 sites dealing with "gastroschisis" it took 0.16 seconds).

Yahoo (www.yahoo.com)

Born at Stanford University (USA) in 1994, is the biggest and most utilized thematic catalogue. Its descriptions are nonetheless very concise. It's linked through a cooperation agreement with Altavista thus allowing transferring to this search engine quests not offering any result with Yahoo. To obtain best results is advisable to choose with the mouse the relevant category or to pick out the national database of interest.

Scientific Search Engines

ArticleSciences (http://articlesciences.inist.fr)

Website devoted to search and order scientific articles, realised by INstitut de l'Information Scientifique et Technique of Centre National de la Recherche Scientifique. Although based in France, can be browsed in many languages.

CiteSeer (http://citeseer.ist.psu.edu/)

CiteSeer is a scientific literature digital library and search engine that focuses primarily on the literature in computer and information science. CiteSeer was developed in 1997 at the NEC Research Institute, Princeton, New Jersey, and is now hosted at the Pennsylvania State University's College of Information Sciences and Technology. CiteSeer was the first digital library and search engine to provide automated citation indexing and citation linking using the method of autonomous citation indexing.

ISI HighlyCited (http://isihighlycited.com/)

Search engine aiming to identify individuals, departments and laboratories that have made fundamental contributions to the advancement of science and technology in the period 1981-1999. Subdivided in 21 broad subject categories in life sciences, medicine, physical sciences, engineering and social sciences, the site identifies the 250 most highly cited scientists within each category, and comprise less than one-half of one percent of all publishing researchers.

Online JOurnals Search Engine (www.ojose.com)

Online JOurnal Search Engine is a free scientific search engine enabling to make search-queries in up to 60 different databases by using only 1 search field. Within the site it is possible to find, download or buy scientific publications (journals, articles, research reports, books, etc). A bit complex in its use.

Scirus (http://www.scirus.com/srsapp/)

Scirus is among the most comprehensive scientific research tools on the web. With over 450 million scientific items indexed at last count, it allows researchers to search for not only journal content but also scientists' homepages, courseware, pre-print server material, patents and institutional repository and website information.

SciSeek (http://www.sciseek.com)

Portal aiming to provide a central place through which universities, medical centers, journals, government agencies, corporations and other organizations engaged in research can bring their news to the media. Organized in sections under the title of Science news, Science forums and Free Magazines. Offers links to many free magazines on health care.

Medical Search Engines

Cancernet (http://www.meb.uni-bonn.de/cancer.gov/index.html)

Redistributed by the University of Bonn Medical Center, it allows searching via a WAIS-full-text-index the Cancernet - Database in English and German. Good amount of pediatric surgical oncology items.

CiteLine (www.citeline.com)

Aggregator of medical Web information, offers - with some commercial flavor - a search of global clinical trials intelligence to the pharmaceutical industry and a complete picture of ongoing worldwide drug development activity.

Clinical Trial Finder (http://www.clinicaltrialfinder.com/)

Scope of this site is to match "...investigators with studies. Investigators can find studies that suit them and sponsors have immediate access to suitable investigators. Investigators can apply immediately for a study reducing the time taken for sponsors and doctors to get in touch. Investigators are alerted to new studies in their therapeutic areas allowing sponsors to target investigators specifically for their study". Needs registration.

Doc Guide (http://www.docguide.com)

Very rich site, with some aspects relevant for pediatric surgeons, presents news, clinical cases, Congress Resource Center, presentation of new drugs, online medical dictionary.

Harriett Lane Links (formerly Pediatric Points of Interest) (http://derm.med.jhmi.edu/poi/index OLD Nov2005.cfm)

Specialized search engine managed by the Johns Hopkins University, Baltimore, USA. The Harriet Lane Links provide an edited collection of pediatric resources (6,285 links) on the WWW. Maintained and edited at the Johns Hopkins University, this site attempts with rather a good result to catalogue, review and score existing links to pediatric information on the Internet.

Health on the Net Foundation (http://www.hon.ch/)

Swiss based non-profit private Foundation aimed to "...promote the effective and reliable use of the new technologies for telemedicine in healthcare around the world." HON is now presented as "...one of most respected not-for-profit portals to medical information on the Internet" featuring, among other items, two widely used medical search tools, MedHunt© and HONselect© and the HON Code of Conduct for the provision of authoritative, trustworthy Web-based medical information. The search for "Pediatric Surgery" made through these tools retrieves 98 pediatric surgical sites subscribing to the HONcode, 150 sites visited and described by HON and 5484 sites and pages automatically retrieved by a robot. The sites retrieved by the system are really many, but unfortunately not always completely focused on the request, having sometime only a very slight pertinence with pediatric surgery.

MedExplorer (http://www.medexplorer.com/)

General search engine with some sections of interest for pediatric surgeons. Noteworthy are the nutritional section, presenting a detailed database on infants' different foods. Updated world Congresses and Conferences program. Worth of a visit the "Humour" section, displaying jokes with medical flavor or "unusual statistics" such as the percentage of British fluid intake that is tea (42%).

MEDLINEplus (http://medlineplus.gov/)

Official US Government site run by the world's largest medical library, the National Library of Medicine, offering authoritative and up to date medical information based on extensive information from the National Institutes of Health and other trusted sources on over 750 diseases and conditions, as well a Medical Encyclopedia including pictures and diagrams, Dictionaries with spellings and definitions of medical words, Information on drugs, health information from the media, and links to thousands of clinical trials.

MedMark (http://www.medmark.org/peds/pds2.html)

A search engine developed in Korea by the MedRIC (Medical Research Information Centre), covers a good amount of pediatric surgical items (although mostly neurosurgical) and offers a list of medical search engines.

PubMed (http://www.ncbi.nlm.nih.gov/PubMed/)

PubMed, a service of the National Library of Medicine, provides access to over 17 million MEDLINE citations back to the 1950's and additional life science journals. PubMed includes links to many sites providing full text articles and other related resources. PubMed is a search and retrieval system that integrates information from databases at NCBI. These databases include nucleotide sequences, protein sequences, macromolecular structures, whole genomes, and MEDLINE, through PubMed. Together with MEDLINEplus, this is one of the most authoritative and reliable specialist search engines available on the Net.

Navigate in Internet without a search engine is like crossing the ocean without a boat: but also the choice among the different engines undergoes a "geopolitical" stratification, with Google being the leader worldwide but with some exceptions. According to an analysis performed by Alexa (www.alexa.com), a company specialised in collecting and publishing web information and statistics, Yahoo is the preferred search engine in India and Japan, LiveSearch in Colombia, Salvador and Paraguay, Rambler in Kazakistan, Naver in South Korea, Yandex in Russia and Baidu in China. Also in the Internet era Chinese do not forget their poetic heritage: "Baidu" is the title of a poem written more than 800 years ago during the Song Dynasty. The poem compares the search for a retreating beauty amid chaotic glamour with the search for one's dream while confronted by life's many obstacles: "…hundreds and thousands of times, for her I searched in chaos, suddenly, I turned by chance, to where the lights were waning, and there she stood." Baidu, whose literal meaning is hundreds of times, represents persistent search for the ideal. By the way, the site is written fully in Chinese.

How to perform a search on a search engine?

First of all, it is mandatory to choose the proper key words and the most suitable search engine. As a general rule, for a very uncommon keyword is better to resort to robotic indexes, while for wider topic a thematic index or better a specialized search engine will give a less cumbersome number of web matches. To give a rough idea of the results that can be obtained with search engines, Table 129.6 presents the results of a search trough general and specialized search engines, conducted on a wide pediatric surgical argument such as the Wilms' tumor, a less common one as the gastroschisis and a definitely unusual one as the pentalogy of Cantrell, together with a request about "Pediatric Surgery " in general.

The search for a site with one of those search engines can be simple or advanced, using more than a simple keyword: the more detailed the choice of key words, the best the results. Important notice: not all search engines work in the same way, then not all the following rules can apply to all engines (what changes is in particular the use of wildcards).

1. Simple search requires entering the more significant keyword / words, and usually provides a long list of addresses in decreasing order of relevancy. For example, if we introduce "surgical treatment of appendicitis" we'll have a substantial amount of documents containing whatever of these words. This search can be extended or refined with the use of wildcards. In such way are defined the symbols * and ? , used to stand for one (?) or more (*) not specified characters in a word. For example, entering "child*" will give as a result "child", "children", "childhood", "childcare", "childish", etc.; entering "surg*" → "surgery", "surgical", "surgeons", etc; entering "surgeon?" → "surgeon" and "surgeons", and likewise "p?ediatric" → "paediatric" and "paediatric"; "tumo?r" → "tumor" and "tumour" (please note that a wildcard can stand also for no characters at all).

2. Advanced search is performed with exactness, boolean logical and complement operators (from George Boole, author in 1847 of the treaty on "Logical Theory of the Binary Systems"). Among these:
   - AND: all terms joined by this operator must be present, also if separated. If we type for example pediatric AND surgery the search will give back all documents containing both these terms, also if one dealing with the pediatric neurology department and the other with the dental surgery department of a hospital. If we want to search exactly for "pediatric surgery" we must enter our request in this very way, i.e. including the words within inverted commas ("…").

Table 129.6: Results given by a search through general and specialized search engines on pediatric surgical topics

	General search engines (results x 1000)			Specialized search engines		
	Google	Yahoo	Altavista	PubMed	Scirus	Article sciences
Wilms' tumor	685	1.190	182	8.729	75.555	1.677
Gastroschisis	86	278	275	1.299	12.328	536
Cantrell's pentalogy	6.7	19.4	15.7	76	1.175	0
Pediatric surgery	1.320	23.300	20.400	10.812	847.316	14.397

Typing two or more keywords without any operator in between gives (usually) the same results than using AND. In some searchers AND is replaced by the sign +, or can be left unexpressed.

- OR: with this operator the search will give back all the documents containing at least one of the terms. It is a very useful operator when dealing for example with a pathology known under different names: "Wilms' tumor" OR nephroblastoma (please note the use of the wildcard "?" to extend the search to both terms "tumor" and "tumour", and the use of inverted commas to link this word to "Wilms'". Otherwise the search would give back all the documents containing the word "Wilms" and "tumor", also if in totally different contexts).
- NOT: this operator excludes all documents containing the marked keyword. To avoid misunderstanding by the system the better form is AND NOT. Searching for example for documents dealing only with omphalocele (known also as exomphalos) and not with gastroschisis, the advanced query will be: omphalocele OR exomphalos AND NOT gastroschisis. In some searchers NOT is replaced by the sign: –
- NEAR: This operator acts as the "and", searching for all specified keywords, but gives back as result only documents in which keywords are separated only by few in-between words (default being usually 10, with the option in some searchers to change this value). If we seek for documents dealing with the treatment of omphalocele, our request will be: omphalocele NEAR treatment.
- ( ): round brackets are used to join two or more keywords under the same operator. The query: Toddlers NOT neonates OR newborns will give back all documents containing the words "Toddlers" or "newborns", excluding only the word "neonates". This is obviously a rather senseless result: if we want to include in our search only toddlers excluding all babies under one month of age, proper query will be: Toddlers NOT (neonates OR newborns). All right, it sounds a bit crazy, but who said that computers are simple and brainy?

Which Pediatric Surgical sites are worth a visit?

Just to offer Pediatric Surgeons surfing the Web an edited guide a sort of an index of virtual pediatric surgical information, we will present some selected sites (written in English), divided in four categories according to their prevailing features: (1) Educational mostly text; (2) Educational mostly images; (3) On line journals; (4) Structured indexes of links.[37-39]

Educational-mostly Text

E-medicine (www.emedicine.com): E-Medicine (a US company privately held launched in 1996) is one of the largest clinical knowledge base available on the Net, covering some 7,000 diseases and disorders and containing an Image Bank of nearly 30,000 multimedia files. The evidence-based content provides current practice guidelines in 62 medical specialties; for Pediatric Surgery look under "Pediatrics". Subchapter on "General Surgery" is unfortunately still empty, but plenty of pediatric surgical pathologies -schematically but comprehensively treated- can be found in the subchapters "Urology", "Gastroenterology" and "Neonatology".

Multilingual glossary of medical terms (http://allserv.rug.ac.be/~rvdstich/eugloss/welcome.html): Project financed by The European Commission (DG III) and executed by the University of Gent (Belgium), it offers glossaries in which are discussed 1830 technical and popular medical terms (with cross-references between them) in nine languages: English, Dutch, French, German, Greek, Italian, Spanish, Portuguese and Danish.

Neonatology on the web (www.neonatology.org): Private-owned site run by a Cedars-Sinai Medical Center physician, features some utilities useful also for pediatric surgeons, such as: (1) General reference materials (Tables and charts commonly used in routine neonatal intensive care; (2) Medications for Neonates (Formulary for neonates, with dosing guidelines by gestational age and weight and references); (3) Teaching Files and Guidelines (an extensive list of links to teaching files and guidelines for neonatal-perinatal medicine); (4) Neonatal Drips calculator.

OMIM - Online Mendelian Inheritance in Man (http://www.ncbi.nlm.nih.gov/sites/entrez?db=omim): This database is a catalogue of human genes and genetic disorders developed for the Net by the U.S. National Center for Biotechnology Information (NCBI). The database contains textual information, pictures, and reference information, as well as the OMIM Morbid Map, a catalogue of genetic diseases and their cytogenetic map locations arranged alphabetically by disease. A visit to the site it's a must for all pediatric surgeons dealing with gene-related pathologies (from Adenomatous polyposis to Wilms' tumor).

Pediatric Surgery Update (http://home.coqui.net/titolugo): Humberto Lugo-Vicente's website is by far the most known and complete among those devoted to Pediatric Surgery in the Net. The volumes of the Journal, appeared in July 1993, cover a wide array of topics; the Pediatric Surgery Handbook for residents is possibly the most complete in the web; well worth of interest are the section on "New techniques in pediatric surgery" and the challenge to the skills of readers in "What is your diagnosis" section.

The Pull-thru Network (http://www.pullthrough.org/): The Pull-thru Network, a chapter of The United Ostomy Association, Inc., is a non-profit support and resource organization dedicated to the families of children who have had or will have a "pull-through" type surgery. The site hosts a full-text quarterly newsletter intended to report items of interest with regard to imperforate anus, cloaca, VATER association, urinary incontinence, Hirschsprung's disease, spinal and renal anomalies, as well as a glossary of medical terms, online terms, surgeries, and abbreviations.

The Hasbro Children's Hospital Pediatric Surgery Handbook (http://bms.brown.edu/pedisurg/Handbook.html): Site designed by the Warren Alpert Medical School of Brown University, it presents a practical handbook dealing with pediatric surgical technicalities such as the choice of catheters and g-tubes, nutritional and fluids intake calculations, trauma management, preoperative care.

Vesalius (http://www.vesalius.com/welcome.asp): Defined as "The Internet resource for surgical education" this site is organised in "Clinical Folios", a collection of graphical educational narratives on surgical anatomy and procedures designed for online reference and study, whose contents are arranged by topic. Narratives are an ordered series of related images, animations, or short videos linked by descriptive text that together explain the key steps in a surgical procedure or the anatomy relevant to one or more surgical procedures; Thumbnails are pages that provide an index of the principal images and text paragraphs in a Narrative; Transparencies are short interactive programs or movies that present a layered or rotational view of surgical anatomy; Discussions are text-based summaries of the epidemiology, etiology, diagnosis, and treatment associated with an underlying condition.

Educational-mostly Images

Leading symptoms in pediatric surgery (http://www.kco.unibe.ch/daten_e/startmenue/login.html): An instructional program for undergraduate and postgraduate study in medicine of the Institute for Medical Doctrine (IML) and the university clinic for pediatric surgery of the Inselspital, Bern, created by Prof. Georges L Kaiser, offers some 1700 pictures and schematics and 20 videos relating to clinic, radiology and situations during surgery illustrate 27 key symptoms in pediatric surgery. Requires free registration.

Pediatric Radiology and Pediatric Imaging (http://paediatricradiology.com/)
The site, partly sponsored by the Radiological Society of North America's Research and Education Foundation, is an extremely rich pediatric radiology and pediatric imaging digital library. It features imaging appearances of 402 (!) common pediatric diseases covered by 1,886 cases; needless to say that a huge amount of these cases are of surgical interest.

The Hasbro Children's Hospital Pediatric Surgery Image Bank (http://bms.brown.edu/pedisurg/Brown/IBCategories.html)
Visual counterpart of the Handbook before presented, it offers a wide choice of images on various pediatric surgical topics from CDH to NEC, from benign liver tumors to congenital lung lesions.

Virtual Children's Hospital Correlapaedia (http://www.virtualpaediatrichospital.org/providers/CAP/CAPHome.shtml)
"Correlapaedia", a site developed at University of Iowa College of Medicine, is a correlative encyclopedia of

pediatric imaging, surgery and pathology. Its goal "...is to create for the medical apprentice a collection of patient stories in which imaging and pathology plays a key role in diagnosing and managing surgical diseases in children. By reviewing these stories, it is hoped the medical apprentice will be able to add them to their memory and be able to recall them when needed in the future to aid in their diagnosis and treatment of patients."Fifty six clinical stories beautifully illustrated in their imaging, surgical and pathological aspects are organized by age, organ and clinical presentation.

Online Journals

Annals of Improbable Research (http://www.improbable.com/): As an exception to the rule of selecting only sites of pediatric surgical interest, we recommend a visit to this journal although (unfortunately?) no pediatric surgeons are, at least for the moment, among the contributors. The visit is particularly worthwhile in case of depression after a heavy workday or in case of lack of inspiration for further studies. It will be then possible to have details on "The gentle art of political taxidermy", or on "Alteration of the platelet serotonin transporter in romantic love," or else how "carefully collecting, classifying, and contemplating which kinds of containers his patients chose when submitting urine samples". The list of the IgNobel prizes awarded by the Journal boasts gems as "The collapse of toilets in Glasgow Public Health" or "The Relationship Among Height, Penile Length, and Foot Size" as well as "The Effects of Unilateral Forced Nostril Breathing on Cognition" (by the way, all these papers before being awarded the IgNobel prize have actually been published!).

European Journal of Pediatric Surgery (http://www.thieme.de/ejps)
Full text is available from issue 3/2000. Subscribers of the printed journal can easily register to get free access to the full text online version. Abstracts are available for free.

Free Medical Journals (http://www.freemedical-journals. com/htm/special.htm): Site promoting free access to medical journals, now totaling over 900 titles subdivided in 96 specialties (Pediatric Surgery unfortunately not among them; Pediatrics 28 journals, Surgery 17 journals). The home page offers good functionality, with the options of viewing journal sites by specialty and by language. It also has a separate listing of journals that are new to the online world.

Journal of Pediatric Surgery (http://www.jpedsurg.org/index.html): Full text is available starting with the September 2000 issue. Tables of contents and abstracts before January 2000 will be added to the site incrementally during the first quarter of 2001. Access to full text is complimentary for a limited period.

Pediatric Surgery International (http://www.springerlink. com/content/101176/): Abstracts only available for volume 12 (1997); full text available from volume n. 13 onwards (1998).

Structured Links

General Pediatrics (http://www.generalpaediatrics.com/): The site is an award-winning digital library that identifies and organizes high quality, authoritative General Pediatrics WWW sites. Information is available on almost 400 common pediatric problems, some of them of surgical interest, plus policy statements, clinical practice guidelines, consumer health information and more.

Martindale's Health Science Guide - 2003 (http://www.martindalecenter.com/HSGuide.html): Guide edited by the University of California at Irvine, in a midst of a wealth of medical links (135,500 MedicalCases and Grand Rounds; 62,300 Teaching Files; 1,295 Courses / Textbooks; 1,735 Tutorials; 420 Journals; 4,410 Databases) it is possible to find something interesting under the heading "Pediatrics/ Anesthesiology and Surgery Center".

Pediatric Surgery on the Internet: Problems and Perspectives

"Is the truth out there?"[40] is the provocative question raised by the observation that Internet information on pediatric surgery, as well as in all other medical domains, varies significantly in quality. Access to medical information via the Internet has the potential to speed the transformation of the patient physician relationship from that of physician authority ministering advice and treatment to that of shared decision making between patient and physician: however, barriers impeding this transformation include wide variations in quality of content on the Web, potential for commercial interests to influence online content, and uncertain preservation of personal privacy.[41] According to Chen et al 75.7% of 141 websites searched for information on various pediatric surgical pathologies contained accurate information, although 93.1% of these were incomplete.[40] A multi-institutional review appeared in JAMA says that most of times health information we consult in Internet is, even in the best pages, difficult to find or understand, inaccurate and incomplete. It concludes that only 1 out of 5 web pages that appear to be useful has important information. Although only the most renowned sites were evaluated, investigators assume that only 45%, in average, affords accurate information and that 53% of times they offer contradictory information about the same subject.[42] Same conclusions are drawn by Minzer et al. looking for information about infantile hemangiomas on the Net: they found only few sites accurately depicting the full disease spectrum from innocuous to severe.[43] Still more pessimistic is the conclusion of the study of Corpron et al, simulating parents' search of information for a child affected by ambiguous genitalia: out of 300 sites retrieved by search engines, only 5 (1.6%) of accessible pages offered appropriate medical information to parents.[44] The situation becomes even worse when the patient bypasses his physician seeking a treatment directly on the Net: a custom that leads to easily predictable complications, going from eye lesions caused by contact lenses purchased over the Internet,[45] to lithium intoxication caused by an Internet self-prescribed "dietary supplement".[45-46]

On the other hand the average patient, although agreeing on the importance of using technology for health-information delivery, still prefers to receive information from health-care staff by face-to-face contacts, and also access to physicians who do internet or e-mail consults is generally low and did not increase between 2001 and 2003, despite growth in internet access and in other internet-related activities; it seems therefore that Internet will not overthrow the traditional relationship between a patient and his doctor.[47,48]

What will possibly be overthrown, on the contrary, is the traditional printed medical journal. It is actually easily foreseeable that the journal of the future will be only electronic, will have a less volatile cost structure, will be supported more by services than by content and will be less able to rely on subscription revenues.[49] Since anyone can publish in the Net online, electronic journals will develop with new peer-review concepts: editors, reviewers, and authors will need to adjust to the use of this information technology. Online publication in Pediatric Surgery will increase as printed form of actual journal joins the cyberspace domain. Cyber citations as proposed by the American Psychological Association or Modern Language Association have yet to be standardized by the American Medical Association to be used as bibliographical style. Authors that use online references will need to keep printed or digital file copy of such articles, since there is no way to avoid drastic changes or movement done to this domain address.[50]

Internet evolution can worsen the gap (digital divide) between developed and developing countries also in the medical field, as it was observed in the 4th World Congress of Medicine in Internet, held in Heidelberg (Germany) in 1999. Among the important conclusions arrived in that congress, it is self-evident, today more than ever, that the difference and the gap between rich and poor countries may become too wide to be crossed on account of the new technologies in information and telecommunications. The group of experts on this subject was able to define the following concepts: (1) Internet is seen by Occident as a means to improve sanitary attention as well as the training and updating of their professionals and public in general. (2) Developing countries are lagged in attaining and using this new technology. (3) This situation will be almost impossible to reverse, unless the economical condition of those countries changes. Colleagues living in these countries have begun to connect to Internet only recently, although Internet diffusion also in these countries is increasing at enthusiastic pace, and also African adolescents utilize the Internet for health information seeking purposes.[51]

At the other end of the spectrum, in the USA, next generation of Internet is in the near future. Meaningfully named "Internet2", this collaboration project among more than 150 universities throughout the USA working in concert with both the government and the private industry, has the ambitious goal of enabling a new generation of applications, recreating a leading edge research and education network capability and transferring new capabilities to the global production Internet (www.internet2.edu.).

REFERENCES

1. Wulkan ML. Computers and the paediatric surgeon: a primer. Semin Paediatr Surg 2000;9:2-5.
2. DeCou JM, Timberlake T, Dooley RL, et al. Virtual reality modeling and computer-aided design in paediatric surgery: applications in laparoscopic pyloromyotomy. Paediatr Surg Int 2002;18:72-74.
3. Günther P, Tröger J, Holland-Cunz S, Waag KL, Schenk JP. Computer-assisted operational planning for paediatric abdominal surgery. 3D-visualized MRI with volume rendering. Radiologe 2006;46:689-97.
4. Postec F, Bossard D, Disant F, Froehlich P. Computer-assisted navigation system in paediatric intranasal surgery. Arch Otolaryngol Head Neck Surg 2002;128:797-800.
5. Lehmann CU, Kim GR, Lehmann HP. Reducing the paper load: computer-based patient records. Semin Paediatr Surg 2000;9:19-23.
6. Schubiger G, Weber D, Winiker H, et al. Die computerunterstutzte Krankengeschichte: eine Arbeitsplatzanalyse. Schweiz Med Wochenschr 1995;125:841-85.
7. Hayden RT, Patterson DJ, Jay DW, et al. Computer-assisted bar-coding system significantly reduces clinical laboratory specimen identification errors in a pediatric oncology hospital. J Pediatr 2008;152: 219-24. Epub 2007 Oct 25.
8. Buick RG, O'Donnell B, McAllindin A. Computer analysis of micturating cystourethrograms in children. J Paediatr Surg 1982;17:48-51.
9. Sakaniwa M, Sawaguchi S, Ohkawa H, et al. Computerized analysis of anorectal manometry. Prog Paediatr Surg 1989;24:21-32.
10. Schuster T, Joppich I, Schneider K, et al. A computerised vector manometry study of the so-called ectopic anus. Paediatr Surg Int 2000;16:8-14.
11. Dimitriou G, Greenough A, Davenport M, et al. Prediction of outcome by computer-assisted analysis of lung area on the chest radiograph of infants with congenital diaphragmatic hernia. J Paediatr Surg 2000;35:489-93.
12. Mogilner JG, Eldar S, Sabo E, et al. Computer-assisted image analysis can aid the prognostication of advanced-stage neuroblastomas. J Cancer Res Clin Oncol. 2000;126:285-90.
13. Wheatley JM, Rosenfield NS, Heller G, et al. Validation of a technique of computer-aided tumor volume determination. J Surg Res 1995;59:621-26.
14. Vijayan V, El Tan C. Computer-generated three-dimensional morphology of the hepatic hilar bile ducts in biliary atresia. J Paediatr Surg 2000;35:1230-35.
15. Puglisi RN, Whalen TV, Doolin EJ. Computer analyzed histology of ischemic injury to the gut. J Paediatr Surg 1995;30: 839-44.
16. Chi CL, Street WN, Ward MM. Building a hospital referral expert system with a Prediction and Optimization-Based Decision Support System algorithm. J Biomed Inform 2008;41:371-86.
17. The World Factbook CIA, Washington, 2008, at https://www.cia.gov/library/publications/the-world-factbook/
18. Bricolo F, Gentile DA, Smelser RL, Serpelloni G. Use of the computer and Internet among Italian families: first national study. Cyberpsychol Behav 2007;10:789-97.
19. Ferraro G, Caci B, D'Amico A, Di Blasi M. Internet addiction disorder: an Italian study. Cyberpsychol Behav 2007;10:170-75.
20. Naito A. Internet suicide in Japan: implications for child and adolescent mental health. Clin Child Psychol Psychiatry 2007;12:583-97.
21. Lugo-Vicente HL. Role of Internet in Paediatric Surgery http://home.coqui.net/ titolugo/review.htm.
22. Srinivas M, Inumpudi A, Mitra DK. The Internet and the paediatric surgeon. Paediatr Surg Int 1998;14:208-11.
23. Whalen TV. The Internet: past, present and future. Semin Paediatr Surg 2000;9:6-10.
24. Wulkan ML, Smith SD, Whalen TV. Paediatric surgeons on the Internet: a multi-institutional experience. J Paediatr Surg 1997;32:612-14.
25. Elliot SJ, Elliot RG. Internet List Servers and Paediatrics: Newly Emerging Legal and Clinical Practice Issues. Paediatrics 1996;97:399-400.
26. DeVille K, Fitzpatrick J. Ready or not, here it comes: the legal, ethical, and clinical implications of E-mail communications. Semin Paediatr Surg 2000;9:24-34.
27. Sterling B. Short History of the Internet. http://www.forthnet.gr/forthnet/ isoc/short.history.of.internet
28. Tarczy-Hornoch P. NICU-Net: An Electronic Forum for Neonatology. Paediatrics 1996;97:398-99.
29. NCSA - A Beginner's Guide to HTML. http://www.ncsa.uiuc.edu/ General/ Internet/WWW /HTMLPrimer.html#A1.10.1
30. De Ville KA. Internet Listservers and Paediatrics: Newly Emerging Legal and Clinical Practice Issues II. Paediatrics 1996;98:453-54.
31. Jan RL, Wang JY, Huang MC, et al. An internet-based interactive telemonitoring system for improving childhood asthma outcomes in Taiwan. Telemed JE Health 2007;13: 257-68.
32. Rangel SJ, Narasimhan B, Geraghty N, et al. Development of an internet-based protocol to facilitate randomized clinical trials in paediatric surgery. J Paediatr Surg 2002;37:990-94.
33. Beals DA, Fletcher JR. Telemedicine and paediatric surgery. Semin Paediatr Surg 2000;9:40-47.
34. Inumpudi A, Srinivas M, Gupta DK. Telemedicine in paediatric surgery. Paediatr Surg Int 2001;17:436-41.
35. Robie DK, Naulty CM, Parry RL, et al. Early experience using telemedicine for neonatal surgical consultations. J Paediatr Surg 1998;33: 1172-76.

36. HON Foundation. Evolution of Internet use for health purposes- May-Jul 2000 http://www.hon.ch/Survey/ResPoll/res_poll0.html.
37. Lugo Vicente H. Internet resources and web pages for paediatric surgeons. Semin Paediatr Surg 2000;9:11-18.
38. Parigi GB, Carachi R, Zachariou Z. Paediatric Surgeons Websurfers Bulletin. Eur J Paediatr Surg 2001;11:211-15.
39. D'Alessandro DM, Kreiter CD. Improving usage of paediatric information on the Internet: the Virtual Children's Hospital. Paediatrics 1999;104:55.
40. Chen LE, Minkes RK, Langer JC. Paediatric surgery on the Internet: is the truth out there? Paediatr Surg 2000;35:1179-82.
41. Winker MA, Flanagin A, Chi Lum, et al. Guidelines for medical and health information sites on the internet: principles governing AMA web sites. American Medical Association. JAMA 2000;283:1600-06.
42. Berland GK, Elliott MN, Morales LS, et al. Health Information on the Internet. Accessibility, Quality, and Readability in English and Spanish. JAMA 2001;285:2612-21.
43. Minzer-Conzetti K, Garzon MC, Haggstrom AN, Horii KA, Mancini AJ, Morel KD, Newell B, Nopper AJ, Frieden IJ. Information about infantile hemangiomas on the Internet: how accurate is it? J Am Acad Dermatol 2007;57:998-1004.
44. Corpron CA, Lelli JL Jr. Evaluation of paediatric surgery information on the Internet. J Paediatr Surg 2001;36:1187-89.
45. Fogel J, Zidile C. Contact lenses purchased over the internet place individuals potentially at risk for harmful eye care practices. Optometry 2008;79:23-35.
46. Pauzé DK, Brooks DE. Lithium toxicity from an Internet dietary supplement. J Med Toxicol 2007;3:61-62.
47. Välimäki M, Nenonen H, Koivunen M, Suhonen R. Patients' perceptions of Internet usage and their opportunity to obtain health information. Med Inform Internet Med 2007;32:305-14.
48. Sciamanna CN, Rogers ML, Shenassa ED, Houston TK. Patient access to US physicians who conduct internet or e-mail consults. J Gen Intern Med 2007;22:378-81.
49. Anderson KR. From paper to electron: how an STM journal can survive the disruptive technology of the Internet. J Am Med Inform Assoc 2000;7:234-45.
50. Aruzen MA. Cyber Citations: Documenting Internet Sources Presents Some Thorny Problems. Internet World Sept 1996;72-74.
51. Nwagwu WE. The Internet as a source of reproductive health information among adolescent girls in an urban city in Nigeria. BMC Public Health 2007;20;7:354.

APPENDIX 1

Glossary of computer and Internet terms

ALU	Arithmetic Logic Unit	A special chip performing all calculations in the motherboard
ARPANET	Advanced Research Project Agency Network	Military network, forefather of Internet
ASCII	American Standard Code for Information Interchange	Numerical code to express letters, digits, symbols, etc.
Backbone		High-speed network linking main computers
Baud		Speed of data transmission by a modem. It is roughly equal to one bit per second (bps)
beamer		Peripheral to be connected to a computer to project the monitor on a wall or a screen (e.g., for slides presentations, interactive sessions, etc.)
BIOS	Basic input/output system	Special chip on the motherboard issuing booting instructions to the computer in 3 phases: (1) System operations test (hardware verification); (2) hardware activation and I/O devices connections; (3) OS test and loading
bit	Binary digIT	Cipher expressed in a binary system
Boot program		Program starting automatically at the switching on of the computer, arranging CPU and peripherals
Bounce		What happens to e-mailing not properly addressed and/or lost in the net, consequently "bouncing" back to the sender
Bps	Bit per second	See Baud
byte		Set of 8 bits - basic unit of measurement of data in computer technology
Cache memory (primary, secondary)		"Hidden" service memory used to temporarily store frequently accessed data to be transferred from the RAM memory to the processor, in order to increase computing speed.
CAD	Computer Aided Design	Software dedicated to the industrial and scientific planning and design
CAI	Computer Assisted Instruction	Teaching system based on interactive learning through a computer program
CD-R	Compact Disk - Readable	A drive allowing to write your own audio and data CD-ROM's. These data cannot be erased or rewritten
CD-ROM	Compact Disk - Read Only Memory	A large capacity read-only media similar to audio compact disk
CD-RW	Compact Disk - Readable Writable	The same as CD-R, but the disk can be erased and rewritten
CERN	Conseil Européen Recherche Nucléaire	Birthplace of the WWW
Clock		Internal timer of the computer, synchronizing all the CPU operations, with a frequency measured in MHz or GHz
COM (1,2,3...)		Abbreviation indicating a serial port and its progressive number
CPU	Central Processing Unit	The "heart" of a computer that performs instructions as directed by the OS and programs
DAT	Digital Audio Tapes	Magnetic support for backup of large amount of data
Default		Parameter or value assigned automatically by the system failing specifications by the user
Display resolution		Number of pixels, or dots, used to display the image on the monitor, usually expressed as width by height.
DNS	Domain Name System	A DNS server is a computer used to translate machine names into IP address
Domain		The last part of an Internet address: .com, .edu, etc.

Contd...

Contd...

Download		To copy a file from an host system to a computer
DSL	Digital Subscriber Loop	A family of technologies capable of transforming ordinary phone lines into high-speed digital lines at speeds up to 1.2 Mbps, ADSL (Asymmetric Digital Subscriber Line), HDSL (High data rate Digital Subscriber Line) and VDSL (Very high data rate Digital Subscriber Line) are all variants of xDSL. DSL is limited by availability and distance from telephone Central Offices.
DVD-ROM		Very-high-capacity read-only media (audio or video) can hold from 9 to 17 GB.
EDP	Electronic Data Processing	
EIDE	Enhanced Integrated Drive Electronics	Technology for manufacturing disk drives. EIDE drives are slower but cheaper than SCSI drives
e-mail	Electronic mail	
FAQ	Frequently Asked Questions	Collection of answers to common questions posed by users of a newsgroup, a freeware program, etc.
FD	Floppy Disk (Drive)	A type of removable media of a standard an all PC
Freeware		Software downloadable for free from the Internet
FTP	File Transfer Protocol	Protocol used to transfer files from computer to computer. The most known is Adobe.
GB	Giga Byte	One billion (1,073,741,824 or 2^{30}) bytes
GHz	GigaHertz	Frequency of the clock - Billion of impulses per second
GIF	Graphic Interchange Program	Format developed in the 1980's by CompuServe to be used to transfer graphic images of a photographic quality
Gopher		User-friendly menu system used to navigate Internet
GUI	Graphical User Interface	Interface using icons to be clicked with a mouse (e.g., the one used with Windows)
HD	Hard Disk (Drive)	A form of permanent storage for programs and data usually made up by several spinning platters each one with read and write heads.
HIS	Hospital Information System	
Host		Public access site
HTML	HyperText Markup Language	System of text tags (plain text tagged with handles <text>) specifying features of the document, used to prepare pages to be published on the WWW
HTTP	HyperText Transport Protocol	Protocol used to transmit pages on the Web
HTTPS	HyperText Transport Protocol Security	Protocol of security allowing to transmit data between two computers in the Web preventing unauthorised access to third parties
Hypertext		Variety of media such as text, pictures, video, audio files
I/O	Input/Output	
IP address	Internet Protocol address	Numeric address of a computer connected to the Internet
IRC	Internet Relay Chat	Method of setting up a chat group in which people connected to Internet can participate in a conference
ISDN	Integrated Services Digital Network	A digital data service with transfer speeds of 64 Kbps or 128 Kbps.
ISOC	Internet Society	Professional organization defining the technical rules and protocols to run the Internet
ISP	Internet Service Provider	Commercial or institutional firm providing access to Internet
Java		Programming language allowing Web sites to load computer programs into the user's Web browser
KB	Kilo Byte	One thousand (1024 or 2^{10}) bytes
Kbps	Kilo Byte per second	Transmission speed of a modem

Contd...

Contd...

LAN	Local Area Network	Network interconnecting computers in the same environment (office block, hospital, etc.)
LCD	Liquid Crystal Display	display device made up of any number of color or monochrome pixels arrayed in front of a light source or reflector
Listserver		Server dedicated to the management of a e-mailing list
Logon/Logoff		To connect/disconnect to an host system
LPT (1,2,3...)		Abbreviation indicating a parallel port and its progressive number
MB	Mega Byte	One million (1,048,576 or 2^{20}) bytes
MFLOPS	Mega FLOating Point Second	Millions of instructions with floating point processed per second
MHz	MegaHertz	Frequency of the clock - Million of impulses per second
MIME	Multipurpose Internet Mail Extension	e-mail standard supporting the transfer of Hypertext
MoDem	Modulator Demodulator	A device that converts signal coming from source from digital to analogic and viceversa, allowing data to be transmitted over the phone lines. Used to connect to the Internet through a provider.
motherboard		Large printed circuit board housing the circuitry to make the whole machine run
MS-DOS	Micro Soft - Disk Operating System	Operating System created for the first personal computer
Netiquette	Net-etiquette	Set of a good-sense rules to behave politely on the net (in a mailing or a chat list, for example)
Network		Communication system linking two or more computers, up to the several millions of computers interlinked through Internet
Newsgroup		Usenet conference
OCR	Optical Character Reader	Utility used jointly with scanners to interpret a text
OMIM	Online Mendelian Inheritance in Man	Free service of the National Center for Biotechnology Information at Johns Hopkins University (USA) containing articles on over 8000 genetic conditions
OS	Operating System	The main program, such as Windows or MacOs, connecting and regulating all computer activities and running all other programs
Parallel Port		A 25-hole port used to connect printers and scanners
PC	Personal Computer	
Peripheral		A device not pertaining to the central core of a computer
Ping		Program able to trace the route of an e-mail between two computers
Pixel	Pictures element	The basic element of a digital picture
POP	Post Office Protocol	Protocol used to transfer e-mail messages between the user and the mail server
Port		Inlet/outlet socket, usually located on the back of the PC box, used to connect peripherals to the CPU. See also LPT, COM and USB.
Program		A series of instructions that the computer can read to perform a particular task (writing a text, playing a CD-ROM, surfing Internet, etc.)
Prompt		Request from the host system to input something (a password, a query, etc.)
Protocol		Set of rules according to which the networked computers send and receive data
RAM	Random Access Memory	Working short-term memory of a computer used to store programs and data
README file		File usually hosted in a FTP site explaining the contents of the site and how to use it
Removable media		Any type of permanent storage that can be removed such as FD, Zip or Jaz drive

Contd...

Contd...

ROM	Read Only Memory	Permanent memory that performs basic tasks on a computer. The BIOS is an example of ROM.
Scanner		Device used to input in the computer digitized images taken from a slide, a picture, a book, etc. The market offers flat scanners, used mostly for pages and pictures, and slide scanners. Useful complement to a scanner is an OCR program, to recognize a scannerized text
SCSI	Small Computer System Interface	Technology used to interface at a high velocity peripherals with the motherboard
Serial port		A 9 or 25 pin port used to connect peripherals, such an external modem.
Server		Computer able to host and automatically allocate websites (or information or files) on the net
Shareware		Software downloadable from the Internet for a nominal fee to be paid to the author of the program
Site		See Website
SMTP	Simple Mail Transfer Protocol	Protocol used to transfer e-mail messages between the user and the mail server
Spam, spamming		Unwanted solicitation or advertisement e-mailed through a listserver
SPF	Standard Picture Frame	
Streamer		I/O peripheral used to write and read data on magnetic tapes or DAT.
Sysadmin	System Administrator	Person in charge of the management of a system (HIS, LAN, host system, etc)
TB	Tera Byte	One thousand of billions (1,099,511,627,776 or 2^{40}) bytes
TCP/IP	Transmission Control Protocol / Internet Protocol	The communication protocol used in Internet to transfer files from a network to another. The heart of the Internet.
Toggle key		Key using a toggle system to switch ON or OFF a particular circuit (e.g., the BLOC NUM key, used alternatively to activate and deactivate the number keypad)
Upload		To copy a file into an host system from a computer
URL	Uniform Resource Locator	Univocal name of an site available on the Internet
USB	Universal Serial Bus	A new type of serial port through which it is possible to connect multiple devices. Its main feature is that this can be done while the computer is on.
WAIS	Wide Area Information Services	Extensive index and catalogue created at the outset of Internet
Webmaster		Person in charge of the management of a site
Website		Set of information to be published in Internet, composed by text, picture, audio, video, organized in various parts called "pages"
WLAN	Wireless local area network	linking of two or more computers without using wires, also for Internet connection
WORM	Write Once Read Many	Name of a CD that can be written only once by a CD-R drive and read as many times as desired
WWW	World Wide Web	Commonly called the Web. Access to hypertext on the Internet through the HTTP protocol
WYSWYG	What You See is What You Get	Expression used to define interactive programs using pointer mouse
XML	Extended Markup Language	The proposed successor to HTML

APPENDIX 2

How to avoid computer troubles: tricks and suggestions

Problems Caused by Improper Use

- A potentially severe problem is to change inadvertently the computer configuration. To avoid it, not to "play" with the many applications in the Control Panel if you do not know exactly what you are doing. In particular, do not mess up files in the operating system or in the applicative software in program files.
- Do not leave files in disorder in the HD, but rather create a rational subdivision with appropriate sub-folders in the "My Documents" folder.
- Do not let old e-mail to clog your e-mail box, but rather delete it once read.

Problems Caused by Breakdowns

- The file on which you are working is contained in the volatile RAM until you do not save it on a disk. A blackout or a problem in the computer will delete everything you have written on the computer after the last save: hence the opportunity to save often your file (say, every 5 to 10 minutes). There is also the option of an automatic save after a selected interval.
- If your electricity supply is unreliable it is advisable to connect the computer to an UPS system (Uninterrutable Power Supply); otherwise, save still more often.

Problems Caused by Software

- Is not unusual (particularly with Windows) a crash in a program, with the ensuing message "This program has executed an invalid operation and will be aborted" and loss of all your work since last save. It is almost always a non-worrying and self-solving problem, once switched off and on the computer, provided that the work has been saved recently (see above). Strongly advisable to save before any multitasking application.
- HD faults are much more dangerous, since all data are contained there; to avoid the risk of losing all one's own work, it is mandatory to backup all data either in a second HD on the same computer, or better in an external HD, or a CD-DVD.
- Magnetic disks are by their nature faint, and a heavy magnetic field can delete them completely; more permanent are laser-written data on a CD-DVD.

Problems Caused by Virus

- One of the least appreciable features of Internet is the possibility to get a virus in one's own computer while surfing the web. A virus is a malicious program whose sole intent is to cause problems on a computer, created by "virtual terrorists" for merely destructive purposes. A virus is self-spreading through infected mailing or flash drives, and is able to interfere with the computer in an unpredictable way, from simple files alteration till complete destruction of the HD content.
- Virus can be of various types. (1) *Programs* - Do not open ".exe" e-mail attachments; beware of attachments sent by unknown persons, or having a double extension, such as: "message_for_you.txt.vbs" (where .txt = text, or .gif .jpg = images are inoffensive extension, the second, hidden extension vbs = visual basic script; .pif = program information file; .exe = executable; .com = command, are programs). For no reason a file has two extensions, if not to use the first to conceal the second: a two-extension file is therefore positively a virus. (2) *Trojan Horses:* as the name suggests, these virus steal in the infected computer and allow their creator, a hacker, to surreptitiously seize control of the computer, unknown to the owner himself. (3) *Macro Viruses:* virus concealed in a Word or Excel file containing a macro (executable program embedded in a file). The only defence is to deactivate all macros before opening a file
- The list of known virus is available at: http://www.viruslist.com/
- To check this threat the market offers many anti-virus programs that are absolutely indispensable once connected to the Net. Highly recommendable are anti-viral programs able to monitor each access file that can become part of computer system whenever downloaded from Internet. Protection against viruses offered by these programs is satisfactory on condition that they are kept updated at least weekly (much better automatically every day), downloading appropriate files from the sites of the software houses producing antiviral software. Free antivirus is available at www.tucows.com or free.grisoft.com/doc/help/us/.
- If you run a windows OS, use often the "Windows Update" tool to download patches used to avoid "script" type virus to enter the system.

Problems Caused by Improper Use of e-mail

- The ISP stores e-mail messages until the electronic box owner retrieves the message. Files can be attached to messages, but avoid over-dimensioned attachments: attachments under 500 Kbyte do not pose any problem, up to 1-2 MByte are tolerable, over 2 Mbyte are meant to clog many e-mail boxes if not large-sized (such as g-mail).
- If a heavy attachment has to be sent, it is advisable to split it in smaller files to be sent with different mailings. Remember also that usually commercial ISP allot a limited amount of memory in the mailing box (2 to 8 MB average): it is therefore mandatory to read regularly one's own e-mail and to empty the mailing box at regular intervals, to avoid the risk of missing messages finding the box full.
- Avoid agreeing with chain mailing, petitions, and appeals: usually they are groundless or positively deceitful, mostly related to urban legends. For an update on this topic see Urban Legends Reference Pages at www.snopes.com.
- Mailing chains, as well as mailing lists, can divulge considerable amounts of e-mail addresses that are the pabulum for the e-mail degeneration known as "spamming", i.e. unsolicited and unauthorized advertising through e-mail. Refrain from answering to these annoying intrusions in your computer, because this just helps the spammer to verify that your address is correct. If you are able to trace the origin of the spamming you can send a message to the ISP from where this originated (technically difficult). To prevent e-mail misuse, avoid to spread liberally addresses of your mailing list: if a message must be sent to many people, write their addresses in the "Bcc" (blind carbon copy) field of the e-mail browser, in order to keep these addresses unknown to third parties.

Problems Caused by Internet Frauds

- Being Internet a mirror of human nature, it is not unlikely to meet with swindlers while surfing the Web and using imprudently e-commerce, particularly if through sites of doubtful reputation. Avoid entering in Internet credit card codes or other sensible data if you are not in protected mode. This is a system, offered to the customers by all reliable providers, that codes messages in order to avoid unauthorized access to the data transmitted. A protected site can be recognized by its URL, starting with "https://" (see glossary) instead of "http://". Most browsers highlight protected mode with the icon of a closed padlock in the navigation bar.

CHAPTER 130

Pediatric Surgery in Europe: Problems and Perspectives

Gian Battista Parigi

HISTORICAL AND INSTITUTIONAL BACKGROUND

The Union of European Medical Specialists (UEMS) was founded on 20th July 1958, one year after the Treaties of Rome, signed the 25th March 1957, established the European Economic Community (EEC) – with the quality as the main issue tackled, trying to obtain from the European Commission and member States a high level of training for the future medical specialists of the Common Market countries (Belgium, France, Germany, Luxembourg, Italy, Netherlands).[1]

In the following years the EEC, that with the Treaty of Maastricht in 1993, changed its name in European Union (EU), progressively enlarged to include Denmark, Ireland and the United Kingdom (1/1/1973), Greece (1/1/1981), Spain and Portugal (1/1/1986), Austria, Finland and Sweden (1/1/1995), Cyprus, Czech republic, Estonia, Hungary, Latvia, Lithuania, Malta, Poland, Slovakia, Slovenia (1/5/2004) and eventually Bulgaria and Romania (1/1/2007), raising the total number of EU Countries to 27, hosting a population just a bit short of half a billion inhabitants.

In the meanwhile UEMS, preceding the European unification process, opened to the EFTA–non EU Countries (Iceland, Norway and Switzerland), as well as to the Countries in the "waiting list" to enter EU, thus becoming Associate Members in the General Council of the Union before achieving the status of Full Member. Most of associate Members become, in recent years, Full Members; today, on top of Countries in the waiting list to enter EU, Associate Membership has been offered also to Countries outside the geographical boundaries of Europe, raising the total number to 5 (Azerbaijan, Croatia, Georgia, Israel, Turkey).

Since 1962, when the process of building Europe was still at its beginning, the UEMS created Specialist Sections for each of the main disciplines recognized and practised in at least three of the member Countries. Objectives of the sections were to defend at international level the title of Specialist and his professional status in society; to study, promote and defend the quality of the comparatively high level of specialist care given to the patients; to contribute to the creation and maintenance of solidarity amongst the European Specialists, particularly the specialists in the same field; to study, promote and defend before the international authorities, the free movement and the moral and material interests of European Specialists.[2]

Specialist Sections increased in time to a total number of 38, Pediatric Surgery (PS) among them, together with 7 Multidisciplinary Joint Committees (Table 130.1)—enlarged their field of interest creating in the early 1990s the European Boards, working groups of the Sections aiming to guarantee optimal care in the field of the speciality concerned by bringing the training of medical specialists to the highest possible level, as well as dealing with CME / CPD issues, the assurance of quality in specialist medicine and the defence of the autonomy of practice of medical specialities and specialists; among them the European Board of Pediatric Surgery (EBPS) is the one dealing with pediatric surgical issues. Every Section is ruled by a General Council, meeting at least once a year and composed by two National Delegates for each of the member Countries, elected four-yearly by the relevant

Table 130.1: UEMS Sections and Boards	
1. Allergology	24. Otorhinolaryngology
2. Anesthesiology	25. Pediatrics
3. Cardiology (Specialist Division of Pediatric Cardiology)	26. Pediatric Surgery
	27. Pathology
4. Cardiothoracic Surgery	28. Physical and Rehabilitation Medicine
5. Child and Adolescent Psychiatry	29. Plastic, Reconstructive and Aesthetic Surgery
6. Clinical Neurophysiology	30. Pneumology
7. Dermatovenereology	31. Psychiatry
8. Endocrinology	32. Public Health
9. Gastroenterology	33. Radiology
10. Geriatrics	34. Radiotherapy
11. Gynecology and Obstetrics	35. Rheumatology
12. Infectious Diseases	36. Surgery
13. Internal Medicine	37. Urology
14. Medical Biopathology	38. Vascular Surgery
15. Nephrology	**Multidisciplinary Joint Committees**
16. Neurology	• Intensive Care Medicine
17. Neurophysiology	• Pediatric Urology
18. Neurosurgery	• Emergency Medicine
19. Nuclear Medicine	• Hand Surgery
20. Occupational Medicine	• Immune Mediated Diseases
21. Ophthalmology	• Pain Medicine
22. Orthopedics	• Sports Medicine
23. Oro-Maxillofacial Surgery/Stomatology	

National Scientific Society; the Council elects among its members the President, the Secretary/Treasurer and six Executives, meeting usually at least twice a year to discuss executive matters.

In order to define aims and limits of PS, after a long gestation period and confrontation with the central UEMS offices, in 1995, the Pediatric Surgical Section of the UEMS issued a statement under the title of "The Scope of Pediatric Surgery" (SPS - Table 130.2). This review article will compare the ideal contents of this document with the factual situation in Europe, taking into account the points covered in the document – namely Children, Pediatric Surgery and Pediatric Surgeons – emphasising problems and perspectives that our Speciality is facing.

CHILDREN

The first point of the SPS states that "…the field of pediatric surgery encompasses the surgical care of the growing individual … from before birth up till the final stages of development." Letting aside the problem about which upper age limit to consider of "pediatric" interest, variously indicated in Europe from 14 to 18 years according to the different national regulations and diplomatically overcome in the SPS with the formula of "growing individual"—thus saving both our specificity and national peculiarities and… jealousies, one of the most powerful obstacles to the real unification of Europe—let us face first the main question: how many are those "growing individuals", in Europe ? And, moreover, which is the trend in the natality in our Continent ?

Europe is sometimes indicated as "the Old Continent": looking at some of the demographic indicators presented in Table 130.3, with the notable exception of Turkey, this definition sadly sounds more than appropriate, particularly if European data are compared with those of India detailed at the bottom of the table. Eleven countries present a population growth rate with the "minus" sign (should we speak of a "population extinction rate" ?), mirroring a birth rate × 1000 inhabitants of less than 10 new Europeans a year in 14 countries. Ireland and Turkey are the only two countries in which 0-14 years-old inhabitants ratio is over 20%, in other words in which at least one inhabitant out of five is less than 14 years old; Latvia

Table 130.2: The Scope of Pediatric Surgery

1. **Pediatric surgery**
   The field of pediatric surgery encompasses the surgical care of the growing individual. It includes management and perioperative care from before birth up till the final stages of development.

2. **Pediatric surgical centers**
   Pediatric surgery should be provided in pediatric surgical units based in centers where a full range of medical and surgical facilities for the care of the sick child are available. Most of these centers should provide postgraduate training in pediatric surgery and research facilities. The pediatric surgical unit should be headed by a trained pediatric surgeon.

3. **Pediatric surgeon**
   A pediatric surgeon is a surgeon specifically trained in the care of children.

4. **Specialist pediatric surgery**
   Specialist pediatric surgery should be performed in a pediatric surgical center or in a specialized center with possibilities to provide adequate care to children.

5. **Training of surgeons, other than pediatric surgeons**
   Surgeons taking care of children should have had adequate training in a pediatric surgical unit. They should also continue to have regular exposure to this type of patients. Moreover, they should stay informed about new developments in the field of pediatric surgery.

6. **Hospital**
   All children should be treated in a hospital environment appropriate for their age group. Children should not be admitted to hospital if this can be avoided.

7. **Referral advice**
   Children should be treated by practitioners experienced in this field. If the expertise is not available, the child should be referred to a centre as defined at article 2.

---

is at stand at the other end of the scale, with only one inhabitant out of seven (13.6%) younger than 14 years. If we eventually have a look at the "young/old population ratio", i.e. the number of young people (< 14 years old) for every one old people (> 65 years old), we can observe that in 16 out of 27 (!) European countries the "pyramid age" describing the age distribution of a population has turned upside down with less than one "under 14" for every "over 65" (0.69 to 1 for Italy), while on the other end of the scale Turkey present a 3.6 to 1 ratio and India a 6.2 to 1 ratio. Possibly no other indicator is more striking in emphasising such a radical difference in the demographic composition.[3]

Another striking difference within Europe emphasised in Table 130.3 is the huge difference in infant mortality ratio among the western and eastern part of the continent. Although this differentiation is now considered "politically incorrect" and seen somewhat with impatience in the hallways of the European commission, it is nevertheless a crude fact that average infant mortality in the former 15 EU countries is 4.38 × 1000, while in the new 12 countries average ratio more than doubles to 9.28 × 1000, with a worrying two-digits figure in Bulgaria and Romania (19.1 and 24.6 × 1000 respectively). The chances for a Swedish newborn to survive his first year of life are 9-fold greater than those of his Romanian mate: we simply cannot limit ourselves to emphasize the difference, we must work to reduce and ultimately to cancel that difference.

What about future? From a demographic point of view, European perspectives for next years are somewhat dark, at least according to the projections presented in Tables 130.4 and 130.5 and in Figs 130.1 and 130.2. Table 130.4 shows the demographic trend in Italy in the years 1992/96 and 2002/06[4]: natural balance of the population is in the negative since 1993, with a slight tendency to an increase in the very last years. Total population is slowly increasing only thanks to the immigration input, that in 2003 accounted on the population balance (+ 609, 580 immigrants) more than the natural increase (+ 544, 063 live births). These data emphasize two huge demographic problems, typical not only to Italy but to Europe as a whole:

Table 130.3: Paediatric population in UEMS Countries and in India – Demographic data

	Population	Population growth rate	Birth rate x 1000 pop.	% 0-14 years	Male 0-14	Female 0-14	Total 0-14 years	Live births per year (x 1000)	Children x woman years	% > 65 years	Infant mortality ratio x 1000 live births	Young to old ratio
Austria	8,199	0.077	8.69	15.1	633	603	1,236	71.2	1.37	17.5	4.54	0.86
Belgium	10,392	0.12	10.29	16.5	873	836	1,709	106.9	1.64	17.4	4.56	0.95
Bulgaria	7,322	-0.83	9.62	13.9	521	496	1,017	70.4	1.39	17.4	19.16	0.80
Croatia	4,493	-0.03	9.63	16.0	368	349	717	43.3	1.41	16.9	6.6	0.95
Cyprus	788	0.52	12.56	19.1	80	76	156	9.9	1.8	11.8	6.89	1.62
Czech R.	10,228	-0.07	8.96	14.1	738	698	1,436	91.6	1.22	14.7	3.86	0.96
Denmark	5,468	0.31	10.91	18.6	520	494	1,014	59.7	1.74	15.4	4.45	1.21
Estonia	1,315	-0.63	10.17	15.0	101	95	196	13.4	1.41	17.5	7.59	0.86
Finland	5,238	0.12	10.42	16.9	449	433	882	54.6	1.73	16.4	3.52	1.03
France	64,057	0.58	12.91	18.6	6,063	5,776	11,839	827.0	1.98	16.2	3.41	1.15
Germany	82,400	-0.03	8.2	13.9	5,894	5,590	11,484	675.7	1.4	19.8	4.08	0.70
Greece	10,706	0.16	9.62	14.3	789	742	1,531	103.0	1.35	19	5.34	0.75
Hungary	9,956	-0.25	9.66	15.3	785	741	1,526	96.2	1.33	15.4	8.21	0.99
Ireland	4,109	1.14	14.4	20.8	442	413	855	59.2	1.86	11.7	5.22	1.78
Italy	58,147	0.01	8.54	13.8	4,121	3,874	7,995	496.6	1.29	19.9	5.72	0.69
Latvia	2,259	-0.64	9.43	13.6	157	150	307	21.3	1.28	16.7	9.16	0.81
Lithuania	3,575	-0.28	8.87	14.9	273	259	532	31.7	1.21	15.8	6.68	0.94
Malta	401	0.41	10.28	16.7	34	32	66	4.1	1.51	13.8	3.82	1.21
Netherlands	16,570	0.46	10.7	17.8	1,505	1,436	2,941	177.3	1.66	14.4	4.88	1.24
Norway	4,627	0.36	11.27	19.0	450	430	880	52.1	1.78	14.8	3.64	1.28
Poland	38,518	-0.04	9.94	15.5	3,070	2,906	5,976	382.9	1.26	13.3	7.07	1.17
Portugal	10,642	0.33	10.59	16.5	914	837	1,751	112.7	1.48	17.3	4.92	0.95
Romania	22,276	-0.12	10.67	15.6	1787	1696	3,483	237.7	1.38	14.7	24.6	1.06
Slovakia	5,447	0.14	10.65	16.4	456	435	891	58.0	1.33	12.2	7.12	1.34
Slovenia	2,009	-0.06	9	13.7	141	133	274	18.1	1.26	16	4.35	0.86
Spain	40,448	0.11	9.98	14.4	3,005	2,826	5,831	403.7	1.29	17.8	4.31	0.81
Sweden	9,031	0.15	10.2	16.4	759	717	1,476	92.1	1.66	17.9	2.76	0.92
Switzerland	7,554	0.38	9.66	16.1	630	584	1,214	73.0	1.44	15.8	4.28	1.02
Turkey	71,158	1.04	16.4	24.9	9,034	8,703	17,737	1167.0	1.89	6.9	38.33	3.61
Un. Kingdom	60,776	0.27	10.67	17.2	5,349	5,095	10,444	648.5	1.66	15.8	5.01	1.09
UEMS countries	578,109	0.12	10.43	16.4	49,941	47,455	97,396	6.029.48	1.50	15.67	7.47	1.04
India	1,129,866	1.6	22.69	31.8	188,208	171356	359,564	25.636.66	2.81	5.1	34.6	6.24

Table 130.4: Demographic trends in Italy 1992-1996 and 2002-2006

Year	Live births	Natural balance	Immigrants	Total population
1992	575,000	30,178	172,886	56,960,300
1993	552,000	2,456	180,645	57,138,489
1994	536,000	−20,848	150,937	57,268,578
1995	526,000	−29,139	93,557	57,332,996
1996	536,000	−21,016	148,997	57,460,977
2002	538,198	−19,195	346,523	57,321,060
2003	544,063	−42,405	609,580	57,888,245
2004	562,599	15941	558,189	58,462,375
2005	554,022	−13,282	302,618	58,751,711
2006	560,010	2118	377,458	59,131,287

Table 130.5: Fertility rate per country observed in 1998 and expected in 2020

Position 1998	Position 2020	Country	Fertility Rate 1998	Fertility Rate 2020
1.	4.	Turkey	2.90	2.10
2.	1.	Israel	2.88	2.68
3.	2.	Moldavia	2.50	2.40
4.	5.	Cyprus	2.38	2.08
5.	6.	Iceland	2.10	1.90
6.	3.	USA	2.06	2.14
7.	22.	Ireland	1.93	1.50
8.	7.	Norway	1.86	1.86
9.	11.	France	1.78	1.80
10.	14.	Finland	1.75	1.75
11.	12.	United Kingdom	1.75	1.80
12.	8.	Denmark	1.71	1.85
13.	16.	Canada	1.70	1.70
14.	17.	Luxembourg	1.69	1.70
15.	18.	Netherlands	1.60	1.70
16.	13.	Belgium	1.56	1.75
17.	10.	Sweden	1.50	1.83
18.	23.	Switzerland	1.49	1.50
19.	24.	Armenia	1.45	1.45
20.	9.	Greece	1.37	1.83
21.	19.	Slovenia	1.34	1.70
22.	15.	Spain	1.33	1.70
23.	20.	Austria	1.32	1.50
24.	28.	Germany	1.26	1.35
25.	29.	Russian Federation	1.26	1.26
26.	26.	Estonia	1.24	1.44
27.	25.	Italy	1.21	1.45
28.	27.	Lettonia	1.13	1.41
29.	21.	Bulgaria	1.04	1.50

1. Immigration is becoming the main demographic input to Europe. Considering also that immigrant families have a birth rate much higher than indigenous families, this phenomenon will soon modify the population composition, with all the enormous amount of adaptation problems that this implies.

2. Actual Italian generation, a bit more than half a million newborns a year, is the "product" of the previous generation, that of the 1970s, composed by roughly a million newborns a year: what will happen when this generation, "halved" in relationship to the one of 30 years ago (mean age of an Italian primipara being now 28.3 years), will enter the parental age? Figure 130.1 gives a graphical answer to this question, emphasising the dramatic drop in pediatric population that Italy will experience in the next two decades.

European situation as a whole will not be much better, as detailed in the Table 130.5 and Fig. 130.2. Here is tabled and graphically expressed the total fertility rate in European countries as well as some other countries world-wide: according to the fact the level of "growth 0" is reached when the fertility rate (= number of children per woman) is > 2,1, is immediate the observation that all European Countries will be well below that danger level.[4,5]

PEDIATRIC SURGERY

The aphorism stating that "… a child is not simply a little adult…" is well known and possibly also overindulged in pediatric area, but it seems still completely unknown (or forgotten ?) by general

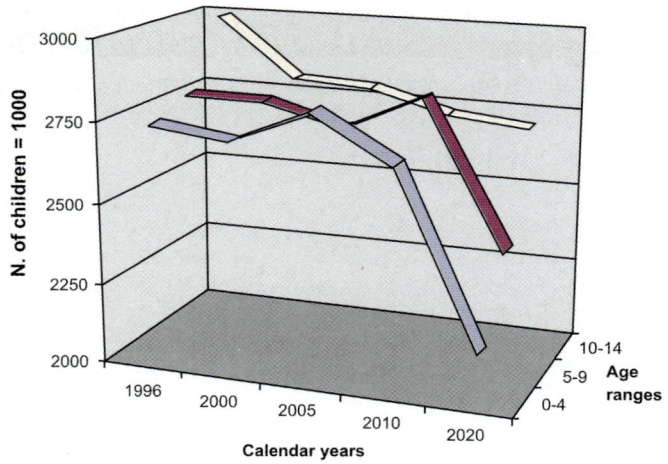

Fig. 130.1: Demographic evolution in Italian population 0-14 years from 1996 to 2020

Denmark, Netherlands and Belgium, PS is not even recognized as an independent speciality, although this shared status does not mirror in common situations. Our Danish and Norwegian colleagues are struggling for "independence" against state regulations aiming to reduce medical specialities to a minimum – and consequently not recognizing the uniqueness of expertise of a pediatric surgeon, comparing him to a surgeon "tout court", while Belgium has temporarily solved the problem introducing a "certification of competence in PS" to be awarded only to those surgeons particularly trained to deal with children.

On the other hand, also in countries in which PS is officially recognized there are "fights" about definition of the field of competence of a pediatric surgeon. Matter of debate are usually borderline pathologies involving particular organs or apparatuses in children, such as pediatric neurosurgery or pediatric orthopedics. Table 130.6 summarizes the situation in some European countries, inferred from the number of subspecialties whose clinical experience is mandatory during training in PS.[6] At the bottom of every column is indicated the number of countries in which that particular subspecialty is dealt with in PS practitioners and by general surgeons in particular. In the SPS is underlined the need that : "All children should be treated in a hospital environment appropriate for their age group ... by practitioners experienced in this field ". Situation in Europe on this issue is far to be uniform. In some countries, namely

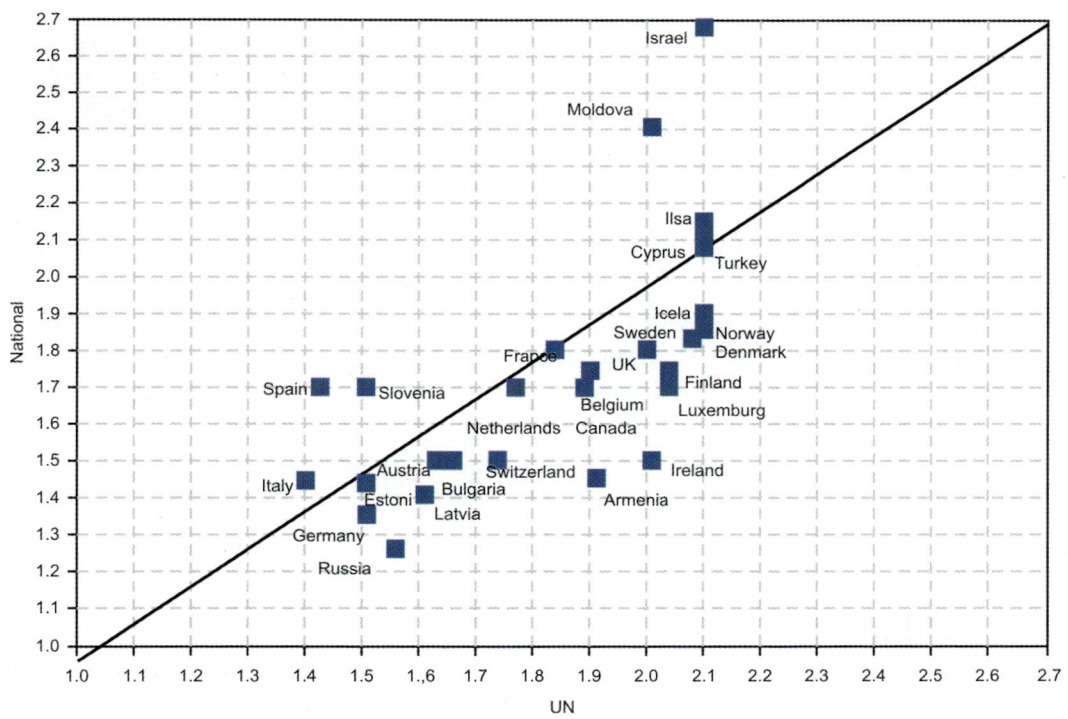

Fig. 130.2: Total fertility rate expected in 2020 in national and UN projections

Table 130.6 - Subspecialties included in pediatric surgery									
+ = included; ± = optional; – = not included									
Country	Abdominal	Oncological	Thoracic	Head and neck	Vascular	Neuro-surgery	Plastic surgery - burns	Trauma-tology	Urology
Austria	+	+	+	+	+	+	+	+	+
Belgium	+	+	–	+	–	–	–	–	+
Croatia	+	+	+	–	–	–	+	+	+
Denmark	+	+	+	+	–	–	–	–	+
Finland	+	+	+	±	+	±	+	+	+
France	+	+	+	±	±	±	±	+	+
Germany	+	+	+	+	+	+	+	+	+
Greece	+	+	+	±	–	–	±	+	+
Hungary	+	+	+	+	–	–	+	+	+
Ireland	+	+	+	+	+	±	–	–	+
Italy	+	+	+	+	+	–	±	±	+
Netherlands	+	+	+	+	+	–	–	+	±
Norway	+	+	+	±	±	–	+	±	+
Poland	+	+	+	±	+	+	+	+	+
Portugal	+	+	+	+	–	+	+	±	+
Spain	+	+	+	+	+	±	+	±	+
Sweden	+	+	±	+	±	±	±	±	+
Switzerland	+	+	+	+	+	+	+	+	+
Turkey	+	+	+	+	–	±	±	+	+
Un. Kingdom	+	+	+	+	+	±	–	–	+
Europe	20	20	18.5	16.5	11.5	8.5	12.5	13.5	19.5

Centers; optional subspecialties are counted as 0.5. Abdominal, Oncological, Thoracic, Urology, and Head and Neck Surgery constitute the core of PS and are dealt with by pediatric surgeons in most if not all countries, while Vascular Surgery, Plastic Surgery - Burns, Traumatology and Neurosurgery are performed by our colleagues in a minority of countries, with Austrian and Swiss as the more "broad spectrum" of all, dealing with all subspecialties (but not without problems with other involved specialties, at least in Austria). To solve "conflicts of jurisdiction" between PS and Urology about the issue of Pediatric Urology the UEMS has created since 2002 a Multidisciplinary Joint Committee in which representatives of Urology and PS Sections, together with the European Society of Pediatric Urology (ESPU), meet regularly to settle incoming problems.

Just as an example, according to the data of the Italian Ministry of Health, in 1998, the percentage of children admitted in pediatric departments on the total of children hospitalized was as high as 89.7% for neonates, reducing to 71.1% for toddlers 1 to 4 years old and quickly dropping to 44.5% for children 5-14 years old. Table 130.7 details were these children are admitted: on the total, in Italy less than two-thirds of them are admitted "...in a hospital environment appropriate for their age group..." as requested in the SPS and in the first article of the "Declaration of

Table 130.7: Distribution % per ward of admission of infants and children < 14 years old - Italy 1998 - n = 959.826 patients			
Pediatric wards	%	Non-pediatric wards	%
Pediatrics	46.1	ENT	8.7
		Orthopedics -Traumatology	7.8
Neonatology	10.7	General Surgery	7.7
		Infectious Diseases	1.2
Pediatric Surgery	6.1	Ophthalmology	1.1
		Internal Medicine	0.5
Children's' neuropsychiatry	1.0	Other wards	9.1
Total	**63.9**	**Total**	**36.1**

Pediatric Surgery" that the World Federation of Associations of Pediatric Surgery (WOFAPS), approved in the Kyoto meeting the 7th April, 2001. Actually, inappropriate admission of infants and children in adult departments seems to be a problem very common in many countries around the world, according to the words of the President of the WOFAPS, Jay Grosfeld, that in his presidential address at Washington meeting of October 8th, 1999: stated: "…one of the greatest threats to pediatric surgery in the next few years is the potential loss of leadership role in the surgical care of infants and children. In some places, pediatric surgery has remained provincially repressed by other groups with a conflict of interest such as general surgical departments and pediatric subspecialists who grow in numbers often well beyond the needed workforce requirements".[7]

PEDIATRIC SURGEONS

Definition of the optimal number of Pediatric Surgeons per number of people served is still an unsettled problem. Moreover, further confusion comes from the different ways in different countries to define a "Pediatric Surgeon": fully trained independent surgeon at consultant's level or just member of the staff of a PS department, possibly not yet fully independent? Legislation also in different European Countries varies substantially, particularly according to the level of clinical "independence" of the staff members from the Chief of Department, rather total in the British system and formally rather nil in other countries. This observation partially explains the huge differences than can be observed in Table 130.8, summarizing the last available data (1999 - updating process ongoing) on the pediatric surgical centers and manpower in some European Countries.[8]

For example, is striking the difference between Ireland, credited with only 4 Pediatric Surgeons (consultants), and Italy that boasts 440 staff surgeons, only 57 of who are Chief of Department. Empirical evaluation adopted by the BAPS indicates as optimal the numbers of 1 consultant Pediatric Surgeon every 500,000 inhabitants, of 1 Pediatric Surgical Center

Table 130.8: Centers and manpower of pediatric surgery in Europe

Country	Specialty recognized	Pediatric surgical centers	Under 14 (x 1000) / center	Pediatric surgeons	Under 14 (x 1000) / pediatric surgeon
Austria	yes	9	152	60	23
Belgium	no	14	125	20	87
Croatia	yes	4	197	51	15
Denmark	no	1	982	6	164
Finland	yes	3	316	45	21
France	yes	27	408	150	73
Germany	yes	78	162	250	51
Greece	yes	13	130	118	14
Hungary	yes	14	127	75	24
Ireland	yes	3	259	4	194
Italy	yes	57	142	440	16
Netherlands	no	6	481	23	125
Norway	yes	3	291	10	87
Poland	yes	56	137	180	43
Portugal	yes	11	153	75	22
Spain	yes	42	139	309	19
Sweden	yes	4	418	26	64
Switzerland	yes	8	157	45	28
Turkey	yes	55	362	139	143
Un. Kingdom	yes	39	291	83	137
Total	-	447	213	2160	44

Country	Training centers in pediatric surgery	Population (x 1000) / training centers	Under 14 (x 1000) / training centers	Length of training (core + specialist)	Selection exam for specialist training	Total trainees	Trainees/ surgeons ratio
Austria	9	904	152	5+2	no	?	?
Belgium	3	3394	583	4+2	no	?	?
Croatia	4	1169	197	3+2	no	7	0.14
Denmark	1	5356	982	6+2	no	3	0.50
Finland	3	1719	316	5+2	yes	4	0.09
France	27	2184	408	3+3	yes	100	0.67
Germany	29	2831	437	6+6	yes	80	0.32
Greece	4	2677	424	3+3	no	40	0.34
Hungary	14	728	127	2+3	yes	12	0.16
Ireland	3	1211	259	3+4	yes	10	2.50
Italy	16	3546	505	2+3	yes	175	0.36
Netherlands	7	2258	412	6+2	no	3	0.13
Norway	3	1480	291	6	no	4	0.40
Poland	21	1839	365	1+5	yes	120	0.67
Portugal	5	1984	337	2+3	yes	27	0.36
Spain	19	2061	308	2+3	yes	38	0.12
Sweden	4	2228	418	3+2	no	15	0.58
Switzerland	8	907	157	6+6	yes	5	0.11
Turkey	22	2982	906	5+2	yes	?	?
Un. Kingdom	39	1516	291	2+6	yes	32	0.39
Total	241	2094	394	-	-	675	0.31

Table 130.9: Training centers in paediatric surgery in Europe

every 2,500,000 inhabitants and the optimal ratio of 1:1 trainee to consultant. Substantial differences among countries are immediately evident, with huge overcrowding of medical doctors in some countries and a lack of trainees in others: thus, Greece has roughly a 40% of unemployed trained pediatric surgeons, Italy some 20%, Germany some 14%, Spain some 10%, Italy an UK and Netherlands. On the other hand, in UK a training program perhaps too long (6 years) and the demographic shift determines a shortage of pediatric surgeons, while in Portugal mean age of pediatric surgeons is over 40 years thus prompting the need of young colleagues. Moreover, this country as well as others (France, UK) are used to host trainees from former colonies and "export" there pediatric surgeons once trained.[9]

"WORK IN PROGRESS" AND PERSPECTIVES

This striking variability among European Countries, once more highlighted by differences in training policies and number of training centers summarized in Table 130.9, prompted the Section of Pediatric Surgery of the UEMS to set up a "peer review system" aiming to harmonize performances and training in PS throughout Europe at the highest standard reasonably attainable. This system is based on four activities: (1) Site visit of training centers; (2) European Register of Pediatric Surgeons and European examination; (3) CME/CPD fostering policies; (4) European Syllabus on Pediatric Surgery.

SITE VISIT OF TRAINING CENTERS

In 1997, the EBPS appointed visiting commissions to check the level of training in relevant PS Centers throughout Europe. Since then, twenty training centers have been awarded the European Certificate (Table 130.10). These site visits are performed in two days, the first spent visiting the Institution with all the facilities, laboratories, library, etc. and the second day spent interviewing the trainees, inspecting their

Pediatric Surgery in Europe: Problems and Perspectives

Table 130.10: UEMS approved training centers in Europe

#	Country	Location
1.	Austria	Graz, Universität Klinik 6-7/4/1997
2.	Spain	Madrid, Hospital Infantil Universitario "La Paz" 12-13/5/1997
3.	Denmark	Copenhagen, Rigshospitalet 8-10/12/1998
4.	Portugal	Porto, Hospital de San Joao 11-12/12/1998
5.	France	Paris, Hôpital Robert Debré 21/10/1999
6.	Germany	Köln, Kliniken der Stadt 7/1/2000
7.	Spain	Barcelona, Hospital Sant Joan de Deu 30-31/3/2000
8.	Germany	Heidelberg Mannheim, Universität 1-2/12/2000
9.	France	Marseille, CHU "La Timone" 15/12/2000
10.	Hungary	Budapest - Szeged - Pécs, Hungarian Universities Consortium for Training in Pediatric Surgery 30/04/2001
11.	Netherlands	Amsterdam, Emma Kinderziekenhuis AMC - VU Amsterdam 7-8/9/2001
12.	Germany	Berlin, Universität Humboldt - Charité 29-30/11/2002
13.	France	Nantes, CHU Mère-Enfant 28/3/2003
14.	Netherlands	Rotterdam, Sophia Children's Hospital 23/4/2004
15.	Turkey	Ankara, Hacettepe University 22/10/2004
16.	Turkey	Istanbul, Cerrahpasa Medical Faculty, Istanbul University 27/1/2005
17.	France	Lille, Hopital "Jeanne de Flandre" 1/12/2005
18.	Czech Republic	Prague, 2nd Medical School, Charles University 26/4/2006
19.	Poland	Warsaw, Children's Memorial Health Institute 12/9/2006
20.	Switzerland	Bern, Universität, Inselspital 27-28/4/2007.

logbooks as well as obtaining details regarding their views on gaining employment after the completion of their training.

An accreditation from the Board, although still devoid of any legal value, it is now recognized as a mark of excellence within the pediatric surgical community: a clue about the esteem in which the certificate is hold comes from the request of centres outside the geographical boundaries of Europe to be visited by the EBPS Committee. First of these "intercontinental" Site Visits will be held in 2008.

EUROPEAN REGISTER OF PEDIATRIC SURGEONS AND EUROPEAN EXAMINATION

The EBPS set up an European Register of Pediatric Surgeons, involving the Certification of Pediatric Surgeons from European Countries. This task was accomplished through a process that in the past was addressed to established Pediatric Surgeons (grandfather clause), trained before 1993, requested to present their application form to be scrutinized by a body organized by the National Scientific Societies to ensure that the applicants were bona fide pediatric surgeons who had undergone training in their own country. These forms were further scrutinized by the Executive Council of the EBPS in January 1997, and a bit more than 1000 colleagues entered the Register, now published on the Section's website.[10]

To allow younger colleagues to be registered also after the "grandfather clause" was no more active, it was designed a full process of European Examination, again with the expressed goal of setting a standard of excellence, setting a bench mark which most pediatric surgeons should strive to achieve. The EBPS Register has not yet legal status but ensures a high standard of candidates who have completed their pediatric surgical training. Since 2005, the European Examination is organized in two parts, hold at least twice a year. Part one is a Multiple Choice Questionnaire with 100 questions in ten sections to be answered. All trainees are eligible to sit this Part, that is valid for up to five years. Candidates successful in Part one can sit for the Part two, subdivided in four events each lasting 45 minutes: (1) Clinical Examination - to include one problem based major case and 2-3 short cases; (2) Neonatal Surgery Oral Examination; (3) General Pediatric Surgery Oral Examination; (4) Genitourinary Surgery Oral Examination. Knowledge of basic sciences will be tested in this examination, including clinically applied physiology, anatomy, biochemistry and embryology. In addition, the candidate will be expected to be familiar with antenatal management of pediatric surgical conditions and to understand the relevance of the genetic basis of its causation. Part two exam, lasting two days, is hold in a training center usually chosen between those already approved (Table 130.10). Since the beginning, in 1999, to the last examination in Budapest in 2007, 77 candidates successfully passed the examination and become Fellows of the European Board of Pediatric Surgery

(FEBPS). Although devoid of any legal value, this Fellowship is a mark of excellence that should ideally distinguish all and only those Pediatric Surgeons whose level of professional value meets the demanding standards set by the European Board.

Wishing to offer also to colleagues non EU-citizens the possibility to challenge themselves with the European Examination since 2006, the Board decided to open the application to candidates from all over the world: successful ones will be awarded the European Board Certification (EBC), being the Fellowship for legal reasons reserved to EU citizens.

CME FOSTERING POLICIES

There is a strong tradition of continuing medical education (CME) in the medical profession and the most powerful motivating factors are positive ones: doctors' awareness of their responsibility for safe medical performance, recognition of peers, collective emphasis on the quality of medical practice. CME has its definite place in the so-called "Quality Agenda", based on the three items of :

1. Quality Improvement – a continuous striving to provide better practice;
2. Quality Assurance – a process applied to the confirmation or continuing fitness to practice (audit, performance review);
3. Quality Control – a wholly distinct area, related to medical regulation, in which doctors who have been identified as having difficulties with their practice are assessed and appropriate action is instituted.

Continuous Medical Education is the most effective form of quality improvement now available and the new password in the field of medical updating, fostered by UEMS since 1993 with the publication of the European Charter on CME, followed in 1998 by the EBPS guidelines for CME (published in the Section website at the URL http://www.uemspaedsurg.org/CME.htm) and in 1999 by the establishment of EACCME, the European Accreditation Council for CME, operational since 2000. Main aim of this body is "… to harmonize and improve the quality of specialist medical care in Europe… by improving quality of CME and accessibility to CME for the medical specialists in Europe" by means of transfer of CME credits (the units of evaluation of CME) in case of migration of a specialist within Europe, between European countries, between different specialties and between the European credit system and comparable systems outside Europe (such as the ABMS – American Board of Medical Specialities). CME activities are classified in three categories:

1. External formally planned CME (Scientific Congress, EACCME registered or not, Courses, Workshops, Seminars and distance learning programs).
2. Internal CME, Hospital based (Postgraduate meetings, Research meetings, Department meetings, Hospital grand rounds, Journal club, Audit meetings) or independent based (Reading medical literature, medical writing, editorial or refereeing work, Internet learning, self assessment examination, medical audiotapes and videos).
3. Other CME activities can be visits to specialized units, preparation and delivery of formal lecture or seminar, preparation and delivery of audit report, publication or presentation of scientific papers or books, teaching, postgraduate examination work.

Adequate completion of CME requirements is mandatory for all Pediatric Surgeons registered into the European Register of Pediatric Surgeons in order to maintain their status of FEBPS.

EUROPEAN SYLLABUS OF PEDIATRIC SURGERY

Being fully within the mission of EBPS to give an expert and authoritative advice, although not legally binding, on what and how has to be taught in a training course in Pediatric Surgery, in January 2006 the Executive Committee decided to prepare a Syllabus on Pediatric Surgery, to stand as reference document for all training centers throughout Europe on which are the contents of Pediatric Surgery, what is essential and what not essential, which fields are mandatory and which just optional, and how should be organized the training. An "ad hoc" Committee, created in full synergy with the European Pediatric Surgeons' Association (EUPSA), prepared the draft that, after four major revisions and two years of work involving all the National Scientific Societies of Europe, it is now ready for publication and will be presented at the IX European Congress of Pediatric Surgery to be held in Istanbul in June 2008.

EUROPEAN WORKING TIME DIRECTIVE (EWTD)

Organization of Training Centers in Europe had recently to be significantly modified according to the rules imposed by the EWTD. This directive states that every European worker (trainees included) cannot work more than 8 hrs per day = 48 hrs per week over 6 working days; in hospitals up to 10 hrs per working day are possible = 60 hrs maximum per week; within 1 working day a minimum time of rest of 45 min has to be assured; after 1 working day minimum time of continuous rest is 11 hrs, thus meaning that no night duty is possible after a working day; after night duty the trainee has to leave the hospital and rest for a minimum of 11 hrs. Born originally as "protection of the clinical personnel against overwork for the benefit of patient"— a really critical issue in some cases in which training of young doctors was including up to 80-100 hrs per week. The solution imposed by the EWTD has actually entailed severe consequences on the training of competent surgical specialists.[11] Among these, it has been emphasized a reduced presence of trainees (only 150-160 days per year instead of > 200 days); a reduced participation of trainees in clinical care as well as in attendance to the OR (30-40% fewer operations than before); impossibility to follow a patient's full clinical history from admission to discharge; available time taken up predominantly by routine work; structured training reduced, with impaired participation in educational seminars, teaching rounds, etc.

WHAT ABOUT FUTURE?

Future development of our specialty in the EU needs to seek an harmonization between what imposed by the EWTD and the concept of Continuous Professional Development (CPD), slowly but steadily overcoming the one of CME, and defined as "…the educative means of updating, developing and enhancing how doctors apply the knowledge, skills and attitudes required in their working lives… the UEMS therefore believes that CPD is essential for ensuring high standards of medical practice".[12] The task now facing UEMS is to define the desired outcomes of CPD - both the maintenance of safe standards of practice, and encouraging the achievement of the highest quality standards; to determine the processes required to achieve these outcomes, making CPD more readily available and making involvement in CPD more effective and verifiable; to agree on structures and funding sources, specific to each country's health care structure, that will support the implementation of CPD for all specialist doctors, pediatric surgeons among them. In this process, the new organization of work determined by the EWTD with a closer supervision of the senior staff on the trainees will might help to avoid pitfalls and secure the continuous medical care of our little patients,[13] and the possibilities offered by long distance web-based learning might replace traditional structured theoretical education.

New approaches and techniques for old concepts: to keep as high as possible the level of care that we are daily called upon to offer to our children.

REFERENCES

1. Carachi R. The UEMS Specialist Section in Paediatric Surgery. Eur J Pediatr Surg 1999;9:132-37.
2. UEMS Statutes (www.uems.net)
3. CIA World Factbook, 2008 edition (https://www.cia.gov/library/publications/the-world-factbook/index.html)
4. Istituto Italiano di Statistica, 2008 report (http://demo.istat.it)
5. European Statistical Office, 2008 report (www.eurostat.eu)
6. Driller C, Holschneider AM. Training in pediatric surgery- A comparison of 24 countries in Europe and other countries around the world. Eur J Pediatr Surg 2003; 13: 73-80.
7. J Grosfeld, XXXII Executive Committee Meeting WOFAPS, 8/10/1999, Washington.
8. UEMS Paediatric Surgery Handbook (http://www.uemspaedsurg.org/Handbook.htm)
9. European Board of Paediatric Surgery Manpower Committee - unpublished data.
10. www.uemspaedsurg.org/Register.htm
11. Ladd AP. Pediatric surgery fellowship compliance to the 80-hour work week J Pediatr Surg 2006;41:687-92.
12. UEMS- The Basel Declaration. 20-10-2001. (www.uems.net/documents)
13. Potts S. The surgeon in training - European qualifications. Eur J Pediatr Surg 2005;15:374-75.

Index

A

Abdominal tuberculosis 646
  clinical presentation 648
    acute abdomen 650
    gastrointestinal involvement 649
    mesenteric lymphadenitis 649
    peritoneal tuberculosis 648
    varied presentation 650
  differential diagnosis 655
  incidence 646
  investigations 651
    colonoscopy 654
    hematological tests 651
    laparoscopy 654
    Mantoux test 651
    percutaneous peritoneal biopsy 654
    radiology 651
    serological tests 651
  pathogenesis 647
  pathology 647
  treatment 655
    laparotomy 655
    medical treatment 655
    surgery 656
Abnormalities of larynx 1287
Abnormalities of the testis 532
Achalasia cardia 363
  clinical presentation 364
  etiopathophysiology 363
  historical background 363
  investigations 364
    barium swallow 364
    CT scan chest 365
    esophageal manometry 364
  management 365
    dilatation 365
    Heller's cardiomyotomy with anti-reflux procedure 365
    laparoscopic/thoracoscopic repair 366
  results 367
Acid-base disturbances 60
  base excess 61
  blood pH 61
  chemical and physiological regulation of the pH body 61
  disturbances in acid-base balance 61
  pH calculation 61
  relation between pH and $PaCO_2$ 62
  standard biocarbonate 61
Adrenal androgen excess 1410
Adrenal disorders 1404
  Cushing's syndrome 1405
    ACTH dependent causes 1406
    ACTH independent causes 1406
    diagnostic evaluation 1407
    ectopic ACTH production 1406
    etiology 1406
    management 1408
    medical management 1409
  disorders associated with excess of adrenocortical hormones 1405
  physiology and metabolism 1404
Adrenal insufficiency (Addison's disease) 1410
  causes 1410
  clinical features 1410
  evaluation and diagnosis 1411
  management 1411
Agarwal's growth curves 39
Alimentary tract duplications 659
  cervical and thoracic duplications 660
  colonic duplications 667
  duodenal duplications 664
    duplications associated with pancreatitis 665
  embryology 660
  gastric duplications 663
  ileal and jejunal duplication 665
  oral and lingual duplications 660
Alkaline solutions 59
Amoebic liver abscess 930
  clinical features 931
  diagnosis 931
  epidemiology 930
  pathology 931
  results and complications 932
  treatment 931
    abscess drainage 932
    antimicrobial therapy 931
Analytical blot transfer techniques 25
Anatomy of bronchial tree 230
Angelman syndrome 28
Anion gap 62
  serum osmolality 62
  serum osmolar gap 62
Anomalies associated with anorectal malformations 825
  cardiovascular anomalies 831
  gastrointestinal anomalies 831
  genital anomalies 830
  genitourinary malformations 826
    management of lower urinary tract dysfunction 828
    management of urologic anomalies 828
  skeletal anomalies 829
    spinal anomalies 829
  spinal cord anomalies 830
    caudal regression syndrome 830
Anorectal malformation: anatomy and physiology 776
  anatomy 781
  antomic considerations 784
    ARM and sacral agenesis 784
    poor continence in high ARM 784
    problems of common wall in ARM 785
  concept of de Vries and Pena 783
  embryology 777
    conventional theory 777
    theory of Chatterjee and Roy 778
    theory of Van der Putte 779
  history 776
  physiology 785
    bowel motility 785
    propulsive force 785
    resistance at the outlet 785
    sensation 785
Anorectal malformations current perspectives 874
  antenatal detection 875
  continence 881
  etiology 875
  incidence 875
  investigation 879
  Krickenbeck classification 877
  management 880
    laparoscopic assisted anorectal pull-through 880
    laparoscopic technique 881
    repair in the neonatal age 880
  rectal atresia 879
  research in anorectal malformations 881

Anorectal malformations: Pena's perspectives 816
   colostomy 816
   limited PSARP 818
      indications 818
      procedure 818
   posterior sagittal anorectoplasty (PSARP) 819
   timing of the definitive repair 817
   utility of PSARP 817
      scientific basis of PSARP 817
Anorectal malformations:diagnosis and management 787
   classification 787
   diagnosis and investigations 790
      antenatal diagnosis 790
      assessment after colostomy 802
      assessment of sphincters and its nerve supply 803
      assessment of sphincters with magnetic resonance imaging 804
      clinical evaluation in female 793
      clinical evaluation in male 792
      dye study of fistula 801
      invertogram 793
      neonatal assessment 790
      preliminary assessment of associated anomalies in neonatal period 802
      ultrasound examination 801
   magnitude of the problem 787
Anterior encephalocele 1152
   prognosis 1159
   treatment 1158
Antibiotics 199
   exact mode of action 199
      disruption of the cell membrane 199
      interference with cell wall synthesis 199
      interference with nucleic acid synthesis 199
      interference with protein synthesis 200
   pharmacokinetics of antibiotis 200
Apert's syndrome 120
Appendicitis 596
   anatomic and histologic basics 596
   appendiceal neoplasms 608
   clinical symptoms and diagnosis 598
      clinical examination 601
         CT scan 603
         diagnostic laparoscopy 604
         laboratory -chemical analysis 602
         MRI 603
         nuclear medicine 604
         ultrasonography 602
   complication 610
   current calssification of appendicitis according to histological basis 609
      acute appendicitis 609
      focal appendicitis 609
      gangrenous appendicitis 609
      neurogenic appendicitis 609
      perforating appendicitis 609
      phlegmenous and ulcerophlegmenous appendicitis 609
      recurrent appendicitis 609
   differential diagnosis 604
   epidemiological facts 596
   pathogenesis 608
   postoperative care 613
   postoperative complications 613
   prognosis 613
   therapy 610
      non-surgical therapy 612
      surgical therapy 610
Arrested hydrocephalus 1141
Ascariasis lumbricoides 678
   clinical manifestations 678
      appendicular ascariasis 679
      intestinal ascariasis 678
      pancreatic biliary involvement 679
      peritoneal ascariasis 680
   etiology 678
   pathogenesis 678

B

Baker's cyst 1315
Barium studies 136
   hypertrophic pyloric stenosis 136
Barium study 417
Barrett's esophagus 404
Barrett's esophagus (BE) 350
Barrett's mucosa 350
Beckwith-Wiedemann locus 30
Bezoars in children 671
   classification 671
      iniobezoars (coirbezoars) 672
      pactobezoars 671
      pharmacobezoars 671
      phytobezoars 671
      pseudobezoars 672
      rare forms 672
      trichobezoars 671
   clinical presentation 673
   complications 675
   etiology 672
      associated partial congenital obstructions 672
      diabetic gastroparesis 672
      intraluminal obstruction 672
      neuropsychiatric disorders 672
      postgastroplasty 672
      postpartial gastrectomy 672
      trichotillomania and trichophagia 672
      uremia 672
   investigations 673
   non-operative treatment 674
      dissolution with enzymatic digestion 674
      endoscopic retrieval 674
      ESWL fragmentation 675
      gastroscopy with laparoscopically assisted fragmentation 675
      suction and lavage 674
      with-holding feeding 674
   operative removal 675
      enterotomy and direct extraction 675
      gastrotomy 675
      milking of bezoars into caecum 675
      Rapunzel syndrome 675
   pathogenesis 672
Bilateral iliac occlusion 301
Biliary atresia 5, 1003
   complications 1008
      biliary lakes 1009
      cholangitis 1008
      malignancies 1009
      portal hypertension 1008
   diagnosis 1005
      duodenal drainage test 1006
      imaging 1005
      liver function tests 1005
      nuclear scanning 1006
      percutaneous needle biopsy 1006
      peroperative cholangiogram 1006
   etiology and pathogenesis 1003
   pathology 1004
   prognostic factors 1009
   surgical management 1006
      surgical technique 1007
Biocompatible polymer matrices 1484
Blood components 82
   cryoprecipitate 87
   fresh frozen plasma (FFP) 86
   granulocyte transfusions 86
   indications for red cell transfusions 83

infants and older children 84
   symptomatic children with Hb
      < 7 g/dL 84
modified components 87
   gamma-irradiated blood
      products 87
   saline-washed red blood cells
      and platelets 87
   use of special filters and
      leucocyte depleted blood 87
neonates 83
   Hb < 10 g/dL in infants with
      failure to thrive 84
   Hb < 10 g/dL, if symptomatic 83
   Hb < 13.0 g/dL, in
      cardiopulmonary disease 83
   physiologic anemia of infancy 83
   replacement of Iatrogenic blood
      loss 64
platelet transfusion 85
red blood cells (RBCs) 82
transfusion of the RBC product 84
Blot transfer techniques 25
Blount's disease 1312
Body surface area (BSA) method 56
Bone and joint infections 1319
   acute hemantogenous
      osteomyelitis 1319
      differential diagnosis 1320
      investigations 1320
      pathogenesis 1320
      surgical treatment 1321
      treatment 1320
   Brodie's abscess (bone abscess) 1321
      differential diagnosis 1322
      treatment 1322
   chronic 1322
      diagnosis 1322
      treatment 1323
   Garre's chronic sclerosing
      osteomyelitis 1323
      sickle cell disease 1323
   hemophilic arthropathy 1327
      laboratory investigations 1328
      radiologic features 1328
      treatment 1328
   infectious arthritis 1324
      relevant anatomy 1324
   neonatal osteomyelitis 1321
   osteomyelitis by unusual
      organisms 1323
      Salmonella osteomyelitis 1323
      syphilitic osteomyelitis 1323
      treatment 1324
      tubercular osteomyelitis 1324
   pyogenic arthritis 1324
      clinical features 1325

      differential diagnosis 1326
      evaluation of pus 1326
      imaging studies 1325
      pathogenesis 1325
      restoration of function 1326
      source of infection 1324
      splinting the joint 1326
      sterilization of the joint 1326
      synovial fluid analysis 1325
      treatment 1326
   sequelae of septic arthritis 1326
      clinical features 1327
      diagnosis 1327
      pathology 1326
      treatment 1327
   subacute osteomyelitis 1321
Bowel management 899
   management 901
      constipation 902
      continent catheterizable
         channel 904
      enema 902
      loose stools and diarrhea 902
      pseudoincontinence 901
      teamwork 902
   preliminary assessment 899
      fecal incontinence 900
      indications 899
      objectives 900
      physical causes of fecal
         incontinence 900
      pseudoincontinence 900
      real fecal incontinence 900
   results 904
Brain tumors 150
   cerebrospinal fluid studies 151
Breast development and pubic hair
      changes in various sexual
      maturity stages (SMR)
      in girls 46
Bronchiectasis 471
   clinical features 472
   etiology and pathogenesis 471
   investigations 472
      bronchoscopy 473
      CT scan 473
      routine blood tests 472
      skiagram chest 473
   management 474

C

Caloric expenditure method 56
Canada Cronkhite syndrome 774
Cardiogenic shock 79
   after load reduction 80
   cardiac obstructive shock 80

   cardiac temponade 80
   inotropic agents used in cardiogenic
      shock 79
   therapy 79
Cat-eye syndrome 826
Caudal anesthesia 113
Caudal regression syndrome 826
Causes of hyperkalemia 52
Causes of hypokalemia 53
Cell sourcing in tissue engineering 1484
Central dogma of molecular biology 22
Cervical esophageal duplications 662
Cervical esophagostomy 398
Chest wall deformities 510
   cardiopulmonary effects 510
   classification 511
   excavatum and pectus carinatum 513
   pectus carinatum 512
      clinical relevance 513
      historical background 512
   pectus excavatum 511
      clinical relevance 512
      historical background 511
   Poland's syndrome 516
   results and complications 516
   sternal defects 517
      cervical ectopia cordis 518
      cleft or bifid sternum 518
      thoracic ectopia cordis 517
      thoracoabdominal cordis 518
   surgical technique for pectus 513
Chiari malformations 1143
Childhood epilepsy 149
Childhood obesity 1415
   assessment 1415
   complications 1418
   etiology 1415
   evaluation 1416
   management 1418
Choledochal cyst 1013
   associated conditions 1021
      disorders of pancreatic duct and
         common channel 1022
      intrahepatic bile duct
         dilatation 1021
   classification 1014
   clinical presentation 1015
   complications and outcome 1022
   differential diagnosis 1017
   embryology 1013
   etiology 1013
   investigations 1016
   surgery 1019
      biliary reconstruction 1020
      choice of operative procedure
         1019
      complete excision 1019

    laparoscopic cyst excision 1021
    mucosectomy 1020
    staged procedure 1020
Chronic lung abscess 475
Chylothorax 491
    antenatal chylothorax 491
    investigations 492
    medical treatment 492
    postnatal chylothorax 491
    surgical treatment 492
Cleft lip and palate 1201
    anatomical and clinical features of clefts 1205
        lip and alveolar cleft 1205
        palate cleft 1207
    associated anomalies 1203
    embryology 1201
    epidemiology and incidence 1203
    genetics and etiology 1202
    prenatal diagnosis 1208
    preoperative preparation 1211
    presentation 1208
    presurgical orthondontics 1211
    terminology, classification and recording 1204
Cleft lip repair 1211
Cleft palate repair 1214
Clinical applications of laser in pediatric surgery 1514
Clinical manifestation of potassium disturbances 53
Clinical relevance of post-transplant anti-HLA and non-HLA antibodies 979
Cloaca 821
Club sandwich 653
CME fostering policies 1562
Colon patch esophagoplasty 426
    advantages 426
    disadvantages 426
    preoperative preparation 426
    surgical technique 427
        postoperative care 427
Common eye problems in children 1239
    congenital anomalies 1239
        acquired ptosis 1241
        acute glaucoma 1240
        congenital cataract 1239
        congenital ptosis 1240
        pseudoptosis 1242
        strabismus (squint) 1243
        surgical management of ptosis 1242
        surgical protocol 1242
    inflammatory disorders 1249
        orbital cellulitis 1251
        routes of infection 1251
        uveitis 1249
    miscellaneous disorders 1253
        vitamin A deficiency 1253
    neoplastic disorders 1247
        retinoblastoma 1247
    physical and chemical trauma 1244
        blunt injury 1245
        chemical injuries 1244
        corneal abrasion 1245
        corneal ulcer 1246
        foreign body 1244
        penetrating injury 1245
        red eye 1246
        subconjunctival hemorrhage 1246
        thermal burns 1245
    proptosis 249
    refractive disorders 1253
        astigmatism 1253
        hyperopia 1253
        myopia 1253
Common radiological procedures in pediatric surgery 131
    anorectal malformations 133
        plain radiography 134
    intravenous urography 133
        contraindications 133
        indications 133
    micturating cystourethrography (MCU) 132
        contraindications 132
        indications 132
    radiation protection 131
    retrograde urethrography (RGU) 132
    ultrasound 134
        computed tomography 134
        magnetic resonance imaging 134
    water soluble intravenous contrast media 131
        ionic contrast 131
        nonionic contrast 131
Complications following PSARP 833
    classification 836
        manometry 838
        physical examination 838
    defecation problems 834
    early and late complications 833
    other complications after PSARP treatment 838
    treatment of postoperative complications 839
    results of the treatment of chronic constipation following PSARP 839
    secondary operations following PSARP 840
Computer 1518
    calculations 1526
    data recording and retrieving 1526
    functions 1521
    images processing and CAD 1525
    mass storage devices 1522
        magnetic disks 1522
        magneto-optical disks (MOD) 1523
        optical disks 153
        removable memory devices 1523
    text processing 1525
    types 1519
        mainframe 1520
        personal computer 1520
        supercomputer 1519
Congenital adrenal hyperplasia 1411
    diagnosis 1413
    management 1413
    role of surgery 1413
    types 1412
Congenital and developmental abnormalities of the cervical spine 1301
    Klippel-Feil syndrome 1301
        treatment 1301
    torticollis 1301
        differential diagnosis 1302
        treatment 1302
Congenital and developmental anomalies of the knee 1310
    bow legs and genu varum 1310
        Blount's disease 1311
        internal tibial torsion 1311
        rickets 1312
    genu valgum 1312
Congenital and developmental disorders affecting foot 1315
    calcaneovalgus deformity 1317
    clubfoot 1315
        pathology 1315
        treatment 1316
    congenital vertical talus 1317
        pathology 1317
        treatment 1318
    pes cavus 1319
    pes planus (flatfoot) 1318
Congenital and developmental disorders of the hip 1308
    developmental dysplasia of hip (DDH) 1308
        Barlow's test 1309
        diagnosis 1309
        Ortolani's test 1309
        pathology 1309
        radiographic examination 1309
        treatment 1310

Congenital and developmental disorders of thoracolumbar spine 1305
  scoliosis 1305
    evaluation 1305
    imaging 1305
    non-structural 1305
    structural 1305
    treatment 1306
  spondylolysis and spondylolisthesis 1307
    treatment 1308
Congenital anomalies of the larynx and trachea 1273
  laryngomalacia 1274
  vocal cord paralysis 1275
    management 1276
  unilateral laryngeal paralysis 1278
Congenital anomalies of the trachea 1287
  tracheal stenosis 1290
    acquired tracheal stenosis 1291
    congenital tracheal stenosis 1290
    diagnosis 1291
    radiologic evaluation 1291
    surgical management 1291
    tracheal resection and reanastomosis 1296
  tracheomalacia 1287
  vascular compression 1288
    anomalous subclavian artery 1289
    double aortic arch 1289
    innominate artery compression 1288
    pulmonary artery dilation 1290
    pulmonary artery sling 1290
    right aortic arch 1289
Congenital anomalies of urinary tract 30
Congenital disorders of hand 1303
  congenital amputations 1304
  congenital trigger thumb 1304
  constriction ring syndrome 1304
  macrodactyly 1304
  polydactyly 1304
  syndactyly 1303
Congenital esophageal stenosis 377
Congenital hemangioma 1088
  chemotherapy 1091
    interferon-alpha 1091
    vincristine 1091
  diagnostic evaluation 1089
  laser therapy 1092
  surgical excision 1092
  treatment for specific lesions 1093
    subglottic hemangioma 1093
    visceral hemangiomas 1094
  treatment of ulcerations 1090

Congenital pouch colon 847
  associated anomalies 851
  classification 848
  clinical presentation 849
  complications 854
  embryogenesis 847
  histopathology 848
  incidence and epidemiology 847
  investigations 850
  management 851
  prognosis 856
  rare variants 854
  results 855
Congenital pouch colon (CPC) 878
Conjoined twins 1349
  anesthetic management 1357
  classification 1350
    asymmetrical conjoined twins 1352
    craniopagus twins 1352
    ischiopagus twins 1352
    pygopagus twins 1352
    thoracopagus twins 1350
    xiphopagus twins 1350
  ethical considerations 1355
  incidence and etiology 1350
  obstetrical management 1352
  postnatal evaluation 1354
  prenatal diagnosis and evaluation 1352
  preoperative planning 1356
  results of surgery 1360
  surgical considerations 1358
    cardiovascular system 1358
    central nervous system 1359
    gastrointestinal system 1359
    genitourinary system 1359
    hepatobiliary pancreatic system 1358
    omphalocele 1359
    skeletal system 1360
  timing of surgical separation 1356
Corrosive strictures 378
Couinaud's studies 949
Craniosynostosis 1193
  diagnosis 1197
  differential diagnosis 1197
  multiple suture involvement 1196
  nonsyndromic 1193
    brachycephaly 1194
    plagiocephaly 1193
    scaphocephaly 1193
    trigonocephaly 1194
  surgical management 1198
  syndromal 1195
    Apert's syndrome 1196
    Crouzon's syndrome 1195

Crohn's colitis 752
Crohn's disease 650, 741
  clinical manifestations 742
    extraintestinal manifestation 742
    gastrointestinal manifestation 742
    growth abnormalities and nutritional deficiencies 742
  diagnosis 743
    endoscopy 743
    history and physical examination 743
    laboratory assessment 743
    radiology 743
  epidemiology 741
  etiology 741
  medical and nutritional management 744
    nutritional therapy 745
    pharmacologic therapy 744
  pathology 742
  prognosis 749
  small and large bowel recurrence and complications 750
  surgical management 745
    bowel resection 746
    indications for operation 745
    management of abscesses 748
    management of extraintestinal manifestations 749
    management of granulomatous colitis 747
    management of intestinal fistulas 747
    management of perianal disease 747
    stricturoplasty 747
    surgical approaches 746
Crohn's ileitis 752
Crouson's syndrome 120
Currarino syndrome 30, 825
Current status in pediatric surgery 15
Cushing's syndrome 1406
Cushing's ulcer 578
Cystic hygroma 1104
  presentation and clinical course 1104
  treatment 1105
Cytokines and cytokine gene 982

D

Dandy-Walker malformation 1084
Day care surgery 115
Dehydration 54
  degree or dehydration 55
  diarrhea 55
  rehydration 55
    oral rehydration solutions 55
  types 54

hypertonic dehydration 54
hypotonic dehydration 54
isotonic dehydration 54
water intoxication 55
Dermoids and dermal sinus tracts of the spine 1187
Development of pain in the fetus and the neonate 123
Development of sexual organs and pubic hair in boys 46
Developmental milestones 42
Diaphragmatic pinchcock 351
Diastematomyelia 1184
Direct and indirect allorecognition 974
Diseases of the gallbladder in children 909
  anatomy and embryology 909
  cholecystectomy 914
  clinical features 913
  congenital anomalies of the gallbladder 909
  incidence and etiology 911
  inflammatory conditions of the gallbladder 910
  laparoscopic cholecystectomy in children 914
  miscellaneous conditions 915
    biliary dyskinesia 915
    gallbladder torsion 915
    polypoid lesions and adenomyomatosis 916
Disorders of the umbilicus 523
  clinical disorders of the umbilicus 523
    omphalomesenteric remnants 524
    umbilical granuloma 523
    umbilical hernia 525
    umbilical infections 523
    urachal remnants 524
  embryology 523
  reconstructions of the umbilicus 526
  surgical uses of the umbilicus 526
Distal hydrocele 531
Distributive shock 78
DNA polymerase 31
DNA topoisomerase 31
Duhamel technique 713
Duhamel's procedure 717
Duhamel's pull-through 717
  complications 722
  indications 718
  preoperative evaluation 718
    barium enema 718
    baseline evaluation 718
    rectal biopsy 718
  preoperative preparation for pull-through 719
  procedure 719
Duhamel's pull-through using staplers 1450
  management 1450
  precautions while stapling 1454
  problems and complications of staplers 1454

E

Effect of hypothermia and hypoxia 150
Electrolytes in pediatric surgery 50
  calcium 53
    hypercalcemia 54
    hypocalcemia 53
  chloride 54
  potassium 51
    hyperkalemia 52
    hypokalemia 53
  sodium 50
    clinical management 51
    hypernatremia 51
    hyponatremia 51
    syndrome of inappropriate antidiuretic hormone secretion 51
    treatment 51
Electrophoresis 31
Empyema thoracis 495
  antibiotic therapy 502
  bacteriology 496
  clinical presentation 498
  complications 506
    bronchopleural fistula (BPF) 506
    empyema necessitans 506
  differential diagnosis 498
  etiology 496
  interventional radiology 503
  investigations 496
    blood investigations 498
    radiologic evaluation 499
  long-term effects 507
  pathophysiology 497
  physical examination 498
  surgical treatment 503
    decortication 504
    lobectomy and pneumonectomy 505
    open drainage 504
    rib resection 503
    video-assisted thoracoscopic surgery (VATS) 504
  thoracentesis 502
  treatment 501
  tube thoracostomy 502

Encephaloceles 1148
  associated pathology 1150
  classification 1148
  clinical presentation 1150
  embryology 1148
  investigations 1154
  treatment 1156
Encephaloceles through the cranial vault 1158
Encysted hydroceles 531
Endogenous inflammatory mediators in shock 68
Endogenous vasoactive mediators in shock 67
Endonuclease 31
Erb-Duchenne palsy 1300
Esophageal achalasia 379
Esophageal atresia 362
Esophageal perforation 432
  clinical features 433
  etiology 432
    extraluminal causes 432
    intraluminal causes 432
  investigations 433
    CT scan 434
    plain X-ray 433
  pathology 432
  treatment 434
    conservative management 434
    debridement and drainage 434
    esophageal diversion and exclusion 435
    esophagectomy and replacement 435
    operative intervention 434
    primary closure and drainage 434
    primary closure with buttress 434
Esophageal replacement with colon 382
  colon interposition 384
    advantages 384
    contraindications 388
    preoperative work up 385
    recent alterations 388
    technical aspects 385
  follow up 390
  routes of esophageal replacement 383
    retrohilar route (westerston operation) 384
    retrosternal (substernal) 384
    transhiatal (mediastinal) route 384
  timing for esophageal replacement 382
    for the corrosive group 383
    for the TEF group 382
  worldwide experience 389

Esophageal strictures 369
   clinical presentations 371
   diagnosis 371
   method of dilatation 372
   prevention 373
   treatment 372
Esophagitis 331
Esophagoscopy 222
   complications 227
   contraindications 227
   indications 222
      diagnostic 222
      therapeutic 224
   instrumentation 226
      flexible esophagogastroscope 226
      rigid esophagogastroscope 226
Ethics in pediatric surgery 215
   euthanasia for other cases 220
   intersex 218
      female pseudohermaphrodite 218
      male pseudohermaphrodite 219
      true hermaphrodites 219
   multiple deformities 217
   neonates 217
   neural tube defects 218
   pediatric malignancy 219
      chemotherapy 220
      euthanasia 220
   prenatal diagnosis 216
   rights of patients 216
Ethics in research 220
   animal experiment 220
   embryo research 220
Euchromatin 31
European register of pediatric surgeons and European examination 1561
European syllabus of pediatric surgery 1562
European working time directive (EWTD) 1563
Evolution of pediatric surgery 10
Ewing's sarcoma 142

F

Fallopian tubes 650
Fanconi's syndrome 53
Features of the pediatric musculoskeletal system 1299
Fecal incontinence and constipation 889
   anatomy 889
   anorectal malformations 896
   history and clinical examination 891
      anorectal manometry 892
      biochemical examination 891
      MRI anorectal region 893
      radiology 891
   investigations 891
   medical management 894
      constipation 894
      fecal incontinence 894
   myelodysplasia 897
   normal anatomy and physiology 889
   normal defecation 890
   surgical management 895
      antegrade continence enema (ACE) 895
      artificial sphincter 896
      colonic resection 895
      dynamic graciloplasty 896
      stomas 896
   treatment 893
FG syndrome 825
Fluid in pediatric surgery 48
   basal metabolic rate 49
   body weight 50
   fluid balance 48
   intake and output charts 50
   laboratory data 50
   maintenance fluid therapy 49
   physical assessment 49
Fluid management in hypovolemic shock 73
Fluorescence in situ hybridization (FISH) 28, 32
Foley's catheter 719, 803
Foreign bodies of the airway and esophagus 1263
Formation of a chimeric molecule of DNA 24
Functional esophageal disorders 377
Fungal infections in pediatric surgical patients 210
   diagnosis 212
   diagnostic criteria for disseminated fungal infection 212
      definitive criteria 212
      likely criteria 212
   epidemiology 210
   fungi 210
   fungal infection of urinary tract 212
   risk factors and pathogenesis 211
      broad-spectrum antibiotics and fungal translocations 211
      burns 211
      central venous access 211
      immunosuppression 211
      nutritional support 211
   treatment and prophylaxis 213
      5-fluorocytosine 214
      amphotericin-B 213
      fluconazole 214
      itraconazole 214
      ketoconazole 213
      miconazole 214
      nystatin 213
Future aspects and research 1488

G

Gardner's syndrome 773
Gastric transposition 409
   advantages 411
   age for gastric transposition 410
   complications 417
      early complications 417
      immediate complications 417
      late complications 417
   disadvantages 411
   follow-up 417
   postoperative complications 415
   postoperative results 419
      acidity 420
      feeding 419
      growth and development 419
      pressure profile and manometry studies 419
      quality of life 419
      rare serious complications 420
   precautions 418
   route for transposition 411
   surgical procedure 411
      operative technique 412
      postoperative care 415
      staged procedure 411
Gastric tube esophageal replacement 391
   choice of esophageal replacement: colonic graft, gastric tube or total gastric transposition 394
   complications 403
      early postoperative complications 403
      late complications 403
   indications 393
   operative technique 396
   optimal time 394
   postoperative care 402
   preoperative preparation 395
   surgical anatomy-practical consideration for GTER technique 392

Gastric volvulus 570
   clinical presentation 571
   complications 571
   differential diagnosis 573
   investigations 572
      contrast studies 572
      plain radiograph 572
      ultrasonography 572
   management 573
   mortality 574
   predisposing factors 570
      primary gastric volvulus 570
      secondary gastric volvulus 570
Gastroesophageal reflux disease 354
Gastroesophageal reflux following repair of esophageal atresia 348
Gastroesophageal reflux in association with specialized conditions 346
Gastroesophageal reflux in children 329
   clinical picture 334
   diagnosis 338
   hiatus hernia 333
   investigations 335
      endoscopy and biopsy 337
      esophageal manometry 336
      pH monitoring 336
      radiography 336
      scintigraphy 337
   operative techniques 341
      Boix-ochoa procedure 343
      laparoscopic techniques 345
      Nissen fundoplication 341
      operative treatment 344
      special situations 343
      THAL fundoplication 342
   pathology and pathogenesis 333
      relevant anatomy and physiology 329
   treatment 339
Gastrointestinal bleeding 575
   GI bleeding in infants 577
   GI bleeding in neonates 575
   GI bleeding in older children 577
      arterio-venous malformation 578
      erosive gastritis 578
      peptic ulcers 577
      portal hypertension 578
      tropical jejunitis 578
   GI bleeding in the pediatric population 575
Gastrostomy tube 397
Gene isolation 23

Genetics of HLA 970
   HLA class I genes 970
   HLA class II genes 970
   HLA class III genes 970
Genitography 135
   contraindications 135
   indications 135
   technique 135
      catheter technique 135
      flush technique 135
GER in the neurologically impaired child 347
Goldenhar's syndrome 1255
Graft rejection 980
   acute rejection 980
   chronic rejection 981
   hyper-acute rejection 980
Grob's modification 717
Growth and development in pediatric surgical practice 34
Guidelines for platelet transfusion 85
Gynecological operations for cases with anorectal malformations 822
Gynecological problems in children 1370
   clinical anatomy 1372
   common gynecological problems in children 1373
      congenital disorders 1373
      endocrine disorders 1379
      inflammatory disorders 1376
      neoplastic disorders 1377
      psychosomatic disorders 1380
      traumatic disorders 1377
   embryology 1370
   examination of the adolescent 1373
   examination of the premenarchial child 1372
   gynecological examination of the newborn 1372

H

Hashimoto's disease 153
Head injuries in children 264
   etiology 264
   management 268
      indications of CT scan 269
      indications of hospitalization for children with head injury 269
      modified Glasgow coma scale 268
      objectives 268
      treatment of raised ICP 269

   mechanisms 264
   pathophysiology 264
   prognosis 270
   sequelae 270
   types 264
      birth injuries 264
      brain contusion or laceration 267
      diffuse axonal injury 266
      diffuse brain swelling 267
      hematomas 266
      pediatric concussion syndrome 267
      skull fractures 265
Heller cardiomyotomy 365
Hemangiomas 1079
   hemangiomas of infancy 1081
      lumbosacral hemangiomas 1086
      multiple cutaneous hemangiomas 1086
      pathogenesis 1081
      patterns of presentation and problematic anatomic locations 1083
      periocular and orbital hemangiomas 1085
      presentation 1082
      subglottic hemangiomas 1086
      tip of nose, lip and ear hemangiomas 1085
      ulceration 1082
      visceral hemangiomas 1087
Hepatic hemangiomas 918
   cavernous hamangiomas in adolescents and adults 924
   clinical features 920
      antenatal 920
      postnatal 920
   diagnosis 920
   epidemiology and prevalence 918
   histological and immunohistochemical features 918
   historical aspects 918
   management 921
      hepatic arterial ligation 922
      hepatic artery embolization 923
      hepatic resection 923
      transplantation 923
Hepatobiliary scintigraphy 165
Hepatobiliary scintigraphy in pediatric patient 163
   imaging of the spleen 166
   liver transplantation 166
   normal findings 163
   persistent hyperbilirubinemia 164

Herniotomy 532
Heterochromatin 32
Heteropagus twinning 1364
   clinical features 1365
   embryology 1364
   investigations 1367
   management 1367
   nomenclature 1366
   prognosis 1368
Heterozygote 32
Hirschsprung's disease 6, 30, 317, 666, 681, 825, 1433
   associated anomalies 683
   clinical presentation 684
   diagnosis 686
   early complications 690
   etiology and pathogenesis 682
   incidence 682
   initial management 685
   intestinal neuronal dysplasia 692
   long-term complications 690
   molecular genetics 682
   open versus laparoscopic pull-through 692
   pathology 683
   staged versus primary pull-through 691
   treatment 687
   ultrashort segment 691
Hodgkin's lymphoma 950
Holiday and segar method 56
Homologus chromosome 32
Hospital ethics committee 220
Hybridization 25
Hydatid disease 936
   clinical features 939
      asymptomatic presentation 939
      symptomatic presentation 939
   diagnosis 940
      imaging techniques 940
      immunologic techniques 941
   drug therapy 942
      contraindications 942
      indications 942
   epidemiology 936
   life cycle 936
      mode of transmission 937
   pathology 938
   surgical management 943
      conservative operation 944
      indications 943
      inscision and exploration 944
      operative procedures 944
      preparation for operation 944
      radical operation 946
   treatment 942

Hydrocephalus 1117
   antenatally detected hydrocephalus 1127
   clinical presentation 1121
   CSF flow 1119
   differential diagnosis 1123
   etiology and classification 1120
      environmental 1120
      impaired venous drainage 1121
      overproduction of CSF 1121
   goals of management 1127
   investigations 1123
   medical management 1128
   pathophysiology 1119
   physiology of CSF formation 1118
   surgical management 1130
      contraindications 1131
      indications 1131
Hyperaldosteronism 1409
   causes 1409
   clinical features and diagnosis 1409
   management 1410

I

Idiopathic primary intussusception 581
   clinical picture 581
      signs 582
      symptoms 581
   etiology 581
      primary intussusception 581
      secondary intussusception 581
   investigations 582
   pathology 581
   prognosis 586
   treatment 582
   types 581
Imaging of the cardiovascular system 155
Imaging of the gastrointestinal tract 160
   gastroesophageal reflux 160
   GI bleed 163
   Meckel's diverticulum 161
Imaging of the lung 153
   inflammation and infection 155
Imaging of the musculoskeletal system 158
   avascular necrosis of femoral head 159
   bone cysts and fibrous dysplasia 160
   osteomyelitis 158
   septic arthritis 159
   trauma 159

Imaging of the thyroid 152
   chronic lymphocytic thyroiditis 153
   hyperthyroidism 152
   normal thyroid gland 152
   subacute (de Quervain's) thyroiditis 153
   thyroid nodule 152
Immune profiling predictive value of HLA antibodies 981
Indian scenario in pediatric surgery 16
Indications for MR in children 138
Infantile hypertrophic pyloric stenosis 564
   anatomy 564
   associated anomalies 565
   complications 568
   diagnosis 655
   differential diagnosis 565
   etiology 564
   incidence 565
   operative management 566
   postoperative care 568
   preoperative management 566
   surgical technique 567
      laparoscopic pyloromyotomy 567
Inguinal hernia and hydrocele 527
   clinical presentation 528
   complications 531
   embryology and anatomy 528
   epidemiology 527
   hydrocele 531
   management 529
      operative procedure 530
      surgical management 529
Intercellular adhesion molecules 262
Internet 1529
   general search engines 1536
      indexing robots 1536
      thematic indexes 1536
   medical search engines 1537
      cancernet 1537
      citeline 1537
      clinical trial finder 1538
      doc guide 1538
      harriett lane links 1538
      health on the net foundation 1538
      medexplorer 1538
      MEDLINE plus 1538
      MedMark 1538
      PubMed 1538
   need to get connected with internet 1530
      hardware 1531
      software 1531
      telephone line 1530
      wireless connection 1530

scientific search engines 1537
    article sciences 1537
    cite seer 1537
    ISI highly cited 1537
to find an e-mail address on the internet 1535
    consult a paper directory 1535
    consult an on-line directory 1535
uses 1531
    discussion lists 1532
    e-mail 1531
    file transfer/usenet/telnet 1532
    www 1533
Intestinal obstruction 633
  acute jejunoileitis 641
  adhesive intestinal obstruction 643
  diagnosis 635
  etiology 633
  historical aspects 633
  investigations 635
    laboratory evaluation 635
    radiologic investigations 635
  obstruction due to roundworm infestation 642
  paralytic ileus 641
  pathophysiology 634
    colonic obstruction 635
    simple mechanical intestinal obstruction 634
    strangulation obstruction 634
  postoperative intussusception 643
  treatment 639
    intestinal obstruction in childhood 640
    operative treatment 640
Intracellular and extracellular fluid composition 48
Intracranial shunting 1140
Intranet 1527
  computer-based patient records 1528
  computer-assisted diagnosis/expert system 1528
  medical intranet 1528
Intrathoracic stomach 430
Intrathoracic trachea 235

J

Jejunal interposition as a substitute of esophagus 422
  long-term results 424
  technique of the operation 422
  timing of operation 422
Jejunal loop 423

K

Kasabach-Merritt phenomenon 1095
Kawasaki disease 156
Kelly's clump 719
Klein-Waardenberg syndrome 826
Klippel-Feil deformity 662
Klumpke's palsy 1301
Kocher's clamps 717
Kyoto declaration 3

L

Langerhans' cell 950
Laryngeal clefts 1284
Laryngeal webs and atresia 1285
Laser in fetal surgery 1516
Laser interaction with tissues 1512
Lasers with surgical application 1513
  argon 1513
  Co2 1513
  dye 1513
  holmium 1513
  KTP 1514
  Nd: YAG and Ho: YAG 1513
  organizing a laser set-up 1514
Legg-Calve-Perthes disease 1328
Lembert's sutures 664
Level of HLA matching in transplantation 973
Ligament injury 296
  schemes for assessing ligament injury 297
Lipomyelomeningocele 1185
  complications 1186
  investigations 1186
  manifestations 1185
    cutaneous syndrome 1185
    neurological manifestations 1186
    orthopedic manifestations 1186
    urologic manifestations 1186
  pathogenesis 1185
Liver resection in pediatric liver transplantation 962
Liver resections 949
  complications 962
  indications 949
    benign liver tumors 952
    malignant liver tumors 950
    trauma 953
    tumors 950
  respectability of liver tumors 955
  surgical anatomy and imaging 952
  techniques 956
    central venous pressure 957
    exposure 956
    inflow occlusion 956
    parenchymal transection 957
    preparation 956
    total vascular exclusion 957
  types 958
    left trisectionectomy 959
    right hemihepatectomy 959
  postoperative management 961
Liver transplantation 5, 988
  indications 989
    assessment 989
  living related donors 994
  long-term survival and quality of life 998
  medical follow-up and late complications 998
  medical management 995
    anti-infection agents 996
    immunosuppression 995
  results 999
  retransplantation 998
  split liver transplantation 994
  surgical complications 996
  surgical technique 990
Lower extremity musculoskeletal trauma 1342
  distal femoral epiphyseal injury 1344
  fracture neck femur in children 1342
    reduction in extension 1342
    reduction in flexion 1342
  fractures of the femoral shaft 1343
    imaging 1343
    mechanism of injury 1343
    treatment of femoral shaft fractures 1343
  fractures of tibia and fibula 1344
    classification 1344
    evaluation 1345
    imaging 1345
    mechanism of injury 1344
    treatment 1345
Lumbar epidural blockade 114
Lumboperitoneal shunts 1140
Lung anomalies 448
  acquired lung abnormalities 460
    bronchiectasis 462
    bullous lung disease 461
    lung abscess 460
  congenital disorders 450
    bronchogenic cysts and lung cysts 456
    congenital cystic adenomatoid malformation 450

pulmonary agenesis, aplasia
and hypoplasia 458
pulmonary sequestration 454
embryology 448
lung tumors 465
metastatic lung tumors 468
primary lung tumors 465
normal anatomy 449
mass lesions in the fetal
thorax 449
Lymphangiomas 1103
classification and pathology 1103
presentation and clinical course
1103
treatment 1103

M

Magnetic resonance imaging 137
special applications 139
Main groups of antibiotics 200
aminoglycosides 201
antifungal therapy 202
antiviral therapy 202
cephalosporin 200
glycopeptides 201
imidazoles 202
macrolides 201
other beta lactams 200
carbapenems 201
meropenem 201
monobactems 200
penicillin 200
quinolones 201
sulphonamides 202
Making recombinant DNA 23
Management of portal
hypertension 1044
distal splenorenal shunt (DSRS)
1046
central splenorenal shunt 1047
mesoatrial shunt 1048
mesocaval shunt 1048
portocaval H-Graft shunt 1049
selective shunting 1046
side-to-side shunt 1048
investigations 1044
imaging studies 1045
laboratory studies 1045
management of acute variceal
bleeding 1045
endoscopic sclerotherapy 1045
pharmacologic treatment 1045
pathophysiology 1044
shunt and non-shunt options 1046
non-shunt therapy 1046
shunt therapy 1046

Management of terminal illnesses 238
anesthetic care 247
Campbell and Duff's schema-cost
benefit analysis 239
characteristics 239
chronic course with short life
expectancy 239
palliative care from time of
diagnosis 239
treatment available, uncertain
prognosis 239
components of palliative care 242
decision making 242
disclosure 242
DNR order 243
procedural aspects 242
ethical issues 239
hastening death 240
interventions around a child's
death 249
focus on religious beliefs of the
family 249
need for formal training 238
pain relief 243
pain assessment 243
palliative care 241
home care 241
hospice care 241
respite care 242
patterns of death 241
postdeath interventions 250
psychosocial support 247
caregiver grief 248
parental grief 248
sibling grief 248
surgical care 247
symptom control 245
anorexia 246
anxiety and delirium 246
bleeding 247
constipation 246
convulsions 247
depression 246
dyspnea 246
fatigue 246
feeding 246
fever 246
nausea and vomiting 246
Marfan's syndrome 1255
Martin's modification 718
McCune-Albright syndrome 1385
Meckel's diverticulum 161, 423, 578,
587, 659, 668
anatomy 587
clinical presentation 588
gastrointestinal bleeding 589
inflammation 591

intussusception 589
obstruction 589
volvulus and other causes of
obstruction 590
embryology 587
histology 588
heterotopic mucosa 588
tumors 588
history and incidence 587
investigations 591
technetium scanning 591
surgical management 592
Medical causes of conjugated jaundice
1002
Metabolic acidosis 63
Microcephaly 1163
antenatal diagnosis 1166
approach to the microcephalic
infant 1166
etiology 1163
outcome 1167
Miller-Deiker syndrome 28
Modern pediatric surgery 14
Molecular biology and the pediatric
surgeon 21
Molecular genetics of Hirschsrung's
disease 1433
clinical presentation and
classification 1433
diagnosis 1433
endothelin type B receptor
pathway 1439
genetic counseling 1442
genetic etiology 1434
modifying genes and interaction
between signaling
pathways 1441
ret proto-oncogene and HSCR 1436
ret receptor tyrosine kinase
pathway 1435
treatment and complications 1434
Monteggia fracture-dislocations 1341
Moya moya disease 150
Muscle injury 295
Muscular cuff 738
Mustard-senning operation 156

N

Nanotechnology 1504
application of nanotechnology in
medicine 1504
clinical laboratory diagnosis
1505
drug and biomolecular delivery
system 1507
imaging 1504
history 1504

Neck anomalies 1222
  congenital lesions 1222
    first cleft defects 1223
    second cleft and pouch defects 1224
    third cleft and pouch defects 1225
Nelaton catheter 398
Neonatal liver abscess 932
Nerve blocks 115
  biliary atresia 118
  bowel artesia 116
  bronchoscopy 117
  congenital diaphragmatic hernia 117
  congenital hypertrophic pyloric stenosis 115
  craniosynostosis 119
  esophageal atresia and tracheosophageal fistula 116
  inguinal hernia 116
  liver tumors 119
  neurosurgery 117
  penile block 115
  thoracic surgery 119
  trauma 118
Nerve injury 292
  classification 292
    axonal injury with endoneurial scarring 293
    isolated axonotmesis 292
    neuroma in continuity 293
    neuropraxia 292
  tests of peripheral nerve function 293
  nerve repair 293
Nissen fundoplication 346
Non-Hodgkin's lymphoma 175
Normal pressure hydrocephalus 1141
Northern blotting 26
Nuclear imaging in pediatric oncology 140, 141
  brain tumors 145
  endocrine tumors 145
    adrenal carcinoma 145
    carcinoids and pheochromocytoma 145
    thyroid cancer 145
  hepatoblastoma 144
  Langerhans' cell histiocytosis 144
  leukemia 146
  lung cancer 146
  lymphoma 141
  neuroblastoma 143
  osteogenic sarcoma and Ewing's sarcoma 142
  soft tissue sarcomas 143
  Wilms' tumor 144
Nuclear imaging in the evaluation of pediatric brain 146
  abscess imaging 147
  blood-brain barrier defects imaging 146
  cerebral metabolism 149
  cerebral perfusion 147
  receptor specific radiopharmaceuticals 149
  SPECT measurement of brain perfusion 147
  technetium-99m-hexamethylene propylamine oxime 147
  tumor imaging 147
Nuclear medicine 140

O

Ondine's curse 683
One port laparoscopically assisted appendectomy 1463
Open reading frames 26
Operative management of high anorectal malformations 809
  colostomy 809
  complications 812
  congenital pouch colon and ARM 810
  posterior sagittal anorectoplasty 810
  postoperative management 810
  results 812
Operative management of low anorectal malformations and single stage perineal repair 805
  anal cutback 805
  anal transposition 806
  anterior sagittal anorectoplasty 806
    advantages 809
    anatomical basis 806
    complications 808
    indications 806
    postoperative care 808
    results 809
    technique 807
  limited posterior sagittal anoplasty 806
  YV anoplasty 805
Opioid and non-opioid analgesics 244
Orbital lymphangioma 1112
Ovarian cysts 1381
  clinical features 1381
  complications 1381
  differential diagnosis 1382
  investigations 1382
  management 1382
  indications 1382
  peripubertal ovarian cysts 1384
  prognosis 1384
  treatment of pubertal ovarian cyst 1385

P

Pain assessment 123
  design issues 124
    abilities of patients 125
    associated medical and psychological issue 125
    needs and desires of the family 125
    severity of pain 125
    technical aspect 125
    type and site of surgery planned 125
  inhibition of central hypersensitization 129
    concept of pre-emptive analgesia 129
  postoperative analgesia 128
  regional administration 127
    caudal block 128
    local infiltration 127
    penile block 127
    peripheral nerve blocks 127
  therapeutic modalities for pain management 125
    nonopioid analgesics 125
    opioids 125
    oral route 125
    parenteral medication 126
    patient controlled analgesia 126
    peridural administration 127
    peridural narcotics 127
    regional anesthesia/analgesia 127
    side effects 127
    use of opioids in analgesia 126
Pancreas and intestinal transplantation 1058
  cadaveric donor operation 1059
  diagnosis of rejection 1063
  graft-related complications 1062
    anastomotic leaks and fistulas 1062
    graft thrombosis 1062
    intrapancreatic abscesses 1062
    pancreatic exocrine sweating 1062
    pancreatitis 1062
  pancreatic donor graft 1059

pancreatic graft preservation 1060
patient selection 1058
postoperative management and
  monitoring 1061
    immunosuppression 1061
    infection and thrombosis
      prophylaxis 1061
    monitoring the graft 1061
preoperative patient evaluation 1059
recipient operation 1060
Pancreatic pseudocyst 1026
  clinical presentation 1027
  complications 1027
  etiology 1026
  intervention 1029
    edoscopic drainage 1029
    morbidity and mortality 1031
    percutaneous drainage 1029
    surgical treatment 1030
  investigations 1027
    blood investigations 1027
    computed tomography scan
      1028
    plain skiagram 1027
    ultrasonography 1028
  management 1028
    conservative medical treatment
      1029
    observation 1028
  pathophysiology 1026
Pancreatitis 1033
  complications 1040
    due to pancreatic damage 1041
    due to the inflammatory process
      1040
  etiopathogenesis 1031
  investigation and diagnosis 1036
    biochemical investigations 1036
    radiological investigations 1036
  medical management 1038
  presentation 1035
  prognosis 1041
  resuscitation and supportive
    treatment 1039
  surgical management 1040
Papillon-Lefevre syndrome 927
PCR cycle 27
  denaturation of template 27
  DNA synthesis by a thermostable
    DNA polymerase 27
  primer annealing 27
Pediatric abdominal trauma 272
  diagnostic peritoneal lavage 274
  imaging 273
  laboratory investigations 273

management 274
  damage control surgery 276
  emergency laparotomy 275
  indications for operation 275
  laparoscopy 276
  nonoperative management 275
  resuscitation 274
management of specific organ
  injuries 276
  extra-hepatic biliary tract 278
  gastrointestinal tract 281
  kidney 282
  liver 276
  pancreas 280
  spleen 278
  ureter, bladder and urethra 283
mechanisms of injury 272
Pediatric anesthesia 103
  anesthetic considerations 103
  fasting 104
  inhalational agents 105
    desflurane 106
    halothane 105
    isoflurane 105
    nitrous oxide 106
    sevoflurane 106
  intravenous agent 106
    ketamine 107
    neuromuscular blocking
      agents 107
    opioids 107
    propofol 106
    thiopentone 106
  local anesthetics 108
  management of anesthesia 108
    intravenous fluids 110
  monitoring 108
  pharmacological interventions 111
  postoperative pain management
    110
  premedication 105
  preoperative assessment 104
  prostaglandin synthetase
    inhibitors 111
    contraindications to PSI 112
    paracetamol dosing in
      children 112
    rectal 112
    weak opioids 112
Pediatric bronchoscopy 229
  bronchoalveolar lavage 231
  care of hopkins rod lens telescope 231
  disinfection of bronchoscope 231
  flexible fiberoptic
    bronchoscopy 232

indications 230
  diagnostic 230
  therapeutic 230
pediatric airway anatomy 229
rigid bronchoscopy 232
therapeutic bronchoscopy 233
  foreign body 234
virtual bronchoscopy 236
Pediatric burns 307
  burn wound healing 312
    epithelialization 312
    immunological response to burn
      injury 312
  classification 309
    agents causing burn 309
    depth 309
    extent of burn 310
  complications 319
    burn wound sepsis 319
    gastrointestinal complications
      319
    orthopedic complications 319
    pulmonary complications 319
  emergency room management 312
    airway and breathing 312
    circulation and intravenous
      access 313
    escharotomy and fasciotomy 313
    investigations 313
  epidemiology 307
    age and sex 307
    incidence 307
  fluid resuscitation in pediatric
    burns 314
    calculation of the
      requirements 314
    place of colloid 314
    place of whole blood 314
    urine output monitoring 314
  hypermetabolic response and
    nutrition 318
    hypermetabolic response 318
    nutrition 318
  infection control 315
  long-term complications 319
    contractures 319
    hypertrophic scar 319
  rehabilitation 319
  mortality 308
  pathophysiology 308
  problems in resuscitation 315
  surgical management of the burn
    wound 315
    deep second degree and third
      degree burns 316

first degree burn 315
    superficial second degree burn 315
    wound coverage 316
  time of occurrence 308
  types 307
Pediatric interventional radiology 168
  pediatric angiography 168
  pediatric nonvascular procedures 175
    aspiration and drainage 176
    biopsy procedures 176
  pediatric vascular interventions 169
    angioembolization 169
    angioplasty 171
    intravascular foreign body retrieval 174
    new applications 174
    thrombolysis 171
  pediatric venography 169
  procedures related to gastrointestinal tract 177
    dilatation procedures 177
    percutaneous gastrostomy (PG) 177
    removal of foreign bodies 177
Pediatric laparoscopy 1455
  indication 1455
    diagnostic laparoscopy in trauma 1460
    laparoscopy in acute abdomen 1455
    laparoscopy in ascites 1460
    laparoscopy in chronic abdominal pain 1457
    laparoscopy in cryptorchidism 1461
    laparoscopy in gastrointestinal bleeding 1457
    laparoscopy in oncology 1459
    laparoscopy in pathologies of liver and biliary tree 1458
    laparoscopy in trauma 1460
Pediatric larynx and trachea 1265
  anatomy 1267
    characteristics 1267
  embryologic development 1265
  laryngeal framework 1268
    cricoid cartilage 1268
    laryngeal cartilages 1268
    laryngeal ligaments and membranes 1269
    laryngeal musculature 1270
    laryngeal vessels and nerves 1270
    thyroid cartilage 1268
  physical examination 1272
    auscultation 1272
    general examination 1272
    nose and oral cavity 1272
    palpation 1272
  radiologic evaluation of the upper airway 1272
    airway fluoroscopy 1273
    frontal (AP) radiographs 1273
    lateral radiographs 1273
  symptoms and diagnosis of laryngeal abnormalities 1271
Pediatric otolaryngology 1257
  ear 1257
    acute otitis media (AOM) 1257
    chronic suppurative otitis media 1257
    deafness in children 1259
    otitis media with effusion 1258
  nose 1259
    catarrhal child 1260
    developmental abnormalities 1259
    epistaxis 1260
    septal deviation in children 1260
    sinusitis in children 1261
  throat 1261
    adenoidectomy 1261
    stridor and airway management 1262
    tonsils and adenoids 1261
Pediatric surgeon and the computer 1518
Pediatric surgery 3
  age group for a pediatric surgical patient 5
  function 4
  recent advances 5
  scope 4
  training in pediatric surgery 5
Pediatric surgery in the nineteenth century 12
Pediatric surgery on the internet: Problems and perspectives 1542
Pediatric surgical specialty in India 6
  challenges 7
  national scenario 7
  teaching and training 7
Pediatric trauma 253
  abdominal trauma 260
  anatomical and physiological differences in children 253
  definitive care 258
  emergency treatment 258
  fractures 260
  head trauma 258
  history 256
  non-accidental injury 261
  primary and secondary brain injury 258
  primary survey 256
    airway and cervical spine control 256
    breathing 256
    circulation and hemorrhage control 257
    disability 257
    exposure 257
    resuscitation 257
    standard investigations 257
  psychological aspects of trauma 260
  secondary survey 258
  thoracic trauma 259
    cardiac tamponade 259
    flail segment 259
    major hemothorax 259
    open pneumothorax 259
    tension pneumothorax 259
  trauma scores 261
    injury severity score 261
    revised trauma score 261
  immune dysfunction 261
Pediatrics surgery in Europe 1552
Peptic stenosis 378
Peptic ulcer 351
Percutaneous transhepatic cholangiography (PTC) and percutaneous transhepatic biliary drainages (PTBD) 177
Peritonitis in children 544
  anatomy and function of the peritoneal cavity 544
  clinical presentation of peritonitis 549
    clinical presentation in infants and small children 549
    physical examination 549
  factors influencing peritoneal inflammation and infection 547
    bacterial virulence 547
  laboratory and radiographic investigations 550
  local response to peritoneal injury or infection 545
    cellular response 546
    changes in blood flow and vascular permeability 546
    fibrin deposition and mechanical sequestration 546
    peritoneal healing 547
meconium peritonitis 556
peritonitis 549
peritonitis in children 559

peritonitis in newborns 558
primary peritonitis 551
    clinical history and investigations 551
    peritonitis in children with nephrotic syndrome and hepatic cirrhosis with ascites 552
secondary peritonitis 554
    management 554
systemic response to peritoneal injury or infection 548
    effects on pulmonary function 548
    effects on tissue metabolism 549
    hypovolemia and hemodynamic changes 548
tertiary peritonitis 557
tuberculous peritonitis 553
    clinical manifestations 553
    treatment 554
Persistent cloaca 857
  antenatal detection 862
  associated malformations 862
    tethered cord 863
  classification 858
    Hendren's description of various cloacal anomalies 858
    Holschneider classification 859
    Pena's description 859
  clinical presentation 860
  cloacal exstrophy 871
  complications 869
  embryology 857
  investigations 863
  postoperative care 869
  treatment 864
    associated pouch colon 868
    colostomy 864
    definitive repair of cloacal malformations 864
    drainage of the hydrometrocolpos 864
    operative procedure 866
    perineal urethrovaginoplasty 866
    posterior sagittal anorectovaginourethroplasty 868
    principles of surgery 865
    repair of high cloacal malformations 866
    total urogenital sinus mobilization (TUM) 866
    vaginal reconstruction 868
Persistent hyperinsulinemic hypoglycemia of infancy 1051

clinical presentation 1052
complications 1055
  late complications 1056
  postoperative 1055
  preoperative 1055
differential diagnosis 1052
embryology 1051
epidemiology 1052
etiopathogenesis 1051
investigations 1052
  blood investigations 1052
  histopathology 1053
  imaging studies 1053
medical treatment 1053
pathophysiology 1052
prognosis 1056
surgical treatment 1054
Pet imaging in pediatrics 167
Peutz-Jeghers syndrome 774
Physiological jaundice 1002
Picibanil (OK-432) in lymphangiomas 1108
  adverse reactions 1110
    major 1110
    minor 1110
  contraindications 1109
  launch of OK-432 1108
  mechanism of action in lymphangioma 1108
  OK-432 in lymphangioma 1108
  precautions 1109
  results 1110
Pierre Robin sequence 1209
Pleuro-peritoneal shunt 493
Poland's syndrome 516
Polyacrylamide gel electrophoresis 26
Polymerase chain reaction 26
Polymorphisms in renal graft outcome 982
Polyposis syndromes 771
  Canda-Cronkhite syndrome 774
  diagnosis 772
  Gardner's syndrome 773
  hamartomatous polyposis 773
    gross and microscopic 774
    juvenile polyposis 773
    juvenile retention 773
  management 772
  neoplastic polyposes 771
    bone tumors 772
    dental lesions 772
    desmoid tumors 772
    endocrine gland lesion 772
    eye lesions 771
    liver and biliary tree tumors 772
    skin lesions 772
  Peutz-Jeghers syndrome 774
  Turcot's syndrome 773

Porto-enterostomy 5
Posterior cloaca 823
Postoperative care in pediatric surgery 180
  initial assessment 181
  monitoring 181
  transport to intensive care unit 180
Potassium containing solutions 59
Povidone iodine gel alcohol 207
Prader-Willi syndrome 28
Preoperative fluid needs 60
Pre-transplant evaluation of antibodies 976
  anti-donor antibodies 976
  flow cytometric crossmatch (FCXM) 977
  panel reactive antibodies 977
Primary neonatal pull-through 813
Principles of lung resection 437
  anatomy of the lungs 437
  bronchial vessels 440
  inflammatory myofibroblastic (Pseudo) tumor of the chest 447
  posterolateral thoracotomy 441
  pulmonary resection in children 441
    left upper lobectomy 446
    right lower lobectomy 446
    right middle lobectomy 445
    right upper lobectomy 445
  pulmonary vessels 439
    left pulmonary artery 440
    pulmonary veins 440
    right pulmonary artery 439
Prognosis in patients with occipital encephaloceles 1158
Prophylaxis 202
  antibiotic resistance 203
  intrapartum prophylaxis 203
  timing of antibiotic prophylaxis 203
Pulmonary artery catheterization 183
  common problems of postoperative care 184
    cardiovascular 188
    clotting 185
    endocrine 187
    hyperglycemia 185
    hypothermia 187
    metabolic problems 184
    pulmonary 189
    renal 186
  infection 193
  neuromuscular blockade 196
  pain management 195
  pressure support ventilation 190
    atelectasis 191

extubation 192
high frequency oscillation ventilator (HFOV) 191
nitric oxide (NO) 192
obstructed endotracheal tube 193
reintubation 193
use of nonendotracheal PEEP 191
work of breathing (WOB) 191
total parenteral nutrition (TPN) 196
ventilator management 190
Pulmonary tuberculosis in children 478
  children at risk 478
  clinical features 479
  complications 486
  follow up 486
  investigations 480
    acid fast bacilli (AFB) staining 480
    antitubercular drugs 485
    directly observed therapy 484
    enzyme-linked immunoassay test 481
    erythrocyte sedimentation rate 480
    extrapulmonary TB 484
    imaging studies 482
    Mantoux test 481
    medical treatment 483
    multidrug resistant TB 484
    mycobacterium culture 481
    nucleic acid techniques 481
    tuberculosis and HIV 484
  pathophysiology 479
  physical examination 480
  prevention 489
  prognosis 490
  role of surgery 487
    endobronchial tuberculosis 487
    post-tuberculosis pulmonary destruction 488
    pre-operative management 487
  tubercular bacilli 479
Pyogenic liver abscess 925
  clinical features 928
  diagnosis 928
  epidemiology 925
  etiology 925
    biliary tract diseases 925
    distant sepsis 927
    intra-abdominal sepsis 926
    structural liver lesions 927
    trauma 927
  pathology 928
  results and complications 930
  treatment 929
    antibiotic therapy 929
    open surgical drainage 930
    percutaneous drainage 930

R

Rare pediatric hernias 534
  complications 542
  femoral hernia 534
    repair 535
  incisional hernia 536
  internal hernias in the abdomen 540
    hernias through mesenteric or omental defect 540
    hernias beneath a mesenteric or peritoneal fold 541
  Littre's hernia 535
  lumbar hernia 537
    associated anomalies 538
    hernia through the inferior lumbar triangle 538
    hernia through the superior lumbar triangle 537
  Richter's hernia 535
  spigelian hernia 537
  ventral hernia 536
    moderate sized defects 536
    phantom hernia 536
    primary repair of the defect 536
Rectal ectasia 884
  classification 884
    primary rectal ectasia 884
    secondary rectal ectasia 884
  clinical presentation 885
  differential diagnosis 886
  embryology and pathophysiology 884
  investigation 886
  prognosis 888
  treatment 886
    medical management 886
    surgical treatment 887
Rectovestibular fistula 820
Recurrent hernia 532
Regional anesthesia in children 112
  complications 113
    prevent 113
    treatment 113
Relief of postoperative pain in children 123
Ringer's lactate (isotonic) 58, 72
Robotic pediatric surgery 1468
  camera holder robots 1470
  future direction in robotic surgery 1478
  history of robotic surgery 1468
  master-slave robots 1472
  neurosurgery robots 1471
  orthopedic robots 1471
  rational for robotic surgery 1469
  robotic pediatric surgery 1474
  types of robotic systems 1469
  urology robots 1471
Role of distribution factor 57
Role of ECF and ICF 57
Rules for determining primary acid-base disorders 62

S

Saccular cysts and laryngocele 1284
Salient characteristics of vector 24
Schwann's cell 292
Scleroderma 377
Scope of pediatric surgery 1554
Septic shock 74
  cardiovascular support—role of vasopressors 76
    dobutamine 76
    dopamine 76
    epinephrine 76
    norepinephrine and isoproterenol 76
  management of complications related to septic shock 78
    adult respiratory distress syndrome 78
    disseminated intravascular coagulation 78
    gastrointestinal, renal and cardiac related complications 78
  newer management strategies in septic shock 77
    activated protein C 77
    angiotensin II 78
    antiendotoxin antibody 77
    antithrombin III 77
    anti-TNF antibody 77
    high volume hemofiltration (HVH) 78
    intravenous immunoglobulin 77
    lenercept 77
    nitric oxide synthase inhibitor 77
    pentoxyfyline 78
    recombinant granulocyte colony stimulating factor (Rh G-CSF) 78
    tissue factor inhibitor 77
    vasopressin 78
  nutritional support in septic shock 77
  pathophysiology 75
    clinical features 75
    investigations 75

renal support in septic shock 77
role of steroids in management of septic shock 77
therapy 76
    antibiotics 76
    fluid therapy 76
Sequencing of DNA by Sanger's method 26
Shock in children 65
    classification of shock 69
        cardiogenic shock 69
        distributive shock 69
        hypovolemic shock 69
        septic shock 69
    diagnosis and monitoring of shock 69
    hypovolemic shock 72
        monitoring 74
        therapy of hypovolemic shock 72
    invasive monitoring 70
        arterial blood gas analysis 71
        CPV measurement 70
        pulmonary artery Swan-Ganz catheter 71
        therapeutic approach 71
    monitoring the patient of shock 70
    pathogenesis and multisystem effect of shock 66
        biochemical mediators in shock 67
        complement activation 67
        inflammatory mediators in shock 67
        myocardial depressant factor 68
        nitric oxide 67
    pathophysiology 65
        compensated shock 65
        decompensated shock 66
        irreversible shock 66
    systemic effect of shock 68
        cardiac 68
        coagulation abnormalities 68
        endocrine 68
        hepatic and gastrointestinal tract 68
        renal 68
        respiratory 68
Short bowel syndrome 618
    clinical sequelae 619
    etiology 618
    long-term outcome 629
    medical management 622
        acute phase management 622
        control of diarrhea 623
        management of complications 624
        nutritional support 622
    morbidity and mortality 629
    physiological changes 620
        adaptation 620
        mechanisms and mediators 621
    recent advances 630
    surgical therapy 624
Shunt complications 1135
Shunt insertion 1133
Shunt systems 1131
Sickle cell disease 927
Sigmoid colon 719
Single nucleotide polymorphism (SNP) 28
Site visit of training centers in Europe 1560
Soave's (Boley scot) endorectal pull-through 723
    complications 728
        early 728
        late 729
    indications 723
    outcome and comparison between different procedures 729
    postoperative care 728
    preoperative evaluation for diagnosis 724
        anorectal manometry 724
        barium enema 724
        baseline investigations 724
        rectal biopsy 724
    redo for soave-redo pull-through 730
    scientific basis of endorectal procedure 723
    single-stage procedure 725
    surgical procedure 724
    surgical technique 726
    two-stage procedure 725
        advantages 725
    three-stage procedure 725
        advantages 725
        disadvantages 725
Soft tissue trauma 286
    management of traumatically amputated parts 288
    mechanism of trauma 286
        blunt trauma 286
        penetrating trauma 286
    skin and subcutaneous tissue injury 286
        clinical type 286
        condition of wound 287
        mechanism of wound 287
        wound assessment 287
    treatment plan 288
        general measures 288
        wound closure 292
Southern blotting 26
Specific consideration in pediatric surgery 115
Specific prophylaxis in pediatric surgery 204
    antimicrobial prophylaxis for urinary tract infections 205
    appendectomy 206
    asplenia/splenectomy 205
    bacterial endocarditis 204
    intravascular catheters 204
    pediatric colorectal surgeries 207
    pediatric GI surgery 206
    pediatric neurosurgical procedures 206
    pediatric oral surgery 206
    pediatric thoracic surgical procedures 206
    pediatric transplantation surgery 207
    prophylaxis related to the specific surgical interventions 206
        clean cases 206
        clean contaminated cases 206
        contaminated cases 206
        dirty cases 206
Spina bifida 1168
    associated anomalies 1176
    classification 1170
        spina bidifa occulta 1171
        spina bifida aperta 1171
    clinical examination 1174
        evaluation of other regions 1175
        general assessment 1174
        local examination 1174
    clinical features 1174
    embryology 1169
    etiology 1170
    investigations 1177
    management 1177
    multidisciplinary care 1180
    postoperative care 1179
        postoperative complications 1179
    prenatal diagnosis 1173
    preoperative care 1178
    role of folic acid 1170
Spina bifida occulta 1182
Spinal anesthesia 114
Spleen 1066
    embryology and anatomy 1066
        abnormal 1067
        normal 1066
    indications for splenectomy 1069
        hematologic disorders 1069
        splenic lesions 1071
    operative techniques 1073

physiology 1068
    abnormal 1069
    normal 1068
postsplenectomy sepsis 1073
trauma 1071
Staging of shock 71
Stem cell therapy 1491
    areas of research 1491
    autologous stem cell transplantation 1496
    classification 1493
    ethical issues 1496
    future applications 1499
    historical background 1491
    mesenchymal stem cells 1495
    recent research 1478
    sources of human stem cells 1493
    stem cell 1491
    stem cell culture 1497
    stem cell transplantation 1497
Strategies to replace tissue loss 1483
Streeter's dysplasia 1304
Subglottic hemangioma 1286
Subglottic stenosis 1279
    acquired subglottic stenosis 1279
        diagnosis 1280
        endoscopic evaluation 1280
        endoscopic management 1281
        management 1281
        pulmonary function test 1281
        radiologic evaluation 1280
        tracheostomy 1281
        voice analysis 1281
    congenital subglottic stenosis 1279
Surgery for pediatric morbid obesity 1421
    current bariatric surgery procedures 1426
    emerging procedures and future research 1426
    factors in patient decision making 1424
    indications for surgery 1422
    overview of bariatric surgery 1424
    pathophysiology 1421
    preoperative counseling 1424
    role of bariatric surgery in children and adolescents 1422
Surgery of occipital encephalocele 1157
Sushruta 6
Swenson's operation 713
Swenson's pull-through 709
    age at Swenson's procedure 710
    comparison with other procedures 713
    complications 712
        early 712
        late 712
    laparoscopy 712
    outcome 713
    preoperative assessment and preparation 709
    relative contraindications 710
    reoperations 713
    staged versus single stage 714
    surgical procedure 710
        abdominal part of the procedure 711
        anal dilatation 710
        anal part of the procedure 711
        transanal dissection for single stage Swenson's procedure 711
Synovial injury 297

T

Tendon injury 295
    management 295
    tendon repair 296
Tethered cord syndrome (TCS) 1182
    clinical features 1182
    functional and metabolic impairment 1182
    investigation 1184
    primary TCS 1182
    treatment 1184
Tetralogy of Fallot repair 156
Thal fundoplication 357
    follow-up 361
    long-term results 362
    postoperative care 361
    reoperation for recurrent GER 361
    results 361
    special situations 361
    surgical technique 359
Thoracic duct 400
Tonicity of solutions 58
Tools for assessment of growth and nutritional status 34
    arm circumference 35
    growth in head circumference 35
    head circumference 34
    head circumference in pre-term babies 38
    infancy-childhood adolescence 34
    intrauterine assessment 34
    large head 38
    length/height growth 38
    skin fold thickness (SFT) 35
    small head 38
    stature (length/height) 34
    weight 35
Topical agents in pediatric surgery 207
Torticollis 1230
    classification 1231
        investigations and differential diagnosis 1231
    clinical features 1231
    complications 1234
    etiology 1230
    natural history and secondary effects 1232
    pathophysiology 1230
    postoperative care 1234
    treatment 1233
        operative treatment 1233
Total colonic aganglionosis 696
    definitive operation 697
    diagnosis 696
    ileostomy 696
    results 699
Total parental nutrition 262
Townes-Brocks syndrome 825
Tracheoesophageal fistula (TEF) 136
Transanal endorectal pull-through 733
    complications 737
        early 737
        late 737
    contraindications 734
    follow-up 737
    indications 733
    outcome 737
    preoperative assessment 734
    preoperative preparation 734
    redo tept 738
    surgical technique 735
Transfusion in disease states requiring multiple transfusions 88
    hemolytic disease of the newborn 88
    hemophilia 88
    oncology patients 89
    sickle cell disease 88
    thalassemia 88
Transhiatal ophagectomy 400
Transplant immunogenetics 969
Transplant tolerance and molecular therapeutics 984
Traumatic brain injury 150
Traumatic hemobilia in children 321
    clinical presentation 321
    investigations 321
        angiography 322

contrast enhanced of
    CT scan 322
endoscopic retrograde
    cholangiopancreatography
    322
MRI and MR angiography 322
radionuclide scans 322
ultrasonography and color
    Doppler 322
upper GI endoscopy 322
management 322
    angiographic embolization 323
    non-surgical treatment 323
    surgical management 323
pathophysiology 321
Treatment of humoral refection 982
Tumors of the adrenals 1410
Turcot's syndrome 773, 775
Types of liver graft 963
    living donor liver graft 963
    monosegmental grafts 964
    split-liver graft 963

U

Ulcerative colitis 758
    clinical manifestations 760
        extraintestinal manifestation
            760
        gastrointestinal manifestation
            760
    diagnosis 761
        clinical examination 761
        endoscopy 761
        laboratory assessment 761
        radiology 761
    epidemiology 759
    etiology 759
    medical and nutritional
        management 762
    pathology 759
    surgical management 763
        indications for operation 763
        surgical approaches 763
    surgical outcome 766
Ultrasound 135
    cranial sonography:equipment and
        technique 135
    special applications 136
Umbilical hernia 525
Umbilical ring 525
Upper extremity musculoskeletal
    trauma 1332
    elbow injuries in children 1333

forearm fractures 1340
    classification 1340
    complications 1341
    mechanism of injury 1340
    treatment 1341
fracture of radial neck 1340
    classification 1340
    evaluation 1340
    imaging 1340
    mechanism of injury 1340
    treatment 1340
fracture of the lateral condyle 1339
    complication 1339
    evaluation 1339
    imaging 1339
    mechanism of injury 1339
    treatment 1339
fracture of the lateral epicondyle
    1339
fracture of the medial condyle 1338
fractures of the medial epicondyle
    1337
    classification 1337
    complications 1338
    evaluation 1337
    imaging 1338
    mechanism of injury 1337
    treatment 1338
injuries of the shoulder region 1332
    classification 1332
    clavicle fractures 1332
    complications 1333
    evaluation 1332
    imaging 1333
    management 1333
    mechanism of injury 1332
pulled elbow 1339
supracondylar fracture of humerus
    1334
    classification 1334
    complications 1336
    evaluation 1334
    imaging 1335
    mechanism of injury 1334
    treatment 1335
transcondylar fracture 1337
Urogenital sinus with normal rectum
    822

V

Vaginal anomalies and reconstruction
    1387
    approach to a high vagina 1391
        passerini-Glazel procedure 1392

posterior sagittal approach 1394
pull through vaginoplasty 1391
approach to a low vagina 1390
    cutback vaginoplasty 1390
    flap vaginoplasty 1390
classification 1387
    vaginal agenesis 1388
skin flaps 1395
    expanded skin 1398
    full thickness skin grafts 1396
    myocutaneous flaps 1396
surgical principles for vaginoplasty
    1388
    vaginoplasty 1389
vaginal substitution 1395
Variant Hirschsprung's disease 701
    hypoganglionosis 704
    immature ganglia 704
    internal sphincter achalasia 705
    intestinal neuronal dysplasia 702
    smooth muscle cell disorders 705
Vascular anomalies 1099
    arteriovenous malformations 1099
        classification and pathology
            1099
        presentation and clinical course
            1101
        treatment 1102
Vascular injuries in children 298
    assessment 299
    characteristics of pediatric injuries
        298
    iatrogenic injuries 300
        peripheral vascular access 302
        umbilical artery catheters 300
    imaging modalities 299
        digital subtraction
            arteriography 300
        Doppler studies 299
    mechanisms of trauma 298
    prevention 306
    traumatic injuries 303
        blunt injuries 304
        compartment syndrome 304
        penetrating injuries 303
    truncal injuries 304
        abdominal injuries 305
        cervicothoracic injuries 304
Vascular injury 290
    diagnosis 291
    mechanism 291
    physical examination 291
    ultrasonic flow detection 291
    vessel repair 292
Vascular rings 374

Vascular tumors 1095
Ventilatory support in children 90
　applied respiratory physiology 90
　　airway resistance 91
　　pulmonary compliance 91
　　time constants 91
　　work of breathing 91
　care of the patient of ventilator 100
　　care of the unconscious patient 100
　　care of the ventilator aspects of the patient 100
　care of the ventilator 100
　　breathing system 100
　complications of ventilation 99
　　barotrauma (rupture of lung parenchyma) 99
　　repeated extubation 99
　　volutrauma 99
　endotracheal tube or tracheostomy 99
　indications 98
　　ICU indication 98
　　postoperative 98
　　preoperative 98
　mode of ventilation 94
　　basic modes 94
　　modes that allows patient machine interaction 95
　　modes to increase FRC 94
　　modes useful for children 97
　　modes useful in weaning 96
　permissive hypercapnia 99
　role of muscle relaxant analgesia and sedation 99
　understanding the ventilator 91
　　anatomy 91
　　physiology 92
　ventilatory strategy 98
　　choosing the right ventilator and the mode of ventilation 98
　weaning 101
Ventriculoatrial shunt 1139

W

Waardenburg's syndrome 683
Webster's article 776
Weil-Marchesani syndrome 1255
Wilms' tumor 30
Work in progress and perspectives in Europe 1560
World Federation of Associations of Pediatric Surgeons 3
World Medical Association Declaration of Geneva (1985) 215